FOUNDATIONS OF NURSING PRACTICE

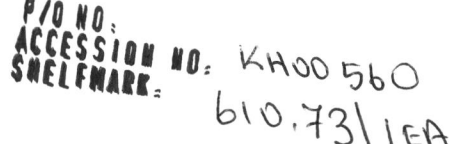

FOUNDATIONS OF NURSING PRACTICE

A Nursing Process Approach

edited by

Julia M. Leahy, PhD, RN

Senior Associate
The Chauncey Group International
Subsidiary of Educational Testing Service
Princeton, New Jersey
Formerly Associate Professor
The Long Island College Hospital School of Nursing
Brooklyn, New York

Patricia E. Kizilay, EdD, RN, CS, FNP

Associate Professor of Nursing
Coordinator, Graduate Program
Brenau University
Gainesville, Georgia

W.B. SAUNDERS COMPANY
A Division of Harcourt Brace & Company

Philadelphia London Toronto Montreal Sydney Tokyo

W.B. SAUNDERS COMPANY
A Division of Harcourt Brace & Company

The Curtis Center
Independence Square West
Philadelphia, Pennsylvania 19106

Library of Congress Cataloging-in-Publication Data

Foundations of nursing practice: a nursing process approach / [edited by]
    Julia M. Leahy and Patricia E. Kizilay.—1st ed.

    p.   cm.

  ISBN 0–7216–3881–3

  1. Nursing. I. Leahy, Julia M. II. Kizilay, Patricia E.
    [DNLM: 1. Nursing Process. 2. Nursing Care. WY 100 F7713 1998]

  RT41.F585 1998   610.73—dc21

  DNLM/DLC   97–9768

Foundations of nursing practice: a nursing process approach   ISBN 0–7216–3881–3

Printed in the United States of America.

Last digit is the print number: 9   8   7   6   5   4   3   2   1

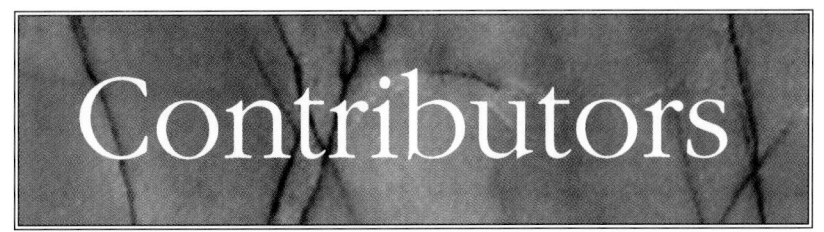
Contributors

Chapter Authors

Cheri Ackert-Burr, MSN, BAEd, RN, CNOR, CRCST

Association of Operating Room Nurses
International Association of Hospital Central Services
and Materials Management
Kingwood, Texas
The Perioperative Experience

Elizabeth N. Arnold, PhD, RN, CS-P

University of Maryland School of Nursing
Baltimore, Maryland
Concepts of Basic Communication

Nancy Berger, MSN, RNC

Quality Resource Specialist—Patient Education
Newark Beth Israel Medical Center
Newark, New Jersey
Bowel Elimination

Judy Bradberry, PhD, RN, NCMT

Associate Professor
Brenau University
Gainesville, Georgia
Sexuality

Nancy J. Brent, RN, MS, JD

Nancy J. Brent Attorney at Law
Chicago, Illinois
Legal Implications in Nursing

John D. Brinsko, BS, IHIT

Corporate Safety and Health Manager
Ferguson Harbour, Inc.
Hendersonville, Tennessee
Physical and Biological Safety

Vicki Brinsko, RN, BA, ADN, CIC

Infection Control Practitioner
Vanderbilt University Medical Center
Nashville, Tennessee
Physical and Biological Safety

Lisa D. Brodersen, CCRN, MA

Research Consultant
Iowa Heart Center
Staff Nurse, Cardiac Surgical and Trauma ICU
Mercy Medical Center
Des Moines, Iowa
Sensory Stimulation

Verna Benner Carson, PhD, RN, CS-P

Formerly, Associate Professor of Psychiatric Nursing
University of Maryland School of Nursing
Baltimore, Maryland
National Director of Behavioral Health
Staff Builders Home Health and Hospice
Lake Success, New York
Spirituality

Michele C. Clark, PhD, MSN, RN

University of Texas School of Nursing at Galveston
University of Texas Medical Branch
Galveston, Texas
Community-Based Care

Barbara Jaffin Cohen, EdD, MEd, BSN, RN

Professor and Director, Department of Nursing
College of Mount Saint Vincent
Riverdale, New York
Urinary Elimination

Dina McDade Culpepper, MSN, RN, CCRN

Assistant Professor
Department of Nursing
Brenau University
Gainesville, Georgia
Fluid-Gas Transport: Oxygenation

Kathleen T. Flaherty, MA, RN, CRRN

Assistant Professor, Department of Nursing
College of Mount Saint Vincent
Riverdale, New York
Urinary Elimination

Michelle L. Foley, RN, C, MA

Senior Nursing Instructor
Charles E. Gregory School of Nursing
Raritan Bay Medical Center
Old Bridge, New Jersey
Bowel Elimination

Terry K. Golden, BSN

Crestview Nursing Facility
Grady Hospital
Atlanta, Georgia
Implementation

Mary Barb Haq, PhD, RN, CS

Associate Professor
Seton Hall University College of Nursing
Visiting Nurse
Patient Care, Inc.
South Orange, New Jersey
Cultural Competency in Nursing

Stephen Paul Holzemer, PhD, RN

Dean and Professor
School of Nursing
The Long Island College Hospital
Brooklyn, New York
Chair, Council of Community Health Services
National League for Nursing
New York, New York
Health, Illness, and Health Care Systems

Bettyann Hutchisson, BSN, RN, CNOR, CRCST

The Methodist Hospital
Houston, Texas
The Perioperative Experience

Esperanza Villanueva Joyce, EdD, RN

Texas A & M University
Corpus Christi, Texas
Stress and Adaptation

Ide Katims, PhD, RN

Assistant Professor
Department of Nursing
State University of New York
New Paltz, New York
Values and Ethics in Nursing Practice

Patricia E. Kizilay, EdD, RN, CS, FNP

Associate Professor of Nursing
Coordinator, Graduate Program
Brenau University
Gainesville, Georgia
Stress and Adaptation

Nursing Diagnosis
Implementation
Evaluation
Concepts of Basic Communication

Virginia Klunder, RNC, MA, CCRN

Educational Consultant
Family Health Resources
Jackson Heights, New York
Adjunct Clinical Instructor
New York University
New York, New York
Infancy Through Adolescence

Dorothy M. Lanuza, PhD, RN, FAAN

Loyola University of Chicago
Chicago, Illinois
Stress and Adaptation

Julia M. Leahy, PhD, RN

Senior Associate
The Chauncey Group International
Princeton, New Jersey
Formerly Associate Professor
The Long Island College Hospital
School of Nursing
Brooklyn, New York
Introduction to the Nursing Process
Assessment
Planning
Administering Medications

Sandra Beth Lewenson, EdD, RN

Associate Professor of Nursing
Lienhard School of Nursing
Pace University
Pleasantville, New York
Introduction to Nursing

June M. Burgess Lewis, RN, BSN, MSN

Assistant Professor
Brenau University
Gainesville, Georgia
Thermoregulation

Jennifer M. Loeper, MS, RN

Director, Clinical Services
Optage
St. Paul, Minnesota
Mobility

Veta H. Massey, PhD, RN

Dean of Nursing
Baptist Memorial College of Health Sciences
Memphis, Tennessee
Theories and Models of Nursing Practice

Maria A. Mendoza, EdM, RN, CS, ANP, GNP

Nurse Practitioner
Jacobi Medical Center
Bronx, New York
Fluid-Gas Transport: Oxygenation

Christine Miaskowski, PhD, RN, FAAN

Professor and Chair
Department of Physiological Nursing
School of Nursing
University of California
San Francisco, California
Rest and Comfort

Patricia Nutz, MSN, RN

Instructor
School of Nursing
St. Francis Hospital
New Castle, Pennsylvania
Administering Medications

Linda Williamson Perez, RNC, MS, CSNP

Nurse Manager, Psychiatry
New York Methodist Hospital
Adjunct Professor, School of Nursing
Long Island College Hospital
Team Leader—Mental Health Specialist
Vice President
LJM Training Associates
Brooklyn, New York
Self-Esteem and Self-Concept

Carol J. Scales, PhD, RN

Assistant Professor
Lander University
Greenwood, South Carolina
Young and Middle Adulthood

Margot M. Schoeps, RN, MS, CS

Psychiatric Clinical Nurse Specialist for Burn Unit,
Adult Critical Care, ER, Trauma Center
Westchester County Medical Center
Clinical Instructor, Psychiatry and Clinical Ethics
New York Medical College
Valhalla, New York
Loss, Death, and Grief

Lisa K. Anderson Shaw, MSN, RNC, MA

Clinical Faculty, Medical Surgical Nursing
University of Illinois at Chicago College of Nursing
Clinical Specialist, Medical Surgical Nursing
University of Illinois Medical Center
Adjunct Faculty, Department of Medical Education,
Clinical Ethics
University of Illinois College of Medicine
Chicago, Illinois
Hygiene

Kim Sherer, BSN, RN, MN

Nursing Chair
Northern Oklahoma College
Tonkawa, Oklahoma
Nutrition

Patricia Albano Slachta, PhD, RN, CS, CETN

Clinical Nurse Specialist, Wounds and Skin
The Queen's Medical Center
Associate Professor
Hawaii Pacific University
Honolulu, Hawaii
Skin Integrity

Betty Patterson Tarsitano, PhD, MSN, RN

Formerly, Clinical Professor
College of Nursing
University of Illinois at Chicago
Chicago, Illinois
Providing Essential Information to Clients

Poldi Tschirch, PhD, RN

Assistant Professor, School of Nursing
The University of Texas
Galveston, Texas
Community-Based Care

Saundra L. Turner, MSN, EdD, BA, BSN, FNP

Assistant Professor
Joint Faculty, Community Nursing and Family
Medicine
Medical College of Georgia
Augusta, Georgia
The Family

Linda J. Ulak, EdD, RN, CCRN, CS

Associate Professor
College of Nursing
Seton Hall University
South Orange, New Jersey
Circulation

Daria Virvan, RN, MSN, CS

Town Center Psychiatric Associates
Rockville, Maryland
Concepts of Basic Communication

Lorraine Mackoviak Wheeler, MSN, RN, CS

Private Practice Consultant
Wheeler & Wheeler Consulting
Santa Fe, New Mexico
The Older Adult

Keeta P. Wilborn, RN, MSN

Assistant Professor
Brenau University
Gainesville, Georgia
Hydration: Principles of Fluid-Gas Transport

Beth A. Yates, BSN, MSN, RNCS

Assistant Professor
Brenau University
Gainesville, Georgia
Staff Nurse
Scottish Rite Children's Medical Center
Atlanta, Georgia
Concepts Basic to Development

Gallery Essay

Nancy Burden, RN, BS, CPAN, CAPA

Director
Morton Plant Mease Trinity Outpatient Center
New Port Richey, Florida
Unit VIII Gallery Essay

Mary Ann Coletta, RN, CRNH

Hospice of Naples, Inc.
Naples, Florida
Unit VI Gallery Essay

Maryann R. Dono, RN, MA, CPN

Course Coordinator, Parent Child Health Nursing
School of Nursing
Saint Vincent's Hospital and Medical Center
New York, New York
Unit I Gallery Essay

Anna Mae P. Dougherty, RN

Chaplain, National Association of Catholic Chaplains
Catholic Health Initiatives
St. Agnes Medical Center
Philadelphia, Pennsylvania
Unit VII Gallery Essay

Susan Rowen James, MSN, RN

Coordinator of Nursing of Children and Assistant Professor
Curry College
Milton, Massachusetts
Pediatric and Adolescent Medicine
Falmouth, Massachusetts
Unit IV Gallery Essay

Ronnie E. Leibowitz, RN, MA, CIC

Formerly, Veterans Affairs Medical Center
New York, New York
Unit V Gallery Essay

Judy Selfridge-Thomas, MSN, RN, CEN, FNP

Department of Emergency Medicine
St. Mary Medical Center
Long Beach, California
Unit II Gallery Essay

Beth Smith, RN, ANP

DuPage Community Clinic
Wheaton, Illinois
Unit III Gallery Essay

Critical Thinking Exercises

The Critical Thinking Exercises that appear at the end of every chapter were contributed by Cathy Dyches, MSN, Brenau University, Gainesville, Georgia.

Community-Based Care Boxes

The Community-Based Care boxes were coordinated by Karen Martin, MSN, RN, FAAN, Martin Associates, Omaha, Nebraska. The Individual Community-Based Care boxes were written by the following people:

Terry Brandt, BSN, RN

Covenant Home Health Care
Milwaukee, Wisconsin

Heather M. Buxton, BSN, RN, MS, CRNI

Independent Nurse Consultant
Venango, Pennsylvania

Lori E. Delfosse, BSN, RN

Covenant Home Health Care
Milwaukee, Wisconsin

Daniela Eichelberger, BSN, RN

Covenant Home Health Care
Milwaukee, Wisconsin

Sandra J. Elsea, BSN, MN

Nebraska Health Connection and County Health Department
Omaha, Nebraska

Catherine R. Glasser, BSN, RN, MBA

Interim HealthCare
Omaha, Nebraska

Lisa A. Gorski, MS, RN, C

Covenant Home Health Care
Milwaukee, Wisconsin

Laurie Grothman, BSN, RN, OCN

UPC Home Health Care
Milwaukee, Wisconsin

Dawn L. Johnson, RN, MN

Covenant Home Health Care
Milwaukee, Wisconsin

Dawn Jourdan, BSN, RN

Interim HealthCare
Omaha, Nebraska

Greg Kamens, RN, ADN

Covenant Home Health Care
Milwaukee, Wisconsin

Cynthia A. Kildare, ADN

Interim HealthCare
Omaha, Nebraska

Donna J. Knobel, BSN, RN, OCN

Covenant Home Health Care
Milwaukee, Wisconsin

Patricia A. Koller, MSN, RN, CCRN

Covenant Home Health Care
Milwaukee, Wisconsin

Karen S. Martin, MSN, RN, FAAN

Martin Associates
Omaha, Nebraska

Donna M. Metoff, MSN, RN

Covenant Home Health Care
Milwaukee, Wisconsin

Barbara J. Sylvester, RN, BBA

Covenant Home Health Care
Milwaukee, Wisconsin

Patricia Varga, BSN, RN

Covenant Home Health Care
Milwaukee, Wisconsin

Laurie A. Wagner, BSN, RN

Interim HealthCare
Omaha, Nebraska

Julie A. Wood, BSN, RN

Covenant Home Health Care
Milwaukee, Wisconsin

Case Study

The case studies that appear within the Nursing Process chapters of the text were contributed by Jane Cox Wrenn, Student, Brenau University, Watkinsville, Georgia

Procedure

Some of the procedures that appear in Chapter 21 were contributed by the following:

Nancy Frets, BSN, RN

Northeast Georgia Medical Center
Gainesville, Georgia

Barbara Hall, MSN, RN

The Chauncey Group International
Educational Testing Service
Princeton, New Jersey

Barbara Hodgson, RN

Cancer Institute
St. Joseph's Hospital
Tampa, Florida

Tracy A. Ortelli, RN, MS, CCRN

The Chauncey Group International
Educational Testing Service
Princeton, New Jersey

Brenda M. Reap-Thompson, MSN, RN

The Chauncey Group International
Educational Testing Service
Princeton, New Jersey

Photographs

Photographs that appear within the text were taken by Ansel Horn, Impact Visuals.
Photographs for the Unit VI Gallery Essay were taken by Michael Ragan, Adelia Parker, Philip Prien, and Kristen Petersen.

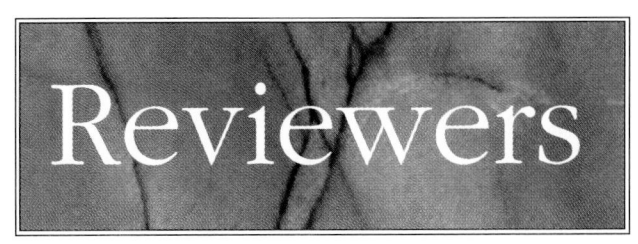

Reviewers

Rebecca Lynn Agnew, MSN, RN

Mercy Hospital School of Nursing
Pittsburgh, Pennsylvania

Diane S. Aschenbrenner, MS, RN, CS

The Johns Hopkins University School of Nursing
Baltimore, Maryland

Alyce Smithson Ashcraft, MSN, RN, CS, CCRN

ADN Instructor
Blinn College
Bryan, Texas

Ann W. Baker, PhD, RN

Assistant Professor
Medical College of Ohio School of Nursing
Toledo, Ohio

Marlene Beauregard, RN

Program Nurse, Brain Injury Adult Unit, and Sexual Health
Counselor
Glenrose Rehabilitation Hospital
Edmonton, Alberta, Canada

Linda Becker, MSN, RN, C

St. Clair County Community College
Marine City, Michigan

Roxanne Bell, PhD, RN

College of West Virginia
Beckley, West Virginia

Margaret W. Bellak, RN, MN

Indiana University of Pennsylvania
Indiana, Pennsylvania

Nancy Berger, MSN, RNC

Newark Beth Israel Medical Center
Newark, New Jersey

Wendy Blackburn, MAEd, BScN, RN

Nurse Clinician, Acquired Brain Injury Program
Parkwood Hospital
London, Ontario, Canada

Mary M. Bliesmer, DNCSc, BSN, RN, MPH

Associate Professor, School of Nursing
Mankato State University
Mankato, Minnesota

Elizabeth Muncey Blunt, MSN, MSEd, RN, ANP-C

Allegheny University of the Health Sciences
Philadelphia, Pennsylvania

Diane M. Booth, MSN, RN

Professor of Nursing
Golden West College
Huntington Beach, California

Linda Dennis Brandon, MEd, RN, MS

Instructor
Riverside School of Professional Nursing
Newport News, Virginia

Margie A. Charasika, MSN, RN

Jefferson Community College
Louisville, Kentucky

JoAnna Christiansen, MSN, RN

East Arkansas Community College
Forrest City, Arkansas

Vonna Roles Cranston, RN, MS, CNS

Department of Nursing
University of South Dakota
Vermillion, South Dakota

Kathryn Dexheimer, MSN, RN

Visiting Nurse Association
Kansas City, Missouri

Julie Doyon, MScN, RN

Clinical Nurse Specialist
Clinical Assistant
University of Ottawa
Ottawa, Ontario, Canada

Chris Easton, RN, MA, MS, CETN

Director, Health Sciences and Nursing
Hartnell College
Salinas, California

Bonita Fae Fador, MSN, RN

Instructor, ADN Program
Belmont Technical College
St. Clairsville, Ohio

Joyce Feldman, MSN, RN, CHE, CPHQ

Morristown, New Jersey

Cheryl Forchuk, PhD, MScN, RN, BA

University of Western Ontario
London Health Sciences Centre
London, Ontario, Canada

Roberta Pecoraro Gates, MSN, CS

Division of Nursing
Darton College
Albany, Georgia

Jean J. Gendreau, MEd, BSN, RN

Formerly, Faculty
Good Samaritan Hospital School of Nursing
Cincinnati, Ohio

Michele A. Gerwick, MSN, RN

Associate Professor
Indiana University of Pennsylvania
Indiana, Pennsylvania

Mona J. Gulino, BSN, RN, MA

Associate Professor
Nassau Community College
Garden City, New York

Carla Guppy, MPT

Senior Physical Therapist
St. Vincent's Hospital and Medical Center of New York
New York, New York

Milly Gutkoski, BSN, MN, RNC

Formerly, Montana State University College of Nursing
Bozeman, Montana

Charlene C. Gyurko, BSN, RN, MPA

Ivy Tech State College
Gary, Indiana

Mary Ann Haeuser, MSN, RN-C, FNP

Dominican College School of Nursing
San Rafael, California

Bonnie A. Hall, MScN, RN

Clinical Nurse Specialist, Geriatrics
Queensway-Carleton Hospital
Nepean, Ontario, Canada

Diane Hahn Heide, BSN, RN, C

Mercy Hospital
Port Huron, Michigan

Nancy S. Hogan, PhD, RN, CS

University of Miami School of Nursing
Coral Gables, Florida

Lou Ella Humphrey, MSN, EdD, RNCS

Associate Degree Nursing Program
Texarkana College
Texarkana, Texas

Frances S. Izzo, MSN, RN, CS

Associate Professor, Nursing Department
Nassau Community College
Garden City, New York

Susan S. Johnson, MSN

Guilford Technical Community College
Jamestown, North Carolina

Carolyn S. Jones, MAEd, MSN

Craven Community College
New Bern, North Carolina

Roseann Kaminsky, MSN, RN, BSEd

Lorain County Community College
Elyria, Ohio

Marion E. Keen, MSN, RN, ADN, AGS

Good Samaritan Hospital School of Nursing
Cincinnati, Ohio

Kathy J. Keister, MS, RN

Doctoral Student
Frances Payne Bolton School of Nursing
Case Western Reserve University
Cleveland, Ohio

Elizabeth Jean Kowal, BScN, RN, BA

Licensure Preparation Consulting Services
Edmonton, Alberta, Canada

Joan Masters, MA, RN, MBA

Bellarmine College
Louisville, Kentucky

Pat McMahon, MSN

Good Samaritan Hospital School of Nursing
Cincinnati, Ohio

Joanne Melhaff, BSN, MA, MS, RN

University of South Dakota
Vermillion, South Dakota

Christine A. Misener, BSN, RN, MALS

Associate Professor of Nursing
Suffolk County Community College
Selden, New York

Sharon E. Moran, BSN, RNC, MPH

Assistant Professor of Nursing
Hawaii Community College
University of Hawaii
Hilo, Hawaii

Patricia J. Nervino, MS, RN

Maurine Church Coburn School of Nursing
Monterey Peninsula College
Monterey, California

Patricia L. Newland, RN, MS, AAS

Associate Professor
Broome Community College
Binghamton, New York

Patricia A. O'Leary, DSN, RN

Middle Tennessee State University School of Nursing
Murfreesboro, Tennessee

Netha O'Meara, MSN, RN, BS

Doctoral Candidate
Wharton County Junior College
Wharton, Texas

Bonnie Nelson, MSN, RN

Medical College of Ohio School of Nursing
Toledo, Ohio

Donna Y. Ortega, MSN, RN

Professor of Nursing, Health and Human Services Division
Community College of Denver
Denver, Colorado

Glenda Paisley, BScN, RN, BA

Royal Alexandria Hospital School of Nursing
Edmonton, Alberta, Canada

Alice R. Pappas, PhD, RN

Associate Professor
Baylor University School of Nursing
Dallas, Texas

Linda P. Picklesimer, MSN, RN

ADN Nursing Division
Greenville Technical College
Greenville, South Carolina

Bonna Stover Powell, MA, RN, CPNP

Assistant Professor
Marycrest International University
Davenport, Iowa

Margaret Prydun, PhD, RN

Houston Baptist University
Houston, Texas

Charlotte A. Richmond, MSN, RN

Associate Professor
University of Texas Health Science Center
San Antonio, Texas

Gill Robertson, MS, RD

Freelancer
Sun Prairie, Wisconsin

Donna N. Roddy, MSN, RN

Chattanooga State Technical Community College
Chattanooga, Tennessee

Mary E. Sampel, MSN, RN

Associate Professor
Saint Louis University
Saint Louis, Missouri

Lisa K. Anderson Shaw, MSN, RNC, MA

University of Illinois College of Nursing
University of Illinois Medical Center
Chicago, Illinois

Kathleen Smid, MScN, RN

Clinical Nurse Specialist, Geriatrics
Riverside Hospital of Ottawa
Clinical Assistant
University of Ottawa School of Nursing
Ottawa, Ontario, Canada

Cheryl Smith, MSN, RNC, AAN

DeKalb County Board of Health
Decatur, Georgia

Mary Margaret Spica, BSN, MS, CSE

The Christ Hospital School of Nursing
Cincinnati, Ohio

Beth Ann Stevenson, BSN, MS, CS

Ohio Department of Health and Capital University
Columbus, Ohio

Judy A. Taylor, MSN, RN

Formerly, Assistant Professor of Nursing
University of Alabama School of Nursing
Birmingham, Alabama

Carroll Thorowsky, BScN, RN, MSA

Policy Consultant
Alberta Health Government of Alberta, Canada
Edmonton, Alberta, Canada

Carole J. Petrosky Vozel, PhD, MSN, RNC, ADN

Western Pennsylvania Hospital School of Nursing
Pittsburgh, Pennsylvania

Mary Ann Wehmer, MSN, RN, CNOR

University of Southern Indiana
Evansville, Indiana

Jean Marie Miller Wortock, MSN, BAN, ARNP

St. Petersburg Junior College
St. Petersburg, Florida

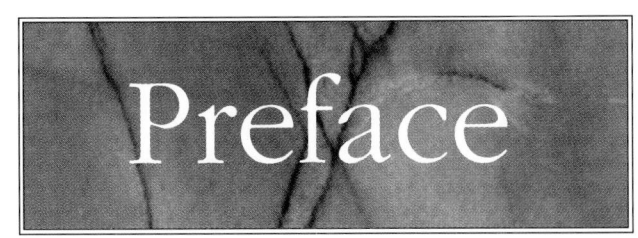

Preface

Nurses are facing the challenges of working in a health care environment that is undergoing a tremendous transformation. They are treating their clients in more diverse settings, from acute and chronic care institutions to community-based care environments. Nurses are working in such varied settings as occupational health centers, consumer advocacy organizations, ambulatory care centers, hospice, and home care. Economics have forced nurses to provide more efficient and creative nursing interventions than ever before. As a result, nurses are expanding their focus from providing care to clients with acute illnesses to attending to clients requiring health maintenance or promotion of health in coping with chronic disease states.

This evolution in health care delivery requires that nurses be able to determine the health of each client, to care for diverse populations, and to intervene effectively with acutely or chronically ill clients. Also, in delivering nursing care, nurses must consider more than just the identified problem. They must consider the psychological and sociocultural patterns of the client that can greatly affect the state of his or her health. Nurses must develop a different paradigm about health care delivery that views the client as a consumer. The public has become better informed about health care issues and seeks a more active role in attaining high-level wellness.

This textbook, *Foundations of Nursing Practice: A Nursing Process Approach,* is designed to introduce the beginning student to the practice of nursing within a rapidly changing health care environment. Because the body of knowledge needed to practice in today's world is expanding rapidly, this textbook is a compilation of chapters written by experts in the field. These specialists present the student with the basic concepts necessary to master subsequent content in the nursing curriculum.

Foundations of Nursing Practice: A Nursing Process Approach is organized using the nursing process as a framework for presenting content related to the care of clients with complex needs in diverse settings. The nursing process itself is viewed as the framework for interacting with clients in need of assistance to maintain or improve their level of health. We recognize that as the nurse interacts with a client, the nursing process is not a linear activity but an iterative one. The beginning student needs to be provided with a method for learning how to apply nursing theory. We present the nursing process as the structure for gathering data, developing a plan of care that is accurate and individualized to the client, and evaluating the client's attainment of expected outcomes.

Throughout the text, concepts of critical thinking, cultural competency, growth, and development have been incorporated. Care of the elderly, community practice, research, and collaborative practice have been emphasized as they support the holistic practice of the nurse. The nurse as teacher, collaborator, and communicator is emphasized for the student.

Special Topic Boxes

Community-Based Care. Community-Based Care boxes integrate special content applicable to nonhospital settings, teaching students to adapt their knowledge and skills to ensure continuity of care.

Health Promotion and Prevention. Health Promotion and Prevention boxes present information that reflects the emphasis on promotion and prevention in health care today.

Elderly Care. Elderly Care boxes focus on how to modify skills to meet the special needs of this growing population.

Clinical Insight. Clinical Insight boxes show students examples of how content applies to real clinical situations and demonstrate the importance of professional publication and research.

Diversity Issues. Diversity Issues boxes emphasize the importance of evaluating the cultural practices and beliefs of each client and explain the implications that these have on the care they receive.

Nursing Diagnosis. Nursing Diagnosis boxes provide possible nursing diagnoses related to client needs, including examples of related factors.

Key Text Features

Critical Thinking Exercises. Critical Thinking Exercises have been developed and are included at the end of each chapter to assist the student in developing an ability to assimilate concepts of critical thinking and to develop clinical decision-making skills.

Case Studies. Client Case Studies are incorporated to provide an illustration of theory to clinical practice.

Unit Opening Photo Galleries. Each unit is introduced with a short vignette written by a nurse practicing in a particular setting. The piece presents a day in the life of the nurse in the setting and is accompanied by photos.

Learning Objectives. Each chapter is introduced with a list of Learning Objectives that address the key points of the chapter. Students can use them as a framework for review, and instructors, for student assessment of knowledge and abilities.

Key Terms. Key Terms begin each chapter of the text. These terms are boldfaced when defined in the chapter, and a Glossary is provided at the back of the text for easy study.

Study Questions. Multiple-choice Study Questions conclude each chapter. Test items are designed to appropriately prepare students for the state boards. Answers and rationales are provided at the back of the text.

Bibliography. A Bibliography appears at the end of each chapter to provide additional reference materials for students and instructors.

Chapter Highlights. Chapter Highlights recap the major emphasis of the chapter and correlate with the chapter objectives.

Chapter Summary. The Chapter Summary ties together the main ideas of the chapter, as well as transition to the Chapter Highlights.

Teaching and Learning Package

Instructor's Manual. This provides creative teaching ideas for classroom, laboratory, and clinical site.

Study Guide. This features exercises that test students' understanding of the material covered in the main text. An easy-to-use study disk gives students practice in answering boards-style questions.

Transparencies. These reproduce superb illustrations from the text to help clarify important content and visually enhance classroom lectures and discussions. Available to adopters of the text.

Test Manual. This contains a wide range of multiple-choice questions that enable the student to easily customize tests to his or her needs. Available to the adopters of the text.

Examaster. This is a computerized test-generation tool. Uses instructor criteria to select from the questions provided, from questions adapted by instructors, and from questions that instructors themselves write. Available to the adopters of the text.

Acknowledgments

This book is the culmination of an extensive effort taking many years to complete and not possible without the work of many dedicated individuals—primarily, the contributing chapter authors, the mainstay of the book. They provided their valuable knowledge and expertise, ensuring a text superior in content and currency. The extensive time and effort exerted writing, revising, and updating their chapters is indicative of their high level of professional commitment.

We also want to recognize the contributions of the reviewers, who provided the chapter authors with valuable recommendations, making a project of this magnitude a reality. The multiple perspectives presented by this diverse group from different geographical areas and practice settings offer a broader presentation of nursing practice and portray a profession that is rich with creativity and inventiveness.

The staff at W.B. Saunders Company has provided tremendous assistance throughout the course of this endeavor. They brought this project from its initial conceptual framework to the reality of this textbook. First and foremost, we express our appreciation to Thomas Eoyang, Vice President, Editor-in-Chief, who had vision and supported this project. Developmental Editors Rosanne Hallowell and Terri Ward both provided guidance throughout the development of this book with the assistance of Rachel Hubbs. Rachel Bedard was a continual part of the developmental process, bringing great ability. Special thanks to our Copy Editor, Blair Davis, who had the task of checking all of the book's editorial details while maintaining consistency throughout the text. Production Manager, Linda R. Garber, made it possible to get the book completed. Additional Saunders staff who did an outstanding job are Illustration Specialist Rita Martello, Designer Ellen Zanolle, Illustrator Sharon Iwanczuk, and Marketing Manager Jean Rodenberger.

A special acknowledgment goes to our photographer, Ansell Horn, RN, who took the photos in the text and acted as a special consultant. Also, we are truly grateful to St. Vincent's Hospital and Medical Center, New York City, and their staff who graciously opened up their doors and allowed us to use their facility to shoot the photos.

Brief Contents

Detailed Contents

Special Features

PROCEDURES

SAMPLE NURSING CARE PLANS

CASE STUDIES

COMMUNITY-BASED CARE

CLINICAL INSIGHT

FOCUS ON THE ELDERLY

HEALTH PROMOTION AND PREVENTION

NURSING DIAGNOSES

Unit ✦ I

INTRODUCTION TO NURSING PRACTICE

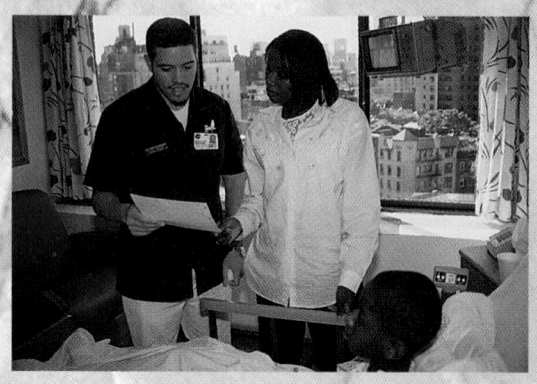

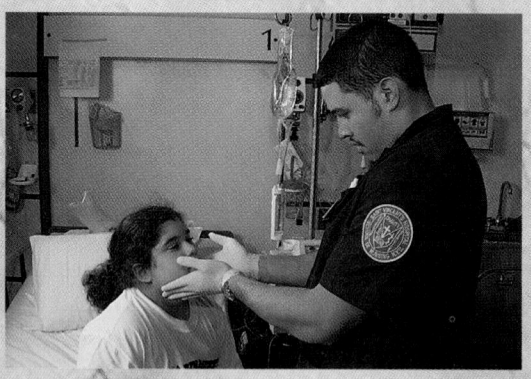

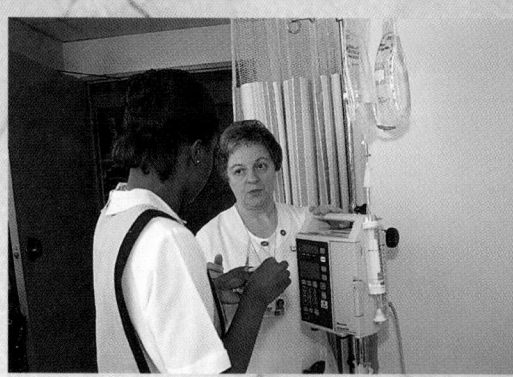

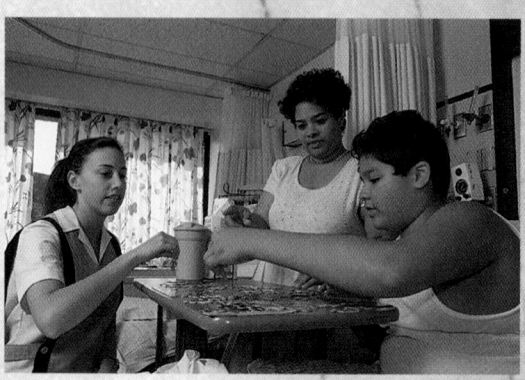

Each semester I enter the classroom to be met by the eager minds and hearts of my students, who are anxious to learn how to care for society's littlest ones. They are motivated and determined to do all they can for the children but often fear their efforts will not be enough.

Each student presents a great responsibility and a great challenge to an instructor. How do I reach each one of them, unique from all others? Before long, I see students cuddling and rocking a seriously ill infant, wiping a tear from the eyes of a crying toddler, explaining patiently to an anxious 3-year-old what is going to happen to him, or playing a game with a frightened 6-year-old, too old to admit he is afraid. The students have learned so much and come so far while experiencing a myriad of emotions—joy at the birth of a newborn or sorrow at the death of another. I have watched them develop their skills, a deep compassion, and a sense of caring.

Teaching is both rewarding and difficult. An effective nurse educator must be knowledgeable and skillful while being open-minded and creative. In today's society, this is not an easy task. The knowledge required of the nurse educator is forever expanding. Technology, especially computerization, can enhance and complement the nurse educator's role. The student of today, reflective of society, is very diverse in age, cultural background, lifestyle, and life experiences. The nurse educator needs to possess keen observational skills to recognize the individualized needs of his or her students and to meet these needs in a caring and sensitive manner.

Nurse education is indeed a responsibility and a challenge, but with it comes a wonderful sense of satisfaction—seeing one's own love of nursing children mirrored in the hands and hearts of the nursing student.

It is extremely rewarding to touch so many lives, helping each student to succeed in his or her own way, hoping and, in some instances, knowing you have made a difference.

Maryann R. Dono, MA, RN, CPN
Course coordinator of Parent Child Health Nursing at Saint Vincents Hospital and Medical Center, School of Nursing, New York City. Her professional career has spanned more than 37 years, focusing on pediatric nursing—the past 30 years working with students. She also coordinates the computerized educational programs that facilitate student learning throughout the curriculum.

Chapter 1

INTRODUCTION TO NURSING

SANDRA B. LEWENSON, EdD, RN

KEY TERMS

✦

advanced practice
   nurse
certification
clinical nurse specialist
licensure
modern nursing
   movement
nurse clinician
nurse practice act

nurse practitioner
nursing centers
professional
   organization
registration
suffrage
voluntary accreditation

LEARNING OBJECTIVES

✦

After studying this chapter, you should be able to

✦ Identify key political, social, and economic factors that influenced the development of the modern nursing movement

✦ Describe the educational pathways into professional nursing practice

✦ Describe the evolution of the definition of nursing

✦ Identify the variety of health care settings

✦ Define the role of the advanced practice nurse

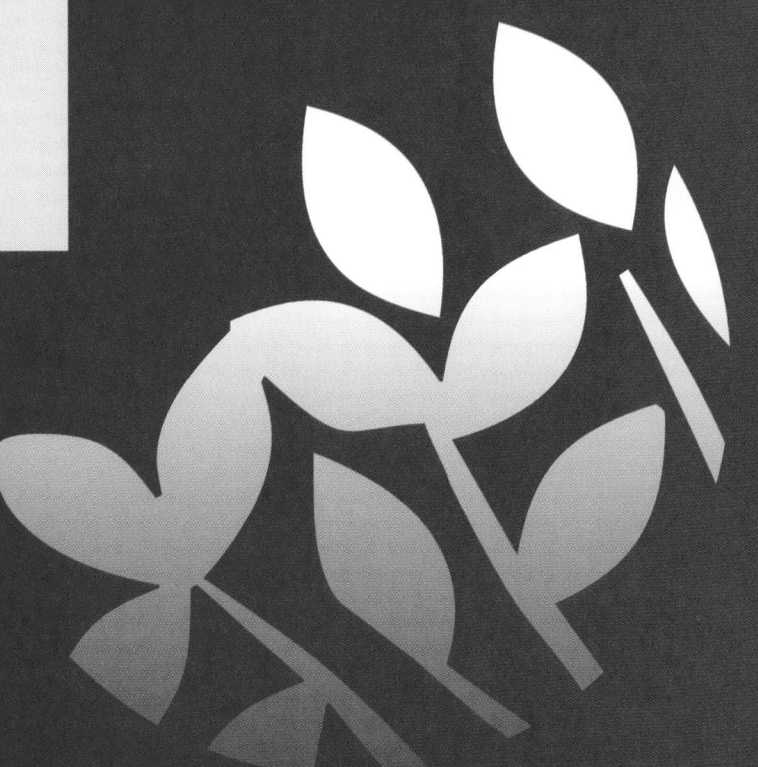

Historians believe that every nurse must have a working knowledge of the founding of the modern nursing movement that began in 1873. Too often, faculty teach, students learn, and nurses practice, oblivious of the strong legacy of political and social activism that pioneer leaders in nursing left behind. The struggles registered nurses face today both in education and practice have plagued our nursing ancestors for over 100 years. Conditions similar to those that nurses faced earlier this century in communities, hospitals, and schools of nursing remain today and offer insight into future professional growth.

This chapter introduces the reader to the foundation of nursing education and practice. It traces nursing's history, highlighting its affiliation with the women's movement at the beginning of the 20th century and follows the movement through the development of nursing education and practice in the latter half of the century. Over time, the profession has evolved, refining its definitions of nursing, offering a variety of educational pathways, creating practice specialties, and assuring the public of the quality of nursing education and practice.

The Founding of the Modern Nursing Movement

Nursing's roots lie deep within the woman movement* that began during the first Woman's Rights Convention held in Seneca Falls, New York in 1848. During this convention, women suffragists such as Elizabeth Cady Stanton (1815–1893) and Lucretia Mott (1793–1880) affirmed the notion that ". . . all men and women are created equal" (*Report of the Woman's Rights Convention,* p. 7). These leaders argued for woman **suffrage** and firmly believed that equality between the sexes could not be achieved until women could vote. Moreover, these visionary leaders believed that with that right came the responsibility to become educated and make informed choices. The woman movement not only signified women's struggle to become enfranchised but also endorsed a women's right to an education.

A few years preceding the Seneca Falls convention, women had little opportunity for an education. Only a handful of schools had opened where women could attend, and even fewer schools were concerned about the educational value of the curriculum. Emma Willard (1787–1870), one of the early celebrated female educators of the 19th century, founded one of the first schools for women. Willard established the Troy Female Seminary in 1821, which was followed 2

years later by the founding of the Hartford Female Seminary for young women in Hartford, Connecticut by another noted author and educator, Catherine Beecher (1800–1878). The Hartford Female Seminary offered women education and training as teachers (Cott, 1987; Lord, 1873; Rudolph, 1971; Solomons, 1985; Waite, 1990).

Women's schools rose in popularity during the mid-1800's. Society soon learned to value women's education as a way of preparing educated mothers who could provide the appropriate home life to raise moral and ethical American citizens (Cott, 1987).

Educators, such as Willard and Beecher, and later, Mary Lyons (1797–1849) and Matthew Vassar (1792–1858), contributed to the changing landscape of expanding educational opportunities for women. Women learned not only how to be moral caretakers of their families but also how to teach and thus to financially support themselves.

The new profession of nursing grew out of this educational tradition. During the late 19th century, newly opened nurses' training schools found a ready supply of interested candidates among educated, middle-class women. Many of these women were single and sought economic independence. They found that the new profession of nursing afforded them the opportunity to find a meaningful and financially rewarding occupation. At the same time, the country moved from an agrarian economy to an industrial one, fought a civil war, and experienced a shift in role expectation of men and women. With those social, political, and economic events, women found opportunity in the emerging nursing profession (Lewenson, 1993).

By 1865, following the Civil War, the United States was ready for health care reform. Many middle-class women had spent the war years as volunteers in hospitals fighting the filth, disease, and unsanitary conditions. These conditions were found to have caused higher morbidity and mortality rates than the wounds received in battle (Moore, 1866; Rosenberg, 1987). At the end of the war, many of these women refused to resume the reticent role they had previously held.

Only a few years prior to the Civil War, England experienced the hardships of war in the Crimea, from which the famed Florence Nightingale (1820–1910) emerged as the founder of the **modern nursing movement.** So widespread was her success at reducing the casualty rate merely by promoting the idea of clean air, clean linen, properly prepared food, and emotional support, that Americans turned to England's heroine for help during the Civil War.

Volunteer nurses during the Civil War such as Clara Barton (1821–1912), Sojourner Truth (1797–1883), Harriet Tubman (1820?–1913), and Dorothea Dix (1802–1887), although untrained in nursing care, instituted in military hospitals many of Nightingale's ideas. However, following the war, American women sought to reform the deplorable conditions found in civilian hospitals and again sought Nightingale's help

---

*At the beginning of the 20th century, the women's movement as we refer to it in the later half of the 20th century was known as the "woman movement."

in establishing the early nurses' training schools in America.

Nightingale, proclaimed a heroine by her English compatriots, had been awarded a large sum of money to establish a nurse training school in London. Nightingale tested her ideas about nursing at the school that she founded at St. Thomas Hospital in England on June 24, 1860.

In addition to instituting her beliefs about the art of nursing, Nightingale asserted that nurses, almost all of whom were women, should be responsible for the education of other nurses. This revolutionary idea dictated that nurses, not physicians, take charge of nursing.

A 1908 editorial that appeared in the newly published *The American Journal of Nursing (AJN)* explained that Nightingale's ". . . brilliant essence lay in her taking from men's hands a power which did not logically or rightly belong to them, but which they had usurped, and seizing it firmly in her own, from whence she passed it on to her pupils and disciples (Editorial Comment, 1908, pp. 333–334).

Although Nightingale's beliefs faced strenuous opposition from physicians and hospital boards (Cook, 1913; Stewart, 1948), her ideas found great support among America's social reformers who saw the opening of nurse training schools as a way to improve civilian hospitals in the United States. Supporters acknowledged that newly trained nurses influenced by Nightingale successfully reduced mortality rates and improved the quality of hospital care (Lewenson, 1993).

Opening of Nurses' Training Schools

Prior to the Civil War, several attempts to begin a nurses' training school had been started, such as that by New York physician Valentine Seaman in 1798, and later by Philadelphia physician Joseph Warrington, who founded the Philadelphia Lying-In Charity in 1828. By the 1860's, other physicians recognized the direct contribution of nursing care to the well-being of patients. Wanting better care for the female patients she treated, Ann Preston (1813–1872), another Philadelphia physician, started The Woman's Hospital in 1861.

One of the early successes in the establishment of a nurses' training school was the New England Hospital for Women and Children. Marie Zakrzewska (1829–1902), a physician, recognized the contributions of a training school and opened one at the hospital she had founded. In September 1872, Linda Richards (1841–1930), distinguished as one of America's first nurse-trained nurses and an early nursing leader, graduated from this school (Kalisch & Kalisch, 1986; Richards, 1915).

Until 1873, most nurse training schools were opened by physicians. However, in 1873 at New York City's infamous Bellevue Hospital, social reformer Louisa Lee Schuyler (1837–1926) opened one of the first Nightingale-inspired nurses' training schools in America. Angered by the inexcusable filth and inadequate care found in the hospital, Schuyler, a philanthropist and activist in the Women's Central Association of Relief, adapted Nightingale's ideas about nursing education and formed the training school for nurses at Bellevue Hospital in New York City (North, 1882).

The same year that Bellevue's nurse training school opened, the Connecticut Training School for Nurses in New Haven, Connecticut and the Boston Training School for Nurses at Massachusetts General Hospital opened as well. Although the training program in Connecticut was initiated by a committee of male physicians, the schools that opened in New York and Boston were started by socially active women ". . . who sought ways to advance women and prepare them for self-support (Dock & Stewart, 1931, p. 155).

Women of the late 19th century saw great opportunity for social reform and personal fulfillment in the newly emerging profession of nursing. Nursing presented a way for women to become self-sufficient in a world that offered few opportunities to do so. Simultaneously, hospital administrators and hospital boards recognized the financial value gained by opening a training school. Nursing schools offered hospitals a cheap source of labor that provided care to patients. Students, under the direction of faculty and a nursing superintendent (the head of the school) applied Nightingale's principles of sanitation and thus provided a safer environment in which patients could recover (Burgess, 1928).

Immediately following the success of these early training programs, Nightingale-inspired nurse training schools proliferated throughout the United States. The number of schools increased from 15 in 1880 to over 2155 in 1926 (Burgess, 1928). Some schools opened for educational purposes and prepared young women in the art and science of nursing. However, most hospital boards found that opening a training program provided a fresh source of good, cheap labor that could provide the hospital with nursing services. Hospitals hired few, if any, graduate nurses because nursing care was so readily and inexpensively provided by students. Graduates from training programs had to find work elsewhere, usually as private duty nurses or as public health nurses.

One of the early nursing pioneers who spoke out against the misuse of nursing students was Louise Darche (1852–1899), an 1885 Bellevue Training School graduate and one of the founding members of the American Society of Superintendents of Training Schools for Nurses (forerunner of the National League for Nursing Education [NLNE], and the National League for Nursing [NLN]). Outraged by the blatant abuse, Darche (1894) warned potential nursing students to beware of such practices when selecting a school. Darche wrote of the numerous hospitals that "had been started with a view to providing a system of cheap nursing for small hospitals" (pp. 667–668). She urged that those interested in attending nursing school should apply to schools connected with large hospitals that could "supply a sufficient number and variety of cases to offer ample opportunity for practically observing and noting the signs and circumstances of different diseases" (pp. 667–668).

The Founding of Professional Nursing Organizations

The American Society of the Superintendents of Training Schools for Nurses (Becomes the National League for Nursing Education in 1912 and the National League for Nursing in 1952)

By 1893, social, political, and economic conditions affecting nursing promoted the establishment of one of the first **professional organizations** for women, the NLN. Challenging the economic forces that had previously directed the fledgling profession, pioneer nursing leaders assumed the responsibility of assuring the public that students received appropriate educational experiences to work as trained nurses (Darche, 1894; Report of the Committee for the Study of Nursing Education, 1923; Robinson, 1946; Stewart, 1948).

Isabel Hampton Robb (1860–1910), one of the founders of the NLN and an 1883 graduate from Bellevue Training School in New York, spoke in June 1893 at the Nurses' Congress at the World's Columbian Exposition held in Chicago. At the Congress, Robb urged other superintendents of nurses' training schools to organize and to establish educational standards in nursing. Other nursing leaders who spoke at the Congress, such as Louise Draper, advised those present to consider the importance of establishing two national nursing organizations: one for superintendents concerned about educational standards and the other for all trained nurses concerned about the working conditions.

Following the first meeting of the NLN held in New York City in 1894, the superintendents met annually until 1952. (Following 1952, the NLN met biannually.) The superintendents met each year to promote fellowship and collegiality and to advance both educational and professional standards of nursing.

They advocated reforms such as a uniform curriculum for all schools, shorter working hours, and an increase in the number of years in nurses' training, and they established an organization for trained nurses (see next section).

The Associated Alumnae of the United States and Canada (American Nurses Association in 1911)

By 1900, single women without personal wealth searched for a means of providing their own financial security. Simultaneously, American women caught up by the spirit of volunteerism and social activism actively sought a change in their social roles. Many of these women, better educated than their earlier counterparts, found the new profession of nursing appealing and exciting. Nursing had discarded its earlier image of unfit and untrained women, usually drunkards and prisoners, for the image of trained, competent nurses. The "new profession" of nursing offered a career and opportunity for social activism (North, 1882).

Women entered nurse training schools and willingly endured the hardships of the life they found there. Following graduation, however, these same students, now nurses, found few job opportunities in the hospitals that had trained them. Most hospitals used students for nurses rather than hire graduates. Undaunted by this harsh economic reality, trained nurses worked as private duty nurses or as public health nurses. Nursing directories developed, allowing a family or physician to hire a trained nurse as a private duty nurse. Training schools, as well as physicians and other entrepreneuring people, formed these lucrative directories; however, abuse raged and nursing leadership felt compelled to support the working graduate nurse.

Lavinia Dock (1858–1956), a nursing leader and staunch woman suffragist, argued for reform in nursing and supported the founding of a second national organization, the Nurses' Associated Alumnae of Training Schools of the United States and Canada in 1896. This second national nursing organization reorganized in 1911 as the American Nurses Association (ANA), which continues to serve the profession as of 1997.

Nursing's second national organization was formed by the increasing number of alumnae associations that graduates from nurse training schools had opened. The alumnae of training schools found the work of a private duty nurse isolating and lonely. Used to the rigorous training and the esprit de corps from their nurses' training school days, graduates expressed a need to join together for fellowship and support. By 1888, alumnae associations had begun to form in several of the training schools and served as the foundation for the Nurses' Associated Alumnae of the United States and Canada. The number of hospital nurse training schools had increased between 1880 and 1897, and the number of graduates increased from 157 to 471. By 1900, the number of graduate nurses increased to 3456 (Burgess, 1928, p. 35).

Along with the political and economic issues such as control of nursing directories, these alumnae associations concerned themselves with broader issues related to job satisfaction, financial security, professional credentialing, and academic accreditation of schools. They advocated the passage of state registration laws and argued for the use of trained nurses in the military (Davis, 1912; Kalisch & Kalisch, 1986).

Nurse alumnae associations fulfilled a need among trained nurses, and membership steadily rose. By 1898, there were 23 nurses' alumnae associations that grew in number to over 142 in 1912. The estimated number of individual members rose to between 17,000 and 20,000 individual graduate nurse members. Each member represented the working graduate nurse and found political strength in numbers. Together, the alumnae had a greater opportunity to address the issues that confronted the profession (Burgess, 1928).

The NLN and the ANA, although separate organizations, worked together in improving the personal and professional life of their members. In 1900, both groups started the *AJN*. The journal provided a forum for nurses to learn and to express their opinions. Topics included patient care, nurses' registration, suffrage, and foreign affairs. Between 1901 and 1912, the NLN and the ANA formed a coalition called the American Federation of Nurses (AFN). The AFN enabled American nurses to join the National Council of Women and the International Council of Women, whose activities centered on the political, social, and economic rights of women (Lewenson, 1994).

The National Association of Colored Graduate Nurses and the Concerns of Women of Color in the Nursing Profession

The National Association of Colored Graduate Nurses (NACGN) started in 1908 under the leadership of Martha Franklin (1870–1968) and served an important role in nursing until 1952 when it affiliated with the ANA. Franklin examined the racially biased practices found in American nursing. She concluded that the exclusion of African-American women from most nurse training schools, the restrictive membership requirements in some state nurses' associations that further precluded membership in the ANA, and the unequal pay and job opportunities warranted the founding of the NACGN (Carnegie, 1991; Thoms, 1929).

The NACGN opened its membership to all African-American nurses whether trained or untrained; however, only registered nurses who graduated from a 3-year training program were entitled to the rank of full membership in the organization. The NACGN served an important need for many nurses, and membership grew from 125 nurses in 1912 to over 500 nurses by 1920 (Hine, 1989; Johns, 1925).

Between 1908 and 1951, the members of the NACGN worked hard to reverse discrimination in education, practice, and professional activities. Mabel Staupers (1890–1990), former executive secretary of the NACGN, sought an integrated nursing world and worked toward the dissolution of the NACGN in 1951 and the acceptance of African-American nurses into the ANA. Staupers (1985) argued that health and illness were not subjected to racial barriers, so nurses should work together to make the world "become increasingly better" (p. 144).

National Organization for Public Health Nursing

Like the NLN and ANA, the NACGN supported the vast public health movement that swept America at the beginning of the 20th century. Increased interest in the health of communities led to the opening of a new field in nursing called public health nursing and the formation of a new organization called the National Organization of Public Health Nursing (NOPHN) in 1912. Unlike the NLN and the ANA, in which membership could be attained through state associations, the NOPHN permitted individual members to join and thereby alleviated the racial barriers that nurses found in several states. Prior to the founding of the NOPHN, NACGN members had already established a working relationship with Lillian Wald (1867–1940), founder of the Henry Street Settlement (1893). Both the NOPHN and the NACGN organizations worked together to improve the health of all citizens living in rural and urban centers. African-American public health nurses mostly worked in black communities where they focused on a wide range of activities such as teaching about health and caring for newborns and the sick. However, those who worked in these communities confronted higher mortality rates, greater levels of poverty, and too few health care facilities than did those who worked in white communities (Buhler-Wilkerson, 1992; Hine, 1989; Kalisch & Kalisch, 1986).

As trained nurses responded to the increasing needs of all communities, the number of newly specialized public health nurses proliferated. Visiting nurse associations opened, and visiting nurses, also known as district nurses and public health nurses, brought the care of trained nurses into the home (see Unit I opening page). Wald and her colleagues started the Henry Street Nurses Settlement on the Lower East Side of New York City in 1893. The Henry Street nurses lived at the settlement house and brought their nursing services to the neighborhood. These public health nurses visited families in their homes, factories, and schools; they established well-baby centers and encouraged neighborhood women to attend the health teaching classes run at the settlement house. They cared for the sick and instructed the well on the importance of sanitary health care behaviors (Buhler-Wilkerson, 1992; The Committee for the Study of Nursing Education, 1923/1984; Craven, 1889/1984; Rothman, 1990).

The NOPHN formed in 1912 to accommodate the increasing number of public health nurses and rising number of visiting nurse associations. Nursing leaders believed that the formation of the NOPHN would provide the essential control of standards and practice of public health nursing. In 1952, in keeping with other nursing organizations whose special interests could be better served in a larger, more powerful organization, the NOPHN dissolved and joined the NLN (Fitzpatrick, 1975).

Organized Nursing and Political Rights

By 1912, registered nurses exercised their political voice within the four professional nursing organizations described previously (ANA, NLN, NOPHN, and NACGN). Each of these organizations represented a constituency interested in improving the quality of nursing education and practice. Organizations provided nurses an opportunity to meet and develop standards for education and practice. However, as nurses advocated control within their profession, women in the larger society did not have the right to vote. Until 1920, women had none of the political rights afforded to men; therefore, they sought other means by which to gain control of their personal and professional lives.

At the beginning of the 20th century, organizations served as a way for women to establish collective power. Nursing, like other women's groups at the time, organized powerful coalitions. Collectively, trained nurses developed a strong voice and politically advocated state nurse registration and social legislation supporting health care reforms. Nurses knew that without a strong organization, they stood politically, economically, and socially isolated. Through professional organizations, nurses expanded and created new meanings for nursing.

In 1952, American nursing underwent a period of self-examination and reorganization. The NLN and the ANA emerged as the two leading organizations in the country representing nurses in education and practice. Since 1952, the profession has grown in numbers and scope as nursing has kept pace with the health care delivery system. Between 1873 and the first quarter of the 20th century, the nursing profession promoted the changing role of women and sought reform in nurses' education and the delivery of care; during the second half of the 20th century, nursing has had to reexamine

education, scope of practice, and nursing's value to society. Although advances have been made since 1873, many of the issues discussed in the 1990s originated in earlier periods, such as the profession's ability to assure the public quality health care.

Varying Entry Levels Into Practice

Nursing education has continued to change and adapt to the needs of society since the opening of the first nurses' training school in 1873. The multiple levels of entry into practice, such as the diploma, associate degree, baccalaureate and master's degree levels have created confusion and dissension among the leaders in nursing. Early debates in nursing education centered around the efficacy of the apprenticeship model found in the diploma schools as compared with nursing education taught in universities. In 1953, some educators advocated a collegiate education for nurses, while others saw the technical role filled by graduates of the newly created community colleges (Bridgeman, 1953; Brown, 1948; Fondiller, 1986; Montag, 1991). The issues surrounding the level of entry into nursing practice remain as we move into the 21st century and foster an ongoing discussion among nursing professionals and the public.

Nevertheless, regardless of the continuing debate, nursing education exists within several educational arenas and graduates registered nurses with a variety of degrees (Fig. 1–1). To become a registered nurse, one can follow different pathways. One of the oldest models, although decreasing in popularity, is that of the hospital-based diploma program. In this model, a student enters the program and graduates with a diploma from the hospital. The hospital, rather than an institution of higher education, provides the education and grants the degree. Graduates of a diploma program are eligible to take the National Council Licensure Examination (NCLEX™) and become a registered nurse (RN).

Another pathway into nursing practice is through a junior or community college. The student graduates from this type of program with an associate degree and also is able to sit for the NCLEX™.

A 4-year college or university offers another entry level into practice, and students at this level graduate with a bachelor's degree and also take the NCLEX™. Many 4-year colleges and universities offer an RN-Bachelor of Science in Nursing (BSN) upper-division program for RNs who already have a diploma or an associate degree in nursing. Changes in the job market, such as the downsizing of hospitals and the increasing number of nursing roles in the community, have led to more and more interest in the BSN. The baccalaureate degree is considered essential in some

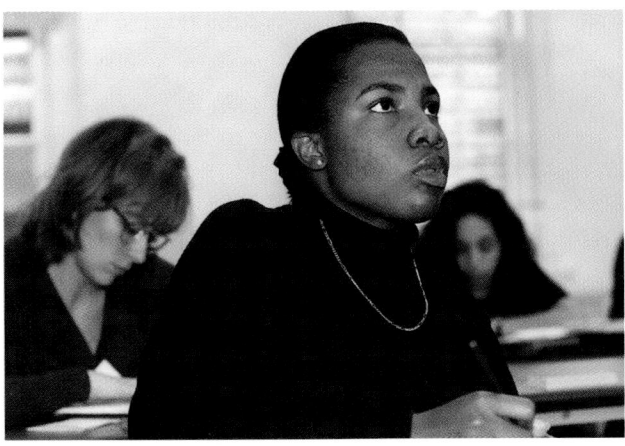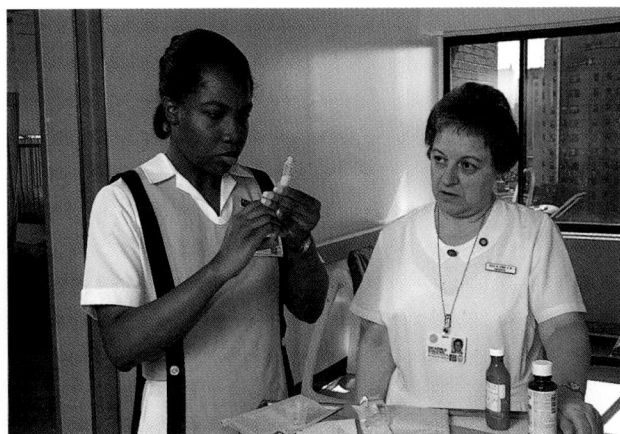

✦ Figure 1–1

Nursing education takes place within several educational arenas and includes classroom as well as hands-on clinical instruction. To become a registered nurse, one can attend a hospital-based program, a junior or community college program, or a 4-year college or university program. Many institutions have developed programs that can accommodate the schedules of adult learners with work and family responsibilities, with weekend and evening classes and long-distance computerized learning. All graduates take the National Council Licensing Exam (NCLEX™) to become registered nurses.

clinical settings, and many argue that it should be the entry-level degree into practice.

To compound the issue further, some educators believe that a minimum degree in nursing should be at the graduate level. Some innovative programs have formed that offer entry into practice at the master's and doctoral levels. Graduates from programs who offer a master's degree or doctoral degree as the first degree in nursing prepare their graduates to sit for the NCLEX™.

Graduates from each of the different entry-level programs take the same NCLEX™ to become RNs. Although each state regulates the licensure of RNs, the NCLEX™ is a national examination, and reciprocity is granted from state to state. Until very recently, the NCLEX™ was given as a paper-and-pencil examination at a few specified times during the year. Now the NCLEX™ is given as a computerized adaptive test at a variety of sites around the country, throughout the year. In addition, the advanced technology of computerized testing has altered the design of the NCLEX™ and allows the test-taker to move through the examination at his or her own speed and difficulty level.

Debates regarding the variety of entry levels into practice and attempts to delineate competencies pertinent to each educational level continue. However, the profession has difficulty in defining competencies specific to each level, and disagreement about entry educational requirements has characterized this issue for many years. The NLN has representation from the various educational levels of entry that serve on a variety of NLN governing boards and policy-making committees. The NLN fosters debate among nurse educators, nursing service representatives, and public members, thus facilitating a broader discussion about articula-

tion, competencies, and common core accreditation criteria.

Another level of practitioner is the licensed practical nurse (LPN) or licensed vocational nurse (LVN). The LPN or LVN graduates from a program that is usually 1 year in length and, following graduation, must pass a state licensing examination. The NLN also has an educational council for the LPN, offering educators in these programs the opportunity to meet and support the education and practice of the LPN.

Educators recognize the importance of higher education and have argued for statewide articulation agreements between the varying educational settings, affording students and graduates opportunity and advancement. Graduates of an LPN program may articulate with an RN program offered at the baccalaureate level, graduate, and continue on for advanced degrees in nursing at the master's or doctoral level. The diploma and associate degree graduate may decide to advance his or her skills and knowledge and enter a baccalaureate degree program.

Many colleges and universities have developed nontraditional programs for the adult learner, such as the RN completion program. Often, this type of program enables RNs to obtain a bachelor's degree while working and raising a family. Many nontraditional programs use advanced technology and offer distance and computerized learning programs. Scheduling weekend and evening classes, providing external degree programs, and granting credits for life experience provide a variety of higher educational opportunities.

At the master's level, graduates are finding more and more opportunities to gain their advanced degrees through similar nontraditional methods. Nurses are able to move into the advanced practice roles of the clinical nurse specialist, nurse clinician, and the

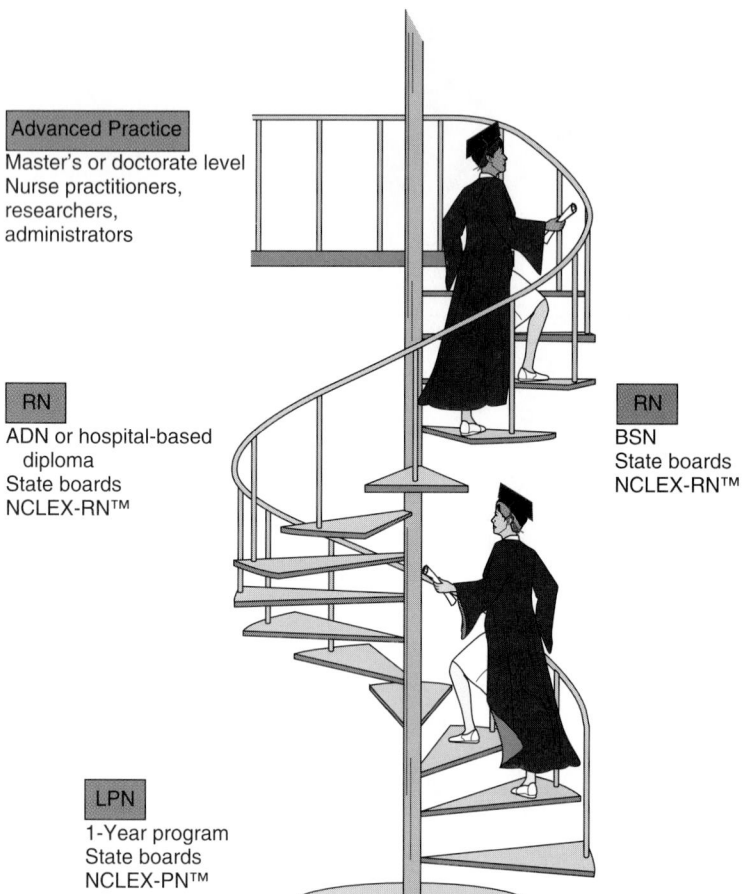

Advanced Practice
Master's or doctorate level
Nurse practitioners,
researchers,
administrators

RN
ADN or hospital-based
  diploma
State boards
NCLEX-RN™

RN
BSN
State boards
NCLEX-RN™

LPN
1-Year program
State boards
NCLEX-PN™

❧ **Figure 1–2**
Professional opportunities for nurses increase with
education advancement.

nurse practitioner through the educational systems. Advanced degrees in nursing prepare the advanced practitioner, as well as administrators and educators.

Trends in the early 1990s indicate that enrollment in nursing education is rising (Fig. 1–2). There was an 8.4% increase in baccalaureate education and a 3.5% increase in associate degree programs. Other trends indicate that the number of men in nursing is increasing. Since the modern nursing movement, the number of men in nursing has been limited. Few schools in the United States allowed men in their programs, and until 1965, political barriers prohibited men from serving as nurses in the armed forces (Gomez, 1994). Although the number of men in nursing is increasing and the historical barriers to the profession have been removed, nursing in America has suffered from a "cultural lag" (Bullough, 1994, p. 267). The cultural lag is attributed to the fact that people are not yet aware of the increasing opportunities in nursing. However, more men will enter the nursing profession, albeit slowly, as the pay and status of nurses improve. Interestingly, while the numbers of men remain low, their influence in the profession has risen, specifically in some of the more lucrative positions such as nurse anesthetist and advanced practice nurse (Bullough, 1994; Louden & Post, 1994).

◆ Accreditation

For over 100 years the nursing profession has worked toward assuring the public of the quality of nursing education and practice by offering a wide variety of programs and services. Since 1952, the NLN has offered a program of voluntary accreditation that has been approved by the Federal government and by other specialized accrediting organizations. Voluntary accreditation is a collegial process involving the evaluation of educational programs by peers, thereby assuring the public of a supply of qualified nursing professionals. The NLN bases its accreditation program on the belief that specialized accreditation maintains and enhances educational quality, ensures program improvement, and contributes to the improvement of nursing practice (National League for Nursing, 1990). While NLN accreditation is voluntary, programs must be state approved before they fit the eligibility criteria for accreditation. Each state board of nursing sets its own standards to evaluate nursing programs. Governmental regulation of nursing from state to state varies according to each state board of nursing. In addition, the Federal Department of Education publishes regulations that accrediting bodies and programs accredited by these bodies must comply with to be approved and to receive Federal funding.

In the 1990s, the higher education community instituted the use of outcome measures as a means of ensuring quality education and monitoring public funds. Similarly, to fulfill the nursing community's public accountability, in 1991 the NLN incorporated outcome measures in the accreditation criteria of nursing programs.

During the accreditation process, nursing programs undergo a period of intense self-study that they describe in a self-study report. The report usually includes a description of a program's philosophy and mission, program outcomes, organization and structure, faculty, student body, library facilities, support staff, and evaluation plan.

Educational institutions with programs in nursing seek the voluntary specialized accreditation that the NLN offers because it fosters development, revision, and improvement of nursing programs. Through a process of consensus building among faculty, students, administrators, and the public, **voluntary accreditation** affords a system of external peer review. Accreditation forces the profession to examine nursing education programs in light of the demands of health care reform.

The move toward increasing specialization and advanced nursing practice makes the need for voluntary accreditation even more pressing. Peer review is essential in ensuring the quality of graduates of new programs on the master's level, such as those preparing nurse practitioners, nurse anesthetists, and nurse-midwives.

Specialty organizations have formed to accommodate specific clinical areas, and some have assumed the responsibility of voluntary specialized accreditation. The American Association of Nurse Anesthetists and the American College of Nurse Midwives have a recognition role and thus develop standards of practice and criteria used to accredit such programs. The National Organization of Nurse Practitioner Faculty has developed standards to be used for accreditation.

Advanced Nursing Practice

Advanced practice nurse (APN) is an umbrella term that refers to graduates of master's programs with a specialty in a particular area of nursing practice. **Nurse practitioners, clinical nurse specialists, nurse clinicians,** certified nurse-midwives, and nurse anesthetists are among those designated as APNs. However, with increasing Federal attention and money focused on nurse practitioners, more and more graduate programs are offering a nurse practitioner track in graduate studies. Federal grant money is becoming increasingly available to graduates of such programs, and a demand for greater funding is being voiced

(Louden *et al.,* 1994). Each year the number of nurse practitioner programs increases, as can be seen in Figure 1–3.

Master's programs in nursing offer concentrations in specialty areas such as adult health, family health, aging, midwifery, community health, psychiatric mental health, school health, and women's health. According to *Nursing Datasource 1994,* Vol. I, "of the 11,219 master's students enrolled in an 'advanced clinical practice' program, 27% were concentrating in adult health/medical-surgical (p. 19)." A total of 11.5% of master's students were enrolled in a community health program, and 10.8% were enrolled in a psychiatric/mental health program (*Nursing Datasource 1994,* Vol. II). In master's programs offering the advanced graduate degree, a strong theoretical base is taught in combination with skills used in assessing, teaching, researching, and counseling.

Advanced practice nurses apply specialized knowledge in a variety of settings from acute care hospitals, community-based nursing centers, or birthing centers, or within an independent practice (American Association of Colleges of Nursing, 1994).

Nurse practitioners, as well as other APNs, provide primary health care to clients. Primary health care, often the entry point into the health care system for many people, is oriented toward health promotion and illness prevention–type activities in the community and health care facilities. Nurse practitioners may provide health care teaching to families, do physical assessments on elderly members of the community, care for individuals with urinary tract infections or stable diabetes, or offer well-baby care and immunizations in the home or clinic setting.

Some APNs provide more specialized services required in secondary- or tertiary-type care settings, such as community hospitals or larger teaching hospitals affiliated with medical schools. APNs such as clinical nurse specialists function in a variety of areas in acute care settings, such as pediatrics, obstetrics, and adult health, specializing in areas such as cardiology, oncology, and diabetes (Bullough & Bullough, 1990; 1992–93 Update, 1993).

Advanced practice nurses find themselves in a precarious position when faced with political barriers and economic roadblocks. Slowly, state laws that govern prescriptive authority, nurse practice acts, and reimbursement privileges have changed to allow advanced practitioners of nursing greater opportunity to expand their nursing practice and to be paid for it directly (1992–93 Update, 1993).

Barriers to direct reimbursement are also being lifted in many states as more states enact legislation that enables the nurse practitioner to be reimbursed by Medicaid. The battle of obtaining third party reimbursement remains as another barrier to the APN, but changes are being made, and in 1993, over 24 states had mandated third party reimbursement for nurse practitioners.

A third obstacle to the APN is the **nurse practice act** and its defined legal scope of nursing practice. In

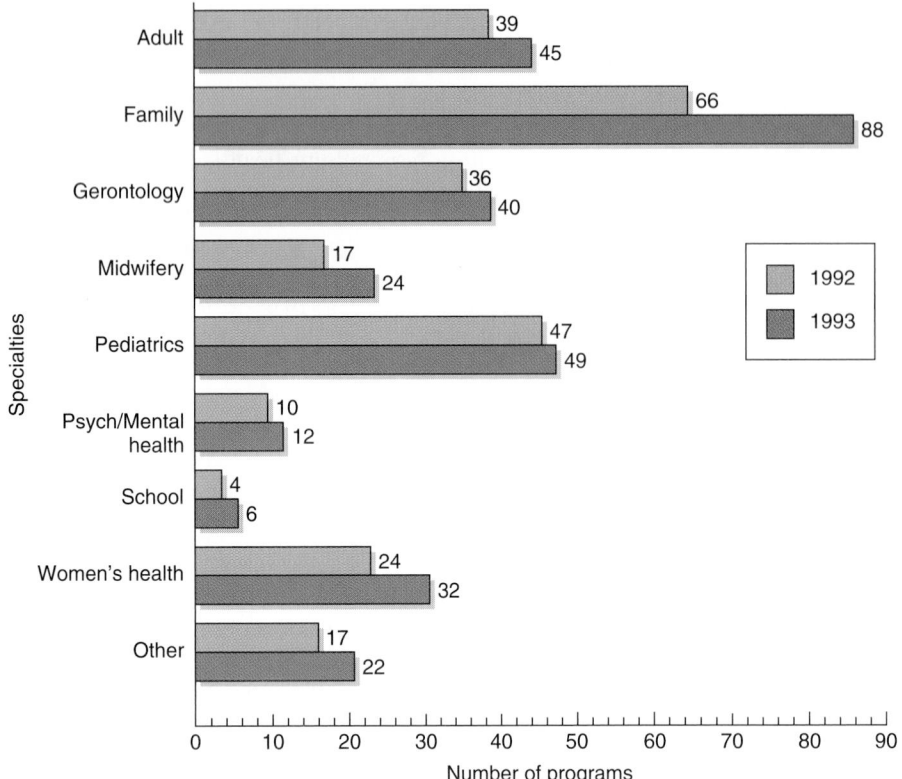

Figure 1–3
Nurse practitioner programs are now offered through 136 master's degree programs in the United States.

some states, nurse practitioners are regulated by both boards of nursing and boards of medicine. Nurse practitioners and their functions are often defined under a broad nurse practice act, and this has spurred debates in nursing about separate licensure.

The nursing profession has faced a long history of barriers to practice that persist late into the 20th century. In 1903, the year that one of the first nurse practice acts was passed in the United States, Ida Giles (1903–1993), president of the American Society of Superintendents of Training Schools for Nurses, argued that there was a "crying need" for unity among nurses to demand state **registration** acts that would protect the rights and privileges of nurses. Until state registration laws were passed at the beginning of the 20th century, anyone could call himself or herself a nurse, even if he or she had not graduated from a nursing program. Paramount to all nurse practice acts was the protection of the public from unqualified practitioners.

Definitions of Nursing

Nursing's rich historical background has set the stage for changes in nursing. Definitions of nursing continue to evolve, and no one definition fits a comprehensive explanation of nursing.

Nightingale (1860/1969) said that nursing "ought to signify the proper use of fresh air, light, warmth, cleanliness, quiet, and the proper selection and administration of diet" (p. 8). Furthermore, Nightingale dispelled the notion that all women could nurse or that nursing was so easily understood. She explained that little was known about what constituted good nursing for the care of either the sick or the well and noted the complexity of elements that enter into the work. Nursing included the elements of providing proper ventilation, warmth, cleanliness, and quiet.

Clara Weeks published one of the first textbooks written by a nurse in 1885 (2nd edition, 1899). According to Weeks, nursing includes not only the "execution of the physician's order" (p. 15) but also the "administration of food and medicine, and the more personal care of the patient, attention to the condition of the sick-room, its warmth, cleanliness, and ventilation, the careful observation and reporting of symptoms, and the prevention of contagion."

At the about the same time that Weeks wrote her text on nursing, nursing leaders struggled with the regulation of untrained and unqualified persons claiming to be nurses. To overcome the misrepresentation to the public and legitimize the profession of nursing within a legal framework, nursing leaders struggled to obtain state registration legislation. Without regulatory laws that would legally define a nurse, anyone could claim to be one. The first registration law passed in

North Carolina in 1903, and since that time, state nurse practice acts reflect the changing defining characteristics of the nurse.

In 1933, nursing educator Bertha Harmer wrote that the "spirit, the art and the knowledge or science of nursing are the three essential elements of nursing" (p. 6). Harmer explained that the application of the scientific method and scientific spirit was necessary if nursing was to be an applied science. Students were to learn how to adjust to new situations and be able to problem solve for themselves. A few years later, Harmer and nursing leader Virginia Henderson (Harmer & Henderson, 1939) wrote a more concise definition that included the idea of health promotion and disease prevention. Harmer and Henderson defined nursing as "that service to the individual that helps him to attain or maintain a healthy state of mind or body; or, where a return to health is not possible, the relief of pain and discomfort" (p. 2).

In 1937, the ANA also defined professional nursing and the professional nurse. In the ANA definition (Harmer & Henderson, 1939, p. 3), professional nursing was described as a blending of

> intellectual attainment, attitudes and mental skills based upon the scientific medicine, acquired by means of a prescribed course in a school of nursing, affiliated with a hospital, recognized for such purposes by the state and practiced in conjunction with curative and preventive medicine by an individual licensed to do so by the state.

A professional nurse was defined as "one who has met all legal requirements for registration in a state and who practices or holds a position by virtue of her professional knowledge and legal status" (p. 3).

Harmer and Henderson (1962) continued to define nursing and the nurse's unique function. Their definitions were later adopted by the International Council of Nurses. In Harmer and Henderson's later work (1962, p. 4) the nurse's role was described as being to

> assist the individual (sick or well) in the performance of those activities contributing to health, or its recovery (or to a peaceful death) that he would perform unaided if he had the necessary strength, will or knowledge. It is likewise her function to help the individual gain independence as rapidly as possible.

Throughout the 20th century, the definition of nursing changed as nurses and nursing moved toward increasing authority and independence. The need to control the regulatory laws of each state and to define the professional role within its professional nursing organizations continued as the social, political, and economic world changed. Newer definitions grew from earlier ones and were influenced by nursing's need for autonomy and independence.

By 1973, New York State passed an act that served as a model for many other states. After a long legislative battle against strong medical and hospital lobbies, a definition emerged that described the independent role of the nurse. New York State law defined nursing as the "diagnosis and treatment of human responses to actual or potential health problems through such means as case finding, health teaching, and counseling."

The ANA had progressed from its earlier 1937 definition of nursing to a later, more prescriptive, definition in 1955. In 1965, the ANA's Committee on Education issued a position paper asserting the independent nature of nursing that identified and elaborated on care, cure, and coordination as components of professional nursing. The 1965 position paper (p. 106) made the following statements about nursing:

> [it is] a helping profession and, as such, provides services which contribute to the health and well-being of people.
>
> Nursing is a vital consequence to the individual receiving services; it fills needs which cannot be met by the person, by the family, or by other persons in the community.
>
> The essential components of professional nursing are care, cure, and coordination. The care aspect is more than "to take care of," it is "caring for" and "caring about" as well. It is dealing with human beings under stress, frequently over long periods of time. It is providing comfort and support in times of anxiety, loneliness, and helplessness. It is listening, evaluation, and intervening appropriately.
>
> The promotion of health and healing is the cure aspect of professional nursing. It is assisting patients to understand their health problems and helping them to cope. It is the administration of medications and treatments. And it is the use of clinical nursing judgement in determining, on the basis of patients' reactions, whether the plan for care needs to be maintained or changed. It is knowing when and how to use existing and potential resources to help patients toward recovery and adjustment by mobilizing their own resources.
>
> Professional nursing practice is this and more. It is sharing responsibility for the health and welfare of all those in the community, and participating in programs designed to prevent illness and maintain health. It is coordinating and synchronizing medical and other professional and technical services as these affect patients. It is supervising, teaching, and directing all those who give nursing care.

In 1980, the ANA adopted a definition similar to the one passed in New York State. The ANA promoted the acceptance of New York State's legal definition of nursing and similarly defined nursing as the diagnosis and treatment of human responses to actual or potential health problems (American Nurses Association, 1980).

The ANA's landmark *Nursing: A Social Policy Statement,* published in 1980, offered nursing a detailed explanation of the profession's social contract with society. It described the social context within which the nursing profession thrives and receives its authority. According to the documents, "a profession acquires recognition, relevance, and even meaning in terms of its relationship to that society, its culture and institutions, and its members" (p. 3). Nursing helps society in the area of health. Historically the profession is health oriented and has contributed "toward the evolution of a health-oriented system of care" (p. 5). To meet the social contract with society, nursing developed codes of ethics and standards of practice.

In 1995, the ANA published an updated social policy statement entitled *Nursing's Social Policy Statement*. In this newer social policy statement, the definition of nursing integrates the recent research on the science of caring and identifies the following as four essential features of contemporary nursing practice (p. 6).

* Attention to the full range of human experiences and responses to health and illness without restriction to a problem-focused orientation
* Integration of objective data with knowledge gained from an understanding of the patient or group's subjective experience
* Application of scientific knowledge to the processes of diagnosis and treatment
* Provision of a caring relationship that facilitates health and healing

Standards of Nursing Practice

As nursing education accommodates and changes to meet the needs of students and the health care requirements of the communities they serve, standards of care are employed. Standards of care were developed within the professional organizations representing specialty areas that proliferated since the 1960's. The ANA concerns itself with issues affecting the practice and welfare of professional nursing, such as developing of standards of nursing practice, defining qualifications of nursing, promoting significant nursing legislation, developing a database of national nursing resources, and promoting the welfare of nurses (Fondiller, 1986). The ANA articulates and strengthens the "social contract that exists between nursing and society" (American Nurses Association, 1980, p. 8).

In 1973, the ANA published a *Standards of Practice* that was used by the profession until it was revised in 1991. The challenges faced by nurses in all specialty areas brought about by increasing health care costs, competition, and regulation, have forced the ANA to find new ways to define nursing practice and develop patient outcomes in more measurable ways than before (American Nurses Association, 1991). Standards need to be developed and revised continually to accommodate the fast-paced changes in health care. The ANA (1991, p. vi) defines standards as "broad statements that address the full scope of nursing practice." They are to be used in conjunction

with the developing practice guidelines in the *Standards of Clinical Nursing Practice*. For further description of these standards, see Chapter 7.

Licensure

In each state, the nurse practice act provides a legal definition of nursing, defines the scope of practice, identifies who can practice, delineates the regulatory agency that administers over the profession, and prescribes criteria for education and **licensure** of nurses. Each state board of nursing determines and administers the criteria for licensure in that state. State licensure requires the passage of the NCLEX™, and reciprocity exists between states.

Certification

Several specialty organizations offer their members **certification** that recognizes performance at a higher level of achievement (Fondiller, 1986). The ANA began a certification program in 1973 and in 1989 established the American Nurses Credentialing Center (ANCC). Boards of Certification at the ANCC develop examinations, determine passing rates, fix eligibility requirements, and certify those who succeed. Certification is designed to promote and enhance the health of the public. Eligibility for certification is reserved for nurses who have met specific requirements in education and functional practice in a specialized area and receive endorsement from peers. Certification examinations are based on national standards set by an organization such as the ANA Congress for Nursing Practice.

While certification attempts to ensure the public's health, because it does not ensure equitable backgrounds for practitioners, certification raises many questions as to its reliability. Educational requirements for certification differ as a result of the many specialty organizations that offer certification. This wide variability creates confusion among practitioners and consumers of health care as to the level of competency. Addressing this concern, the ANCC has announced to prospective candidates that in 1998, a baccalaureate or higher degree in nursing will be required of all generalist examinations.

In the case of the APN, certification requirements vary as well, leading to confusion on the part of consumer and practitioner. Concerned for the viability of certification, the American Association of Colleges of Nursing (AACN) has argued for a uniform certification process and, in the case of the APN, urges as a requirement the "completion of a graduate degree in nursing" (American Association of Colleges of Nursing, 1994). Requiring the graduate degree is central to developing uniform certification requirements that will reflect the width and breadth of a professional knowledge base. Master's degree programs with tracks in advanced practice nursing will provide a curriculum that uses professional standards and clearly defined core competencies.

Evolution of the Nursing Profession

Throughout history, nursing has adapted to the needs of society. At the beginning of the 20th century, nursing leaders in education and practice struggled to develop the role of the RN. During the late 1800s and early 1900s, nurses worked mostly in private homes as private duty nurses or in the community as public health nurses (Table 1–1). By the 1930s, the needs of society changed as the United States found itself in the throes of an economic depression. Nursing jobs in the private and community sector all but disappeared. Moreover, too many nursing programs had opened and far too many nurses had graduated. Nurses, formerly independently employed, found themselves in sharp competition for the few jobs that were available. As a result, nurses lost their income and place to practice (Lynaugh, 1993).

By mid-century, hospitals had become the major employer of nurses and for years to come dominated both the professional and educational settings. Influenced by a shortage of practicing nurses in the late 1940s and early 1950s, hospitals institutionalized the use of unskilled workers to supply nursing care. Nursing leaders turned to educational solutions, such as the associate degree in nursing, to resolve the problem brought on by the increased demand for nurses in the 1950s. Studies of nursing by the national organizations allowed the profession to examine more closely educational and practice sites (Baer, 1993).

Intensive care units, requiring the watchful supervision of the nurse, opened in the 1950s due to an increase in the number of hospitalizations and an increasing acuity level of those hospitalized (Fairman, 1992). By the 1960s, nurses found themselves working in expanded roles in a variety of health care settings. The roles of educator, caregiver, change agent, advocate, and researcher emerged as nurses provided care in hospitals, communities, and schools. In the 1960s, many nursing leaders argued for one entry level into practice at the baccalaureate level. Although the debate continues in the 1990s, the position of APN, which demands a high level of professional expertise to meet the health care needs of society, bypasses the question of entry by requiring a graduate degree in nursing to practice.

Nursing continues to evolve to meet the increasing demands of a highly technical work environment, shorter hospital stays, the downsizing of hospitals and the loss of professional nursing jobs, the increasing acuity of patients in the home, the increasing social awareness for primary health care and cost containment, and the profession's need to continually adapt.

Practice Settings

Community

To meet the changing demands of health care in this country in the 1990s, nurse educators project an increasing community-based focus (Fig. 1–4). People across the life span spend most of their lives at home in the community. Consumers requesting health care information to make informed decisions are seeking partnership relationships with health care professionals that require nursing to respond. Greater access to primary care in the community affords individuals, families, and communities the opportunity to learn and practice health-promoting and illness-preventing behaviors.

Health care needs in the community have been affected by changes in the early discharge pattern of hospitals, which provide tertiary care for the acutely ill. Patients now spend fewer days in the hospital, which means that many return home in a more acute stage than ever before. This change creates a greater demand for more specialized community health nursing interventions (Bullough & Bullough, 1990).

In 1991, *Nursing's Agenda for Health Care Reform* (American Nurses Association, 1991) was published to accommodate changes in health care. Nursing's proactive agenda for the delivery of health care necessitated

Table 1–1	
EVOLUTION OF THE NURSING PROFESSION	
Late 1990s	Increased community-based focus in nursing; downsizing in hospitals
Early 1990s	Increased enrollments in nursing education (*e.g.,* in baccalaureate and associate degree programs)
1960s	Nurses in expanded roles in various health care settings (*e.g.,* hospitals, communities, schools)
1950s	Hospitals became the major employer of nurses
1930s	Economic depression in United States—Nursing jobs in private and community sector almost disappeared
Late 1800s and early 1900s	Nurses worked mainly in private homes as private duty nurses or in the community as public health nurses

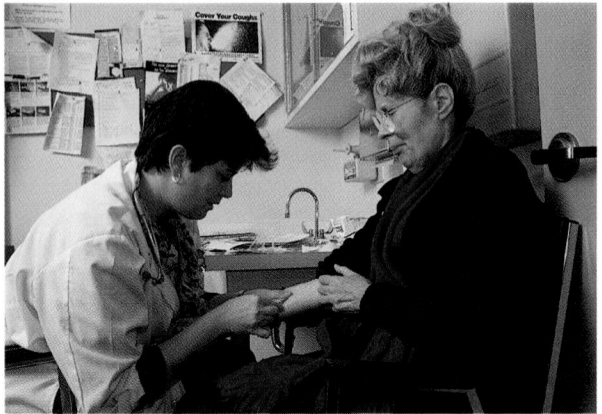

❧ Figure 1–4
Today's nursing curriculum is being redesigned so that graduates will be prepared to practice in community as well as hospital settings. According to *Nursing's Agenda for Health Care Reform* (American Nurses Association, 1991), nurses will assume greater roles in the delivery of primary health care services in a variety of settings, including community outreach programs and nurse-operated nursing centers.

a reassessment of the kind of practitioner that will be needed. Nurses will assume greater roles in the delivery of primary health care services in a variety of settings outside of the traditional institutions. Increases in nurses having autonomous practice, dealing with third party reimbursement, and seeking recognition by the public as health care professionals demand that nurses be better prepared to cope with these issues. *Nursing's Agenda for Health Care Reform* promotes changes in the relationship between clients and health care professionals, requiring a more informed client to assume greater responsibility for his or her care. Nurses working with clients as individuals, families, and communities need skills that will allow them to think critically, work with diverse cultural and ethnic communities, and work with an ever-increasing aging population. Reforms in health care demand that nurses be educated in a new paradigm.

Today's visionaries call for a redesigned curriculum at all educational levels so that graduates will be prepared to practice in the community. Along with these changes, nursing educators and practitioners have had to adapt as well to the changing dynamics of student populations. Throughout the mid-20th century, nursing students entered a nursing program directly out of high school; however, by the 1990s, the trend is that students enter nursing at an older age, as a second career, and often from diverse cultural and ethnic backgrounds. This heterogeneity allows for a broader understanding of the communities in which nurses serve and fosters a wider interpretation of nursing, thus promoting a revolutionary change in both education and practice (*Vision for Nursing Education,* 1993).

The move toward providing primary health care in the community has led to a movement by nurses to open **nursing centers.** Nursing centers are organized and administered by nurses providing a wide variety of nursing services. Nurses are the primary care providers in these settings (Lockhart, 1995). Several categories of centers are found in the community. Some are run by independent nurse practitioners, APNs who offer a variety of health-promoting and health-restoring services. Others are founded in community outreach programs and are often institutionally based, such as university-run nursing centers run by faculty of the university. Nursing centers afford nurses a place to practice autonomously as well as provide educational experiences for students.

Hospitals

Although hospitals continue to be the place where individuals receive acute care, it is predicted that acute-care hospitals will become a collection of intensive care units, and the home care industry will expand to provide more care in the home (*Vision for Nursing Education,* 1993). Hospitals, however, continue to provide medical and nursing care to people and therefore provide career opportunities for nurses. Hospitals offer 24-hour nursing care in a variety of specialty areas such as obstetrics and maternity, pediatrics, and adult medical-surgical units. Increasing acuity levels and shorter hospital stays have moved the emphasis of hospitalization to specialty units providing acute care.

In the 1980s, as a way of containing escalating health care costs, the concept of diagnosis-related groups (DRGs) was introduced. Loosely defined, DRGs set limits on the number of days someone could be hospitalized based on a particular procedure or disease entity. Using DRGs means that patients are sent home quicker but often in a more acute stage than ever before. Although home care agencies have adjusted to the increasing acuity level found in the home, subacute care is becoming a new practice setting for nurses (Andreola & O'Neill, 1995; Ginsburg, 1995; Huey, 1995).

Subacute care is defined by The Joint Commission on the Accreditation of Healthcare Organizations (Andreola & O'Neill, 1995, p. 4) as

> goal-oriented, comprehensive, inpatient care designed for someone who has had an acute illness, injury, or exacerbation of a disease process. It is rendered immediately after, or instead of, acute hospitalization to treat one or more specific, active, complex medical conditions or to administer one or more technically complex treatments, in the context of a person's underlying long-term conditions and overall situation.

Subacute care offers services that fall between those of traditional nursing and the intensive care unit. Subacute care uses a team of interdisciplinary professionals who work together on a specifically defined program, regardless of whether the subacute unit is located in the hospital or in a long-term care facility (Andreola & O'Neill, 1995).

Economics have influenced the rise of subacute care units as a result of reimbursement schedules. According to some reports, treatment of at least 62 DRGs within a subacute care setting would lead to a savings of approximately 9 billion dollars a year (Huey, 1995). As a result of such findings, hospitals are seeking ways to provide care to the segment of people who still have acute health care needs following a hospital discharge, and they are opening subacute care settings to accommodate this group. Long-term care facilities, which traditionally provide skilled nursing care to the chronically ill and elderly, are also responding to the need and are opening subacute care units.

Long-Term Care Facilities

Long-term care provides a range of services "that address the health, social, and personal care needs of persons who are unable to care for themselves because of a physical or mental impairment caused by a chronic condition" (Reif & Estes, 1982, p. 151). Nurses constitute the majority of professionals working in this setting and provide most of the services that are needed.

The patient population in long-term care facilities traditionally has been the elderly and the chronically ill requiring skilled nursing care. The expected rise in an older population in the United States correlates with projected increase in the use of long-term care facilities by this age group (Reif & Estes, 1982). Gerontological nurses, nurses who specialize in aging, must be aware of issues surrounding aging, such as how ageism, developmental changes, and chronicity affect the care of the elderly. Moreover, long-term care nurses need a solid understanding of the social, political, and economic ramifications of aging and how they influence nursing care.

Summary

Nurses will find opportunities to practice in a variety of health care settings; however, as we move into the 21st century, these settings will change. What we know as practice sites today will shift to accommodate the social, economic, and political climate of the period. Therefore, it is important for nurses to keep abreast of the social, political, and economic factors that will influence where and how they practice in the future. Not unlike their early predecessors at the end of the 18th or 19th century, nurses today will need to keep politically involved, keep abreast of the times, and keep their voices heard within the professional nursing organizations and the political system.

■   ■

CHAPTER HIGHLIGHTS

✦

✦ The modern nursing movement in the United States occurred in the late 19th century, just as the country sought hospital reform, women wanted economic freedom, and newly opened nurses' training schools recruited qualified candidates. During this period, nursing supported women's right to receive an education, to work, and to vote.

✦ Graduates from nurses' training schools at the end of the 19th and beginning of the 20th centuries organized professional nursing organizations to assure the public of quality nursing education and practice and to advocate the rights of trained nurses. Nursing organizations worked to establish state registration laws throughout the country.

✦ Many educational pathways into nursing practice exist in the late 20th century. Prospective RNs are educated within many types of educational programs and then are eligible to take the NCLEX™ to become RNs. Although each state regulates the licensure of RNs, the NCLEX™ is a national examination, and reciprocity from state to state is granted.

✦ The definition of nursing has evolved over time. The ANA defines nursing as the diagnosis and treatment of human responses to actual or potential health problems.

✦ Licensure of nurses exists at the state level. The nurse practice act in each state provides the legal definition of nursing and prescribes the criteria used to grant state licensure.

✦ Advanced practice nurses, such as nurse practitioners, clinical nurse specialists, nurse clinicians, nurse-midwives, and nurse anesthetists, provide primary health care to individuals, families, and communities. APNs work in a variety of settings that include independent practice, community-based nursing centers, and acute care institutions.

✦ In the late 20th century, nurses will assume greater roles in the delivery of primary health care services in a variety of settings outside of the traditional institutions. Having an independent practice, dealing with third party reimbursement, and seeking public recognition require nurses to be better educated when serving individuals, families, and communities.

Study Questions

1. The NLN was formed for the purpose of controlling nursing

a. directories
b. education
c. licensing
d. certification

2. The NOCGN started as a result of racial

a. opportunity
b. diversity
c. inequity
d. equality

3. Outcome measures in accreditation ensure

a. reliability
b. stability
c. quality
d. validity

4. An important function of the nurse practice act is to

a. protect the public
b. educate nurses
c. ensure quality
d. define procedures

5. Licensure for nurses is granted by each

a. hospital
b. school
c. country
d. state

Critical Thinking Exercises

1. Describe what a young woman entering nursing in 1776, 1930, and 1997 could expect in her education and in her working conditions after graduation.

2. In 1997, clients are being admitted to acute care facilities sicker and being discharged earlier. Nurses are also finding more employment in community and home health care settings. How might this influence the education and preparation of nurses in the year 2000?

References

American Association of Colleges of Nursing. (1994). *AACN urges national standard for certifying advanced practice nurses: Position statement calls for standardized certification process by year 2000.* Washington, DC: American Association of Colleges of Nursing.

American Nurses Association. (1965). Committee on Education definition of nursing. *American Journal of Nursing, 65,* 106.

American Nurses Association. (1980). *Nursing: A social policy statement.* Kansas City, MO: American Nurses Association.

American Nurses Association. (1991). Nursing's agenda for health care reform. Washington, DC: American Nurses Association.

American Nurses Association. (1995). *Nursing's social policy statement.* Washington, DC: American Nurses Publishing.

American Nurses Association. (1991). *Standards of clinical nursing practice.* Washington, DC: American Nurses Publishing.

Andreola, N. M., & O'Neill, S. P. (1995). Subacute: A hot new trend on the shifting horizon of healthcare. *Nursing Spectrum, 7A*(3), 4–5, 7, 10.

Baer, E. (1993). Toward professional maturity, 1945–1952. In N. Birnbach, & S. Lewenson (Eds.), *Legacy of leadership: Presidential addresses from the Superintendents' Society and the National League for Nursing Education 1894–1952* (pp. 357–367). New York: National League for Nursing Press.

Benson, E. (1990). Nineteenth century women, the neophyte nursing profession. In V. Bullough, B. Bullough, & M. Stanton (Eds.), *Florence Nightingale and her era: A collection of new scholarship* (pp. 117–118). New York: Garland Publishing.

Benson, E. (1986). Nursing and the World's Columbian Exposition. *Nursing Outlook, 34* (2), 88–90.

Bridgeman, M. (1953). *Collegiate education for nursing.* New York: Russell Sage Foundation.

Brown, E. L. (1948). *Nursing for the future.* New York: Russell Sage Foundation.

Buhler-Wilkerson, K. (1992). Caring in its "proper place": Race and benevolence in Charleston, SC, 1813–1930. *Nursing Research, 41,* 13–16.

Bullough, V. (1994). Inquiry, insights, and history: Men in nursing. *Journal of Professional Nursing, 10* (5), 267.

Bullough, B., & Bullough, V. (1990). *Nursing in the community.* St. Louis: C.V. Mosby.

Bullough, V., Bullough, B., & Stanton, M. (Eds.) (1990). *Florence Nightingale and her era: A collection of new scholarship.* New York: Garland Publishing.

Burgess, M. A. (1928). *Nurses, patients, and pocketbooks: Report of a study of the economics of nursing conducted by the Committee on the Grading of Nursing Schools.* New York: Committee on the Grading of Nursing Schools.

Carnegie, E. (1991). *The path we tread: Blacks in nursing, 1854–1984.* Philadelphia: J. B. Lippincott.

The Committee for the Study of Nursing Education. (1984). *Nursing and nursing education in the United States.* New York: Macmillan. (Original work published 1923.)

Cook, E. (1913). *The life of Florence Nightingale* (Vol. 1). London: Macmillan.

Cott, N. (1987). *The grounding of modern feminism.* New Haven: Yale University Press.

Craven, D. (1984). *A guide to district nurses.* London: Macmillan. (Original work published 1889.)

Darche, L. (1894). Employments for women. No. 2. Trained nursing. *The Delineator: A Journal of Fashion, Culture and Fine Arts, 82,* 667–668.

Darche, L. (1949). Proper organization of training schools in America. In I. Hampton (Ed.), *Nursing of the sick 1893.* New York: McGraw-Hill. (Original work published 1894.)

Davis, M. E. P. (1912). Organization, or why belong. *American Journal of Nursing, 12* (6), 474–477.

Dietz, L. D., & Lehozky, A. R. (1967). *History and modern nursing* (2nd ed.). Philadelphia: F. A. Davis.

Dock, L. L. (1991). Directories for nurses. First and second annual conventions of the ASSTSN. (Reprinted in N. Birnbach, & S. Lewenson (Eds.) (1991) *First words: Selected addresses from the National League for Nursing 1894–1933* (pp. 87–90). New York: National League for Nursing Press.

Dock L., & Stewart I. (1931) *A short history of nursing: From the earliest times to the present day* (3rd ed. revised, pp. 146–152). New York: G. P. Putnam's Sons.

Fairman, J. (1992). Watchful vigilance: Nursing care, technology, and the development of intensive care units. *Nursing Research, 41*(1), 56–60.

Fitzpatrick, L. (1975). *The National Organization for Public Health Nursing, 1912–1952: Development of a practice field*. New York: National League for Nursing.

Fondiller, S. (1986). The American Nurses Association and National League for Nursing: Political relationships and realities. In R. White (Ed.), *Political issues in nursing: Past, present, and future* (Vol. 2, pp. 119–143). Baltimore: John Wiley & Sons.

Giles, I. (1993). *Address of President Ida Giles, Tenth annual convention of the Superintendents' Society, 1903, Pittsburgh, Pennsylvania*. (Reprinted in N. Birnbach, & S. Lewenson (Eds.). (1991). *First words: Selected addresses from the National League for Nursing 1894–1933*. New York: National League for Nursing Press.) (Original work published 1903.)

Ginsburg, E. (1995). Addressing the needs of patients not ready to return home. *New York Times,* January 1.

Gomez, A. (1994). Guest editorial: Men in nursing: An historical perspective. *Nurse Educator, 19*(5), 13–14.

Hampton, I. (1991). Introduction. In N. Birnbach, & S. Lewenson (Eds.), *First words: Selected addresses from the National League for Nursing 1894–1933*. New York: National League for Nursing Press.

Hampton, I. (1949). *Nursing of the sick 1893*. (New York: McGraw-Hill. (Reissue of J. S. Billings, & H. M. Hurd (Eds). (1894). Part III, Nursing of the sick. In *Hospitals, dispensaries and nursing: Papers and discusssions in the International Congress of Charities, Correction, and Philanthropy. Section III, Chicago, June 12–17th, 1893*. Baltimore: Johns Hopkins Press.

Harmer, B. (1933). *Text-book of the principles and practice of nursing* (2nd ed.). New York: Macmillan.

Harmer, B., & Henderson, V. (1939). *Textbook of the principles and practice of nursing* (4th ed.). New York: Macmillan.

Harmer, B., & Henderson, V. (1962). *Textbook of the principles and practice of nursing* (5th ed.). New York: Macmillan.

Hine, D. C. (1989). Racism, status, and the professionalization of black nurses. In D. C. Hine (Ed.), *Black women in white*. Bloomington, IN: Indiana University Press.

Huey, F. (1995). Subacute: Breaking the market barrier for skilled nursing. *Nursing Spectrum, 7A*(3), 3.

Johns, E. (1925). A study of the present status of the negro woman in nursing [Letter to Ethel Johns from Petra Pinn, President of the National Association of Colored Graduate Nurses, dated November 15, 1925]. Pocantico, NY: Rockefeller Archive Center, Record Group. RAC, RC, RG 1.1, Series 200, Box 122, Folder 1507, Appendix I.

Kalisch, P. A., & Kalisch, B. J. (1986). *The advance of American nursing* (2nd ed.). Boston: Little, Brown & Co.

Lewenson, S. (1994). "Of logical necessity . . . They hang to together": Nursing and the woman's movement, 1901–1912. *Nursing History Review, 2,* 99–117.

Lewenson, S. (1993). *Taking charge: Nursing, suffrage, and feminism, 1873–1920*. New York: Garland.

Lockhart, C. A. (1995). Community nursing centers: An analysis of status and needs. In B. Murphy (Ed.), *Nursing centers: The time is now*. New York: National League for Nursing.

Lord, J. (1873). *The life of Emma Willard*. New York: Appleton.

Louden, D., & Post, D. (1994). Executive summary. In *Nursing datasource 1994: Volume I. Trends in contemporary nursing education*. New York: National League for Nursing Press.

Louden, D., Zemokhol, R., & Jones, D. (1994). Executive summary. In *Nursing datasource 1994: Volume II. Graduate education in nursing advance practice nursing*. New York: National League for Nursing.

Lynaugh, J. (1993). Toward economic stability, 1929–1944. In N. Birnbach, & S. Lewenson (Eds.), *Legacy of leadership: Presidential addresses from the Superintendents' Society and the National League for Nursing Education 1894–1952* (pp. 215–229). New York: National League for Nursing Press.

Montag, M. L. (1991). *T. C. and the creation of the associate degree programs in nursing* [Unpublished paper delivered at the First Emeriti-Sponsored Seminar of 1991–92 held at Teachers College, Columbia University, New York].

Moore, F. (1866). *Women of the war: Their heroism and self-sacrifice*. Hartford, CT: S. S. Scranton & Co.

Munson, H. (1934). *The story of the National League for Nursing Education*. Philadelphia: W. B. Saunders.

National League for Nursing. (1990). *Policies and procedures of accreditation for programs in nursing education*. New York: National League for Nursing.

Nightingale, F. (1969). *Notes on nursing: What it is, and what it is not*. New York: Dover Publications. (Original work published 1860.)

North, F. (1882). A new profession for women. *The Century Illustrated Monthly Magazine, 25*(1), 39.

Nursing datasource 1994: Volume I. Trends in contemporary nursing education. (1994). New York: National League for Nursing Press.

Nursing datasource 1994: Volume II. Graduate education in nursing advanced practice nursing. (1994). New York: National League for Nursing.

Nutting, A. (1993). Address of President M. Adelaide Nutting, Fourth annual convention of the Superintendents' Society, 1897. In N. Birnbach, & S. Lewenson (Eds.), *Legacy of leadership: Presidential addresses from the Superintendents' Society and the National League for Nursing Education 1894–1952* (pp. 25–33). New York: National League for Nursing Press. (Original work published 1897.)

Pearson, L. (1993). 1992–93 Update: How each state stands on legislative issues affecting advanced nursing practice (1993). *The Nurse Practitioner: The American Journal of Primary Health Care,* 5th annual update. *18*(1)23–28.

Progress and reaction [Editorial comment]. (1908). *American Journal of Nursing, 8,* 333–334.

Reif, L., & Estes, C. L. (1982). Long-term care: New opportunities for professional nursing. In L. Aiken, & S. Gortner (Eds.), *Nursing in the 1980s: Crisis, opportunities, challenges* (pp. 147–181). Philadelphia: J. B. Lippincott.

Report of the Committee for the Study of Nursing Education. (1984). *Nursing and nursing education in the United States*. New York: Garland. (Original work published 1923.)

Report of the Woman's Rights Convention. Reprint, Eastern National Park and Monuments Association. Washington, DC: U.S. Department of the Interior. (Original work published 1848.)

Reverby, S. (1985). The search for the hospital yardstick: Nursing and the rationalization of hospital work. In J. W. Leavitt, & R. L. Numbers (Eds.), *Sickness and health in America: Readings in the history of medicine and public health* (2nd ed., pp. 206–216). Madison, WI: University of Wisconsin Press.

Richards, L. (1915). *Reminiscences of Linda Richards* (2nd ed.) Boston: Whitcomb & Barrows.

Robinson, V. (1946). *White caps: The story of nursing.* Philadelphia: J. B. Lippincott.

Rosenberg, C. E. (1987). *The care of strangers: The rise of America's hospital system.* New York: Basic Books.

Rothman, N. (1990). Toward description: Public health nursing and community health nursing are different. *Nursing and Health Care, 11*(9), 482–483.

Rudolph, F. (1971). Emma Hart Willard. In E. T. James, J. Wilson James, & P. S. Boyer (Eds.), *Notable American women 1607–1950: A biographic dictionary* (Vol. 3, pp. 610–613). Cambridge, MA: The Belknap Press of Harvard University Press.

Sklar, K. K. (1973). *Catherine Beecher: A study of American domesticity.* New Haven: Yale University Press.

Solomon, B. M. (1985). *In the company of educated women: A history of women and higher education in America* (pp. 14–26). New Haven: Yale University Press.

Staupers, M. (1985). Story of the National Association of Colored Graduate Nurses. In D. C. Hine (Ed.), *Black women in the nursing profession: A documentary history* (p. 144). New York: Garland.

Stewart, I. (1948). *The education of nurses: Historical foundations and modern trends* (pp. 84–87, 93–95). New York: Macmillan.

Tao, D. (1992). Louise M. Darche. In V. Bullough, L. Sentz, & A. P. Stein (Eds.), *American nursing: A biographical dictionary* (Vol. 2, pp. 75–77). New York: Garland.

Thoms, A. (1929). *Pathfinders: A history of the progress of the colored graduate nurses.* New York: Kay Printing House.

Vision for nursing education. 1993. New York: National League for Nursing.

Waite, R. (1990). Emma Hart Willard. In A. Zophy, & F. M. Kavenik (Eds.), *Handbook of American women's history* (pp. 662–663). New York: Garland.

Weeks, C. S. (1899). *Text-book of nursing* (2nd ed.). New York: Appleton.

Bibliography

Birnbach, N., & Lewenson, S. (Eds.). (1991). *First words: Selected addresses from the National League for Nursing 1894–1933.* New York: National League for Nursing Press.

Birnbach, N., & Lewenson, S. (Eds.). (1993). *Legacy of leadership: Presidential addresses from the Superintendents' Society and the National League for Nursing Education 1894–1952* (pp. 357–367). New York: National League for Nursing Press.

Bullough, V., Bullough, B., & Stanton, M., (eds.). (1990). *Florence Nightingale and her era: A collection of new scholarship.* New York: Garland.

Carnegie, E. (1991). *The path we tread: Blacks in nursing. 1854–1984.* Philadelphia: J. B. Lippincott.

Hine, D. C. (1989). *Black women in white: Racial conflict and cooperation in the nursing profession, 1890–1920.* Bloomington, IN: Indiana University Press.

Kalisch, P. A., & Kalisch, B. J. (1986). *The advance of American nursing* (2nd ed.). Boston: Little, Brown & Co.

Lewenson, S. (1993). *Taking charge: Nursing, suffrage, and feminism, 1873–1920.* New York: Garland.

Melosh, B. (1982). *"The physician's hand." Work, culture, and conflict in American nursing.* Philadelphia: Temple University Press.

Reverby, S. (1987). *Ordered to care: The dilemma of American nursing, 1850–1945.* Cambridge, MA: Cambridge University Press.

Rosenberg, C. E. (1987). *The care of strangers: The rise of America's hospital system.* New York: Basic Books.

Waite, R. (1990). Emma Hart Willard. In A. Zophy, & F. M. Kavenik (Eds.), *Handbook of American women's history* (pp. 662–663). New York: Garland.

Chapter 2

THEORIES AND MODELS OF NURSING PRACTICE

VETA MASSEY, PhD, RN

KEY TERMS
♦

concept	nursing
environment	person
health	proposition
model	theory

LEARNING OBJECTIVES
♦

After studying this chapter, you should be able to

♦ Identify the importance of theory in nursing

♦ Describe the relationship of theory to practice and research

♦ Identify four types of theories

♦ Examine concepts important to nursing

♦ Explore interdisciplinary theories that are used by nurses

♦ Discuss the history and evolution of nursing theory

♦ Describe selected nursing theories and their relationship to the nursing process and to client needs

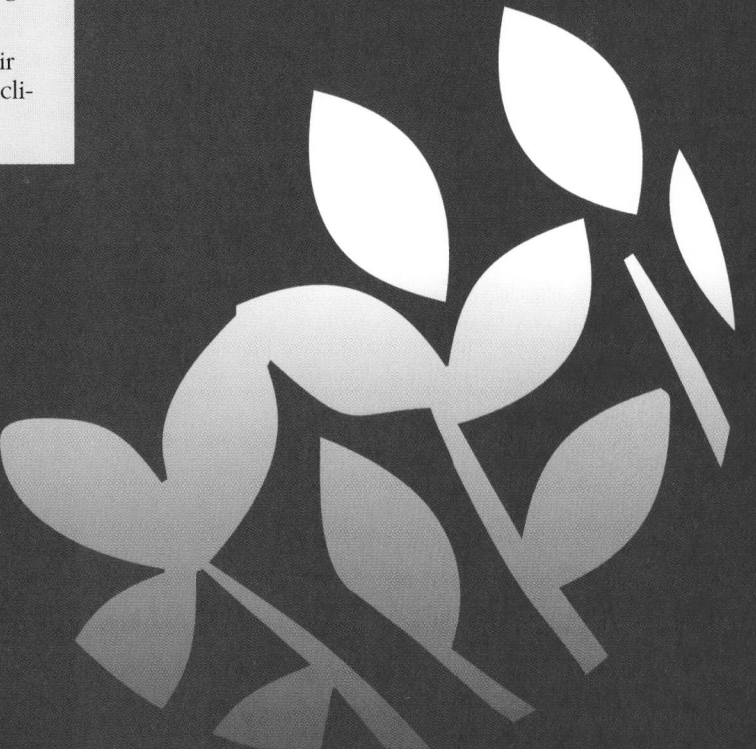

Overview of Theory

Practicing in today's health care delivery system requires that the nurse make decisions that are based on knowledge and scientific rationale. As technology continues to expand and the acuity level rises for clients in the hospital and at home, a strong theoretical knowledge base assumes greater importance. Nursing theory is necessary for nurses to make valid decisions and to demonstrate nursing's unique contributions to care. A profession is built on a specialized body of knowledge, and for nursing to establish itself, nursing theory is essential. Theory helps avoid a random approach to client care and guides the nurse in making pertinent observations, analyzing deviations from normal, and planning nursing care activities.

A **theory** consists of a set of interrelated concepts and propositions that explain some aspect of our reality. It provides a window through which one may view a part of the world. It is a pattern or blueprint that helps organize some phenomenon. Successful theories differentiate a particular phenomenon from similar, related phenomena in terms of content, processes, context, and goals. *Content* is the knowledge embedded in the phenomenon. *Processes* define the methods and practices. *Context* refers to the environment in which the phenomenon is found, and *goals* relate to the unique purpose of the phenomenon (Barnum, 1994). According to Torres (1990, pp. 6–9), theories have the following basic characteristics:

1. Theories can interrelate concepts in such a way as to create a different way of looking at a particular phenomenon.
2. Theories must be logical in nature.
3. Theories should be relatively simple yet generalizable.
4. Theories can be the basis for hypotheses that can be tested.
5. Theories contribute to and assist in increasing the general body of knowledge within the discipline through the research implemented to validate them.
6. Theories can be utilized by the practitioners to guide and improve their practice.
7. Theories must be consistent with other validated theories, laws, and principles but will leave open questions that need to be investigated.

Relationship of Theory to Practice and Research

These characteristics outline the direct relationships that theories have with practice and research. Nurses use theories to direct decisions made in daily work situations and to plan interventions that are supported by rationale. Nurse researchers also use theories to derive hypotheses that can be tested with scientific studies. When nursing research is grounded in theory, the results contribute to the body of knowledge that is unique to nursing. When theories are supported through use in practice and research, their usefulness is demonstrated and their validity intensifies. Thus, the use of nursing theory is essential to guide practice and research, and nursing practice and research contribute to the development and support of theory.

Types of Theory

Depending on its level of development and use, a theory may be descriptive, explanatory, predictive, or controlling (Fig. 2–1). A *descriptive* theory simply describes or delineates the phenomena of interest. When little is known about an area or event, the first type of theory is likely to be descriptive and will identify the characteristics and dimensions of the situation. After descriptive theories have been supported, *explanatory* theories may be developed. These theories will outline or explain the relationships among the characteristics and dimensions of a phenomenon. When explanatory theories have been tested and validated, predictive theories may emerge. *Predictive* theories are used to predict cause and effect relationships among the dimensions of a phenomenon. Finally, after a predictive theory has received considerable support, it may evolve into a *controlling* theory, which provides for control of the phenomenon.

Theories related to smoking may provide an example of a way in which the development of theories occurs. Several years ago, scientists proposed theories that described the effects of cigarette smoking. As research and scientific observations supported these descriptions, the theories evolved into explanations about the relationships between smoking and lung cancer, heart disease, and other chronic illnesses. After these relationships received validation, theories began to predict that people who smoked would have a higher incidence of lung cancer, heart disease, and other chronic illnesses. Now that these predictive theories have been supported in practice and with scientific evidence, theories have evolved that delineate ways to control the occurrence of lung cancer, heart disease, and other chronic illnesses that result from smoking.

Concepts, Propositions, and Models

As stated previously, theories consist of interrelated concepts and propositions. **Concepts** are mental images or ideas to which a label or meaning is attached. Torres (1990) classifies concepts as empirical, inferen-

Theory development: Effects of cigarette smoking

✦ **Figure 2–1**
Theories about the effects of
cigarette smoking serve to
illustrate the way in which
scientific theories are developed
and used.

tial, or abstract, depending on the degree to which they can be observed in the world. *Empirical* concepts are those that can be readily observed, such as a chair or desk. *Inferential* concepts, such as pain or blood pressure, are indirectly observable, while abstract concepts, such as stress or health, are not observable. *Abstract* concepts are more difficult to clearly understand and communicate to others. Some concepts may be abstract in one situation and empirical in another. For example, the concept of person is abstract when it refers to all people because all people cannot be observed. However, when the concept of person refers to a specific individual, it is empirical because one individual can be observed.

In a theory, concepts are linked together by **propositions,** which are statements that specify and clarify the relationships among the concepts (Hickman, 1995). For example, many theories propose that health is affected by the environment. A theory may be diagrammed as a **model,** a symbolic representation that uses a minimal number of words to express the abstract concepts and propositions. Most models are schematics, which convey the concepts and propositions through the use of boxed words, arrows, and other symbols. A model may be mathematical and use letters, numbers, and mathematical symbols.

·· ✦ ··
Concepts Important to Nursing
··

Nursing theories describe the relationships among the concepts of interest to the profession. Most nursing theorists agree that there are four concepts important

to nursing—person, health, environment, and nursing care activities. However, each theorist may define the concepts and the relationships among the concepts in very different ways. These differences will become evident when the various nursing theories are discussed later in this chapter.

Person refers to the recipient of care and may be an individual, family, group, or community. The term *patient* or *client* is frequently used to designate the person. This concept is viewed as being central to the profession and may be considered as the most important. The person varies from one nursing situation to another, requiring the nurse to be versatile, knowledgeable, and adept at critical thinking.

Health is the goal of nursing and is defined in many different ways by various groups and individuals. The American Nurses Association (ANA) (1980) defines health as "a dynamic state of being in which the developmental and behavioral potential of an individual is realized to the fullest extent possible" (p. 5). Thus, health can change drastically throughout life and may vary from day to day. It is more than and different from the absence of disease and may exist independent of pathophysiological conditions that have been labeled as diseases. A person may be diagnosed with a disease but may be considered healthy.

Environment is all the conditions and circumstances affecting the person and is the setting in which nursing care activities occur. The environment surrounds each individual, and there is constant interaction between the person and the environment. This concept was first emphasized by Florence Nightingale, and it is receiving renewed interest today. It is essential for the nurse to consider the ramifications of environmental factors on health.

The ANA (1980) defines **nursing** as the "diagnosis and treatment of human responses to actual or potential health problems" (p. 9). To fulfill this function, many activities are employed. *Nursing care activities* include all of the actions taken by nurses while interacting with and for clients. These actions range from the technical tasks, such as bathing and bed making, to the complex critical thinking transactions required when using the nursing process.

Relationship of Theory to the Nursing Process

The nursing process is a problem-solving approach used by nurses in many different practice settings. Its specific steps—assessment, diagnosis, planning, implementation, and evaluation—are particularly helpful to students. (See Chapters 7–12 for specific information on the nursing process.)

Theory may be viewed as the knowledge necessary for practice, while the nursing process is a method of applying theory to or using content in practice. Skillfully using the nursing process is the art of nursing, the ability to use knowledge effectively in practice (Torres, 1986). Consequently, to demonstrate the art of nursing, a nurse must also exhibit the science of nursing and vice versa. The theory and knowledge base cannot be separated from their application through the nursing process. To completely and thoroughly assess a client; accurately derive nursing diagnoses; and plan, implement, and evaluate nursing care activities, a nurse must have a solid theoretical knowledge base. Theories from other disciplines as well as nursing theories may be included in the knowledge base.

Interdisciplinary Theories

Systems Theory

Systems theory is used by several disciplines as a way to explain interactions and changes that result from interactions. A system consists of interrelated components known as subsystems and is also part of a suprasystem. Each component has a function, and the system has a purpose. The world is seen as a hierarchy of systems, with each system having one or more suprasystems and subsystems (Kenney, 1990). For example, a family may be viewed as a system consisting of mother, father, son, and daughter as subsystems and community, city, and state as suprasystems. In addition, an individual may be viewed as a system consisting of neurological, cardiovascular, and gastrointestinal subsystems and family, community, city, and state suprasystems.

All living systems are open systems and are surrounded by a semipermeable boundary through which there is exchange of energy and information between the system and its environment. The boundary acts like a filter and regulates the rate and flow of interchanges. Systems that have frequent interchanges are known as very open systems while those with little interchange are said to be relatively closed systems. In times of crisis, systems may tighten their boundaries and become less open than usual.

The information, matter, and energy that the system receives from the environment provide input for the system. The system uses, organizes, and transforms the input in a process known as throughput and releases information, matter, and energy as output into the environment. Output that returns to the system as input is called feedback. Because of these interactions, change in one part of the system affects the entire system and results in rebound changes (Leddy & Pepper, 1993). Figure 2–2 illustrates how systems theory can be used to examine a nursing school.

Systems theory can be used to guide the nursing process when caring for an individual, family, or community. If used, it would guide the nurse to assess and analyze all subsystems, input, throughput, output, and feedback. Planning would take into consideration ways in which interventions directed toward one part of the system would affect and change the entire system. Evaluation would be directed toward measuring the impact on all components of the system. Several of the nursing theories discussed later in the chapter are based on systems theory.

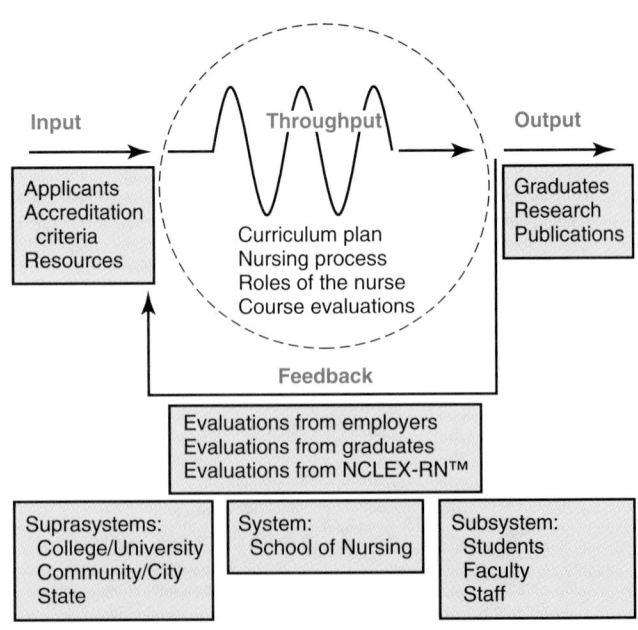

❥ Figure 2–2
A systems model may be used to examine the functions and relationship of a school of nursing in relation to the community of which it is a part.

Needs Theory

Abraham Maslow outlined a hierarchy of human needs theory that has gained a large following from several disciplines. His theory is based on several assumptions:

1. Certain internal and external, physical and psychological needs are common to all people.
2. Human needs can be arranged in a hierarchical order, with basic needs being the first that must be met.
3. Needs that have not been met create tension, which motivates an individual to meet specific needs.
4. When a need is completely met, an individual is no longer aware of the need and it no longer motivates behavior.
5. The dominant needs that motivate an individual will vary throughout his or her life.

Figure 2–3 demonstrates Maslow's Hierarchy of Needs Model.

Needs theory is frequently used by practicing nurses when employing the nursing process. Assessment, diagnosis, planning, implementation, and evaluation of physiological needs must take place before higher-level needs are considered. If no problem is found with physiological needs, then safety needs are examined. Belonging needs are not assessed until all physiological and safety needs are met. In this way, the nurse can use the nursing process to ascend the hierarchy and focus attention on the lowest level in which needs are identified.

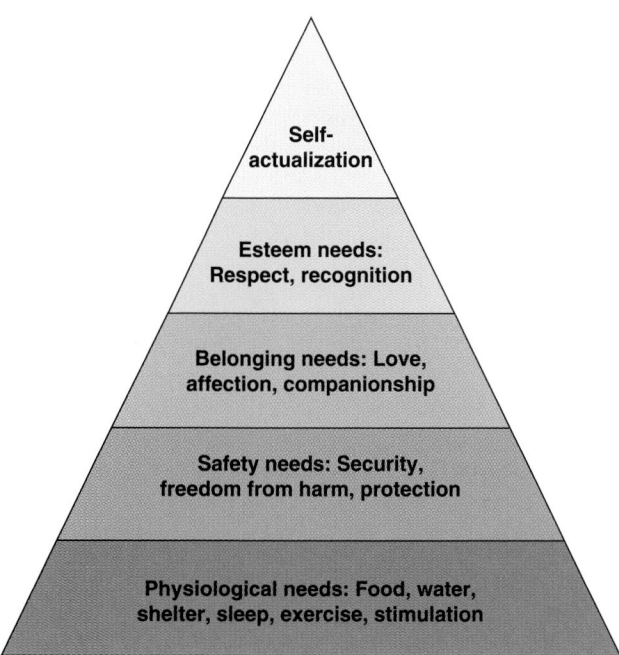

❦ **Figure 2–3**
Maslow's Hierarchy of Human Needs.

Health Belief Model

As stated earlier, a theory may be diagrammed as a model. Rosenstock (1966) outlined the theoretical elements of the health belief model in an attempt to aid understanding of why and under what conditions people take action to prevent or detect disease. The model includes two categories of variables: a psychological state of readiness to take action and the extent to which a particular action is believed to be beneficial. He defined the state of readiness as the individual's perceived susceptibility to a condition and the perceived seriousness of that condition. People's perceptions vary widely; they are subjective beliefs and may have no basis in fact.

The extent to which action is believed to be beneficial is viewed in conjunction with existing barriers to that action. An individual may believe that a certain activity will help prevent or detect a condition but at the same time may see that activity as expensive, painful, or inconvenient. Thus, if one believes an action to be very beneficial with few negative aspects, the likelihood of taking that action is high. If one believes an action to be only somewhat beneficial while having several negative aspects, the possibility of action is low.

Rosenstock (1966) also suggested that a cue to action, a trigger to set off an appropriate behavior, appeared to be necessary. The cue could be internal, such as experiencing pain or indigestion, or external, such as a news story or a reminder card from the doctor. If the individual's perceptions of susceptibility and severity were relatively low, an intense cue would be needed to trigger an action. On the other hand, if the individual's perceptions of susceptibility and severity were high, a relatively mild cue might be sufficient to stimulate an action. For example, a woman who thinks she is not susceptible to breast cancer may not examine her breasts even though her best friend is diagnosed with breast cancer, while a woman who believes she is very susceptible to breast cancer will examine her breasts when she sees a brochure about breast cancer. Figure 2–4 illustrates how the health belief model could be applied to mammography.

The health belief model is particularly useful when using the nursing process to promote health. It leads the nurse to assess the client's beliefs about a particular condition and about activities related to prevention or early detection of that condition. This information is used to plan the health promotion program. For example, if assessment reveals that a client believes that she is susceptible to breast cancer and that breast cancer is serious but has not had a mammogram because of the expense, planning and implementation of the health promotion program should be aimed toward interventions that would enhance the perceived benefits and reduce the perceived barriers rather than education about the likelihood and consequences of breast cancer. See Chapter 5 for additional information on health models and their use in nursing practice.

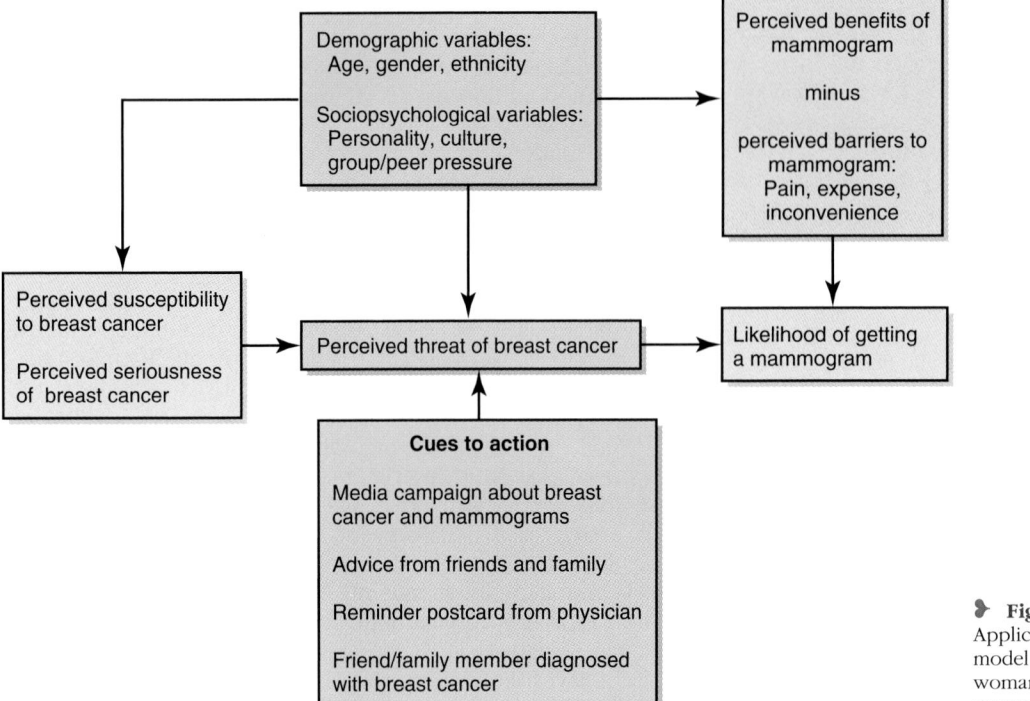

❧ **Figure 2–4**
Application of the health belief model to understanding of a woman's decision to undergo mammography.

Developmental Theories

Several theorists are associated with a variety of developmental frameworks. Freud is credited as being one of the first theorists to examine the psychosocial development of children. Erikson built on Freud's theory and extended the concept of development to cover the life span rather than limiting it to childhood. He outlined eight developmental stages that individuals experience between birth and death. According to Erikson, each stage has an associated task that must be resolved during the stage for the person to successfully progress to the following stages. If the task is not resolved, a person may have difficulty later in life. See Chapters 15 to 18 for more details on developmental theories and their use in practice.

Other developmental theorists have generated frameworks that apply to the development of families. These viewpoints examine changes and interactions that take place within the family unit over time. The family is seen as having a life cycle that begins with the marriage of the couple, proceeds through the birth and launching of the children, and ends with the death of both spouses. The assumption is made that all families progress through stages based primarily on the age of the first child. Each stage has associated tasks and goals that the family should accomplish. These theories have been criticized because they do not consider unusual events or diverse family compo-

sitions. See Chapter 19 for additional information on family theories and their use with the nursing process.

Stress/Adaptation Theories

Theories related to stress and adaptation have originated in many disciplines and have influenced several nursing theorists. Stress may be seen as both a cause and an effect and as having physiological and psychological components. Major life events are described as stress and may cause illnesses. Regardless of whether the life events are perceived as joyful or sad, they are stressful, and illness may result, especially when numerous major life events occur within a limited time span.

Selye (1974) describes stress as the body's nonspecific response to any demand made on it. He uses the term *stressor* to refer to any nonspecific demand requiring adaptation. The body's reactions to stressors became known as the general adaptation syndrome, which consists of three phases: (1) the alarm reaction; (2) the stage of resistance; and (3) the stage of exhaustion (Fig. 2–5). During the alarm phase, the body shows the changes characteristic of the fight or flight response, and the individual is mobilized for defense. Resistance ensues as the body adapts to the stressor. If the body continues to be exposed to the stressor, adaptation energy is exhausted, and the individual dies.

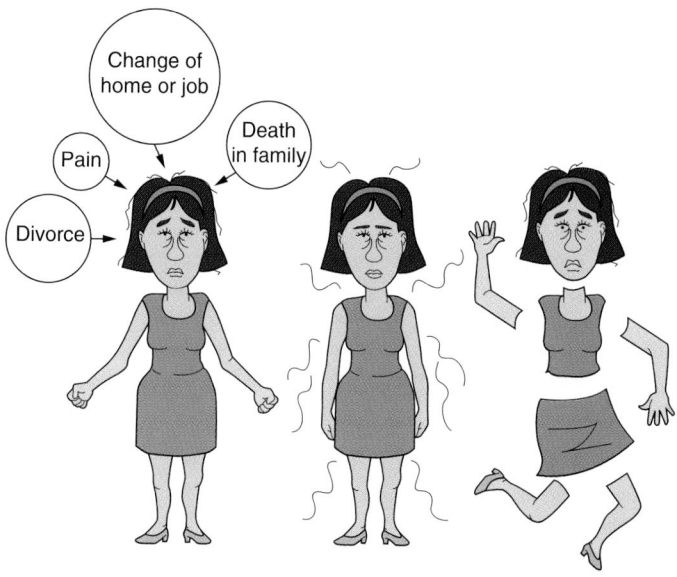

Phase 1:
Alarm reaction
Body mobilizes against
stressors with
fight-or-flight
response

Phase 2:
Resistance
Body adapts to
stressors

Phase 3:
Exhaustion
With continued
exposure to
stressor, adaptation
energy is
exhausted—
eventual outcome
is death

❧ **Figure 2–5**
General adaptation syndrome, consisting of the initial alarm
reaction, followed by resistance and eventual exhaustion.

Lazarus and Folkman (1984) view stress in relation
to cognitive appraisal and coping. Whenever an event
occurs, it undergoes primary and secondary appraisal.
With primary appraisal, the individual may categorize
the event as irrelevant, benign-positive, or stressful. If
the event is judged to be stressful, it is then classified
as harm/loss, threat, or challenge. In harm/loss events,
some damage to the person has occurred. Threat
events concern harms or losses that are anticipated,
while challenge appraisals focus on the potential for
gain or growth. Threat and challenge are not mutually
exclusive, and one event may be appraised as containing both threat and challenge. For example, beginning
nursing school holds potential for gaining new knowledge and skills; at the same time it creates the possibility of not performing as well as one would like.

When an event has been judged as threat or challenge, secondary appraisal becomes necessary. During
this appraisal, the individual evaluates what can be
done to manage the situation. This is a complex process that takes into account which coping options are
available, the likelihood those coping options will succeed, and the likelihood that a certain strategy can be
used. Theories related to stress and adaptation are
particularly valuable to nursing because illness is usually stressful to the client and family. See Chapter 6 for
specific ways stress theories are used with the nursing
process.

Nursing Theories

History and Evolution of Nursing Theory

Nursing theory originated with the work and writings of Florence Nightingale. However, until the
1950s, nursing was primarily based on theories from
psychology, sociology, and the physical sciences. Between the time of Florence Nightingale and the early
1950s, there was a dearth of nursing practice theory.
In the mid-1950s, with the publication of Hildegard
Peplau's book *Interpersonal Relations in Nursing*
(1952) and the journal *Nursing Research* and the advent of graduate nursing programs, interest blossomed
in developing nursing theories.

The 1960s witnessed the birth of several nursing
theories along with a surge in scientific research, conferences, and publications. In 1960, Faye Abdellah developed her typology of 21 nursing problems that focus on the physical, biological, and psychosocial
needs of the patient (Abdellah *et al.*, 1960). The following year, Ida Jean Orlando (1961) published her
Nursing Process Theory, which outlined principles to
guide nursing practice and the nurse-patient relationship. Three years later, Ernestine Wiedenbach (1964)

published the Helping Art of Clinical Nursing theory detailing her three principles of helping—inconsistency/consistency, purposeful perseverance, and self-extension. Also in 1964, Lydia Hall presented her Core, Care, and Cure theory representing the interactions among the patient, the body, and the disease. In 1966, Virginia Henderson refined her definition of nursing and proposed 14 components of basic nursing care. In 1969, Myra Levine proposed her conservation theory that espoused four principles to conserve energy, structural integrity, personal integrity, and social integrity. All of these early nurse theorists made critical contributions to the theoretical foundation for nursing practice.

The 1970s might be called the heyday of nursing theory. Many of the nursing theories used today were spawned during this decade and have continued to evolve. Details about these theories are given later in this chapter. Theory development was stimulated by the publication of articles and books on theory, national conferences on theory development, and nursing education accreditation requirements for conceptual frameworks. Nursing was striving to be recognized as a profession, and the generation of nursing theory was perceived as a crucial step.

The 1980s and 1990s have witnessed the refinement of several nursing theories and the origination of others. However, some of the theories developed in this period have been limited to specific practice areas rather than encompassing the entire clinical arena. For example, Ramona Mercer's theory of Maternal-Role Attainment (Bee *et al.,* 1994) and Kathryn Barnard's theory of Parent-Child Interaction (Baker *et al.,* 1994) deal only with the area of parent-child nursing. In addition, there has been a growing acceptance of the philosophy of holism and the value of personal, subjective experiences. Indeed, this seems to be the wave of the future, as nursing is concerned with the whole, unique individual and not just selected parts of the person. With acceptance of this philosophy, qualitative research is leading to the generation of grounded theory in nursing. An example of this is Joy Johnson's (1991) grounded theory of Adjustment Following a Heart Attack. Her theory evolved from in-depth interviews with 14 people who had experienced a heart attack.

Florence Nightingale's Environmental Theory

Florence Nightingale is credited as being the first nurse theorist, even though she did not use current terms such as *concept* and *theory.* Her book, *Notes on Nursing: What It Is and What It Is Not,* was first published in 1859 and continues to serve as a foundation for nursing practice.

Nightingale (1859/1946) viewed nursing as more than the administration of medicines and application of treatments. The nurse's control of the environment is the main theme throughout her writings. Nurses

should properly use fresh air, light, warmth, cleanliness, and quiet to help the patient recover.

Ventilation, especially with fresh air and without drafts, is of primary importance. Ventilation must be sufficient to remove effluvia (vapors) discharged from excreta and the diseased body. In fact, all substances discharged from the body should be immediately taken from the room to prevent the effluvia from endangering the patient. While ensuring adequate ventilation and fresh air, it is also essential to guard against the loss of heat and prevent chilling. If body heat is lost, warmth may be restored by using proper bedclothes and hot bottles.

Next in importance is the value of light, particularly sunlight. Light is essential to health and recovery from illness. Sunlight helps purify the air and makes the room more cheerful. Both body and mind degenerate without sunlight. If possible, the client should be placed so that he or she has a view from the bed or at least can see the sky and sunlight.

The greater part of nursing consists of preserving cleanliness. Fresh air will not be beneficial in a room where scrupulous cleanliness is not observed. Dusting must be done with a damp cloth to remove the dust and not just move it around. The skin must be kept clear of excretions, so the nurse should never postpone attending to the client's cleanliness. The nurse's hands should also be washed frequently.

Intermittent, sudden noise is to be avoided, especially during a client's first sleep. If one is awakened out of first sleep, it is almost certain there will be no more sleep. Whispered conversations in the room or hallway should be avoided, as they create excitement and uncertainty in the client. A firm, light step will disturb the client less than will walking on tip-toe.

Nightingale's theory is mainly concerned with the need for a safe and protective environment. The main physiological needs addressed are the needs for sleep and air. Psychosocial needs are addressed by an emphasis placed on the importance of occasional variety and her view that recovery is enhanced by the effect of beautiful, colorful objects. Growth and development needs are not considered in this theory. The relationship of Nightingale's theory to the nursing process is presented in Table 2–10.

Hildegard Peplau's Interpersonal Relations Theory

Hildegard Peplau (1952/1991) states that nursing has a serial and goal-directed nature that requires certain steps and actions between the nurse and the client. Nursing is an interpersonal process that is often therapeutic, in that people benefit from the interaction. Nursing is a human relationship between the one who is in need of health services and the nurse who has been educated to respond to the need. The nurse-client relationship has four overlapping phases—orientation, identification, exploitation, and resolution.

During the orientation phase, an individual seeks

assistance because of a felt need. A health problem has emerged, and professional help is sought. This is the first step in a dynamic learning experience from which personal and social growth should result. Orienting the client to recognize the problem and the extent of need is a complex task. The client is engaged as an active partner by encouraging participation in identifying and assessing the problem. When a client seeks assistance for a felt need, there is tension and anxiety present. The nurse must help the client use the energy from the tension and anxiety for positive action directed toward understanding the problem. The nurse should also help reduce anxiety and tension by orienting the client to the environment and procedures to be done.

During the identification phase, the client understands the situation and responds to the nurse, who can supply the needed help. Clients become cheerful and optimistic as they identify with nurses who are cheerful and optimistic. The client and the nurse clarify preconceptions and expectations of each other. The nurse uses professional education and skill to help the client learn how to make use of the nurse-client relationship.

During the phase of exploitation, the client makes full use of the services offered and explores all possibilities. At the same time, new goals, such as going home and returning to work, are identified. There is shifting back and forth as the client tries to strike a balance between dependence and independence.

As needs are met and energy is directed toward the new goals formulated during exploitation, the patient enters the phase of resolution. Dependent behavior is fully relinquished. However, resolution is more psychological than physiological, so medical recovery and the wish to terminate the relationship do not always coincide. The nurse must ensure that needs for psychological dependency are met, or the associated

anxiety may be converted into vague physical symptoms.

Throughout the four phases of the nurse-client relationship, the nurse functions in several roles. These roles are presented in Table 2–1.

Peplau's theory (1952/1991) is mainly concerned with the need for growth and development and with psychosocial needs. She views nursing as a force that promotes movement of the personality in becoming more creative and productive. The physiological needs are secondary to the psychosocial needs, and it is the psychological environment that needs to be safe and protective. Peplau states that "the nursing process is educative and therapeutic when nurse and patient can come to know and to respect each other, as persons who are alike, and yet, different, as persons who share in the solution of problems" (p. 9). The relationship of her theory to the nursing process is presented in Table 2–10.

Martha Rogers' Science of Unitary Human Beings

Martha Rogers developed one of the most abstract conceptual systems of nursing theory. Unitary human beings are irreducible wholes that cannot be understood when reduced to parts. The environment also has a unitary nature that is irreducible. The concept of field is used as a means of looking at people and their environments as wholes. Human beings and their environments are viewed as dynamic, infinite energy fields (Rogers, 1986).

An energy field is always open and has a pattern, the distinguishing characteristic, which is perceived as a wave. The nature of the pattern is continuously changing. Each human energy field pattern is unique and is integral with its unique environmental energy field pattern. The concept of four-dimensionality, a nonlinear domain without space and time limitations, characterizes human and environmental energy fields. It is a way of seeing humans and their world. Thus, the unitary human being and the environment are both defined as "an irreducible, four-dimensional energy field identified by pattern and manifesting characteristics that are different from those of its parts" (Rogers, 1986, p. 5). Manifestations of field patterning are observable, and increasing diversity of field patterning is characteristic of change.

Rogers (1986) derived three principles of homeodynamics from her conceptual system. These principles propose the nature and direction of change and are presented in Table 2–2.

Rogers' Science of Unitary Human Beings (1986) is concerned with the need for a safe and protective environment, which is seen as an energy field that is infinite and integral with the human energy field. Rogers' conceptual system is also concerned with growth and development needs. Aging is a developmental process continuous from conception through the dying process. Field patterns become increasingly di-

Table 2–1
ROLES OF THE NURSE IN INTERPERSONAL RELATIONS THEORY

ROLE	DEFINITION
Resource person	Provides knowledge and answers specific questions about the health problem
Teacher	Uses a combination of roles to develop the client's interest in medical information
Leader	Gives direction during the present problem
Surrogate	Acts as substitute figure that the client imagines the nurse to be, such as mother or aunt
Counselor	Facilitates self-directed actions that arise within the client

Table 2–2

PRINCIPLES OF HOMEODYNAMICS

PRINCIPLE	DEFINITION
Resonancy	The continuous change from lower to higher frequency wave patterns in energy fields; movement toward increasing complexity
Helicy	The continuous and innovative increasing diversity of field patterns characterized by nonrepeating rhythmicities; changes in life processes are irreversible
Integrality	The continuous mutual human and environmental field interaction; changes in life processes occur at the same time in both fields

verse and change more rapidly. Physiological and psychosocial needs cannot be considered separately in this theory, as it would be against the concept of the unitary human being. The relationship of Rogers' theory to the nursing process is presented in Table 2–10.

Dorothea Orem's Self-Care Deficit Theory

Dorothea Orem (1991) began theorizing about nursing in 1958 and has continued to refine her theory. She proposes that the self-care deficit theory of nursing is a general theory that contains three subtheories: (1) the theory of self-care, (2) the theory of self-care deficit, and (3) the theory of nursing system. The general theory involves relationships between the concepts of self-care, self-care agency, therapeutic self-care demand, self-care requisite, self-care deficit, and nursing agency. These concepts are defined in Table 2–3.

The theory of self-care proposes that people perform actions to control factors that affect their own development to enhance life, health, and well-being. They also perform these actions for dependent family members. Self-care requisites are of three types: (1) those universally required for all human beings, (2) those required because of developmental processes, and (3) those that arise from an individual's health status.

The theory of self-care deficit identifies the object of nursing as human beings with limitations in self-care. Self-care is affected by an individual's health-related limitations in knowing what to do or how to do it. Nursing is necessary when there is a deficit present or when a future deficit can be anticipated. *Deficit* stands for the relationship between the actions

one would take and the actions one is capable of taking.

The theory of nursing system establishes the relationship between the client and the nurse. Three types of nursing systems are identified: (1) wholly compensatory, (2) partly compensatory, and (3) supportive-educative. If a client is totally unable to engage in self-care activities, the wholly compensatory nursing system is required. If the client can perform some but not all of the self-care activities required, the partly compensatory nursing system is necessary. The supportive-educative nursing system is used when the client can perform all self-care actions required but needs support and guidance with decision-making, behavior control, or acquiring skills and knowledge.

Orem's theory (1991) is concerned with growth and development needs, which she identifies as developmental self-care requisites. The theory is also concerned with physiological and psychosocial needs, which are identified as health-deviation self-care requisites. The need for a safe and protective environment is one of Orem's eight universal self-care requisites. The relationship of her theory to the nursing process is presented in Table 2–10.

Table 2–3

CONCEPTS IN OREM'S SELF-CARE DEFICIT THEORY

CONCEPT	DEFINITION
Self-care	Learned, goal-oriented activity directed to self or the environment in the interest of maintaining life, health, development, and well-being
Self-care agency	The capability that enables individuals to determine and meet their requirements for action to regulate their functioning and development
Therapeutic self-care demand	Everything required by an individual in relation to meeting all known self-care requisites
Self-care requisite	The goal of self-care; the reason for which self-care is undertaken
Self-care deficit	When self-care agency is unable to meet therapeutic self-care demands
Nursing agency	The capabilities of persons educated as nurses that empower them within an interpersonal relationship to help persons meet therapeutic self-care demands

Table 2-4

CONCEPTS IN ROY'S ADAPTATION MODEL

CONCEPT	DEFINITION
Stimuli	
Focal	Stimulus immediately confronting the system
Contextual	All other factors in the situation that affect the focal stimulus
Residual	Internal and external factors whose effect on the focal stimulus is unclear
Coping mechanisms	
Regulator subsystem	Neural, chemical, and endocrine processes
Cognator subsystem	Perceptual/information processing, learning, judgment, and emotion
Adaptive modes	
Physiological	Senses, fluids and electrolytes, neurological, and endocrine
Self-concept	Psychological and spiritual
Role function	Roles in society
Interdependence	Interactions related to love, respect, and values
Responses	
Adaptive	Promote integrity and goals
Ineffective	Threaten survival, growth, reproduction, and/or mastery

with pain, residual stimuli might include previous experiences with pain and pain experiences of others that have been related to the client. All of the stimuli constitute the person's adaptation level, which represents the ability to respond positively.

As inputs, the stimuli and adaptation level are processed through the coping mechanisms, which are categorized as the regulator subsystem and the cognator subsystem. The regulator subsystem responds automatically through neural, chemical, and endocrine processes. For example, the postoperative client who has pain will experience many effects from the input to the nervous and endocrine systems that cause chemical, neural, and hormonal changes. The cognator subsystem responds through four cognitive-emotive channels — perceptual/information processing, learning, judgment, and emotion. The client who is in pain would selectively attend to the pain, gain insight about the pain, employ problem-solving and decision-making activities, and utilize emotional defenses to seek relief from the anxiety associated with the pain.

The responses that result from the regulator and cognator subsystems can be observed in four adaptive modes known as the physiological, self-concept, role function, and interdependence modes (see Clinical Insight Box). Behavior in the physiological mode is seen in the physiological activity of the senses, fluids and electrolytes, neurological function, and endocrine function. Basic to physiological integrity are the needs for oxygenation, nutrition, elimination, activity and rest, and protection. The self-concept mode focuses on the psychological and spiritual aspects of the person and the need to know who one is so that one can

Sister Callista Roy's Adaptation Model

Sister Callista Roy began development of her theory while she was a graduate student, and she has continued to examine and test the theoretical propositions as the model has evolved. Her theory is based on concepts from systems theory and adaptation theory, and she describes the recipient of nursing care as a holistic adaptive system (Roy & Andrews, 1991). Concepts from Roy's model are summarized in Table 2-4.

Inputs to the system are called stimuli and may be internal or external. Three types of stimuli are identified — focal, contextual, and residual. The focal stimulus is the stimulus that is immediately confronting the system, such as pain in the postoperative client. Contextual stimuli are all other objects or events in the situation that contribute to the effect of the focal stimulus. In the postoperative client with pain, contextual stimuli might be the temperature of the room and the presence or absence of significant others. Residual stimuli are the internal and external factors whose effects on the focal stimulus are unclear. For the client

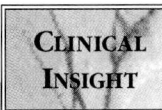

CLINICAL INSIGHT

Fawcett and Knauth conducted a factor analysis of the Perception of Birth Scale, which was developed to measure women's perceptions of their labor and delivery experience. The scale had been used to represent adaptation within the framework of the Roy Adaptation Model. The results of the data analysis suggested that the scale reflects the coping mechanism. Perception of birth is viewed within the Roy Adaptation Model as a mediating factor between the focal stimulus, such as cesarean birth, and responses in the four adaptive modes, such as pain (physiological mode), self-esteem (self-concept mode), functional status (role function mode), and feelings about the baby (interdependence mode). The Perception of Birth Scale appears to be a useful instrument for assessing a woman's perception of the birth experience.

Fawcett, J., & Knauth, D. (1996). The factor structure of the Perception of Birth Scale. *Nursing Research, 45,* 83–86.

exist with a sense of unity. The role function mode focuses on the roles an individual holds in society and the need to know who one is in relation to others so that one can act. The interdependence mode focuses on interactions related to love, respect, and value and the need to feel secure in nurturing relationships.

After processing the stimuli and adaptation level through the coping mechanisms, the person makes a response through the adaptive modes. These responses demonstrate how well the person is adapting and may be classified as adaptive or ineffective. Adaptive responses promote the integrity and goals of the person and contribute to growth, reproduction, mastery, and survival. Ineffective responses do not promote integrity and threaten survival, growth, reproduction, and/or mastery.

Roy's model (1991) speaks to the physiological needs in the regulator subsystem and the physiological mode. The psychosocial needs are addressed in the cognator subsystem and the self-concept, role function, and interdependence modes. The need for growth and development is a goal of adaptation and is achieved through adaptive responses. The stimuli come from the internal and external environment; thus, a safe and protective environment is important. The relationship of Roy's theory to the nursing process is presented in Table 2–10.

Madeleine Leininger's Culture Care Theory

While working with disturbed children, Madeleine Leininger became aware that children from various cultures responded differently to nursing interventions (see Box 2–1). This led her to propose that culture was the link to understanding care of persons from different backgrounds. She combined her experience in nursing with her doctoral study in cultural anthropology to examine the concepts of care and caring. Nursing is considered to be synonymous with caring, which is viewed as the central dominant focus of nursing. Care is dependent on culture, which is essential to understanding people and nursing (Reynolds & Leininger, 1993).

Leininger wanted to examine what is universal and what is diverse about culture care around the world. This broad view was essential to study variations and similarities among cultures. The purpose of developing the theory was to determine culture care diversities and universality to generate nursing knowledge. The goal was to provide culturally congruent nursing care to improve care and lead to health or well-being.

Two kinds of caring are believed to exist in every culture and are identified as generic caring and professional caring. Generic caring is the basic expression of human caring and includes home remedies and folk care. The generic caring behaviors need to be identified to determine the ways in which they are beneficial. Professional caring is learned, practiced, and transmitted knowledge obtained through formal and informal education. It includes psychomotor skills, communication, and other psychosocial techniques. Generic care and professional care are needed to provide culturally congruent care.

In addition to generic and professional care, several other factors are seen as influencing the well-being of individuals and communities. These factors include the world view (the way people look at their world), religion, kinship, cultural values, economics, technology, language, ethnohistory (past events that are people centered and explain human life within a culture), education, political, and environmental context. If all of these factors are not considered, the nurse will have only fragmented knowledge about culture care.

Leininger proposes three modes (Table 2–5) to guide nursing decisions and actions when providing culturally congruent care. These modes are not interventions but are guides to help nurses understand how to intervene with clients.

Leininger's theory is primarily concerned with the need for a safe and protective environment. The environmental context is a broad concept that refers to the totality of events in different sociocultural settings. The environmental context influences culture care and the well-being of clients. Psychosocial needs, from a cultural viewpoint, are also of primary concern and greatly influence well-being. The theory specifically discusses the psychosocial factors of religion, kinship, technology, values, politics, economics, and education. Physiological needs and the need for growth and development are only addressed in broad terms, such as care being an essential human need to help people keep healthy and grow. The relationship of Leininger's theory to the nursing process is shown in Table 2–10.

Box **2–1**

LEININGER'S THEORY OF CULTURE CARE DIVERSITY AND UNIVERSALITY

Culture is a major concept in Leininger's Theory of Culture Care Diversity and Universality. Humans are cultural beings, and nurses provide care to people of different cultures. However, nurses may not practice from a culture perspective. For care to be effective, nursing must be based on transcultural knowledge. Cultural differences and similarities between nurses and patients will always exist, and culturally congruent care can only occur when the nurse knows and uses cultural values. Nursing care based on culture is a critical factor in promoting health or aiding recovery from illness.

Table 2–5

LEININGER'S MODES TO GUIDE NURSING IN GIVING CULTURALLY CONGRUENT CARE

MODE	DEFINITION
Cultural care preservation or maintenance	Those assistive professional actions that help people of a particular culture retain relevant care values so they can maintain well-being, recover from illness, or face handicaps or death
Culture care accommodation or negotiation	Those assistive professional actions that help people of a particular culture adapt to or negotiate with others for a beneficial health outcome
Culture care repatterning or restructuring	Those assistive professional actions that help clients change their lifeways for different, more beneficial health care patterns while respecting their cultural beliefs and values

Imogene King's Conceptual Framework and Theory of Goal Attainment

Imogene King (1981) utilized systems theory as a way to organize her conceptual framework for nursing. She identified three dynamic, interacting systems—personal systems, interpersonal systems, and social systems. The theory of goal attainment was derived from the framework. *Nursing* is defined as a process of human interactions leading to goal attainment. The goal of nursing is to help individuals and groups attain health.

Personal systems are individuals. There are selected concepts that are relevant for understanding individuals (Table 2–6). These concepts are interrelated and cannot be separated. For example, the space-time dimensions of the environment influence the other four concepts; behavior reflects perceptions of self and body image; the way in which persons grow and develop influences perceptions.

Human beings interact in several types of interpersonal systems such as dyads (two individuals interacting), triads (three interacting individuals), and groups (four or more individuals interacting). There are additional concepts that are relevant for understanding interpersonal systems (see Table 2–6).

Groups with common goals and interests create social systems. The family, church, school, work, and peer group are examples of social systems that influence people as they grow and develop. Concepts that are relevant for understanding social systems are summarized in Table 2–6.

From this open systems conceptual framework, King (1981) derived a theory of goal attainment that describes the nature of nurse-client interactions that lead to achievement of goals. The concepts of interaction, perception, communication, transaction, role, stress, space, and time are used in the theory. It is proposed that nurse-client interactions are characterized by

1. Communication—information is exchanged
2. Transactions—needs of nurse and client are shared
3. Perceptions—of nurse and client and the situation
4. Self—in role of client or nurse
5. Stressors—influencing each person and the situation in time and space

Nursing is defined as "a process of human interactions between nurse and client whereby each perceives the other and the situation; and through communication, they set goals, explore means, and agree on means to achieve goals" (p. 144).

King's conceptual framework (1981) is concerned with the need for growth and development. It is a main concept in the personal system. The need for a safe and protective environment is also part of King's conceptual framework, as the systems are in constant interaction with the environment. Psychosocial needs are addressed by the concepts of self, body image, communication, role, and stress. Physiological needs are a factor if they are related to a goal. The relationship of King's theory to the nursing process is presented in Table 2–10.

Betty Neuman's Systems Model

Betty Neuman (1982) based her model on systems theory and stress theory. The model is based on the client's reaction to stress. Health is synonymous with wellness and is seen as the condition that results when all parts are in harmony with the whole. The environment is the internal and external forces surrounding an individual at any point in time. There is constant reciprocal motion between an individual and the environment. Stressors are defined as disrupting forces, either noxious or beneficial, operating within or on the system.

The client is an open system in interaction with the environment. The interaction results in the environment adjusting to the individual or the individual adjusting to the environment. This interaction-adjustment process contains the factors that create the flexible line of defense that serves as a protective buffer for preventing stressors from breaking through the line. Factors in the flexible line of defense include

Table 2–6

CONCEPTS RELEVANT TO KING'S FRAMEWORK AND THEORY OF GOAL ATTAINMENT

CONCEPT	DEFINITION
Personal Systems	
Perception	A representation of reality; a process of organizing, interpreting, and transforming information subjectively to give meaning to an experience
Self	An open system that is dynamic and goal oriented; the sum total of all one can call one's own; a person's inner world
Growth and development	Cellular and behavioral changes that are a result of genetic inheritance, experiences, and an environment conducive to helping persons move toward maturity
Body image	The personal, subjective picture one has of one's body; results from others' reactions to self
Space	Exists in all directions and exists to the extent that it is perceived by an individual; culture dictates behavior related to space
Time	The duration between the occurrence of two events; based on a person's perceptions of the movement of life events
Interpersonal Systems	
Interaction	A series of verbal and nonverbal goal-directed behaviors that occur between two or more persons
Communication	The structure of symbols and signs that brings meaning and order to interactions; an interchange of thoughts and opinions
Transaction	A process of interaction to achieve goals that are valued; results in a reduction of tension and stress
Role	Behaviors expected from a person occupying a social position
Stress	A dynamic state of interaction between the person and environment to maintain balance for growth, development, and performance
Social Systems	
Organization	Social unit that has structure, functions, and resources to achieve goals; composed of individuals with prescribed roles and positions
Authority	Power to make decisions that influence the behavior of self and others; resides in the person who provides rewards and sanctions, who has special knowledge and skills, or who provides leadership
Power	The process whereby people are influenced by others; it is situational, dynamic, and goal directed
Status	The position of one person in a group as perceived by others in the group; it is situational, depends on position, and is reversible
Decision-making	A purposeful process in which one choice is selected from several alternatives in an attempt to achieve a goal

developmental state, age, gender, physiology, sociocultural background, and cognitive skills. Interventions of primary prevention focus on strengthening the flexible line of defense to prevent a stressor from disrupting the system.

At the center of the system is a central core consisting of basic factors such as genetic responses and the mechanism for maintaining a normal body temperature. Surrounding the central core are the flexible lines of resistance, which are the internal factors that help defend against stressors. Mobilization of white blood cells and the immune response are examples of the flexible lines of resistance. Surrounding the flexible lines of resistance is the normal line of defense. Factors included in the normal line of defense are lifestyle and usual coping patterns.

When a stressor causes a disruption, interventions of secondary prevention are given, depending on symptoms that are exhibited. Secondary prevention focuses on using the person's resources and strengthening the internal lines of resistance. If the individual does not return to the previous level of wellness, interventions of tertiary prevention are needed. In tertiary prevention, emphasis is on mobilizing energy resources.

Neuman's model (1982) is primarily concerned with the need for a safe and protective environment. Consideration of the environment is critical because the client is in constant interaction with the environment, which consists of all the factors affecting and affected by the individual. The need for growth and development, physiological needs, and psychosocial needs are all factors or variables affecting the flexible line of defense and determine the client's reaction to stressors. The relationship of Neuman's model to the nursing process is presented in Table 2–10.

Margaret Newman's Health as Expanding Consciousness

In the development of her theory, Margaret Newman (1986) was influenced by her mother's struggle with amyotrophic lateral sclerosis, her own interactions with Martha Rogers, and Bohm's theory of implicate order. She came to realize that her mother, though physically incapacitated, was not "ill." While a student in Martha Rogers' seminar in graduate school, she was stimulated by Rogers' views on the unitary nature of human beings in constant interaction with the environment and by Rogers' statement that health and illness are expressions of the life process, with one being no more important than the other. Bohm's theory of implicate order helped Newman comprehend the underlying, unseen pattern of life and the interconnectedness of all that exists.

Expanding on Rogers' viewpoint that health and illness express life in its totality, Newman eliminates all dichotomies. Opposites include each other—health includes disease and disease includes health. This synthesis of health and disease yields a new concept—pattern of the whole. Health as pattern of the whole is regarded as the interpretation of the underlying pattern of person-environment. Objective manifestations of health, such as vital signs and laboratory values, reflect the person-environment interaction and help us see and understand the pattern. Pattern recognition is critical and requires one to move from looking at parts to looking at patterns.

Patterns have relatedness, movement, diversity, and rhythm. The pattern has diverse parts that are constantly moving in relation to each other. Rhythm, or waves of energy, identifies the pattern. One person's reality is only a tiny portion of the total pattern in time-space. The important factor is the relationship among all the parts, the process through which the parts are continually being integrated into an ever-changing whole. According to Newman (1986, p. 17)

> The shift is from treatment of symptoms to a search for patterns; from viewing pain and disease as wholly negative to a view that pain and disease are information; from seeing the body as a machine in good or bad repair to seeing the body as a dynamic field of energy within other fields; from seeing disease as an entity to seeing it as a process.

The total person-environment pattern is seen as a network of consciousness. Consciousness is defined as "the informational capacity of the system: the capacity of the system to interact with its environment" (Newman, 1986, p. 33). An individual does not have consciousness—the individual is consciousness. Life evolves toward increasing complexity and higher levels of consciousness. This process of evolving consciousness is the process of health. The highest level is absolute consciousness where only love exists.

Newman's theory is concerned with the need for growth and development as individuals are identified by their patterns of consciousness. The need for a safe and protective environment is central to the pattern of the person-environment and cannot be considered apart from the whole. Physiological and psychosocial needs are considered as manifestations of person-environment interaction. The relationship of Newman's theory to the nursing process is shown in Table 2–10.

Rosemarie Parse's Theory of Human Becoming

Rosemarie Parse's theory has evolved since 1974 and was influenced by experiences that led her to the conclusion that clients behaved according to their own reality. In developing her theory, Parse synthesized concepts from Rogers' Science of Unitary Human Beings and from existential phenomenology. The concepts synthesized from Rogers are helicy, integrality, resonancy, energy field, openness, pattern and organization, and four-dimensionality. The concepts synthesized from existential phenomenology are subjectivity, intentionality, coconstitution, coexistence, and situated freedom (Bunting, 1993).

Subjectivity refers to the individual as a conscious being who is able to encounter the world, relate to it, and grow from the relationship. In this relationship, the person confers meaning on all experiences, thereby creating the reality of self and world. *Intentionality* means that the individual is consciously open to, involved with, and present to the world. *Situated freedom* refers to the belief that a person chooses experiences and the responses that he or she has to the experiences. Each experience and situation is related to the previous choices made by that individual. *Coexistence* means that life is an experience of being with others, and one's perceptions result from interaction with others. *Coconstitution* means that reality is made up of all the elements of a situation and the meaning assigned by an individual to that situation. The ability of the person to shape the environment, to choose meaning, to take responsibility, to shape patterns of relating and existing, and to transcend the present is central to Parse's theory.

Parse's theory (Bunting, 1993) contains nine major concepts that are processes in which people actively engage. The concepts are defined in Table 2–7.

Human beings are in open, mutual, constant interchange with the environment. Health is seen as a process of the individual relating to the universe. Health is lived experiences, a synthesis of values, a continuously changing process that a person cocreates. Nursing focuses on the health of persons in interrelationships with their environments. The nurse seeks to enhance the quality of life as perceived by the

Table 2–7

CONCEPTS IN PARSE'S HUMAN BECOMING THEORY

CONCEPT	DEFINITION
Imaging	Knowing in all the ways one can know; creating reality that includes images of the past and the future along with the present
Languaging	Communicating through verbal and nonverbal channels
Valuing	Living cherished beliefs while integrating the new
Connecting-separating	The rhythmical process of simultaneously moving closer to some elements and farther from others, yet always becoming more diverse
Revealing-concealing	Simultaneously revealing part of self to another while choosing to conceal other parts
Enabling-limiting	Each choice simultaneously enables new possibilities while limiting others
Powering	The drive and force behind change and creativity
Originating	Creating new patterns of interrelationships and ways of being in the world
Transforming	Changing views as experiences shed light on what is known; a continuous process that leads to increasing diversity and transcending

individual and family and guides the choosing of alternatives.

Parse's theory (Bunting, 1993) is concerned with the need for growth and development as the person is transforming and transcending and becoming. The need for a safe and protective environment could be inferred by the interrelationship of humans with their environment. Physiological and psychosocial needs cannot be considered separately in this theory. The nursing process is not accepted by Parse. Consequently, Parse's theory is not included in Table 2–10. Dimensions of practice include illuminating meaning, synchronizing rhythms, and mobilizing transcendence. The processes for nursing practice according to Parse are

1. Explicating—using languaging to clarify what is happening

2. Dwelling with—giving self over in the interhuman cadence of connecting-separating

3. Moving beyond—propelling toward the "possibles" in transforming and transcending

Jean Watson's Theory of Human Care

In developing her theory, Jean Watson (1985) was influenced by Eastern philosophy and her phenomenological-existential orientation. Health is viewed as harmony within the mind, body, and soul and the congruence between the self perceived and the self experienced. Illness is disharmony or turmoil within the inner self or soul. An inner soul that is in disharmony can lead to illness, which can cause disease. Nursing's goal is to help clients achieve harmony, which in turn produces self-knowledge, self-healing, and self-care processes. This goal is pursued through human care transactions and the caring process.

Caring is seen as the moral ideal of nursing in which there is high concern for human dignity. Transpersonal human caring transactions require personalized giving-receiving behaviors and responses derived from a scientific, professional, ethical, esthetic, and creative base. Both the nurse and the client are in a process of being and becoming; both bring unique life histories and phenomenal fields. The phenomenal field is the individual's perspective in the world that can be known only to that person. The caring transaction helps develop spiritual essence, self-knowledge, and self-healing for both the nurse and the client.

Human care requires enabling actions that allow others to solve problems and grow. The combination of interventions is called carative factors and are summarized in Table 2–8.

Watson's theory (1985) is concerned with the need for growth and development. Transpersonal caring is viewed as a means whereby one moves toward a higher sense of self and greater harmony. Psychosocial needs and physiological needs are addressed on a very abstract level and are described as striving toward actualization of one's spiritual self and establishing harmony within the mind, body, and soul. The need for a safe and protective environment is addressed by

Table 2–8

WATSON'S TEN CARATIVE FACTORS

Humanistic-altruistic system of values
Faith-hope
Sensitivity to self and others
Helping-trusting human care relationship
Expressing positive and negative feelings
Creative problem-solving caring process
Transpersonal teaching-learning
Supportive, protective, and/or corrective mental, physical, and spiritual environment
Human needs assistance
Existential-phenomenological-spiritual forces

the eighth carative factor. The relationship of Watson's theory to the nursing process is presented in Table 2–10.

Dorothy Johnson's Behavioral System Model

Dorothy Johnson (1980) used systems theory as a framework for her nursing theory. She views the client as a behavioral system rather than seeing the client as a biological system, as do many physicians. Most people experience times of crisis or illness that disturb the system balance, and nursing is the force that supplies assistance during these times.

The behavioral system as a whole is composed of all the ways of behaving that characterize each person's life. These ways of behaving form a functional unit that determines the interaction and the relationship between the individual and the environment. Subsystems have evolved to carry out special tasks for the system as a whole. Each subsystem has a set of behavioral responses that are developed through maturation, experience, and learning. A disturbance in the functioning of one subsystem will have an effect on the other subsystems and the whole system. Each subsystem must be protected from noxious influences, nurtured from the environment, and stimulated to grow and develop.

Johnson (1980) identified seven subsystems and the function of each. They are defined in Table 2–9.

In addition to function, each subsystem has structure. Problems arise when there are disturbances in the structure or function of the subsystems. Nursing is the external force that acts to preserve the integration of the patient's behavior at an optimal level. The goal is to restore behavioral system balance and stability at the highest possible level.

Johnson's theory (1980) is concerned with the need for growth and development as the subsystems evolve through maturation, experience, and learning. The need for a safe and protective environment is also a concern because system malfunctions are usually caused by a sudden environmental change. Physiological and psychosocial needs are addressed through the seven subsystems. The relationship of Johnson's theory to the nursing process is shown in Table 2–10.

Summary

This chapter introduced the characteristics of theories and described the interrelationships among theory, research, and practice. Descriptive, explanatory, predictive, and controlling theories were identified. Concepts, propositions, and models in relation to theory were defined. Person, health, environment, and nursing care activities were presented as the four concepts most important to nursing.

Several interdisciplinary models and theories used in nursing were described. These included systems theory, needs theory, health belief model, developmental theories, and stress/adaptation theories. The history and evolution of nursing theory from Florence Nightingale to the present were outlined. Details were included for 12 nursing models and theories. Each model and theory was discussed in relation to the need for growth and development, need for safe and protective environment, physiological needs, psychosocial needs, and the nursing process.

Table 2–9

JOHNSON'S SUBSYSTEMS OF THE BEHAVIORAL SYSTEM MODEL

SUBSYSTEM	DEFINITION
Affiliative	Forms the base for all social organization, intimacy, and social bonds
Dependency	Succoring behavior that elicits a nurturing response
Ingestive	Determines when, how, what, in what amount, and under what conditions one eats and drinks; may not be consistent with the biological requirement
Eliminative	Determines when, how, and under what conditions one eliminates wastes; influences the biological acts of elimination
Sexual	Originates with gender role identity and behaviors expected by and learned from the cultural setting
Aggressive	Promotes protection and preservation of self
Achievement	Attempts at mastery or control of the self or environment

CHAPTER HIGHLIGHTS

♦

♦ A strong, theoretical knowledge base is important for the nurse to be able to make sound decisions.

♦ Practicing nurses use theories to plan interventions backed by scientific rationale; nurse researchers use theories to derive hypotheses to be tested.

♦ A theory may be categorized as descriptive, explanatory, predictive, or controlling.

♦ Concepts paramount to nursing include person, health, environment, and nursing care activities.

♦ Interdisciplinary theories useful to nurses include

Table **2–10**

NURSING THEORISTS AND THE NURSING PROCESS

THEORIST	ASSESSMENT	DIAGNOSIS*	PLANNING	IMPLEMENTATION	EVALUATION
Nightingale	Focus on the environment: ventilation, warmth, noise, light, cleanliness	Altered protection Ineffective thermoregulation Social isolation Sleep pattern disturbance	Set goals based on environmental changes needed	Aimed at placing the person in the best position in the environment	Note changes in the client's condition and determine if goals have been met
Peplau	Focus during the orientation phase with the client's participation in identifying the problem	Anxiety Knowledge deficit Powerlessness Decisional conflict	Takes place during identification phase as the patient and nurse clarify expectations	During exploitation phase, the client uses the services available	During resolution phase, dependent behavior is relinquished, and the relationship is terminated
Rogers	Focus on the human and environmental energy fields and manifestations of field patterning	Altered growth and development Relocation stress syndrome Altered family processes Sleep pattern disturbance	Active participation of the client within the environmental field to set goals aimed toward health	Seeks to promote the integrality of human and environmental energy fields and field patterning	Note changes in the field patterning and integrality
Orem	Focus on identifying self-care deficits	Self-care deficit Altered parenting Altered growth and development Knowledge deficit	Determine self-care requisites and type of nursing system required	Wholly compensatory Partly compensatory Supportive-educative	Self-care agency restored
Roy	Focus on behavior and stimuli	Altered role performance Hopelessness Impaired adjustment Ineffective coping	Determine adaptive response that is desired	Alter the focal, contextual, and/or residual stimuli	Adaptive behavior restored
Leininger	Focus on generic and professional care as well as world view, religion, kinship, values, economics, technology, language, ethnohistory, and environmental factors	Impaired adjustment Altered health maintenance Impaired home maintenance management Ineffective management of therapeutic regimen	Establish care goals that are culturally congruent with the client	Culture care preservation or maintenance Culture care accommodation or negotiation Culture care repatterning or restructuring	Well-being is maintained, recovery from illness, and/or face handicaps or death
King	Focus on perceptions, self, growth and development, body image, role, and stress	Powerlessness Altered growth and development Body image disturbance Impaired verbal communication	Interaction with client to set goals	Nurse-client interactions to implement mechanisms to attain goals	Goal attainment

Table 2–10

NURSING THEORISTS AND THE NURSING PROCESS
(Continued)

THEORIST	ASSESSMENT	DIAGNOSIS*	PLANNING	IMPLEMENTATION	EVALUATION
Neuman	Focus on stressors, coping patterns, and resources	Health-seeking behaviors Activity intolerance Ineffective denial Ineffective thermoregulation	Strengthen flexible line of defense, normal line of defense, or flexible lines of resistance	Primary prevention Secondary prevention Tertiary prevention	Equilibrium restored Steady state maintained
Newman	Focus on client-environment interaction to search for the underlying pattern of the whole	Sleep pattern disturbance Fatigue Decisional conflict Altered sexuality patterns	Enter into a partnership with client with goals for mutual growth	Being with the client and interacting rather than doing	Higher levels of consciousness achieved
Watson	Focus on the phenomenal field and the client's condition of spirit	Spiritual distress Personal identity disturbance Self-esteem disturbance Body image disturbance	Coparticipate in the transpersonal care transaction	Utilize the ten carative factors and enabling actions	Harmony between mind, body, and soul is achieved
Johnson	Focus on the structure and function of the subsystems	Altered patterns of urinary elimination Impaired social interaction Social isolation Sexual dysfunction	Achieve behavioral system balance at highest level possible	Impose regulatory or control mechanisms, change structural units, or fulfill functional requirements of the subsystems	Behavioral system balance restored

*Examples from the North American Nursing Diagnosis Association (NANDA) that are consistent with the theory.

systems theory, needs theory, health belief model, developmental theories, and stress/adaptation theories.

✦ Nursing theory originated with Florence Nightingale but made little progress before the latter half of this century.

✦ Nursing theories useful to nurses include Florence Nightingale's Environmental Theory, Hildegard Peplau's Interpersonal Relations Theory, Martha Rogers' Science of Unitary Human Beings, Dorothea Orem's Self-Care Deficit Theory, Sister Callista Roy's Adaptation Model, Madeleine Leininger's Culture Care Theory, Imogene King's Conceptual Framework and Theory of Goal Attainment, Betty Neuman's Systems Model, Margaret Newman's Health as Expanding Consciousness, Rosemarie Parse's Theory of Human Becoming, Jean Watson's Theory of Human Care, and Dorothy Johnson's Behavioral System Model.

Study Questions

1. Which of the following clients would require Orem's wholly compensatory nursing system?

   a. newly diagnosed diabetic teenager
   b. anesthetized woman in surgery
   c. paraplegic man in rehabilitation
   d. newly delivered mother

2. What are the four concepts most important to nursing?

   a. care, culture, nursing process, and healing
   b. growth and development, safe and protective environment, physiological needs, and psychosocial needs
   c. nutrition, oxygenation, fluid, and elimination
   d. person, health, environment, and nursing care activities

3. During which phase of Peplau's nurse-client relationship does implementation occur?

   a. orientation
   b. identification
   c. exploitation
   d. resolution

4. In using Roy's Adaptation Model to care for a mother who has just delivered her baby, what is the focal stimulus?

   a. the birth
   b. the delivery room
   c. the doctor
   d. the father

5. Which of the following theorists has developed a nursing theory that emphasizes culture?

   a. Leininger
   b. Parse
   c. Rogers
   d. Watson

Critical Thinking Exercises

1. Mr. C. is 39 years old and has just been diagnosed with terminal lung cancer. He is married and has two children ages 4 and 8. Use one theory to explain how the concepts of person, environment, and health might apply in this situation.

2. How can nursing theories be used in practice? Choose one of the following situations and discuss how nursing theory might be used in the situation.

   a. acute care of a surgical client
   b. long-term care of a chronically ill emphysema client
   c. client receiving home health care for acquired immunodeficiency syndrome
   d. immunization clinic at the public health department
   e. psychiatric care of a schizophrenic client at an acute care facility

References

Abdellah, F. G., Beland, I. L., Martin, A., & Matheny, R. (1960). *Patient-centered approaches to nursing.* New York: Macmillan.

American Nurses Association. (1980). *Nursing: a social policy statement.* Kansas City, MO: American Nurses Association.

Baker, J. K., Borchers, D. A., Cochran, D. T., Kaltofen, K. G., Orcutt, N., Peacock, J. A., Terry, E. G., Wesolowski, C. A., Yeager, L. A. (1994). Kathryn E. Bernard: Parent-child interaction model. In A. Marriner-Tomey (ed.) *Nursing theorists and their works* (3rd ed.). St. Louis: Mosby.

Barnum, B. J. S. (1994). *Nursing theory: Analysis, application, evaluation* (4th ed.). Philadelphia: J. B. Lippincott.

Bee, A. M., Legge, D., & Oetting, S. (1994). Ramona T. Mercer: Maternal role attainment. In A. Marriner-Tomey (ed.). *Nursing theorists and their work* (3rd ed.). St. Louis: Mosby.

Bunting, S. (1993). *Rosemarie Parse theory of health as human becoming.* Newbury Park, CA: Sage.

Fawcett, J., & Knauth, D. (1996). The factor structure of the Perception of Birth Scale. *Nursing Research, 45,* 83–86.

Hall, L. (1964). Nursing: What is it? *Canadian Nurse, 60,* 150–154.

Henderson, V. (1966). *The nature of nursing.* New York: Macmillan.

Hickman, J. S. (1995). An introduction to nursing theory. In

J. B. George (Ed.), *Nursing theories: The base for professional nursing practice* (4th ed.). Norwalk, CT: Appleton & Lange.

Johnson, D. E. (1980). The behavioral system model of nursing. In J. P. Riehl, & Sr. C. Roy (Eds.), *Conceptual models for nursing practice* (2nd ed., pp. 207–216). New York: Appleton-Century-Crofts.

Johnson, J. L. (1991). Learning to live again: The process of adjustment following a heart attack. In J. M. Morse, & J. L. Johnson (eds.). *The illness experience.* Newbury Park, CA: Sage.

Kenney, J. W. (1990). Overview of selected models. In P. J. Christensen, & J. W. Kenney (Eds.), *Nursing process application of conceptual models* (3rd ed., pp. 20–52). St. Louis, MO: C. V. Mosby.

King, I. (1981). *A theory for nursing.* New York: John Wiley & Sons.

Lazarus, R. S., & Folkman, S. (1984). *Stress, appraisal, and coping.* New York: Springer.

Leddy, S., & Pepper, J. M. (1993). *Conceptual bases of professional nursing* (3rd ed.). Philadelphia: J. B. Lippincott.

Levine, M. E. (1969). *Introduction to clinical nursing.* Philadelphia: F. A. Davis.

Neuman, B. (1982). *The Neuman Systems Model application to nursing education and practice.* Norwalk, CT: Appleton-Century-Crofts.

Newman, M. A. (1986). *Health as expanding consciousness.* St. Louis, MO: C. V. Mosby.

Nightingale, F. (1946). *Notes on nursing: What it is and what it is not.* London: Harrison and Sons. (Original work published 1859.)

Orem, D. E. (1991). *Nursing concepts of practice* (4th ed.). St. Louis, MO: Mosby-Year Book.

Orlando, I. J. (1961). *The dynamic nurse-patient relationship.* New York: G. P. Putnam's Sons.

Peplau, H. E. (1952/1991). *Interpersonal relations in nursing.* New York: Springer.

Reynolds, C. L., & Leininger, M. (1993). *Madeleine Leininger: Culture care diversity and universality theory.* Newbury Park, CA: Sage.

Rogers, M. E. (1986). Science of unitary human beings. In V. M. Malinski (Ed.), *Explorations on Martha Rogers' science of unitary human beings* (pp. 3–8). Norwalk, CT: Appleton-Century-Crofts.

Rosenstock, I. M. (1966). Why people use health services. *Milbank Memorial Fund Quarterly, 44*(Suppl.), 94–127.

Roy, Sr. C., & Andrews, H. A. (1991). *The Roy Adaptation Model: The definitive statement.* Norwalk, CT: Appleton & Lange.

Selye, H. (1974). *Stress without distress.* Philadelphia: J. B. Lippincott.

Torres, G. (1990). The place of concepts and theories within nursing. In J. B. George (Ed.), *Nursing theories the base for professional practice* (3rd ed.) (pp. 1–12). Norwalk, CT: Appleton & Lange.

Torres, G. (1986). *Theoretical foundations of nursing.* Norwalk, CT: Appleton-Century-Crofts.

Watson, J. (1985). *Nursing: Human science and human care.* Norwalk, CT: Appleton-Century-Crofts.

Wiedenbach, E. (1964). *Clinical nursing: A helping art.* New York: Springer.

Bibliography

Allmark, P. (1995). A classical view of the theory-practice gap in nursing. *Journal of Advanced Nursing, 22,* 18–23.

Arndt, M. J. (1995). Parse's theory of human becoming in practice with hospitalized adolescents. *Nursing Science Quarterly, 8,* 86–90.

Artinian, N. T. (1994). Selecting a model to guide family assessment. *DCCN: Dimensions of Critical Care Nursing, 13*(1), 4–13.

Billings, J. R. (1995). Bonding theory—tying mothers in knots? A critical review of the application of a theory to nursing. *Journal of Clinical Nursing, 4,* 207–211.

Bunting, S. (1993). *Rosemarie Parse: Theory of human becoming.* Newbury Park, CA: Sage.

Conway, J. (1994). Reflection, the art and science of nursing and the theory-practice gap. *British Journal of Nursing, 3*(3), 114–118.

Duldt, B. W. (1995). Integrating nursing theory and ethics. *Perspectives in Psychiatric Care, 31*(2), 4–10.

Evans, C. L. S. (1991). *Imogene King: A conceptual framework for nursing.* Newbury Park, CA: Sage.

Fawcett, J. (1995). *Analysis and evaluation of conceptual models of nursing* (3rd ed.). Philadelphia: F. A. Davis.

Fawcett, J. (1993). *Analysis and evaluation of nursing theories.* Philadelphia: F. A. Davis.

Fontes, H. C. (1994). Maps: Understanding theory through the use of analogy. *Nurse Educator, 19*(1), 20–22.

Forchuk, C. (1993). *Hildegard E. Peplau: Interpersonal nursing theory.* Newbury Park, CA: Sage.

Frey, M. A., Rooke, L, Sieloff, C., Messmer, P. R., & Kameoka, T. (1995). King's framework and theory in Japan, Sweden, and the United States. *Image: Journal of Nursing Scholarship, 27,* 127–130.

Frey, M. A., & Sieloff, C. L. (Eds.). (1995). *Advancing King's systems framework and theory of nursing.* Thousand Oaks, CA: Sage.

Hart, M. A. (1995). Orem's Self-Care Deficit Theory: Research with pregnant women. *Nursing Science Quarterly, 8,* 120–126.

Hartweg, D. L. (1991). *Dorothea Orem: Self-care deficit theory.* Newbury Park, CA: Sage.

Kappeli, S. (1994). Why not practice-based theory? *Clinical Nursing Research, 3*(1), 3–6.

Kelly, L. S. (1995). Parse's theory in practice with a group in the community. *Nursing Science Quarterly, 8,* 127–132.

Kite, K., & Pearson, L. (1995). A rationale for mouth care: The integration of theory with practice. *Intensive and Critical Care Nursing, 11*(2), 71–76.

Levine, M. E. (1995). The rhetoric of nursing theory. *Image: Journal of Nursing Scholarship, 27,* 11–14.

Lutjens, L. R. J. (1991). *Callista Roy: An adaptation model.* Newbury Park, CA: Sage.

Lutjens, L. R. J. (1991). *Martha Rogers: The science of unitary human beings.* Newbury Park, CA: Sage.

Macrae, J. (1995). Nightingale's spiritual philosophy and its significance for modern nursing. *Image: Journal of Nursing Scholarship, 27,* 8–10.

Marchione, J. (1993). *Margaret Newman: Health as expanding consciousness.* Newbury Park, CA: Sage.

Marckx, B. B. (1995). Watson's theory of caring: A model for implementation in practice. *Journal of Nursing Care Quality, 9*(4), 43–54.

Marriner-Tomey, A. (1994). *Nursing theorists and their work* (3rd ed.). St. Louis, MO: C. V. Mosby.

McElmurry, B. J. (1995). Theory in nursing research. *Research in Nursing and Health, 18,* 377.

Mercer, R. T. (1995). *Becoming a mother: Research on maternal role identity from Rubin to the present.* New York: Springer.

Neuman, B. (1995). *The Neuman Systems Model* (3rd ed.). Norwalk, CT: Appleton & Lange.

Norgan, G. H., Ettipio, A. M., & Lasome, C. E. M. (1995). A program plan addressing carpal tunnel syndrome: The utility of King's Goal Attainment Theory. *American Association of Occupational Health Nursing Journal, 43,* 407–411.

O'Connor, N. (1993). *Paterson and Zderad: Humanistic nursing theory.* Newbury Park, CA: Sage.

Orem, D. E. (1995). *Nursing: Concepts of practice* (5th ed.). St. Louis, MO: C. V. Mosby.

Parker, M. E. (Ed.). (1991). *Nursing theories in practice.* New York: National League for Nursing.

Parker, M. E. (Ed.). (1993). *Patterns of nursing theories in practice.* New York: National League for Nursing.

Parse, R. R. (Ed.). (1995). *Illuminations: The human becoming theory in practice and research.* New York: National League for Nursing.

Reed, K. S. (1993). *Betty Neuman: The Neuman systems model.* Newbury Park, CA: Sage.

Reynolds, C. L., & Leininger, M. M. (1993). *Madeleine Leininger: Cultural care diversity and universality theory.* Newbury Park, CA: Sage.

Roy, C. L. (1995). Developing nursing knowledge: Practice issues raised from four philosophical perspectives. *Nursing Science Quarterly, 8,* 79–85.

Schmieding, N. J. (1993). *Ida Jean Orlando: A nursing process theory.* Newbury Park, CA: Sage.

Scott, H. (1994). Why does nursing theory fail in practice? *British Journal of Nursing, 3*(3), 102–103.

Selanders, L. C. (1993). *Florence Nightingale: An environmental adaptation theory.* Newbury Park, CA: Sage.

Thomas, L. W. (1995). A critical feminist perspective of the health belief model: Implications for nursing theory, research, practice, and education. *Journal of Professional Nursing, 11,* 246–252.

Wesley, R. L. (1995). *Nursing theories and models* (2nd ed). Springhouse, PA: Springhouse Corporation.

Wright, P. S., Piazza, D., Holcomb, J., & Foote, A. (1994). A comparison of three theories of nursing used as a guide for the nursing care of an 8-year-old child with leukemia. *Journal of Pediatric Nursing, 11*(1), 14–19.

Chapter 3

VALUES AND ETHICS IN NURSING PRACTICE

IDE KATIMS, RN, PHD

KEY TERMS

◆

accountability	justice
autonomy	nonmaleficence
beneficence	paternalism
confidentiality	privacy
deontology	utilitarianism
ethical dilemma	values
ethics	veracity
informed consent	virtues

LEARNING OBJECTIVES

◆

After studying this chapter, you should be able to

◆ Discuss the roles that values and ethics play in nursing practice

◆ Understand how ethical principles relate to nursing activities

◆ Compare and contrast three major ethical approaches relevant to nursing

◆ Use an ethical decision-making framework

◆ Synthesize the various ethical perspectives through application utilizing a case study

Values can be defined as deeply held beliefs that provide reference points as we make judgments and set priorities in daily life. Values give direction to people's lives and shape practical decisions and actions that mark who each person is. They refer to the things people deem worthy, standards by which people judge the worth of things, as well as standards by which people judge themselves and others. Because values guide us in deciding what is important, what is good, and what is right, our value system has significant moral implications. For example, if a person deeply values self-reliance, he or she will believe that it is morally imperative that people assume responsibility for their own lives and well-being. He or she will be motivated to be self-sufficient. Dependence, in oneself or in others, would be judged indefensible. It would be difficult for this individual to support social policy such as public assistance programs that he or she thinks would foster dependence.

Formation of Personal and Professional Values

For the most part, people do not set out to learn values. Rather, as members of families, religious communities, or cultural groups, values are etched into the larger mosaic of people's socialization and development. Thus, all of us come to the practice of nursing with an already established set of personal values. These would be our political and religious orientations, our attitudes regarding family and social responsibility, our judgment in terms of the worth of people and things, and our general outlook in life, to name a few. But like all professions, nursing has its own value system. Being socialized into a profession means taking on, to a personally comfortable level, the set of values that the profession champions (Table 3–1).

Since nursing is a publicly recognized practice of caregiving, its value system is shaped over time by public expectation and nursing's own understanding of its social mission of care. Because of this, nursing's value system closely approximates the values of the society within which nursing has evolved. For example, freedom is deeply valued in American society. Correspondingly, the notion of **autonomy** (the client's rights to self-determination) is central to nursing within this culture, as reflected in *A Patient's Bill of Rights* (Fig. 3–1) and the *Rights of Home Care Consumers* (see box). In contrast, Asian cultures highly value family decision-making and the benefits of harmonious human relationships. Nurses in Asian societies would view the notion of individual rights as only of secondary importance.

Table 3–1

ESSENTIAL PROFESSIONAL VALUES IN NURSING: COMPARISON OF THE AMERICAN, CANADIAN, AND INTERNATIONAL CODES OF ETHICS

The following are essential values of the profession of nursing. Many of these essential values are found within nursing's codes of ethics. Three codes and the nursing values they address are identified here.

Valuing Caring

The professional value of caring is not mentioned in the code of ethics. Caring, however, can be considered a professional value that has great ethical consequences: Nursing practiced with a caring attitude, as opposed to an uncaring attitude, is more likely to be an ethical practice in terms of protection and advocacy for the client, in terms of a committed effort to meet the needs of the client, and in terms of the quality of the nurse-client relationship.
* Show concern for the welfare of others
* Act with compassion and authenticity
* Commit to the nurse-client relationship

Valuing Equity

* Act with fairness and justice
* Provide clients with equitable access to nursing services*

Valuing Respect for Persons

* Have respect for life†
* Prize clients' individual rights and privacy*,†,‡
* Honor human dignity and unique qualities*,†,‡
* Honor clients' values, customs, and beliefs*,†

Valuing Quality Service to Clients

* Restore health and alleviate suffering†
* Promote health and prevent illness†
* Advocate for and protect clients*,†,‡
* Meet the social and health needs of the public*,†

Valuing Professional Competence

* Maintain theoretical knowledge, clinical skills, and competency in nursing care*,†,‡
* Assume responsibility for personal growth and professional development†
* Be accountable for your actions and decisions*,†
* Contribute to nursing's body of knowledge*,†
* Uphold nursing's standards of practice*,†
* Embody nursing values and ethics in practice and place trust in nursing‡
* Maintain standards in personal conduct†

*American Nurses' Association, 1985.
†International Council of Nurses, 1972/1989.
‡Canadian Nurses Association, 1991.

A Patient's Bill of Rights

1. The patient has the right to considerate and respectful care.

2. The patient has the right to obtain from his physician complete and current information concerning his diagnosis, treatment, and prognosis in terms the patient can be reasonably expected to understand. When it is not medically advisable to give such information to the patient, the information should be made available to an appropriate person in his behalf. He has the right to know, by name, the physician responsible for coordinating his care.

3. The patient has the right to receive from his physician information necessary to give informed consent prior to the start of any procedure and/or treatment. Except in emergencies, such information for informed consent should include but not necessarily be limited to the specific procedure and/or treatment, the medically significant risks involved, and the probable duration of incapacitation. Where medically significant alternatives for care or treatment exist, or when the patient requests information concerning medical alternatives, the patient has the right to such information. The patient also has the right to know the name of the person responsible for the procedures and/or treatment.

4. The patient has the right to refuse treatment to the extent permitted by law and to be informed of the medical consequences of his actions.

5. The patient has the right to every consideration of his privacy concerning his own medical care program. Case discussion, consultation examination, and treatment are confidential and should be conducted discreetly. Those not directly involved in his care must have the permission of the patient to be present.

6. The patient has the right to expect that all communications and records pertaining to his care should be treated as confidential.

7. The patient has the right to expect that within its capacity a hospital must make reasonable response to the request of a patient for services. The hospital must provide evaluation, service, and or referral as indicated by the urgency of the case. When medically permissible, a patient must be transferred to another facility only after he has received complete information and explanation concerning the need for and alternatives to such a transfer. The institution to which the patient is to be transferred must first have accepted the patient for transfer.

8. The patient has the right to obtain information as to any relationship of his hospital to other health care and educational institutions insofar as his care is concerned. The patient has the right to obtain information as to the existence of any professional relationships among individuals, by name, who are treating him.

9. The patient has the right to be advised if the hospital proposes to engage in or perform human experimentation affecting his care or treatment. The patient has the right to refuse to participate in such research projects.

10. The patient has the right to expect reasonable continuity of care. He has the right to know in advance what appointment times and physicians are available and where. The patient has the right to expect that the hospital will provide a mechanism whereby he is informed by his physician or a delegate of the physician of the patient's continuing health care requirements following discharge.

11. The patient has a right to examine and receive an explanation of his bill, regardless of source of payment.

12. The patient has a right to know what hospital rules and regulations apply to his conduct as a patient.

❧ **Figure 3–1**
A patient's bill of rights. (Reprinted with permission of the American Hospital Association. Copyright © 1992.)

◆ Values Conflict

As with social and personal values, the professional values of nursing constitute a matrix of deep convictions that guide daily practice. Despite consensus on what constitutes values *concerns* for nursing, values *conflicts* exist. For example, while all nurses would agree that it is imperative to support a client's autonomy, they might disagree whether autonomy is the most important value that must take precedent over everything else. Consider the situation in which a nurse supports a frail elder person's right to make decisions regarding his own care, and he insists on returning home to the care of his daughter. Would the nurse have the obligation to support the elder's decision based on respect for his autonomy and disregard the undue burden imposed on the daughter who must provide the care?

Nurses' value conflicts almost always arise from their relationships with clients, other health care team members, and their employers. Institutional rules may differ from, or even contradict, the values of professional nursing. In the case of the elder returning home to the care of his daughter, even if the nurses decide that it is in the best interest of the client and his daughter to have the man stay an extra day at the hospital, hospital utilization guidelines may deny this leeway. The nurses would end up doing second best for the client and his family. Even seemingly trivial nursing decisions and actions in daily practice are often values issues and are morally significant because all together they may not measure up to nursing's long-held professional values.

In another area of values conflict, a nurse may

RIGHTS OF HOME CARE CONSUMERS

With the 1987 Budget Reconciliation Act of 1987, clients' rights specific to home health care services were introduced. Sabatino (1990) categorized the rights of home care consumers into five areas:

1. **Informational rights.** Right to full information regarding the home health agencies, sources and destinations of referrals, cost, and identity of personnel

2. **Participation and control rights.** Right to participate in planning and evaluating care, have access to medical records, consent to or refuse treatment, and be taught self-care skills

3. **General civil rights and protection.** Freedom from intrusions of fundamental rights such as respect, dignity, privacy, confidentiality, and nondiscriminatory treatment

4. **Remedial rights.** Right to have problems arising from home health care services identified and resolved, including being given information on the formal procedure for complaints

5. **Quality rights.** Right to safe, timely, and professional care, including having continuity, provided by qualified and competent personnel

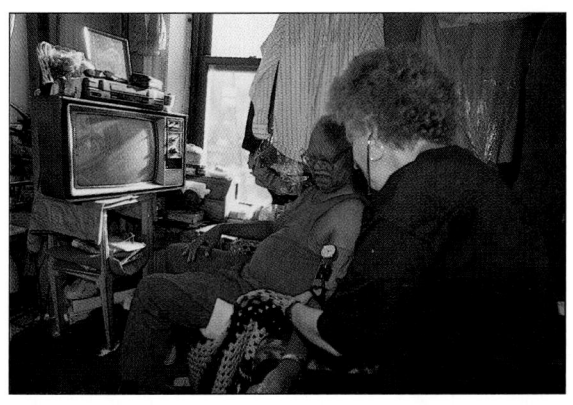

simultaneously hold values viewpoints that are at odds with one another. For example, a nurse can believe that all clients should receive care for as long as there is a need, and, at the same time, believe that clients should respond to nursing care (e.g., by learning whatever the nurse is trying to teach them in a timely manner and changing their behavior to reflect this teaching) to be deserving of more care. How, then, should nurses decide what constitutes right action (Table 3–2)?

This is why we turn to the study of ethics. It teaches us ways of understanding questions regarding values and questions of "what ought we to do." While there is often no right or wrong answer to ethical questions, the study of ethics introduces us to a host of ethical standards and rationales on which we can construct personally and professionally satisfactory answers.

Moral Values and Ethics

Ethics can generally be viewed as a philosophical inquiry into the nature and reason of morality. American philosopher John Dewey offers that ethics is "an account of human action" (1969, p. 1) and that the goal of ethical deliberation is to judge human action. Another philosopher suggests that ethics concern the combined study of values and obligations (Attfield, 1987). Yet another defines ethics as "a discipline that tries to understand rationally (as opposed to understanding in ways that are aesthetic, religious, economic, patriotic, etc.) how we ought to resolve various kinds of values conflicts" (Cooper, 1993, p. 3). *The central tenets of ethics, therefore, are judgments of good, right, or just; our moral duty and obligation relative to these judgments; and the use of moral principles or ethical theories by which to anchor our moral viewpoints.*

The Need for Ethics

The terms *morals* and *ethics* have similar meaning, the former derived from Latin and the latter from Greek (Dewey, 1969). There have been some attempts to differentiate morals from ethics, with the former attributed to religious beliefs and the latter, to self-reflective analysis of the goodness or badness of human conduct (Kelly & Joel, 1995). There is, however, no consensus that morals and ethics are indeed different things.

THE VALUES CLARIFICATION PROCESS

Values conflicts are common experiences of nurses. When faced with difficult choices (*e.g.*, nurses' obligation to clients versus their obligation to employers), nurses often are unclear about what they actually value. To be clear about what we actually do value and to act consistently when we carry out our professional duties, we can turn to values clarification strategies. Based on the classic works of Raths and colleagues (1972) and Simon and coworkers (1978), seven steps are identified in the valuing process:
• Choose freely
• Choose from alternatives
• Choose after considering consequences
• Prize and cherish one's choice
• Publicly affirm one's belief
• Act on the value choice
• Develop consistency in using this value to guide decisions and actions

Ethical precepts and theories help us put our values quandary into a philosophical perspective and show us the moral significance of seemingly ordinary events.

Consider the issue of why nurses should wear on their clothing a small plastic card on which their name and photograph are imprinted when they are at work. By this identification badge, nurses inform clients, family members, and other members of the health team who they are. Should nurses be required to wear an identification badge, or should their rights to privacy and free choice entitle them either to comply or not? Should government regulations and employers mandate that wearing an identification badge be a condition of practice or employment? If so, who is being protected: clients, the hospital itself, the nursing profession, or other members of the health care team? What values are implied by the act of clear identification: the nurses' acknowledgement of accountability and responsibility for their own actions? Why would such an acknowledgement be important to the health and safety of clients?

A concrete event like wearing an identification badge can thus possess a series of ethical implications. With so many perspectives to consider, how should one make sense of the multitudes of ethical concerns? Should some ethical concerns take precedent over others? Indeed, depending on different forms of ethical thinking—known as ethical theories—some ethical concerns are emphasized over others. For example, one type of ethical thinking is primarily concerned with what is good for the entire profession of nursing. In this case, one would argue that it is good for the profession of nursing that all nurses are required to wear identification badges, regardless of the wishes of individual nurses. Another type of ethical thinking is concern foremost with the nurse's own sense of personal accountability, which makes it morally good for the nurse to identify himself or herself. The former emphasizes the benefit for a group, while the latter honors the moral person who acts on one's own behalf. Different ethical theories, therefore, have their own points of focus and characteristic foundational principles to support their conclusions. Some common ethical issues in nursing practice today are listed in Table 3–3.

Ethical Theories

Each ethical theory presents a certain kind of thinking about what is right and ought to be done, as well as specific moral rules that guide judgment, standards, and conduct. Each ethical theory has its own system of moral reasoning, emphasizes specific values, and demands that these values be given top priority in all ethical decisions.

Three major forms of ethical thinking are of relevance to nursing: (1) deontology, (2) utilitarianism, and (3) values-oriented ethics. The first two are

Table 3–3

SURVEY OF COMMON ETHICAL ISSUES IN PRACTICE

A survey conducted by the American Nurses' Association's Center for Ethics and Human Rights in June 1994 listed ethical issues commonly confronting nurses (in order of frequency):
- Cost containment issues that jeopardize patient welfare
- End-of-life decisions
- Breaches of patient confidentiality
- Incompetent, unethical, or illegal practices of colleagues
- Pain management issues
- Use of advanced directives
- Informed consent for procedures
- Access to health care
- Issues in the care of persons with HIV/AIDS
- Providing "futile" care

AIDS = acquired immunodeficiency syndrome; HIV = human immunodeficiency virus. From Scanlon, C. (1994). Ethics survey at nurses' experience. *The American Nurse*, November/December, 22.

known as "normative" ethics, because they attempt to give authoritative standards, or norms, for human conduct. The third does not prescribe norms but instead emphasizes a person's morality, virtue, and sense of goodness and care.

Normative Ethics

Deontology

According to deontological thinking, human beings have the freedom, thoughtfulness, and sensibility to act in a moral manner. After self-reflective thinking, an individual is capable of deciding what he or she *ought* to do to be a moral person. Because of these human characteristics, people possess intrinsic worth and human dignity. Unconditional *respect* for the *person* as a human being constitutes the central motif of this ethical perspective.

Because of this fundamental respect for the person's capacity and will to make moral decisions, **deontology** holds that a person's action is right if it follows moral rules, such as being fair, being honest, and intending to do good and not to do harm. A person's action is wrong, without exception, if it violates these rules. Even if the consequences of the action turned out to be negative, the action is still considered ethically right if the original motive is consistent with moral precepts. For example, if a client asks the nurse to promise to tell the truth regarding her diagnosis and prognosis, the nurse is then duty-bound to keep this promise. If it turns out that the client is greatly distressed by the information, the

Table 3-4

DEONTOLOGY

The nurse is duty-bound to act under moral rules that establish the right or wrong:
- Duty to honor a patient's autonomy
- Duty to promote good and well-being
- Duty to be just or fair
- Duty to do no harm
- Duty to tell the truth
- Duty to keep promises and confidentiality

The individual is important. My primary responsibility is to support the interest of my client as an individual.

Examples of Application to Health Care

A person has free will and self-determination and can refuse any medical or nursing treatment or procedure

nurse is still ethically right to have told the truth, as he or she has promised the client. Breaking a promise, lying to the client, or depriving the client of information, even with the intention of shielding him or her from emotional distress cannot be morally justified. In practice, the nurse should, of course, only disclose the distressing information at the appropriate time and in the appropriate place. He or she should do so with skill, compassion, and care. The nurse should also use to the fullest extent the sustaining and caring nurse-client relationship that has been established, as well as the client's own support system. Fundamental respect for the person calls for no less care and preparation.

Another perspective on respect for the person addresses whether human beings can be used to achieve some desirable goal. The German moral philosopher Immanuel Kant (1724–1804) admonished: "Act in such a way that you treat humanity, whether in your own person or in the person of any other, never simply as a means, but always at the same time as an end" (1948, p. 96). A analogy may be helpful here. Suppose one sees a beautiful tree rising magnificently 50 feet into the sky. One can respect and admire the tree as a tree (as an end in itself) or as potential first-quality lumber for building a house (as the means to an end). This Kantian moral rule prescribes that we treat people with the utmost respect because of human dignity and worth (the person being an *end* in himself or herself). The person must never be used as a *means* to achieve other goals outside the final consideration of the person's dignity and worth. For example, one might question the ethics of researchers offering substantial sums of money to entice people to participate in medical experiments. The experiment may indeed lead to scientific breakthroughs, but if it does not directly benefit the research subjects themselves, and if the monetary reward is large enough so that people find it difficult to turn it down, the decision to subject themselves to the risks of medical experimentation may not be truly voluntary. The researchers may have violated the ethical precept of respect for persons. The

ANA Code for Nurses

1. The nurse provides services with respect for human dignity and the uniqueness of the client, unrestricted by considerations of social or economic status, personal attributes, or the nature of health problems.

2. The nurse safeguards the client's right to privacy by judiciously protecting information of a confidential nature.

3. The nurse acts to safeguard the client and the public when health care and safety are affected by the incompetent, unethical, or illegal practice of any person.

4. The nurse assumes responsibility and accountability for individual nursing judgments and actions.

5. The nurse maintains competence in nursing.

6. The nurse exercises informed judgment and uses individual competence and qualifications as criteria in seeking consultation, accepting responsibilities, and delegating nursing activities to others.

7. The nurse participates in activities that contribute to the ongoing development of the profession's body of knowledge.

8. The nurse participates in the profession's efforts to implement and improve standards of nursing.

9. The nurse participates in the profession's efforts to establish and maintain conditions of employment conducive to high-quality nursing care.

10. The nurse participates in the profession's efforts to protect the public from misinformation and misrepresentation and to maintain the integrity of nursing.

11. The nurse collaborates with members of the health professions and other citizens in promoting community and national efforts to meet the health needs of the public.

♦ Figure 3–2

ANA Code for Nurses. (Reprinted with permission of the American Nurses' Association [1976, 1985]. *Code for nurses with Interpretative Statements.* Kansas City: American Nurses' Association.)

Values from Canadian Nurses Association Code of Ethics for Nursing

Health and well-being: Nurses value health and well-being and assist persons to achieve their optimum level of health in situations of normal health, illness, injury, or in the process of dying.
1. Nurses provide care directed frirst and foremost toward the health and well-being of the client.
2. Nurses recognize that health is more than the absence of disease or infirmity and assist clients to achieve the maximum level of health and well-being possible.
3. Nurses recognize that health status is influenced by a variety of factors. In ways that are consistent with their professional role and responsibilities, nurses are accountable for addressing institutional, social, and political factors influencing health and health care.
4. Nurses support and advocate a full continuum of health services, including health promotion and disease prevention initiatives, as well as diagnostic, restorative, rehabilitative, and palliative care services.
5. Nurses respect and value the knowledge and skills other health care providers bring to the health care team and actively seek to support and collaborate with others so that maximum benefits to clients can be realized.
6. Nurses foster well-being when life can no longer be sustained by alleviating suffering and supporting a dignified and peaceful death.
7. Nurses provide the best care circumstances permit even when the need arises in an emergency outside an employment situation.
8. Nurses participate, to the best of their abilities, in research and other activities that contribute to the ongoing development of nursing knowledge. Nurses participating in research observe the nursing profession's guidelines, as well as other guidelines, for ethical research.

Choice: Nurses respect and promote the autonomy of clients and help them to express their health needs and values and to obtain appropriate information and services.
1. Nurses seek to involve clients in health planning and health care decision-making.
2. Nurses provide the information and support required so that clients, to the best of their ability, are able to act on their own behalf in meeting their health and health care needs. Information given is complete, accurate, truthful, and understandable. When they are unable to provide the required information, nurses assist clients in obtaining it from other appropriate sources.
3. Nurses demonstrate sensitivity to the willingness/readiness of clients to receive information about their health condition and care options. Nurses respect the wishes of those who refuse, or are not ready, to receive information about their health condition.
4. Nurses practice within relevant legislation governing consent or choice. Nurses seek to ensure that nursing care is authorized by informed choice and are guided by this ideal when participating in the consent process in cooperation with other members of the health team.
5. Nurses respect the informed decisions of competent persons to refuse treatment and to choose to live at risk. However, nurses are not obliged to comply with clients' wishes when doing so would require action contrary to the law. If the care requested is contrary to the nurse's moral beliefs, appropriate care is provided until alternative care arrangements are in place to meet the client's needs.
6. Nurses are sensitive to their position of relative power in professional relationships with clients and take care to foster self-determination on the part of their clients. Nurses are sufficiently clear about personal values to recognize and deal appropriately with potential value conflicts.
7. Nurses respect decisions and lawful directives, written or verbal, about present and future health care choices affirmed by a client prior to becoming incompetent.
8. Nurses seek to involve clients of diminished competence in decision-making to the extent that those clients are capable. Nurses continue to value autonomy when illness or other factors reduce the capacity for self-determination, such as by providing opportunities for clients to make choices about aspects of their lives for which they maintain the capacity to make decisions.
9. Nurses seek to obtain consent for nursing care from a substitute decision-maker when clients lack the capacity to make decisions about their care or did not make their wishes known prior to becoming incompetent, or for any reason it is unclear what the client would have wanted in a particular circumstance. When prior wishes of an incompetent client are not known or are unclear, care decisions must be in the best interest of the client and based on what the client would want, as far as is known.

Dignity: Nurses value and advocate the dignity and self-respect of human beings.
1. Nurses relate to all persons receiving care as persons worthy of respect and endeavour in all their actions to preserve and demonstrate respect for each individual.
2. Nurses exhibit sensitivity to the client's individual needs, values, and choices. Nursing care is designed to accommodate the biological, psychological, social, cultural, and spiritual needs of clients. Nurses do not exploit clients' vulnerabilities for their own interests or gain, whether this be sexual, emotional, social, political, or financial.
3. Nurses respect the privacy of clients when care is given.
4. Nurses treat human life as precious and worthy of respect. Respect includes seeking out and honoring clients' wishes regarding quality of life. Decision-making about life-sustaining treatment carefully balances these considerations.
5. Nurses intervene if others fail to respect the dignity of clients.
6. Nurses advocate the dignity of clients in the use of technology in the health care setting.
7. Nurses advocate health and social conditions that allow persons to live with dignity throughout their lives and in the process of dying. They do so in ways that are consistent with their professional role and responsibilities.

Confidentiality: Nurses safeguard the trust of clients that information learned in the context of a professional relationship is shared outside the health care team only with the client's permission or as legally required.
1. Nurses observe practices that protect the confidentiality of each client's health and health care information.
2. Nurses intervene if other participants in the health care delivery system fail to respect client confidentiality.
3. Nurses disclose confidential information only as authorized by the client, unless there is substantial risk of serious harm to the client or other persons, or a legal obligation to disclose. Where disclosure is warranted, both the amount of information disclosed and the number of people informed is restricted to the minimum necessary.
4. Nurses, whenever possible, inform their clients about the boundaries of professional confidentiality at the onset of care, including the circumstances under which confidential information might be disclosed without consent. If feasible, when disclosure becomes necessary, nurses inform clients what information will be disclosed, to whom, and for what reasons.
5. Nurses advocate policies and safeguards to protect and preserve client confidentiality and intervene if the security of confidential information is jeopardized because of a weakness in the provisions of the system, e.g., inadequate safeguarding guidelines and procedures for the use of computer databases.

Fairness: Nurses apply and promote principles of equity and fairness to assist clients in receiving unbiased treatment and a share of health services and resources proportionate to their needs.
1. Nurses provide care in response to need regardless of such factors as race, ethnicity, culture, spiritual beliefs, social or marital status, gender, sexual orientation, age, health status, lifestyle or the physical attributes of the client.
2. Nurses are justified in using reasonable means to protect against violence when they anticipate acts of violence toward themselves, others, or property with good reason.
3. Nurses strive to be fair in making decisions about the allocation of services and goods that they provide, when the distribution of these is within their control.
4. Nurses put forward and advocate the interests of all persons in their care. This includes helping individuals and groups gain access to appropriate health care that is of their choosing.
5. Nurses promote appropriate and ethical care at the institutional/agency and community levels by participating, to the extent possible, in the development, implementation, and ongoing review of policies and procedures designed to make the best use of available resources and of current knowledge and research.
6. Nurses advocate, in ways that are consistent with their role and responsibilities, health policies and decision-making procedures that are fair and comprehensive, and that promote fairness and inclusiveness in health resource allocation.

Accountability: Nurses act in a manner consistent with their professional responsibilities and standards of practice.
1. Nurses comply with the values and responsibilities in this *Code of Ethics for Registered Nurses* as well as with the professional standards and laws pertaining to their practice.
2. Nurses conduct themselves with honesty and integrity.
3. Nurses, whether they are engaged in clinical, administrative, research, or educational endeavours, have professional responsibilities and accountabilities toward safeguarding the quality of nursing care clients receive. These responsibilities vary but are all oriented to the expected outcome of safe, competent and ethical nursing practice.
4. Nurses, individually or in partnership with others, take preventive as well as corrective action to protect clients from unsafe, incompetent or unethical care.
5. Nurses base their practice on relevant knowledge, and acquire new skills and knowledge in their area of practice on a continuing basis, as necessary for the provision of safe, competent and ethical nursing care.
6. Nurses, whether engaged in clinical practice, administration, research or education, provide timely and accurate feedback to other nurses about their practice, so as to support safe and competent care and contribute to ongoing learning. By so doing, they also acknowledge excellence in practice.
7. Nurses practise within their own level of competence. They seek additional information or knowledge; seek the help, and/or supervision and help, of a competent practitioner; and/or request a different work assignment, when aspects of the care required are beyond their level of competence. In the meantime, nurses provide care within the level of their skill and experience.
8. Nurses give primary consideration to the welfare of clients and any possibility of harm in future care situations when they suspect unethical conduct or incompetent or unsafe care. When nurses have reasonable grounds for concern about the behaviour of colleagues in this regard, or about the safety of conditions in the care setting, they carefully review the situation and take steps, individually or in partnership with others, to resolve the problem.
9. Nurses support other nurses who act in good faith to protect clients from incompetent, unethical or unsafe care, and advocate wotk environments in which nurses are treated with respect when they intervene.
10. Nurses speaking on nursing and health-related matters in a public forum or a court provide accurate and relevant information.

Practice environments conducive to safe, competent, and ethical care: Nurses advocate practice environments that have the organizational and human support systems, and the resource allocations necessary for safe, competent and ethical nursing care.
1. Nurses collaborate with nursing colleagues and other members of the health team to advocate health care environments that are conducive to ethical practice and to the health and well-being of clients and others in the setting. They do this in ways that are consistent with their professional role and responsibilities.
2. Nurses share their nursing knowledge with other members of the health team for the benefit of clients. To the best of their abilities, nurses provide mentorship and guidance for the professional development of students of nursing and other nurses.
3. Nurses seeking professional employment accurately state their area(s) of competence and seek reasonable assurance that employment conditions will permit care consistent with the values and responsibilities of the code, as well as with their personal ethical beliefs.
4. Nurses practise ethically by striving for the best care achievable in the circumstances. They also make the effort, individually or in partnership with others, to improve practice environments by advocating on behalf of their clients as possible.
5. Nurses planning to participate in job action, or who practise in environments where job action occurs, take steps to safeguard the health and safety of clients during the course of the action.

Figure 3–3
Canadian nursing code of ethics. (From *Code of ethics for registered nurses.* [1997]. Ottawa, Ontario: Canadian Nurses Association. Reprinted with permission from the Canadian Nurses Association.)

International Council of Nurses Code for Nurses—Ethical Concepts Applied to Nursing

The fundamental responsibility of the nurse is fourfold: to promote health, to prevent illness, to restore health, and to alleviate suffering.

The need for nursing is universal. Inherent in nursing is respect for life, dignity, and right of man. It is unrestricted by considerations of nationality, race, creed, color, age, sex, politics, or social status.

Nurses render health services to the individual, the family, and the community and coordinate their services with those of related groups.

Nurses and people
The nurse's primary responsibility is to those people who require nursing care.

The nurse, in providing care, promotes an environment in which the values, customs, and spiritual beliefs of the individual are respected.

The nurse holds in confidence personal information and uses judgement in sharing this information.

Nurses and practice
The nurse carries personal responsibility for nursing practice and for maintaining competence by continual learning.

The nurse maintains the highest standards of nursing care possible within the reality of a specific situation.

The nurse uses judgement in relation to individual competence when accepting and delegating responsibilities.

The nurse when acting in a professional capacity should at all times maintain standards of personal conduct that would reflect credit upon the profession.

Nurses and society
The nurse shares with other citizens the responsibility for initiating and supporting action to meet the health and social needs of the public.

Nurses and co-workers
The nurse sustains a cooperative relationship with co-workers in nursing and other fields.

The nurse takes appropriate action to safeguard the individual when his care is endangered by a co-worker or any other person.

Nurses and the profession
The nurse plays the major role in determining and implementing desirable standards of nursing practice and nursing education.

The nurse is active in developing a core of professional knowledge.

The nurse, acting through the professional organization, participates in establishing and maintaining equitable social and economic working conditions in nursing.

❧ **Figure 3–4**
International nursing code of ethics. (From International Council of Nurses. [1972]. *Code for nurses.* Geneva, Switzerland: International Council of Nurses. Reproduced with permission from the International Council of Nurses, approved by the Council of National Representatives in 1973 and reaffirmed in 1989.)

contemporary professional values in nursing place a great deal of emphasis on people's rights to be a dignified person. The ethics of respecting persons is at the heart of all ethics of autonomy.

Deontological Ideals and Nursing Values

People's right to be treated with respect and to have their human worth and freedom honored puts certain obligations on nurses. For example, nurses ought not to restrain clients, either by physical or chemical means, without full medical justification. If the nurse must do so, the least restrictive means must be used. Another example is that it is a nurse's obligation to provide a client every opportunity to make choices about his or her own care, or to give formal consent prior to medical and nursing procedures. It is also a nurse's obligation to teach a client self-care strategies and give relevant information, so that a client can live, to the greatest extent possible, an independent and dignified life.

For a client to be able to exercise the rights of a fully autonomous individual, nurses must act with justice and fairness, respect the client's privacy, maintain confidentiality with regard to information pertaining to the client, be truthful when communicating with the client, and generally act in such a way as to do good and not do harm. These are all ethical principles of the deontological tradition (Table 3–4).

These deontological ideals are reflected in nursing's professional codes of ethics (Figs. 3–2 to 3–4). According to the American Nurses' Association (ANA) *Code for Nurses* (ANA, 1985), the nurse is expected to provide services "with respect for human dignity and the uniqueness of the client," "to safeguard the client's right to privacy," and "to safeguard the client . . . when [their] health care and safety" are at issue (p. 1). The code also details nurses' duties toward themselves in terms of self and professional development. Highly valuing accountability, the ANA code urges nurses to "maintain competence in nursing" and "to participate in the profession's efforts to implement and improve standards of nursing" (p. 1).

Critique of the Deontological Perspective

Although ethical principles serve as moral guideposts, they are not always able to provide guidance in highly complex contemporary situations in nursing and health care. The deontological disregard for consequences of actions could pose a problem in actual decision-making. Furthermore, all ethical precepts are viewed as equally important. When competing and equally obligatory ethical principles come into conflict in clinical situations, deontological ethics give no guidelines as to how one should prioritize them. Given the complexity of modern ethical problems in the field of health care, conflicts between moral rules are common. Consider this scenario: A 13-year-old girl tells the nurse caring for her in a family practice clinic that she suspects that she has contracted a sexually transmitted disease. She says that she is afraid to tell her mother that she is sexually active. After the interview, the girl's mother takes the nurse aside and inquires about the nature of her daughter's concerns. Here, the teenager's right to privacy and confidentiality is pitted against her mother's right to know. Both parties have just claims. The duty to safeguard information is inherent in the nurse-client relationship, yet the girl's mother has the duty and the right to make decisions regarding her child's health care. This situation represents an **ethical dilemma,** a situation in which all options for resolution are equally unsatisfactory.

In this scenario, the nurse most likely needs to turn to the facts of the clinical situation itself to help balance the possible benefit or harm for both the client and her mother. If the nurse betrays the teenager's trust, the teenager may not return to receive follow-up treatment and the nurse would have caused her real harm. Because of this, the client's right to privacy and confidentiality might very well outweigh the mother's autonomy and right to know. Although the mother's rights are violated, the nurse can mitigate harm by encouraging the teenager and her mother to have a more open relationship so that the teenager can share the information herself. In addition, the family practice clinic might publicize such confidentiality policies and the rationale behind them. The point is that deontological principles alone are unable to give a clear sense of whether the rights of the teenager or the mother ought to take priority (Table 3–5).

Utilitarianism

Whereas deontological thinking informs people of what they ought to do, **utilitarianism,** as an ethical theory, focuses instead on what constitutes *"good."* Variations in the meanings of good within utilitarian thinking range from the narrowest hedonist view of self-centered pleasure to higher-order good that represents outcomes of social actions that bring great benefit to people. In contemporary nursing ethics, the notion of good includes human experiences that are universally valued or sought; for example, enjoyment of good health and access to health care.

Utilitarianism has only one ethical principle—the principle of *utility* or the principle of "greatest happiness." Derived from the work of British philosophers Jeremy Bentham (1748–1832) and John Stuart Mill (1806–1873), utilitarianism values actions and decisions that produce the greatest quantity of happiness for the greatest number of people (Table 3–6). Em-

Table 3–5
NORMATIVE ETHICAL THEORIES: MAJOR POINTS OF CONTRAST
Deontology
• Grounded in the idea that a rational person has the capacity and will to be moral • The rightness or wrongness of a person's action must be considered in terms of its moral significance alone • Ethical principles that serve as standard; *e.g.,* principle of autonomy (self-determination) and principle of beneficence (to do good)
Utilitarianism
• Grounded in the idea that right action is one that brings about the greatest good and the least amount of harm for the greatest number of people • Only actions that are most likely to produce good consequence are right • Sole ethical principle that serves as standard: principle of utility (conducive to bring about desirable outcomes)

phasis is not placed on a person's motives and intentions. An action is right if it brings about increased happiness or benefit and wrong if it decreases people's happiness or benefit.

When applied to health care, protection of people's health is considered a worthwhile end product of human action. For example, various states' public health law requires people who have pulmonary tuberculosis in the infectious stage to comply with treatment, if not voluntarily, then by forced compliance. Here, unlike deontological theory, a person's free will and self-determination give way to the protection of large groups of people. Another example that illustrates this mode of ethical thinking is the mandatory immunization of children to ensure that the community does not have to bear the cost of treating diseases and human mortality. Families do not have the choice as to whether they want to have their children immunized, even though immunization carries some risk of complications. A further example is the mandatory drug testing of people who drive buses and operate trains, so that passengers are protected from injury and wrongful death.

Critique of the Utilitarian Perspective

Few people will find mandatory treatment of people spreading tuberculosis bacilli, immunization of children, or drug testing of bus drivers morally repugnant. Utilitarian thinking, however, also philosophically supports some decisions in health care based on cost-benefit analysis. The rationale is that resources, no matter how limited, ought to be stretched to benefit as many people as possible.

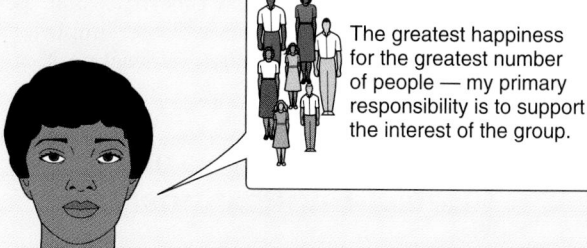

Table 3-6

UTILITARIANISM

Concern with the consequences or end product of our actions: An action is right if it brings increased happiness or benefit for those concerned; an action is wrong if it decreases people's happiness or benefit
- The principle of utility
- The principle of the greatest happiness for the greatest number of people

The greatest happiness for the greatest number of people — my primary responsibility is to support the interest of the group.

Examples of Application to Health Care

- Mass immunization of children, voluntarily or involuntarily
- Random drug testing of people operating buses or trains

In health care, when economic feasibility is pitted against the intrinsic value of certain clinical decisions and practices, utilitarianism may cause moral discomfort. For example, screening mammography for breast cancer has been proven a successful strategy for cancer prevention and therefore has intrinsic value as a clinical procedure (Fig. 3–5). Appropriate guidelines for its use are debated by health care professionals. Concerns surrounding screening mammography center on (1) the appropriate age for screening, (2) whether screening should occur every 1 or 2 years, and (3) whether the procedure should be available to high-risk women who are younger than the common screening age (Breen & Brown, 1994). These are all questions that seek balance between benefit and cost.

When older women alone are entitled to routine mammography, a much smaller number of examinations will be conducted. Because older women are generally at higher risk for breast cancer, routine mammography will detect a higher number of breast cancers relative to the number of examinations given, as opposed to the number of breast cancers that may be picked up if the examination were applied to a large general population of women of all ages, at both high and low risk for breast cancer.

One may feel morally comfortable with a mammography screening program that exclusively targets the population most at risk and is cost-effective because the mammography screening program can return so many more positive results. But what happens to the small number of younger women who do not belong to the high-risk group, who did not receive routine, periodic mammography screening, and who ended up developing breast cancer? These few outside-of-the-majority-group individuals did not benefit from the opportunity of early diagnosis.

The "good" and "usefulness" of screening mammography for a large number of women are unquestioned. The guideline for its use is desirable for the

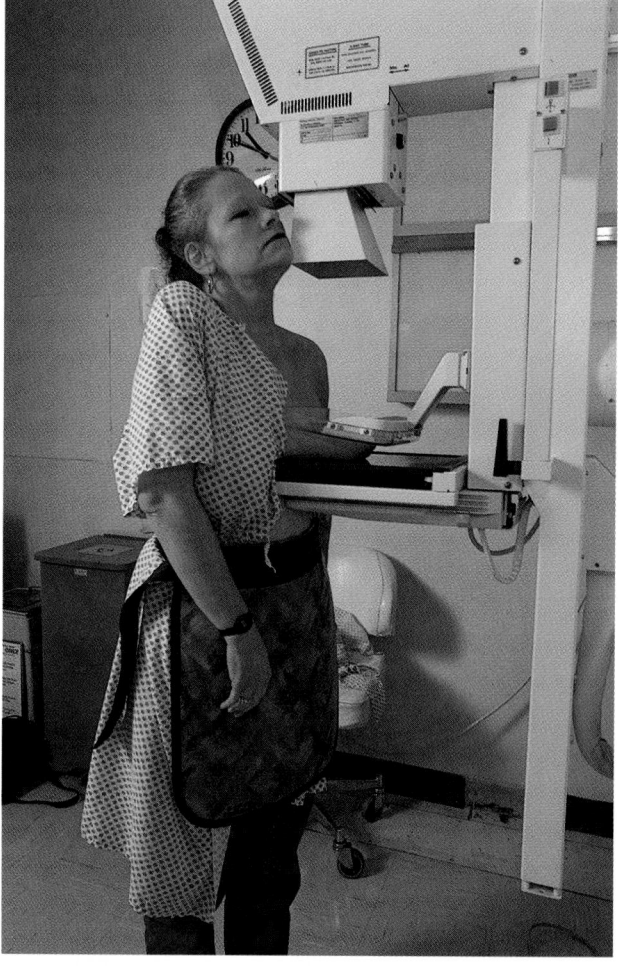

❧ Figure 3–5
Who should undergo routine screening mammography for breast cancer? This is a controversial question (utilitarianism vs. ethics) because the decision is based partly on economic considerations.

community too. Its cost-effectiveness makes the program cheaper to support. Thus, from a utilitarian viewpoint, it satisfies the principle of utility. The ethical goal of achieving the greatest amount of benefit extended to the largest number of women possible is met. According to utilitarian theory, the minority group has no just claim. Herein lies the weakness of utilitarian thinking.

Ethical Principles and Clinical Implications

In clinical practice, it is not always practical to refer to entire ethical theories for decision-making. Nurses often look toward narrower, more specific ethical principles to guide their judgment and decisions, many of which have both deontological and utilitarian roots. Examples are principles of autonomy, beneficence, nonmaleficence, justice, and utility.

The Principle of Autonomy

The term **autonomy** originally referred to political independence of states and nations. In health care it

CONTRASTING CULTURAL EXPECTATIONS:
WHETHER TO DISCLOSE A DIAGNOSIS
OF CANCER

In Western cultures, especially the United States, where the principles of autonomy and individual rights are supreme values, it would be morally indefensible for nurses and physicians to withhold information on the diagnosis of cancer to spare the client emotional distress. Health care providers have no moral authority to act paternalistically on a presumption that their client would prefer to be ignorant of the diagnosis.

By contrast, the Confucian tradition in Asian cultures, *e.g.,* Japan, nurtures a more paternalistic approach. Trusting that health care providers will act for the client's good, the withholding of information regarding a diagnosis of cancer aims to reduce the psychological burden of the fear of death and to allow physicians and nurses to give hope (Takahashi, 1990; Morioka, 1991).

Transcultural ethics is an ethical approach that says that there are universal ethical truths that span all cultures (Kikuchi, 1996). These universal ethical truths center on natural human needs, such as the need for health. If nondisclosure of a diagnosis of cancer prevents a client from seeking appropriate treatment, then it is not morally justifiable to withhold this information. If, on the other hand, the client is at the terminal stage of cancer, and treatment is only palliative, then, if culturally preferred, nondisclosure of this information may be morally justifiable. In most cases, family members are informed of the diagnosis, and the decision to withhold the information may be at their request.

has come to mean a self-directing freedom and moral independence in which an individual is free to choose and implement his or her own decisions. Autonomy can be defined as "a cluster of notions including self-determination, freedom, independence, liberty of choice and action. In its most general terms, autonomy signifies control of decision-making and other activity by the individual. It refers to human agency free·of outside intervention and interference" (Collopy, 1988, p. 10). This view of the person is consistent with the deontological tradition. An autonomous person is assumed to possess an inner capacity for self-governance, as well as to be free of coercive restraint. Autonomy also implies that the person will use a stable set of values and beliefs in making reasoned decisions and choices, rather than submitting to capricious impulses. Edge and Groves (1994) summarize the three basic features of autonomy: (1) the ability to decide, (2) the power to act upon decisions, and (3) a respect for the individual autonomy of others. Depending on the individual's values and beliefs, outcomes of decisions vary greatly from person to person. For example, a person may believe that it is never reasonable to choose to end one's life, while another may believe that suicide is permissible if he or she is fully aware of all implications.

The concept of autonomy binds nurses and clients in a very special way. Consistent with this respect for clients' autonomy or right of self-determination, nurses ought to refrain from interfering with the clients' rights to choose, to decide, to accept, or to reject. **Paternalism** is the deliberate restriction of people's autonomy by health care professionals based on the idea that they know what is best for the clients. In some instances, it is justifiable; *e.g.,* when a client must be involuntarily hospitalized, such as in the case of a mentally ill person who is disoriented and is a danger to himself or herself. Paternalism, in this case, is keeping the client from harm.

In a more subtle form of paternalism, health care workers may justify infringing on people's autonomy by the professional goal of promoting what is "good." An example of this is the mandated childhood immunization program. Here, utilitarian thinking is in operation, where good or right action is justified by the consequence of producing the greatest good or benefit for the community.

Informed consent, by contrast, is marked by "disclosure, understanding, voluntariness, competence, and permission giving" (Edge & Groves, 1994, p. 32). In a clinical situation, this means that a nurse is obligated to ensure that (1) a client is given appropriate information, (2) he or she is able to understand the information, and (3) the client agrees to a treatment voluntarily. Factors that may interfere with the client's autonomy in terms of informed consent include extreme anxiety and fear. The client may be temporarily rendered incapable of making a decision, may not understand the information being given, or could be unable to weigh rationally the risks and benefits of a procedure. In such a case, a client cannot give true informed consent. Thus, informed consent is closely associated with the notions of self-determination, non-interference, and free choice. It is a key element of autonomy. The ANA *Codes for Nurses* (1985), as well as the American Hospital Association's Bill of Patient's Rights (see Fig. 3–1), clearly articulate these standards for the nurse-client relationship.

The Principle of Veracity

Closely associated with autonomy and informed consent is the principle of **veracity.** Veracity—the duty to tell the truth—is part of the respect we owe to persons. If a person fails to be truthful, he or she in effect misleads others, debases their hopes and life plans, and restricts their autonomy. From a deontological standpoint, the nurse's failure to act with veracity in a nurse-patient relationship constitutes unethical interference. In practice, however, nurses must use their clinical judgment to choose the best approach to disclose information and the most appropriate time to do so (see box).

There are three levels of veracity: (1) fully disclosing information, (2) withholding information, and (3) giving false information. Full disclosure of information is always morally preferable. From a client's perspective, truthfulness is the clearest means to being informed. Giving false information or lying to clients, on the other hand, is almost always morally indefensible. Whether the middle course, withholding information, is morally justifiable depends on the situation. For example, should a nurse disclose information on all of the side effects of a medication, including those unusual and rare, to a client? A nurse may make a clinical judgment, after careful assessment, that the client is capable only of absorbing a few critical pieces of information at that particular time. In this case, only information essential to his or her care, including the major and common side effects of the medication, should be given. Additional information may confuse the client, induce great anxiety, or even cause him or her to reject the medication, which may be critically needed. It is morally permissible, on utilitarian grounds, that some information be withheld from the client, as long as the client benefitted from the consequence of the nurse's action. The terms of the principle of utility are met. But the nurse must be judicious about balancing utility, beneficence, and paternalism. As a general rule, the client should have as much information as possible.

The Principle of Confidentiality

Privacy and confidentiality are related concepts. In the course of caring for a client, nurses get to know many things about that person: medical diagnoses (including those vulnerable to social stigma such as acquired immunodeficiency syndrome and mental illnesses), prescribed medications, lifestyle, pain, hopes, and other intimate details. **Privacy** refers to the client's rights, and **confidentiality,** the nurse's corresponding duty, to protect this personal information.

The client must feel that he or she and the nurse are in a relationship of trust and confidence for such information to be shared. In a multidisciplinary health care environment, information about the client often must be communicated to other health care professionals. Such disclosure should aim only at creating appropriate services for the client. In any event, the client ought to be well aware of the referrals made on his or her behalf to other health care providers.

The core element of individual autonomy is a person's ability to control information about himself or herself. To respect clients' privacy and need for confidentiality is to honor the clients as autonomous individuals. From a deontological viewpoint, the breaching of confidentiality represents a serious threat to a client's autonomy. It is no less of a moral wrong from a utilitarian perspective. Because the consequence of breaching confidentiality harms clients, the nursing profession itself, and society in general (Edge & Groves, 1994), the greatest good for all is better served if nurses respect the principle of confidentiality. The breaching of confidentiality undermines the nursing profession's ability to fulfill its social mission because of the inevitable gradual erosion of public trust. Exceptions are situations in which a nurse learns that a third party may be endangered, such as a child being neglected or abused. In this case, the nurse has not only an ethical but also a legal obligation to disclose the confidential information.

The Principles of Beneficence and Nonmaleficence

Beneficence and nonmaleficence have to do with actions that befit professional practice (Appelbaum & Lawton, 1990). **Beneficence** means "doing good," while ***nonmaleficence*** refers to refraining from doing harm. These ethical principles serve as the moral anchor of the Hippocratic Oath, in which the physician pledges to use his or her skill to benefit the sick and never to use his or her art with a view toward injury and wrongdoing. Such sentiments are also appropriate for nursing practice.

In deontological thinking, beneficence calls for a positive duty—one that carries an obligation to act, to promote the welfare of clients, or to remove harm from the client's way. The problem facing nurses, however, is how to determine the limits of beneficence beyond what might be considered due care. Imagine confronting Jack, a 35-year-old client who had quadriplegic paralysis, drank alcohol to excess, and was irresolute in his effort to assume serious responsibility for his own life and self-care. After months of providing home care services and helping him acquire equipment, such as an electric wheelchair and a computer, with which he could be restored to some degree of independence, Jack continued to be unmotivated. While the nurses were deeply attuned to his despair, they questioned their professional obligation to this patient. Was one more month, week, or one last home visit due him?

From the utilitarian perspective, due care—a reasonable and accommodating level of care that, at minimum, conforms to professional standards—is the most effective use of health care and human resources because resources can be stretched to serve the largest number of clients. A nurse may go beyond the basic requirements of practice to assist the client, but it is not a breach of duty if such action does not take place.

Nonmaleficence, the duty to cause no harm, is a much clearer concept and easier to incorporate into the overall moral duties nurses have toward clients. This ethical principle follows from basic ethical considerations of respect for persons and protection of individuals from harm. Appelbaum and Lawton (1990), suggest, however, that nonmaleficence "does not mean avoiding harm altogether. . . . The sense of nonmaleficence is the avoidance of harm unless the action promises a greater good" (p. 39). For example, a nurse who changes the bandage of a severely burned client inflicts pain, but since the procedure ultimately brings about healing, the nurse meets the terms of nonmaleficence. By contrast, if a nurse gives a wrong medication to a patient, even if unintended, the nurse causes harm and has failed to act with nonmaleficence. Here, as with the principle of beneficence, both deontological and utilitarian thinking are reflected.

The Principle of Justice

The moral focus of the principle of **justice** is on the community. There are three vantage points from which the principle of justice can be examined: fairness, equality, and the state of being deserving. The first two are rooted in deontological ethical theory, the last in utilitarianism.

The notion of fairness suggests impartiality and should ideally guide a moral community toward the right ways to distribute social benefits and goods, such as education, employment opportunities, wealth, and health care. In reality, in community decision-making, various groups with varying health needs vie for health care resources. A reasonable community with a strong moral impulse will not allocate resources based on self-interest, special interest, or other forms of gross inequity. There will be reasoned debate, cooperation, and consideration for one another's needs, a form of justice that is acceptable to all.

Justice can also be viewed as equality, suggesting the condition of equal access or equal opportunity. Inherent is a fundamental respect for all people, the idea of which is of clear deontological origin. Whether there should be universal access to health care has been an issue of intense debate for a number of years in the United States.

Nurses and the profession of nursing should assume the role of active participants in the debate regarding fairness and equality. They should also be a visible force in community decision-making, acting as advocates for clients.

Lastly, justice can be interpreted as a state of being deserving. From this standpoint, justice is giving to people what they need or desire based on some agreed on criteria of worth. In health care, where there are not enough resources to meet the needs of all people, individuals vie for the attention of nurses and physicians in a busy hospital ward, an intensive care bed, a hemodialysis machine, a home health aide, or an organ for transplant. Individuals become "worthy" to receive health care resources because they meet some criteria according to the logic of health care. Their deserving quality may be based on

1. Demonstration of health care needs. For example, a diagnosis of heart attack will secure a bed in the intensive care unit for a person.
2. The ability to pay for the desired services. For example, a person may purchase costly cosmetic surgery.
3. Social worth as a person, such as being a person who must rear children. For example, community resources are devoted to programs that support families and parenting efforts.
4. The ability to respond to treatment or health care. For example, in medical triage, emergency medical attention is given first to victims of disasters most likely to survive and not the most seriously injured.
5. Some common good. For example, all people with pulmonary tuberculosis, from the rich to the homeless, are treated, so that they are prevented from spreading the infectious disease to their neighbors and coworkers. The concern here is not so much for the clients with pulmonary tuberculosis, but for the good of the public.

Justice, linked to the criterion of being deserving, has the same goals as the principles of utility and beneficence. The role of the nurse in this context is to balance carefully the deontological perspective of respecting the needs all people and the utilitarian perspective of how best to utilize scarce resources for some deserving individuals.

Values-Oriented Ethics

Another approach to ethical thinking is **values-**oriented ethics. While normative ethics prescribe what is good, values-oriented ethics put the emphasis on the responsibility of doing the right thing on the actor's personal character and his or her determination to act morally. Instead of asking "What ethical principle do I use to guide my action?" the question becomes "How should I act in this situation if I have the capacity to act morally?" Personal moral strengths such as courage, pride, wisdom, care and compassion, and self-respect, are important elements of values-oriented ethics.

Brody (1988) proposes that personal moral strengths and virtues illuminate and strengthen normative ethics. For example, without compassion, the ethical principle of beneficence is untenable. Without a

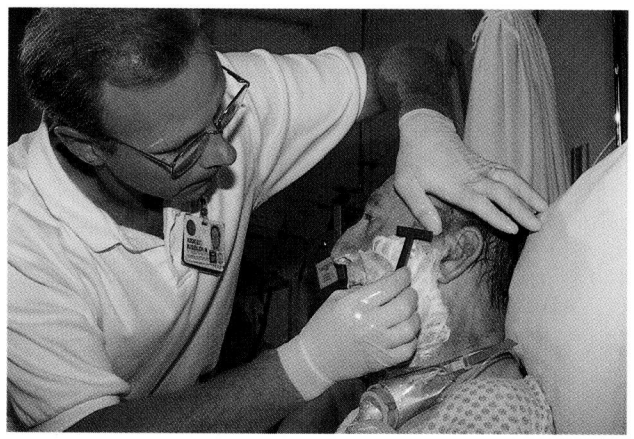

✦ Figure 3–6
Providing physical care demonstrates the "virtue of caring." Swanson (1993, p. 354) defines caring as "a nurturing way of relating to a valued other toward whom one feels a personal sense of commitment and responsibility."

provides physical care to a client. That means that the caring quality of the nurse's attentiveness, touch, voice, commitment, skills, and competence can be recognized and felt by the client (Fig. 3–6). Usually clients are much more likely to be receptive to health teaching or even to an uncomfortable procedure if these are provided by a nurse who is caring, compassionate, and understanding (Table 3–7).

Virtues also emphasize practical judgment and nonextreme actions that attempt to balance all relevant facts of a situation. To determine what is good and right, nurses must try to understand the context of a nursing problem, identify all individuals involved in a situation, and deliberate—with honesty, caring and compassion, and fairness and beneficence—the course of action that benefits the client and his or her family. The final decision, grounded in caring and consistent with respect for persons, must be focused on people's need to live a fruitful and meaningful life.

sense of fairness, one is unable to live by the principle of justice.

Two types of values-oriented ethics are relevant for nursing practice. They are virtue ethics based on nursing caring and the moral sense inherent in nursing practice.

Virtue Ethics Based on Caring

Virtue may be defined as "a human strength" that "helps us live as we 'ought to' " (Cooper, 1993, p. 23). The classical conception of virtue emphasizes practical wisdom and actions that are moderate. To the ancient Greeks, extreme emotion and action were considered vices. They reasoned that a virtuous person has the practical wisdom and ability to balance relevant facts and adopt a moderate course of action that considers all important facts in a situation. Thus, virtues are not abstract concepts that exist in the minds of people. They are instead human traits of compassion, courage, wisdom, and so forth, exhibited by people in concrete situations. For example, courage is not saying "I am brave" but is expressed as the act of rescuing another person in extremely dangerous conditions.

Based on who the individuals are, they may aspire to certain unique virtues. For the clergy, they may cultivate the virtue of faith; for lawyers, the virtue of fairness; and for nurses, the virtue of caring.

Nurse scholars who wrote about caring in nursing (the classics of which include Watson, 1979, 1985; Benner & Wrubel, 1989) offer it as a foundational concept in nursing. Swanson (1993) defines caring as "a nurturing way of relating to a valued other toward whom one feels a personal sense of commitment and responsibility" (p. 354). The key elements of Swanson's definition are (1) nurturing, (2) relating, (3) valuing another, and (4) providing individualized attention. Because virtues are expressed through human conduct, nursing caring should be evident when the nurse

The Moral Sense Inherent in Practice

The moral sense inherent in practice comprises three aspects. The first relates to the significance of ordinary nursing activities. These activities, such as monitoring clients' vital signs, fluid and electrolyte balances, side effects of medications, and so forth, seem far removed from concerns of ethics and virtues. However, nursing activities are directed toward the goal of

Table **3–7**
A NURSE REFLECTS
"Caring? I am not sure I know how to define it. I do know that, as a nurse, I want to do the best for my patients. To give the highest quality care, to be in tune with their needs and emotions. But at the same time, I keep my own goals for them in mind. "Perhaps this sense of great concern I have for my patients is caring. Like Mr. M. over there in the end room, he has been so withdrawn—even when his wife is visiting. I am concerned about his emotional state as well as his physical condition. Even if it is only for a few seconds, I look in on him: just to smile and say hello . . . I know he appreciates it; it is in his eyes. "We have been having a very difficult time getting Mr. M. to take his medication, but he does try for me. I know he likes to add a little honey to his water, so that is what I bring with his medication. It's just a simple thing, but I want him to know that I *care* about whether or not he takes his medicine. "My own goal for Mr. M. is also a big part of caring for him. Getting him stabilized, getting him home, getting him back to the things that he loves. . . ."
C. T., September 1994, personal communication.

producing positive health outcomes (Packard & Ferrara, 1988), which makes nursing activities both "good" and "worthwhile." Thus, even ordinary nursing activities have moral significance.

The second aspect of the moral sense in practice relates to the nurse's commitment to excellence in relation to these ordinary nursing activities. Day-to-day nursing activities characterized as "just the performance of tasks" can be approached with knowledge, skill, thoughtfulness, and caring. Consider the administration of medication: Instead of merely passing out the pill to a client, the nurse can crush it and sweeten it with honey so the client will find it easier to swallow, or the nurse can bring apple juice with the pill because that is the client's preference. The nurse's knowledge and skill to ascertain correct dosage and to watch for intended as well as unintended effects of the medication also demonstrate a commitment to excellence.

Self-imposed attempts to achieve excellence allow the nurse to enjoy the satisfaction of having given his or her best effort. With this realization, a firm moral habit of mind develops, a condition that Bishop and Scudder (1987) call "moral autonomy." *Moral autonomy* refers to an internal moral compass that directs an individual to do what is right without constant external reinforcements and reminders.

The third aspect of the moral sense in practice relates to the role of the nurse. Nurses are located in a unique "in-between" position in health care. This in-between stance (1) has nurses implementing physician-prescribed treatments; (2) places nurses next to the client and family, allowing them to be intimately aware of their needs; (3) requires nurses to maintain order in the nursing unit; and (4) demands that nurses enforce hospital and other policies (Bishop & Scudder, 1987).

Nurses often find themselves squarely in the midst of **ethical dilemmas** where there are competing interests and diverse goals. Because of the complexity of contemporary ethical issues, there is the need to make cooperative decisions involving all parties. Nurses may be in the best position to foster joint decisions that represent a consensus about the best course of action.

Consider this example: A young woman farm worker brought her 2-year-old child with febrile convulsion into the rural health clinic. The child was immediately hospitalized. On the second day, as soon as the child's fever subsided somewhat, the mother removed the child from the hospital against medical advice. Did the mother have the right to remove the child? Was the child's health and life endangered? The physicians, nurses, and social workers were extremely concerned and debated reporting the woman to the local Child Protective Services for medical neglect. The nurses at the hospital also made a referral to the public health nurses. After locating the family, a public health nurse discovered that the child was indeed quite ill. The mother was very distressed, and she was trying all sorts of folk remedies in hopes of bringing the child's fever down. She was afraid to bring him back to the hospital because they were illegal immigrants. She saw the hospital and hospital staff as the "authorities" and was fearful that they would deport the family.

The public health nurse immediately obtained care for the child, but she was acutely aware of the fear, anxieties, and social issues that were involved. Without deliberate intent to harm him, the mother nevertheless had jeopardized the safety of her child. To assist this family, the cooperation of health care providers and social and legal services is necessary.

Critique of Values-Oriented Ethics

The benchmark for values-oriented ethics is what a moral person and a "good" nurse might do in a similar situation. Morality therefore depends in part on tradition and past experiences. This becomes problematic when traditional views of what is good provide no answers for emerging situations and new issues.

The appeal to a person's inner capacity to act wisely, moderately, and appropriately according to the specifics of a situation may not be as easy as it seems. Some people do not have the practical wisdom to consider all variables to balance and counter-balance the particulars of a moral dilemma. While the strength of values-oriented ethics is its grounding in people's real life events, its weakness is the unpredictability of human judgment.

Case Study and Ethical Decision Making Process

The Ethics Committee

Many institutions have ethics committees. Their membership includes physicians, nurses, the clergy, attorneys, and lay representatives. The purposes of these committees vary from institution to institution. In general, they are concerned with

1. Issues of patient care that presents as ethical dilemmas
2. The institution's ability to protect the rights and interests of clients in general
3. The development of institutional policies and educational programs on ethical issues

Clinical Ethics Consultation

Bedside clinical ethics consultations are performed by physicians, nurses, and other health care professionals who are both clinicians and experts in health care ethics. Clinical ethicists focus primarily on client situations where ethical dilemmas block clinical decision-making. Clinical ethicists examines the client and interviews family members and members of the health care team. Their role is to mediate values conflicts between the parties involved in the ethical problem.

Mrs. E. is a 69-year-old woman who has a diagnosis of Alzheimer's disease. A widow of 10 years, she lives in a small second-floor apartment in an apartment complex in a small college town. Her only living relative is a 42-year-old son who lives 100 miles away in a major city. Prior to her diagnosis, Mrs. E. was a vivacious, free-thinking individual who valued independence and her own brand of eccentricity: she prided herself on always doing things her own way. She loved to travel and enjoyed the arts. Her favorite activity was to take long car drives, meandering through country roads.

Now moderately cognitively impaired, Mrs. E. can no longer take care of herself. Neighbors who had previously helped and the personal care attendant placed in the home 3 hours a day have been subjected to Mrs. E's frequent rages, mostly as a result of her intense frustration over the fact that she cannot locate personal and household things and she forgets why she had entered a room.

The home care nurse has two other major concerns. First, Mrs. E. is on a cardiac medication that she is to take once a day in the morning, usually observed by the personal care attendant. From the number of pills left in the bottle, the nurse realizes that Mrs. E. may have been taking additional doses during the day. When inquired, Mrs. E. claims that she takes her medication in the morning only, but it soon becomes evident that she does not really know the time of day, and has mistaken afternoons for additional mornings. The second major concern is Mrs. E.'s driving. When the personal care attendant leaves in the early afternoon, Mrs. E. takes her car out. While she always manages to return to the parking lot, Mrs. E. is unable to locate her apartment. Neighbors see her wandering around the apartment complex and notify the manager, who collects her and brings her back to her home. The nurse suggests to Mrs. E. that she should give up driving. Mrs. E. is adamant that she will continue to do what she enjoys the most and that she will surrender her car keys, worn around her neck, to no one.

Mrs. E.'s son, remembering his mother as a fiercely independent and vibrant woman, is reluctant to work with the nurse. He concedes that his mother would perhaps benefit from living in a more structured and supervised environment, but he indicates that he does not have the will to force his mother to give up the car or the apartment.

Framework for Ethical Decision-Making

STEP ONE. Describe the context, the clinical, social and ethical issues, and the parties involved.

Mrs. E., age 69, has a diagnosis of Alzheimer's disease. Her cognitive ability is decreasing, but she continues to insist on independence. The problematic clinical and social issues:

- Lives alone
- Son lives 100 miles away
- Three hours only with personal care attendant daily
- Cognitive impairment is increasing

- Inappropriate self-administration of medication
- Driving may endanger others, but she refuses to give up the activity

STEP TWO. State the problem(s) in ethical terms.

- Should the client have the right to full independence (as desired by her) when she may jeopardize her own well-being and the well-being of others?
- Are there moral justifications for restricting the client's rights?

STEP THREE. Articulate the desired goals and objectives of the client, the nurse, and involved others. Describe how the desired goals and objectives impact on the others involved in this problem, including conflicts with applicable laws and regulations and legal ramifications.

- The desired goal of client is to continue to be independent, including driving.
- The desired goal of client's son is not to interfere.
- The desired goals of the nurse are to

  Protect Mrs. E.'s physical well-being by providing more intense supervision for activities of daily living, by preventing her from self-administering medication, and by preventing her from driving

  Protect the safety of the public by preventing Mrs. E. from driving

  Support the legal rights of the state to revoke Mrs. E.'s license, as she is no longer competent to drive

  Support Mrs. E.'s dignity and self-determination in all other aspects of her life as long as she poses no danger to herself and to others

STEP FOUR. Determine the client's decision-making capacity, and the parties who should participate in making the decision. Search for evidence of client's and family's prior wishes, such as advanced directives and proxies.

- Mrs. E.'s decision-making capacity should be restricted only to issues related to activities of daily living
- Mrs. E.'s son is unwilling to be a participant
- There are no documented prior wishes, advanced directives, or proxies
- The nurse, in consultation with the health care team, has to make a decision regarding the protection of Mrs. E.'s physical well-being and the safety of the public

STEP FIVE. List as many as possible nursing intervention options and the ethical principles and values that justify the various options. Consider what ethical principles and values have been prized and what have been sacrificed.
Options:

- Move Mrs. E. out of her apartment against her will to a supervised setting, which is unsatisfactory because this would constitute drastic interference with Mrs. E.'s autonomy. Nonmaleficence and beneficence are prized; autonomy is sacrificed.

- Increase the hours of the personal care attendant, which may conflict with the criteria of the home care agency and third party reimbursement guidelines. The principle of justice in terms of the distribution of scarce resources is at work. If Mrs. E. receives additional services, she is deserving because of her needs. But it is also justifiable to say that she has received her fair share, even though it may not be enough. In this case, the principle of utility is prized.
- Control Mrs. E.'s medication by locking it up or entrusting it to a neighbor. Administration will be under direct observation. Mrs. E.'s autonomy is severely restricted. The principle of beneficence (doing good) is utilized to justify violating Mrs. E.'s autonomy.
- Assist the state in revoking Mrs. E.'s driver's license. The car key is kept from Mrs. E. As before, Mrs. E.'s autonomy is severely restricted. The principle of beneficence is utilized. In addition, the principle of utility supports action that furthers the public good.

STEP SIX. Propose a range of acceptable options that are consistent with your personal values and the professional values of nursing.

Acceptable options are the third and fourth ones listed under "Step Five." The unacceptable option is the first one. The second option, increasing the personal care attendant hours, can be negotiated with the home care agency. The professional values of nursing mandate that Mrs. E.'s autonomy, to the greatest extent possible, should still be respected.

STEP SEVEN. Make decisions, take action, and evaluate ethical outcomes.

Mrs. E.'s plan of care is revised to incorporate options 3 and 4. The nurse will continue to work with Mrs. E. and her son to explore safety and supervision issues. While the nurse can no longer honor Mrs. E.'s autonomy to make decisions regarding driving and the use of medication, the nurse should never confuse this with Mrs. E.'s right to do things according to her preferences, to the extent that she is capable.

Discussion

The principle of autonomy has guided decision-making in health care in the United States for the last two decades. Autonomy is premised on the deontological view of respect for the person, humanity, and the human condition. Despite diminishing cognitive ability, Mrs. E. has to be fully respected and honored as a person. In fact, her vulnerability immediately imposes a duty on the nurse to protect her dignity and rights. Does this stretch to the protection of Mrs. E.'s autonomy in terms of her wishes to live independently in her apartment and to drive a car? Here, we need to separate the issues of respect for the person and the person's moral authority to make independent decisions.

Respect for Mrs. E. as a person relates to attention to her inherent worth and uniqueness as an individual. Despite her cognitive impairment, the nurse continues to address Mrs. E. as she prefers to

be addressed and to talk with her with openness and honesty about her anxiety and fear regarding the progressive lost of control and independence. Mrs. E. is treated with consideration, kindness, respect, and most of all, with empathy—the kind of treatment all people would desire for themselves. These are the ethical goals of nursing that have roots in deontological thinking.

Privacy and confidentiality, also themes of respect for persons, are important for clients who are cognitively impaired. Just because Mrs. E. wanders lost in the apartment complex under the gaze of her neighbors does not mean that Mrs. E. forfeits her rights to privacy and confidentiality. Indeed, Mrs. E.'s activities of daily living, other than her driving and wandering, should be safeguarded by the nurse as strictly private. Enlisting the help of the apartment manager and neighbors to return her safely to home is necessary but is just that. In recruiting the cooperation of the neighbors, information about Mrs. E.'s personal habits and health problems divulged should be limited to the essential minimum.

Mrs. E.'s driving, however, poses a different challenge to the traditional notion of autonomy. Self-determination should rightly be confined to decisions and actions that affect only oneself. If Mrs. E.'s driving negatively affects the health and safety of other people in the larger community, not to mention her own, one questions the degree to which Mrs. E. has the right to decide as she wishes. Her autonomy must be balanced against the autonomy of others who share the roadways with Mrs. E. Certainly, nurses have no moral obligation to support client behaviors that would jeopardize others or to become involved in promoting those inappropriate behaviors. In fact, it is morally incumbent on nurses to prevent an incompetent individual from harming himself or herself and others, as in the case of Mrs. E.'s driving. However, while the nurse can no longer honor Mrs. E.'s autonomy to make this decision, the nurse should never confuse this with Mrs. E's right to do things according to her preferences in her daily activities, such as choice of clothing, food, or a ride in someone else's car.

Because of the issue of safety, one could question the adequacy of Mrs. E.'s care and supervision. Only 3 hours of personal care attendant service per day are given to Mrs. E., despite the fact that she could use more. However, health insurance policies in part regulate the amount of service to which Mrs. E. is entitled. Availability of personal care attendants is also at issue. Twenty-four–hour supervision may just not be possible, despite her need. Nurse and personal care attendant time can thus be considered a scarce resource and must be stretched to serve as many people as possible. This utilitarian moral viewpoint does not take into consideration the consequences of Mrs. E.'s inadequate supervision.

Mrs. E.'s unintended misuse of medication is a major concern. The past debate on ethics suggested that health care providers have been far too paternalistic toward those to whom they give care. The discussion has focused on the need to restrict such paternalism, emphasizing the rights of clients to determine the specifics of their care based on their own values and desires. The client's responsibilities and obligations as a care recipient are underscored. However, all this is untenable for a cognitively impaired client. In the case of Mrs. E., she does not have the capacity to recognize the time of day to use her medication appropriately. The nurse must manage Mrs. E.'s immediate environment in such a way that limits Mrs. E.'s access to her medication. Whether the nurse comes daily to administer the medication, asks a neighbor to do so, or locks up the bottle and gives the key to the personal care attendant, paternalistic action is demonstrated. Failure of the nurse to act paternalistically, however, could cause harm and violate the principle of nonmaleficence. The clinical judgment and ethical decision that underpin the nurse's chosen action require the human virtues of reasonableness, practical wisdom, and common humanity. The decision also depends on the nurse's own moral sense of what excellent nursing practice is about: the protection and advocacy of the client's well-being.

✦

Summary

Values and ethics play a major role in nursing practice. They are deeply held convictions and beliefs that shape people's interpretation of what constitute the "good," the "just," and what "ought to be done." Ethical considerations not only are given to morally problematic, crisis situations but also must be applied to seemingly ordinary events, because nursing practice represents actions that are taken and decisions that are made over time. Thus, all actions and decisions have moral significance as well as ethical implications for the nursing profession and for client well-being.

Three major approaches of ethical thinking are of relevance to nursing practice. They are deontology, utilitarianism, and values-oriented ethics. The first two are traditional ethical theories that inform us of norms that should govern our duties and obligations to one another, such as attentiveness to personal autonomy, justice, and beneficence. The third represents a way of ethical thinking that is of utmost importance to nursing from the perspective of care. Values-oriented ethics focuses on the nurse as actor and insists on a perspective of care, of morality, and of excellence in practice.

■ ■

CHAPTER HIGHLIGHTS

✦

✦ Personal and professional values, as well as the knowledge of ethics, guide nurses in making judgments and setting priorities in nursing practice.

✦ Ethical principles draw nurses' attention to issues of client autonomy, information disclosure, privacy and confidentiality, beneficence and nonmaleficence, and justice.

✦ While moral justification from the perspective of deontology is always grounded in the respect for the person, utilitarianism is based on calculation of the amount of benefit for large groups of people. Virtues-oriented ethics place the responsibility to act morally—to do the right thing—on the nurse. By accepting this challenge, a nurse must cultivate a personal moral strength, a sense of caring, and an awareness of his or her central position in the health care team.

✦ Ethical decision-making is a systematic process. Ethical problems, nursing goals, and a range of acceptable options that are consistent with the nurse's personal and professional values can be identified.

Study Questions

1. A central theme of utilitarianism is

   a. respect for the person
   b. people's free will and self-determination
   c. the greatest good for the largest number of people
   d. equal access to health care services

2. Which of the following ethical concepts is *most* consistent with the beliefs of deontology?

   a. autonomy
   b. utility
   c. justice
   d. paternalism

3. Under what condition can the client's autonomy be restricted?

   a. when the client does not understand the English language
   b. when the client's rights clash with the rights of a community
   c. when the nurse knows what is more beneficial to the client
   d. there is no condition under which the client's autonomy can be restricted

4. The *first* step in the ethical decision-making process is

   a. for the nurse to consider his or her own ethical beliefs
   b. to determine the client's decision-making capacity
   c. to gain an overall understanding of the situation
   d. to determine which ethical principles to use

5. The *second* step in the ethical decision making process is

   a. to state the problem in ethical terms
   b. to consult a clinical ethicist
   c. to determine the client's decision-making capacity
   d. to bring the case to the ethics committee

Critical Thinking Exercises

1. A client tells you in a "confidential" psychiatric interview that she is having homicidal thoughts about her husband. What are the ethical and legal implications for the nurse who conducted the interview?

2. You go in to check on a client with acquired immunodeficiency syndrome, and the client is obviously in cardiac arrest. The client is currently a full code status. The nurse who is with you does not want to try to resuscitate the client due to fear of contracting acquired immunodeficiency syndrome. What would be the ethical and legal implications for your actions?

References

American Nurses' Association. (1985). *Code for nurses*. Washington, DC: The American Nurses' Association.

Appelbaum, D., & Lawton, S. V. (1990). *Ethics and the professions*. Englewood Cliffs, NJ: Prentice Hall.

Attfield, R. (1987). *A theory of value and obligation*. New York: Croom Helm.

Benner, P., & Wrubel, J. (1989). *The primacy of caring*. Menlo Park, CA: Addison-Wesley.

Bishop, A. H., & Scudder, J. R. (1987). Nursing ethics in an age of controversy. *Advances in Nursing Science, 9*(3), 34–43.

Breen, N., & Brown, M. L. (1994). The price of mammography in the United States: Data from the national survey of mammography facilities. *The Milbank Quarterly, 72*(3), 431–450.

Brody, J. (1988). Virtues ethics, caring, and nursing. *Scholarly Inquiry for Nursing Practice, 2*(2), 87–96.

Canadian Nurses Association. (1991). *Code of ethics for nursing*. Ottawa, Ontario, Canada: Canadian Nurses Association.

Collopy, B. (1988). Autonomy in long term care: Some crucial distinctions. *Gerontologist, 28* (Suppl.), 10–17.

Cooper, D. (1993). *Value pluralism & ethical choice*. New York: St. Martin's Press.

Dewey, J. (1969). *Outlines of a critical theory of ethics*. New York: Greenwood.

Edge, R. S., & Groves, J. R. (1994). *The ethics of health care: A guide for clinical practice*. Albany, NY: Delmar Publishers.

International Council of Nurses. (1989). *Code for nurses*. Geneva, Switzerland: International Council of Nurses. (Original work published 1972.)

Kant, I. (1948) *Immanuel Kant, groundwork of the metaphysics of morals* (H. J. Paton, Trans.). London: Hutchinson University Library.

Kelly, L. Y., & Joel, L. A. (1995). *Dimensions of professional nursing* (7th ed.). New York: McGraw-Hill.

Kikuchi, J. F. (1996). Multicultural ethics in nursing education: A potential threat to responsible practice. *Journal of Professional Nursing, 12*(3), 159–165.

Morioka, Y. (1991). Informed consent and truth telling to cancer patients. *Gastroenterologia Japonica, 26,* 789–792.

Packard, J. S., & Ferrara, M. (1988). In search of the moral foundation of nursing. *Advances in Nursing Science, 10*(4), 60–71.

Raths, L. S., Simon, S. B., & Harmin, M. (1972). *Values clarification: A handbook of practical strategies for teachers and students*. New York: Hart Publishing.

Sabatino, C. P. (1990). Client-rights regulations and the autonomy of home-care consumers. *Generations, XIV*(Suppl), 21–24.

Simon, S. B., Howe, L. W., & Kirschenbaum, H. (1978). *Values clarification*. New York: A & W Visual Library.

Swanson, K. M. (1993). Nursing as informed caring for the well-being of others. *Image, 25*(4), 352–357.

Takahashi, Y. (1990). Informing a patient of malignant illness: Commentary from a cross-cultural viewpoint. *Death Studies, 14,* 83–91.

Watson, J. (1979). *Nursing: The philosophy and science of caring*. Boston: Little, Brown & Co.

Watson, J. (1985). *Nursing: Human science and human care*. Norwalk, CT: Appleton-Century-Crofts.

Bibliography

Beauchamp, T., & Childress, J. F. (1989). *Principles of biomedical ethics*. New York: Oxford University Press.

Bayer, R. (1988). Toward justice in health care. *American Journal of Public Health, 78,* 583–588.

Bishop, A. H., & Scudder, J. R. (1996). *Nursing ethics: Therapeutic caring presence*. Boston: Jones and Bartlett.

Callahan, D. (1987). *Setting limits: Medical goals in an aging society*. New York: Simon and Schuster.

Carter, M. A. (1993). Ethical framework for care of the chronically ill. *Holistic Nursing Practice, 8*(1), 67–77.

Cooper, M. A. (1991). Principle-oriented ethics and the ethic of care: A creative tension. *Advances in Nursing Science, 14*(2), 22–31.

Dula, A., & Goering, S. (Eds.). (1994). *It just ain't fair: The ethics of health care for African Americans*. New York: Prager Press.

Eliason, M. J. (1993). Ethics and transcultural nursing care. *Nursing Outlook, 41,* 225–228.

Fry, S. T. (1989). The role of caring in a theory of nursing ethics. *Hypatia, 4*(2), 89–103.

Haddad, A. M., & Kapp, M. B. (1991). *Ethical and legal issues in home health care*. Norwalk, CT: Appleton & Lange.

Hall, J. K. (1996). *Nursing ethics and law*. Philadelphia: W. B. Saunders.

Minogue, B. (1996). *Bioethics: A committee approach*. Boston: Jones and Bartlett.

Mohr, W. K. (1996). Ethics, nursing, and health care in the age of "Re-form". *N&HC: Perspectives on Community, 17*(1), 16–21.

Noddings, N. (1984). *Caring: A feminine approach to ethics and moral education*. Berkeley: University of California Press.

Pence, T., & Cantrall, J. (1990). *Ethics in nursing: An anthology*. New York: National League for Nursing.

Chapter 4

LEGAL IMPLICATIONS IN NURSING*

NANCY J. BRENT, RN, MS, JD

KEY TERMS

✦

advance directive	legal liability
criminal law	nurse practice act
law	tort

LEARNING OBJECTIVES

✦

After studying this chapter, you should be able to

✦ Define key legal terms used in the chapter as they relate to nursing practice

✦ Describe the various ways that nursing practice is regulated

✦ Explain the concept of legal liability in nursing practice

✦ Identify proactive solutions to specific areas of potential liability of the nurse that may minimize or eliminate liability for the nurse

✦ Compare and contrast the rights of a nurse as a health care provider with those of the client

The practice of any profession cannot occur in isolation, and nursing is no exception. In fact, many societal factors impinge on the practice of nursing, including ethics, economics, religion, and law. Nursing's relationship with the law is relatively young, however. It was not until the 1940s that the law began to hold nursing legally accountable for the care it provided clients (Brent, 1997). From that time forward, however, the law and nursing practice continued to develop their demanding relationship with each other. Today, there is no question that nursing practice is a profession that is accountable to itself, to those to whom care is provided, and to the law.

This chapter provides the reader with a beginning understanding of the law as it relates to nursing practice. An overview of selected areas of the law encountered in the practice of nursing is presented, including the sources and types of law and the regulation of

nursing practice. Selected legal liability concerns for the nurse also are analyzed. Factors that affect the nurse's legal liability are highlighted. Client rights and the concomitant legal responsibilities of the nurse also are identified.

Sources of Law

The **law** is a system composed of general rules governing conduct and the procedures for resolving disputes when the rules are not followed (Pozgar, 1996, p. 2). Law comes from many different sources. Table 4–1 provides a summary of the sources of law and examples of how those laws affect the nurse and nursing practice.

Table 4–1

SOURCES OF LAW

TYPE OF LAW	ORIGIN	GOVERNS	EXAMPLE
Constitutional	State or Federal constitution	Organization of state and Federal government; limits power of state and Federal government; grants individuals specific rights and responsibilities (*e.g.,* freedom of speech, due process)	State board of nursing (a government agency) cannot discipline a nurse for a violation of the nurse practice act without specific due process protections (*e.g.,* notice of charges)
Statutory	State or Federal legislative bodies (*e.g.,* state assembly, Congress)	Passage of state and Federal laws, respectively, that affect entire nation or entire state (Federal laws supersede state laws if the two conflict)	State child abuse and neglect laws mandate a nurse to report suspected abuse and neglect to an identified state agency; Federal Americans With Disabilities Act prohibits employers from discriminating against qualified employees with disabilities
Administrative	State and Federal agencies through specific hearings and rule-making procedures	Decisions and rules concerning the particular state or Federal statute the agency is responsible for administering and enforcing	State Department of Public Health sets requirements for reporting of communicable diseases; Federal Department of Health and Human Services decides (after a hearing) that a state did not properly adhere to Medicare requirements
Judicial (also called "decisional")	State or Federal court decisions	Interpretation of all of the laws mentioned here and resolution of disputes among parties (*e.g.,* two individuals, an individual and a hospital) using past case decisions as a guide ("precedent")	State court opinion holds a particular provision of a state statute unconstitutional; Federal court decision supports a breach of contract by hospital

Data from Black, H. C. (1991). *Black's law dictionary* (6th ed.). St. Paul, MN: West Publishing Company.

Table 4–2

TYPES OF LAW

CATEGORY NAME	PURPOSE OF LAW	EXAMPLE
Private law	Controls relationships between private individuals and private organizations	Torts (*e.g.,* professional negligence where a client sues a hospital and a nurse for a client care injury); contracts (*e.g.,* nurse has an employment contract with a home health care agency)
Public law	Regulates relationships between the government and its agencies and the individual	Criminal law (*e.g.,* nurse charged with the crime of illegal possession of a controlled substance); administrative law (nurse is disciplined by state board of nursing due to violation of nurse practice act and registered nurse license placed on probation)
Common law	Recognizes, affirms and enforces rules and customs of society through judicial decisions	Right of privacy (*e.g.,* state court holds that a nurse invades the privacy of a client when sharing information about the client's diagnosis at client's neighborhood picnic); foreign relations issues (Federal courts)
Civil law	Regulates disputes between individuals and/or individuals and groups by providing money (*e.g.,* for damages or as compensation) when injury is caused by another	Nurse sues a physician for defamation of character when the physician calls her incompetent in front of coworkers, and jury awards a verdict of 1 million dollars in favor of nurse
Criminal law	Protects society by defining criminal behavior and punishing those whose conduct violates established rules (*e.g.,* fine, imprisonment, death); crimes are defined as a misdemeanor (less serious) or a felony (more serious)	Nurse who abuses elderly patient is charged with crime of aggravated battery of a senior citizen, found guilty, and sentenced to 2 y in prison (a felony)
Substantive law	Creates, defines, and regulates rights and responsibilities of parties in civil, criminal, and administrative law	State criminal law defines the offense of aggravated battery of a senior citizen
Procedural law	Sets requirements for specific manner of proceeding when specific substantive law is violated	State criminal procedure establishes arrest and trial requirements when individual is charged with a crime

Data from Black, H. C. (1991). *Black's law dictionary* (6th ed.). St. Paul, MN: West Publishing Company; Brent, N. J. (1997). *Nurses and the law: A guide to principles and applications.* Philadelphia: W. B. Saunders; Guido, G. W. (1997). *Legal issues in nursing* (2nd ed.). Stanford, CT: Appleton & Lange.

Types of Laws

The sources of law are further categorized into particular groups or types of laws. All of the types of law also influence nursing practice. Table 4–2 summarizes the types of laws and provides examples of their existence in nursing.

It is important for the reader to note that the categories of laws listed in Table 4–2 are not necessarily mutually exclusive. For example, the criminal law is an example of public law. Separating the types and examples is helpful in providing an organization to the many separate, yet often overlapping, examples of laws.

Regulation of Nursing Practice

Nurse Practice Acts

Every state in the United States has the ability to exercise its "police powers." Among other things, a state's police power is used to ensure that its citizens receive nursing care from competent registered nurses or licensed practical (or vocational) nurses. As a result, every state legislature has passed practice acts that regulate the practice of health care providers in that particular state. These practice acts include, among other requirements, the necessity of nurses, physicians, dentists, and other health care providers to be licensed in that state before they can practice their profession (Inglis & Kjervik, 1993).

Nurse practice acts are administered and enforced by a governmental body or agency, that power having been delegated by the state legislature to the agency. For nurse practice acts, a board of nursing (or similar title) ensures compliance with the nurse practice act and its rules and regulations.

Nurse practice acts vary from state to state, because each state has the power to define what nursing practice is in that particular state, as well as the other specific provisions in the act. Even so, some common provisions seen in nurse practice acts include (1) a definition of the scope of nursing practice; (2) the regulation of educational programs of nursing in the state; (3) rights of the nurse licensee if a disciplinary action is taken against the nurse; and (4) the licensure requirements one must meet before being able to obtain a license to practice nursing in that state (American Nurses Association, 1990).

Licensure

A license grants the owner the permission to carry out a particular business, to exercise an identified privilege, or to practice a particular trade or profession (Black, 1991). When granted by a governmental agency, like a board of nursing, the license indicates to the public that the licensee has gone through the licensure process established by the agency and has met minimal competency standards to ensure the public's health, safety, and welfare (Reaves, 1993).

Although the licensure process for nursing practice may again vary from state to state, most states require that certain educational requirements (*e.g.,* graduation from an accredited nursing education program) be met and that the nurse successfully pass the National Council Licensure Examination (NCLEX™) for registered nurses or for practical nurses.

It is important to note that all states in the United States require individuals who practice as a registered nurse or a licensed practical nurse to be licensed in the state ("mandatory licensure"). However, there are some limited exceptions to that requirement. For example, nursing students enrolled in a bona fide, accredited nursing education program need not be licensed to practice nursing during the time they are going through their educational program. As long as the students' practice of nursing is part of the clinical and academic requirements of their education and the students are supervised and guided by the nursing faculty in that program while practicing nursing, a license is not required. On completion of the program, the graduate nurse would be required to obtain his or her license to practice nursing.

Registration

In the early 1900s, nurse practice acts were "permissive," meaning that if one wanted to practice nursing, the only requirement to do so was to "register" with the state agency administering and enforcing nursing. If an individual did register, he or she could use the initials "R.N." after his or her name. If a person decided not to register with the state agency, the person could still practice nursing, but could not use the title "R.N." (Springhouse Corporation, 1992).

Because all states in the United States now require a license to practice nursing, registration is not an option for a person *legally* to practice nursing or practical nursing. As a result, registration does not have the same meaning that it did in the early 1900s. Today, *registration* or *registered* is often defined as being equivalent to the term *licensure* or *license* in many nurse practice acts (Illinois Nursing Act of 1987).

Credentialing

Credentials are defined as the documentary evidence of an individual's authority, most often appearing in the form of letters, licenses, or certificates (Black, 1991). A registered nurse who has graduated from a baccalaureate program in nursing and passed the NCLEX would have the following credentials:

Mary J. Smith, B.S.N., R.N.

Because credentials entitle a person to assert authority and, in the case of nursing, to practice nursing *legally*, most nurse practice acts contain provisions that prohibit the use of credentials that are regulated specifically by the act (*e.g.,* "Registered Nurse," "Licensed Practical Nurse"). If an individual uses any credential governed by the act that he or she does not have, he or she can be charged with a crime (usually a misdemeanor) and, if found guilty, he or she can be punished in accordance with the state's criminal laws.

Certification

Certification is a formal process conducted by a private professional or trade organization that recognizes exceptional competence in a particular area of practice (Reaves, 1993; Redd & Alexander, 1997). In 1992, an estimated 225,000 registered nurses in the United States were certified, representing at least 35 different nursing specialties (Redd & Alexander, 1997).

In nursing, the certification process requires the registered nurse to meet certain educational, experiential, and clinical practice prerequisites. For example, the American Nurses' Credentialing Center, requires that specific criteria in clinical practice be met, as well as additional education beyond one's basic nursing educational program, before a registered nurse can sit for its many certification examinations (American Nurses' Credentialing Center, 1995). Beginning in 1998, the American Nurses Association (ANA) would require a bachelor's degree in nursing for any candidate sitting for the generalist certification examination. If the previously mentioned Mary Smith successfully obtained certification in the specialty of rehabilitation nursing, she would have the following credentials:

Mary J. Smith, B.S.N., C.R.R.N.

It is important to note that certification implies but does not guarantee competence and expertise over and above the criteria required for licensure. Even so, the decision to become certified is a voluntary one. However, some nurse practice acts *require* certification by a recognized national certifying body before a registered nurse can obtain a license for, or simply practice, that nursing specialty. Advanced nurse practitioners—including nurse anesthetists, nurse midwives, nurse practitioners, and clinical nurse specialists—are required in many states to obtain certification in their specific area of practice as a condition of licensure.

Accreditation

The process of rating educational programs in nursing is vital to ensure that graduates of nursing programs are adequately prepared to provide competent nursing care to the public. In addition, graduation from an accredited nursing educational program is an almost certain way of meeting a state's nurse practice act requirement of graduation from an "approved" program of nursing education to sit for the licensure examination or obtain a license to practice nursing in that state through endorsement or reciprocity. Even so, there is no legal requirement that a nursing education program be accredited. Moreover, accreditation is a voluntary process.

The accreditation of nursing educational programs is done through private organizations. Since 1952, the National League for Nursing (NLN) has been one of the leaders in this process in the United States. Although the NLN continues to accredit nursing programs, there is speculation that other private professional groups, such as the American Association of Colleges of Nursing, are developing an accreditation process to fill the continuing need for accreditation of nursing education programs.

Implications for the Registered Nurse

Because the potential for liability exists for the nurse if he or she does not practice in accordance with the state nursing practice act and its rules and regulations, it is important for the registered nurse to be familiar with the nursing practice act in his or her state. This familiarity must begin with the specifics concerning initial licensure and extend to all areas of the act, especially in view of the registered nurse's specific area of practice. Moreover, the registered nurse needs to be familiar with the reasons he or she may be disciplined for alleged violations of the act (*e.g.,* breach of nurse-client confidentiality, unprofes-

sional conduct) and the concomitant rights provided to the registered nurse during any disciplinary action by the board of nursing or other regulatory agency (*e.g.,* right to an attorney, right to notice of the allegations). Because the board or state agency is an arm of the state, specific state and Federal constitutional protections are required to be afforded to the registered nurse who faces a disciplinary action by the regulatory authority.

Familiarity with the other regulatory processes that impinge on nursing practice is also essential for the registered nurse. Credentialing, certification, and accreditation, whether mandatory or voluntary, all impact on nursing practice in various ways. For example, if a nurse working in rehabilitation nursing does not possess certification as a rehabilitation nurse and is sued for professional negligence, the lack of certification will most probably be raised by the plaintiff at trial. If the lack of certification as a rehabilitation nurse sways the jury so significantly that a verdict is returned against the nurse, the need for certification, even if a voluntary process, becomes clear. The registered nurse must be ever vigilant in assessing the respective effects of these regulatory processes on nursing practice from a legal and professional perspective.

Legal Liability for Nurses

Legal liability can be defined as an obligation one is bound in law or justice to perform. When the obligation is not performed or is performed in an unacceptable manner, a court or other tribunal can enforce liability between the parties (Black, 1991). As presented in Tables 4–1 and 4–2, a registered nurse's liability can be based in many sources of laws and in many types of laws. Several areas of liability for the nurse are discussed.

Criminal Law

Criminal law is composed of state and Federal statutes that define criminal offenses and corresponding fines and/or punishment (Black, 1991). Under the **criminal law,** a nurse may be charged with a crime that is a felony, the most serious type of crime. If found guilty of a felony, the criminal is usually sentenced to death or to more than 1 year in state prison (Black, 1991). Felonies may also be classified by class (*e.g.,* A, B) or by degree (*e.g.,* first, second) with varying sentences. Examples of felonies include murder and possession of a controlled substance.

In contrast, a misdemeanor is a crime that carries a sentence of less than 1 year of imprisonment in a local jail or a fine (LaFave & Scott, 1986). Misdemeanors may also be classified by class or by degree. Examples of misdemeanors include reckless conduct and practicing a licensed profession without a valid license.

Because criminal laws exist to protect society, when an alleged violation of criminal law occurs, it is the state, through its state attorney general or local attorney general, that brings the action against the individual defendant or defendants. *Intent* to carry out the felony or misdemeanor is an essential element of every crime that must be proven by the state. In addition, the state must prove its case "beyond a reasonable doubt" (LaFave & Scott, 1986).

Although the registered nurse can face liability for alleged violations of the criminal law, a more common area of potential liability for the nurse is in tort law.

Tort

A **tort** is a civil wrong, other than a breach of contract, in which the law provides a remedy by allowing an injured person to seek damages from the person whose conduct caused the injury (Keeton, 1984). Two types of torts of importance to the registered nurse are negligence and professional negligence/malpractice.

Negligence

Negligence is defined as "conduct which falls below the standard established by law for the protection of others against unreasonable risk of harm" (Keeton, 1984, p. 7). The risk of harm in negligence also includes the forseeability of the risk of harm. In other words, the injury that occurs when a person is negligent is an injury that could be anticipated by the defendant (the person causing the harm) because at the time of injury, a reasonable likelihood existed that it could take place (Keeton, 1984).

The conduct of the defendant is measured by an objective standard called the "ordinary, reasonable and prudent person" standard (of care). When a jury must decide if a defendant has been negligent, it measures the defendant's conduct with this standard of care by determining if the conduct was what an ordinary, reasonable, and prudent person would have done in the same or similar circumstances. If the jury decides the defendant's conduct was in conformity with this standard, they return a verdict in favor of the defendant. If, however, the defendant's conduct did not conform to this standard, then a verdict is returned against the defendant and in favor of the plaintiff (the person who brings the suit).

In any negligence action, there are four essential elements that must be met by the plaintiff to prove that the defendant was negligent (Keeton, 1984):

1. Duty—At the time of the injury, a duty existed between the plaintiff and the defendant
2. Breach of duty—The defendant breached his or her duty (of care) to the plaintiff
3. Causation—The breach of the duty was the proximate cause (or legal cause) of injury to the plaintiff

4. Injury—The plaintiff experienced injury, damages, or both that are recognized by law and can be compensated for by law

Negligent conduct can include acts of commission as well as acts of omission. For example, a mechanic may repair car brakes in a negligent manner that, when the driver cannot stop the car, causes an accident and injuries to the driver. Alternatively, the mechanic may fail to make necessary repairs on car brakes after the driver brings the car in for an inspection, resulting in a subsequent accident and injuries to the driver.

Unlike violations of the criminal law, the negligent defendant does not *intend* or *want* to cause the injury or damages sustained by the victim. Rather, the person causing the injury or damages has failed to meet his or her duty to identify and avoid forseeable and unreasonable risks of harm to which he or she has exposed another.

It is important to keep in mind that the concept of individual or personal liability requires that each individual is responsible for his or her own behavior, including his or her negligent behavior. For example, it would be unsuccessful for the mechanic who repaired the car brakes in a negligent manner to try to defend his actions by stating that his boss told him to repair the brakes negligently.

Professional Negligence/Malpractice

Professional negligence involves the actions of professionals, including registered nurses, that fall below the standard of care for the specific professional group. The standard has generally been referred to as including "a standard minimum of special knowledge and ability" (Keeton, 1984, p. 185).

Because professionals are individuals with education, training, skill, and expertise that nonprofessionals do not possess, people who seek their professional advice or services rely on that advice when making whatever decisions they are faced with and expect the services to be provided in a nonnegligent manner.

Clients and their families rely on the registered nurse to provide nonnegligent care and other professional services. When a client suffers an injury or damages, the nurse's conduct is compared with that of other ordinary, reasonable and prudent *professional nurses* in the same or similar situations in the same or a similar community. It is important to note that the "same or a similar community" portion of the nurse's standard is not exactly as it sounds.

Rather than the nurse's conduct being compared with that of other nurses in the same geographic community where the nurse practices, the "community" for comparing the nurse's conduct has become a national one. The ease with which information can be shared throughout the United States—indeed the world—and the technological advances in health care and the use of national (now computerized) licensing examinations are all factors that no longer justify a true local community standard for evaluating an allegedly negligent nurse's conduct.

The standard of conduct of the registered nurse involved in a lawsuit is established through the use of an expert witness. Both the registered nurse (the defendant) and the injured client (the plaintiff) use their own expert witness. The role of the expert witness in the trial process is to educate the jury as to the applicable duty of the nurse in the situation in which the client was injured so that the jury can decide whether the nurse's conduct conformed to that standard.

Because the standard of conduct is a national one, the expert witness for both of the parties to the suit can be from the same city or state where the nurse practices, or the expert witness can be from another state. In either case, after the expert witness has testified, the jury must decide if the nurse defendant was professionally negligent or if his or her conduct met the standard required in the situation.

Intentional and Quasi-Intentional Torts

Unlike negligence and professional negligence, the intentional and quasi-intentional torts have as an essential element the requirement that the injury suffered by the victim was "intended" by the wrongdoer. *Intent* means either that the wrongdoer had a specific plan to cause a specific outcome that unlawfully affects the rights of another (for *intentional torts*) (Keeton, 1984, p. 34; Restatement of Torts, 1997) or that a person voluntarily caused another person's right to be adversely affected (for *quasi-intentional torts*) (Brent, 1997).

✦ **Assault and Battery.** An assault occurs when a person puts another person in fear of a harmful or an offensive contact (Keeton, 1984). For this intentional tort to be actionable (*i.e.,* able to be brought to court), the victim must be aware of the threat of harmful or offensive contact. For example, if a nurse in an emergency department comes toward a client with leather restraints and threatens to place the client in those restraints immediately, an allegation of assault against the nurse by the client may be possible.

A battery, in contrast, is defined as an unpermitted, actual contact with one's body, an extension of one's body (*e.g.,* a shirt), or anything attached to it (*e.g.,* a purse) (Keeton, 1984). With this intentional tort, the person who experiences the unpermitted contact *need not* be aware that the unpermitted touching has taken place. A common example of a battery in health care is when a surgical procedure is performed on an anesthetized client without his or her consent. However, a battery can also occur during the delivery of client care, as illustrated in Figure 4–1.

As the definitions of assault and battery illustrate, several ways for the nurse to avoid allegations of assault and battery include never threatening a client, obtaining the consent of the client before nursing pro-

Battery

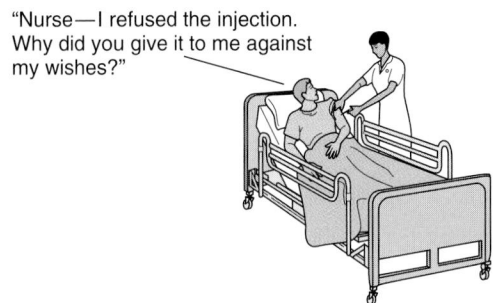

"Nurse—I refused the injection. Why did you give it to me against my wishes?"

✦ **Figure 4–1**
An example of the intentional tort of battery.

cedures are undertaken, and never forcing treatment on a client.

✦ **Invasion of Privacy.** This quasi-intentional tort takes place when an individual's private affairs are unreasonably intruded into by the defendant (Keeton, 1984). Invasion of privacy can take many forms, but two of interest to the nurse include using someone's picture or name for one's own commercial advantage without the person's consent and unreasonably intruding into a person's private and personal affairs or matters.

An example of the first type of invasion of privacy action might be when a health care facility or its nursing staff takes pictures of clients in a new wing of the facility. The pictures taken of the clients are full face, front shots (not photographs in which the clients have their backs to the camera). The facility does not obtain the consent of the clients to take the photographs or to use the photographs to promote business for the new wing. In such a circumstance, any clients who can be identified in the photographs can sue the facility for an invasion of privacy.

An example of the second type of invasion of privacy action might be when a client's care is observed by others, including nursing and medical students, without the client's consent or when photographs of the client are shown at a scientific meeting without his or her consent to use the photographs for that purpose.

A good way to avoid any liability for an invasion of privacy suit filed by a client is to always obtain the informed consent of the client for any photographs taken, especially when the client can be readily identified in the photograph, and for any observers who will be watching care being provided to the client. Consent for observers can be easily accomplished by telling the client that observers will be present and then asking if that is agreeable. If the client agrees, consent has been obtained. If, in contrast, the client does not want observers present, then they should not be allowed to watch any client care procedure, as the client has refused his or her consent for the observation.

❧ **False Imprisonment.** This intentional tort happens when an individual's freedom of movement is unlawfully restricted, regardless of the length of time that restriction exists (Keeton, 1984). In addition, the person who is falsely imprisoned must be aware of the confinement and have no means of escaping from the confinement, whether because of a physical barrier (*e.g.,* a locked door) or by force (*e.g.,* a security officer standing at an open door out of the room) (Keeton, 1984).

False imprisonment in health care can take place whenever a client is not allowed to leave a health care facility when there is no *legal* justification to detain the person (*e.g.,* an against medical advice discharge, when a client refuses care and is competent to make that decision). It can also occur when a posey belt, leather restraints, or other restraining devices are used on clients without a clinical need to do so, as illustrated in Figure 4–2.

Avoiding liability for false imprisonment requires that nursing staff restrict a client's freedom of movement only when there is a legal and clinical reason to do so; *e.g.,* a client attempts to injure himself or herself after abusing drugs. Careful documentation of the need for the restriction is necessary, as is contacting the physician and others included in the facility's policies and procedures.

The nurse should also remember that if a client gives consent for a restriction of his or her freedom to move about (*e.g.,* when a psychiatric client feels he or she may lose control and asks to be restrained or secluded until he or she regains control of his or her behavior), there can be no liability for false imprisonment. However, the nurse should carefully document these circumstances in the medical record to avoid a later allegation by the client that cannot be defended.

❧ **Defamation.** The quasi-intentional tort of defamation takes place when something *untrue* is said (slander) or written (libel) about a person, resulting in injury to that person's good name and reputation (Keeton, 1984). For example, a nurse may make a defamatory statement about a client by telling individuals in the community that the client has a diagnosis

of acquired immunodeficiency syndrome (AIDS) when that diagnosis is not true (*Wyatt v. St. Paul Fire & Marine Insurance Company,* 1994). Alternatively, a nurse may be defamed when a physician falsely accuses him or her of being incompetent in front of clients and visitors.

A defense against allegations of defamation is truth. In the two examples given here, if it were true that the client's diagnosis was AIDS and it were true that the nurse was incompetent, no liability for defamation (slander) would be possible. Other defenses include consent of the person to speak or write about the otherwise defamatory information, and privilege. *Privilege* means that even though information about a person might be defamatory if shared with another, in some instances the law protects the person sharing that information if in fact he or she is required to do so. In the case *Judge v. Rockford Memorial Hospital* (1958), the appeals court found no defamation of a nurse when a director of nursing at the nurse's place of employment responded to a request by a prospective employer for a written reference. The director of nursing's letter stated that she would not hire the nurse again because of a concern about narcotics loss whenever the nurse worked a shift at the hospital. The court held that the director of nursing had a legal duty to inform the prospective employer of this information. Because the information was privileged, no liability for defamation could be found.

Legal Boundaries, Legal Concepts, and Nursing Safeguards in Nursing Practice

In addition to the laws that regulate nursing practice and govern liability, other factors impinge on a registered nurse when delivering care to clients. These factors include where and how the nurse provides nursing care.

Employee Guidelines

Most registered nurses work as employees in a particular hospital, home health care facility, or clinic. As a result, the nurse must understand that another theory of liability—*respondeat superior*—is important to keep in mind when providing nursing care within an employer-employee relationship.

Respondeat Superior

Respondeat superior is a Latin term meaning "let the master answer" (Black, 1991). Simply put, this legal doctrine states that an employer will be held vicariously (indirectly) liable for any negligent acts of an employee if the alleged negligent act occurred dur-

False imprisonment

"Mr. X—I am going to restrain you so that you can't leave."

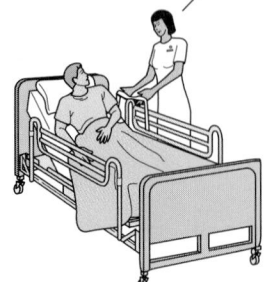

❧ **Figure 4–2**
An example of the intentional tort of false imprisonment.

ing the employment relationship and was within the scope of the employee's responsibilities. In health care, the ramification of this doctrine is that the employer (*e.g.,* a hospital) can be sued for the alleged professional negligence of a nurse employee in addition to the nurse employee being sued. In most instances, under this doctrine, the registered nurse's potential liability for a client injury may also be that of his or her employer.

If the registered nurse practices nursing in accordance with the client care policies and procedures established by the employer, functions within his or her job description and job responsibilities, and provides care consistent with standards of care in a nonnegligent manner, the potential for liability for both the nurse and the employer can be minimized. However, all client injuries cannot be avoided. If an injury does occur and the client sues the nurse and his or her employer under a negligence theory for that injury, the employer and the nurse employee can vigorously defend the suit, knowing that the nurse adhered to the legal requirements affecting the provision of client care.

Standards of Care

Adherence to standards of care by the registered nurse is an essential part of providing nonnegligent client care. If the nurse cares for a client as other ordinarily reasonable nurses would in the same or similar circumstances, the nurse is clearly meeting the standard of care in that situation.

Knowledge of what the standards of care are in a particular client care situation is easy to obtain. Professional associations, such as the ANA, the American Association of Operating Room Nurses, and the American Association of Critical Care Nurses all publish standards of care for those respective specialty areas in nursing. Additional information concerning standards of care can be obtained through continuing education programs, reading journal articles, and participating in regular updates on new practice issues and techniques.

Nursing Competence

Nursing competence can be defined as possessing the suitable skill, knowledge, and experience necessary to provide adequate nursing care. The requirement of nursing competence includes the mandate that the nurse not only know what his or her abilities to perform nursing care are but also identify areas in which skill, knowledge, and experience are not present. Unfortunately, liability for a client injury often occurs because the registered nurse does not possess the required skill, knowledge, and experience to provide nonnegligent care. Table 4–3 lists some of the common injuries suffered by clients and what nursing competencies are required to avoid those injuries (see also Fig. 4–3).

Table 4–3

COMMON CLIENT INJURIES INVOLVING NURSES

SITUATION	NURSING COMPETENCIES REQUIRED	HOW LIABILITY MAY BE AVOIDED
Client falls out of bed, breaking hip	Assessment of client's mental and physical status, knowledge of policies and procedures concerning client restraint; assessment of client's safety needs; knowledge of client's diagnosis and medications	Side rails of bed up; call button within reach of client; frequent monitoring of client; obtain order for posey belt or other restraint if clinically necessary
Nurse administers wrong medication to client	Knowledge of and experience in proper medication administration; knowledge of specific medication administered to client	Adherence to proper medication administration requirements; listening to client comments concerning medication (*e.g.,* "This doesn't look like my usual pill")
Nurse is working on unit that is understaffed, and client is not monitored as ordered	Knowledge of client care requirements; understanding of client-nurse ratios; assessment of safety issues presented by understaffing; knowledge of policies for reporting client care issues in facility	Identify problems with understaffing as soon as possible; contact immediate nurse manager for help in resolving problem; reassign client care duties to cover care until resolution occurs
Physician order is unclear, resulting in client receiving wrong treatment	Knowledge of client diagnosis and usual treatment modalities; knowledge of policies and procedures for clarifying unclear orders; knowledge of how orders are to be written in facility	Obtain clarification from physician before treatment instituted; seek help from nurse manager if clarification does not occur

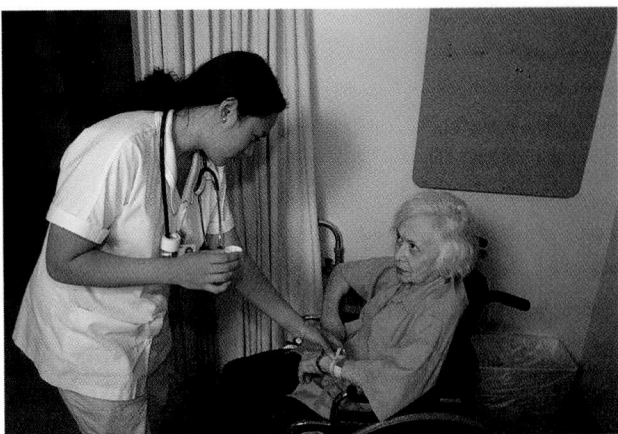

◆ Figure 4–3
Nurse checking client's wristband before administering medication.

Physician Orders

Physician orders are an essential part of nursing practice. The physician is responsible for the medical care and treatment of the client. When a physician determines that a client needs a particular medication, treatment, or surgery, those needs are written in the client's medical record as orders. The nurse is responsible for carrying out the orders of the physician in a timely and nonnegligent manner.

If, however, the nurse determines that an order is unclear, that the order may harm a client (*e.g.,* the physician orders a medication to which the client is allergic), or the order is otherwise of concern to the nurse, he or she must immediately clarify the order with the physician who wrote it (Fig. 4–4). If there is no resolution to the nurse's questions about the order (either because the physician cannot be located or because after talking with the physician, the order remains as it was written), the nurse should then contact the nurse manager for further clarification as to what the next step should be. Under no circumstances should the nurse proceed to carry out the order until clarification is obtained, unless, of course, the client may be forseeably harmed by the delay. For example, in a code situation, the importance of quick intervention to attempt to save the client's life is the first priority.

Most often, the resolution of the nurse's concerns about a physician order can be obtained with the help of the nursing administration. It may be that a call from the nurse manager will resolve the uncertainty. Or, the nurse manager may need to contact his or her nurse manager so that a resolution can be worked out with the physician's immediate superior. It is clear that although others may also be held liable for an incorrect order that results in harm to a client, the nurse surely can be held responsible for carrying out an order that would have been questioned by other reasonably prudent nurses in the same or similar circumstances.

Documentation of Care

The documentation of client care is legally required by a number of sources, including accrediting agencies, state licensing laws for health care delivery systems, and state nurse and medical practice acts. Requirements for medical record contents include the client's medical history, reports of diagnostic and other laboratory results, client or family teaching, and client care (Roach & The Aspen Law Center, 1994).

The accurate and complete documentation of quality nonnegligent client care can be the nurse's "best defense" against allegations of professional negligence. On the other hand, if the documentation of client care contains errors, reflects a nonadherence to standards of care, or is nonexistent, the documentation can be used to attempt to prove that negligent nursing care was provided (Brent, 1997). Although it is not a complete list of documentation guidelines, Box 4–1 includes many helpful rules for the nurse when documenting the client care record.

Computerized documentation in some form in health care delivery is becoming more and more common. The nurse who uses the computer to document client care must be familiar with the facility's policies and procedures concerning the proper procedures to follow when documenting in the electronic medical record (EMR) (Fig. 4–5). Additional guidelines that must be followed when using the EMR include

• Using only the user identification code, name, or password given to the nurse when documenting in the EMR
• Never lending the access identifier to another nurse
• Using the correct client code when documenting his or her care
• Maintaining the privacy and confidentiality of documented information printed from the computer

Client Teaching

Client and family teaching is an inherent role of the nurse. Instructions to the client or his or her family

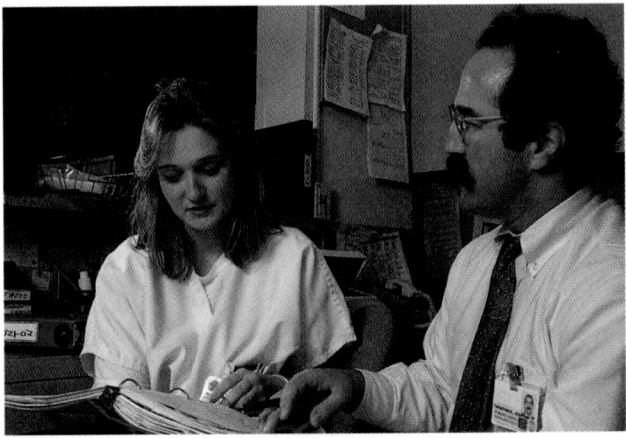

◆ Figure 4–4
Nurse clarifies unclear order with physician.

Box 4–1

DOCUMENTATION PRINCIPLES FOR THE NURSE

Document care given, medication administered, and treatments done as soon as possible after completion

Entries should be objective, factual, and complete

Date and time every entry following facility policies and procedures

Do not leave any blank spaces in narrative charting, on flow sheets, or on check lists

Document any calls made to others on the health care team (*e.g.*, physician, supervisor), including time called, information shared, and instructions or changes in orders given

Document any client care interventions and the client's response to those interventions (*e.g.*, "Client stated he was in less pain after receiving the medication ordered")

Sign name and title after each entry and use initials only pursuant to facility policies (*e.g.*, on the medication administration record)

When a documentation error is made in the client record, follow facility policies carefully in correcting the error (*e.g.*, drawing one line through the error, initialing and dating the line, and then providing the correct information)

Consent for or refusal of treatment must be documented following facility policies and procedures

Client and family teaching should be documented, including what was taught, how the client's understanding of the information was evaluated, and who was present during the teaching

The use of correct spelling, punctuation, and grammar is essential

Any additions to the client record (*e.g.*, a late entry or additional information not remembered at the initial time of documentation) should be done pursuant to facility policy (*e.g.*, marked as "Late entry" and dated at the time of documentation)

Data from Roach, W. & The Aspen Law Center (1994). *Medical Records and the Law,* (2nd ed.). Gaithersburg, MD: Aspen Publishers; and Brent, N.J. (1997). *Nurses and the Law: A Guide to Principles and Applications.* Philadelphia: W.B. Saunders.

and/or the family what could happen if the client did *not* follow the information shared during the process of teaching. In *LeBlanc v. Northern Colfax County Hospital* (1983), a nurse in the emergency department did not tell the client that if pain did not subside, it might mean that he was bleeding internally and he might die if he did not return for help. The client did die after delaying his return for several days. The family filed a suit against the hospital, alleging that the client care instructions given to Mr. LeBlanc by the nurse were inadequate. The trial court dismissed the case, but the appeals court reversed the decision and remanded (returned) the case back to the trial court.

Client Confidentiality

Confidentiality is defined as including a special relationship between two persons (*e.g.*, nurse and client) in which information shared between those two persons will not be shared with a third party who is not directly involved in the client's care (Annas, 1992). In addition, confidentiality includes the concept of testimonial privilege; that is, the person receiving information within a confidential relationship is not legally able to disclose the information in a court or other judicial proceeding without the consent of the individual who shared it (Annas, 1992).

Confidentiality is an important right of all clients. Nurses are bound to protect client confidentiality by most nurse practice acts, by ethical principles and standards (*e.g.*, The Code For Nurses), and by institutional and agency policies and procedures. However, some clients are provided with additional confidentiality protections. Those receiving treatment for mental illness, drug and alcohol use, and sexual assault are examples of some clients who are further protected through state and Federal statutes governing the release of specific treatment information and treatment records.

Regardless of the type of client that the nurse is caring for, he or she must maintain the confidentiality

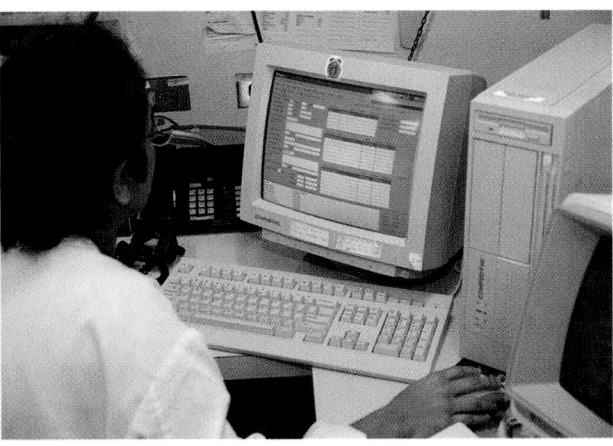

✦ **Figure 4–5**
Nurse enters client care information into EMR.

may take place as the client is nearing discharge from the facility, in the client's home, or during a clinic visit. Regardless of the setting in which the teaching takes place, the nurse doing the instruction must ensure that it is done completely, in a language the client or family can understand (*e.g.*, not "medicalese," in the primary language of the client), and that the nurse can document his or her assessment of the client's understanding of the subject matter presented.

Moreover, the nurse must share with the client

of the client and the client's treatment record. The nurse must not talk about clients in public areas of the health care facility or agency. Revealing a diagnosis to a third party, which occurred in the *Wyatt* case discussed earlier in this chapter, is also a breach of client confidentiality. Treatment records should not be released to any third party without the client's written consent and only after the facility or agency's policies and procedures on release of client information are complied with. If the nurse works in a facility or agency that uses the Electronic Medical Record (EMR), he or she must be certain that any printouts concerning client information are carefully discarded to avoid a breach of confidentiality if those discarded pages may be read by someone not entitled to the information. Any testimony given by a nurse in a judicial or administrative proceeding should be done only after the nurse consults with the attorney for the facility and/or an attorney of the nurse's choice.

Risk Management

The process of risk management involves "identifying, evaluating and minimizing" the potential liability that inherently exists in providing health care (University Hospital Consortium, 1992, p. 3). Once the potential liabilities are identified and evaluated, an affirmative, proactive plan can be put into place to reduce or eliminate the liability that might result if the risk is ignored.

The specific risk management plan identified depends on the risk identified (*e.g.,* injuries to clients in the operating room, injuries to visitors). Regardless of the particular potential liability involved, risk management solutions—including education of nursing and other staff, monitoring of the identified risk(s), better identification of similar risks, and, along with quality assurance, suggestions of how to improve client care—are then evaluated to ensure that the plan has indeed minimized or eliminated the identified liability.

In a health care facility, risk management may be carried out by a risk management department (in a large facility) or by one risk manager. Depending on the size of the risk management department, additional responsibilities might include purchasing liability insurance for the hospital and the health care providers and managing liability claims (University Hospital Consortium, 1992).

Nurses play an important role in helping the risk manager or risk management department manage liability claims by providing vital information concerning difficulties experienced in the provision of nursing care that may give rise to liability. They provide this information to the risk manager through the use of incident or occurrence reports.

Incidence Reports

Incident or occurrence reports request information from nursing staff and others involved in the client care situation that is identified as potentially causing liability for the facility and/or staff. Some of the more common information requested on the incident or occurrence form includes data concerning the client (*e.g.,* name, age, diagnosis), a factual description of the incident, any injuries experienced by those involved, and the outcome of the situation (West *et al.,* 1994).

A successful risk management program requires that good policies and procedures be in place for the nurse to refer to when he or she needs to notify the risk manager of a potential risk. The policy should include, among other things, that (1) the incident or occurrence reports are confidential and privileged information and should not be copied, placed in the chart, or have any reference made to them in the client's record; (2) they must be filled out completely, accurately, and factually; (3) the reports should not be used as a way to punish staff for their conduct but rather as a means of identifying and improving client care; (4) the incident report is *not* a substitute for a complete entry in the client's record concerning the incident; and (5) specific documentation guidelines—like those for documenting in the client's record—should be followed when filling out an incident or occurrence report.

Professional Liability Insurance

Professional liability insurance is usually purchased by the nurse or his or her employer to provide coverage for specific professional activities listed in the insurance policy. For example, if a client is allegedly injured due to a nurse's negligent care and the provision of client care is an example of the kind of professional activity covered in the policy, the insurance company will represent (defend) the nurse in a suit filed by the client.

The policy of insurance is a contract between the insured (*e.g.,* the nurse) and the insurer (*e.g.,* the company offering the insurance protection). As a result, it is important that the nurse be knowledgable about the coverage he or she has under the insurance contract. Information such as the amount of coverage provided, the nurse's obligations under the contact of insurance (*e.g.,* notification of insurance company when suit is filed, cooperation with insurance company), and any professional activities *not* covered in the policy (*e.g.,* criminal allegations) are just a few of the areas that must be carefully evaluated by the nurse.

Careful evaluation of these and other issues concerning professional liability insurance is also important for the student nurse to undertake at the onset of his or her educational program in nursing.

Contracts

A contract is a voluntary agreement (written or oral, express or implied) between at least two persons that creates an obligation to do or not do something and that creates enforceable rights or legal duties (Black, 1991). Contracts affect many areas of nursing practice. The previous discussion of professional liability insurance is one example of how a contract delineates the respective rights and responsibilities of the nurse and the insurer. Likewise, the nurse employee-employer relationship is governed by established employee handbooks and client care policies and procedures that create obligations, rights, and duties between those two parties.

When a nurse undertakes the care of a client, whether in a hospital or in the client's home, a contractual relationship is formed. Among other things, the nurse agrees to provide competent nursing care in a legally and ethically acceptable manner, and the client agrees to accept that care, follow the nursing regimen recommended, and to pay for the services rendered.

Contracts also regulate the nurse-client relationship when special types of contracts, such as advance directives (*e.g.,* living wills) are executed by clients that reflect their decisions concerning care. These types of contracts and the nurse's responsibilities are discussed in the "Client Rights" section of this chapter.

Contracts are vital for those nurses who start their own business or who are hired by health care delivery systems as independent contractors. For example, a nurse who works for a home health care agency on a *per diem* basis, as opposed to an employee basis, has a contract with the agency specifying hours of work, pay rates, and other rights and responsibilities between the two parties.

Good Samaritan Laws

A good samaritan law is passed by a state legislature to encourage nurses and other health care providers to provide care to a person when an accident, emergency, or injury occurs, without fear of being sued for the care provided. The need for such a law exists because most states do not require that a health care provider give care at the scene of an accident or other emergency. Good samaritan laws vary from state to state. The law may be in the form of a statute specifically dealing with good samaritan protection or it may be part of a practice act (*e.g.,* nursing or medical).

Regardless of the form of the good samaritan law, its protection lies in the inability to sue the nurse or other health care provider for negligence in the care provided at the scene of the accident or during the emergency, even if further injury occurred due to the health care provider's care. Called immunity from suit, this protection usually applies only if all of the conditions of the law are met (*e.g.,* the health care provider receives no compensation for the care provided) and the care given is not wilfully and wantonly negligent. Wilful and wanton negligence is also usually defined in the law, but it generally means providing care in a manner that is an "extreme departure from ordinary care" (Black, 1991, p. 718).

The Nursing Student

Responsibilities

The student of nursing has many responsibilities during his or her years of study. First and foremost, the student must be clear about the responsibilities he or she has to the client to whom care is provided. A student of nursing *can* be sued for alleged negligent care provided to a client during the course of his or her years of study.

The standard of care that is applied to the student is not what other ordinary, reasonable, and prudent *student nurses* would have done in the same or similar circumstances in the same or similar community. Rather, the standard of care utilized is that of the *graduate* professional nurse in the same or similar situation (University Hospital Consortium, 1992). As a result, the student must be well prepared for any clinical assignment, request supervision from his or her clinical instructor when needed, and ask for a change in a client care assignment if not fully prepared to provide the care in a safe manner (Brent, 1997).

The nursing student also has the responsibility to conform to the mandates of the state nurse practice act. This responsibility includes performing nursing care within the scope of nursing as defined in the act. In addition, if the student is employed by a health care facility as a nurse's aide or in another capacity (*e.g.,* during the summer), the student must be careful to carry out client care that is within his or her current job description, not what can be done while in a formal nursing educational program. For example, a student nurse could not legally pass medications while working as an aide. To do so would expose the student to charges of practicing nursing without a license, which is a criminal offense.

Some of the other responsibilities that the student of nursing possesses include not discriminating against clients; maintaining client privacy and confidentiality; reporting any unsafe practitioners, abusive health care providers, or others whose misconduct is observed to the clinical instructor; and following the policies and procedures of the institution in which the student's clinical experience occurs.

Rights

Nursing students, like students in other educational, professional programs, possess rights as they progress through their educational program. Whether in a private or public (*e.g.,* state university program) academic setting, the student nurse's relationship with the educational program is governed by many laws, including contract law (*e.g.,* the student handbook), constitutional law (*e.g.,* due process protections for students in public institutions), and statutory law (*e.g.,* the Americans With Disabilities Act). These laws confer specific rights on the student.

For example, if a nursing student in a nursing program in a private school was dismissed from the school in violation of the student handbook, he or she could sue the institution for a breach of contract (the handbook). A qualified applicant to a nursing program who is denied admission to the program due to a disability can sue the school for a violation of the Americans With Disabilities Act.

Nursing students also possess other rights. Those rights include reasonable supervision while in the clinical area, privacy, confidentiality of student records and information, and freedom from discrimination on the basis of a protected class (*e.g.,* race, gender).

No right exists without concomitant responsibilities. The nursing student must carefully review any and all materials that govern the student-academic institution relationship. It is essential to obtain clarification when requirements or obligations in those materials are unclear. When a difficulty arises, the student should share his or her concerns with the student's academic advisor or the faculty member involved as soon as possible. If no resolution occurs on an informal level, the student should use the grievance procedures established by the academic institution for a formal resolution of a particular problem.

✦ Client Rights

Consumers of health care (clients) possess specific rights in their relationship with health care delivery systems and health care providers. Two specific rights, the right of informed consent and rights in relation to death and dying, are particularly important.

Informed Consent

The legal right of consent for treatment was firmly established in the 1914 case *Schloendorff v. Society of New York Hospitals*. In this landmark case, Justice Cardozo held that "every human being of adult years and sound mind has a right to determine what will be done with his own body . . ." (p. 93). Several years after the *Schloendorff* case, another case, *Salgo v. Leland Stanford Jr. University Board of Trustees* (1957), mandated that a physician had a duty to disclose to the client "any facts necessary to form the basis of an intelligent consent by the patient to proposed treatment" (p. 181).

Courts across the country have established what information must be shared with the client for his or her consent to be informed. That information is listed in Box 4–2.

Although the courts clearly look to these criteria in determining whether informed consent from a client was obtained, the law also allows for a physician's professional judgment in determining, for example, that informing a particular client of a certain material risk may not be in that client's best interest. So long as the physician documents his or her decision in the medical record as to why a particular element was not

---

Box 4–2

ELEMENTS OF INFORMED CONSENT

Client diagnosis

Name of procedure, test, medication

Explanation of procedure, test, medication, including reason for recommending

Anticipated benefits of the recommended regimen (but no guarantees)

Material risks of procedure, test, medication

Alternatives to recommended regimen, if any

Prognosis if recommended regimen refused

Data from Meisel, A. (1989). *The right to die.* Vol. I. NY: John Wiley & Sons (with 1994 Cumulative Supplement, No. 2); LeBlang, T., W. E., Peters, J. D., Fineberg, K., *et al.* (1986). *The law of medical practice in Illinois.* Rochester, NY: The Lawyers Cooperative Publishing Company. (with September 1993 Supplement)

---

discussed with the client and that decision is in accordance with the standard of care, the physician's decision will be upheld by the courts.

There is a presumption in the law that every adult, including the elderly client and the psychiatric client, possesses decision-making capacity and can therefore make informed consent choices. If a physician or other health care provider believes that an adult *lacks* decision-making capacity, an evaluation of the client by a neurologist, a psychiatrist, or other specialists must take place and an opinion must be rendered that the client is unable to make treatment choices before his or her right of informed consent is not honored.

Informed consent for medical procedures must be obtained by the physician, surgeon, or other medical practitioner performing the treatment or procedure, as illustrated in Figure 4–6. In most states, when a nurse is involved in the informed consent process for medical procedures, he or she is only witnessing the signature of the client on the informed consent form, pursuant to the policies and procedures in the health care facility.

For nursing care and procedures, the nurse should be involved in obtaining the informed consent of the client. Likewise, advanced nurse practitioners—nurse anesthetists, nurse midwives, and nurse practitioners—often obtain the informed consent of the client for the care they provide by sharing with the client the elements in Box 4–2.

Generally, there are only two instances in which the informed consent of the adult client is not needed. One instance is when an emergency is present and delaying treatment for the purpose of obtaining informed consent would result in injury or death to the client. For example, when a client is brought to the emergency department after a serious accident and is

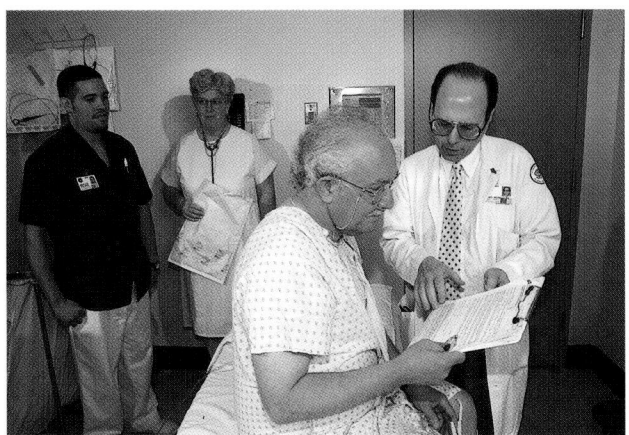

❧ Figure 4–6
Client signs informed consent form for medical treatment after physician provides required information.

unconscious and bleeding profusely, surgery is immediately done without the client's consent to save his or her life.

The second instance in which informed consent is not necessary to obtain is when the client waives his or her right to give informed consent. Some clients prefer *not* to be informed of the details of a particular treatment or surgery. The decision by the client not to be given the information legally required must be completely documented by the physician or nurse in the medical record.

Because minors (those under the age of 18) are seen by the law as lacking decision-making capacity, the parents or legal guardian of the minor provides informed consent for the minor. Some minors, however, are seen by the law as more "mature" and therefore able to provide their own consent for treatment. Minors who are married or emancipated from their parents and those seeking treatment for sexually transmitted diseases are some of the exceptions to the general rule that the parents provide consent for treatment for their children. Regardless of whether it is the parent, legal guardian, or the minor providing consent for treatment, the same information in Box 4–2 must be provided so that an informed choice concerning treatment can be made.

If a client has been determined by a court to be unable to make decisions for himself or herself, that person is declared *incompetent* or *under a legal disability.* If the incompetent person is found unable to make decisions concerning health care, a personal guardian is then appointed by the court to make all of those decisions for the incompetent person (also called the ward).

Some states have passed statutes that establish a decision-making process without resort to the courts when an individual cannot make treatment decisions. These "health care surrogate" or "family" decision-making statutes are diverse. Even so, they generally provide that on the determination by a physician that a person lacks decision-making capacity and that no

advance directive exists, a list of individuals who can make treatment decisions for that person is included in the law. The physician must ask the first person on the list, if available, and continue down the list in the order in the statute. An example of that order might be

* Spouse
* Adult child
* Parents
* Brother or sister
* Adult grandchild

Advance Directives

Another manner in which a client can ensure that his or her choices concerning treatment will be shared with health care providers is through the use of an advance directive. The Patient Self-Determination Act (PSDA) (1991), a Federal law passed by Congress to educate clients about treatment decisions and help health care providers dialogue with clients about those choices, defines an **advance directive** as a written document recognized by state law that provides directions concerning the provision of care when the person is unable to make his or her own treatment choices. Common examples of advance directives include the living will and the durable power of attorney for health care. Table 4–4 compares these two types of advance directives.

Implications for Nurses

The nurse must protect the client's legal right to provide a voluntary, informed decision concerning treatment. To do so, the nurse must be knowledgeable about the laws in his or her state that govern informed consent and the utilization of advance directives. A knowledge of the health care facility's policies and procedures concerning informed consent is also necessary, as is following those policies and procedures.

If a client raises questions or concerns about a treatment decision with the registered nurse, the nurse should explore those concerns and share whatever information is obtained from the client with the nurse manager and the client's physician. Factual and complete documentation of the discussion in the client's medical record is also necessary.

Under the PSDA, a client's advance directive must be made a part of his or her medical record, and the physician must be notified of its presence so that orders can be written consistent with the client's wishes. Because the nurse is often the first health care provider the client meets when he or she begins the role of a client, the nurse's legal responsibility under the PSDA can easily be met by complying with these requirements.

Last, the nurse must be certain that any treatment decisions made are made by a person legally authorized to do so. This is especially important when working with a health care agent, a surrogate, or a

Table 4–4

TYPES OF ADVANCE DIRECTIVES	
LIVING WILL	**DURABLE POWER OF ATTORNEY FOR HEALTH CARE**
May be called natural death document	May be called health care proxy/agency
Client not able to make own treatment decisions before document becomes effective	Client not able to make own treatment decisions before document becomes effective
Client's condition must be "terminal," in "persistent vegetative state" and/or "permanently unconscious," certified by physician	Client's condition not required to be "terminal," in "persistent vegetative state" and/or "permanently unconscious," but any treatment decision must be ordered by physician
Governs removal of "life-sustaining" treatment only	Governs removal of "life-sustaining" treatment as well as continuing treatment; provides many treatment options for client based on predetermined choices
Defines what "life-sustaining" treatment can be withdrawn or withheld	
Usually directed to health care provider; no agent appointed	Health care agent or proxy appointed in document who informs health care provider of treatment decisions based on choices in document

Data from *Refusal of treatment legislation: A state by state compilation of enacted and model statutes.* (1995). New York: Choice In Dying, Inc. (with regular updates).

guardian. To avoid liability for not working with the authorized decision-maker, the nurse can refer to the facility's policies and procedures governing consent. An additional resource is the nurse manager or risk management department.

Death and Dying
Right of Informed Refusal

A logical extension of the client's right to informed consent is the right of informed refusal for treatment. The US Supreme Court, in the landmark case *Cruzan v. Director, Missouri Department of Health* (1990), held that a competent adult (one with decision-making capacity) has a constitutional right to refuse treatment—even life-sustaining treatment—due to the 14th Amendment to the US Constitution's protection of liberty; *i.e.,* to be free from unwanted treatment. One type of treatment that is often refused by a client is cardiopulmonary resuscitation (CPR).

Do Not Resuscitate Order

External cardiac massage is one type of treatment that a client can refuse. In fact, health care delivery systems of all kinds have developed policies to guide the physician and other health care providers when a client or the legal representative no longer desires external cardiac massage as an acceptable form of treatment. The policies should include the following parameters (Brent, 1997; President's Commission, 1983):

* A written order must be present for do not resuscitate (DNR) status
* Any DNR order must be reviewed or renewed on a regular basis

* Specific guidelines must be given as to when and under what circumstances an oral DNR order is acceptable
* Specific requirements must be given regarding to whom an oral DNR order can be given (*e.g.,* only a registered nurse with another registered nurse witnessing the verbal order)
* The client or the legal representative must provide informed consent for the DNR status
* Both DNR and CPR must be clearly defined so that other treatment not refused by the client will be continued

Organ Transplant

Like the decision to refuse CPR, a client may also determine that an organ transplant is not a form of treatment that is desired; therefore the option to accept an organ transplant can be refused.

The client also has the right to donate his or her own organs for transplantation when death occurs. The informed choice to donate an organ for transplantation can take place with the use of a written document signed by the client prior to death (*e.g.,* a will, donor card, or an advance directive). If this process of providing informed consent for donation is not completed, then the Uniform Anatomical Gift Act (UAGA) (Uniform Laws Annotated, 1989), a law in all states, would control the donation of any organ.

If no directions concerning organ donation were provided by the client prior to his or her death, the Uniform Anatomical Gift Act provides a list of individuals who can provide informed consent for the donation of any organ. Like the health care surrogate statutes discussed earlier, the list includes the spouse, adult children, and parents of the deceased, and the people listed must be contacted in the order stated in the statute.

Autopsy

An autopsy is a medical examination of the body after death for the purpose of determining the cause of death. An autopsy is required by state law in certain circumstances, including the sudden death of a client and a death that occurs under suspicious circumstances.

If an autopsy is not required by law, the decision to have an autopsy voluntarily performed after the death of a family member or loved one is often a difficult one. Many individuals possess strong feelings concerning whether they want to have an autopsy performed. As a result, they have provided instructions orally or in an advance directive or other written document for the health care agent or others to follow concerning this decision.

If no oral or written instructions were given by the decendent, state law determines who has the authority to consent for any autopsy requested on a voluntary patient. Often, the decision rests with a surviving relative or next of kin who has the right to make decisions for the disposal of the body.

Health Care Provider–Assisted Suicide

The issue of physician-assisted suicide has resulted in a major legal, ethical, and moral controversy concerning the role of health care providers in aiding clients to end their life when suffering from a terminal or incurable disease. Clearly, legal support exists for a client to refuse life-sustaining treatment and for health care providers to honor the client's voluntary and informed decision by withdrawing or withholding treatment for which there is no consent. However, the legal support for health care provider–assisted suicide, where the health care provider takes an active role in aiding the client to die (*e.g.,* by providing the medication needed to cause the client's death or by actually administering a lethal dose medication), is less clear. In fact, in many states, assisting *anyone* to commit suicide is a criminal offense.

Moreover, many health care provider professional associations, including the ANA, have adopted position statements strongly rejecting a health care provider's participation in assisted suicide (ANA, 1994). The ANA's opposition is based on the ethical foundations of the profession and the ANA's *Code For Nurses With Interpretive Statements* (1985).

Nurses must carefully evaluate any role they may consider in assisted suicide. Participating in open and supportive discussions in the workplace with colleagues and others, including ethics and legal consultants, can help the nurse analyze the many legal, moral, and ethical issues associated with health care provider–assisted suicide. Active participation on the health care facility's policy and procedure committees concerning pain control, consent and refusal of treatment, and end-of-life care can result in guidelines for the health care provider that promote client decision-making in a supportive and caring environment. In

addition, membership on the home care agency or hospital's ethics committee is another way in which the role of the health care provider in this complex matter can be explored.

The Supreme Court heard arguments early in 1997 concerning Washington and New York states' respective laws on physician-assisted suicide (*Compassion in Dying v. State of Washington,* 1996; *Quill v. Vacco,* 1996). The nurse should review the decision of the US Supreme Court in this matter.

Client Testamentary Wills

A testamentary will is a document executed according to state law by which a person (the testator) makes a disposition of his or her real property (*e.g.,* a house) and personal property (*e.g.,* furniture), to take effect after his or her death (Black, 1991). Because most state laws require that the signature of the testator on the will be witnessed by at least one person, the nurse caring for a client in the hospital or a home health care nurse may be asked to witness a client's signing of the will. Most health care facilities, however, have specific policies that prohibit the nurse or other health care provider who provides care to the client from witnessing the signing of this legal document.

If no facility, agency, or state law prohibits against a nurse acting as a witness to a client's will, the nurse's role as a witness is to attest to two conditions: (1) that the client signed what he or she acknowledged was his or her will; and (2) that the client appeared to be of sound mind and understood what he or she was signing (Black, 1991).

The nurse who has witnessed a client's testamentary will or any other legal document must also document the event and the factual circumstances surrounding the signing in the medical record. Information to document in the nurse's note includes who was present, any significant comments by the client, and the nurse's observations of the client's conduct during the process.

If the nurse prefers not to be a witness to a client's signing of his or her testamentary will, the nurse should feel comfortable in explaining that preference to the client and not act in that capacity.

Other Selected Legal Issues Affecting the Nurse

Controlled Substances

The administration of controlled substances is an area of nursing practice fraught with many legal issues. Because narcotics and other controlled substances are heavily regulated by Federal and state laws, the nurse must constantly and consistently adhere to facility policies and procedures concerning their administration. The proper documentation of controlled substances when given to a client, the careful counting of narcotics on each shift, using the correct procedure for any narcotic substance that is wasted, and the judicious control of narcotics storage keys are just a few of the areas of concern for any nurse administering controlled substances.

Occupational Safety and Health Act

The Occupational Safety and Health Act (OSHA) of 1978 requires an employer to provide a healthful and safe workplace for its employees and to comply with workplace regulations promulgated by the Occupational Safety and Health Administration. The Administration has been active in protecting health care workers' rights under the Act. For example, in 1991, the Administration passed its universal precautions regulations (Bloodborne Pathogen Standard) to protect health care workers from undue exposure to bloodborne contagious diseases, including human immunodeficiency virus and hepatitis. Among other things, the regulations require that employers offer the hepatitis vaccine to new employees at no cost to the employee within 10 days of starting work; that employers require the use of universal (standard) precautions and the use of personal protective equipment, such as gowns, gloves, and masks; and that employers supply this equipment to their employees.

Another important protection that the Act provides to employees is the ability to report confidentially working conditions that violate the Administration's requirements to the local administration office. The Act also provides that an employee who does report unhealthy or unsafe working conditions cannot be retaliated against by the employer (*e.g.,* be fired) (29 C.F.R. Section 1977 [1990]).

Sexual Harassment

Sexual harassment in the workplace is prohibited by state and Federal laws. The Equal Employment Opportunity Commission (EEOC), the Federal agency empowered to investigate claims of discrimination, including sexual harassment, defines sexual harassment as *unwelcome* conduct of a sexual nature where (1) submission to or the rejection of the conduct is the basis of an employment decision ("*quid pro quo* harassment"), or (2) where the conduct is so "severe" or "pervasive" that it affects the employee's conditions of employment and "creates an abusive or hostile work environment" ("hostile environment harassment") (Cooper, 1993, p. 6).

Most employers have policies and procedures to handle concerns or complaints about sexual harassment. If the nurse believes he or she is being subjected to unwelcome sexual conduct, those concerns should be reported immediately to the person identified in the employer's policies. If an investigation and resolution by the employer does not occur in a manner consistent with the employer's policy, the nurse may need to consult with an attorney to fully evaluate his or her options in the circumstances.

It is also important for the nurse not to be involved in any conduct that might be seen as sexually harassing by other employees. Sexually suggestive jokes, touching, pressuring a coworker for a date, and open displays of sexually oriented photos or posters are examples of conduct that could be considered sexual harassment by another worker (Cooper, 1993).

✦

Summary

There is no question that a myriad of legal concerns exist in the practice of nursing. The nurse who is knowledgeable about the law and how it affects nursing practice is a step ahead of those colleagues who are not aware of the legal issues faced in health care delivery. By practicing nursing with a proactive, critical approach to the legal issues that exist on a daily basis, the nurse can avoid liability for careless, unknowledgeable actions. The beginning nurse can take a proactive approach by remembering the importance of (1) maintaining the registered professional nurse license in good standing; (2) documenting clearly and consistently; (3) adhering to standards of nursing practice; (4) acting as a client advocate; and (5) knowing institutional or agency policies and procedures. Liability can never be completely avoided, however. Even so, if the nurse practices his or her profession in a thoughtful, caring, and knowledgeable manner, the law can be an added benefit to the nurse and to the client for whom care is provided.

◼   ◼

CHAPTER HIGHLIGHTS

✦

- ✦ The types and sources of law that affect nursing practice include statutory law, constitutional law, private law, and administrative law
- ✦ The regulation of nursing practice rests with the state nurse practice act and the state agency empowered to administer and enforce the act
- ✦ Licensure, certification, and credentialing are also ways in which nursing practice is regulated.
- ✦ Nursing practice may bring with it liability in the areas of criminal law and tort law, including professional negligence, defamation, and false imprisonment
- ✦ Adherence to standards of care and maintaining competence in one's area of practice are important steps in reducing liability for negligent care

✦ The careful and complete documentation of client care in the medical record is one's best defense against allegations of professional negligence

✦ Active involvement in the facility's risk management plan, including the use of incident reports, is essential for the nurse.

✦ Student nurses possess specific rights and concomitant responsibilities during their nursing education program

✦ The nurse must protect the client's rights of informed consent and informed refusal for treatment

✦ Administering controlled substances in a manner consistent with state and Federal laws regulating narcotics and other substances is essential

✦ The Occupational Safety and Health Act (1978) protects the nurse's right to a healthful and safe workplace

✦ Sexual harassment in the workplace should not be tolerated, nor should the nurse engage in conduct that might be considered sexual harassment by colleagues.

Study Questions

1. Failing to provide care considered standard for a client would be classified as

   a. malpractice
   b. negligence
   c. a misdemeanor
   d. reckless conduct

2. An example of assault is

   a. restraining a client's arm prior to having an intravenous inserted
   b. restraining an infant's arms after he or she had a cleft lip repaired
   c. restraining a client who wants to leave the hospital against medical advice
   d. placing a psychiatric client in seclusion who has been throwing objects around the unit

3. Which of the following situations would be considered a violation of a client's confidentiality?

   a. informing the physician that the client has had a history of a sexually transmitted disease
   b. allowing a client's family to read the client's chart when they request to do it
   c. providing information about the client's history to other staff members during a change-of-shift report
   d. completing a referral form for a mental health consultation about the client's medical history

4. The responsibility for obtaining an informed consent rests with the

   a. physician
   b. charge nurse
   c. supervisor
   d. family member

5. If a nurse were charged with theft of a narcotic substance, this would be considered

   a. a tort
   b. reckless conduct
   c. a felony
   d. malpractice

Critical Thinking Exercises

1. Sally Nurse administers Demerol to Mr. B. and leaves the room without raising the bed's siderails. Discuss this act in relation to the four factors of negligence.

2. Nancy Nurse charts "client found on floor complaining of pain in hip, bed in low position, siderails down. No medications given in the last 24 hours. Physician notified and orders noted" versus "client apparently fell to floor, called physician, and x-rays obtained." Compare the two entries for legal implications.

References

American Nurses Association. (1985). *Code for nurses with interpretive statements*. Washington, DC: American Nurses Association.

American Nurses Association. (1994). *Position statement on assisted suicide*. Washington, DC: American Nurses Association.

American Nurses Association. (1990). *Suggested state legislation: Nursing Practice Act, Nursing Disciplinary Diversion Act, Prescriptive Authority Act*. Kansas City, MO: American Nurses Association.

American Nurses' Credentialing Center. (1995). *Certification catalogue*. Washington, DC: American Nurses' Credentialing Center.

Annas, G. (1992). *The Rights of Patients*. (2nd ed.). Totowa, NJ: Humana Press.

Black, H. C. (1991). *Black's law dictionary* (6th ed). St. Paul, MN: West Publishing Company.

Bloodborne pathogen standard, 29 C.F.R. 1910.1030 (1991).

Brent, N. J. (1997). *Nursing and the law: A guide to principles and applications*. Philadelphia: W. B. Saunders.

Compassion in Dying v. State of Washington, 79 F. 3d 790 (en banc), *reb'q en banc by full court denied*, 85 F. 3d (9th Cir. 1996), *cert. granted sub. nom, Washington v. Glucksberg*, 65 U.S.L.W. 3254 (U.S. October 1, 1996) (No. 96-110).

Cooper, C. (1993), Sexual harassment: Preventive steps for the healthcare practitioner. *Annals of Health Law, 2*, 1–33.

Cruzan v. Director, Missouri Department of Health, 497 U.S. 261 (1990).

Illinois Nursing Practice Act of 1987, 225 ILCS 65/3(h) (1987).

Inglis, A. B., & Kjervik, D. K. (1993). Empowerment of advanced practice nurses: Regulation reform needed to increase access to care. *The Journal of Law, Medicine & Ethics, 21*, 193–205.

Judge v. Rockford Memorial Hospital, 150 N.E. 2d 202 (Ill. App. Ct. 1958).

Keeton, W. P. (Ed.). (1984). *Keeton and Prosser on the law of torts*. (5th ed.). St. Paul, MN: West Publishing Company. (With updated pocket parts).

LaFave, W., & Scott, A. (1986). *Criminal law*. (2nd ed.). St. Paul, MN: West Publishing Company. (With 1995 pocket parts).

LeBlanc v. Northern Colfax County Hospital, 672, P. 2d 667 (New Mexico 1983).

Occupational Safety And Health Act (OSHA), 29 U.S.C. Sections 651–678 (1978).

Patient Self-Determination Act (PSDA), 42 U.S.C. 1395cc(f) (1) and 43 U.S.C. 1396(a) Supp. 1991; 42 U.S.C. 4206 (3); 4751 (4) (1991).

Pozgar, G. (1996). *Legal aspects of health care administration* (6th ed.). Gaithersburg, MD: Aspen Publishing.

President's Commission for the Study of Ethical Problems in Medicine and Biomedical Research. (1983). *Deciding to forgo life-sustaining treatment: Ethical and legal issues in treatment decisions.* Washington, DC: US Government Printing Office.

Quill v. Vacco, 80 F. 3d 716 (2d Circ. 1996), *cert. granted,* 65 U.S. L. W. 3254 (U.S. October 1, 1996) (No. 95-1858).

Reaves, R. (1993). *The law of professional licensing and certification* (2nd ed.). Montgomery, AL: Publications For Professionals.

Redd, M. L., Alexander, J. W. (1997). Does certification mean better performance? *Nursing Management, 28,* 45–49.

Roach, W., & the Aspen Law Center. (1994). *Medical records and the law* (2nd ed.). Gaithersburg, MD: Aspen Publishers.

Salgo v. Leland Stanford Jr. University Board of Trustees, 317 P.2d 170 (1957).

Schloendorff v. Society of New York Hospitals, 105 N.E. 92 (1914).

Springhouse Corporation (1992). *Nurse's handbook of law & ethics.* Springhouse, PA: Springhouse Corporation.

Uniform laws annotated, master edition. Vol. 8A. (1989).

University Hospital Consortium. (1992). *Nursing-legal survival: A risk management guide for nurses.* Oak Brook, IL: University Hospital Consortium.

West, S., Walsh, K., & Youngberg, B. J. (1994). Risk management program development. Youngberg, B. (Ed.), In *The risk manager's desk reference.* Gaithersburg, MD: Aspen Publishers.

Wyatt v. St. Paul Fire & Marine Insurance Company, 315 Ark. 547, 868 S.W. 2d 505 (1994).

Bibliography

The American Association of Nurse Attorneys. (1989). *Demonstrating financial responsibility for nursing practice.* Baltimore, MD: The American Association of Nurse Attorneys.

Rothstein, M. (1990). *Occupational safety and health law* (3rd ed.). St. Paul, MN: West Publishing Company.

Hafemeister, T., & Hannaford, P. (1996). *Resolving disputes over life-sustaining treatment: A health care provider's guide.* Williamsburg, VA: National Center for State Courts.

Spielman, B. (Ed.). (1996). *Organ and tissue donation: Ethical, legal and policy issues.* Carbondale, IL: Southern Illinois University Press.

Sovereign, K. (1994). *Personnel law* (3rd ed.). Englewood Cliffs, NJ: Prentice Hall.

Chapter 5

HEALTH, ILLNESS, AND HEALTH CARE SYSTEMS

STEPHEN PAUL HOLZEMER, PhD, RN

LEARNING OBJECTIVES

♦

After studying this chapter, you should be able to

♦ Define the concepts of health and illness according to the perspectives related to the health-illness continuum, levels of prevention, wellness, and holism

♦ Explore the difference between the needs of the individual and the needs of society

♦ Identify the various settings where health care services are delivered

♦ Examine the critical components of health care reform

♦ Investigate the impact of economics on health care delivery

♦ Evaluate the importance of continuity of care in providing health-related services

♦ Speculate on the directions health care will take in the future and the adaptations that will be necessary for health care providers working in future health care systems

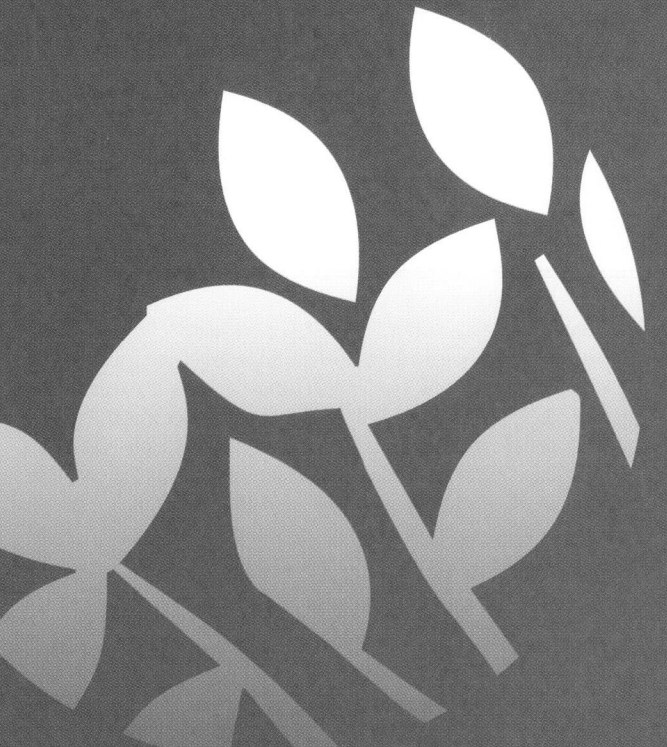

The meaning of terms like *health* and *illness* may seem obvious, but these words do not mean the same thing to everyone. The way in which people understand health and illness varies from culture to culture and from generation to generation, even from one period in a person's life to another. Ideas about health and illness have shaped the image and activities of the nursing profession for hundreds of years (Bishop & Scudder, 1991; Dolan, 1978). Although *health* and *illness* are relative terms, they have always related to the functioning of the physical, psychological, emotional, spiritual, and cultural needs of clients. This chapter reviews concepts that are basic to the meaning of health and illness: the health-illness continuum; the primary, secondary, and tertiary levels of prevention; high-level wellness; and holistic care.

When illness meant an early death, nurses comforted the sick with little more than touch and implementation of basic hygiene. As physicians delegated more technical tasks to the well-trained but not necessarily educated nurse, nurses began to be seen as essential assistants in the increasingly sophisticated health care system. The new respect afforded nursing as a professional, educated discipline has encouraged nurses to become primary care providers and to develop their own vision of the meaning of health and illness (Bishop & Scudder, 1990, 1991; Kalisch & Kalisch, 1986). As nurses provide more care to clients, using theories and frameworks that express what is important about nursing care, the profession will continue to evolve. In the future, some nurses will continue to provide direct care, whereas others will provide more care management and supervision.

The essence of the profession of nursing is the important role the nurse plays as an escort to the client maneuvering through the health care system. The nurse is privileged to be with clients during some of the most private experiences of their passage from birth to death. The nurse has the responsibility of meeting client needs as they relate to health and illness on a 24-hour basis. The nurse remains central to safe and effective care of clients in the roles of client advocate, educator, and care provider. Increasingly, nurses are seen as client-centered specialists rather than as technological specialists.

Nursing has a key role in allocating health care resources by examining the needs of the individual versus the needs of society. The relationship between the needs of individuals and those of the general population (society) is the driving force in the creation of health care systems. Health care systems in which nurses work include hospitals, private homes, hospice facilities, long-term care settings, and quick care settings like surgi-centers, ambulatory care settings, and public health departments.

Health care systems are affiliating in new and different ways. New constellations of services are being developed, with cost-effectiveness as the primary concern. Health care partnerships are developing, whereas independent, stand-alone facilities, like isolated hospitals, reflect a model of the past. Hospital chains and other types of service relationships are becoming the norm for providing all levels of health care. Health care reform also involves changes in access to and participation in health care services. The family physician no longer makes independent decisions about referrals to specialists. The economics of managed care, the expense of high and low technology, the existing multitier systems of care, and issues such as rationing of health care services and continuity of care are all important topics in the health care arena today. All care providers must "reengineer" their skills and knowledge base to meet the needs of clients in changing care delivery models.

Health and Illness

The concepts of **health and illness** have limited meaning when examined in isolation. These concepts are connected and have meaning only in terms of the actual experiences of individuals, families, groups, and communities, who may thrive and survive or wither and die. A newborn may be viewed as the picture of health; a family experiencing divorce may be a reflection of an ill relationship. Groups of young adults with radical and prejudicial beliefs are seen as ill, whereas communities rebuilding after civil unrest represent a healthy response to an unhealthy situation. Individuals and communities themselves may feel "healthy" or "sick," depending on various conditions.

Health and illness are concepts rooted in a historical context. Each generation of Americans and each health crisis have made unique demands on the health care system. During the polio epidemic in the early part of this century, supportive care was all that could be provided until a vaccine was discovered. Then there was tremendous pressure not only to immunize people against this disease but also to research and provide immunization for other common diseases. Likewise, when the Women's Movement of the 1960s and 1970s was in full swing, the medical establishment was forced to acknowledge that women often had received less refined health care services than men. The growing attention to women's health needs is slowly reducing this imbalance. Recently, care of people with acquired immunodeficiency syndrome (AIDS) has become an important concern. Despite negative feelings about certain sexual behaviors and drug use, the society as a whole has pressured for research into a cure for this disease. As topics of concern change over time—from polio to women's health care to acquired immunodeficiency syndrome—health care systems change with them (Carroll *et al.,* 1994; Friedman, 1994; Pan American Health Organization, 1994), requiring providers to adapt to these changes.

Historically, care for the ill was given in the home.

The visiting nurse or the family physician's being called to the home represents a classic image of the past. With industrialization and the explosion of technology in health care, services were shifted to hospitals, where it was believed the quality of care would improve because services were centralized. Centralization of care had both benefits and drawbacks. Strangers provided care once given only by family members. The most intimate aspects of care from birth to death were redefined within the sterile confines of the growing medical industrial complex, and health became a medical problem.

Issues of health as well as the systems in which we receive health care continue to change. After years of centralization, health care delivery systems are being redirected toward community-based models. Changes in how Americans value health-related and illness-related services are being reconceptualized in discussions about health care reform and the economics of health care (Ceslowitz, 1993; Smith, G. R., 1994). The public and health care professionals are returning to the basic questions of who should receive care and who will pay for services. The unique part of the current debate is the involvement of the consumer in discussing how resources will be used. Consumers are being empowered to take part in discussions with care providers about what care they want to receive (Healthy America, 1992; Rabkin *et al.*, 1994). Continuity of care, discussed later in this chapter, is emerging as a critical component of the current health care debate.

Models of Health and Illness

Health-Illness Continuum

A linear diagram of health and illness as polar opposites suggests that people are at any one time *either* healthy *or* ill. The *health-illness continuum* is such a model in which health and illness are viewed as opposites. They are at one end or the other in a one-dimensional design, or at one fixed point between the extremes. This view suggests that birth is when one is healthiest and death follows the most severe episode of illness. The problem with this model is that certain events are not explained very completely or accurately. People's response to health and illness is more complex.

People can show characteristics of both health and illness at the same time, and the best nursing interventions are those that are generated from an understanding of how these concepts relate to each other within the unique experience of the client. The two case examples here provide insight into the relationship between health and illness. In these examples, Mr. Taylor and Ms. Clerka experience health and illness very differently.

CASE STUDY Mr. Taylor Needs Health Teaching

Bruce Taylor, age 73 years, is seemingly the picture of good health. He exercises regularly and chooses foods low in salt and fat content. Mr. Taylor lectures to older people about proper nutrition. One afternoon, Mr. Taylor comes to the clinic complaining of being lightheaded (vertigo) and is slightly disoriented. His nursing history reveals that he has self-administered daily enemas for months to keep his bowels regular. Laboratory serum evaluation reveals mild electrolyte imbalance. Mr. Taylor experiences a specific deficit in knowledge about how his behavior is affecting his health status.

Many people might consider Mr. Taylor to be healthy on the whole. Yet, although he shows many positive health behaviors, his bowel regimen reflects a potentially serious problem. His nurse was correct to complete a full nursing assessment, uncovering a significant area for health teaching and supportive care. The nurse must support his healthy behaviors while trying to help him improve other, less healthy behaviors. The plan on which Mr. Taylor and his nurse agree to work focuses on both healthy and unhealthy behaviors.

CASE STUDY Ms. Clerka Is Dying

Mary Clerka, age 30, has decided to stop treatment for uterine cancer, which has metastasized to multiple organ systems. Ms. Clerka has proceeded to make plans to have her two children placed in foster care. She has communicated with other family members during her illness and now feels "ready to die." Ms. Clerka has completed a will and has named her mother as her health care proxy. Her mother knows what Mary wants done for her physically if she can no longer direct her care.

Ms. Clerka is gravely ill physically and seemingly close to death. Close examination of her behavior suggests that she is approaching death in a healthy way. Planning for her children's care, communicating with her family, and stating that she feels ready to die are behaviors that indicate a high level of health in the midst of physiologic collapse. Ms. Clerka is using the rest of her life in a smooth transition to death. The nurse and Ms. Clerka work together to make this type of transition possible. The nurse and Ms. Clerka are maintaining as healthy a state as possible as death approaches.

Levels of Prevention

Leavell and Clark (1965) developed a classic scheme for understanding the disease model. They separated the idea of **illness** into the period before (prepathogenesis) and during (pathogenesis) an infectious process. Three levels of prevention were identified, which included interventions that theoretically would halt or slow down the disease process. According to this model, the goal of health is to prevent the client from moving toward disability and death. A strength of this model is that it categorizes interventions that nurses and others can use to prevent, as well as to treat, illness. Also, ideas about prevention can be applied not just to individuals but also to social problems like poverty and violence (Zwerdling, 1994). One of the limitations of the model is that it reinforces the misconception that death and disability can be postponed indefinitely.

Primary prevention services relate to health promotion activities and specific protection from disease or illness. Health promotion activities include concerns of nutrition, personal hygiene, environment, and living habits. Specific protection (from illness) includes activities such as immunization, drug therapy (to prevent complications), and environmental protection (Leavell & Clark, 1965). Primary prevention is reflected in the activities that prevent the ill state. Nurses use primary preventive activities when they teach a specific part of the population to decrease their salt intake because of a pattern of cerebrovascular accidents (stroke) in this group. Hopefully, this would result in many people in this group completely avoiding disease.

Secondary prevention focuses on the early diagnosis and prompt treatment of disease. Secondary prevention is effective early in the disease process. Diagnostic tests and pharmacotherapy to treat illness and surgery to prevent complications are examples of secondary prevention. Disability limitation is also considered to be in this level of prevention. Every effort to catch disease early in its development and limit its negative effects occurs through secondary prevention activities. Nurses use these principles when they encourage women over the age of 40 to obtain periodic mammograms and when they actively screen for hypertension in a community in which strokes are common. They also use these principles when they encourage clients to take antihypertensive medications as prescribed and to report certain symptoms to their primary care nurse immediately.

Tertiary prevention is represented by rehabilitative services. These interventions assist the person to function at his or her highest or most advanced level of functioning. Tertiary prevention assumes that full recovery to the previous completely well state is uncommon. The nurse implements tertiary prevention activities to help the person return to the closest preillness state possible. For a client who has experienced a stroke, for example, therapeutic exercises and the use of a walker might allow for a 65% return in mobility, whereas providing no support would result in a steady and progressive loss of function.

Wellness

Ardell (1977) introduced a new blueprint for what is called high-level wellness. The idea that self-responsibility, nutritional awareness, stress management, physical fitness, and environmental sensitivity all contributed to wellness is key to Ardell's model (Fig. 5–1). Today, what we call "comorbidity" or "cofactors" in illness reflects this earlier thought—that illness often occurs because of multiple problems. The idea of **wellness** suggests that the infectious agent or microorganism does not necessarily have the central role in the disease process. The concept of wellness relates to a view in which all aspects of illness and health are interrelated (Fig. 5–2).

Ardell's writing about wellness in the late 1970s paralleled a time of social change in which the importance of the client as a decision-maker was just beginning to emerge. Contemporary concerns related to wellness are receiving increasing attention from health care professionals as well as the public. Today, clients should be considered full partners in health care decisions, ranging from health promotion (Stockhausen,

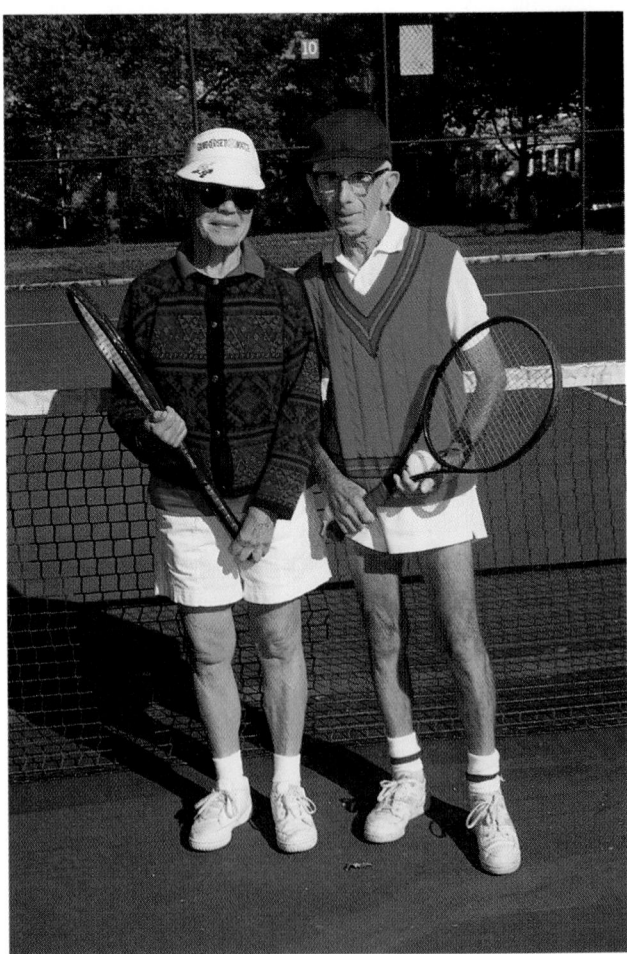

❥ **Figure 5–1**

Examples of high-level wellness; the man is 85 years of age, and the woman is 78.

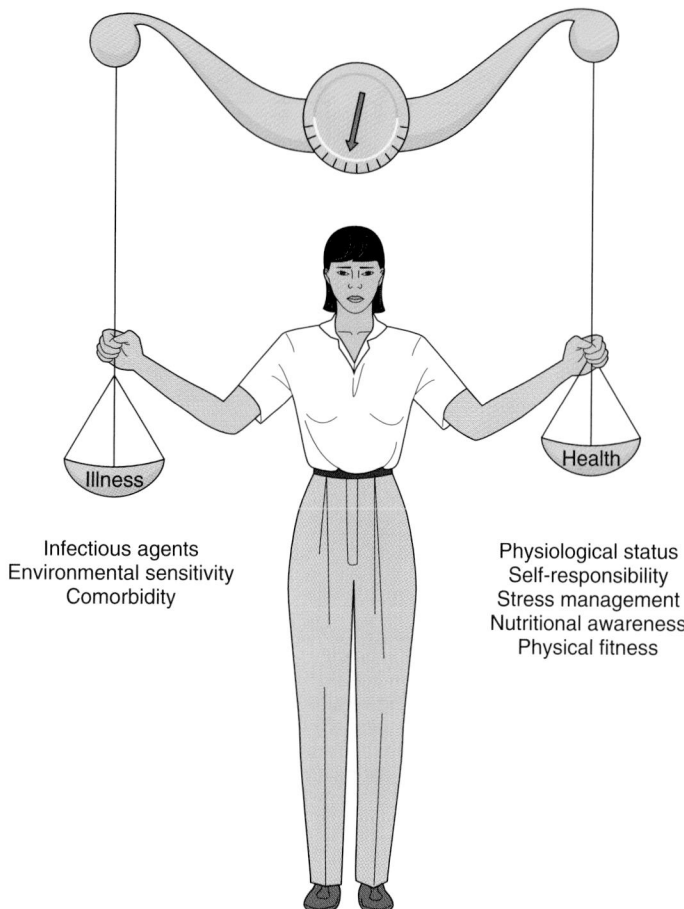

✦ **Figure 5–2**
The balance of wellness in an individual can be tipped toward
health or illness by many factors, of which an infectious agent
may be only one.

1994) to coping with chronic and/or terminal illness
(Wright *et al.,* 1993).

Together, nursing and the public need to explore
the many factors that relate to problems like the prevalence of stroke and homicide among African-Americans (US Department of Health and Human Services,
1995); the lack of first trimester prenatal care among
Hispanics, Native Americans, and Inuits; and suicide
among Native Americans, Inuits, and whites. Ongoing
assessment of wellness can assist in resolving problems and making sound health-planning decisions.

Holistic View of Health

Early medical research focused on individual microorganisms that caused disease. The advent of antibiotics was one factor that reinforced this idea. Rapid
advances in medical technology focused attention on
mechanical and scientific aspects of health care. What
was seen to have value was quantifiable, and looking
at health and illness concerns more broadly (holistically) seemed unscientific and imprecise. The medical
model of health care matched the medication to the
infection and took a narrower view of what was important to investigate in relation to illness. Objective
data (data that can be obtained and confirmed by

instrumentation) were seen as more valuable than
subjective data.

However, it is being recognized again that subjective and objective measurements are both important
components of data collection. The nurse's level of
experience often helps in deciding which measurements are most important to collect, especially in an
emergency. If the client is diaphoretic (sweating), has
a diagnosis of diabetes, reports feeling cold and
clammy, and is not eating properly, the nurse would
not initially take the person's temperature, thinking
that the sweating is from a fever. The sum of symptoms would guide the nurse to obtain a blood glucose
measurement to explore the possibility of a hypogly-
cemic reaction.

The benefits of providing nursing care from a holistic view and addressing the individual are more than
just physical. For example, if a client complains of a
stomach ache and lack of appetite the night before
surgery, the astute nurse would consider the emotional anxiety of the client as an important piece of
data. The level of nursing care is more comprehensive
when it includes the physical, psychological, spiritual,
and cultural aspects of the client's health.

Nurses have always enjoyed the opportunity to
focus on the holistic care of clients. The art and sci-

Activation of the nursing process

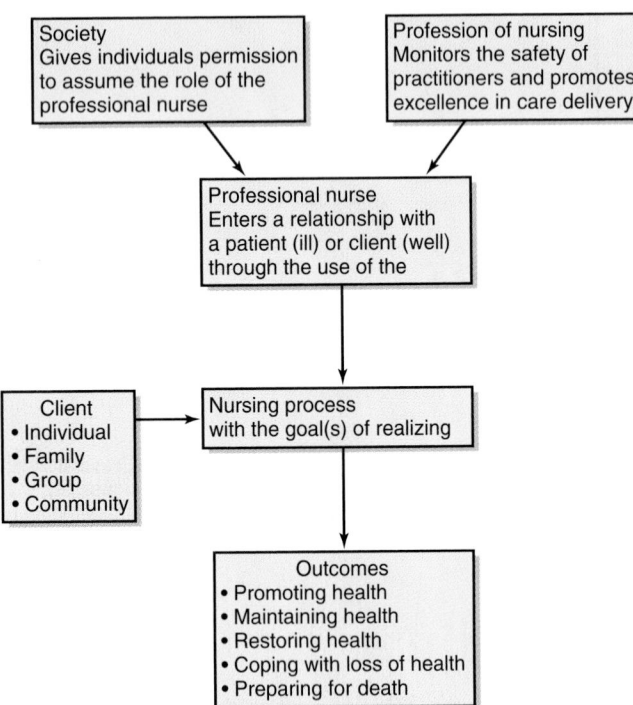

❧ Figure 5–3
Relationship among the concepts of health and illness and the
nursing process.

ence of nursing demand an all-encompassing view of
the recipient of nursing services. Figure 5–3 shows
the relationship among the concepts of health and
illness and the way nurses care for others. The relationship between "society" and the profession of nursing is actualized in the nurse's day-to-day care of individuals.

The client and the nurse enter into a purposeful
relationship referred to as the nursing process. This is
necessary to realize health-related goals. The outcomes are those that society sanctions and considers
appropriate in the nurse-client bond and are reflected
in the law (nurse practice acts). The nursing process is
key to a holistic view of health and illness because it
requires a comprehensive approach to a total plan of
care. It clearly defines nursing's responsibility in a
nursing care plan, as well as in interdisciplinary plans
of care with other providers.

Needs of the Individual Versus Needs of Society

Stereotype of Normal

In many parts of the world, the predominant race,
religion, or common belief system determines what is
considered the ideal or normal. A stereotype of nor-

mal reflects the largest or most powerful group in the
society. The average characteristics of the dominant
groups, although not inclusive of all people, result in
a stereotypic definition of health and illness.

In the early days of the United States, people of
European descent provided the model of what was
considered normal. Native Americans, actually the
largest segment of the population, were not part of
the standard-setting process in developing health care
services. In fact, as history shows, their needs were
ignored from a Western medical perspective. Euro-
pean-based medicine and traditional Native American
cures seemed incompatible.

Defining Individual and Societal Needs

In the current health care arena, the question of
just "who is the client" is being asked. At times, the
answer is the individual, and at other times, the answer is the society as a whole. Owing in part to this
questioning, the health care needs of individuals are
no longer necessarily met at the expense of society at
large (Callahan, 1990). For example, societies plagued
by poor nutrition and low immunization rates among
their children are seen as having more significant
problems than the expensive medical needs of an isolated few. The wisdom of transplanting organs into
very sick individuals is being questioned when the
same resources might be more efficiently used in preventive measures that could stop these illnesses from
occurring.

Individual needs are pressing when they occur,
yet the long-term "health" of society can have more
wide-ranging and devastating consequences. Because
of this, issues such as gun control, human immunodeficiency virus infection, and domestic abuse must be a
part of our thinking about our national, or even
global, "health" (Callahan *et al.,* 1994; Centers for Disease Control, 1993; Riley, 1994; Yu, 1994). The morbidity and mortality associated with community violence and communicable diseases not only affects
individuals and families in the present but also change
the future of the community forever. A healthy society
must include medical, social, and legal resources to
meet people's needs.

Respect for Culturally Diverse Groups

Problems in health care occur when the needs of
certain individuals are not considered in the overall
plan when developing services. In this country, for
example, women have been excluded from many research protocols. This means that in many cases, their
reaction to drugs or treatments still is not known. People of various cultural groups may also not be given
as much health care attention as the major group in
society. The nursing care provided to these clients
may be inappropriate—or worse, detrimental—to

them. Lack of respect for cultural diversity can cause physical, emotional, and spiritual distress because the care that is provided is not care that is meaningful to the client.

It is important for nurses to respect the needs of culturally diverse groups when making plans of care (refer to Chapter 36 for a detailed discussion of cultural diversity). When members of the health care team demonstrate respect for **cultural diversity,** it is more likely that health care resources will be used by the people who need them. People from different cultures, races, religions, and backgrounds should be made to feel welcome by care providers (Fig. 5–4). This can be achieved if the caregiver shows respect for the client's unique health beliefs and considers these beliefs when developing the person's plan of care (Geissler, 1994; Spector, 1991).

Nurses must learn to be comfortable with different cultural groups. A nurse, whether of Irish, Chinese, or Egyptian ancestry, needs to make every effort to care for others in a way that celebrates their uniqueness. Respect for cultural diversity is not the same as holding the beliefs of another as true, but the nurse must respect those views as important. For example, a nurse with atheistic beliefs should not have trouble caring for a religiously observant Jew. A nurse who values the use of blood products in health care should be able to support the beliefs of a Jehovah's Witness who refuses a blood transfusion. Nurses are culturally competent when they allow their client's beliefs to mold and direct the care they provide, within accepted standards of practice.

Concerns about cultural diversity are reflected in the changing values and beliefs about health care and the services that are provided. Changes in health care services should be more inclusive of different peoples' needs (Andrews & Boyle, 1995). Changing values and beliefs are centered on the categories of the meaning of health and illness, who should receive care, and who should decide who is provided with health care services.

The values and beliefs of people are reflected in the systems of health care that they develop, as well as other activities in which they are involved (Thomas, 1991). An important role for nurses as individuals, as well as the profession as a whole, is to make sure that the needs of culturally diverse groups are discussed and provided for whenever possible. Although it is not realistic for nurses to expect that every cultural belief will be considered in every health care decision, people from different cultures should have confidence that nursing care will at least entertain their unique concerns and that the nursing profession will promote acceptance of diversity.

✦ Health Care Delivery Systems

The **health care delivery systems** that nurses help create are located in many different settings. At one time, high-technology care was always provided in the hospital, and people knew that they would have to go to the hospital if they wanted a certain level of care. Today, the setting in which care is delivered is not always clearly defined. Clients receive care in hospitals, their homes or residences, hospices and long-term care facilities, quick-care settings, and private physician's offices. These services are increasingly being integrated in an attempt to save money, provide quality care, and case-manage clients (Fig. 5–5).

Hospital Care

Until recently, the most impressive type of health care service was provided by the hospital. The hospital system of care was developed for the convenience of the health care provider, who could treat many more clients because they were located in one place. Moving sick people to the hospital may have improved many of the technical aspects of care delivery at the cost of more personal aspects, such as having individuals and their families understand the experience of suffering and death. The shift in care today is back to providing as much care as possible outside of the hospital to decentralize care delivery. The once-elegant hospital facilities are now seen as expensive artifacts within an increasingly cost-effective care delivery system.

Home Care

The primary site for care delivery in the early 21st century will be the person's place of residence. This "home care" is provided wherever the person lives, whether in sheltered spaces, long-term care facilities, or elsewhere. Some professionals feel that an attractive aspect of home care is the possibility of using family members as caregivers. An assumption often is made that the family member will provide care that is necessary. However, it is important for the nurse to assess

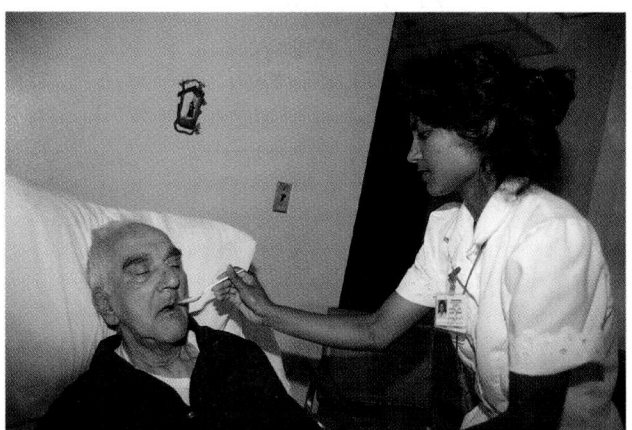

❧ **Figure 5–4**
The nurse reaches past racial and cultural differences to assist the client.

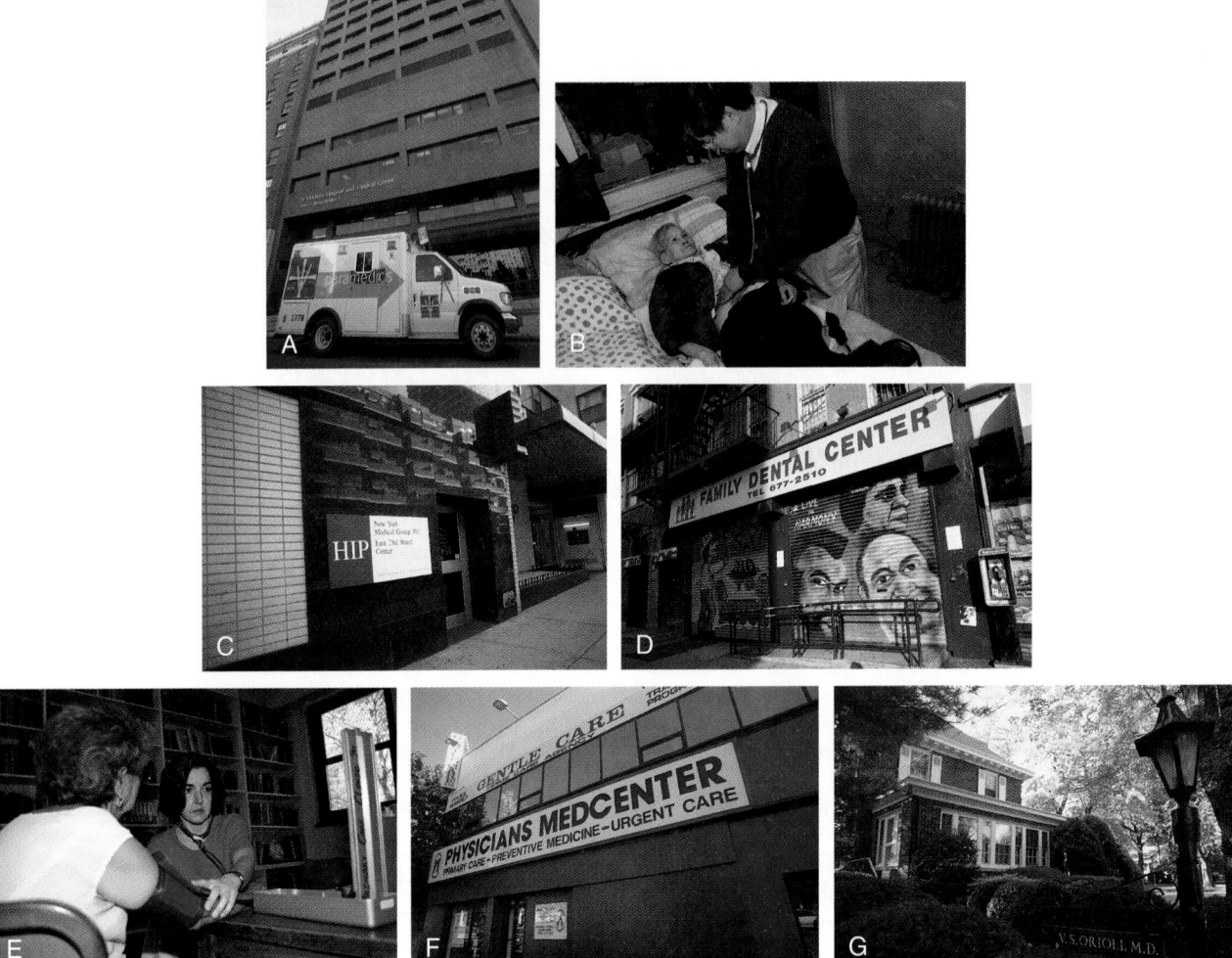

❧ **Figure 5-5**
Available health care delivery systems include hospital (*panel A*), client's home (*panel B*), health maintenance organization (*panel C*), dental clinic (*panel D*), long-term care facility (*panel E*), quick care medical center (*panel F*), private physician's office (*panel G*).

whether there is a family member who is both willing and able to care for the person who is sick. In addition, the nurse should be careful to assess for caregiver stress or burnout. Family members serving as caregivers need training, support, and at times respite (relief) from this role. Some family members may be reluctant to accept the caregiver role if support is not available. Many potential problems in providing home care services are being studied (Dee-Kelly *et al.,* 1994; Dellasega *et al.,* 1994; O'Donnell & Sampson, 1994).

Many women, the primary lay caregivers in the home, are considered members of the "sandwich generation" (see Chapter 17)—they care for their children and for their parents or older relatives at the same time. This caregiver is "sandwiched" between competing claims for care. Researchers have only recently begun to explore the effects of the stress of caring for both generations (Brody, 1994; Stein *et al.,* 1994). Nurses who are themselves in the sandwich generation may experience even more care-related stress as

they care for strangers professionally and then return to care for family and others. Little is known about the relative stress experienced by male nurses compared with female caregivers.

Hospice Care

Providing supportive care for the dying person and his or her family and caregivers is the goal of hospice care. Pain management is often one of the key aspects of hospice services. Ensuring a pain-free death can be one of the most significant acts in allowing the individual to approach death with limited fear. Hospices also provide respite care for the family or caregivers of the dying person. Hospice care allows caregivers to take a break from the stresses of ongoing caregiving and allows them to focus on their need for support to accept the impending death (Martin *et al.,* 1990).

Hospice care can be delivered in a person's home, in a residence such as a nursing home, or in a high-technology hospital-hospice center. Wherever it is provided, hospice care is intended to support the person's journey toward death, however it unfolds. Sometimes there is a misconception that hospice care is only for people who seem fully prepared for death or for those who will die soon. Although some reimbursement mechanisms limit the time for which someone can obtain hospice services, these services can be provided for varying lengths of time.

Long-Term Care

Long-term care is often provided in nursing homes, group residences, or rehabilitation facilities. Long-term care is for clients with a partial or complete deficit that makes long-term supportive care necessary. In the past, long-term care used to mean supportive care provided until death. Today, if someone recovers from a condition so that he or she can provide more self-care, that person would be discharged from the long-term care facility to a lower-skilled facility or their residence, whichever is appropriate and available. Later, if self-care abilities decline, the client might enter the long-term care facility again.

Quick Care (Surgi-Centers, Emergi-Centers)

Specialized health care is also increasingly delivered in convenient locations that provide quick and less costly services. Following the model of eye examination offices, skilled care is being provided in neighborhoods and other convenient locations that offer the advantage of lower-cost overhead. These facilities were developed to provide a narrow scope of services at a lower cost (to the provider) than the cost of equivalent care in the hospital. Consumers, however, may actually pay more for quick care because of the convenience of services.

An emergi-center provides both basic and sophisticated first aid and saves the person with a health emergency a trip to an overcrowded and more expensive hospital center. People can also obtain quick care from surgi-centers. Like the emergi-center, surgi-centers provide care outside of a hospital. This type of facility focuses on minor surgical procedures. Follow-up care is often provided in the facility but can be referred elsewhere.

Follow-up care is an important part of service. Clients need to understand that further care will probably be necessary after the emergency is handled. A criticism of quick care settings is that, without the ongoing interpersonal relationship that develops between a client and a primary care provider, follow-up is difficult, and care can be fragmented. Quick care centers are more highly specialized than ambulatory care centers, whereas ambulatory care is considered more comprehensive with regard to providing multiple services.

Ambulatory Care

Ambulatory care is care provided in many settings without admitting the client to a hospital. Previously, this type of care was associated with outpatient clinics. The new ambulatory care system makes it possible to avoid the cost of hospitalization while providing more than health teaching and simple procedures. Many types of complex medical-surgical procedures that were once restricted to the hospital are now being done on an outpatient basis.

In the not-too-distant past, the majority of health care procedures were performed on an inpatient basis. Hospitals had hundreds of beds and a few outpatient clinics. Today the trend is toward fewer inpatient beds and many ambulatory care sites in the community. These sites are located where clients can reach them conveniently. They are affiliated with health care systems and, like all services, may be integrated with similar or different types of services.

Public Health Departments

Individual states protect the health of the public through the operation of public health departments. Some public health departments are restricted to illness prevention and health maintenance activities, such as pest control and nutrition programs for pregnant and newly delivered mothers. Collection of vital statistics and prevention of communicable disease (*e.g.,* sexually transmitted disease, tuberculosis) are typical responsibilities of state departments of health. In addition, some health departments provide skilled home care and specialty clinics for a variety of illnesses. The mission and scope of services for departments of health are set by the state legislature, in response to the needs of the community.

Vertical and Horizontal Integration of Services

Stand-alone health care services are a thing of the past. Current and future systems of care will rely on innovative partnerships to diversify their services and better meet the needs of the public. ***Vertical integration of services*** refers to a number of different levels of service that are related. A hospital, nursing home, clinic, and home care department may be associated to improve patient care; for example, after discharge from the hospital, the client would be referred to a specific nursing home and from there to a specific clinic for ambulatory care, while receiving help from the home care department in his or her residence. ***Horizontal integration of services*** relates to a cluster of similar services that are connected. A set of hospitals, for example, may share the costs and use of a magnetic resonance imaging machine or other ex-

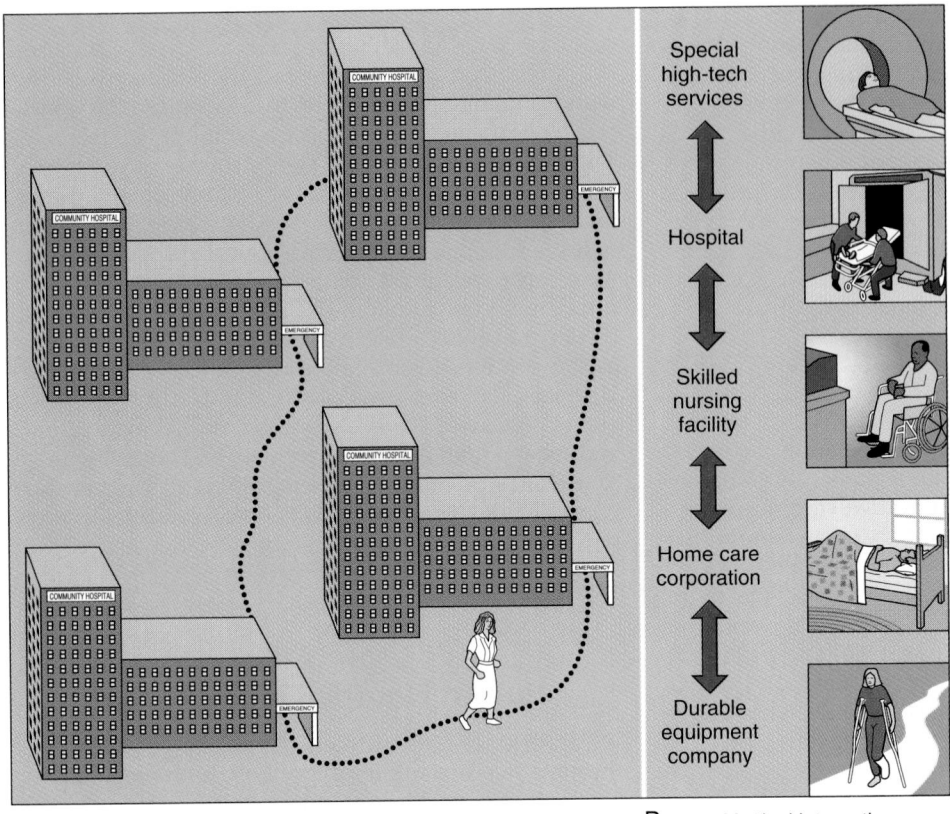

A   Horizontal integration

B   Vertical integration

✦ **Figure 5–6**
Health care services are increasingly integrated both horizontally and vertically to better meet clients' needs and to share resources efficiently.

pensive technological equipment. Figure 5–6 shows both types of integrated services.

Both methods of integration are intended to control the use of resources and the way clients are referred. This control suggests that clients will receive the care they need more efficiently. There is little debate that the use of human and material resources can be more efficient when those resources are shared. The concerns surrounding proper referral are less clear. In the event that a group of integrated health care delivery providers does not offer a service, it is unclear how clients would get the care they need. Mechanisms should be in place to ensure referral out of the system when care is not available within the system.

The fiscal viability of services is a major concern of all care delivery systems no matter how they are organized. Nurses at all levels of practice must share the concern that cost savings not be pursued at the expense of quality health care. Health care systems are undergoing reform across the country. Health care reform, once thought to be impossible without Federal legislation, is evolving spontaneously in every area of health care delivery. All aspects of the business of providing health care are being reconsidered with an eye toward how best to make improvements (Kissick, 1994) while keeping the bottom line of costs under control.

Health Care Reform and the Role of Gatekeeper Services

Three key issues in **health care reform** in this country are access to services, client participation in services, and the shifting role of gatekeeper in the care delivery system. Access to services has been most frequently discussed, but concerns about participation and gatekeeping are receiving increasing attention. Access to and participation in services are strongly affected by the kinds of care society values. American society values high-technology care that mirrors the major causes of disease. Specialized cardiac, cancer, and trauma facilities exist to provide the latest technological treatments for these diseases.

The major ethical principle that should guide all discussions of health care reform is the principle of distributive justice. Distributive justice is concerned with whether society offers health care services fairly to all its members and whether services are made available in a way in which people can participate in them. The principle of distributive justice should direct who decides who will have health care services in the United States. A basic minimum of care should be established despite some clients' ability to pay for more care. For example, basic care may be seen as hospitalization in a four-bed room, allowing clients with additional money to buy private accommodations if they want them.

Access to Services

Access to services relates primarily to whether the services are affordable, available (location), and culturally appropriate for those who need them. *Affordability* suggests that the services can be paid for without undue hardship. If a person is unable to pay for some other basic need such as food or housing because of medical bills, then the medical expenses would be considered a hardship. Some people are labeled medically indigent because they cannot afford health care services. Contemporary discussions about access to basic health care demand that basic services be provided to all (Solomon & Blacker, 1993).

Services are *available* when the person can get to them using a reasonable amount of resources, such as energy, time, and money. A person who needs services should be able to get them without undue disruption in his or her life. For example, needing to take off 2 days from work to travel 500 miles for a particular basic health service (such as a mammogram) indicates that the service is not readily available. Of course, it is expected that more obscure or highly specialized services will be available only in certain centralized locations. A client who needs the services of a specialist in cancer therapy, for example, may need to travel long distances for services. The public needs to decide what services should be available to all people, in both rural and urban settings.

Basic health care services such as immunizations and primary health care should be readily available to everyone. How the public and local, state, and Federal governments will make basic health care available to everyone is not clear. Issues of availability surface when people do not have the resources to obtain services they need. Even though services cannot be duplicated everywhere, it seems unjust when people cannot get basic services because they do not have child care, money for transportation, or knowledge of where services are located.

Another key component of access to services is their cultural acceptability, as discussed earlier in this chapter. Nurses should strive to maintain cultural competence in care delivery so that people can get the care they need in a way they can accept. Nurses who are not in advanced practice may have limited influence in the affordability and availability of services, but they have total influence over providing nursing care that is culturally sensitive.

Participation in Services

In many ways, the concept of participation in services is even more crucial than access to them. When health care systems are being developed, potential clients can provide suggestions for creating the type of services they will use. For people of orthodox Jewish belief, for instance, participation may hinge on availability of services at certain hours of the day or on certain days of the week. Single mothers may need day care services to be free to keep appointments. People with debilitating problems may need special group support services to be able to participate in care. Although it is important to see the client in the central role of decision-making, it is not always clear how to evaluate the client for the competence or ability to negotiate the care system (Berenson, 1994).

Nursing has a special responsibility to help clients participate in services. Nurses and other providers have the job of anticipating what the person will need to complete a course of treatment or stay in a program of services. It is unethical for nurses to assist a client to develop a plan of care when the client obviously will be unable to participate in the services. Common solutions to helping clients participate in care include providing assistance with transportation, making day care services available, supporting flexible hours of operation, providing language translators, and, at times, supplying basic needs like food and clothing. Nurses collaborate with other health care services and personnel to assist the client.

Control of Gatekeeping

The function of **gatekeeping** is to control who gets health care services. The action of gatekeeping refers to allowing entry into and exit from an area of care. In health care, the gatekeeper decides who will be admitted and discharged from the hospital, home care, or ambulatory care service.

The gatekeeper, once exclusively the physician and, to a lesser degree, the health care administrator, is responsible for deciding who receives health care. Although physicians and administrators will continue to hold key positions in gatekeeping, the field of players is expanding. Gatekeeping functions are now being shared with other primary care providers, such as advanced practice nurse practitioners (Madden & Ponte, 1994), and the insurance industry (Griffin, 1994). Insurance companies play an increasingly major role in identifying who will receive care because they authorize reimbursement.

Many people cannot afford to supplement their health care coverage with their own out-of-pocket money for very long. Insurance companies are becoming the primary negotiators in deciding what services will be covered by their clients' health care plans. Nurses educated for advanced practice roles, such as clinical nurse specialists, nurse midwives, nurse practitioners, and nurse anesthetists, are increasingly assuming roles that require the provision of high-quality care at a reasonable cost.

The list of gatekeepers is growing; the trend is movement away from one provider and toward decision-making care teams. Shared gatekeeping means that many people are involved in how resources are allocated. The role of the consumer in making health care decisions is assuming priority and should expand even more in the future (Bradley, 1992; Faherty, 1993; National League for Nursing, 1990).

Economics of Health and Illness

The *economics of health and illness* relate to the cost of health care and how we make health care fiscal decisions. Health expenditures represent over 13% of the gross domestic product of the United States. Private health care costs, paid for by consumers, represent about 52% of costs. The government or public sector pays for approximately 44% of health care. Nonpatient revenues pay for a little more than 4% of costs (US Bureau of the Census, 1993). Sixty-five percent of consumers rely on insurance to pay for their health care. Thirty-five percent of Americans have to pay out of pocket for health care because they do not have sufficient insurance (US Bureau of the Census, 1993). The United States pays more than any other country for a system of health care that offers no care or limited care for millions of people.

Because of the expense of the current health care system, people often wait until they are ill before seeing a physician or other primary care provider. Although it is cheaper not to seek care initially, it is more expensive in the long run to treat an illness after it has begun. Many people do not have the money to get care early in the course of an illness when complications could be avoided. These people come into the health care system gravely ill, with multiple, complex physiologic, emotional, cultural, and spiritual needs.

Part of the reason that health care in this country is so expensive is that it began as a fee-for-service system. People paid for services either individually or through insurance. The more services that were needed, the higher the cost grew. The debate about what services were really necessary never occurred because whatever care people received was reimbursed. The rapidly developing high-technology market of drugs and equipment has become too expensive for most to afford, but people expect this care to be available for them when they become sick.

Many Americans (an estimated 14% of the population) are not covered by health insurance at all. Although uninsured individuals and families can be of any race, income, level of education, and age, the most vulnerable people are men or women who are African-American, have less than 12 years of education, are unemployed, are between 18 and 24 years of age, and are from households with an income below $20,000 (US Bureau of the Census, 1993). Although the profile of the typical uninsured or underinsured person may change over time, the impact of this group on the health care system will always be of concern. Often the only avenue for care for this group has been the public, municipal hospital system, and in many locations services at such hospitals are being severely reduced.

People who do not have the disposable income to purchase health care services because they are unemployed or uninsured often use health care services inappropriately. They may use public hospital emergency departments for their primary medical care. However, because of the nature of emergency departments, they do not obtain preventive care there; instead, they go to the emergency department only when they are quite ill.

Clients who delay care often need more resources than if they had been treated earlier for their health care problem. Clients who cannot afford to enter the health care system earlier cost the overall system more when they finally get the care they need—if it is not too late to be effective. The nursing profession needs to support the reexamination of economic trends while making sure people get the nursing care that they need (Baer & Gordon, 1994). All nursing care needs to be rendered with an eye toward fiscal responsibility and just provision of care. Nurses need to be active in the fiscal affairs of health care delivery (Barnum, 1994).

Managed Care

Managed care is an ongoing attempt to meet the health care needs of groups of people in cost-effective ways. A hallmark of managed care is the prevention of illness or at least the prevention of complications. Because the resources needed to keep people well or to minimize the morbidity of illness are much less than those needed to treat a full-blown illness, a certain amount of resources is preallocated for preventive health care. Care is provided within these limits. The cornerstone of managed care is quality assurance. Making sure that an expected outcome occurs in the best interest of the client suggests that quality services have been provided. Managed care occurs efficiently and safely when services are appropriate, are provided in a cost-efficient way, and result in the desired health-related outcomes (Eckholm, 1995; Kongstvedt, 1993; Shapiro & Blyweiss, 1994).

An example of how managed care works is evident in the following case study on Mrs. Luchias, who is confused and unable to take her medication properly. Mrs. Luchias needs someone to assist her at home or someone to create a system that will provide care for her if she cannot care for herself. The nurses who have been caring for her are aware that sending Mrs. Luchias home into an unsafe environment would constitute a negligent act. The nurses understand that a simple intervention may enable her to go home.

Mrs. Luchias Is Not Ready for Discharge

Mrs. Luchias is unable to be discharged from the hospital because she is unable to take her prescribed medication (for a pulmonary infection) by herself. She does not have any family members to assist her at home. Because Mrs. Luchias is essentially well otherwise, the hospital nursing staff set up a phone support service with Mrs. Luchias and the home care department.

The plan is for a volunteer from the home care agency to call Mrs. Luchias to remind her when to take her medication. The public health nurse makes an evaluation and determines that the phone support intervention is sufficient to maintain the plan for Mrs. Luchias to stay at home. Mrs. Luchias' need for a home health aide is decreased to 4 hours every other week to escort her to ambulatory care visits with her primary care nurse practitioner.

In this scenario, Mrs. Luchias was able to go home from the hospital 2 days earlier because of the appropriate, efficient, and effective nursing intervention. Her care was managed in a way that took into consideration concerns of cost-effectiveness and quality of care and safety. If Mrs. Luchias' needs had been different, the proper nursing intervention would have been to keep her in the hospital.

Managed care sometimes demands an individualized approach to care, although a certain standard of care should be appropriate for a number of clients. The role of the nurse in managed care is to make care decisions that are in the client's best interest.

Effective managed care situations may provide a number of different plans of action in the event that changes in the client's needs or available resources occur. In Mrs. Luchias' situation, the nurse was able to set up three action plans. The first plan was the previously described phone follow-up program conducted by the agency. In the event that the nurse was unable to continue with the first plan, the second plan consisted of daily contact from a neighbor and the rabbi from Mrs. Luchias' synagogue. The third plan was established when Mrs. Luchias said she was willing to pay for a private phone answering/message company to call her to remind her to take her medication.

The success in treating Mrs. Luchias leads the nursing staff to consider implementing this approach to care with a larger aggregate of people who are like Mrs. Luchias. The principles of the phone follow-up program now become part of the discharge plan of many other clients. The cluster or aggregate of clients like Mrs. Luchias will receive the same level of care, with individual evaluation of results. Cost savings can be predicted because many people will get the same level of care. Staff will be able to make better use of their resources and pay closer attention to how their chosen intervention works with individual people. A cluster of clients will be managed in the same way without neglecting their individual needs.

Identification of patterns in care delivery has generated care delivery protocols called care maps or standard plans of care (Fig. 5–7). The idea is to identify a list of activities that reflect a typical course for an illness or condition. Care providers follow the standard plan and assume that care will be delivered more efficiently and cost-effectively. The only problem with this approach surfaces when a client does not respond like the average client. When using care maps, nurses must be aware that they are responsible for providing care according to the individual needs of the client—not a predetermined recipe of care. If the care map does not meet the client's nursing care needs, it should not be used.

Expense of High-Technology and Low-Technology Care

Generally speaking, the higher the technology used in health care, the higher the cost. A teaching project to prevent hypertension, which can be considered a low-technology intervention, costs less than medication required to treat the disease or surgery that would follow a cerebrovascular accident. No one denies the importance of low-technology care like prevention activities, but these options are often seen as less urgent than high-technology care, especially if one cannot afford both types of care.

Nursing has always been in the vanguard concerning its contribution to low-technology care. The image of the nurse caring for a sick person with little more than a comforting touch is the archetypal symbol of low-technology care. The advent of the technological revolution in health care has changed the expectations of both clients and professionals about the type of care that people need.

Like many other health care professionals, nurses have been seduced by the glamor of high technology. For some, it seems that nothing significant is done for the client unless a machine is used. For example, a client often would not want a practitioner to use his or her intuitive skill to suggest that an upset stomach is due to work-related stress. Many clients link a "reliable" and accurate diagnosis with findings from a technological process, such as results from an upper gastrointestinal roentgenogram. Therefore, high-technology interventions are usually included when making a diagnosis.

It is important for nurses to accept some responsibility for the current fascination with high-technology nursing and medical care. In part, high technology helps to secure nurses' position in the care delivery setting. More than 80% of nurses work in hospitals, where high-technology flourishes (National League for Nursing, 1994). Unfortunately, some health care administrators do not see nursing as essential for the delivery of high-technology care and feel that nurses

The Long Island College Hospital
MULTIDISCIPLINARY ACTION PLAN

DAY 1

MD: _____

DIAGNOSIS: Neonatal Sepsis
(34 weeks to full term)

DATE: _____

PATIENT PROBLEM AND NURSING INTERVENTION	EXPECTED PATIENT OUTCOME AND/OR DISCHARGE OUTCOME	ASSESSMENT/EVALUATION*		
1. THERMOREGULATION	1. STABLE THERMOREGULATION			
A. Place under radiant warmer with ISC	A. Maintain warmth	A.	A.	A.
B. Record axillary temperature q 30 minutes until stable, then q 8; report temperature >100°F or <97°F	B. Temperature stable	B.	B.	B.
C. Give sponge bath when axillary temperature stabilizes at >98°F	C. Axillary temperature stable, bath given	C.	C.	C.
D. Transfer to incubator when temperature stabilizes at >98°F and work-up is complete	D. Transfered to incubator	D.	D.	D.
E. Neutral thermic range for infant is WNL See chart	E. Temperature within range	E.	E.	E.

* If the expected patient outcome is observed, the nurse signs his or her name in the assessment column. If the outcome is not observed, the nurse signs with an asterisk (*) and describes the outcome in the progress notes. The three assessment columns represent the three 8-hour shifts.

❥ **Figure 5–7**
Portion of a standard plan of care for newborn with neonatal sepsis. Care maps, or standard plans of care, are increasingly used to ensure that care is delivered efficiently and cost-effectively while not neglecting any client's individual needs. (ISC=infant servo-control [radiant warmer]; WNL=within normal limits.)

are too expensive to be cost-effective care providers in these settings.

In the interests of cost containment, some nurses are being replaced by cheaper, unlicensed technicians who complete discrete tasks at a lower cost. One technician may be responsible for several tasks, such as taking vital signs, completing an intake and output sheet, running electrocardiograms, and bathing clients. Although nurses are resisting this trend, it is occurring, and it is not clear what impact the proliferation of technological workers will have on nursing. It does appear, though, that hospitals will look to the nurse to supervise the care provided by unlicensed assistive personnel.

The use of skilled technicians in the clinical area has been the norm in military nursing, where one nurse may supervise many medics or corpsmen. If this is the future of professional nursing, then nursing will evolve into a more administrative role, at least in the acute care hospital setting. The future of direct patient care by nurses may well be in community-based care, where a greater number of less acutely ill clients will receive care. However, nurses do need to respond

flexibly to health care trends so they can be players in health care decisions (Porter-O'Grady, 1994).

Multiple-Tier Systems of Care

A system in which all people have access to and could participate in the same level of health care would be considered a one-tier system. In many societies, however, **multiple-tier systems of care** exist (although they may be an unpopular topic of discussion). Different levels of care have sometimes been established, based on gender, race, ability to pay, or other reasons. Multiple-tier systems indicate that ethical problems may exist in the way that care is being delivered. In America, many levels of care exist, although some people deny that this is so. Variable care options exist because some clients are unable to pay for certain services or because of discrepancies in the services that are available to clients in, say, urban versus rural settings.

For some people, the level of care that they receive is related to their ability to pay. Basic services may be available to all people, while specialized services may be available only to the few who can pay extra. One example of this is in the field of plastic or reconstructive surgery. Resetting a facial fracture after a car accident would be seen as an essential service for anyone who experienced this injury. Cosmetic surgery to enhance beauty, on the other hand, would probably be restricted to people who could afford to pay for it. In this example, both levels of care service are not (and would not) be available to all. Although it may be unfortunate, it is not considered unethical to restrict people with less money from undergoing procedures to improve their beauty.

Sometimes, however, the differences in levels of care raise serious ethical concerns. For instance, insurance policies often state where a client can go for hospitalization, but different hospitals may provide different levels of care. For discussion purposes, consider that there is a way to rate Hospital A and Hospital B according to the differences in the skill of their nursing staffs. Hospital A has well-educated nurses who are certified in their specialties and work hard to make sure that the nursing assistants complete their tasks carefully. In client surveys, 98% of clients rate their nurses as very good to excellent. Hospital A is located in an inner-city area and serves mainly people without insurance. Hospital B has nurses who do not attend continuing education classes, who are not certified, and who do not take their supervision responsibilities seriously. Only 24% of clients in this hospital find the nursing care to be very good to excellent. Hospital B is located in an affluent suburb of the city and is the designated hospital for many private hospital insurance plans.

In this example, better nursing care can be found at Hospital A. The differences in levels of nursing care are related to the expertise of the professional staff— not the client's ability to pay. Whatever causes the development of different levels of care, the nurse should make sure that basic care is provided in a safe and comprehensive way.

Professional associations like the American Nurses Association and the National League for Nursing set standards for the profession and provide the public with information about what level of nursing care to expect. Consumer ratings of services, publication of accreditation reports, and release of client satisfaction surveys are ways to assure high standards of performance for nursing and other professional groups in every health care setting.

Overt Versus Covert Rationing of Health Care Services

The fact that health care services are rationed is denied by many care providers or is at least thought to be a recent development. In fact, health care services have been rationed since the beginning of care delivery. Whenever the need for services is greater than the availability of services, rationing occurs. The fear that rationing might be life threatening makes the topic unpopular and controversial. Although not every act of rationing is life threatening, the act of rationing can have a great impact on the person's ability to get health needs met.

The rationing of preventive services may not appear to be life threatening when it occurs, so the public might easily tolerate the rationing. With this type of rationing (covert rationing), it takes months, or even years, for effects to be seen. A good example of covert rationing is reduction of funding to prevent cigarette smoking. The savings are obvious and immediate; however, years later, those who began smoking or who did not quit, as well as those in the environment who suffered from second-hand smoke, will show the effects in lung disease and cancer.

Overt rationing is a clear and more immediate type of rationing. Less health care teaching about sexually transmitted diseases in poor neighborhoods results in a rapid rise in venereal disease rates. Less police protection in various areas of a city can be linked immediately to changes in crime statistics. What is most important from a nursing perspective is for people to understand that obvious and disguised forms of rationing both occur and that they often have more serious consequences for vulnerable populations. Nurses have an ethical duty to protest if rationing of health care puts clients in danger.

Continuity of Care

Continuity of care is a way of providing clinical quality management. Appropriateness of care, efficiency of services, and effectiveness of interventions are all monitored in the process of addressing continuity of care (Connors, 1992). Continuity of care monitors services to decrease duplication (Goodwin, 1994). Ensuring that care is provided without interruption is also a way to conserve resources. The following example reflects how continuity of care assists with resource management.

CASE STUDY | **Ms. Daret Receives Continuous Care**

Ms. Daret has been sent home from the hospital following foot surgery. The nurse visits her daily for dressing changes until the wound has almost healed. Although the nursing visits are no longer necessary, Ms. Daret's nurse calls her every 2 weeks to assess her condition. During one phone call, the nurse notices that Ms. Daret sounds confused. After contacting her physician, the nurse visits Ms. Daret and discovers that the client has low blood sugar. After immediate health-related teaching, Ms. Daret agrees to see her physician monthly for blood glucose analysis. After two such office appointments, the nurse makes monthly home visits for 4 months.

Ms. Daret receives continuous care although the intensity of care changes. Sometimes she needs to see the nurse daily; other times she needs to see her physician monthly. The health care team members adjust the type and level of service provided to the needs of Ms. Daret. At times, client needs and provider services fluctuate. Continuity of care means that although the need for services varies, the supervision to be sure services are adequate is maintained (Holzemer *et al.,* 1995).

CASE STUDY **Mr. Ferguson Uses Care Facilities Improperly**

Mr. Ferguson has foot surgery and is discharged home after arrangements are made with the visiting nurse service for dressing changes. After the wound is healed, services are discontinued. Mr. Ferguson becomes confused one day, falls outside the home, and cuts his foot. He decides not to call his doctor or nurse unless the wound becomes infected. A week later, Mr. Ferguson goes to the local emergency department because his foot is red, warm, and very tender. He is admitted to the hospital with a generalized infection.

In this scenario, Mr. Ferguson and the health care team members who care for him did not approach his care from a perspective that reflected continuity of care. Although not every accident or problem can be prevented, a closer relationship between the care providers and Mr. Ferguson may have allowed for better communication and better use of services. The use of services in a continuous way might have prevented the infection that led to hospitalization. If a friendly visitor program or a phone assessment project had been in place, Mr. Ferguson's care would have remained continuous.

The care provider and the client may not always carry an equal level of responsibility for continuity of care (Rheaume *et al.,* 1994). Clients who are unfamiliar with health care services and procedures need frequent teaching, support, and encouragement. A critical component of continuity of care includes an ongoing assessment by the nurse of how the client is coping with his or her role and responsibilities. Nurses and other providers must always be thinking about how best to reach clients with unusual problems in their care. A seamless continuum of care should be the goal of both the client and the nurse (Boston, 1994).

Continuity of care is closely associated with the concept of risk management. Risk management identifies patterns of problems and relies on early intervention to resolve them. When the nurse is in a continuous relationship with the client, the nurse will see potential problems quickly and can attempt to resolve them immediately. If the nurse can keep the nurse-client relationship in a state of continuous evaluation, any physical, psychosocial, or spiritual problems that

do develop can be managed more quickly and effectively (Bishop & Scudder, 1990; Boykin & Schoenhofer, 1993; Gordon, 1994).

Future Directions in Health Care Delivery and Work Reengineering

If the changes in health care delivery in the past 20 years have provided a lesson, it may well be that we must reconsider our rigid adherence to professional roles and boundaries. All care debates have been reduced to an informed discussion about what the client realistically needs and who can safely provide those services.

Care providers no longer ask whether the client has a legitimate voice in making health care decisions. Care providers and recipients share decision-making responsibility, except in the rarest of situations. Children, people with mental health disruptions, and those under the influence of drugs that impair their judgment are among those who need someone else to make their health care choices. People who are able to make decisions are asked to designate a health care proxy in the event that their ability to decide becomes diminished.

Many health care managers predict future trends in the industry with varying degrees of success. Without the aid of a crystal ball, guesswork may well be useless. Instead of guessing, nurses should adopt a proactive strategy of preparing for whatever future trends in health care occur (Fauk & Bower, 1994; Langfitt, 1991). Engaging in the health care political arena and observing for changes can usually alert the professional to change as it unfolds. Nursing must simultaneously participate in the changing scope of practice while protecting its professional integrity (National League for Nursing, 1994; Sherer, 1994). Figure 5–8 suggests one way to recognize the signs of change in the health care system.

Contemporary standards of practice should address current health and illness trends as they relate to the role of the nurse (American Nurses Association, 1991). When new or recurring health problems are identified, the process of adapting the health care system to those problems begins. Using a process similar to the nursing process, the health care community performs assessment, makes a diagnosis, constructs a plan, implements it, and evaluates what was done to resolve the problem. Based on the evaluation, the standards of practice may then be redefined. Therefore, standards of practice evolve continuously, rather than remaining static or fixed.

The meaning of health will continue to unfold as people come to view themselves as part of a changing society trying to stay well (Riley, 1994). Nurses will remain key players in the maintenance of health so

Methods to prepare for future trends in health care

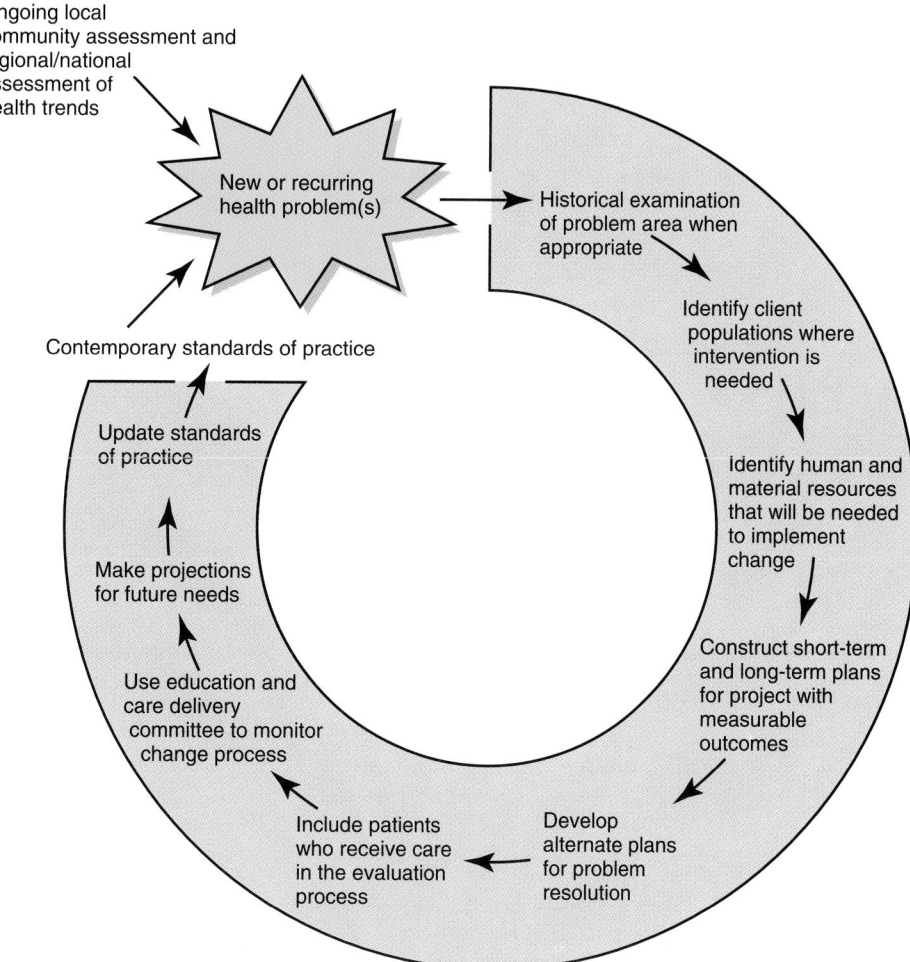

♪ Figure 5–8
Anticipating, preparing for, and participating in changes in health care systems are ongoing responsibilities of nursing as a profession.

long as they cooperate with other team members, stay flexible in work situations, and continuously educate themselves for a changing future in health care (Curtin, 1994; deTornyay, 1992, 1993; Porter-O'Grady, 1994) in health care. Nurses must actively pursue ongoing education to secure their position in a rapidly unfolding, economically volatile health care system (Dessau & Fischbuch, 1992; Oermann, 1994; Taylor *et al.*, 1994). As the needs of the health care system change, so will the educational needs of the nurse.

Summary

Health care systems are changing in the United States, and nurses, like other health care providers, are concerned about their place in the evolving systems of care. In the past, care was usually delivered in centralized places, with a few key people deciding what care was to be delivered. Today, care is provided in multiple, decentralized settings by various personnel. In nursing, advanced practice professionals are making

more and more decisions about what care people will receive.

People have their own ways of understanding the meaning of health and illness, and nurses must be respectful of cultural beliefs in providing appropriate health care services. Helping people to participate in their care, in a cost-effective way, involves making services accessible and available when the client needs them, not when the provider wants to provide them. Nursing is in a position of increasing influence in helping clients to make their health care needs known.

CHAPTER HIGHLIGHTS
✦

✦ The personal meaning of health and illness is different for everyone; although there are similarities among cultures and groups, it is important for the nurse to appreciate and try to comprehend the various ways in which people think about and act in relation to health and illness and to respond with therapeutic nursing interventions.

✦ Thoughts about health and illness have generated models for understanding these concepts. The health-illness continuum, levels of prevention, high-level wellness, and the holistic model of health are examples of some of these concepts.

✦ Today, nursing generally approaches the concepts of health and illness from a holistic perspective; nurses are concerned with both objective and subjective signs of health and illness for the body, mind, and spirit.

✦ Concepts of health and illness are also a reflection of how resources are allocated; debate is ongoing about the needs of the individual versus the needs of society. Cultural awareness is key to meeting the needs of clients; culture influences how clients get their health care needs met.

✦ Health care is provided in many settings; the nurse is responsible for assessing these sites for safety, availability of caregivers, and the ability to move the client into and out of care systems as necessary. Health care services are often integrated in vertical or horizontal systems to decrease cost and provide for smooth referral.

✦ Health care reform is occurring throughout the United States; key aspects of reform relate to access to care, ability to participate in care, and control over gatekeeping (deciding who will get care).

✦ The economics of health care have led to the development of many systems to decrease costs; managed care is a system that tries to combine cost containment with quality of care. The appropriateness of using high-technology versus low-technology care is a concern in managed care because it is sometimes not clear which interventions are best.

✦ A multitier system of care exists in America and is complicated by the rationing of health care resources; the only way a multitier system of care can function ethically is for all basic services to be made available to all who need them; the existence of overt and covert rationing of resources suggests that problems exist in how resources are provided to the public.

✦ Continuity of care suggests that the care clients need will be available to them; their needs are continuously being assessed for either an increase or a decrease in the level of services required.

✦ Although the future of health care is uncertain, nurses must be ready to adapt to change. Nursing's future depends on how well it will reeducate its practitioners, educators, and teachers for the future.

Study Questions

1. The most important step for the nurse to remember when discussing health and illness concerns with the client is to
   a. ask the family of the client to define concepts of health and illness
   b. validate the meaning of health-related concepts with the client
   c. search the literature for recent definitions of health and illness
   d. use the interpretation of health-related concepts found in the hospital mission statement

2. Frequently, the needs of the individual compete with the needs of society because
   a. not enough resources are available to meet every need
   b. some people have unreasonable needs
   c. no resources exist that could improve health outcomes
   d. most individuals cannot identify what they need

3. The primary reason that various settings exist to provide health care is that
   a. health care planners prefer multiple sites to attract clients to services
   b. government public health laws require options in service location
   c. people have changing needs for health care services
   d. nurses and physicians prefer certain settings over other settings for care delivery

4. The major conflict in the ongoing health care reform is between the concepts of
   a. justice and distribution of services
   b. professional autonomy and payment for services
   c. state licensure and management of outcomes
   d. cost and quality of care

5. Continuity of care means that services will be administered
   a. in a way that guarantees reimbursement
   b. at the same intensity without interruption
   c. according to a predetermined plan
   d. as they are necessary

Critical Thinking Exercises

1. Mrs. G. comes to the clinic complaining of chest pain on exertion. She is overweight and does not exercise. She is a single mother of two children, ages 19 and 17 years. She has not had a Papanicolaou smear in 10 years and does not perform breast self-examination. Discuss the primary and secondary nursing care you would give Mrs. G.

2. Health care reform affects access, ability to participate, and who will receive health care. Discuss the factors in your community that affect those three aspects of care.

References

American Nurses Association. (1991). *Standards of clinical nursing practice.* Kansas City, MO: American Nurses Association.
Andrews, M. M., & Boyle, J. S. (1995). *Transcultural concepts in nursing care.* Philadelphia: J. B. Lippincott.

Ardell, D. B. (1977). *High-level wellness: An alternative to doctors, drugs and disease*. Emmaus, PA: Rodale Press.

Baer, E. D., & Gordon, S. (1994). Money managers are unraveling the tapestry of nursing. *American Journal of Nursing, 94* (10), 38–40.

Barnum, B. S. (1994). Realities in nursing practice: A strategic view. *Nursing & Health Care, 15,* 400–405.

Berenson, R. A. (1994). Can a managed care market work? *Postgraduate Medicine, 96* (4), 55–57.

Bishop, A. H., & Scudder, J. R. (1991). *Nursing: The practice of caring*. New York: National League for Nursing Press.

Bishop, A. H., & Scudder, J. R. (1990). *The practical, moral, and personal sense of nursing*. Albany, NY: State University of New York Press.

Boston, C. (1994). If it ain't broke . . . break it! *Journal of Nursing Administration, 24* (1), 16–17.

Boykin, A., & Schoenhofer, S. (1993). *Nursing as caring: A model for transforming practice*. New York: National League for Nursing Press.

Bradley, V. (1992). Healthy America: Practitioners for 2005. *Journal of Emergency Nursing, 18,* 365–367.

Brody, E. M. (1994). Women as unpaid caregivers: The price they pay. In E. Friedman (Ed.), *An unfinished revolution: Women and health care in America*. New York: United Hospital Fund.

Callahan, D. (1990). *What kind of life: The limits of medical progress*. New York: Simon & Schuster.

Callahan, C. M., Rivara, F. P., & Koepsell, T. D. (1994). Money for guns: Evaluation of the Seattle gun buy-back program. *Public Health Reports, 109,* 472–477.

Carroll, M., Cheek, J. E., & Craig, A. (1994). Hantavirus pulmonary syndrome: Interim guidelines for health care providers. *The IHS Primary Care Provider, 19* (4), 61–65.

Centers for Disease Control and Prevention (1993). *Surgeon General's report to the American public on HIV infection and AIDS*. Washington, DC: Centers for Disease Control and Prevention.

Ceslowitz, S. B. (1993). Managed care: Controlling costs and changing practice. *Med-Surg Nursing, 2* (5), 359–366.

Connors, H. R. (1992). Case management: Within and beyond the walls. In National League for Nursing. *Perspectives in nursing 1991–1993* (pp. 113–120). New York: National League for Nursing Press.

Curtin, L. L. (1994). Learning from the future. *Nursing Management, 25* (1), 7–9.

Dee-Kelly, P. A., Heller, S., & Sibley, M. (1994). Managed care: An opportunity for home care agencies. *Nursing Clinics of North America, 29,* 471–481.

Dellasega, C., Dansky, K., King, L., & Stricklin, M. L. (1994). Use of home health services by elderly persons with cognitive impairment. *The Journal of Nursing Administration, 24* (6), 20–25.

Dessau, L., & Fischbuch, M. (1992). *Academic health centers & the community: A practical guide for creating shared visions*. Hamilton, Ontario, Canada: Dixon Desktop Publishing.

deTornyay, R. (1992). Reconsidering nursing education: The report of the Pew Health Professions Commission. *Journal of Nursing Education, 31,* 296–301.

deTornyay, R. (1993). Nursing education: Staying on track. *Nursing & Health Care, 14* (6), 302–306.

Dolan, J. A. (1978). *Nursing in society: A historical perspective*. Philadelphia: W. B. Saunders.

Eckholm, E. (1995, January 29). A hospital copes with the new order. *The New York Times,* section 3, pp. 1, 7.

Faherty, B. (1993). Now is the time to advocate. *Nursing Outlook, 41* (6), 248–249.

Fauk, C. D., & Bower, K. A. (1994). Managing care across department, organization, and setting boundaries. In K. Kelly (Ed.), *Health care rationing: Dilemma and paradox* (pp. 161–176). St. Louis: C. V. Mosby.

Friedman, E. (Ed.). (1994). *An unfinished revolution: Women and health care in America*. New York: United Hospital Fund.

Geissler, E. M. (1994). *Pocket guide to cultural assessment*. St. Louis: Mosby-Year Book.

Goodwin, D. R. (1994). Nursing care management activities: How they differ between employment settings. *The Journal of Nursing Administration, 24* (2), 29–34.

Gordon, S. (1994, June). Inside the patient-driven system. *Critical Care Nurse* (Suppl). 3–6, 8, 10, 14–28.

Griffin, G. C. (1994). "We don't have a healthcare crisis in this country" . . . yet. *Postgraduate Medicine, 94* (3), 15–16, 23–25.

Healthy America: Practitioners for 2005. (1992). *Journal of Allied Health, 21* (4), 3–22.

Holzemer, S. P., Rothenberg, R., & Fish, C. (1995). Continuity of care. In P. Kelly, S. Holman, R. Rothenberg, & S. P. Holzemer (Eds.), *Primary care of women and children with HIV infection: A multidisciplinary approach*. Boston: Jones and Bartlett.

Kalisch, P. A., & Kalisch, B. J. (1986). *The advance of American nursing* (2nd ed.). Boston: Little, Brown & Co.

Kissick, W. L. (1994). Fix the healthcare system without making it worse. *Postgraduate Medicine, 95* (7), 71–74.

Kongstvedt, P. R. (1993). *The managed health care handbook* (2nd ed.). Gaithersburg, MD: Aspen Publishers.

Langfitt, T. W. (1991). *Healthy America: Practitioners for 2005*. Durham, NC: The Pew Health Professions Commission.

Leavell, H. R., & Clark, E. G. (1965). *Preventive medicine for the doctor in his community* (3rd ed.). New York: McGraw-Hill.

Madden, M. J., & Ponte, P. R. (1994). Advanced practice roles in the managed care environment. *The Journal of Nursing Administration, 24* (1), 56–62.

Martin, J. P., Hughes, A. M., & Franks, P. (Eds.). (1990). *AIDS home care and hospice manual* (2nd ed.). San Francisco: Visiting Nurses and Hospice of San Francisco.

National League for Nursing. (1994). *1994 nursing data review*. New York: National League for Nursing Press.

National League for Nursing. (1990). *Position statement: Consumer access to nursing services*. New York: National League for Nursing Press.

O'Donnell, K. P., & Sampson, E. M. (1994). Home health care: The pivotal link in the creation of a new health care delivery system. *Journal of Health Care Finance, 21* (2), 86.

Oermann, M. (1994). Reforming nursing education for future practice. *Journal of Nursing Education, 33* (5), 215–219.

Pan American Health Organization. (1994). Strengthening the health infrastructure through disease control: The polio eradication study. *Bulletin of the Pan American Health Organization, 28* (3), 277–279.

Porter-O'Grady, T. (1994). Working with consultants on a redesign. *American Journal of Nursing, 94* (10), 33–37.

Rabkin, J., Remien, R., & Wilson, C. (1994). *Good doctors & good patients: Partners in HIV treatment*. New York: NCM Publishers.

Rheaume, A., Frisch, S., Smith, A., & Kennedy, C. (1994). Case management and nursing practice. *Journal of Nursing Administration, 24* (3), 30–36.

Riley, M. W. (1994). Changing lines and changing social structures: Common concerns of social science and public health. *American Journal of Public Health, 84* (8), 1214–1217.

Shapiro, E., & Blyweiss, D. J. (1994). Making managed care work for you. *Postgraduate Medicine, 95* (3), 67–70, 75.

Sherer, J. L. (1994). Job shifts. *Hospitals & Health Networks, 68* (19), 64, 66, 68.

Smith, G. R. (1994). Power and health care reform. *Journal of Nursing Education, 33* (5), 194–196.

Smith, S. S. (1994). Outpatient care surveyed. *Public Health Reports, 108,* 592–593.

Solomon, J. E., & Blacker, R. A. (1993, October). The road to reform: Clinton's health care proposal. *Health Care Law Newsletter,* 1–12.

Spector, R. E. (1991). *Cultural diversity in health and illness* (3rd ed.). Norwalk, CT: Appleton & Lange.

Stein, R. E., Bauman, L. J., & Jessop, D. J. (1994). Women as formal and informal caregivers of children. In E. Friedman (Ed.), *An unfinished revolution: Women and health care in America.* New York: United Hospital Fund.

Stockhausen, L. J. (1994). Clinical strategies for health promotion. *Journal of Nursing Education, 33* (5), 232–235.

Taylor, T. E., Barrick, C. B., & Harrell, F. H. (1994). Preparing students for health care reform: An innovative approach for teaching leadership/management. *Journal of Nursing Education, 33* (5), 230–232.

Thomas, R. R. (1991). *Beyond race and gender: Unleashing the power of your total work force by managing diversity.* New York: American Management Association.

US Bureau of the Census. (1993). *Statistical abstract of the United States* (113th ed.). Washington, DC: US Bureau of the Census.

US Department of Health and Human Services. (1995). *Prevention '93/'94: Federal programs and progress.* Washington, DC: US Government Printing Office.

Wright, J., Henry, S. B., Holzemer, W. L., & Falknor, P. (1993). Evaluation of community-based nurse case management activities for symptomatic HIV/AIDS clients. *Journal of the Association of Nurses in AIDS Care, 4* (2), 37–47.

Yu, M. (1994). Gene therapy for HIV/AIDS. *The AIDS Reader, 4* (5), 145–148.

Bibliography

American Association of Colleges of Nursing. (1995). *A model for differentiated nursing practice.* Washington, DC: American Association of Colleges of Nursing.

American Nurses Association. (1995). *The ANA basic guide to safe delegation.* Washington, DC: American Nurses Association.

Anderson, E. T., & McFarlane, J. M. (1996). *Community as partner: Theory and practice in nursing* (2nd ed.). Philadelphia: J. B. Lippincott.

Bullough, V. L., & Bullough, B. (1984). *History, trends, and politics of nursing.* Norwalk, CT: Appleton-Century-Crofts.

Cohen, E. L. (1996). *Nurse case management in the 21st century.* Philadelphia: C. V. Mosby.

Cohen, E. L., & Cesta, T. G. (1993). *Nursing case management: From concept to evaluation.* Philadelphia: C. V. Mosby.

Holman, S., Sorin, M. D., Crossette, J., & LaChance-McCullough, M. L. (1994). A state program for postpartum HIV counseling and testing. *Public Health Reports, 109,* 521–529.

Holzemer, S. P. (1995). CCHS confronts issues in community-based and managed care. *NLN Update, 1* (1), 5.

National Association of County Health Officials. (1993). *Core public health functions.* Washington, DC: National Association of County Health Officials.

National League for Nursing. (1993). *A vision for nursing education.* New York: National League for Nursing Press.

Newell, M. (1996). *Using nursing case management to improve health outcomes.* Gaithersburg, MD: Aspen Publications.

Pew Health Professions Commission. (1993). *Contemporary issues of health professions education and workforce reform.* San Francisco: Pew Health Professions Commission.

Pew Health Professions Commission, California Primary Care Consortium. (1995). *Interdisciplinary collaborative teams in primary care: A model curriculum and resource guide.* San Francisco: Pew Health Professions Commission.

Rawnsley, M. (1990). Of human bonding: The context of nursing as caring. *Advances in Nursing Science, 13* (1), 41–48.

Reinhardt, U. E. (1996). Economics. *Journal of the American Medical Association, 275* (23), 1802–1804.

Schaef, A. W., & Fassel, D. (1988). *The addictive organization.* San Francisco: Harper.

US Department of Health and Human Services. (1994). *Clinician's handbook of preventive services.* Washington, DC: US Government Printing Office.

US Public Health Service. (December 1994, January 1995). *Prevention report.* Washington, DC: US Public Health Service.

Williams, A., & Wold, J. L. (1996). Healthcare for the future: Caring for populations in alternative settings. *Nurse Educator, 21* (2), 23–26.

Zwerdling, M. (1994). The health care delivery system in the year 2000: Nursing care for the societal client. *Nursing & Health Care, 15,* 422–424.

Chapter 6

STRESS AND ADAPTATION

ESPERANZA VILLANUEVA
JOYCE, EdD, RN

DOROTHY M. LANUZA, PhD,
RN, FAAN

PATRICIA E. KIZILAY, EdD, RN,
CS, FNP

KEY TERMS

✦

adaptation
anxiety
autonomic nervous
    system
biofeedback
burnout
coping
crisis
cultural adaptation
feedback
homeostasis
homeostatic
    mechanisms
maturational crisis

negative feedback
overshoot
physiological
    homeostasis
positive feedback
psychological
    homeostasis
set point
situational crisis
social adaptation
stress
stress responses
stressors

LEARNING OBJECTIVES

✦

After studying this chapter, you should be able to

✦ Distinguish between stressors and stress responses

✦ Describe the concept of adaptation

✦ Discuss the concept of stress

✦ Discuss the nursing diagnoses appropriate for the anxious person

✦ Discuss planning for the person experiencing stress

✦ Describe nursing interventions useful for the person in stress

✦ Discuss crisis intervention

✦ State how to evaluate the management of stress

✦ Discuss the implications of stress, adaptation, and crisis for nurses

✦ Define the concept of homeostasis

✦ Explain biofeedback

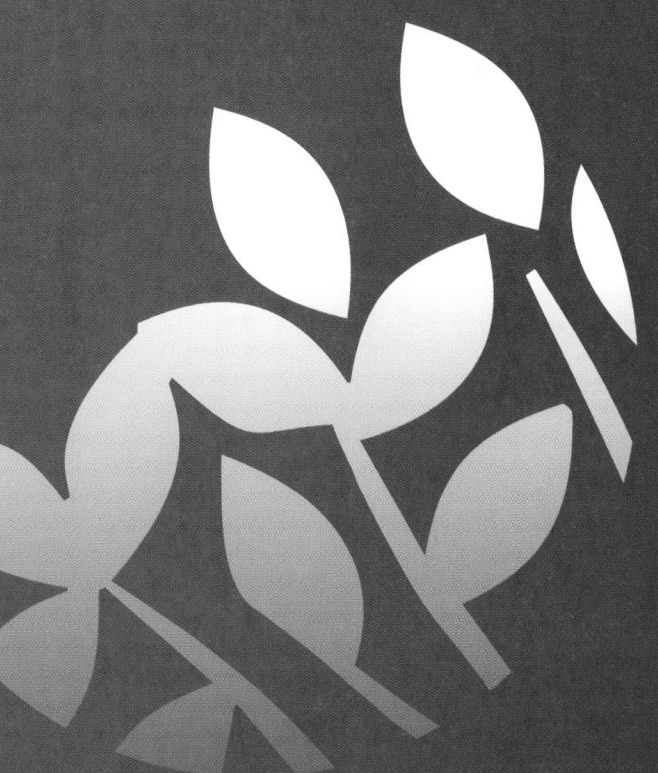

Stress is a universal feeling. All persons have experienced uncomfortable emotional and bodily changes that reflect its presence. Nurses are taught to observe for psychophysiological stress responses in themselves and their clients. Today, students are taught to use the nursing process to reduce the negative effects of stressors.

In the 1950s, the late Hans Selye (1956) described the specific effects of stressors on the physiology and body chemistry of animals. Selye linked stress with certain diseases (*e.g.,* gastric and duodenal ulcers, endocrine disorders, and high blood pressure). Soon it became clear that stress could bring on many physical and mental illnesses in humans. Although it is difficult to define and measure, the concept of stress remains a cornerstone in the study of health and disease.

Stress

In this chapter, **stress** is considered to be the process of adjusting to circumstances that disrupt, or threaten to disrupt, a person's equilibrium (Lazarus & Forlman, 1984; Selye, 1982). The problem of defining stress is distinguishing between sources of stress and responses to stress. For example, a man notices a lump in his groin. His father had recently died of bowel cancer. The man becomes irritable and angry but does not seek help. The source of stress is the lump in the groin, and the response is irritability. Events and situations (such as the lump in the groin) to which people must adjust are sources of stress. Stress responses are the physical, psychological, and behavioral reactions (such as nausea, nervousness, and tiredness) that people display in times of stress (see later).

The experience of stress depends on the circumstances in which the stress occurs and on each person's physical and psychological characteristics. Stress is not a specific occurrence; it is a process. Understanding the process of stress requires attention to three areas:

* Sources of stress
* Factors that make people more or less sensitive to stressors
* Differences among stress responses

Stressors

Stressors are agents or factors that place a strain on the person and challenge the adaptive capacities of an organism or person. They can be helpful or harmful, depending on the individual, the situation, the intensity, and the person's coping responses. Examples of stressors are

* Pathological changes caused by disease or injury
* Trauma (*e.g.,* injury, burns, assaults, electric shock)

* Inadequate food, warmth, protection
* Unmet basic needs (*e.g.,* hunger, sexual desires)
* Planned therapeutic programs (*e.g.,* dieting, physical therapy, psychotherapy)
* Disruptive social and family relationships
* Conflicting social and cultural expectations
* Normal changes in physiological function (*e.g.,* puberty, menstruation, pregnancy, menopause)
* Anticipated stressful events (*e.g.,* an important social event, an examination, a courtroom hearing, a painful diagnostic test)
* Imagined threats of injury (*i.e.,* sources of stress do not have to be based in reality)
* Natural disasters (*e.g.,* earthquakes, floods)
* Attacks by bacteria, viruses, or parasites
* Social isolation
* Competitive sports
* Geographic relocation (even a welcome change of residence or travel)
* War and social unrest
* Activities of everyday life (*e.g.,* entertaining, driving on a freeway)
* Positive situations that nonetheless bring momentous change (*e.g.,* marriage, having a baby, graduation from college)

The absence of stressors can be harmful in that it results in boredom and lack of personal growth.

Stress Responses

Stress responses are physiological and psychological reactions to stress. Physiological stress responses include reactions such as changes in cardiovascular function, increased gastric secretion, tremor, and loss of sphincter control. Psychological responses include such reactions as anxiety and depression and the use of defense mechanisms such as denial or repression. The manner in which an individual responds to stress situations is mediated by personality, perception of the stressor, and resources for coping. Whether our stress responses are successful or not, they are means of defending us from stressors.

Physiological Defenses

Several types of physiological defenses exist. Two examples are the unbroken skin and intact immune system that protect us against the onslaught of viral and bacterial stressors. Other physiological defenses include genetic makeup, nutritional status, and general physical condition. For example, an infection may develop more readily in a malnourished person who receives a cut than in a well-nourished, well-exercised individual who receives a more serious injury.

Psychological Defenses

The ability to respond adaptively to stress depends on previous experience with the stressor, formal education, support systems, intellectual capabilities, tendency toward anxiety, lifestyle, and economic status.

Coping means responding adaptively to stress. Lazarus and Forlman (1984) described five models of coping:

* Information seeking from ourselves and from others
* Direct action (*e.g.,* walking away from a tense situation or confronting a person with whom you are having a disagreement; by using direct action, you deal directly with the stressor)
* Inhibition of action (*e.g.,* not pounding your fist on the table even though you are very angry; by inhibiting your action, you protect yourself from unhelpful responses)
* Seeking social support from significant others or other appropriate sources
* Use of intrapsychic defense mechanisms

People learn new coping responses throughout their lives. Coping measures help us resist and master stressors. Once we master a stressor by using a particular coping response, that coping skill becomes part of our stress response, and we are likely to use it again in a similar situation. Coping responses may be grouped into three major types, depending on the ways they help us deal with stressful situations. They are responses that (Pearlin, 1884)

* Change the situation from which a potentially stressful experience arose
* Control the meaning of the situation before it can elicit a stress response
* Control the stress reaction after it has developed

Theoretical Models of Stress

Recent developments in the field of stress owe a great deal to the pioneering work of scholars such as Hans Selye, Thomas Holmes, Richard Rahe, and Richard Lazarus.

Selye's General Theory of Stress

In 1950, Selye published *The Physiology and Pathology of Exposure to Stress* (Selye, 1950), which described his theory of stress and influenced stress research. Selye's model emphasized the physiological components of stress, particularly the body's attempts to deal with stressors by means of adaptive hormones. Stress was defined as a physiological phenomenon. Selye defined a nonspecific response as one that affects most, if not all, of a system's agents that place demands on it. For example, exposure to extreme heat or cold acts as a specific stressor to which the body adapts by either shivering (in the case of cold) or perspiring (in the case of heat). Although the specific responses to these stressors are different (shivering vs. perspiring), heat and cold are nonetheless similar in that they promote a nonspecific response. They force the total body (*i.e.,* nervous system, skin, blood vessels) to return the organism to its previous state of balance.

On an emotional level, the body also responds nonspecifically to stressful events. These events can be perceived as either joyful or distressing. For example, a stress response can be as powerful at a person's wedding as at a loved one's funeral. In both cases, the body responds as a whole, nonspecifically, to specific events.

Selye concluded that stress plays a role in every disease process, regardless of cause. He noted that most diseases are characterized by only a few specific signs and symptoms, such as weight loss, fatigue, malaise, aches and pains, and gastrointestinal upsets. Selye called this phenomenon the general adaptation syndrome (GAS) and suggested that certain hormones, called adaptive hormones, are released during stress responses.

According to Selye, the GAS appears whenever an organism is subjected to long-continued stress. Some manifestations include adrenal gland stimulation, release of adrenocortical hormones, and lymph gland atrophy (shrinkage). Stressors that cause GAS are nonspecific and include trauma, infection, burns, severe cold, and emotional upsets.

In addition to the body's systemic response to stress, Selye proposed that the body also adapts to local stressors. He named this local response the local adaptation syndrome (LAS). LAS takes place within a single organ or specific area, such as with inflammation.

Selye suggested that both the GAS and the LAS develop in three distinct stages: (A) alarm, (B) resistance, and (C) exhaustion. These three phases are elaborated in Figure 6–1.

Selye theorized that adaptation plays a role in every disease and that faulty adaptation can cause disease. Selye named these "derailments" of the adaptive syndrome the diseases of adaptation and indicated that these "derailments" are not caused by any specific pathogen but instead are a direct result of a faulty response to a stressor. Usually, adaptation involves a balance of defense and submission on the part of the body. However, when the body overdefends itself, excessive proinflammatory hormones are released, and such problems as arthritis, allergy, and asthma develop. When the body underdefends itself, excessive antiinflammatory hormones are released, and overwhelming infection or ulcers result.

Holmes and Rahe's Model Relating Life Change to Illness

In the 1960s, Thomas Holmes and Richard Rahe (1967) began studying the relationship between

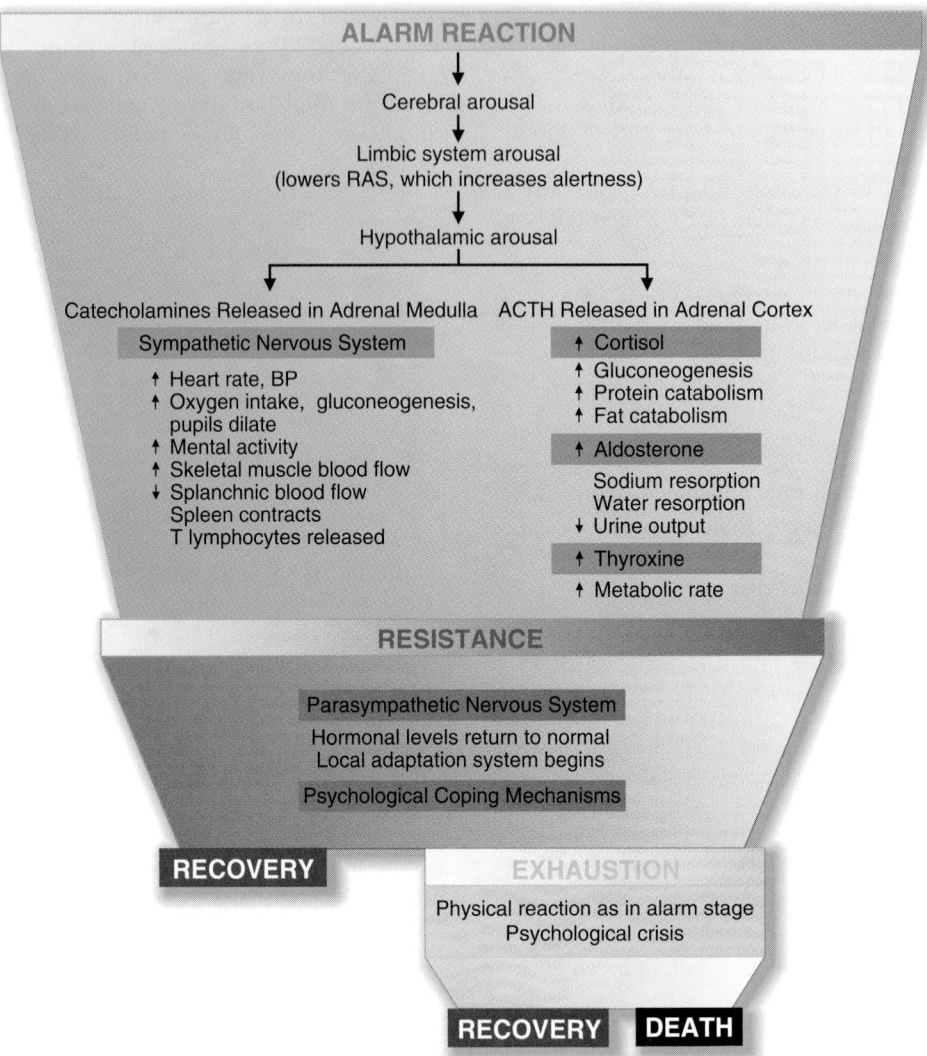

PHYSICAL OR PSYCHOLOGICAL STRESSOR

ALARM REACTION

Cerebral arousal

Limbic system arousal
(lowers RAS, which increases alertness)

Hypothalamic arousal

Catecholamines Released in Adrenal Medulla

Sympathetic Nervous System
- ↑ Heart rate, BP
- ↑ Oxygen intake, gluconeogenesis, pupils dilate
- ↑ Mental activity
- ↑ Skeletal muscle blood flow
- ↓ Splanchnic blood flow
  Spleen contracts
  T lymphocytes released

ACTH Released in Adrenal Cortex

- ↑ Cortisol
  - ↑ Gluconeogenesis
  - ↑ Protein catabolism
  - ↑ Fat catabolism
- ↑ Aldosterone
  - Sodium resorption
  - Water resorption
  - ↓ Urine output
- ↑ Thyroxine
  - ↑ Metabolic rate

RESISTANCE

Parasympathetic Nervous System

Hormonal levels return to normal
Local adaptation system begins

Psychological Coping Mechanisms

RECOVERY   **EXHAUSTION**

Physical reaction as in alarm stage
Psychological crisis

RECOVERY   **DEATH**

Figure 6–1
The general adaptation syndrome. (From Black, J. M., & Matassarin-Jacobs, E. [1993]. *Luckmann and Sorensen's medical-surgical nursing: A psychophysiologic approach* [4th ed., p. 46]. Philadelphia: W. B. Saunders.)

change and illness. Change is a form of stress requiring both psychological and physical adaptations. Adapting to change consumes a person's energy beyond that needed to maintain a "steady state" of life.

Holmes and Rahe developed the Social Readjustment Rating Scale (SRRS), a ranking of major life events according to life change units (LCUs) (Fig. 6–2). The death of a spouse, for example, is worth 100 LCUs (and ranks highest as a stressor), whereas a vacation is worth only 13 LCUs. By obtaining life change scores from thousands of people, Holmes and Rahe explored the link between the amount of change in a person's life and subsequent illness. They discovered that the higher a person's life change score was, the greater was the likelihood that an illness would subse-

quently develop. The SRRS provides a general impression of the stressors in a person's life. The more stressors a person experiences in a short period (1–2 years), the more likely that physical illness, mental disorders, or other stress responses will follow. Does this mean that you can predict the stress problems in a person's life just by using the SRRS? No. Many people with high scores on the SRRS do not subsequently experience serious problems. In addition, low scores do not guarantee a life free of the dangers of stress. Why? One reason is that mediating factors, such as how the individual perceives and copes with each stressor, play an important role in determining the impact stressors have on each individual. The Lazarus model attempts to explain this further (Fig. 6–3).

Rank	Life event	Life change units	Your score	Rank	Life event	Life change units	Your score
1	Death of spouse	100	_____	23	Son or daughter leaving home	29	_____
2	Divorce	73	_____	24	Trouble with in-laws	29	_____
3	Marital separation	65	_____	25	Outstanding personal achievement	28	_____
4	Jail term	63	_____				
5	Death of close family member	63	_____	26	Wife begins or stops work	26	_____
6	Personal injury or illness	53	_____	27	Begin or end school	26	_____
7	Marriage	50	_____	28	Change in living conditions	25	_____
8	Fired at work	47	_____	29	Revision of personal habits	24	_____
9	Marital reconciliation	45	_____	30	Trouble with boss	23	_____
10	Retirement	45	_____	31	Change in work hours or conditions	20	_____
11	Change in health of family member	44	_____	32	Change in residence	20	_____
12	Pregnancy	40	_____	33	Change in school	20	_____
13	Sex difficulties	39	_____	34	Change in recreation	19	_____
14	Gain of new family member	39	_____	35	Change in religious activities	19	_____
15	Business readjustment	39	_____	36	Change in social activities	18	_____
16	Change in financial state	38	_____	37	Mortgage or loan less than $10,000	17	_____
17	Death of close friend	37	_____				
18	Change to different line of work	36	_____	38	Change in sleeping habits	16	_____
19	Change in number of arguments with spouse	35	_____	39	Change in number of family get-togethers	15	_____
20	Mortgage over $10,000	31	_____	40	Change in eating habits	15	_____
21	Foreclosure of mortgage or loan	30	_____	41	Vacation	13	_____
				42	Christmas	12	_____
22	Change in responsibilities at work	29	_____	43	Minor violations of the law	11	_____
						TOTAL	

Scoring

Add up your score. If your total for the year is under 150, you probably will not have any adverse reaction. A score of 150–199 indicates a problem, with a 37% chance you will feel the impact of stress with physical symptoms. From 200–299, you qualify as having a "moderate" problem, with a 51% chance of experiencing a change in your health. A score of over 300 could really threaten your well-being.

❧ **Figure 6–2**

Social readjustment rating scale. (Adapted from Holmes, T. H., & Rahe, R. H. [1967] The social readjustment rating scale. *Journal of Psychosomatic Research, 11* [2], 213. With permission from Elsevier Science.)

✦ Adaptation

Adaptation is the adjustment of an organism to changes in its environment. Adaptation is the ultimate goal of coping and can be viewed as long-term coping (Fig. 6–4). Whenever people encounter stressors from any source, they attempt to adapt to them. If adaptation is successful, balance is maintained or restored. If adaptation is faulty, people become ill and must adapt to illness. Adaptation is of vital concern to nurses, who manage the adaptive changes that illness forces on people.

Adaptation includes the whole range of protective responses, from the simplest motor action to the most complex interaction. Human adaptation is more complicated: We respond to the environment with our bodies, intellects, and emotions.

Levels of Adaptation

Human adaptation occurs at four levels: (1) psychological, (2) physiological or biological, (3) sociocultural, and (4) technological. In daily life, these four levels are interrelated.

Psychological Level of Adaptation

Psychological adaptation involves adjusting our attitude toward a psychologically stressful situation so

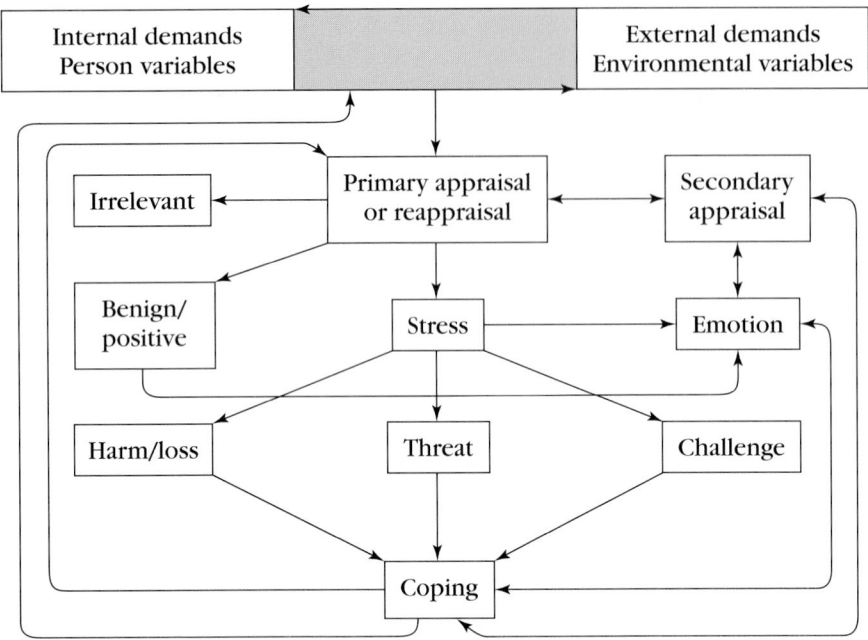

✦ **Figure 6–3**
Lazarus stress and coping paradigm.
(From Trygstad, L. [1984]. *Stress and
coping in psychiatric nursing*
[unpublished dissertation]. San Francisco:
University of California at San Francisco
Medical Center.)

that we can cope with it. Coping behavior is always purposeful but may not always seem appropriate. We adapt to stressors to the best of our ability at the time. To accomplish this, we might use defense mechanisms (*e.g.,* denial of the problem) or learn new behaviors (*e.g.,* relaxation techniques). Psychological adaptation can be healthy or unhealthy.

In trying to adapt to a stressful situation, some individuals may adapt in a manner that may temporarily work to relieve anxiety and physiological discomfort but ultimately may not be in their best interest. For example, a person with anorexia nervosa has adapted in a harmful way and needs professional help.

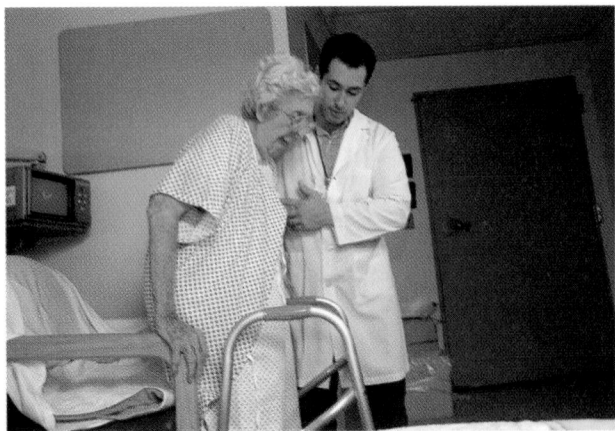

✦ **Figure 6–4**
Client learns to cope.

Physiological Level of Adaptation

Physiological or biological, adaptation involves compensatory changes that occur within the body in response to increased or altered demands made on the body.

Consider Judy. She realizes that since she entered the nursing program she has become sedentary and has decided to make a lifestyle change by taking an exercise class. In the beginning, she experienced muscular soreness, aching, and exhaustion. She continued to follow the recommended schedule, increasing her efforts a little every day and eventually was able to exercise for a longer time. Her muscles, heart, and lungs gradually increased in strength and functional efficiency, adapting to the additional demands placed on them. As frequently happens with exercise, the immediate stress seems negative, but the long-term benefits are positive.

The body's reaction to invading microorganisms illustrates physiological adaptation to stress. We resist attacks by stressors such as viruses and bacteria by becoming immune to them. This involves having the infectious disease and overcoming it or being inoculated against it.

In physiology, adaptation is sometimes described as a decrease in the intensity of a sensation resulting from stimulation or continuous responses. Olfaction provides a good example of adaptation. For instance, when we come into contact with a noxious odor, we are immediately offended. If we remain in contact with this odor (stimulation), however, we become accustomed to it rather quickly. Gradually, the intensity of the sensation decreases until we no longer notice the odor.

Sociocultural Level of Adaptation

Social adaptation is the adjustment of an individual's actions and conduct to the norms, conventions, beliefs, and pressures of various groups. Families, professional societies, labor unions, social clubs, and sororities are a few examples of the wide assortment of groups that demand our involvement and commitment. **Cultural adaptation** means adjustment of an individual's behavior to the concepts, ideas, traditions, and institutions of a culture. Examples of cultural groups include racial groups, geographical groups (*e.g.,* American, European), and certain religious groups.

As an illustration of sociocultural adaptation at the group level, consider your own experience as a student preparing to become a professional nurse (Fig. 6–5). When you first entered your nursing program, you were exposed to a new set of ethics, to a new vocabulary, and to certain standards of performance. All of these demands perhaps seemed overwhelming at first. Gradually, you began to adapt by learning to speak the language of nursing. You should be adopting more and more the values that you were taught, and as time goes on, you will certainly gain the confidence necessary to function effectively in the nursing role.

In addition to adapting at the group level, nurses are continually called on to adapt at the cultural level. Indeed, nurses may experience cultural shock as their nursing practice brings them into contact with various cultural groups. Also, nurses frequently work with people who are poverty stricken. For the student nurse who has been raised in a middle-class or professional-class home and neighborhood, the first contacts with severe poverty may be devastating and disturbing. Not all students psychologically survive the challenge of working with very poor people who are ill. Those who do adapt use various coping mechanisms. Some mechanisms, such as developing a hardened at-

titude or burning out, may be unhealthy. Other students use healthy adaptation. For example, they talk with classmates, discuss the problems of the people in their care with their instructor, develop plans of action with a social worker, face the fact that they may sometimes feel inadequate in the face of so much suffering, and finally begin to set realistic goals for themselves and for those in their care. In time, with experience and personal growth, the student who successfully adapts can work with very poor people and feel accepting and empathic but not shocked and disillusioned.

Technological Level of Adaptation

Technology, an outgrowth of culture, has allowed us to modify and change our surrounding environment and to control many of the stressors that are a natural part of that environment. Unfortunately, modern technology has also created new stressors to which we must adapt (*e.g.,* water, air, and noise pollution).

Health care technology has evolved at a tremendous rate over the past decades. As a result, we are making strides in understanding and gaining control over disease, pain, and death. Serious philosophical, ethical, and legal dilemmas have evolved as a result of our technological adaptation. These complex dilemmas serve as stressors to which we must adapt. For example, with increasing use of radioactive materials, we must be concerned with disposal of radioactive waste in the environment.

Some important questions that have evolved as a result of our technological adaptation include How do we control medical waste? How should technology be used? How do we provide health care for all individuals? and Who should control health care decisions?

Characteristics of Adaptation

All adaptive mechanisms are used to attempt to maintain optimal physical and chemical conditions within the system or organism. The process of maintaining a fairly steady internal environment is called **homeostasis.** Adaptation is a dynamic process. Individuals do not passively submit to environmental or internal stressors. Such internal stimuli as hunger and thirst result in our actively seeking food and water. When external stressors (*e.g.,* fires, battle conditions, extreme weather, an attack by an animal or another person) threaten us, we can flee from them, block them from consciousness (*e.g.,* by fainting), or actively struggle against them.

When individuals adapt to change or to stress, they tend to adapt as total organisms. In other words, adaptation embraces all levels of human experience: physiological, psychological, sociocultural, and perhaps even technological. Thus, when you became a nursing student, you probably had to adapt physiolog-

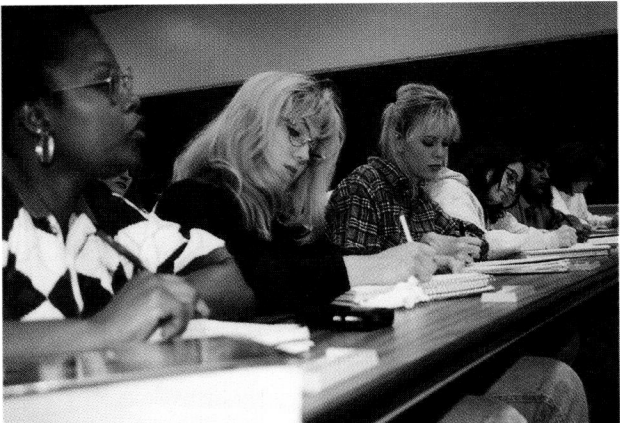

Figure 6–5
Student in class preparing to become a professional nurse.

ically to the greater workload, to the long hours of study, and to the muscular exertion required for lifting and moving people. You had to adapt intellectually to the new and different subject matter and emotionally to the responsibilities and problems of giving care. At the sociocultural level, you had to adjust to the ethics, norms, and subculture of the nursing profession. At the technological level, you had to learn to operate new equipment.

Adaptive mechanisms operate within the limitations of that individual's genetic makeup, general physical condition, intelligence, and emotional stability. For example, people cannot flap their arms and fly away from danger like birds, nor can they remain submerged in water indefinitely like fish. We must adapt within the confines of human nature or through technological innovations (*e.g.,* use of an airplane or scuba diving equipment). Adaptive responses are much more limited in number and scope at the physiological level than they are at the social and psychological levels. For instance, blood sugar, oxygen content, and internal body temperature can fluctuate only within certain narrow limits and still be consistent with life. On the other hand, many adaptive solutions are available in emotional or social difficulties. Even in these circumstances, however, the number of possible solutions is finite.

Time is an important factor in adaptation. The individual who has sufficient time can adapt better to stress than can the individual who must adapt quickly. For example, the body is able to adapt to gradual blood loss. Individuals with a slowly bleeding peptic ulcer can lose quite a bit of blood without symptoms of shock because blood loss occurs over a prolonged period. The body adapts less adequately to rapid blood loss. Consequently, persons experiencing sudden hemorrhage from trauma may suffer shock, as evidenced by rapid pulse, low blood pressure, and restlessness. If the body is unable to compensate quickly and appropriate emergency measures are not taken swiftly, the shock may become irreversible, and death may result.

Adaptability varies from individual to individual. Flexible individuals who respond readily to change and who use a wide range of compensatory mechanisms are more adaptable. They are more likely to survive stressful situations and change than are individuals who react to life challenges in a rigid, limited manner. Physical illnesses challenge people's adaptive capabilities. People with incapacitating diseases, such as severe heart problems, may be called on to change their occupation and lifestyle. These changes may be demanded of them at a time in their lives when they are least able to make sweeping modifications. Unless these individuals are given reassurance and guidance in planning the future, they may be unable to adapt to a new way of living.

Adaptation makes us less sensitive to some stimuli and more sensitive to other stimuli. For example, when we are listening to a lecture that has great interest or importance for us, we focus on what the speaker is saying. We may not notice that the person sitting next to us is whispering or coughing. We become selective in our attention.

Adaptive responses may be adequate to meet stress or to change and reestablish homeostatic balance, but adaptive mechanisms may also be inadequate, excessive, inappropriate, or stressful in themselves. Inflammation, for example, can serve adequately as an adaptive function but can also be inadequate, so that the body is overwhelmed by the invading organisms. An inflammatory process can also be excessive and inappropriate. If, for example, the irritant is not a dangerous microbe but a harmless pollen, then inflammation acts as an excessive and inappropriate adaptive mechanism. In this case, inflammation is not aiding the individual but instead is creating unnecessary pathological changes that do not serve any protective purpose.

Although it is usually helpful, adaptation itself can be stressful. For example, although inflammation is useful, it is also stressful because it causes physiological changes that result in heat, swelling, and pain. These uncomfortable symptoms demand a response and therefore are stressful.

✦ Homeostasis

For an organism to preserve its life, it must adapt satisfactorily to change and keep a degree of internal stability in the face of a variable and stressful environment. Living organisms have developed internal mechanisms for automatically maintaining balance despite constant threats to equilibrium that may lead to disequilibrium. These mechanisms are called **homeostatic mechanisms,** and they operate at all levels of life, regulating biological functioning and counteracting change and imbalance. Homeostasis is quite complex. An imbalance in one system (*e.g.,* the cardiovascular system) can cause disequilibrium in other systems (*e.g.,* the renal and adrenocortical systems). Returning the ill person to homeostatic balance is the ultimate goal of all nursing care.

Cannon (1967) viewed homeostasis as a type of dynamic equilibrium. His use of the term *homeostasis* was applied mainly to systems related to the fight-or-flight response associated with emotional arousal and the self-regulation of such internal physiological processes as

• Body temperature
• Blood pressure
• Blood glucose concentration
• Water and electrolyte balance
• Hydrogen ion (pH) balance

- Muscle tone
- Blood oxygen and carbon dioxide levels

Physiological Homeostasis

Physiological homeostasis is the maintenance of a relatively stable and constant internal equilibrium. Homeostatic balance is the basis for health, whereas homeostatic imbalance is the basis for disease. The internal environment is composed primarily of extracellular fluid (ECF), which is found outside cells. The ECF provides all cells with the same environment of (Guyton 1991)

- Nutrients
- Glucose
- Fatty substances
- Amino acids
- Oxygen

Cell function depends on internal equilibrium. If it becomes physiologically unbalanced, the individual becomes ill. Severe physiological imbalance that remains uncorrected leads to death.

Maintenance of Physiological Homeostasis

To maintain physiological homeostasis, the body must meet basic physiological requirements for oxygen, water, and nutrients, including electrolytes and tissue-building materials. The body must also have the appropriate mechanisms for using these elements under varying conditions. For example, pulmonary ventilation increases during exercise to accommodate the need for more oxygen. Providing additional oxygen depends on healthy lungs and adequate circulation of blood. In addition, the body must be able to store certain basic nutrients; for example, glucose is stored as glycogen for use during periods of exercising or fasting. Finally, to remain in balance, the body must be able to eliminate waste products and quantities in excess of basic requirements. For instance, if a person takes in certain water-soluble vitamins in excess of what is needed, the body excretes the excess, thereby avoiding toxic build-up of these substances.

Homeostasis also depends on physical integrity, so the body must be kept whole and in good repair. Mechanisms that protect the body from injury, such as blinking an eye, or that repair damage, such as blood clotting to prevent bleeding, promote physical integrity.

Furthermore, homeostasis depends on sociocultural and behavioral factors. Malnutrition, drug addiction, and air pollution, for example, upset physiological balance by altering the body's chemical balance. Certain emotional states, such as fear, anxiety, or hostility, as well as psychological conditions, such as depression or irregular behavioral patterns of rest and activity, affect physiological balance.

Mechanisms of Physiological Homeostasis

Homeostatic regulators control numerous physiological processes, including those involved in

- Water, sodium, hydrogen ion (pH), potassium, calcium, and phosphate balance
- Regulation of blood oxygen and carbon dioxide levels
- Body temperature regulation
- Control of blood pressure

Major Regulators of Physiological Homeostasis

The major homeostatic regulators are the nervous and endocrine systems. Because the nervous system and endocrine system complement one another in promoting homeostasis, the two systems are often called the neuroendocrine system. All healthy systems and organs work together to maintain a balance. All systems in the body are involved in homeostatic regulation:

- The cardiovascular system pumps oxygen and nutrients to cells and removes carbon dioxide and other waste products from them.
- The respiratory system controls the exchange of oxygen and carbon dioxide.
- The gastrointestinal tract is the route of intake for fluids and electrolytes, important for regulating fluid and electrolyte balance.
- The concentration of glucose in the blood is primarily regulated by the liver, kidneys, and pancreas.
- The kidneys regulate fluid balance and the ECF concentrations of hydrogen, sodium, potassium, phosphate, calcium, and other ions and excrete and/or reabsorb many byproducts of carbohydrate, fat, and protein metabolism (Fig. 6–6).

Psychological Homeostasis

Psychological homeostasis is a state of equilibrium characterized by a satisfying self-concept, emotional balance, and smooth interactions with the environment. People with consistently good mental health may have had a stable psychological environment from infancy onward and thereby developed the capacity to trust and love others early in life. Typically, a person who is in a state of emotional balance has

- A harmonious relationship with the environment
- A stable environment (*e.g.,* a safe and relatively comfortable living situation, adequate food)
- Life experiences that are consistent with the individual's self-concept or self-image
- Healthy relationships (*i.e.,* the ability to love and experience love, as well as to maintain close and supportive relationships with significant others)

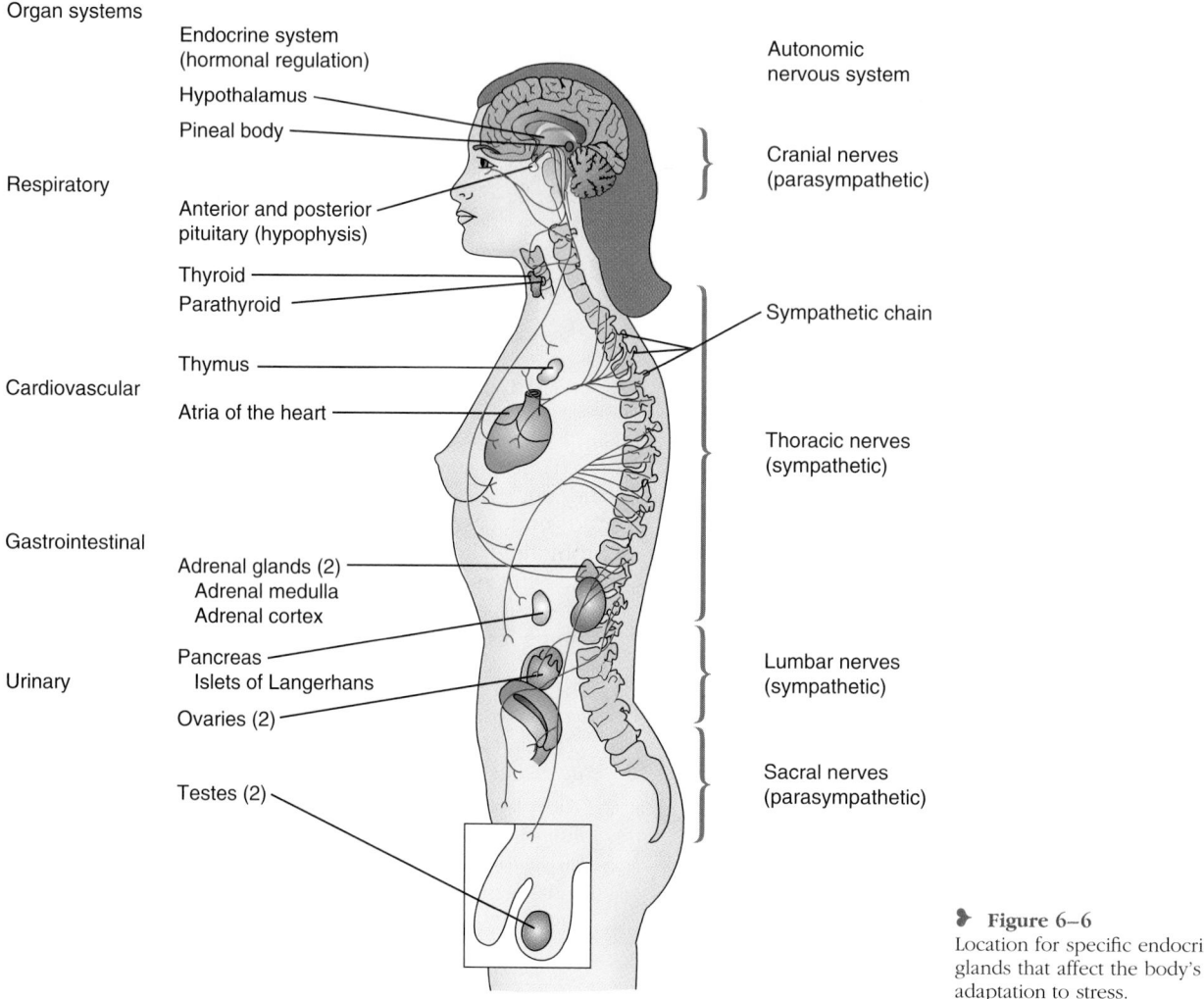

Organ systems

Endocrine system
(hormonal regulation)

Hypothalamus

Pineal body

Respiratory

Anterior and posterior
pituitary (hypophysis)

Thyroid
Parathyroid

Cardiovascular

Thymus

Atria of the heart

Gastrointestinal

Adrenal glands (2)
Adrenal medulla
Adrenal cortex

Pancreas
Islets of Langerhans

Urinary

Ovaries (2)

Testes (2)

Autonomic
nervous system

Cranial nerves
(parasympathetic)

Sympathetic chain

Thoracic nerves
(sympathetic)

Lumbar nerves
(sympathetic)

Sacral nerves
(parasympathetic)

❯ Figure 6–6
Location for specific endocrine
glands that affect the body's
adaptation to stress.

- Work or study that is interesting and fulfilling
- A sense of interdependence with others
- Good physical health
- Adequate economic means
- Enjoyable creative and recreational outlets
- A sense of hope for the future

On the other hand, when people view themselves negatively, a state of disequilibrium, or imbalance, may be experienced. They usually feel out of step with the environment and perceive other people— even friends—as remote and distant. Emotional disequilibrium can be triggered by many factors, such as:

- A sense of loss of control
- A threat to self-image
- Failing a major examination
- Losing a job
- Being reprimanded by a supervisor

- Having a serious argument with a loved one
- Being hospitalized

The person's coping skills play an important role in returning the emotional equilibrium.

Autonomic Nervous System

The **autonomic nervous system** (ANS) is a portion of the nervous system consisting of the sympathetic and parasympathetic systems, and it operates without conscious control. The ANS is composed of two major divisions: the sympathetic, or thoracolumbar, and the parasympathetic, or craniosacral, systems, which usually affect the body in opposite ways. For example, parasympathetic stimulation increases gastrointestinal motility, whereas sympathetic stimulation decreases gastrointestinal motility.

Under stressful conditions, the sympathetic nervous system initiates a series of physiological responses that may be grouped together as the "fight or flight" response (Cannon, 1967). This response makes the individual more alert and prepared to fight or flee. The parasympathetic nervous system has an opposite effect and often exerts its major influence during periods of rest. When the body is in homeostatis, the parasympathetic division is more dominant, but the sympathetic division supplies sufficient input to maintain the balance. Under extreme stress, the sympathetic nervous system predominates and enables the individual to gather the necessary energy for battle or flight.

Normal Deviations

The concept of homeostatic balance represents an ideal, but every self-regulating system incorporates some deviation or error from what is optimal or normal for that system. Control can be achieved only through adjustment of the error.

Compensation

Homeostatic mechanisms preserve the integrity of the body by balancing stressors and compensating for change. The main objective of a homeostatic mechanism is to minimize the difference between how a system should behave ideally and how it is behaving in reality. Blood pH, glucose, and electrolyte levels and body temperature are all maintained by homeostatic compensatory mechanisms.

Compensatory Growth

Cell proliferation and organ and tissue hypertrophy (enlargement) also illustrate the compensatory nature of homeostasis. For example

- Red blood cell count gradually rises in response to increased demands for oxygen.
- Muscle hypertrophies in response to vigorous and prolonged exercise.
- The spleen and lymphatic organs enlarge when infectious organisms invade the body.
- When a kidney is severely damaged or removed, the remaining kidney increases in size to perform the work of both kidneys.
- If hardened arteries (arteriosclerosis) increase the workload of the heart, the left ventricle enlarges to overcome increased arterial blood vessel resistance and to maintain adequate circulation.

Self-Regulation

Homeostatic mechanisms automatically attempt to correct any deviation from what is normal for the individual. However, only a healthy individual enjoys the privilege of a body that is self-regulating. When severe illness strikes, physiological homeostatic mechanisms lose their automatic corrective responses. At this point, the health care team attempts to regulate the physiological functions by

- Administering intravenous fluids or medications
- Using technological devices such as hypothermia blankets and ventilators
- Performing surgical procedures

Homeostatic mechanisms maintain a system in controlled limits through feedback loops and the exchange of information and energy with the internal or external environment. If too much or too little of a substance (*e.g.,* blood glucose) is present, homeostatic mechanisms initiate changes to return that substance to a point within a normal range.

Feedback is a process that feeds some of the output of a system back into the system as input. The input of information influences the behavior of the system and its subsequent output. Feedback may be negative or positive. Negative feedback inhibits change, whereas positive feedback encourages or stimulates change.

Negative feedback is feedback that leads to beginning a series of changes that attempt to correct any radical change from the norm, either toward excess or deficiency. To understand how negative feedback operates within the body, we use models and analogies, such as comparing a home heating system that is regulated by a thermostat with biological regulator mechanisms.

Thermostat-Like Negative Feedback Mechanisms

Many negative feedback systems are thermostat-like in their operation. Thermostat-like regulators are distinguished by two features. First, these mechanisms operate by correcting deviations from a predetermined goal or set point. The **set point** is the optimal level or concentration above or below which the negative feedback system will inhibit or enhance the output. For example, low hormone concentrations result in negative feedback signals that lead to stimulation of further hormone secretion. The second feature of thermostat-like regulators is that they appear to have the following components:

- A receptor, which receives input from the internal or external environment
- A central integrator (*e.g.,* thermostat), which senses a deviation from the set point
- An effector, which attempts to correct the deviation

Whenever the system detects an error or deviation, it activates responses to correct the deviation and return to the set point. Although set points may change in response to pathological processes and overwhelming stress, normal fluctuations in physiological variables also occur. For example, operating by negative feedback, the hypothalamic thermostat keeps the body temperature steady at a set point of approximately 37.0°C (98.6°F), despite environmental conditions. Another illustration of thermostat-like control and set points is a theory of weight regulation, which states that body weight and fat are maintained at a genetically predetermined or preferred level. The body automatically balances food intake, physical activity, and metabolism to sustain the weight at which an individual functions most comfortably.

Rangelike Negative Feedback Mechanisms

Other negative feedback mechanisms, such as those involved in the control of blood glucose and hormone levels, are characterized by a set point that fluctuates within a range of normal limits. The controls of blood glucose and hormone levels are set points that operate within a range, depending on the time of day and other factors (*e.g.,* diet, time of meals).

The negative feedback mechanism for blood glucose operates within the normal range of approximately 80 to 100 mg/dl. Blood glucose rises rapidly following a meal and causes an increase in insulin in the bloodstream. As the blood glucose level returns toward the normal range, insulin secretion is inhibited. Hormone levels are controlled by negative feedback.

Positive Feedback Mechanisms

Positive feedback is a response to stimuli that results in intensifying the initiating stimuli, leading the organism away from the normal state. It tends to be disruptive for biological systems. The original error or imbalance is repeated or intensifies the problem. Continued positive feedback causes an uncontrolled, increasing deviation from the norm that can only be tolerated for a limited time. Severe injury, illness, or even death may result unless the positive feedback is corrected.

Although most homeostatic mechanisms are based on negative feedback, cyclic changes in female reproductive hormones are an example of the positive type of system. This positive feedback mechanism produces a sudden rise of luteinizing hormone, thus triggering ovulation and the formation of the corpus luteum, which secretes progesterone, a hormone that inhibits luteinizing hormone secretion. Note that the positive feedback cycle breaks after a certain point.

Homeostatic Fluctuations

Homeostatic mechanisms always fluctuate to some degree. When an error is detected in a homeostatic system, the system tries to correct the error. A time lag may exist between the moment the error is detected and the moment corrective action is started. As a result, the system may **overshoot,** or overcompensate, during attempts at self-correction to achieve homeostasis. After another time lag, the system readjusts and overshoots in the opposite direction. Overshooting in opposite directions creates fluctuations as the system attempts to correct itself and return to a normal range. Some overshooting is unavoidable because homeostatic systems continually adjust to new stressors. If a homeostatic system is not too badly disturbed, it returns to its former status. If a system is severely disturbed, it may either break down entirely or go on to a new balance. In the latter case, the system will stabilize but at a different set point or range. If the fluctuations increase in magnitude, unstable changes develop and may cause the system to lose its self-correcting mechanism, and the organism is threatened.

Limitations of Homeostatic Mechanisms

All self-regulating homeostatic mechanisms have limitations. Rapid growth and change, severe stressors, reduction in adaptive energy, or damage to the system leads to one or all of the following consequences: (1) a continued but inadequate performance of the mechanism, leading eventually to an overdriven system; (2) interruption of the mechanism; and (3) a complete breakdown of negative feedback control, resulting in death. Negative feedback mechanisms typically disintegrate in conjunction with uncontrolled positive feedback.

Failure of Homeostatic Mechanisms

When compensatory reactions are inadequate, the result can be an overdriven system. For example, with blood glucose regulation, levels must remain within certain limits; if these limits are exceeded, glucose is converted to glycogen and stored in the liver. Abnormal glucose excretion leads to such compensatory mechanisms as a craving for sweets, increased urinary output, and thirst. In cases of severe insulin deficiency, the diminished entrance of glucose into the cells leads to the inability of the body to function.

Interruptions of Homeostatic Mechanisms

Some diseases interrupt and thereby disrupt homeostatic mechanisms. Cancer, for example, appears to disrupt the normal regulation of cell division. The physical crowding of cells that inhibits the further growth of cells is impaired in malignant cells, and instead they multiply in an uncontrolled and uncoordinated manner. Lack of negative feedback on abnormal cell division apparently causes proliferation of malignant cancer cells.

◆
Crisis

A **crisis** is a disequilibrium in a steady state, occurring when the usual problem-solving strategies are ineffective. Obstacles to life goals produce periods of disorganization and disturbance typically called crises. Furthermore, because crises are not everyday events, people usually have not developed problem-solving methods for dealing with them. During this chaotic period, people may frantically try to solve the problem through trial and error.

Characteristics of Crises

Characteristics of crises include the following

- Crisis is a universal experience. Crises develop among individuals of all races, cultures, and socioeconomic levels.
- A crisis is usually time limited. It typically is resolved (it is hoped, with success) within 4 to 6 weeks.
- Almost all crises develop in a predictable manner.

Crisis exists on a continuum. It begins with the potential crisis state, then proceeds through precrisis, immediate crisis, and intermediate and advanced crisis states before developing into a full crisis state. Anyone is susceptible at the potential crisis state. At full crisis, however, individuals at risk are those who have failed at all attempts to solve their problems, who believe all available problem-solving resources have been used, and who do not obtain relief from their stress (Brownell, 1984; Caplan, 1964; Infante, 1982).

Developmental Phases of a Crisis (Caplan, 1964)

1. Immediate crisis—when a serious problem or threat develops, people become increasingly tense as they attempt to use their usual problem-solving techniques.
2. Intermediate crisis—people grow more upset with each failure of their usual coping methods, and they enter a state of disequilibrium.
3. Advanced crisis—as tensions continue to build, people mobilize all internal and external resources to restore equilibrium. At this stage, the problem may be reevaluated and attacked from a new angle, or the problem may be distorted and viewed as unsolvable.
4. Full crisis state—if the problem is not resolved, emotional pressures continue to build, and people become completely disorganized or immobilized because of severe anxiety or depression.

If people survive a crisis either by solving the problem or by adapting to it, emotional growth may have occurred. On the other hand, people who do not satisfactorily "work through" a crisis will find it more difficult to deal with future problems. Ultimately, the resolution of a crisis (for better or for worse) depends on the individual's perception of life, coping mechanisms, and the available resources (*e.g.,* significant others, health care professionals, a minister). Crises may be categorized as maturational or situational.

Maturational Crisis

A **maturational crisis** is a predictable, stressful event that occurs during each person's developmental process and for which the person has no coping skills. Severe stress at each stage of development interferes with mastery of developmental tasks. In infancy, childhood, adolescence, and adulthood, events that may lead to crises are usually related to family and peer relationships. For example, at approximately 2 years of age, children are expected to learn to control their bladder and bowel functions. They learn that they can please their parents if they are successful but may earn their displeasure if they are not. They have no previous experience with mastery of their sphincters, do not know how to gain control as expected at this stage of development, and begin to feel a great deal of stress as they face this maturational stage. They are in a maturational crisis. As they learn to control elimination, they will solve the crisis of this stage and will not experience another maturational crisis until the next developmental stage. Because individual growth occurs in stages, it is possible to anticipate maturational events that may create disequilibrium and thus assist the individual in dealing with the crisis of each stage. Expected maturational events include

- First day of school
- First date
- Marriage
- Childbirth
- Death of a parent

Situational Crisis

A **situational crisis** is usually a sudden, unexpected stressful event that happens to an individual at any point in life and that cannot be controlled by the individual. Situational crises usually cannot be predicted, and anticipatory guidance cannot be offered. Early identification and intervention, however, can assist the individual to cope with the crisis. Self-help groups, such as rape crisis centers, have been developed to assist individuals to cope with specific events that precipitate a situational crisis. Examples of situational crises include

- Sudden death of a family member
- Severe family discord
- Spouse or child abuse
- Serious accidents
- Military combat
- Loss of a limb
- Loss of a job with severe financial ramifications
- Rape or attempted rape
- Natural disasters (*e.g.,* tornadoes)

- Disasters caused by people (*e.g.,* forest fires)
- Divorce

In each of these situations, people suffer abrupt interruptions in the normal routine of life, and disequilibrium occurs.

Crises tend to occur in cycles, with one crisis following another. For example, people who have been involved in serious automobile accidents are usually hospitalized. Hospitalization may threaten a person's job and financial stability. If the person is married, the spouse may be forced to work overtime, thus disrupting family cohesiveness. Consequently, serious behavioral problems may develop in the children. Thus, as the old saying goes, "troubles never come singly."

People undergoing crisis are often highly susceptible to the influence of other individuals in their environment. Thus, the individuals in crisis are usually quite responsive to crisis intervention by others.

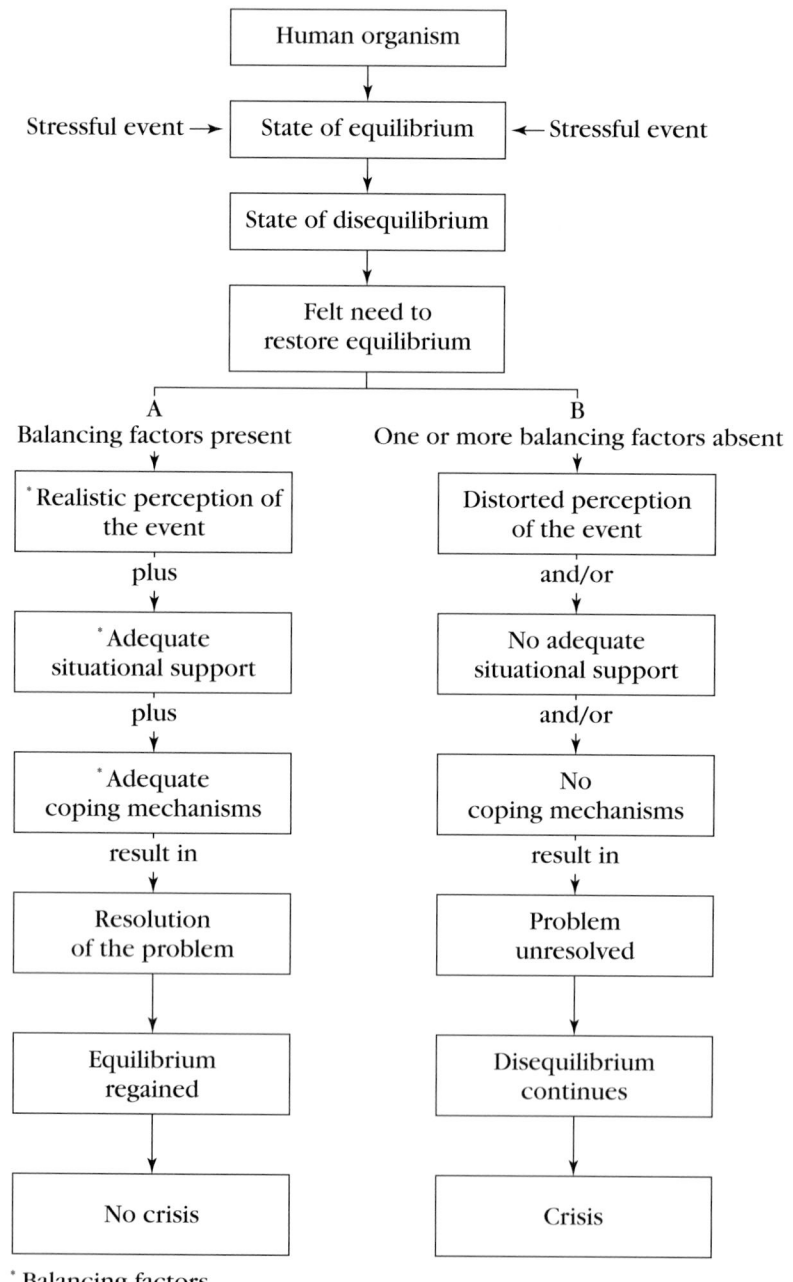

* Balancing factors

✦ **Figure 6–7**
Paradigm: The effect of balancing factors in a stressful event. (From Aguilera, D. C., & Messick, J. M. [1998]. *Crisis intervention: Theory and methodology* [8th ed.]. St. Louis: C. V. Mosby.)

Crisis Intervention

Reactions

People in crisis display typical psychological and physiological reactions. Immediate reactions to a critical problem include fear, anxiety, anger, panic, the drive to act, and heightened tension. All these responses suggest an emergency, with activation of the fight or flight mechanism. Within hours to days after the onset of a crisis, a person may become confused, depressed, immobilized, and unable to make decisions. These responses are not helpful and in fact prevent satisfactory resolution of the problem.

Coping With Potential Crises

Personal problems, even serious ones, do not have to culminate in a crisis. Crises are preventable. According to Aguilera (1990) and Aguilera and Messick (1984), whether a situation develops into crisis depends on three factors: (1) the individual's perception of the problem or event, (2) available situational supports, and (3) coping mechanisms.

Note in Figure 6–7 that if a person undergoing a stressful event perceives the situation realistically and has adequate situational support (*e.g.,* significant others with whom to discuss the problem) and adequate coping mechanisms (*e.g.,* ways of reducing tension by expressing anger or frustration), the problem will probably be resolved, and crisis averted. On the other hand, if one or more factors are missing, the problem may not be resolved, and a crisis could develop.

The Nursing Process As It Applies To Stress

Assessment

Nurses help people appraise and cope with the stressors in their lives. To do so, we must assess people's perceptions of and vulnerability to stressors, responses to stressors, and coping resources. In addition, we must plan nursing interventions to help people cope with stress responses and stress-related illnesses. The more we understand the underlying dynamics of stress, the better we can prevent harmful stress responses or stress-related psychophysiological disorders in ourselves and others. The ultimate goal of stress management is to adapt to stressors.

People with inadequate defenses and coping mechanisms suffer severe stress responses and even illness. Individuals with strong natural defenses do not perceive most stressors as major or even moderate. Still other people have fewer natural defenses but are willing to develop and experiment with new coping skills. By using new coping skills, these individuals may emerge from a stressful situation with a sense of mastery that they carry over to new situations.

Stressors

Stressors challenge the adaptive capacities of an individual. They place a strain on the person, resulting in a stress response and, possibly, illness. Stressors may be perceived by an individual as minor, moderate, major, or overwhelming. The magnitude of the stressor depends on the individual's unconscious and conscious perception and cognitive appraisal of the event. Thus, for one person, flying in an airplane is a minor stressor, whereas for another person it is an overwhelming stressor.

As Lazarus pointed out, it is not the major problems and life changes that are overwhelming for most people. Rather, it is the everyday hassles that finally push us to the breaking point.

Part of assessment is determining the cause of the precipitating event that led to the individual's request for help. By listening to the client's description of the "last straw," you can assess the critical issues that are problematic to the person. Clues about stress reactions come from behavioral stress responses; that is, from changes in how people look, act, or talk. Emotional responses usually show up in facial expressions or other nonverbal communications. For example, perspiration, a shaky voice, tremors, and spasms in facial or other muscles may be indicators of physiological stress responses. Posture and position can also provide information about stress. A person who is fully dressed but is curled up in bed in a fetal position, with face covered, window blinds drawn, and door closed is physically signaling a stress reaction. As people attempt to escape stressors, unusual behaviors may be observed. Some people quit their jobs, drop out of school, run away from home, or attempt suicide to escape stressors.

When collecting your data during assessment, remember that mind and body continuously interact with each other. Distressing physiological symptoms trigger anxiety and other emotions, which in turn trigger more distressing physical symptoms (Hopping, 1980; Seyle, 1956; Selye, 1982; Smith, 1990).

Physiological Responses to Stressors

Major physiological responses to stressors include

- Increased heart rate
- Increased oxygen intake
- Increased serum glucose levels
- Decreased inflammatory and immune responses
- Pupil dilation
- Reduced peristaltic action
- Increased alertness
- Changes in blood pressure
- Immunological responses

- Hormonal responses
- Gastrointestinal responses
- Sensory responses
- Renal system changes

When stressors are less than overwhelming, homeostasis, or physiological balance, is usually restored. When the stress is overwhelming, however, physiological mechanisms go awry, and disease or death results. Today, this response most often occurs in situations that are unrelated to survival. See Box 6–1 for assessment guidelines related to homeostasis.

Human beings must maintain homeostasis to survive on all levels, from the cellular level to the entire human organism. Any assessment tool that can measure changes from the individual's normal range of responses and behaviors is a tool that can help in assessment of homeostasis.

Psychological Responses to Stressors: Anxiety

Anxiety is apprehension, dread, foreboding, or uneasiness that is not related to an identifiable source of danger. When we perceive that we must confront a major stressor, we prepare for fight or flight, a series of physiological responses. The emotional components of fighting or fleeing are anger or rage and anxiety or fear. As nurses, we deal with both anger and anxiety in people. Of these two, the more common emotional response to life's stressful demands is anxiety, and nurses work daily with anxious people.

Anxiety differs from fear. Although we experience the same feelings with fear as with anxiety, our feelings stem from different sources. With fear, the source

of danger is recognized and can be identified. With anxiety, it is not. Both anxiety and fear arise in the same part of the brain, and both cause the fight or flight response. Other distinctions between anxiety and fear are as follows:

- Anxiety is concerned with the future; fear is concerned with the present.
- Anxiety is vague in character; fear is definite.
- Anxiety is the result of psychological conflict; fear is the result of a specific threat to biological integrity.
- Anxiety does not always make sense; fear is rational.

Anxiety varies with an individual's perception, which in turn depends on a person's psychosocial makeup, education, degree of maturity, and life experience. Generally, anxiety makes us feel uncomfortable. Such feelings are usually a mix of physical and mental states. We are aware of feeling nervous or uneasy. We may also experience various physiological reactions. As uncomfortable as anxiety is, we usually cannot identify its exact cause, and the confusion is all the more distressing. People experience anxiety in certain situations and not in others, and a situation may provoke anxiety in a person one time but not another time. In this case, the meaning of the situation for the person has changed, probably because of reappraisal.

Causes of Anxiety

Generally, situations of frustration, conflict, or stress that threaten the physical or mental security of an individual produce anxiety. Because illness is physically as well as mentally taxing, sickness produces anxiety. Hence, ill people are usually uncomfortable emotionally as well as physically.

Physiological threats are recognized more easily than threats to a person's mental well-being. For instance, life-threatening physiological disorders have distinct manifestations. Infections or injury have obvious signs and symptoms. Identifying psychological threats, however, is more difficult. We must remember to be as sensitive to the anxiety that a sick person experiences as we are to signs of physical disease.

Communication of Anxiety

People may communicate their anxiety both verbally and nonverbally. A person's voice may shake or break, pitch may change, and speed may fluctuate. A tense posture, nervous movements, sweat, or a "wide-eyed" appearance hint nonverbally at anxiety, and, like a bad cold, anxiety can spread from one person to another. One anxious person can make others anxious. An anxious nurse can communicate anxiety to coworkers and to those receiving care.

Assessment of Anxiety

Anxiety, or lack of anxiety, can be assessed by analyzing its intensity, appropriateness, duration, and

---

Box 6–1

ASSESSMENT GUIDELINES— HOMEOSTASIS

To assess whether a client is able to maintain normal physiological homeostasis, you may note whether the client

- Has sufficient basic physiological requirements (oxygen, food, water, and electrolytes)
- Has adequate function of body systems
- Has normally functioning processes that protect the body from injury and that repair the body when physical damage has occurred
- Has a satisfying self-concept
- Is emotionally balanced
- Has relatively harmonious interactions with the environment, including others in society
- Can compensate for variations from normal and optimal conditions

somatic symptoms. *Ataraxia* is a state in which anxiety is absent or so minimal that it does not affect the individual. *Well-being* is a state of being relaxed, comfortable, and happy; it usually follows a satisfying experience; the mild anxiety that sometimes exists with a feeling of well-being is believed to be healing. What we normally think of as anxiety can be viewed on a numerical scale:

(+1) Mild anxiety—mild anxiety is a low level of anxiety that is useful. It increases perception, puts the person in a state conducive to learning, and encourages problem solving.

(+2) Moderate anxiety—at its lower levels, moderate anxiety heightens productivity and abilities. At higher levels, it may cause a person to use selective inattention, being unaware of ongoing activities but noticing those pointed out by an observer.

(+3) Severe anxiety—severe anxiety is not useful and requires intervention. It consumes most of a person's energy, and it inhibits physical recovery. It prevents a person from noticing what is going on and from being able to respond appropriately.

(+4) Panic—Panic is a frightening, violent, overpowering anxiety that causes a person to lose control. It is a critical state that needs intervention; it cannot be endured for long. During panic, people distort situations and events, they cannot comprehend them rationally, and they cannot maintain goal-directed activity.

As our level of anxiety increases, we become increasingly unable to understand what is happening to us and what is expected of us. Because the extremely anxious person easily misunderstands what is said, remember to keep your communication with anxious people clear and brief. Repeating statements is helpful because anxious people tend to forget easily. Nonverbal movements may aid in clarifying communication. Remember also that the anxious person needs an opportunity to discuss feelings with a calm, nonjudgmental person.

Assess the appropriateness of anxiety, and remember that appropriate anxiety serves a useful, adaptive purpose. Students, for example, tend to lack the appropriate motivation to study unless they are mildly anxious, but excessive anxiety has a disintegrative effect. It can immobilize the person or lead to panic, making appropriate goal-directed behavior impossible. On the other hand, apathy or the absence of anxiety also makes goal-directed behavior impossible.

Assess the duration of the person's anxiety. Most people can tolerate even intense levels of anxiety for brief periods, but our bodies cannot tolerate severe anxiety for sustained periods. Sustained anxiety can lead to chronic physical or mental illness or both if the condition is not controlled by self-help measures or professional intervention. When working with an anxious individual, gear questions to the length of time the person has been feeling anxious. Is being anxious a chronic state, or is the person's anxiety related to a specific individual or situation?

Assess the somatic symptoms that anxiety generates: Some of these physiological effects are anorexia, nausea, vomiting, abdominal cramps, and diarrhea. In addition, people may feel flushed, perspire excessively, or experience chest pain. Some individuals urinate more often. Anxiety can produce dysmenorrhea and frigidity in women. Men may become impotent. In some instances, aching muscles or joints, backache, and headache are also attributable to anxiety. Each individual experiences different somatic reactions to anxiety. Sustained or chronic anxiety, however, eventually causes disease by keeping the body in an abnormal state.

Stress-Related Psychophysiological Disorders

Physical or mental illness develops if (1) a person's defenses are overwhelmed by stressors, (2) a person is unaware of the significance of a stress response and chooses to deny or ignore it; (3) a person is either unwilling or unable to engage in self-help activities; or (4) a person overuses defense mechanisms. For example, some people pass through a period of denial and psychological withdrawal when exposed to major stressors (*e.g.,* death of a loved one). These responses are temporarily helpful during the early phases of grief, but they are harmful if the grief goes unresolved after a long period. See Box 6–2 for advice on assessment.

Nursing Diagnosis

Many nursing diagnoses relate to stress, but Anxiety is the most common. Anxiety, fear, dread, and panic are all important factors in several nursing diagnoses. The two most important nursing diagnoses you may make for anxious individuals are Anxiety and Fear.

Box 6–2

ASSESSMENT GUIDELINES—ANXIETY

When assessing a client for stress, it is important to assess for such factors as the following:

• Stressors impinging on the individual (the SRRS [see Fig. 6–2] can be a valuable assessment tool for such purposes)
• Presence of maturational crises
• Presence of situational crises
• Physiological responses to stressors
• The level of anxiety (ranging from ataraxia to panic)
• Presence or history of stress-related psychophysiological disorders

Anxiety may be the first part of the nursing diagnosis for an anxious individual, or it may be the second part of the nursing diagnosis. In fact, the word *anxiety* need not appear in a nursing diagnosis statement every time you observe signs and symptoms of anxiety in a person. The individual may have another problem that requires nursing intervention, one for which anxiety is one of many defining characteristics; for example,

- Fluid Volume Excess
- Social Interaction, Impaired
- Denial, Ineffective
- Decisional Conflict (specify)
- Sensory/Perceptual Alteration (specify)
- Thought Processes, Altered
- Pain
- Anticipatory Grieving
- Violence, Risk for
- Post-Trauma Response
- Rape-Trauma Syndrome (all types)

Anxiety can also alter a person's life in ways that create difficulties and can therefore lead to other defining characteristics. For example, anxiety may serve as

- An internal cue to which some persons respond
- A mental factor
- A mental status change
- An internal risk factor
- A basis for feelings of inadequacy
- Evidence of alterations in mood

Nursing Diagnoses Related to Stress and Adaptation

In addition to nursing diagnoses related to characteristics of anxiety, the following nursing diagnoses may be used for stress and adaptation:

- Nutrition: Less Than Body Requirements, Altered
- Constipation
- Colonic Constipation
- Diarrhea
- Breathing Pattern, Ineffective
- Communication, Impaired Verbal
- Social Isolation
- Role Performance, Altered
- Parenting, Altered
- Altered Parenting, Risk for
- Sexual Dysfunction
- Sexuality Patterns, Altered
- Family Processes, Altered
- Family Coping, Ineffective
- Family Coping, Compromised
- Individual Coping, Ineffective
- Noncompliance
- Fatigue
- Sleep Pattern Disturbance
- Health Maintenance, Altered
- Breastfeeding, Ineffective
- Self-Care Deficit: Bathing/Hygiene
- Self-Care Deficit: Dressing/Grooming
- Self-Care Deficit: Toileting
- Body Image Disturbance
- Personal Identity Disturbance

Planning

For any nursing diagnosis, planning means identifying expected outcomes. The main outcome for any nursing diagnosis is that the person adapts to the new environment, as evidenced by diminished psychological or physical symptoms. When planning, you must identify the specific psychological or physical symptoms experienced by the individual client. These include any defining characteristics for this nursing diagnosis that are experienced by the client.

In assisting the client to control stressors, the nurse should plan for the healthiest possible outcomes. In general, as independently as possible, the person should be able to

- Deal with the stressful problem
- Deal with the feelings engendered by the problem
- Reduce the physiological arousal of stress (Trygstad, 1980)

Who helps ensure outcomes? Resources include the client, the client's significant others, community resources, and the nurse.

The Client

As much as possible, individuals must make decisions so they can increase their sense of control over their own health care. The nurse must be judicious, however, because urging decision-making before a person is ready can lead to increased, possibly intolerable, levels of stress. The ultimate goal is to have the person independently managing stress. The nurse must plan to teach the person to use all the resources available to manage stress.

Significant Others

A strong, supportive network of significant others can help a person deal with life's difficulties. A significant other may be a parent, a spouse, a child, a best friend, or a pet. Encourage individuals to confide in those close to them. Help those who are lonely to reach out and bring new people into their lives. When feeling anxious, talking with an empathic person, perhaps one who has been through a similar experience, is beneficial.

The effects of social support on stress have been heavily researched. The results imply that social support is a powerful modifier of potentially negative stress effects. In addition, social support facilitates coping with life's demands. Research indicates that individuals with social support have less somatic (physical) illness, increased mental health, (Cobb, 1976) and longer lives (Syme & Berkman, 1979).

Community Resources

Help your client to understand that, when in need of information concerning a specific problem, it is wise to seek out appropriate resources (*e.g.,* a professional counselor or an organization devoted to helping people with certain problems). For some people, a religious affiliation is a source of comfort. For others, personal growth groups, assertiveness training, encounter groups, and other self-help organizations prove useful.

The Nurse

The nurse assists the individual in planning for stress management by helping to strengthen ties with significant others, making referrals to community resources, and teaching the client to manage stress. Obviously, the optimal time for planning occurs before a person becomes hospitalized as a result of stress. To teach stress management after a person has suffered a stroke or some other health-related problem is, in many ways, too late. Plan to teach stress management before the person becomes hospitalized. To accomplish this goal, you must regard the nurse's role as extending beyond the health care facility. Nurses are role models. People look to nurses for examples of healthy lifestyles.

You do not have to be in a formal setting or in a therapeutic relationship to teach stress management. First, plan to teach stress management by example. If you look fit and exude vitality and enthusiasm, people will notice and may want to imitate you in diet, exercise patterns, and so on. You can also be available as a significant other to those around you who are feeling stressed. Associates will listen to your recommendations for stress control if you seem to have your own life and health under control.

CASE STUDY   **John Jacobs Has Heart "Palpitations"**

One month ago, John Jacobs, a nurse manager for a large intensive care unit, was seen by the nurse practitioner for heart "palpitations" and a "fluttery feeling" in his chest. These symptoms first occurred when he was working at his high-pressure job, and he feared he was "having a heart attack."

The nurse practitioner ruled out any physical causes for Mr. Jacobs' symptoms but did note that he was 25 lb overweight and had slightly high blood pressure. Assessment findings for Mr. Jacobs included the following:

* 35-year-old, slightly obese male
* Height, 68 in; weight, 180 lb
* Skin intact, warm, and ivory in color
* Temperature, 36.7°C; blood pressure, 150/98; pulse, 76; respirations, 24
* Complains of being "very tired lately" and suffering from daily headaches for past 3 weeks
* States that he loves his job but has been under increased stress during the past 2 months because of the demands of his new position within the hospital

---

The Sample Nursing Care Plan for Mr. Jacobs (p. 120) describes possible expected outcomes and nursing interventions.

Implementation

Nursing interventions, if appropriate and timely, aid the body in adapting and returning to homeostatic balance. Some helpful interventions include the following:

* Assess the client's perception of the situation
* Monitor physical and psychosocial responses to the situation
* Identify the client's coping mechanisms
* Establish a supportive, caring relationship with the client
* Encourage the client to discuss feelings about the situation
* Listen to and accept the client's feelings
* Assist the client to look at alternative ways to cope with the situation
* Refer the client to appropriate resources, as needed
* Provide relaxation and comfort measures, such as a back rub
* Teach the client general relaxation techniques

Some stress responses may be so disturbing that they demand the person's attention; examples include heart palpitations, difficulty breathing, nausea, and loss of appetite. One disturbing psychological response is severe anxiety or panic. If responses of this magnitude develop, the aware person uses and develops self-help measures to counter and control stress reactions, thereby reducing the chance of developing an acute or chronic illness. Three methods of stress management, identified by Trygstad (1980), are as follows:

* Deal with the problem by identifying the source of the problem, changing the situation, changing your perception, and changing your response.
* Deal with the feelings engendered by the problem by identifying, acknowledging, experiencing, and expressing feelings.
* Reduce the physiological arousal of stress by resting, engaging in physical exercise, relaxing, eating properly, smoking less, and using relaxation techniques.

These essentials of stress management apply to one's own life and to work with people who are experiencing stress responses.

Dealing With the Problem

The first step in handling a stressor is to identify its source. Identification helps reduce the powerlessness we often feel while in the grip of a stress response. It is often possible to pinpoint the source of a stressor by asking a few general self-assessment questions. For example, ask yourself, or have the person you are caring for ask, the following:

* Is the stress related to work, to home, or to a relationship? Are too many demands being made at home, on the job, or at school?

SAMPLE NURSING CARE PLAN

CLIENT EXPERIENCING ANXIETY

Nursing Diagnosis	Anxiety, related to change in role functioning
Expected Outcomes	Client will demonstrate ability to deal with job stressors in a healthier manner, as evidenced by limiting work to 40 hours/week
	Client will deal with anxiety in a healthier manner, as evidenced by identifying his anxious feelings and taking steps to deal with them
	Client will demonstrate reduced physiological arousal in work setting, as evidenced by blood pressure below 145/90, other vital signs within normal limits

Nursing Intervention	**Rationale**
1. Discuss with client the potential sources of his job-related stress.	1. Identifying potential sources of stress will help the client to begin problem solving and develop coping strategies.
2. Once specific sources of stress have been identified, assist client in deciding how to change situation (e.g., delegating minor tasks, eliminating superfluous tasks).	2. The client will be in better control, and anxiety will decrease when he is not feeling overwhelmed with his job.
3. Assist client in identifying his own anxiety by asking him to identify the feeling, its source, and his responses to the feeling.	3. Once the source and coping skills are identified, he can develop more coping skills to help with future stressors.
4. Assist client in acknowledging his feeling and accepting this as a common experience that can be dealt with appropriately.	4. By acknowledging the feeling, the client will be able to process it and utilize appropriate coping skills and stress reduction techniques.
5. Teach appropriate ways to deal with anxiety (*e.g.,* be aware of the feeling, take a break from the anxiety-provoking situation, seek support persons, use coping skills that have been helpful in the past).	5. When a client knows how to deal with the feeling appropriately, it will not overwhelm him if it recurs.
6. Teach exercises to improve general physical fitness (*e.g.,* aerobic exercises).	6. Exercise increases muscle tone, decreases anxiety, and increases potential for weight reduction.
7. Teach progressive relaxation exercise to be performed for 20 minutes each day.	7. This helps the client control tension, leading to decreased heart rate and blood pressure, creating mental and emotional calmness.
8. Teach about low-sodium, low-cholesterol, 1400-calorie diet.	8. This will help with weight reduction and enhance the ability to deal with stress.
9. Teach to avoid caffeine, alcohol, sugar, and preservatives.	9. These foods may magnify stress responses.
10. Discuss biofeedback training as a potential means of learning to control stress.	10. This will help to control blood pressure and heart rate by conscious control and self-regulation.

Is it impossible to get enough rest?
Is the possibility of a serious illness a concern?

• Has a distressing situation occurred recently that has not been adequately resolved?

• Are there events coming up in the future that are anxiety provoking?

• Are many life changes going on at one time?

If the answer to one or several of these questions suggests a possible source, then take the second step and deal with the stressor. You can try to change the situation, and if change is not entirely possible, at least alter your perception of the situation and your response. For example, if you feel overwhelmed with your studies, changing the situation by quitting school is rarely appropriate. Instead, change your perception of the problem and your response. When you feel overburdened, look at each assignment separately rather than as one large mountain of work, and tackle each task one at a time. Develop a reasonable schedule. Make small but important changes in your situation by eliminating superfluous tasks. Also you might apply for a scholarship or loan so that you do not have to work in addition to going to school.

If a person for whom you are providing care feels overburdened with responsibilities at home, suggest a change in the situation by delegating tasks. If the person feels guilty about delegation, point out that no one person should assume all the housekeeping tasks. In this way, you help change the person's self-perception as a martyr who must shoulder all the burdens of home alone. The person's response to housework may also change after requesting help without feeling guilty.

Recognizing stressors and acting on them early, instead of denying them and allowing them to grow, are essential to mental and physical health.

Dealing With Feelings

Feeling "stressed" can manifest itself in anxiety, frustration, anger, or other emotions. The first step in handling feelings of stress is assessment. What feeling is being experienced? What is its source? It is not always easy for people to identify what they are feeling at a particular time or why they are feeling as they do. Therefore, encourage self-assessment. Specifically look at what happened to precipitate the feeling. Did a friend make an unkind remark? Did the person fail a major examination or make a mistake at work? What somatic responses accompanied the feeling (*e.g.,* upset stomach, tears, palpitations)? Under what circumstances did the feeling dissipate (*e.g.,* did the person discuss the problem with a friend who helped him or her to see the humorous side of the situation)?

Once the feeling has been identified, it is important for the person to acknowledge it. For instance, if you feel very angry with a client who is not complying with your instructions, you need to acknowledge to yourself that you are angry. Acknowledging anger can be difficult. The idealized view of nursing is that nurses are always kind and helpful and never irritated or angry. In reality, we all become angry at times, and that anger needs to be acknowledged and expressed in an appropriate way.

For example, imagine that you are taking care of Mr. Jones, who suffers from severe arthritis. Mr. Jones sometimes expresses his anger, frustration, and pain by leveling harsh criticisms at the nurses. Today you are taking care of Mr. Jones, and he is in a bitter mood. As you give him his bath, you can feel yourself becoming angrier as he becomes more caustic. Finally, with your stomach in knots, you excuse yourself for a minute and leave the room. You realize that you must help Mr. Jones deal with his frustrations, but first you must deal with your own! You take a few deep breaths and try to relax. You review in your mind what you have learned about pain and the many ways people try to cope with it. You may take time to talk with your instructor or other nurses who care for Mr. Jones. As you discuss how you feel, you sense that your anger is decreasing. Soon you feel able to return to Mr. Jones. In time, as you work with Mr. Jones and grow to know him and as he comes to trust you, it may be possible to help this person express his feelings more appropriately.

Reducing the Physiological Arousal of Stress

General Methods of Stress Reduction

Poor physical condition lowers our resistance to stressors and makes us more vulnerable to serious stress responses. Peak physical condition, on the other hand, means stamina, the necessary reserves to withstand an attack of stressors, and protection against unpredictable periods of life change. Exercise not only works toward physical fitness but also relieves stress and tension. Keeping fit is one of the best self-help mechanisms for coping with stress.

Because certain foods seem to magnify stress responses, dietary changes can help manage stress. Substances such as caffeine, alcohol, sugar, preservatives, and certain food flavorings and colorings can cause adverse psychophysiological responses. For example, too much caffeine increases blood pressure, causes tachycardia, and induces "nervousness." Excessive alcohol can have serious short- and long-term effects on mind and body. Good nutrition strengthens that first line of defense against stress.

Cigarette and pipe smoking also can increase stress responses. Nicotine increases epinephrine and norepinephrine secretion, which results in increased heart rate, blood pressure, and oxygen consumption. To control stress responses, smokers need to stop smoking or at least to control smoking by modifying the amount smoked per day.

Behavioral coping strategies such as time management (*e.g.,* getting a part-time vs. a full-time job) can assist in decreasing stress levels. Stress also can be dissipated through relaxation exercises, controlled breathing techniques, or meditative approaches, such as yoga, Zen, or transcendental meditation.

In progressive relaxation, the client is taught first to tense and then to relax groups of voluntary muscles in a systematic manner: first the feet, then the lower legs, then the thighs, and so on up to the trunk and arms to the face. This process helps the person learn to control tension in the muscles, thus leading to reductions in heart rate and blood pressure and creating mental and emotional calmness.

Forms of personal recreation, such as reading, listening to music, or taking walks, are also practical methods for dealing with stress.

Biofeedback Training

Biofeedback training uses the concept of feedback to help individuals monitor and control automatic physiological functions (*e.g.,* blood pressure, heart rate). Within the past decade, the concept of feedback has been applied with considerable success to the behavioral regulation of the so-called involuntary biological functions (hence, the term *biofeedback*). Scientists now believe that with biofeedback training, people may learn to self-regulate such body functions as blood pressure and heart rate. As a result, people can learn to avoid disease.

Biofeedback training is a scientifically planned program that trains selected subjects to control one or more "involuntary" functions. Biofeedback training involves

1. Attaching the subject to electronic monitoring equipment
2. Monitoring a particular physiological function (*e.g.,* heartbeat)
3. Feeding back selected information about that function (*e.g.,* increases or decreases in heart rate) to the subject by pictures, sounds, and so on
4. Rewarding the person for learning to control that function

Biofeedback training is used by some clinicians to treat hypertension, lower back pain, tension headache, and insomnia when these symptoms are caused by anxiety and muscle tension.

Guided Imagery

Guided imagery is a method of enhancing relaxation and comfort by suggesting that a person relax and picture himself or herself in a certain pleasant scene; experience sights, sounds, smells, and other sensations associated with the scene; and feel the comfort and relaxation associated with the scene and experiences. At first, the nurse guides the person in this imagery, but after learning the method, the individual may independently concentrate on the pleasant image and experience reduced anxiety without the nurse's guidance. Similar techniques can also be used to help a person control pain and other unpleasant sensations.

Guided imagery involves the following steps:

1. Begin the session with the person lying in bed or seated in a chair.
2. Ask the person to assume a position as comfortable as possible—one in which the person might even fall asleep.
3. Sit near the person and speak slowly and soothingly as you provide guidance in the person's thought processes.
4. Try to elicit images that are pleasant, relaxing, and associated with positive physical sensations.

One example of an image is the following scenario. Picture yourself on a warm fall evening. You are in a wagon on its way home from a hay ride. You are dressed in comfortable clothing and are lying back against a soft pile of hay, looking up at the vast black sky with its millions of stars and its huge harvest moon. You are there among many friends, and all of you have been singing old songs. Now it is mostly quiet as one friend plays a guitar. As the two horses pulling the wagon slowly plod toward home, the wagon below you sways slightly as it moves along the

road. You smell the odor of hay mixed with a slight smell of the horse, and it is very pleasant out there in the warm, fresh air. Every now and then you hear a wheel creak and feel a soft breeze blow across your face and feel yourself so relaxed and so happy. The wagon transports you slowly through the night toward home, and you are at peace with your friends and all the world. You are rocked gently and you feel your eyelids grow heavy with sleep. As you ride along, so relaxed, so pleasant, your eyelids grow heavier and heavier, and you feel yourself floating pleasantly. You begin to fall asleep and as you sleep, you have very, very pleasant dreams.

Managing Stress Reduction

Despite the benefits of these self-help measures, keep in mind that the mechanisms for reducing stress can promote stress as well. For example, if a person embarks on an exercise program to regulate stress, the novelty of exercise to the unprepared body can be jolting. Likewise, an extreme change in diet can be physiologically upsetting. Self-help mechanisms used for reducing stress must be applied in moderation.

Help persons who are under stress to assess their lifestyles and coping responses. Help people engage in self-care and make lifestyle changes to control stress and prevent stress-related disorders.

Coping with Actual Crisis

Crisis intervention begins with an initial assessment of the individual and the circumstances that led to the crisis. Next, armed with knowledge about the person and precrisis events, the nurse plans and prescribes proper intervention. At this point, the intent is simply to return the individual to a precrisis state rather than to make major changes in the person's character and lifestyle.

Now the stage is set for actual intervention. According to Aguilera (1984) crisis intervention should help the individual to

• Understand the nature of the crisis, the nature of the events that precipitated the crisis, and the relationship between the two
• Examine conscious feelings concerning the crisis as well as feelings that the individual may have suppressed
• Reenter the social world if the person has retreated from others because of grief or depression.

After crisis intervention, resolution of the crisis begins. Crisis management should include planning. At this point, the nurse reinforces coping responses that the person successfully used to reduce tension and anxiety in the past. The nurse also helps the individual develop new coping skills to deal with the present crisis. Newly learned coping strategies used for the present crisis can then be incorporated into the body's defense system for future use, preferably long before a situation reaches another crisis state.

To help the person develop these new coping strategies, appropriate referrals to other professionals or agencies can be of assistance for the immediate crisis. Federal, state, and community organizations such as the American Red Cross help people deal with major crises, such as floods and hurricanes. Other sources of assistance are more available for help on a day-to-day basis. The client should understand that such sources of assistance will often be available in the future to prevent another crisis from arising. You might, for example, refer the person to sources of assistance for food, shelter, employment, child care, medical care, and so forth, as needed by the individual. You can also help the individual in dealing with stress. Skills that will remain useful as a means of helping to cope in the future include guided imagery and other relaxation techniques.

Once serious illnesses develop, individuals must reach out beyond self-help to the health care professional. At this point, drug therapy, hospitalization, physical therapy, crisis intervention, or psychotherapy may be needed. Within the therapeutic setting—be it a hospital, clinic, or home—it is hoped that people will learn coping skills they can incorporate into their lifestyles once the illness is under control. Beyond this point, unchecked stress could lead to chronic physical or mental illness and even death.

Caring for Hospitalized Persons

When stressors cause illness, the illness in itself becomes a stressor. When illness is so serious that hospitalization is required, hospitalization compounds the stress of illness. As a result, the person faces escalating psychological and physiological stressors.

Volicer and Bohannon (1975) studied specific causes of stress responses in hospitalized people. The Hospital Stress Rating Scale measures stress caused by hospitalization (Table 6–1). Note the similarities between this assessment tool and the one developed by Holmes and Rahe (see Fig. 6–2). According to Volicer and Bohannon, the greater the magnitude of stress scale events reported, the greater the number of problems described by the subjects of the study on discharge (e.g., increased pain and slower recovery).

Cohen (1991) and Lazarus and Forlman (1984) extensively studied how people cope with illness and hospitalization. They presented five major coping tasks for the ill person:

- Reduce harmful environmental conditions and enhance prospects of recovery
- Tolerate or adjust to negative events and realities
- Maintain a positive self-image
- Maintain emotional equilibrium
- Continue satisfying relationships with others

Several nursing interventions help the hospitalized person master coping tasks. First, help the person reduce harmful environmental conditions within the care facility and thus enhance prospects of recovery. For many people, a hospital is a frightening place filled with unfamiliar people. Take time to orient the individual to the facility's schedule for meals, visitors, physician's rounds, nursing routines, and religious services. Introduce the individual to roommates. Support the person and significant others.

Also reduce iatrogenic problems (i.e., problems that arise as a result of treatment, medication, or hospitalization). For example, so often nurses and other health care workers forget that rest promotes healing. Medications, treatments, and even surgery cannot replace rest as a vital therapeutic intervention. Yet the schedule for routine nursing care and meals in many health care facilities completely overlooks this need. It is not unusual for a hospitalized person who has been awake, restless, and anxious all night and who finally falls asleep at 4:30 A.M. to be awakened at 5:00 A.M. to be weighed or have vital signs checked. This schedule benefits the facility, not the person. Therefore, keep these factors in mind and try to work for the convenience and comfort of the person in your care.

Help the person adjust to the realities of current health status. The hospitalized person often experiences fears—real or imagined. Recognize these fears, accept them, and help the person cope with them. The nurse, by acting as a sounding board, can allay fears and soften reality. Talking things out not only provides catharsis for the individual but also gives the nurse valuable information and insight into the person. Discussion also provides the person with insight into himself or herself and perhaps a greater sense of control.

Help the person maintain a positive self-image. Remember that the hospitalized person frequently is dependent, an uncomfortable status for most adults. Be prepared to give additional emotional support as needed (Fig. 6–8). While hospitalized, people often feel a loss of identity. For example, we view ourselves as individuals on the basis of the clothes we wear, our diet, our daily routine, and the like. Often residents in a hospital wear the same hospital gown, almost everyone eats a regular diet, and an entire ward of clients is expected to go to sleep and wake up at the same time every day. To help affirm a person's identity, talk with respect and warmth. When permitted, allow the person to wear regular clothes, read until sleepy, or sleep late some mornings. These interventions reinforce the person's self-image and help speed recovery.

Assist people in maintaining emotional equilibrium by helping them cope with the hospital experience. For example, most people are nervous when they must undergo a crucial diagnostic test or an uncomfortable procedure. Some people fear that they will lose control or experience intolerable pain. Take time to explain what will happen during tests and procedures and how they can cooperate and assist. Allow clients to verbalize questions and concerns.

Help clients continue to have satisfying relationships with others by encouraging them to relate to the

Table 6-1

HOSPITAL STRESS FACTORS

FACTOR	STRESS SCALE EVENTS	ASSIGNED RANK
1. Threat of severe illness	Thinking your appearance might be changed after your hospitalization	17
	Being put in the hospital because of an accident	24
	Knowing you have to have an operation	32
	Having a sudden hospitalization you were not planning to have	34
	Knowing you have a serious illness	46
	Thinking you might lose a kidney or some other organ	47
	Thinking you might have cancer	48
2. Loss of independence	Having to eat at different times than you usually do	02
	Having to wear a hospital gown	04
	Having to be assisted with bathing	07
	Not being able to get newspapers, radio, or television when you want them	08
	Having a roommate who has too many visitors	09
	Having to stay in bed or the same room all day	10
	Having to be assisted with a bedpan	13
	Not having your call light answered	35
	Being fed through tubes	39
	Thinking you may lose your sight	49
3. Unfamiliarity of surroundings	Having strangers sleep in the same room with you	01
	Having to sleep in a strange bed	03
	Having strange machines around	05
	Being awakened in the night by the nurse	06
	Being aware of unusual smells around you	11
	Being in a room that is too cold or too hot	16
	Having to eat cold or tasteless food	21
	Being cared for by an unfamiliar doctor	23
4. Problems with medications	Having medications cause you discomfort	28
	Feeling you are getting dependent on medications	30
	Not getting relief from pain medications	40
	Not getting pain medication when you need it	42
5. Lack of information	Thinking you might have pain because of surgery or test procedures	19
	Not knowing when to expect things will be done to you	25
	Having nurses or doctors talk too fast or use words you cannot understand	29
	Not having your questions answered by the staff	37
	Not knowing the results or reasons for your treatments	41
	Not knowing for sure what illnesses you have	43
	Not being told what your diagnosis is	44
6. Separation from spouse	Worrying about your spouse being away from you	20
	Missing your spouse	38
7. Separation from family	Being in the hospital during holidays or special family occasions	18
	Not having family visit you	31
	Being hospitalized far away from home	33
8. Isolation from other people	Having a roommate who is seriously ill or cannot talk with you	12
	Having a roommate who is unfriendly	14
	Not having friends visit you	15
	Not being able to call family or friends on the phone	22
	Having the staff be in too much of a hurry	26
	Thinking you might lose your hearing	45
9. Financial problems	Thinking about losing income because of your illness	27
	Not having enough insurance to pay for your hospitalization	36

Adapted from Volicer, B. J., *et al.* (1977). Medical-surgical differences in hospital stress factors. *Journal of Human Stress, 3,* 3. Reprinted by permission of Opinion Publications, Inc., and the author.

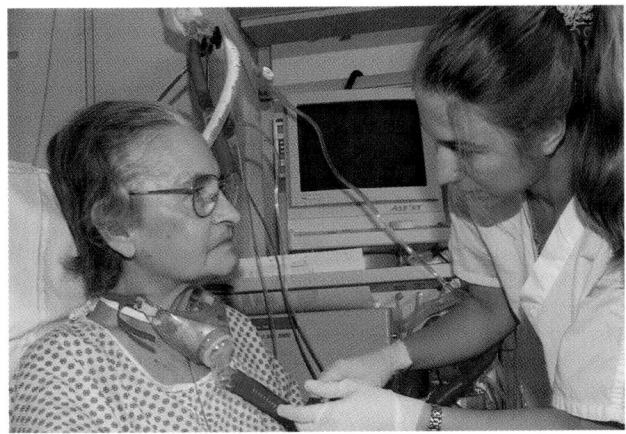

✦ **Figure 6–8**
Nurse gives support to client in addition to providing care.

staff, to roommates, and to their significant others. Remember to support significant others as well as the hospitalized individual. Encourage friends and family to visit, and plan your interventions around their visits. By showing compassion, understanding, and concern for the person's significant others, you reinforce those valuable relationships.

Evaluation

Evaluation means comparing actual with expected outcomes. To evaluate whether the individual has been able to adapt adequately, you must look for evidence that the specific psychological and/or physical symptoms have been decreased or no longer exist. For example, when comparing current status of the person with your baseline assessment, you may find that the person who previously complained of feeling lonely, being unable to sleep, and having a decreased appetite no longer voices these complaints.

Nursing evaluation includes assessing the degree to which the interventions were effective in assisting the person to reduce anxiety or stress. With effective interventions, the person should have taken measures to reduce identified sources of stress, and the person's anxiety should be reduced to a moderate level. Physiological measurements of stress (*e.g.*, pulse and blood pressure readings) should be within the normal range or approaching normal limits. Perhaps more important, the person should have new coping skills necessary to be able to manage future stress independently.

✦ Implications for Nurses

Stress of Caring for Ill People

As we have said, illness is stressful for most people. Because ill people look to the nurse to reduce stress, alleviate pain, give comfort and support, and

provide selfless service, caring for the sick is also demanding and stressful (Fig. 6–9). Many nurses work a lifetime without becoming physically exhausted and emotionally drained. Others burn out early in their career and either leave the nursing profession or continue to work in nursing but without enthusiasm or interest. What causes a person who was once excited about being a nurse to gradually become indifferent or even callous to the needs of sick people?

Burnout

What is professional burnout, what are its causes, what are its signs, and how can you prevent it from damaging your career? **Burnout** is a condition of physical and emotional exhaustion experienced as a result of job stressors related to caring for the ill and the troubled. Burnout is described by Maslach as "a syndrome of emotional exhaustion, depersonalization, and reduced personal accomplishment that can occur among individuals who do 'people work' of some kind. It is a response to the chronic emotional strain of dealing extensively with other human beings, particularly when they are troubled, ill or having personal problems" (Maslach, 1982).

If being idealistic and working with people puts a person at risk for developing burnout, nurses are clearly vulnerable. People who enter the nursing profession tend to be idealistic and altruistic. When you ask nursing students why they want to be a nurse, the answer is often "I want to help people." However, if the idealistic student graduates and finds it impossible to apply what has been learned in the classroom, disillusionment results. When workloads are too heavy, demands are too great, and nursing care suffers, ideals clash head on with reality. The resulting disappointment and failed personal expectations are the breeding ground for burnout in nurses.

Signs of Burnout

In the early stages of burnout, nurses recognize that they are not performing up to standard but may

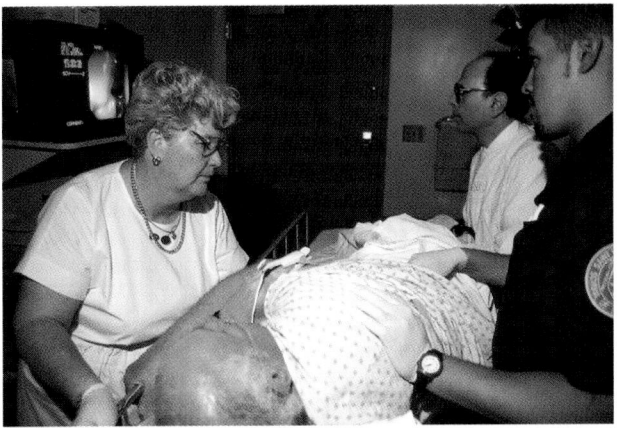

✦ **Figure 6–9**
Nurses often find themselves in stressful situations as they provide care.

not understand why. They may not realize that over-work can produce not only physical exhaustion but also emotional exhaustion. Because nurses have high expectations for themselves, they sometimes blame themselves rather than the work situation for an emotional "slump." Self-blame and guilt brewing inside the person may later erupt in numerous self-destructive ways.

Behavioral indicators of burnout include decreased productivity and quality of job performance, frequent mistakes or acts of poor judgment, forgetfulness, reduced attention to detail, preoccupation, reduced creativity, loss of interest, absenteeism, and lethargy. Some physical signs of burnout are elevated blood pressure, increased muscle tension, slumped posture, tension headache, upset stomach, change in appetite, and restlessness. Emotional indicators include irritability, depression, withdrawal, emotional outbursts, hostile and aggressive behavior, paranoia, and feelings of worthlessness (Schneider, 1982).

Burnout results from the hopelessness and helplessness that people feel when they try to achieve the unachievable. Signs of burnout indicate that the exhausted persons are trying to protect themselves from further psychological exhaustion.

Preventing Burnout

Preventing burnout requires many of the same coping skills we use to combat reactions to any stressor. Recognition of the problem is a first step, followed by self-help measures (including use of available sources of support) and, if necessary, professional counseling. To care for others, you must first care for yourself. To help others deal successfully with life's demands, you must practice stress management in your own life.

Summary

Theories of stress, homeostasis, and crisis have laid the groundwork for nurses to work effectively with clients who are having difficulty adapting to stress or coping with a crisis. Examining the concepts of stress, stressors, and stress responses allows the nurse to identify causes of stress and plan interventions to assist the client to manage stressful situations. By identifying levels of anxiety and planning nursing care accordingly, the nurse assists in stress reduction. Knowing the effects of negative and positive feedback on equilibrium is useful for nurses as they assist the client to return to a state of balance. Nurses need to be able to identify clients who are likely to have a situational or maturational crisis, evaluate the situation, and intervene and/or determine appropriate referrals. Finally, nurses must be able to honestly appraise their own equilibrium and responses to stress. Realistic self-appraisal and lifestyle patterns foster emotional health, thus providing a model for clients.

CHAPTER HIGHLIGHTS

✦ Stressors are sources of stress, and the *stress response* refers to reactions to stress.

✦ *Adaptation* refers to the adjustment that is made to stress. The nurse needs to assess stressors and crises that are affecting the client, including responses to stressors, level of anxiety, and psychophysiological disorders. Then the nurse and client should collaborate to deal with the stressors and the feelings engendered by the problem and reduce the physiological arousal to stress. Stress reduction interventions can be evaluated by noting what measures the client has taken to reduce identified stressors, reduce anxiety, change physiological measurements, and develop new coping skills.

✦ Selye defined stress from a physiological focus and developed the theory of the General Adaptation Syndrome (GAS) and the Local Adaptation Syndrome (LAS). Holmes and Rahe developed an instrument to quantify social stressors, and Lazarus emphasized cognitive appraisal for dealing with stress.

✦ Crisis theory, including the disequilibrium that occurs when previous coping strategies are ineffective, is described. Crisis intervention involves making appropriate referrals and assisting the client to develop new, effective coping strategies.

✦ Homeostasis should be assessed using biological, psychological, social, and cultural measurements. Mechanisms of homeostasis are compensatory, self-regulatory, primarily negative feedback processes; they exhibit some degree of deviation, and they have limitations. The mechanisms work together to regulate a single physiological process. Homeostatic mechanisms can be disrupted when the system is interrupted by illness, is overdriven, or completely breaks down from accelerated positive feedback.

✦ To maintain physiological homeostasis, the body must have and be able to store adequate amounts of oxygen, water, and nutrients. Elimination of excess in the form of waste products is essential.

✦ Psychological equilibrium is having a positive self-image and emotional balance and being at peace with the environment. Disequilibrium is manifested by negative self-perception and feeling out of step with people and the environment.

✦ Biofeedback training is educating an individual to become aware of and control certain involuntary physiological variables.

✦ Nurses must practice stress management and healthy lifestyle behaviors to deal with the stresses of life and set an example for clients.

Study Questions

1. Which of the following is a biofeedback technique?

    a. being aware of involuntary cues
    b. seeking support of a friend
    c. being aware of stress
    d. going to the nurse at work when ill

2. Sam, age 4 years, will start school for the first time tomorrow. For what would you assess Sam that would require new coping skills?

    a. signs of anxiety
    b. signs of psychophysiological responses
    c. signs of situational crisis
    d. signs of maturational crisis

3. All but one of the following is important when assessing a client's potential for crisis. Which of the following would *not* be included in your assessment?

    a. perception of event
    b. mental status
    c. support systems
    d. coping skills

4. Which of the following combinations of foods may magnify stress?

    a. apples, carrots, cereal, milk
    b. caffeine, alcohol, sugar, preservatives
    c. strawberries, broccoli, pepper, bagels
    d. bread, water, eggs, tomatoes

5. When a person is experiencing positive feedback

    a. he or she is returning to a normal state of homeostasis
    b. he or she is moving away from a normal state of homeostasis
    c. his or her blood hormone levels are being kept within normal limits
    d. he or she is recovering from an illness

Critical Thinking Exercises

1. Mr. G., 25 years of age, fell from a tree while hunting and is admitted with a C4 fracture. He is paralyzed from the neck down. He has two children, ages 2 and 3. He is recently divorced. His occupation is a United Parcel Service driver. Discuss the adaptation process of Mr. G.

2. Mr. F. is 35 years old and has a 4-year-old daughter and a 7-year-old son. His wife was killed in a car wreck last year. He is a nurse who currently works in the intensive care unit 11:00 A.M. to 7:00 P.M. He is beginning to make mistakes, call in sick frequently, and miss critical details. Discuss what is happening to Mr. F.

References

Aguilera, D. (1990). *Crisis intervention: Theory and methodology* (6th ed.). St. Louis: C. V. Mosby.

Aguilera, D., & Messick, J. M. (1984). *Crisis intervention: Theory and methodology* (4th ed.). St. Louis: C. V. Mosby.

Brownell, M. J. (1984). The concept of crises: Its ability for nursing. *Advances in Nursing Science: Crisis Intervention, 6* (4), 10–21.

Cannon, W. B. (1967). *The wisdom of the body: Revised and enlarged edition.* New York: W. W. Norton.

Caplan, G. (1964). *Principles of preventive psychiatry.* New York: Basic Books.

Cobb, S. (1976). Social support as a moderator of life stress. *Psychosomatic Medicine, 38* (5), 300–314.

Cohen, G. S. (1991). Anxiety and general medical disorders. In C. Salzman, & B. D. Lebowitz (Eds.). *Anxiety in the elderly.* New York: Springer.

Guyton, A. C. (1991). Functional organization of the human body and control of the "internal environment." In *Textbook of Medical Physiology* (8th ed, pp. 2–8). Philadelphia: W. B. Saunders.

Holmes, T. H., & Rahe, R. H. (1967). The social readjustment rating scale. *Journal of Psychosomatic Research, 11* (2), 213–218.

Holroyd, K. A., & Lazarus, R. S. (1982). Stress, coping, and somatic adaptation. In L. Goldberger, & S. Breznitz (Eds.). *Handbook of stress: Theoretical and clinical aspects.* New York: Free Press.

Hopping, B. (1980). Physiological response to stress: A nursing concern. *Nursing Forum, 19* (3), 259–269.

Infante, M. S. (1982). *Crisis theory: A framework for nursing practice.* Reston, VA: Reston Publishing.

Lazarus, R. S., & Forlman S. (1984). Coping and adaptation. In W. D. Gentry (Ed.) *Handbook of behavioral medicine.* New York: Guilford Press.

Maslach, C. (1982). *Burnout: The cost of caring.* Englewood Cliffs, NJ: Prentice Hall.

Pearlin, L. (1984). *Stress and coping mechanisms.* American Women's Medical Association.

Schneider, S. (1982). Curing burning while you work. *Nursing Life, 2* (5), 38–43.

Selye, H. (1982). History and present status of the stress concept. In L. Goldberger, & S. Breznitz (Eds). *Handbook of stress: Theoretical and clinical aspects.* New York: Free Press.

Selye, H. (1950). *The physiology and pathology of exposure to stress: A treatise based on the concepts of general adaptation syndrome and the disease of adaptation.* Montreal: Acta.

Selye, H. (1956). *The stress of life.* New York: McGraw-Hill.

Selye, H. (1974). *Stress without distress.* Philadelphia: J. B. Lippincott

Smith, W. H. (1990). Hypnosis in the treatment of anxiety. *Bulletin of the Menninger Clinic, 54* (2), 209–216.

Syme, S. F., & Berkman, L. F. (1979). Social networks, host resistance, and mortality: A nine year follow-up study of Almeda county residents. *American Journal of Epidemiology, 109* (2), 186–204.

Trygstad, L. (1980). Simple new ways to help anxious patients. *RN, 43,* 28–32.

Trygstad, L. (1984). *Stress and coping in psychiatric nursing* [Unpublished doctoral dissertation]. San Francisco: University of California at San Francisco Medical Center.

Volicer, B. J., & Bohannon, M. W. (1975). A hospital stress rating scale. *Nursing Research, 24* (5), 352–359.

Bibliography

Benner, P. E., & Wrobel, J. (1989). *The primacy of caring: Stress and coping in health and illness.* Menlo Park, CA: Addison-Wesley.

DeLaune, S. C. (1991). Effective limit setting. How to avoid being manipulated. *Nursing Clinics of North America, 26* (3), 757–764.

Dellasaga, C. (1990). Coping with caregiving. Stress management for caregivers of the elderly. *Journal of Psychosocial Nursing and Mental Health Services, 28* (1), 15–16, 19–22.

Easton, S. (1990). Learn to relax and counter stress. *Occupational Health, 42* (6), 172–174.

Goldstein, D. S. (1990). Neurotransmitters and stress. *Biofeedback and Self-Regulation, 15* (3), 243–271.

King, J. V. (1988). A holistic technique to lower anxiety: Relaxation with guided imagery. *Journal of Holistic Nursing, 6* (1), 16–20.

Koontz, E., Cox, D., & Hastings, S. (1991). Implementing a short-term family support group. *Journal of Psychosocial Nursing and Mental Health Services, 29* (5), 5–8, 10.

Kunkler, J., & Whittick, J. (1991). Stress-management groups for nurses: Practical problems and possible solutions. *Journal of Advanced Nursing, 16* (2), 172–176.

McKerracher, B. (1990). How to lend support in a crisis. *Nursing, 20* (11), 62–64.

Nolan, M. R., et al. (1990). Stress is in the eye of the beholder: Reconceptualizing the measurement of career burden. *Journal of Advanced Nursing, 15* (5), 544–555.

O'Connell, K. A. (1991). Why rational people do irrational things. *Journal of Psychosocial Nursing and Mental Health Services, 29* (1), 11–14.

Pasquali, E. A. (1990). Learning to laugh: Humor as therapy. *Journal of Psychosocial Nursing and Mental Health Services, 28* (3), 31–35.

Sadow, D., & Ryder, M. (1990). Anxiety reduction. Lessons that benefit students and patients. *Journal of Psychosocial Nursing and Mental Health Services, 28* (9), 29–30.

Swayze, S. (1991). Helping them cope. *Journal of Psychosocial Nursing and Mental Health Services, 29* (5), 35–37.

Young, R. F., & Kahana, E. (1987). Conceptualizing stress, coping, and illness management in heart disease caregiving. *Hospice Journal: Psychosocial and Pastoral Care of the Dying, 3* (2/3), 53–73.

Unit ✦ II

THE NURSING
PROCESS

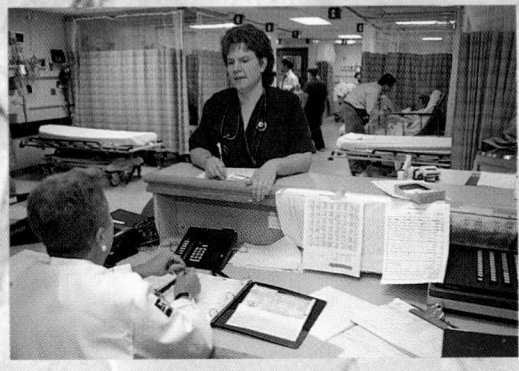

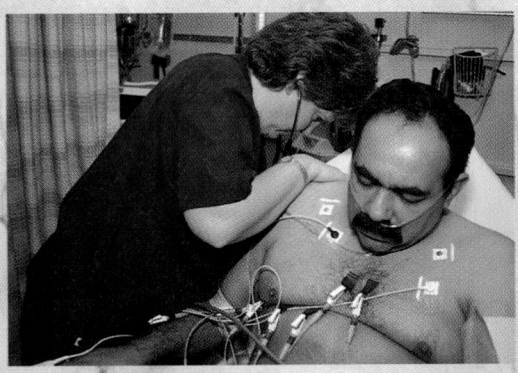

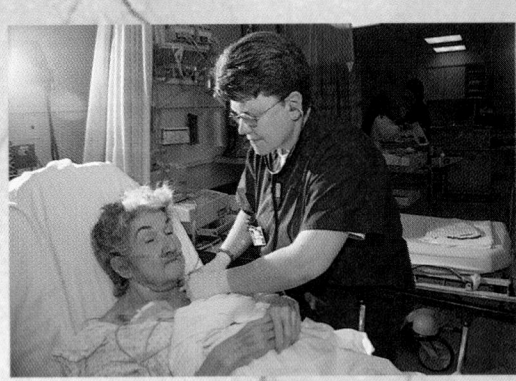

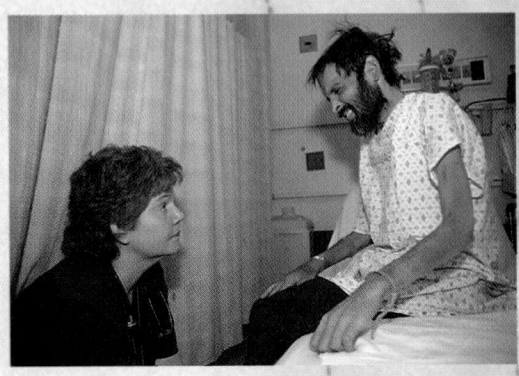

Frequently, I am asked "How do you do what you do?" Often, my answer is simply "I don't know," but I do know that for me, being an emergency nurse is the essence of nursing. I knew as a student nurse that the emergency department was where I could be the nurse I wanted to be, incorporate all my nursing skills, and make nursing a reality.

Emergency nursing is a multidiversified specialty, with opportunities ranging from clinical bedside nursing to flight nursing to acting as a clinical specialist or nurse practitioner. Today's emergency nurses are action oriented and well prepared. They possess the ability to thrive in a constantly changing environment while simultaneously providing compassionate nursing care to clients who are scared, hurting, or dying or have no other place to seek health care. Emergency nursing combines quickly and accurately assessing clients, reaching to comfort someone in crisis, and providing the connection between reality and what a client or family fears.

Emergency nurses care for clients of all ages and socioeconomic groups. They are confronted daily with new aspects of common illnesses, share in the joy at the beginning of a new life, and are present at the end of another life. For myself, there is nothing that equals easing a client's pain or fears, seeing a child smile after I have helped mend his hurt, knowing I played a part in saving a life, or having a client say, "I don't know how you do this, but I'm glad you do."

Judy Selfridge-Thomas, RN, MSN, CEN, FNP
An emergency nurse for more than 20 years, Judy Selfridge-Thomas fulfills the roles of clinical nurse, clinical nurse specialist, department manager, and nurse practitioner. She currently practices as a nurse practitioner in an emergency department in Long Beach, California.

Chapter 7

INTRODUCTION

TO THE

NURSING

PROCESS

✦

JULIA M. LEAHY, PhD, RN

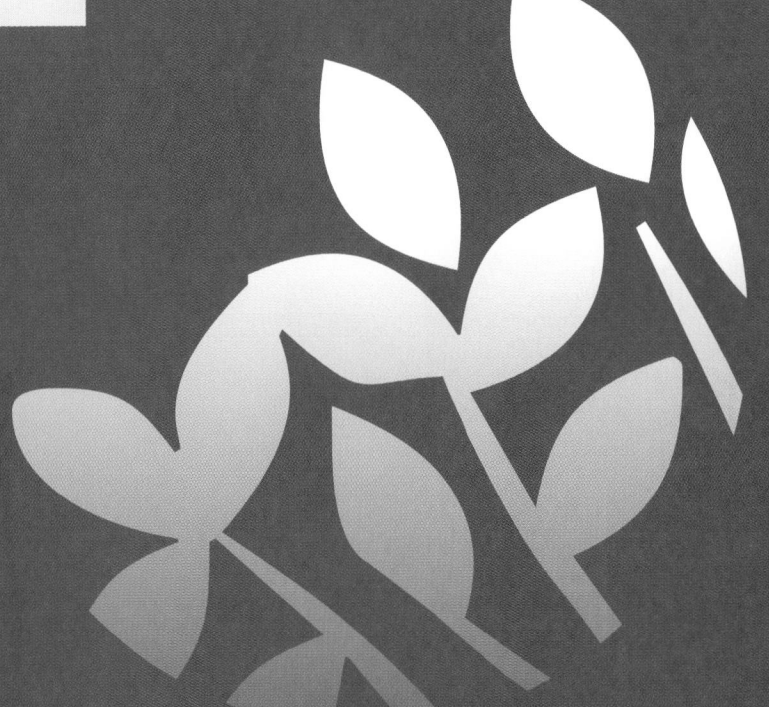

The practice of nursing involves the provision of comprehensive nursing care to clients based on knowledge from the biological, physical, and social sciences. Integral to the practice of nursing is the nursing process, an activity that facilitates the nurse's interaction with clients in an effort to assist clients to maintain and restore health. Through this method, nurses assess the client's health status, identify relevant nursing diagnoses and other health care problems, plan appropriate nursing intervention or collaborate with other health care providers, implement the plan of care, and evaluate the outcomes of care (Fig. 7–1).

The primary intent for using this process is to provide individualized, holistic, quality nursing care to clients and families. The nursing process, as described in these six chapters, primarily refers to the independent responsibility of the nurse in providing client care. It has been derived from the scientific method and adapted as an organized, systematic method for identifying client concerns and problems (nursing diagnoses), choosing expected client outcomes, determining interventions to resolve these problems, and evaluating achievement of expected outcomes following provision of nursing care.

✦ Historical Perspective

Before the 1950s, nurses learned the practice of nursing primarily from an apprentice model, working in staff positions as part of their training. Their practice was predominantly based on the physician's prescriptions for specific medical diagnoses. Knowledge of nursing solely reflected the medical model. Independent nursing practice was only evident in the provision of hygiene and comfort.

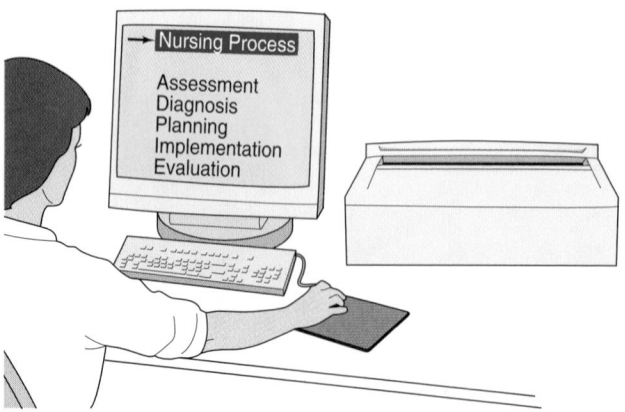

✦ **Figure 7–1**
The nursing process includes assessment (collection of data), diagnosis (analysis of the data), planning (developing a care plan), implementation of the plan, and evaluation of whether the plan worked.

In the 1950s, nursing leaders began to define the role of the nurse in terms of an autonomous profession. These authors articulated a profession based on the science of nursing that has the human being as the focus of nursing care. Hall in 1955 was the first to use the term ***nursing process*** to describe the independent role of nurses in caring for clients (George, 1980). Since then, a variety of descriptions of nursing practice and nursing diagnosis have emerged. Phases of the nursing process were delineated in a variety of ways.

Johnson (1959) described nursing practice as assessing client situations, making decisions, implementing a prescribed course of action, and evaluating those actions. Wiedenbach (1963) identified three components of nursing practice: observation of the client's behavior, ministration of help that the client needs, and validation that nursing actions were helpful. Knowles (1967) described nursing in terms of discovery and delving (involving assessment of client data), deciding on a plan of care, doing (or implementing), and discriminating (or evaluating) the client's actions.

In 1967, the first comprehensive book on nursing process was written by Yura and Walsh, who identified the four steps of assessing, planning, implementing, and evaluating. These authors considered nursing diagnosis as the logical end of the assessment process. Nursing diagnosis was first identified as a separate phase of the nursing process by Durand and Prince (1966) and Rothberg (1967). Gebbie and Lavin (1975) participated in the formulation of the first national conference on classification of nursing diagnosis. This group formally became the North American Nursing Diagnosis Association (NANDA) in 1982 and continues to meet every 2 years to define and classify relevant nursing diagnoses.

The American Nurses' Association (ANA) incorporated the components of the nursing process into the *Standards of Nursing Practice,* first published in 1973 and subsequently revised in 1991. By doing this, the ANA legitimatized the nursing process as a primary activity of nursing practice (Table 7–1). The nursing process was further legitimatized in 1972 with the legislation of the revised New York State Nurse Practice Act, which identified registered nursing practice as the diagnosis and treatment of human responses to illness. Many states subsequently changed their nurse practice acts. In 1980, the ANA stated that "nursing is the diagnosis and treatment of human responses to actual or potential health problems" (ANA, 1980).

In 1982, the National Council of State Boards of Nursing adopted a new blueprint for the nurse licensure examination that replaced the five-part examination representing the medical model of medicine, surgery, pediatrics, obstetrics, and psychiatry. The blueprint incorporates the five-part nursing process as one of the main organizing concepts. This further focused the practice of nursing as an independent professional activity that is collaborative with other health care professions.

Table 7–1

AMERICAN NURSES' ASSOCIATION STANDARDS OF CLINICAL NURSING PRACTICE

STANDARD	
1. Assessment	The nurse collects client health data
2. Diagnosis	The nurse analyzes the assessment data in determining diagnoses
3. Outcome identification	The nurse identifies expected outcomes individualized to the client
4. Planning	The nurse develops a plan of care that prescribes interventions to attain expected outcomes
5. Implementation	The nurse implements the interventions identified in the plan of care
6. Evaluation	The nurse evaluates the client's progress toward attainment of outcomes

Adapted from American Nurses' Association. (1991). *Standards of nursing practice.* Washington, DC: ANA.

Box 7–1

CHARACTERISTICS OF THE NURSING PROCESS

1. Goal directed
2. Systematic and organized
3. Dynamic and always changing
4. Widely applicable to clients, families, and groups
5. Adaptable to changing client situations
6. Interpersonal and interactive
7. Widely useful in conjunction with multiple nursing models

• **It is interactive in nature.** Although the nursing process appears sequential when viewed as a linear progression from one step to another, each step interacts with another. Expert, experienced nurses learn to appreciate the interrelatedness of the nursing process, as they are able to use instinct to recognize patterns of human response and to use analytic skills to solve problems that are not familiar or recognizable (Benner, 1984). The beginning nurse needs to learn the steps of the nursing process in the identified sequence to incorporate and develop skills required for expert practice. With experience, however,

Characteristics of the Nursing Process

The nursing process uniquely defines the practice of nursing. It has characteristics that describe its usefulness to the profession of nursing and that significantly affect client care. Kenney (1995) has defined several characteristics (Box 7–1). In addition, the characteristics of the nursing process can be identified as follows:

• **It distinguishes the nursing model from the medical model.** The nursing process is an activity that has been derived from the problem-solving method and is similar to those activities involved with the medical model. Several authors have shown that the differences are not in the steps involved as much as in the focus and the language (Henderson, 1987; McHugh, 1991). Physicians diagnose medical conditions; plan medical or surgical interventions; treat, cure, or surgically remove a disease process; and evaluate the effectiveness of these therapies. Nurses identify individual, family, or community responses to actual or potential health problems for which the nurse is accountable; identify those interventions that will modify or change these responses; and evaluate the effectiveness of nursing interventions in achieving stated outcomes. Nurses are focused more on health promotion and maintenance as opposed to curing and treating specific diseases (Fig. 7–2).

Problem solving: Nursing process versus medical model

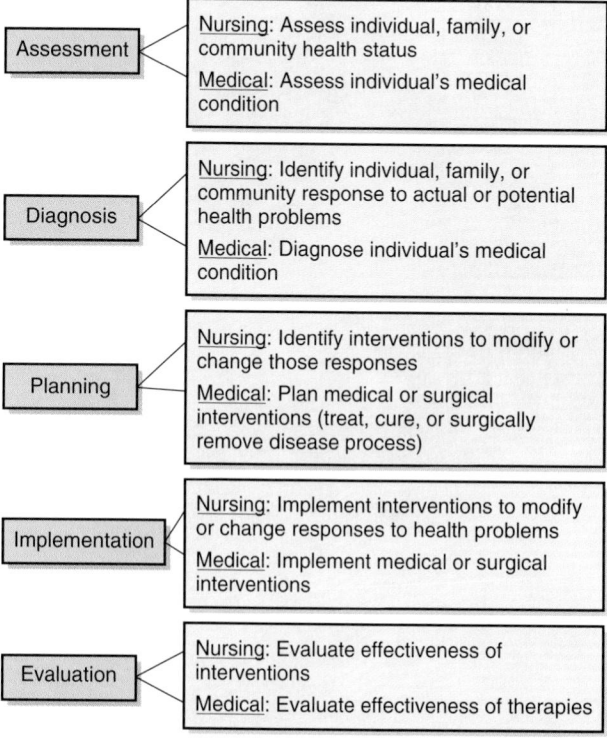

Figure 7–2
As a problem-solving method, the nursing process parallels medical decision making.

these skills become a natural part of the nurse's interaction with clients and the steps overlap and merge. For example, while providing an intervention for one problem, the experienced nurse may also assess for the emergence of new problems or the resolution of old problems.

- **It incorporates principles of problem solving.** Problem solving has evolved from the scientific method of identifying problems, collecting data, developing hypotheses, making a plan of action, testing the hypothesis, and evaluating the results of the action. In the nursing process, the nursing diagnosis is the hypothesis, and nursing actions are implemented to test resolution of the nursing diagnosis. Problem solving may also involve trial and error until a satisfactory solution is found, or it may be based on intuition, a common practice among expert nurses (Benner, 1984).

- **It encourages the use of creativity and critical thinking.** Creativity involves the ability to generate multiple problem-solving alternatives that go beyond usually expected actions. Developing individualized plans of care for clients requires the nurse to use creativity to identify alternative activities or adapt care for a specific environment. Planning care for the client in the home will require using different methods that are more applicable in that setting. Critical thinking is the mental activity that involves reasoning to solve problems. An individual can analyze how

language is used, make multiple assumptions about possible causes, formulate hypotheses about how to solve the problem, evaluate alternatives to solve the problem, and make conclusions in an effort to justify decisions and to determine the best choice of action (Bandman & Bandman, 1988). Making a hypothesis that a new nursing action will be more effective than a previously acceptable action and then evaluating the outcome of the action requires critical thinking. New practices emerge from this type of thought practice.

- **It helps in making sound clinical judgments.** Clinical judgment involves pulling together a multitude of skills to judge what courses of action to take in specific clinical situations. Nurses make judgments about aspects of client care based on their assessment of the client's health status and an indepth knowledge about a variety of care modalities. Selecting those interventions that are applicable in a particular situation requires that the nurse evaluate the situation and make a sound clinical judgment.

- **It is applicable in multiple settings.** Nurses practice in a variety of clinical settings, from the traditional acute care hospital–based environment to community-based settings, including home care and ambulatory care facilities. Regardless of the clinical practice area or the age and/or acuity of the clients, nurses function in a variety of roles and assume multiple responsibilities (Fig. 7–3A–D).

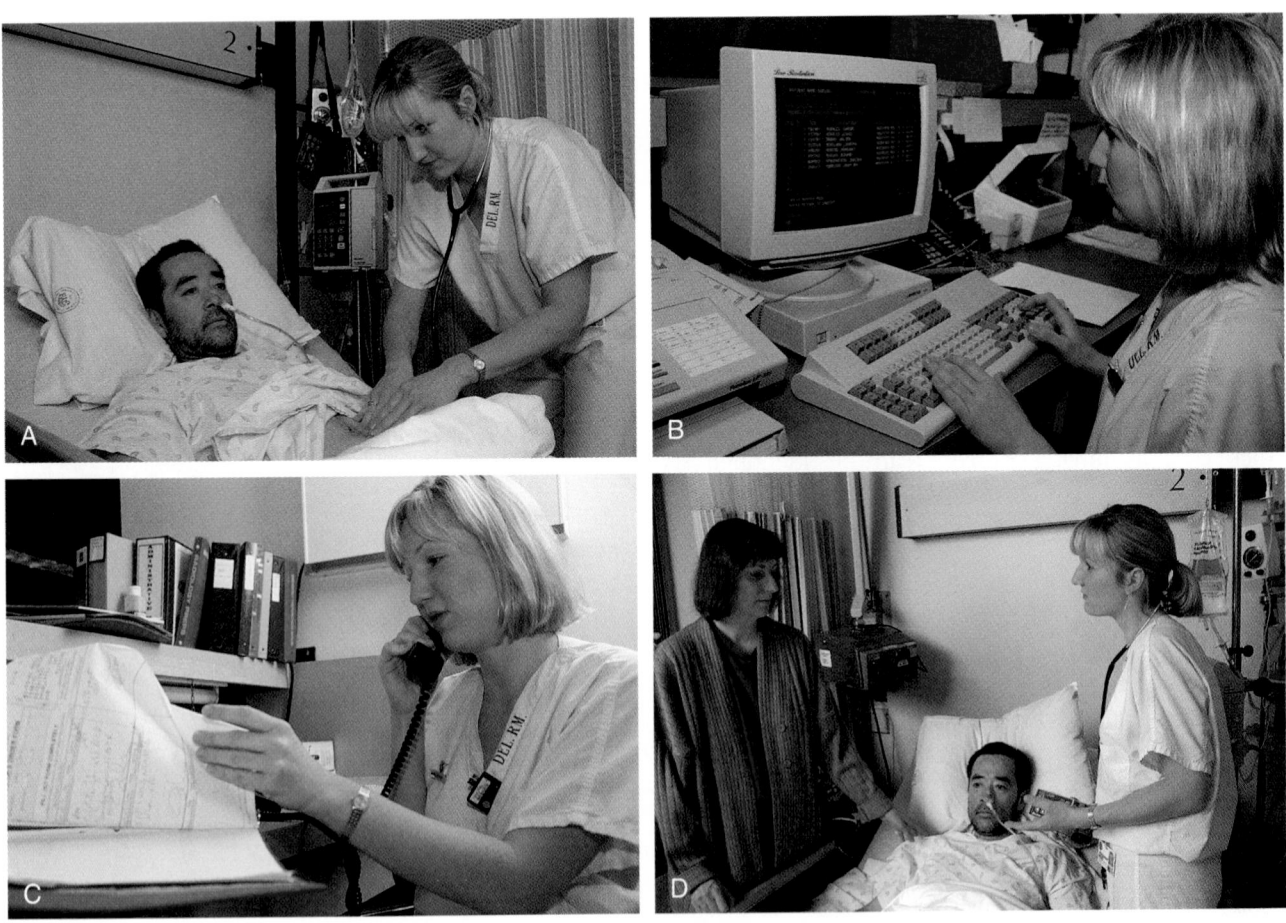

❧ **Figure 7–3**
The nurse's roles include *(panel A)* accurate assessment, *(panel B)* careful diagnosis, *(panel C)* planning in collaboration with the client and other health care personnel, and *(panel D)* implementation and evaluation of nursing actions.

Through the structure of the nursing process, nurses can assess the health care needs of clients and provide appropriate interventions applicable to the setting.

Components of the Nursing Process

The nursing process is a deliberate, organized, systematic activity that is used by nurses to carry out their professional roles when interacting with clients (Kenney, 1995). The nursing process for the independent nursing role is a five-step process that is sequential and repetitive throughout all phases of the nurse-client relationship. These steps include assessment, diagnosis, planning, implementation, and evaluation. A brief description of each step follows.

Assessment

Assessment is the organized, purposeful collection and validation of data about the client's health status, including the client's strengths and weaknesses. The collection of a database is essential to determine the client's health status. The database includes the nursing history, the physical examination, diagnostic test results, developmental considerations, and psychosocial development. The assessment phase is an essential part of the nursing process that guides the remaining steps. From the assessment, the nurse will identify relevant nursing diagnoses, determine appropriate client outcomes, and design a comprehensive plan of care. Data collection is an ongoing activity throughout all phases of the nursing process.

Nursing Diagnosis

Diagnosis involves the analysis of the assessment data to determine the client's responses that are amenable to nursing intervention, the clustering of data into distinct patterns, and the formulation of appropriate nursing diagnoses. After all of the data about the client are collected, the nurse begins to sort through the data to identify patterns that are amenable to nursing intervention. From these patterns, a nursing diagnosis emerges. The nursing diagnosis is a statement of the client's actual or potential health problem and the factor or etiology that is contributing to the problem. The current approved list of nursing diagnoses by NANDA generally serves as a primary guide for writing nursing diagnoses.

Planning

In the **planning** phase, the nurse systematically and deliberately determines an individualized nursing care plan that considers the holistic nature of the client. Following the collection of a database and the identification of the nursing diagnoses, the nurse works with the client (if feasible) to develop a mutually acceptable plan of care to resolve, limit, or prevent the problems that were identified. For each nursing diagnosis, the nurse selects measurable and observable expected outcomes to be achieved by the client following nursing intervention. These outcomes, or goals, are usually specific statements about the behaviors to be achieved by the client. The nurse establishes priorities of care and develops a plan of care. In some health care settings, standardized plans of care, or care maps, are now being used, either in conjunction with or instead of individual nursing plans of care.

Implementation

Implementation involves putting into action the nursing strategies (often referred to as nursing orders or nursing actions) that were identified in the nursing plan of care. These actions help clients achieve their expected outcomes relative to restoring health, preventing disease or illness, promoting wellness, or coping with an altered health state. As the nurse implements planned activities, ongoing assessment of the client continues to determine the need for any modification of the care plan or additional nursing diagnoses. Documentation of these actions is an integral component of the implementation phase.

Evaluation

Evaluation is the process of determining the extent to which expected outcomes are achieved by the client. By collecting additional data, the nurse identifies client responses to nursing actions and estimates the degree to which objectives or client outcomes have been attained. Modification of the plan of care reflects the changing health status of the client.

A summary of the nursing process is presented in Table 7–2. To show the steps of the nursing process with a particular client, the following chapters discuss the case of Mrs. C., a client who has suffered a fractured hip.

Purposes of the Nursing Process

The nursing process serves multiple purposes. Primarily, the nursing process is a directed activity that is designed to restore and promote the client's optimal state of wellness and to support the client's quality of life in situations in which wellness cannot be achieved (Yura & Walsh, 1988). This purpose emphasizes the roles of the nurse in health promotion, health maintenance, health restoration, and palliative support.

Kenney stated that the systematic methodology of

Table 7–2

OVERVIEW OF THE NURSING PROCESS

PHASE	ACTIVITIES
Assessment	Obtain a nursing history
	Interview the client and significant others
	Perform a physical examination
	Review results of diagnostic studies
Diagnosis	Identify cues
	Cluster data into patterns
	Identify gaps in data
	Determine client responses to health problems
	Formulate relevant nursing diagnoses
Planning	Establish priorities of care
	Identify expected outcomes
	Select appropriate nursing interventions and actions
	Collaborate with client and/or family
	Write the nursing plan of care
Implementation	Perform interventions and actions as identified in the plan of care
	Continue to assess the client
	Revise the plan of care as needed
	Document nursing actions in the record
	Communicate nursing actions to other health care professionals
Evaluation	Reassess the client after care is rendered
	Compare the client's response to stated outcomes
	Modify the plan of care as needed

the nursing process "unifies, standardizes, and directs nursing practice" (1995, p. 11). Through this practice method, nurses are able to function in roles that serve other purposes:

- To promote continuity of care
- To ensure clear documentation of care rendered
- To provide care that is individualized to the client
- To facilitate an open, interactive nurse-client relationship
- To ensure quality of care rendered
- To validate the accountability of nursing practice
- To verify the health care needs of clients
- To encourage collaborative interaction with other health care members
- To encourage client involvement in relevant health care decisions

Summary

The nursing process is a dynamic process that provides the nurse with a structure to approach client care. The structure provides the nurse with the framework for assessing clients and planning care to meet expected outcomes. The structure remains constant across clients, medical diagnoses, health care environments, and the level of nursing practice.

CHAPTER HIGHLIGHTS

✦

- ✦ The nursing process is a deliberate, purposeful activity that provides a framework for interacting with clients. Its goals are the maintenance, restoration, and promotion of health or the provision of palliative support for terminally ill clients.

- ✦ The nursing process is composed of five steps: assessment, diagnosis, planning, implementation, and evaluation. These steps are interrelated, as the activities involved overlap.

- ✦ Assessment is the organized, purposeful collection and validation of data about the client's health status. This is an essential step to determine the client's health status, strengths, and weaknesses.

- ✦ Diagnosis involves the analysis of the assessment data to determine the client's responses that are amenable to nursing intervention and for which the nurse is accountable and responsible as an independent professional.

- ✦ Planning is the systematic, deliberate determination of an individualized nursing care plan that considers the holistic nature of the client.

- ✦ Implementation involves putting the nursing care plan into action. Continual assessment of the client and documentation of nursing activities are integral components of this phase.

- ✦ Evaluation is the process of determining the extent to which stated outcomes are achieved by the client.

- ✦ The primary purpose of the nursing process involves the provision of individualized, quality nursing care to clients.

Critical Thinking Exercises

1. Ms. S. is hospitalized for a new cord injury of C8. Discuss how you would implement the nursing process with her.

2. Mr. T. is homeless and visits your clinic because he began coughing up blood. Discuss the variations in the use of the nursing care you would use with Mr. T.

References

American Nurses' Association. (1980). *Nursing: A social policy statement*. Washington, DC: ANA.

American Nurses' Association. (1973). *Standards of nursing practice*. Kansas City, MO: ANA.

American Nurses' Association. (1991). *Standards of nursing practice*. Washington, DC: ANA.

Bandman, E. L., & Bandman, B. (1988). *Critical thinking in nursing*. Norwalk, CT: Appleton & Lange.

Benner, P. (1984). *From novice to expert*. Menlo Park, CA: Addison-Wesley Publishing.

Durand, M., & Prince, R. (1979). Nursing diagnosis: Process and decisions. In A. Marriner (Ed.), *The nursing process: A scientific approach* (2nd ed.). St. Louis: C. V. Mosby.

Gebbie, K., & Lavin, M. (1975). *Classification of nursing diagnosis*. St. Louis: C. V. Mosby.

George, J. (Ed.) (1980). *Nursing theories: The base for professional nursing practice* (2nd ed.). Englewood Cliffs, NJ: Prentice-Hall.

Henderson, V. (1987). Nursing process—a critique. *Holistic Nursing Practice, 1*(3), 7–18.

Johnson, D. E. (1959). A philosophy of nursing. *Nursing Outlook, 8*(April), 198–200.

Kenney, J. W. (1995). Relevance of theory-based nursing practice. In P. J. Christensen, & J. W. Kenney (Eds.) *Nursing process: Application of conceptual models* (4th ed.). St. Louis: C. V. Mosby.

Knowles, L. (1967). *Decision-making in nursing: A necessity for doing: ANA Clinical Sessions, 1966*. New York: Appleton-Century-Crofts.

McHugh, M. K. (1991). Does the nursing process reflect quality care? *Holistic Nursing Practice, 5*(3), 22–28.

Rothberg, J. J. (1967). Why nursing diagnosis? *American Journal of Nursing, 67*(5), 1040–1423.

Wiedenback, E. (1963). The helping art of nursing. *American Journal of Nursing, 63*(11), 54.

Yura, H., & Walsh, M. B. (1967). *The nursing process: Assessing, planning, implementing, and evaluating*. New York: Appleton-Century-Crofts.

Yura, H., & Walsh, M. B. (1988). *The nursing process: Assessing, planning, implementing, and evaluating* (5th ed.). Norwalk, CT: Appleton & Lange.

Bibliography

Alfaro-LeFevre, R. (1994). *Applying nursing process: A step by step guide*. Philadelphia: W. B. Saunders.

Alfaro-LeFevre, R. (1995). *Critical thinking in nursing*. Philadelphia: W. B. Saunders.

Benner, P. E., Tanner, C. A., & Chesla, C. A. (1996). *Expertise in nursing practice: Caring, clinical judgement and ethics*. New York: Springer.

Bullough, B., & Bullough, V. (1994). *Nursing issues in the nineties and beyond*. New York: Springer.

Calladine, M. (1996). Nursing process for health promotion using King's theory. *Journal of Community Health Nursing, 13*(1), 51–57.

Doegnes, M. E., Moorhouse, M. F., & Burley, J. T. (1995). *Application of the nursing process and nursing diagnosis: An interactive text for diagnostic reasoning*. Philadelphia: F. A. Davis.

Ellis, J. R., & Hartley, C. L. (1995). *Nursing in today's world: Challenges, issues, and trends* (5th ed.). Philadelphia: J. B. Lippincott.

Facione, N. C., & Facione, P. A. (1996). Externalizing the critical thinking in knowledge development and clinical judgement. *Nursing Outlook, 44*(3), 129–136.

Jones, R. A. P., & Beck, S. E. (1996). *Decision making in nursing*. Albany, NY: Delmar Publishers.

Murray, M. E., & Atkinson, L. D. (1994). *Understanding the nursing process* (5th ed.). New York: McGraw-Hill, Health Professions Division.

Wilkinson, J. M. (1996). *Nursing process: A critical thinking approach* (2nd ed.). Menlo Park, CA: Addison-Wesley.

Chapter ✦ 8

ASSESSMENT

JULIA M. LEAHY, PhD, RN

LEARNING OBJECTIVES
✦

After studying this chapter, you should be able to

✦ Define basic terminology identified at beginning of the chapter

✦ Compare subjective and objective data

✦ Describe the purposes of a nursing history

✦ Describe the components of a nursing history

✦ Describe the purposes of an interview in obtaining data from the client

✦ Identify sources of client data

✦ Describe a nursing physical examination

✦ Define the four skills used during a physical examination

✦ Describe the importance of collecting data from diagnostic studies

✦ Describe the different types of diagnostic data

✦ Describe the role of the nurse during diagnostic studies

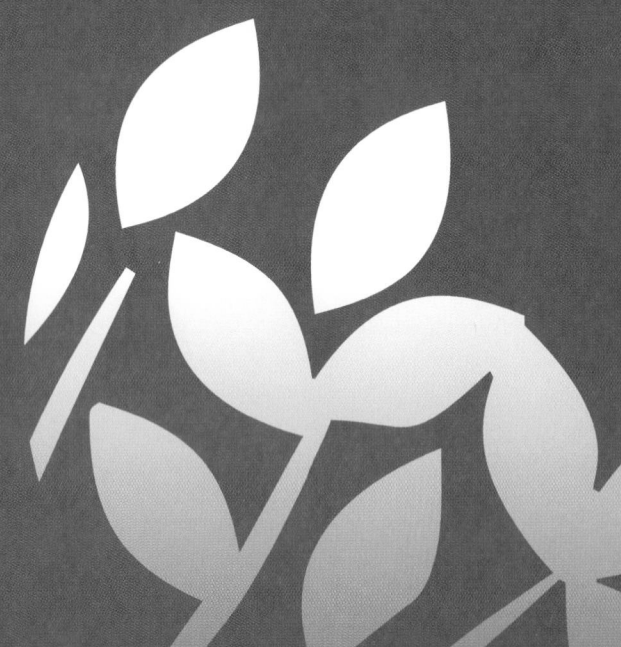

Assessment is the organized, purposeful collection and validation of data about the client's health status, including the client's strengths and weaknesses. Data collection is both the first step of the nursing process and an ongoing component of the remaining phases of the nursing process (Fig. 8–1).

Assessment guides the steps of the nursing process. The nurse obtains the initial database through an indepth collection of *pertinent* information about the client. The primary focus of the assessment process is the *client's responses* to health care concerns; these concerns may be physiological, psychological, sociocultural, or spiritual in nature (Christensen & Kenney, 1995). A well-constructed database reflects the holistic nature of the individual client and enables the nurse to identify relevant nursing diagnoses, to determine appropriate client outcomes, and to design a comprehensive plan of care.

The database includes all the relevant information about the client, including

* Nursing history
* A comprehensive physical examination
* Past and present medical history
* Laboratory and other diagnostic test results
* Input from family and significant others

The nurse collects data using a systematic process, which enables the nurse to gather all the pertinent and appropriate information about the client and to avoid errors related to missing data.

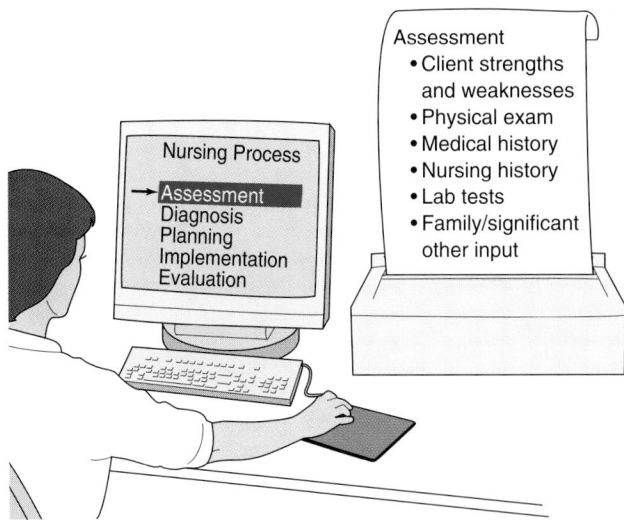

❧ Figure 8–1
Assessment is both the first step of the nursing process and an ongoing part of the four steps that follow. Data are collected regarding the client's health status from a variety of sources.

Data Collection

Types of Data

Data that the nurse collects about the client can be either subjective or objective. **Subjective data** are pieces of information that only the client can report and that cannot be verified by another. Having pain, feeling sad, and experiencing hot or cold are examples of subjective data. These data are frequently called symptoms or covert data. Symptoms are uniquely described by each individual, and comparisons are sometimes difficult. Pain is one type of subjective data that the nurse may attempt to quantify. The client is asked to rate the pain on a scale of 0 (no pain) to 10 (severe pain). Consider the following example:

> It is 1 day after an adult client has undergone an open reduction and internal fixation of a fracture of the hip. The client complains of pain and tells the nurse that the pain is a 7 on a scale from 0 to 10. One hour after receiving narcotic analgesic medication for the pain, the client tells the nurse that the pain is now a 2.

By doing this, the nurse can compare changes in the level of pain and determine whether measures taken to reduce pain are effective. In this example, the nurse can determine that the client received relief from the medication. Because symptoms can only be experienced by the client, the nurse must be careful to document these data as reported by the client. The nurse's judgments, feelings, or interpretations should not be included in the documentation and communication of these symptoms.

Objective data can be observed by the nurse or can be measured by an appropriate method or instrument. These data can be verified by another person, and many can be judged by acceptable standards. Examples of objective data include blood pressure measurements, appearance of the skin, and the response of the pupils to light. When the nurse records the client's vital signs and includes specific numerical references based on protocols that are standard, objective data about the client are being documented. In the client's record, the nurse should document the specific behaviors observed as objective data and the feelings described by the client as subjective data (Fig. 8–2). This allows for accurate comparison over time and between observers.

Sources of Data

The Client

The nurse's primary source of data for the assessment is the client. Usually, the client is the most reliable source of needed information for the nursing database. It is assumed that the information provided by the client is accurate and trustworthy. Because the client is seeking health care, information is usually shared willingly with the nurse and health team mem-

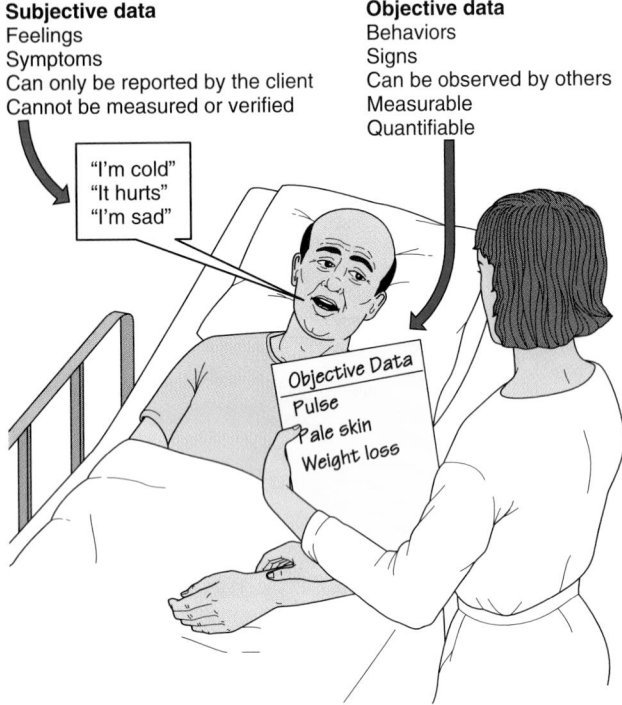

Subjective data
Feelings
Symptoms
Can only be reported by the client
Cannot be measured or verified

"I'm cold"
"It hurts"
"I'm sad"

Objective data
Behaviors
Signs
Can be observed by others
Measurable
Quantifiable

Objective Data
Pulse
Pale skin
Weight loss

❧ **Figure 8–2**
Both subjective and objective data are carefully recorded by the nurse.

bers. Occasionally, the client may be unable to provide reliable data because of illness, diminished mental ability, emotional distress, or age. A client who is having severe shortness of breath may have difficulty speaking and concentrating. An individual with a psychological dysfunction may distort reality and provide unreliable information. Young children may have a limited understanding of their health problem. It is important for the nurse to provide the client with the opportunity to give information, to document the information received from the client, to determine the deficient or erroneous areas in the database, and to seek alternative sources of information, if needed.

Significant Others

Significant others include family members, friends, and support persons who know the client well and can provide additional data related to the client's health status. When the client is unable or has a limited capacity to provide data, significant others help the nurse to complete and verify the nursing history. Very young children may not be able to provide any information because of limited vocabulary. School-age children may be able to describe subjective feelings but might be limited with regard to specific factual information. Adults who are comatose might present a problem for health care workers if no significant other is available to provide important information. The nurse should indicate in the record the name and relationship of the significant other who is being inter-

viewed and the perceived reliability of this source in giving accurate data.

The Client's Medical Record

The medical record is a source of past and current information about the client's personal data, such as age, finances, insurance, religion, and occupation, and health status. The client's medical record is multidisciplinary, containing information provided by various members of the health team, including physicians, physical therapists, dietitians, social workers, and radiology personnel. Notations by health team members indicate their evaluation of the client's response to care, the client's progress toward achieving the goals of care, and their prescriptions or suggestions for treatment measures. The record also includes reports of laboratory and other diagnostic tests, consultations, referrals to social service or a visiting nurse agency, and reports of operative procedures. The information provided by these sources assists the nurse in developing, implementing, and evaluating the nursing plan of care.

Records of previous admissions and prior health prevention or maintenance activities provide the nurse with additional data about the client's health status and medical problems. Information about the client's previous medical or surgical problems and patterns of response to treatment are essential components of the database.

Other Health Care Professionals

The nurse is a member of an interdisciplinary team that works collaboratively to assist the client in maintaining or restoring health. Members of the team may include physicians, social workers, pharmacists, physical therapists, inhalation (or respiratory) therapists, dietitians, home care providers, and others. Interactions among members of the interdisciplinary team can occur formally at client care conferences or informally when the need arises.

Health Care Literature

Health care and nursing literature resources are a good source of information about client problems and alternative care methods. Specific information about illness; diagnostic procedures; the relationship of age, culture, and psychosocial attributes with illness; and treatment modalities can guide the nurse in completing a comprehensive and detailed assessment. The literature can also provide the nurse with the means for validating inferences made about the client's database.

Components of the Database

Nursing History

The **nursing history** is a detailed description of the client's health status. The nurse obtains a nursing history through a planned, systematic interview with the client. Ideally, this interview should occur at the time the client enters the health care system for the first time, whether that is when the client is admitted to the hospital or when the client first visits an ambulatory care setting. The nursing history provides the nurse with an initial database to plan care and to determine expected outcomes of care for the client.

The nursing history should contain the following information (Box 8–1) about the client, based on the guidelines presented by Iyer and colleagues (1995):

• Biographical client profile: Such information includes age, marital status, and occupation. For children, birth date, information about other family members, and parent's name and work numbers are to be included.

• Source of information: Generally, the client is the primary source of data. If the client is unable to provide the information because of illness, limited mental ability, or age, then family or significant others are appropriate sources of data.

• Chief complaint: Description of current problem for which client is seeking assistance, including the history of the present illness. For children, have the parent or guardian describe the child's current problem or the reason for seeking health care.

• Past medical and surgical history: Include a listing of previous illnesses, surgical procedures, and allergies. For children, a listing of immunizations and childhood illnesses in addition to any pertinent data about the child's prenatal development and status at birth should be included.

• Family history: A history of the illness and cause of death of immediate family members (parents, siblings, children) can determine the client's risk factors for disease. A family tree diagram that includes age and health or age and cause of death of family members is included. For children, include information about the family dynamics, including who is the principle caretaker, whether any recent family crisis has occurred, and who disciplines the child.

• Medication history: List all medications taken by the client, including the dosage, frequency of administrations, duration of therapy, and time of last dose. This should include over-the-counter drugs and oral contraceptives.

• History of alcohol and tobacco use: Describe the usual patterns, including amount per day, type, age started, and age stopped (if applicable).

• Social history: Description of the client's occupation, income, medical insurance, living environment, spiritual patterns (including religious orientation and observance, values, and diet modifications), and support systems (availability of family or significant others). For children, information about the child's friends, play activities, and schooling is important.

• Patterns of daily living: Details of the client's personal data can include developmental patterns (level of development), activities of daily living (eating, grooming, dressing, sleep/rest pattern, activity, and elimination), preferences for types of health care services, and type of health practices used.

• Transcultural issues: Data related to culturally based health beliefs and practices are an important aspect of the health history. Included are the individual's beliefs about the causation of illness, the stigma attached to illness symptoms, the meaning of the illness to the client and family, and the individual's usual methods for healing and treatment (Jarvis, 1996). Refer to Chapter 36 for a more detailed discussion about the importance of cultural influences on health care.

The nurse generally follows a specified guide within an identified framework. Examples of structured frameworks are presented later in this chapter.

Interview

The **interview** is an interactive communication process that involves a mutual or reciprocal exchange of information between the nurse and the client. During the interview, the nurse must develop refined communication and interaction skills to identify those responses by the client that require nursing intervention. The interview requires an organized, logical, and systematic format to focus on the behavior, needs, and attitudes involving the client's health status.

The interview provides the nurse with these opportunities:

• To introduce the client to the health care setting
• To establish a therapeutic relationship with the client through an open dialogue
• To obtain information about the client's health care concerns and expectations required for identification of nursing diagnoses and planning
• To allow the client to participate in setting priorities of goals for care
• To determine those areas requiring special attention during other components of the assessment (Iyer *et al.,* 1995)

There are three segments of the interview: introduction or orientation, working phase or body, and termination.

Introduction

Before beginning the interview, the nurse should become familiar with the client's history and current

---

Box **8–1**

ELEMENTS OF A NURSING HISTORY

• Biographical client profile
• Source of information
• Chief complaint
• Past medical and surgical history
• Family history
• Medication history
• History of alcohol and tobacco use
• Social history
• Patterns of daily living
• Transcultural issues

health problem, if possible. This assists the nurse in focusing the interview. The nurse should have an organized sequence of questions and interview techniques that address the client's specific health care concerns. The nurse should also be familiar with the data collection format to be used to streamline the interview process and to avoid irrelevant or inappropriate conversation. While each health care setting may have a structured format that varies in style and format, the nurse will find that there is consistency in the type of questions that are being asked during a nursing history interview.

Before beginning the interview, the nurse should also consider the setting of the interview and the environmental factors that could affect the process. A quiet setting that affords the client with privacy will enhance the exchange of information between the client and the nurse. If a private room or area is not available, the nurse should limit the number of individuals within hearing distance. Family and significant others should be asked to leave the interview setting, unless the client prefers that they remain in attendance. The client should be assured of confidentiality of the information, since information about personal aspects of the client's life will be asked. This means that only those health care team members involved in the care of the client will have access to the data collected. The nurse should sit close enough to the client to facilitate the exchange of information. The closeness of the nurse to the client should primarily depend on the client's preference for personal space distance.

Ideally, the interview should be scheduled at a time that is convenient to both the client and the nurse. The client should be relaxed and free from pain and distractions. Obtaining useful and pertinent data requires that the client concentrate on the interview questions. The nurse needs to be aware of the client's health status at the time of the interview and determine how much time and effort the client can expend at any one time. Several sessions may be required for clients who are severely ill. If so, the nurse needs to determine which information is a priority for immediate assessment and which information can be delayed until a later time. Consider the following example:

> An adult client comes to the emergency department in acute distress, reporting severe chest pain. The client is breathing rapidly, the blood pressure is low, and the pulse is rapid and irregular. The history reveals that the chest pain began about 1 hour ago and the client has no history of heart disease.

In this situation, the nurse must focus the interview on the client's immediate problem and the need to relieve chest pain and resolve the cardiac problems. When the client's condition stabilizes, the nurse can then perform a more detailed collection of history. The nurse determines priorities even during the interview by identifying which information is imperative to obtain immediately and which information can be obtained at a later time.

After determining that the client is comfortable and the setting is appropriate, the nurse should initiate the interview with an introduction and then tell the client the purpose of the interview, including a brief description of the information to be obtained. The client's initial contact with the nurse is very important, especially if this is the client's first experience with the health care system. The nurse should maintain a professional demeanor and be respectful of the client to create an atmosphere of trust conducive to a therapeutic nurse-client relationship. Failure to do this will have a detrimental effect on the other phases of the interview. To show interest and concern for the patient, the nurse should speak to the client directly, use the client's name, and maintain eye contact.

Body, or Working Phase

During the body of the interview, the nurse gathers the necessary information about the client's past and present health status. The nurse should begin the interview with the client's current complaint or concern and proceed according to the identified format. The focus of the interview should be on the subjective data, as expressed by the client. The nurse should use communication skills during the interview that include both verbal and nonverbal techniques that facilitate the acquisition of the database. Developing skill in using these techniques effectively requires that the nurse

- Learn these techniques
- Incorporate these techniques into daily practice
- Record in writing or by audio or videotape the interactions with clients
- Analyze his or her own techniques when responding to the client to determine the degree of success in using these techniques (Stuart & Sundeen, 1995).

✦ Verbal Techniques. Verbal communication during the interview process requires a conscious effort on the part of the nurse. To be effective, the nurse should use language that the client will understand and use verbal techniques that are

1. Simple and understandable by the client
2. Precise in meaning
3. Relevant to the current situation
4. Adaptable to the client's needs
5. Deemed credible by the client

During the interview, the nurse uses two types of questioning methods: open-ended and closed questions. **Open-ended questions** require the client to give more detailed answers and not simply answer yes or no. The nurse uses open-ended questions to elicit information from the client about feelings, concerns, opinions, and perceptions and to allow for validation of both subjective and objective data. Because open-ended questions can elicit lengthy answers, the nurse needs to keep the conversation focused on the topic of concern and to allow adequate time for the interview. **Closed questions** are appropriate for the nurse to use when obtaining specific factual information. Questions beginning with "what," "how," and "which" tend to elicit explanations, whereas those beginning with "why" can put the client in a defensive position.

Table 8–1 compares closed and open-ended questions. When asking a client a series of questions, the nurse should present one question at a time, allowing the client the opportunity to respond specifically to that question. Using multiple questions together can be confusing for the client and should be avoided. Furthermore, asking more than one question at once gives the client the choice of which question to answer, thus allowing some questions to go unanswered.

Another verbal interviewing technique for the nurse to use during the interview is reflection. The nurse's interpretation or perception of a client's behavior or verbal response is repeated or rephrased. Restating the client's answer in the form of a question encourages the client to expand on, clarify, or verify the response previously given. Reflection of feelings involves informing the client about feelings that the nurse perceives the client is having. This is done to assist the client in focusing on these feelings and making him or her more aware of them. It also allows the nurse to assess the client's response to this reflection and to judge whether the interpretation was accurate.

Frequently, clients want the nurse to validate and to give approval to their perceptions and feelings. Nurses should avoid expressing their own opinions, giving advice beyond that which is within the nurse's present role, and providing false reassurance about the future outcome of the client's condition.

✦ **Nonverbal Techniques.** A variety of nonverbal techniques can facilitate or hinder the communication process and its effect on the nurse-client relationship. Nonverbal messages often have a greater impact than verbal ones and are accepted more readily by the receiver. The use of these techniques reflects the nurse's insight about the relationship between nonverbal "body language" and therapeutic interaction with the client. How a message is received by the client depends primarily on the nonverbal technique utilized with the verbal statements.

Nonverbal techniques include a variety of body language maneuvers, including gestures, facial expressions, body positions, tone of voice, use of touch, and appearance, as well as silence and active listening. Nonverbal techniques that contradict what is stated verbally may cause confusion.

Body language reveals important information about the client. The client's facial expression should be consistent with the verbal message. If the client is conveying information about a rewarding occupation, the nurse should expect to observe a facial expression that is consistent with this perception. If, however, the client appears sad or smirks while talking, then the nurse might conclude that there is a mismatch between the verbal and nonverbal message. The nurse should also be aware that some clients might have an inappropriate expression or laughter, be unable to maintain eye contact, or appear restless and irritable because of nervousness, anxiety, boredom, disinterest, or preoccupation with something else. The nurse may then use verbal techniques to point out these observations and to verify the accuracy of these perceptions.

Silence is an important tool for the nurse when interviewing the client. By remaining silent at certain points during the interview, the nurse encourages the client to express his or her feelings, despite feeling awkward. It may also help the client to gain insight into behavior. The nurse needs to allow time for the client to respond appropriately and completely to questions posed and not fill in the silent periods with additional questions or useless conversation. Silence also conveys acceptance of the client's feelings, beliefs, and values.

Another important skill for interviewing is the use of active listening, which is essential for obtaining an understanding of the client (Stuart & Sundeen, 1995). Developing the skill of listening enables the nurse to focus actively on both the content and the intonation of the client's responses (Fig. 8–3). This involves listening to the verbal component of the message, identifying the existence of nonverbal cues in the client's body language, and carefully interpreting the significance of both (Iyer *et al.,* 1995). To listen effectively, the nurse must exert effort to give full attention to the client and to avoid daydreaming. When listening, the nurse should be observant of the client's body language, which can provide clues about the client's true feelings and emotions. The nurse can identify what areas in the database need additional exploration and validation. (See Chapter 13 for more discussion of active listening.) Table 8–2 summarizes therapeutic and less therapeutic techniques.

Termination

The interview concludes when the database is completely obtained or when the nurse determines that the client is not able to continue. Informing the

Table 8–1	
COMPARISON BETWEEN CLOSED AND OPEN-ENDED QUESTIONS	
CLOSED QUESTIONS	**OPEN-ENDED QUESTIONS**
Did you take something for the pain?	What did you do for the pain?
Are you feeling sad?	How do you feel about this?
Do you get along with your children?	Describe your relationship with your family.
Is your job rewarding?	Tell me about your job.

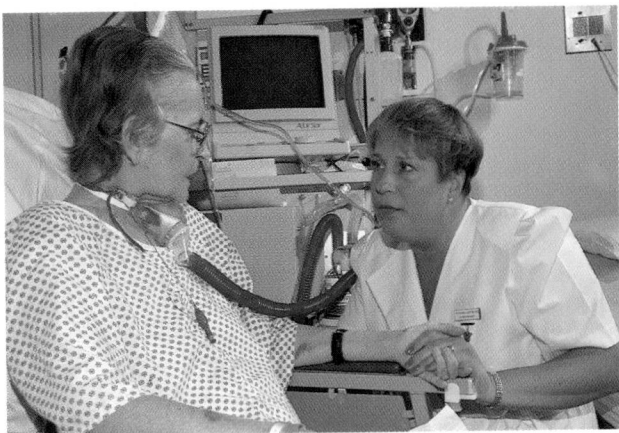

✦ **Figure 8–3**
Active listening involves focusing completely on the client's words and expressions.

client that the interview will be ending shortly prepares the client for the conclusion. At this point, no new material should be introduced by the nurse. The nurse should summarize the main points of the database. The client is provided with the opportunity to clarify or negate the nurse's descriptions. The client can be asked, "What additional information would be helpful to planning your care?" This allows the client the option of introducing any new topic of concern. The nurse should allow enough time for the client to answer this question.

The client is informed about what to expect after the interview. Any subsequent procedures or treatments that are planned are explained to the client. The roles of the nurse, especially in maintaining confidentiality, are reviewed to reassure the client and to promote the client's understanding of the health care system.

Physical Examination

During the physical examination, the nurse collects information about the client's objective or overt physical signs. Unlike the physician's examination that is geared toward identification of disease, the nurse performs a physical examination to identify the client's response to disease, to establish an initial database for later comparison, and to validate subjective data presented by the client during the interview (Iyer *et al.,* 1995).

Techniques

The nurse uses the techniques of inspection, palpation, auscultation, and percussion when performing the physical examination. With each type of technique, the nurse should explain to the client the purpose and procedures involved.

Inspection refers to the close, visual observation of the client, first of the individual as a whole, and

Table **8–2**	
INTERVIEWING TECHNIQUES	
THERAPEUTIC TECHNIQUES	**EXAMPLES**
Using silence	Remaining silent to encourage the client to verbalize feelings
Restating	Client: "I don't feel well. I feel sick to my stomach." Nurse: "You feel sick to your stomach."
Offering general leads	"Go on." "And then."
Reflecting	"How do you feel about this?" "What do you think the problem is?"
Exploring	"Could you tell me more about how this occurred?"
Seeking clarification	"Are you having second thoughts about having surgery?"
Encouraging comparison	"Tell me about any similar experiences." "How does this pain compare with the previous pain?"
Making observations	"You seem tense." "You seem sad when telling me this story."
Consensual validation	"Let's see if we both mean the same thing."
Summarizing	"Let me review what you have told me."
LESS DESIRABLE TECHNIQUES	**EXAMPLES**
Reassuring	"Don't worry about that."
Challenging	"How can you feel that way?!"
Advising	"I think that you should do this."
Giving approval	"I'm glad that you feel this way."
Rejecting	"Let's not discuss this now."
Interpreting	"I think that you mean. . . ."

then of the separate body systems. Inspection is the first technique that the nurse uses when performing the physical assessment. The nurse examines the size, shape, appearance, color, movement, and symmetry of body parts. This type of observation requires careful and systematic evaluation of the client using the senses of sight, hearing, and smell. Refer to Table 8–3 for examples of the type of observations that can be made by the use of the senses. While the nurse generally uses the unaided eye, special equipment is often utilized when performing inspection. Such equipment may include a flashlight to inspect body cavities, a tape measure to identify the length or circumference of a body area, an otoscope to visualize the ear canal,

Table 8-3

OBSERVATION: USE OF THE SENSES

SENSE	TYPE OF OBSERVATION
Sight	Abrasions, bleeding, braces, burns, casts, cleanliness, crutches, crying, cyanosis, dentures, drainage, ecchymosis, edema, eyeglasses, gait, hearing aids, frowning, moles, pregnancy, scars, scratches, shivering, skin color, tatoo, twitching, ulcerations, urine, vomiting, walker, warts, yawning
Hearing	Banging, blood pressure, bruit, burping, coughing, crying, expressions of pain, gargling, gasping, gurgling, harsh cough, heart rate and rhythm, hoarseness, hyperactive or hypoactive bowel sounds, laughing, moaning, sighing, sneezing, tone of voice, wheezing, whispering, yawning
Touch	Coarseness, coldness, dryness, edema, goosebumps, hardness, heat, lumps, masses, moisture, pulsation, relaxation, roughness, skin texture, smoothness, softness, swelling, temperature, tension, tremors, warmth, wetness
Smell	Alcohol, axillary odor, bleeding, breath or body odor, disinfectants, feces, foot odor, gas, onion, purulent drainage, tobacco, urine, vomitus

From Iyer, P. W., Taptich, B. J., & Bernocchi-Losey, D. (1995). *Nursing process and nursing diagnosis* (3rd ed., p. 61). Philadelphia: W. B. Saunders.

and an ophthalmoscope to visualize the interior of the eye (Fig. 8–4*A*).

Palpation refers to the use of touch to determine temperature, texture, size, shape, pulsation, consistency, and movement. The hands and the fingers are the primary tools for palpating specific parts of the body. The back or dorsum of the hand is particularly useful to determine variations in temperature, because the skin there is thinner and more sensitive to temperature fluctuations. The fingertips are useful for fine tactile assessment of texture and size because of the concentration of nerve endings there (Fig. 8–4*B*). The palmar or ulnar surface of the hand is sensitive to vibration and therefore is useful to evaluate phenomena such as abdominal movements. Light palpation with the dominant hand is generally used when examining body parts. Deeper palpation is used to evaluate abdominal organs and should be used with caution to avoid any trauma to organs and tissues.

Auscultation involves the sense of hearing for listening to sounds produced by various organs and systems. While some sounds are audible by the unaided ear, the nurse uses a stethoscope to hear deeper body sounds. A stethoscope consists of an amplifying mechanism, such as a diaphragm (mainly for high-frequency sounds such as heart, lung, and bowel sounds) or a bell (for low-frequency sounds such as heart murmurs), connected to earpieces by plastic or rubber tubing. The ear tips should be large enough to fit snugly into the ear canal. The slope of the earpieces should point forward toward the nose. The nurse uses a stethoscope to assess blood pressure, heart sounds, breath sounds, and bowel sounds and to determine frequency, intensity or loudness, quality (such as crackles or wheezes in the lungs), and duration of these sounds (Fig. 8–4*C*).

Percussion is done by striking a body surface with short, sharp blows of the fingers or striking a nondominant finger with the dominant finger to produce sound to determine the size, position, and density of the underlying parts (Fig. 8–4*D*). Sounds that are produced by percussion may be described as flat, dull, resonant, hyperresonant, and tympanic. Flat sounds are heard when the nurse percusses an abnormally solid part and are low pitched. Dull sounds are short and moderately high pitched, with little resonance and have a thudlike quality. Resonant sounds are elicited over cavities, such as an air-filled lung, and are moderate to loud high-pitched sounds. Hyperresonant sounds are very loud and high pitched. Tympanic sounds are loud and drumlike, such as sounds heard over a gas-filled stomach.

Approaches

The nurse uses an organized, systematic method when performing the physical examination on the client. The method that is selected depends on a number of factors, including the preference of the nurse, the philosophy of the institution, and the condition of the patient. Some examples of structured frameworks are presented in Table 8–4. Other approaches that the nurse may use are the head-to-toe or body systems approach. A head-to-toe assessment begins at the head and systematically progresses down the trunk to the feet. A systems approach provides the nurse with a focus on the functioning of each system rather than each body part.

A combination of approaches may be used. In the following case study about Mrs. C., a combined head-to-toe and systems approach is used.

CASE STUDY — Assessment of Mrs. C.

Mrs. C., a 79-year-old woman, is admitted to the orthopedic floor following repair of her fractured left hip. Mrs. C. is a retired elementary school teacher with a college education. She lives with her husband in a one-story home. Her four children are grown, married, and in good health. One son lives close by, and the other children live in neighboring states. Mrs. C. is active in her church and community and drives her own car.

Source of information: Client and family.

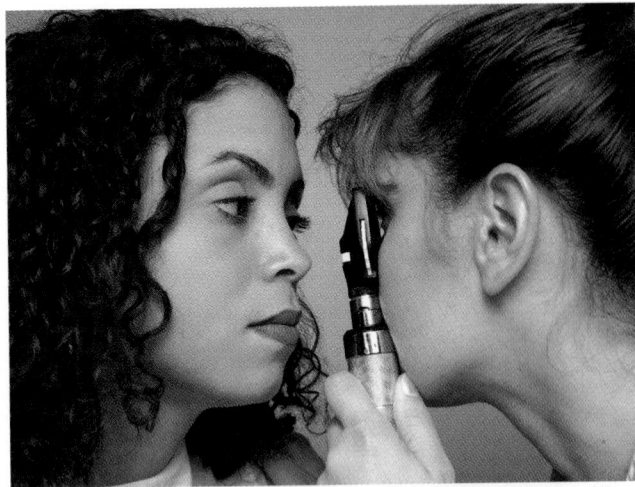

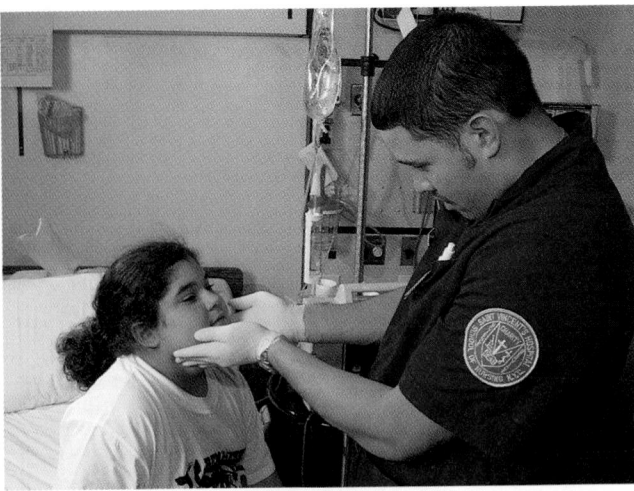

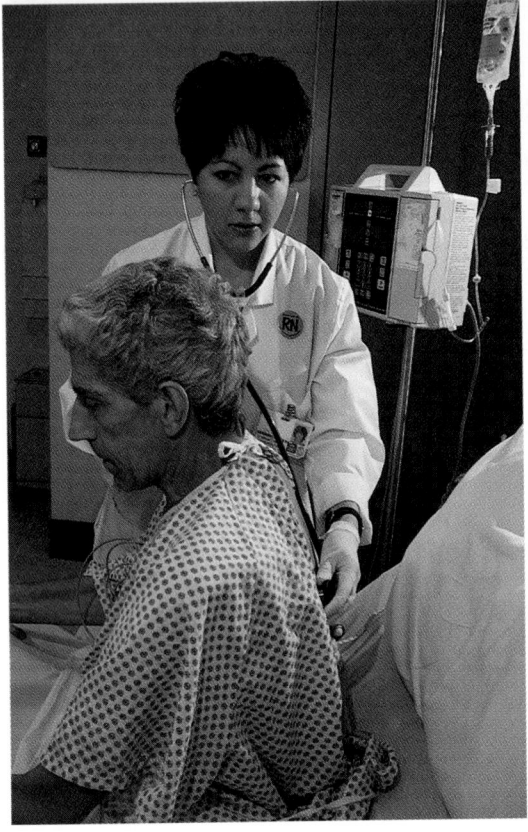

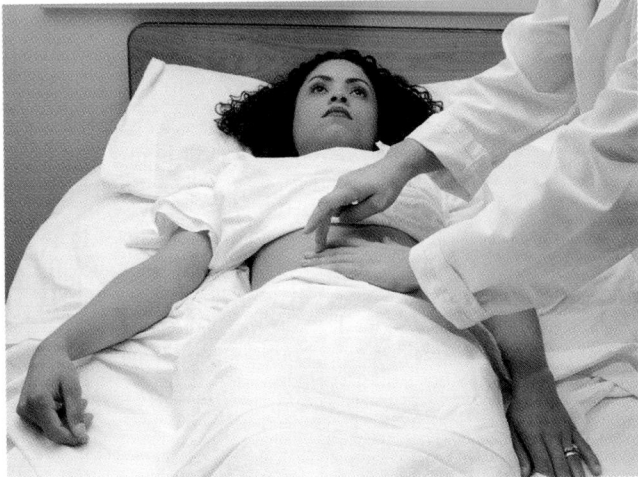

❧ Figure 8–4
A, An ophthalmoscope is used to *inspect* the interior of the eye.
B, Fingertips are used in *palpating* lymph nodes. *C,* The nurse
auscultates deep body sounds with a stethoscope. *D, Percussion*
determines the size, position, and density of body parts.

General Health

States health is good. No history of chronic illnesses
or disease. Exercises regularly and eats a good diet.
Nonsmoker.

Illnesses

Pneumonia requiring hospitalization in 1989. Chest
pain and palpitations, 1991. Electrocardiography indicated old anterior myocardial infarction. Cardiac
catheterization was normal. No history of tuberculosis, diabetes, asthma, bronchitis, hypertension, gastrointestinal problems, or cancer.

Operations

Abdominal hysterectomy, 1974.

Psychosocial

Apprehension and concern expressed over possible
decreased physical ability and independence.
Doesn't want to be a burden on husband and children.

Current Medications

- Procardia XL, 30 mg, taken orally (PO) daily
- Baby aspirin, PO daily
- Metamucil, 1 t, PO, as needed

Allergies

Percocet causes rash and pruritus.

	Table 8–4

EXAMPLES OF STRUCTURED ASSESSMENT FRAMEWORKS

GORDON'S FUNCTIONAL HEALTH PATTERNS	ROY ADAPTATION MODEL	HUMAN RESPONSE PATTERNS
Health-perception–health-management patterns: Describe client's perceived pattern of health and well-being and how health is managed	*Physiological mode:* Includes behaviors related to oxygenation, nutrition, elimination, activity and rest, skin integrity, the senses, fluid and electrolytes, neurological function, and endocrine function	*Exchanging:* Cardiac, peripheral, oxygenation, nutrition, elimination, skin integrity, physical regulation
Nutritional-metabolic patterns: Describe pattern of food and fluid consumption relative to metabolic need and pattern indicators of local nutrient supply	*Self-concept mode:* Describes beliefs and feelings that one holds about oneself, including one's concerns about physical self, personal self, spiritual self, and self-esteem	*Communicating:* Ability to read, write, and understand English or any other languages
Elimination pattern: Describes patterns of excretory function relative to bowel, urine, and skin.	*Role function mode:* Describes actions taken in relation to the performance of specific roles that the client assumes in life, whether primary, secondary, or tertiary	*Relating:* Relationships, socialization
Activity-exercise pattern: Describes pattern of exercise, activity, leisure, and recreation	*Interdependence mode:* Involves the close relationships of the client that involve the willingness and ability to love, respect, and value others and that include the ability to accept and respond to love, respect, and value given by others	*Valuing:* Religious preferences and practices, spiritual values, cultural practices
Cognitive-perceptual pattern: Describes sensory-perceptual and cognitive pattern		*Choosing:* Coping, participation in health regimen
Sleep-rest pattern: Describes patterns of sleep, rest, and relaxation		*Moving:* Activity, sleep pattern, recreation, self-care ability, health maintenance
Self-perception–self-concept pattern: Describes self-concept pattern and perceptions of self		*Perceiving:* Body image, self-concept, self-esteem, sensory perception, meaningfulness
Role-relationship pattern: Describes pattern of role engagements and relationships		*Knowing:* Current health problems, past medical history, mental status
Sexuality-reproductive pattern: Describes client's patterns of satisfaction and dissatisfaction with sexuality pattern; describes reproductive patterns		*Feeling:* Pain, loss and grief, emotional status
Coping–stress-tolerance pattern: Describes general coping pattern and effectiveness of the pattern in terms of stress tolerance		
Value-belief pattern: Describes patterns of values, beliefs (including spiritual), or goals that guide choices or decisions		

Data from Gordon, M. (1993). *Nursing diagnosis: Process and application* (3rd ed.). New York: McGraw-Hill; Roy, S. C. (1984). *Introduction to nursing: An adaptation model* (2nd ed.). Englewood Cliffs, NJ: Prentice-Hall; Iyer, P. W., Taptich, B. J., & Bernocchi-Losey, D. (1995). Nursing process and nursing diagnosis (3rd ed.). Philadelphia: W. B. Saunders.

Immunizations

Current, including pneumovax and influenza.

Physical Assessment

(Combined Head-to-Toe and System Approach)

General Inspection

State of consciousness: Alert and oriented to time, person, and place. Responses are immediate and appropriate. Able to understand and follow commands.

Any outstanding signs: Grimacing facial expression and groaning with movement of lower body.

General: Temperature, 97.6°F, pulse, 78, respiration, 20, blood pressure (BP), 110/60, weight, 145 lb, height, 5 ft 4 in. Skin pink, warm, and dry. No pigmentation, rashes, or lesions.

Head

Vision: Visual acuity not tested. Wears glasses for reading and driving. Conjunctiva clear, without pallor. Pupils equal, react to light and accommodation. Extraocular muscles intact. Red reflex present bilaterally.

Hearing: No lesions of the external ear. No inflammation, discharge, or pain bilateral pinnas and tragus. Hearing is good.

Mouth: No lesions on the lips. Buccal mucosa, tongue, and gums are pink and moist. No lesions or masses. Upper and lower dentures. No hoarseness; clear speech.

Face: Symmetrical. No edema. Denies frontal or maxillary pain.

Neck: Full range of motion without pain. No lymphadenopathy. Trachea midline. Thyroid nonpalpable. Carotids 2+, no bruits. No jugular venous distension.

Trunk

Respiration: Respirations, 20 per minute and regular. Chest expands symmetrically. Breath sounds are diminished at bilateral lower bases. No pain or dyspnea with breathing. Denies dry or productive cough.

Circulation: Apical pulse, 78 beats per minute and regular. S_1S_2 (first 2 heart pounds) normal. Point of maximal intensity is the fifth left intercostal space in the midclavicular line. No lifts, heaves, or thrills. No murmurs, rubs, or gallops. The peripheral pulses—carotids, radial, femoral, dorsalis pedis, and posterior tibial—are present, full, and equal. BP 110/60. Brisk capillary refill.

Gastrointestinal: Rounded. Lower abdominal scar. Soft and nontender. Bowel sounds present in all quadrants. No palpable masses. Daily bowel movements are usually soft and brown. Denies rectal bleeding or drainage.

Genitourinary: Foley catheter present and secured to leg. Draining light yellow urine. No genital inflammation or discharge.

Hydration: Skin smooth with elastic turgor. Mucous membranes pink and moist.

Extremities

Movement: Color pale. Sensory intact. No edema of the feet and ankles. Peripheral pulses 2+ throughout. Dressing over left hip incision clean and dry. No lesions or inflammation. Nails are pink, with brisk capillary refill.

Laboratory and Diagnostic Test Results
Preoperatively

Complete blood count, medical profile, bleeding times (prothrombin time [PT] and partial thromboplastin time [PTT]), blood type and screen, and urinalysis (all studies were normal except the serum potassium of 3.1 mg)

12-Lead electrocardiogram, normal sinus rhythm, old anterior infarct

Chest x-ray, no evidence of infiltrate or cardiomegaly

Postoperatively

Hemoglobin and hematocrit (10.2 g/33.1 g).

Oxygen saturation, 97%

Data from Gulanick, M., Kloop, A., Galanes, S., *et al.* (1994). *Nursing care plans: Nursing diagnosis and interventions* (3rd ed.). St. Louis: Mosby–Year Book. Case study written by Jane Wrenn, BSN.

···

Developmental Considerations

The nurse must remember that a child is different from an adult, both physically and behaviorally. Knowledge of normal growth and development is essential. Because children are frequently anxious and upset about the physical examination, the parent is usually present and may assist the nurse as needed. School-age children and adolescents may prefer their privacy and should be asked if the parent is to be present.

Infants are totally dependent on adults for their basic needs and usually do not react negatively to touch. The parent may assist by holding the infant (Fig. 8–5). Keep the infant warm and use a soft voice when talking to the infant. If the infant cries, use a pacifier. Listen to the heart and lungs while the infant is quiet, and perform procedures that might distress the infant last.

Toddlers are attempting to become more independent in their search for autonomy, making them difficult to examine. Since they like to say "no," do not give them a choice when there is none. Instead, tell them what will be done and how, using language that they will understand. Try to make a game out of the examination.

Preschoolers are learning to develop initiative in doing activities and are therefore frequently cooperative and willing to become involved in designated tasks. However, these children fear body injury and may see illness as punishment for doing something

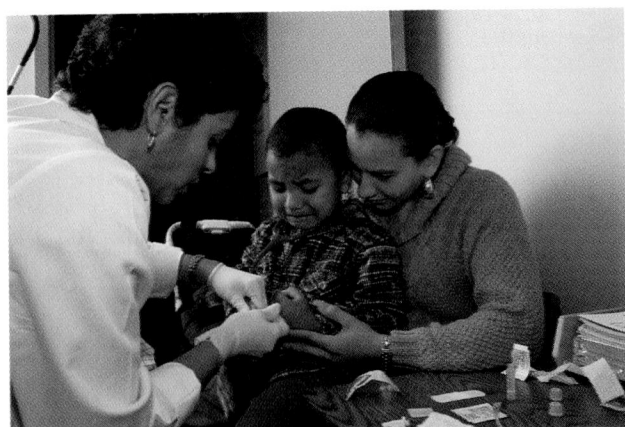

❧ **Figure 8–5**
By providing reassurance to the child, the parent assists the nurse in obtaining a blood sample.

bad. Explain in clear terms the steps of the examination and allow the child to play with equipment that is not sharp. Tell the child how cooperative he or she is as the examination progresses, but do not give the child a choice if there is none. Approach the examination as a game with the child.

The school-age child is interested in mastering tasks and winning approval from adults. A sense of accomplishment is important for him or her. Let the child undress independently and ask the child if he or she wants the parent present. Explain the procedures involved with the examination and let the child listen to his or her heart or bowel sounds to enlist cooperation.

Adolescents tend to be self-conscious and value peer group acceptance. They prefer to be examined without the presence of parents. They are not to be treated as children but require careful and respectful interaction. The teenager's progress from early to late adolescence and his or her evolution toward independent adulthood guides the selection of developmentally-based therapeutic interventions.

The elderly adult has a steady decline in normal body functions and may be slow in moving. This does not indicate a decrease in intellect or mental status. The nurse should give frequent explanations of what is being done to allay the client's anxiety. Pace the examination according to the client's physical ability level. Do not rush the client, and provide rest periods as needed.

Assessing the client's developmental level is an important component of the data collection process. The reader is referred to Unit IV for a more extensive description of growth and development.

Diagnostic Studies

Diagnostic tests are an integral component of the assessment of the client and provide important additional information about the client's medical status. Every client will have some type of diagnostic procedure done during a health care assessment. The most frequent diagnostic test performed on individuals is blood and urine testing. The importance of diagnostic studies explains the frequency of their use when nurses seek information about the client's physical status.

Nursing Considerations

The nurse plays a significant role when a client is to have a diagnostic procedure performed. The client needs to be informed about the procedure and its purpose for assessment and treatment. The nurse uses the results of these tests as part of the database for the identification of nursing diagnoses and for the planning and implementation of nursing care. Although there may be specific policies and procedures about diagnostic studies within each institution, there are some general guidelines that nurses should follow before, during, and after the procedures.

✦ **Before the Test.** The client gives consent for treatment on admission to the health care institution. This may be sufficient for many procedures that are performed, such as most blood and urine tests and some x-ray procedures. Some tests are considered invasive and require a separate, additional written consent from the client. The physician is responsible for explaining the procedure and obtaining the consent. The consent indicates that the client has been informed of the procedure, its purpose, and any possible risks or complications.

The nurse is responsible for ensuring that the client has adequate knowledge of the procedure and for reinforcing the physician's instructions. Many tests require special preliminary preparation, such as restrictions in diet and fluids, enemas, and medications. The nurse instructs the client about any test preparation. If the client is to prepare for the procedure at home, written instructions or a pamphlet may be useful to ensure that the client follows the correct steps. The nurse should be aware that the client may be nervous about the test and the potential outcomes and will require emotional support to ease anxiety.

✦ **During the Test.** Many procedures require the assistance of the nurse. The client may need to be placed in a special position or to have vital signs monitored. The nurse needs to assess the client frequently during the procedure and compare these results with baseline data. The physician should be informed of any deviation from the client's normal pattern, which may indicate that the procedure should be temporarily halted or that a specific medication should be given to the client. The nurse should be primarily concerned with the client and the client's reaction to the procedure.

The client may also need emotional support during the procedure. The nurse should offer reassurance or assistance by talking to the client, holding the client's hand, or having the client place attention on a focal point. If the procedure is painful or uncomfortable, the client should be instructed to breathe slowly and deeply. The client's physical and mental welfare is the primary concern for the nurse. The nurse may also be responsible for assisting the physician during the procedure and for care of specimens following the procedure.

✦ **After the Test.** Following the procedure, the nurse should be concerned primarily with the client. If the client had an invasive procedure, the client's reaction to the procedure, including the vital signs, should be assessed and compared with baseline data and recorded. The frequency of these assessments depends on the type of diagnostic procedure performed and the client's overall physical and mental status. The nurse should clearly inform the client about these posttreatment procedures and their rationales. The comfort needs of the client should be a priority for the nurse. Assuming a relaxing position, receiving pain medication, being provided with warmth, and having visits from family and significant others are some of the important needs of the client after a diagnostic procedure. Many hospitals have units that are specially designed as cooperative care units where family members or significant others are actively involved in the posttreatment care of the client.

The nurse needs to document in the client record the date and time of the procedure, the type of procedure performed, any medication that was administered before or during the procedure, whether a specimen was obtained, and the client's response to the procedure. If a specimen was obtained, the nurse should ensure that it is properly labeled and sent to the appropriate laboratory for analysis. Fluids that are withdrawn or aspirated should be noted on the fluid balance sheet as output. The nurse should be careful to avoid contact with any blood or body fluids by wearing gloves while handling specimens and following universal precautions.

Types of Diagnostic Studies

A variety of diagnostic studies can be performed on a client. Many require minimal, if any, preparation, whereas others are considered invasive and require specific protocols before, during, and after the procedure. The nurse is responsible for being knowledgeable about the diagnostic study and the required nursing interventions.

✦ **Blood.** The most common type of diagnostic studies are those that are performed on blood. Generally, a venipuncture is performed by puncturing a vein with a needle (Fig. 8–6). A specimen of blood is aspirated from the client's vein and collected in a small vial. The type of vial that is used depends on the blood test to be performed. Some tubes contain a small amount of a prescribed preservative that is essential for specific tests. Although most blood specimens are obtained by a laboratory technician, the

nurse is responsible for explaining the procedure to the client. Many blood tests require that the client be in a fasting state, having no food or fluid for a specified period of time. The nurse should be aware of the client's state during this fasting period and make arrangements to ensure that the blood drawing is not delayed.

Blood studies can be generally classified as follows:

Hematological studies, which involve the analysis of blood and blood-forming products. The most common hematology test is the complete blood count, which calculates the amount of blood cells present in the blood and is a basic screening test. Results include the hemoglobin, hematocrit, red blood cell count, white blood cell count, and platelet count. Frequently, the WBC is analyzed for specific types of cells.

Chemistry studies, which involve the analysis of the chemical components of the blood to assist in the diagnosis and treatment of a wide range of diseases. Examples of blood chemistry studies include serum electrolyte values, which include sodium, potassium, and chloride; tests of blood sugar; and tests of a variety of enzymes that provide information about the status of the kidney and liver in particular.

Microbiology studies, which involve the testing of the blood for the presence of microorganisms. Blood cultures are done when the client is suspected of having bacteremia or septicemia to identify the causative organism and determine appropriate medication to administer.

✦ **Urine.** Urine is another body fluid that is frequently analyzed. Urine is produced by the kidney and contains thousands of substances (although the main components are urea and sodium chloride), dissolved in water. The composition of urine depends on the function of the nephrons in the kidney and its ability to filter blood and excrete waste products. There are several types of urine specimens:

* A single, random specimen: A specimen of urine that is obtained at an unspecified time.

* A single, timed specimen: A specimen of urine that is obtained at a prescribed time to test for the presence of a substance in the urine in relation to a specific event, such as a meal.

* A long-term, timed specimen: A specimen of urine that is collected over a period of time—usually 24 hours. This type of urine testing allows the evaluation of the kidney's ability to excrete a particular substance over a 24-hour period.

The most common type of urine test is the urinalysis, which identifies the various properties of urine, including color, odor, specific gravity, pH, and components of glucose, protein, ketones, and blood. Urine, normally a sterile, or bacteria-free, body fluid, can be tested for the presence of bacteria to identify a possible genitourinary infection. Other urine tests are used to evaluate a variety of metabolic processes or to identify possible disease conditions.

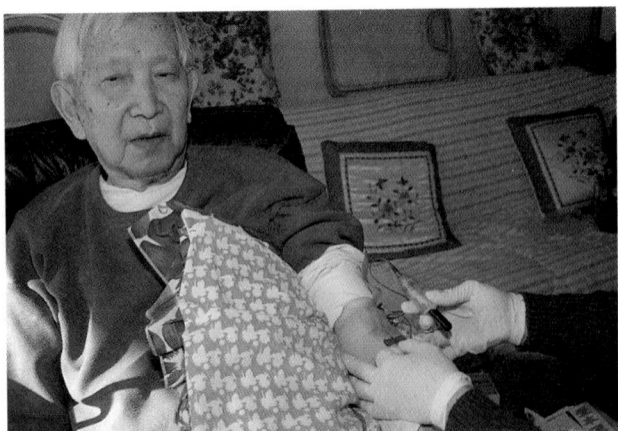

✦ **Figure 8–6**
Blood and urine testing are the two most common diagnostic procedures.

✦ **Other Body Fluids.** Other body fluids or outputs, including feces, spinal fluid, and wound drainage, are sources for examination. Although these fluids are tested less frequently than blood and urine, they are important sources of information to assist in the diagnosis and treatment of many diseases. Their collection usually involves special nursing techniques or occurs in conjunction with a procedure performed by a physician, such as a lumbar puncture. The nurse is responsible for obtaining the specimen using proper technique and for sending the specimen to the appropriate laboratory for analysis. Universal precautions should be followed for specific body fluids.

✦ **Radiography.** Radiography procedures involve the use of x-rays that penetrate a body part and produce an image on a photographic film or on a screen, which is a fluoroscopy. X-rays provide information about the size, shape, and density of a body organ or part. Fluoroscopy allows for direct observation of the function of deep body structures during a diagnostic procedure. These procedures usually involve the use of a contrast medium, which is either ingested orally by the client or injected in the client's vein. Examples of specialized radiographic procedures included an upper gastrointestinal series, a barium enema, a mammogram, and an intravenous pyelogram. These procedures are discussed in more detail in related chapters.

✦ **Endoscopy.** Direct visualization of an internal organ or cavity is performed using an endoscope. The endoscope is usually flexible, although some may be rigid. Rigid endoscopes have a specialized lens within the tube that permits visualization of the intended organ or cavity. It also allows the physician to obtain a biopsy specimen for examination, to remove a foreign body, or to excise a diseased part. Those body organs or cavities most frequently endoscoped are the lung, upper gastrointestinal tract, colon, bladder, and joints. Insertion of an endoscope into the peritoneal cavity through the abdominal wall, termed a laparoscopy, has facilitated advances in surgical procedures and reduced lengthy hospitalizations. Removal of a gall bladder using a laser beam that is directed through a laparoscope has drastically decreased surgical complications and length of stays.

The nurse should ensure that the client is fully informed and has signed the informed consent prior to the endoscopy. The type of preparation that is required varies according to the specific procedure. The client may receive a tranquilizer or sedative prior to the endoscopy. After the procedure, the client's vital signs should be checked frequently. In addition, the nurse should assess the client for the presence of pain, hemorrhage, and swallowing ability (if an oral endoscopy was performed).

✦ **Electrical Impulse Procedures.** These procedures involve the recording of electrical impulses on a graph or an oscilloscope. The most common type of this procedure is an electrocardiogram, which records the electrical impulses generated by and transmitted through the heart. An electroencephalogram records the electrical impulses of the brain, and an electromyogram records those in selected muscles. For each of these procedures, electrodes are placed over specified areas of the body. These electrodes sense these impulses and transmit them for recording on ruled graph paper. These procedures are valuable tools to assist in the diagnosis of heart, brain, or muscle diseases. The client needs an explanation of the procedure that should include instructions for the client to remain still during the test. The nurse should inform the client that he or she will not receive an electric shock from the electrodes. Generally, there is no specific preparation for these procedures. In some instances, certain medications may need to be withheld prior to an electroencephalogram.

✦ **Ultrasonography.** Ultrasonography is defined as a noninvasive procedure that uses high-frequency sound waves that penetrate and bounce back according to the density of the organ or tissue. These sound waves are produced by a transducer that is placed externally over the area of the body to be evaluated and that converts the reflected waves to an image, which is then produced on a viewing screen. Generally, no specific preparation is required. A pelvic ultrasonography requires the ingestion of large volumes of water just prior to the procedure, and an abdominal ultrasonography may require that the client abstain from food and fluid for several hours before the procedure.

◆ Data Validation

The database frequently needs to be validated with alternate sources to ensure that the data are valid and correct. The nurse's intuition may indicate that, while the client describes a health problem, another problem is of concern but is not being verbalized. When a client states that he or she has no postoperative pain but is grimacing and looks tense, the nurse should inquire further into the situation. Other clients may not be forthright in providing information that is necessary to differentiate between health care problems. This requires that the nurse obtain additional information from other sources. Adolescents who are fearful of parental response may not admit certain events that led to a crisis situation. In other cases, the severity of the illness may temporarily cloud a client's memory or judgment.

Any time that the nurse believes that data are either missing or inaccurate, he or she should pursue other methods for validating the database. These methods may include interviewing the client further, interviewing family or significant others, obtaining old medical records, or contacting other health care professionals.

Summary

The assessment phase of the nursing process provides the nurse with all of the information about the client that is needed to identify goals, determine priorities of nursing diagnoses, and plan care. As the first step in the nursing process, the nurse builds the database, from which the plan emerges. The assessment data provide the basis for analyzing the client's health care status and determining actual and potential problems requiring intervention. The assessment phase of the nursing process provides the necessary information for the analysis phase of the nursing process, during which the nurse makes an interpretation of the data. This interpretation then supports the nursing diagnoses that are identified.

CHAPTER HIGHLIGHTS

♦ Assessment is the organized, purposeful collection and validation of data about the client's health status, including the client's strength and weaknesses. The database includes the nursing history, the physical examination, diagnostic studies, developmental considerations, and psychosocial development.

♦ The primary source of data is the client. When the client is unable to give information, the client's family or significant others provide the database. Additional sources of data include the client's family, significant others, and the client's medical record.

♦ Subjective data can only be obtained from the client and relayed to the nurse. Objective data can be observed or measured by the nurse and other members of the health care team.

♦ The interview, which is essential for collection of the nursing history, is an interactive communication process that involves a mutual exchange of information between the client and the nurse and that facilitates the establishment a therapeutic relationship with the client.

♦ Communication techniques used during an interview include both open-ended and closed questions. Open-ended questions elicit information about feelings, emotions, opinions, and perceptions and allow for validation of both subjective and objective data. Closed questions are appropriate for obtaining specific factual information. A variety of nonverbal techniques, specifically silence and

listening, facilitate and enhance the interview process.

♦ The nursing examination provides the opportunity for the nurse, through the techniques of inspection, palpation, percussion, and auscultation, to collect data about the client's physical health status. Some approaches to examination include the head-to-toe, body systems, functional health pattern, and the human response pattern approaches.

♦ When approaching the client and when collecting data, the nurse must consider the developmental and psychosocial aspects of the client.

♦ Diagnostic studies are an integral component of the database and provide important additional information about the client's medical status. The nurse plays a major role before, during, and after the diagnostic procedure.

Study Questions

1. The nurse collects all of the following data from a client. Which piece would be considered subjective data?

   a. pulses in the client's foot are palpable
   b. client's skin is warm to the touch
   c. client has periods of nausea before meals
   d. client's breathing pattern is regular

2. Which of the following *best* describes the purpose of a nursing history?

   a. it is a component of the assessment phase of the nursing process
   b. it provides the nurse with an initial database to plan care for the client
   c. it primarily includes information about the client's current health care problem
   d. it is an informal process that involves communicating with the client

3. Which of the following statements about an interview is true?

   a. it should be conducted in a quiet setting that affords the client privacy
   b. it should be completed at a time that is convenient for the nurse
   c. it should focus primarily on the client's past medical history
   d. it should take no longer than 15 minutes to complete

4. When a nurse is determining the temperature or texture of a client's skin, which of the following assessment techniques is being used?

   a. inspection
   b. auscultation
   c. percussion
   d. palpation

5. A diagnostic test that involves direct visualization of an internal organ is an

   a. x-ray
   b. endoscopy

c. ultrasonogram
d. electrical impulse procedure

Critical Thinking Exercises

1. Decide whether the following data are subjective or objective and discuss how they might be used in the assessment process:

   a. auscultated wheezing and rhonchi throughout lung fields
   b. coughing up green-tinted sputum
   c. temperature 101°F
   d. white blood cell count, 30,000
   e. history of frequent colds
   f. verbalizes chest pain on inspiration

2. Ms. G. tells you that her husband has died and both of her daughters have moved out within the last 3 months. Discuss variations in interview techniques you might use.

References

Alfaro, R. (1994). *Applying nursing diagnosis and nursing process* (3rd ed.). Philadelphia: J. B. Lippincott.

American Nurses' Association (1995). *Nursing: A social policy statement* (2nd ed.). Washington, DC: ANA.

Christensen, P. J., & Kenney, J. W. (1995). *Nursing process: Application of conceptual models* (4th ed.). St. Louis: C. V. Mosby.

Gordon, M. (1993). *Nursing diagnosis: Process and application* (3rd ed.). St. Louis: Mosby-Year Book.

Iyer, P. W., Taptich, B. J., & Bernocchi-Losey, D. (1995). *Nursing process and nursing diagnosis* (3rd ed.). Philadelphia: W. B. Saunders.

Jarvis, C. (1996). *Physical examination and health assessment* (2nd ed.). Philadelphia: W. B. Saunders.

Murray, M. E., & Atkinson, L. D. (1994). *Understanding the nursing process* (5th ed.). New York: McGraw-Hill, Health Professions Division.

Roy, S. C. (1984). *Introduction to nursing: An adaptation model* (2nd ed.). Englewood Cliffs, NJ: Prentice-Hall.

Stuart, G. W., & Sundeen, S. J. (1995). *Principles and practices of psychiatric nursing* (5th ed.). St. Louis: Mosby-Year Book.

Bibliography

Burke, L. J., & Murphy, J. (Eds.). (1995). *Charting by exception applications: Making it work in clinical settings.* Albany, NY: Delmar Publishers.

Crow, R. A., Chase, J., & Lamond, D. (1995). The cognitive component of nursing assessment: An analysis. *Journal of Advanced Nursing, 22*(2), 206–212.

Fuller, J., & Schaller-Ayers, J. (1994). *Health assessment: A nursing approach.* Philadelphia: J. B. Lippincott.

Morton, P. E. (Ed.). (1995). *Nurse's clinical guide to health assessment.* Springhouse, PA: Springhouse.

Newell, R. (1994). *Interviewing skills for nurses and other health care professionals: A structured approach.* New York: Routledge.

North, S. D., & Serkes, P. C. (1996). Improving documentation of initial nursing assessment. *Nursing Management, 27*(4), 30, 33.

Thompson, J. M., & Wilson, S. F. (1996). *Health assessment for nursing practice.* St. Louis: C. V. Mosby.

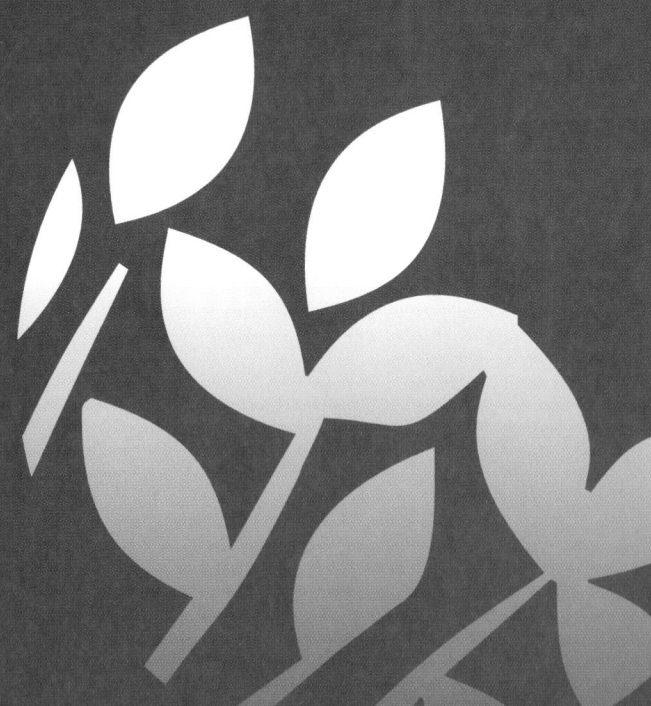

Chapter ✦ 9

NURSING DIAGNOSIS

PATRICIA E. KIZILAY, EdD, RN, CS, FNP

KEY TERMS
✦

clinical reasoning
collaborative problem
cue
data clustering
data validation
diagnosing
error of commission
error of omission

health problem
medical diagnosis
nursing diagnosis
problem, actual
problem, potential
problem, risk
synthesis

LEARNING OBJECTIVES
✦

After studying this chapter, you should be able to

✦ Define the term *nursing diagnosis*

✦ Define the basic terminology identified in the chapter

✦ Discuss the advantages of using a nursing diagnosis

✦ List the advantages of using the North American Nursing Diagnosis Association–approved list of nursing diagnoses

✦ Identify the steps in the process of making a nursing diagnosis

✦ Identify the essential parts of a diagnostic statement

✦ Describe the one-part, two-part, and three-part statements used in writing a nursing diagnosis

✦ Compare nursing diagnoses and collaborative problems

✦ Identify the difference between a nursing diagnosis and a medical diagnosis

✦ List the common errors in writing a nursing diagnosis

✦ Describe ways to validate a nursing diagnosis

Nursing diagnosis is the step of the nursing process that enables the nurse to identify those client problems that are the responsibility of the nurse. The assessment data are examined to determine what client responses will be amenable to nursing intervention. The nursing diagnoses that are derived from these data are the basis for planning, implementing, and evaluating the nursing care plan and the client's health status (Fig. 9–1).

In 1966, Hammond identified the need for nurses to be competent in information-seeking strategies and to have a sound foundation of theoretical knowledge to conduct a search for cues and evaluate evidence, resulting in an accurate diagnosis. Aspinall (1976) described nursing diagnosis as the "weak link" in the nursing process and later proposed a decision tree to guide nurses in making accurate nursing diagnoses (Fig. 9–2).

The American Nurses' Association (ANA) included nursing diagnosis as a function of professional nursing in *Standards of Practice* in 1973. In 1980, the ANA issued a *Social Policy Statement,* which defined nursing as follows: "NURSING is the diagnosis and treatment of human response to actual or potential health problems."

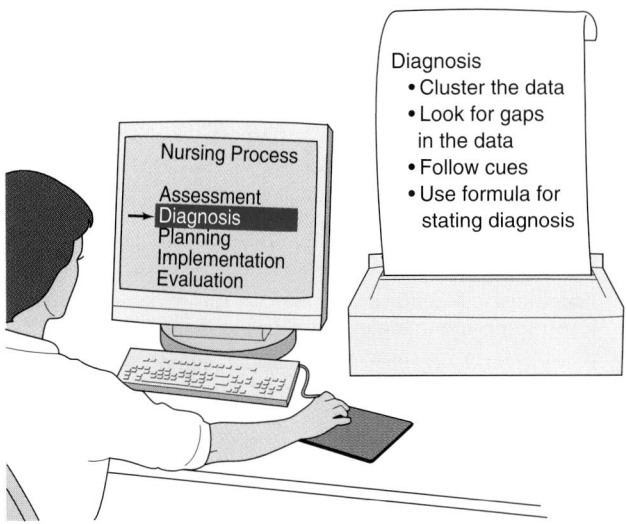

❥ Figure 9–1

Diagnosis is the second step of the nursing process. Diagnosis allows the nurse to identify client problems that are of concern to the nurse and provides the basis for planning, implementation, and evaluation.

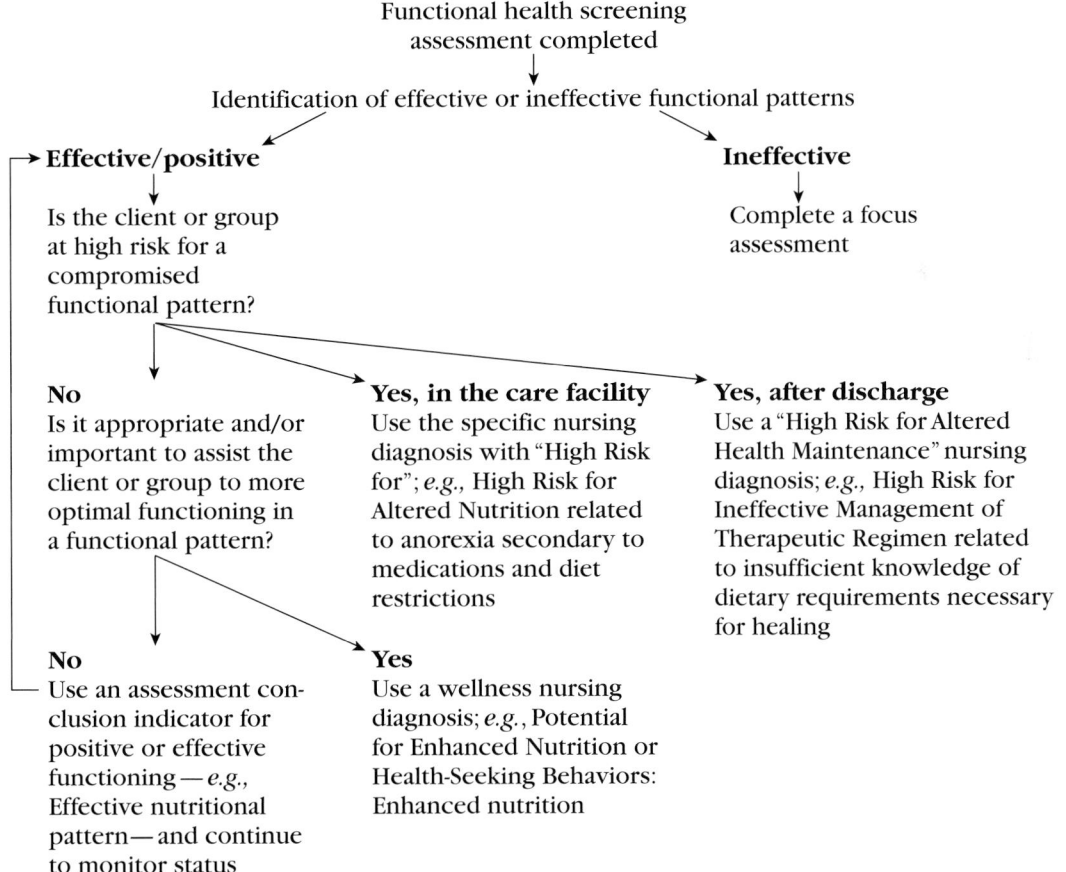

❥ Figure 9–2

Decision tree for nursing diagnoses. (Adapted from Carpenito, L. J. [1997]. Nursing diagnosis: Application to Clinical Practice [7th ed.]. Philadelphia: Lippincott-Raven.)

In 1973, the First National Conference on Classification of Nursing Diagnosis was held in St. Louis. This was the beginning of a national effort to recognize, standardize, and classify problems that nurses can treat. The group has been renamed the North American Nursing Diagnosis Association (NANDA). It meets every 2 years and has appointed a task force to

* Gather information and disseminate it (through the Clearinghouse for Nursing Diagnosis)
* Encourage educational activities (at the regional and state level) to promote implementation of nursing diagnosis
* Promote and organize activities to continue the development (classification and testing) of nursing diagnosis (Carpenito, 1992)

The process of arriving at a nursing diagnosis involves decision making based on intuitive reasoning, experience, and a sound theoretical foundation in the biological and social sciences. The diagnosis phase involves four steps: data analysis, synthesis, nursing diagnosis, and validation.

Data Analysis

During the data analysis step, the data are separated and critically examined for health problems. **Health problems** are deviations from or variations in the well-being of a client. Areas needing further assessment, or incongruencies in the assessment, are identified.

Gaps in the Data

A gap in the assessment data is a lack of information that is needed to determine patterns and specific approaches to client problems. The question must be asked: "What additional information is needed to develop a comprehensive base for the nursing diagnosis?" It may not be necessary to gather all of the assessment data initially. Some data may be obtained at a later date. For instance, a sexual history or a comprehensive family history may be deferred on the initial interview with a client. There may be some information that a client is reluctant to share in the first assessment but may share more openly when a trusting relationship is established.

Conflicting information needs to be clarified so that the appropriate nursing diagnosis may be made. For instance, a client may report that no alcohol has been consumed. Yet the laboratory test reveals a high concentration of alcohol in the blood. This incongruency needs to be clarified before proceeding with the nursing diagnosis. On further assessment, the information obtained may reveal that the client has a history of alcohol abuse. In this situation, a nursing diagnosis regarding the addiction is necessary. Conversely, the client may have just attended a party and consumed alcohol for the first time in the past 12

months. In this instance, no further plan for intervention is necessary.

Cues

A **cue** is a piece of data that is significant or that will influence decision making. Cues from the nursing assessment, such as rhonchi on auscultation of the lungs or elevated temperature, and data available from other sources, such as the client reporting a cough, are analyzed to determine whether the client's response is an isolated incident or indicates a pattern. Some data gathered will not lead to a nursing diagnosis. In the previous example, the cues indicate the need to gather data regarding a problem with the lungs.

Synthesis

Synthesis is the clustering or linking together of cues resulting from the data analysis to determine which cues can be clustered together to form a pattern. There may be multiple cues that need to be clustered to form a single entity. Theiele and colleagues (1986, p. 319) describe clinical situations "as a series of pieces, or cues, much as the pieces of a puzzle . . . (and) fitting together of these cues to form the total picture is called linking." The patterns are determined by the theoretical base that is used.

Theoretical Models

Theoretical models have been developed to explain and guide nursing actions. A description of these models can be found in Chapter 2. Some of the more common models used for determining patterns were identified in Table 8–4. It is important to realize that patterns can be identified in one or more areas in any of these models. NANDA has identified nine patterns of human response, which are believed to be the beginning of a taxonomy or classification system for nursing diagnosis. Gordon (1982) has identified eleven functional health patterns that may be used to cluster the data. Roy's adaptation model (1984) would facilitate clustering the data in patterns to fit the adaptive modes in situations of health and illness. **Data clustering** is organizing information gained during assessment into categories that can be used to determine a client's strengths and health problems.

Several other important theorists have provided methods for identifying patterns. Orem (1985) organizes data by seven areas in which there can be self-care deficits. Neuman (1982) identifies disruptions in the physiologic, psychologic, sociocultural, or developmental spheres. King (1987) defines areas of care according to how the client perceives, thinks, desires, decides, and identifies goals. Once the patterns have

Box 9–1

NORTH AMERICAN NURSING DIAGNOSIS ASSOCIATION–APPROVED NURSING DIAGNOSES

Activity Intolerance

Activity Intolerance, Risk for

Adaptive Capacity: Intracranial, Decreased

Adjustment, Impaired

Airway Clearance, Ineffective

*Anticipatory Grieving

Anxiety

Aspiration, Risk for

Body Image Disturbance

Body Temperature, Risk for Altered

*Bowel Incontinence

Breastfeeding, Effective

Breastfeeding, Ineffective

Breastfeeding, Interrupted

Breathing Pattern, Ineffective

Caregiver Role Strain

Caregiver Role Strain, Risk for

*Chronic Low Self Esteem

*Chronic Pain

*Colonic Constipation

Communication, Impaired Verbal

Community Coping, Ineffective

Community Coping, Potential for Enhanced

Confusion, Acute

Confusion, Chronic

Constipation

*Constipation, Colonic

*Constipation, Perceived

Decisional Conflict (Specify)

Decreased Cardiac Output

Defensive Coping

Denial, Ineffective

Diarrhea

Disorganized Infant Behavior

Disorganized Infant Behavior, Risk for

Disuse Syndrome, Risk for

Diversional Activity Deficit

Dysfunctional Grieving

Dysfunctional Ventilatory Weaning Response

Dysreflexia

Energy Field Disturbance

Environmental Interpretation Syndrome, Impaired

Family Coping: Compromised, Ineffective

Family Coping: Disabling, Ineffective

Family Coping: Potential for Growth

Family Process: Alcoholism, Altered

Family Processes, Altered

Fatigue

Fear

Fluid Volume Deficit

Fluid Volume Deficit, Risk for

Fluid Volume Excess

Functional Incontinence

Gas Exchange, Impaired

Grieving, Anticipatory

Grieving, Dysfunctional

Growth and Development, Altered

Health Maintenance, Altered

Health Seeking Behaviors (Specify)

Home Maintenance Management, Impaired

Hopelessness

Hyperthermia

Hypothermia

Incontinence, Bowel

Incontinence, Functional

Incontinence, Reflex

Incontinence, Stress

Incontinence, Total

Incontinence, Urge

Individual Coping, Ineffective

Infant Feeding Pattern, Ineffective

Infection, Risk for

Injury, Risk for

Knowledge Deficit (Specify)

Loneliness, Risk for

Management of Therapeutic Regimen: Community, Ineffective

Management of Therapeutic Regimen: Families, Ineffective

Management of Therapeutic Regimen: Individual, Effective

Management of Therapeutic Regimen (Individuals), Ineffective

Memory, Impaired

Noncompliance (Specify)

Nutrition: Less than Body Requirements, Altered

Nutrition: More than Body Requirements, Altered

Nutrition: Risk for More than Body Requirements, Altered

Oral Mucous Membrane, Altered

Organized Infant Behavior, Potential for Enhanced

Pain

Pain, Chronic

Box continued on following page

Box 9–1

NORTH AMERICAN NURSING DIAGNOSIS ASSOCIATION–APPROVED NURSING DIAGNOSES
(Continued)

Parent/Infant/Child Attachment, Risk for Altered

Parental Role Conflict

Parenting, Altered

Parenting, Risk for Altered

*Perceived Constipation

Perioperative Positioning Injury, Risk for

Peripheral Neurovascular Dysfunction, Risk for

Personal Identity Disturbance

Physical Mobility, Impaired

Poisoning, Risk for

Post-Trauma Response

Powerlessness

Protection, Altered

Rape-Trauma Syndrome

Rape-Trauma Syndrome: Compound Reaction

Rape-Trauma Syndrome: Silent Reaction

*Reflex Incontinence

Relocation Stress Syndrome

Role Performance, Altered

Self Care Deficit
  Bathing/Hygiene
  Dressing/Grooming
  Feeding
  Toileting

*Self Esteem, Chronic Low

Self Esteem, Disturbance

*Self Esteem, Situational Low

Self-Mutilation, Risk for

Sensory/Perceptual Alterations (Specify) (visual, auditory, kinesthetic, gustatory, tactile, olfactory)

Sexual Dysfunction

Sexuality Patterns, Altered

*Situational Low Self Esteem

Skin Integrity, Impaired

Skin Integrity, Risk for Impaired

Sleep Pattern Disturbance

Social Interaction, Impaired

Social Isolation

Spiritual Distress

Spiritual Well-Being, Potential for Enhanced

*Stress Incontinence

Suffocation, Risk for

Sustain Spontaneous Ventilation, Inability to

Swallowing, Impaired

Thermoregulation, Ineffective

Thought Processes, Altered

Tissue Integrity, Impaired

Tissue Perfusion, Altered (Specify Type) (renal, cerebral, cardiopulmonary, gastrointestinal, peripheral)

*Total Incontinence

Trauma, Risk for

Unilateral Neglect

*Urge Incontinence

Urinary Elimination, Altered

Urinary Retention

Violence, Risk for: Self-directed or directed at others

---

* These are duo-referenced for ease and speed in locating the correct diagnosis. From North American Nursing Diagnosis Association (1997). *Nursing diagnoses: Definitions & classification 1997–1998.* Philadelphia. Reprinted with permission, Nursecom, Inc.

---

been established within the framework of a theoretical model, the nursing diagnosis can be written.

◆
Nursing Diagnosis

Nursing diagnosis is a clinical judgment about individual, family, or community responses to actual health problems, situations in which the client is at risk for health problems (deviations or variations in the well-being of a client), and situations in which there is a potential for either health problems or enhanced wellness.

The focus of a nursing diagnosis includes problems that are primarily treated by nurses and problems that may be treated by health care professionals in other disciplines. There are three types of problems: actual, risk, and possible.

* **Actual problems** are existing responses that occur as the result of a medical condition; *e.g.,* ineffective breathing pattern, spiritual distress, dysfunctional grieving, altered parenting, activity intolerance

* **Risk problems** are concerns that are risks for the client; *e.g.,* there may be a risk for injury related to immobility or a sensory-perceptual deficit

* **Potential problems** are concerns that have not been verified or validated; *e.g.,* the nurse may suspect that a client is depressed but needs additional information to confirm

the concern; therefore, there may be a diagnosis of Self-Esteem Disturbance, Possible

Nursing diagnosis provides the basis for the selection of nursing interventions to achieve those outcomes for which the nurse is accountable (NANDA, 1990). For example

* Individual: Health Maintenance, altered, related to increased food consumption
* Family: Family Coping, Ineffective, related to loss of job and income
* Community: Knowledge Deficit related to environmental pollution

Many schools, health care organizations, and regulatory organizations use the standard NANDA list of nursing diagnoses as an effective means of facilitating implementation and documentation of nursing care plans. NANDA meets every other year to explore and evaluate the current list and facilitate the development of an updated list of nursing diagnoses. The NANDA list (Box 9–1) has several advantages: It provides common terminology for nurses to use; common terminology will facilitate computer use; and it provides a method for justifying and reimbursing nursing activities rather than activities related to the medical diagnosis.

Writing the Nursing Diagnosis

Nurses find that writing the diagnostic statement is a challenge, and practice is needed to be able to write an accurate statement. Each client has unique responses; therefore, the diagnoses must be individualized. The nurse uses **clinical reasoning** to analyze the data and make diagnoses. Clinical reasoning is the process by which collected data are analyzed and diagnostic statements are made. Nursing diagnoses may be written in one-, two-, or three-part statements. One-part statements are used for wellness and syndrome diagnoses. Two-part statements are used for actual responses, situations that place the client at risk for a response, and situations that lead to a potential response. Three-part statements are used for actual diagnoses. Box 9–2 illustrates the use of each type of statement.

The first part of the diagnostic statement identifies the human response that is a concern to the nurse. It is based on the assessment data and obtained from the NANDA list. This part of the diagnostic statement indicates the focus for changes that need to occur in the client as a result of nursing interventions. Modifiers can be used to clarify the type of response or the degree to which the human response is present. Modifiers are identified in Table 9–1. The outcomes, long-

---

Box 9–2

TYPES OF DIAGNOSTIC STATEMENTS

Part I	Related to	Part II	As evidenced by	Part III
Human response (individual, family, or community) Suggesting a change that needs to occur in client *(may add)*		**Contributing factors** Environmental Physiological Psychological Sociocultural Spiritual		**Reinforcement or clarification** Signs or symptoms Medical diagnosis
Modifier (type or degree of response)				

One-Part Statements

* Wellness nursing diagnosis
  Potential for Enhanced Organized Infant Behavior
  Potential for Enhanced Community Coping
* Syndrome nursing diagnosis
  Rape-Trauma Syndrome
  Relocation Stress Syndrome

Two-Part Statements

* Risk nursing diagnosis
  Injury, Risk for, related to lack of awareness of hazards
* Potential nursing diagnosis
  Potential Body Image Disturbance related to reports of isolating behaviors of husband after surgery

Two-Part Statements Continued

* Actual nursing diagnosis
  Skin Integrity Impaired, related to prolonged immobility
  Altered Nutrition: Less than Body Requirements related to inability to feed self

Three-Part Statements

* Actual nursing diagnosis
  Skin Integrity, Impaired, related to prolonged immobility secondary to fractured pelvis, as evidenced by a 2-cm sacral lesion

Adapted from Carpenito, L. J. (1992). *Nursing diagnosis: Application to clinical practice.* Philadelphia: J. B. Lippincott.

Table 9—1

NURSING DIAGNOSIS MODIFIERS

MODIFIER	DESCRIPTION/DEFINITION	EXAMPLE
Altered	A change from the usual or optimal well-being for a particular client	Body Temperature, Altered
Risk for	The individual is at risk for a problem	Infection, Risk for
Ineffective	Not producing the desired effect; not capable of performing satisfactorily	Thermoregulation, Ineffective
Decreased	Smaller; lessened; diminished; less in size, amount, or degree	Decreased Cardiac Output
Impaired	Made worse, weakened; damaged, reduced; deteriorated	Swallowing, Impaired
Deficit	Amount or quantity that is less than necessary, desirable, or usable	Diversional Activity Deficit
Excess	Amount or quantity that is more than necessary, desirable, or usable	Fluid Volume Excess
Dysfunctional	Abnormal; impaired or incomplete functioning	Sexual Dysfunction
Disturbance	The state of being agitated, interrupted, or interfered with	Sleep Pattern Disturbance
Acute	Severe, but of short duration	Acute Urinary Retention
Chronic	Lasting a long time; recurring; habitual, constant	Chronic Pain
Less than	A smaller amount	Nutrition: Less Than Body Requirements, Altered
More than	A larger amount	Nutrition: More Than Body Requirements, Altered
Anticipatory	Occurring in advance	Anticipatory Grieving
Compromised	To lay open to danger; to endanger the interests of	Family Coping: Compromised, Ineffective

term goals, or objectives are usually based on the first part of the diagnostic statement. These are discussed in later chapters.

The second part of the diagnostic statement reflects the relationship of the first and second parts of the diagnostic statement by identifying the contributing factors. These include the environmental, physiological, psychological, sociocultural, and spiritual factors that may be causing or contributing to the human response. Medical diagnoses are not to be used in a "related to" statement. The more precise this part of the statement is, the more accurate the interventions will be. The nursing interventions, orders, and actions discussed in later chapters are derived from the second part of the diagnostic statement.

The third part of the diagnostic statement is not always necessary. In this part, the signs and symptoms, or the medical diagnosis, may be used to reinforce or clarify the second part of the diagnostic statement.

It is important for the nurse to know why the human response is occurring so that interventions to prevent, alleviate, or minimize a response can be planned. Guidelines that are important to consider when writing the diagnostic statement are found in Table 9–2. The nursing diagnosis is not a statement of all of the conclusions or client problems identified at the end of the assessment phase of the nursing process. There may be medical problems that would not be applicable to a nursing diagnosis for which nurses could not intervene. These would be collaborative problems.

Collaborative Problems

Collaborative problems occur in relation to specific pathology identified by another health care provider. They are certain physiologic complications that nurses monitor to detect the onset of further complications or changes in status of the complications. These represent situations in which the primary responsibility of the nurse is to diagnose and manage changes in the client's status using the medical diagnosis to formulate a nursing diagnosis and determine interventions. For example, a client who has undergone surgery with a medical diagnosis of a fractured pelvis would have the

	Table 9–2
GUIDELINES FOR WRITING A NURSING DIAGNOSIS	
STEPS IN WRITING A DIAGNOSIS	**ACTIONS TO AVOID**

1. Write a statement
  a. Of the client's response rather than the nursing need
  b. That is legally advisable
 	
  c. That does not contain value judgments
 	
  d. That expresses the related factor in terms that can be changed
  e. That does not include medical diagnosis in parts one and two
  f. That is clear and concise
  g. That is in terms that provide direction for nursing interventions
2. Write a list of diagnoses using the NANDA list of approved nursing diagnoses a. that reflect the client's current health status
3. Be sure that the two parts of the statement
  a. Do not mean the same thing
  b. Are connected with "related to"
	a. Nursing needs; *e.g.,* change dressing, check blood pressure
	b. Legally inadvisable statements; *e.g.,* fear of beatings by spouse; ineffective family coping related to indifference to parenting
	c. Value judgments; *e.g.,* noncompliance related to failure to keep appointments; inadequate coping related to limited intellectual ability
	
	a. Reversing the parts of the statements
	b. Using single cues in the first part of the statement

Data from Iyer, P. W., Taptich, B. J., & Bernocchi-Losey, D. (1991). *Nursing process and nursing diagnosis* (2nd ed.). Philadelphia: W. B. Saunders.

following collaborative problems during the postoperative period:

Potential complications
  Avascular necrosis of the femoral head
  Compartment syndrome
  Displacement of hip joint
  Fat emboli
  Hemorrhage/shock
  Peroneal nerve palsy
  Pulmonary embolism
  Venous stasis thrombosis

The nursing diagnosis would be

Fear related to anticipated dependence

Pain related to trauma, incision, and muscle spasms

Self-Care Deficit related to activity restrictions

Risk for Constipation related to immobility

Risk for Sensory/Perception Alteration, Kinesthetic, related to age, immobility, and pain

Risk for Management of Therapeutic Regimen: Individual, Ineffective, related to insufficient knowledge of restrictions, home care, follow-up care, and support services

Medical Diagnosis

As mentioned in Chapter 7 (see Fig. 7–2), medical diagnoses should not be confused with nursing diagnoses. *Nursing diagnosis* is not a new term for medical diagnosis, and the terms cannot be used interchangeably. A **medical diagnosis** describes a specific pathophysiological condition, which usually requires medication, surgery, or radiation. A medical diagnosis usually does not vary from one client to another. A nursing diagnosis describes the effect of symptoms and pathophysiology on the client's lifestyle and activities. An example of the difference between the medical and nursing diagnoses for a client suffering from decreased mobility is found in Table 9–3.

Sources of Error

A common error that nurses make is to state all of the client problems as a nursing diagnosis. There are two other types of errors commonly made by nurses when making diagnostic statements: errors of commission and errors of omission. An **error of commission** occurs when the nurse "overdiagnoses" a client or when nonexistent health problems are diagnosed. For example, the nurse determines that a client has a bowel movement every other day and writes a diagnosis of constipation, when in fact this may be normal for this client. If the nurse had assessed the client further, then information about the client's bowel habits would have been revealed and the diagnosis would not have been made. An **error of omission** occurs when the nurse fails to identify a health care problem.

Table 9–3

DIFFERENCE BETWEEN MEDICAL AND NURSING DIAGNOSIS

MEDICAL DIAGNOSIS	NURSING DIAGNOSIS
Data are gathered to determine a. What limitations are present and to make a medical diagnosis of one of the following: Fracture Osteoarthritis Cerebrovascular accident b. The need for surgery, medications, rehabilitation, physiotherapy	History taken for recent events, current activities, and demands on daily living that are altered by changes in: a. Internal resources involving physical and emotional strength, which could result in a nursing diagnosis such as Self-care deficit: Nutrition, Less than Body Requirements related to decreased mobility b. Relationships with external resources—persons and things that could result in the following nursing diagnosis: Social Isolation related to decreased mobility

Adapted from Carnevali, D. L., Mitchell, P. H., Woods, N. F., & Tanner, C. A. (1984). *Diagnostic reasoning in nursing.* Philadelphia: J. B. Lippincott.

Table 9–4

DIAGNOSIS OF MRS. C.

CUE CLUSTERS	NURSING DIAGNOSIS	RELATED FACTORS
Client reports pain a "9" on a scale of 1–10; client grimaces when shifting positions; profuse sweating, altered vital signs—pulse, 98; BP, 128/86	Pain (high priority)	Trauma Recent orthopedic surgery Limited mobility
Client is unable to position self comfortably in bed; client unable to perform ADL; ambulation is difficult	Physical Mobility, Impaired (high priority)	Trauma/surgery Pain/discomfort Anxiety Weakness
Family member states that left foot is cool and pale	High Risk for Deep Vein Thrombosis (high priority)	Surgical procedure Immobility
Client states that abdomen is bloated; unable to pass gas; bowel sounds are sluggish	Risk for Constipation (low priority)	Immobility Pain Narcotics Decreased fluid intake
Client's intravenous site is erythematous and occluded; operative site draining serosanguineous fluid; client has a low-grade temperature of 99.7°F	Infection, Risk for (high priority)	Surgery Intravenous device Foley catheter Immobility
Client unable to bathe, dress, toilet, transfer, and ambulate without assistance	Self Care Deficit (low priority)	Surgery Pain Immobility
Client frustrated with gait training using walker; client asking many questions; client and family members express concern about discharge and home care	Knowledge Deficit of Therapeutic Regimen and Discharge (low priority)	New condition Lack of knowledge of home care, assistive devices, and support services
Husband states concerns about caring for client at home; husband concerned his own health will suffer	Caregiver Role Strain (low priority)	Client will need assistance with ADL at home; husband is elderly and has health problems; husband has insufficient knowledge of home care and support services

ADL = activities of daily living; BP = blood pressure.
Case study diagnoses for Mrs. C. were written by Jane Wrenn, BSN.
Data from Gulanick, M., Kloop, A., Galanes, S., *et al.* (1994). *Nursing care plans: Nursing diagnosis and interventions* (3rd ed.). St. Louis: Mosby-Year Book.

For example, for a client with multiple complaints, the nurse might decide that the client is always complaining and fail to collect the necessary data to make the accurate diagnoses.

Errors usually occur as the result of incomplete data collection, incorrectly clustered data, or incorrectly interpreted data. Lack of clinical knowledge may result in critical data not being collected.

The diagnoses for Mrs. C., whose case is assessed in Chapter 8, are illustrated in Table 9–4.

Validation

Before the nursing diagnosis can be finalized, it is important to confirm its accuracy. There must be adequate data to support the diagnosis. Also, the cues should be consistent with the client's responses and form a pattern. If the data and cues are consistent with the nursing diagnosis, then the following questions need to be answered:

1. Will nursing interventions modify the diagnosis?
2. Would other nurses using the data write the same nursing diagnosis?

The **data validation** step is finalized when the nursing diagnosis is discussed with the client, unless the client's condition negates the possibility of a discussion. Agreement between the client and the nurse is essential. If there is no consensus between the nurse and the client, the nurse needs to continue the discussion until an agreement can be reached.

Computer Assistance

Computers are used to interpret data collected during the assessment phase, to assist the nurse in arriving at a diagnosis, and to recommend outcomes in a program known as *computer-assisted diagnosis* (CAD) (Iyer *et al.*, 1991). With CAD, a list of nursing diagnoses is generated from the data entered, and the nurse can accept or reject diagnoses from the list. The advantage of using computer-generated diagnoses is that it helps to avoid errors of omission, providing diagnoses that the nurse may overlook.

Summary

Analysis follows the gathering of data during the assessment phase of the nursing process. It involves clustering the data, conducting further assessment as necessary, and clarifying conflicting information. After this is done, the nurse can determine patterns and synthesize the data. Clustering of the data is based on the model of nursing practice used.

The diagnosis is written as a client-oriented statement based on the analysis of the data. The diagnostic statement is then validated, checked for errors, and modified as the client's health status changes.

CHAPTER HIGHLIGHTS
✦

✦ Nursing diagnosis is the step of the nursing process in which the assessment data are analyzed and synthesized to make a diagnostic statement. The diagnostic statement is the basis for planning, implementing, and evaluating the nursing care plan.

✦ A nursing diagnosis is the statement of an actual or high risk for a health problem that can be treated with an independent nursing intervention.

✦ The problem statement identifies that aspect of the client where change is needed. Subjective and objective data initially identify the problem. The etiology identifies the factors that maintain the unhealthy state and suggests appropriate nursing interventions.

✦ The diagnostic process includes analysis and interpretation of data. The nurse must validate and cluster data to identify client's health problems, health risks, and strengths.

✦ Nursing diagnoses are written for the physical developmental, intellectual, emotional, social, and spiritual dimensions of the client, to develop a plan of care that will help the client and family to adapt to changes resulting from illness or a change of lifestyle.

✦ The following are *not* nursing diagnoses and should not appear in the diagnostic statement: medical diagnosis, medical pathology, diagnostic tests, treatments, equipment, therapeutic client needs, therapeutic client goals, a single sign or symptom, and invalidated nursing inferences.

✦ Diagnostic errors can occur by either commission or omission. Errors of commission occur when there is incomplete data collection, incorrect clustering of data, overdiagnosis, or diagnosis of a nonexistent health problem. Errors of omission occur when the nurse fails to identify a health problem or there is incomplete data collection, incorrect data clustering, or improper interpretation of data.

✦ Nursing diagnoses are written in one-, two-, or three-part statements. Each diagnostic statement should be clear, concise, client centered, related to one problem, and based on reliable and relevant assessment data.

✦ The development of a taxonomy of nursing diagnoses is ongoing. A valid taxonomy would define the independent scope of practice, facilitate nursing research, and clarify communication among nurses and other health professionals.

Study Questions

1. Rape trauma syndrome

    a. is not a nursing diagnosis
    b. is a one-part nursing diagnosis
    c. is the first part of a two-part nursing diagnosis
    d. is the first part of a three-part nursing diagnosis

2. Gaps in the data collection are evident in all but one of the following situations

    a. there is a lack of information needed to make a nursing diagnosis
    b. multiple nursing diagnoses can be made
    c. conflicting information needs to be clarified
    d. the client is reluctant to share information

3. The purpose of theoretical models in nursing diagnosis is to

    a. cluster the data
    b. guide the search for cues
    c. structure the interview
    d. guide nursing actions

4. The group that has made the largest contribution to developing nursing diagnoses is

    a. ANA
    b. National League for Nursing
    c. NANDA
    d. National Organization of Nurse Practitioner Faculties

5. Which of the following would not be part of a nursing diagnosis?

    a. subjective data
    b. objective data
    c. value judgments
    d. modifiers

Critical Thinking Exercises

1. Develop a three-part nursing diagnosis based on one of the following data sets:
    Set A: Client complaining of pain in right foot that worsens with walking over 50 ft, dorsalis pedis and posterior tibialis pulse obtainable only with Doppler, right foot cool and pale, shallow pale ulcer on heel where client hit it 2 weeks ago.
    Set B: Client sitting upright using accessory muscles to breathe, respirations 40 and shallow, lung sounds diminished with rales noted halfway up lungfields, neck veins distended; client has history of anterior myocardial infarction 2 years ago.

2. Discuss how nursing and medical diagnoses are related.

References

American Nurses' Association. (1980). *Social policy statement.* Kansas City, MO: American Nurses' Association.

American Nurses' Association Congress on Practice. (1973). *Standards of practice.* Kansas City, MO: American Nurses' Association.

Aspinall, M. J. (1976). Nursing diagnosis: The weak link. *Nursing Outlook, 24*(7), 433–436.

Carnevali, D. L., Mitchell, P. H., Woods, N. F., & Tanner, C. A. (1984). *Diagnostic reasoning in nursing.* Philadelphia: J. B. Lippincott.

Carpenito, L. J. (1992). *Nursing diagnosis: Application to clinical practice.* Philadelphia: J. B. Lippincott.

Gebbie, K., & Lavin, M. A. (1974). Classification of nursing diagnosis. *American Journal of Nursing, 74,* 250–253.

Gordon, M. (1982). *Nursing diagnosis: Process and application.* New York: McGraw-Hill.

Hammond, K. R. (1966). Clinical inference in nursing: A psychologist's viewpoint. *Nursing Research, 15,* 27–38.

Iyer, P. W., Taptich, B. J., & Bernocchi-Losey, D. (1991). *Nursing process and nursing diagnosis* (2nd ed.). Philadelphia: W. B. Saunders.

King, I. M. (1987). King's theory of goal attainment. In R. R. Parse (Ed.), *Nursing science: Major paradigms, theories and critiques.* Philadelphia: W. B. Saunders.

Neuman, B. (1982). *The Neuman systems model: Applications to nursing education and practice.* New York: Appleton-Century-Crofts.

North American Nursing Diagnosis Association. (1990). *Proceedings of the Ninth Conference.* St. Louis, MO.

Orem, D. E. (1985). *Nursing: Concepts of practice.* New York: McGraw-Hill.

Roy C. (1984). *Introduction to nursing: An adaptation model* (2nd ed.), New York: Prentice-Hall.

Taylor, S. G. (1991). The structure of nursing diagnosis from Orem's theory. *Nursing Science Quarterly, 4*(1), 24–32.

Theiele, J. E., Baldwin, J. H., Hyde, R. S., *et al.* (1986). An investigation of decision theory: What are the effects of teaching cue recognition? *Journal of Nursing Education, 25*(8), 319.

Bibliography

Anderson, J. E., & Briggs, L. L. (1988). Nursing diagnosis: A study of quality and supportive evidence. *Image, 20*(3), 141–144.

Cassmeyer, V. L. (1989). Using physiology and pathophysiology in the nursing diagnostic process. *Journal of Advanced Medical Surgical Nursing, 1*(3), 1–10.

Dobrzyn, J. (1995). Components of written diagnostic statements. *Nursing Diagnosis, 6*(1), 29–36.

McGillan, P. M. (1990). Assessment and care planning for autonomy in practice. *Provider, 16*(6), 37–38.

Putzier, D. J., & Padrick, K. P. (1984). Nursing diagnosis: A component of the nursing process and decision making. *Topics in Clinical Nursing, 5*(4), 21–29.

Weber, G. J. (1991). Nursing diagnosis: A comparison of textbook approaches. *Nurse Educator, 16*(2), 22–27.

Wolley, N. (1990). Nursing diagnosis: Exploring factors which may influence the reasoning process. *Journal of Advanced Nursing, 15*(1), 110–117.

Chapter 10

PLANNING

JULIA M. LEAHY, PhD, RN

LEARNING OBJECTIVES

◆

After studying this chapter, you should be able to

◆ Define basic terminology related to planning

◆ Describe guidelines used to set priorities of care

◆ Define expected client outcomes

◆ Describe characteristics of an outcome statement

◆ Describe the types of domains for classifying outcome behaviors

◆ Define the three components of a well-written outcome statement

◆ Describe guidelines for selecting appropriate nursing interventions

◆ Describe characteristics of appropriate nursing interventions

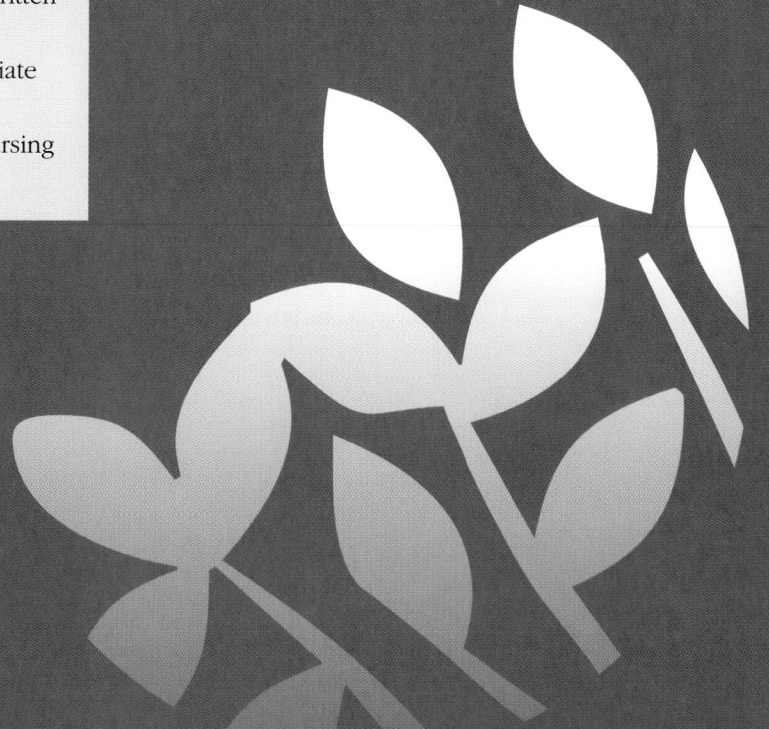

Planning involves the systematic and deliberate determination of an individualized **nursing plan of care** that considers the client as a holistic human being. After the nurse collects the database, interprets the findings, and identifies the relevant nursing diagnoses, then he or she develops a mutually agreeable plan of care that should be done in collaboration with the client to resolve, limit, or prevent those problems identified from the data analysis (Fig. 10–1). The plan should include the expected outcomes to be achieved by the client and those interventions that will assist the client in achieving these outcomes.

This phase of the nursing process includes establishing priorities of care, identifying outcomes to be demonstrated by the client, selecting appropriate nursing interventions, and writing the plan of care. These activities require a collaborative effort with the client and family as well as other members of the health care team. When the nurse involves these individuals in this part of the nursing process, he or she is encouraging compliance with the plan. Clients are more likely to carry out planned activities when they have input into developing them. The client is primarily involved in adapting or adjusting to health problems and demonstrating those outcomes of health maintenance or promotion (see Box 10–1).

An effective plan is one that has three major characteristics (Niziolek & Shaw, 1991). First, it should reflect collaborative practice among the multidisciplinary care providers (Fig. 10–2), including other nurses,

---

> **Box 10–1**
>
> ## PLANNING
>
> * Establish priorities
> * Identify outcomes
> * Select nursing interventions
> * Write the plan of care

---

physicians, dietitians, physical therapists, and respiratory therapists, to name a few. Second, there should be evidence that the nurse has set priorities of the client's needs by determining which problems should be addressed first. Third, nursing care that is identified should be specifically directed to those outcomes that the client should achieve after care is rendered. The actions that the nurse has identified should reflect the client's abilities and goals.

The nurse should develop an individualized plan of care for each specific client. Data from the assessment provide the basis for selecting nursing activities. When the nurse on a geriatric unit considers that the client usually takes a bath in the evening and provides for access to the tub room prior to sleep, then individual planning is occurring. When the nurse on a pediatric unit learns that a child prefers to eat bananas with his cereal and notifies the kitchen of this dietary request, individual planning is occurring. While there are common, prescribed interventions for designated health care problems, the nurse should be flexible in applying these interventions to individual client situations. By doing this, the nurse demonstrates consideration of the holistic nature of the client.

Writing the plan of care is an integral part of nursing practice. Including this plan in the formal record of the client demonstrates that nursing care is being provided and evaluated. The documentation of nursing care provides evidence of the nurse's professional accountability; that is, the record indicates actual care rendered by the nurse in response to the client's needs or identified problems.

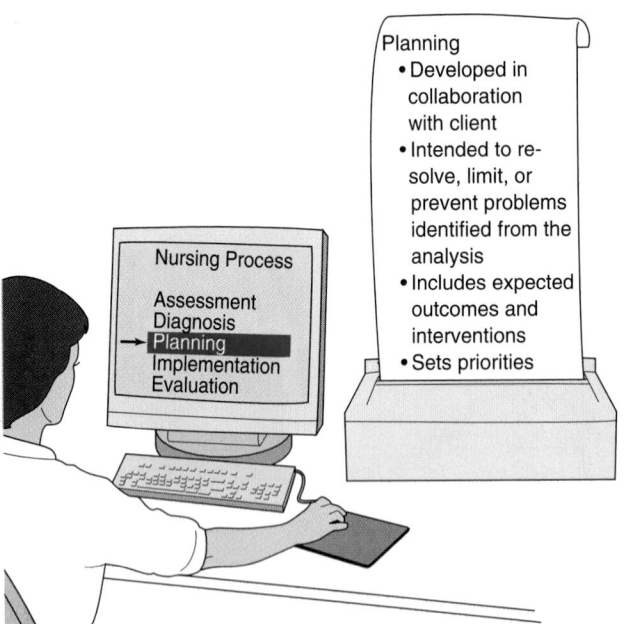

Planning
• Developed in collaboration with client
• Intended to resolve, limit, or prevent problems identified from the analysis
• Includes expected outcomes and interventions
• Sets priorities

Nursing Process
Assessment
Diagnosis
→ Planning
Implementation
Evaluation

❧ **Figure 10–1**
Planning is the third step of the nursing process and includes establishing priorities of care, identifying client outcomes, determining appropriate nursing interventions, and developing the nursing plans of care.

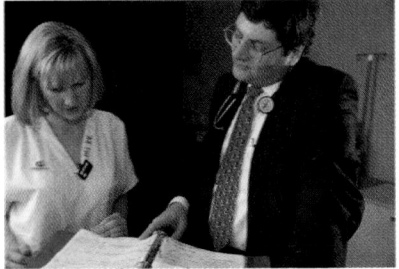

❧ **Figure 10–2**
Team collaboration is an essential part of planning.

When to Plan

Planning occurs at various points along the nurse-client relationship and continues through all phases of the relationship. Initial planning occurs when the client first enters the health care setting seeking intervention. Following an initial assessment of the client's health status, the nurse makes an initial plan of care to meet preliminary problems. The plan reflects the need to meet the client's initial health care problems and should be flexible to be revised as the client's status changes. If the client is initially seen in the emergency department, then the initial plan of care deals with the emergency situation but should consider the need for follow-up by the nurse. If the client is seeking health maintenance assessment, as in an annual physical examination, then the plan should primarily focus on measures to maintain the client's current physical health.

Ongoing planning represents the continued interactions between the client and the nurse (Fig. 10–3). Frequently, this involves multiple nurses who interact with the client at various points in time. In a hospital setting, nurses provide input into the client's plan of care during each shift and on each day that the client is hospitalized. In a community setting, such as a home setting, each home visit requires the nurse to reevaluate the plan as needed. Consider the client who has diabetes mellitus and requires close monitoring of the blood glucose. The client has a monthly appointment in an ambulatory care setting for evaluation of his or her progress in controlling the blood sugar. Each interaction with the client requires that the nurse identify outcomes and plan interventions for the next month as part of the ongoing provision of nursing care.

The last type of planning is referred to as discharge planning and usually suggests the need to plan for the client's discharge from a hospital or acute care environment. Discharge planning considers the termination of the relationship with the client and the transfer of that relationship to another health care setting, such as long-term care or home environments. In today's health care environment, many clients are either being discharged from a hospital after a very short period or are receiving surgical treatments in an ambulatory surgical center, making discharge planning even more imperative. Many clients assume the responsibility for their own care and require detailed instructions as part of their discharge planning. The discharge plan considers those activities that will be required after discharge and the resources available for the client. For some clients, referrals to other health care professionals, such as visiting nurses, social workers, physical therapists, or dietitians, may be required.

Setting Priorities

Once the nurse has identified the nursing diagnoses that pertain to the client, the determination of priorities begins. The nurse must select those nursing diagnoses that are of prime concern and that require immediate intervention. This does not mean that other diagnoses must be ignored or delayed until resolution of more priority diagnoses. Setting **priorities** simply means deciding which needs or problems require immediate action and which ones could be delayed until a later time because they are not urgent.

The following guidelines have been identified (Christensen, 1995) for setting priorities:

1. **Those problems that involve actual or life-threatening concerns are considered prior to actual or potential health-threatening concerns.** Threats to respiratory or cardiac function are a higher priority than problems that are not life threatening or are not directly related to the current illness. Consider the following example: Mr. Thompson is an 85-year-old resident of a long-term care facility who comes to the emergency department in acute respiratory distress because of advanced cardiac failure. Fluid is accumulating in his lungs. He has a history of cerebrovascular accident (stroke) and has been bedridden for the past month. He has a small open pressure sore on his sacrum. In the emergency department, the nurse assesses that he has a tendency to be incontinent. When the nurse reviews the data about Mr. Thompson, he or she should set priorities of the nursing diagnoses as follows:

    Ineffective gas exchange related to the presence of fluid in the lungs

    Altered patterns of urinary elimination related to incontinence

    Risk for infection related to the presence of an open skin lesion

2. **Consideration must be given to time constraints and to the human and material resources available.** These factors affect the extent to which certain diagnoses

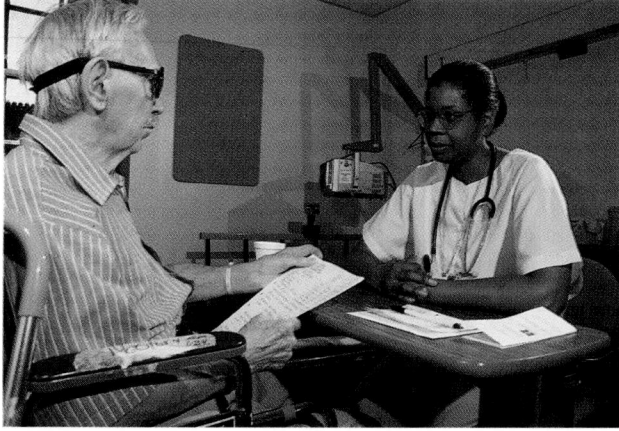

✦ Figure 10–3
Presenting a care plan to a client.

can be dealt with. Limited staff, equipment, and supplies can reduce the number of diagnoses that can be treated at any given time. Infrequent contact with clients who are seen in an ambulatory care setting limits nursing interventions to more crucial, high-priority diagnoses. In these situations, the nurse needs to be creative in identifying alternative methods of providing nursing care. Sometimes it is important to consider those problems that can be resolved within a short time to provide the client with a sense of accomplishment or resolution. For example, when a client needs to learn a new skill, such as self-administration of insulin, making important strides in learning the procedure provides positive feedback in attaining independence in performance.

3. **Those diagnoses that the client identifies as important must be given high priority and consideration by the nurse.** The nurse should value and elicit the client's input into this process. A high-priority diagnosis that a client should lose weight is dependent on the client's willingness to lose that weight. In other situations, the nurse is confronted with a client who may be complaining of one problem and not be aware of a more serious problem. The nurse must deal with the problem identified by the client first before pursuing one that he or she has identified. For instance, a client who comes to an ambulatory health center complaining of pain in the foot may be totally unaware of an abdominal mass, which may not be causing as much difficulty as the foot pain. Even though the abdominal mass may be a sign of an intestinal tumor, the nurse must provide measures to relieve the foot pain before proceeding with measures focused on the abdominal mass.

4. **Priority-setting is guided by theories, models, and principles that provide the standard of comparison for evaluating the list of nursing diagnoses.** For example, one theory frequently used to set priorities is Maslow's hierarchy of needs (1968), with levels of physiological needs, safety, love and belonging, self-esteem, and self-actualization (see Chapter 2 for more detailed discussion). For example, needs of oxygen and fluid are considered a higher priority than the need for self-esteem. The more basic needs are met before moving to other needs in the hierarchy. Use of standards, models, and theories guides the decision-making ability of the nurse and gives direction for individualizing nursing care.

Determining Client Outcomes and Objectives

Once the priorities are set, then the nurse, in collaboration with the client, identifies the expected outcomes for the client. An **outcome** is a statement of the behavior or human response that is expected after provision of nursing care. It may involve the prevention, modification, or correction of the behavior stated in the nursing diagnosis. The identified outcome provides the direction for selecting and evaluating nursing interventions.

When determining outcomes, standards determined by legal authorities (state nurse practice acts), professional organizations (such as the American Nurses Association [ANA] standards for nursing practice [1991]), and the institution must be applied. The nurse is responsible for being aware of these standards and following appropriate statutes and guidelines.

A variety of different terms have been used to describe client outcomes. Examples include **goals** and *client* or *behavioral objectives*. Although these terms may be used interchangeably, it is suggested that goals or objectives are broader than outcomes (Alfaro, 1990) and that outcomes represent a more specific behavior to be obtained by the client. If the goal is that a client will be free of pain, an additional statement beginning with "as evidenced by" would clearly state that specific outcome associated with the goal.

Outcomes should relate directly to the nursing diagnosis and its etiological factor. Outcome statements indicate the specific human response or behavior that the client is to achieve after nursing intervention and that will resolve the specific problem that the client is experiencing.

Outcome statements should have the following characteristics:

- Be focused on the client, for it is the client who must achieve the designated outcome. Outcomes should focus on the behavior of the client that is to be achieved. The outcome statement should specifically relate to the human response pattern identified in the nursing diagnosis. Starting outcomes with the phrase "the client" ensures that the focus is on the client and not the nurse or health care team. For example, if the client has a problem with urinary incontinence, the outcome statement should speak to achieving some control of urination.

- Be concise and explicit. The statement should be clear to members of the health care team to promote continuity of care. Terms or phrases that may be confusing or leave doubt about the specific behavior to be achieved should be avoided. Only acceptable terminology should be used to ensure consistency across all health team members.

- Reflect a mutual agreement between the client and the nurse. The desired outcome should be decided by both the client and the nurse, if possible. The outcome is more likely to be achieved if the client is in agreement with it. There are times when the client, because of physical or mental illness, is unable to participate actively in this process. The client's family or significant others should be consulted if possible. For example, a client who is comatose and unable to respond verbally to questions would be unable to provide consent to necessary treatments. As soon as the client's condition improves, outcomes and the plan should be adjusted to reflect this change of status.

- Be observable and measurable. Effectiveness of the nursing care plan is determined by the evaluation of the client's responses after care is rendered. An outcome that describes a specific observable, measurable response facilitates the evaluation process. For example, instead of "Client will walk independently in 3 days," a more specific outcome might be "Client will walk 50 yards without assistance in 3 days." By being more specific in describing the exact behavior to be achieved, there is little confusion about the goal of care.

- Be realistic. Consideration must be given to the client's

physical abilities, growth and development, mental status, and usual coping abilities. Outcome statements should reflect the client's capabilities and limitations (Christensen, 1995). It would be very important to note that a client who is learning to walk is paralyzed as a result of a cerebrovascular accident (or stroke).

- Have a specified time limit. The outcome statement should contain the time frame for achievement of the objective. This may range from a short time frame (such as "within 4 hours") to a longer time frame ("within a week"). The time frame that is identified provides the basis for evaluating the effectiveness of care. Depending on the type of behavior to be achieved, the nurse may identify points of time along the way, which serve as mileposts for evaluating progress towards the end result.

The factors involved in outcome statements are illustrated in Figure 10–4.

Outcome Domains: Cognitive, Affective, Psychomotor

Outcomes may be classified by the action of the verb in the statement, according to the following domains: cognitive, affective, and psychomotor (Bloom, 1956). These domains relate to the type of response that the client is to achieve—how the client will think, feel, or act after the plan is implemented or after teaching is given.

The cognitive domain includes those outcome statements that describe a specific knowledge level. A hierarchial list of six classes of cognitive functions (Bloom, 1956) includes:

- Knowledge: Ability to recall specific factual information from memory

- Comprehension: Demonstrates an understanding of factual information that can be expressed in client's own words
- Application: Ability to use the new information in specific situations to solve a problem
- Analysis: Ability to discriminate between aspects or parts of a situation
- Synthesis: Ability to develop new patterns from existing ones to draw a conclusion
- Evaluation: Ability to appraise a situation for its merit and value

Consider the following example of an outcome statement in the cognitive domain:

> Nursing diagnosis: Knowledge Deficit about procedures to perform self-monitoring of blood glucose
> Outcome: Client will describe the steps used when performing self-monitoring of blood glucose after receiving instruction about the procedure

The affective domain includes those outcome statements involving changes in attitudes, beliefs, values, or feelings. A hierarchical list of five classes (Krathwohl *et al.,* 1964) includes

- Receiving: Demonstrating an awareness of values, beliefs, attitudes, and feelings
- Responding: Demonstrating an interest in receiving pleasure or interest from received phenomena
- Valuing: Demonstrating behavior that reflects a held value
- Organizing: Demonstrating an ability to determine interrelationships among values and to decide the importance of these values
- Characterizing by a value or value complex: Demonstrating behavior that is consistent with perceived values

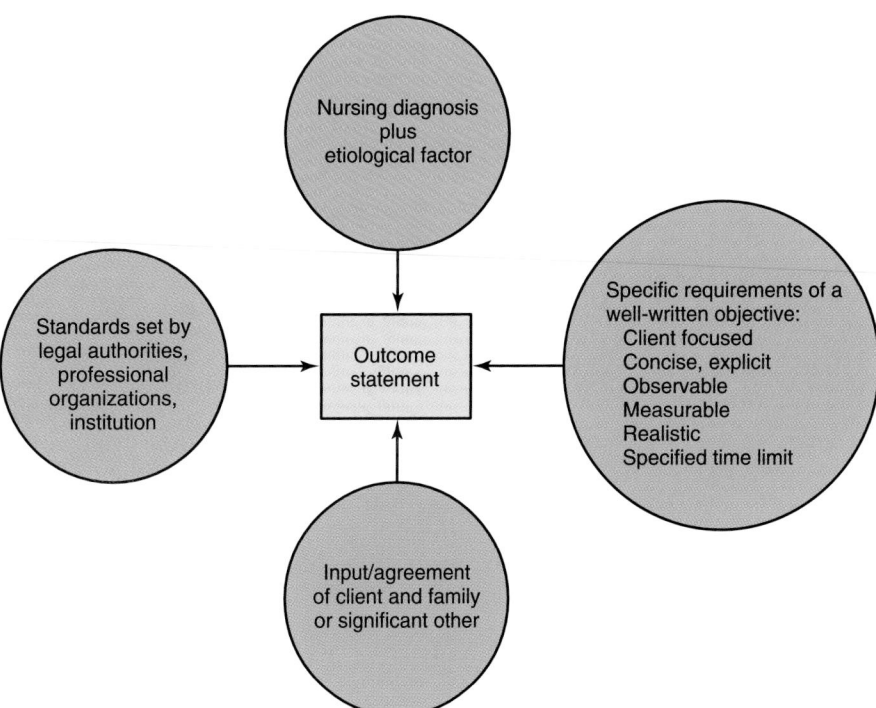

♣ **Figure 10–4**
Identifying expected client outcomes.

Consider the following example:

> Nursing diagnosis: Noncompliance in performing self-monitoring of blood glucose related to fear of sticking self with a needle
>
> Outcome: Client will accept responsibility for performing self-monitoring of blood glucose by demonstrating willingness to perform the procedure

The psychomotor domain focuses on those behavioral responses that involve some type of a motor skill. Seven major classes of psychomotor skills (Simpson, 1966; Urbach, 1970) include:

* Perception: Knowledge of objects and relations through the senses
* Set: Having mental, physical, and emotional readiness to perform an action
* Guided response: Ability to act under the guidance of an instructor or through trial and error
* Mechanism: Developing confidence and proficiency through performance of action
* Complex overt response: Performance of activity with smooth, efficient, and automated performance
* Adaptation: Ability to adjust the performance of an action when challenged with a new situation
* Origination: Ability to construct new procedures based on knowledge of past actions

Consider the following example:

> Nursing diagnosis: Altered Health Maintenance related to failure to perform self-monitoring of blood glucose correctly
>
> Outcome: Client will demonstrate correct procedure for performing self-monitoring of blood glucose

A variety of verbs may be used to identify the domain that is being considered. Table 10–1 provides a suggested list of verbs that represent each of the three domains. In addition to these domains, outcome

statements may describe a specific physiological response that is desired. For example, for the nursing diagnosis, "Risk for Impaired Skin Integrity related to decreased mobility," the following outcome statement may be identified: "Client will have no evidence of skin breakdown at time of discharge."

Long-Term Versus Short-Term Outcomes

When writing an outcome statement, the nurse should evaluate the time that would be required to achieve the outcome. Some outcomes require a longer time to be achieved, whereas other outcomes could be achieved as the client progresses toward the final outcome. A long-term outcome would then reflect the behavior to be achieved at the end, whereas short-term outcomes reflect the points along the way.

The need to have a long-term outcome with short-term outcomes depends on the type of nursing diagnosis that has been identified and the situation in which the client is found. Chronic or subacute health care problems necessitate long-term outcomes more frequently than do acute or episodic problems. For example, the client who has a leg ulcer requiring daily dressing changes might have a long-term outcome such as "the client's ulcer will heal completely within 3 months." Several short-term outcomes might be set to mark certain milestones of the healing process.

Writing the Outcome Statement

An outcome statement should be derived from and relate directly to the nursing diagnosis. Therefore, a well-written outcome statement should include:

* The client, who is the subject or recipient of nursing intervention and is therefore the primary focus of the outcome. (In situations where the client has a primary caregiver, then the caregiver may become the subject of the outcome.)
* A task that includes a verb in conjunction with the specific response or behavior that is expected.
* A criterion that identifies either a condition under which the client is to accomplish the task; a time frame for when the task is to be completed; or a criterion for how well the task is to be performed.

Outcome statements do not need to include all three types of criteria, but at least one is needed to be able to judge achievement of the outcome. Generally, a time limit is included for evaluating the speed for completion of the outcome and for distinguishing between a short-term or a long-term expectation. Examples include

* Nursing diagnosis: Altered Nutrition: More Than Body Requirements related to excessive food intake and limited exercise
  Long-term outcome: The client (subject) will lose (task) 5 lb (criterion) within 1 month (criterion)
  Short-term outcome: The client (subject) will begin to par-

Table **10–1**
EXAMPLES OF VERBS USED IN OBJECTIVES CLASSIFIED BY THEIR DOMAIN

DOMAIN	ACTION VERBS/BEHAVIORS
Cognitive	Define, describe, identify, list, state, give examples, predict, differentiate, modify, relate, show, use, create, organize, plan, tell, write, compare, contrast
Affective	Express a desire, appreciate, accept responsibility, show an awareness or sensitivity
Psychomotor	Perform, demonstrate, use, apply, locate, follow, operate, walk

ticipate *(task)* in an exercise program by walking 1 mile per day *(criterion)*

• Nursing diagnosis: Risk for Altered Health Maintenance related to lack of knowledge of diabetic self-care.
Long-term outcome: The client *(subject)* will demonstrate knowledge of diabetic self-care *(task)* by having blood sugar levels over time within expected levels *(criterion)*
Short-term outcome: The client *(subject)* will demonstrate *(task)* correct *(criterion)* procedure for self-administration of insulin *(task)* after receiving instruction about the procedure *(criterion)*

The outcome statement will provide the nurse with the specific basis for evaluating care that is provided. By including a criterion with the task to be achieved, the nurse plans for the evaluation of the care rendered. Knowing when and how the behavior is to be demonstrated guides the selection of nursing strategies and the implementation of the plan of care. The formal, written plan should reflect these specific outcome criteria, and the nurse should document progress toward achieving this outcome.

Determining Nursing Interventions

After the outcome statements have been identified, the nurse then must determine which nursing actions or interventions will be most helpful in achieving the expected outcome. Nursing **interventions** are those actions performed by the nurse that are aimed at the prevention, maintenance, and restoration of a client's health. Although these actions should be related to the nursing diagnosis, it is the etiology, or the "related to" section, that prescribes the specific actions to be selected. The factor that is deemed responsible for the health problem should become the focus of the care plan. For example, immobility is caused by a variety of conditions, such as fractures, postoperative status, paralysis or hemiparalysis, weakness, and impaired mental status. The actions that the nurse selects to improve the client's mobility status depend primarily on the cause of the immobility.

Actions that are selected also reflect the nursing model that guides practice in the situation at hand. If the Roy Adaptation Model (Roy, 1984) guides practice, actions selected will be aimed toward assisting the client in adapting to environmental stressors. The Orem (1995) Self-Care Model focuses actions toward fostering self-care on the part of the client. It is important that the nurse be knowledgeable about the model that is used in the institution. Student nurses will find that schools of nursing frequently have identified a specific nursing model that guides the curriculum. This model not only provides the framework for the presentation of the course content but also describes how nurses interact with and provide care to clients.

The process for determining which interventions to select should follow certain guidelines:

1. **Identify possible interventions that are based on sound scientific rationale.** The rationale for nursing practice is grounded in science and in nursing theory, which is an ever-changing body of knowledge. The foundation of nursing practice is the development of a knowledge base that reflects science, nursing theory, and the behavioral sciences. New research findings suggest new or revised methodologies to support practice. Nurses need to be aware of these findings and adjust nursing practice accordingly. An example of changing practice involves the use of even, gentle massage over bony prominences, once believed to be an essential component of skin care in an immobilized client (Kozier *et al.,* 1989; Taylor *et al.,* 1989). It is now believed that even gentle massage may damage tissue underlying skin, making an individual more prone to pressure ulcers (US Department of Health and Human Services, 1992).

2. **Consider a wide variety of possible nursing interventions.** The more diverse the approach that is taken, the more likely the client will be able to achieve the identified outcome. Incorporating several actions, combining physiological and psychosocial approaches, and using independent nursing measures when implementing the physician's orders are techniques that the nurse can employ to ensure achievement of the expected outcome. For example, for a client who is anorexic because of cancer chemotherapy, the nurse might examine multiple methods to increase the client's appetite, including both pharmacological and nonpharmacological methods.

3. **Determine which interventions are appropriate and related to the identified outcome and the etiology of the nursing diagnosis.** Because the etiology of nursing diagnoses varies in relation to the individual client's needs and health care problems, the nurse must consider the individual nature of the client and the situation when selecting nursing interventions. Interventions cannot be the same for all clients with similar health problems. What works for one client will not necessarily be helpful for another. Similarly, what works in one setting, such as a hospital, will not necessarily work in another, such as the client's home. Determining what will best assist the individual client to meet his or her needs and resolve his or her health problems is the guiding principle for selection of nursing actions. When making these decisions, the nurse must use critical thinking to make sound clinical judgments. Also, actions that are selected should not be in conflict with those of other health team members, including the physician.

4. **Standards of nursing practice should serve as a guide for evaluating the appropriateness of selected nursing interventions.** Standards such as those defined by the ANA or those determined by the health care setting are appropriate resources for the nurse. Nurses are accountable for their practice and must follow those standards as outlined by these official agencies and institutions. Some of the standards (ANA, 1991) address the following:
    a. Nursing interventions should provide a safe and therapeutic environment and protect the client from sustaining any injury or suffering any emotional response.
    b. Nursing interventions should include teaching-learning methodologies when appropriate. These include assessment of the client's learning needs, determining the client's readiness to learn, identifying the client's outcomes after teaching, preparing an individualized teach-

ing plan for the client, and evaluating the teaching plan in terms of outcomes to be achieved after teaching is presented.

c. Nursing interventions should include the utilization of appropriate resources, such as financial resources or constraints, type and availability of equipment, and presence of adequate human resources.

Figure 10–5 illustrates some of the factors involved in determining appropriate nursing interventions.

Following these guidelines does not necessarily guarantee that clients will resolve their health care problem and demonstrate the expected outcome. Nurses must continually consider the possibility of revising the plan and incorporating alternate measures into the care plan. New measures as evidenced by research should be considered and evaluated.

✦ Writing Nursing Orders

When developing a plan of care, interventions or activities that the nurse identifies as being appropriate in a given situation are termed **nursing orders,** which include not only independent nursing activities that nurses are legally permitted to provide but also those nursing actions that involve implementation of the physician's orders. Nursing orders are designed to address the specific client health problem, in terms of the nursing diagnosis, and are targeted to meet the

expected outcome that has been defined. Nursing orders are frequently referred to as nursing interventions. Whereas a physician may prescribe an analgesic to be administered to a client when necessary for relief of pain, the nurse will identify in the care plan those activities that involve the implementation of that order. For instance, providing the client with relaxation techniques to ease pain or administering the analgesic before the client complains of severe pain or begins a specific activity are examples of nursing orders that are within the scope of nursing practice.

When writing the list of nursing orders, the nurse should follow certain guidelines:

1. **There should be a separate list of nursing orders for each nursing diagnosis and client outcome.** These nursing orders should be specifically intended to achieve the expected client outcome. For example, if the nursing diagnosis is Pain related to swelling of extremity that is in a cast, then the nursing orders should speak to actions that will decrease the swelling in an effort to alleviate the pain.

2. **There should be a sufficient number of nursing orders to address each nursing diagnosis.** Although the minimum number of nursing orders is not etched in stone, usually two to six orders are deemed to be sufficient (Fayram & Christensen, 1995). The actual number that would be adequate depends on whether the outcome would be achieved with the number of orders listed.

3. **Nursing orders should be dated and signed by the nurse to indicate when the orders were written and**

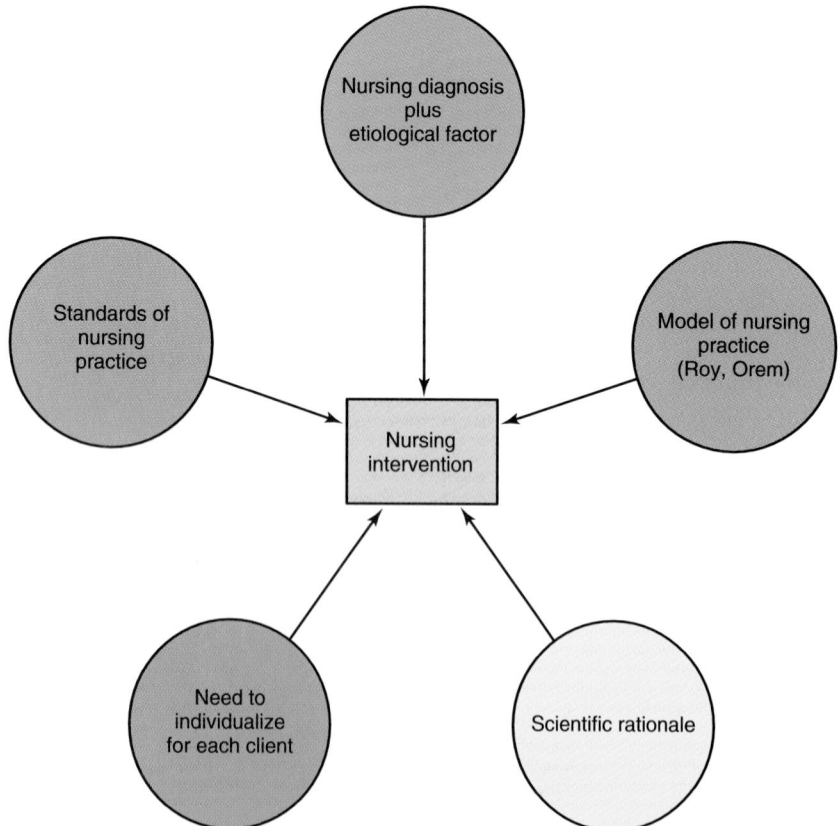

❧ **Figure 10–5**
Identifying appropriate nursing interventions.

to verify the accountability of the nurse. Nursing orders should be initiated on the client's admission to the hospital or health care unit. When the nurse identifies the actions to be accomplished, a notation should be made by the nurse as to the date on which the orders were prescribed.

4. **Nursing orders should be documented in ink.** The client's medical record is a legal document and, as such, should be recorded in ink. Erasures should not be made; errors are usually handled by the nurse striking out the error with one line and signing his or her name.

5. **Nursing orders should include specific actions that are to be implemented and should indicate the individual who is to carry out the action.** Nursing orders should include those that involve ongoing assessments (such as vital signs), milestones for when to evaluate care and make changes, and required teaching that should be provided to the client. Although the nurse is the primary provider of nursing activities, there are times when the client, a family member, or a member of the health care team will be the care provider. Providers (if not the nurse) and their responsibilities should be indicated clearly on the plan.

6. **Nursing orders should be revised and updated as the client's health status changes.** As each change is made, it should be dated and signed by the nurse making the change. For example, if a client's pain is not relieved with a selected nonpharmacological action, then the nurse should indicate on the plan that action is to be discontinued and a new one instituted in its place.

7. **Nursing orders should incorporate the physician's orders and identify all nursing actions related to the implementation of physician orders.** A client's care reflects a combination of dependent, interdependent, and independent nursing actions. For every physician order, there are numerous independent nursing actions. These actions should be clearly listed in the plan of care.

8. **The nursing plan of care should be part of the client's permanent record to document the provision of nursing interventions and the achievement of client outcomes.** The plan of care is a permanent record of the care provided to the client. It demonstrates the accountability of the nurse in providing appropriate and quality care to the client.

9. **All entries on the nursing plan of care should be done using appropriate and acceptable terminology and abbreviations** (see Table 11–2).

Writing the Nursing Care Plan

Documentation of the nursing plan of care in a formal record provides a clear and concise method for ensuring continuity of care. A written plan keeps all members of the health care team informed about the identified client outcomes or goals, the selected nursing interventions, and the client's progress toward achieving those outcomes.

Although the nursing plan of care may take various forms, there are three basic components: nursing diagnoses, client outcomes, and nursing interventions. For each nursing diagnosis, there should be at least one client outcome. A list of nursing interventions should then follow each outcome. Each intervention

should be clear and concise so that all members of the health team will be able to implement them as written.

Formats for Plans of Care

Although there are common aspects of care plans, nurses will find a variety of formats that can be utilized. Typically, care plans have at least a three-column format, one column each for the nursing diagnosis, the client outcome, and the list of nursing interventions. Types of nursing care plans include:

1. **Individually constructed plans of care:** These plans of care are developed from scratch for each client and are time consuming for the nurse to develop. They usually consist of a three-column format, including the nursing diagnosis, expected outcomes, and nursing interventions. The care plan for the case study of Mrs. C is provided in Table 10–2.

2. **Standardized or institutionalized plans:** These plans are usually prepared formats that can be used as guides for implementing nursing interventions for common, recurring nursing diagnoses. These formats provide for making changes that are individualized for the client yet assist the nurse in maintaining acceptable standards of nursing practice. These care plans are available either on paper or on computer and are kept as part of the client's permanent health record. Frequently these care plans are based on the medical diagnosis, such as for clients with myocardial infarction, or on a nursing diagnosis, such as for clients with impaired gas exchange. Standardized care plans provide a structure for determining the care to be provided to the client. The nurse is able to make the interventions flexible by making changes, such as noting specific time frames or making additions to those already included. These plans reflect standards of care that are determined for the health problem and the clinical environment. The standards of care are agency dependent and are not part of the client's medical record but serve as the basis for developing the standardized plan of care.

3. **Critical pathways:** These are plans that incorporate a multidisciplinary approach to client care. Critical pathways, or interdisciplinary care maps, are an outgrowth of managed care and allow for all health care disciplines to provide input into the care of the client. Institutions that use critical pathways have eliminated nursing plans of care, as the pathway becomes the primary documentation of client care. However, critical pathways follow the framework of the nursing process, requiring assessment, problem identification, interventions, and evaluation.

4. **Kardex care plans:** These care plans (Fig. 10–6) are usually smaller, compact versions of the more detailed care plan in the client's record. These plans are part of a kardex file that includes an overview description of the client's health status, the prescribed physician's orders for medications and treatments, and the client's ability to perform self-care and activities of daily living. A component of the kardex is a compact version of the client's nursing care plan. In many institutions, these kardexs are kept as the permanent record. Nurses should be aware of the institution's policy regarding kardex care plans. These are the only care plans that may be written in pencil.

5. **Student care plans:** These care plans are more detailed

Table **10–2**

PLAN OF CARE FOR MRS. C.

NURSING DIAGNOSIS	OUTCOME STATEMENT	INTERVENTIONS
Pain	The client will experience relief or reduced pain to be able to rest comfortably or participate in care	1. Assess the seven characteristics of pain (quality, location, severity, onset, duration, precipitating/ameliorating factors) 2. Teach client pain scale and have her rate pain from 1 to 10 3. Observe for other pain indicators, such as increased pulse and blood pressure, diaphoresis, and facial grimaces 4. Administer prescribed analgesics and monitor for relief in 30 min 5. Implement alternative comfort measures if needed (reposition with pillows and blanket rolls, therapeutic touch, or guided imagery) 6. Assess any unrelieved or sudden pain 7. Notify physician of unrelieved pain
Impaired Physical Mobility	The client will walk the length of the hall and back by day three; the client will maintain full range of motion (ROM) in all unaffected joints; the client will regain optimal mobility before discharge.	1. Position client in proper alignment in bed 2. Assist client to perform ROM in bed with unaffected extremities 3. Provide trapeze for bed and instruct client how to use it 4. Use thromboembolic disease stockings (TEDS) and sequential compression devices (SCDs) if ordered by physician 5. Assist client to follow the physical therapist's instructions regarding transfer, ambulating, use of walker 6. Assist with use of elevated bedside commode and chair
Risk for Deep Vein Thrombosis (DVT)	The client will remain free of DVT in lower extremities, indicated by warm, pink skin and good capillary refill and pulses	1. Monitor client for signs or symptoms of decreased tissue perfusion in left lower extremity (weak or absent pulses, prolonged capillary refill, increased pain or numbness, and coolness) 2. Examine TEDS or SCDs for proper fit and application 3. Assess for DVT by having client dorsiflex foot 4. Inform physician immediately if altered tissue perfusion is suspected
Risk for Infection	The client will be free of infection during recovery, verified by normal body temperature, normal white blood cell count (WBC) and healing incision	1. Wash hands before and after each client contact 2. Monitor vital signs 3. Assess client for signs and symptoms of infection (erythema, edema, pain, or purulent drainage at operative site, intravenous site, and foley catheter) 4. Use aseptic technique for dressing changes and when starting intravenous line 5. Monitor WBC as ordered by physician 6. Note sputum characteristics if client has productive cough 7. Teach client to turn, cough, and deep breathe
Risk for Constipation	The client will maintain her regular bowel elimination during hospitalization (Mrs. C. has a stool every day)	1. Assess bowel function by auscultating and palpating abdomen 2. Ask client when was last bowel movement 3. Provide plenty of oral fluids and encourage and assist client to drink 4. Assist with ROM and ambulation 5. Provide regular time and privacy for patient to have bowel movements 6. Administer stool softener if ordered by physician 7. Keep accurate record of bowel elimination

Table 10-2

PLAN OF CARE FOR MRS. C.
(Continued)

NURSING DIAGNOSIS	OUTCOME STATEMENT	INTERVENTIONS
Self-Care Deficit	The client will be able to perform self-care activities within own capabilities before discharge to home	1. Assess client's ability to perform activities of daily living (ADL), observing strengths and weaknesses 2. Help client to acknowledge level of dependence in activities that require assistance 3. Determine which adaptive equipment is needed to assist client to perform self-care 4. Teach client proper use of adaptive equipment; reinforce the physical therapist's instructions to client on transfer and ambulation 5. Collaborate with client on the best way to perform ADL, such as bathing, dressing, toileting, given new limitations 6. Provide constructive feedback, encouragement, and praise as client works to attain prior independence 7. Communicate with nursing staff and collaborative team to provide continuity of care 8. Initiate necessary referrals for assistive devices, home care, and physical therapy
Knowledge Deficit of therapeutic regimen and discharge	Client will understand plan of care during hospitalization; client will verbalize the correct understanding of the discharge instructions	1. Initiate teaching and discharge planning on hospital admission 2. Teach client, husband, and other support persons principles and rationale for care of client with fractured hip 3. Initiate referral to social worker 4. Provide written discharge instructions before day of discharge 5. Answer client's and family's questions concerning care during hospitalization and discharge
Caregiver Role Strain	The client's husband and family will be able to verbalize an understanding of the discharge instructions; caregiver states that the formal and informal support systems are adequate to provide rest for him	1. Establish relationship with husband, children, and client; encourage open, effective communication 2. Evaluate husband's understanding of client's care and his role 3. Assess husband's health status 4. Encourage husband to discuss feelings and concerns about wife's condition and his increased responsibilities 5. Evaluate family resources and support system 6. Encourage involvement of children 7. Initiate referral to social worker

Data from Gulanick, M., Kloop, A., Galanes, S., *et al.* (1994). *Nursing care plans: Nursing diagnosis and interventions* (3rd ed.). St. Louis: Mosby-Year Book. The plan of care for Mrs. C. was written by Jane Wrenn, BSN.

Please Use Pencil	**CLIENT CARE PLAN**				**TREATMENTS**
Activity	bedrest	Diet	soft ↑ calorie		5/20 O₂ via nasal cannula @ 2 L/min
Bath	bed	Fluids	1000 cc 8 shift		Daily weights
TPR	q 4h	Intake/Output	✓		
BP-P	q 4h	Physical Limitations			
S&A		Allergies	hay fever		
SPECIAL EQUIPMENT AND THERAPY					
Commode at bedside					
Incentive spirometer at bedside					

(front)

EMOTIONAL ASPECTS	**TEACHING GOALS**
Refer to American Lung Association for participation in support group.	Breathing exercises Use of medications Dangers of alcohol and tobacco use
FAMILY PROBLEMS	**POST DISCHARGE PLANNING**
Client lives alone. No relatives or support system in this area.	Refer to: ① O₂ supplier for home ② Visiting Nurse Service ③ meals on wheels
IMMEDIATE GOAL: Maintain client airway today.	LONG RANGE GOAL: Client will self administer meds. by discharge.
CLIENT NEEDS	**APPROACH**
Gas exchange	Elevate head of bed, monitor vital signs, resume activity slowly.
Nutrition - less than body requirements	Assess diet habits, give frequent oral care, provide small frequent feedings
SURGERY AND DATE	
	CONSULTATIONS Pulmonary Medicine
DIAGNOSIS Pneumonia	COMPLICATIONS COPD
ADM. DATE 5/20/98 — AGE 65 — BIRTH DATE 4/20/33 — RELIGION Catholic	CRITICAL — DATE ANOINTED
ROOM # 102 — CLIENT'S NAME Johnson, Jim	IPA — DOCTOR Smith

(back)

❧ **Figure 10–6**
A kardex care plan.

than the care plans that are used by health care institutions. Because students are in a learning situation, practice with all phases of the nursing process is a major component of the course requirements. Student care plans are designed to facilitate this learning experience. Assessment data are summarized in the first section of the plan. The main part of the care plan usually consists of a five-column format: nursing diagnosis, client outcome, nursing interventions list, scientific rationale for each intervention, and evaluation of client outcome. Most of the care plans illustrated in this text emphasize diagnoses, interventions, and rationales to assist the student.

Summary

Planning involves determining priorities among the nursing diagnoses, then identifying the expected outcomes for each nursing diagnosis and writing the nursing orders or interventions that relate directly to resolving the problem. Planning occurs during the initial contact with the client, as part of the ongoing relationship with the client, and prior to discharge, or termination, from a health care environment. Priorities need to be determined so that emergency or critical problems are given immediate attention. Expected outcomes are those behaviors that the client is expected to attain after nursing intervention. Nursing interventions, or orders, are the activities designed to resolve the nursing diagnosis and achieve the outcome identified. A variety of care plans are used and are agency based as to specific type.

CHAPTER HIGHLIGHTS

✦

✦ Planning is the systematic and deliberate determination of a individualized nursing care plan that considers the holistic nature of the client. After determining nursing diagnoses during the analysis phase, the nurse develops a mutually agreeable care plan in conjunction with the client, if feasible.

✦ Planning occurs at various points during the nurse-client relationship. An initial plan is completed on the first contact with the client. Ongoing planning reflects that continued relationship with the client. Discharge planning refers to the type of planning when the client is to be terminated from one health care environment, such as a hospital.

✦ After identifying nursing diagnoses for the client, the nurse determines which diagnoses require more immediate intervention. This process is called prioritization. Problems that involve actual or life-threatening concerns are considered prior to actual or potential health-threatening concerns.

✦ The nursing care plan includes the expected outcomes that are to be achieved by the client. An expected outcome is a statement of the behavior or human response that is expected after provision of nursing care. The outcome statement should provide direction for the prevention, modification, or correction of the behavior that is stated in the nursing diagnosis.

✦ Outcome statements should be focused specifically on the client, be concise and explicit, reflect a mutual agreement between the nurse and the client, be observable and measurable, be realistic, and have a specified time limit or target date.

✦ A well-written expected outcome statement includes the client as the object of the outcome; the task of the response or behavior that is involved; and a criterion that specifies either a condition, a time frame, or criteria for how well the task is to be performed.

✦ Outcome statements are classified according to the domain of the verb in the statement: cognitive domain involves a specific knowledge level; affective domain involves changes in attitudes, beliefs, values, or feelings; psychomotor domain involves responses that require a motor skill; and physiological domain involves changes in some type of bodily function.

✦ Nursing orders are those actions or interventions performed by the nurse, which the nurse is accountable for providing. These actions are aimed at the prevention, maintenance, and restoration of the client's health and are determined mainly by the etiology of the nursing diagnosis.

✦ When writing nursing orders, the nurse should identify all possible interventions based on sound scientific rationale, consider a wide variety of possible nursing interventions, determine which interventions are appropriate and related to the identified outcome and the etiology of the nursing diagnosis, and follow standards of nursing practice as defined by such agencies as the ANA and by the health care institution.

✦ Interventions should be consistent with the medical plan of care, be individualized to the client and the situation, provide a safe and therapeutic environment, include any teaching-learning methodologies, and include the utilization of appropriate financial and equipment resources.

✦ Nursing interventions include activities that reflect the independent practice of nurses as identified in the nursing care plan, as well as those activities that are dependent on the physician's prescriptions for medications and treatments.

✦ The nursing care plan should be documented in

the formal record of the client to ensure continuity of care and to verify the accountability of the nursing staff. Although the care plan format may vary greatly, it should include a list of nursing interventions for each identified expected outcome.

Study Questions

1. When setting priorities of care, first priority is given to problems that

   a. require extensive use of time and resources
   b. are identified by the client
   c. involve a life-threatening event
   d. are mandated by the standard of care

2. Which of the following outcomes would be described as being in the cognitive domain?

   a. client will express a desire to enroll in a weight-reduction program
   b. client will have a blood sugar level within a range of 120 to 130 mg/dl
   c. client will demonstrate an ability to perform self-monitoring of blood glucose
   d. client will identify the signs and symptoms of hypoglycemia

3. Which of the following would be considered a dependent nursing intervention?

   a. administer acetaminophen 650 mg, every 4 hours for temperature above 101°F (38.3°C)
   b. ausculate lung sounds every 2 hours
   c. provide instructions on prescribed low-sodium diet
   d. reposition client every 2 hours while in bed

4. Which of the following is a plan of care that is developed through a multidisciplinary approach?

   a. kardex care plan
   b. critical pathway plan
   c. standardized care plan
   d. computerized care plan

Critical Thinking Exercises

1. Develop a long-term and a short-term goal for the following client: Mr. Gastrop has had a gastric bypass and is experiencing postoperative nausea and vomiting 1 month after surgery.

2. Develop interventions for the following diagnosis and outcome: Diagnosis: Altered Tissue Perfusion (Cardiopulmonary) related to coronary artery disease, as evidenced by chest pain at rest. Short-term goal: client will not experience chest pain in the morning while performing activities of daily living. Long-term goal: client will have adequate perfusion at discharge, as evidenced by absence of chest pain while walking hallways.

References

Alfaro, R. (1990). *Applying nursing diagnosis and nursing process* (2nd ed.). Philadelphia: J. B. Lippincott.

American Nurses Association. (1991). *Standards of clinical nursing practice*. Washington, DC: American Nurses Association.

Atkinson, L. D., & Murray, M. E. (1995). *Clinical guide to care planning: Data to diagnosis*. New York: McGraw-Hill.

Bloom, B. (1956). *Taxonomy of educational objectives: The classification of educational goals. Handbook I: Cognitive domain*. New York: David McKay.

Christensen, P. J. (1995). Planning: Priorities and outcome identification. In Christensen, P. J., & Kenney, J. W. (Eds.), *Nursing process: Application of conceptual models* (4th ed.). St. Louis: Mosby-Year Book.

Christensen, P. J., & Kenney, J. W. (1995). *Nursing process: Application of conceptual models* (4th ed.). St. Louis: C. V. Mosby.

Fayram, E. S., & Christensen, P. J. (1995). Planning: Strategies and nursing orders. In Christensen, P. J., & Kenney, J. W. (Eds.), *Nursing process: Application of conceptual models* (4th ed.). St. Louis: Mosby-Year Book.

Iyer, P. W., Taptich, B. J., & Bernocchi-Losey, D. (1995). *Nursing process and nursing diagnosis* (3rd ed.). Philadelphia: W. B. Saunders.

Kozier, B., Erb, G., & Bufalino, P. M. (1989). *Introduction to nursing*. Menlo Park, CA: Addison-Wesley.

Krathwohl, D., Bloom, B., & Masia, B. (1964). *Taxonomy of educational objectives: The classification of educational goals. Handbook II: Affective domain*. New York: David McKay.

Maslow, A. (1968). Toward a psychology of being (2nd ed.). New York: Van Nostrand-Reinhold.

Murray, M. E., & Atkinson, L. D. (1994). *Understanding the nursing process* (2nd ed.). Philadelphia: W. B. Saunders.

Niziolek, C., & Shaw, S. M. (1991). Professional practice: Whose plan—whose care? *Journal of Professional Nursing, 3* (May–June), 145.

Orem, D. E. (1995). *Nursing: Concepts of practice* (5th ed.). St. Louis: C. V. Mosby.

Roy, S. C. (1984). *Introduction to nursing: An adaptation model*. Englewood Cliffs, NJ: Prentice-Hall.

Simpson, E. J. (1966). *The classification of educational objectives: Psychomotor domain*. Urbana, IL: University of Illinois Press.

Taylor, C., Lillis, C., & LeMone, P. (1989). *Fundamentals of nursing*. Philadelphia: J. B. Lippincott.

Urbach, F. (Ed.). (1970). *The psychomotor domain of learning*. Paper presented at Teaching Research, Salishan, Oregon. The Department of Higher Education, Monmouth, Oregon.

US Department of Health and Human Services. (1992). *Preventing pressure ulcers: A patient's guide*. Rockville, MD: Public Health Service.

Bibliography

Ball, M. J., Hannah, K. J., Newbold, S. K., & Douglas, J. V. (Eds.). (1995). *Nursing informatics: Where caring and technology meet* (2nd ed.). New York: Springer-Verlag.

Carlson, J. H., Craft, C. A., McGuire, A. D., & Popkess-Vawter, S. (1991). *Nursing diagnosis: A case study approach*. Philadelphia: W. B. Saunders.

Carpenito, L. J. (1995). *Nursing diagnosis: Application to clinical practice*. Philadelphia: J. B. Lippincott.

Daly, J. M., Maas, M., McCloskey, J. C., & Bulecheck, G. M. (1996). A care planning tool that proves what we can do. *RN, 59*, 26–29.

Eggland, E. T., & Heinemann, D. S. (1994). *Nursing documentation: Charting, recording, and reporting.* Philadelphia: J. B. Lippincott.

Ferri, R. S. (Ed.). (1994). *Care planning for the older adult: Nursing diagnosis in long term care.* Philadelphia: W. B. Saunders.

Greenwood, D. (1996). Nursing care plans: Issues and solutions. *Nursing Management, 27,* 33, 37–40.

Jones, R. A. P., & Beck, S. E. (1996). *Decision making in nursing.* Albany, NY: Delmar Publishers.

Marrelli, T. M., & Hilliard, L. S. (1996). *Home care and clinical paths: Effective care planning across the continuum.* St. Louis: C. V. Mosby.

Newell, M. (1996). *Using nursing case management to improve health outcomes.* Gaithersburg, MD: Aspen Publishers.

Taptich, B. J., Iyer, P. W., & Bernocchi-Losey, B. J. (1994). *Nursing diagnosis and care planning* (2nd ed.). Philadelphia: W. B. Saunders.

Windle, P. E. (1994). Critical pathways: an integrated documentation tool. *Nursing Management, 25,* 80F.

Chapter 11

IMPLEMENTATION

PATRICIA E. KIZILAY, EdD, RN, CS, FNP

TERRY K. GOLDEN, BSN

KEY TERMS

✦

change of shift report

confidentiality

dependent nursing action

implementation

independent nursing action

interdependent nursing action

narrative notes

nursing action

nursing care conference

nursing care rounds

problem-oriented record

protocol

source-oriented record

LEARNING OBJECTIVES

✦

After studying this chapter, you should be able to

✦ Understand the meaning of the key terms in this chapter

✦ Describe dependent, independent, and interdependent nursing interventions

✦ Describe the skills needed to provide competent nursing care

✦ Discuss the use of labels for nursing interventions

✦ Identify the factors to be considered when selecting a nursing intervention

✦ Identify the variables influencing implementation

✦ Identify the steps in the preparation phase of implementation

✦ Identify the difference between protocols and guidelines

✦ Identify the purposes and legalities of charting

✦ Identify the abbreviations commonly used on charts

✦ Identify the similarities and differences of different documentation systems: computer records, problem-oriented records, and source-oriented records

✦ State the importance of accurate documentation of nursing actions

✦ State the importance of data collection in the implementation phase of the nursing process

✦ Describe the change of shift report

✦ State the importance of confidentiality

The implementation phase of the nursing process involves actually providing the client with planned care through interventions or orders that are identified in the planning phase. In addition to being classified as implementation, these strategies may be identified as nursing actions, activities, interventions, orders, treatments, or therapeutics. Implementation focuses on providing safe, individualized care using nursing actions necessary to meet the goals, and expected outcomes are identified in the nursing care plan. The purpose of the implementation phase of the nursing process is to assist clients in achieving the identified expected outcomes related to restoring health, preventing disease or illness, promoting wellness, or facilitating coping in an altered health state (Fig. 11–1).

Just as the use of nursing diagnoses has created an awareness of the value of a standardized language in the nursing process, some nurses agree that there is a need for similar language for interventions and outcomes. Outcomes and goals focus on client behaviors, whereas nursing interventions focus on nurse behaviors. For example, outcomes and goals for the client may be to select an exercise program based on interest and time constraints. Interventions from the nurse would be to provide a variety of exercise programs that are low in cost due to financial limitations of the client.

Since 1987, a group of nurses at the University of Iowa has been working on a taxonomy of nursing interventions that will include the direct treatments that nurses perform for clients. In 1989, the American Nurses' Association (ANA) issued the following statement: "Nursing must be able to name itself and to describe what it does in order to function effectively in a world where computerized information is used to establish everything. . . . Until nurses can name what they do and assign a computer code to that name, we may be neither reimbursed nor recognized as a profession with unique skills and knowledge."

Implementation is carried out by the client and the nurse and may involve other health professionals or caregivers in a variety of health care settings. The health status of the client determines the degree of participation of the client, the nurse, and the other participants. Implementation fosters client advocacy and coordination among health care team members. Bulechek and McCloskey (1992a) define a nursing intervention, or **nursing action,** as "any direct care treatment that a nurse performs on behalf of a client which includes nurse-initiated treatments, physician-initiated treatments, and performance of daily essential functions" (p. xii).

Data collection continues and plans are modified during this phase. All activities are documented according to the documentation system in place at the agency where implementation takes place.

Types of Nursing Actions

Three categories of nursing actions are used in implementing a plan: independent, dependent, and collaborative (interdependent).

Independent Nursing Actions

An **independent nursing action** is one that is initiated by the nurse based on nursing knowledge and skills (Fig. 11–2). These actions are the result of the assessment of client needs and may be initiated without the direction or supervision of another health care professional. The actions are determined by nursing diagnoses, and nurses are held legally accountable. Mundinger (1980), for example, describes positioning clients: "knowing why, when and how to position clients and doing it skillfully makes the function an autonomous therapy" (p. 4). Every time a nurse teaches a client about a diagnosis, how to take a medication, or special measures to take in preparation for and after a procedure, the nurse is functioning as an independent practitioner. The whole realm of activities involved in the nurse's role as client advocate is considered entirely independent practice.

Dependent Nursing Actions

Dependent nursing actions are those carried out according to specific routines, under the supervision of a physician, or as the result of an order by a physician. The activity is usually related to the client's

✦ **Figure 11–1**
Implementation is the fourth step of the nursing process and is influenced by many factors, such as client and nurse characteristics and the particular diagnosis.

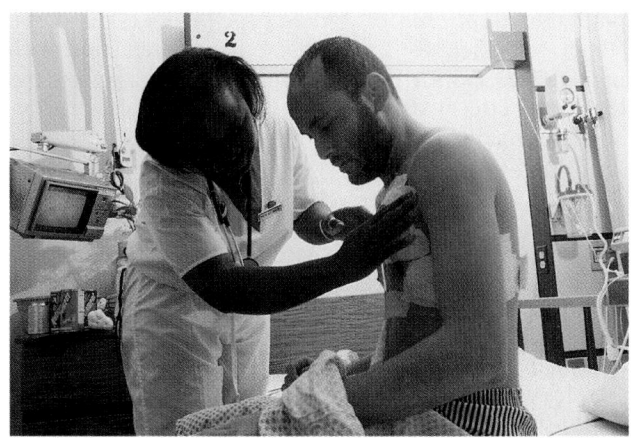

♪ Figure 11–2
Nurse checking dressing and chest tube.

disease. For example, a medication may be prescribed. In addition to giving the medication to the client, the nurse's other dependent actions would be to monitor the client for side effects and to take any precautions necessary when administering the drug, such as monitoring blood pressure or administering the drug before or after meals. Dependent nursing interventions generally are related to medications, treatment modalities outside the scope of nursing, and surgery.

Collaborative, or Interdependent, Nursing Actions

Collaborative, or **interdependent, nursing actions** are performed either as the result of a joint decision by a nurse and another health team member or as a joint action with another team member. Working with a physical therapist to provide physical exercises to a client who is bedridden provides a clear example of interdependent nursing practice. Planning a teaching session about a diabetic diet with the dietitian further demonstrates this type of nursing role.

Some health care facilities are placing more emphasis on an interdisciplinary approach to patient care. In some institutions, the team makes rounds together and discusses patient needs. The team often includes a physician, nurse, dietitian, clinical pharmacologist, and dentist, plus other specialists that may be indicated, such as a speech therapist, physical therapist, occupational therapist, respiratory therapist, social worker, or psychologist. The ANA describes collaboration as "true partnership, in which the power of both sides is valued by both, with recognition and acceptance of combined spheres of activity and responsibility, mutual safeguarding of legitimate interests of each party, and a commonality of goals recognized by both parties" (1980, p. 7).

The type of nursing actions that a nurse implements falls on a continuum between dependent and independent nursing interventions. In more technical,

acute-care–focused situations, the nurse is involved in a higher percentage of dependent activities. This is evident in intensive care of emergency units, where nurses function in high-technology environments, interacting with clients requiring immediate physiological treatments and interventions. A staff nurse may be in the middle of the spectrum, spending 50% of the day in an independent role and portions performing dependent or collaborative interventions. A nurse practitioner, in contrast, may spend 100% of the day in an independent role.

♦ Selecting a Nursing Intervention

Many factors need to be considered when selecting a nursing intervention. Bulechek and McCloskey (1992a, p. 8) have identified the following:

* The desired client outcome
* The characteristics of the nursing diagnosis
* The research base associated with the intervention
* The feasibility of implementing the intervention successfully
* The acceptability to the client
* The capability of the nurse

The terms used in Table 11–1 can assist nurses in writing nursing actions using common terminology. When these factors are addressed, the steps in implementation can be considered.

♦ Factors Influencing Implementation

Factors that may influence implementation can be related to the client, the nurse's level of expertise, utilization of research findings, or circumstances at the location where the care is implemented (Fig. 11–3).

Client

Implementation may need to be modified based on the client's previous responses to the intervention; developmental stage; and social, psychological, or cultural background. The client may be unwilling to participate in the care being given, or the client's ability to participate may change.

Nurse

The nurse's level of expertise, creativity, willingness to provide care, and available time may affect nursing actions. Nursing actions must be consistent

Table 11–1

ACTION WORDS USED IN NURSING INTERVENTION LABELS

TERM	MEANING
Administer	Direct the movement or behavior of, having charge of (also see Manage)
Assist	Help
Care	Pay close attention; give protection; be concerned about
Counsel	Give advice
Enhance	Make greater; augment; increase (also see Promote)
Facilitate	Make easier; assist; help
Maintain	Continue or carry on; support
Manage	Direct the movement or behavior of; have charge of (also see Administer)
Modify	Change slightly or partially
Monitor	Watch and check
Promote	Advance (also see Enhance)
Protect	Shield from injury (also see Take precaution)
Provide therapy	Have a therapeutic nature; heal
Reduce	Lessen; diminish
Restore	Reinstate; bring back to normal or unimpaired state
Support	Sustaining; strengthening
Take precaution	Take care beforehand against a possible danger (also see Protect)
Teach	Instruct; educate
Train	Instruct in a particular skill

Adapted from Bulecheck, G. M., & McCloskey, J. C. (1992). *Nursing interventions: Essential nursing treatments* (2nd ed.). Philadelphia: W. B. Saunders.

with the *Standards of Practice* (ANA, 1973) and the statutory guidelines, or the nurse may be charged with negligence. Nurses are responsible for knowing the legal and ethical dimensions of practice and are morally and legally accountable for their practice.

Research

The quality of nursing care is enhanced by including research findings into professional practice. Recent findings can be attained by attending conferences and continuing education workshops and by reading professional journals.

Nursing Unit

If the nursing unit is constantly understaffed or does not have adequate supplies, then nursing interventions will be affected.

Protocols and Standing Orders

Protocols and standing orders are primarily institution based and therefore vary from agency to agency.

Protocols

A **protocol** is a written plan indicating the nursing actions to be accomplished in specific situations. Examples of situations in which protocols would occur are

* Admissions: Steps to follow when a client is admitted, such as having forms signed, having laboratory work completed, and transferring the client to the hospital unit
* Discharges: Informing clients of follow-up appointments, giving enough doses of medication until they can get to a pharmacy, and providing instructions about care when the client arrives at home after hospitalization
* Referrals: In clinics, there may be protocols for determining when a nurse can manage the client's care and when a client should be referred to a physician

Standing Orders

A standing order is a written statement about rules, regulations, policies, or orders regarding client care. It empowers the nurse to initiate actions under certain circumstances that usually require an order or supervision of a physician. The standing order is carried out by the nurse for a particular type of client unless it is canceled by the physician. Some of these situations may be:

* Medication administration: In emergency situations, as on a coronary care unit, if certain electrocardiogram changes occur in a client, there may be a standing order to administer an antiarrhythmia medication
* Routine admission orders: Laboratory tests such as a complete blood count, hemoglobin, hematocrit, and urinalysis may be ordered for every client
* Notification of family if client's condition changes: Some physicians give a standing order that when the client's condition deteriorates, family members are to be notified

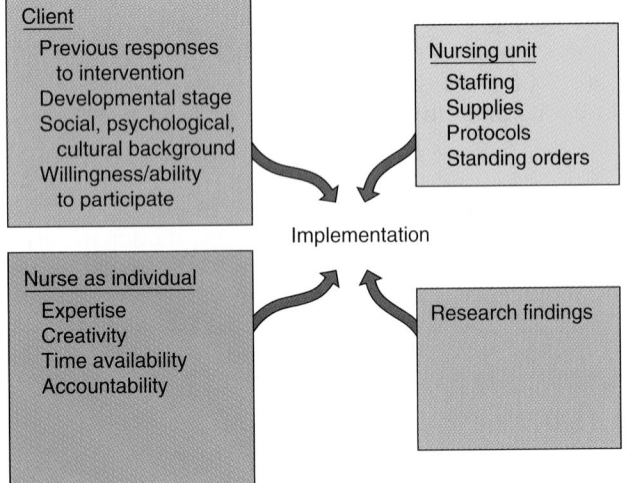

❧ **Figure 11–3**
Factors that may influence the implementation of nursing interventions.

Steps in Implementation

Three steps of implementation were identified by Fayram (1995): preparation, the actual implementation, and postimplementation.

Preparation

During this step, the nurse prepares for the actual implementation of the plan. This step consists of knowledge of the plan, validation of the plan, the knowledge and skills required by the nurse to implement the plan, preparation of the client, and preparation of the environment:

- Knowledge of the plan: The nurse must be acquainted with the plan that has been developed to interact with the client. The nurse should become familiar with the plan by reading the chart and listening to verbal reports from other nurses and members of the health team.

- Validation of the plan: The client, the nurse, and other health team members participate in validating the plan. The nurse uses previous experience and knowledge, together with client records to determine if the plan is current. Fayram (1995, p. 188) recommends asking the following questions:
    1. Is the plan relevant based on the client's status and concerns at this point in time?
    2. Have priorities changed or remained the same?
    3. Is the plan safe and based on sound rationale, including legal and ethical aspects?
    4. Is the plan individualized?
  Based on the findings, the plan may need to be modified. If a client is in pain, then the nurse might defer implementing a teaching plan and deal with the client's comfort. A plan to alleviate postoperative discomfort may not be necessary or relevant a few days after surgery. When a client chooses not to participate in nursing care, the nurse must be flexible in preparing to implement the plan.

- Knowledge and skills required of the nurse to implement the plan: The nurse's ability to carry out the plan must be assessed. The following questions can help the nurse to determine if he or she possesses the necessary knowledge and skills to carry out the plan.
    1. Do I have the knowledge needed?
    2. Do I have the skills needed?
    3. Is there support available while I carry out the plan?
    4. Are there resources nearby for me to use?
  If the answer to these questions is "no," the nurse should not attempt to implement the plan. The appropriate action for the nurse to take would be to:
    a. Get assistance from another nurse
    b. Research the necessary knowledge or skills
    c. Observe another nurse carrying out the procedure

- Preparation of the client: The client should be informed of the plan to be implemented *before* any nursing actions take place. Aspects of the plan related to nursing actions, expected client responses, client responsibilities, and expected outcomes should be discussed before beginning to implement the plan. Other aspects of preparing the client are providing privacy, protecting the client physically when necessary, and protecting the client's sense of modesty.

- Preparation of the environment: The environment needs to be prepared prior to implementing the plan to ensure prompt and efficient implementation. Preparing the environment involves
    1. Gathering the necessary resources; *e.g.,* equipment, audiovisual materials, personnel
    2. Providing adequate lighting
    3. Minimizing distractions and interruptions
    4. Turning down volume of radios or televisions
    5. Providing a quiet room to meet with the client and/or family members
    6. Considering seating arrangements that are conducive to your goals

Actual Implementation

During the actual **implementation,** the nurse carries out the care plan for the client. Nursing care is client focused and outcome oriented to meet the physical and psychosocial needs of the client.

Client-Focused Implementation

Client-focused implementation means individualizing care based on the biological, psychosocial, and spiritual aspects of the individual client. Some ways to individualize implementation are to

- Explain the procedure based on the client's cognitive level
- Use communication that is appropriate for the age of the client
- Act as a client advocate
- Encourage the client to participate actively in the plan
- Protect the rights of the client
- Collaborate with other health professionals
- Include the client and caregivers in planning

When the client is involved in the implementation, the nurse's role shifts to that of facilitator. The nurse ensures that safe, outcome-oriented care is provided by preparing the client thoroughly and by being available to assist and support the client while the plan is being implemented.

Outcome-Oriented Implementation

Outcome-oriented actions are compatible with the goals and objectives of the plan. It is possible to meet several goals and objectives at once, using time reasonably while meeting the needs of the client. For example, during a bath or dressing change, it may be possible to implement part of a teaching plan.

There are several nursing actions used by the nurse when carrying out the care plan. The nurse should be able to identify at least one specific nursing action for each nursing diagnosis. Each action requires theoretical knowledge and clinical skills. Actions that are part of nursing responsibilities include:

- Assisting the client with activities of daily living
- Counseling the client about his or her illness and treatment plan
- Teaching the client about self-care measures (Fig. 11–4)

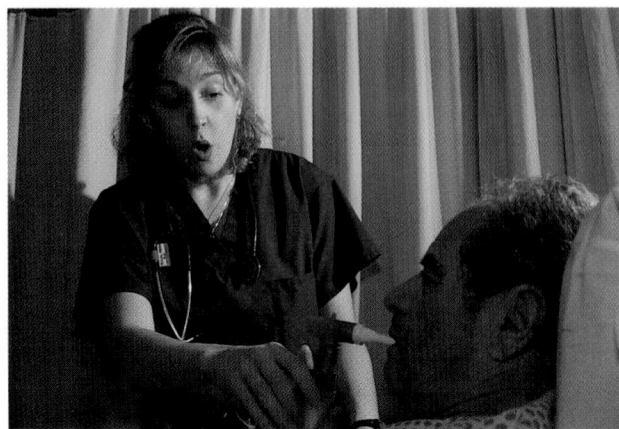

✦ **Figure 11–4**
Teaching use of incentive spirometer.

* Providing care to achieve therapeutic goals for the client by
    1. Reducing or counteracting adverse reactions to treatment, medications, or diagnostic tests
    2. Preventing illness
    3. Promoting health
    4. Preparing for procedures and using correct techniques in performing the procedures
    5. Initiating life-saving measures
* Providing an environment that facilitates meeting the client's health care goals
* Supervising and evaluating other staff members

Physical and psychological safety must be provided for the client. Physical safety can be provided by using appropriate techniques, getting assistance when needed, and maintaining safe surroundings. Psychological safety is provided through the use of interpersonal skills (see next section).

Skills Needed

Efficient implementation of care, using the appropriate intellectual, interpersonal, and technical skills, enhances the provision of competent care to the client. When competent care is provided, the client's trust and confidence in the nurse increase, and the nurse-client relationship is enhanced.

✦ **Intellectual Skills.** The intellectual skills that are essential to provide safe, intelligent nursing care are

* Creativity, which involves solving problems by establishing new relationships, planning nursing strategies, and changing nursing actions to provide improved and more efficient nursing care
* Critical thinking, which includes problem solving, selecting and organizing relevant information, and making judgments that enable nurses to make unbiased decisions quickly
* Decision making

✦ **Interpersonal Skills.** Interpersonal skills are any activities that people use when communicating with

each other. They may be verbal or nonverbal and include

* Accepting the client's values and lifestyle
* Conveying knowledge, attitudes, feelings, and interest
* Active listening, which requires responses on the part of the listener
* Counseling the client or caregiver
* Making a referral
* Providing support

✦ **Technical Skills.** Technical skills include the ability to do simple and complex nursing procedures. They are frequently referred to as the "hands on" activities of the intervention phase and include activities such as assessing vital signs, bandaging, administering injections, moving and positioning clients, and suctioning a tracheostomy.

Ongoing Data Collection

During the implementation step, ongoing data collection is important to determine the client's physical, psychosocial, and spiritual responses to nursing actions. *Nurses need to be cognizant of dramatic or subtle changes in a client's condition or in his or her responses to nursing measures.* This is done by

* Interacting with the client
* Measuring outcomes
* Observing responses

Findings are used to update and revise the care plan and indicate whether to proceed with the intervention or to make adjustments.

Postimplementation

After the implementation is completed, there are two parts to the postimplementation step. The first involves *closure with the client* and includes

* Summarizing nursing actions
* Clarifying information
* Answering questions
* Identifying the client's response

The second part of this phase is *leaving the client safe and comfortable.* Examples of nursing actions that might be appropriate are

* Raising side rails
* Placing the call button within reach
* Removing and disposing of equipment
* Documenting actions and the client's response
* Verbally communicating with other staff members

The nursing interventions for the case study of Mrs. C. are provided in Table 11–2.

Table **11–2**

NURSING INTERVENTIONS FOR MRS. C.

NURSING INTERVENTIONS	RATIONALE/NURSING CONSIDERATIONS
Nursing Diagnosis: Pain	
1. Assess the seven characteristics of pain (quality, location, severity, onset, duration, precipitating/ameliorating factors)	**1.** It is important to assess each complaint thoroughly to provide the proper intervention
2. Teach the client the pain scale and have her rate pain from 1 to 10	**2.** Pain is subjective; the pain scale allows the pain to be quantified and validated
3. Observe for other pain indicators, such as increased pulse and blood pressure, diaphoresis, and facial grimaces	**3.** These signs and symptoms may confirm that the client is experiencing pain; some clients will not admit to hurting for many different reasons; therefore, these indicators can be an objective approach to diagnosing pain
4. Administer prescribed analgesics and monitor for relief or possible adverse side effects within 30 min of administration	**4.** Drugs are absorbed and metabolized differently for each individual; the nurse must monitor for the desired/adverse effect of the analgesic (if medication does not relieve pain, it may be necessary to notify the physician for a higher dose or different medication)
5. Implement alternative comfort measures if needed (*e.g.,* reposition with pillows and blanket rolls, therapeutic touch, or guided imagery)	**5.** Pain may be relieved through measures that decrease pressure on bony prominences, reduce tension, and provide distraction
6. Assess any unrelieved or sudden pain	**6.** Sudden or unrelieved pain may be indicative of a hip dislocation
7. Notify physician of unrelieved pain	**7.** The physician may need to change pain medication or order x-rays
Nursing Diagnosis: Physical Mobility, Impaired	
1. Position client in proper alignment in bed	**1.** Proper alignment helps the client to rest more comfortably and helps prevent injury to the operative hip
2. Assist client to perform ROM in bed with unaffected extremities	**2.** This helps to avoid the complications of bedrest—decreased muscle tone and venous pooling
3. Provide trapeze for bed and instruct client how to use it	**3.** A trapeze allows the client to position herself, allowing for increased comfort, exercise of upper body, and increased independence
4. Use elastic stockings (TED) and SCDs if ordered by physician	**4.** TED and SCD promote venous blood return to the heart, thereby decreasing risk of DVT or embolus
5. Assist client to follow the physical therapist's instructions regarding transfer, ambulating, use of walker	**5.** This will reinforce the instructions from the physical therapist, provide continuity of care, and be less confusing for the client and family (this requires a collaborative effort between nursing and physical therapy to ensure that the client is being taught the same techniques)
6. Use elevated bedside commode and chair	**6.** Elevated devices prevent hip flexion greater than 90 degrees, which may cause dislocation and injury to repaired fracture
Nursing Diagnosis: Potential for Constipation	
1. Assess bowel function by auscultating and palpating abdomen	**1.** Hypoactive bowel sounds indicate decreased peristalsis of small intestine; constipation usually occurs in colon and cannot be detected through auscultation
2. Ask client when was last bowel movement	**2.** Bowel movements are not necessary every day
3. Provide plenty of oral fluids and encourage and assist client to drink	**3.** Fluid helps make stool softer and defecation easier
4. Assist with ROM and ambulation	**4.** Immobility fosters constipation
5. Provide regular time and privacy for patient to have bowel movements	**5.** The negative psychological aspect of having a bowel movement is diminished if privacy is maintained

Table continued on following page

Table **11–2**

NURSING INTERVENTIONS FOR MRS. C.
(Continued)

NURSING INTERVENTIONS	RATIONALE/NURSING CONSIDERATIONS
Nursing Diagnosis: Potential for Constipation	
6. Administer stool softener if ordered by physician	**6.** A stool softener makes defecation easier by decreasing the amount of straining to pass stool
7. Keep accurate record of bowel elimination	**7.** Recording the client's bowel movements on a graphic sheet communicates whether further nursing interventions need to be implemented
Nursing Diagnosis: Self Care Deficit	
1. Assess client's ability to perform ADL	**1.** Strengths and weaknesses can be observed to evaluate the client's needs
2. Help client to acknowledge level of dependence in activities that require assistance	**2.** Client may need time to accept the new physical limitation due to trauma and surgery
3. Determine which adaptive equipment is needed to assist client to perform self-care	**3.** This makes it easier and safer for the client to perform ADL
4. Teach client proper use of adaptive equipment; reinforce the physical therapist's instructions to client on transfer and ambulation	**4.** Collaboration and communication among staff members makes it less frustrating for the client
5. Collaborate with client on the best way to perform ADL, such as bathing, dressing, toileting, given new limitations	**5.** Working with the client to divide ADL into steps reduces frustration, fosters learning, and provides greater independence
6. Provide constructive feedback, encouragement, and praise as client works to attain prior level of independence	**6.** This type of communication is more productive and increases client self-confidence
7. Initiate necessary referrals for assistive devices, home care, and physical therapy	**7.** Initiate referrals early in hospitalization to ensure that the necessary arrangements are in order for discharge
Nursing Diagnosis: High Risk for Deep Vein Thrombosis	
1. Monitor client for signs or symptoms of decreased tissue perfusion in left lower extremity (*e.g.,* weak or absent pulses, prolonged capillary refill, increased pain or numbness, and coolness)	**1.** Two serious complications of DVT are pulmonary embolism and phlebitis; they can be caused by immobility or bedrest, which puts a client with a hip fracture at high risk
2. Examine TEDS or SCDs for proper fit and application	**2.** TEDS that are too small or applied incorrectly may restrict blood return and cause clot formation; remove b.i.d. and check skin condition
3. Assess for pain by having client dorsiflex foot	**3.** Calf pain, a sign of DVT, may be elicited by dorsiflexion of the foot (positive Homan's sign)
4. Inform physician immediately if altered tissue perfusion is suspected	**4.** Tissue necrosis occurs quickly in tissue without an adequate blood supply; pulmonary embolus can be life threatening
Nursing Diagnosis: Risk for Infection	
1. Wash hands before and after each client contact	**1.** This is the single most important method to prevent the spread of infection
2. Monitor vital signs	**2.** Increased temperature and pulse can be clinical manifestations of underlying infection
3. Assess client for signs and symptoms of infection (*e.g.,* erythema, edema, pain, or purulent drainage at operative site, intravenous site, and foley catheter)	**3.** Report any signs or symptoms to the physician so that antibiotic therapy may be initiated
4. Use aseptic technique for dressing changes and when starting an intravenous line	**4.** Aseptic technique reduces the risk of transferring pathogens to areas of entry
5. Monitor white blood cells as ordered by physician	**5.** Elevated white blood cells are the body's defense against harmful organisms

Table **11–2**

NURSING INTERVENTIONS FOR MRS. C.
(Continued)

NURSING INTERVENTIONS	RATIONALE/NURSING CONSIDERATIONS
Nursing Diagnosis: Risk for Infection	
6. Note sputum characteristics if client has productive cough 7. Teach client to turn, cough, and deep breathe	6. Yellow or green sputum suggests a respiratory infection, a complication of bedrest and age 7. This simple exercise is effective in preventing a respiratory infection
Nursing Diagnosis: Knowledge Deficit of Therapeutic Regimen and Discharge	
1. Initiate teaching and discharge planning on hospital admission 2. Teach client, husband, and other support persons principles and rationale for care of client with fractured hip 3. Initiate referral to social worker 4. Provide written discharge instructions before day of discharge	1. Assess client's readiness and ability to learn to determine the best teaching method 2. These persons provide majority of care after discharge and will benefit learning how best to assist client 3. The social worker can organize the needed resources for home care (*e.g.,* physical therapy, home health, Meals on Wheels) 4. This provides time for learning, reinforcement, evaluation, and questions from client and family
Nursing Diagnosis: Caregiver Role Strain	
1. Establish relationship with husband, children, and client; encourage open, effective communication 2. Evaluate husband's understanding of client's care and his role 3. Assess husband's health status 4. Encourage husband to discuss feelings and concerns about wife's condition and his increased responsibilities 5. Encourage involvement of children	1. Open, effective communication will allow this family to explore concerns about client's situation 2. The husband's appraisal of the situation will be more accurate with an increased understanding of the client's care after discharge 3. Is the client's husband physically and mentally able to assist client when discharged to home? 4. Allowing the husband to verbalize will help him to see the situation more clearly and explore options to help relieve burden 5. Encouraging the children to devise a schedule will assist their parents in initial home care

ADL = activities of daily living; b.i.d. = twice a day; DVT = deep vein thrombosis; ROM = range of motion; SCD = sequential compressive device; TEDS = thromboembolic disease stockings.
Data from Gulanick, M., Kloop, A., Galanes, S., *et al.* (1994). *Nursing care plans: Nursing diagnosis and interventions* (3rd ed.). St. Louis: Mosby–Year Book. The case study nursing interventions for Mrs. C. were written by Jane Wrenn, BSN.

◆ Communicating Nursing Care

Effective communication is essential for coordination and continuity of care. It enables health care professionals to complement and supplement each other's services and avoid omissions and duplications. The primary means of communication are

- Recording
- Reporting
- Conferring

Recording is the written legal documentation of pertinent information regarding assessment, diagnosis, planning, implementation, and evaluation of the nursing process; it is often called "charting" by health care providers. *Reporting* is oral (sometimes on audiotape), written, or computer-based communication to inform other health care professionals. For example, the laboratory data communicates pathology or results of blood work, or the nurse may communicate the client's responses to activities during the shift. *Discussing,* or *conferring,* is a face-to-face way to share information, clarify a problem, or develop a strategy for problem resolution.

Recording

The Client Record or Chart

The client's record is a legal document that provides a comprehensive picture of the client's ongoing health status and the care given by members of the health care team. The record, written in ink, is composed of several different forms containing pertinent information that has been entered by various health care professionals. The forms are usually placed in a binder in an area that is easily accessible to all health care providers.

The client record serves several purposes:

- Audit: Charts may be reviewed to determine the quality of care provided and the competence of the providers
- Care planning: The client's baseline data of responses to the treatment plan are current and available so that the care plan can be modified
- Communication: Health care professionals who interact with the client at different times are able to communicate with each other
- Education: Nurses can learn about clinical manifestations of a particular problem, the most effective treatment plans, and factors that affect meeting the treatment goals
- Historic document: Records may be valuable in providing pertinent data on client responses in the future based on the data available on a current chart
- Legal document: Client records are legal documents that may be used as evidence in court proceedings, implicating or absolving health practitioners charged with improper care, or for injury or accident claims made by clients; the best defense against litigation is accurate reporting of facts
- Research: The record may be used to learn about the most effective ways to recognize and treat clients with similar health problems

✦ **Confidentiality.** Nurses are responsible for maintaining **confidentiality** of information about their clients. Clients give information to nurses based on trust and the understanding that the information will not be disclosed to other clients or visitors. Disclosing information about a client without the client's consent is grounds for a lawsuit. Staff members who are directly involved with the client are the only persons who have legitimate access to the client's record. Under special conditions, other health professionals may have access to the records for a specified purpose, such as data gathering, research, or continuing education. This is acceptable as long as the records are used for the purpose specified.

The nurse is responsible for knowing the location of the records at all times and that they are properly stored when the client leaves the health care agency. Nurses are responsible for protecting the records from unauthorized readers, such as other clients or visitors.

✦ **Nursing Entries on Charts.** Nurses make various types of entries on client records, depending on the type of problem and the client care situation (Fig. 11–5). Nursing documentation includes

- Brief, comprehensive nursing assessment: Obtained from the nursing history, physical examination, and other related information.
- Individualized, current care plan: Developed from the nursing diagnosis and problem list; revisions to care plan can be computer generated, handwritten, or a combination of both.
- Narrative notes: Documentation on the **narrative notes** includes nursing notes, integrated progress notes, flow sheets, preprinted checklists, and dictated reports; they can be computer assisted or computer generated. Examples of computer-assisted records are certain types of medication sheets and vital signs records.
- Flow sheets: Often referred to as "shorthand" progress notes or "abbreviated progress notes." Graphic formats that allow documentation of those variables or parameters that are unique to the client or to the nursing case management of the client.
- Graphic sheets: Also called the clinical record or the graphic observation record, graphic sheets record data that include temperature, pulse, blood pressure, and respirations.
- Medication records: Include recording of medications and responses of the medication (*e.g.,* dosage, route, time, date, name of the patient, any allergic reactions). If narcotics are given, these records show any relief, who gave the medication, and if any of the narcotic was wasted. (There are separate forms for narcotics.)
- Discharge summary

It is important to select essential and complete information to enter in the client's record. Essential information to be included in the client's record is

- A change in behavior
- Changes in physical functioning
- Physical signs or symptoms that
  1. Are severe; *e.g.,* pain
  2. Are recurrent or persistent
  3. Are abnormal; *e.g.,* elevated blood pressure
  4. Change in severity
  5. Indicate complications
  6. Cannot be relieved by prescribed measures
  7. Indicate faulty health beliefs and practices
  8. Are known danger signals
- Nursing interventions provided and the client's responses
- Visits by other health team members

Guidelines for Documentation

Nurses are responsible for documenting the elements of the nursing process. The record should indicate realistic outcomes that reflect the current standards of nursing practice. For discharge planning, the record must indicate thorough preparation of the client for managing care and treatments on leaving the hospital.

There are three areas to consider when documenting nursing actions: content, format, and timing.

✦ **Content**
- Avoid derogatory terms and stereotypes. According to documentation standards, documentation should reflect an ap-

EMOTIONAL ASPECTS	TEACHING GOALS
FAMILY PROBLEMS	**POSTDISCHARGE PLANNING**
Lives with husband, visits daily	
IMMEDIATE GOAL:	**LONG-RANGE GOAL:**
Reduce pain, prevent complications	
CLIENT NEEDS	**APPROACH**
Comfort	Assess pain, administer P.R.N. medications, evaluate response
Prevent complications	Perform ROM activities to extremities frequently
	Ambulate in hall as tolerated
	Use TED stockings
Prevent constipation	Provide foods high in bulk; offer fluids frequently; ambulate

SURGERY AND DATE

9/17/97   Open reduction/Internal fixation Ⓛ hip

CONSULTATIONS
Orthopedic

DIAGNOSIS	**COMPLICATIONS**
Fractured Ⓛ hip	

ADM. DATE	AGE	BIRTHDATE	RELIGION	CRITICAL	DATE ANOINTED
9/16/97	79				

ROOM #	CLIENT'S NAME		IPA #	DOCTOR
	Mrs. C.			

❧ **Figure 11–5**
Nursing entry on chart.

propriate writing style, suitable choice of words, correct spelling, legible writing, and an organized plan. A professional health care provider should never use derogatory terms or stereotype a client. Personal feelings and comments should always be omitted from documentation and public conversation.

- Avoid value judgments such as "average," "normal," "good," or "sufficient." They are subject to individual interpretation.
- Avoid generalizations—do not overgeneralize documentation or be too vague in charting. This leaves room for assumptions or inappropriate interventions.
- Document all consultation and visits by other health care providers.
- Document the nursing response to questionable medical orders. Factually note the date and time a physician was notified and the physician's response. Identify any nursing supervisors or administrators who are notified.
- Enter information concisely and accurately in a factual manner.
- Note problems as they occur; delete or update problems when appropriate.
- Record findings—not the interpretation of findings.

❦ **Format.** There are many different forms that may require entries by the nurse. Some of these are the progress note, medication record, vital signs sheet, and intake and output record. It is important when making entries to

- Chart on the proper forms.
- Use correct grammar and spelling and write legibly.
- Use approved symbols and abbreviations (Box 11–1).
- Enter the date and time of each entry.
- Chart entries chronologically. Never skip lines. Draw a single line through blank spaces so that no entry can be made in that area by another person.
- Sign all entries with your first initial, last name, and title.
- Never use dittos, erasures, or correcting fluids. If a correction is needed, a single line should be drawn through the incorrect statement, the words "error" or "mistaken entry" should be printed beside the entry, and it should be signed and dated. The entry should then be rewritten correctly.
- The client's name and identification number should be written on each page prior to making any entries.
- The color ink and the type of pen used should be consistent with agency policy.

❦ **Timing.** Proper recording of the time nursing actions occur is imperative to the accuracy of the client record. Some agencies use 12:00 A.M. to 11:59 A.M., then 12:00 P.M. to 11:59 P.M. Other agencies use a 24-hour cycle, where 1:00 P.M. becomes 1300. When making entries, it is important to remember

- *Never* to document an intervention before it is performed.
- To document interventions as soon as possible after they

are carried out. The more seriously ill the client is, the more significant it is to keep documentation current.

- To follow agency policies regarding documentation and modify documentation when changes in the client's status require more frequent documentation.
- To include the time of the entry and the time of the interventions for each entry. This becomes important when there are legal issues about the client.

Types of Records

Several types of records are used in different agencies: source-oriented and problem-oriented records, charting by exception, and focus charting. The advantages and disadvantages of these types of records are shown in Table 11–3.

Nursing Kardex

The nursing Kardex (see Fig. 10–6) provides information that is needed for the daily care of the client. It is a flip-over card kept in a file at the nurses' station. Nurses refer to the Kardex frequently throughout each shift and at the change-of-shift report. The Kardex is updated on an ongoing basis to provide pertinent current information concerning the client's care plan. Unlike all other written records, it is usually written in pencil and erased as appropriate. The following information is usually found in the Kardex:

- Demographic data
- Primary medical diagnoses
- Current physician's orders
- Nursing care plan
- Nursing orders
- Scheduled tests and procedures
- Safety precautions needed for the client
- Diet orders
- Factors related to activities of daily living

Source-Oriented Records

Source-oriented records are the traditional narrative charting method that is used in many institutions and agencies. Professionals in each discipline keep data on their own separate form. Entries such as physicians, nurses, and physical therapist, appear in chronological order, with the current entries at the front of the chart. The number of entries depends on the acuity of the client but there is at least one entry by nursing on each shift. Nursing documentation includes assessment data, implementation of nursing and medical orders, and the client responses to medical and nursing interventions. Table 11–4 describes types of forms and information to be recorded on each.

Box **11–1**

COMMONLY USED ABBREVIATIONS AND SYMBOLS IN NURSING RECORDS*

Assessment Data

abd	abdomen
ADL	activities of daily living
AMB	ambulatory
ax	axillary
BP	blood pressure
BSA	body surface area
BX	biopsy
CC	chief complaint
C&DB	cough and deep breath
C/O	complains of
DOA	dead on arrival
DOE	dyspnea on exertion
Dx	diagnosis
ER	emergency room
F	Fahrenheit
GI	gastrointestinal
GU	genitourinary
H/O	history of
HPI	history of present illness
HR	heart rate
ICU	intensive care unit
imp	impression
LLL	left lower lobe
LLQ	left lower quadrant
LMP	last menstrual period
LOC	level of consciousness
lt or Ⓛ	left
LUL	left upper lobe
LUQ	left upper quadrant
NAD	no apparent distress
neg	negative
NG	nasogastric
OTC	over the counter
P	pulse
PE	physical examination
per	through, by way of, each
PERRLA	pupils equal, round, and reactive to light and accommodation
PMH	past medical history
R	respiration
RLL	right lower lobe
RLQ	right lower quadrant
RML	right middle lobe
R/O	rule out
ROM	range of motion
ROS	review of systems
rt or Ⓡ	right
RUL	right upper lobe
RUQ	right upper quadrant
Rx	treatment
sib	sibling
SOB	shortness of breath
Sx	symptoms
T	temperature
TPR	temperature, pulse, and respiration
VS	vital signs
WNL	within normal limits
⊕	positive
⊖	negative

Diagnostic Studies

ABG	arterial blood gases
BE	barium enema
BSR	basal metabolic rate
BUN	blood urea nitrogen
CAT or CT	computed (axial) tomography
CBC	complete blood count
CNS	central nervous system
CPK	creatinine phosphokinase
C&S	culture and sensitivity
CSF	cerebrospinal fluid
CVP	central venous pressure
CXR	chest x-ray [film]
D&C	dilatation and curettage
DIFF	differential [blood count]
ECF	extracellular fluid
ECG or EKG	cardiogram
ECT	electroconvulsive therapy
EEG	electroencephalogram
EMG	electromyogram
FEV	forced expiratory volume
FRC	functional residual capacity
GYN	gynecological
Hb	hemoglobin
Hct	hematocrit
ICF	intracellular fluid
ICP	intracranial pressure
Ig	immunoglobulin
IOP	intraocular pressure
IVP	intravenous pyelogram
IVU	intravenous urogram
lytes	electrolytes
NMR	nuclear magnetic resonance
MRI	magnetic resonance imaging
PEG	pneumoencephalography
PET	positron emission tomography
pH	hydrogen ion concentration (alkalinity and acidity)
PKU	phenylketonuria
PM	post mortem
ppm	parts per million
RBC	red blood cells
spec	specimen
UA	urinalysis
UGI	upper GI
US	ultrasound
WBC	white blood cells

Elements, Measures, Formulations, Symbols

C	Celsius (centigrade)
cc	cubic centimeter
Cl	chloride
cm	centimeter
CO	carbon monoxide
CO_2	carbon dioxide
D_5W	5% dextrose in water
dl	deciliter
D/W	dextrose in water
elix	elixir

Box continued on following page

Box 11–1

COMMONLY USED ABBREVIATIONS AND SYMBOLS IN NURSING RECORDS*
(Continued)

Elements, Measures, Formulations, Symbols		Orders	
ft	foot	$\overline{a}$	before
gm or g	gram	a.c.	before meals
gr	grain	ad lib	as desired
gtt	*guttae* (Latin) drops	agit	shake
h	hour	A.M.	morning
H_2O	water	AMA	against medical advice
in	inch	aq	water
K	potassium	aq dest	distilled water
kcal	kilocalorie (food calorie)	b.i.d.	two times daily
kg	kilogram	BM	bowel movement
L	liter	BP	blood pressure
m	meter	BRP	bathroom privileges
mEq	milliequivalent	$\overline{c}$ or $\overline{C}$	with
Mg	magnesium	cath	catheter, catheterize, catheterization
mg	milligram	CBR	complete bed rest
min	minute	CPR	cardiopulmonary resuscitation
ml	milliliter	dc or disc	discontinue
mm	millimeter	dil	dilute
µg or mcg	microgram	DNR or no code	do not resuscitate
µm or mcm	micrometer		
N	nitrogen	DSD	dry sterile dressing
Na	sodium	Dx	diagnosis
NaCl	sodium chloride; salt	HS	hour of sleep
O_2	oxygen	IM	intramuscularly
oz	ounce	I&O	intake and output
ppm	parts per million	IPPB	intermittent positive-pressure breathing
sp gr	specific gravity	IU	International Unit
supp	suppository	IV	intravenous(ly)
susp	suspension	IVp	intravenous push
tab	tablet	K/O	keep open (IV)
tbsp	tablespoonfull	noct	at night
tinct	tincture	non rep	do not repeat
tsp	teaspoonfull	NPO	nothing by mouth
U	unit	NS or N/S	normal saline
wk	week	O_2	oxygen
wt	weight	o.d.	daily
µ	micron	OD	right eye
/	per	OOB	out of bed
>	greater than	OS	left eye
<	less than	OT	occupational therapy
≥	greater than or equal to	OU	both eyes
≤	less than or equal to	$\overline{p}$	after
≈	approximately equal to	P&A	percussion and auscultation
±	plus or minus; very slight trace	pc	after meals
↑	increase	P.M.	afternoon
↗	increasing	p.o.	by mouth
↓	decrease	post-op	postoperative
↘	decreasing	pre-op	preoperative
1°	primary; first-degree	prep	preparation
2°	secondary to; second-degree	p.r.n.	as needed
3°	tertiary; third-degree	PT	physical therapy
=	equal to	pt	patient
≠	unequal to	q	every
♀	female	q.a.d.	every other day
♂	male	q4h	every 4 hours
°	degree	q.i.d.	four times a day
@	at		

Box **11–1**

Commonly Used Abbreviations and Symbols in Nursing Records*
(Continued)

Orders

q.s.	quantity sufficient
rep	may be repeated
s̄ (S)	without
SC or Sq	subcutaneous
sig	write on label
sol	solution
s.o.s.	if necessary
stat	immediately
T&C	type and crossmatch
t.i.d.	three times a day
TPN	total parenteral nutrition
up ad lib or	up as desired
UAL	
VS	vital signs
WC	wheelchair
X	times

Diseases

AIDS	acquired immunodeficiency syndrome
ASHD	arteriosclerotic heart disease
ASCVD	arteriosclerotic cardiovascular disease

Diseases

BPH	benign prostatic hypertrophy
CA	cancer
CAD	coronary artery disease
CHF	congestive heart failure
COPD	chronic obstructive pulmonary disease
CVA	cerebrovascular accident
DM	diabetes mellitus
FUO	fever of unknown origin
Fx	fracture
HIV	human immunodeficiency virus
HTN or ↑ BP	hypertension
IDDM	insulin-dependent diabetes mellitus
MI	myocardial infarction
PVD	peripheral vascular disease
STD	sexually transmitted disease
TB or tbc	tuberculosis
TIA	transient ischemic attack
URI	upper respiratory infection
UTI	urinary tract infection

* These are some of the most commonly used abbreviations and symbols. However, it is wise to check for any particular preferences that an institution might have.

Problem-Oriented Records

Problem-oriented records parallel the nursing process. They are organized around client problems rather than information from the various disciplines. All disciplines work together to generate a master problem list and collaborate on a plan of care. The main categories of this system are

- Database: Information is integrated and recorded by health care workers in all disciplines with a consistent format, using the same database and progress notes. Data are more accessible and focus on the individual client's needs.

- Problem list: The problem list contains all the actual or potential problems that require attention. They may be identified by individual health care providers or collaboratively at case conferences. The status of each problem may be active, being resolved, or inactive. As the client's condition improves, problems may be removed from the list. When the problem is resolved, the date of resolution is placed next to the problem.

- Plan: Once the problem has been identified, a plan of care must be developed. This may consist of medical orders, nursing interventions, treatments, and education. The plan should be written according to outcome criteria, and specific orders to accomplish the plan should be written.

- Progress notes: Progress notes are used to document the client's response to the plan. Narrative entries from all disciplines are present, and evaluation of the client's re-

sponses toward outcomes can be measured. The frequency of recording varies, depending on the setting and the institutional policies. The format for progress notes is specific. The acronym *SOAP* was originally used and stands for

    S—Subjective data
    O—Objective data
    A—Assessment
    P—Plan

Later, the original version was modified to *SOAPIE,* and *SOAPIER.* The additional letters stand for

    I—Implementation
    E—Evaluation
    R—Revision

An example of each of these formats can be found in Table 11–5. It is not necessary to include every component each time an entry is made. If there is no objective data, the "O" can be omitted, or revisions may not be necessary; thus the "R" can be omitted.

Focus Charting

This form of organizing nurses' notes has three components: a focus label; organization into the categories of data, action, and response; and flow sheets for documenting the data. Focus charting, or focus notes, according to Lampe (1988), are used to

Table **11—3**

Systems of Record Keeping Used to Document Client Care

SYSTEM	ADVANTAGES	DISADVANTAGES
Source-oriented records	Easy access to forms and documentation by each discipline	Fragmentation of documentation according to the provider No clear definition of problem or interdisciplinary approach to management Lack of integrated documentation of client's response Inconsistent documentation of interdisciplinary teaching Difficulty auditing record Notes are not organized into topics, which makes it difficult to retrieve data
Problem-oriented records (SOAP and SOAPIER)	Quality care is facilitated Multidisciplinary approach to client and data Collaboration is encouraged Learning is increased Evaluation is easily performed Research is facilitated	Education of disciplines may be lengthy and costly Some disciplines may resist multidisciplinary charting Does not solve the problem of fragmented care Difficult to determine what goes into parts of the note May be redundant with nursing care plan
Focus charting	Information in distinct columns Key words make it easy to locate information about particular aspects of client's care Format provides complete brief description of each focus	Data from notes and flow sheets may be redundant
Charting by exception	Changes in client's status easily found on flow sheet Normal findings documented concisely Printed guidelines lead to consistency Data are recorded immediately	Implementation requires major change in many agency documentation systems System may not support a lawsuit
Computer-generated charting	Sorts data into categories Easy to read Displays provide structure for data to be included in progress notes Progress notes from all disciplines are integrated	Categories may be limited May be difficult to individualize an entry Different screens are needed to document different data

SOAP = subjective data, objective data, assessment, plan; SOAPIER = subjective data, objective data, assessment, plan, implementation, evaluation, revision.
Data from Iyer, P. W., Taptich, B. J., & Bernocchi-Losey, D. (1995). Nursing process and nursing diagnosis (3rd ed.). Philadelphia: W. B. Saunders.

- Expand on flow sheet data to record unusual or unexpected events
- Document client responses
- Document discharge plans
- Describe the status of a client when he or she is transferred or discharged
- Describe the psychosocial or emotional needs of the client

Charting by Exception

Charting by exception was developed to streamline charting and reduce the time nurses spend on documentation. Flow sheets that contain medical and nursing diagnoses are used to document findings and interventions for each 24-hour period. Check marks are used when there are no significant findings, and asterisks are used to indicate that there are significant findings, which are elaborated on in the narrative section of the chart.

Computer-Assisted Records

There are various types of computer-assisted records. Some systems generate a flow sheet for each shift that defines the dependent and independent

Table 11–4

EXAMPLES OF FORMS AND INFORMATION IN SOURCE-ORIENTED RECORDS

FORM	INFORMATION TO BE RECORDED
Forms with Documentation by Nurses	
Activity flow sheet	Activities and safety measures Bathing and skin care Diagnostic tests and treatments Diet and eating patterns Elimination Isolation
Graphic sheet	Temperature Pulse Respiration Blood pressure Intake and output
Medication sheet	Name of each medication Dosage of each medication Route of administration Time of administration Name and initials of nurse administering the medication
Nursing admission assessment	Information gathered during the nursing history and findings on the physical assessment
Nurse's notes	Description of important observations of the client Client complaints Coping mechanisms Responses to nursing interventions Statements that identify nursing measures Client's progress toward achieving short- and long-term goals
Forms Used by Health Care Workers in Other Disciplines	
Admission sheet	Client's name, address, date of birth, hospital identification number, age, sex, religion, occupation, insurance coverage Date, time, and reason for admission Attending physician
Medical history and physical examination form	Medical diagnoses Family history Health history Results of physical examination Plan of treatment
Miscellaneous forms	X-ray and laboratory reports Consultation findings Results from physical, respiratory, or radiation therapy
Physician's order sheet	Orders for medication and treatments
Physician's progress notes	Client's responses to medical treatment Interpretation of pathological findings

nursing activities for each client, including the appropriate client outcomes and nursing interventions. Nurses initial the actions that have been implemented. Nurses' notes are handwritten in the format described in the source-oriented record. Other systems use the problem-oriented method. A prioritized problem list is generated at the client's bedside, and the nurse selects the diagnoses, client outcomes, and nursing interventions. They may be simple statements or detailed descriptions of care given. The system sorts the information into the SOAPIE format. Another approach involves selecting data from displays to build the progress notes. The nurse chooses from structured screens, allowing documentation of current data and the opportunity to add new findings. Progress notes from all disciplines are integrated. There may be different screens to document different data, such as charting the administration of medications or sending the client for a laboratory test.

Reporting

Reporting is a method nurses use to communicate specific information to a person or group of people, either orally or in writing.

Change-of-Shift Report

The **change-of-shift report** is the report most frequently given by nurses. The purpose of the report is to provide continuity from one shift to the next. It is an oral report, given either face-to-face or by an audiotape recording (Fig. 11–6). A complete report is important, as it demonstrates the nurse's accountability to the client.

The report should be concise and should be given quickly and efficiently, without idle chatter or gossip. The nurse discusses the client and family in a nonjudgmental manner and avoids labels when describing client behavior. Value judgments are not conducive to establishing working relationships between staff members and the client and may cause staff members to form prejudicial opinions about a client.

The face-to-face report provides the opportunity for the listener to ask questions and clarify information. However, this method can be very time consuming. The guidelines identified here can be helpful to nurses when preparing and presenting reports (Hesse, 1983; Smith, 1986):

- Follow a particular order when reporting about more than one client
- Identify the client by name, room number, and bed number
- Give the client's reason for admission and medical diagnosis
- Identify the tests and procedures performed in the last 24 hours and indicate their results

		Table 11–5
EXAMPLES OF PROGRESS NOTES USING SOAP AND SOAPIER		

Nursing Diagnosis: Sensory Perceptual Alteration related to impaired vision.

	SOAP	**SOAPIER**
1300	S: "I can't see. Everything is blurred." O: Right eye bandaged following surgery. Cannot wear corrective lens for left eye because of bandage. A: Client will need assistance with activities and mobility. P: Encourage client to ask caregiver for assistance.	S: "I can't see. Everything is blurred." O: Right eye bandaged following surgery. Cannot wear corrective lens for left eye because of bandage. A: Client will need assistance with activities and mobility. P: Encourage client to ask caregiver for assistance. I: Give instructions to caregiver and client. Discuss environmental hazards with the caregiver. E: Client is reluctant to express needs to the caregiver. R: Support the client in assuming a dependent role.

SOAP = subjective data, objective data, assessment, plan; SOAPIER = subjective data, objective data, assessment, plan, implementation, evaluation, revision.

- Note any significant changes, improvement, or worsening of the client's condition
- Present client changes using a nursing process format: assessment data, nursing diagnosis, planning, interventions, and evaluation
- Provide exact, factual information
- Do not include unremarkable measurements unless a change has taken place; *e.g.,* only report a normal blood pressure reading if the client previously had high blood pressure
- Report the client's emotional responses that need to be addressed before any interventions can take place

Telephone Report

A telephone report is a way that health professionals frequently communicate with each other.

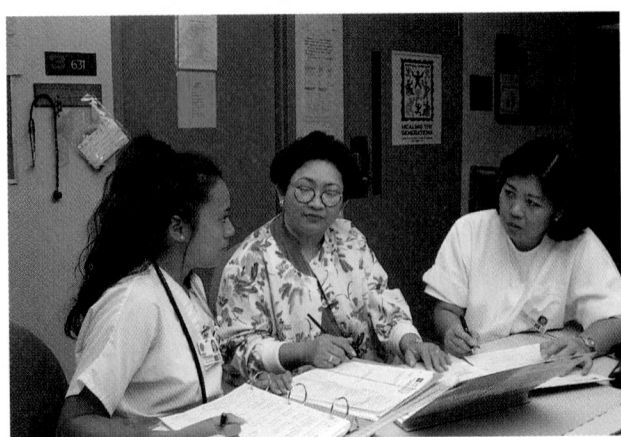

♦ **Figure 11–6**
Change of shift report.

Nurses may inform physicians about changes in a client's condition, relay information about a transfer, or receive test results in a telephone report. Since there may be no permanent documentation of this communication, it is imperative that the reports be made carefully with clear and concise information. Information concerning the client must be verified by repeating the messages clearly and precisely. Nurses should always be courteous when communicating with other health team members. Courtesy conveys a sense of professionalism and promotes cooperation among the health team.

♦ Conferring

Nurses may need to meet in groups to discuss client problems and explore possible solutions. Nursing care conferences and nursing care rounds are two ways that nurses most commonly confer.

Nursing Care Conference

The **nursing care conference** is a meeting of a group of nurses, often including the client, family members, and other health professionals, to discuss problems a client may be having. It allows each nurse to express opinions about possible solutions. Other health professionals, such as a nurse practitioner, dietitian, physical therapist, and social worker, may be invited to offer their expertise about a particular problem.

Conferences are most effective when there is a climate of respect for those who express values, opinions, and beliefs that seem different. This involves listening with an open mind and respecting each contribution, even when it is different from your own.

Nursing Care Rounds

During **nursing care rounds** a group of nurses visits clients at the bedside. The purposes of this are to

* Gather information that will assist in planning nursing care
* Give clients the opportunity to discuss their care
* Evaluate nursing care that is given

The advantages of nursing care rounds are that the clients can participate in a discussion of their care, and the nurse can actually see the client while the report is being given. To facilitate client participation, nurses need to use language that is understood by the client—not medical terminology.

♦

Summary

During implementation, the focus is on providing safe care to meet the outcomes identified in the care plan. Implementation is carried out by independent, dependent, and collaborative (interdependent) nursing actions. Intellectual, interpersonal, and technical skills are needed by the nurse.

Communication among nurses and between nurses and other health care providers is essential for coordination and continuity of care. It is important that the information be complete and accurate. Entries on the client record must be done in a timely manner on the proper forms. Oral communication gives nurses and other health care providers the opportunity to exchange information, explore problems, and discuss solutions.

■ ■

CHAPTER HIGHLIGHTS

♦

* Implementation is putting the nursing strategies identified in the nursing care plan into action. The nurse uses cognitive, interpersonal, and technical skills to implement the nursing care plan. There are three types of interventions: dependent, independent, and interdependent.

* Selecting nursing interventions requires consideration of many factors that lead to labeling of nursing actions.

* Reassessing and validating the care plan is an ongoing process during the implementation phase. Nursing care is modified as the client's condition and health care needs change.

* Implementation methods fall into the following categories: assisting with activities of daily living, counseling and teaching, providing care to achieve therapeutic goals, facilitating the client's attainment of health care goals, and supervising other personnel.

* Nurses are accountable for all of their actions. The nurse must be knowledgeable about the procedure being implemented, when it is needed, how to do it, and the expected outcome. Nursing actions to achieve therapeutic goals include compensation for adverse reactions, preventive measures, correct techniques for administering care, preparing clients for procedures, and lifesaving measures.

* The implementation phase of the nursing process includes the documentation of all nursing activities and client responses. Written records ensure the transmission of information about a client to all health care workers. They are a source of educational, research, and statistical data and allow audit of client care standards. Record entries should be brief, accurate, legible, chronologic, written on consecutive lines, and appropriately signed.

* The client record is the only legal document that provides a comprehensive picture of the care given to the client. Because the client record is a legal document admissible as evidence in a court of law, erasures or "white outs" are not permitted, standard terms and abbreviations must be used, and the nurse must sign his or her legal name.

* Health team members must communicate effectively with each other to provide coordinated, high-quality care. The Kardex record is widely used for easy access to current data about clients. Reports about clients need to be concise and pertinent and must include significant changes in the client's condition or therapy. Nurses share information by conferring during nursing care conferences, nursing care rounds, and nursing reports.

Study Questions

1. Implementation is carried out by

   a. the nurse and the physician
   b. the client and the physician
   c. the physician and the family
   d. the client and the nurse

2. When administering a medication, it is the responsibility of the nurse to monitor the client for side effects; this would be an example of

   a. an independent nursing action
   b. an interdependent nursing action
   c. a dependent nursing action
   d. a collaborative nursing action

3. All but one of the following is considered essential information to be entered in the client record

   a. physical signs and symptoms
   b. changes in behavior
   c. visits by friends
   d. visits by health team members

4. Records where professionals from each discipline keep data on separate forms are known as

   a. problem-oriented records
   b. source-oriented records
   c. focus charting
   d. charting by exception

5. A potential complication for a medical diagnosis would be considered

   a. a collaborative problem
   b. a dependent nursing problem
   c. an independent nursing problem
   d. a nonnursing problem

Critical Thinking Exercises

1. A client who has been diagnosed with new-onset diabetes mellitus who is prescribed insulin and blood sugar monitoring is assigned to your care. Discuss the types of interventions for this client.

2. Write a sample nurses' note entry for a client who fell while trying to get up. You did not witness the fall.

References

American Nurses' Association. (1989). *Classification systems for describing nursing practice* [Working Papers]. Kansas City, MO: American Nurses' Association.

American Nurses' Association. (1980). *A social policy statement*. Kansas City, MO: American Nurses' Association.

American Nurses' Association Congress on Practice. (1973). *Standards of practice*. Kansas City, MO: American Nurses' Association.

Bulechek, G. M., & McCloskey, J. C. (1992a). Defining and validating nursing interventions. *Nursing Clinics of North America, 27,* 2.

Bulechek, G. M., & McCloskey, J. C. (1992b). Nursing Diagnoses, interventions, and outcomes. In G. M. Bulechek, & J. C. McCloskey (Eds.), *Nursing interventions: Essential nursing treatments* (2nd ed.; pp. 1–20). Philadelphia: W. B. Saunders.

Fayram, E. (1995). Implementation. In P. J. Christensen, & J. W. Kenney (Eds.), *Nursing process* (4th. ed.). St. Louis: C. V. Mosby.

Hesse, G. (1983). A better shift report means better nursing care. *Nursing 83* **[Canadian Edition],** *13,* 65.

Iyer, P. W., Taptich, B. J., & Bernocchi-Losey, D. (1995). *Nursing process and nursing diagnosis* (3rd ed.). Philadelphia: W. B. Saunders.

Lampe, S. (1988). *Focus charting*. Minneapolis: Creative Nursing Management.

Mundinger, M. O. (1980). *Autonomy in nursing*. Germantown, MD: Aspen.

Smith, C. E. (1986). Upgrade your shift reports with the three R's. *Nursing 86, 16,* 63–64.

Bibliography

Buckley-Womack, C., & Gibney, B. (1987). A new dimension in documentation: The PIE method. *Journal of Neuroscience Nursing, 19*(5), 256–260.

Bulechek, G. M., Kraus, V. L., Wakefield, B., & Kowalski, D. K. (1990). An evaluation guide to assist with implementation of nursing diagnosis. *Nursing Diagnosis, 1*(1), 18–23.

Hartman, D., & Knudson, J. (1991). Documentation: A nursing data base for initial patient assessment. *Oncology Nursing Forum, 18*(1), 123–130.

McCloskey, J. C., Bulechek, G. M., Cohen, M. Z., Craft, M. J., Crossley, J. D., Deneny, J. A., Glick, O. J., Kruckenberg, T., Maas, M., Prophet, C. M., & Tripp-Reimer, T. (1990). Classification of nursing interventions. *Journal of Professional Nursing, 6*(3), 151–157.

Ponder, P. M., (1990). The nursing process and computers. *Point of View, 27*(1), 14–15.

Chapter ✦ 12

EVALUATION

PATRICIA E. KIZILAY, EdD, RN, CS, FNP

KEY TERMS
✦

concurrent audit
criteria
nursing audit
outcome evaluation

quality assurance
    program
retrospective audit
standard

LEARNING OBJECTIVES
✦

After studying this chapter, you should be able to

✦ Understand the key terms listed at the beginning of the chapter

✦ Describe the purpose of evaluation

✦ Describe the relationship of evaluation to the other steps of the nursing process

✦ Evaluate the client outcomes identified in the nursing care plan

✦ Modify the nursing care plan based on the client's responses

✦ Explain the relationship between nursing care plans and quality assurance programs

✦ Discuss the five steps of the evaluation process

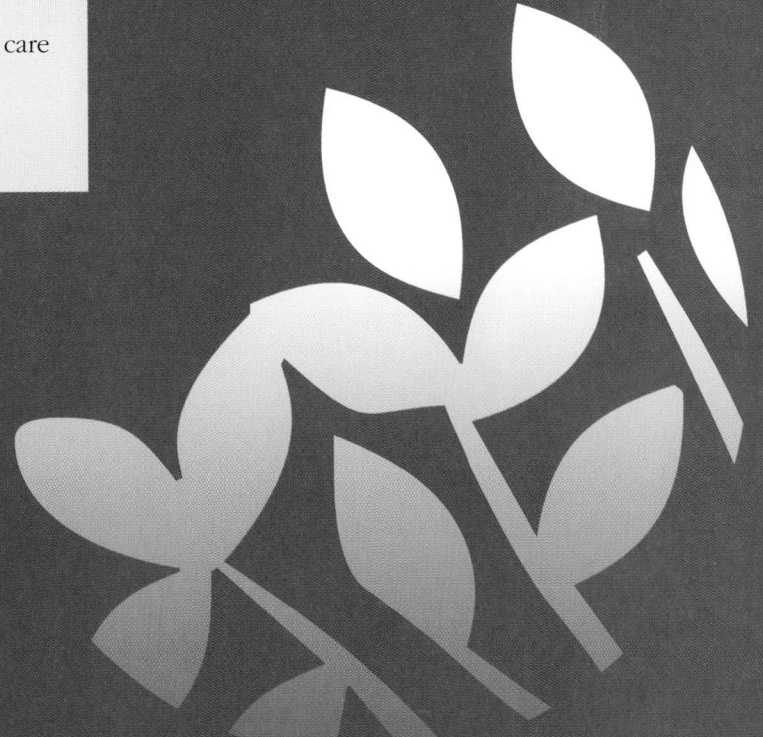

201

Evaluation is an integral part of nursing. It is needed to plan care for clients. Evaluation is identified as the final phase of the nursing process; however, it is ongoing and formal. It assists the nurse in identifying nursing actions that are effective or ineffective and enhances the scientific base of professional nursing practice. Knowledge of health, pathophysiology, and evaluation methods is necessary for an effective evaluation. Evaluation helps identify the effectiveness of nursing actions and enhances the scientific basis of nursing practice (Kenney, 1995). Patterson (1988) defines evaluation as an assessment that determines the meaning and importance of the nursing actions. It includes making judgments about both the quality and appropriateness of nursing care based on comparisons between the current practices in nursing service and predetermined clinical indicators (Fig. 12–1).

Traditionally, nurses were evaluated by supervisors on attributes such as dependability, punctuality, leadership, and organization in addition to clinical skills. Currently, standards of care have been established, and nurses determine their capability to meet those standards. To accomplish this, nursing care to individuals and the care delivered at agencies must be evaluated.

Nursing care of consumers is evaluated by the achievement of outcomes through effective use of the nursing process in the clinical area. The consumer may be the client, the client's family member, or the community.

Nurses may be evaluated by the administration based on the standards set for nurses in a particular institution. This may include the areas of complementary values of the institution and the nurse, experience and qualifications for a particular role, and congruence between the needs for the nurse's development and institutional needs.

Evaluation in the Nursing Process

Although evaluation has been identified with the last phase of the nursing process, evaluation is an important part of each phase. It occurs whenever a nurse interacts with a client. Evaluation can be conducted during any phase of the nursing process or at the end of the process to determine whether the client outcomes identified in a plan of care have been met. The initial assessment serves as a baseline for determining the client's progress and comparing changes in the client's responses. Nursing diagnoses identify the client's health concerns and the areas to be evaluated. The outcomes formulated during the planning phase of the nursing process are the criteria used to determine improvement in the client's status. During the implementation phase, nurses provide nursing actions to appraise client responses and to judge the effectiveness of the plan. The most important act of evaluation performed by nurses is determining that the outcomes are achieved. **Outcome evaluation** is the collection and analysis of data about client responses. Evaluation of nursing care includes five steps:

1. Identifying the outcome criteria that will be used
2. Collecting data related to the criteria identified
3. Comparing the client's response with the criteria and determining whether outcomes were achieved
4. Relating nursing actions to client outcomes
5. Modifying the nursing care plan

Evaluating nursing care is a complex task. It is difficult to separate the contributions of nurses from those of other health care professionals. For example, the nursing action for a client with a fractured hip might be to assist the client to ambulate for 15 minutes twice a day (Fig. 12–2). An outcome would be to increase the distance the client would ambulate by a specific date. The client may also be going to physical therapy every day. The outcome may be met, but is it because of the nursing action, the physical therapy treatment, or the combination?

Purpose

The major purpose of evaluation is to determine the client's progress toward meeting specified outcomes that will be used as a guide to direct future nurse-client interactions. Another important purpose is to judge the effectiveness of the nursing process. If nursing actions are performed caringly, competently,

Evaluation
- Identify outcome criteria
- Collect data related to criteria
- Compare client's response to criteria
- Relate nursing actions to client outcome
- Modify nursing care plan as needed

Nursing Process
Assessment
Diagnosis
Planning
Implementation
→ Evaluation

❧ **Figure 12–1**
Evaluation is the fifth and final step of the nursing process. However, evaluation is also ongoing throughout the nursing process.

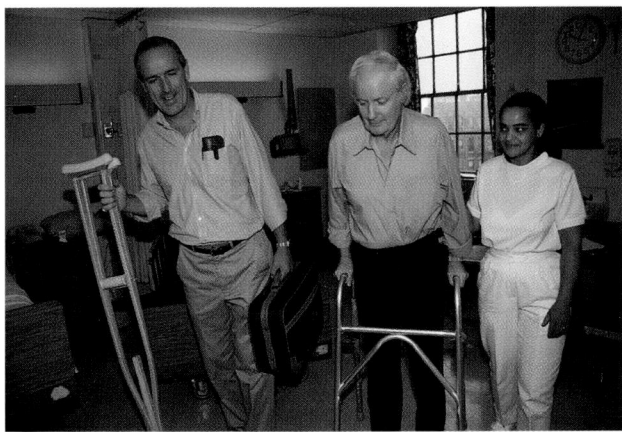

✦ **Figure 12–2**
The nurse and the physical therapist may both use client ambulation as an intervention.

and creatively, but the client does not move toward the desired outcome, the actions are meaningless. Nurses are accountable for designing and implementing accurate care plans and judging the effectiveness of their nursing actions. Both the client's progress and the nursing actions are evaluated. These actions demonstrate accountability for nursing practice.

Criteria and Standards

The terms *criteria* and *standards* are often used interchangeably, but their meanings are different.

✦ **Criteria.** Kenney (1995) describes **criteria** as measurable qualities, attributes, or characteristics that specify skills, knowledge, or attitudes that influence a client's behavior. Examples of each are

   Skill—return demonstration of a dressing change or blood sugar monitoring

   Knowledge—verbalizing information about how to determine the amount of insulin to give

   Attitude—client's indifference about taking insulin, which may result in noncompliance

They are written in nursing care plans to describe the expected behaviors that result from acceptable levels of performance of the nurse and the client.

✦ **Standards. Standards** are written rules for clients and nurses that indicate acceptable levels of performance by nursing staff and other health care workers that a client may expect. They are established by custom, authority, or general consent. In 1973, the American Nurses' Association (ANA) established *Standards of Nursing Practice* describing essential actions of the nursing process (see Table 7–1). These standards provide the framework for judging the quality of nursing care delivered. They contain broad general statements that have been modified by most specialty groups to reflect their teaching and clinical expertise.

Outcomes

The nature of the outcome determines what type of data collection is appropriate to support outcome achievement. Following is a list of the types of outcomes to be evaluated.

✦ **Cognitive Outcomes.** Cognitive outcomes involve increasing the client's knowledge and can be evaluated by having the client repeat information or having the client apply the new knowledge to a situation. For example, the client will repeat the dangers of alcohol consumption after viewing a videotape.

✦ **Psychomotor Outcomes.** Psychomotor outcomes describe the achievement of skills and can be evaluated by having the client demonstrate the skill. For example, the client will walk to the end of the room on crutches three times today.

✦ **Affective Outcomes.** *Affective outcomes* refer to changes in the client's attitude, beliefs, or values and are somewhat difficult to measure. Conversation and observations of the client's behavior are used to determine whether these outcomes have been achieved. For example, the client will verbalize feelings of loss 2 days after her mastectomy.

✦ **Physical Changes.** Physical changes may be the desired outcome. To evaluate this type of outcome, the nurse uses physical examination skills and compares the data with data acquired earlier. For example, the client's blood pressure will be no higher than 110/80 in 3 days.

The time needed to complete the outcome varies. Short-term outcomes require immediate action and should be accomplished prior to discharge. Intermediate outcomes are short-range actions directed toward meeting the long-range outcomes. Long-term outcomes indicate the overall direction for actions of the health team and may not be achieved prior to discharge (Doenges *et al.,* 1989). An in-depth discussion of outcomes is found in Chapter 10.

Measuring Outcome Achievement

The nurse measures outcome achievement by collecting and analyzing data about the client's responses to nursing interventions.

✦ **Data Collection.** Both subjective and objective data are important, but it is preferable to collect objective data to determine nursing actions. The data collected must be recorded accurately and concisely and can be obtained from the following sources:

* Client interview
* Direct observation
* Physical examination

- Review of documents
- Significant others
- Nursing staff
- Other hospital employees

Katz and Green (1992) have identified four reasons to collect data:

- To validate that things are happening as planned
- To provide a basis for change and improvement
- To provide a rationale for increasing, decreasing, or maintaining resources
- To provide a basis for developing thresholds for evaluation to use in determining trends of care

Evaluation of the client takes place by

- Continuously assessing the nursing actions; for example, is the client comfortable after repositioning?
- Comparing client responses with outcomes; for example, if the outcome is to decrease weight by 0.5 lb each day, the nurse must determine if the client lost 0.5 lb in the last day.
- Determining client's lack of progress; in the previous example, if the client has not lost 0.5 lb per day, the nurse must evaluate the outcome to determine if it is realistic.

Depending on the outcome, modifying the nursing care plan may be the appropriate action.

✦ **Continuously Appraising and Reassessing the Nursing Actions.** Client responses to nursing actions are continuously appraised and reassessed. When implementing nursing actions, the nurse observes the client's response, reviews the client's chart and note changes, checks on the client and family's compliance with the therapeutic regimen, and assesses the client's understanding of any information given.

✦ **Comparing Client Responses With Outcomes.** Client responses are compared with the client's outcomes to determine the extent to which the outcomes have been met. The nurse judges the effects of the nursing actions on the client and family, compares the client's ability with those stated in the objectives, and enters the information on the client record. If the outcomes are easily met, the plan may be moving too slowly or at just the right pace. The nurse then decides on the progress the client is making toward meeting the outcomes. The outcomes may be

- Completely met: The client responded as expected
- Partially met: The short-term outcome, but not the long-term outcome, was met or some but not all of the short-term or long-term outcome criteria were met
- Not met at all

If the outcomes are only partially met or not met at all, the nurse needs to collect data to determine what happened.

The following situation gives examples of outcome achievement:

> **CASE STUDY** — **Mary Jones Has a Nursing Diagnosis of Nutrition Less Than Body Requirements**
>
> Mary Jones has a nursing diagnosis of Nutrition, Less Than Body Requirements, Altered, related to low self-esteem. The long-term outcome is: The client will gain 20 lb in 10 weeks. The short-term goal is: The client will eat a 2000-calorie diet every day. The outcome criterion is: The client will gain 2 lb a week. One week later, the nurse and Ms. Jones meet to evaluate the outcomes. Following are some examples of what might occur. If the outcome is met: The client has gained 2 lb. For an outcome partially met, the finding might be: The client has gained 1 lb. If the outcome is not met, the finding may be: The client has lost 0.5 lb.

✦ **Determining the Client's Lack of Progress.** The client's lack of progress toward achieving outcomes is determined. Client responses are evaluated and recorded in the chart and the nursing care plan. The nurse determines whether to change the outcomes or revise the nursing actions.

In the previous case study, for the outcome partially met, an option would be to change the outcome to 1 lb a week and adjust the long-term outcome accordingly. The nurse would be fostering the client's self-esteem by acknowledging the client's success. For the outcome not met, it might be desirable to change the nursing diagnosis to alteration in self-concept and plan outcomes for that diagnosis before trying the deal with the alteration in nutrition, or it may be necessary to change the nursing action, such as having the nurse sit with the client during meals, increasing the caloric intake, or decreasing the exercise regimen of the client.

In the Case Study evaluation of Mrs. C., some modifications of the care plan were necessary (Table 12–1).

✦ **Modifying the Nursing Care Plan.** The care plan is modified when the client's condition changes or when outcomes have not been adequately met. All phases of the nursing process should be reviewed when revisions are necessary.

Assessment. Update the assessment data. Inaccurate or incomplete data affect all the subsequent phases of the nursing process. New data may invalidate existing data, resulting in new nursing diagnoses, outcomes, and nursing actions.

Nursing Diagnoses. Revise the nursing diagnoses. If additional data have been obtained, a new nursing diagnosis may be needed. The nurse needs to determine whether the problem was reflected correctly in the nursing diagnosis.

	Table **12–1**

EVALUATION OF MRS. C.

NURSING DIAGNOSIS	OUTCOME STATEMENT	MET/ UNMET	MODIFIED OUTCOME
Pain	The client will experience relief or reduced pain to rest comfortably or participate in care	Met	The client will require less medication to control pain
Physical Mobility, Impaired	The client will walk the length of the hall and back by day 3; the client will maintain full range of motion in all unaffected joints	Met	The client will regain optimal mobility before discharge; the client will walk the hospital hall three times daily with minimal assistance
Risk for DVT	The client will not develop DVT in her lower extremities, indicated by warm, pink skin, good capilliary refill and pulses	Met	
Infection, Risk for	The client will be free of infection during recovery, verified by normal body temperature, normal white blood cell count, and healing incision	Met	The client will be cognizant of the signs and symptoms of infection post discharge
Potential for Constipation	The client will maintain her regular bowel elimination during hospitalization	Met	
Self Care Deficit	The client will be able to perform self-care activities within own capabilities before discharge to home	Partially met	The client will have assistance with dressing and wound care when discharged
Knowledge Deficit of Therapeutic Regimen and Discharge	The client will understand plan of care during hospitalization; the client will verbalize the correct understanding of the discharge instructions	Met	The client will be able to apply knowledge during recovery at home; the client will know who to call for assistance with a question
Caregiver Role Strain	The client's husband and family will be able to verbalize an understanding of the discharge instructions; the caregiver will state that the formal and informal support systems are adequate to provide rest for him	Unmet	The client's son and daughter-in-law will be responsible for helping the client meet unmet needs; the family will grow stronger in their commitment to each other

DVT = deep venous thrombosis.
Data from Gulanick, M., Kloop, A., Galanes, S., *et al.* (1994). *Nursing care plans: Nursing diagnosis and interventions* (3rd ed.). St. Louis: Mosby–Year Book. The case study evaluation of Mrs. C. was written by Jane Wrenn, BSN.

Planning. Change the goals and outcome criteria to reflect other changes in the nursing care plan. The nurse and the client need to determine (1) if the outcome criteria are realistic and (2) that the priorities have remained the same (Fig. 12–3). Delete criteria that are no longer appropriate. New outcomes and actions are established mutually by the client and the nurse and are noted in the Kardex, chart, and nursing care plan.

Implementation. New nursing actions should reflect the revised outcome criteria. The nurse must ascertain (1) that the actions selected were carried out, (2) whether the nursing actions were related to the outcomes, and (3) that they were the best ones to reach the outcome. If the actions are unclear or unreason-able for the resources available, the actions may not have been implemented.

✦ Factors Influencing Outcome Attainment. Client, nurse, and health care system variables can have a positive or negative impact on outcome attainment.

* Client variables—if the outcome is to decrease anxiety, a visit from the clergy may have a positive outcome on reducing a client's anxiety, whereas news of a serious illness may result in a negative outcome
* Nurse variables—inadequate assessment by the nurse does not provide enough information and results in a negative outcome, whereas a comprehensive assessment increases the likelihood of a positive outcome
* Health system variables—a negative outcome may occur if laboratory test results are delayed, resulting in a delay in

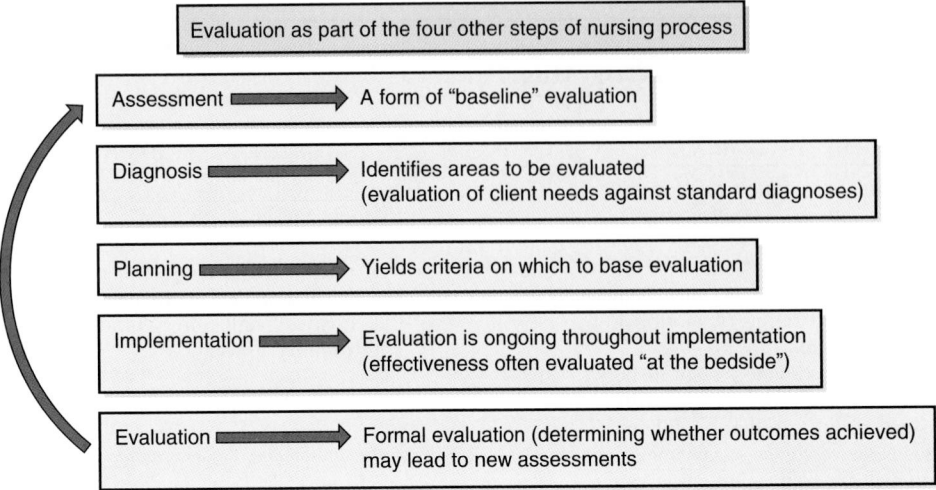

Figure 12–3
Evaluation is not only the final step of the nursing process but also an integral part of each of the other four steps.

treatment, whereas timely return of the results tests increases the likelihood of a positive outcome.

Once these variables are known, the nurse can reinforce the positive factors by using them in future interactions and deal with those variables that are likely to create problems.

When the outcomes are achieved, the nurse may decide that the problem no longer exists or that the problem exists even though the outcome was achieved.

Quality Assurance

Quality assurance programs involve the planned and organized evaluation of the nursing care given to groups of clients. Their goal is to promote excellence in nursing practice. The scope of the program may vary from a small program implemented on one nursing unit, to an institutional program, to one encompassing a state or country.

Agency evaluation is usually referred to as *quality assurance,* which involves nursing audits and standard guidelines. The process ensures that the institution delivers quality patient care. Activities should focus on the priorities that have the greatest impact on results and influence the balance between quality of care and cost containment.

Consumer pressure for evaluation of health care resulted in the passage of legislation in 1972. Congress mandated professional monitoring of health services for Medicare, Medicaid, and Maternal-Child Health Program recipients.

In 1975, the ANA developed a quality assurance program. In 1991, the ANA revised the original standard to reflect current practice. The standards describe nursing care and are used to guide nursing interventions. They provide the structure for evaluating the quality of nursing care. Katz and Green (1992) describe quality assurance as a process or orderly series of activities for ensuring conformity with requirements and complying with written standards. They have identified the most important activities to be evaluated as

- High volume: Those activities that occur frequently or involve large numbers of clients and staff, such as clients using emergency clinics for routine problems. These clients could be served efficiently in clinics or out-of-hospital facilities.

- High risk: Those activities that will cause harm if they are performed or omitted, such as medication administration. If a medication is administered in an incorrect dose—either too much or not enough—it will cause harm to the client.

- Problem prone: Those activities or situations that are problems for the client or staff, such as a client with decubitus ulcers. This is an ongoing problem for affected staff and clients. There are many treatments available, but the problem is difficult to treat. The healing process takes a long time, and clients are uncomfortable.

- High cost: Those activities that are expensive or that are small in cost but of sufficient volume to drain resources, such as laboratory tests and radiological studies. Often, costly studies are done or are repeated when less-expensive studies could reveal the data needed for effective intervention with the client.

Nursing Audit

The **nursing audit** is the process for studying quality assurance. It assists nurses in assessing the quality of services provided. It is important to know when to collect the data for a nursing audit. The two types of audits are

- **Concurrent audit:** This audit takes place when the nursing actions or the client responses occur. A time is established to determine whether the changes in the client behavior described in the outcome have occurred. At the designated time, the nurse collaborates with the client and others who may be involved to evaluate the client's ability to demonstrate the desired behaviors.

Table 12–2

CRITERIA FOR A NURSING AUDIT

CRITERIA	DESCRIPTIVE STATEMENT
1. Application and execution of physician's legal orders	Medical diagnosis complete Medical orders complete, current, and executed promptly Evidence that nurse understood the cause and effect Evidence that nurse took medical history into account
2. Observations of symptoms and reactions	Related to the course of this disease Related to the course of this disease in this client Related complications due to therapy Vital signs Client's attitude toward his or her condition Client's response to the course of his or her disease
3. Supervision of the client	Evidence that initial nursing diagnosis was made Safety and security of client Support the client in reactions to conditions and care Continual assessment of the client's condition and capacity Nursing plans updated based on assessment Interaction with significant others considered
4. Supervision of other caregivers (excluding the physician)	Care is taught to client, family, and other nursing personnel Physical, emotional, and mental capacity to learn is considered Continual supervision is available to those who are taught Support available to caregivers
5. Reporting and recording	Facts needed for future care are recorded Essential facts are reported to the physician Facts reported have been evaluated Client and caregiver instructed on what to report to the physician Continuity of care is evident in the record
6. Application and execution of nursing procedures and techniques	Administration and/or supervision of medications Personal care Nutrition Fluid balance and elimination Sleep Physical activity and exercise Treatments and rehabilitation Recreation and diversion Prevention of complications
7. Promotion of physical and emotional health by direction and teaching	Plans for emergencies evident Emotional support of client and family Teaching prevention Evaluating the need for resources (*e.g.,* spiritual, social service, and physical or occupational therapy) Action taken where needs are identified

---

• **Retrospective audit:** These audits occur after the services to a client have been discontinued. Usually the information is obtained from the client's hospital record. Occasionally, the information may be obtained by a telephone interview or a questionnaire mailed to the client. A nursing audit is designed to be objective and methodical. Tinubu (Nursing audit. Unpublished paper, Teacher's College, Columbia University, New York, 1976) identified the following purposes for the nursing audit:

To develop tools for evaluating, verifying, and improving the quality of nursing practice

To provide a basis for educational programs for clients and staff

To provide a means for evaluating and improving nursing records

To reveal strengths and weaknesses in nursing care when measured against standards

To reduce the incidence of legal complications of medical or nursing practice arising from incomplete or inaccurate records

❥ **Audit Criteria.** The criteria developed for the nursing audit must reflect the mission and goals of the organization where the care is being rendered. The audit must be personalized by the system that is using it. Phaneuf (1966) identified seven general functions, listed in Table 12–2, that may serve as the basis for an audit.

Professional Standards Review Organizations

Professional Standards Review Organizations (PSROs) were created in the 1970s as the forerunner of the Professional Review Organizations (PROs). The purpose of the PROs includes the following:

1. To ensure that all health care reimbursed from Federal funds is necessary
2. To ensure that care meets professional standards
3. To require that care be provided economically in an appropriate setting (Iyer *et al.*)

Joint Commission

The Joint Commission on the Accreditation of Healthcare Organizations (JCAHO) is the most active organization in evaluating the quality of health care. In 1983, it identified the essential requirements for an acceptable client care evaluation:

- Objectivity: Measurable standards and criteria must be established prior to the evaluation
- Clinical soundness: The standards and criteria must reflect optimal care of the client that is achievable by the caregivers with the expertise and resources available
- Efficiency: Professional nursing time must be used when necessary, and nonprofessional time should be allocated to those parts of a program requiring no clinical judgment
- Flexibility: Variations from standards and criteria are permitted when reported with good cause
- Documentation: Decisions and evaluations must be written and signed and reported to the person responsible for quality care
- Action-orientation: Confirmed deficiencies must be analyzed, and appropriate corrective interventions must be implemented

The JCAHO (1989a) evaluates a facility's outcomes to guarantee that resources are used effectively. During the same year, the JCAHO (1989b) identified clinical indicators as the quantitative measure that can be used to evaluate client care and support services. The indicators can be used to evaluate nursing diagnoses and interventions related to outcome criteria. The JCAHO has identified the following factors as determinants of quality client care:

- Accessibility
- Timeliness
- Effectiveness
- Appropriateness
- Efficiency
- Continuity
- Privacy
- Confidentiality
- Participation of client and family
- Environmental safety

In 1990, the JCAHO defined standards as patient-focused guidelines for care, focusing on outcomes. The standards provide the basis for information needed to care for a client skillfully.

Summary

Evaluation is an ongoing process used to determine the effectiveness of nursing care to individuals and groups of clients. Based on the findings, nursing care plans may be modified. Quality assurance results may be compared with institutional standards but are frequently compared with regional and national standards. National standards for nursing practice are set by the ANA and the JCAHO.

The results of evaluation and quality assurance contribute to a knowledge base that assists professional nurses to maintain excellence in nursing practice.

CHAPTER HIGHLIGHTS

✦

✦ Evaluation determines to what extent the goals stated in the nursing care plan have been met

✦ The nurse and the client measure the level of goal attainment and modify the nursing care plan accordingly

✦ If the nursing care plan needs to be modified, all of the steps in the nursing process need to be checked for accuracy

✦ Projected outcomes are stated in behavioral terms to describe the desired effects of nursing actions and determine when and how the goals will be met

✦ Evaluation findings are recorded on the nursing care plan to inform the staff of the client's level of outcome achievement

✦ Decisions about how well an outcome was achieved and supporting data about the client's response are noted, and the entry is signed and dated

✦ Quality assurance programs evaluate excellence in nursing and health care by using outcome, structure, and process standards focusing on the client, the nurse, and the institution

Study Questions

1. Nursing care is evaluated through

   a. time management
   b. efficient use of equipment
   c. outcome data
   d. team cooperation

2. A consumer of health care may be all but one of the following

   a. the community
   b. the client's family
   c. the client
   d. the health provider

3. Evaluation occurs

   a. at the end of the nursing process
   b. whenever a nurse interacts with a client
   c. whenever a nurse interacts with a health care provider
   d. at the end of each shift

4. Which organizations have developed guidelines and standards for quality assurance in nursing practice?

   a. ANA and National League for Nursing (NLN)
   b. NLN and JCAHO
   c. ANA and JCAHO
   d. JCAHO and American Medical Association

5. When an outcome is completely met

   a. the short-term outcome, but not the long-term outcome, was met
   b. both the short-term and long-term outcomes were met
   c. the short-term outcome was not met, but the long-term outcome was met
   d. the short-term and long-term outcomes were not met

Critical Thinking Exercises

1. You develop a goal for Mr. Waltz to be able to walk 2 miles a day twice a week in 1 month. The client returns to the clinic and states that he is walking 1 mile once a week. State the changes in the nursing plan you would implement.

2. Discuss how evaluation of the nursing care plan affects quality assurance.

References

American Nurses' Association. (1973). *American Nurses' Association Standards of Practice*. Kansas City, MO: American Nurses' Association.

American Nurses' Association. (1975). *A plan for implementation of the Standards of Practice*. Kansas City, MO: American Nurses' Association.

Doenges, M. E., Townsend, M. C., & Moorhouse, M. F. (1989). *Psychiatric care plans: Guidelines for patient care*. Philadelphia: F. A. Davis.

Iyer, P. W., Taptich, B. J., & Bernocchi-Losey, D. (1991). *Nursing process and nursing diagnosis* (2nd ed.). Philadelphia: W. B. Saunders.

Joint Commission on the Accreditation of Hospitals (1983). *Accreditation manual for hospitals*. Chicago: The Joint Commission on the Accreditation of Hospitals.

Joint Commission on the Accreditation of Healthcare Organizations (1989a). *Accreditation manual for hospitals*. Chicago: Joint Commission on the Accreditation of Healthcare Organizations.

Joint Commission on the Accreditation of Healthcare Organizations (1992). *Accreditation manual for hospitals*. Chicago: Joint Commission on the Accreditation of Healthcare Organizations.

Joint Commission on the Accreditation of Healthcare Organizations (1989b). Characteristics of clinical indicators. *Quality Review Bulletin, 15*(11), 330–339.

Katz, J., & Green, E. (1992). *Managing quality: A guide to monitoring and evaluating nursing services*. St. Louis, MO: Mosby–Year Book.

Kenney, J. W. (1995). Implementation. In P. J. Christensen & J. W. Kenney: *Nursing process* (4th ed.). St. Louis, MO: C. V. Mosby.

Patterson, C. H. (1988). Standards of patient care: The Joint Commission's focus on nursing quality assurance. *Nursing Clinics of North America, 23*(3), 625–637.

Phaneuf, M. (1966). The nursing audit for evaluation of patient care. *Nursing Outlook, 14*(6), 51–54.

Bibliography

Castledine, G. (1987). The nursing process evaluated. *Geriatric Nursing and Home Care, 7*(1), 8.

Goldmann, R. C. (1990). Nursing process components as a framework for monitoring evaluation activities. *Journal of Nursing Quality Assurance, 4*(4), 17–25.

Hanson, M. H., Kennedy, F. T., Dougherty, L. L., & Baumann, L. J. (1990). Education in nursing: Evaluating clinical outcomes. *Journal of Continuing Education in Nursing, 21*(2), 79–85.

Lillesand, K. M., & Korff, S. (1983). Nursing process evaluation: A quality assurance tool. *Nursing Administration Quarterly, 7*(3), 9–14.

Pont, M. (1986). Last but not least . . . evaluation of the quality of care. *Nursing Times, 82*(41), 54–55.

Stanley, B. (1984). Evaluation of treatment goals: The use of goal attainment scaling. *Journal of Advanced Nursing, 9*(4), 351–356.

THE COMMUNICATION PROCESS

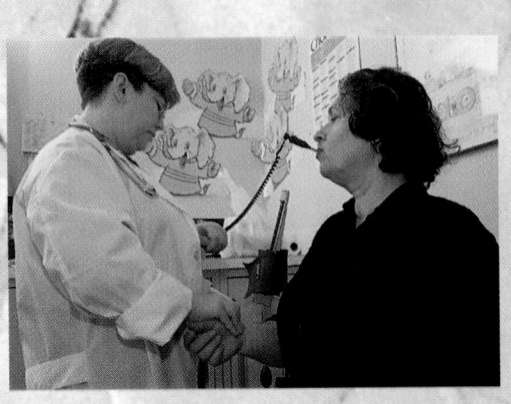

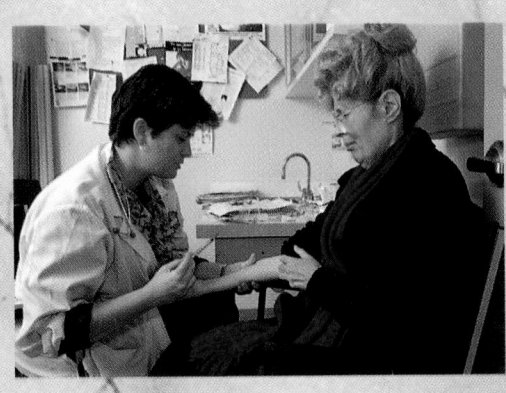

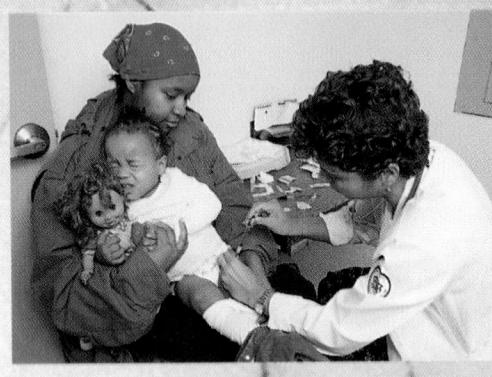

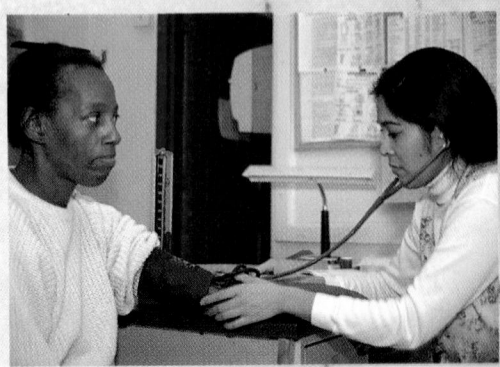

I have been a nurse practitioner for 17 years—the past 4 years at Dupage Community Clinic in Wheaton, Illinois. While in this position, I have provided primary health care to a homeless and low-income population. Although part of my role as a nurse practitioner is diagnostic and therapeutic, much of what I do in treating and preventing disease is through health education.

No matter what setting one practices in, the most important aspect of health education is viewing each client as an individual and creatively presenting the information in a way that is understandable and suitable to the client.

This approach requires the assessment of many factors, such as age, sex, educational level, cultural background, language, living conditions, family, and other support systems. These all play an important role in providing the proper treatment. For example, I can't tell a client from one of the local shelters who has a sprained ankle to go home, put his or her foot up and apply ice. He or she has no home and no ice and often walks quite a distance for a meal and overnight shelter.

At Dupage Community Clinic, we see people of many different cultures from all over the world. Some of our clients have no knowledge of basic health care issues. They are refugees from places where there is little food, sanitation, and health care. In this situation, you must begin with the fundamentals of health care. We also see people who were practicing physicians in their native countries and therefore have an advanced understanding of health care. It is very important to assess (consider) a client's level of existing health care knowledge before proper treatment can begin.

It can be very frustrating to health care providers to spend time doing health teaching while sensing a disbelief that it can produce results regarding how the client is feeling. Many people come to us only wanting a pill to cure their ills. However, it is incredibly satisfying when that same client returns a month later for a follow-up, after having adhered to the recommended changes, and sees visible results. All without a pill!

Educating our clients is an important responsibility. It should not get lost in the paperwork and other busyness of our practices.

Beth Smith, RN, NP

Beth Smith has been a nurse practitioner for the past 17 years. She has been working for the last 4 years at the Dupage Community Clinic in Wheaton, Illinois. The Dupage Community Clinic provides free primary health care to the homeless and low-income populations.

Chapter 13

CONCEPTS
OF BASIC
COMMUNICATION

✦

ELIZABETH ARNOLD, PhD, RN, CS

DARIA VIRVAN RN, CS, MSN

PATRICIA E. KIZILAY, EdD, RN, CS, FNP

KEY TERMS

✦

active listening
attending behaviors
body language
context
decoder (receiver)
educational groups
encoder (sender)
feedback
group
group cohesion
group culture
group dynamics
group goals
group process
group roles
group therapy
human reduction
language
leadership
maintenance roles
message
nontherapeutic communication techniques

nonverbal communication
paralanguage
personal space
positive listening
primary groups
secondary groups
sensory channel
support groups
talking
task groups
task role
therapeutic rapport
therapeutic relationship
 orientation phase
 termination phase
 working phase
unconditional positive regard
verbal communication
work groups
written communication

LEARNING OBJECTIVES

✦

After studying this chapter, you should be able to

✦ Identify the tasks associated with each of the three phases of the therapeutic relationship
✦ List the six elements of communication
✦ Identify how Peplau and Travelbee contributed to an understanding of the nurse, the client, and communication
✦ Identify the elements of body language and paralanguage
✦ Contrast therapeutic and nontherapeutic communication techniques
✦ List seven guidelines for the appropriate use of therapeutic techniques of communication
✦ Identify appropriate uses of communication in all phases of the nursing process
✦ Define what is meant by a group and contrast the nature of primary and secondary groups
✦ Identify different types of groups used in health care settings
✦ Define selected concepts related to group dynamics
✦ Describe how group process parallels the nursing process

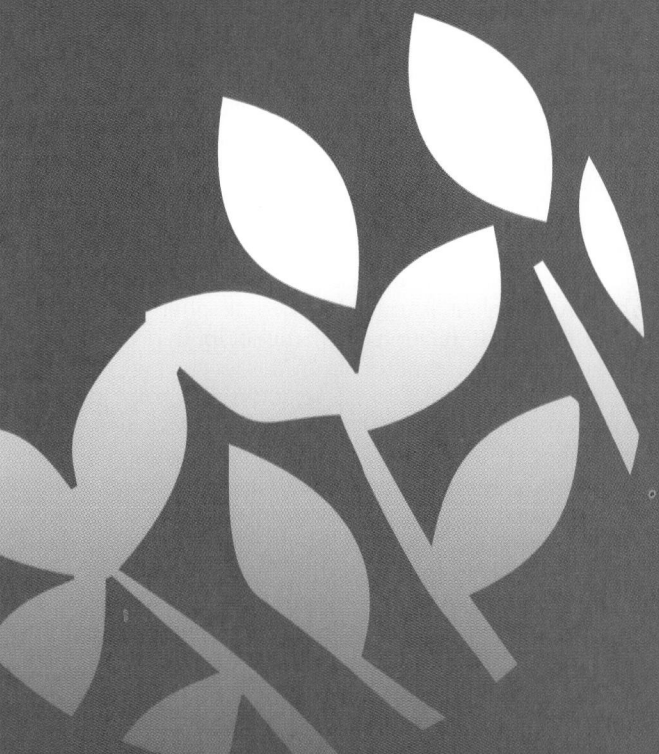

This chapter will orient you to beginning theories, principles, and techniques of therapeutic communication related to the nurse-client interactions with individuals and groups. Because you will be expected to use therapeutic communication techniques to work with individuals and groups throughout your professional life, it is vital that you begin to learn these skills early in your student experience. As beginning students, you will engage in a variety of experiences, directly with forethought or indirectly as part of the educational process. Like most skills you learn in nursing, you will continue to develop skill and will gain mastery of these techniques as you practice them in the clinical setting.

Practicing before you try the skills with actual clients and groups will help you to be more confident and lead to better outcomes. Interactions with clients, nurses, other health professionals, and families or caretakers is ongoing in the nurse's work environment. Your clinical conferences and group assignments will run more smoothly with an understanding of group dynamics and group process. In health care settings, effective group and individual communication is essential for optimal functioning.

The Therapeutic Relationship

A **therapeutic relationship** is a helping relationship. Nurses are helpers, and clients are those seeking help. A therapeutic relationship is personal, client focused, and aimed at realizing mutually determined goals.

In a therapeutic relationship, individuals who are seeking help bring their own life experiences, intelligence, achievements, values, beliefs, and motivations for change to the relationship. Nurses bring experience, understanding, and skills. The nurse and client can be viewed as unique systems that intersect on a common ground: the therapeutic nurse-client relationship.

A therapeutic relationship is not a social relationship. Although it is true that people often help each other in social relationships, the help that occurs in social relationships differs from that occurring in therapeutic relationships. Social relationships may involve an infinite range of nonspecific helping activities, such as driving a neighbor to the dentist or helping a person who is using a cane to push a grocery cart. Social helping such as this may result in the helper deriving more satisfaction from the interaction than the person being helped. Helping is often only a small part of a social relationship.

The help that occurs in the therapeutic relationship is the central activity of the relationship. The therapeutic relationship remains focused on eliciting the client's feelings, thoughts, and values and centers on achieving the client's goals.

Another difference between the social relationship and the therapeutic relationship is that the social relationship is more reciprocal, with both persons sharing personal beliefs, feelings, and opinions with each other. This is not true of the therapeutic relationship. Although the nurse may share some feelings with the client, this is not reciprocal sharing, and it is done only when appropriate for the benefit of the client.

For example, Mr. Jones is 84 years old and is reminiscing about his life. Nurse Blue is listening to him. Mr. Jones says, "I was never allowed to make my own choices because I had to obey my father." If Nurse Blue is truly therapeutic, which of the following replies would she make?

* "That's infuriating! I couldn't have lived like that!"
* "You felt restricted because ideas were different than they are now?"
* "People were so narrow-minded then. Thank goodness things have changed."

The first and third choices are excellent examples of social responses and represent the way people most often talk and support each other. However, it is the second response that is focused on the client and that is attempting to elicit further information and feelings that might lead to the client's being helped. In this case, the nurse has no helpful reason for sharing personal feelings with the client. Therefore, the second example is the therapeutic response.

Elements of the Therapeutic Relationship: The Nurse, the Client, and Communication

Three elements are present in all phases of the therapeutic relationship: the nurse, the client, and communication. As an element of the therapeutic relationship, the nurse is a helper who is trained in skills that facilitate client growth; the client is the person seeking help with personal growth; and communication is the meaningful interaction between the two that leads to growth. Before we discuss theories about the interactions among these three elements, let us discuss the elements of communication.

Elements of Communication

A widely accepted model for the communication process is depicted in Figure 13–1. This model consists of the following six elements:

Encoder (sender): This person initiates a transaction to exchange information, convey thoughts and feelings, or engage another.

Message: This is the content that the sender wishes another person (the receiver) to receive in the process of communication. The message must be encoded in a language of symbols or cues that are understandable to both sender and receiver.

Sensory channel: This is the means by which a mes-

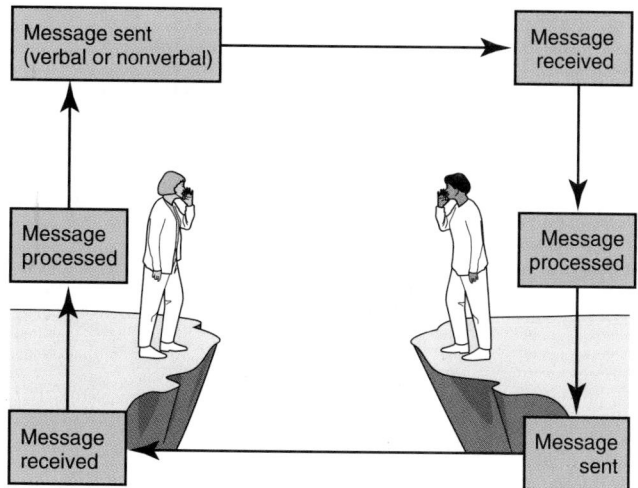

Figure 13–1
The six elements of communication.

sage is being sent. The three primary routes are the visual, auditory, and kinesthetic channels. Using these three channels, a wink, a tone of voice, or a hand gesture can all effectively convey a message without benefit of words.

Decoder (receiver): This is the person to whom the message is being aimed. This person must be able to decode the message sent so it is a clearly understood thought. If the message that the sender intends is what the receiver understands, then clear and effective communication has occurred.

Feedback: This is the process by which effectiveness of communication is determined.

Context: This is the condition under which a communication occurs.

Feedback is a process that is so important to communication that it deserves additional attention. Four types of feedback exist: internal, external, positive, and negative.

Internal feedback is a mechanism of self-perception. When we communicate, an inner critical assessment of what we have said or done is triggered. For example, if we make a verbal blunder, we react self-consciously after realizing our mistake. If, however, we communicate clearly what we meant, we feel pleased and satisfied with the effort.

External feedback is received from another or others, such as an audience. The response to the message sent gives information about how effectively we transmitted the message.

Positive feedback affirms our efforts to communicate by rewarding and reinforcing successful communication. If our messages are met with a smile or exclamation of relief, we feel good and continue to use those communication behaviors.

Negative feedback is a return message that our original message was poorly transmitted or received. This feedback tells us that modification is needed. However, there is more to negative feedback than just

a message telling us that our original message was garbled. Negative feedback may also be judgmental and can send us a negative opinion that has resulted from the message. For example, let us compare positive and negative feedback that might be received in response to the same message:

> Jill: "I can't meet with you as we had planned."
>
> Pat (providing positive feedback): "I'm sorry you can't make it—maybe some other time."
>
> Krista (providing negative feedback): "I'm sorry you think you can never eat lunch with me again. If you were a friend you'd find some time."

In both cases, the feedback given provided us with clear information about how the message was interpreted by the receiver.

It is important to note that both sender and receiver can seek feedback and clarify and qualify the message as necessary. For example, consider the following interaction between Mrs. Charl and her nurse, Mrs. Joanes, as Mrs. Joanes is completing Mrs. Charl's treatment:

> Mrs. Charl: "I felt so much better after my treatment yesterday."
>
> Mrs. Joanes (insulted that her treatment was being compared unfavorably with a treatment given by another nurse and seeking clarification): "Are you saying that you feel worse today after this bath than you felt yesterday, after the treatment Miss Lewis gave you?"
>
> Mrs. Charl (understanding that Mrs. Joanes has misunderstood): "Oh, not at all. I wasn't comparing her treatment to your treatment. I was comparing how I felt yesterday, before her treatment, with how I felt after her treatment. I had blood all over me from the accident and I felt so much better after it was cleaned off."

Had Mrs. Joanes not clarified what Mrs. Charl meant by "better," she might have left the interaction with negative feelings about Mrs. Charl and about her own ability to give a treatment. Suppose Mrs. Joanes had not sought clarification. The interaction might still have been saved by the process of seeking feedback. For example, it might have gone like this:

> Mrs. Charl: "I felt so much better after my treatment yesterday."
>
> Mrs. Joanes (obviously hurt): "I see."
>
> Mrs. Charl (seeking feedback): "What I said seems to bother you. Can you tell me what I said that upset you?"
>
> Mrs. Joanes: "When you say you felt better after Miss Lewis gave you a treatment than you feel today after your treatment I guess my feelings got a little hurt. I suppose I'm being childish, but I did think that I had done a good job."

With the receipt of this feedback about how her message was perceived, Mrs. Charl can clarify, as in the first interaction.

With these two examples, you can see how disruptive it can be to an interaction, and even to a relationship, if an unclear message is not clarified by seeking and receiving feedback or correction. It is unfortunate that the client had to be the one to seek feedback and to clarify in this situation, because this should be done by the nurse.

The nurse bears responsibility for keeping communications clear and therapeutic, and there are a number of ways to do this.

Factors That Influence Basic Communication

Developmental Differences

Communication techniques must be appropriate for the client's stage of development, or communication can be diminished. Examples of how to apply therapeutic techniques to children, adolescents, and adults of all ages have been provided in Box 13–1. For additional information on specific developmental stages, see Chapters 15 through 19.

Cultural Differences

Clients from different cultures may or may not speak a different language but most often have differing customs, values, mores, and social structures, all of which can affect communication. Obviously, the more you understand about the culture of your client, the better you will be able to communicate. Learning crucial words and sentences can be very helpful, as can having a translator write out cards with bilingual sentences. However, understanding the nonnative client requires more than just learning a few new phrases. You must be aware of any personal biases to avoid stereotyping and labeling clients. Respect for the client's experience and acceptance of the differences that exist between you can help to establish a safe, therapeutic environment in which maximum communication can occur.

Gender Differences

Men and women communicate differently, and understanding those differences enhances therapeutic relationships. Deborah Tannen, a linguistics professor, popular author, and communication expert, pointed out that men and women have different styles of intimacy and independence. According to Tannen, men seek dominance in a hierarchical structure to be dependent and subordinate but do not need to dominate. Intimacy to women means a free sharing of thoughts, hopes, and feelings. Men avoid such sharing to preserve personal freedom (Tannen, 1990).

The Hearing Impaired

Those who are hearing impaired have special problems to be overcome. Hearing loss can range from mild to profound. Clients may have been deaf or hard of hearing since birth, or they may have lost all of part of their hearing at a later time as a result of trauma, illness, or aging. The greatest incidence of

---

BOX 13–1

THREE PHASES OF COMMUNICATION AT VARIOUS DEVELOPMENTAL STAGES

Opening Phase

Nurse with child: "Let me sit with you for 15 minutes and read a story."

Nurse with adolescent: "I'd like to eat lunch with you."

Nurse with adult: "Let's walk to the cafeteria together."

Working Phase

Nurse with child: "I'm sorry, I can't give you a 'kissen' because I don't know what a kissen is. Is it like a hug and kiss?"

Nurse with adolescent: "I didn't understand what you meant. Can you say that in different words?"

Nurse with adult: "Let me repeat back to you what I think I heard you say."

Nurse with child: "Then what happened at school?"

Nurse with adolescent: "Please continue what you were saying."

Nurse with adult: "And . . . . ?"

Nurse with child: "You said you like your friend Laura the best. Can you tell me more about Laura?"

Nurse with adolescent: "You said you get more satisfaction out of helping out at the flower shop. I'd like to hear more about that."

Nurse with adult: "These dreams you mentioned, what are they like?"

Nurse with child: "You said you hate all of your brothers. Tell me about Melvin first."

Nurse with adolescent: "You've briefly mentioned two suicide attempts. For now, I'd like to focus on just what was going on with you at the time of the first attempt."

Nurse with adult: "Let's return to the last point that you made and talk more about that."

Terminating Phase

Nurse with child: "Okay, we agreed that you will take your medicine when the cartoons are over."

Nurse with adolescent: "In the past half hour we have talked about several possible ways you could handle this. There are . . ."

Nurse with adult: "When we first met, you were afraid you were never going to get over your depression. As we progressed, you began to take charge of your life. Now you are . . ."

---

hearing loss occurs in individuals 65 years of age and older.

Because hearing is especially important in decoding spoken messages, its loss presents a challenge to both nurse and client. The client with a profound hearing loss may have an inability to speak clearly or may have an excellent speaking ability, usually depending on whether the hearing loss occurred before or after speech was mastered. If speech is not understandable, the nurse will have difficulty decoding the client's messages.

If some residual hearing remains, the client usually wears a hearing aid. To increase communications with persons with hearing aids, be certain the aid is fine-tuned to the correct volume for the client, that the batteries in the aid are fresh, and that the aid is turned on.

For clients with aids or those who are unable to hear even with an aid, it is helpful if the nurse follows some basic guidelines:

* Assess the profoundly hearing impaired client for sign language skills. If the client uses signing, ascertain whether the client needs a sign language interpreter and obtain one, if available and necessary.
* Ensure that the client can see you as you speak by providing adequate lighting and by standing in front of the client.
* As you speak, enunciate words clearly as you would for any hearing person (*e.g.*, do not say "Jeet" when you mean "Did you eat?"), but do not exaggerate lip movements.
* When the client cannot understand you by reading your lips, try gestures, pantomime, or writing notes.
* Always have plenty of paper and pens available for notes.

Do not shout at a client who is hearing impaired. This can be painful to the ear canal and can actually result in additional loss of residual hearing. If the client has no residual hearing, he or she will not be able to hear you even if you do shout. Also, shouting causes distortion in your facial features that can prevent the client from reading your lips.

The Visually Impaired

Visually impaired clients receive messages via speech effectively but lose nonverbal communications such as facial expressions, body posture, hand gestures, and nods or shakes of the head. Visually impaired clients need support to negotiate new environments, and the nurse should describe new places to provide orientation.

Touch is often important to prevent feelings of isolation. Other senses should also be used, as necessary, to maximize communication, just as is true with sighted individuals.

The Dying

Clients who are dying have special communication needs. Depending on the cause of impending death and the stage of dying, the client may be fearful, in pain, and unable to communicate or totally calm, oriented, and able to participate.

Soft voice tones, gentle touch, and soft lighting may increase the client's comfort and reduce anxiety. Also, it is often comforting to have significant others near when possible and desired by the client. They may be needed to interpret for the client.

Respect, empathy, acceptance, and flexibility are particularly important qualities for the nurse to bring to the interaction. Dying is private, and the nurse should accede to the client's wishes as much as possible. Remind family members and friends that hearing is the last sense to be lost before death is final, so they may continue to speak to the client even when a response is not possible.

Personal Distances

We all have a **personal space** (a private zone or "bubble" around our body that we believe is an extension of ourselves and belongs to us). We carry this space with us at all times wherever we go. Except for a very select number of other persons whom we allow to enter this space at certain times, we tend to be uncomfortable if others enter this space at all. Therefore, we behave in ways to prevent this from happening. At certain times and in certain situations, the space grows larger, and to maintain comfort, most people must stay even farther away from us than usual.

The size of this space appears to be at least partially culturally determined and can vary considerably from culture to culture. Persons within each culture respect each other's personal space and use culturally determined body language signals to help maintain appropriate distances from each other. Although individuals vary in their need for space, in our own Western culture, most persons maintain similar distances from each other according to their relationships and to the activities involved. As an example, two men who are strangers on opposing teams might grapple together on a football field when they would never think of allowing their bodies to come into contact in the shower after the game. See Figure 13–2 for the generally accepted levels of personal space in our culture as these might be seen in nursing situations.

In our culture, if one person feels that a second person is coming too close, the first person tends to back away to maintain the desired distance between the two. In fact, backing away should not be necessary, and any subtle movement of the body in the backward direction should send the same signal—"stop. You are getting into my bubble." The second person should read this body language, stop approaching the person, and back off slightly to adjust the distance between the two to a more comfortable level. Consider this when you approach a client who is in bed. Remember that the mattress prevents the client from backing away from you and be aware of subtle client movements, such as tucking in of the chin or a tensing of the muscles, that indicate discom-

Personal Space

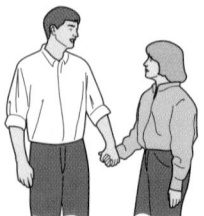

Intimate distance
0.0–1.5 ft
Close physical contact

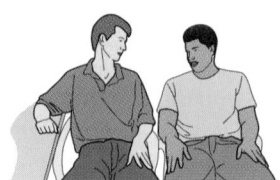

Personal distance
1.5–4.0 ft
Less intimate contact

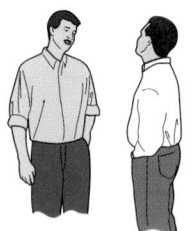

Social distance
4–12 ft
Conversational/
social contact

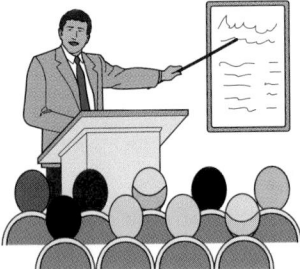

Public distance
12 ft or more
Reserved for
impersonal contact

❥ **Figure 13–2**
Four levels of personal space.

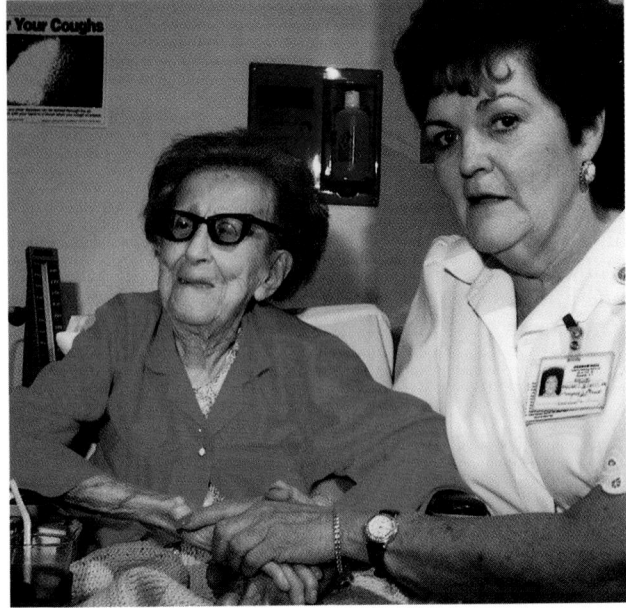

❥ **Figure 13–3**
Nurse comforts older client by holding her hand.

fort as you approach and interact with the client. Usually, the edges of the mattress are the client's outermost boundaries in such a case.

Touch

Nurse-client touching is an issue that requires much sensitivity on the part of the nurse. Because nursing is a hands-on profession, it is our daily practice to touch persons often and intimately. However, we must constantly be aware that touch has many meanings to our clients. It may indicate such things as agreement, caring, loving, or even sexual desire.

Many clients are hungry for a hand clasp or other form of human touch and will demonstrate this by reaching out to you. Most desire or feel neutral about such touching as a pat on the arm during the course of normal conversation. However, clients who have been physically or sexually abused tend to see uninvited touch as a boundary violation.

If a client has not indicated a specific desire to touch or be touched, you should assess the client's feelings about touch before using it. A rule of thumb is to ask permission before touching. It is easy to ask, "May I touch your arm?", and asking can avoid possible problems. In certain settings, it is appropriate to say, "I'd like to give you a hug. May I?" (Fig. 13–3).

Touch may be accepted more or less readily in different situations. A nurse's hug, for example, may be greeted with relief by a family member in a hospice when support is needed most, whereas it would probably be looked on as a violation of personal space in an initial meeting with a client in a clinic. Touch has different meanings within different communications. It can soothe or disturb us to our very depths. Therefore, it must be used judiciously based on assessment of the client's needs and wishes.

Phases of the Therapeutic Relationship

Therapeutic relationships develop and evolve over a period of time. The time may be brief, or it may extend over weeks, months, or even years. Regardless of the length of time, three distinct phases to the relationship exist: the orientation phase, the working phase, and the termination phase. Because relationships are fluid, the phases flow into each other, but each phase may be recognized by the tasks associated with it.

Orientation Phase

During the **orientation phase** of the therapeutic relationship the nurse and client make an agreement that they will be working together to solve one or more of the client's problems. This phase represents an oral contract between nurse and client. It signals the initiation of a working relationship. This part of the relationship is the basis for the work they will do together in the future.

As you enter into a relationship with a client, it is helpful to be aware of the personal feelings that can arise at these times. Both nurse and client may experience anxiety and discomfort during this phase. As the nurse, you may feel inadequate. The client may feel unsure about you and may need to know that you are willing and able to help.

A primary goal of the orientation phase is the establishment of trust. Trust is enhanced when the nurse connects with the client in a respectful and nonintrusive manner that conveys personal consideration and concern.

Your consideration and concern give the client confidence in you. It is not necessary that you know all there is to know about everything. That would be impossible. Anyone knows that no one human being knows everything. If you try to pretend that you know more than you do, you will fool no one, and the client's trust in you will drop precipitously.

Honesty and enthusiasm are helpful in establishing trust. These two traits are shown in responses such as, "I don't know the answer right now, but I will ask and let you know in an hour" or "I can't promise I can help solve your problem, but I can listen and I do care."

Trust is also promoted when the nurse establishes confidentiality as a ground rule for the relationship. However, you must be careful with promises about confidentiality. Sometimes, in a desire to have the client trust us, we are tempted to promise complete confidentiality and then are placed in a dilemma when the client confides something that must be told to others for the client's protection or for the protection of others. For example, what would you do if you pledged unconditional confidentiality to a client only to have her confide that she has a gun and is contemplating shooting her son and then committing suicide? If you do not tell someone, you are left alone to deal with the possibility of two deaths. If you do tell, you have broken your word and violated the client's trust.

Recall from Chapter 3 that confidentiality may be regarded as an ethical obligation to share health care information about a person only with other persons who have a need to know the person's health status. The phrase "only with other persons who have a need to know the person's health status" is key.

Do not promise that you will never tell anyone about anything that occurs between you and your clients. You may safely promise that you will maintain respect for client privacy and will not share anything with anyone else unless another person has a need to know. It is important to tell your clients that you cannot maintain confidentiality if doing so would endanger the health and well-being of themselves or others.

Such a pledge should make clients feel that you will protect them and not allow them to hurt themselves or others. If clients feel safe, they will feel a sense of trust, and the relationship will be reinforced.

During the orientation phase, the nurse is responsible for establishing the ground rules for the relationship. If you will be meeting with a client a number of times, it is important to specify clearly where, when, and for how long each meeting will be. For example, Mrs. Flynn, a primary nurse, might say, "As your primary nurse, I will be following your care very carefully and would like to meet with you routinely throughout your stay here in the hospital. Would you agree to meet with me every weekday for 15 minutes, between 10:15 and 10:30, here in your room? I will not be here on weekends, but Mr. Carlsong can meet with you on Saturdays and Sundays at the same time."

As you establish meeting times and places, honesty and achievability are paramount. Do not promise what you may not be able to do. It is better if the client can rely on meeting with you for 15 minutes each day than for you to promise 30-minute sessions that may not be possible.

At any time after your initial contact, you may begin to feel a bond with the client. This bond, termed **therapeutic rapport,** is a special bond that exists between nurse and client because they have established a sense of trust and a mutual understanding of what will occur in their relationship with each other.

It is during the orientation phase that the nursing process begins. At this stage, the nursing process consists of collecting assessment data, making preliminary nursing diagnoses, and formulating an initial plan of care.

Working Phase

Once rapport has been established with the client and the therapeutic relationship has been structured, the **working phase** (middle phase) of the relationship begins. In the working phase, the nurse participates actively in further client assessment and in examining and exploring data found. Covert client feelings, values, beliefs, and attitudes are sought out and examined.

Often during this phase, initial nursing diagnoses are corrected, or additional nursing diagnoses are formulated. However, the working phase of the therapeutic relationship is mainly a time for completing nursing outcomes. The nurse responds to the client. It is a time when the nurse presents information to the client and helps to validate and clarify client understandings. Rather than directing a client, the nurse attempts to help him or her become self-directed. It is a time when the client can formulate, try, and test solutions to his or her emotional problems. Evaluation also occurs in this phase of the relationship, and, when necessary, the plan is revised.

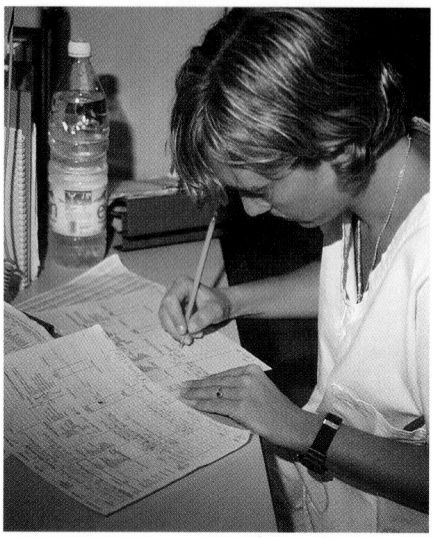

❄ **Figure 13–4**
Nurse documenting nursing care.

Termination Phase

The **termination phase** of the therapeutic relationship occurs near the end of the relationship when the work of the client and nurse is coming to a close. The termination itself should not be abrupt and unexpected because it is acknowledged from the beginning of the relationship. Recall the example given in the orientation phase, in which the primary nurse, Mrs. Flemming, said, "As your primary nurse, I will be following your care very carefully and would like to meet with you routinely throughout your stay here in the hospital." This was not a meaningless pleasantry. It was a way of clarifying exactly when the relationship would end. The nurse did not say she wanted to meet with the client "every weekday" and leave it at that. No one should have interpreted her offer to meet with the client as extending beyond the hospital stay. Therefore, the nurse was saying, in effect, "I will be meeting with you only until you are discharged." Such communications help to set up clear expectations from the onset of the relationship.

Although the end of the relationship is planned, it is still often difficult to end a meaningful interaction. Both nurse and client understand that this phase precedes a possibly permanent separation, and both may experience anxiety, sadness, and a sense of loss.

The client's reaction to the termination is determined by the meaning assigned to it, the length of the relationship, and how or whether outcomes were achieved. Clients may display denial and regret and may engage in acting-out behaviors (inappropriate or unexpected client behaviors that communicate a message to the nurse about the client's true or subconscious feelings and concerns). Acting-out behaviors frequently seen in the termination phase include refusal to talk during meetings with the nurse, missing appointments with the nurse, and increased forgetful-

ness. At such times, the nurse may help the client to recognize feelings about saying good-by while pointing out positive changes that have occurred during the relationship. It may be helpful to offer support and express optimism for the future. At the same time, it is important to be clear about ending the relationship without offering false hope for continuation. This is often uncomfortable for the new nurse but offers the client clear boundaries and expectations.

Theories Concerning the Nurse, the Client, and Communication

Several theorists have provided us with a better understanding of the nurse, the client, and communication and of the interaction among these elements in a therapeutic relationship. Here we look only at selected examples.

Hildegard Peplau

Hildegard Peplau, a psychiatric nurse and one of the first nurse theorists, identified the following six roles assumed by the nurse (in relation to the client) within a therapeutic relationship (Peplau, 1952):

* The stranger: This role is shared by both nurse and client entering into the therapeutic relationship. The nurse offers the client respect, interest, and acceptance in a nonpersonal manner. The client is assumed to be emotionally intact unless conflicting evidence arises.
* The resource: In the resource role, the nurse helps the consumer-client to negotiate the health care system by providing care and offering answers to specific questions.
* The teacher: In the role of teacher, the nurse educates the client and helps him or her understand and use experiences within the health care system.
* The leader: In the leader role, the nurse helps the client, as follower, to contribute to and participate in a democratic nursing process.
* The surrogate: As a surrogate parent figure, the nurse helps the client to resolve interpersonal problems that need to be safely worked out in the presence of an understanding other. The nurse provides the client with a corrective interpersonal experience.
* The counselor: In the counselor role, the nurse helps to integrate both reality and the client's emotional responses associated with illness into the total life experience.

Peplau believed that a nurse who related with a client in a healthy way could provide a corrective interpersonal experience for the client. She believed that the experience of a positive relationship with the nurse would allow for healthier relationships with others. She encouraged nurses to promote trust in their relationships by relating to their clients in an authentic manner by sharing feelings and thoughts appropriately. For example, note how Miss Brown, a baby's nurse, shares her feelings with the baby's father, Mr. Dunne, when he learns that his infant daughter has died of sudden infant death syndrome. He is red eyed and shaking but unable to verbalize his feelings:

> Miss Brown (making eye contact with Mr. Dunne): "This is a hard time for you."
>
> Mr. Dunne: Starts to cry but remains silent.
>
> Miss Brown (wiping her eyes): "I feel very sad too, Mr. Dunne. It doesn't seem fair to lose a baby without warning."

Peplau noted that closeness in a therapeutic relationship builds trust, increases the client's self-esteem, and leads to new personal growth for the client (Peplau, 1952).

Joyce Travelbee

Joyce Travelbee pointed out that the nurse is a human being who is vulnerable to stereotypes, labels, and generalizations. Travelbee noted that it is not possible for a stereotype (of a nurse) to relate to another stereotype (of a client) in a human way. Take, for example, Miss Lois, a nurse working with elderly clients. Miss Lois believes that older people are less mentally astute and have poorer hearing than younger people. She also thinks that nurses are poorly paid and that elderly people should be grateful for whatever nursing care they receive. Miss Lois is assigned to care for Mr. Allan, an alert 76-year-old man who is recovering from a stroke that impaired his mobility. Miss Lois enters his room, and the following dialogue takes place:

> Miss Lois: "Hi, Mr. Allan, it's time for us to take our walk today."
>
> Mr. Allan: "I think I can use the walker alone this morning."
>
> Miss Lois (in an aside to another nurse): "This guy is crazy if he thinks I'm going to lose my license over this." (to Mr. Allan): "No, sweetie, I'm going to help. Now let's get this show on the road. I have eight other people to take care of this morning."

Not only has Miss Lois failed to relate to Mr. Allan as another human being who is deserving of respect and consideration, but also she has rendered other nurses vulnerable to being labeled as callous, rude, and insensitive.

Travelbee noted that one nursing goal is to change the distorted beliefs others have about nurses and nursing. According to Travelbee, the client is the help seeker whose overt and covert needs are the focus of the therapeutic relationship. She proposed that understanding the individual client's experience is paramount and that individuals cannot be known if their uniqueness is not appreciated. The task for the nurse, then, is to see the individual "with fresh eyes" and without labeling or stereotyping (Travelbee, 1966).

An important component of Travelbee's theory concerns the process of **human reduction** (Travelbee, 1966). This term is synonymous with the word *dehumanization*. The term refers to viewing the client as other than a human being. Viewing the client as an illness ("the heart attack in 210"), a task ("the bed bath and dressing change on Team B"), or a stereotype ("all amputees") are three examples of human reduction. It is only in overcoming assigned labels that nurses and clients can relate humanly and a therapeutic relationship be established.

Travelbee believed that the human-to-human relationship allows nurses to help individuals and families cope with illness and to find meaning in the experience. She recognized that each interaction has differences and similarities that prohibit forming rigid rules of action but that do permit the nurse to develop skill as a communicator (Travelbee, 1966).

Types of Communication

There are generally two types of communication: verbal and nonverbal. Each type has several components.

Verbal Communication

Verbal communication is the use of words to convey messages. This type of communication is achieved by writing or speaking in a code mutually understood by sender and receiver. The tool of verbal communication is language. **Language** is a set of words that have meanings that are comprehensible within a group. However, the fact that a word has a definition does not guarantee that its meaning will be interpreted in the same way by all group members. For example, in the English language, the word *hot* could mean "very warm," "stolen," or "attractive to members of the opposite sex." It is important, therefore, to validate meaning between nurse and client.

Talking is the act of verbalizing symbols to convey thoughts, feelings, or ideas. It is a skill so taken for granted that we feel helpless to communicate without it.

Written communication transfers a thought or spoken symbol into printed form. Being able to communicate accurately and clearly in writing is critical for nurses (*e.g.,* in documenting nursing care). It can be especially useful in communicating with clients who are unable to hear or speak clearly, if at all. If you communicate with clients by writing, you should communicate as clearly as if you were speaking to the person. For example, it is important that you use clear language, use an appropriate vocabulary, and speak at the client's level of understanding. Correct spelling is vital to clear written communication. Here are two examples of correct and incorrect written communication:

Correct: "Are you having trouble breathing?"

Incorrect: "Are your respirations labored or are you experiencing any other form of dyspnea?"

Correct: "Are you hoarse?"

Incorrect: "Are you horse?"

Obviously, in the first example, the language in the incorrect case is at too high a level of understanding for most laypersons and could lead to a breakdown in communication. The spelling error in the second example might not only cause the message to be misunderstood, but it could also cause the client to lose faith in the abilities of the nurse who cannot spell correctly.

When communicating with clients in writing, you should ensure that your printing is large enough and dark enough to be legible, that the room lighting is conducive to reading, and that the client is wearing reading glasses, if needed. Clients with visual defects could be completely frustrated if they cannot see, hear, or speak.

Nonverbal Communication

Nonverbal communication is the set of behaviors that convey messages either without words or by supplementing verbal communication. Nonverbal communication consists of body language, paralanguage, and any other means by which we communicate with each other without the use of words. As health care professionals, we are mainly concerned with body language and paralanguage.

Body language refers to nonverbal communication behaviors that are accomplished by how we move our bodies or body parts, present ourselves to the world, and use the personal space around us. Thus, personal appearance; conscious and unconscious changes in facial expressions, body posture, and gestures; the distances we maintain from others; and how we touch others are among the common body language behaviors we use and observe daily.

Paralanguage refers to nonverbal components of spoken language. These components give speech its rhythm and humanness and include stress, accent, pitch, pause, intonation, rate, volume, and quality.

As nurses, we frequently look at nonverbal behavior when we assess and evaluate our clients. Take, for example, the case of Mr. Goldmann. His body language shows that he is red faced, sweating profusely, clenching and unclenching his fists, and pacing the length of the hall. His paralanguage consists of mumbling inaudibly most of the time, with occasional outbursts of loud sounds resembling "Phah!" When asked what is troubling him, he shouts answers such as, "I'm fine. You don't have to concern yourself with me!" Obviously, his verbal message clashes with the way he says it and with all of his other nonverbal messages. Most nurses would surmise that this client is truly angry and agitated despite his protests. Similarly, a client who is sitting calmly and who has no readable facial expressions but who laughlingly tells you that he is "furiously angry" is providing verbal and nonverbal cues that do not match. The nurse who assesses clients who demonstrate incongruent verbal and nonverbal behaviors should make further inquiries to determine their actual emotional status.

Nursing Attitudes That Promote Communication

Before making an attempt to enter into a therapeutic relationship, it is helpful to know the nursing attitudes that facilitate effective therapeutic communication. These are sometimes referred to as responsive characteristics.

Awareness

Awareness of clients is necessary before human relationships with them are possible. Showing awareness is acknowledging the presence of clients. It is best demonstrated by displaying attending behaviors.

Attending behaviors show that the nurse is paying attention to what the client is saying. The nurse demonstrates attending behaviors, for example, by facing the client, leaning toward the client, using appropriate eye contact, keeping eyes open with eyebrows raised, and maintaining an open body posture, a body position in which the arms and legs are uncrossed.

Acceptance, Respect, and Unconditional Positive Regard

Acceptance is an openness to the unique qualities and attributes of individual clients. Acceptance does not mean condoning inappropriate client behaviors. It means that clients are accepted for the persons they are, even if their behavior is undesirable.

Respect is more than an attitude of acceptance. It also includes valuing, highly regarding, or esteeming clients for what they are.

Unconditional positive regard, coined by the psychologist Carl Rogers, describes respect that is not dependent on the client's behavior. For example, as nurses, many of us can value and care for clients because their humanity warrants our care.

This is appropriate because nurses should not be critical, derogatory, or judgmental. We should understand the client's imperfections as part of the total picture, and those behaviors that are undesirable can be understood to be coping mechanisms that the client needs at the time. Many clients struggle with dehumanizing aspects of illness and dependency. Nurses empower clients by showing respect and by appreciating their humanness without ridiculing or demeaning them.

Another reason why the nurse should not judge

the client is simply that the client should not view the nurse as a judge. Judgment by the nurse sets up a relationship in which the client seeks to please the nurse. This diverts attention from the real business at hand, which is to focus on the client's health and growth.

Empathy

Empathy is the accurate perception of the client's feelings. It is the experience of "being in the other person's shoes" without taking on the client's feelings or thoughts. Empathy is not sympathy, wherein the nurse feels sorry for the client. Rather, it is a sense of "being with" the client.

Relatedness

Relatedness is the experience of recognizing similarities between nurse and client and the forging of emotional connections based on them. Relating to clients helps to establish human-to-human ties that make communication possible.

Caring

Caring is feeling a personal interest in the client's welfare. By investing ourselves in the client, we consciously decide to take emotional risks and give of our skills, compassion, and experience. Such concern can be draining, and the nurse must continually assess personal psychic energy and emotional resources to prevent exhaustion.

Objectivity

Objectivity is a reality-based sense of the communication process that allows the nurse to attend to the client's thoughts and feelings over his or her own. To be truly objective does not rob the nurse of warmth or feelings for the client, but it does require the nurse to attach an evaluative component to the relationship. Thinking about the client objectively allows the nurse to understand client experiences and to identify areas of difficulty so the client can be guided toward developing appropriate problem-solving skills.

Protectiveness

Protectiveness leads the nurse to shield the fragile and vulnerable client while he or she recovers from illness. A fine line exists between protectiveness and fostering dependence. Protectiveness is a caring attitude that should be judiciously used while continuing to evaluate the client's capacity to defend the self.

Genuineness

Genuineness is the ability of the nurse to be honest, open, and sincere in self-presentation. The phrase "what you see is what you get" describes the demeanor of a genuine person. It is important not to confuse being genuine with being totally self-disclosing or casually spontaneous, as one would be with friends or family.

Openness

Being open with a client reflects the ability and willingness of the nurse to be real, genuine, and emotionally accessible. Openness does not mean that boundaries are violated. It means that the nurse chooses what to share with the client and shares it in an authentic manner. When the nurse is open with a client, the client tends to lower defenses and to relate more honestly with the nurse.

Professional Closeness or Distance

A delicate balance exists between maintaining the objectivity and firm boundaries associated with professional distance and the warmth, openness, and availability associated with professional closeness.

Nurses should be accessible to the clients, but the therapeutic relationship is not a friendship. Friendships are social rather than therapeutic relationships. This does not mean, however, that nurses must be impersonal or treat clients with indifference.

Professional closeness and distance vary throughout the relationship as nurses and clients come together as strangers, work on mutual goals, and proceed to termination. New nurses may feel uncomfortable with attempts at maintaining professional closeness and distance. A good rule to follow is to become invested without being engulfed. This guideline translates to caring about clients and allowing yourself to know their concerns but not taking their thoughts, feelings, or attitudes as your own.

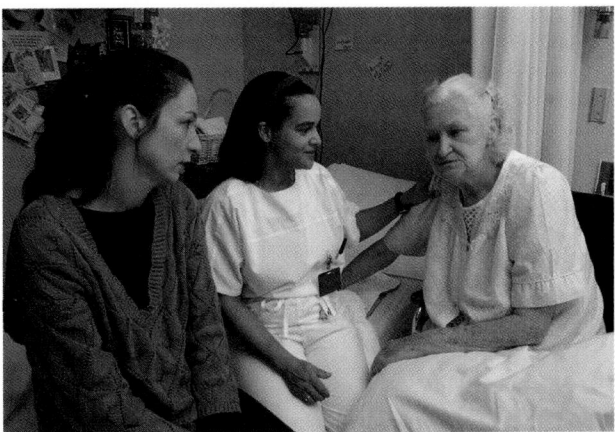

♦ Figure 13–5
Nurse spends time visiting with older client and daughter.

Sense of Humor

Many have questioned the appropriateness of the use of any form of humor in a therapeutic relationship. Surely, we must avoid certain types of "humor" such as morbid humor, humor based on sarcasm, or humor that degrades anyone. This type of material is not funny and is beneath us as professionals. However, we must be open to laugh at ourselves and at the humorous situations that can arise. Being a role model of this openness and demonstrating the appropriate use of humor can be therapeutic for clients, just as it is for ourselves.

Thus, appreciation of the humor in life can be a desirable attitude for the nurse. However, the ability to use humor therapeutically is a talent that not all nurses possess. Nurses who are comfortable with the sensitive use of humor can sometimes use it to put clients at ease, defuse emotionally loaded situations, or simply inject a light note into an otherwise difficult day. Such nurses must assess each client's readiness for humor. If the client perceives levity as a put-down, it is much better to maintain a more serious demeanor.

Although clients can appreciate wit as much as anyone, they must first feel that the nurse is trustworthy, dependable, and on their side.

Action-Oriented Characteristics

In addition to the responsive attitudes discussed previously, the nurse who is to be effective in therapeutic communications must possess three action-oriented characteristics. These characteristics must be used with the responsive attitudes if they are to be effective without alienating the client.

Concreteness

Concreteness refers to communicating concerns in specific and personal language. The nurse can help the client be concrete by role modeling concreteness and by asking the client to remain in the "here and now" during discussions.

The concrete nurse discourages vague or general references to events and seeks information as explicitly as possible. For example, rather than inviting a client to "tell me all about yourself," the nurse might ask the client to "tell me how that affects you personally at this time." Concreteness helps keep communications clear and helps the client cope with experiences in measurable terms.

Immediacy

Immediacy requires direct attention to the specific dynamics existing within the relationship between the nurse and client. If a nurse has difficulty working with a client or if tension exists in the relationship, it is easier to ignore the conflict and avoid the client. However, this models avoidance for the client and provides no assistance in negotiating human relationships.

To practice immediacy, the nurse speaks with the client to attempt to elicit information about what is interfering with their interactions. For instance, if the nurse had previously reminded the client that it was nearing time for terminating their relationship and the client refused to talk to the nurse after that, the nurse might say, "I've noticed that we've been pretty quiet around each other since our last meeting. I wonder what's going on between us that makes it difficult for us to talk." Note that the nurse does this without focusing on the client or the nurse. Rather the focus is on what is occurring between the two.

Confrontation

Confrontation is the process in which the nurse sensitively points out inconsistencies in a client's behavior. Confrontation is not angry, attacking, or demeaning. Nor should it be used before trust is established. In a therapeutic relationship, the nurse uses confrontation to enlighten the client about inconsistencies in verbal and nonverbal behaviors. For example, the nurse might say, "Your jaw is clenched tight and you are wringing your hands, but you told me you were calm. Now I am wondering what it is you really feel."

Techniques That Enhance Therapeutic Communication

Maximizing therapeutic communication requires the use of techniques that encourage clients to open up and speak more freely. A number of such therapeutic techniques of communication are generally considered helpful for nurses to use. However, inappropriate use of these techniques can turn them from therapeutic techniques to nontherapeutic techniques, so it is helpful to know what to do and what not to do when using them. Some guidelines follow:

- Individualize each technique to your client's level of understanding. For example, you might tell a 30-year-old man, "I'd like some private time with you to focus on some of your personal issues and concerns," whereas, you'd ask a 6-year-old boy, "Can we talk a while, Timmy?"
- Vary the therapeutic techniques used. Particularly avoid using any one type of technique repeatedly. For example, saying, "I see" shows acceptance of what the client is saying and is therapeutic. However, saying "I see" after everything the client says will quickly show that you are not giving a thoughtful response to each utterance. Too many "I see's" (or any other therapeutic technique) can be maddening.

• Use paralanguage appropriately to convey your intended meaning. For example, you may say something generally considered to be therapeutic, such as "I see," but say it sarcastically, icily, or in some other way so as to be nontherapeutic. Another nurse may say something generally considered to be nontherapeutic but say it so warmly and with such caring that it is actually therapeutic for the client. Two nurses may say the exact same words, and one is seen as a helpful nurse, whereas the other is not. In such cases, it may be paralanguage that makes the difference.

• If you are using therapeutic techniques correctly, your client will be doing most of the talking as you listen and guide the interaction. If you find that you are doing most of the talking, something is wrong and you need to pause and reflect about how to get back on track.

• You will probably make mistakes in talking with clients and say some things that are not the best possible responses. In fact, there may be times you will want to bite your tongue off because you said something so nontherapeutic. However, if you have a genuinely therapeutic relationship with the client, the relationship will be able to withstand an error or two.

• As you enter the clinical area to talk with a client for the first time, relax and realize that most clients want very much to talk to you.

• Any specific technique of communication might be used at any time, according to the client and the situation, but some techniques tend to be more helpful at the beginning of an interaction and some tend to be more helpful in the middle or at the end of an interaction.

One Technique That Must Occur Throughout the Interaction: Active Listening

Listening is how we receive spoken and other auditory information. Listening is an integral part of communication. **Positive listening** is simply understanding the auditory messages sent by a sender. It can be tremendously comforting to be listened to when we are lonely, frightened, and doubtful. In **active listening,** the nurse takes an active part by eliciting details from the client and by inviting the client to think more about what is being said. It goes beyond positive listening.

Active listening is a means of "being with" the client and indicating acceptance and agreement. It is an art. It is the key to therapeutic interaction. To use it, you must understand and use all of the other therapeutic techniques of communication.

Techniques Often Helpful at the Beginning of an Interaction

Offering Self

Offering self is a technique in which the nurse offers to stay with the client and either talk or just sit quietly. In offering self, the nurse clearly establishes parameters for the amount of time offered; for example, "I have 20 minutes available to talk with you at 1 o'clock today" or "I'll stay with you while you wait for the surgeon."

In some cases, it is therapeutic to give the person a choice about your offer; for example, "Would you like to meet with me for 20 minutes at 1 o'clock today?" However, some persons, such as those who are depressed, very much need to have you with them but will tend to reject your offer. Others should not be asked to make decisions about anything because it raises their anxiety level. As you learn more and more about such persons and their individual needs, you will learn who can be asked and who should just be told that you are there for them. Until you do know, or if you are ever in doubt, it is always safe to offer without allowing a choice.

Offering self can be very helpful when you are talking with someone who seems unable to express his or her thoughts or who does not want to talk at the moment. You can say something like, "It is okay if you don't feel like talking right now, I'll just stay here with you for 10 minutes." Be sure that if you say you will stay for a period of time, you do follow through and stay for as long as you said you would. This helps establish you as someone who can be trusted.

Providing Broad Openings

Early in a meeting with a client, it may be useful to provide a broad opening. In this case, the nurse invites the client to select a topic for discussion. Here too, it is therapeutic to set some parameters in regard to what you are willing to discuss. For example, in most instances, it would not be helpful for the client to discuss personal information about you or for you to engage in social-level small talk with the client. Therefore, it is not always appropriate to say, "We can talk about anything you like." It is better to say, for example, "We can discuss any issues of concern to you." The latter is a very broad opening that still focuses on the client.

Making an Observation

In making an observation, the nurse acknowledges that something or someone exists or has changed in some way. The nurse makes an observation without appearing to judge either positively or negatively. When the observation pertains to the client, this technique may be termed *giving recognition.* However, the term *recognition* is less desirable because it may be misconstrued to mean that the client is receiving approval or praise from the nurse. The acknowledgment made by the nurse who is making an observation should open up communication about the subject at hand but not provide the client with any specific positive reinforcement.

Suggesting Collaboration

Suggesting collaboration is a technique in which the nurse offers to work together with the client. This technique is useful in beginning a relationship with a client because it establishes that the nurse and client will work together as a team. Initially, the work may be to discuss some of the issues of concern to the client. Later, as problems are identified and nursing diagnoses made, the work may be to establish and meet client outcomes. At all times, the work focuses on the client.

Techniques Often Helpful as an Interaction Progresses

Providing Silence

Providing silence in a therapeutic manner is allowing the verbal conversation to stop to provide a time for quiet contemplation of what has been discussed or for formulation of thoughts about how to proceed. This can also provide a time for tension reduction when the interaction has been concerned with powerful issues and when emotions have been particularly deep.

Many persons are uncomfortable with silence and will talk continuously about nothing just to break it. This is obviously not a therapeutic approach for the nurse to take. If you find that you are uncomfortable with silence, think about what is going on during the silence, and use it constructively to think about what you will say next. You will find that, with practice, you can become more and more comfortable with silence.

Accepting Messages

Accepting messages is a way of providing feedback to acknowledge to the client that the nurse has heard and understood what has been said. The acknowledgment is done in a manner that is neutral in tone, without the nurse agreeing, disagreeing, or providing any judgments about the message. The accepting may be done verbally or nonverbally. Your method of accepting messages should be brief and should allow the client to continue on with a train of thought without any real interruption.

Providing General Leads

In ordinary social communications, people are used to taking turns in communicating. Therefore, after your clients have spoken for a while, they may hesitate because they are uncertain whether it is appropriate to continue, or they may try to draw you into the conversation to give you "your turn." It is the nurse's task to keep clients focused on their own issues and to ensure that they continue to feel comfortable discussing them. To do this, you may use the technique of providing general leads. General leads are brief interjections that let clients know that they are on the right track and should continue. The leads provided should not cause real interruptions in the train of thought as they urge clients forward.

Exploring

As clients are talking, they may mention something that you believe is significant enough to warrant further attention. If they have brought the subject up and have not indicated that further discussion is undesirable, it is appropriate to attempt to delve into the matter in greater detail. To do this, the nurse uses the technique of exploring. To explore, you ask the client to describe something in more detail or to discuss it more fully.

When you use exploring with clients, be careful not to use the nontherapeutic technique of probing. That is, if your client gives any indication that further discussion is off limits, honor this and use another technique, such as providing a general lead to get the client to continue with what he or she was saying.

Focusing

Often as clients are talking with nurses, they come to a point at which they provide a great deal of meaningful information in a very short amount of time. It may seem that several topics seem worth exploring, but, of course, this cannot all be done at once. In such instances, it is helpful to select one subject to explore further and to keep the other subjects in mind for future discussion. Selecting one subject for exploration from among several is termed *focusing*.

For example, an adult client might say, "My sister died when I was 7. She was only 4 years old. My alcoholic father had been drinking and killed her in an automobile accident. My mother was so grief stricken and felt so guilty that she had failed to prevent the accident that she had to have several series of electroshock treatments for depression. It seems she was always away in the hospital." How do you decide which point to explore? You may decide to focus on how the client felt about losing a sibling at the age of 7, about having a father who was an alcoholic, about the fact that the death was the father's fault, about the absences of the mother during her hospitalizations, or about how one or more of these factors affected the way the others in the family related to the client.

If you focus on any one point, you can always return to other points at a later time. You might prepare the client for this by making an observation, focusing, and then requesting further exploration in the future. For example, you might say, "You have given me a great deal to think about, and much of it seems worth talking about [making an observation]. For now, I'd like to hear what went on with you at the time of your sister's death [focusing], and later on, perhaps we can explore some of the subsequent events [requesting further exploration in the future]."

Techniques Often Helpful in Keeping Communication Clear

Asking for Clarification

Sometimes clients say things that lack clarity, have more than one specific meaning, or are simply vague. These types of messages can garble communication. When this is the case, a number of techniques can be used to help clarify the message for both the nurse and the client. The most straightforward technique is asking for clarification. Simply let the client know that you are not certain about what was said, and, if necessary, request that the client clarify anything that is obscure. If the client does not understand what was unclear, you may have to tell the person how it could be clarified for you. For example, if you are unsure whether the client said "The thing I liked best in that country was the prints" or "The thing I liked best in that country was the prince," you may have to ask the client to spell the word—*prints* or *prince*—or define it.

Restating

Another way to clarify is to use the therapeutic technique of restating. This is paraphrasing what the client has said. To do this, you take the client's words and alter them so that the meaning is the same as what you understand the client's meaning to be but in somewhat different words. You may feed this back to the client in the form of a statement or a question and provide the client the opportunity to agree that this was the intended message or to disagree and to clarify further.

Seeking Consensual Validation

Sometimes, when a certain term used by a client has been unclear, the nurse can use the technique of seeking consensual validation to help ensure that both client and nurse agree on the meaning of the term. For example, a female client might say, "I'm blue." The client might mean that her skin is literally blue from cold or that she is feeling sad. In such a case, the nurse might believe one meaning of the word to be the one intended and seek to verify whether this was, in fact, the client's meaning. For example, the nurse might ask, "When you used the word *blue,* I believe that you meant "sad" or "depressed." Is that correct?" The client then has the opportunity to agree or disagree and to clarify further.

Placing Events in Time or Sequence

Often in describing an event or a series of events, clients fail to relate the story in strict chronological order. This can make the client's message about the occurrence difficult to follow. When this happens, the nurse can ask the client to explain more about when the event occurred (placing the event in time) or to explain the sequence of a series of events (placing events in sequence).

Techniques That Can Help the Client Gain Increased Self-Awareness

Verbalizing the Implied

With the technique of verbalizing the implied, the nurse understands the words that the client has said but believes that the words have an underlying meaning that was hinted at but not voiced specifically. The nurse verbalizes this underlying message. The client may then verify that the message the nurse received was indeed true. This frees the client to discuss with the nurse some underlying feelings that had not been voiced before.

It is always possible, however, that the client did not mean to imply anything more than the actual words expressed. Verbalizing the implied allows the client to clarify if the nurse has an inaccurate perception of the communication.

Encouraging Assessment of Emotions

It is important for people to be in touch with their own feelings. Too often, to cope with overwhelming feelings, clients wall themselves off from all emotions. This can be very unhealthy. To help clients get back in touch with their feelings, the nurse can use the technique of encouraging assessment of emotions. To do this, the nurse asks clients to focus on their feelings and asks them how they feel.

Translating into Feelings

Sometimes clients find it difficult or impossible to express their feelings verbally using appropriate terms for common emotions. The nurse can help the client by translating their messages into verbal expressions of feelings. The nurse should always be open to correction if the client finds the translation to be inaccurate.

Reflecting

Reflecting is a technique whereby questions and statements are reflected back to the client to assist him or her in thinking about them and coming to a conclusion. This helps the client gain confidence in making assessments and decisions and encourages the client's self-reliance.

There are two forms of reflection. One form is used when the client asks a question and the question is turned around and reflected back to the client. For example, the client might ask, "Do you think I have been making enough progress to go home this weekend?" and the nurse might reflect back with, "Do *you* think you have?" This shows that the nurse values the client's opinion.

The second form reflects back to the client some of the client's own words. This should not be confused with parroting, in which all of the client's words are directed back, without thought on the part of the nurse. With reflection, however, the nurse does think about the message and selects the word or words that are important for the client to think about. This requires active involvement on the part of both client and nurse. For example, the client might say, "I have always hated my brother." With parroting, the nurse would reply, "You have always hated your brother." With reflection, the nurse might reply, "Hated?" and suggest that the client think about that word and perhaps reconsider it or discuss it further. Alternatively, the nurse might reflect back with the word, "Always?" and cause the client to think back to a time when perhaps no hard feelings existed toward the brother.

Encouraging Comparison

To help clients integrate new experiences into what they know of life and to help them learn, the nurse can encourage comparison. To do this, the nurse may ask the client to compare or contrast a certain experience with some other experiences in life.

Techniques Helpful When Contact With Reality Is Impaired

Encouraging Descriptions of Perceptions

Sometimes clients perceive things that others do not. It is helpful if the nurse can ask the client to describe such perceptions and the emotions attached to them. This is the technique of encouraging descriptions of perceptions. This technique is suitable when working with clients who have hallucinations of various types.

It is not recommended that you attempt to communicate with a client who is actively hallucinating. If you know that this is happening, wait until the hallucination has ended.

Voicing Doubt

Sometimes clients have a misperception of reality. You know that it is nontherapeutic to disagree with clients because it strengthens their resolve to convince you that they are correct. So what do you do when clients tell you they see something that is not there and ask whether you also see it? One thing you can do is use the therapeutic technique of voicing doubt. To do this, you do not agree or disagree. You accept the fact that they have perceived something that you have not perceived, but you let them know that you have difficulty understanding how their perception could be real. You do not doubt them, but you do doubt the reality of their perception.

For example, thousands of persons have reported seeing unidentified flying objects. Are all of these persons hallucinating? Such persons, regardless of what they have perceived, should understand that it is difficult for you to believe that flying saucers exist because you have never seen one. They should also be made to understand that, although you may question the validity of their perceptions, you still accept them as persons worth. Therefore, it is always the reality of the perception that is questioned and never the person's truthfulness about the perception. Say, for example, "I just can't believe such a thing could be," not "I just can't believe you."

Presenting Reality

When faced with situations in which clients are with you when a misperception of reality occurs, you can be the person who can help these clients identify what is real and what is not. This is termed presenting reality. Presenting reality can be very reassuring to some persons. To use this technique, as with voicing doubt, you accept the fact that they have perceived something that you have not perceived, but you let them know that you did not have a similar perception. You might say, for example, "It must be very frightening for you to see a dead person over there on the pool table, but I don't see anything there."

If something in the environment is obviously being misperceived, it is therapeutic to try to make a correction about that as well. For example, someone might hear sounds coming from a nearby room and believe that others are in there talking. You could present reality by saying, "A radio is playing in there. That might account for the voices that you heard."

Techniques That Often Are Helpful Near the End of an Interaction

Encouraging Formulation of a Plan of Action

Once you are into the working phase of the relationship and you and the client have identified problems, diagnoses, and desired outcomes, you need to encourage formulation of a plan of action. Note that in using this technique, you encourage the client to formulate the plan. It is much more therapeutic and much more likely to be successfully carried out if the plan comes from the client rather than from you or others.

To encourage formulation of a plan of action, you ask the client to consider in advance what might be the best thing to do in a future situation should the occasion arise. The situation that is anticipated might be one that the client has never experienced, or it might be one that the client has experienced but was not able to handle successfully. This allows the client to think things out in advance and to be prepared.

This technique may also be used near the end of a relationship in which the client has had an opportunity to try out a plan and has not been successful. After evaluating with the client what went wrong, the nurse might suggest formulation of a new plan of action. This helps the client to see that new approaches can be tried.

Summarizing

One therapeutic technique that might be done at intervals is summarizing. Most often, the nurse summarizes by briefly stating, in an orderly manner, what has been discussed. One usually thinks of this as a final activity, but if a client presents a great deal of data to you or you and the client have discussed many options, it is often helpful to summarize briefly at opportune times. Such summaries help ensure that you and the client are in agreement about what went on and what decisions were made. They also help to ensure that you covered all of the information you both wanted to discuss. As a final activity in a longer-term relationship, summarizing can help bring closure as you terminate.

Techniques That Impair Therapeutic Communication

Before you begin to learn about therapeutic techniques, it is imperative that you understand what not to do. This is true because so many ways to say things exist that you cannot be given specific words or phrases that will always be helpful to all people in all situations at all times. You can only be given generally accepted guidelines and examples, and you must practice your therapeutic techniques within these guidelines using your own words. It is difficult to know which of your own words might be hurtful or merely less than helpful, unless you have a good grasp of what should not be done.

It is vital that you recognize nontherapeutic techniques so that you can avoid them as you begin to practice using therapeutic techniques.

Nontherapeutic communication techniques impair the flow of communication in what would otherwise be a progressive movement toward client growth. Some nontherapeutic techniques thwart communication by undermining the nurse, for example, by calling into question the nurse's honesty or by diminishing trust in the nurse. Other nontherapeutic techniques thwart communication by undermining the client. Nontherapeutic techniques that undermine the client are those that are demeaning, those that reinforce or strengthen irrational ideas or beliefs, those that tend to raise client anxiety levels, and those that tend to block the flow of ideas between client and nurse. Some nontherapeutic techniques block communication in more than one way.

Communication in the Nursing Process

Communication is essential for all parts of the nursing process. Both you and the client are communicating throughout the process, and accurate verbal communication and proper interpretation of nonverbal communication will lead to successful outcomes.

Assessment

Clients may communicate a great deal with body language and paralanguage. Messages sent by these means can be important in the overall assessment of the client. Examples of the general areas you may assess follow.

Body Language

Personal Appearance

A rapid assessment of the client's general appearance gives an initial impression of factors as varied as social standing, self-esteem, and emotional status. The person who has not attended to personal appearances may be indicating a lack of wherewithal to do so, a lack of desire to do so, a lack of ability to do so, or a lack of time to do so. We must, of course, be careful about making judgments based on external appearances. It is always useful to validate impressions with additional data.

Facial Expressions

Assessing a client's eyes and facial movements can yield valuable information. A client can communicate pain, fear, anger, sadness, happiness, contentment, or excitement with the eyes and with facial muscular activity. When you assess these areas, note whether the movements are voluntary or involuntary (winks or smiles vs. tics or twitches). Note whether the client can focus and maintain eye contact. Observe the eyes for redness, clarity, and tearing and the face for the raising and lowering of eyebrows or the presence of a smirk, smile, or frown.

Reading facial expressions is not an exact science. For example, you note a client's eyes are red rimmed and teary and see that he has difficulty making eye contact with you. Use your observations of facial expressions as cues to let you know where further assessment might be needed.

Body Posture

Body posture and stance can also provide cues to an individual's physical and emotional state. To assess body posture, note whether the person is standing straight, is slumped, or is hunched over. An erect posture usually signifies a feeling of fitness and confidence. A slump often occurs in persons who are physically exhausted, weak, or emotionally depressed. A hunching with forearms crossed over the abdomen may indicate guarding of a painful abdomen.

Gestures

Observe the types of gestures used by your clients. Some clients talk with their hands by gesturing while they speak. Emphatic gestures often convey messages of urgency. The urgency may be an expression of distress or of great happiness or excitement. Urgent hand gestures may represent the conversion of pent-up emotional energy into physical energy. Urgent hand gestures can be read as a sign that the person has strong needs to be heard or as a means of client coping when the person is unable to adequately convey messages verbally. It is important to understand what gestures mean within different cultures to avoid misunderstanding when communicating with persons from diverse backgrounds.

Paralanguage

An understanding of paralanguage can help us understand the content and the client's mood. Some examples of paralanguage are as follows.

Stress

Stress refers to the part of a word, phrase, or sentence that is highlighted by changing pitch or elongating the syllable. Words that are stressed are generally the more important words. For example,

"Nice to meet you" (with no particular stress)

"*Nice* to meet you"

"Nice to *meet* you" and

"Nice to meet *you*"

all have slightly different meanings because of the way stress is used.

Accent

Accent refers to the different pronunciation of syllables used by some speakers of a language. Accent can cause a loss of clarity. Seek to clarify what has been said by asking the person to repeat what was said, say it in different words, or write out the troublesome phrase.

Pitch

Pitch refers to how high or low the voice is. Men's voices are usually pitched lower than those of women. Children's voices are usually pitched higher than voices of adults. In any individual, changes in pitch can alter the meaning of the content of a message. We all know that the pitch rises at the end of a question (interrogative sentence) and stays the same or lower when we make a statement (declarative sentence). Thus, "You have tuberculosis" and "You have tuberculosis?" are very different in meaning.

Pause

Pauses punctuate speech with periods of silence or nonword sounds. For example, "Let me see . . ." or "Hmmm, I believe you are right." Often a pause indicates that the person is still considering whether to share something with you or to reflect on the words to be used to tell something. Pauses should be respected and the person given adequate time to complete the communication.

Intonation

Intonation is the variety of stress and pause patterns within a phrase or sentence. Persons often use one intonation when giving a formal speech and other intonations when communicating with a superior at work or with a close friend.

Rate

The rate of speech refers to how many syllables are spoken per unit of time. Increased rate of speed may indicate anxiety, nervousness, or agitation.

Volume

Volume is the loudness and intensity associated with the speaking voice. Intensity is a measure of forcefulness and can convey a message about the speaker's emotions. Generally, a loud voice indicates anger or frustration. Changes in volume (either up or down) may also occur in anxiety.

Quality

Voice quality is a measure of clarity, hoarseness, or nasality of the speaker's voice. Physical and emotional conditions can cause a change in voice quality. Voices often become husky with deeply felt emotions, harsher with anger, and more nasal with a cold.

Nursing Diagnosis

Once the assessment is completed, the nursing diagnoses are formulated. These diagnoses must be communicated to the client and other nurses involved in caring for the client. The nursing diagnoses must be communicated in writing to all who are involved with care of the client, as well as communicated verbally. The diagnoses are recorded on the client's chart.

Planning

This phase requires collaboration with all persons involved in caring for the client, including the client and significant others involved in the care of the client. It is important during this step to assess the nonverbal responses of the client. It is equally important to have input from other members of the health team and significant others to determine whether the plan is realistic. If the plan is not accepted by the client and other health team members, implementation will not be effective and outcomes will not be met.

Implementation

The nurse and the client use both verbal and non-verbal communication during the implementation phase of the nursing process. Effective verbal communication with the client assists the client to understand the care being administered and enhances the care delivered. It provides an opportunity for the client to tell the nurse what aspects of the implementation are effective and what difficulties are being experienced. Accurate written communication for other health professionals is essential so that continuity of care can take place. Implementation is usually done by more than one person, so it is important for each person to have an accurate description of what the implementation is and how the client is responding.

Evaluation

Evaluation is dependent on the verbal and non-verbal cues of the client, as well as observations by the nurse. The client's response will indicate whether and to what extent the outcome is being met. From that data, the nurse determines if revisions to the plan are necessary and what they should be. Results of the evaluation are communicated verbally and in writing to colleagues and verbally to the client.

Communication in Groups

Group communication is important in nursing. Developing good group communication skills and having a basic understanding of group dynamics are critical to successful living (Johnson & Johnson, 1989). People are social animals. Life is a cooperative enterprise involving an unending series of negotiations within and between groups. Socialization into the larger society occurs through membership in a number of different groups. Groups offer a slightly different approach to self-awareness. In a group, a person learns to combine experiences in new and different ways. Group communication provides a structural framework for many aspects of our activities of daily living. Self-esteem, social status, and work performance all reflect communication with others as a member of one or more groups. Throughout life, our values and attitudes reveal the groups to which we belong.

As beginning students, you will engage in a variety of group communication experiences, directly with forethought or indirectly as part of the educational process. Your clinical conferences and group assignments will run more smoothly with an understanding of the group dynamics and processes underlying their accomplishment. As you interact with client, family, and professional groups, group communication concepts of norms, cohesion, goals, and role functions will take on new meaning.

The Nature of Groups

A **group** is two or more individuals who share one or more common characteristics and meet on a regular basis in face-to-face interactions to achieve a common goal. Much of what we know about group life and the impact it has on the behavior of individuals developed from the work of Kurt Lewin and his colleagues. His findings suggest that life experience, viewed in a structured setting that allows feedback, reflection, and examination by others, provides experiential learning that is impossible individually. Lewin (1951) visualized the group as a "dynamic whole" in which change in any part of the group system necessarily affects other parts. He maintained that the essential component of group effectiveness is the active interdependency of group members on one another. The value of the collective good will that emerges in the group serves as the catalyst for wanting to achieve group goals.

Characteristics of Groups

Groups differ from other combinations of unrelated people in several important ways:

* Unity of purpose
* Face-to-face interactions over a span of time
* Shared meanings and characteristics
* Interdependency of individuals
* Unique role relationships and norms

Most important is the concept of shared purpose. People join together because of common interests in achieving similar goals. Without a common purpose in mind, the group will disintegrate because there is little reason to stay together. The group develops a **"group culture"** or set of common characteristics that help facilitate goal achievement. Shared characteristics might involve a common ethnic heritage, a similar health problem, or the need to complete a group project for a grade. Interactions occur on a regular basis. Group conversations occur within a certain format, they are related to the accomplishment of group goals, and they take place over time. In a group, members intentionally influence, and are influenced by, others in the group. A unity of purpose draws individuals together in face-to-face interaction.

During the course of the group's life, emotional bonding develops from the shared meanings. The result is that members become socially interdependent as they strive to reach common, agreed-on goals. The group is held together through these interrelated elements and by norms regulating the behaviors of group members and defining specific role relationships.

Primary and Secondary Groups

Groups are classified as primary and secondary. **Primary groups** are naturally occurring formations with informal structures. Membership is automatic or spontaneously chosen. Primary groups include family, friends, and social groups. **Secondary groups** are formations specifically developed by people for the purpose of achieving identified goals.

Primary Groups

Primary groups consisting of family and close friends are the most basic group formations. These informal groups do not always have identified prescribed goals, yet in each is a distinct unity of purpose and interdependency among its membership that has meaning and distinguishes members from nonmembers. A person can be a member of several social groups simultaneously. They are an important source of social and emotional support to people.

Characterized as a long-term informal group structure, family groups exist throughout a lifetime, ideally providing nurturance and support. Membership automatically begins at birth. Older members of the family introduce the younger members of the group to the cultural heritage and social mores. Parents teach their children the group culture in a fundamental way through their overall communication style and parenting approaches. The ways members of family groups interact with each other significantly affect the productivity and emotional satisfaction of the family unit. Implicit and explicit social norms learned in the family group continue to operate throughout the individual's life, affecting human responses with others outside the family group. Many individual communication problems can be traced to behavioral responses originally learned within the family group that are not applicable and are poorly understood outside it.

Acknowledging the membership of an individual client within a larger family group is an important dimension of nursing care that can mean the difference between successfully achieved or failed treatment goals.

Secondary Groups

As the child's world enlarges to include more than family, socialization into the larger society becomes necessary, which stimulates the formation of secondary groups. Secondary groups have a formal structure and purpose. They meet for a variety of interpersonal and work-related goals. From a social perspective, people seek to recreate or build on the sense of belongingness a family represents in school and civic life. Sororities, fraternities, and civic groups such as the Masons or Junior Chamber of Commerce expand group memberships beyond those of the family unit.

Group membership can also serve as a buffer for unsatisfactory family relationships. When membership in a family group becomes too difficult for individual members, the alienated member often seeks membership in one or more other intimate social groups to compensate for the deficiency. Positive use of group membership to augment or substitute for deficient family relationships includes membership in boys' clubs, Big Sisters, and Scouts.

In therapeutic and work groups, members join together as a unit to achieve specific goals. They have a more structured format and specific, identified purposes. Group purposes relate to broadened interpersonal functioning, problem solving, information giving, or task accomplishment. Members join together as a unit to achieve specific goals. Usually, a designated leader assumes primary responsibility for the overall functioning of the group. Specified meeting times related to the achievement of objectives are identified. Members are not likely to meet on a regular basis socially outside the group experience.

Educational groups have goals related to information exchange. Some educational groups are highly structured and require attendance and participation. For example, some classes have laboratory groups or discussion groups as part of the course requirements. Other educational groups form spontaneously to complete a project or provide practical information and support. The purpose of the secondary group determines the structure and influences the quality and focus of group communication.

◆ Group Dynamics and Group Process

In the study of group life, there are two important considerations: group dynamics and group process. **Group dynamics** are the conscious and unconscious forces or emotional flow operating in a group and facilitating or impeding the group process and progression toward goal achievement. The naturally progressive phases of group development constitute **group process.** An understanding of both concepts plays an important role in determining successful group communication.

Concepts Related to Group Dynamics

Effective group dynamics depend on the establishment of clear goals, group norms that support goal achievement, a healthy balance between the group's tasks and its maintenance, and the development of group cohesion. Structural factors such as a pleasant and private environment, timing, and interpersonal sensitivity for members' needs influence the dynamics of the group.

Group Goals

An established group goal is the foundation of the group's existence. It gives meaning and direction to the group's efforts. **Group goals** are the outcomes or end results that the group seeks to achieve through its common effort. Group goals differ from personal goals in that they are broader. They represent a collective aim; they are not necessarily the same as the goals of individual group members. In a group, each member is expected to contribute to the overall group goal.

Goals vary from group to group, depending on the personal and collective resources of the individuals composing the group, the nature of the group, and other external factors, such as time and institutional support. Individuals join groups because they or others believe that certain goals can be achieved better collectively than alone. Achievable goals in line with individual values that are reinforced through support and encouragement and rewarded by those in power are likely to stimulate greater group participation. Two prerequisites for successful goal achievement are that goals be clearly stated and that goals be accepted by the group members as valid and achievable. The leader who allows full presentation of facts and maximal involvement of the group members in the development of group goals is more likely to find that group members work effectively toward goal achievement.

Group Roles

Group roles support the goals and affect the functioning of the group. **Group roles** are sets of behaviors that individuals display in relation to the expectations of the rest of the group members (Wilson & Hanna, 1990). The roles people take in groups can be formal; for example, chairperson or secretary. They also can be informal, fulfilling a function needed for goal achievement.

Benne and Sheats (1948) described three types of informal role functions observed in group dynamics: task, maintenance, and self-centered goals. **Task role** functions are important because they promote task accomplishment. Task role functions help the group stay focused on the task and directly assist the group in achieving its identified goal. **Maintenance roles** are equally important because they support member involvement.

Group maintenance role functions are the role functions that help build and maintain group morale. Group members assuming maintenance role functions draw attention to the relational aspects of group life needed to nourish and support members as they labor to achieve the group task. Examples of group maintenance role functions include seeking to reduce conflict, encouraging compromise, and keeping the channels of communication open among members. Because group maintenance functions relate to the emotional life of the group, they require interpersonal sensitivity and good interpersonal communication skills.

Group task and maintenance role functions are very much interrelated. A healthy balance between task and maintenance role functions provides a rewarding atmosphere in which members work together to achieve common group goals. Group members assume different role functions at different times. Self-centered roles are not functional for the group. They distract from task accomplishment and group maintenance functions; they mire the group in personal conflicts and they neglect group goals.

Group Cohesion

Group cohesion is an important dynamic characteristic of effective groups. The word *cohesion* is a Latin derivative of a word meaning "sticking together." **Group cohesion** refers to all of the positive values that people see as part of the group climate. A positive group climate is perceived as cooperative and ego enhancing. People are attracted to groups that provide companionship and practical or emotional support. They choose groups in which they can have status as a member of the group and personal satisfaction with goal achievement.

Cohesion is measured by the degree to which the group satisfies an individual's need for belonging. In a group with high cohesion, members feel relaxed and are more willing to share ideas and feelings.

A lack of group cohesion decreases group productivity, satisfaction, and frequency of comments. People are afraid to express their ideas openly for fear of criticism. Most people do not want to waste their time and effort in a competitive environment with people they dislike and at the risk of being subjected to criticism.

Allowing dominating or blocking members to sabotage the group goals by default, that is, by not confronting their actions, prevents cohesion from developing.

Several ways to foster positive group cohesion exist. Cohesion develops from a trusting relationship. A group in which an individual's contributions are valued and accepted in a cooperative atmosphere encourages people to disclose their ideas and to commit their resources to accomplishing group goals. Ideally, the leader and other members consider the impact of their communication on the other person.

Concepts Related to Group Process

Group process refers to "the stages of development of a group and the characteristics of each stage" (Corey, 1990). Many theorists believe that the group process offers a microcosm of life relationships. Groups grow and develop from simple beginnings to emerge as complex, productive forces during the middle working phase of group life, and they cease to exist when goals are achieved. In the process of developing, groups form their own identities.

Different theoretical models of group development are presented in Table 13–1. In each of these models is an initial introductory stage in which members come together and tentatively explore what member-

Table 6–1

PHASES OF GROUP DEVELOPMENT

Tuckman	Forming	Storming	Norming	Performing			
Sarri and Galinsky	Origin phase	Formative phase	Intermediate phase	Revision phase	Intermediate phase II	Maturation phase	Termination
Bennis and Shepard	Dependence (authority relations)			Interdependence (personal relations)			
	Dependence-flight			Enchantment-flight			
	Counterdependence-flight			Disenchantment-flight			
	Resolution-catharsis			Consensual validation			
Yalom	Early Formative			Advanced Group			
	Orientation		Conflict	Development of	Recurrent problems		Termination
	Hesitant participation		Dominance	cohesion	Subgrouping		
	Search for meaning		Rebellion		Self-disclosure		
					Conflict		
	Stormy and Emotionally Intense						
Bach (analytic approach)	Members test out group situation	Look to conductor and center hopes on him or her	Regression—playing out family roles	Role playing becomes more fanciful	Emotional discharge results	Take more serious view of selves as group; see structure and function	Deep analytical interpretations
Schultz	Inclusion	Control	Affection				
Gibbs	4 Modes of Activity						
	Acceptance	Data flow	Goal	Control			

Adapted from Arnold, E., & Boggs, K. (1989). *Interpersonal relationships: Professional communication skills for nurses.* Philadelphia: W. B. Saunders, p. 272.

---

ship in the group will mean for each of them. This stage is followed by a second conflictual stage, marked by greater assertiveness, conflict, and the establishment of operating procedures. Once group norms are established to the satisfaction of the group, the actual work of the group on task accomplishment begins. When the group task is complete, members take stock of their achievement, determine the need for follow-up or referral, and disband.

Types of Groups Found in Health Care Settings

In health care settings, nurses use structured groups with clients, families, and other health care professionals to accomplish the goals of professional nursing practice. The group's purpose determines its classification.

Therapeutic Groups

Therapeutic groups offer people a format for increasing self-esteem and taking charge of their lives. Through group interactions, clients learn to handle frustration, anger, and conflicts constructively in a nonthreatening environment.

Task (Work) Groups

Task groups, or **work groups,** are designed to further the goals of an organization. They exist as the official communication unit in many health care settings. Examples of task groups within health care settings include standing committees, ad hoc task forces, and "quality circles." A standing committee is an established committee usually made up of elected members and designed to accomplish the goals of the organization. Examples of standing committees include professional standards committees and administrative councils. Ad hoc task forces are temporary committees established for the purpose of performing a certain task. Quality circles are unit-based task forces formed to resolve administrative and clinical problems.

Input from task groups often forms the nucleus for important changes within a work organization. Shared governance represents a participative management approach heavily dependent on group communication. Participative management relies on group decision-making for strategic planning and implementation of its goals. Health care settings using participative management in group formats experience higher levels of productivity and employee morale. With participative management, the work group functions as an integrated unit linked by shared history, vision, and values and a collective commitment to achieving tangible outcomes. Workers involved in the decision-making process in matters related to their work world feel that they have the capacity to improve their immediate work environment. They are more likely to take an active interest in doing their work and to have pride in their organization. Employees actively involved in participative management report greater satisfaction with their work (Napier & Gershenfeld, 1989; Sashkin, 1984).

Educational Groups

Educational groups are developed to teach participants skills and provide information. They are a modified form of the work group. Study groups, training seminars, aerobics classes, and adult education courses are examples of groups formed for educational purposes. Unlike primary groups, group meetings are scheduled, and the group life is time limited, even when the group is informally structured.

Support Groups

Support groups are formed by people who have experienced a similar problem. Individuals learn that they are not alone in experiencing a particular problem. Members help each other by sharing their experiences and telling each other how they are managing and coping with situations that occur because of the problem.

Group Leadership

A leader provides guidance and direction to a group. The task of the group leader is to guide the group process by maintaining rapport and moving the group process forward to facilitate goal accomplishment.

Leadership Development

Leadership is both a position and a role. Usually, there is a formally designated leader in charge of the group. This is the "position" aspect, and the leader is referred to as the appointed leader. Leaders also emerge within the group and are referred to as emergent leaders. Emergent leadership can be highly effective when it is shared, when it is sanctioned by the leader, and when it fits the temporary needs of the group. It can be highly disruptive when it occurs because the designated leader fails to take charge of the group or lacks the communication skills to respond effectively to the members' needs. Emergent leader-

ship that is competitive rather than collaborative with the designated leadership can sabotage group goals.

Leadership can be viewed in several ways. The first, referred to as the Great Man or trait theory, assumes that leaders are born, not made. The difficulty with this theory is that people with different personal traits are excellent leaders. Leadership can be learned, as evidenced by the fact that many individuals who were not identifiable as leaders in their youth emerge as highly effective leaders when circumstances force them to become leaders in adult life.

Another way of looking at leadership is to describe different styles of leadership. Styles of leadership can vary from individual to individual and according to the situational needs of the group's members.

Strategies for Effective Group Communication

Effective groups focus on the task yet reflect a healthy balance between task and relationship maintenance. Goals are well defined and understood by all members. Effective groups have a basically cooperative atmosphere marked by open communication, respect for differences, participative management of objectives, and a sense of cohesion. Progress reports show clear progression toward stated group goals.

A cooperative group atmosphere does not develop spontaneously. It is the result of much hard work. Members of effective groups choose to develop individual goals in ways that are complementary to or compatible with the identified group goals. Team sports offer a good example. The goal of the individual team member, as well as of the team as a whole, is to win as many games as possible. In a cooperative group atmosphere, the norms support each participant's efforts to achieve the common goal. The teammates of the individual who makes the winning score are just as excited as if they were personally making it. The successful effort of one member brings them closer to the team goal of winning the game. Although the skills and personal resources of each individual member are judged and valued as different, they are all vitally important to the successful achievement of the whole.

The group leader can stimulate greater discussion and commitment to group goals by using focused or open-ended questions. For example, the leader might use one or more of the following comments to draw out member reactions:

We talked a great deal about _____. Which ideas seem most relevant to you?

Would anyone like to react to what John just said?

We've covered much ground today. Is there anything you think we haven't considered yet?

Barriers to Effective Group Interactions

Groups have identified agendas related to the accomplishment of task objectives. They frequently also have unidentified agendas that relate to the emotional aspects of task or group life. It is the unexplained agenda that consumes energy and can sabotage legitimate group goals. Unidentified agendas can relate to power, jealousy, mind reading, or overcoming personal insecurities. Such agendas can interfere with the achievement of apparently straightforward group goals. Sometimes, a legitimate misunderstanding of the motives of others occurs that also needs to be clarified before the work of the group can progress.

Understanding the underlying dynamics that cause people to act in ways that are directly opposed to the goals of the group and to their own self-declared interest helps the leader.

Hidden agendas are expressed in a variety of ways. For example, silence can be productive when it occurs when people are thinking about the issue under discussion. Or the silence can be a reflection of escalating anxiety and resistive anger. One way of determining the nature of silence is to make the observation that the group seems silent and wait for a response. If none is forthcoming, the leader might ask, "Does this mean that everyone is in agreement?" Usually, the group will respond at this point, and the points of conflict will be out on the table for group discussion and resolution.

Uncomfortable as the process of confrontation is for group members and their leader, failure to resolve important emotional responses to the group process can negatively affect group outcomes. Individual member attitudes can have an impact on group dynamics in ways that sabotage group goals.

Steps in the Decision-Making Process

Three sequential steps exist in the decision-making process. The first is diagnosis of the problem in need of a solution. Accurate diagnosis of the problem serves as the foundation for assessing the resources and maturity level of the system regarding its ability to resolve the problem. This involves open discussion with the group and a climate that allows members to freely pose and answer questions. The amount of time available to resolve the problem, how important group members perceive the resolution of the problem to be, and the level of acceptance of the consequences of proposed solutions are considered.

The clarity of problem identification is significantly related to the second step in the decision-making process, identification of alternative solutions. This step can take time because it involves brainstorming ideas. All ideas are given equal weight initially, and group members are encouraged to express all of their thoughts and feelings about the problem, even if they seem far-fetched. The key element is that the ideas must relate to the problem under discussion. Without this norm, group discussions can become tangential to the accomplishment of the group goal.

Once sufficient ideas have been generated, the group turns to an analysis of possible alternatives. Group members realize that there are a number of alternative solutions to the problem but that some will result in more desirable outcomes based on what is known about the problem at the time. The focus shifts from equal consideration of all ideas to further discussion of the most promising ones. The outcome of the decision-making process is the final selection of the most desirable solution and a call for commitment to its implementation. After implementation, the group can focus on further revisions and refinement of the original decision.

Group Process as a Parallel to the Nursing Process

In many ways, the group process developmentally parallels the nursing process. Both have an initial assessment phase in which the group explores the nature of the problem, develops a diagnostic statement, and determines the activities necessary to resolve it. Within the group, the members plan what activities will be needed to achieve group goals and who will be responsible for carrying out the functions. Together, group members develop a plan of action. Although this is an informal process in many groups, the developmental process is similar to the planning phase of the nursing process. In the working or implementation phase of the group, group members implement their plan so that most of the actual interventions related to task accomplishment take place. The termination phase of group life parallels the evaluative segment of the nursing process. When the work of the group is complete, group members evaluate their progress and goal achievement, make necessary modifications, and terminate the group.

Summary

Communication is essential for delivering accurate and effective nursing care. The nurse uses verbal, nonverbal, and paraverbal communication when interacting with clients and health team members, individually and in groups. Understanding the communication patterns of clients and collaborating with clients and their significant others, health team members, and group members enhances all aspects of the nursing process. This facilitates trust and optimal delivery of nursing care.

CHAPTER HIGHLIGHTS
✦

✦ Three phases of the therapeutic relationship exist: the orientation phase, the working phase, and the termination phase.

✦ The six elements of communication are the encoder, the message, the sensory channel, the decoder, feedback, and context.

✦ Nurses must develop effective communication skills to work with clients of different ages, cultures, and genders who present with various health problems.

✦ Nurses can prepare for client interactions by knowing which techniques are helpful at the beginning, middle, and end of an interaction.

✦ Body language is a form of nonverbal communication that consists of alterations in personal appearance, changes in facial expression and body posture, use of gestures and touching, and maintenance of personal distance.

✦ Paralanguage is a form of nonverbal communication that consists of elements of stress, accent, pitch, intonation, rate, volume, and quality.

✦ Nontherapeutic communication techniques should be recognized so they can be avoided.

✦ Many responsive characteristics exist that a nurse may demonstrate to facilitate effective communication.

✦ Groups are composed of two or more individuals who share one or more common characteristics and meet on a regular basis to achieve a common goal.

✦ The main types of groups encountered in health care settings are therapeutic groups, support groups, task groups, and educational groups.

✦ Primary groups are naturally occurring groups in which membership is automatic; secondary groups are specifically developed for the purpose of achieving identified goals.

✦ Therapeutic communication is an integral part of all phases of the nursing process.

✦ Phases of group development parallel the steps of the nursing process.

✦ Concepts important to an understanding of group dynamics are goals, roles, norms, and cohesion.

Study Questions

1. Which of the following is true of a therapeutic relationship?

   a. it is focused on nonspecific helping behaviors
   b. it is client focused
   c. it is a reciprocal relationship
   d. help is a small part of the relationship

2. Raising your voice to a person who is hearing impaired

   a. assists the client in hearing you
   b. provides better lip reading for the client
   c. causes additional residual hearing loss
   d. makes your speech clearer to the client

3. In what phase of the therapeutic relationship is trust established?

   a. working phase
   b. termination phase
   c. orientation phase
   d. preorientation phase

4. An example of a secondary group is

   a. family
   b. Boy Scouts
   c. friends
   d. social groups

5. The termination phase of a group parallels what phase of the nursing process?

   a. evaluation
   b. assessment
   c. planning
   d. implementation

Critical Thinking Exercises

1. You are in the termination phase of a therapeutic relationship. The client states "I want you to continue to just visit me." How would you as the nurse respond?

2. You are asked to head a support group based on your expertise of stress management. Discuss how you would assess, describe, and evaluate group communication.

References

Arnold, E., & Boggs, K. (1989). *Interpersonal relationships: Communication skills for nurses.* Philadelphia: W. B. Saunders.

Benne, K. D., & Sheets, P. (1948). Functional roles and group members. *Journal of Social Issues, 4* (2), 41–49.

Corey, G. (1990). *The theory and practice of group counseling* (3rd ed.). Pacific Grove, CA: Brooks/Cole.

Johnson, D., & Johnson, F. (1989). *Joining together: Group theory and group skills* (3rd ed.). Englewood Cliffs, NJ: Prentice Hall.

Lewin, K. (1951). *Field theory in social science* (pp. 146–147). New York: Harper & Row.

Napier, R., & Gershenfeld, M. (1989). *Groups: Theory and experience.* Boston: Houghton Mifflin.

Peplau, H. (1952). *Interpersonal relations in nursing.* New York: McGraw-Hill.

Sashkin, M. (1984). Participative management in an ethical imperative. *Organizational Dynamics, 12* (4), 5–22.

Tannen, D. (1990). *You just don't understand: Women and men in conversation.* New York: Ballantine Books.

Travelbee, J. (1966). *Interpersonal aspects of nursing.* Philadelphia: F. A. Davis.

Wilson, G., & Hanna, M. (1990). *Groups in context: Leadership and participation in small groups* (2nd ed., pp. 154–162). New York: McGraw-Hill.

Bibliography

Bradley, J. C., & Edinburg, M. A. (1990). *Communication in the nursing context* (3rd ed.). Norwalk, CT: Appleton & Lange.

Davis, A. J. (1984). *Listening and responding*. St. Louis, MO: C. V. Mosby.

Masson, R., & Jacobs, E. (1989). Group leadership: Practical pointers for beginners. *Personnel and Guidance Journal, 58* (3), 52–55.

Miller, L. E. (1989). Modeling awareness of feelings: A needed tool in the therapeutic communication workbox. *Perspectives in Psychiatric Care, 25* (2), 27–29.

Purtilo, R. (1990). *Health professional and patient interaction* (4th ed.). Philadelphia: W. B. Saunders.

Redland, A. R. (1988). Working effectively with groups. *Clinical Nurse Specialist, 2* (3), 131.

Selleck, K. J. (1991). Nurses' interpersonal behavior and the development of helping skills. *International Journal of Nursing Studies, 28* (1), 3–11.

Thobaben, M. (1990). Evaluation of the therapeutic nurse-patient relationship. *Home Healthcare Nurse, 26* (7), 8–16.

Topf, M. (1988). Verbal interpersonal responsiveness. *Journal of Psychosocial Nursing, 26* (7), 8–16.

Chapter 14

PROVIDING ESSENTIAL INFORMATION TO CLIENTS

BETTY PATTERSON TARSITANO, RN, PHD

KEY TERMS

✦

affective domain
anxiety
cognitive domain
concrete operational stage
individual learning
knowledge deficit
learning
operations
preoperational thought
psychomotor domain
purposeful learning
readiness to learn
self-active learning
transfer of learning
unitary learning

LEARNING OBJECTIVES

✦

After studying this chapter, you should be able to

✦ Define key terms related to client teaching and learning

✦ Describe the principles of teaching and learning

✦ Describe the domains of learning and their implications for teaching

✦ Describe teaching strategies

✦ Describe the psychoeducative process

✦ Identify the characteristics of a nurse teacher

✦ Describe client-learner characteristics

✦ Describe characteristics of a conducive learning environment

✦ Identify psychological factors that influence readiness to learn

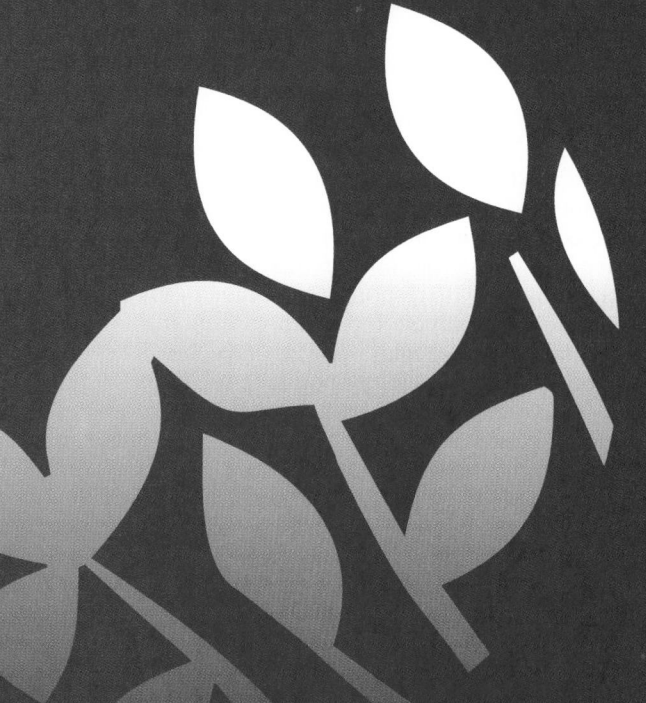

Always a hallmark of nursing practice, client teaching is now considered an integral part of the delivery of safe, quality care in all health care organizations (Beck *et al.,* 1993; Henderson, 1966; McGinnis, 1993; Nightingale, 1932). The purpose of client teaching is to assist the learner in gaining the knowledge and skills needed to achieve optimal outcomes of health, independence, and quality of life. Providing essential information to the client is a process that requires mutual setting of psychoeducative goals by the client and family/significant others with the nurse, independently or collaboratively with other health professionals, depending on the situation.

Impetus for client teaching by nurses stems from formal statements, standards, and mandates found in documents such as nurse practice acts (Rivers, 1991; Rothman & Rothman, 1981), the *Code for Nurses With Interpretative Statements* (ANA, 1985), *A Patient's Bill of Rights* (AHA, 1973), *The Professional Nurse and Health Education* (ANA, 1975), and *Accreditation Manual for Hospitals* (JCAHO, 1996). Client teaching has been shown to be effective in increasing the client's and the family/significant other's knowledge about self-care management (Devine & Reifschneider, 1995; Redman, 1993). The importance of client teaching by nurses is now reflected in job performance evaluations and in the standards of care developed within the particular health care setting (Thoma, 1994).

Increased health care costs and related budget restraints have changed the model for delivery of health care to clients. Unfortunately, as a result, clients are being discharged from the hospital earlier. Early discharge places constraints on the time needed for client teaching. Fewer professional nurses and more nursing technicians are used to administer care in hospital settings (Morse, 1990).

With fewer professional nurses, the number of clients to be taught by staff nurses is greater. The acutely ill client is discharged much earlier in the recovery process. The client's readiness to learn is deterred by decreased energy levels. At the time of discharge, the client and family/significant other may know certain aspects of self-care management. However, they still need to adapt or transfer this learning to the home environment. In response to earlier discharge and in an effort to compete for health care monies, numerous types of home health services have been developed, especially for the elderly population.

Decreased length of hospital stay, cost-containment measures, and increased home health services require that teaching of the client and family/significant other in health care settings be facilitated. The nurse as teacher must be able to assess both the client's and the family/significant other's learning needs and learning ability in a variety of health care settings, especially the home. It is important that the nurse be able to present essential client information within a limited time frame to learners, with consideration of ability, age, education, experiences, and cultural and socioeconomic needs. When teaching the client and family/significant other, the nurse is involved with providing information about the safe and effective use of medications and equipment, potential drug and food interactions, needed follow-up care after hospital discharge, and how to obtain that care. The outcomes of the teaching must be monitored, documented, and communicated to other professionals continuously (Bubela *et al.,* 1990; Foster, 1988; Whitman *et al.,* 1992). Providing client information in a manner understandable to the learner requires that the nurse have a basic understanding of written and oral communication skills (Breeze, 1987; Dixon & Park, 1990; Doak *et al.,* 1985; Miller & Bodie, 1994).

The purpose of this chapter is to help the nurse (1) develop a perspective of the scope and complexity of the nurse-teacher role in providing essential information to the client and family/significant other in health care settings; (2) recognize the application of the nursing process of assessing, diagnosing, planning, implementing, evaluating, and documenting as a systematic and orderly approach to presenting essential information to learners in a timely and effective manner; and (3) consider characteristics or principles of the learning-teaching process relevant to caring for clients and families/significant others in health care settings.

Client Teaching

Effective client teaching is based on principles of teaching and learning. Principles of teaching and learning are concepts or generalizations that serve as guidelines for teachers to assist learners move toward the attainment of mutual goals and health outcomes. Principles applied by the nurse when providing essential client information are derived from different schools of thought about the nature of teaching and learning. Although different principles of learning and teaching are described by psychologists and educators, there is general agreement that learning is essentially a change in behavior owing to experience. Certain conditions must be present for learning to take place.

Principles of Learning Applied to Client Teaching

Providing essential client information effectively requires that the nurse teacher understand basic principles of client teaching and be able to apply them in a variety of health care settings and situations (Gage & Berliner, 1992; Gagne, 1977; Heidgerken, 1965; Knowles, 1990; Slavin, 1991). Learning is unitary, self-active, purposeful, individual, creative, and transferable. Characteristics of learning principles used in client teaching are described in Table 14–1.

Table **14–1**

LEARNING PRINCIPLES AND CLIENT TEACHING

Learning Is Unitary. Learning is considered unitary in that the learner reacts to the whole learning situation rather than to any single stimulus or part of the whole. Unitary learning is not purely intellectual or compartmentalized into definite and concrete parts. It includes attitudes, values, and habits, as well as knowledge and skills. Each learner is a whole person responding intellectually, emotionally, physically, culturally, and spiritually to the total situation. These responses are simultaneous. Each learner responds to the total situation, to the personality of the nurse, doctor, and other health professionals who may come in contact with the learner. These factors influence, positively or negatively, the learner's responses and outcomes. Likewise, the nurse teacher and other professionals apply the unitary learning principle when they no longer refer to the learner as "the cardiac bypass who needs discharge teaching" or "the newly diagnosed diabetic on insulin." The nurse recognizes that each learner is a whole person with psychological strengths and weaknesses and health care experiences that play a role in his or her learning, illness, and recovery.

Learning Is Self-Active. The basic principle of learning is self-activity (Bigge, 1982). Providing information alone does not offer an effective learning experience. Learning does not take place without learner activity. The learner must be actively involved in the process. Self-activity refers to the learner's ability to actually react to or interact with the learning experience. Active learning maximizes application and transfer of learning and changes cognitive, affective, and psychomotor behaviors. Self-activity means more than skeletal movements or manual activity alone. Self-activity includes listening, visualizing, recalling, memorizing, reasoning, judging, thinking, and doing. For example, self-activity in learning is promoted by the nurse when administering a medication. At the time an oral medication is administered, the client, who is alert and ready, listens to the instructions given about the purpose of the prescribed drug; its intended effects; adverse effects for which to observe; the dose and schedule of doses; and the color, size, and shape of the medication. A written teaching aid reinforcing this information is given to the client. To keep the client engaged and involved in the learning process, the next time the medication is administered, the nurse shows the client the medication and asks whether it's the right pill, the right dosage, and the right time for administration. The client asks questions about information in the written teaching aid. On the day of discharge, the client has more questions about the effects of the medication. These questions are answered by the nurse using the written teaching aid. Meaningful learning experiences mutually planned by the client and/or family/significant other facilitate self-activity, which leads to positive outcomes.

Learning Is Purposeful. Self-activity is aroused by a meaningful outcome and is sustained by a feeling of progress toward that outcome. The purposeful learner is active in a certain direction toward a known attainable outcome. Learning is effective to the degree that the learner, with guidance from the nurse, directs activities toward the attainment of meaningful and expected outcomes. Outcomes are influenced by motives. Motives are both physical and psychological conditions within each learner. These motives dispose the learner to act in certain ways. Motives are designated by many terms, such as needs, desires, attitudes, and interests. Motives energize the learner to seek out and engage in experiences that satisfy a need. Because a need must arouse activity, needs are the basis of learning. The learner does not learn unless some need arouses self-activity. Motives govern attention and readiness for learning. If the client is to be motivated toward a specified outcome, he or she must have a state of alertness that corresponds to attentive behavior or attention. Attention is well-motivated behavior directed toward a specific task. Alertness is related to certain physical and mental states, such as sleepiness, fatigue, anxiety, or being under the influence of medications. Alertness is also affected by the learning environment. When essential client information is being provided, alertness must be present in the learner. The learner will not participate in learning activity unless he or she is alert and ready. The level of readiness for learning influences the efficiency of the learning. Readiness for learning is the level at which the learner has the capacity to undertake the learning of specified information (Good, 1959). Past learning experiences, perceptual and motor skills, emotional states, willingness to learn, and the particular situation influence the client's and the family/significant other's readiness to learn. The nurse provides the information when the learner is motivated, ready, willing, and able.

Learning Is Individual. Learning is individual because all activity must be *self*-activity and, therefore, is influenced by the ability, the experience, the attitudes, and the values of the individual learner. Basic to all other considerations, when the nurse provides essential client information, the client and/or family/significant other is to be viewed as a unique learner with individualized needs, characteristics, and problems different from those of others.

Learning Is Creative. The learner responds to a situation not as it appears to others, and not even solely as it exists objectively. The client and/or family/significant other responds to the environment created by the self and behaves in ways that are consistent with the environment that the learner has created. Learning is more than a duplication of an act performed or modeled by someone else; it is the mastery of skills, the acquisition of knowledge, and/or the attainment of understanding. Learning is an organization of all these activities. The behavioral outcome results in a new way of acting for the particular learner. The newly generated behavior is unique and individual. Learning may thus be considered creative. The nurse teacher recognizes this creative behavior.

Table continued on following page

Table 14-1

LEARNING PRINCIPLES AND CLIENT TEACHING
(Continued)

Learning Is Transferable. Transfer of knowledge is the assumption of all learning. The nurse hopes that whatever the client and family/significant other have learned in one context or situation will apply or affect another context or situation. For example, a person who has learned how to self-administer insulin in the hospital will also be able to administer the insulin at home or while traveling. The amount of knowledge that an individual is able to transfer varies. True learning takes place only when the learner acquires a type of information or skill or changes an attitude in response to a real need. Several factors influence the permanency and amount of learning that takes place. For example, transfer of learning is influenced by the conciseness of mutually stated outcomes and by the learner's intellectual capacity, experiences, and willingness to achieve the outcome and to sustain sound activities that lead toward that outcome (Helberg, 1990). Transfer of learning seldom takes place automatically. Transfer is facilitated by the nurse, who plans and promotes transfer by informing the learner of the possibility of transfer. Opportunities to transfer learning in concrete, meaningful situations are provided.

Principles of Teaching Applied to Client Teaching

❧ **Client Teaching Situations Require a Climate Conducive to Teaching and Learning.** A climate that is conducive to a teaching-learning situation in a health care setting has three important aspects: physical comfort; mutual trust, caring, and respect; and resources and support. Whether in the hospital, home, outpatient setting, or doctor's office, factors such as room temperature, lighting, noise, time of day, seating arrangements, and mobility affect the client teaching situation. Physical discomfort and environmental distractions for the teacher and learner are kept to a minimum. Mutual trust, caring, and respectful relationships are fostered by a nurse who is a knowledgeable, sensitive, and attentive listener familiar with the particular situation and health care setting (Fig. 14–1).

In a conducive learning climate, sound resources, such as relevant standardized client information, audiovisual materials, documentation tools, and support from administration, physicians, colleagues, and significant others, are available and used by the nurse teacher. The most reliable sources are selected for providing essential client information (Jackson & Johnson, 1988; Rankin & Stallings, 1990).

❧ **Initial Client Information Is Based on Learning Needs.** The teacher should prioritize learning needs with the learner. Learning is more effective when the learner perceives the need to learn to be important. Once the perceived need is satisfied, the learner is more likely to attend to other important learning needs. High-priority learning needs include essential information about safety, surgery, recovery from surgery, examinations, illness, diet, exercise, medication, coping strategies, and self-care activities at home. Essential information is directed toward achieving meaningful outcomes and begins with the nurse's assessment of what information is needed by a particular individual in a particular situation at a particular time.

The nurse assesses what information is presently available to the learner, the accuracy of the information, the readiness of the learner to receive the information, the time frame needed to present the information, and the time actually allowed for delivery of that information. The nurse builds on the learner's previous accurate knowledge about the particular situation and lays the groundwork for future learning and transfer. When information must be provided and the learner is not ready to receive the information and the time available to teach is shortened by early discharge or a situational crises, the nurse proceeds with steps of the nursing process. The degree to which outcomes are met or not met is documented. Documentation includes a note about the client's status, indicating that further learning is needed before the client can be discharged safely. Documentation is recorded in the official forms of the particular health care agency— nurse's notes, progress notes, and/or discharge notes. The nurse teacher reports the results to other professionals as indicated.

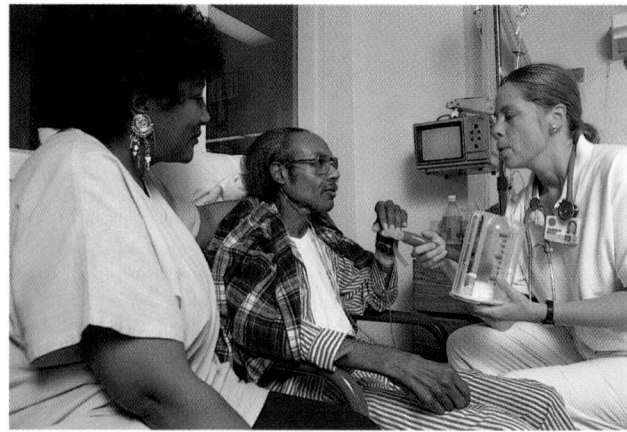

❧ **Figure 14–1**
Caring, sensitivity, and a respectful attitude create a climate that fosters patient learning. The presence of a spouse or other family member can be reassuring to the patient and help to relieve anxiety.

✦ Organized Information Promotes Learning Retention. Standardized information adapted to the learner and presented in an orderly sequence by a reliable source promotes retention and application of learning. Once the nurse has identified the information needed to be taught and the client and/or family/significant other is ready to receive this information, the information is given. Effective delivery of client information requires the nurse teacher's recognition of the psychological effects of teaching (Cormier *et al.,* 1984). How the teacher delivers information influences the learner's attainment of goals. Effective client teaching is facilitated when the information provided is consistent and accurate.

Following are some guidelines for effective client teaching:

* To promote consistency and accuracy in delivery, standardize client information. Standardized client information includes the purpose of the information, the type of information to be given, characteristics of the audiovisual materials, learner characteristics, and the content to be taught.

* Personalize all teaching. Standardized information is personalized for the client when the nurse uses personal pronouns such as "you" in the instruction. Personalized standardized information adapted to the particular situation and setting and to the capabilities of the client, the family/significant other, and the teacher fosters the learner's self-activity in the psychoeducative process.

* Provide direction for learning by giving a brief overview of the information and its purpose, describing what the information is about and what its value may be for the learner.

* Use audiovisual materials pertinent to the purpose of the instruction to enhance learning. Visual materials should correspond with the verbal information given.

* Recognize psychological factors that may or may not enhance learning, such as fear and anxiety. The teacher seeks the learner's reaction to the information provided. The amount of information given is paced according to the level of anxiety or fear present. Teaching strategies are adjusted accordingly. The learner's reaction should be documented in the nurse's notes.

* For effective presentation, use simple language, speak clearly, use repetition, and limit the amount of information given at one time. Be sure that the information is specific, brief, and accurate.

* Establish a sequence from easy to difficult content to aid the learner's understanding. Information is organized and presented in a step-by-step approach that is meaningful to the learner. Because of time constraints, the most important information is given first.

* If possible, give a short presentation containing all relevant information rather than a long presentation.

* Remember that the importance or relevancy of the content, the time available for the presentation, and the emotional and physical state of the learner influence whether the information is best presented all at once or in a sequence.

* For effective presentation of client information, take into consideration the learner's level of vocabulary, education, and comprehension. Comprehension is dependent on reading skills rather than on educational or grade levels completed.

* Present information clearly in terms and words that are familiar to the client and the family/significant other. The language used should be nontechnical and free from jargon. If technical language is used, terms are defined in everyday language or examples are given so that the learner can understand.

* Reinforce the purpose of the information with a final summary.

* Repeat goal-directed information as indicated. The teacher confirms when outcomes are met or not met by using measurable criteria.

* Remember that learning is enhanced when the learner becomes aware of attaining new information and improving skills. The learner needs time to assimilate and integrate the instruction given.

* Document what has been learned by the client. This serves as a guide for further reinforcement or advancement of the instruction as indicated.

* Present information in a sensitive and friendly but authoritative manner.

* As nurse teacher, you must know what client information to provide and when and how to provide it. Multiple factors influence when, what, and how information is to be provided, including characteristics of both the teacher and the learner; the learner's physical and mental ability, anxiety level, experiences, education, age, gender, cultural practices, and primary language; the usefulness of the information to the learner; the importance of the specific information; the time available for teaching; reinforcement and evaluation; the teacher's familiarity with the content; and the particular situation.

✦ Domains of Learning: Implications for Teaching

Three domains of learning that are used frequently in client teaching are cognitive, affective, and psychomotor. When one learns, one is thinking, feeling, and doing. Thinking, feeling, and doing are domains or types learning. The domains are related but distinct. Learning is a unified process in which the person learns as a total system.

Classification of learning into domains or types of learning determines emphases. Specific objectives belong in one domain rather than another. The objectives define and order behaviors in terms of complexity, communication specific long- and short-term goals with specific outcome criteria that are measurable. Specified measurable outcomes facilitate the evaluation of the degree to which goals are met. When providing client teaching, the nurse must decide on which domain the learner needs to focus his or her attention.

Cognitive Domain

The **cognitive domain** involves learning behaviors concerned with knowledge, comprehension, application, analysis, synthesis, and evaluation. *Knowledge* involves recalling previously learned information. For example, the client recalls the purpose of his or her medication, Coumadin (warfarin sodium). *Comprehension* is knowledge beyond the capacity of recall without relating it to other material or seeing its implications. For example, the client recalls two hazards of taking Coumadin (bleeding and bruising). *Application* is the ability to use the information in new and concrete situations. Before taking Coumadin, the client reports the occurrence of bleeding gums when brushing the teeth to the physician. *Analysis* is the ability to break down the information into its component parts so that the organizational structure of the information can be comprehended. The client differentiates the presence of bleeding gums since taking Coumadin with the absence of bleeding gums prior to taking Coumadin. *Synthesis* is the ability to put parts together to form a new whole. The client explains the action of Coumadin on the blood clotting mechanism and the relationship to bleeding. *Evaluation* is making conscious value judgments for a given purpose, depending on one's ability to organize and determine the relevance of the information. The client appraises the success of his or her ability to report hazards related to Coumadin while at home.

Behavioral changes in the cognitive domain are based on objectives that begin with the learner recalling and recognizing essential client information. The process continues with comprehending the essential information, applying the knowledge that is comprehended, analyzing situations concerned with this knowledge, synthesizing this knowledge into new organizations, and evaluating the value of the knowledge for given purposes (Bloom, 1956). The knowledge could include terminology, facts, trends, principles, rules, generalizations, criteria, and theories related to procedures, tests, treatments, medications, the disease process, safety measures, and self-care.

The major intellectual process of learning knowledge involves memory. Remembering begins with recall and recognition. Retention and retrieval are phases directly concerned with memory. The learner is expected to store information in the memory for later recall. Memory consists of short- and long-term phases. Short-term memory retains information long enough for processing. Long-term memory permanently stores the information.

Aids to memory include (1) summarizing important information and the structure of what is to be remembered, beginning with basic factual elements through increased abstraction; (2) deciding how the information relates to what is already known; and (3) dividing what must be learned into small sets of logical sequence (Weinrach & Boyd, 1992).

The nurse's assessment of the client's cognitive ability is an essential step in the teaching-learning process. Any deficits in cognitive ability that may hinder client learning and goal attainment should be documented.

Affective Domain

The **affective domain** consists of learning behaviors dealing with expression of feelings, interests, attitudes, values, appreciation, and methods of adjustment. Affect involves an internal process that influences the learner's interaction with the environment. This process begins with the learner receiving stimuli, responding to stimuli on request, valuing an activity, organizing values into a single whole, and characterizing values into a single whole (Krathwohl et al., 1956).

Receiving stimuli is the learner's passive awareness of a particular activity developing toward more active attention. *Responding* on request is the learner willingly participating in a learning activity and taking satisfaction in that participation. *Valuing* is the learner's acceptance of the activity and his or her voluntarily seeking ways to respond to the learning, ranging from simple acceptance of an activity to a more complex level of commitment. The learner *organizes* by comparing, relating, synthesizing, and prioritizing different values. Conflicts between values are then resolved by the learner, who builds an internally consistent value complex into a single whole. This whole becomes a *characterization* of the learner. The characterization is in agreement with the learner's overt behavior. The behavior is persistent and predictable.

Changing values, attitudes, and feelings, such as accepting cessation of smoking, following diet restrictions, and taking medications, usually takes longer than increasing knowledge in the cognitive domain. A change in affective behaviors takes place slowly. Client teaching in complex, threatening situations may begin with the affective domain. The affective domain is closely related to the learner's readiness to learn. The initial step of learning in the affective domain depends solely on the teacher for evoking the attention and awareness of the learner. The teacher must first establish a trusting relationship. The learner must want to change the given behavior.

Psychomotor Domain

The **psychomotor domain** emphasizes motor and procedural skills (Fig. 14–2). Psychomotor learning is concrete and the easiest to measure (Harrow, 1979). According to Simpson (1972), psychomotor learning begins with the learner's perceptions and develops through a series of activities called set; guided response; mechanism, and a complex overt response. *Perception* is the becoming aware of objects by way of the sense organs. *Set* is preparation or readiness for a

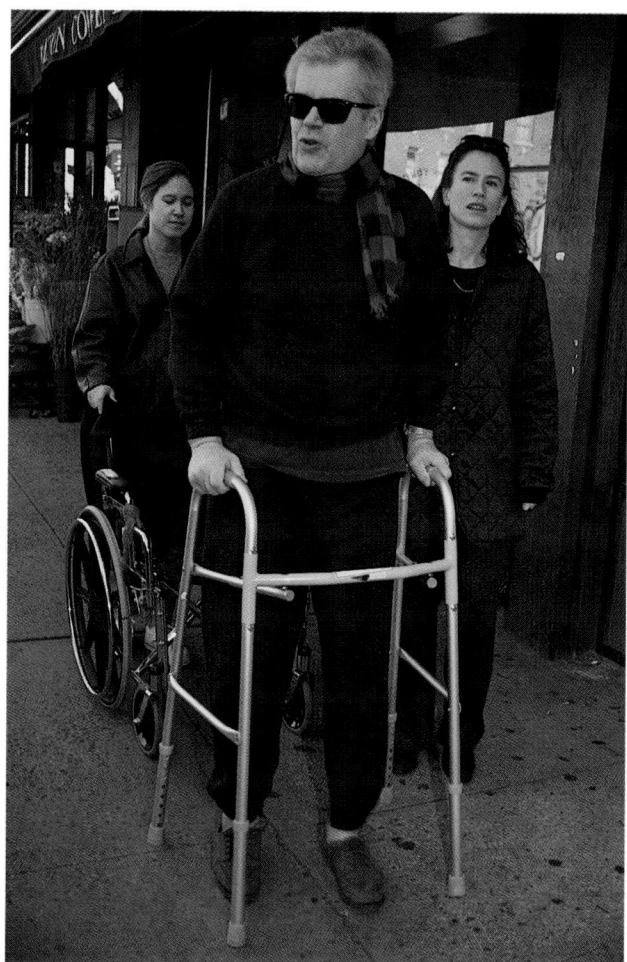

✦ **Figure 14–2**
Teaching outside ambulation using a walker employs the psychomotor domain of learning behaviors. The teacher demonstrates how to perform the skill using a series of steps. The learner then demonstrates with coaching from the teacher, and practice is encouraged. Psychomotor learning is concrete and easy to measure.

particular kind of experience. **Guided response** is the overt act of the learner under the guidance of the teacher. The learner has a model or criteria against which he or she can judge his or her performance. *Mechanism* is the learned response becoming habitual. *Complex overt response* is performance of an act requiring a movement pattern with fine coordination, certainty, adaptation to a new situation, and **origination,** new ways of manipulating materials out of understanding, ability and skills developed *in the psychomotor area.*

In psychomotor learning, the teacher demonstrates to the learner how to perform a skill using a series of steps. A return demonstration by the learner with coaching from the teacher is given. Errors are identified. Correct activities are then reinforced. Practice is recommended until mutual satisfaction as to performance level is reached.

Characteristics of the Nurse Teacher

Whether novice or expert, the nurse teacher must be perceived by the client learner as being competent, trustworthy, and supportive. Before client teaching, the nurse should assess how confident the client is about possessing the information to be presented and should be aware of his or her own attitude that is being conveyed to the learner. For instance, is the nurse inflexible or relaxed and willing to listen (Hanak, 1986)?

The competent nurse teacher has knowledge of the procedural, sensory, and factual aspects of the subject to be taught and conveys this knowledge with consideration of the learner's levels of anxiety and fear. The competent teacher is familiar with the content of audiovisual materials provided to the learner. The audiovisual materials are used in consideration of the learner's reading ability and vocabulary. The competent teacher distinguishes between lack of ability and lack of understanding caused by age or by cultural, ethnic, or religious differences.

The trustworthy teacher delivers accurate and reliable information in a dynamic manner. The supportive teacher is attentive and friendly, with genuine positive regard for the learner. To enhance the learner's belief in the nurse teacher's competence, the teacher dresses for the role, clarifies the teacher role as indicated, and delivers the information that was mutually agreed on, using sound teaching strategies. To increase the learner's belief in the trustworthiness of the nurse as teacher, the nurse delivers essential information that is accurate and reliable. The supportive teacher uses good communication skills, both verbal and nonverbal, promoting positive interactions (Spees, 1991; Streiff, 1986). The competent nurse documents outcomes of teaching in the nurse's notes and communicates the results to other professionals as indicated.

Characteristics of the Learner

After the purpose and type of essential information to be provided and the unique characteristics of the learner are specified, client teaching is initiated. Assessment of client characteristics enables the nurse teacher to determine if the client (1) can learn, (2) cannot learn or is not ready to learn, and/or (3) needs adjustments or upgrading of present knowledge (Rakel, 1992).

The client's readiness to learn, learning ability, and attitudes toward learning are influenced by several factors, including age, gender, level of maturity, level of anxiety and fear, intelligence, educational

Table 14-2

BARRIERS TO LEARNING

- Pain
- Fatigue
- Anxiety
- Decreased coping abilities
- Experiences with illness
- Previous hospitalization
- Personal values and priorities
- Support systems
- Impaired memory
- Job or school experiences
- Future plans

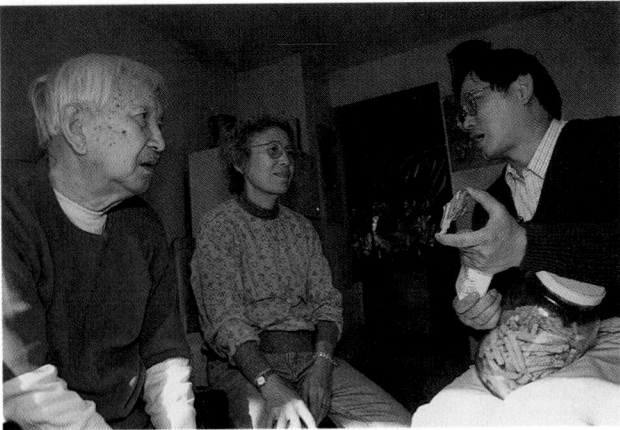

❥ **Figure 14-3**
While providing information in a home care setting, this nurse compares traditional and Western remedies. Culture influences how health, illness, and pain are perceived. The nurse must take cultural variations into account to effectively communicate with patients and their families.

background, current level of knowledge, socioeconomic status, lifestyle, cultural differences, primary language, and available support systems (Davis *et al.*, 1990; Gilbert, 1993; Jubeck, 1994; Opdyce *et al.*, 1992). Assessing the learner's characteristics before teaching saves time and effort by helping to establish learning priorities and allowing teaching strategies to be tailored to the individual's learning needs and capabilities. Characteristics of the learner that may be barriers to the teaching-learning process should be documented. Barriers to learning are listed in Table 14-2.

❥ **Psychological Factors.** Learners respond to health care situations, especially in hospital settings, with varying levels of anxiety and fear. The client and family/significant other may be too anxious or fearful to hear what is being taught (Lierman *et al.*, 1994).

Uncertainty in stressful situations may be related to the learner's perceived loss of personal control. Providing accurate standardized information tailored to the individual and to the particular situation promotes the client's and/or family/significant other's sense of control and may facilitate participation in the learning process and attainment of positive outcomes (Breemhaar & van den Borne, 1991).

In the initial steps of the nursing process, important concerns of the client and family members should be addressed first, because anxiety, fear, and uncertainty generated by those concerns may interfere with the learner's ability to process essential information effectively. Coping preferences of the client and/or family/significant other in stressful situations vary. Events may be perceived as being threatening or as being challenging (Lazarus & Folkman, 1984). Learning readiness and positive outcomes are enhanced by personalized, structured information that is paced, accurate, and consistent, in consideration of the learner's anxiety and fear (Davis, *et al.*, 1994; Melnyk, 1994; Tarsitano, 1992).

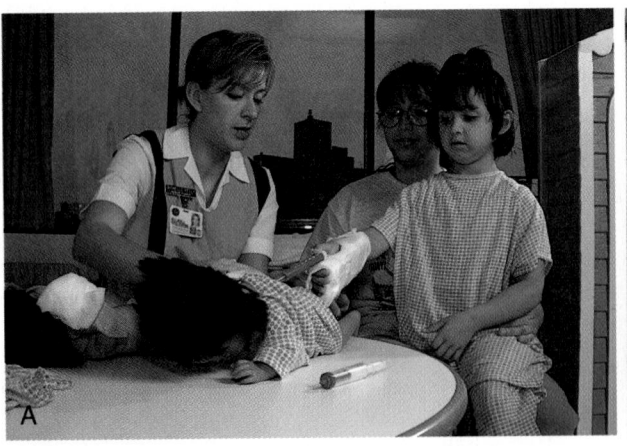
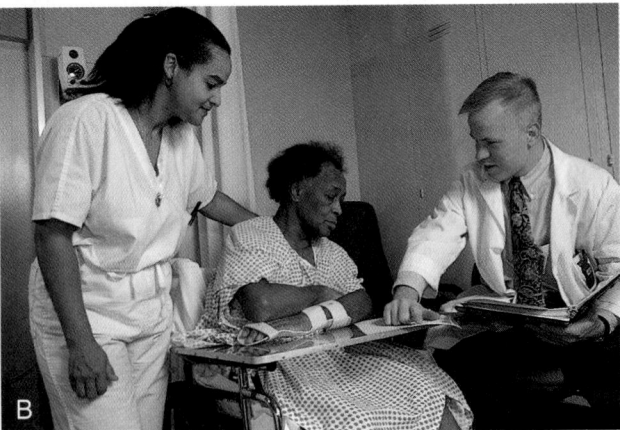

❥ **Figure 14-4**
The nurse's approach to teaching differs from one age group to another. *A*, The nurse teaches a young child, using a doll to demonstrate. Sitting on her mother's lap puts the child more at ease and thus makes her more open to understanding the nurse. *B*, The nurse and nutritionist use visual aids to explain dietary modifications to an older patient. A well-lighted room that is free from distractions facilitates learning.

❧ **Physiological Factors.** Essential information is presented in consideration of the learner's physiological changes. Physiological problems such as pain, fatigue, and change in sleep patterns related to the disease process may interfere with the learner's ability to concentrate. Neurological problems such as memory, hearing, and visual impairment; aphasia; organic-brain syndrome; and loss of fine motor coordination and muscle strength may impair learning capability.

❧ **Cultural Factors.** Illness, pain, and health care practices are perceived differently from culture to culture (Fig. 14–3). Cultural diversity includes differences in ethnicity, religious practices, socioeconomic status, gender preferences, and aging (Capers, 1992). The key to success in providing essential information to the client is first to assess the individual's belief about how to maintain health, prevent illness, and treat disease (Germain, 1992; Tripp-Reimer, 1989).

When the nurse teacher is from a culture different from that of the client and family/significant other, communication problems may arise. Understanding cultural differences between the learner and the teacher helps the nurse teacher tailor teaching to the

---

Table 14–3

DEVELOPMENT STAGE AND IMPLICATIONS FOR CLIENT TEACHING

INFANT

At this stage, learning is not health focused. The nurse teacher makes the infant feel as secure as possible and provides familiar comfort objects from home.

TODDLER

The nurse includes parents in the teaching process. Play, practicing motor skills, and sensory experiences are used to teach about procedures. Use simple commands; offer picture books and tapes that describe health experiences; use slow, simplified speech and verbs, nouns, and adjectives that have meaning that the child shares with others. Provide an opportunity to imitate what was taught. Teaching sessions are brief. When a behavior is necessary, a choice is not given to the toddler.

PRESCHOOLER

Cognitive development is in the preoperational stage. When the nurse provides information, the parents and/or significant others are involved. Information is provided using visual symbols and sensory experiences, such as a drawing, doll, teddy bear, and/or model or diagram. Preschoolers are given only as much as they can handle. Opportunities to repeat information that has been learned are given. Teaching sessions are brief. Role playing, imitation, and play are used.

SCHOOL-AGE

Cognitive development is in the concrete operational stage. School-age children are ready for direct formal learning from the nurse. They welcome sensory, factual, and procedural information. They are able to learn about safety rules for activities, injury control, first aid, exercise regimens, how equipment works, stress control, and illness prevention. They seek clarification of information. Repetition and summarization are useful methods for reinforcing. Younger school-age children may need the presence of parents during teaching sessions. Teaching sessions should be 30 minutes in length and no more than 2 days apart. A sense of success is fostered by the nurse through systematic instruction in skills and tasks that promote self-care management.

ADOLESCENT

Cognitive development is in the stage of formal operations, where the learner pays close attention to details and carefully analyzes new problems and situations. The nurse teaches about self-care skills, home care management, manipulation of equipment for medical treatment, accident prevention, environmental safety, sexuality, obesity, pregnancy, venereal disease, substance abuse, and AIDS. Verbal and written materials, complex models, and diagrams are used as indicated. The adolescent participates in planning how needs will be met and, when possible, is allowed autonomy for scheduling teaching sessions.

YOUNG AND MIDDLE-AGED ADULT

Cognitive development has achieved its full capacity. Learning is motivated when information is meaningful and applicable. Both young and middle-aged adults need to be involved with planning and directing learning. Client information should be meaningful and presented with consideration of lifestyle changes, cognitive abilities, energy levels, and hearing and seeing acuity.

OLDER ADULT

Cognitive development may be affected by motivation, interest, decreased speed response, and less efficient short-term memory. Fragmented sleep cycles contribute to fatigue and inability to concentrate. Information should be relevant to existing life needs. Allow longer response time. Provide opportunities for recall.

TEACHING OLDER ADULTS

- Assess for fatigue, pain, hunger, anxiety
- Assess for visual acuity
- Assess hearing; check for hearing aid; face the client if loss is present
- Keep sessions short
- Teach at a time when the person is able to concentrate
- Keep explanations simple and concrete
- Teach in a quiet, well-lighted room free from distractions
- Encourage the client to ask questions

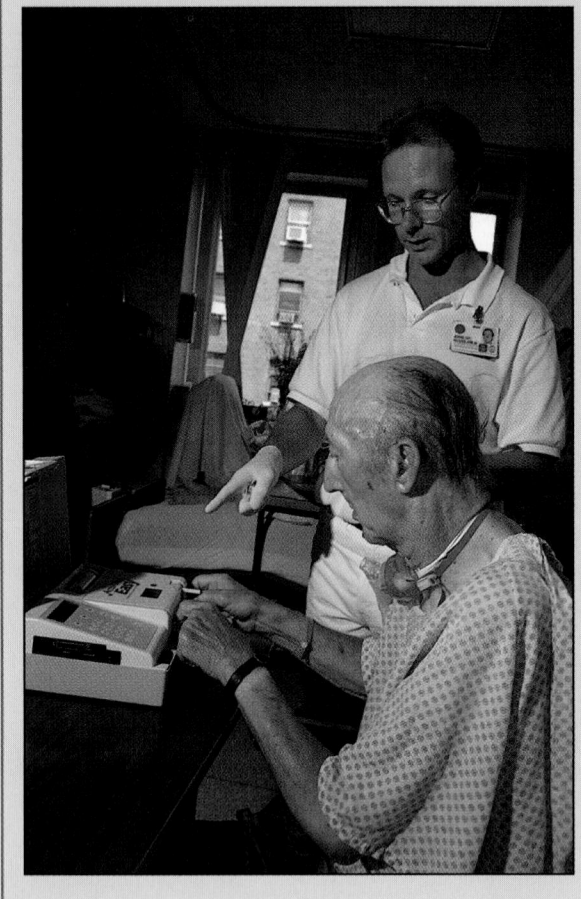

client's and family/significant other's beliefs and practices. Effective communication of essential client information requires the nurse teacher to be aware that learning is often culturally based. How the person prefers to learn is unique in each teaching-learning situation.

✦ **Developmental Factors.** Developmental tasks involve biological, cognitive, and psychosocial factors that influence readiness to learn at a particular stage of life (Bowers *et al.*, 1992; Erikson, 1963; Ginsburg & Opper, 1979; Havighurst, 1967). Developmental tasks may arise from a combination of these factors, such as physical maturation, pressure of cultural processes, and/or values, interests, needs, and aspirations (Fig. 14–4). See Unit IV for further discussion of growth and development. Task achievements are identified by age ranges such as, child, adult, or older adult, rather than by actual chronological age. The actual age of the learner may vary.

The teaching moment or learning readiness is based on the learner's willingness and ability to make use of the information taught. Readiness to learn is limited by the degree of maturity of the learner at the time the learning situation is encountered. The learner's physical maturation and abilities, psychosocial capacity, and cognitive ability are important considerations when providing essential client information. Developmental learning characteristics and teaching implications are found in Table 14–3.

Infants, toddlers, and preschoolers depend primarily on parents and significant others for learning. School-age children are ready for direct formal learning from the nurse. Adolescents can participate in planning how learning needs will be met. Young, middle, and older adults need to be involved with the planning and directing of learning. The older adult can learn skills that help maintain independent functioning as fully as possible (Williams, 1992). Certain teaching tips are helpful when providing essential client information to the elderly (see box).

Characteristics of Setting

Client teaching may take place in a number of different settings. Providing essential information to the client and family/significant other is expected in any practice area in which nurses administer nursing care, including hospital settings, physicians' clinics, ambulatory care, home health care agencies, and the community (DeMuth, 1989; Diehl, 1989; Miner, 1990, Ruzicki, 1989). As mentioned earlier, the setting must provide an environment conducive to learning. Whatever the setting—hospital, home, outpatient settings—the learner's preference for room temperature, lighting, noise, time of day, seating arrangements, and mobility status can affect the teaching-learning process. Characteristics of the client, the family/significant other, and the nurse influence the selection of teaching strategies for learning in a particular setting.

Application of the Nursing Process to Client Teaching

Client teaching is an interactive process between the client and family/significant other and the nurse or, when indicated, other health professionals. The nursing process of assessment, analysis, planning, implementation, evaluation, and documentation assists the nurse teacher in determining the client's and the family/significant other's learning needs, interests, and problems, including readiness to learn.

Using the nursing process, the nurse assesses the client by reviewing the chart and by interviewing the client and significant others. Nursing diagnoses related to teaching and learning are listed, and priorities are determined. The nurse then sets outcomes with specified measurable criteria collaboratively with the learner. The nurse plans meaningful learning experiences with the learner that will aid in achieving mutually set outcomes and evaluating the degree to which the outcomes are met in a particular health care situation.

Each step of the process is documented in the nurse's notes (Fig. 14–5) and communicated orally to other nurses and professionals as indicated. Today, client teaching and documentation of the teaching by nurses are considered reasonable standards of care. Documentation includes both the nursing intervention, such as what was taught, and the outcome, such as what was or was not learned. Failure of nurses to meet this standard can serve as grounds for lawsuits (Fiesta, 1994).

Teaching-learning interventions are adapted to each learner, implemented, evaluated, and documented accordingly. Essential client information (sensual, procedural, and/or factual) is selected and presented by the nurse. The process is psychoeducational, because the information is provided by the nurse in consideration of both learning and emotional needs. The psychoeducational process is structured, flexible, and adapted to the particular learner and health care situation. Communication skills are directed toward motivating the learner to become actively involved in the learning process to achieve positive health outcomes. Providing essential client information requires that the nurse have an understanding of the basic principles of client teaching and learning as well as of the nursing process (Fig. 14–6).

Assessment

In the initial assessment phase of the nursing process, objective and subjective data are collected to determine the client's and the family/significant other's needs, learning ability, learning limitations, and readiness to learn. Assessment provides the nurse with data that identify emergency and safety needs, important client concerns, and health problems. Priorities of nursing diagnoses are set accordingly. Emergency and safety needs, as well as important concerns identified by the client, should be met first.

The nurse collects data that influence the learning process. Data collection includes assessment of physiological, psychological, developmental, cultural, and socioeconomic factors. During physical assessment, the nurse determines the client's levels of anxiety and fear, energy, comfort, visual and hearing acuity, sense of personal control, psychomotor skills and coordination, developmental tasks achieved, cognitive ability, and prior learning experiences. While interviewing, the nurse explores what the client and family/signifi-

---

Nursing Notes

Patient: *J. K. Boer.*

10/23 **S.**   *"I need to know more about this blood pressure medicine before going home."*

   O.   *Wears hearing aid in left ear and glasses for reading.*

   A.   *Knowledge deficit regarding hydrochlorothiazide related to lack of exposure.*

   P.   *Oral and written instruction about medication regimen, purpose, dosage, side effects, food and drug interactions was given. Gave a teaching booklet listing drug facts.*

   E.   *May need further instruction due to hearing deficit. Learning environment noisy. Not able to state name of medication and side effects.*

                                                                                            Maria West, RN

10/27.   *On discharge, medication instruction reviewed again. Client able to state name of medication (i.e., hydrochlorothiazide), purpose, dose, schedule, food and drug interactions, and adverse effects. Instructed to keep appointment with MD. Provided list of adverse effects with instructions to call MD if effects occur.*

                                                                                            Maria West, RN

✦ **Figure 14–5**
Written verification that teaching took place must always be included in the nursing notes or discharge notes. The nursing notes shown here use the SOAPE format.

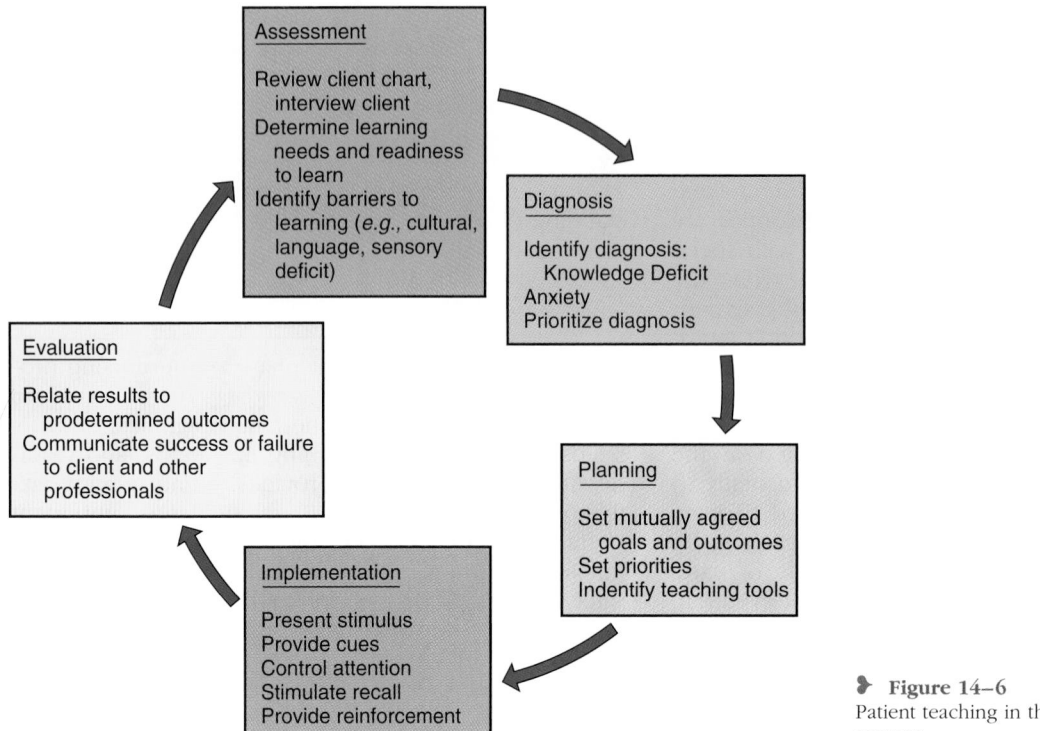

Assessment

Review client chart,
    interview client
Determine learning
    needs and readiness
    to learn
Identify barriers to
    learning (*e.g.*, cultural,
    language, sensory
    deficit)

Diagnosis

Identify diagnosis:
    Knowledge Deficit
Anxiety
Prioritize diagnosis

Evaluation

Relate results to
    prodetermined outcomes
Communicate success or failure
    to client and other
    professionals

Planning

Set mutually agreed
    goals and outcomes
Set priorities
Indentify teaching tools

Implementation

Present stimulus
Provide cues
Control attention
Stimulate recall
Provide reinforcement

❥ **Figure 14–6**
Patient teaching in the context of the nursing process.

cant other want to learn and what the client already knows (Fig. 14–7).

While interviewing and performing the physical assessment, the nurse observes facial expressions, personal hygiene, and body language. Learning capabilities, barriers to learning, and what essential information is needed are documented in the nurse's notes and communicated to other health care team members as indicated. Characteristics of the teaching-learning environment are also considered. Available meaningful teaching resources are identified.

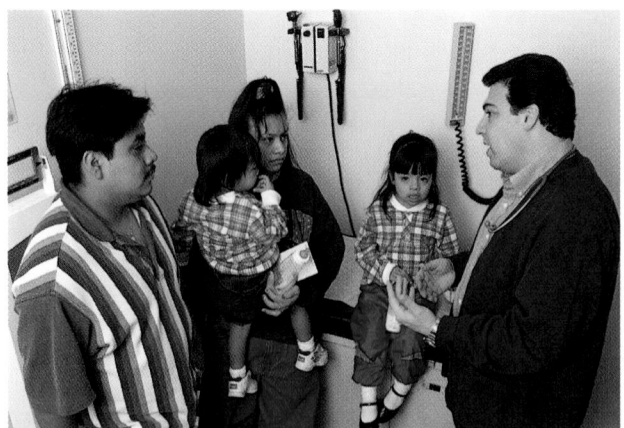

❥ **Figure 14–7**
The nurse explores what the patient and family want to learn and what they already know. Teaching-learning interventions are adapted to the particular learners and the health care situation.

Nursing Diagnosis

Once data collection is completed, the nurse organizes and analyzes the data to form nursing diagnoses related to learning needs, such as knowledge deficit and anxiety. Knowledge deficit can be applied to deficits in all three learning domains (cognitive, affective, and psychomotor). For example, knowledge deficit may be related to the prescribed plan of treatment (cognitive), the potential for recovery from illness (affective), or the self-administration of insulin (psychomotor). The client and/or significant other may be experiencing knowledge deficit as demonstrated by the following characteristics:

* Verbalization of inadequate information or of inadequate recall of information about health problems, procedures, and home self-management
* Verbalization of misunderstanding or misconception of information
* Request for information
* Inadequate follow-through of instruction
* Inadequate performance on a test
* Inadequate demonstration of a skill

Factors associated with knowledge deficit are:

* Cultural or language barriers
* Inattention
* Intellectual limitations
* Ineffective coping related to pain, anxiety, or lack of social support

- Lack of exposure to accurate information
- Lack of motivation to learn
- Lack of readiness to learn
- Memory loss or sensory deficits
- Pathophysiological states associated with illness

See the accompanying box for examples of nursing diagnoses for knowledge deficit.

Nursing diagnoses that may occur with knowledge deficit are:

- Ineffective coping related to anxiety, pain, or lack of social support
- Noncompliance related to inadequate or inaccurate knowledge, altered thought processes, decreased motivation, or inadequate resources
- Impaired home maintenance management related to insufficient knowledge
- Impaired communication related to physical condition or language barrier
- Impaired physical mobility related to activity intolerance, perceptual/cognitive impairment, limited strength, or severe anxiety

Before presenting client information, the nurse examines both objective and subjective data for characteristics that indicate the presence of anxiety. Anxiety is a vague, uneasy feeling, the source of which is often nonspecific or unknown to the individual. Defining characteristics that indicate that the client may be experiencing anxiety are (Kim *et al.,* 1993):

- Increased heart rate
- Increased blood pressure
- Pupil dilation
- Restlessness
- Poor eye contact
- Insomnia
- Uncertainty
- Trembling
- Increased urinary frequency
- Narrowed perceptual field
- Poor appetite
- Distress
- Apprehension
- Increased tension

> **SPECIFIC KNOWLEDGE DEFICIT DIAGNOSES**
>
> - Knowledge deficit (digoxin) related to memory loss
> - Knowledge deficit (fiber diet) related to lack of exposure to accurate information
> - Knowledge deficit (insulin administration) related to anxiety

---

> **SPECIFIC ANXIETY DIAGNOSES**
>
> - Severe anxiety related to controlled ventilation
> - Moderate anxiety related to anticipated transfer to nursing home
> - Severe anxiety related to uncertain surgical outcome

Related factors include:

- Unconscious conflict about essential values and goals of life
- Threat to or change in health status
- Socioeconomic status
- Role functioning
- Change in environment
- Change in interaction patterns
- Situational and maturational crises
- Unmet needs

Examples of nursing diagnoses for anxiety can be found in the accompanying box.

In the process of providing essential information to the client, the nurse takes into account the learner's level of anxiety, pacing the presentation of information and providing structure to the situation as indicated. Documentation of anxiety levels observed and action taken is made in the nursing notes.

Planning

The psychoeducative plan provides structured client information (sensory, procedural, and/or factual) to the learner. The plan takes into account nursing diagnoses related to the client's and the family/significant other's learning needs and anxiety levels. The information to be presented is identified. The pace of the presentation depends on the anxiety level of the learner.

Mutually agreed on outcomes with achievable, measurable criteria are specified, usually in writing. Priorities are set. Safety needs are met first. The teaching plan is initiated when the learner is physically able to listen and ask questions. The structured plan effectively assists the individual learner in attaining mutually set learning outcomes within a reasonable amount of time and with a reasonable amount of effort.

The information to be taught is tailored to the client and/or family, taking into account characteristics of the nurse teacher, the learner, and the particular setting. The overall goal is to promote positive health behaviors. The plan guides the nurse in the teaching-learning process. The plan identifies available teaching tools (*e.g.,* audiovisuals, anatomical models, hand puppets, pamphlets, transparencies), suggested methods for intervention, and educational objectives based on learning domains and developmental levels of the learner. The plan provides guidelines to the nurse on how, when, and where to record the results of the teaching event, beginning from assessment to evaluation and starting from admission through discharge.

An example of a standardized care plan is given to use when teaching a client and/or family about a medication (see Nursing Care Plan 14–1). The content of the plan is adjusted to the learning needs of the learners as indicated by assessment.

NURSING CARE PLAN

THE CLIENT WITH CHEST PAIN

Situation: Mr. J. is a 63-year-old who was admitted to the hospital because of chest pain. His electrocardiogram and enzymes were normal. His blood pressure stabilized at 160/98. He will be discharged on a hypertensive medication. He has never taken any medication before this hospitalization.

Nursing Diagnosis: Knowledge deficit related to prescribed medication owing to lack of exposure.

Expected Outcomes: Following teaching by the staff nurse, at the time of discharge the client and/or family/significant other will be able to state orally the name of the medication; the dose and schedule of doses; the color, size, and shape of the medication; its intended effects; and side effects and adverse effects for which to be alert and actions to be taken.

Action	Rationale
1. Greet client and family/significant other by name. Speak clearly and distinctly. Introduce yourself with your title. Explain what you will be doing.	1. Establishes rapport and initiates a trusting relationship
2. Ask about important concerns. Summarize information.	2. Clarifies the client's expectations and helps the nurse match the information to be provided.
3. Assess the client's readiness to learn about the medication by determining functional, cognitive, and sensory abilities such as memory, vision, hearing, tactile stimulation, and sense of smell and taste; ability to read aloud from client education material; cultural barriers; anxiety level; and learning climate.	3. Provides a baseline assessment for the purpose of making nursing diagnoses related to learning needs and anxiety level to implement a teaching plan tailored to the client and the particular setting.
4. Set mutually agreed on learning outcomes with the client and family/significant other.	4. Learning is effective when it is directed to expected achievable outcomes.
5. Provide the client with information explaining the purpose of the medication; its intended effects; adverse effects and actions to take when they occur; the dose and schedule of doses; and the color, size, and shape of the medication.	5. A well-informed client can help prevent medication errors and other adverse effects.
6. Show the client the medication and ask him if it's the right pill and right dosage. Ask him what time he's to receive his medication	6. The learner becomes actively involved and moves toward achieving the outcome. Meaningful visual aids reinforce the instruction and promote attention.
7. At discharge, verify the client's and/or family/significant other's understanding of his prescription. Ask him the name of the medication. Ask why he is taking the medication. What adverse effects are reasons to contact his MD? How will his activities be affected by the medication? Give the client a list of the adverse effects with instructions to call his MD if the effects occur. Instruct the client to keep his appointment with the MD.	7. The client should have written information about the medication and keep his scheduled appointment with the MD to prevent medication error and check on health status.
8. Evaluate the degree to which the stated outcomes were achieved. Document what was taught, when the information was taught, and whether the outcomes were met or not met in the client's record. Use the term "teach" or "instruct" when describing the process.	8. Evaluation and documentation provide continuity of care. Use of the term "teach" when documenting client education serves as written evidence that nurses spend time teaching their clients.

c. checks with other professionals
d. assesses the client's and family/significant other's understanding of adverse effects

2. The nurse applies the unitary learning principle when he or she refers to the client as

a. the cardiac bypass who needs discharge teaching
b. the new diabetic mother in room 426
c. Mrs. Jones, who was just discharged home
d. Jane, the cardiac, in room 504 who was just admitted

3. When teaching the client and family/significant other, the nurse should

a. document what was taught and the outcomes achieved
b. consider safety needs last
c. limit sessions to 30 minutes
d. ignore the presence of anxiety

4. Following a teaching session on heart medications, the nurse asks Miss J. to explain the purpose of the heart medication she is taking. The nurse is attempting to

a. evaluate the degree to which a learning outcome has been achieved
b. plan for time to provide more information
c. organize information to be presented
d. assess learning needs

5. Which of the following learning activities requires the most active participation on the part of the learner?

a. reading a medication pamphlet
b. watching a video film
c. answering questions
d. practicing insulin administration

Critical Thinking Exercises

1. You are going to teach a newly diagnosed diabetic client how to care for her condition at home and prevent complications. What are some of the initial assessment data you would use to support a diagnosis of "knowledge deficit?"

2. Mr. T. is living in a low-income apartment complex and receives food stamps and Medicare. He is to be discharged with a diagnosis of post–coronary artery bypass surgery. What would be some of the interventions and strategies you would use for teaching Mr. T. as his home health nurse?

References

American Hospital Association. (1973). *A patient's bill of rights.* Chicago: American Hospital Association.

American Nurses' Association. (1975). *The professional nurse and health education.* Kansas City, MO: American Nurses' Association.

American Nurses' Association. (1985). *Code for nurses with interpretative statements.* Kansas City, MO: American Nurses' Association.

Anderson, C. (1990). *Patient teaching & communicating in an information age.* Albany, NY: Delmar Publishers.

Beck, L., *et al.* (1993). Use of the code of ethics for accountability in discharge planning. *Nursing Forum, 28*(3), 5–12.

Bigge, L. (1982). *Learning theories for teachers.* New York: Harper.

Bloom, B. S. (1956). *Taxonomy of educational objectives: Book I: Cognitive domain.* New York: David McKay.

Bowers, A. C., *et al.* (1992). *Clinical manual of health assessment* (4th ed.). St. Louis: Mosby–Year Book.

Breemhaar, B., & van den Borne, H. W. (1991). Effects of education and support for surgical patients: The role of perceived control. *Patient Education and Counseling, 18,* 199–210.

Breeze, W. (1987). Educational readiness in hospitalized adults. *Today's OR Nurse, 9*(7), 28–32.

Bubela, N., *et al.* (1990). Factors influencing patients' informational needs at time of hospital discharge. *Patient Education and Counseling, 16,* 21–28.

Capers, C. F. (1992). Teaching cultural content: A nursing education imperative. *Holistic Nursing Practice, 6*(3), 19–28.

Cormier, L. S., Cormier, W. H., & Weisser, R. J. (1984). *Interviewing and helping skills for health professionals.* Monterey, CA: Wadsworth Health Science Division.

Davis, T. C., *et al.* (1990). The gap between patient reading comprehension and readability of patient education materials. *Journal of Family Practice, 31,* 533–538.

Davis, T. M., *et al.* (1994). Preparing adult patients for cardiac catheterization: Informational treatment and coping style interactions. *Heart and Lung, 23*(2), 130–139.

DeMuth, J. (1989). Patient teaching in the ambulatory setting. *Nursing Clinics of North America, 24*(3), 645–653.

Devine, E. C., & Reifschneider, E. (1995). A meta-analytic analysis of effects of psycho-educational care in adults with hypertension. *Nursing Research, 44*(4), 237–245.

Diehl, L. N. (1989). Client and family learning in the rehabilitation setting. *Nursing Clinics of North America, 24*(1), 257–264.

Dixon, E., & Park, R. (1990). Do patients understand written health information? *Nursing Outlook, 38*(6), 278–281.

Doak, C. C., *et al.* (1985). *Teaching patients with low literacy skills.* Philadelphia: J. B. Lippincott.

Erikson, E. H. (1963). *Childhood and society* (2nd ed.). New York: W. W. Norton.

Fiesta, J. (1994). Premature discharge, *Nursing Management, 25*(4), 17–20.

Foster, S. D. (1988). The role of education in discharge planning. *Maternal Child Nursing, 13*(6), 403.

Gage, N., & Berliner, D. (1992). *Educational psychology* (5th ed.). Boston: Houghton Mifflin.

Gagne, R. M. (1977). *The conditions of learning* (3rd ed.). New York: Holt, Rinehart, & Winston.

Germain, C. P. (1992). Cultural care: A bridge between sickness, illness and disease. *Holistic Nursing Practice, 6*(3), 1–9.

Gilbert, M. D. (1993). Caring for culturally diverse patients. *R.N. 10,* 44–45.

Ginsburg, H., & Opper, S. (1979). *Piaget's theory of intellectual development* (2nd ed.). Englewood Cliffs, NJ: Prentice-Hall.

Good, C. (1959). *Dictionary of education.* New York: McGraw-Hill.

Hanak, M. (1986). *Patient and family education: Teaching programs for managing chronic disease and disability.* New York: Springer.

Harrow, A. J. (1979). *A taxonomy of the psychomotor domain: A guide for developing behavioral objectives.* New York: David McKay.

Havighurst, R. J. (1967). Development tasks and education (2nd ed.). New York: David McKay.

Heidgerken, L. (1965). *Teaching and learning in schools of nursing: Principles and methods* (3rd ed.). Philadelphia: J. B. Lippincott.

Helberg, J. (1990). Information needs in home care: A review and analysis. *Public Health Nursing, 2*(1), 65–71.

Henderson, V. (1966). *The nature of nursing: A definition and its implication for practice, research, and education.* New York: Macmillan.

Jackson, J., & Johnson, E. (1988). *Patient education in home care.* Rockville, MD: Aspen.

Johnson, J. E., *et al.* (1978). Sensory information, instructions on a coping strategy, and recovery surgery. *Research in Nursing and Health, 1,* 4–17.

Joint Commission on the Accreditation of Healthcare Organizations. (1996). *Accreditation manual for hospitals: Nursing services.* Oak Brook Terrace, IL: The Joint Commission on the Accreditation of Healthcare Organizations.

Jubeck, M. E. (1994). Teaching the elderly: A common sense approach. *Nursing 1994, 5,* 70–71.

Kim, M. J., *et al.* (1993). *Pocket guide to nursing diagnoses* (5th ed.). St. Louis: Mosby–Year Book.

Knowles, M. (1990). *The adult learner: A neglected species* (4th ed.). Houston, TX: Gulf.

Krathwohl, D. R., *et al.* (1956). *Taxonomy of educational objectives: Book II: Affective domain.* New York: David McKay.

Lazarus, R., & Folkman, S. (1984). *Stress, appraisal and coping.* New York: Springer.

Lierman, L. M., *et al.* (1994). Effects of education and support on breast self-examination in older women. *Nursing Research, 43*(3), 158–163.

McGinnis, J. M. (1993). The role of patient education in achieving national health objectives. *Patient Education and Counseling, 21,* 1–3.

Melnyk, B. M. (1994). Coping with unplanned childhood hospitalization: Effects of informational interventions on mothers & children. *Nursing Research, 43*(1,), 50–55.

Miller, B., & Bodie, M. J. (1994). Determination of reading comprehension level for effective patient health-education materials. *Nursing Research, 43*(2), 118–119.

Miner, D. (1990). Preoperative outpatient education in the 1990's. *Nursing Management, 21,* 40–44.

Morse, G. (1990). Resurgence of nurse assistants in acute care. *Nursing Management, 21*(3), 34–36.

Nightingale, F. (1932). *Notes on nursing: What it is, and what it is not.* New York: Appleton.

Opdyce, R. C., *et al.* (1992). A systematic approach to educating elderly patients about their medications. *Patient Education and Counseling, 19,* 43–60.

Padilla, G. V., *et al.* (1981). Distress reduction and the effects of preparatory teaching films and patient control. *Research in Nursing and Health, 4,* 375–387.

Rakel, B. A. (1992). Interventions related to patient teaching. *Nursing Clinics of North America, 27*(3), 397–422.

Rankin, S. H., & Stallings, K. D. (1990). *Patient education: Issues, principles, practices* (2nd ed.). Philadelphia: J. B. Lippincott.

Redman, B. K. (1993). *The process of patient education* (7th ed.). St. Louis: Mosby–Year Book.

Rivers, O. (1991). Staff perception of responsibilities to provide patient education in the hospital setting. *Journal of Health Care Education and Training, 6*(12), 8–12.

Rothman, D., & Rothman, N. (1981). The legal basis for patient education practice in nursing. In B. K. Redman (Ed.), *Issues and concepts in patient education.* New York: Appleton-Century-Crofts.

Ruzicki, D. A. (1989). Realistically meeting the educational needs of hospitalized acute and short-stay patients. *Nursing Clinics of North America, 24*(3), 629–637.

Simpson, E. J. (1972). The classification of educational objectives in the psychomotor domain. In *Contributions of behavioral science to instructional technology: The psychomotor domain.* Mt. Ranier, MD: Gryphon Press.

Slavin, R. E. (1991). Educational psychology: Theory into practice (3rd ed.). Boston: Allyn & Bacon.

Spees, C. M. (1991). Knowledge of medical terminology among clients and families. *Image, 23*(4), 225–229.

Streiff, L. (1986). Can clients understand our instructions? *Image, 18*(2), 48–52.

Tarsitano, B. J. (1992). Structured preoperative teaching. In G. Bulechek & J. McCloskey (Eds.), *Nursing interventions: Essential nursing treatments* (2nd ed.). Philadelphia: W. B. Saunders.

Thoma, G. B. (1994). Evolution of a patient education program in a rural hospital. *Nursing Management, 25*(1), 46–48.

Tripp-Reimer, T. (1989). Cross-cultural perspectives on patient teaching. *Nursing Clinics of North America, 24,* 597–604.

Weinrach, S. P., & Boyd, M. (1992). Education in the elderly: Adapting and evaluating teaching tools. *Journal of Gerontology Nursing, 18,* 15–20.

Whitman, N. I., *et al.* (1992). *Teaching in nursing practice: A professional model* (2nd ed.). Norwalk, CT: Appleton-Lange.

Williams, A. S. (1992). Adaptive diabetes education for visually impaired persons. Teaching nonvisual diabetes self-care. *Journal of Home Health Care Practice, 4*(3), 62–71.

Bibliography

Brown, S. (1990). Studies of educational interventions and outcomes in diabetic adults: A meta-analysis revisited. *Patient Education and Counseling, 16,* 189–215.

Freiberg, K. L. (1983). *Human development: A life-span approach* (2nd ed.). Monterey, CA: Wadsworth Health Science Division.

Hathaway, D. (1986). Effect of preoperative instruction on postoperative outcomes: A meta-analysis. *Nursing Research, 35,* 269–274.

Kruger, S. (1991). The patient educator role in nursing. *Applied Nursing Research, 4*(1), 19–24.

Unit ✦ IV

APPLICATION OF THE NURSING PROCESS TO NORMAL GROWTH AND DEVELOPMENT

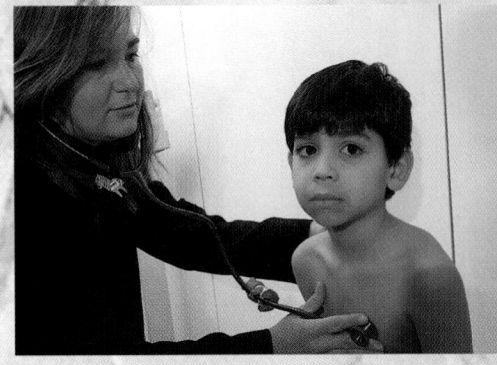

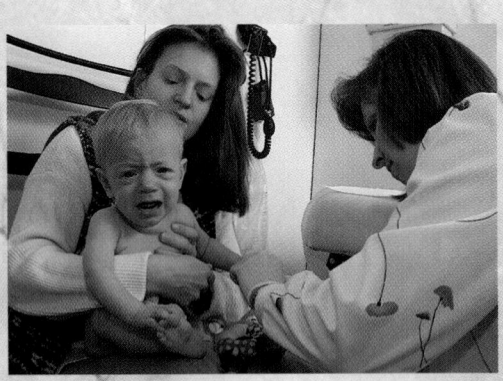

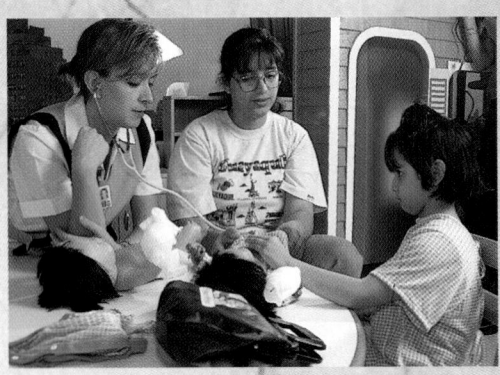

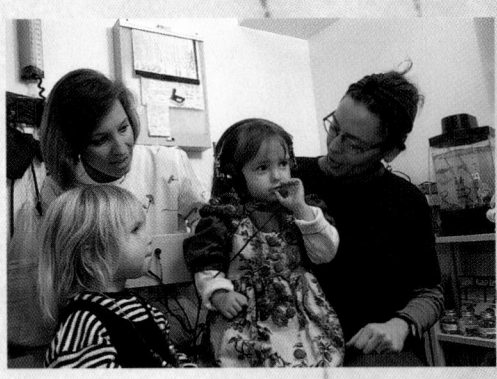

People often ask me how I can regularly work with ill children. They believe that seeing children sick or in pain must be a devastating experience for a nurse. When I think of pediatric nursing, however, two important themes come to my mind— resiliency and magic. The interaction between these two makes the nursing of children a gratifying and challenging experience.

Many children are resilient— even the most severely ill or those who are exposed to the most adverse environmental conditions. Resiliency is a concept that describes how children are able to withstand long-term emotional consequences of serious illness or adversity. An ongoing nursing challenge is to help children use their unique resiliency factors to cope with pain, fear, and anxiety. Actively incorporating supportive families in the child's care is a most important action that bolsters resiliency in children. Play, which is part of the fabric of children's lives, can distract children from pain and can help them achieve a measure of control over a variety of unpleasant situations.

Being an effective pediatric nurse requires a sense of fun and a willingness to play with children. Don't be afraid to work a child's magical view of life into nursing care. Be willing to be sprinkled with pretend fairy dust by a child who wants to be sure that you will give an immunization gently. Don't be afraid to "blow a kiss" to someone who needs a "boo-boo" made better. Explain things in automotive language to the child who says he is a 16-wheeler truck today. Encourage children to safely play with medical equipment and decorate the equipment to make it more interesting to play with. Being able to use a child's magical approach to life to enhance resiliency is a challenge unique to pediatric nursing. It makes working with children always a new and exciting experience.

Susan Rowen James, RN, MSN
With nearly 30 years of experience as a pediatric nurse, clinical specialist, and educator, Susan James currently practices in a pediatric/adolescent ambulatory care setting in Falmouth, Massachusetts. She is also an assistant professor of nursing at Curry College in Milton, Massachusetts, teaching nursing of children and community health.

Chapter 15

CONCEPTS BASIC TO DEVELOPMENT

BETH A. YATES, RN, MSN, PCNS

KEY TERMS

✦

cephalocaudal
cognitive development
development
developmental tasks
faith development
growth
holistic care

moral development
proximodistal
psychosexual development
psychosocial development

LEARNING OBJECTIVES

✦

After studying this chapter, you should be able to

✦ Understand growth and development and related terms

✦ Identify and explain the principles of growth and development

✦ Discuss the normal growth and development patterns throughout the life span

✦ Identify major growth and development theorists and compare the different theories

✦ Discuss the major theorists in relation to psychosocial, cognitive, spiritual, and moral development

✦ Recognize factors that can alter the growth and development process

✦ Use growth and development in developing a nursing care plan

✦ Apply knowledge of multiple theories of development in performing nursing care

For years, the focus has been on illness and system reviews to solve people's health problems. Health care is now being considered from a different perspective. The focus is shifting to health promotion, wellness, and the whole person. To practice holistic care, the nurse needs to consider the physical, cognitive, social, moral, and spiritual aspects of a person's life. All these areas combine to make up the whole person and cannot be separated for individual treatment.

Nurses care for individuals of all ages and at all stages of growth and development. This chapter is intended to help the nurse realize the importance of growth and development when caring for clients, whether they are 1 month or 72 years old. As one ages, one never stops growing or developing physically, emotionally, spiritually, socially, and cognitively. Developmental growth continues throughout the entire life span.

This chapter looks at some developmental theorists who have studied humanity and development over the past several decades. The theories being discussed are related to psychosexual, psychosocial, cognitive, moral, and religious development. Each aspect of development studied considers at least one theorist's opinion. These developmental theories are useful because they give guidelines for developing nursing care on an individual basis according to the client's developmental level. It is important to remember that a developmental theory does not consider individualism. Therefore, it is important to stress that the theories studied should be considered only as guidelines for use in nursing care.

In addition, most theorists focus on one aspect of the whole person, such as cognitive, social, moral, and so forth. There are some theorists who study only a particular period of life rather than the entire life span. Therefore, when assessing growth and development, it is necessary to consider several theorists.

Growth and development principles are also explored. These principles are important because they supply the nurse with predictable age-related data.

There is less written about adult stages of growth and development than about children. When studying adult developmental stages, the emphasis is placed primarily on the psychosocial aspects of aging rather than on the biological changes that occur during this period of a person's life.

Understanding growth and development principles and theories can broaden the nurse's knowledge and understanding of findings during an assessment and can help with expected behaviors and approaches. This chapter looks at a variety of developmental theories and developmental expectations at different periods throughout the life span.

Growth and Development Principles

Because every person is unique, growth and development occur at an individual rate. However, growth and development are predictable to some extent, because they proceed in an orderly and sequential manner. Both are influenced by a person's genetic makeup and interactions within a family and a community at large.

A developmental assessment should be an integral part of all nursing assessments. It is a means of evaluating a person based on the expected behaviors for his or her particular age. If the developmental assessment indicates that the person is not responding at the appropriate age level, further assessment should be done. Continual evaluations are necessary, because each individual grows and develops at his or her own pace.

Growth refers to a measurable increase in size or maturity. Physical growth is often evaluated using a standardized chart or scale. These measurements allow the nurse to determine whether the child is growing according to a standard norm for his or her age level. **Development** refers to an increase in complexity of function or to qualitative changes. Qualitative changes refer to functional, psychosocial, and cognitive aspects of growth. Growth occurs with development, and one is needed for the other.

Development is considered to follow **cephalocaudal, proximodistal,** and simple to complex patterns. Cephalocaudal development refers to a directional growth from head to toe. Cephalocaudal growth is dependent on the neuromuscular functions of the individual. Examples of cephalocaudal growth include the child learning to control the head before the trunk or extremities, being able to hold the head erect before standing, and controlling hand movement before being able to put the feet in the mouth.

Proximodistal growth refers to development from near to far. When considering near to far, look at the midline or center (proximal part) of the body and go outward to the periphery. This growth is exemplified by the maturing nervous system. The central nervous system develops before the peripheral nervous system. Examples include an infant being able to control the shoulders before mastering the hands and grasping with the whole hand before manipulating the fingers.

Growth from simple to complex occurs in all areas of development, including fine motor, gross motor, language, and social development. This development is known as differentiation. Examples of simple to complex development include the child crawling before standing, standing before walking, saying words before combining words to make sentences, and playing alone before interacting with others.

Factors That Influence Growth and Development

Remember that growth and development begin with conception and do not end until death. Growth and development are influenced by family dynamics, cultural beliefs, differences in health practices, and child-rearing expectations. Involving the family with health care and understanding the developmental needs of infants, children, and adults are important aspects of nursing today.

Many environmental factors influence growth and development. The external environment usually begins with the family and then extends to peers, school, and eventually the community at large. Examples of some factors that can influence growth and development include:

* Biological—central nervous system development and the onset of puberty
* Historical—family role expectations and child-rearing practices
* Life events—the birth of a sibling and the death of a loved one

In recent decades, having both parents employed outside the home has become more common. This can further broaden the environment in the early years of life. Children are exposed to caregivers outside the home because they are in day care at an earlier age.

There has been much debate concerning whether genetic makeup or environmental factors are stronger influences over growth and development. Most theorists believe that a combination of the two actually determines the end results. The genes help determine what a person is capable of accomplishing, but it is the environment that builds and molds these capabilities.

Often growth and development are thought of in terms of children. However, one of the fastest growing population segments in the United States today is the age group around 85 years. This rapidly growing elderly population is causing more adjustments in middle-aged adults. These adults are concerned not only with their own growing children and families but also with their elderly parents. It is important to assist families in understanding the developmental changes taking place in their growing and changing children, along with the developmental changes occurring in their elderly parents. By assessing the whole family, the nurse can identify problems that interfere with a healthy, coping attitude. The nurse can help family members realize that they are not alone and that solutions and support are available.

When looking at the individual theories, it is important to remember that no single theory covers all aspects of individual growth and development. The nurse must be familiar with a number of theories to care for a client as a whole being.

COMMUNITY BASED CARE

GROWTH AND DEVELOPMENT ASSESSMENT

When nurses work in community settings, they must assess their client's growth and development and other holistic needs quickly and accurately to be able to intervene effectively. Usually, these nurses work independently and see individuals and families who vary markedly in age, developmental stage, and other characteristics. Nurses increase the accuracy and speed of data collection related to growth and development by using

1. Agency forms: Many agencies have standardized, comprehensive assessment forms, which nurses complete during initial visits with diverse clients. It is the nurse's responsibility to determine what sections of the form are to be completed if the client's inability or unwillingness to provide all data and time constraints do not permit completing the entire form.

2. Specialized tools: By evaluating admission data, nurses identify cues or patterns that suggest the need for more specific assessment. For example, when an infant's weight falls below the normal weight curve on a growth grid, the nurse may use the Denver Developmental Screening Test. Bindings help the nurse select the most appropriate interventions and can be shared with the infant's parents, physician, and others if a referral is indicated. As another example, when an older person seems discouraged, the nurse may use the Geriatric Depression Scale. Findings can also help the nurse provide appropriate health teaching and referrals for further evaluation, counseling, and support or social groups.

3. Automation: Some community settings have automated point-of-care documentation systems that simplify assessment. Nurses who carry a laptop computer use it to complete their new referral's admission assessment and even specialized assessments.

Conception to Birth

Growth and development begin with conception. During intrauterine life, the developing fetus grows and becomes a viable infant. All organs are formed and differentiated during the first 3 months of uterine life.

While in the uterus, the fetus is vulnerable to external environmental threats. The placenta protects the growing fetus and provides the nutrients and blood supply needed for growth. Because the blood supply is part of the mother, it is affected by the mother's activities. Environmental factors such as illness, drugs, alcohol, and smoking can cause problems with the developing fetus.

During later intrauterine life, the fetus continues to

grow, and all organ systems, including the neurological and cardiac systems, mature. Nutritional stability is of great importance to the pregnant woman, because the fetus is completely dependent on the mother. Maternal health, through early prenatal care, is essential to help ensure a healthy newborn.

Developmental Theorists and Their Theories

Sigmund Freud's Theory of Psychosexual (Psychoanalytical) Development

Sigmund Freud was a psychoanalyst who studied personality development (Thomas, 1979). Freud studied neurotic adults, not children. He believed that an individual's personality consisted of three parts—id, ego, and superego. According to Freud, certain parts of life were not remembered; these parts were identified as the unconscious mind. The unconscious stored items that could not be recalled but affected one's behaviors.

According to Freud, the id is the part of the mind concerned with self-gratification. The id can get what it wants without realizing any consequences. The ego is the part of the mind that puts restraints on the id. The ego is known as the reality part of the mind, or the conscience. The superego represents the moral development of the mind. The superego is developed from the ego and is concerned with what is right and wrong. Morals and prejudices are determined from the superego.

Freud's five stages of personality development emerged from the beliefs of the unconscious mind. Each stage relates to a body part that brings pleasure or gratification. These body parts are known as erogenous zones. Freud believed that each stage builds on the previous stage. The stages developed by Freud cover the period from infancy through early adulthood.

Oral Stage

The first stage of personality development is called the oral stage and occurs from birth to approximately 18 months of age. This stage is concerned primarily with id gratification. The erogenous zones or body parts that give pleasure are the mouth, lips, tongue, and teeth. Pleasure is gained through sucking, swallowing, chewing, and biting. During this period, infants explore their environment by putting everything in their mouths (Fig. 15–1).

Anal Stage

The anal stage is Freud's second stage and occurs from 18 months to 3 years of age. During this period, the erogenous zone is the anal area. The primary fo-

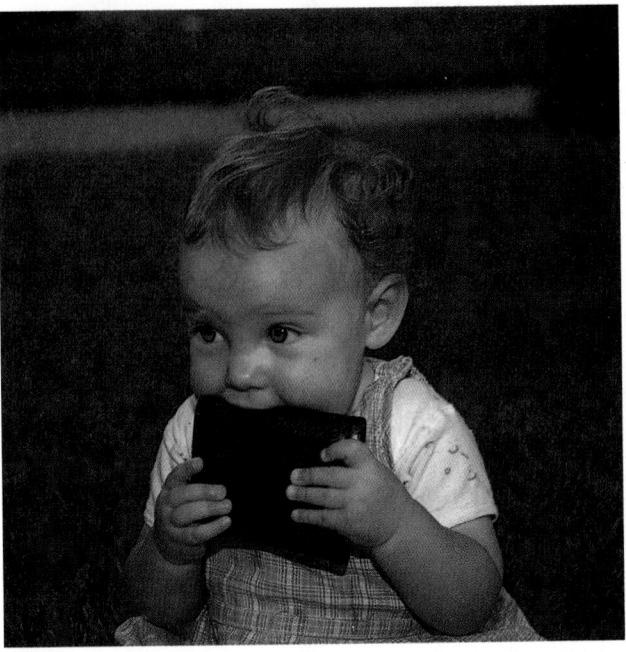

➤ Figure 15–1

An infant explores her environment by putting objects into her mouth. Infancy (birth to 18 months) is Freud's oral stage of personality development.

cus during this stage is toilet training. According to Freud, a conflict occurs between holding on and letting go. The holding-on principle occurs not only with toilet training but also with life situations such as parental control. This conflict of control is considered to be resolved when the child is successfully toilet trained.

Phallic Stage

The third stage of personality development, from 3 to 6 years of age, is identified as the phallic stage. This is the period when the Oedipus or Electra complex occurs. The genitals are the major focus or erogenous zone during this period of development. This is a time when children are learning the differences between the sexes. Conflicts occur while children are learning the roles and relationships of these sex differences by observing their fathers and mothers. This is a very stormy period in the child's development. The conflict is resolved when the child is able to identify with the same-sex parent.

Latency Stage

The period from 6 to 12 years of age is known as the latency stage. This is a period when things are quiet and calm. The child continues to identify with the same-sex parent, with little conflict occurring. During this time, the child is preparing for the last stage.

Genital Stage

The last stage is called the genital stage, which occurs from 12 to 20 years of age. This period begins

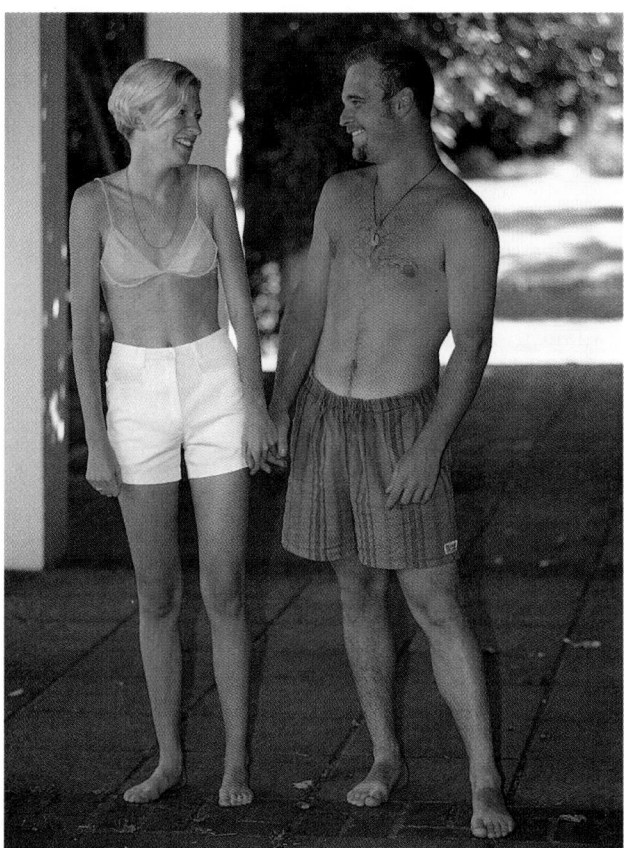

❥ **Figure 15–2**
A young couple holding hands.

with the maturation of the reproductive organs and the production of sex hormones. The genital organs become the erogenous zone and the major source of both pleasure and conflict. The child is preparing for the formation of lasting relationships, a career, and eventually marriage (Fig. 15–2). See Table 15–1 for a summary of Freud's theory.

Erik Erikson's Theory of Psychosocial Development

Erikson studied personality development and expanded on Freud's theory. He believed that personality development is influenced not only by psychosexual drives but also by the social and cultural influences of a society. The child's physical interactions with significant others, particularly early caregivers, play an important role in development. He believed that positive interactions with the environment were necessary for the child to develop a healthy personality.

Erikson (1950) described eight stages or key conflicts that an individual must master during critical growth periods. Each stage has either a favorable or an unfavorable outcome. Progression from one stage to the next stage depends on satisfactory resolution of the previous stages. Erikson also believed that the conflicts faced in early stages continue to reappear throughout life. Therefore, if a person has not successfully resolved an earlier stage, he or she will have difficulty dealing with that type of situation in later years. For example, an individual who did not develop a sense of trust as an infant may have difficulty trusting a spouse after marriage. Erikson believed that the first three stages were the most important for the development of a healthy personality.

Erikson differed from most theorists in his definition of outcomes. Most theorists believe that a stage is either completed or not completed. Erikson identified two separate outcomes for each stage, one positive and one negative. The negative outcome is more than simply the absence of a positive outcome.

Infancy (Trust Versus Mistrust)

A sense of trust must be developed during infancy. This trust is the first and most important stage of development and is the foundation for all other

		Table **15–1**
FREUD'S STAGES OF PSYCHOSEXUAL DEVELOPMENT		
STAGE	**APPROXIMATE AGE**	**CENTER OF FOCUS**
Oral	Infancy 0–18 mo	Mouth is the chief source of pleasure
Anal	Toddlerhood 1½–3 y	Control of bodily excretions provides gratification
Phallic	Preschool 3–6 y	Genitalia exploration, masturbation, and sexual curiosity result in pleasurable sensations; identifies with same-sex parent by end of stage
Latency	School-age 6–12 y	Quiet sexual period; energy is directed toward physical and mental growth
Genital	Adolescence and adulthood 12–20 y	Pleasure derived from genital function and heterosexual relationships

stages to build on. This sense of trust is acquired by having a quality caregiver. The caregiver can be the mother or another significant person in the infant's life. Trust is obtained by having the infant's needs for food, warmth, comfort, and security met. The infant's needs must be met with both affection and a caring attitude. If the needs are met but there is no affection, the infant may still develop a sense of mistrust.

The caregiver should not try to anticipate the infant's needs at all times but must allow the infant to signal needs. If an infant is not allowed to signal a need, he or she will not learn how to control the environment. Erikson believed that a delayed or prolonged response to an infant's signal would inhibit the development of trust and lead to mistrust of others.

Toddler (Autonomy Versus Shame and Doubt)

The child focuses on independence between the ages of 1 and 3 years. At this age, the child is able to be more independent because of physical maturity and complete myelination of the spinal cord. Physical changes allow the child to have more control of fine and gross motor movements, speech, and bowel and bladder function. Areas of independence occur in feeding, dressing, locomotion, and toileting. A sense of autonomy occurs when the child receives encouragement from the parents, learns to do achievable tasks independently, and feels good about these accomplishments. Doubt occurs if the child is not allowed to become independent and remains dependent on the caregiver. If forced to remain dependent, the child will doubt first his or her abilities and then himself or herself. Doubt can also occur if the parent's expectations are too high and the child is unable to perform tasks at the expected level.

Gaining independence often means that the child has to rebel against the parent's wishes. Saying things like "no" or "mine" and having temper tantrums are common during this period of development. Being consistent and setting limits on a child's behavior are the necessary elements. Shame will occur if parents do not allow the child to learn and make mistakes without frequent criticism. Parental guidance must maintain a delicate balance that keeps the child within his or her limits but also allows growth and control over areas ready to be mastered.

As children go through this period of rapid discovery and change, routines become important to their sense of stability. Nurses need to be aware that a hospitalized child has lost all the routines that define his or her existence. This disruption frequently leads to regression and increased feelings of dependency in the child.

Preschool (Initiative Versus Guilt)

The child is now beginning to learn right from wrong and is beginning to develop a conscience. The child is also learning prejudices, biases, and socially acceptable behavior patterns.

According to Erikson, a sense of initiative is achieved as the child gains confidence while exploring and actively interacting with the environment. From this confidence, the child is able to accomplish tasks and gain satisfaction in activities. The child uses all the senses—sight, hearing, feeling, and smelling—to explore the world.

A sense of guilt and loss of confidence occur if the child attempts to perform beyond his or her capabilities and fails. The child feels guilty because he or she believes that the actions were inappropriate. According to Erikson, these guilty feelings will lead the child to develop an unhealthy personality. Therefore, parental setting of limits is an important element during the preschool years.

Middle Childhood (Industry Versus Inferiority)

Erikson believed that middle childhood was the stage of accomplishment. The child focuses on his or her achievements and the recognition gained through these accomplishments. The child enjoys doing projects that he or she can complete independently. It is a time when the child must meet the demands of school. The child must be able to meet the demands of teachers and parents and at the same time feel accepted by peers (Fig. 15–3). During this time, the child begins to move toward peers and friends and away from parents for support. The child also begins to develop special interests that reflect his or her own developing personality instead of the parent's.

One important role for the parents during this period is to prepare the child for school. Upon entering school, the child realizes that he or she is not good at all things. It is important for the child to realize that all children have inadequacies in some areas. Therefore, the child needs adult guidance in finding and developing strengths. The parent must provide praise for the child's accomplishments to build the child's self-confidence. If the child's accomplishments are met with a negative response, the child will develop a sense of inferiority and will lack self-worth.

Adolescence (Identity Versus Role Confusion)

Adolescence is a period of major physical changes. The adolescent is very much aware of these changes and is very concerned with the way he or she appears to others. Adolescents are also trying to learn who they are by trying out different roles within the safety of peer groups. Peer pressures and expectations are very influential on the adolescent. To belong to or be a part of a group is more important than pleasing parents. Therefore, it is common to rebel against parental ideals.

Intimate relationships with the opposite sex occur, and the adolescent is also determining which career or occupation to pursue. Role confusion occurs when the

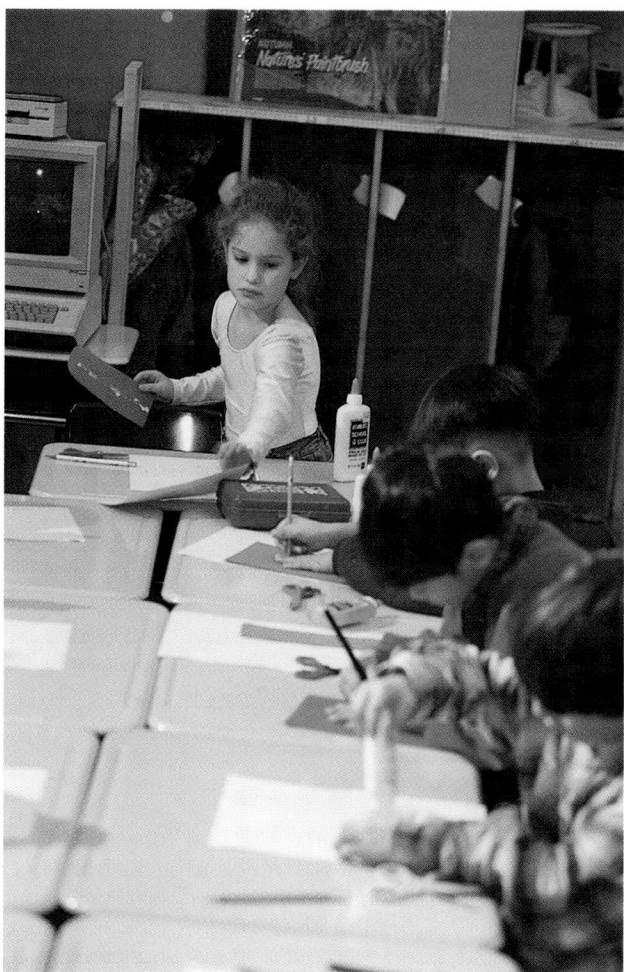

♦ Figure 15–3
According to Erikson, the tasks of middle childhood include achieving a sense of independent accomplishment and gaining peer acceptance.

adolescent is unable to see himself or herself as separate or unique from others and does not establish a direction or career goal in life.

Young Adulthood (Intimacy Versus Isolation)

From about 20 to 40 years of age, the adult makes commitments to others. These commitments occur in all aspects of personal life, such as marriage and work. With personal commitment comes the development of intimate relationships. Intimate relationships lead to marriage, and the person develops a sense of belonging. Fear of commitment in either career goals or marriage or fear of intimacy results in the person being alone and isolated.

Middle Adulthood (Generativity Versus Stagnation)

During this time of life, most people see themselves as productive and creative. The adult is con-

cerned with raising children and what the world will hold for the next generation. The person's career is at its peak, and parenting is a high priority. The adult becomes interested in community activities, wants to make a contribution to the outside world, and is less self-centered. He or she has many life experiences to draw on to assist in resolving conflicts. The generative adult is able to accept the changes that occur in life.

If a person becomes self-absorbed and interested only in his or her own welfare, that person can become stagnated. Stagnated adults hate the changes associated with aging. Characteristics of stagnation are rebellion and withdrawal; such a person is often described by others as "hard to get along with." Stagnated individuals consider themselves old, feel sorry for themselves, and feel that they have nothing to offer the next generation.

Late Adulthood (Ego Integrity Versus Despair)

Late adulthood is the period of old age. The adult reminisces about past life experiences, viewing them in a positive manner. This adult needs to feel good about accomplishments, see successes in life, and feel that he or she has made a contribution to society. Knowledge gained throughout life is passed on to the generations to come (Fig. 15–4).

If the person thinks that life was wasted or sees only failures instead of accomplishments, he or she will feel despair. The individual in despair is disgusted with life, tends to set unrealistic goals, and is overly concerned with weaknesses. See Table 15–2 for a summary of Erikson's theory.

Jean Piaget's Theory of Cognitive Development

Jean Piaget was a well-known theorist in the study of cognitive development from infancy through adolescence. He believed that children progress through a

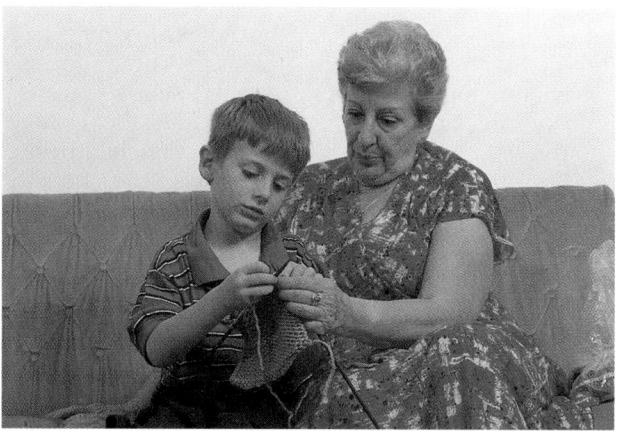

♦ Figure 15–4
An older adult guides a child through craft activity, sharing knowledge gained through life.

Table **15–2**

ERIKSON'S EIGHT STAGES OF PSYCHOSOCIAL DEVELOPMENT

STAGE	APPROXIMATE AGE	GOALS OF TASKS
Trust vs. mistrust	Infancy 0–1 y	Learns to trust others as basic needs are met
Autonomy vs. shame and doubt	Toddler 1–3 y	Learns to become independent in speaking, feeding, dressing, locomotion, and toileting
Initiative vs. guilt	Preschool 3–6 y	Attempts and masters new activities; very active and imaginative
Industry vs. inferiority	Middle childhood 7–12 y	Learns to do activities well and develops a feeling of self-worth through achievements
Identity vs. role confusion	Adolescence 13–20 y	Development of a personal identity and a career goal
Intimacy vs. isolation	Young adulthood 20–40 y	Develops intimate, lasting relationships and a career commitment
Generativity vs. stagnation	Middle adulthood 40–65 y	Productive in career, commitment to community, and concern for parenting and guiding the next generation
Integrity vs. despair	Late adulthood 65 y–death	Satisfied with self and life accomplishments and accepts the inevitability of death

series of mental stages in an orderly, sequential manner. As with the theorists discussed earlier, Piaget also believed that each stage builds on the previous stages (Piaget & Inhelder, 1969). Piaget identified four major stages in the development of logical thinking.

Sensorimotor Stage

The first stage is identified as the sensorimotor stage and occurs from birth to 24 months of age. This particular stage is further divided into six substages. The first substage, from birth to 1 month, is termed the reflexive stage. The infant responds to the environment with reflexive actions, such as sucking or grasping an object. There is no awareness of self or of the existence of the outside environment.

As the child gets older, the reflexive behavior is replaced with voluntary imitative acts. These imitative behaviors happen during the second substage, called primary circular reactions, and last until the child is about 4 months old. During this time, the child begins to recognize familiar faces and objects. The child focuses mainly on his or her own body but soon becomes bored when left alone.

As children continue to mature, they move into the third substage, which is termed secondary circular reactions. This substage occurs from 4 to 8 months of age. The child replaces the imitative acts with intentional behaviors. Activities include a social smile, reaching for objects, shaking a rattle, and searching briefly for objects hidden from sight. Increased activity occurs with increased eye-hand coordination.

The fourth substage is identified as coordination of secondary schemata and occurs from 8 to 12 months of age. During this stage, the infant builds on the imitative and intentional behaviors learned in the previous stages. Now the child is beginning to realize the cause and effect of relationships and can anticipate a result. Therefore, movements become purposeful, with a goal in mind. During this substage, the infant focuses mainly on what is seen. Because of the infant's increased development and motor skills, he or she is able to explore more of the environment. Another concept that occurs around 8 months of age is stranger anxiety. The child becomes very anxious when taken from his or her mother or significant caregiver. The value of this information when caring for a child this age is to realize the importance of having the parent present as much as possible when performing treatments or tests.

The fifth substage is tertiary circular reactions and occurs from 12 to 18 months. At this age, the child is able to separate himself or herself from the environment. Therefore, the child is also able to separate from his or her parents more easily. Cause-and-effect reactions are beginning to develop. The child continues to repeat actions over and over again because he or she cannot yet readily transfer knowledge to new situations. Object permanence—the realization that something out of sight still exists—is also developing. The child in this stage of development will look for an object that has been hidden from sight. The child can understand simple commands but cannot reason. Therefore, a nurse caring for a 2-year-old or younger child needs to realize that it is useless to attempt to reason with this child.

The sixth substage is identified as orientation of new means and occurs from 18 months to 2 years of age. During this period, the child continues to combine all previous learning. This is when the concept of object permanence is achieved. Now the child not only looks where an object has been hidden but also explores other hiding places. A child at this age understands simple words and can anticipate actions or events in relationship to the spoken word. For example, the word *ba-ba* can mean bottle, or *bye-bye* can mean going for a ride in a wagon. During this time, the child loves to play games such as peek-a-boo or this little piggy.

Preoperational Stage

From 2 to 7 years of age is the preoperational stage. This stage is divided into two substages. The first is the preconceptual substage, which occurs from 2 to 4 years. The main characteristic of this period is the development of language. Speech is egocentric and telegraphic. Egocentric speech occurs when the child talks just for fun and cannot see another's point of view. With telegraphic speech, few words are needed to express a thought. For example, when a child wants to use the potty, he or she may say something like "go potty." These two words express a whole sentence. The child gets frustrated when trying to explain an idea if that idea is not understood by others. For this reason, a thorough assessment is necessary on admission to the hospital to discover the child's words for using the bathroom, eating, or a favorite toy.

Piaget identified several concepts that occur during this period of the child's life. One concept common to the preconceptual substage is centration. Centration means that the child can focus on only one thing at a time. A child this age cannot make decisions based on two things. Therefore, the nurse should not give such a child a choice, because it can be frustrating.

Animism is another concept used during this substage. Animism means that all inanimate objects are given living meaning. For example, a child this age will scold the floor or a table if the child hurts himself or herself on the object.

Two other concepts that Piaget identified during this substage are global organization and irreversibility. The first means that if any part of an object or situation changes, the whole thing has changed. For this reason, rituals are important, and absence of familiar routines can be upsetting to a hospitalized child. The nurse may find a child refusing to eat because of the absence of a favorite dish or cup. The second term, irreversibility, means that the child cannot think backward, or reverse a situation. Therefore, one should try to be positive and avoid statements such as "stop that." Instead, use phrases such as "write only on the paper."

A child this age is just beginning to express the need for independence. This need, combined with

lack of social skills, often leads to conduct that is frustrating to the caregiver. Typical behaviors include negativism and saying "no" to virtually everything.

The second substage during the preoperational stage is initiative. At this stage, the child begins to see relationships between things. A child can describe objects and events according to how they are used. Thoughts are understood in relation to what is seen, heard, felt, or smelled. In other words, the senses are used to explore and understand the world. Thus, when the nurse is explaining situations or treatments to a child, they should be described in terms of what the child will see, hear, feel, taste, or smell.

Concrete Operations

The third stage is known as the concrete operations stage and occurs from 7 to 11 years of age. According to Piaget, it is not enough to watch or to be taught. Children must be able to handle and manipulate objects. This hands-on experience is necessary to enhance development. School is a prominent influence in the child's life. A child learns to classify objects according to similarities and learns reversibility. The child is now able to see from another's point of view. Thinking is concrete and in a systematic order. By the end of this stage, the child's mental capacity has developed to the point that he or she is able to think through a task and understand it without actually having to perform the task.

Formal Operations

The last stage identified by Piaget is formal operations, which occurs from 11 to 15 years of age. At this time, the child is able to think in abstract terms. Deductive reasoning is used, and the child attempts to solve hypotheses. A child this age is flexible and can learn to make logical conclusions. Piaget believed that the framework is in place by adolescence, and children continue to grow and build on this framework throughout adulthood. See Table 15–3 for summary of Piaget's theory.

Lawrence Kohlberg's Theory of Moral Development

Moral development follows cognitive development, according to Kohlberg (1984). His theory of moral development is closely aligned with Piaget's levels of cognitive development. Kohlberg (1968, p. 490) stated that "moral judgements tend to be universal, inclusive, consistent, and based on objective, impersonal, or ideal grounds." Thomas (1979, p. 364) further explained Kohlberg's definition of moral judgement as "universal, [it] applies in all situations, and is founded on ideal convictions."

Moral development is just one other aspect of the holistic being. It is also influenced by one's family, cultural background, and environmental experiences.

Table **15-3**

PIAGET'S STAGES OF COGNITIVE DEVELOPMENT

STAGE/SUBSTAGE	APPROXIMATE AGE	COGNITIVE BEHAVIORS
Sensorimotor stage	0–2 y	
Reflexive (substage 1)	0–1 mo	Reactions are primarily reflexive in nature
Primary circular reactions (substage 2)	1–4 mo	Reflexive activity changes to imitative pleasurable behaviors centered mainly on the body
Secondary circular reactions (substage 3)	4–8 mo	Behaviors become intentional, are repeated because of pleasure received, and extend beyond self to the environment
Coordination of secondary schemata (substage 4)	8–12 mo	Child becomes aware of cause-and-effect relationships; has a goal in mind
Tertiary circular reactions (substage 5)	12–18 mo	Continues to strive for new goals and begins to learn object permanence
Orientation of new means (substage 6)	18–24 mo	Begins to understand the environment and anticipates events; object permanence is achieved
Preoperational stage	2–7 y	
Preconceptual (substage 1)	2–4 y	Has difficulty separating fantasy from reality; rapid increase in language development, using telegraphic speech
Initiative (substage 2)	4–7 y	Less egocentric, continues to increase language skills, uses senses to understand the world
Concrete operations stage	7–11 y	Understands conservation, reversibility, and classification of objects; has logical thought patterns; can do mental operations; is aware of others' viewpoints
Formal operations stage	11–15 y	Has the ability to think abstractly, can solve hypotheses; continues throughout adult life

Through growth and experience, the child begins to internalize these beliefs until they become part of the child's own value system. See Table 15–4 for a summary of Kohlberg's theory.

Preconventional or Premoral Level

Kohlberg (1968) identified three levels of moral development, each of which has two stages. The first is the preconventional or premoral level, which coincides with the preconceptual level of cognition and occurs from 2 to 7 years of age. During this time, morals are thought to be motivated by punishment and reward. If the child is obedient and is not punished, then he or she is being moral. This first stage is called the punishment and obedience orientation. At this age, the child does not think about what is right or wrong. The child sees actions as either good or bad. If the child's actions are good, the child is praised; if the child's actions are bad, the child is punished.

The second stage is the naive instrumental orientation. During this stage, the child sees the rewards received for good actions as greatly exceeding the fear of punishment for wrong behavior. Therefore, choices are made to meet the child's own needs. It is during this period that the child learns prejudices and biases through the teachings of the parent or significant other.

Conventional Level

The second level identified by Kohlberg is the conventional level, which coincides with the concrete operations level of cognition and occurs from 7 to 11 years of age. During this period of development, the child is concerned with conforming to the rules, pleasing others, and being loyal to family, peers, or even the nation. Stage three is identified as the good boy, nice girl orientation. That is, if a child is good or nice, the behavior is right. Behaviors that meet with the approval of and please or help others are considered moral. A child this age can usually judge an action by its intentions rather than by its consequences. This is in contrast to earlier years, when consequences were the primary consideration.

Table 15–4

KOHLBERG'S SIX MORAL STAGES

LEVEL/STAGE	APPROXIMATE AGE	CHARACTERISTICS
Level I: Preconventional (pre-moral)	2–7 y	
Stage 1: Punishment and obedience orientation		Socially acceptable behavior is moral, and if behavior is punished, it is wrong
Stage 2: Naive instrumental orientation		Acts to meet own interest and needs; right is what is fair
Level II: Conventional	7–11 y	
Stage 3: Good boy, nice girl orientation		Motivated by living up to expectations of family and peers
Stage 4: Law and order orientation		Upholds laws and rules of society or religious organizations
Level III: Postconventional or Autonomous	12 y–adulthood	
Stage 5: Social contract orientation		Obeys laws to protect the rights of others and chooses moral principles to live by; can work toward changing laws
Stage 6: Universal ethical principle orientation		Must respect the dignity of others, regardless of personal or societal beliefs

The fourth stage is called the law and order orientation. The child obeys rules of conduct and laws because of his or her respect for the authoritative power carried.

Postconventional or Autonomous Level

The final level of moral development is the postconventional or autonomous level. It has also been called the principle level of moral development. This level coincides with the formal operations stage of cognition and occurs from age 12 to adulthood.

Stage five is identified as the social contract orientation. The child believes that behavior is good or correct based on individual rights and standards. A child this age also considers whether an action is legal. At the same time, the child is beginning to see that laws can be changed under certain circumstances.

The universal ethical principle orientation is the sixth and last stage. Kohlberg believes that this stage is rarely achieved. An individual must believe in equality for all, regardless of the beliefs of others or of society.

A person's morals evolve through each of the six stages. At some point, these concepts are internalized as an individual's personal moral code, but the evolution never really stops. As a person continues to grow, more life experiences continue to affect the individual's moral code.

Kohlberg's theory has been criticized as being gender biased. For example, Carol Gilligan (1982) stated that Kohlberg's studies were biased because the populations were mostly male and did not account for sex differences. She believes that men and women make moral judgments in different ways.

Carol Gilligan's Theory of Moral Development

Carol Gilligan began studying moral development with Kohlberg. Gilligan saw male and female moral views as being different. She believed that the female viewpoint was not represented in Kohlberg's work. Therefore, she decided to investigate moral development from the female perspective.

Gilligan's theory attempts to distinguish between male and female concepts of morality. Men and women see morals differently. Male moral concepts are based on obligations, rights, and justice. Women tend to temper these "justice concepts" with an awareness of the importance of caring and responsibility within relationships.

Gilligan identified the morals of women as developing an ethic of care (1982, p. 74). In her theory of moral development, Gilligan identified three levels. See Table 15–5 for a summary of Gilligan's theory of moral development.

Table 15–5	
GILLIGAN'S THEORY OF MORAL DEVELOPMENT	
LEVEL	FEMALE MORAL CHARACTERISTICS
1: Selfishness	Caring for self, excluding all others
2: Goodness	Caring for others, excluding self
3: Ethic of caring	Balance between caring for self and others

Level 1: Selfishness (Caring for Oneself)

The focus in level one is on oneself. The person is self-centered and wants to please only herself. The main outcome is to care for the self. The individual eventually begins to feel selfish and is then ready to move on to level two.

Level 2: Goodness (Caring for Others)

In level two, after recognizing her selfishness, the individual is able to move from caring for self to caring for others. This person begins to feel responsible for the actions of others and excludes her own self-care. The main focus in level two is not hurting others and neglecting one's own needs.

Level 3: Ethic of Caring (Caring for Self and Others)

In level three, the woman realizes that both her personal needs and the needs of others are important. The woman realizes that she must find a balance between the selfishness level and the goodness level. Gilligan believes that the combination and balancing of these two levels is what women's morals are all about. Gilligan states that the two main concepts that balance the needs of self and caring for others are caring and responsibility (Fig. 15–5). Gilligan believes that if one's own needs are not met, one cannot care for others.

Robert Havighurst's Theory of Developmental Tasks

The developmental tasks theory refers to certain tasks that are completed from infancy to death. Every person is faced with certain problems or dilemmas that must be mastered at certain periods of his or her life. Havighurst (1972) believed that in order for the child to live and grow, learning must take place. Behaviors that are learned are called **developmental tasks.** These developmental tasks are learned throughout life. If the task is completed successfully, the person will be happy in his or her own eyes and in society's eyes. A foundation is built as tasks are completed. Completing tasks at one level enables the person to move on to new tasks at the next level. If the person is unsuccessful in achieving these developmental tasks, he or she will be unhappy and unaccepted by society and will have difficulty in later tasks.

Havighurst identified six stages of development that occur throughout the life span. Each of these six stages has from six to ten tasks that must be learned. Havighurst believed that the developmental tasks in each stage are influenced by the individual's physiological growth and capabilities, cultural or societal beliefs, and psychosocial influences.

The stages of development are infancy and early childhood (birth to 5 years), middle childhood (6 to 12 years), adolescence (13 to 17 years), early adulthood (18 to 30 years), middle age (31 to 54 years),

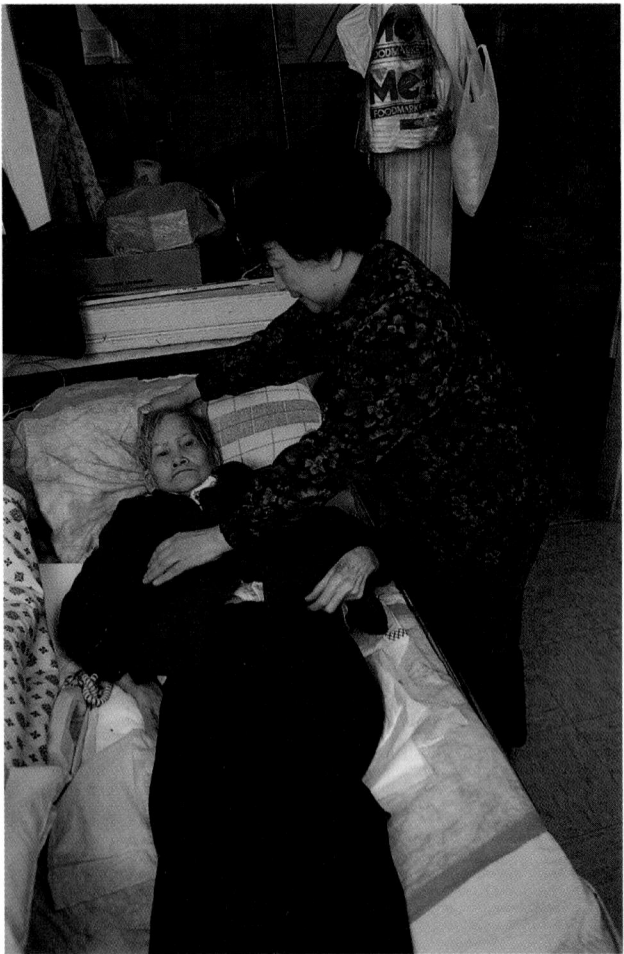
Figure 15–5
Caring for aging parents is one of the tasks of middle adulthood. Women who care for aging parents often find it difficult to balance their own needs and the needs of others. Carol Gilligan explores this dilemma in her theory of the moral development of girls and women.

and later maturity (55+ years). The individual tasks for each stage are listed in Table 15–6.

James Fowler's Theory of Faith Development

Fowler believes that faith is what one uses to define the meaning of life and to make life worth living. Fowler defines faith as follows (1981, p. 4):

Faith is not always religious in its content or context. . . . It is one way of finding coherence in and giving meaning to the multiple forces and relations that make up our lives.

His theory of faith development is closely related to the moral, cognitive, and psychosocial theories of Kohlberg, Piaget, and Erikson. He has divided the process into seven stages (stages 0 through 6) that range

from infancy through adulthood. The stages are not age specific, but because new ideas, thoughts, and behaviors are added to what already existed, each stage must be taken in sequence. Table 15–7 describes each stage and the approximate age at which he expects it to occur.

Fowler believes that faith development is not present in the infant period of growth. During toddlerhood, faith is mainly an imitative act. By the time the child is a preschooler, he or she usually has taken on the faith of the parents.

During the school years, the child has a strong interest in faith and beliefs. The child begins to ask many questions and begins to wonder about the validity of his or her religion and beliefs.

As the child becomes an adolescent, he or she is more aware of spiritual disappointments. The child begins to modify personal beliefs and practices and to form in his or her own mind what to believe. A child

Table 15–6

HAVIGHURST'S DEVELOPMENTAL TASKS

INFANCY AND EARLY CHILDHOOD (BIRTH–5 y)	EARLY ADULTHOOD (18–30 y)
Learning to walk Learning to take solid foods Learning to control the elimination of body wastes Learning sex differences and sexual modesty Forming concepts and learning to describe social and physical reality Getting ready to read	Selecting a mate Learning to live with a marriage partner Starting a family Rearing children Managing a home Getting started in an occupation Taking on civic responsibility Finding a congenial social group
MIDDLE CHILDHOOD (6–12 y)	**MIDDLE AGE (31–54 y)**
Learning physical skills necessary for ordinary games Building wholesome attitudes toward oneself as a growing organism Learning to get along with age-mates Learning an appropriate masculine or feminine social role Developing fundamental skills in reading, writing, and calculating Developing concepts necessary for everyday living Developing conscience, morality, and a scale of values Achieving personal independence Developing attitudes toward social groups and institutions	Assisting teenage children to become responsible and happy adults Achieving adult social and civic responsibility Reaching and maintaining satisfactory performance in one's occupational career Developing adult leisure-time activities Relating oneself to one's spouse as a person Accepting and adjusting to the physiologic changes of middle age Adjusting to aging parents
ADOLESCENCE (13–17 y)	**LATER MATURITY (55 y–d)**
Achieving new and more mature relations with age-mates of both sexes Achieving a masculine or feminine social role Accepting one's physique and using the body effectively Achieving emotional independence from parents and other adults Preparing for marriage and family life Preparing for an economic career Acquiring a set of values and an ethical system as guide to behavior; developing an ideology Desiring and achieving socially responsible behavior	Adjusting to decreasing physical strength and health Adjusting to retirement and reduced income Adjusting to death of a spouse Establishing an explicit affiliation with one's age group Adopting and adapting social roles in a flexible way Establishing satisfactory physical living arrangements

From Havighurst, R. (1972). *Developmental tasks and education* (3rd ed.). New York: Longman. Reprinted by permission of Addison-Wesley Educational Publishers Inc.

Table 15–7

FOWLER'S STAGES OF SPIRITUAL DEVELOPMENT

STAGE	APPROXIMATE AGE	DESCRIPTION OF TASKS
0: Undifferentiated	0–3 y	A presage of faith based on infant's self-concept and interactions with the environment
1: Intuitive/projective	4–6 y	Influenced by a vivid imagination and beliefs of parents; imitative behavior without understanding
2: Mythical/literal	7–12 y	Understanding faith through role playing and biblical stories; can see others' points of view and fairness
3: Synthetic/conventional	13–17 y	Questions others' values and beliefs (family and peers) and develops a better understanding for self
4: Individuative/reflective	18–29 y	Accepts and internalizes own beliefs and attitudes
5: Conjunctive/midlife	30 + y	Truth emerges from one's own beliefs and the integration of others' beliefs
6: Universal	?	Belief in love and justice for all and an existence in the future

this age tends to compare his or her beliefs with those of peers and others and then determine what he or she believes from his or her own perspective.

As young adulthood is reached, a person needs to begin to take responsibility for his or her own beliefs. Some people do not reach this stage until just short of middle age, and some never reach it. At this stage, a person's search for self-identity is no longer bound or limited by the beliefs of significant others.

The sixth stage, usually reached at around age 30 or 40, involves integrating a person's own beliefs with the views of others into an understanding of truth. A person also becomes aware of the inconsistencies of his or her own beliefs.

In the last stage, actually reached by very few people, the inconsistencies encountered earlier are overcome, and a total trust in the principles accepted is developed.

◆ Relevance to Nursing

An understanding of the theories of growth and development is important for all nurses, but each theory has limitations. The theories are based on developmental norms of a population group and make no allowances for individual differences. Therefore, the theories should be used only as guidelines and should be individualized for every client. In addition, most theorists focus on only one aspect of the individual. The nurse needs to remember that a combination of several theories and factors such as culture, social status, and education is necessary to understand and evaluate the whole person.

When performing nursing care, the nursing process should be used to identify client problems and nursing interventions. The nurse must always include a developmental assessment as part of the nursing process. Some possible nursing diagnoses could be:

- Ineffective coping related to loss of independence or loss of peer relationships
- Diversional activity deficit related to lack of age-appropriate toys or immobility
- Knowledge deficit related to hospitalization or lack of understanding of illness and limitations

By understanding growth and development principles and theories, the nurse will have a better idea of a person's capabilities. This is important not only with children but also with adult and elderly clients. If the client's developmental level is assessed, part of health teaching can focus on the developmental needs of clients.

For example, a nurse is assigned to care for a 2½-year-old hospitalized for a tonsillectomy. The nurse should remember that this child is in the preconceptual stage of cognitive development. Therefore, the nurse knows that the development of speech is one characteristic of this age, along with irreversibility. The nurse should know the specific words the child uses, such as the word for medicine. The nurse should be positive when approaching the child and say "it is time to take your medicine" rather than "do you want to take your medicine now?"

Another example would be a school-age child who is admitted to the hospital because of a fractured femur and is in traction. With a knowledge of psychosocial development, the nurse should remember that the most important people in this child's life are the peer group. Because this child is in traction, she cannot go anywhere to participate in appropriate activities. Therefore, it is important to have other children visit the child's room or to move the child's bed to where she can be an active participant in activities. Other suggestions would be to encourage phone calls to friends and to make sure that the child's teacher is aware of her hospitalization. Often a teacher will have the whole class write to a hospitalized child. Receiving an envelope with letters from her class at school will brighten this child's day.

The nurse also needs to avoid stereotyping based on a person's age. An elderly person may be hospitalized for many reasons. Elderly clients can feel helpless and depressed because of worry about how they will manage after going home. Remembering Havighurst's and Erikson's theories, the nurse assesses the client's previous level of functioning and helps this person cope with the lifestyle changes needed on discharge from the hospital. If the client has a positive outlook on life and feels good about earlier levels of developmental achievements, he will be able to get through this adjustment easier. If the client has a feeling of despair, the nurse will have to help the client refocus on strengths and earlier accomplishments. By focusing on these positive aspects, the client will be able to see his life in a more positive manner and will have a more positive attitude about the present situation.

✦ Summary

Nurses must work with entire families, not just individuals, when caring for clients in the hospital or community. A better understanding of growth and development principles enables the nurse to plan better nursing care. Care can now be holistic by being based not only on a client's physical needs but also on the client's developmental needs.

CHAPTER HIGHLIGHTS
✦

✦ Growth is quantitative, whereas development is qualitative in nature.

✦ Growth proceeds from cephalocaudal, proximodistal, and simple to complex.

✦ Each age period revolves around different tasks that need to be accomplished.

✦ Most theories predict a progressive and sequential pattern of development.

✦ Developmental theories should be used as guidelines for delivering holistic nursing care.

✦ Several theories must be considered to deliver holistic nursing care.

✦ Growth and development are influenced by the environment, family dynamics, cultural beliefs, differences in health practices, child-rearing expectations, and genetic makeup.

Study Questions

1. According to Piaget, language development is the main characteristic during the

   a. sensorimotor stage
   b. preconceptual stage
   c. initiative stage
   d. concrete operations stage

2. According to growth and development theorists, growth and development progresses

   a. in only one direction, simple to complex
   b. the same for all children
   c. in a predictable, sequential manner
   d. in a measurable sequence for infants

3. On admission to the hospital, a nursing assessment should include

   a. a physical assessment
   b. a history of present signs and symptoms
   c. a developmental assessment
   d. all of the above

4. The best way to prepare a 15-year-old for a painful procedure is to

   a. be honest when explaining the procedure
   b. allow the adolescent to freely discuss and ask questions about the procedure and any concerns he or she may have
   c. explain in detail how painful the procedure is going to be so there are no surprises
   d. a and b

5. A 4-year-old child has been admitted to the hospital for asthma. The doctor has ordered an x-ray of the child's chest. The best way for the nurse to prepare the child for this procedure is to say that

   a. the doctor wants to look at his or her lungs to see if they are working OK
   b. a large machine is going to take a picture of his or her lungs to see how they are working
   c. this will not hurt and Mommy can stay during the whole procedure
   d. the doctor and nurses will take good care of him or her

Clinical Thinking Exercises

1. You are caring for a preschool child with asthma and a teenager with asthma. Using developmental, moral, psychosocial, and faith theories, compare and contrast how your nursing care would differ for the two clients.

2. A 22-year-old female client has just been diagnosed with a cervical spinal cord injury. She is now a quadraplegic.

Discuss the possible impact of this injury on her moral, psychosocial, and faith development.

References

Erikson, E. (1950). *Childhood and society* (2nd ed.). New York: Norton.

Fowler, J. W. (1981). *Stages of faith: The psychology of human development and the quest for meaning.* New York: Harper & Row.

Gilligan, C. (1982). *In a different voice: Psychological theory and women's development.* Cambridge, MA: Harvard University Press.

Havighurst, R. S. (1972). *Human development and education* (3rd ed.). New York: Langmans, Green.

Kohlberg, L. (1968). Moral development. In *International encyclopedia of the social sciences.* New York: Macmillan.

Kohlberg, L. (1984). *The psychology of moral development.* San Francisco: Harper & Row.

Piaget, J., & Inhelder, B. (1969). *The psychology of the child.* New York: Basic Books.

Thomas, R. M. (1979). *Comparing theories of child development.* Belmont, CA: Wadsworth.

Bibliography

Campbell, J. M. (1992). Parenting classes: Focus on discipline. *Journal of Community Health Nursing, 9*(4), 197–208.

Frick, S. B. (1987). Integrating growth and development content into practice: A nursing process framework. *Nurse Educator, 12*(1), 30–33.

Gillis, A. J. (1990). Nurses' knowledge of growth and development principles in meeting psychosocial needs of hospitalized children. *Journal of Pediatric Nursing: Nursing Care of Children and Families, 5*(2), 78–87.

Holaday, B. (1993). Adolescent literature as a means of studying growth and development. *Journal of Nursing Education, 32*(2), 93–95.

Jansen, M. T., Dewitt, P. K., Meshul, R. J., Krasnoff, J. B., Lau, A. M., & Keens, T. G. (1989). Meeting psychosocial and developmental needs of children during prolonged intensive care unit hospitalization. *Child Health Care, 18*(2), 91–95.

Kohlberg, L., & Kramer, R. (1969). Continuities and discontinuities in childhood and adult moral development. *Human Development, 12,* 93–120.

MacLean, T. B. (1992). Influence of psychosocial development and life events on the health practices of adults. *Issues in Mental Health Nursing, 13*(4), 403–414.

McCool, W. F., & Susman, E. J. (1990). The life span perspective: A developmental approach to community health nursing. *Public Health Nursing, 7*(1), 13–21.

Miller, A. (1985). When is the time ripe for teaching? *American Journal of Nursing, 85,* 801–804.

Orr, J. (1991). Piaget's theory of cognitive development may be useful in deciding what to teach and how to teach it. *Nurse Education Today, 11*(1), 65–69.

Penrose, W. O. (1979). *A primer on Piaget.* Bloomington, IN: Phi Delta Kappa Educational Foundation.

Piaget, J., Wolff, P. H., Spitz, R. A., Lorenz, K., Murphy, L. B., & Erikson, E. H. (1972). *Play and development.* New York: W. W. Norton.

Pontious, S. L. (1982). Practical Piaget: Helping children understand. *American Journal of Nursing, 82*(1), 114–117.

Robison, C. (1987). Preschool children's conceptualizations of health and illness. *Child Health Care, 16*(2), 89–96.

Sullivan, B. (1991). Growth enhancing interventions for nonorganic failure to thrive. *Journal of Pediatric Nursing: Nursing Care of Children and Families, 6*(4), 236–242.

Whaley, L. F., & Wong, D. L. (1991). *Nursing care of infants and children* (4th ed.). St. Louis: Mosby.

Chapter 16

INFANCY THROUGH ADOLESCENCE

VIRGINIA KLUNDER, RNC, MA, CCRN

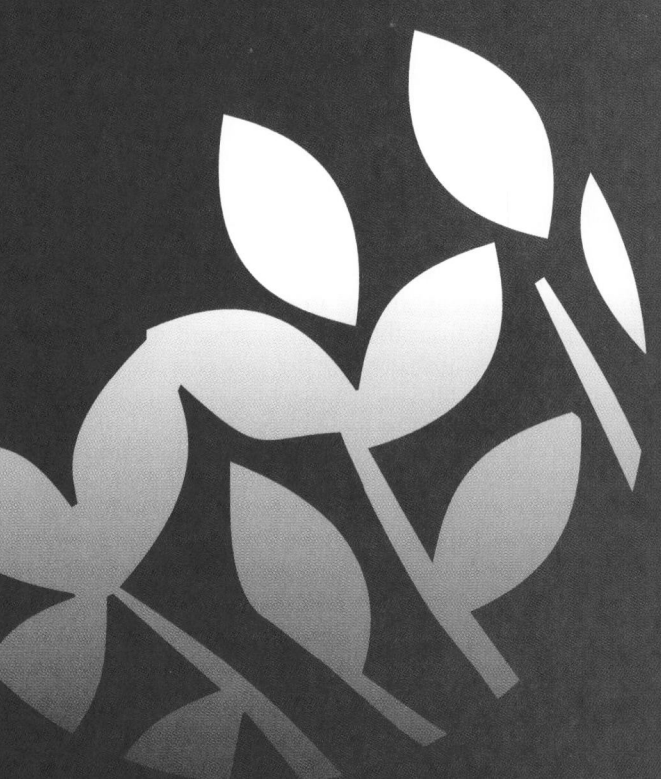

Every child deserves to be born healthy; have a nurturing family and dependable friends; experience joy and self-esteem; live in an environment free of undue risk of injury, abuse, and violence; and have access to coordinated health-promoting and preventive care. As we enter the next millennium, nurses play a pivotal role in realizing the vision of the national initiatives *Bright Futures: Children's Health Charter* (Green, 1994) and *Healthy Children 2000* (1992). To provide children in America with what they deserve, nurses need to incorporate the nursing process into a developmental and family-centered approach to primary and secondary health care from infancy through adolescence. It is important for nurses to understand stages of growth and development when observing the behavior of children, their parents, and others who interact and provide care for them. By using a nursing process approach to understanding normal growth and development, nurses can recognize health, health alterations, and risks to health that provide a basis for **anticipatory guidance** and for adapting care for children of different ages. Thus, nurses who know at what age an infant is likely to crawl can teach parents and caregivers the importance of continuous supervision and childproofing the home.

Principles of growth and development help to establish a comprehensive care plan. For instance, knowing that 8-month-old infants can pull themselves up to a standing position but lack motor coordination requires that nurses place them in cribs with the side rails pulled up to the highest position to prevent falling.

Genetics and the quality of prenatal and postnatal care decide growth and development. Although many aspects follow distinct patterns, the importance of individual differences in children should be considered. Arnold Gesell, a psychologist and physician, founded the Child Development Clinic at Yale University. Gesell formulated the atlas of developmental patterns— guidelines we commonly use today when assessing growth and development in children (Gesell & Ilg, 1946). Gesell's landmark research concluded that physiological growth and development proceed in predictable directions (Fig. 16–1). **Cephalocaudal development** proceeds from the head downward through the trunk, the legs, and then to the feet. For instance, a newborn infant lifts its head when lying prone and subsequently develops the ability to sit, crawl, and then stand as development proceeds. **Proximaldistal development** progresses from the center of the body outward. Thus, an infant gains muscular control of the upper arm and forearm before that of the hands and fingers. Motor development proceeds from general to specific **(gross motor development** to **fine motor development).** For example, an infant can shake a rattle before being able to hold a cup and drink from it.

We also credit Gesell with the term *maturation,* which refers to the way in which developmental

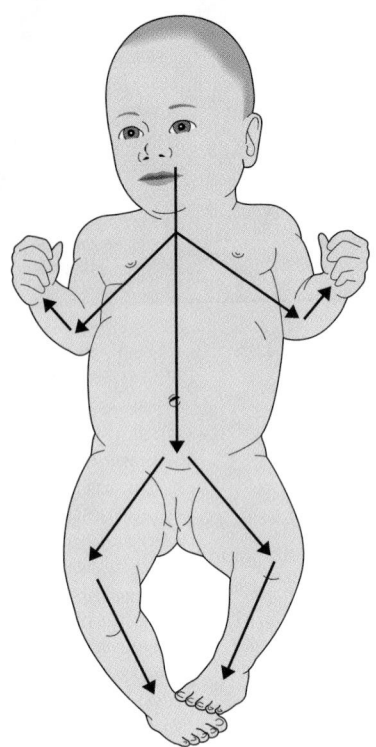

> **Figure 16–1**
Development proceeds from head to foot (cephalocaudal) and from the center to the extremities (proximodistal).

change occurs when an individual's genetic timetable shows readiness for the change to happen. In other words, walking at 10 months versus 14 months may have more to do with genetics than environment and opportunity. Likewise, knowing that children seldom achieve readiness for potty training before 18 months can help prevent disappointment caused by starting training earlier. These examples of readiness are part of what nurses recognize as developmental norms. Using information in this chapter will help nurses incorporate principles of growth and development into the nursing process when caring for the neonate, infant, toddler, preschooler, school-age child, and adolescent. By following these guidelines, nurses are doing their part in guiding children toward a healthy and bright future.

The Neonatal Period (Birth–28 Days)

Approximately 266 days after conception, a new human being emerges into the outside world. The period of floating in a warm fluid-filled amniotic sac and having all needs supplied through the umbilical cord ends at birth. Adjusting to extrauterine life is a developmental stage common to all newborns, whether full term or premature. Assessments begin immediately after birth.

Physiological Adaptation

The shift from intrauterine to extrauterine existence requires the newborn to conform immediately to its new environment. Critical adaptations are the initiation of breathing, adjustments in the circulatory system, and **thermoregulation** (regulation of body temperature). If these vital adaptations fail to occur, the newborn's survival is at serious risk.

Breathing

At birth, circulation and exchange of oxygen and carbon dioxide transfer from the umbilical cord to the heart and lungs. Clamping the cord allows the stump to dry and fall off, forming the navel in 1 to 2 weeks. Newborns generally breathe spontaneously and cry within seconds after birth. This happens because the **chemoreceptor reflexes** become sensitive to the buildup of carbon dioxide in the blood; therefore, it is not necessary to slap newborns to start them crying. Amniotic fluid that is in the lower breathing passages at birth quickly absorbs through the capillary beds that line the surface area of the lungs. Suctioning the mouth and nose after delivery of the head removes some accumulated products of conception, such as blood, mucus, and amniotic fluid, before the newborn takes its first breath.

Circulation

Within the heart, circulation of blood changes as the structures that aid fetal circulation are no longer needed. The **foramen ovale,** a connection between the right and left atria, functionally closes shortly after birth with a tissue flap that is held in place by a high-pressure gradient on the left side of the heart. The **ductus arteriosus,** a fetal shunt or opening between the aorta and pulmonary artery, gradually closes within a few weeks after birth. Because immaturity exists in the microcirculation, neonates exhibit **acrocyanosis,** a bluish tinge to the hands and feet. This phenomenon disappears within 2 to 4 weeks. Despite low levels of vitamin K–dependent blood clotting factors, bleeding episodes are rare. Nonetheless, newborns routinely receive vitamin K intramuscularly shortly after birth to offset any potential bleeding problems.

Thermoregulation

Because of an immature nervous system, the neonate's thermoregulating mechanism does not raise or lower body temperature through shivering or sweating. Consequently, the neonate is vulnerable to its surroundings. Neonates also lack subcutaneous fatty tissue, which normally provides a layer of insulation. Placing a neonate in direct contact with the mother's skin or in a preheated environment, such as an open warming unit, can help stabilize core body temperature after birth.

Psychosocial and Cognitive Adaptation

Neonates build on their motor, sensory, and reflex capacities to learn about and act on their world. Each experience leads to more complex behavior. The central nervous system (brain and spinal cord) is one of their most immature organ systems. The brain stem, which helps to regulate respiration, heartbeat, blood pressure, coughing, sneezing, swallowing, and postural reflexes, is more developed than the rest of the brain. Less well developed is the cerebellum, which coordinates balance and vision, and the cerebral hemispheres, which control learning, thought, and memory. Because of cerebral immaturity, nurses recognize neonates as reflexive (Table 16–1). Growth of the cerebrum occurs slowly throughout childhood.

Sleep

Sleep is the major activity of neonates throughout the first few weeks of life. Sleep states range from (1) regular sleep, in which neonates are at full rest; to (2) periodic sleep, in which bursts of rapid shallow breathing are interspersed with deep slow respirations; to (3) irregular sleep, in which periods of irregular breathing, rapid eye movements, facial grimacing, and

Table 16–1

SOME REFLEX ACTIVITIES OF NEONATES

REFLEX	DESCRIPTION
Rooting	Directs mouth toward source of any facial stimulation and begins sucking movements
Sucking	Uses tongue and lips to take in food or liquid to the back of the mouth when object touches mouth
Grasping	Very tight contraction of hand muscles around an object, allowing neonate to support own weight
Moro (startle)	Swings arms and legs out, then rapidly back in, to hug oneself into a curled ball when startled
Babinski	Toes fan up and out in response to stroking of the sole of foot
Tonic neck	Extends arm and leg on one side in fencing posture when head is turned to that side when lying supine

limb movements occur. Awake behaviors range from (1) drowsiness; to (2) alert inactivity; to (3) alert activity, during which neonates move their body, head, or limbs; to (4) crying.

Communication

Neonates are able to set up a communication system with their parents soon after birth. Within weeks, parents learn to recognize differences in their newborn's cries—to distinguish those that mean "I'm hungry" from those that mean "I'm wet." Likewise, neonates soon know whether their messages are getting through to their parents by the activity carried out when they are picked up.

Sensation

Neonates perceive the world through various senses—they react to heat and cold, touch, and pain. They can hear and recognize complex stimuli. Although their pupils widen in darkness and narrow in brightness, research in the area of visual acuity concludes that neonates are often myopic and astigmatic at birth. Everything they see beyond 8 in (20 cm) is a blur (Mehler & Dupoux, 1994). The fact that newborns flinch at sharp odors has established the presence of smell at birth, and some research demonstrates distinction to various tastes (Aslin & Pisoni, 1980).

Learning

Like children of any age, neonates can get bored with what is going on around them. As they become familiar with a stimulus, their reaction decreases. This process, called **habituation,** is thought to be one of the best signs of neonatal learning (Brazelton, 1973). For instance, a newborn startles when hearing a dog bark for the first time, but after days of repeated exposure to the barking dog, the newborn sleeps through the stimulus. As reflexive behavior decreases, the psychosocial and cognitive aspects of the neonate develop more rapidly, as seen in subsequent stages of development.

Nursing Process for Neonates

Assessment

The assessment phase of the nursing process begins with an initial contact with the neonate and family. Whether in the hospital, birthing center, ambulatory care setting, or home, nurses gather subjective and objective data through observation and interview. These data help to create a mutually agreeable and realistic plan of care. Collecting, verifying, and communicating data are nurses' primary responsibilities during this phase of the nursing process. Neonates discharged less than 48 hours after birth should have a home or health care visit during the first week of life.

Physiological Assessment

The Apgar Scoring System

The **Apgar scoring** system assesses physiological status at birth using a numerical scale for five different parameters. Nurses assess heart rate, color, muscle tone, reflex irritability, and respiratory effort at 1 minute and at 5 minutes after birth. Neonates with low scores may require resuscitative measures. The Apgar scoring system is depicted in Table 16–2.

Respiration, Circulation, and Temperature

Measure respiration, heart rate, and temperature after birth until all are stable and during all subsequent health care visits. Blood pressure is not routinely assessed unless you suspect a cardiac or renal problem. Obtain less invasive parameters first, such as respiration and heart rate, while neonates are at rest. Then perform more invasive procedures that are likely to cause the heart rate and respiration to increase, such as temperature and blood pressure. Assess the respiratory rate by observation or auscultation. Count the number of respirations for 1 full minute. Neonatal breathing patterns are often irregular, with rates that vary between 35 and 50 breaths per minute. During

Table 16–2

THE APGAR SCORING CHART			
SIGN*	**0**	**1**	**2**
Heart rate	Absent	Slow (<100)	Fast (>100)
Respiratory effort	Absent	Slow, irregular	Good, crying
Muscle tone	Flaccid	Some flexion of extremities	Well flexed
Reflex irritability	No response	Weak cry or grimace	Vigorous cry
Color	Blue, pale	Body pink, extremities blue	Completely pink

*Each sign is rated in terms of absence or presence from 0 to 2; highest overall score is 10.

their first days, neonates cough, sneeze, and yawn a great deal as they clear their air passages of fluids and mucus. Breathing can be noisy, rapid, shallow, irregular, or periodic. Neonates use abdominal muscles, rather than the diaphragm for respiration.

Auscultate the heart rate in the apical area of the chest for 1 full minute. The average apical heart rate at rest is 120 to 160 beats per minute (bpm) and is regular. During sleep, the heart rate may drop below 100 bpm, and during crying, may exceed 180 bpm. Blood pressure is variable but characteristically low during this period—approximately 78/54 mmHg.

Measure the neonate's temperature by the axillary route. The normal axillary temperature ranges from 97 to 99°F (36.1–37.2°C.) Place the bulb of an oral glass thermometer deep into the pocket of the axilla, and hold it in place for at least 10 minutes to get a correct reading. Follow individual instructions when using electronic equipment. Normal body temperature may not stabilize for 24 hours after birth.

Weight and Length

Weigh neonates shortly after birth. Properly balance an infant scale and place the neonate in the center of it unclothed. Keep a hand suspended close to the neonate to prevent falling (Fig. 16–2). The average neonate weighs 7 lb, 8 oz (3400 g) at birth. Weight loss of up to 10% of the birth weight occurs within the first few days, but it is regained within 10 to 14 days.

Measure the head-to-heel length shortly after birth. Position the neonate flat or recumbent on the back on a firm surface and extend the lower extremities. The soles of the feet should be perpendicular to the flat surface. Then measure from the top of the head to the soles of the feet using an accurate tape measure (Fig. 16–3A). The average length of a neonate is 20 in (50 cm).

Head Circumference

The neonate's head may initially be misshapen at birth as a result of molding that occurs during passage

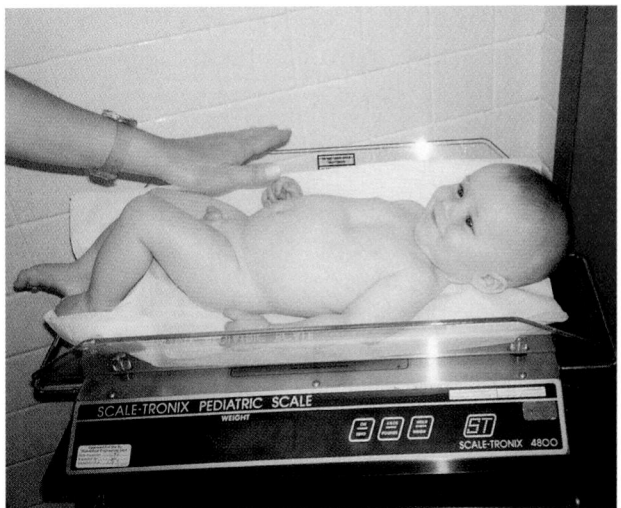

✦ **Figure 16–2**
Infant being weighed on scale.

through the birth canal. Repeated measurements may be indicated until the head regains its symmetry— usually within a week. Measure the head circumference at the most prominent part of the occiput directly above the eyebrows with an accurate tape measure (Fig. 16–3B). The average head circumference is 14 in (35 cm) at birth. Palpate for the anterior and posterior **fontanelles.** Fontanelles form at the junctions of unfused skull bones. Placing the neonate in an upright position allows for the most accurate assessment of the fontanelles. They usually feel soft, and you may observe them pulsating. The fontanelles should be flat along the surface line of the skull and should not feel tense in a calm neonate. Fontanelles vary in size. The diamond-shaped anterior fontanelle is several centimeters larger than the triangular posterior fontanelle.

Chest Circumference

Obtain the chest circumference while the neonate is recumbent. Place the tape measure around the chest
text continued on page 282

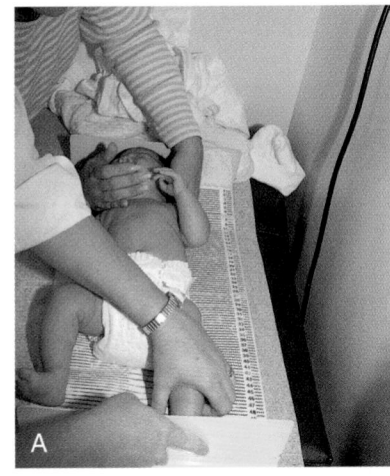
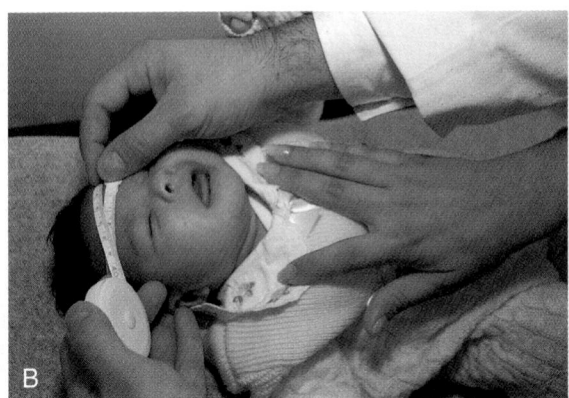

✦ **Figure 16–3**
A, Length is measured by laying a tape alongside the infant. B, The head circumference is measured at the largest point.

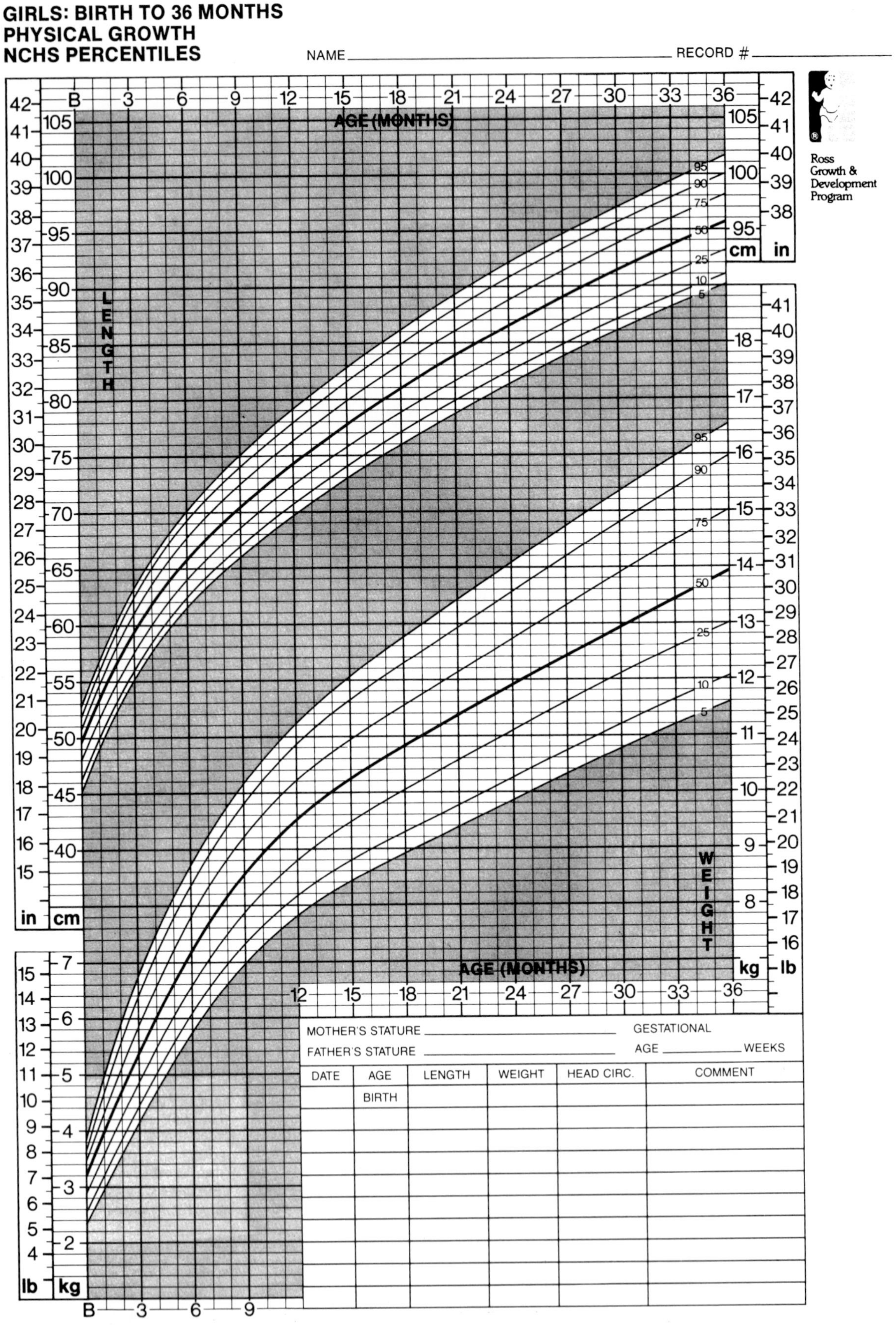

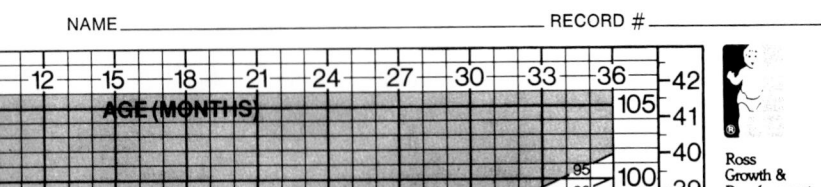

GIRLS: BIRTH TO 36 MONTHS
PHYSICAL GROWTH
NCHS PERCENTILES

NAME _____ RECORD # _____

Ross
Growth &
Development
Program

A

❯ Figure 16–4

Anthropometric charts for girls from birth to 36 months *(panel A)* and boys from 2 to 18 years *(panel B).* (Adapted from Hamill, P. V. V., Drizd, T. A., Johnson, C. L., Reed, R. B., Roche, A. F., & Moore, W. M. (1979). Physical growth: National Center for Health Statistics percentiles. *American Journal of Clinical Nutrition, 32,* 607–629, American Society for Clinical Nutrition. Data from the Fels Longitudinal Study, Wright State University School of Medicine, Yellow Springs, Ohio. Copyright 1982 Ross Laboratories.)

MOTHER'S STATURE _____ GESTATIONAL
FATHER'S STATURE _____ AGE _____ WEEKS

DATE	AGE	LENGTH	WEIGHT	HEAD CIRC.	COMMENT
	BIRTH				

BOYS: 2 TO 18 YEARS
PHYSICAL GROWTH
NCHS PERCENTILES

NAME_____ RECORD #_____

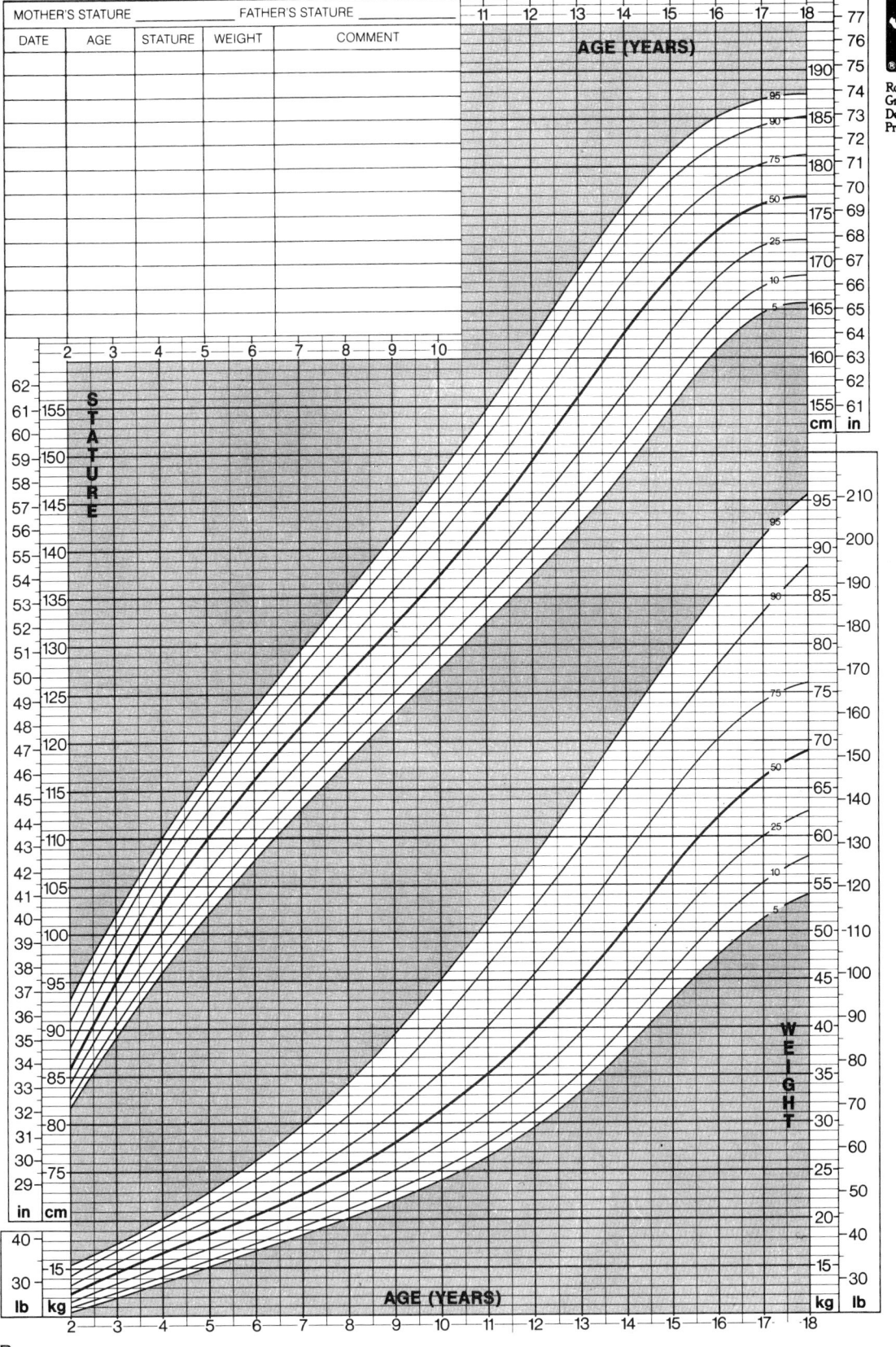

B

❧ Figure 16–4
(Continued)

at the nipple line midway between inspiration and expiration. Generally the chest circumference is about 1 in (2.5 cm) less than the head circumference. The measurement occasionally is equal to the head circumference but should never exceed it. The transverse and anteroposterior diameters are approximately equal in size.

Perform these assessments at each health care visit and record the parameters on standard growth charts, also known as **anthropometric charts.** Comparing these data with previous serial measurements determines the neonate's growth pattern (Fig. 16–4).

Motor Development

Generally neonates lie with the head to one side when in the prone position. The pelvis is high, and the knees tuck up under the abdomen. By 28 days of age, neonates lift their heads from this position for a short period. When supine, they exhibit the tonic neck reflex, as described in Table 16–1. Their heads completely lag when in a sitting position. Although neonates in general assume an abducted and flexed position when sleeping, during wakeful active times, you can observe uncoordinated periods of movement involving all four extremities. Any organized movements during this period are usually a result of functional reflexes.

Nutrition, Digestion, and Elimination

By assessing the neonate's sucking ability, a nurse can indirectly estimate nutrition. Eating is the second major activity that neonates experience. Although they are seldom hungry immediately following delivery, neonates can be put to the mother's breast because they experience a short period of alertness, and they demonstrate a strong sucking reflex during this time. However, within 30 minutes, they will get drowsy and fall asleep. After 2 to 4 hours they awake and demonstrate signs of hunger through the rooting and sucking reflexes (see Table 16–1). Neonates tend to suck slowly in the first few days of life but pick up speed as they become more skillful (Pollitt *et al.,* 1991). They also pause frequently and stare at the parent—this in turn elicits some form of parental response, such as smiling, talking, or singing. These behaviors become important in establishing infant-parent bonding. Before milk production begins in the postpartum mother, the breast-feeding neonate will receive a thin yellow serous fluid while suckling. This fluid, called **colostrum,** contains water, minerals, vitamins, and maternal antibodies, among other substances.

Assess digestion and elimination during the first day of life. Peristaltic bowel sounds are generally present within 2 hours of birth but may be irregular. At birth, the neonate's lower intestine is filled with a greenish-black sticky substance called **meconium.** This first stool normally passes within the first 24 hours of life, with subsequent stools turning a lighter golden yellow color. If meconium is not passed within 24 hours of life, the neonate needs further evaluation of the gastrointestinal tract. The number and consistency of stools vary from infant to infant and differ based on the type of feeding.

General Appearance

Always observe the neonate's resting appearance prior to any physical contact during examination. Generally, neonates abduct and flex both arms and legs. Their heads appear large in proportion to the remainder of the body—approximately one fourth of the total body length (see Figure 16–7). Their necks are short and chubby, and the abdomen is soft and protuberant.

Skin

Assess the skin for color, rashes, birthmarks, jaundice, hydration status, and birth trauma. Color may vary according to racial background, pigmentation, and physiological changes. **Vernix caseosa,** a white cheesy substance, covers the skin at birth. This substance protects the skin in utero. **Lanugo,** a fine, downlike hair, may also be present on the skin, especially the back, shoulders, and ear pinnae. Erythema toxicum, a transient newborn rash, is sometimes seen and is a normal neonatal variation. The rash has white vesicles with a red macular base and is differentiated from **milia,** which are small white papules found on the face and upper torso. Locate size, color, and distribution of any birthmarks. "Stork bites" or capillary hemangiomas may be present on the nose, neck, forehead, and eyelids and often disappear after several months. **Mongolian spots** are large, irregular, dark pigmented areas generally found on the posterior lumbar region of infants of Asian, African, or Native American descent. They are often mistaken for ecchymotic areas. Assess for physiological jaundice by depressing the bridge of the nose and observing the color. Neonates exhibit a yellow color if jaundice is present. Jaundice results from the metabolism of bilirubin and is often seen after 24 hours of age—if jaundice is present before 24 hours after birth, it is considered pathologic. Assess hydration status by palpating the texture and tone of the skin. Neonatal skin is soft and quickly returns to the original position when pinched. Observe for birth trauma in the form of ecchymosis, abrasions, or lacerations (especially to the brow, face, and scalp) from the use of forceps during delivery. Palpate the scalp for the presence of edema. **Caput succedaneum,** which is a soft tissue edema, or **cephalhematoma,** which indicates bleeding between the bone and periosteum, may result in scalp swelling. Both occur as a result of passage through the birth canal.

Psychosocial and Cognitive Assessment

Assessment of neonatal psychosocial and cognitive development focuses on testing and observing functional reflexes, innate behaviors, and sensory functions. This assessment also serves as a useful indicator of neurological functioning at birth. The absence or prolongation of these behaviors beyond the period for which they are expected may indicate alterations in neurological development.

Neonates are thought to have about 70 distinct functional reflexes (see Table 16–1) at birth (Illingworth, 1986). Some have immediate survival value, such as the rooting reflex that enables a neonate to locate a nipple for feeding. Other reflexes serve as a foundation for future mental development, and yet others have no value that can be determined.

Observe for innate neonatal behaviors including periods of sucking, crying, sleeping, and activity. Sucking is generally a reflexive behavior and is not an indicator of hunger. Research studies of neonatal **non-nutritive sucking** reveal that the more neonates suck, the more alert and attentive they are to their surroundings (Mehler & Dupoux, 1994). Assess the parents' feelings regarding the use of pacifiers or thumb sucking. Pacifiers are often used to soothe a crying baby. If a pacifier is not used, neonates often find a way to suck on their fingers. Rhythmic sucking is comforting and in some cases may lull the newborn to sleep.

Crying is the manner in which neonates respond to a stimulus. Their cry is strong and lusty. It may take time before parents can distinguish crying patterns. Assess how parents react to crying. Parents frustrate easily when they cannot determine an apparent cause for the crying. This places neonates at risk for **child maltreatment syndrome** when parents cannot deal with the added stress of excessive crying and lash out physically.

Observe the neonate's sleeping pattern. Recognize that neonates sleep approximately two thirds of the day intermittently but have increasingly longer periods of sleep during the night hours as they mature.

Assess sensory perception by introducing some change into the environment and then observing its effect on the neonate's physiological behavior. For instance, presenting a loud noise or flashing light may elicit crying, head turning, or even sucking at a faster pace, indicating that hearing and vision are present. For smell and taste, hold a cotton swab soaked with an aromatic solution near the nose and provide distinctive tasting solutions through a nipple. Neonates' reactions will be similar to those of adults. Newborns are capable of withdrawing a body part when touched and of increasing their activity level when cold. These indicators show evidence of sensation, especially to pain and discomfort.

The nursing process continues after an assessment is performed, with the nurse analyzing the data and then organizing them into a framework in which human responses (nursing diagnoses) are generated. A plan of care is then developed in conjunction with the family to establish realistic goals and appropriate interventions. The next section presents a plan of care for the normal neonate.

Diagnosis, Planning, Intervention and Evaluation

Some common nursing diagnoses for this age group are presented here, along with the planned outcomes, nursing interventions, and appropriate evaluations. See the Nursing Diagnosis Box for possible nursing diagnoses for this age group.

Nursing Diagnosis

Airway Clearance, ineffective, related to excessive mucus and fluid accumulation after delivery

Planning

The outcome criteria for this diagnosis would include

The neonate will maintain a patent airway and exhibit a respiratory rate within normal limits (35–50 breaths per minute)

Intervention

Suction mouth and nasopharynx with bulb syringe as needed

Position on side with head maintained in a neutral position, especially after feedings

Keep oxygen and suction equipment nearby for use in the event of respiratory distress

Obtain Apgar score at 1 and 5 minutes after birth and continue to monitor respiratory rate as indicated by newborn's status

Notify health care provider of deviations from normal respiratory status

---

NURSING DIAGNOSES FOR NEONATES

Airway clearance, Ineffective, related to excessive mucus and fluid accumulation after delivery

Thermoregulation, Ineffective, related to newborn transition to extrauterine environment

Risk for Injury related to lack of awareness secondary to maturational age

Risk for Nutrition: Less Than Body Requirements, Altered, related to developmental helplessness and parental knowledge deficit

Family Processes, Altered, related to birth of newborn and change in the family unit

Evaluation

Airway remains patent and the respiratory rate is between 35 and 50 breaths per minute.

Nursing Diagnosis

Thermoregulation, ineffective, related to newborn transition to extrauterine environment

Planning

The outcome criteria for this diagnosis might be stated as follows:

The neonate will maintain a temperature between 97°F (36.1°C) and 99°F (37.2°C)

The parents will verbalize measures to avoid heat loss in the neonate

Intervention

Assess axillary temperature initially every 30 minutes until stable, then every 4 to 8 hours.

If temperature is less than 97°F (36.1°C):
   Assess for environmental sources of heat loss (*e.g.,* drafts, vents, cold objects)
   Wrap in blankets and place stockinette cap on head or place next to mother's skin and cover both with blanket
   Notify health care provider if hypothermia persists for more than 1 hour
   Assess for complications of cold stress (*e.g.,* hypoxia, hypoglycemia, respiratory acidosis)

If temperature is greater than 99°F (37.2°C):
   Assess environment for thermal gain (*i.e.,* ambient temperature >80°F [26.7°C])
   Loosen blankets and remove cap
   Notify health care provider if hyperthermia persists for more than 1 hour

Initiate health teaching to parents regarding
   Why newborn is vulnerable to temperature fluctuations
   Sources of environmental heat loss, including
      a. Evaporation—loss of heat when moisture on skin changes to vapor (dry newborn well)
      b. Convection—loss of heat as air circulates over skin (avoid drafts)
      c. Conduction—loss of body heat when skin is in contact with cool surface (warm objects that will be touching newborn)
      d. Radiation—loss of body heat to cool surfaces without direct contact (place crib away from walls and windows)
   How to check the newborn's temperature for when the baby is sick, irritable, or feels hot to touch

Evaluation

Temperature remains between 97°F (36.1°C) and 99°F (37.2°C)

Parents verbalize understanding of potential sources of heat loss

Parents demonstrate proper use of a thermometer

Nursing Diagnosis

Risk for Injury related to lack of awareness secondary to maturational age

Planning

The outcome criteria for this diagnosis could be listed as follows:

Neonate will remain free from injury

Parents will verbalize understanding of ways to keep newborn safe

Intervention

Assess parents' knowledge base regarding injury prevention and related safety issues

Implement and teach parents the infant safety guidelines provided in Table 16–3

Advise parents regarding how to seek help in an emergency

Teach parents cardiopulmonary resuscitation

Evaluation

Remains free from injury

Parents verbalize and return demonstrate appropriate safety measures

Nursing Diagnosis

Risk for Altered Nutrition, Less Than Body Requirements related to developmental helplessness and parental knowledge deficit

Planning

The outcome criteria for this diagnosis may be phrased as follows:

The neonate will retain feedings and begin to gain weight after 10 to 14 days

Intervention

Assess parental feeding preference (*e.g.,* breast or bottle)

Assess the strength of sucking and ability to coordinate with swallowing

Offer intake to neonate in accordance with preference:
   Breast-feeding initially every 1 to 3 hours on demand
   Bottle-feeding initially 2 to 3 oz every 3 to 4 hours or on demand

Assist breast-feeding and bottle-feeding mothers with positioning and technique during initial feedings

Avoid supplementing feedings with water unless indicated

Encourage father to participate in bottle-feeding

Encourage father to assist breast-feeding mother with relaxation, positioning, and emotional support

Table 16–3

CHILD SAFETY GUIDELINES

AGE	COMMON INJURY	PREVENTION STRATEGIES
Infancy	Motor vehicle crash	Use infant car restraints that meet safety standards Infants weighing <20 lb (9.1 kg) face rear in center back seat of car (never in passenger front seat because of danger of airbag deployment) Install restraint and secure infant appropriately according to manufacturer's guidelines
	Falls	Never leave child unattended on bed, changing table, or other high place Keep cribs away from windows; put mattress in lowest position Use safety gates at top and bottom of staircases
	Burns/scalds	Never hold child while handling hot foods, liquids, or cigarettes Keep water heater temperature at 110–120°F (43.3–48.9°C) Test water prior to bathing Use outlet covers; keep electric cords out of reach Use sunscreen with sun protection factor ≥30; expose to sun gradually
	Drowning	Hold on to infant at all times during bath Never leave unattended while bathing or near water
	Choking/suffocation	Avoid propping bottles for feeding Keep small objects out of reach Keep plastic bags and balloons out of reach Check all toys for loose parts Avoid tying pacifier around neck Keep cribs away from drapery and dangling cords Learn cardiopulmonary resuscitation (CPR)
	Poisoning	Use cabinet latches on all low cabinets Keep house plants out of reach Keep syrup of ipecac handy Post poison control center phone number by the telephone
Toddler	Motor vehicle crash	Switch to toddler car restraint when child weighs >20 lb (9.1 kg) Avoid placing children <12 years of age in front passenger seat to avoid injuries from airbag deployment Hold child's hand when crossing street Begin teaching proper street crossing and safety rules Set a good example when crossing streets
	Falls	Continue infant guidelines Switch to youth bed when child can climb over crib rails or leave the rails down Install window guards on windows that open more than 4 in
	Burns/scalds	Continue infant guidelines Avoid placing hot objects in child's reach Restrict child from cooking areas Cook on back burners of stove and turn pot handles inward Avoid using table cloths Keep matches/lighters out of reach Begin teaching the meaning of "hot"
	Drowning	Supervise continually in bath and near lakes, ocean, rivers, and pools Begin teaching water safety and swimming Keep away from toilets and buckets of water
	Choking	Continue infant guidelines Cut table foods well and instruct not to talk or run while eating Avoid feeding hard candies, peanuts, raw vegetable sticks, raisins, and frankfurters
	Poisoning	Continue infant guidelines Use cabinet latches on all high and low cabinets Avoid taking pills in child's presence

Table continued on following page

Table **16–3**

CHILD SAFETY GUIDELINES
(Continued)

AGE	COMMON INJURY	PREVENTION STRATEGIES
Preschool	Motor vehicle crash	Continue toddler guidelines Use regular car safety restraints for children ≥40 lb or 4 years of age
	Falls	Continue toddler guidelines Supervise playground activities Ensure padded ground in playground areas Use approved helmet and knee and elbow pads for bicycling and skating
	Burns/scalds	Continue toddler guidelines Teach stop, drop, roll, and cool in event of flame burns Practice home fire safety drills
	Choking	Instruct not to talk or run while eating Instruct to chew food well Learn CPR
	Poisoning	Continue toddler guidelines
School Age	Motor vehicle crash	Continue use of car safety restraints Most at risk for pedestrian injury Stress street crossing safety guidelines Stress bicycling, skating, and motorized vehicle safety
	Falls	Continue preschool guidelines
	Burns/scalds	Continue preschool guidelines
	Drowning	Continue supervision when in and around water Teach swimming and proper diving guidelines if not already done
	Choking	Continue preschool guidelines Learn CPR
	Poisoning	Monitor for signs of depression or despondency, which may lead to intentional ingestion
	Firearm injury	Store all guns unloaded and out of reach Install trigger latches on all firearms Have child attend hunting safety classes if appropriate
Adolescence	Motor vehicle crash	Monitor for signs of alcohol use and counsel to avoid drinking and driving Instruct teen to avoid riding with an impaired driver Continue to stress safety restraint use Have teen attend driver education classes
	Falls	Instruct regarding proper use of protective gear to prevent sports-related injuries
	Burns	Instruct regarding dangers of smoking and smoking in bed
	Drowning	Instruct regarding dangers of diving into unknown (shallow) bodies of water to prevent head injury Stress attending boating/coast guard safety course
	Choking	Continue stressing not talking while eating, especially if alcohol impaired Learn CPR
	Poisoning	Continue school-age guidelines
	Firearm injury	Continue school-age guidelines

Burp newborn to remove swallowed air in the middle and at the end of feeding

Position newborn on the right side after feeding to prevent aspiration

Observe for 6 to 10 wet diapers per day

Observe for passing of stool according to infant's established pattern

Evaluation

Tolerates feedings well

Shows a pattern of weight gain after 10 to 14 days

Has 6 to 10 wet diapers per day

Passes stool within normal pattern

Nursing Diagnosis

Family Processes, Altered, related to birth of newborn and change in the family unit

Planning

The outcome criteria for this diagnosis would include

Parents will demonstrate positive attachment behaviors with neonate

Siblings will adjust to newborn

Intervention

Encourage parents to see and hold infant as soon after delivery as possible

Assess parents' initial response to newborn (*e.g.*, note behaviors of making eye contact, talking to newborn, touching or stroking newborn)

Identify to parents specific behaviors of infant (such as sucking and rooting behaviors), initial alertness, and attention to human voice

Encourage parents to talk about the labor and delivery experience

Encourage rooming in if feasible

Observe the reciprocity of attachment cues between newborn and parents

Report to health care provider any behaviors that may represent inadequate attachment processes

Allow sibling visiting and participation in care of newborn if feasible

Explain to siblings (within their level of understanding) physical differences and developmental needs of newborn (*e.g.*, not a plaything, needs complete care)

Encourage parents to spend individual time with siblings at home

Evaluation

Parents demonstrate attachment behaviors soon after birth and continue throughout neonatal period

Siblings express positive interest in newborn

Nursing Process For Infants (1 Month–1 Year)

Assessment

As the infant progresses in the first year of life through a period of rapid physical growth and psychosocial and cognitive advances, nurses use assessment skills to monitor progress from reflexive to purposeful behavior and the achievement of developmental milestones. In addition to physical growth parameters, assessment in the areas of nutrition, dentition, sleep and activity, and immunizations are areas that nurses explore when promoting optimal health during infancy. Assessments of well infants should routinely be performed at 2, 4, 6, 9, and 12 months of age.

Physiological Assessment

Steady and proportional growth during infancy is more relevant than the absolute amount of growth during this time period. Obtaining serial anthropometric measurements during infancy helps to identify growth problems early on. Measurements of weight, length, and head and chest circumference are obtained at all health care visits, recorded on growth (anthropometric) charts, and compared with previous data (see Fig. 16–4). Vital signs are measured at each health care visit.

Respiration, Circulation, and Thermoregulation

Obtain respiration, heart rate, and temperature during health care visits using techniques described for neonates. Assess blood pressure if you suspect a cardiac or renal problem. Use a newborn- or infant-sized cuff on the upper limbs or an infant-sized cuff on the lower limbs and an electronic blood pressure device, if possible, for the most accurate measurement. Alternatively, palpate the nearest pulse distal to the cuff and record the systolic pressure reading at the point impulse returns. Blood pressure at 6 months of age averages 90/53 mmHg or 90/palpation. By the end of the neonatal period, respiratory, circulatory, and thermoregulatory variations of that period stabilize. Although respiratory patterns remain diaphragmatic in character throughout infancy, the rate and depth vary less, with the rate averaging about 30 breaths per minute. The average heart rate at rest during infancy ranges from between 100 and 150 bpm. There is no longer any evidence of acrocyanosis. Circulation to the distal extremities is evidenced by pink, warm hands and feet that have a capillary refill time of less than 2 seconds. Although temperature remains stable during infancy, great care must still be taken to prevent cold stress.

Weight and Length

Weight increases from an average of 7 lb, 12 oz (3.5 kg) to 22 lb (10 kg) in the first year of life. More than 50% of healthy infants double their birth weight by 4 months of age, with formula-fed infants gaining slightly faster than breast-fed infants. By their first birthday, infants triple their birth weight (Lowrey, 1986). During the first year of life, infants increase their birth length by approximately 10 in (25 cm) or 50% of their birth length. Female infants tend to be smaller on the average than male infants, although the rate of height increase is associated with size at birth and nutritional status. Obtain weight and length using the method described for neonates.

Head Circumference

With infancy being a period of rapid brain growth, the head circumference measurement becomes one of the most important parameters to obtain. Studies have shown that there is essentially no head circumference variation in relation to race, nationality, or geographic location. However, male infants have a slightly larger (< 1 cm) measurement than female infants. Head circumference growth correlates strongly with weight and chest circumference (Illingworth, 1986.) A 4-inch (10 cm) increase in head circumference occurs within the first year of life. Palpate for the anterior and posterior fontanelles. Whereas the anterior fontanelle is present, the posterior fontanelle closes at approximately 2 months of age and can no longer be felt. Obtain head circumference and palpate for fontanelles by using the methods described for neonates.

Chest Circumference

By the time infants reach 1 year of age, the general shape of the chest takes on a different form. The transverse diameter becomes 1.25% that of the anteroposterior diameter. The chest circumference equals the head circumference at 9 to 10 months of age, then surpasses it by 1 year. Obtain chest circumference by using the method described for neonates.

Motor Development

As infants mature, the position they take when prone becomes more relaxed. The pelvis lowers as the hips and knees extend. By 3 months of age they can hold their head and shoulders up from a flat plane. When in a sitting position, some head lag may still be present, but this disappears by 5 months. Most infants sit unsupported by 6 months of age, crawl by 9 months, and walk by 13 months. At 4 weeks, their hands remain mostly closed, but by 3 months the hands are open most of the time. Gross motor coordination and eye-hand coordination improve gradually; by 9 months, infants reach out and grasp objects with a degree of accuracy. Prior to 9 months, grasping is accomplished through the use of fingers and the palm (palmar grasp). By 1 year, the infant begins to grasp with the use of the thumb in opposition to the other fingers (pincer grasp). The latter represents the development of fine motor coordination. For a more comprehensive look at gross and fine motor development in infancy, see Table 16–4.

Denver Developmental Screening Test (Denver II)

The **Denver Developmental Screening Test (Denver II)** assesses development in children between the ages of 3 months and 6 years. The Denver II rates four categories of development: (1) personal-social, (2) fine motor–adaptive, (3) language, and (4) gross motor skills. Although administration of the tool is not considered difficult, it is a standard measure and its validity depends on utilization by trained personnel. Ideally, a Denver II is administered to an infant at 3 to 4 months and again at 10 months. It is administered again later in development. Inform parents that the Denver II is not an intelligence test but a screening tool that assesses development.

Nutrition

Assessing infants' nutritional status involves more than obtaining growth parameters of weight, height, and head and chest circumferences. Continue assessing by obtaining information regarding normal feeding and elimination patterns. Explore parents' attitudes and approaches toward weaning, the introduction of new foods other than breast milk or formula, and their knowledge of healthy and safe feeding practices. Health care professionals do not support the practice of introducing solid or semisolid food into an infant's diet prior to 6 months of age (Bainbridge & Tsang, 1995). Firstly, infants do not have adequate head control or the ability to sit up without assistance before 4 to 6 months of age. Unless supported adequately, the neck flexes in an awkward position for swallowing semisolid foods. Secondly, infants exhibit the extrusion reflex until about 5 months of age. This protective reflex causes any food or foreign object placed in the mouth to be pushed out by the tongue. Finally, the ability of the body to produce adequate amounts of pancreatic amylase and gastric pepsin (enzymes needed to aid digestion of complex carbohydrates and protein) does not develop fully until 9 months of age (Leventhal, 1985).

Assessing for iron deficiency anemia should begin at 4 to 6 months of age when maternal iron stores deplete. "Iron deficiency has been associated with poor growth, an increase in certain infectious diseases and reduced physical and intellectual performance" (Filer, cited in Lifshitz, 1995, p. 57). A nurse should suspect iron deficiency in infants who appear lethargic, pale, and somewhat obese. Parental guidelines for feeding infants are presented in Table 16–5. Use these guidelines to assess parental knowledge regarding infant feeding practices.

Table **16–4**

MILESTONES OF GROSS AND FINE MOTOR DEVELOPMENT IN INFANCY

AVERAGE AGE, *mo*	GROSS MOTOR	FINE MOTOR
1	Turns head from side to side	Grasping reflex present
2	Holds head at 45-degree angle when prone	Holds rattle briefly
3	Begins rolling over	Grasps rattle or dangling objects
4	Slight head lag when pulled to sitting position	Brings objects to mouth
5	No head wobble when held in sitting position	Transfers objects from hand to hand
6	Sits without support	Manipulates and examines large objects with hands
7	Stands while holding on	Reaches for, grabs, and retains object
8	Pulls self to stand	Grasps objects with thumb and finger
9	Crawls backwards	Begins to show hand preference
10	Creeps on hands and knees	Hits cup with spoon
11	Walks using furniture for support	Picks up small objects with thumb and forefinger (pincer grasp)
12	Stands alone easily	Puts three or more objects into a container
12–16	Walks alone easily	Turns two or three pages in a large cardboard book

Table **16–5**

PARENTAL GUIDELINES FOR FEEDING INFANTS AND TODDLERS

AGE	GUIDELINE

Birth to 6 mo	Breast Milk
	    Colostrum, a fluid rich in immune substances, precedes milk production, which will occur within 1–3 d after birth
	    Supplements of fluoride and vitamin D are required for all breast-fed infants
	    Supplements of iron should be added from 4–6 mo of age
	    Will consume amount based on satisfaction (adequacy determined by weight gain, wet diapers, and contentment)
	Formula
	    Iron supplemented formula should be used to promote optimal growth
	    Fluoride may need to be supplemented based on concentration in local water supply if used to prepare formula
	    Should consume 20–24 oz of formula a day

6 mo to 1 y	Breast Milk/Formula
	    Should continue up to 1 y of age
	    Avoid putting infant to bed with a bottle of formula or milk to prevent dental caries
	Solid or Semisolid Foods
	    May begin to add solid foods by 6 mo of age
	    Initial foods should be pureed or finely mashed
	    Introduction of new foods should be done weekly, starting with cereals, then fruits, then vegetables, then meat
	    Toward the end of the first year, finger foods such as cheese sticks, teething crackers, and banana slices may be introduced
	    As the quantity of solid foods increases, formula should be limited to 900 ml (30 oz) daily

Table continued on following page

Table **16–5**

PARENTAL GUIDELINES FOR FEEDING INFANTS AND TODDLERS
(Continued)

AGE	GUIDELINE
6 mo to 1 y	**Cereals** Iron-fortified prepared cereals can be given one or two times daily Supplemental iron can be stopped if infant tolerates iron-fortified cereal **Fruits** Freshly made applesauce, mashed bananas, and pears are generally well tolerated If using commercially prepared fruits, choose specially prepared baby fruits, as others may be loaded with additives such as salt, sugar, and preservatives Limit amount of fruit juice to one 4-oz serving daily due to high sugar content and empty calories Avoid offering fruit juice at bedtime in a bottle to prevent dental caries **Vegetables** Mashed or well-cooked carrots, peas, and squash are generally well tolerated If using commercially prepared vegetables, choose those specially prepared for babies, as others may be loaded with additives such as salt, sugar, and preservatives Commercially prepared vegetable juices should be avoided, as they often contain excessive amounts of salt **Meats, Fish, Poultry, Eggs, and Cheese** Trim excessive fat from meats, fish, and poultry Avoid fried foods Blenderize or food process to puree foods or cut into tiny bite-size pieces for easy consumption Avoid commercially prepared meat and vegetable combinations, as they are low in protein Introduce eggs and fish toward the end of first year and in small amounts, as many infants are allergic to them Cheese can be substituted for a serving of meat and used as a finger food
1 y to 36 mo	**Liquids** Cow's milk may be added after 1 y of age and should be limited to 600 ml (20 oz) daily Avoid the use of low-fat or skim milk products, as the fat that dairy foods provide is needed for proper brain development All liquids should be offered in a cup because there is no longer a developmental indication to continue with bottle-feeding Continue to avoid large amounts of fruit juice (especially apple), as this may produce diarrhea **Solid Foods** As the toddler becomes more mobile, eating becomes less important, and an erratic appetite ensues Finger foods should predominate at this time Foods can be prepared in small pieces for easy handling by the toddler Certain types of foods should not be offered because of their high aspiration potential (*e.g.,* raisins, peanuts, frankfurters, raw vegetable sticks, and hard candies) Recognize that the toddler will not eat an adequate amount of solid foods if given the opportunity to "fill up" on bottles or cups of milk and juice (24 oz should be an adequate amount of liquid consumed daily in a healthy toddler's diet)

Dentition

A difficult period for infants is when the **deciduous** (primary) **teeth** erupt. In assessing dentition, nurses not only observe the normal developmental pattern but also look into the physiological responses of infants' "teething" experience. The lower central incisors are the first teeth to erupt, followed closely by the upper central incisors. The crown of these teeth breaks through the periodontal membrane somewhere around 6 to 8 months. Physiological responses to this process vary from infant to infant, with some experiencing minimal discomfort, with symptoms including drooling, biting on hard objects, and an increase in finger sucking, and others demonstrating periods of irritability and difficulty sleeping. Teething is not responsible for respiratory infections, rashes, fever, or diarrhea. Instruct parents to report symptoms of this nature to their health care provider. Assessing oral hygiene practices should begin in infancy, with the nurse determining the parents' knowledge level regarding prevention of dental caries.

Sleep and Activity

Patterns of sleep and activity vary among infants. By the end of the first year, infants sleep a total of 13 to 14 hours per day. By 3 to 4 months, most infants develop a nighttime sleeping pattern lasting from 8 to 10 hours. The remainder of the time will be divided into napping periods during the day. Most infants need no encouragement to be active in movement. As infants become more aware of their surroundings, they achieve great pleasure by discovery in their newfound mobility. Parents often have questions regarding behaviors they find abnormal; for example, frequent nighttime crying spells or prolonged daytime napping. Nurses can uncover parental behaviors that may contribute to this unwanted infant behavior, such as excessive use of commercial infant seats, strollers, and walkers, which hinder infant movement and thus delay gross motor skills and greater activity.

Immunizations

The decline of infectious diseases in the last half century can be attributed to the worldwide use of immunization. **Immunization** is a process by which resistance to certain infectious diseases is induced through the administration of vaccines. Assessment of immunization status is done by nurses at every health care visit (Fig. 16–5). Instruct parents to carry an immunization record for each child that includes the dates and type of immunizations received. This will help determine the infant's current status and show any further immunizations needed. Table 16–6 lists the current recommended schedule for immunization of infants and children in the United States. The nurse should recognize that immunization schedules often change based on the development of new vaccines or the epidemiology of disease. Contact the local health department for any recent changes in immunization schedules for your geographic area or for a schedule to administer missed vaccines to infants not previously immunized.

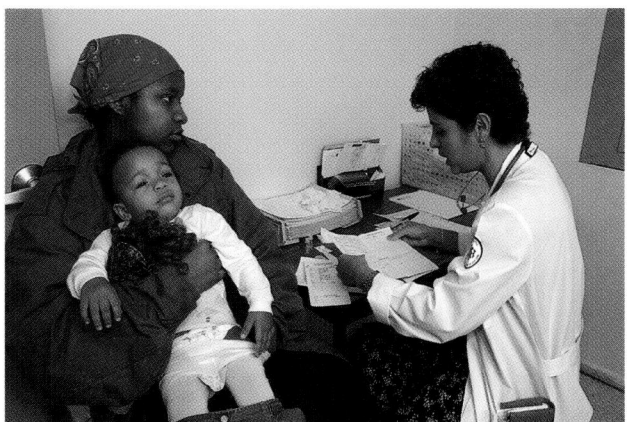

✦ **Figure 16–5**
Review of the immunization schedule should be part of every health care visit.

Psychosocial Assessment

Over the first month of life, infants establish patterns or rhythms of feeding and sleeping, as well as some ability to control their own state of being through nonnutritive sucking. Other activities that help infants to meet their basic needs are generally in place by this time. Parents and infants further the emotional bond by means of communication. A deeper emotional tie begins to emerge as infants become less reflexive and more aware of their surroundings. During their first year, infants discover the boundaries between self and the environment. They differentiate themselves from others. By 2 months of age, their smiles are in response to pleasure rather than reflex actions. At 6 months they show a clear preference for their closest caregiver, and by 8 months they generally respond differently to a stranger. Infants seek pleasure from social games such as peek-a-boo and pat-a-cake and by 1 year begin to enjoy more complex interactive games such as hide-and-seek. Much of their social interactive ability is dependent on the theory of attachment being a lifelong process.

Erikson (1963) describes the psychosocial developmental task at this stage as trust versus mistrust (see Chapter 15). Infants depend on their caregivers to meet their needs for food, warmth, love, and security. If these needs are met promptly and consistently, a sense of trust will develop. If these needs are met at the convenience of others or not at all, a sense of mistrust will develop. Resolution of this task affects development at other stages. Infants have no concept of "waiting." Their initial reaction to stress of any nature is to cry. Crying is their means of communicating during this preverbal stage. An infant gradually learns other means of tolerating stress. Freud (1946) describes an infant's ability to reduce tension through sucking and mouthing objects as the oral stage. Nurses need to recognize these normal infant behaviors when providing care.

Cognitive Assessment

In addition to motor development and psychosocial task achievement, sensory impressions provide the groundwork for infants' knowledge of the world. Improved visual acuity and color discrimination makes the environment more interesting to see and explore. As the mind continues to develop, hearing becomes more discriminating and vocalization proceeds from crying to cooing to laughing. By the end of the first year, infants imitate sounds, comprehend simple commands, and repeat a few simple words such as "Da-Da" and "up" and know what they mean. This sensorimotor stage (Piaget, 1952) unfolds as an infant interacts with the environment. Infants acquire knowledge by perceiving and doing, gaining the ability to prolong or repeat actions they find pleasurable. By the end of the first year, infants recognize objects as distinct and separate from themselves. They will search for objects removed from sight. However, they may

Table 16–6

RECOMMENDED CHILDHOOD IMMUNIZATION SCHEDULE*

	HEPATITIS B (HB)	ORAL POLIOVIRUS (OPV)	DIPHTHERIA, TETANUS, PERTUSSIS (DTP)	HAEMOPHILUS INFLUENZA TYPE B (HiB)	MEASLES, MUMPS, AND RUBELLA (MMR)	VARICELLA-ZOSTER VIRUS (VZV) (CHICKENPOX)
Birth	HB #1 or					
1 mo	HB #1 or HB #2 or					
2 mo	HB #1 or HB #2 or	OPV #1	DTP #1	HiB #1		
4 mo	HB #2	OPV #2	DTP #2	HiB #2		
6 mo	HB #3 or	OPV #3 or	DTP #3	HiB #3 or		
12–15 mo	HB #3 or	OPV #3 or	DTP #4 or	HiB #3 or #4	MMR #1	VZV #1 or
15 mo	HB #3 or	OPV #3 or	DTaP if ≥15 mo			VZV #1 or
18 mo	HB #3	OPV #3 or				VZV #1
4–6 y		OPV #4	DTP #5 or DTaP		MMR #2 or	
11–12 y	HB (catch-up)		Td or		MMR #2	VZV (catch-up)
14–16 y			Td (and every 10 y after that)			

*This schedule of recommended immunizations is based on the 1996 guidelines published by the US Public Health Department and the American Academy of Pediatrics Committee on Infectious Diseases. Wherever the word *or* occurs, it indicates that an acceptable range of time has been indicated for obtaining that particular immunization. The nurse should keep in mind that various preparations of the same vaccine are available and may be administered on a different schedule. In addition, immunization schedules change frequently according to new science and epidemiology.

not be able to find them if moved to another site. This ability will come at a later age. Mandler (1990) and others through their research have challenged Piaget's theories of cognition, suggesting that infants' ability to conceptualize occurs much earlier than previously thought. Because infants need to develop and use their senses, nurses and parents should take every opportunity to provide pleasing sensory stimulation. If an infant is tired or ill, however, overstimulation can hinder cognitive development. Therefore, parents and nurses should continually evaluate infants' emotional and physical states.

Moral and Spiritual Assessment

Pleasure and pain are the indicators that infants utilize to begin associating right from wrong. Cogni-

tively, infants can understand only that their behavior may result in an approving smile or pleasant voice from their parent or, on the other hand, a disapproving frown or scolding. Moral and spiritual development takes on more form as the child grows older.

The nursing process steps of diagnosis, planning, intervention, and evaluation are presented here for some of the most common nursing diagnoses for this age.

Nursing Diagnosis

The Nursing Diagnosis Box lists some of the most common diagnoses for this age group.

Planning

The outcome criteria for these diagnoses would include

Parents will demonstrate understanding of their role in the maintenance of health and wellness in their infant

Infant will exhibit age-appropriate physical growth and psychosocial, cognitive, moral, and spiritual development patterns

Infant will remain free from injury

Parents will verbalize understanding of and demonstrate ways to keep the infant safe

Intervention

Health Maintenance Visits

Instruct parents to keep regularly scheduled health promotion appointments at 2 weeks and at 2, 4, 6, 9, and 12 months of age.

Nutrition

Assess feeding patterns at each health care visit and correlate with serial measurements on the anthropometric charts

Provide anticipatory guidance using suggested guidelines for feeding infants in Table 16–5

Report any deviations from expected findings to the health care provider for further assessment

Assess for expected pattern of tooth eruption

Observe for evidence of dental caries

Encourage parents to start dental hygiene measures early in infancy (*e.g.*, fluoride supplements, avoidance of formula or juice bottle during sleep time, beginning to clean teeth with small soft toothbrush soon after tooth eruption)

Begin dental visits early to avoid fear experienced when infant is older

Sleep and Activity

Assess sleeping patterns and motor or developmental milestones at each health care visit (see Table 16–4)

Administer the Denver II screening tool at 4 and 10 months of age

Report any deviations from normal patterns to the health care provider

Provide parents and caregivers with information on appropriate toys and activities (infants enjoy patting, hugging, and mouthing objects; therefore, toys should be durable, washable, large enough to prevent aspiration, and have smooth edges)

Immunizations

Assess immunization status of infant at each health care visit

Review infant's immunization record with parents to remind them of importance of good record-keeping and adherence to schedule in providing optimal protection

Review expected local and systemic reactions for each immunization given and advice on when to call the health care provider in the event of an untoward reaction

Injury Prevention

Assess parents' knowledge base regarding injury prevention and related safety issues

Implement and teach parents the infant safety guidelines provided in Table 16–3

Advise parents regarding how to seek help in an emergency

Teach parents cardiopulmonary resuscitation or suggest how they can receive training

Anticipatory Guidance

Assess knowledge level regarding common infant health concerns and provide information to dispel any myths (see Table 16–7)

Evaluation

Parents keep all scheduled health maintenance visits

Parents verbalize that age-appropriate dietary, sleep, activity, and play needs are being met

Infant thrives and develops according to expected developmental milestones

Infant remains free from injury

Parents verbalize and return demonstrate appropriate safety measures

Childproofing measures are observed in the home

Nursing Process for Toddlers (1–3 years)

Assessment

Not an infant but not yet a fully developed child, the toddler experiences great strides in mobility and cognitive development far beyond those of physical

Table **16–7**

ANTICIPATORY GUIDANCE IN INFANCY

ISSUE	RATIONALE	GUIDANCE
Thumb sucking or use of pacifier	Sucking is a major pleasure for the infant Benefits such as decreased crying and increased relaxation have been identified by meeting the infant's need for nonnutritive sucking Infants will generally find their fingers or hands to suck on to meet this need without the use of a pacifier As the need for nonnutritive sucking decreases, so does the need for the pacifier or thumb, unless their use is treated as a reinforcement by children's parents to relieve infant distress	Explore parents' feelings regarding the infant's need to use a pacifier If pacifiers are to be used, review safety considerations in their use (*e.g.*, preferably constructed in one piece, have a flange with at least two ventilation holes and be large enough to prevent aspiration, remove from infant when not in use, never secure to infant by tying with a cord around the neck) Thumb sucking is generally abandoned by the age when dental problems may become an issue (when permanent teeth erupt) If a pacifier is used, try removing it around 6 mo of age, when the infant is not yet old enough to remember or miss it for long If pacifiers are used beyond the first year, unless you are meticulous about sterilizing them they can be very unhygienic as the infant toddles around with it; this is a good reason to discontinue pacifier use
Teething	Teething seldom causes discomfort in an infant younger than 4 mo of age At 5 or 6 mo, as the first tooth emerges, drooling, chewing on hard objects, and some irritability may accompany the minor inflammation of the gums Most discomfort is felt by the infant with the eruption of the first molars at age 12–15 mo	Believing that an infant younger than 4 mo of age is irritable for long periods due to "teething" may cause a parent to neglect a real illness Medical attention should be sought for any infant experiencing fever, diarrhea, vomiting, loss of appetite as these are not symptoms of teething Avoid the use of teething gels because they contain anesthetics that may cause untoward effects in the infant if overused Provide something cold to bite on; for example, a frozen gel-filled teething ring
Separation/stranger fear	Around 8 mo of age, infants have sufficient capacity to recognize their primary caregivers and find comfort in their presence Because they have not yet developed the task of object permanence, infants experience great displeasure when their caregivers leave them alone or with an unfamiliar substitute This behavior may continue into toddlerhood	Parents (caregivers) should accustom the infant to new persons, especially those that may be called on to babysit in the future (the more frequent the exposure, the less likely the fear) Give infants opportunity to explore strangers at their own pace to allow a "warm up" period of adjustment Talk to infants when leaving them and greet them when you return. This can aid the development of object permanence and reassure them that you will always return Use a transitional object such as your scarf or a toy to reassure them of your continued presence

growth during this period. As toddlers make progress in mastering their newfound independence, their emotions can swing in a moment from happiness to misery. Parents and caregivers express frustration with the need to encourage independence yet be firm and consistent in setting limits that will ensure their toddler's safety and well-being. These psychosocial and cogni-

tive parameters are essential for a nurse to assess. In addition, recording vital signs and serial measurements of weight, length, and head circumference, as well as nutrition, dentition, sleep and activity, and immunizations during health maintenance visits is relevant. Toddlers are generally screened at 15 months, 18 months, 2 years, and 3 years of age.

Table 16-7

ANTICIPATORY GUIDANCE IN INFANCY
(Continued)

ISSUE	RATIONALE	GUIDANCE
Spoiling/limit setting	When infants' needs are not promptly met or are only met after a period of delay, they become anxious, quicker to fuss or cry, and slower to accept comfort; therefore, the less you meet the infants' needs, the more demanding they become As infants become more mobile toward the latter half of the first year, parents need to set limits to provide for their safety; however, there is no substitute for vigilant parental monitoring	Prompt attention to the crying infant often is greeted by the infant's smile and comfort Delaying attention to the crying infant leads to an encounter with a miserably distressed infant who does not settle down easily, has a stomach full of air from excessive crying, and will most likely start crying again before long Limit setting is done with the older infant through consistent and age-appropriate methods A negative voice and stern eye-to-eye contact may be all that is needed A quiet period for the infant in the playpen may be warranted Parents who express concern over discipline in the infant stage should recognize that the earlier it is started, the easier it is to maintain throughout childhood

Injury prevention	Unintentional injury is the second leading cause of death in infancy
	Common risks associated with this developmental stage include
	  Choking or suffocation
	  Falls
	  Motor vehicle crash injuries
	  Burns
		Parents and caregivers should be instructed in the techniques of CPR
		Home/environmental safety check list should be reviewed with parents
		Review prevention guidelines in Table 16–3

Crying/colic	Periods of crying of up to 2 hours per day are considered normal and part of the infant's temperament Colicky infants are described as those who cry for long periods with legs drawn up, generally for periods in excess of 3 hours daily Colic has no known cause but has been associated with intolerance to cow's milk formula or ingestion of milk products by breast-feeding mothers and passive smoking As infants cry, they swallow more air, distend the abdomen, cry some more, pass flatus, and the cycle continues	Reassurance should be given to parents that the crying period is a source of energy release for the infant Parents should always initially respond to the infant's cry to determine the cause Continuation of long periods of crying should be reported to the health care provider When no cause for the crying episodes can be identified, time of onset should be noted; immediate response to the infant by changing position, massaging the abdomen, swaddling in blanket, taking for car ride, or placing infant in wind-up swing has been successful Avoid smoking near infant Provide, small frequent feedings; burp during and after feeding; have the infant sit upright for half an hour after feeding

Physiological Assessment

Respiration and Circulation

The cardiopulmonary system becomes more stable in toddlerhood, with the heart rate slowing to about 110 bpm and the respiratory rate to 24 breaths per minute at rest. Toddlers are too active for a nurse to count a peripheral pulse accurately, so apical heart rates should be auscultated. Assess blood pressure routinely if you can gain cooperation. Readings average 90/56 mmHg in the 2-year-old child. Use a child-sized blood pressure cuff to obtain the reading.

Weight and Height

During toddlerhood, physical growth continues at a considerably slower pace than in infancy. Because of a decrease in appetite during the second and third year of life, toddlers will only gain about 5.5 lb (2.5 kg) per year. Plump infants become more muscular and lean toddlers. By the time toddlers are 2 years old, their proportions are quite different than those of an infant (Fig. 16–6). Their bodies elongate; this is especially noticeable in the long bones of the legs. As toddlers assume a more upright posture, the characteristic lumbar lordosis and protuberant abdomen is evident. A gain of approximately 3 to 5 in (7.5–12 cm) will occur yearly during toddlerhood. Obtaining weight and height measurements presents a great challenge with this age group. Try a standing-type upright scale initially; however, if the child is not cooperative, attempt to use the infant scale. If all else fails, have the parent hold the child and weigh them both on the upright scale, then reweigh the parent without the child. Subtract the parent's weight from the combined weight to obtain the child's approximate weight. You can generally obtain an upright height measurement from a cooperative toddler. Use the technique described for preschoolers later in this chapter.

Head Circumference

During the second year of life, the head circumference increases approximately 1 in (2.5 cm) but will have reached four fifths of its adult size. The anterior fontanelle closes between 12 and 18 months, completing the most accelerated period of brain growth that will occur during life. Continue measuring head circumference at all health care visits until age 3 years. Assess the anterior fontanelle until it is no longer palpable.

Motor Development

Both gross and fine motor abilities develop rapidly during toddlerhood, allowing performance of such self-care activities as feeding, dressing, and toileting

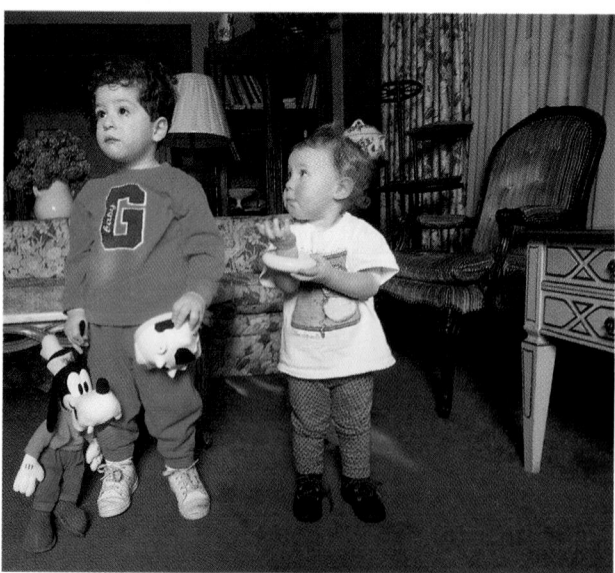

✦ **Figure 16–6**
A 1-year-old child and a 2-year-old child side by side. Note the physical differences.

with minimal assistance. Toddlers can hold a spoon and place it in the mouth correctly. They drink well from a cup. Their gait becomes steady, and they are able to run, jump, and ride a tricycle.

Nutrition

Information regarding the toddler's normal feeding and elimination patterns is gathered in addition to the anthropometric data during a nutritional assessment. Before the age of 2, most toddlers still need help with drinking from a regular glass or cup. Spilling occurs frequently because of poor wrist control. However, by 3 years, most toddlers have this challenge well under control. In addition, they generally feed themselves with minimal assistance.

Care should be taken in assessing the types of foods and fluids that are offered to toddlers and what they actually consume. Excessive intake of milk or juice interferes with proper nutrition, not only by providing inadequate nutrients but also by "filling up" toddlers so their appetite for solid foods is diminished. Research shows that if parents make good nutritious foods available to children and let them choose how much to eat, they are less apt to have problems controlling how much they eat later in life, thereby hindering overeating and obesity (Johnson & Birch, 1994).

Dentition

Most children enter toddlerhood with at least a few of their deciduous (primary) teeth, and by age 3, all 20 teeth should be in place. Over the past 25 years, the number of cavities in primary teeth declined by approximately 75%. This decrease is attributed to improved oral hygiene practices and the use of fluoride. Assessment of oral hygiene practices continues into toddlerhood, with the nurse determining what practices have been ongoing from infancy. Habits that are established early on are important for lifelong dental health.

Sleep and Activity

Assessing toddlers' sleep and activity patterns helps nurses to identify those that vary from normal infancy transition. At 13 months, toddlers are well on their way to sleeping approximately 12 hours at night with two daytime hour-long naps. After 15 months, only one nap is usual during the day. With rapid maturation in motor development, toddlers are full of energy. They work very hard at pushing themselves to their physical limit. Learning to walk and climb requires coordination, and when they get tired, toddlers fall, bump into things, and hurt themselves many times in a day. Getting overtired is a very common problem in toddlerhood. Assess parents' ability to recognize this behavior. An assumption should not be made that toddlers who are still rushing around are not tired. Nurses can guide parents toward more healthful relationships with their young children by teaching them to pick up on signals generated by their active toddlers.

Immunizations

Assessment of immunization status continues at every health care visit throughout toddlerhood (see Table 16–6). A study by Zell and colleagues (1994) found that fewer than half of the 2-year-old children in major American cities received all of the recommended immunizations. This failure to immunize relates directly to the rising rates of certain childhood illnesses such as measles. The local health department should be contacted to provide missed vaccines for toddlers who have not received all scheduled immunizations during infancy.

Psychosocial Assessment

Toddlerhood is a developmental stage of increased activity and awareness. Attachment behaviors that developed during infancy continue unfolding during the toddler years. Only now are prolonged periods of body-to-body contact replaced with visual contact of a familiar caregiver. This allows toddlers to step out and explore their surroundings. In this stage of development, known as autonomy versus shame and doubt (Erikson, 1963), children develop a sense of autonomy if parents provide them with a safe environment in which their needs of curiosity and exploration can be met without undue control or permissiveness (see Chapter 15). Limit setting is important to maintain their safety and well-being. Freud (1946) believed that the toddler's drive for independence and self-control is a pleasure-seeking behavior, and the locus shifts from the mouth in infancy to the anus in toddlerhood (hence the term *anal stage*). Often toilet training can be a battle of wills between parent and toddler. The vague pleasure of "feeling grown up" or being praised by parents for using the potty cannot make toddlers any more ready to use it independently. Signs of readiness involve not only the physical capacity of sphincter control but also the emotional and intellectual ability to perform the task. These concepts are depicted in Box 16–1.

Cognitive Assessment

Intellectual abilities during the toddler years continue to develop through sensory interaction with the environment. By toddlerhood, the physical senses are almost fully developed. The eyes can focus accurately and can perceive color. By 20 months of age, visual acuity is usually about 20/40. The ears can distinguish variations in the pitch and quality of sound, and hearing is as sharp in the 3-year-old child as it is in the adult. Toddlers have the ability to correlate sight with sound, such as a siren with a fire engine. Their sensations of taste and smell are very discriminating, and toddlers will let you know their likes and dislikes.

According to Piaget (1952), the toddler will complete the sensorimotor stage and enter the preconcep-

---

Box 16–1

ASSESSING READINESS FOR TOILET TRAINING

MUSCULAR MATURATION + COGNITIVE MATURITY + CHILD/PARENT MOTIVATION = SUCCESSFUL TOILET TRAINING

Often, toilet training begins with determined parents who want to get the "dirty task" over with long before the child can control the necessary muscles. Three milestones must be reached before successful bowel and bladder training can be achieved. The child must be able to

1. Become familiar with the sensations that indicate the need to eliminate
2. Keep the muscles tightened until he or she is securely on the toilet or potty
3. Loosen the muscles and eliminate at the proper time and place

When a child can eliminate in the potty at a very early age, it usually means that the parent has been "successfully trained" to recognize the child's preelimination cues and can get the child to the potty in time.

---

tual stage of cognitive development. Toddlers display an ability to imitate the behaviors of others through symbolic function. Symbolic function allows them to observe an event, construct a mental image, and later mimic the event. For example, toddlers may imitate the parent sweeping the floor or talking on the telephone. Symbolic thinking manifests also as toddlers play. Two-year-old children are often observed playing with objects for long periods, substituting their real purpose for something else, such as placing a plastic bowl on the head as if it were a hat. Toddlers are curious, stubborn, impulsive, and negative. By asserting a newfound curiosity, they step away from their caregivers, recognizing an ability to explore new objects and territories. However, unable to comprehend most of these actions with forethought of consequence, they often get into trouble. For example, at 15 months, toddlers may be able to creep up a few stairs and will do so given the opportunity but will not be able to think ahead of how to get down, a motor skill they are unable to perform. Because they learn by oral exploration, toddlers put things in their mouths, which places them at risk for poisonings. Unfortunately, this risk is a consequence of normal development. For example, toddlers may attempt to drink an amber-colored cleaning product that resembles apple juice. Even though negative consequences result from this ingestion, the injury may happen again if measures are not taken to "childproof" the environment. Toddlers' memory is very short, so day after day, stubbornness will allow them to trip and tumble over the same step in the house until the repeated experience and gentle parental reminders give it a final resting place in their memory.

Although their vocabulary may grow from 4 words at 12 months to more than 400 words at 36 months, toddlers are not able to understand the spoken word quite as effectively as older children or adults. By 36 months, toddlers are able to produce grammatically correct sentences in the present tense. However, their vocabulary is still quite literal. For example, to expect toddlers to keep a promise, even when they use those words, would be unrealistic. A parent may offer a toddler 5 more minutes to play if he or she promises to then put away the toys. A toddler will gladly say "I promise" and then be totally confused by the parent's anger or disappointment when the "promise" is broken. Toddlers are unable to understand someone else's viewpoint or to put themselves in someone else's place. Because children's moral development is keenly connected with their cognitive abilities, one can observe the beginning of morality during toddlerhood.

Moral and Spiritual Assessment

From 1 to 3 years of age, children are unable to comprehend the concepts of right and wrong. Rather, they behave simply to seek out pleasure and avoid unpleasantness. When a 2-year-old child grabs a toy and yells "mine!" a primitive statement about individual property rights has been expressed. Although this behavior does not fall into any of Lawrence Kolberg's three categories of moral reasoning, the underpinnings for moral development are being tested during toddlerhood. Spirituality has not yet developed in this age group.

The assessment provides the nurse with data to structure into diagnoses, plans, interventions, and evaluations. These steps of the nursing process are illustrated here for some common nursing diagnoses in this age group.

Nursing Diagnosis

The diagnoses listed in the box entitled "Nursing Diagnoses for Infants Through School-Age Children" continue to be the primary nursing diagnoses that the nurse encounters.

Planning

The outcome criteria for these nursing diagnoses might be expressed as follows:

Parents will demonstrate understanding of their role in the maintenance of health and wellness in their toddler

Toddler will exhibit age-appropriate physical growth and psychosocial, cognitive, moral, and spiritual development

Toddler will remain free from injury

Parents will verbalize understanding of ways to keep toddler safe

COMMUNITY-BASED CARE

INFANT AND YOUTH SERVICES

During the infancy stage, the nurse working in the community plays a vital role in well-baby services and in care for infants with illnesses or disabilities. The public health nurse may work in clinics, providing immunizations and teaching about the importance of and schedules for the various immunizations. Frequently, nurses visit high-risk mothers and babies, such as teenage mothers and premature infants. The purpose of these visits is to assess, teach, and monitor health status. Often, referrals to home care agencies are needed for infants with more intensive, skilled care needs, such as those who have hyperbilirubinemia, failure to thrive, or apnea. The home care nurse assesses the infant for progress and potential complications, provide ordered treatments, and provide emotional support and education for the parents.

As children grow to school age, the school nurse participates in assessment, teaching, and routine screening (i.e., vision and hearing) as related to this age group. The nurse may formulate a plan to reduce injuries and increase nutritional status after collecting data such as frequency of school absences relating to injury or illness. The school nurse also participates in care planning for children with special health care needs in collaboration with families, school personnel, and physicians.

As children mature to adolescence, community health and school nurses work together to educate this population. Nurses may evaluate the incidence of teenage pregnancy, substance use, or sexually transmitted diseases. The school nurse may provide health counseling and education for students, parents, and teachers that address these important concerns.

Intervention
Health Maintenance Visits

Instruct parents to keep regularly scheduled health promotion appointments for their toddler at 15, 18, and 24 months and at 3 years of age

Nutrition

Assess toddler's feeding and elimination patterns and correlate with serial measurements on the anthropometric charts

Provide anticipatory guidance using suggested guidelines for feeding toddlers in Table 16–5

Instruct parents not to overcontrol or force feed toddlers; allowing self-regulation helps toddlers to stay in touch with their natural hunger cues

Dentition

Assess for expected pattern of tooth eruption

Observe for evidence of dental caries and baby-bottle syndrome

Encourage parents to continue dental hygiene measures (*e.g.,* fluoride supplements, avoidance of formula or juice bottle during sleep time, beginning to clean teeth with small soft toothbrush soon after tooth eruption, and flossing)

Begin dental visits early to avoid fear experienced when child is older

Sleep and Activity

Assess sleeping patterns and developmental milestones at each health care visit

Report deviations to health care provider

Administer the Denver II screening tool at 3 years of age

Provide parents and caregivers information about appropriate toys and activities for toddlers (push-pull toys, picture books with bright colors, puzzles with large pieces)

Immunizations

Assess immunization status of toddler at each health care visit

Review toddler's immunization record with parents to remind them of importance of good record-keeping and adherence to schedule in providing optimal protection

Review expected local and systemic reactions for each immunization given and advice on when to call the health care provider in the event of an untoward reaction

Injury Prevention

Assess parents' knowledge base regarding injury prevention and related safety issues

Implement and teach parents the toddler safety guidelines provided in Table 16–3

Advise parents regarding how to seek help in an emergency

Teach parents cardiopulmonary resuscitation or suggest how they can receive training

Anticipatory Guidance

Assess knowledge level regarding common toddler health concerns and provide information to dispel any myths (Table 16–8)

Evaluation

Parents keep all scheduled health maintenance visits

Parents verbalize that age-appropriate dietary, sleep, activity, and play needs are being met

Daytime bowel and bladder control is achieved by age 3 years (with occasional accidents)

Toddler thrives and develops according to expected growth and developmental milestones

Toddler remains free from injury

Parents verbalize and return demonstrate appropriate safety measures

Childproofing measures are observed in the home

✦

Nursing Process for the Preschooler (3–6 Years)

Assessment

The preschooler emerges from the toddler years and begins to behave like a "real person." Physical development slows and stabilizes, while maturation of the central nervous system rapidly expands the preschooler's cognitive abilities and increases control and coordination over the body. As with the infant and toddler, assessment of physical growth parameters, nutrition, dentition, sleep and activity, and immunization status should be performed. Health care visits should be made at 3, 4, and 5 years of age.

Physiological Assessment

Respiration and Circulation

The heart rate and respiratory rate decrease slightly during this period. The heart rate averages 90 bpm, while the respiratory rate is approximately 22 breaths per minute. Most children in this age group cooperate for radial pulse measurements. Blood pressure rises to an average of 94/56 for the 5-year-old child. Use a child-sized blood pressure cuff to obtain the reading.

Weight and Height

As their trunks, arms, and legs grow longer, children begin to acquire a body appearance that by the age of 6 years has steadily become more adultlike in appearance (Fig. 16–7). Normally fed children during the preschool years generally gain about 4.5 lb (2 kg) per year and by age 6 weigh approximately 46 lb (21 kg). The potbelly of the toddler disappears as the preschooler's abdominal muscles develop. Steady increases, an average of 3 in (7 cm) per year, occur, resulting in a height of approximately 46 in (117 cm) by age 6 years. Generally, boys appear more muscular, have less body fat, and are slightly taller and heavier than girls throughout childhood. Weigh children in light clothing or in underwear without shoes on a standing-type upright scale. If a height marker is not attached to the scale, height can be obtained with the child standing against a wall on a level surface and barefoot. Mark the height on the wall at the top of the head, then use a tape measure to record the measurement from floor to wall mark.

Head Circumference

Although not measured routinely anymore, preschoolers' skulls reach almost adult proportion by the sixth birthday, when brain capacity reaches approxi-

Table 16–8

ANTICIPATORY GUIDANCE IN TODDLERHOOD

ISSUE	RATIONALE	GUIDANCE
Toilet training	The ability to master control over elimination requires muscular maturation as well as cognitive maturity The toddler needs to understand instructions as well as the purpose for accomplishing this task for which there is no tangible reward other than that of "pleasing" a caregiver Eighty-four percent of 3-year-old children are dry throughout the day, and 66%, throughout the night	Most parents initiate toilet training efforts between 20 and 24 mo Parents should be informed that "successful" toilet training at a very early age is usually because the *parent* is "trained" to recognize the child's readiness and places the child on the potty at the appropriate time Teach parents to keep a record of the toddler's pattern and signals of elimination for several weeks prior to starting Have parents obtain a sturdy potty chair, if possible, so the child can independently sit and get up, or a sturdy step stool to access toilet with adult supervision Have parents dress child in loose-fitting clothing to aid easy access and prevent accidents Inform parents that when the child signals that a bowel movement or voiding may be on the way, they should casually suggest to the child that he or she may want to sit on the potty Encourage parents not to force the child to sit on the potty or to show disappointment if attempts are unsuccessful Explain to parents that accidents will happen and will need to be taken in stride Nagging and punishing a child for being uncooperative or for having "accidents" will mean certain failure, as the toddler will become overwhelmed and confused with what is expected
Temper tantrums	Temper tantrums are commonly seen toward the end of the second year of life Tantrums are the result of excessive frustration; for example, when a child becomes overwhelmed with emotion and feelings of tension, an explosive outburst is a means of release Tantrums often involve screaming, thrashing, and breath-holding spells	Parents should be taught that a temper tantrum is like an "emotional blown fuse," which is not something that the toddler can control Parents need to recognize a balance between a frustration level that their child can tolerate and that is useful for learning and the amount of frustration that will cause the fuse to blow During a tantrum, a parent should be instructed to try to protect child from harm but not to overpower him or her, as this physical restriction may heighten the anger Reassure parents that breath-holding spells, although alarming to watch, do not result in physical harm. The body's natural reflex to breath will allow the child to take in air before any damage can occur
Stress, anxiety, and fear	Toddlers live on an emotional see-saw, with most of the stress and tears arising from the basic contradiction of wanting independence and the desire to be protected and loved by their caregivers Again they need a balance of autonomy yet protection from separation anxiety A toddler begins to feel anxious whenever his own feelings become uncontrollable leading to crying or temper tantrums	Inform parents to recognize cues from the toddler that indicates an impending problem; for example, excessive clinginess, less adventurous behavior, increased shyness Instruct parents to offer more affection, attention, and protection for several days until the toddler regains a normal sense of independence and adventure

Table **16–8**

ANTICIPATORY GUIDANCE IN TODDLERHOOD
(Continued)

ISSUE	RATIONALE	GUIDANCE
Bedtime struggles	As many as 50% of all children between the ages of 1 and 2 y engage in fussing or bedtime struggles lasting for more than an hour Sometimes these struggles are associated with family stress, such as illness or change in normal routines Most times they are caused by continued infancy routines of "being put to sleep" by nursing, rocking, or coddling	Inform parents that they are not alone with this struggle—that is is very common Inform parents that if they continue to coddle, rock, or nurse their toddlers to sleep at this age, it will be harder to institute a different bedtime routine Instruct parents to alter the routine by providing about 20 min of sedentary activity, such as quiet conversation or story-telling Have parents keep a night light on if it makes child more comfortable Tell parents to finish their sedentary time with a pleasant "goodnight," and if child begins to cry and continues for several minutes, they should go back in the room, repeat "goodnight" and leave again; this performance should be repeated every few minutes for as long as it takes toddler to settle down Any sleep problem that persists over several months should be referred to the child's health care provider

Unintentional injuries	Unintentional injury is the leading cause of death and disability in toddlerhood
	Toddlers are especially vulnerable to unintentional injuries due to their activity level, developing motor skills and inability to perceive dangerous situations
	Common risks associated with this developmental stage include
	  Drowning
	  Burns or scalds
	  Motor vehicle injuries
	  Falls
	  Poisoning
		Parents and caregivers should be instructed in the techniques of CPR
		Home and environmental safety checklist should be reviewed with parents and caregivers
		Review prevention guidelines in Table 16–3
		Reinforce with parents and caregivers the importance of vigilant child monitoring and supervision during this highly vulnerable developmental stage

Play activities	Play is the "work" of the young; it helps children to use their muscles and gain mastery over what they think, see, and do—a form of learning Pretending or imaginative play emerges during this period—the toddler reenacts past experiences through retained mental pictures of things seen or heard; for example, a little boy might dip a sock in the dog's water bowl and use it to clean his toy truck after having observed his father wash the car the previous month	Inform parents that providing a safe place, safe toys or other play equipment, and time is all that is needed to promote healthy play activities in the toddler If the toddler gets frustrated, the toys or activities may be too advanced, or he or she may be asking for some assistance or guidance Boredom will ensue if the play space and the activities are not varied from time to time Inform parents that toys need not be expensive; children at this age are content to play with household objects, such as plastic bowls and wooden spoons Instruct parents to be responsible consumers; when purchasing toys, they should (1) inspect them for small pieces or loose parts that may cause a choking hazard, (2) determine if they are age appropriate for their child, and (3) not sacrifice safety and quality for price

Child Development and Proportion

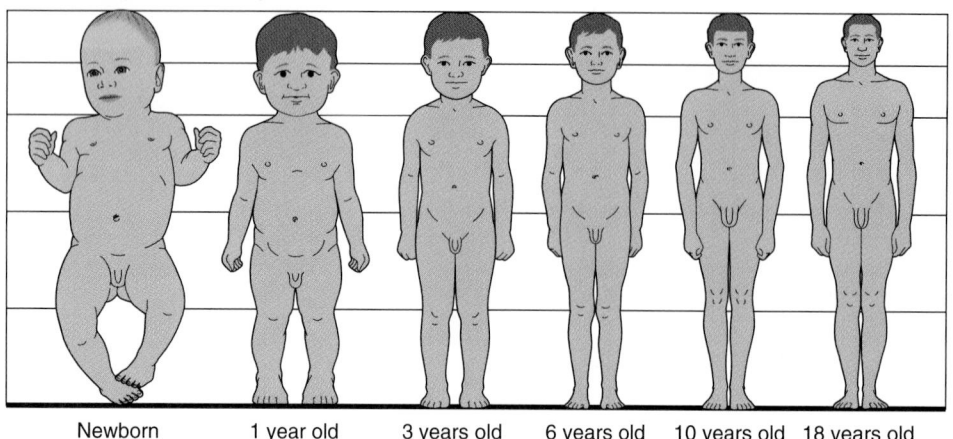

Newborn   1 year old   3 years old   6 years old   10 years old 18 years old

> **Figure 16–7**
> Changes in body proportions over time.

mately 90%. The face grows proportionately more than the cranial cavity, with the jaw widening in preparation for permanent tooth eruption.

Motor Development

As their bodies grow stronger and less top-heavy, and as they develop greater control and coordination over their muscles, preschoolers make great improvements in both gross and fine motor skills. They are able to run, jump, climb, and skip with greater grace and speed. Greater dexterity allows them to button clothing, pour milk into a cup, and cut along a line with a scissor by the time they reach age 4 years. At 5 years of age, preschoolers begin to show permanent preference for using one hand over another. The Denver II is still used as a developmental screening tool during this stage.

Nutrition

As the growth rate slows, so does a child's appetite, along with a need for fewer calories per pound of body weight. Parents often express concern regarding their children's small intake and compensate by offering a diet high in sugared foods and low in nutrients. A nutritional assessment at each visit is necessary to identify nonhealthy eating habits early so that proper guidance can be offered. This way, healthy lifelong nutrition practices can be acquired.

Dentition

Eruption of the deciduous (primary) teeth should be complete by the start of the preschool years. Inspect the oral cavity during each health visit for manifestations of poor oral hygiene and nutrition. Dental caries should not be ignored. Parents often take a complacent attitude toward dental care for their young children because these teeth are "not permanent." However, good habits need to start early in life to establish regular routines that will lead to lifelong dental health. Review with the parent and child brushing,

flossing, fluoride supplementation, and the need for routine dental visits.

Sleep and Activity

A different bedtime routine emerges during the preschool years. Three-year-old children take a longer time falling asleep than toddlers. After retiring to bed, requests for a glass of water, leaving the light on, and one more bedtime story are not uncommon. A favorite toy or blanket is often needed for the child to fall asleep. The average 3-year-old child sleeps about 12 hours each night and occasionally takes a daytime nap but by age 5 only sleeps 11 hours and skips naps altogether. Assessing a preschooler's sleep patterns may uncover sleep disturbances, which occur regularly in this age group. Anticipatory guidance is provided for this and other problems encountered during the preschool years in Table 16–9.

Immunizations

More than 80% of preschool children in the United States have received their full schedule of immunizations. This results from Federal regulations for immunizations prior to school entry. Nonetheless, the nurse should review with the parent at all health care visits the child's immunization record and complete the schedule for any missing dosages and boosters as indicated. Refer to Table 16–6 for the recommended schedule.

Psychosocial Assessment

As preschoolers begin to interact with the social world both physically and symbolically through activity and language, their self-awareness and understanding of others grows appreciably. Their relationships with parents and siblings grow and become more complex; in addition, they begin to explore various social roles with other children as they venture into the neighborhood through play groups, day care, and preschool settings (Fig. 16–8).

Table 16–9

ANTICIPATORY GUIDANCE FOR THE PRESCHOOL CHILD

ISSUE	RATIONALE	GUIDANCE
Aggression	A hostile act may be intended to hurt somebody or to establish dominance and is usually triggered by the social conflicts that arise in the course of cooperative play during the preschool years Children between 2 and 5 years of age who fight the most tend to be the most sociable and competent In many cases, a decline in physical aggression is often accompanied by an increase in verbal aggression, usually in the form of name calling Even in a normal child, aggression can get out of hand and become dangerous Since the 1950s, research has correlated televised violence with aggressive behavior in children	Parents can often reduce aggressive tendencies by the way they act or react to the situation Teach parents to deal with misbehavior by reasoning with the child, reinforcing good behavior, and being consistent in their approach to discipline Spanking causes a child to suffer frustration, pain and humiliation, and it is poor role modeling—the child sees hitting as an acceptable solution to a problem Encourage parents to monitor their child's television viewing by limiting total time allowed for viewing and selecting model shows that are educational and prosocial
Fearfulness	Preschoolers have an inability to distinguish "pretend" from reality as part of normal development Preschoolers have an intense sense of fantasy and are more likely to be frightened by something that looks "scary" than by something that can cause real harm Common fears of this age group include separation from parent, dark, animals, and noises—especially those in the dark Sometimes the anxiety is grounded in reality: for example, a child who was bitten by a dog may fear that the event will happen again	Parents can often reduce fears by instilling a sense of trust and normal caution without being overprotective Teach parents to avoid ridiculing their child but to provide reassurance and encourage open expression of feelings Have parents avoid coercion and logical persuasion, because developmentally, the child is unable to process such statements as "Pet the nice parrot—it won't hurt you," or "Lions are only found in a zoo" Encourage parents to seek out modeling behavior and expose their child to it; by observing fearlessness in other children, their child will gradually overcome the perceived threat
Daycare or preschool	Preschoolers can thrive physically, intellectually, and emotionally in daycare and preschool settings that have small groups, high adult-to-child ratios, and a stable, competent, and involved staff Preschoolers develop best when they have a balance between structured activities and freedom to explore on their own Parents may feel less stress knowing that their child is being well cared for while they are earning the income needed or fulfilling personal achievements	Teach parents strategies for choosing a good program for their child that includes the following: Provides a safe, clean setting Welcomes parents who visit unannounced Has warm and friendly personnel that are responsive to the children Fosters social skills, self-esteem, and respect for others Helps parents improve their parenting skills Teach parents to avoid programs that Employ staff members who are not educated, trained in CPR, or experienced in child care or child education Are not licensed by the state Have no written plan for meals or emergencies Have poor ventilation or lighting or no smoke alarms, fire extinguisher, or first-aid kit

Table continued on following page

Table **16–9**

ANTICIPATORY GUIDANCE FOR THE PRESCHOOL CHILD
(Continued)

ISSUE	RATIONALE	GUIDANCE
Sleep disorders	Approximately one in four preschoolers suffers from either night terrors or night-mares Night terrors are identified by abrupt awakening from deep sleep in a state of panic; the child is not really awake and will quiet down quickly and not remember the incident in the morning Night terrors do not indicate underlying emotional problems and are thought to be an effect of very deep sleep states Nightmares usually come toward the early morning and are vividly remembered by the child Persistent nightmares, especially those that cause fear and anxiety to the child during the day, may indicate excessive stress in the child	Explain to parents that these are common sleep problems in preschoolers Teach parents to enlist a pleasant and relaxed bedtime ritual to share with their child, such as recalling a happy family outing or event Recommend that parents leave a small light on that does not produce shadows on the wall Encourage parents to provide their child with comfort and reassurance each and every time an episode occurs

Unintentional injuries	Unintentional injury continues to be the leading cause of death and disability in preschool children
	Preschoolers are no longer content with their home environment and venture outside of the home, often with less supervision than in previous years
	Common risks associated with this developmental stage include
	    Motor vehicle injuries
	    Burns or scalds
	    Drowning
	    Falls
	    Poisoning
		Parents and caregivers should be instructed in the techniques of CPR
		Home and environmental safety checklist should be reviewed with parents and caregivers
		Review preschooler prevention guidelines in Table 16–9
		Reinforce with parents and caregivers the importance of vigilant child monitoring and supervision

Unless their social world makes it impossible, children enter the preschool years with a positive impression of themselves. Harter and Pike (1984) discover that most preschoolers see themselves as competent with regard to both physical and intellectual skills. However, it is during these years that Erikson (1963) places children in the stage of initiative versus guilt. Unlike the toddler asserting autonomy, preschooler initiative reflects a genuine desire to accomplish a task. However, preschoolers take the risk of feeling guilty when their efforts result in criticism or failure. This guilt may squelch their desire to try new things, and therefore they must learn to regulate this fear and develop courage to take risks. Parents and caregivers can help preschoolers achieve this task by allowing them the opportunity to do new things on their own while providing limits that will help keep them out of harm's way. Observe preschoolers at play and also assess parent-child interactions to evaluate developmental progress.

During the phallic stage (Freud, 1946), boys are said to form sexual attractions to their mothers and girls to their fathers, and both have a competitive relationship with the same-sex parent. Children later learn to deal with guilt and fear by identifying with the same-sex parent, thereby developing a conscience. During the assessment, determine if the child has been asking questions of the parents regarding where babies come from or about sexual differences, and provide guidance for parents.

Cognitive Assessment

The preschool period is a time of momentous cognitive accomplishments. Four-year-old children talk continuously and have a comment about everything. Somewhat correct grammar begins to take shape at approximately age 5. However, Piaget, in labeling this period the preoperational stage, highlights what this

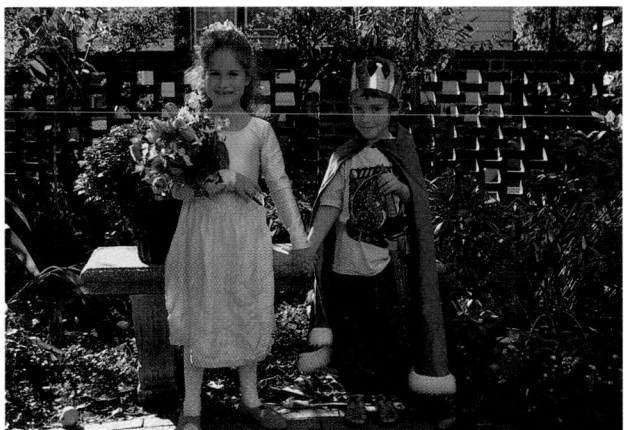

✦ **Figure 16–8**
Preschoolers explore roles and relationships through role play.

period of development lacks; that is, logical thinking. The preoperational stage explains an important finding in preschool development that has implications for parental guidance—understanding the difference between what things appear to be and what they really are. Parents may think that their child is lying, when in fact, the child is truly unable to distinguish between fantasy and reality. Egocentrism plays a part in this behavior as well. When preschoolers are unable to distinguish what goes on in their own head from reality, they become confused and profess only their point of view. This results in behaviors such as talking to themselves and to imaginary playmates and verbalizing how their "bad" thoughts caused a misfortune, such as a family death. Assess language development and counsel parents on the meaning of their child's age-appropriate behavior.

Moral and Spiritual Assessment

According to a recent study (Kantrowitz, 1991), parents are the single most important influence on their children. One of the most important human characteristics that parents teach their children is an ability to distinguish between right and wrong. This principle is part of what preschoolers learn as an underpinning of moral development. In view of egocentricity, many developmentalists feel that preschoolers cannot be taught morals but can be trained to behave. If taught properly—that is, by nonphysical discipline—children can learn from the harmful consequences of their behavior rather than learn to deal with others through aggressive acts. Assess parents' disciplinary style to better educate them in fostering, rather than hindering, their child's moral development.

Religious practices at this stage involve those rituals bestowed on the preschooler by the parents. Therefore, if the parents practice praying and attending religious services, the child will most likely partici-

pate as well without understanding the true spiritual reasons.

Nursing process steps of diagnosis, planning, intervention, and evaluation follow the collection of assessment data.

Nursing Diagnosis

The nurse will find that the diagnoses listed in the Nursing Diagnosis Box are still the most common diagnoses for preschool children.

Planning

The outcome criteria for these nursing diagnoses would include

Parents will demonstrate understanding of their role in the maintenance of health and wellness in their preschooler

Preschooler will exhibit age-appropriate physical growth and psychosocial, cognitive, moral, and spiritual development

Preschooler will remain free from injury

Parents will verbalize understanding of ways to keep preschooler safe

Intervention
Health Maintenance Visits

Instruct parents to keep regularly scheduled health promotion appointments for their preschooler at 3, 4, and 5 years of age

Nutrition

Assess preschooler's feeding and elimination patterns and correlate with serial measurements on the anthropometric charts

Provide a variety of foods in portions that allow child to develop self-feeding skills with a fork and dull knife by age 5 years

Instruct parents not to overcontrol or force feed preschoolers; allowing self-regulation helps child to stay in touch with his or her natural hunger cues

Dentition

Assess for complete set of 20 deciduous teeth

Observe for evidence of dental caries and baby-bottle syndrome

Encourage parents to continue dental hygiene measures (*e.g.,* fluoride supplements, tooth brushing, and flossing)

Continue dental visits every 6 months

Sleep and Activity

Assess sleeping patterns and developmental milestones at each health care visit

Report persistent sleep disturbances to health care provider

Administer the Denver II screening tool at 3 years

Provide parents and caregivers information about appropriate toys and play activities for preschoolers (coloring books and crayons, dolls, trucks and cars, child-sized playhouse, clothes for playing dress-up)

Immunizations

Assess immunization status of preschooler at each health care visit

Review preschooler's immunization record with parents to remind them of importance of good record-keeping and adherence to schedule in providing optimal protection

Review expected local and systemic reactions for each immunization given and advice on when to call the health care provider in the event of an untoward reaction

Injury Prevention

Assess parents' knowledge base regarding injury prevention and related safety issues

Implement and teach parents the preschooler safety guidelines provided in Table 16–3

Advise parents regarding how to seek help in an emergency

Teach parents cardiopulmonary resuscitation or suggest how they can receive training

Anticipatory Guidance

Assess knowledge level regarding common preschooler health concerns and provide anticipatory guidance and information to dispel any myths (see Table 16–9)

Evaluation

Parents keep all scheduled health maintenance visits

Parents verbalize that age-appropriate dietary, sleep, activity, and play needs are being met

Preschooler uses all parts of speech in complete sentences by age 5 years

Preschooler thrives and develops according to expected growth and developmental milestones

Preschooler remains free from injury

Parents verbalize and return demonstrate appropriate safety measures

Childproofing measures are observed in the home

Nursing Process for School-Age Children (6–13 Years)

Assessment

During the school years, children become less dependent on their caregivers as they become more cognitively mature and master more advanced psychomotor skills at a much faster pace than in earlier stages of development. These developments make it possible for older children to become more involved in everyday decision-making and the promotion of their own health. Health promotion visits should be made at ages 6, 8, 10, and 12 years.

Physiological Assessment

School-age children physically develop at a slow and consistent pace. Older school-age children enter a period referred to as the preteen years, during which, especially in girls, the sex hormones become active and secondary sex characteristics appear. The school-age years are the calm before the storm of adolescence.

Respiration and Circulation

Cardiopulmonary functioning becomes more efficient during the school years, with the resting heart rate averaging 65 to 90 bpm, blood pressure stabilizing at 110/70 mmHg, and the respiratory rate decreasing to 18 breaths per minute. Because of development of the heart and lungs during the middle childhood years, children are able to run faster and exercise longer than ever before. Count the radial pulse for 1 minute and use either a child-sized or an adult-sized blood pressure cuff to measure the blood pressure, depending on the circumference of the arm.

Weight and Height

Well-nourished school-age children gain approximately 5 lb (2.25 kg) and grow 2.5 in (6 cm) each year. At 10 years, typical school-age children weigh about 70 lb (32 kg) and measure 54 in (137 cm). They appear slimmer and more muscular than in previous years. As they grow taller, their body proportions change (Lowrey, 1986; see Fig. 16–7).

After age 10, girls generally begin their growth spurt and suddenly appear taller and heavier than boys of the same age. Measure the child using the techniques described for preschoolers.

Head Circumference

The brain has reached approximately 95% of its adult size by age 12, and near-adult head circumference of 21 in (53–54 cm) is reached. Routine measurements are not obtained. Facial bones grow, and sinuses are well formed by age 7 years.

Motor Development

During the school-age years, motor development becomes smoother and more coordinated in children (Fig. 16–9). Boys generally develop stronger gross motor skills related to the activities in which they participate. However, the stereotype of boys running faster, jumping higher, and throwing objects farther than girls is less prominent now that more girls are beginning to participate in similar activities. Girls, on the other hand, usually outperform boys in overall flexibility and dexterity, giving them an edge in gymnastics and fine motor activities such as playing musical instruments. By 10 to 12 years of age, most children demonstrate complex and intricate motor skills similar to those of the adult.

Nutrition

To support steady growth and constant exertion, a school-age child needs approximately 2400 calories each day. Finger feeding often reappears during this stage — just in time for children to eat on the go. Parents need to develop or continue rituals of regular mealtimes, especially at breakfast, so that bad habits do not persist into adolescence. Although sugar has gotten "bad press" over the years as contributing to

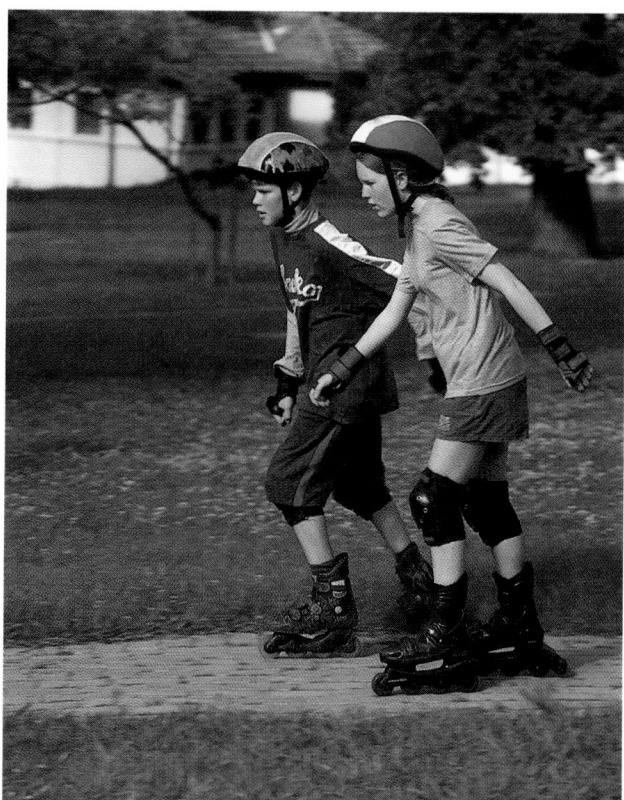

♪ **Figure 16–9**
School-age children make great strides in coordination.

hyperactivity in children, recent studies suggest that neither sugar nor artificial sweeteners adversely affect behavior, mood, or intelligence (Kinsbourne, 1994: Wolraich et al, 1994). Nonetheless, perform a nutritional assessment during the school years to evaluate the substance of meals and snacks. They should include a balance of nutrients that will support energy needs — not just empty calories.

Dentition

During the school years, children lose their deciduous teeth and begin to erupt permanent teeth. Tooth loss begins at age 6 years, and continuous replacement takes place at a rate of four teeth per year for the next 5 years. Assessment starts with an oral inspection at every health care visit and continues with an inquiry of the parents and child about routine dental practices.

Sleep and Activity

School-age children are in constant motion and are busy learning and doing — trying out all the world has to offer. Their increasing physical and mental capabilities permit greater speed, efficiency, and effort. All this energy makes them tired enough to average about 10 hours of sleep per night at age 6 and 9 hours at age 12. Although they may not go to sleep immediately, children are often content with a sedentary bedtime activity such as reading or listening to the radio. Older school-age children sometimes put up a fuss about going to bed at a certain time. Regardless, bedtime problems are rarely observed and are generally associated with the need for persistent bedtime rituals.

Immunizations

Scheduled immunizations are recommended prior to entry into the first grade of school. A nurse should review with the parent at all health care visits the child's immunization record and complete the schedule for any missing dosages and boosters as indicated. Because immunity to the measles, mumps, and rubella vaccines (MMR) may decrease over time, an MMR should be given at entry to middle or junior high school unless two doses were given after the first birthday. Refer to Table 16–6 for the recommended schedule.

Psychosocial Assessment

Children's initiative during the school years brings them in contact with a wealth of new experiences. During these years, children develop new friendships, may acquire a "best friend," and begin to be influenced by same-sex peer groups. However, early on, the family is still the child's major social milieu. With each experience, children spend their energies toward mastery at the risk of feeling incompetent or unproductive. Erikson (1963) refers to this stage as industry versus inferiority. In addition to an expanding interest in music, forming collections, constructing objects, and computer games, team activities are common. School-age children enjoy having parents and siblings present for competitions. However, they are easily embarrassed. For example, if a parent kisses his or her 10-year-old child in front of classmates, the child becomes visibly upset with the parent.

Boys and girls often break down into sex-segregated groups in the school-age years. Freud (1946) describes this as the latency period, in which children have little or no interest in the opposite sex. In the late school-age years, they do think about appearance and looking good to the opposite sex. They may even talk about boyfriends and girlfriends, but usually they really are referring to who talks to whom in the lunch line at school. Awkward feelings with the opposite sex emerge as children begin to develop an interest in one another. This behavior is manifested in boys and girls by fighting, teasing, and harassing one another.

Assess that children are progressing through this stage of development at an age-appropriate pace. Ascertain if parents can work behind the scenes, so as not to embarrass their child in social situations.

Cognitive Assessment

Extraordinary progress in language development occurs during the school years. Not only can children effectively communicate verbally using rules of grammar and proper syntax, but they can print and then later write in script. With the upsurge in personal computer use, many are also learning to use the keyboard effectively. With advanced language skills, their ability to comprehend also expands. School-age children think that they know it all. This trait, which so many parents describe as obnoxious, is called **cognitive conceit.** If children beat their parents at a card game, they take that as proof that they are brilliant and their parents are dumb. Logical reasoning is replacing intuitive thinking at this stage. Nevertheless, the school-age child still cannot figure out the abstract steps of an algebraic equation.

School-age children are in what Piaget (1952) refers to as the stage of concrete operations, in which they have an ability to understand the principle of conservation—they can sort, order, and classify objects. However, they still have limited understanding of abstract concepts. School-age children are capable of understanding another viewpoint as well as knowing that there are exceptions to rules. They are increasingly able to make independent and sound judgments. As parents recognize these abilities in their children and as more and more single-parent households and dual-earner households materialize, a pattern is emerging whereby older school-age children are home alone for several hours after school. Assess these "latchkey children" for their cognitive achievements, along with the parents' ability to recognize their readiness for self-care. Box 16–2 provides self-care readiness guidelines for this age.

Box 16–2

ASSESSING SELF-CARE READINESS IN THE SCHOOL-AGE CHILD

Before being left home alone without adult supervision, children should be able to perform all of the following tasks

- Unlock and open and close and lock doors well enough to enter and exit home
- Hold on to keys without losing them
- Keep self and siblings free of bodily injury
- Tell time
- Know how to access help in an emergency
- Prepare a snack or sandwich
- Safely operate necessary household equipment
- Understand and recall spoken and written instructions
- Be able to take phone messages
- Know not to tell visitors or callers that they are home alone
- Be resourceful and flexible to handle the unexpected
- Stay alone without being afraid or lonely

Moral and Spiritual Assessment

Moral development can be seen as an outgrowth of personality, emotional attitudes, and cultural influences. Piaget (1952) maintains that a child cannot make sound moral judgments until cognitively mature enough to look at situations as another might see them. Because this ability to recognize another person's viewpoint emerges during the school-age years, so does moral development. Kohlberg (1984) classifies young school-age children in the preconventional level of moral development. Like preschoolers, school-age children observe rules to obtain rewards or to avoid punishment. After age 9, children enter the conventional level, in which they begin conforming to norms and society's rules.

McClowry (1995) indicates that discipline is still essential during the school-age years to foster proper social skills. However, toward the middle school years, caregivers should accommodate the child's need to develop negotiation and problem-solving skills as well.

Spirituality begins to take on a deeper meaning during this stage. A child can now take part in religious rituals with a keen understanding and be capable of comprehending the permanence of death.

Once assessment data are collected, the other steps of the nursing process—diagnosis, planning, intervention, and evaluation—can be employed.

Nursing Diagnosis

Some of the most common nursing diagnoses for school-age children are listed in the previous Nursing Diagnosis Box.

Planning

The outcome criteria for these common nursing diagnoses would include

Parents will verbalize and demonstrate understanding of their role in the maintenance of health and wellness in their school-age child

The school-age child will exhibit age-appropriate physical growth and psychosocial, cognitive, moral, and spiritual development

The school-age child will remain free from injury

Parents will verbalize understanding of ways to keep their school-age child safe

Intervention
Health Maintenance Visits

Instruct parents to keep regularly scheduled health promotion appointments for their school-age child at 6, 8, 10, and 12 years

Respect privacy during interviews and physical examinations

Nutrition

Assess child's nutritional status and correlate with serial measurements on the anthropometric charts

Seek appropriate counseling for overweight children

Provide a variety of nutritious foods to allow child to develop good eating habits

Encourage parents to allow child to assist with meal preparation and to have family interaction during mealtime

Instruct parents not to overcontrol food intake; allowing self-regulation helps child to stay in touch with his or her natural hunger cues

Discourage excessive intake of junk foods and empty calories, especially prior to vigorous exercise

Dentition

Assess for expected pattern of tooth eruption

Inspect mouth for evidence of dental and gum disease

Assess ability to perform good oral hygiene while explaining the relationship of plaque to dental and gum disease

Encourage parents to maintain dental visits every 6 months

Sleep and Activity

Assess sleeping patterns at each health care visit

Encourage continuance of schoolwork, hobbies, and other interests

Explore strategies if needed to balance school, peer, and family activities (children at this age often enjoy group games, board games, arts and crafts, video and computer games, and reading)

Immunizations

Assess immunization status at each health care visit

Administer immunizations according to the schedule in Table 16–6

Determine if MMR and any other boosters are needed and if hepatitis and/or varicella zoster virus vaccines are indicated

Review expected local and systemic reactions for each immunization given and advice on when to call the health care provider in the event of an untoward reaction

Injury Prevention

Assess parents' knowledge base regarding injury prevention and related safety issues

Implement and teach parents and children the school-age child safety guidelines provided in Table 16–3

Advise parents regarding how to seek help in an emergency

Teach parents cardiopulmonary resuscitation or suggest how they can receive training

Anticipatory Guidance

Assess knowledge level regarding common school-age child health concerns and provide information to dispel any myths (see Table 16–10)

Evaluation

Parents keep all scheduled health maintenance visits

Parents verbalize that age-appropriate dietary, sleep, activity, social, and emotional needs are being met

Child thrives according to expected growth and developmental milestones

Child demonstrates ability to interact appropriately with peers and parents and other adults

Child remains free from injury

Nursing Process for Adolescents (13–19 Years)

Assessment

The nature of adolescent assessment encompasses important dimensions—especially those surrounding puberty. Rapid skeletal changes, sexual maturation, and emotional development occur early in adolescence. Hormones secreted by the endocrine glands (testosterone in boys and estrogen in girls) contribute to dramatic physical and emotional changes. Although the obvious changes are quite dramatic, they do not

Table **16–10**

ANTICIPATORY GUIDANCE IN SCHOOL-AGE CHILDREN

ISSUE	RATIONALE	GUIDANCE
School anxiety or phobia	Adjusting to grade school is a significant change for a 6-year-old, even if preschool was attended; no longer is the focus play, the sessions are full days, and the expectations are high Major tasks occur in first and second grade as children learn to read and write and have to meet the teachers expectations Competing with schoolmates for the teacher's attention and approval can cause strain and anxiety Children sometimes resist attending school by becoming physically sick—abdominal pain or complaints of headache last until the child is allowed to stay home for the day	Encourage parents to communicate with the child's teacher on a regular basis to stay well informed on progress and to help identify problems early on Have parents spend time each evening reviewing the child's day and homework assignments and provide guidance and security when indicated Inform parents that school adjustments take place not only in first grade but every time there is a change in grade, teacher, classmates, and when other stressful events are happening around the child If continuous anxiety or other school difficulties persist, suggest that the parent have the child evaluated by a health care provider or refer for counseling
Dental problems	As primary teeth shed and secondary teeth erupt, the child is at risk for malocclusion, a condition where the upper and lower teeth malalign, predisposing the child to permanent jaw and dental problems Dental caries are a significant health problem in all age groups; however because school-age children are relied on to independently perform all self-care activities, dental hygiene measures often are neglected Tooth evulsion, or loss due to trauma, occurs commonly in this active age group because children participate in more risky and challenging physical activities than when they were younger, such as contact sports and rollerblading	Orthodontic referrals for braces are usually made during early adolescence after all of the primary teeth are shed; however, in the case of malocclusion, prompt referral should be made as soon as the problem is evident Stress to parents the importance of dental checkups every 6 months and daily oral hygiene measures to prevent formation of dental caries In addition to brushing and using fluoride supplements, school-age children should floss their teeth on a regular basis; nurses can provide instruction and reinforce teaching in this area Instruct parents and children about what to do if a permanent tooth is traumatically knocked out; tell them to hold the tooth by the crown and avoid touching the root; if dirty, rinse under running water, then insert the root end into the socket and seek medical care immediately Always stress the importance of wearing protective gear, including mouth shields, when playing contact sports and other physical activities to minimize injuries

become full blown overnight, and each child's progress through puberty and adolescence is different. In addition to obtaining general assessment parameters, the nurse's role in adolescent health assessment encompasses those aspects of development that pose the greatest risk for this vulnerable population. Motor vehicle injuries, homicide and violent crimes, self-esteem, sexuality, and nutrition issues are paramount for this age group. Although yearly visits are stressed, minimally, the adolescent should be screened at ages 13, 15, and 17. An assessment should be done without

the parent in attendance, but then parents should be interviewed as well, either with or without the teen present. Confidentiality becomes an important factor in the adolescent-nurse relationship.

Physiological Assessment

The physical changes of adolescence signal the end of childhood. A period of rapid growth in height and weight (commonly referred to as the growth spurt) is second only to growth during infancy.

Table 16–10

ANTICIPATORY GUIDANCE IN SCHOOL-AGE CHILDREN
(Continued)

ISSUE	RATIONALE	GUIDANCE
Sleeptalking or sleepwalking	Approximately one in every six children experiences an episode of sleepwalking during the school-age years, with few who walk persistently Sleepwalking and talking occur during the first 1–2 h after onset of sleep and are associated with neurological immaturity or anxiety-provoking daytime experiences Almost all children outgrow this behavior and do not develop persistent sleeping problems	Inform parents of the self-limiting nature of this problem and have them focus on maintaining safety for the child who wanders from bed at night by keeping doors securely locked Guiding the sleepwalking child back to bed before ready may result in the child getting up again during the night; remain with the child until he or she returns to bed or awakens from the trance If these behaviors suddenly develop in the child, have parents try to identify a possible stressor or exciting event that the child recently experienced as the potential cause of the sleep problem Instruct parents to prevent their children from watching action-packed television or videos prior to sleep and to encourage more sedentary activities like reading or playing a card game instead
Sex education	Ideally, the preteen years are the time when parents need to be available to answer their child's questions regarding sex Many parents are extremely uncomfortable discussing sex with their children because they are ignorant about the topic themselves As they enter puberty, older school-age children have many questions about sex and often have no place to get answers; they turn to misinformed peers for information Nurses are in a good position to educate parents and children about sexuality but only after examining their own beliefs and attitudes about such issues	Introduce the subject of sex education to parents of preteens and assess their knowledge and comfort level with the topic Ask parents if they are willing to introduce the topic of sex to their children, and if not, would they allow you to Approach the topic initially from a physiological perspective, informing them about the outward changes that will occur as they go through puberty; then advance to more social and emotional issues when they are ready A matter-of-fact tone should be used when presenting information to children so they can observe the lack of spirited emotion attached to the subject Reinforce to them that no person has a right to touch them in places that make them feel uncomfortable

Changes in body proportions and the attainment of sexual and physical maturity occur (see Fig. 16–7).

Respiration and Circulation

Obtain pulse, respiration, and blood pressure measurements at each visit. The lungs of an adolescent triple in weight during this period, increasing their capacity to breathe more deeply and slowly. Their respiratory rate averages 16 to 18 breaths per minute. The heart doubles in size, and the total volume of blood increases, allowing the heart to beat efficiently at a rate of 82 bpm at rest. Blood pressure remains stable at 120/80. An adult-sized blood pressure cuff is generally used for measurement.

Weight and Height

Obtain height and weight measurements and continue to record them on the anthropometric charts and compare them with previous serial measurements. During early adolescence, children have a noticeable increase in appetite, which contributes to the typical 38-lb (17-kg) weight gain in girls and 42-lb (19-kg) weight gain in boys between the ages of 10 and 14. This weight gain is generally through the accumulation of fat in girls, especially on their legs and hips, and in boys by their becoming more muscular overall. Soon after the onset of weight gain, adolescent height increases are noticeable, approximately 9.5 in (24 cm) for girls and 10 in (25 cm) for boys. There is an orderly progression of skeletal growth from distal to proximal, beginning with growth of the feet. The upper extremities follow a similar pattern. This results in disproportionately large hands and feet, contributing to an adolescent's apparent clumsiness. Assess for idiopathic scoliosis, a common spinal deformity that becomes noticeable during the preadolescent growth spurt.

Puberty

Assess pubertal development and primary and secondary sexual characteristics at each health visit. Puberty begins when the pituitary gland sends a message to the sex glands to begin hormone secretion, resulting in mature sex organs that are capable of reproduction. This process generally takes about 4 years, beginning about 2 years earlier for girls (10.5 years of age) than for boys (12.5 years of age). The precise time at which this event occurs appears to be regulated by multiple factors, including genes, individual health, and the environment.

Primary sex characteristics are those associated di-

rectly with reproduction. In girls, the specific event taken to indicate fertility is **menarche,** or the onset of menstruation, which occurs at a mean age of 12.5 years in the United States. Primary sex characteristics are present when the ovaries discharge eggs, the uterus enlarges, and the vaginal wall thickens in girls (Fig. 16–10). However, menstruation is not the first noticeable pubertal change in girls. Secondary sex characteristics begin first, including breast development. A boy is considered fertile as soon as viable sperm are present. **Spermarche,** or the first ejaculation of seminal fluid containing sperm, often occurs through masturbation or may occur during sleep in a nocturnal emission (a "wet dream") or during sexual intercourse. The timing of the appearance of sperm is highly variable, occurring generally around 13.5 years of age. Enlargement of the testes, seminal vesicles, and prostate gland represents development of primary sex characteristics in boys. Secondary sex characteristics, which develop during this period, include the broadening of the shoulders and the development of body hair, including facial, pubic, and axillary growth. Voice changes occur in both sexes but more promi-

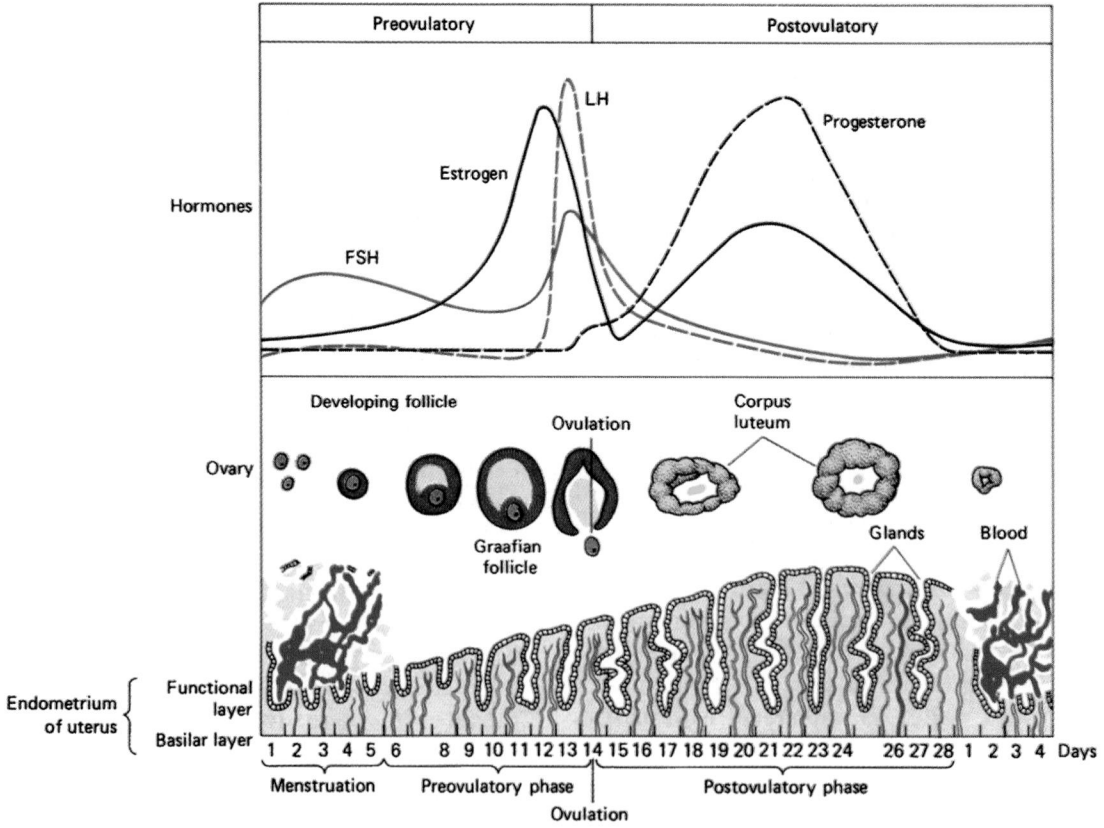

❧ **Figure 16–10**
Hormonal and vaginal changes of the menstrual cycle. (Solomon, E. P., & Phillips, G. A. [1987]. *Understanding human anatomy and physiology* [p 338]. Philadelphia: W. B. Saunders.)

nently in boys. Hormonal changes during this period also cause the oil, sweat, and odor glands of the skin to become much more active. Approximately 85% of all adolescents suffer from acne to some degree because of these changes. Body odor and oilier hair also result from these active glands. See the female-male comparison chart in Table 16–11.

Nutrition

Rapid body changes in puberty require additional nutrients for proper growth and development. Obtaining specific nutrients tends to be more of a problem than obtaining food to eat. Studies show that although typical adolescents skip breakfast, they do consume four or more calorie-laden meals per day. Iron is the most deficient nutrient in adolescents, especially in menstruating girls between 15 and 17 years of age (Baynes & Bothwell, 1990).

Although many adolescents are generally well nourished, some experience periods of overeating and undereating, causing nutritional imbalance. Adolescents are particularly vulnerable to fad foods and diet crazes and are at risk for developing serious eating disorders, including obesity, anorexia nervosa, and bulimia.

In addition to a full nutritional and dietary history, assessing an adolescent for obesity (the most common eating disorder of this period) includes weight, height, and skinfold measurements. No matter what the related cause, obese adolescents can lose weight. When providing counseling, it is important to consider family preferences and economic factors, which can greatly affect the success of a modification program.

With 17 being the average age of onset for **anorexia nervosa,** assessing for this condition is relevant during health visits. Anorexia nervosa is a state of self-imposed starvation seen mostly in white females. Eval-

uate adolescents for this condition who weigh less than 85% of normal for height and weight and who have a distorted view of themselves. Individuals with **bulimia** are also obsessed with their weight and body shape. Occurring again primarily in females, bulimia differs from anorexia nervosa in that adolescents diet for a period and then when extremely famished overeat compulsively, for example binging on a whole box of cookies or a half-gallon of ice cream. Either stomach pain or self-loathing then leads to an episode of purging by self-induced vomiting or excessive use of laxatives. Assessment is more difficult for this condition because individuals may be of normal weight, underweight, or overweight. A nurse should assess the condition of teeth, skin, and hair because regurgitated stomach acids cause extensive tooth decay, nutritional deficiencies, skin problems, and hair loss.

Dentition

Adolescents erupt their second molars at about 13 years and their third molars between 18 and 21 years of age. Dental health is often neglected by adolescents. Dental caries occur in 95% of the teen population. Therefore, perform a careful oral inspection at each health care visit. Observe for upper and lower teeth contact as well. This is the time when orthodontal referrals are made for brace application.

Sleep and Activity

Balancing rest and activity during adolescence poses a great challenge to the youth of America. In addition to school and social activities, many of today's youth hold part-time jobs—not only in summer but also during the school year. Their youthful energy, mature muscle coordination, and well-developed faculties allows their stamina to excel. Nonetheless, 8 to

	Table 16–11

SEQUENTIAL PUBERTAL PHYSIOLOGICAL CHANGES IN ADOLESCENCE

GIRLS	AGE OF FIRST APPEARANCE, y	BOYS
Growth of breasts	8–13	
Growth of pubic hair	8–14	
Body growth	9.5–14.5	
Menarche	10–16	
	10.0–13.5	Growth of testes, scrotal sac
	10–15	Growth of pubic hair
	10.5–16.0	Body growth
	11.0–14.5	Growth of penis, prostate gland, and seminal vesicles; change in voice
	One year after beginning growth of penis	Spermarche
Underarm hair	Two years after appearance of pubic hair	Facial and underarm hair
Increased oil and sweat production		Increased oil and sweat production

9 hours of sleep per night is required. Nurses should ask at what time they retire and awaken each day to determine if enough rest is being obtained. With the roots of inactivity starting in childhood, it is also important for nurses to determine if adolescents are participating in at least 20 minutes of vigorous exercise at least three times each week. Sedentary lifestyles add to health problems seen later in life.

Immunizations

Immunization records should be reviewed during each health care visit to ensure proper coverage, which will continue into adulthood. Between 14 and 16 years of age, tetanus and diphtheria boosters are indicated. Assessing whether an adolescent ever had chickenpox could indicate the need for the newly approved varicella-zoster virus vaccine. Because contracting the varicella virus in adulthood can be life threatening, a series of two shots should be given if administered after the age of 13.

Psychosocial Assessment

Individual responses are quite evident as adolescents meet the challenges of psychosocial adaptation. Family, peers, the school system, the community, and society at large all take their toll on the emerging identity of the adolescent.

Alterations in the family structure resulting in an increase in the divorce rate, single-parent families, and dual-parent employment foster a greater amount of unsupervised time for adolescents, thus increasing their time alone with peers. Some researchers document increases in risk-taking behaviors, such as sexual intercourse and substance abuse, in addition to socialization with deviant peers, during these times (Patterson & Stouthamer-Loeber, 1984). During adolescence, conformity to peer pressure and socialization is very evident. Pressure to go along with the crowd or participate in clique behavior exerts powerful control over the lives of adolescents. Cliques are intimate groups with same-sex members. When cliques get together with other cliques of the opposite sex, a crowd is formed. This somewhat less personal group has much influence on the adolescent.

Early adolescence is a period of sexual self-exploration. According to Freud (1946), this behavior corresponds to the genital stage of psychosexual development, beginning at puberty and continuing until old age. The genital organs become the major source of pleasure. Dating becomes of major importance, with the majority of adolescents having their first date between the ages of 12 and 16. Of some concern is "going steady" at an early age. Problems at home or school and adolescent pregnancy have been linked to this behavior.

The many challenges that a youth must face (*e.g.,* sexual and peer relationships, schooling, and the be-

ginning of long-term decisions concerning the future) begin to shape the true identity of the adolescent. Unfortunately, they bring with them a period of conflict and contradictions. Adolescents who conceive an ideal self-image often fall short of this reality and reach a low point around the age of 13. Self-esteem begins to slowly improve if Erikson's (1963) task of identity versus role confusion is achieved. Adolescents struggle to establish themselves as separate individuals while maintaining some connection with meaningful past experiences and accepting values of a peer group. This is a heavy plate for a young individual to carry. Issues of self-esteem are important to assess in an adolescent, not only to identify stressors but also to determine coping abilities. Adolescents are often considered "moody" and they are said to complain often. Areas to explore with teens include peer relationships and involvement in group activities. Question any concerns they express about body image and being different, such as concerns about acne, fatness, shortness, or delayed puberty. Discuss school adjustment, academic achievement, and future goals. Observe relationships between teens and parents. With suicide being the third leading cause of death in this age group,

---

Box **16–3**

DISTINGUISHING BETWEEN DEPRESSED MOOD AND MAJOR DEPRESSIVE DISORDER IN ADOLESCENTS

Depressed moods are characterized by periods of unhappiness or sadness lasting for a brief or extended period. These episodes often result from failure of the adolescent at an important task or the loss of a significant relationship. Major depressive disorder, on the other hand, is present in youths who experience at least five of the following nine symptoms for at least 2 weeks:

1. Depressed mood or irritability most of the day
2. Reduced interest in pleasurable activities
3. Changes in weight or inability to reach age-appropriate weight norms
4. Sleep-related problems
5. Fatigue or reduced energy levels
6. Decreased ability to concentrate and make decisions
7. Psychomotor agitation or retardation
8. Increased amounts of guilt and worthlessness feelings
9. Repeated episodes of suicidal ideation verbalizing plans or actual suicide attempts

---

Adapted from Petersen, A. C., Compas, B. E., Brooks-Gunn, J., Semmler, M., Ey, S., & Grant, K. E. (1993). Depression in adolescents. *American Psychologist, 48,* 155–168. Copyright ©1993 by the American Psychological Association. Adapted with permission.

assessing the teen for signs of depression becomes paramount. Box 16–3 can help a nurse identify those at high risk.

Cognitive Assessment

The transition to junior high or high school is a crucial element in adolescence, not only from a psychosocial point of view but also from a cognitive one. Teens have the opportunity to get together with old friends, meet new friends, and participate in sports. They also acquire new knowledge, sharpen old skills and master new ones, and begin to examine career choices. Piaget (1952) delineates this behavior as the period of formal operations. Adolescents develop the capacity for abstract thought. For example, they can conceptualize things that do not physically exist. Testing hypotheses and entertaining various solutions to a problem and having a future-minded orientation become commonplace toward the end of adolescence. Nonetheless, Piaget notes that although idealistically they have the capacity to delay immediate gratification for future gain, adolescents often become frustrated with the world.

Schooling can make a decided difference in academic achievement, self-image, and future success of adolescents. Often, poor student achievement is blamed on the family, minority background, socioeconomic status, or genetic factors. However, recent studies controlling for these factors demonstrate that certain schools educate their students much more effectively than others. A central characteristic of these successful schools is that they have clear, high, attainable goals and support from the entire school staff (Page & Valli, 1990). Nonetheless, schools cannot sustain intellectual growth without help from home. Parents' indifference to their adolescents' school performance can have a tremendous negative long-term consequence regarding future schooling and career selection. Although dropout rates continue to decline in the United States for whites (8.9%) and African-Americans (13.6%), Hispanics continue to leave high school before graduating at an alarming rate of 35.3% (US Department of Education, 1992). Socioeconomic status and language seem to be critical factors.

Moral and Spiritual Assessment

Moral and spiritual development serves to mold one's identity and value system. Adolescents are capable of moral reasoning only if they can think abstractly and conceive of universal moral principles. The third and highest level of Kohlberg's (1984) level of moral reasoning, postconventional reasoning, rarely begins prior to age 13 and is generally never fully achieved. This level marks attainment of true morality, when for the first time an individual acknowledges the possibility of conflict between two socially accepted standards and tries to decide between them. This is evident during adolescence as teens constantly challenge the norms of society. Spirituality in adolescence also evolves at an abstract level. Adolescents in contemporary America are less focused on the tangible concept of organized religion than on the conceptual nature of a religious commitment (Steinberg, 1989). This may lead to another area of family tension, as adolescents may temporarily or permanently question or abandon traditional religious practices.

High-Risk Behavior Assessment

Assessing high-risk behavior in adolescence is challenging. Knowing the facts can assist nurses in meeting that challenge. Many significant changes over the past decade have an impact on a recent finding that adolescents' mortality rate has dropped 13%. A dramatic reduction in unintentional injury–related deaths influenced these data. However, although a dramatic positive change has been seen in one area, a negative trend has been observed in the area of interpersonal violence (Sells & Blum, 1996).

Motor Vehicle Fatalities

Motor vehicle death rates for adolescents decreased significantly between 1979 and 1992. Experts contribute this outcome to the enactment of passive restraint laws, reduced speed limits, increasing the national legal drinking age to 21, and safer automobiles (Sells & Blum, 1996). Despite this improvement, most fatal crashes involve alcohol-impaired youths between the ages of 16 and 20, with males accounting for three fourths of these deaths. During a health assessment visit, obtain information regarding adolescents' understanding of motor vehicle injury preventative measures. Determine if they drive and if they have participated in driver's education programs at school. Discuss issues regarding alcohol and drug use by targeting their critical judgment skills. This determines readiness to respond to risk reduction education.

Homicide and Violent Crimes

Approximately 40,000 adolescents between the ages of 15 and 19 died as a result of firearm injuries between 1979 and 1991, with 60% reported as homicides. One contributing factor is the easy availability of lethal weapons that are kept unlocked and often loaded in nearly half of all US homes (Sells & Blum, 1996). Assessing an adolescent's involvement in or knowledge and fears of firearm or other violent activities assists you in providing necessary protection, guidance, and intervention. Question teens and parents regarding the availability of unlocked firearms in the home, and develop educational strategies for each to become responsible adults.

Sexuality Issues

Unfortunately for many adolescents, especially younger ones, their bodies are more ready for sex than their minds. Therefore, the extent of assessment in the area of sexuality at a particular visit generally depends on the adolescent's maturity, stage of development, and experiences with sexual activities.

With teenage pregnancy and the high occurrence of sexually transmitted diseases (STDs) as major problems among adolescents, health assessment becomes paramount in developing a successful care plan. The adolescent pregnancy rate in the United States is the highest of any in the developed world and is an explosive social issue as policy-makers struggle over abortion rights, contraceptives, and sex education in the schools. According to the Centers for Disease Control (1992), the highest rates of the most common STDs—gonorrhea, syphilis, chlamydia, and herpes—occur in 10- to 19-year-old individuals who are sexually active. Even though most cases are not serious if promptly treated, many young people delay medical care and place themselves at risk for life-threatening complications and sterility. In addition, acquired immunodeficiency syndrome and human immunodeficiency virus (HIV) infection rates are rising rapidly among youths of high school and college age because of their high-risk sexual behavior. Question teens regarding relationships with sexual partners and establish their understanding of reproductive anatomy and physiology and STD transmission. Determine the immediacy of need for contraception and information regarding protection from STDs. Actual testing for STDs or pregnancy may need to be performed at this health visit. Papanicolaou smears for detection of cervical cancer should be performed yearly in sexually active girls. Discuss with the adolescent an approach to be taken with parents regarding the information disclosed during your interview. Confidentiality issues and the law vary from state to state. You should be familiar with local laws in your area.

Substance Use and Abuse

Although substance use among adolescents is less today than it was in the 1960s, 1970s, and 1980s, the trend appears to be cyclic and may be on an upswing as we enter the next millennium. Most young people use alcohol, tobacco, and marijuana because it seems like the "grown-up" thing to do, especially because both cigarettes and alcohol are freely available to adults in the United States and therefore also to many young people. Ask adolescents in a nonjudgmental manner what drugs they use, and you will probably get an honest answer. Armed with this knowledge, you can provide appropriate guidance and counseling. Successful outcomes can only be met through careful and realistic planning.

When assessment data have been obtained, the nurse may proceed to the other steps in the nursing process.

> ### NURSING DIAGNOSES FOR ADOLESCENTS
>
> Health Seeking Behaviors (Parental) related to lack of knowledge regarding health promotion
>
> Health Seeking Behaviors (Adolescent) related to lack of knowledge regarding health promotion
>
> Risk for Growth and Development, Altered, related to perceived loss of independence and autonomy
>
> Risk for Injury related to high-risk behavior

Nursing Diagnosis

Some of the most common diagnoses for adolescents are listed in the Nursing Diagnosis Box.

Planning

The outcome criteria for some of these common nursing diagnoses would include

Parents will demonstrate understanding of their role in the maintenance of health and wellness in their adolescent

Adolescent will demonstrate understanding of his or her role in the maintenance of personal health and wellness

Adolescent will exhibit age-appropriate physical growth and psychosocial, cognitive, moral, and spiritual development

Adolescent will remain free from injury

Adolescent will verbalize understanding of personal consequences resulting from engaging in high-risk behaviors (see Nursing Care Plan for the Adolescent)

Interventions
Health Maintenance Visits

Instruct parents and adolescent to seek health care appointments yearly or minimally at 13, 15, and 17 years of age

Respect privacy during interviews and physical examinations

Nutrition

Assess adolescent's nutritional status and correlate with serial measurements on the anthropometric charts

Seek appropriate counseling for underweight or overweight teens

Encourage a diet with a variety of foods in portions that allow for adolescent satiety

SAMPLE NURSING CARE PLAN

NURSING CARE PLAN
FOR THE ADOLESCENT

T. L. is a 14-year-old girl who comes to the school-based clinic requesting birth control pills. She tells the nurse that she has been having unprotected sex with her boyfriend, who is 17 years old, for about a month. She is concerned that if she becomes pregnant, her parents may find out about her having a steady boyfriend.

Nursing Diagnosis:	Health Maintenance, Altered, related to insufficient knowledge of sex-related consequences, as evidenced by engaging in high-risk behavior, choice of birth control method being sought, and reason for seeking pregnancy protection.
Expected Outcomes:	T. L. will not experience an unplanned pregnancy or acquire an STD.
	If sexual activity is continued, T. L. will select and report use of a contraceptive method that reduces the risk of acquiring HIV and other STDs.
	T. L. will report an increase in communication activities with her parents regarding sexuality issues.

Actions	Rationale
1. Establish a trusting relationship with T. L. by being nonjudgmental in your approach and by informing her that her discussion with you will be kept confidential. Do not judge the adolescent by your own beliefs and practices.	1. If adolescents perceive health care personnel as warm, unembarrassed, objective, and reassuring, they will be trusting and honest. Being perceptive of your own beliefs and practices allows a nurse to reduce personal biases when addressing controversial issues.
2. Assess T. L.'s knowledge and attitudes regarding sexuality issues and reproduction. Speak in age-appropriate or slang terms if necessary to convery meaning Ask questions related to Attitudes toward sex, nudity, touching Whether these issues were discussed at home How pregnancy occurs Various methods of birth control How STDs occur	2. Determining how an adolescent views sexuality can help the nurse uncover knowledge deficits, clarify common misconceptions, and help provide accurate information that encourages health-promoting behaviors. Knowing if sexuality issues are discussed in the home setting can help identify an altered parenting issue.
3. Ask T. L. if she wants to have sex with her boyfriend or is she just doing it because she feels trapped into engaging in sex to maintain their friendship. Counsel T. L. to understand that having sex is her choice. Inform her that both partners in a sexual relationship should derive pleasure.	3. Being honest and direct with adolescents will often elicit a truthful response. They will generally admit to engaging in high-risk behavior because of peer pressure. Adolescents need to know that the sign of an adult sexual relationship is that the activity is pleasurable to both partners. Therefore, if the activity is not enjoyable or if one sexual partner is not interested in the other's response, then the relationship should be reconsidered.
Role play with T. L. to help her improve her perspective and to learn how to say no.	Role playing can help the adolescent gain confidence in discussing abstinence, birth control, and STD issues with parents and/or sexual partner.
4. Determine what type of sexual behavior T. L. has engaged in with this partner and any other previous partners. Inform her that she may already be pregnant or have an STD based on self-report of having "unprotected sex." Suggest that T. L. be tested at this time.	4. Providing a gynecological examination, with pregnancy and STD testing to individuals who are sexually active is an important aspect of health promotion.

Nursing Care Plan continued on following page

SAMPLE NURSING CARE PLAN

NURSING CARE PLAN
FOR THE ADOLESCENT
(Continued)

Actions	Rationale
5. Provide T. L. with guidelines for practicing safer sex with relation to pregnancy and STD prevention. Inform her that oral contraceptives will not protect her against human immunodeficiency virus (HIV) infection or other STDs. Have T. L. practice applying condoms on a plastic model.	**5.** Providing information about barrier devices (condoms) in addition to other contraceptive devices will allow the adolescent to make informed choices about protection from pregnancy and disease. An adolescent can ease embarrassment and develop skill in applying condoms on her partner if the technique is practiced routinely in a low-stress environment.
6. Encourage T. L. to speak to her parents about her boyfriend and sex-related issues. Inform her that you are willing to arrange a meeting with them to help facilitate discussion on these issues.	**6.** Open communication can bridge the generational gap between adolescents and parents. Sometimes parents themselves have outdated and inaccurate information about sexuality issues that may have to be clarified.

Instruct parents not to overcontrol the adolescent's dietary choices; allowing self-regulation encourages staying in touch with the teen's natural hunger cues

Discourage excessive amounts of junk foods and empty calories—especially before vigorous exercise

Dentition

Inspect mouth for evidence of dental and gum disease

Assess ability to perform good oral hygiene and explain the relationship of plaque to dental and gum disease

Continue to encourage dental visits every 6 months

Sleep and Activity

Assess sleeping patterns at each health care visit

Encourage continuance of schoolwork, hobbies, and other interests

Explore strategies, if needed, to balance school, peer, family, and work responsibilities

Immunizations

Assess immunization status at each health care visit

Determine if any boosters are needed and if hepatitis and/or varicella zoster virus vaccines are indicated

Review expected local and systemic reactions for each immunization given and advise on when to call the health care provider in the event of an untoward reaction

Injury Prevention

Assess adolescent's and parents' knowledge base regarding injury prevention and related safety issues

Assess adolescent's involvement with high-risk behaviors, such as drug, alcohol, and tobacco use; gang- or violence-related activities; and unsafe sexual practices

Seek appropriate referrals or counseling as needed

Implement and teach age-appropriate safety guidelines provided in Table 16–3

Advise adolescent regarding how to seek help in an emergency

Teach adolescent and parents cardiopulmonary resuscitation or suggest how they can receive training

Sexuality Issues

Assess adolescent's knowledge base regarding sexual activity and transmission of STDs

Provide concrete information about sexuality, function, bodily changes, and STD and pregnancy prevention

Anticipatory Guidance

Assess knowledge level regarding common adolescent health concerns and provide anticipatory guidance and information to correct misconceptions (Table 16–12)

Evaluation

Adolescent keeps all scheduled health maintenance visits

Adolescent verbalizes that age-appropriate dietary, sleep, activity, social, and emotional needs are being met

Adolescent thrives according to expected growth and developmental milestones

Adolescent demonstrates ability to interact appropriately with peers and parents

Adolescent remains free from emotional distress and physical injury

Table **16–12**

ANTICIPATORY GUIDANCE FOR THE ADOLESCENT

ISSUE	RATIONALE	GUIDANCE
Self-esteem and depression	Risk-taking behaviors and suicide are correlated with low self-esteem and body image Adolescents are often too shy or embarrassed to discuss self-esteem issues and hope that the health care provider will introduce the topic for discussion Stress, sadness, and low self-esteem are frequently related to family conflicts, strained peer relationships, school difficulties, and work-related problems Approximately 5000 adolescents commit suicide each year, with nearly 200 attempts for every death	Use a direct approach to discuss sensitive issues with adolescents, such as peer pressure, body image, dating, sexuality, and substance abuse—encourage parents to do the same Teach parents to be "good listeners," by paying attention to their adolescent's interests, likes, dislikes, and feelings without passing judgment Have parents ask for their adolescent's opinion and allow their input into decisions Teach parents that normal behavior for an adolescent includes belonging to a peer group and a desire to be like the rest of the group yet be dissimilar from adults (including wearing unconventional clothing, hairstyles, and jewelry) Encourage parents to foster independence without abandoning discipline, fair household rules, and consistency in their approach Encourage parents to respect privacy Counsel parents in methods to distinguish between normal adolescent depressive moods and true depression (see Box 16–2)
Sexuality	Adolescents have one of the highest rates of STDs, especially chlamydial infection and syphilis. There is also an alarming increase in the rate of HIV in this age group Approximately 1 million pregnancies occur annually in the United States among women 19 years of age and younger, with 20% occurring within 1 month of first intercourse and 50% within the first 6 months	Use general questions regarding pubertal changes to lead into more detailed inquiry regarding specific sexual behaviors or concerns Assist the adolescent to develop strategies for saying "no" to partners who may be pressuring them into having sex Discuss responsible sexual behavior and inform the adolescent who talks about becoming sexually active about contraception and preventing STDs, including HIV infection Provide a pregnant adolescent with information about options prenatal care, and make appropriate referrals Teach parents to become familiar with their adolescent's friends and to be proactive in addressing sexual issues before problems arise
Nutrition	Iron deficiency anemia is the major nutritional deficit in American adolescents, especially in girls, related to poor nutritional intake, rapid growth, and menstrual blood loss Although the average adolescent girl needs about 2200 calories per day and the male, 2800 calories per day, they may put on weight, and some—especially girls—react by focusing on a lifelong struggle to reduce Although anorexia nervosa and bulimia are generally seen in adolescent females, males are also affected and should be screened during health visits	Review with parents the need to observe teens for early signs of nutritional deficiencies and eating disorders, including food binging, obsessing over weight, inactivity or overexercising, and excessive intake of empty calorie or fast foods Review with teens their food likes and dislikes and build dietary recommendations on the preferences that are healthy choices (everyone has a few) Be sensitive to adolescents' need to include some fast food or nonnutritious choices in the diet occasionally Assist teens to develop a healthy body image by offering positive comments about their appearance, including their weight, hairstyle, or makeup application Make appropriate referrals if you suspect or see evidence of eating disorders, including obesity

Table continued on following page

Table **16–12**

ANTICIPATORY GUIDANCE FOR THE ADOLESCENT
(Continued)

ISSUE	RATIONALE	GUIDANCE
Substance use and abuse	More than 90% of high school seniors have used alcohol, nearly 50% have smoked marijuana, and 20% are regular cigarette smokers. Although few teens suffer from hypertension, heart disease, chronic lung disease and cancer, continued use of these substances put them at risk in adult life. In addition, use of mind-altering substances puts them and others at immediate risk for disability or death due to injury Early identification and intervention is crucial to success in preventing or reducing adolescent dependency problems	Early educational drug abuse programs and individual counseling programs for teens should be available in all high schools Assist the adolescent to develop strategies for saying "no" to peers who may be pressuring them into substance use Use a direct approach to discuss substance use and abuse with teens and encourage parents to do the same Follow anticipatory guidance strategies listed under "Self-esteem and Depression" because these may offset potential problems Provide appropriate referrals to drug and alcohol treatment programs if needed
Unintentional injuries	Injuries are the leading cause of death in adolescents, with an estimated 18,000 related to motor vehicle crashes More than 50% of motorcycle deaths occur in the 15- to 24-year-old age category Of the almost 6000 adolescent homicides annually, many are related to gunshot wounds Many adolescent deaths can be correlated with lack of experience and immature judgment, leading to risk-taking behavior and carelessness	Stress to parents that despite the perils of adolescence, most teens enter adulthood mature, healthy, and responsible Assist the adolescent to develop strategies for saying "no" to peers who may be pressuring them into risk-taking behavior Parents and teens should be instructed in the techniques of CPR Review adolescent prevention guidelines in Table 16–3

✦ Summary

Child health is determined by many factors, including physiological, psychosocial, cognitive, environmental, and a confluence of various other determinants. Nurses can either work with these elements to promote health or ignore them and impede health. Having a thorough understanding of normal growth and development and knowledge of how to apply it using a nursing process approach allows nurses to understand the strengths and vulnerabilities of children at different ages. This adds an important dimension to health assessment, planning, and outcome measurement from infancy through adolescence.

Nurses can orient themselves toward successful health promotion strategies for children by incorporating a developmental and family-centered approach into the nursing process. Parents and caregivers play a pivotal role in the health of children. Because parents are not born with "parenting" skills, nurses can empower them by providing anticipatory guidance and age-appropriate health education strategies for promoting and maintaining their children's health. Pro-

viding children with what they so richly deserve, nurses can meet the changing health paradigms for the next millennium straight on. This chapter enables nurses to do just that.

CHAPTER HIGHLIGHTS
✦

✦ After birth, neonates are vulnerable to their surroundings as circulation patterns and oxygen and carbon dioxide exchange transfer from the umbilical cord to the heart and lungs and because of an immature nervous system

✦ Sleep is the major activity throughout the first few weeks of life

✦ Outcome measures for neonates include maintenance of a patent airway and normal respiratory rate and normal core body temperature

✦ Infants normally double their birth weight by 4 months and triple it by 1 year

✦ Infants' motor development proceeds from reflexive to purposeful movements in a cephalocaudal and proximaldistal direction

✦ Outcome measures for infants include exhibiting age-appropriate physical growth and psychosocial and cognitive development

✦ Nursing interventions for infants are geared toward health promotional activities including nutrition, sleep, activity, immunizations, and injury prevention

✦ Toddlers only gain about 5 to 6 lb (2.5 kg) per year; however, their bodies elongate, and they assume a more upright posture, growing approximately 3 to 5 in (7.5–12.0 cm) per year

✦ Both gross and fine motor abilities develop rapidly during toddlerhood, allowing toddlers to perform such self-care activities as feeding, dressing, and toileting with minimal assistance

✦ During the preschool years, height and weight steadily increase, resulting in an approximate height of 46 in (117 cm) and a weight of 46 lb (21 kg) by age 6 years; generally, boys appear more muscular, have less body fat, and are slightly taller and heavier than girls

✦ Preschoolers are able to run, jump, climb, and skip with greater grace and speed, and greater dexterity allows them to button clothing, pour milk into a cup, and cut along a line with a scissors by the time they reach age 4 years

✦ Preschoolers' relationships with parents and siblings grow and become more complex, and they begin to explore various social roles with other children as they venture into the neighborhood through play groups, day care, and preschool settings

✦ Many feel that preschoolers, because they are egocentric, cannot be taught morals but can be trained to behave

✦ Nursing interventions for toddlers and preschoolers are geared toward teaching parents safety guidelines

✦ Well-nourished school-age children gain approximately 5 lb (2.25 kg), grow 2.5 in (6 cm) during each year, and appear slimmer and more muscular than in previous years

✦ After age 10 years, girls generally begin their growth spurt and suddenly appear taller and heavier than boys of the same age

✦ By 10 to 12 years of age, most children demonstrate complex and intricate motor skills similar to those of the adult

✦ School-age children develop interests in music, collecting things, constructing objects, and participating in team activities

✦ Changes in body proportions and the attainment of sexual maturity develop, beginning about 2 years earlier for girls (10.5 years of age) than for boys (12.5 years of age)

✦ Menarche, or the onset of menstruation, occurs at a mean age of 12.5 years and indicates fertility in adolescent girls

✦ Spermarche, or the first ejaculation of seminal fluid containing sperm, is highly variable, occurring generally around 13.5 years of age in adolescent boys

✦ In addition to obtaining physical assessment parameters, a nurse's role in adolescents' health promotion should include assessing their risk for motor vehicle injuries; homicide and violent crimes; and problems with self-esteem, sexuality, substance use, and nutrition.

Study Questions

1. To stimulate the rooting reflex in a neonate, a nurse should

   a. place the tip of a rubber nipple into the newborn's mouth
   b. turn the newborn's head to the right side
   c. stroke the newborn's cheek with a fingertip
   d. rub the bridge of the newborn's nose in a circular fashion

2. A nurse should expect to assess which of these motor activities in a normal 6-month-old infant?

   a. sits on the floor without support
   b. puts three objects into a container
   c. pulls self to a standing position
   d. grasps objects using thumb and forefinger

3. When providing anticipatory guidance during a health promotion visit, which piece of information should a nurse give to a parent of a 3-year-old child?

   a. "Peer group relationships become an important part of your child's playtime activities"
   b. "Potty training efforts can begin as soon as your child's diaper remains dry for at least 2 hours"
   c. "This is the time when you should encourage your child to begin a stamp collection"
   d. "Your child may experience fearful reactions to the dark, animals, and unfamiliar noises"

4. Which of these behaviors, if observed in a school-age boy, indicates achievement of Erikson's task of industry versus inferiority?

   a. continually stares at his image when passing mirrored store windows
   b. cooperatively participates with other children when playing his favorite board game
   c. repeatedly reads to his parents the same passage from a short-story book
   d. periodically verbalizes to his classmates the details of a special family vacation

5. A nurse can expect which of these pubertal changes to occur first in the young girl?

    a. sweat production increases
    b. menstrual periods begin
    c. underarm hair grows
    d. breast buds form

Critical Thinking Exercises

1. Mrs. M. comes to the health clinic with a 7-year-old child and 9-month-old infant. Based on the developmental stages of the children, what risks would you anticipate to educate Mrs. M. on home safety?

2. Parents come to your clinic complaining of moodiness and withdrawal of their adolescent son. Discuss the counseling you would give the parents.

References

Aslin, R. N., & Pisoni, D. B. (1980). Effects of early linguistic experience on speech discrimination by infants: A critique of Eilers, Ganin and Wilson. *Child Development, 51,* 107–112.

Bainbridge, R., & Tsang, R. (1995). Optimal nutrition in low birth weight infants. In F. Lifshitz (Ed.), *Childhood nutrition* (pp. 33–52.) Boca Raton, FL: CRC Press.

Baynes, R. D., & Bothwell, T. H. (1990). Iron deficiency. *Annual Review of Nutrition, 10,* 133.

Brazelton, T. B. (1973). *Neonatal behavioral assessment scale.* Philadelphia: J. B. Lippincott.

Centers for Disease Control, Division of STD/HIV Prevention. (1992). *1991 Annual Report.* CDC: Atlanta.

Centers for Disease Control and Prevention. (1995). Recommended childhood immunization schedule—United States. *Morbidity and Mortality Weekly Reports, 44,* (RR-5), 2.

Erikson, E. H. (1963). *Childhood and society.* (2nd ed.). New York: W. W. Norton.

Filer, L. J. (1995). Iron deficiency. In F. Lifshitz (Ed.), *Childhood nutrition* (pp. 53–60.) Boca Raton, FL: CRC Press.

Freud, A. (1946). *The ego and the mechanisms of defense.* New York: International Universities Press.

Gesell, A., & Ilg, F. (1946). *The child from five to ten.* New York: Harper and Row.

Green, M. (Ed.). (1994). *Bright futures: Guidelines for the health supervision of infants, children and adolescents.* Arlington, VA: National Center of Education in Maternal Child Health.

Harter, S., & Pike, R. (1984). The pictorial scale of perceived competence and social acceptance for young children. *Child Development, 55,* 1969–1982.

Illingworth, R. S. (1986). *The development of the infant and young child—normal and abnormal* (9th ed.). New York: Churchill Livingstone.

Johnson, S. L., & Birch, L. L. (1994). Parents' and children's adiposity and eating style. *Pediatrics, 94,* 653–661.

Kantrowitz, B. (1991). The good, the bad and the difference. *Newsweek, Summer* (special edition), 48–50.

Kinsbourne, M. (1994). Sugar and the hyperactive child. *New England Journal of Medicine, 330,* 355–356.

Kohlberg, L. (1984). *The psychology of moral development.* New York: Harper and Row.

Leventhal, E. (1985). Impact of digestion and absorption in the weaning period of infant feeding practices. *Pediatrics, 207* (suppl).

Lifter, K., & Bloom, L. (1989). Object knowledge and the emergence of language. *Infant Behavior and Development, 12,* 395–424.

Lowrey, G. H. (1986). *Growth and development of children* (8th ed.). Chicago: Yearbook Medical Publishers.

Mandler, J. M. (1990). A new perspective on cognitive development in infancy. *American Scientist, 78,* 236–243.

McClowry, S. G. (1995). The influence of temperament on development during middle childhood. *Journal of Pediatric Nursing, 10,* 160–165.

Mehler, J., & Dupoux, E. (1994). *What infants know: The new cognitive science of early development.* Cambridge, MA: Blackwell Publishers.

Nottleman, E. D., Susman, E. J., Blue, J. H., Inoff-Germain, G., Dorn, L. D., Loriaux, D. L., Cutler, G. B., & Chrousos, G. P. (1987). Gonadal and adrenal hormone correlates of adjustment in early adolescence. In R. M. Learner, & T. T. Foch (Eds.), *Biological-psychological interactions in early adolescence.* Hillsdale, NJ: Erlbaum.

Page, R., & Valli, L. (Eds.). (1990). *Curriculum differentiation: Interpretive studies in US secondary schools.* Albany, NY: State University of New York Press.

Patterson, G., & Stouthamer-Loeber, M. (1984). The correlation of family management practice and delinquency. *Child Development, 55,* 1299–1307.

Piaget, J. (1952). *The origins of intelligence in children.* (M. Cook, Trans.) New York: International Universities Press.

Pollitt, E., Consolazio, B., & Goodkin, F. (1991). Changes in nutritive sucking during a feed in two-day- and thirty-day-old infants. *Early Human Development, 5,* 201–210.

Sells, C. W., & Blum, R. W. (1996). Morbidity and mortality among US adolescents: An overview of data and trends. *American Journal of Public Health, 86,* 513–519.

Steinberg, L. (1989). *Adolescence* (2nd ed.). New York: McGraw-Hill.

U.S. Department of Education. (1992). Dropout rates in the U.S., 1991 (Publication No. NCES 19-129). Washington, DC: U.S. Government Printing Office.

U.S. Department of Health and Human Resources. (1992). *Healthy children 2000.* Boston: Jones and Bartlett.

Wolraich, M. L., Lindgrin, S. D., Stumbo, P. J., Stegink, L. D., Appelbaum, M. I., & Kiritsky, M. C. (1994). Effects of diets high in sucrose or aspartame on the behavior and cognitive performance of children. *New England Journal of Medicine, 330,* 301–307.

Zell, E. R., Dietz, V., Stevenson, J., Cochi, S., & Bruce, R. H. (1994). Low vaccination levels of U.S. preschool and school-age children. *Journal of the American Medical Association, 271,* 833–839.

Bibliography

Aslin, R. N., & Pisoni, D. B. (1980). Effects of early linguistic experience on speech discrimination by infants: A critique of Eilers, Ganin and Wilson. *Child Development, 51,* 107–112.

Bantz, D. L., & Siktberg, L. (1993). Teaching families to evaluate age-appropriate toys. *Journal of Pediatric Health Care, 7,* 111–114.

Barness, A. (1991). *Manual of pediatric physical diagnosis* (6th ed.). St. Louis: Mosby-Year Book.

Behrman, R. E. (1992). *Nelson textbook of pediatrics* (14th ed.). Philadelphia: W. B. Saunders.

Christophersen, E. R. (1994). *Pediatric compliance. A guide for the primary care physician*. New York: Plenum Medical Book Company.

Clinton, H. R. (1996). *It takes a village: And other lessons children teach us*. New York: Simon & Schuster.

Collins, C. (1994). Baby walkers: The question of safety. *New York Times, Nov. 10*, p. C2.

Cole, M., & Cole, S. R. (1993). *The development of children* (2nd ed.). New York: Scientific American.

Coplan, J. (1995). Normal speech and language development: An overview. *Pediatrics in Review, 16*, 91–100.

Dickey, S. B. (1987). *A guide to the nursing of children*. Baltimore: Williams & Wilkins.

Dixon, S. D., & Stein, M. T. (1992). *Encounters with children: Pediatric behavior and development* (2nd ed.). St. Louis: Mosby-Year Book.

Fewell, R. R. (1993). Observing play: An appropriate process for learning and assessment. *Infants & Young Children, 5*, 35–43.

Frick, S. B. (1987). Integrating growth and development content into practice: A nursing process framework. *Nursing Education, 12*, 30.

Gallahue, D. L., & Ozmun, J. C. (1989). *Understanding motor development—infants, children, adolescents, adults* (3rd ed.). Madison, WI: Brown & Benchmark.

Gillis, A. J. (1990). Nurses knowledge of growth and development principles in meeting psychosocial needs of hospitalized children. *Journal of Pediatric Nursing, 5*, 78.

Hart, R., Mather, P. L., Slack, J. F., & Powell, M. A. (1992). *Therapeutic play activities for hospitalized children*. St. Louis: Mosby-Year Book.

U.S. Department of Health & Human Resources. *Healthy Children 2000*. Boston: Jones and Bartlett.

Illingworth, R. (1975). *The development of the infant and young child* (6th ed.). London: Churchill Livingstone.

Illingworth, R. (1983). *The development of the infant and young child* (8th ed.). London: Churchill Livingstone.

Leach, P. (1989). *Your baby & child. From birth to age five*. New York: Alfred A Knopf.

Levine, M. D., Carey, W. B., & Crocker, A. C. (1992). *Developmental-behavioral pediatrics* (2nd ed.). Philadelphia: W. B. Saunders.

Lewis, M., & Volkmar, F. (1990). *Clinical aspects of child and adolescent development* (3rd ed.). Philadelphia: Lea & Febiger.

Lifshitz, F. (1995). *Childhood nutrition*. Boca Raton, FL: CRC Press.

Morrison, G. S. (1990). *The world of child development—conception to adolescence*. New York: Delmar Publishers.

Neinstein, L. S. (1991). *Adolescent health care: A practical guide* (2nd ed.). Baltimore: Urban & Schwarzenberg.

Nugent, K. E. (1989). Routine care: Promoting development in hospitalized infants. *MCN; American Journal of Maternal Child Nursing 14*, 318.

Ogasawara, T., *et al*. (1993). Readiness for toothbrushing of young children. *Journal of Pediatric Nursing: Nursing Care of Children and Families, 8*, 200.

Oski, F. A. (1993). Infant nutrition, physical growth, breast feeding, and general nutrition. *Current Opinion in Pediatrics, 5*, 385–388.

Palfrey, J. S. (1994). *Community child health. An action plan for today*. Westport, CT: Praeger.

Petersen, A. C., Compas, B. E., Brooks-Gunn, J., Semmler, M., Ey, S., & Grant, K. E. (1993). Depression in adolescents. *American Psychologist, 48*, 155–168.

Pollak, M. (1993). *Textbook of developmental paediatrics*. New York: Churchill Livingstone.

Prizant, B. M., & Wetherby, A. M. (1993). Communication and language assessment for young children. *Infants & Young Children, 5*, 20–34.

Rankin, W. W. (1988). The homes in their minds: A child's major field of reference is the home. *Journal of Pediatric Nursing, 3*, 273.

Rudlin, C. R. (1993). Growth and sexual development. *Journal of the American Academy of Physician Assistants, 6*, 25–35.

Rudolph, A. M. (1991). *Rudolph's pediatrics* (19th ed.). East Norwalk, CT: Appleton & Lange.

Ryan-Wenger, N. M. (1993). A taxonomy of children's coping strategies: A step toward theory development. *Journal of Pediatric Nursing: Nursing Care of Children & Families, 8*, 200.

Salkind, N. J. (1994). *Child development* (7th ed.). Fort Worth, TX: The Harcourt Press.

Schilling, L. S., & DeJesus, E. (1993). Developmental issues in deaf children. *Journal of Pediatric Health Care, 7*, 161–166.

Sewell, K. H., & Gaines, S. K. (1993). A developmental approach to childhood safety education. *Pediatric Nursing, 19*, 464–466.

Smith, M. (1993). Pediatric sexuality: Promoting normal sexual development in children. *Nurse Practitioner: American Journal of Primary Health Care, 18*, 37–38.

Spock, B., & Rothenberg, M. B. (1985). *Dr. Spock's baby and child care*. New York: Simon & Schuster.

Suskind, R. M., & Suskind, L. L. (Eds.). (1993). *Textbook of pediatric nutrition* (2nd ed.). New York: Raven Press.

Vargas, A., & Koss-Chioino, J. (1992). *Working with culture: Psychotherapeutic interventions with ethnic minority children and adolescents*. San Francisco: Jossey-Boss.

Vaughan, C., & Litt, F. (1990). *Child and adolescent development: Clinical implications*. Philadelphia: W. B. Saunders.

Wegman, M. E. (1990). Annual summary of vital statistics—1989. *Pediatrics, 86*, 835.

Chapter 17

YOUNG AND MIDDLE ADULTHOOD

CAROL J. SCALES, PhD, RN

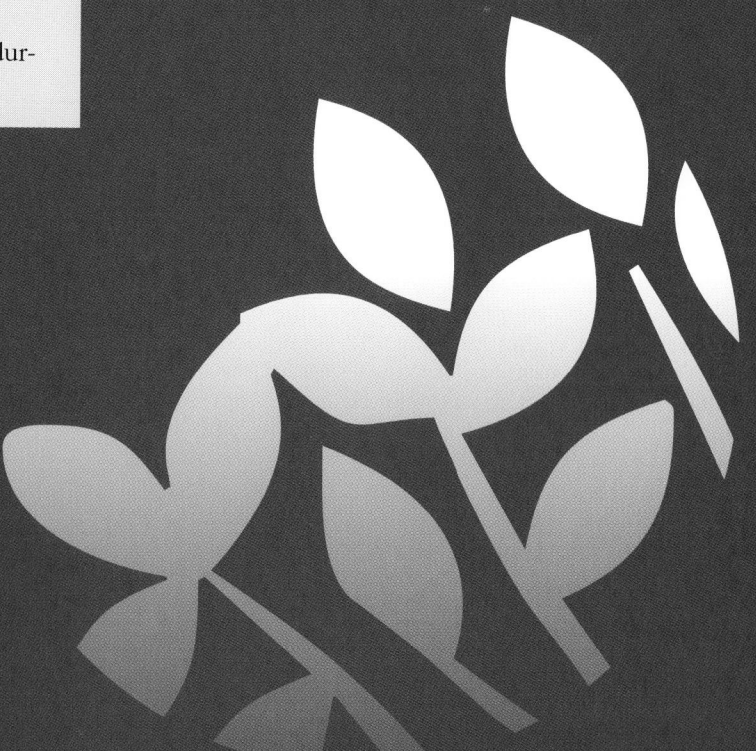

The young and middle adult years are generally healthy and productive for most people. However, the number and complexity of life transitions that occur during this time can affect the individual's ability to cope and can interfere with the maintenance of a healthy lifestyle. Some transitions during this period of life are anticipated, such as selecting an occupation, developing a special relationship with another individual, starting a family, or the death of parents. Some transitions are unanticipated, such as widowhood, terminal illness, or the loss of a child. This results in a dynamic challenge for nursing.

The roles and responsibilities, as well as the needs, of young adults differ from those of middle adults with respect to career, relationships, sexuality, physical health, biological changes, and lifestyle priorities. The nurse should be familiar with these changing needs and design nursing care that is individualized.

The nurse can play an essential role in helping young and middle-aged adults maintain their health and cope effectively with stressors that may occur. Through primary prevention, the nurse can teach individuals how to retain their highest level of ability and personal sense of well-being.

Young and Middle Adulthood Today

In response to improved medical care, better nutrition, control of disease, and changes in lifestyles, people are living longer. As a result of this longevity, the periods of "young" and "middle" adulthood have been extended over the years. Young adulthood today includes 20- to 40-year-olds, and middle adults are individuals 41 to 65 years of age.

With this increased longevity, individuals are resetting the time frames for certain maturational benchmarks and placing a premium on the quality of life. Some middle adults are retiring early from one career to start a second one. Many young couples are postponing starting a family in order to proceed with career or educational plans. However, there are those individuals in young and middle adulthood whose physical health requires the assistance of family and health services. Young and middle adults represent a population of culturally diverse individuals who have varied health care needs. Nurses providing care for young and middle adults must be knowledgeable about a broad spectrum of health issues and able to adapt this knowledge with cultural sensitivity. The nurse may develop a plan of care designed to avoid illness through health education (primary prevention). Care may need to focus on treating an existing disease (secondary restorative care). The nurse may provide tertiary nursing care by helping an individual attain an optimal level of wellness after being ill. As young and middle adults experience their lives, there is a con-

stant shifting in their health status and interpersonal relationships.

Role of the Nurse in Young and Middle Adulthood

The nurse needs to have knowledge and skills from a broad array of clinical perspectives to teach, support, and serve as a role model for healthy behaviors for young and middle adults. Peplau (1957) describes six roles that the nurse may be called on to assume: counselor, socializing agent, manager, health teacher, technician, and mother-surrogate (Box 17–1). In addition, the nurse may be called on to provide spiritual support. Given the comforting nature of nursing and the intimacy of the relationship established between nurse and client, it is not unexpected that the client may turn to the nurse for spiritual support. The nurse may provide spiritual care directly or by engaging ministers, priests, rabbis, or other spiritual resources important to the client.

All these roles are important. However, in the current health care delivery process, the nurse-manager role is particularly valued. The nurse is expected to collaborate with other health care providers in the comprehensive plan of care. Physicians, nurses, social workers, psychologists, community agencies, and governmental agencies must communicate effectively and efficiently to provide the client with the necessary care and service in a cost-effective manner.

Knowledge of crisis intervention theory (Aguilera, 1994) and the nursing skills that accompany its use are

---

Box 17–1

NURSING ROLES IDENTIFIED BY PEPLAU

Mother-surrogate: Provides basic care such as bathing, feeding, protecting.

Technician: Provides competent, efficient, and accurate technical care, such as monitoring vital signs, administering medications.

Health Teacher: Provides information to maintain health or to improve the health situation.

Manager: Deploys resources and manipulates the environment to promote health maintenance or recovery.

Socializing Agent: Assists in connecting the client with social activities that promote physical and emotional health.

Counselor: Uses interpersonal techniques to facilitate the adaptation to difficult or changing life experiences.

Data from Peplau, H. E. (1957). Therapeutic concepts. In *The league exchange*. New York: National League for Nursing.

and bodily functions continues to support the body-mind connection. The nurse should be knowledgeable about techniques that can help adults minimize the effects of stress. Interventions such as visual imaging, muscle relaxation, exercise, and activity diversion are strategies that the nurse can use to help individuals who are experiencing stress (Snyder, 1992). Nurses need to learn and use these independent nursing techniques in their clinical practice.

The nurse must know about group dynamics and be able to use group process skills. At times, the nurse may use the nursing process with an identified group of young or middle adult individuals; the "client" may be more than one person. Such is the case when the nurse works with a family, a group of employees in a company, a parents group, or a preretirement club.

Young Adulthood

The period of young adulthood, from 20 to 40 years of age, is filled with choices and transitions. Decisions about career, living arrangements, marriage, children, and lifestyle are but a few of the choices that are made during this period of life, and with each decision comes transitions in roles and responsibilities. Box 17–3 summarize the developmental tasks of young adulthood.

Physical Development

Young adulthood is frequently referred to as the prime of life. The musculoskeletal, cardiovascular, and endocrine systems are fully developed and are functioning at optimal levels. Regular menses in women signals the body's ability to accommodate the growth and development of a fetus. Having reached sexual maturity in adolescence, men continue their high interest in sexual activity.

This sense of wellness and energy experienced by young adults may cause them to neglect early warnings of potential health problems. They may not feel the need for regular physical checkups, Lifestyles that include poor nutrition, insufficient rest, lack of regular

---

Box 17–2

STEPS IN EFFECTIVE CRISIS INTERVENTION

1. Help the client feel safe
   Set limits on client's aggressive or destructive behavior.
2. Establish a relationship with the client quickly
   Use techniques of active listening, unconditional acceptance, and attention to immediate needs.
3. Assessment
   Clarify the crisis.
   Determine what precipitated the crisis.
   Determine why the client is seeking professional help at this time.
   Assess for suicidal/homicidal potential.
   Determine the level of disruption to client and family.
   Identify previous problem-solving methods.
   Identify resources available to the client.
4. Planning
   Focus on the here and now.
   Use coping strategies not already being used.
   Mobilize available resources.
5. Intervention
   Allow and acknowledge feelings of anger, helplessness, guilt, and powerlessness.
   Explore optional coping mechanisms.
   Discourage lengthy dialogue and rationalizations.
   Help the client gain an intellectual understanding of the problem.
   Reopen social world to minimize sense of isolation.
   Guide the client through the problem-solving process.
6. Evaluation
   Assess the client for diminished level of stress related to the crisis.
   Assist the client to anticipate successful strategies for future crises.

---

beneficial in applying the nursing process to the young and middle adult population. The nurse has to gather information specific to the precipitating stressor, assess the individual's coping abilities, and analyze the assessment information. A working relationship must be established to mutually identify actions that need to be taken and evaluated to determine whether the immediate goals have been met and whether the person feels able to deal with a recurrence. Box 17–2 outlines steps for effective crisis management within a nursing process framework.

Information about the relationship between stress

Box 17–3

DEVELOPMENTAL TASKS OF YOUNG ADULTS

Psychosocial: Develop intimate relationships

Moral: Make judgments based on interpersonal effects and cooperation

Spiritual: Evaluate worldview and examine personal beliefs and values

Educational: Decide on a career and learn to live within new social structures

exercise, smoking, substance abuse, and poor stress management may compromise their physical status over time and make the expected and unexpected events of this life stage more difficult.

A young woman may find that her body is unable to fully support the additional demands of pregnancy as a result of nutritional deficits or the use of harmful substances such as alcohol or drugs. Young men may see career dreams altered as a result of poor physical fitness or dependence on alcohol, drugs, or other ineffective coping mechanisms.

Developmental Tasks and Stages

♦ **Psychosocial Development.** After having successfully used adolescence to develop a sense of individual identity, the young adult is now ready for intimate personal relationships (Fig. 17–1). Focus on the "I am" of adolescence is replaced with the "we are" of young adulthood (Erikson, 1950/1963). The task for the young adult is to use the newly established identity to develop a healthy balance between the need for intimacy and the need for isolation. The result of that balance fosters love. Intimacy is not confined to sexuality, but rather encompasses a broad psychosocial context that includes all aspects of the young adult's life. It is during this time that an individual usually makes a commitment to another person that frequently produces a child. The sense of caring that results from balancing intimacy and isolation may also influence career decisions and community involvement.

♦ **Moral Development.** The young adult is at the "conventional level" of moral development (Kohlberg, 1968). Judgments at this level are based on their interpersonal effect. Young adults have moved beyond judgments based solely on self-interest. They recognize the importance of pleasing significant others and have developed a sense of duty that tends to supersede personal wishes and peer group pressure. Their

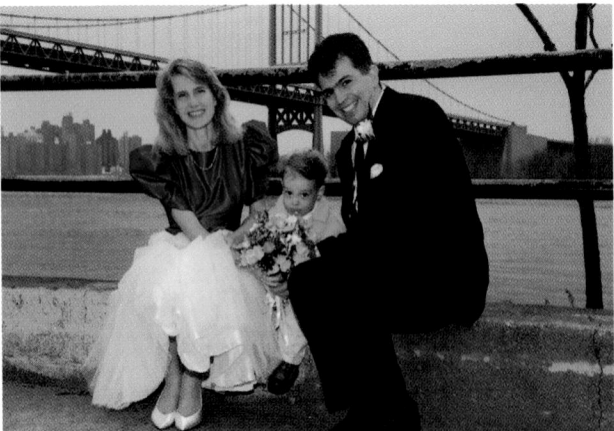

♦ **Figure 17–1**
Developmental tasks of young adulthood include intimacy and commitment, exemplified by the establishment of a family.

morality is one of cooperation (Piaget, 1965). Gilligan (1982) contends that as a result of their socialization process, moral judgment in women develops contextually and is based more on principles of caring than on principles of justice. As gender roles evolve, and more young adults have new parental role models, these differences may converge. More men are performing traditional female roles, such as entering nursing and staying at home with children, and women are assuming heretofore male responsibilities in executive positions and providing essential income.

♦ **Spiritual Development.** In the early part of young adulthood, there may be a tendency to be less active in formal spiritual activities. As a remnant of adolescent identity-seeking behaviors and rebellion against parental values, many younger adults refrain from participating in religious services. Young adulthood is a time of "individuative-reflective faith" (Fowler, 1974), when personal worldviews are critically examined and the meanings of religious symbols and beliefs are evaluated. The success of this process results in an autonomous individual who can be given to a supreme being. As a new family develops, the older young adult may resume participation in spiritual affiliations.

♦ **Educational Development.** The process of living requires learning and growing. Young adulthood is a period of life with many learning needs and few educational opportunities (Havighurst, 1952). Having finished one's formal education, it is now time to decide on a career. Frequently, the early young adult may take several years to become adjusted to the expectations of adulthood. Later learning tasks may include selecting a mate and learning to live within a relationship and manage a home. The arrival of children requires learning child-rearing skills. There are expectations that young adults will become involved in their communities and engage in civic activities. The young adult may wish to identify and join congenial social groups. All these new learning experiences encountered in young adulthood provide the nurse with valuable teachable moments for health education.

In general, young adulthood is a physically healthy period. The body has reached maturation, and biological systems are functioning fully. One's ability for physical activity is at a peak during this period. However, healthy behaviors such as diet, exercise, stress reduction, and regular medical checkups will have an impact not only on maintaining the young adult's current health status but also on sustaining health in later years.

The Nursing Process and the Young Adult Client
Assessment and Nursing Diagnosis

To provide a proper assessment of the young adult, the nurse must have thorough knowledge of the choices and transitions associated with this stage of life. Each stressor has the potential to either disrupt physical or emotional well-being or promote individual growth. The nurse is in a key position to help the young adult minimize the negative effects of life stressors through health education. In caring for the young adult, the nurse should recognize that there is stress associated with each of the following categories. Related nursing diagnoses are highlighted in the accompanying box.

✦ **Career.** It may take several job changes to find a career compatible with financial needs, skills, interests, and mobility. Career decisions may also involve moving away from family and friends and living independently. Each choice requires the individual to assume new and different responsibilities. These changes may precipitate stress (Fig. 17–2). The young adult is now

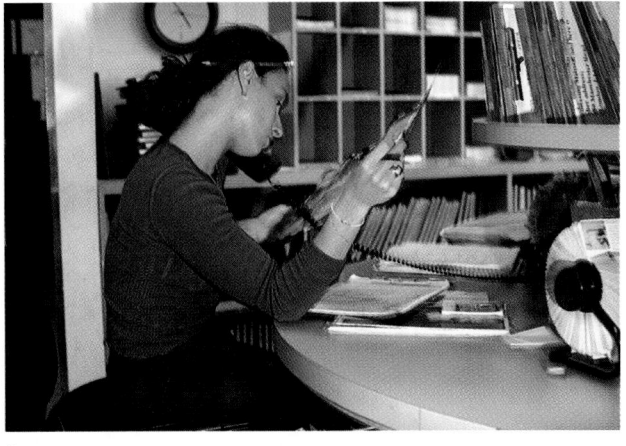

✦ **Figure 17–2**
Job-related stress is common in young adulthood. Career decisions may involve moving away from family and friends, and work pressures may cause conflicts with relationships and family responsibilities. The nurse can help by encouraging open expression of concerns and fears and providing stress-management counseling.

an employee, a fellow worker, a tenant or home owner, a community member, an adult child. Each role demands that the young adult assume new and additional responsibilities. Possible nursing diagnoses include

> Relocation Stress Syndrome
> Powerlessness
> Role Performance, Altered
> Decisional Conflict

Two-career families are now common and may cause additional interpersonal stress. One member may have a higher-paying job or one with more prestige. Career relocations or opportunities for advancement for one member may impose unwanted changes for the other member. When children are involved, issues surrounding child care must also be considered. Many couples are delaying having children to achieve their career goals. Some parents are determining child care responsibilities on the basis of career objectives; a father may stay at home caring for the children while a wife-executive pursues her career. Possible nursing diagnoses include

> Parental Role Conflict
> Home Maintenance Management, Impaired

Although these changes may be stressful for the individual, couple, or family at the time, in general they are growth promoting, and individuals and families adapt. The nurse must be able to help the young adult assess the stress that career decisions may cause and help the individual deal with that stress through growth-promoting interventions. Facilitating open communication among those impacted by this stress is a helpful intervention. Each individual has a chance to express concerns, fears, hopes, and perceived losses to the others, and mutual understanding can ease

---

NURSING DIAGNOSES THAT MAY BE APPLICABLE TO YOUNG ADULT CLIENTS

Diagnoses Related to Career

Relocation stress syndrome

Powerlessness

Altered role performance

Decisional conflict

Parental role conflict

Impaired home maintenance management

Diversional activity deficit

Altered family processes

Impaired social interaction

Diagnoses Related to Sexuality

Risk for infection

Knowledge deficit

Self-esteem deficit

Diagnoses Related to Physical Health

Activity intolerance

Health-seeking behaviors

Altered nutrition: less/more than body requirements

Sleep pattern disturbance

Ineffective denial

Knowledge deficit

Noncompliance

Diagnoses Related to Relationships

Risk for altered parenting

Parental role conflict

Altered role performance

Situational low self-esteem

the stress for everyone. Possible nursing diagnoses include

Diversional Activity Deficit

Family Processes: Alcoholism, Altered

Social Interaction, Impaired

✦ **Sexuality.** Young adulthood is a time when important and intimate relationships are being explored. Never before have sexual relationships borne greater interpersonal responsibility. Unplanned pregnancies and nonfatal sexually transmitted diseases have always been a potential consequence of irresponsible sexual behavior. However, the discovery of fatal HIV/AIDS has placed even greater attention on using protection, specifically condoms, when having sexual intercourse. See Chapter 37 for methods of contraception.

➤ **NURSING TIP**
Ask these assessment questions:
  How frequently are you having sex?
  What methods are you using to avoid becoming pregnant?
  Are you having sex with someone who has ever used IV drugs?
  Have you ever had a sexually transmitted disease (STD), such as syphilis, gonorrhea, chlamydia?
  Have you ever been tested for STDs or HIV/AIDS?

The nurse should recognize the needs of young adults with respect to establishing intimate sexual relationships, provide accurate information about the health risks of certain behaviors, and help identify interventions that can be used to reduce those risks. Possible nursing diagnoses include

Risk for Infection

Knowledge Deficit

Self Esteem Disturbance

✦ **Physical Health.** Young adults tend to be physically active members of the community. They recognize the importance of exercise, and many walk, jog, or bicycle; join health clubs; and engage in competitive sports. Frequently, however, the busy lifestyles of young adults make it difficult to find the time to accommodate a regular program of physical fitness. Possible nursing diagnoses include

Activity Intolerance

Health Seeking Behaviors

Similarly, the constraints of job and family may interfere with maintaining a pattern of healthy nutrition. "Fast food" becomes a convenient, but less than healthy, source of nutrition as individuals and families have less time for meal planning and preparation. A possible nursing diagnosis would be

Nutrition: Less/More Than Body Requirements, Altered

The increasing responsibilities at home and at work can alter the regular sleep patterns of young

adults. Insufficient sleep can result in accidents, irritability that interferes with interpersonal relationships, and impaired performance. Sleep, especially rapid eye movement (REM) sleep, is an essential component to a physically and emotionally healthy lifestyle. Like nutrition, sleep is often neglected as the young adult is adjusting to new responsibilities. A possible nursing diagnosis would be

Sleep Pattern Disturbance

Young adults frequently offer time constraints and a general sense of well-being as reasons for not attending to preventive health care. Routine checkups for physical and dental care and vision screening are particularly important in this age group. Early detection is essential in minimizing the effects of any beginning disease process. The nurse should encourage, support, and facilitate every effort to ensure that young adults have adequate information to make healthy decisions about their well-being. Frequently, the nurse is called on to explain or interpret health information for the young adult and therefore must keep apprised of new information in the health field. Possible nursing diagnoses include

Denial, Ineffective

Knowledge Deficit

Noncompliance

➤ **NURSING TIP**
Ask these assessment questions:
  What kinds of planned exercise do you engage in? How frequently and for how long?
  What do you think is your best weight? Have you lost/gained weight recently? Was that weight change planned? Describe your typical breakfast, lunch, and dinner.
  How much sleep do you require to feel rested? How much sleep are you getting? Do you have any trouble falling asleep or staying asleep?
  How frequently do you do a self-examination of your breasts (females)/testes (males)? When was the last time you saw a physician/nurse practitioner for a physical examination?

✦ **Relationships.** The young adult can choose how to define a relationship, but each decision may bring internal and external pressures. Many young adults are deciding to marry later and placing career and independence goals ahead of making a commitment to an individual or starting a family. They may experience pressure from relatives and friends to conform with the expectation that they "settle down," and they may have to defend their choices.

Young adults who decide to marry, consistent with sociocultural expectations for this period, may also face the pressures of role adjustment. The change from being autonomous to being interdependent and sharing responsibilities can be stressful to the individual and the couple. Becoming truly intimate in a relationship requires adjustment to the needs of the new entity, the couple. Financial, career, recreational, and personal needs compete for limited personal resources and may have to be reprioritized.

Parenthood contributes additional dimensions to a couple's relationship. No matter how much the new baby is wanted by the pair, the baby's arrival changes the couple's relationship. Women experience the physiological and psychological changes of pregnancy. Most women are excited about the prospect of becoming mothers but concerned about being able to meet the additional physical and emotional demands. Most men are proud of the promise of fatherhood but worry about providing financially and emotionally for a growing family. Most couples achieve the equilibrium of a new family as roles shift to accommodate additional responsibilities. Men may have to assume more of the domestic responsibilities and become involved in the direct care of the children to allow women to continue to work outside the home, especially when second incomes are necessary.

The nurse needs to understand the pressures experienced by new parents. Information about normal changes that can be expected during pregnancy can help parents anticipate and minimize the stress they may encounter (Fig. 17–3). The nurse can provide support for the pregnant woman who is feeling physically unattractive and fearful of losing her husband's affection. The nurse can help the husband understand his wife's mood swings as a consequence of physiological changes, so that he will not take them personally. Men can be advised that women may wish to refrain from sexual intercourse late in pregnancy and for a brief period after delivery. This sexual hiatus should not be construed by the husband as personal rejection or disinterest, but rather a normal phenomenon. By working with the parents to develop new ways to adjust, the nurse can help the couple anticipate other lifestyle changes that having a new baby will cause, such as interrupted meal times, disturbed sleep, and curtailed social activities. Nurse-midwives and nurses who teach child-birthing classes are valuable resources for expectant parents.

Young adults may experience unanticipated pregnancy. The couple needs to know about the choices they can make. Adjusting to the arrival of a new baby, deciding to terminate the pregnancy by abortion, or offering the newborn for adoption are options. Private and public community agencies can provide information and counseling to assist individuals in making a decision.

Couples need not be married to confront problems of intimate relationships. Many young adults decide to live together as heterosexual or homosexual couples. They too experience the pressures of having to change to accommodate the needs of another person. Roles and functions within these relationships must be worked out, just as they are in a marriage. Conflicting individual career goals can produce stress. In addition, the young adult's choice of a nontraditional relationship may produce external pressure from family and friends. By understanding the stress inherent in any intimate relationship, the nurse can help

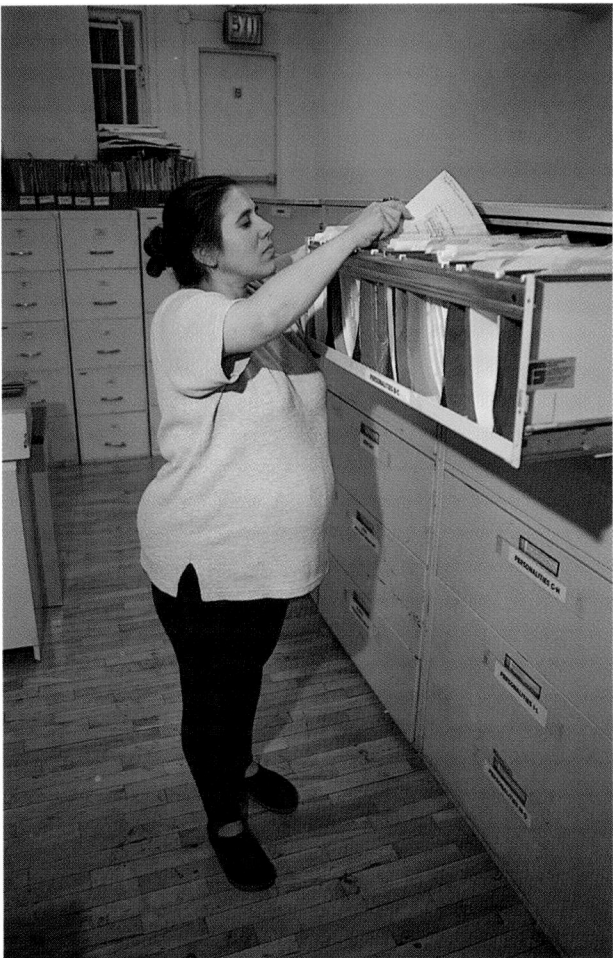

♦ **Figure 17–3**
The nurse can provide anticipatory guidance to first-time parents about normal changes that can be expected during pregnancy. Anticipation of changes in lifestyle after the birth of the baby will also help parents-to-be adjust to their new roles.

nontraditional couples develop strategies to minimize any detrimental effects on health.

Possible nursing diagnoses include

Risk for Altered Parenting

Parental Role Conflict

Role Performance, Altered

Situational Low Self Esteem

Planning, Intervention, and Evaluation

Given the nature and diversity of the choices and transitions confronting the young adult, primary prevention for this population focuses on health education.

Primary Prevention

♦ **Routine Medical Examinations.** Wherever the nurse encounters young adults, emphasis should be given to teaching the importance of regular physical examinations to screen for cancer, coronary artery disease, and other health risk factors. Young adults should get in the habit of seeing their health care provider on a regular basis, having semiannual dental checks, and seeking vision and hearing evaluations at the earliest sign of possible impairment. The nurse should support and facilitate all efforts by a young adult to use primary prevention to maintain a healthy lifestyle. The early detection of actual or potential health problems can have an impact on more serious complications.

❧ **Teaching Self-Examination.** The nurse as educator can instruct young adults in how to do breast self-

HEALTH PROMOTION AND PREVENTION

DO-IT-YOURSELF MONTHLY BREAST SELF-EXAMINATION

In the shower. Raise one arm. With fingers flat, touch every part of each breast, gently feeling for a lump or thickening. Use your right hand to examine your left breast, your left hand for your right breast.

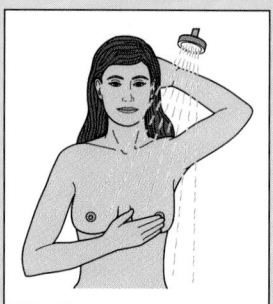

Before a mirror. With arms at your sides, then raised above your head, look carefully for changes in the size, shape, and contour of each breast. Look for puckering, dimpling, or changes in skin texture.

Gently squeeze both nipples and look for discharge.

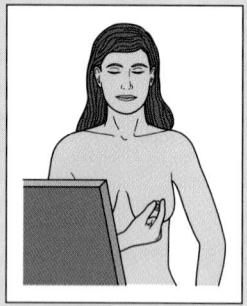

Lying down. Place a towel or pillow under your right shoulder and your right hand behind your head. Examine your right breast with your left hand.

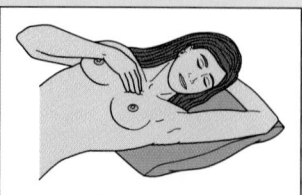

Fingers flat, press gently in small circles, starting at the outermost top edge of your breast and spiraling in toward the nipple. Examine every part of the breast. Repeat with left breast.

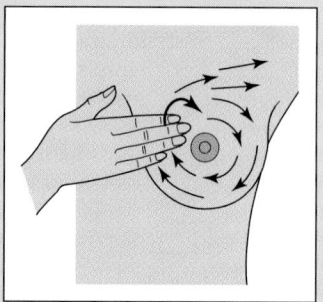

With your arm resting on a firm surface, use the same circular motion to examine the underarm area. This is breast tissue too.

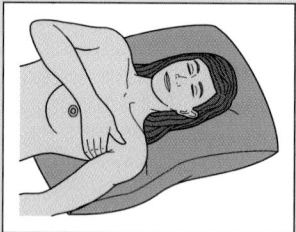

Note: This self-exam is not a substitute for periodic examinations by a qualified physician.

A Three-Step Early Detection Program

Breast cancer, even in very early stages, can be identified easily. You can monitor your own health with a three-step program:

Step 1: Schedule Regular Mammograms

A mammogram is a special breast x-ray that can reveal a small breast cancer up to 2 years before it can be felt. This important test is extremely safe, as modern mammography uses very low amounts of radiation. If you are 40 or older, schedule regular mammograms.

HEALTH PROMOTION AND PREVENTION
(Continued)

Mammography Guidelines

The following **mammography guidelines** for women with no symptoms are based on the consensus of a number of medical organizations:

* An initial screening mammogram between ages 35 and 40 and then every other year to age 49.
* A mammogram every year for women 50 and over.

Your family physician can advise you if this frequency is right for you, and will help you schedule a mammogram. If there are signs or symptoms of breast cancer, your physician may recommend a different program.

Step 2: Examine Your Breasts

You should examine your breasts monthly, several days after your menstrual period, or on the same day every month if you no longer menstruate. Your family physician can show you how to do this. If you find a lump, don't be alarmed. Breast lumps are common, and more than 80% are not cancerous. You should consult your physician, however, for an expert opinion about the lump.

Step 3: See Your Physician Regularly

Self-examination, although important, is not enough. If you are between 20 and 40 years old, your breasts should be examined by your physician at least once every 3 years. If you are over 40, your breasts should be examined every year.

©1987 Albert Einstein Healthcare Foundation, Philadelphia, PA 19141

---

examinations (BSEs), described and illustrated in the box. Basic information about why BSE is important, coupled with actual skill in doing the examination and structured support, can promote adherence to a regular program of BSE (Lierman *et al.,* 1994). Young women should be taught and encouraged to do monthly self-examination of their breasts. Early identification of breast lumps, dimpling, sores, and other unusual changes may make a difference in the kind of treatment used and improve the outcome.

Similarly, medical experts are encouraging men to do routine self-examinations of their testes to identify any changes that might warrant medical attention. Testicular self-examination (TSE) has been less well publicized but is equally as important as breast examination. The nurse working with young adult men can educate them about how to do the examination and its importance (see box).

✦ Recognizing the Symptoms of Communicable Diseases. Nurses can help young adults recognize the signs and symptoms of infectious diseases through health education. Young adults are active members in the community and may become exposed to any number of communicable diseases in the course of school and work.

Respiratory diseases are the most common. The nurse can emphasize the importance of simple but effective health habits such as good hand washing, the use of disposable tissues, and covering the mouth and nose when coughing and sneezing, which may prevent the spread of communicable disease to others. Individuals who are experiencing the signs and symptoms of infectious diseases should understand the importance of self-isolation for the protection of others. Feeling external pressures, young adults may continue to go to school or work, knowing that they are not feeling well, and place others at risk for getting ill. Occupational, school, and hospital nurses particularly should encourage individuals who are not feeling well to remain at home to contain the spread of infection.

✦ Environmental Safety. Young adults should be aware of the hazards associated with their workplaces. Every job involves certain risks, be they harmful chemicals, dangerous equipment, potential for assault, or risk of disease. The federal and local government, as well as the employer, may have safety standards to ensure employee well-being. Young adult employees should be encouraged by the occupational nurse to know and practice these standards to maintain safety in their workplaces.

Young adults are mobile, and preventing vehicular accidents and minimizing injury are important. The simple and automatic use of seat belts in motor vehicles can save lives and reduce injury. An estimated 4000 lives might have been saved in 1987, when only 42% of all passengers used their seat belts (*Healthy People 2000,* 1990). Similarly, accidents resulting from driving while under the influence of alcohol kill not only young adults but also other innocent travelers.

✦ Nutrition, Exercise, and Rest. The nurse can help the young adult recognize the importance of nutrition, exercise, and rest in establishing a healthy lifestyle. Helping the young adult balance the multiple stressors resulting from life choices and transitions involves developing a strategy to meet the individual's

HEALTH PROMOTION AND PREVENTION

TESTICULAR SELF-EXAMINATION

Recommended monthly after warm bath or shower when the scrotal skin is relaxed.

1. Stand in front of a mirror and look for any swelling on the skin of the scrotum.

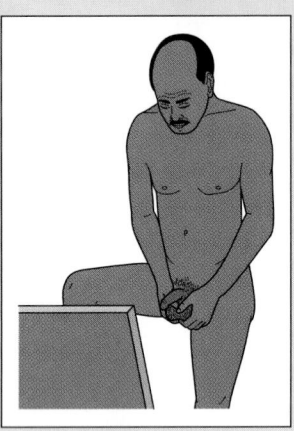

2. Using both hands, with fingers under the scrotum and thumbs on top, gently roll the testicles feeling for any lumps.

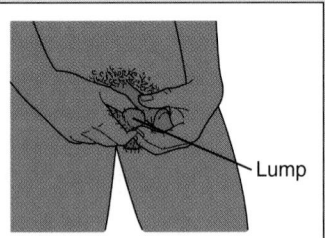

Lump

3. The epididymis, a normal cordlike structure on the top and back of each testicle, is then palpated.

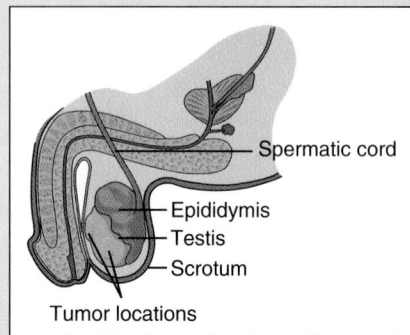

Spermatic cord
Epididymis
Testis
Scrotum
Tumor locations

Testicular cancer almost always occurs in only one testicle and is usually a pea-sized, painless lump. It is highly curable when found early.

Data from Anderson, K. N. (ed.). (1994). *Mosby's medical, nursing and allied health dictionary* (4th ed., p. 1538.). St. Louis: Mosby.

---

need for nutrition, exercise, and sleep. Each young adult is unique in his or her specific requirements, and the nurse individualizes the teaching to include specific risk factors, such as elevated blood cholesterol levels, exercise heart rate, and need for REM sleep to feel rested.

❧ Stress Reduction Techniques. The nurse can build on the young adult's known techniques for relieving stress. Perhaps jogging, a hot bath, reading, gardening, swimming, or some other hobby helps the individual feel refreshed and less stressed (Fig. 17–4). The nurse can introduce the young adult to other stress management techniques, such as picturing himself or herself in a pleasant, restful place or focusing on the tension and relaxation of each set of muscles, working from the top of the body to the feet. Eastern exercises are popular, and groups that teach yoga and

tai chi may help the young adult improve the way he or she manages stress.

As health educator, the nurse can help the young adult with early detection and intervention strategies using routine health checkups, self-examination, recognition of potentially harmful conditions, and stress management.

Secondary Prevention

Adults, especially young adults, have the opportunity to assume responsibility for their health through changes in lifestyle. "Preventing chronic disease depends often on individual decisions—to quit smoking, to drink in moderation if at all, to consume less saturated fat, to increase physical activity" (*Healthy People 2000*, 1990, p. 22).

In addition to the anticipated stressors associated

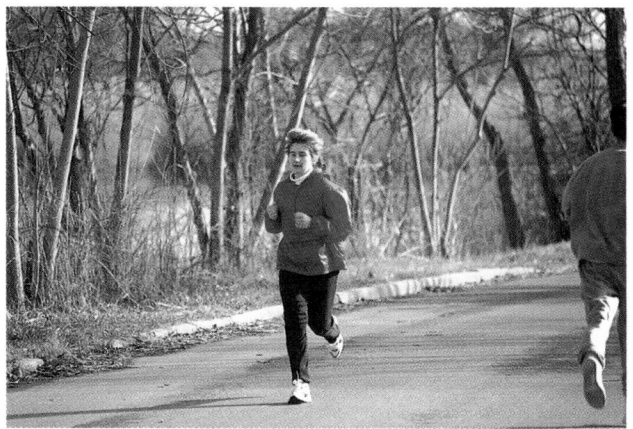

✦ **Figure 17–4**
Jogging and other forms of cardiovascular exercise can help reduce stress. Nurses can also suggest other activities for stress reduction, such as yoga or Tai Chi, reading, gardening or other hobbies, or relaxing in a hot bath.

with transitions in young adulthood, situations may occur that require specific health care intervention. The nursing role in planning, implementing, and evaluating care when disease or accident occurs is directed toward returning the individual to an optimal level of wellness. Unanticipated health stressors may happen at any point in the young adult's life.

✦ **Career.** Once the individual finds a satisfying and rewarding job, there is a tendency to assume that things will continue without incident. However, a number of unanticipated occurrences within the context of an individual's job may result in the need for direct health care intervention. Environmental hazards such as exposure to toxic chemicals, asbestos, and passive smoke may result in respiratory disease or cancer. Accidents on the job, such as burns, falls, and lacerations, may also result in the need for medical attention. Losing, changing, or becoming dissatisfied with a job may impose the need for psychological intervention and resultant medical care. Sustaining a career is an important role function in young adulthood, and situations that threaten a career impose not only physical and psychological hardship on the individual but also financial and health insurance concerns for other members of the family.

✦ **Sexuality.** During young adulthood, sexual functioning is at its peak, and individuals may not always be aware of sex-related health problems that may occur. Public attention has been focused on sexually transmitted diseases (STDs) such as genital herpes, chlamydia, gonorrhea, and syphilis, which are most common in young adults. Of particular concern is HIV/AIDS, which is spreading to the heterosexual population and is the number-one cause of death in 25- to 40-year-olds. Methods of prevention include abstinence, knowledge of partners' sexual and drug use histories, and the use of condoms.

Another unanticipated consequence of sexual ac-

tivity is pregnancy and the choices that have to be made: keeping the baby as a single parent, keeping the baby and marrying the child's father, having an abortion, or offering the infant for adoption. Each choice carries a number of individualized consequences, and the nurse can help the individual or couple consider each consequence thoughtfully and honestly to make the best decision for everyone concerned.

Young adult women are at risk for a number of diseases and disorders associated with the sexual organs, such as cysts, tumors, and inflammations. Problems of infertility are especially stressful for a young couple desiring to start a family. Once pregnant, mis-

COMMUNITY BASED CARE

ANTEPARTUM AND POSTPARTUM SERVICES

Programs that address the needs of pregnant and postpartum women and their newborn infants are offered by many home care agencies. Nurses with specialized knowledge and experience in obstetrical care are an important component of such programs.

Home care for clients discharged after only 24 to 48 hours after delivery is common. In the hospital, there is little time to accomplish all of the necessary teaching related to recovery and well-baby care. Also, potential complications, such as infant jaundice, may not be detected. Early discharge programs consist of assessment of the newborn and the mother and teaching that includes

1. Self-care issues: activity and rest, elimination, emotional aspects of the postpartum period, sexual activity, and family adjustment

2. Infant care issues: bathing, temperature taking, elimination, cord care, jaundice, bottle- or breast-feeding, safety at home and out, when to call the physician

When planning teaching for this population, consider that the multigravida and primagravida have different concerns and priorities. Primagravida concerns include a greater lack of knowledge, anxiety, and uncertainty related to infant care. Breast-feeding is also a common concern. Multigravida teaching includes the need for rest and how to cope effectively with the demands of one or more other children.

Prenatal high-risk care that may also be managed in the home includes

1. Gestational diabetes

2. Tocolytic therapy and monitoring for premature labor

3. Intensive monitoring for women who develop toxemia or preeclampsia

4. Hydration or parenteral nutrition for management of hyperemesis

5. Heparin therapy for thromboembolic complications of pregnancy

carriage and spontaneous abortion may precipitate feelings of grief and loss that can be so disabling as to require medical attention.

Young adult men may also be at risk for sexual performance disorders such as premature ejaculation and early impotence. As with female breast tumors, the effects of testicular tumors can be reduced by early detection. Young adult men should be taught how to conduct a testicular self-examination (TSE) of the scrotum to palpate for any abnormalities.

The nurse should be aware that health problems can occur in young adults related to sexuality and sexual anatomy. Primary prevention is ideal, but early detection and treatment improve the course of most illnesses.

✦ **Substance Abuse.** Alcohol and tobacco continue to be the primary substances abused by young adults. The relaxation and improved socialization effects of these substances, and of illegal drugs such as cocaine, amphetamines, and marijuana, are frequently viewed as being helpful with interpersonal relationships. Unfortunately, continued use of these substances leads to needing more of the substance to get the same psychological and physical effect (tolerance), resulting in physical and psychological dependency. Serious legal and health problems ensue. Substance abuse can cause physical injuries and death as the individual's cognitive abilities and motor skills become impaired.

The nurse can provide information about the consequences of substance abuse for the individual, the family, and the unborn child. If dependency has occurred, the nurse can help the individual recognize the need for treatment and be supportive of the young adult and his or her family during this difficult time. It is important that the nurse help the individual and the family face this problem directly and to seek help from professionals and self-help support groups such as Alcoholics Anonymous (AA). The purpose of AA is to help members stay sober by promoting total abstinence as the only treatment for this illness. The philosophy of AA is contained in the Twelve Steps, which serve as a guide to attaining sobriety (Box 17–4).

✦ **Other Dysfunctions.** In addition to substance abuse, young adults may experience other addictions, such as gambling or compulsive eating. Regular incidents of spousal or child abuse may also occur during this time. Like the Alcoholics Anonymous program, there are peer support groups available in most communities for these problems. Professional therapists, such as psychologists, nutritionists, psychiatrists, counselors, and clinical nurse specialists, treat individuals and couples affected by dysfunctional behaviors.

✦ **Nutrition.** Today's young adult leads a fast-paced life. There seems to be little time to prepare and enjoy a well-balanced and nutritious meal. "Convenience" foods eaten on the go seem to be the nutritional norm. Substantial media attention is given to maintain-

---

Box **17–4**

ALCOHOLICS ANONYMOUS 12-STEP PROGRAM

1. We admitted we were powerless over alcohol—that our lives have become unmanageable.
2. Came to believe that a Power greater than ourselves could restore us to sanity.
3. Made a decision to turn our will and our lives over to the care of God *as we understood Him.*
4. Made a searching and fearless moral inventory of ourselves.
5. Admitted to God, to ourselves, and to another human being the exact nature of our wrongs.
6. Were entirely ready to have God remove all these defects of character.
7. Humbly asked Him to remove our shortcomings.
8. Made a list of all persons we had harmed and became willing to make amends to them all.
9. Made direct amends to such people whenever possible, except when to do so would injure them or others.
10. Continued to take personal inventory and when we were wrong promptly admit it.
11. Sought through prayer and meditation to improve our conscious contact with God *as we understood Him,* praying only for knowledge of His will for us and the power to carry that out.
12. Having a spiritual awakening as a result of these steps, we tried to carry this message to alcoholics and to practice these principles in all our affairs.

The Twelve Steps are reprinted with permission of Alcoholics Anonymous World Services, Inc. Permission to reprint the Twelve Steps does not mean that A. A. has reviewed or approved the contents of this publication, nor that A. A. agrees with the views expressed herein. A. A. is a program of recovery from alcoholism *only*—use of the Twelve Steps in connection with programs and activities which are patterned after A. A., but which address other problems, or in any other non–A. A. context, does not imply otherwise.
From Alcoholics Anonymous (1978). *Twelve steps and twelve traditions.* New York: Alcoholics Anonymous World Services.

---

ing a trim, athletic figure, yet commercial advertisements promote fast foods. For many young women, this mixed message results in a preoccupation with physical appearance and weight, and some take it to the extreme. Young adult women are the most prevalent group to succumb to the eating disorders of anorexia nervosa (an extreme preoccupation with being too fat, although the individual is well below normal body weight) and bulimia (a condition in which the individual binges on a large quantity of food and then purges by vomiting). The nurse can help the young adult recognize unhealthy nutritional habits and substitute healthier choices that still fit within a chosen lifestyle (Table 17–1). Because the young adult has reached body maturation, the nurse can help the indi-

Table 17–1

CALORIES AND FAT GRAMS FOR POPULAR FOODS FROM FAST-FOOD RESTAURANTS

	CALORIES	FAT GRAMS	RESTAURANT
Hamburger	161	8	White Castle
	270	9	Wendy's
	255	9	McDonald's
	270	11	Jack in the Box
	260	10	Burger King
Cheeseburger	200	11	White Castle
	320	13	Wendy's
	305	13	McDonald's
	320	14	Jack in the Box
	300	14	Burger King
French fries	301 (reg)	15	White Castle
	204 (sm)	12	Wendy's
	220 (sm)	12	McDonald's
	220 (sm)	11	Jack in the Box
	372 (med)	20	Burger King
Cheese pizza (2 slices)	506	18	Pizza Hut
	484	14	Godfather's Pizza
	376	10	Domino's Pizza
Baked potato (plain)	290	4	Wendy's
	240	2	Arby's
	130	1	Roy Rogers
Taco (soft chicken)	213	10	Taco Bell
	180	8	Taco John's
Hot dog and roll	310	19	Nathan's
	280	16	Dairy Queen
Roast beef sandwich	260	4	Roy Rogers
	270	11	Hardee's
Chicken nuggets/sticks	270 (6)	15	McDonald's
	236 (6)	13	Burger King
	287 (8)	15	Chick-Fil-A

From Natow, A. B., & Heslin, J. (1995). *The fat counter* (3rd ed.). New York: Pocket Books.

vidual balance nutritional needs with a planned program of regular exercise.

✦ **Physical Health.** Being a young adult provides no insurance against physical disease. Individuals can help improve their health status by altering at-risk behaviors such as smoking and overeating, by performing appropriate self-examinations such as breast and testicular, by having routine medical checkups, and by contacting their health care providers with early symptoms. Being aware of the family health history can provide the young adult with valuable information about early detection and prevention. The nurse can help the individual whose family has a history of heart disease, cancer, or respiratory disease take early steps to minimize the effects of illness by assuming better

health habits and seeking routine preventive health care.

✦ **Relationships.** Young adulthood can be a time of developing new and lasting relationships, but it can also be a time of loneliness, loss, isolation, rejection, and grief. Those wishing to be married may find it difficult to find partners. Relationships thought to be solid and loving may come apart through divorce, separation, or abuse. Couples may find themselves unable to have children or may lose a child to illness or accident, or they may be stressed by an unplanned pregnancy. Early widowhood may find the individual unprepared to manage alone. The young adult's parents may die, causing unexpected feelings of emptiness and abandonment. The status of relationships and the young adult's physical health may precipitate depression and even the consideration of suicide. The nurse needs to be supportive of the individual or young adult couple during these times of transition and loss. A kind, understanding, but realistic approach is most helpful to the young adult.

When unanticipated health needs arise for the young adult, the nurse may need to provide direct nursing care, modify health teaching strategies, and recommend and support follow-up health care. The nurse may also be a young adult, and issues of concern to the client may be of concern to the nurse as well. The nurse may find it difficult or embarrassing to discuss the client's intimate health needs. A professional demeanor and matter-of-fact approach is best used to discuss these personal matters. It is also important for the nurse to be a role model for the client with respect to appropriate health habits. The nurse who smokes will lose credibility in trying to convince a client to stop smoking, and the obese nurse may not be heeded when teaching diet and exercise management.

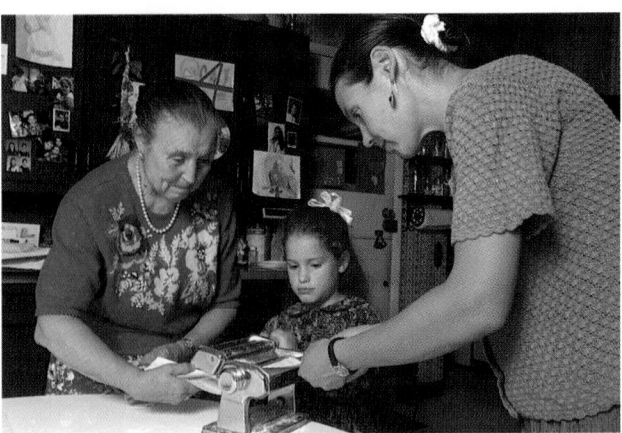

❧ **Figure 17–5**
Middle adults sometimes find themselves "sandwiched" between generations, responsible for the care and well-being of both children and aging parents.

Summary of Young Adulthood

Young adulthood is a period of multiple transitions, each one presenting new challenges. Health habits developed in this period will affect wellness throughout the remainder of life. Young adults who practice prevention and low-risk health behaviors are more likely to sustain their health as they continue to mature. The role of the nurse in this phase is to assist the young adult by keeping him or her fully informed regarding the normal and anticipated changes in this period of life. Should unanticipated health incidents occur during young adulthood, the nurse may provide direct nursing care to minimize the complications of any illness and to help the individual return to his or her optimal level of wellness.

Middle Adulthood

Individuals from 41 to 65 years of age are considered middle adults. Approximately 42% of the population in 2010 will be in their middle adult years (Spencer, 1989). Like people in young adulthood, middle adults are also confronted with many role transitions (Box 17–5). Depending on choices made in their earlier years, some middle adults may be preparing for children to leave home for college, the military, or other independent ventures. Others, having delayed starting a family, may have young children at home. Those who chose to remain single may be pursuing their careers or may be revisiting that earlier decision. This age group has been referred to as the "sandwich generation" (Fig. 17–5). Frequently, they find themselves sandwiched between responsibilities for their children and for their aging parents.

Physical Development

Middle adults experience important physiological changes. The ongoing aging process of body tissues becomes more discernible at this time. There is a general slowing down, as evidenced by diminishing muscular and sensory perceptual abilities. Noticeable physical signs of aging include graying hair; drying and wrinkling of the skin; growth of stiff hair in the noses, ears, and eyebrows of men and hair growth on the upper lips of women; and thinning of scalp hair.

The slowing of metabolism, along with decreased vigor and activity endurance, can result in weight gain and a redistribution of adipose tissue around the middle of the body. The senses of taste and smell may also be altered and affect food choices. Increasingly, salty, sweet, sour, or spicy food may conflict with existing or potential health problems, such as diabetes, hypertension, and peptic ulcer.

Box **17–5**

DEVELOPMENTAL TASKS OF MIDDLE ADULTS

Psychosocial: Give guidance, knowledge, and nurturing to the next generation

Moral: Make judgments based on the good of the community, using internalized universal values

Spiritual: Evaluate life from a philosophical perspective, acknowledging one's own mortality

Educational: Learn about adaptations necessary to move successfully into old age

Changes in the senses may require adaptive devices. Ocular lens inelasticity makes visual focusing difficult without eyeglasses. Bifocals for reading may become necessary. Hearing becomes diminished, impairing socialization and placing the individual at risk for accidents from unheeded alarms. The older middle-aged adult may require a hearing aid to improve acuity.

Men and women experience decreased hormonal production during middle adult years. In women, this hormonal change results in the cessation of menstruation, which usually occurs between the ages of 40 and 55. The physiological process, called menopause, frequently takes several years. The graafian follicles cease to open, the mucous membrane of the uterus is no longer routinely replaced, and the ovaries cease producing estrogen and progesterone. The symptoms resulting from this disturbance in the endocrine balance can include hot and cold flashes, dizziness, insomnia, irritability, and headaches. Psychological responses to menopause vary. Some women view this event negatively and feel that their value (to procreate) has ended. Other women see this as a liberating event, relieving them of concerns about pregnancy.

Men of approximately the same age experience decreased androgen levels (andropause or climacteric). Although fertility may not be impaired, changes in penile erection, ejaculation, and refractory time may occur. Sexual interest and activity may begin to wane slightly during this period. Physical changes noticed by some men may precipitate feelings of loss of masculinity, depression, extramarital affairs, and impotency.

American society places a high premium on youth, which places an additional burden on the middle adult. Efforts to remain youthful in appearance and activity can become a preoccupation for middle-aged adults. A myriad of commercial products (cosmetics, creams, clothing, exercise equipment) and medical treatments and procedures (hair transplants, plastic surgeries, liposuction) are marketed to the middle-aged adult. Some products are valid health and fitness adjuncts and can have positive benefits, but other products prey on the vulnerabilities of aging adults. The nurse can be a valuable consultant by helping the middle adult distinguish between and among these products.

Developmental Tasks and Stages

✦ **Psychosocial Development.** Erikson described the developmental task of middle adulthood as one of "generativity." This term refers to activities that are concerned primarily with establishing and guiding the next generation (Fig. 17–6). Generativity not only involves sharing with one's own children but also extends to concepts such as mentoring in the school and job arenas. Individuals who do not engage in generativity may focus only on themselves, resulting in what Erikson calls "stagnation." The healthy balance between nurturing the next generation and becoming

separated from that process results in a sense of care (Carson, 1989).

✦ **Moral Development.** Middle adults have generally reached higher levels of moral reasoning, where values are more global. Middle adults appreciate a sense of duty and make judgments based on what is best for a community. Some individuals may reach the postconventional level of moral reasoning, having internalized universal moral values such as justice, fairness, and caring as the basis for their decisions.

✦ **Spiritual Development.** Spiritually, the middle adult population provides the base for organized religions. Frequently, younger middle adults return to churches, synagogues, and mosques to provide their children with a religious foundation. With advancing years, the middle adult tends to view life from a more philosophical perspective, recognizing his or her own mortality, and spirituality becomes more valued. Middle-aged adults tend to recognize that their beliefs may represent only a partial view of the truth and may be more accepting of those with differing perspectives.

✦ **Educational Development.** Whereas young adults are viewed as being at their physical peak, middle adult men and women are seen as having the greatest influence on society. Although important demands are placed on middle adults, they are provided with limited educational opportunities to prepare themselves for future life changes (Havighurst, 1952). Education about the physiological changes associated with the aging process could help personal adjustment. Learning about and fostering new interests and activities compatible with physical changes could help the individual approaching older adulthood. Learning about and planning for the possibility of widowhood is important. Roles and functions assumed by the deceased partner will have to be learned. Education can include

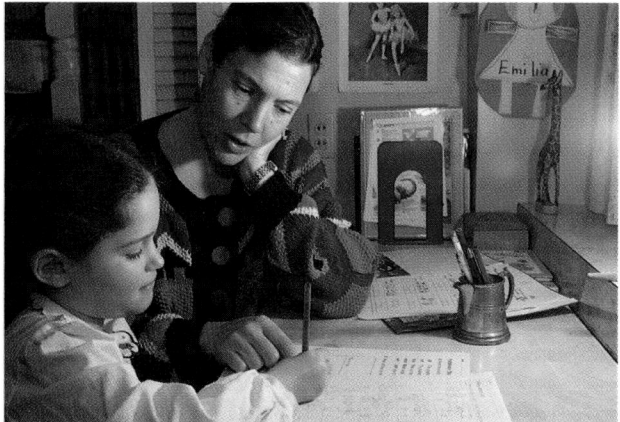

✦ **Figure 17–6**
Generativity is the developmental task of middle adulthood, according to Erikson. Nurturing and guiding the younger generation can be accomplished with one's own children or with other children and adolescents in one's extended family and community.

of life. Nursing diagnoses that may apply in middle adulthood are listed in the accompanying box.

As traditional medical care becomes costly and difficult to access, more middle adults are using alter-

ALTERNATIVE HEALTH PRACTICES

Increasing numbers of clients are using alternative or complementary therapies to promote health, reduce stress, and manage illness. The following is a list of some of the more commonly used complementary therapies.

Acupressure	Hypnotherapy
Acupuncture	Light therapy
Application of heat or cold	Meditation
	Music
Aromatherapy	Naturopathy
Biofeedback	Nutritional supplements
Chiropractic	Osteopathy
Guided imagery	Progressive relaxation
Herbal remedies	Tai Chi
Homeopathy	Therapeutic touch
Humor	Yoga
Hydrotherapy	

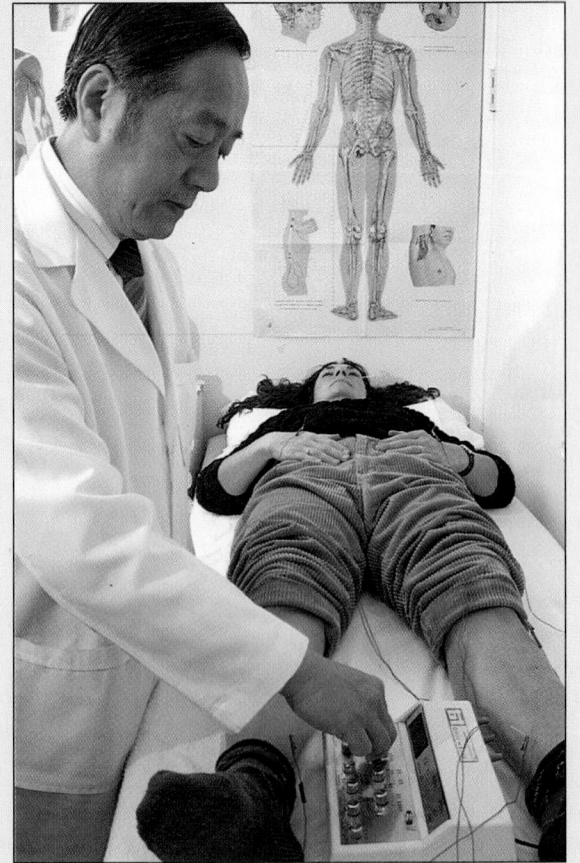

Acupuncture

formal classroom courses in preretirement at a community college or local support, church, or civic group.

In general, health habits and lifestyles begun in young adulthood influence the health of the middle adult. Programs of regular exercise, nutritious eating, stress management, and adequate rest enhance the middle adult's response to the normal aging process. A pattern of regular self-examinations and medical checkups increases the likelihood of early detection of illness. In general, improved medical care, better-informed individuals, and healthier lifestyles make the period of middle adulthood a relatively healthy and productive time of life.

The Nursing Process and the Middle Adult Client

Assessment and Nursing Diagnosis

Nurses working with middle adults are better able to make assessments, analyze and identify problems, plan interventions, and evaluate outcomes when they fully understand the anticipated stressors of this time

native and complementary health alternatives such as practitioners of chiropractic, acupuncture, massage therapy, hypnosis, and naturopathy (see box). The nurse needs to be informed about these practices in planning with the client for optimal wellness.

✦ **Career.** By the early middle adult years, the individual is in the midst of pursuing a selected career. Later in middle adulthood, the individual has achieved status within his or her career and is making plans for retirement. More and more middle adults are retiring from one career only to begin a second. Some may return to school for additional or new education and training; others may turn hobbies into productive employment.

Many middle adults seek the counseling of financial planners to help them prepare for a retirement that will allow them to pursue their interests. Because children may be grown and no longer financially dependent, it is a good time to reassess fiscal resources. Homemakers may choose to return to employment and careers they put on hold while caring for their families. Some working wives may decide to stay at home as the financial responsibility for children ceases. Middle adults may find time to volunteer with community agencies and to become more involved with leisure interests such as gardening, reading, crafts, or other hobbies. For two-career families, one middle adult may decide to retire earlier than the other, requiring role shifts within the relationships. Upon retirement, couples who have had active, independent lives may find that they have more time together. This can be a rewarding discovery, but it can also produce strain on the relationship. The couple may need to become reacquainted, or they may find that they have few common interests.

All these changes can produce stress, and for the physically compromised individual, this may result in illness. A person's career often represents an important aspect of his or her self-esteem. Loss of career status, even by choice, can affect how individuals feel about themselves. The nurse can help the middle adult cope with these anticipated changes related to career by reviewing alternative choices and discussing consequences for the individual and the couple. Thoughtful planning and open discussion help minimize the stress associated with changes in career status.

Possible nursing diagnoses would be

Role Performance, Altered
Self Esteem Disturbance
Knowledge Deficit

✦ **Sexuality.** Middle adulthood is a period of normal physiological change. Women experience menopause, the cessation of menses, during this time. As a result of lower estrogen levels, perimenopausal women may experience weight gain, hot flashes, sweating, fatigue, depression, sexual dysfunction, memory loss, and dizziness. Hormone replacement therapy can reduce these symptoms and provide protection against osteo-

porosis and ischemic heart disease ("Wonder Drug," 1994). However, women who generally feel healthy during menopause and are able to accept menopausal symptoms as normal bodily changes may not require any treatment (Bernhard & Sheppard, 1993).

Some women feel relieved that the potential for pregnancy is over and are able to enjoy sexual activity more fully. Other women view menopause as the end of a productive and useful period. Emotional lability associated with changes in hormones may influence decisions made during this time. Women who feel that they have not reached their potential may decide at menopause to actively pursue unmet personal goals, such as resuming an interrupted career or assuming a new one. These resultant changes in roles, responsibilities, and relationships may cause stress for the individual or the couple.

Men also experience a sexual and emotional change during middle adulthood, sometimes called andropause or climacteric. Men may interpret these changes in sexuality differently. Some men are particularly vulnerable and may seek additional relationships to confirm their sense of masculinity, producing stress for the individual and the couple.

The nurse can help the middle adult recognize the normal physiological sexual changes associated with growing older, adapt to these changes, and continue satisfactory sexual activity. Lubricating adjuncts can alleviate a couple's discomfort from dry intercourse. Changes in foreplay practices may augment the arousal and orgasmic phases of sexual activity. Through increased knowledge of the anatomy, the physiology of sexual functioning, and the psychological importance of sex for the individual, the nurse can minimize any embarrassment associated with discussing sexuality with a client. However, there may be specific sexual issues that the nurse feels are best addressed by a specialist in the area: a gynecologist, a urologist, or a sex therapist. The nurse should help the client seek and use such specialities and encourage honest and open communication about sexual concerns.

Although normal physiological changes occurring in middle adulthood affect sexual intercourse, sexual interest and attraction between individuals do not change. Intimate relations may improve as the pressures of raising a family and developing a career ease. Middle adult couples may have greater opportunity for special times together.

Possible nursing diagnoses related to sexuality in middle adulthood include

Sexuality Patterns, Altered
Anxiety
Adjustment, Impaired

✦ **Physical Health.** A number of physical changes are associated with middle adulthood. Obvious changes apparent to the individual and to observers include graying of hair and/or balding; increased wrinkling of the skin; the need for appliances to enhance the senses, such as glasses and hearing aids; the tendency to gain weight; and loss of muscle tone, resulting in changes in body shape. Changes apparent primarily to the individual may include a decrease in physical strength and a longer exertion recovery time, changes in sleep patterns and food choices, and longer time for memory searches. Rest-producing sleep and good sleep hygiene practices are especially important (see box).

It is never too later to make positive lifestyle changes. Middle adults who did not adopt patterns of regular exercise, nutritious eating, and stress management or who did not decide to stop smoking or reduce alcohol consumption can choose to do so at this point in their lives and experience health benefits.

The nurse can help the middle adult distinguish the normal physical changes associated with aging from those that may indicate the need for medical intervention. Although physical changes may impact the individual's lifestyle and sense of self, the nurse can help the middle adult redefine himself or herself to include a more physically mature self-concept. The nurse can reinforce the preventive teachings of earlier

years to influence the middle adult to decide on a healthier lifestyle.

Possible nursing diagnoses related to physical health in middle adulthood include

> Fatigue
> Health Maintenance, Altered
> Nutrition: More Than Body Requirements, Altered
> Sleep Pattern Disturbance
> Thought Processes, Altered

✦ **Relationships.** Middle adulthood can be a time of important transitions in roles and relationships. Studies of middle-aged men reveal that many undergo tumultuous transitions that are at least as great as those experienced during adolescence (Julian *et al.,* 1992). Typically, men have their strongest intimate relationships in the context of marriage, so the quality of that marital relationship is pivotal in midlife. Changes in marital status associated with separation and divorce are more likely to occur during this time.

Middle adults are affected by the decisions of their adult children. Individuals may decide to relocate to be closer to their children for emotional, physical, or financial reasons. This relocation can result in the additional stress of leaving familiar communities and friends. The separation and divorce of children can also have a direct impact on the middle adult couple, who may find themselves financially and emotionally supporting adult children and grandchildren. In the instance of remarriage, new "step" and "half" relationships are created that may not always blend successfully. Middle adult grandparents may find themselves removed from relationships with grandchildren as a result of separation, divorce, or distance.

Aging parents may require additional financial, physical, and emotional support from middle-aged children. Some middle adult children may bring parents into their own homes for care; others may decide on nursing home placement. The decision about how best to care for a parent is often fraught with complex emotions such as guilt, anger, love, resentment, and fear. Family members may not agree or may have unrealistic expectations about who should provide care. The aging parent may have to be rotated among middle adult children for financial, emotional, and availability reasons. This is disruptive not only for the parent but also for the middle-aged adult child. However the logistics of care are worked out, the middle adult may have to be actively involved in sharing or assuming responsibilities for parents who are living longer.

The latter years of middle adulthood may find the individual widowed. The transition from being a couple to being single again is a difficult one for both men and women. Roles, skills, and functions once assumed by the deceased partner must now be performed by the survivor.

Those individuals who have chosen single status may also find middle adulthood difficult. Friends and coworkers may relocate as a result of job changes,

HEALTH PROMOTION AND PREVENTION

GOOD SLEEP HYGIENE PRACTICES

- Determine individual sleep requirements. Go to sleep at the same time every night for several weeks and sleep until you awaken naturally.

- Establish a consistent pattern of sleep. Go to sleep and wake up at the same time, even on weekends.

- Use your bed and bedroom only for sleeping and other pleasurable activities. Do not eat, watch television, read, or study in bed.

- Evaluate the bedroom environment for lighting, noise level, and temperature conducive to sleep.

- Reduce fluid intake before bedtime to prevent sleep interruption for urination.

- Do not exercise, use alcohol, consume caffeine, or smoke before going to sleep, as these activities stimulate the body. Exercise in the late afternoon or early evening is sleep promoting.

- A warm bath before bedtime is conducive to relaxation and slows metabolism.

- Eat a light snack before bedtime. Hunger interferes with sleep.

- Deal with any problems or concerns, follow up on details of the day, and plan for tomorrow before going to bed. Active thinking impedes sleep.

- Limit daytime naps to 20 minutes.

- If you have difficulty falling asleep after 20 minutes, get out of bed and do something quiet and relaxing and return to bed when tired. Tossing and turning increases stress and is likely to delay sleep.

marital changes, or retirement. Making new friends requires continued effort.

Nurses can help middle adults use healthy coping strategies to address the relational changes associated with this period. The nurse can refer the individual to appropriate support groups for widows and widowers, for retiring individuals, and for the children of aging parents. These groups provide information and networking to help the middle adult cope with particular changes in relationships.

Possible nursing diagnoses related to relationships in middle adulthood include

Spiritual Distress
Social Interaction, Impaired
Role Performance, Altered
Situational Low Self Esteem
Powerlessness
Anticipatory Grieving
Fear

Planning, Intervention, and Evaluation

Primary Prevention

Health education is the primary prevention strategy in the middle adult years. The nurse should support the individual's continued practice of routine self-examinations and medical checkups. Helping individuals anticipate and plan for the physical, biological, social, and psychological changes that may occur during this period is also an important intervention. The nursing role may include referral for specific services: ophthalmologist for vision problems; otologist for hearing problems; physicians for medical concerns; support groups for special circumstances such as Alcoholics Anonymous, Weight Watchers, and children of parents with Alzheimer's disease; community groups such as the YMCA or YWCA for programs of exercise, stress management, and leisure activity; and even financial planners. The nurse needs to be fully aware of the resources in the community to help the middle adult establish a network of services and agencies that can provide assistance in maintaining and restoring health.

Secondary Prevention

The leading causes of death for middle adults are, in order of prevalence, cancer, heart disease, injuries, stroke, suicide, liver disease, and chronic lung disease (*Healthy People 2000*, 1990). All these conditions can be prevented in whole or in part by assuming personal responsibility for lifestyles or social behaviors that affect health. As people learn more about how certain practices are related to fatal conditions, they have the opportunity to choose healthier behaviors.

✦ **Substance Abuse.** Social behaviors can be related to health risk during middle adulthood. Lung cancer is the most common cancer seen in these years, yet it is the most preventable. Over three quarters of lung cancer deaths are related to cigarette smoking. Changing

a lifestyle that includes smoking may contribute substantially to the individual's longevity and the quality of life. Abuse of alcohol is a significant factor in the incidence of unintentional accidents and cirrhosis of the liver. Changing a lifestyle that includes the excessive use of alcohol can reduce the chance of death from accidents and illness.

✦ **Physical Health.** Approximately 100,000 deaths from coronary heart disease and 15,000 deaths from cerebrovascular accident or stroke occur in the middle adult years. High blood pressure or hypertension is an etiological factor in both these disorders. Regular physical examinations and appropriate medications can reduce the risk of heart disease and stroke resulting from high blood pressure.

The individual can assume responsible health practices to improve coronary risk factors. Unhealthy dietary habits, such as the consumption of excess fat and sodium, and alcohol abuse can be changed. Exercise and weight reduction help lower blood pressure. Low- to moderate-intensity exercise for at least 45 minutes five times a week is the most effective for weight control (Grubbs, 1993). Similarly, stress management techniques, such as deep relaxation, guided imagery, and recreational activity, are effective means of reducing hypertension. The tendency to put on weight during middle adult years can also affect mobility by placing additional strain on body joints. Men may choose to join health clubs or engage in sports activities to confront weight gain. To ensure successful weight maintenance, middle adult women need to reduce their daily caloric intake by 200 to 300 calories and adhere to a program of regular exercise. Walking, bicycling, swimming, and aerobics are popular exercises. Middle-aged women who selected exercising with weights reported improved muscular strength and felt better about how their bodies looked (Tucker & Mortell, 1993).

When working with clients whose weight places them at risk for medical problems, the nurse should be mindful that an individual is more likely to participate in programs of exercise, nutrition, and stress management that are convenient and enjoyable. A detailed health assessment and a plan developed collaboratively with the client are most apt to produce desired outcomes.

Sudden death during exercise is a rare but dramatic event. Men older than 40 who have led sedentary lifestyles, people in their 30s with coronary artery disease, and postmenopausal women should consider exercise testing before beginning an exercise program (Sherman, 1993). Exercise immediately after eating puts additional stress on the cardiac system. Every exercise program should begin with warm-ups and conclude with cool-down exercises. Performing exercise in areas where there is a heavy carbon monoxide concentration should be avoided. Although the benefits of exercise outweigh the risks, if possible, exercise should be delayed until at least an hour after awakening. Middle-aged adults should limit exercise programs involving competitive sports. In the heat of competition, important physical symptoms may be disregarded. Ignoring these symptoms may result in serious health problems for the middle-aged adult.

Although rare in this middle adult population, chronic degenerative diseases do occur. Multiple sclerosis or osteoarthritis can devastate an individual's life by necessitating changes in career performance, family functioning, and general independence. Postmenopausal osteoporosis resulting in frequent bone fractures can be treated with estrogen replacement therapy, in addition to dietary calcium supplements. Medication for coronary disease may result in impotence for some men in their middle adult years—a disturbing condition that can be helped medically.

How people react and adjust to learning that they have an acute or chronic disease is highly individualized. The method of coping selected by a person is based on previous successful coping strategies. In a study of men and women who had cardiovascular disease, Badger (1992) found that women reported less disruption in their lifestyles from the disease than did men. The nurse needs to assess each client's previous adaptation to stressful situations, the particular meaning the disease has for the client, and the personal fears that he or she may be anticipating.

✦ **Relationships.** An acute or chronic illness affects family, friends, and community. Roles and responsibilities of family members may have to change to accommodate the functions previously performed by the person who is now ill. Friends may be called on for additional favors, and employers may be called on to create flexible scheduling. An illness in midlife comes at a person's most productive period. Spouses, children, and friends may be overwhelmed at having to become unexpected caregivers. With more complicated medical treatments occurring in the home, family members are expected to balance these additional medical demands with those usually occurring during this time of life. The nurse should recognize that caregivers need support and information. The nurse can help caregivers by including spouses and other family members in planning and deciding on interventions, encouraging the free expression of feelings, and encouraging and facilitating opportunities for socialization to reduce caregiver isolation. By recognizing the individual needs of caregivers and clients, the nurse can facilitate an adjustment to the acute or chronic illness (Foxall et al., 1985).

Individuals who are not prepared for or who are resistant to the changes and transitions of the middle adult years may experience psychological problems. People who feel isolated, uncared for, hopeless, helpless, and worthless may develop a clinical depression. Dysfunctional grief from actual or perceived losses such as death, separation, divorce, or retirement may also result in depression.

The nursing role in secondary prevention continues to include health education and referral, but it may begin to require direct care as individuals experience specific illnesses. The nursing process is aimed at restoring the middle adult to his or her optimal level of wellness and making successful adaptations as they are required. Care needs to be individualized and must take into consideration the client, family, work setting, resources, and future plans. Holistic care for an individual necessitates that the nurse consider all aspects of the client's life that will have an impact on restoring wellness.

A sense of well-being is a subjective or perceived condition. It encompasses contentment, pleasure, happiness, spiritual experiences, and activities that move one toward the ideal human potential (Orem, 1991). In a study of 153 healthy middle-aged women, Hartweg (1993) found that the nurse did not have to generate ideas for the promotion of well-being but simply had to assist women in developing and enhancing those actions that they had already identified in their self-care systems. The client actually defines wellness and the quality of life that he or she desires. The role of the nurse is to help the client establish and maintain habits that protect health into the older adult years.

Summary of Middle Adulthood

The middle years of adulthood are a time of multiple transitions. Roles, relationships, and health habits all have an impact on the wellness of the middle adult. Health habits that stress prevention help the middle adult minimize the risk of illness and move on to older adulthood as a healthier individual. The role of the nurse during this time is to continue to stress health practices that promote well-being, foster early illness detection and intervention, and help restore the ill adult to his or her highest level of wellness.

CHAPTER HIGHLIGHTS

✦ The steps of the nursing process—assessment, diagnosis, planning, intervention, and evaluation—provide a valuable framework for helping young and middle adults cope with anticipated and unanticipated stressors in their lives.

✦ Effective stress management has become an essential factor in the primary prevention of illnesses in young and middle adults.

✦ The nurse's knowledge and skill in crisis intervention techniques can assist young and middle adults in managing stressful transitions effectively.

✦ Although young adults are usually believed to be at their peak physical health, age alone is not sufficient to prevent illness.

✦ After successfully establishing their identity during adolescence, young adults are challenged to commit themselves to others in intimate relationships.

✦ The nurse's primary role among young adults is as educator.

✦ Routine self-examination practices begun in young adulthood can provide early detection of potentially serious health problems.

✦ All leading causes of death for middle adults (cancer, heart disease, injuries, strokes) can be prevented in whole or in part by assuming personal responsibility for lifestyles or social behaviors affecting health.

✦ The multiple, simultaneous demands of the young and middle adult years require the purposeful management of healthy habits (proper nutrition, rest, exercise, relaxation) to minimize the risk to personal health.

✦ Middle adults may find themselves "sandwiched" between the needs of their children and those of aging parents.

✦ Middle adults who anticipate the physical and psychological changes associated with aging and learn effective coping strategies will be better prepared as older adults.

Study Questions

1. Which of the following best describes what Erikson meant by *generativity?*

   a. taking a grandchild to the movies
   b. tutoring children in an after-school program
   c. watching children enjoy themselves playing in the park
   d. watching a neighbor's child while she goes shopping

2. As middle-aged adults develop spiritually, they

   a. become more tolerant of other people's perspectives
   b. are less likely to participate in organized religions
   c. avoid the reality that life is coming to an end
   d. frequently decide to enter the ministry

3. Which of the following is *not* an example of primary prevention by the nurse when working with a young adult?

   a. promoting regular physical and dental checkups
   b. teaching self-examination procedures
   c. explaining the importance of proper diet, exercise, and rest
   d. providing support after a substance-abuse relapse

4. During which phase of the nursing process is the nurse most likely to say to the middle adult, "Tell me about the chest pains you have been feeling?"

   a. assessment
   b. planning
   c. intervention
   d. evaluation

5. Middle adults may find themselves having to provide care for an ailing spouse or a parent. Which of the following is *not* a good strategy by the nurse to help the caregiver and the patient manage care at home?

   a. include family members in decisions about interventions
   b. encourage the free expression of feelings
   c. make arrangements for the caregiver to have relief
   d. take over all decisions about care and treatment

Critical Thinking Exercises

1. Ms. D., age 26 years, is 4.5 months pregnant. She has a 3-year-old daughter, is married, and works full time as a nurse. She is found to be in labor prematurely and is ordered to maintain bed rest for the duration of her pregnancy. Discuss the implications of bed rest for Ms. D.

2. Mr. S., age 55 years, is diagnosed with new myocardial infarction (heart attack). He has smoked two packs per day for 30 years, is married, and works as an air traffic controller. He has two children, ages 19 and 21 years, as well as a grandchild to be born at any time. Discuss the health promotion teaching you would implement for Mr. S.

References

Aguilera, D. C. (1994). *Crisis intervention theory and method* (7th ed.). St. Louis: Mosby.

Anderson, K. N. (ed.). (1994). *Mosby's medical, nursing and allied health dictionary* (4th ed.). St. Louis: Mosby.

Badger, T. A. (1992). Coping, life style changes, health perceptions, and marital adjustment in middle-aged women and men with cardiovascular disease and their spouses. *Health Care for Women International, 13*(1), 43–55.

Bernhard, L. A., & Sheppard, L. (1993). Health, symptoms, self-care, and dyadic adjustment in menopausal women. *Journal of Obstetric, Gynecologic, and Neonatal Nursing, 22*(5), 456–461.

Carson, V. B. (1989). *Spiritual dimensions of nursing practice*. Philadelphia: W. B. Saunders.

Erikson, E. H. (1950/1963). *Childhood and society* (2nd ed.). New York: W. W. Norton.

Fowler, J. W. (1974). Toward a developmental perspective on faith. *Religious Education, 69*(2), 207–219.

Foxall, M. J., Ekberg, J. Y., & Griffith, N. (1985). Adjustment patterns of chronically ill middle-aged persons and their spouses. *Western Journal of Nursing Research, 7*(4), 425–444.

Gilligan, C. (1982). *In a different voice*. Cambridge, MA: Harvard University Press.

Grubbs, L. (1993). The critical role of exercise in weight control. *Nurse Practitioner: American Journal of Primary Health Care, 18*(4), 20, 22, 25–26.

Hartweg, D. L. (1993). Self-care actions of healthy middle-aged women to promote well-being. *Nursing Research, 42*(4), 221–227.

Havighurst, R. J. (1952). *Developmental tasks and education*. New York: David McKay.

Healthy people 2000: National health promotion and disease prevention objectives. (1990). U.S. Department of Health and Human Services, pub. no. 91-50212.

Julian, T., McKenry, P. C., & McKelvey, M. W. (1992). Components of men's well-being at mid-life. *Issues in Mental Health, 13*(4), 285–299.

Kohlberg, L. (1968). Moral development. In *International encyclopedia of social science.* New York: Macmillan.

Lierman, L. M., Young, H. M., Powell-Cope, G., Georgiadou, F., & Benoliel, J. Q. (1994). Effects of education and support on breast self-examination in older women. *Nursing Research, 43*(3), 158–163.

Natow, A. B., & Heslin, J. (1993). *The fat counter.* New York: Pocket Books.

Orem, D. E. (1991). *Nursing: Concepts of practice* (4th ed.). St. Louis: Mosby–Year Book.

Peplau, H. E. (1957). Therapeutic concepts. In *The league exchange.* New York: National League for Nursing.

Piaget, J. (1965). *The moral judgment of the child* (M. Gabain, Trans.). New York: Free Press.

Sherman, C. (1993). Sudden death during exercise: How great is the risk for middle-aged and older adults? *Physician and Sports Medicine, 21*(9), 92–94, 98–99, 101–102.

Snyder, M. (1992). *Independent nursing interventions* (2nd ed.). Albany, NY: Delmar Publishers.

Spencer, G. (1989). *Projections of the population of the United States by age, sex, and race 1988.* Washington, DC: U.S. Department of Commerce, Bureau of Census.

Tucker, L. A., & Mortell, R. (1993). Comparison of the effects of walking and weight training on body image in middle-aged women: An experimental study. *American Journal of Health Promotion, 8*(1), 34–42.

Wonder drug. (1994). *Nursing Times, 90*(4), 32–36.

Bibliography

Edelman, C., & Mandle, C. L. (1986). *Health promotion throughout the life span.* St. Louis: C. V. Mosby.

Levinson, D. J., Darrow, C. N., Klein, E. B., Levinson, M. H., & McKee, B. (1978). *The seasons of a man's life.* New York: Knopf.

Murray, R. B., & Zentner, J. P. (1985). *Nursing assessment and health promotion throughout the life span* (3rd ed.). Englewood Cliffs, NJ: Prentice-Hall.

Sheehy, G. (1977). *Passages: Predictable crises of adult life.* New York: E. P. Dutton.

THE OLDER ADULT

LORRAINE M. WHEELER,
MSN, RN, CS

LEARNING OBJECTIVES

✦

After studying this chapter, you should be able to

✦ Identify demographic trends associated with aging, including gender, racial and ethnic diversity, and marital status

✦ Compare and contrast the aging society to the changes in society at large to include compression of morbidity, employment, retirement, allocation of health care resources, and long-term care

✦ Define the invisible generation and relate the concept of ageism

✦ Describe the changes that occur in the aging body, with an emphasis on systems at risk

✦ Discuss the impact of the aging mind on the aging process

✦ Relate the steps of the nursing process to the care of the older adult

Warning
Jenny Joseph

When I am an old woman I shall wear purple
With a red hat which doesn't go, and doesn't suit me.
And I shall spend my pension on brandy and summer gloves
And satin sandals, and say we've no money for butter.
I shall sit down on the pavement when I'm tired
And gobble up samples in shops and press alarm bells
And run my stick along the public railings
And make up for the sobriety of my youth.
I shall go out in my slippers in the rain
And pick the flowers in other people's gardens
And learn to spit.

You can wear terrible shirts and grow more fat
And eat three pounds of sausages at a go for a week
Or only bread and pickle for a week
And hoard pens and pencils and beer mats and things in boxes.
But now we must have clothes that keep us dry
And pay our rent and not swear in the street
And set a good example for the children.
We must have friends to dinner and read the papers.

But maybe I ought to practice a little now?
So people who know me are not too shocked and surprised
When suddenly I am old, and start to wear purple.

(From selected poems published by Bloodaxe Books
Ltd. Copyright © Jenny Joseph 1992.)

This poem conveys to us a wealth of images and understandings of making the transition to the second half of life. Aging is inevitable. Everyone grows older. This poem challenges us to respond differently to the changes that accompany aging. One of the most dramatic demographic trends affecting America today is the aging of the population.

Demographic Trends

In 1995, there were 32.3 million persons 65 years of age and older in the United States—19.2 million women and 13.0 men. They represented 12.7% of the US population.

The fastest growing segment of the older population consists of those 85 years of age and older. By the year 2000, the number of people over 85 years of age is expected to double to 4.2 million. Between the years 2010 and 2030, the most rapid increase is expected as baby boomers reach age 65. By 2030, there will be about 70 million older persons, more than twice as many as in 1990. The population over 65 years of age is projected to represent 13% of the population in the year 2000 but will be 20% by the year 2030.

We are an aging society. One in eight Americans, or 31 million people are elderly. Most Americans will survive to their elder years. Life expectancy in 1990 is projected to be 75 years, and chances of surviving to age 65 have risen to 80%. As we examine the demographic data, we begin to see that we have relatively more middle-aged and older people than young people, compared with past decades. In 1990, we had as many people 60 years and older as we had children under the age of 14. More and more people in their 50s and 60s have surviving parents, aunts, and uncles. The four-generation family is becoming common.

Compression of Morbidity

In times past, families did not have to consider providing for the needs of the frail elderly. People simply did not live long enough to require assistance for a long time. With advances in science and modern medicine, people living beyond age 85 represent one of the most rapidly growing groups. The *oldest* old is an increasing proportion of the elderly population. In 1990, the 85-and-over group was only 4% of the population. It is now 10%. The Census Bureau had never measured the 85-and-over population separately before 1990. This shift is called the **"compression of morbidity."**

The oldest of the old becoming frail and disabled has a major impact on families and on the health care system of the nation (Bureau of the Census, 1991). A larger population of elderly requires a greater service level for higher incidence of disease and injury.

Racial and Ethnic Diversity

The trends in racial and ethnic diversity are dramatic and have produced a mosaic of cultures in our cities and towns. Minority populations are projected to represent 25% of the elderly population in 2030, up from 13% in 1990. Between 1990 and 2030, the white non-Hispanic population 65 and older is projected to increase by 93%, compared with an average of 396% for all other minorities. This group breakdown is shown in Table 18–1 (Fowles, 1993).

Sociopolitical Policy Issues

Fragmented families, mobility, and emerging retirement patterns of the elderly separate them from family members. Thus, the aging of American society increas-

Table 18–1

PERCENTAGE OF PROJECTED GROWTH IN ELDERLY MINORITY POPULATIONS BETWEEN 1990 AND 2030	
MINORITY GROUP	**PROJECTED GROWTH, %**
Hispanics	555
Non-Hispanic African-Americans	160
Native Americans, Inuits, and Aleuts	231
Asians and Pacific Islanders	639

From American Association of Retired Persons. (1993). *A profile of older Americans.* Washington, DC: American Association of Retired Persons. © 1993, American Association of Retired Persons. Reprinted with permission.

ingly results in the elderly needing more governmental support, which requires the Congress to examine public policy areas and implement legislation to act on these findings. Demographic trends play a significant role in shaping public policy in aging. Consider these factors:

* The elderly will make up an increasingly larger proportion of the US population through the middle of the next century. By 2030, one person in five will be 65 or older.
* Women over age 85 will account for higher proportions of the elderly population.
* Because women marry younger than men and outlive men, most elderly women are widows. Most elderly men are married and live with their wives. Elderly women living alone tend to be poorer and at greater risk of institutionalization than the general elderly population.
* Higher rates of poverty exist among the very old, those living alone, and African-Americans.
* Social Security benefits are and will continue to be the largest single source of income for most elderly people.
* The cost of programs to benefit the elderly has grown rapidly. There will be growing competition as the senior boom and baby boom collide early in the next century, placing enormous pressures on programs that benefit the elderly.

The Economics of Retirement

The declining population of entry-level workers for the balance of the century and the increasing population of elderly people may require revisions and regulations related to older workers and retirement. It may be necessary to provide greater incentives for older workers to remain in the work force longer if we are

to have enough skilled workers to run our businesses and to support those who cannot work.

Allocation of Health Care Resources

The cost of health care in this country has skyrocketed. Because the elderly are major consumers of health care services, this inflation in cost has placed a special burden on this group and on the programs that care for them. It becomes imperative that we find a solution to containing climbing health care costs before the senior boom begins.

Long-Term Care

The number of elderly people needing long-term care is expected to rise sharply in the next several decades because of the growing numbers of people over the age of 85 and the growing numbers of elderly people living alone. The need for public help in providing long-term care is expected to grow because the traditional caregivers—adult women—are increasingly working outside the home and are not as likely to be available for full-time care in the future. Currently, public support for long-term care is very limited and is biased toward medical treatment, institutional care, and away-from-home support and family assistance (Congressional Clearinghouse on the Future, 1985).

The Invisible Generation

We have long thought of ourselves as a nation of youth. One has only to look at media images to believe we are all still in our 20s. Older Americans are generally invisible in our society. The most common treatment of old persons is not to treat them at all. Although older persons participate in virtually all daily activities, they are often absent from printed and audiovisual materials. **Ageism** refers to the discriminatory ways in which older persons are treated. It is an insidious denial of the potential of all individuals and another form of bigotry. Consider the age-old stereotypes in Table 18–2 and reflect on how different the "reframed" responses are.

Another facet of ageism is language use. The words we use often demean, patronize, and further stereotype the older person. Think of what images come to mind as you reflect on the terms in Table 18–3.

How often have you made comments about or perhaps simply had negative thoughts that you kept to yourself regarding older adults?

Table **18–2**

BIASED AND REFRAMED LANGUAGE OF AGING

AGEIST/BIASED	REFRAMED/NOT BIASED
What does an old man like that want with a sports car?	Now that his children are on their own, he can have that sports car that he's always wanted.
That man she's with must be half her age!	Men of all ages find her attractive.
When people get old, they become fault finding, irritable, and demanding.	Some people are more fault finding, irritable, and demanding than others.
Ask my grandmother, I'm sure she'll do it. She always has plenty of time.	Ask my grandmother. She always tries to find time to help others.
I hate the thought of getting older because all getting older means is physical complaints and illness.	Getting old is natural and sure beats dying. I'm going to take care of myself now so I'll feel good later.
All old people are invalids.	Most old people are self-sufficient.
The old are always sick and end up in nursing homes.	Everyone gets sick sometimes, and the elderly are no exception. While older persons are generally more susceptible to disease and injury, few live in nursing homes.
Old people belong on the shelf. They shouldn't take a younger person's job.	No one belongs on the shelf. We all have something to contribute.
What do they have to look forward to? Food stamps and old age relief!	Most older persons live comfortably, but some are poor and wholly dependent on food stamps and social security benefits. They help, but not enough.
Old people should retire. They've lost their skills. They can't do a decent job.	Forced retirement does not make sense for individuals or businesses. Many older persons have valuable skills that can only be acquired over many years.
Retired people just sit and watch life pass them by.	In retirement, many people become involved in activities they didn't have time for when they were working.
Tennis is a game for the young. As with most sports, a 35 year old is over the hill.	Tennis is a sport for all ages. You may slow down as you get older, but by using the strategic expertise developed over the years, you can still play a tough game.
A smart politician goes after the youth vote.	A smart politician does not overlook the power of any segment of voters.
Most older people are socially isolated and lonely.	The degree to which a person is socially isolated is not determined by his or her age.
Most older people are neglected by their families.	Most old people are close to their families.
It's silly for people over 65 to fall in love.	You're never too old to fall in love.
Old people are unable to adjust to change.	Some people are slow to adjust to change.
Most old people are pretty much alike.	All people are individuals who become more unique with age and a lifetime of experiences.

Biopsychosocial Perspective

What does it mean to grow old? We are all growing older from the time we are born. What is normal aging? There are many theories of aging. One theory supports the idea that aging is simply wear and tear on the body. This theory suggests that our body structures and functions inevitably "wear out" from overuse. In contrast, stress adaptation theory describes effects from the residual damage of accumulated stresses. Physical, psychological, social, and environ-mental stressors, both internal and external, contribute to the body giving up. When the body is no longer able to resist the stress, it dies. "Aging, physiologically speaking, it is the decline and fall of practically everything . . . [that] must eventually produce some sort of *clinical debility*" (Johnson, 1985, p. vii). Nursing theorist Rogers explains aging as ". . . not running down, not as disease, but as a *developmental process* that begins at conception" (p. 35).

We do not all age at the same rate or in the same way. Some of us may have healthy hearts but struggle with alterations in the digestive tract. Others may feel

Table 18–3

DEMEANING DESCRIPTORS OF AGING

DESCRIPTORS	EXAMPLES
Patronizing adjectives	Cute, sweet, dear, little
Negative physical description	Crippled, deaf, emaciated, feeble, fragile, frail, gray, doddering, wrinkled
Negative personality description	Cheerless, eccentric, queer, sad, senile, obstinate, foolish, meek
Demeaning labels	Old maid, old codger, old biddy, fuddy duddy, Geritol generation, over the hill, out of date, has been, fading fast
Stereotypical descriptions	Passive, dependent, frivolous, shrewish, nagging

From American Association of Retired Persons. (1986). *Truth about aging, guidelines for accurate communications.* Washington, DC: American Association of Retired Persons. © 1986, American Association of Retired Persons. Reprinted with permission.

a broken spirit while maintaining a youthful body. Some may suffer from psychological problems such as depression. A number of factors contribute to this puzzle: genetics, lifestyle, economics, and education. One person may live actively to near 80 years, bowl three games, and then return home to collapse and die of a massive heart attack. Another's health begins to degenerate soon after retirement when he or she becomes less and less active. What makes the difference? Where is the line between normal aging and the disease process?

Currently, scientists are conducting a longitudinal study to determine answers to these questions. The Baltimore Longitudinal Study on Aging (BLSA) has been ongoing for 35 years (National Institute on Aging, 1993). Begun in the late 1950s, it has over 1100 participants, both men and women. Using these data, scientists have produced over 600 articles and reports that have helped change aging research, clinical practice, and the way we view aging. There are really three overall threads or themes to research with BLSA data:

* Longitudinal changes
* The relationship between health and disease
* Fundamental biology of aging (Fig. 18–1)

This study of transitions helps us to examine the normal aging process and follow its progression into states of "dis-ease" that sometimes, but do not always, accompany aging. Dis-ease is the body's way of alerting us to a disruption with our ease of living. We are "out of sync," out of balance, out of harmony with

ourselves. The findings can be studied from three perspectives: the aging body, the aging mind, and the aging spirit.

The Aging Body

The Integumentary System

Aging skin is frequently one of the first changes noticed as we grow older. Cosmetic changes of aging can be upsetting to us as we watch the force of gravity and aging processes produce flabby and wrinkled skin. Crow's feet and wrinkles are often the first visible signs that the body is changing (Fig. 18–2). Wrinkles occur when the deep layer of the skin, the dermis, loses moisture and elasticity. Factors such as genetic endowment play an important part in this process. Perhaps the most important factor in aging of the skin is exposure to the sun. One has only to look at the faces of those living in sun-belt areas of the country to be reminded of what impact the sun has on wrinkles. Skin that never sees the light of day remains smooth and elastic much longer. While younger women may worry about wrinkles and invest in expensive skin care products, studies have shown that women over the age of 65 tend to dismiss wrinkles as not worth worrying about. Itching may also become more common in older people due to the loss of oils in the skin.

The effects of skin aging are less noticeable in males because men have more oil in the sebaceous glands, which lubricate the skin. In men, hormonal changes account for scalp hair loss. Most men can anticipate some loss of hair, particularly male pattern baldness. Male pattern baldness is a genetic trait that is passed down from mothers or fathers. Graying of the hair is caused by loss of hair pigmentation and also is associated with genetic endowment. Graying is neither harmful nor the sign of a worrisome person. These physical changes are ongoing reminders of a fleeting youth for some people.

The Cardiovascular System

Circulation sets the pace for the aging body. In the BLSA study, participants, moving rhythmically on treadmills, have shown scientists that the older heart *adapts* to the effects of age. The healthier older exercising heart increases its output in a somewhat different but just as efficient manner as the younger heart. However, coronary artery disease does increase as people age. Scientists have learned that exercise screening can be useful in detecting cardiovascular disease in people who have a family history or other risk factors for the disease, such as smoking or elevated cholesterol levels in the blood (National Institute on Aging, 1993).

Women develop cardiovascular disease on average 10 to 20 years later than men, even when carrying

HOW THE BODY AGES

The Baltimore Longitudinal Study of Aging is yielding information on how people age *on the average*. It is important to remember that many people do not conform to these averages.

Lungs: Maximum breathing capacity decreases 40% between ages 20 and 80.

Pancreas: Glucose metabolism declines progressively, as measured by glucose tolerance test.

Blood vessels: Arterial walls thicken; systolic blood pressure increases 20–25% between ages 20 and 75.

Muscles: Muscle mass declines, and with it oxygen consumption during exercise decreases 5–10% per decade. Hand grip strength decreases 45% by age 75.

Bones: Bone mineral is lost and replaced throughout life; loss begins to outstrip replacement around age 35; loss speeds up in women at menopause.

Brain: Memory and reaction time may begin to decrease around age 70.

Eyes: Difficulty focusing on close objects begins in 40s; ability to see fine detail decreases in 70s. From age 50, susceptibility to glare increases, ability to see in dim light decreases, ability to detect moving targets decreases.

Ears: Ability to hear high-frequency tones may decrease in 20s, low-frequency in 60s; men lose hearing more than twice as quickly as women between ages 30 and 80.

Heart: Heart rate during maximal exercise decreases 25% between ages 20 and 75.

> ❧ **Figure 18–1**
> The Baltimore Longitudinal Study on Aging, ongoing over several decades, has yielded information shown here on how the body ages. (From National Institute on Aging, National Institutes of Health. [1993]. *With the passage of time: The Baltimore Longitudinal Study of Aging.* NIH Publication No. 93-3685. Bethesda, MD: National Institutes of Health.)

the same risk factors. Whereas men may suffer a sudden death–type heart attack, women are more likely to develop angina, a condition of chest pain on exertion that indicates that the heart muscle is getting in-

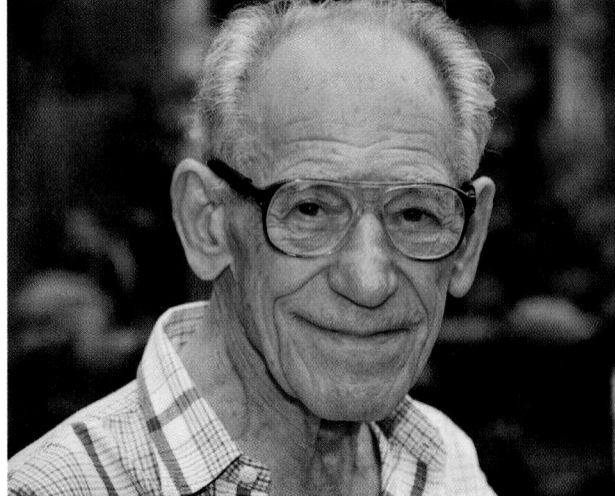

> ❧ **Figure 18–2**
> Wrinkles, a visible sign of aging, occur when the deep layer of the skin loses moisture and elasticity. Genetic factors and sun exposure are important influences on the degree of wrinkling.

sufficient oxygen. It is believed that estrogen protects a woman from cardiovascular disease, making estrogen replacement therapy an important consideration for postmenopausal women. When women do develop heart disease, the outlook is much grimmer than that for men, because women are two to three times more likely to suffer a second heart attack within 5 years of the first than are men.

Although women are less susceptible to heart disease as they grow older, their risk of developing hypertension is actually greater. High blood pressure becomes common in both men and women after age 65. Called the silent killer because it causes no symptoms, high blood pressure damages the kidneys, eyes, blood vessels, and heart. This damage leads to renal failure, blindness, stroke, and heart attack. People with high blood pressure are three times more likely to suffer a heart attack, five times more likely to develop congestive heart failure, and eight times more likely to experience a stroke (National Institute on Aging, 1994).

It is a well-documented fact that high cholesterol levels remain a risk factor for cardiovascular disease. Earlier studies focused only on middle-aged men. Recent studies indicate that people ages 65 to 96 with high cholesterol levels continue to be at an increased risk. Women are more likely than men to have elevated cholesterol levels. Nearly 50% of women over age 55 have high blood cholesterol compared with less than 33% of men of the same age (National Institute on Aging, 1994). The findings point the way to preventive measures, such as a low-fat diet and perhaps cholesterol-reducing drugs well into old age.

Physical Fitness

Physical fitness declines about 5 to 10% per decade on average. The best known measure of physical fitness is oxygen consumption. In older people, during exercise, oxygen use declines. However, older athletes maintain higher levels of oxygen than do older people who are less active. A study of 184 BLSA participants (National Institute on Aging, 1993) showed that a major reason for oxygen decline was decline in muscle mass. Muscle tissue consumes the vast majority of oxygen during exercise, and when it declines, oxygen use also declines. While lean muscle declines with age, the other component of body composition, fat, tends to increase with age.

The BLSA study has shown that across the adult age span, increasing fatness around the abdomen is associated with lower glucose tolerance, increased blood pressure, and shifts in levels of cholesterol and other fats. Moderate weight is linked to a longer life than that for people who are very fat or very thin. A study of BLSA participants shows that those who gained a moderate amount of weight over the years have lived longer in general than those who remain youthfully slim. Findings such as these document how important it is to maintain an exercise program as we grow older (Fig. 18–3) (National Institute on Aging, 1993).

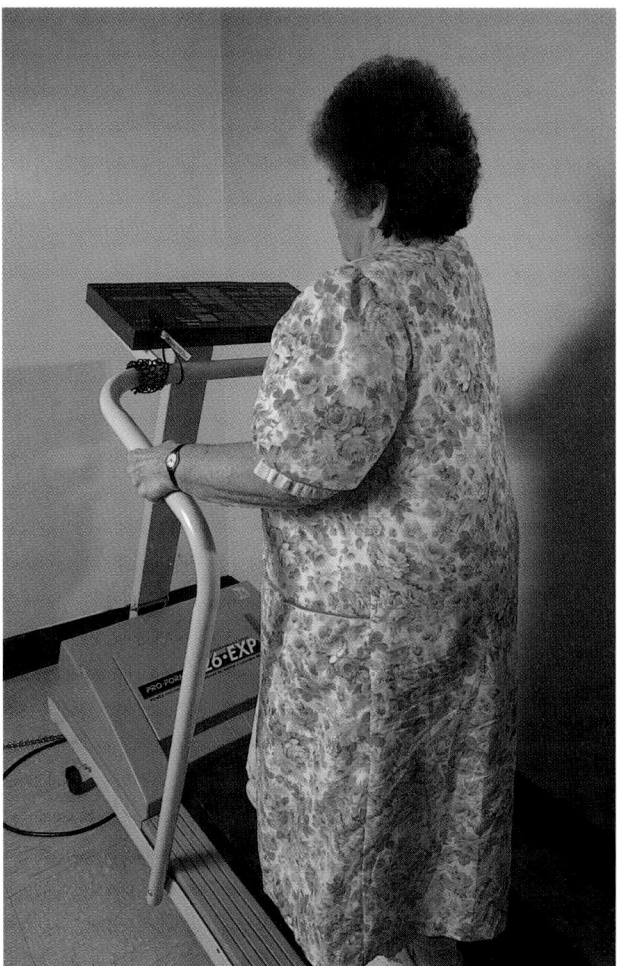

✦ **Figure 18–3**
Physical exercise helps older people maintain health by increasing oxygen consumption and moderating weight. This 83-year-old woman exercises on a treadmill.

Nutrition

High levels of high-density lipoproteins ("good cholesterol") are associated with high vitamin C levels, which seem to protect against plaque build-up in the arteries. Vitamins A, C, and E, known as antioxidants, help rid the body of oxygen free radicals, which are considered harmful. Studies suggest that these vitamins may help protect against heart disease, cataracts, cancers, and other conditions common with advancing age.

As scientists study nutrient intake among those over age 65 years, they find that vitamin B_6, magnesium, and zinc intake is substantially low, although we live in a well-nourished and health-conscious society. Thus, the nurse can encourage increased intake of these nutrients.

The Respiratory System

Lung capacity falls by about 40% between ages 20 and 80. This decline appears to be universal and due purely to aging. Those who smoke or suffer from other diseases will lose lung capacity at a higher rate.

The Musculoskeletal System

Our bones constantly lose cells and replace them throughout life. Around age 35, the rate of bone loss speeds up; the rate outstrips replacement. In women, bone loss speeds up again around the time of menopause. As women age, they lose more than half the density of the top of the femur and 42% of the density of vertebrae in the lower back. While men also lose bone density, it occurs at a slower rate. Ongoing studies focus on differences in bone loss between older and younger men.

We still do not understand why the prevalence of some diseases, like osteoporosis, increase with age. Osteoporosis is a condition characterized by brittle, porous bones that are susceptible to fracture. By age 40 years, men and women begin to lose bone mineral because of decreased ability to absorb calcium. With age, calcium absorption decreases as much as 50%, and healthy bones lose density.

Many people begin to feel old when they awaken to stiff joints in the morning. Arthritis, or inflammation of the joint tissues, is more common in older men and women. When it occurs in women, it is usually more severe. Joints lose flexibility with age and are more subject to accidental injury because of tissue changes in supporting tendons, ligaments, and muscles. This age-related breakdown in connective tissue fibers reduces joint mobility and reinforces the importance of stretching exercises for older people.

Gastrointestinal Changes

Changes in lifestyle, use of medications, and reduced physical activity all contribute to the digestive problems of the elderly. However, changes occurring in the digestive system are relatively minor. Muscles may move more slowly as they propel food through the digestive system. Less stomach acid is produced, and ability to absorb some nutrients is impaired. Use of laxatives can affect absorption of vitamins and minerals. Older persons should eat a diet high in fiber, fruits, and vegetables and limit animal proteins and fats. Moderate intake of salt, sugar, caffeine, and alcohol is recommended. Interestingly, stomach ulcers are twice as common in men than women as we age.

While lung cancer claims the lives of many, cancers of the colon and rectum are high for white males and even higher for black males. Environment, lifestyle, and diet high in fat are linked to a high incidence of colon cancer.

The Urinary Tract

A hidden, embarassing problem many women face as they age is stress incontinence, or the inability to control the passing of urine. Often it occurs following physical exertion such as coughing, sneezing, or lifting. The pelvic floor muscles become weaker with age, particularly in women who are overweight or have borne children.

As many as 80% of men over the age of 50 experience enlargement of the prostate, possibly due to hormonal changes. The prostate gland produces fluid that is needed to transport and nourish sperm. Men may find urination difficult due to enlargement of the prostate. Sometimes older men experience bouts of prostatitis, or inflammation of the prostate gland.

The Aging Mind

While progressive loss of neurons and a general loss of total brain bulk occur with aging, mental capabilities can remain sharp well into old age (see Box). The best insurance against a cloudy old age is to "use it or lose it." While people may slow down a little and may be a bit more forgetful as they age, older adults in general remain as intelligent and creative as ever. One

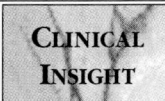

CLINICAL INSIGHT

Research on Aging and the Brain: Three Different Approaches

Changes in Mental Functioning

Memory and problem solving remain strong until at least age 70 and then do not decline in most people. Aging is not linked to declining mental skills.

Health and Disease

Researchers can now pinpoint early markers of when the brain is passing from normal to diseased states. For example, decline in immediate visual memory is an early marker for later developing Alzheimer's disease.

Biological Changes in the Brain

Ongoing studies in brain structure and function use brain scans to determine whether cognitive changes, *i.e.,* visual memory and mental skills, are related to biological changes.

From National Institute on Aging. National Institutes of Health. (1993). *With the passage of time. The Baltimore Longitudinal Study of Aging.* NIH Publication No. 93-3685. Bethesda, MD: National Institutes of Health.

has only to observe older people in shopping malls or senior centers actively engaging in various activities to see clear examples of this.

Dementia and Alzheimer's disease are two conditions that do affect the mental capacity of older Americans. **Alzheimer's disease** is a type of dementia characterized by carelessness, loss of judgment, and loss of interest in everyday living. Alzheimer's disease affects more women than men. This is simply due to the fact that most victims are over the age of 80 years, an age at which women outnumber men two to one. Scientists believe that Alzheimer's disease is most likely caused by a genetic predisposition coupled with an environmental trigger, such as a virus or toxin. People with Alzheimer's may live 15 years or more with brain deterioration as their only illness.

Dementia is cumulative damage from small strokes. These mini-strokes block blood flow to the brain, causing death of brain tissue. These infarcts subsequently cause disability. Risk may be reduced by eating properly, exercising regularly, and maintaining a normal blood pressure. Conditions such as depression, adverse drug reactions, and hypothyroidism may present with dementia-like symptoms, causing many elderly people to be misdiagnosed as suffering from dementia.

The brain, like the heart, may do more adapting and less declining with age than was previously thought. After age 70, vigilance declines sharply in many people, and more time is needed to respond to stimuli. *Vigilance* is described as the ability to respond to infrequent and unpredictable stimuli. For example, an elderly person may have slower reaction times when driving a car. Gender differences show that women do better at remembering words, and men have higher scores when it comes to immediate recall of numbers.

Future studies on the aging brain are aimed at using **magnetic resonance imaging (MRI)** and **positron emission tomography (PET)** for a period of years to learn more about how changes in visual memory and other mental functions are linked to brain structure and function.

The Senses

Hearing

On average, low-frequency hearing begins to fade between the ages of 60 and 70 years. However, different aspects of hearing decline at different rates. Generally, high-frequency tones are the first to become difficult to hear. Men lose their hearing twice as fast as women. Studies show that women on average have more sensitive hearing at all ages.

Vision

Studies of eyesight, cataracts, and contrast sensitivity explore changes with age. Vision tends to decline with age, although the ability to see fine detail changes little until one's 70s. The lens of the eye becomes cloudy and hardens, sometimes leading to cataracts. The ability to distinguish between light and dark declines with age, although scientists believe that contrast sensitivity may be a better gauge of how we actually see. Glare and peripheral vision difficulties are particularly troublesome to older people. Frequently older people do not drive at night because of "night blindness" or problems with headlight glare.

Smell

The sense of smell deteriorates as one ages, requiring modifications in food presentation. Older persons slowly lose the ability to smell and lose the pleasure derived from fragrant scents.

Taste

Taste buds are destroyed by 50% as one ages, causing older persons to lose their appetite and not enjoy eating as they once did.

Touch

As with the other sensory losses of aging, the kinesthetic sense of touch requires more adaptation, as the older person reacts more sensitively to hot and cold.

Sexuality and Aging

Sexual functioning in older adults is one area of great variability. There is sex after 60. It is simply different. Common changes in sexual functioning for men can include delayed and less firm erection, less seminal fluid, and briefer orgasms followed by longer periods before erection is possible. For women, changes occur in the genitalia. Tissues in the vulva become thinner, and a woman will take longer to arouse and to lubricate. Many women report that after menopause, when fear of pregnancy and the distractions of midlife have passed, they become more sexually responsive.

Couples may need to use lubricating creams and lotions to compensate for some of these changes. While age is one factor in loss of libido, psychological factors also play a role. Overwork, family conflict, depression, or fear of impotence may all compound the changing sexual picture as people age.

The main difficulty with a woman's sexuality in later years is not her inability to perform but the unavailability of suitable partners. Because women outlive men by 7 or 8 years, most married women are eventually widowed. The average age of widowhood is 56 years; by the age of 65, 52% of women are widowed. By the age of 75, this figure increases to 68%. At the same time, most older men are still married. Creative aging attempts to transcend the common generalizations of aging as a biological problem and old age as a disease.

Menopause

Whereas age-related changes thus far have been compared between men and women, menopause is one age-related change belonging exclusively to women. When a woman's life expectancy was an average of 51 years, the age of menopause was around 46 years and thought to mark the end of a woman's life. Today, women achieve menopause around age 50 and are expected to live to about age 78. This means that a woman will live one third of her life after menopause; thus, menopause marks a new phase of a woman's life. Many women are not prepared for this transition.

The period leading up to the menopause is called the climacteric. During this period, 75% of women report experiencing hot flashes. Hot flashes, lasting a few minutes, are surges of heat felt in the neck, face, chest, and arms. The flash may be accompanied by sweat, shallow breathing, and a quickened pulse. The skin may turn red. Afterward, a woman may feel chilled and out of breath. As the ovaries begin to cease functioning, their production of estrogen also decreases. The pituitary gland in a compensatory effort begins to release more pituitary hormone and mistakenly sets the body's thermostat too high. Although they can be embarrassing, irritating, and inconvenient, hot flashes are not a debilitating condition. Symptoms often associated with menopause such as irritability, moodiness, loss of skin tone, insomnia, lack of energy, and change in sex drive may not be totally due to menopause. Changes in marital status, changing work patterns, the emptynest syndrome, and the need to care for aging parents may all contribute to the picture.

The Aging Spirit

We are always the same age inside.

—Gertrude Stein

Personality remains stable over the life span. Studies have concluded that despite serious illness, disease, life crisis, and transition, as people age they are no more cranky, no more conservative, and no more prone to complaining about their health than when they were younger (National Institute on Aging, 1993).

Biologists seek to explain aging by describing changes at the cellular and molecular levels. Sociologists describe aging in terms of roles and role theory. Numerous developmental models exist that seek to name and explain psychological issues surrounding the second half of life. Developmental psychologists speak of changes before physical maturity as differentiation of the person and changes after differentiation as aging. A single definition of aging is impossible when one attempts to describe such a complex process (Gress & Bahr 1984).

Generativity Versus Stagnation

Older adults are challenged to grow or die (Erikson, 1963). Using Freud's dynamics as a foundation, Erikson describes specific developmental tasks of older adulthood. Stage VII is depicted as **generativity** versus **stagnation** (Table 18–4). Generativity refers to growth. Stagnation is a sense of staleness. The challenge to the individual is to remain actively involved while evolving new concepts for coping with the larger world (Fig. 18–4). Terms such as *hope, will, purpose, competence, fidelity, love, care,* and *wisdom* complement this stage. Carlsen (cited in Gress & Bahr, 1984, p. 58) speaks of our adult capacity to care:

In youth, you find out what you care to do and who you care to be—even in changing roles. In young adulthood you learn whom you care to be with—at work and in private life, not only exchanging intimacies, but sharing intimacy. In adulthood, however, you learn to know what and whom you can take care of.

Integrity Versus Despair

Aging adults struggle to place closure on their lives. Older age is often a period of intense reflection.

Table 18–4

ERIKSON'S STAGE VII—STAGNATION VERSUS GENERATIVITY

STAGNATION	GENERATIVITY
Boredom	Energy, motivation
Mental decline	Mental growth
Self-absorption	Other-absorption
Obsessive pseudo-intimacy	Promotion of next generation
Narcissistic self-indulgence	Production of offspring
	Care of offspring
	Altruistic and creative acts

From Carlsen, M. B. (1991). *Creative aging: A meaning-making perspective.* New York: W. W. Norton.

Erikson's final stage of adult development is **integrity** versus **despair** (Table 18–5). Integrity is defined as a "sense of coherence or wholeness." It is the ability to keep things together at a time of losses and linkages in every aspect of living. These losses include biological, psychological, and sociological losses. Integrity implies that one has played the roles and met the challenges associated with previous stages. As one finds a way to make life count for something, one becomes part of the ongoing flow or current of all that has occurred before. The gift of this stage is the virtue of wisdom.

Wisdom, as an end-of-life state of mind, prepares us for death, as is summarized in this quote by Peck (cited in Carlsen, 1991, p. 50):

Then might not the human end-point be this: to achieve the ability to live so fully, so generously, so unselfishly that the prospect of personal death looks and feels less important than the secure knowledge that one has built for a broader future, for one's children and one's society, than one ego could ever encompass.

Table 18–5

ERIKSON'S STAGE VIII—INTEGRITY VERSUS DESPAIR

DESPAIR	INTEGRITY
Arousal/anxiety/blocking	Serenity
Pulling in from life	Continuity, openness to life
Decline of perceptual acuity	Growth or maintenance of perceptual acuity

From Carlsen, M. B. (1991). *Creative aging: A meaning-making perspective.* New York: W. W. Norton.

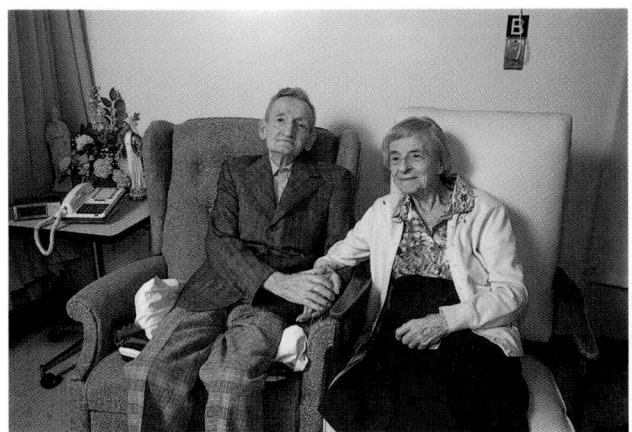

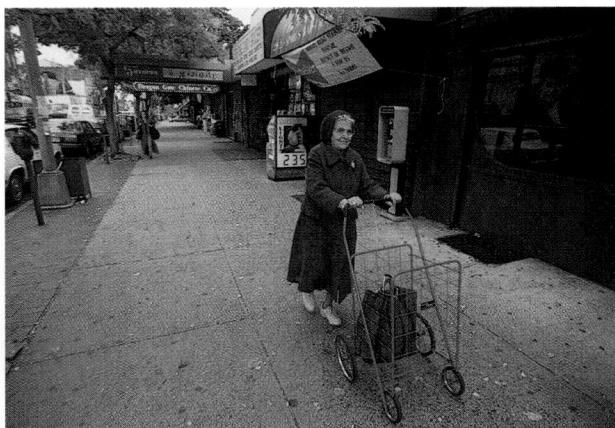

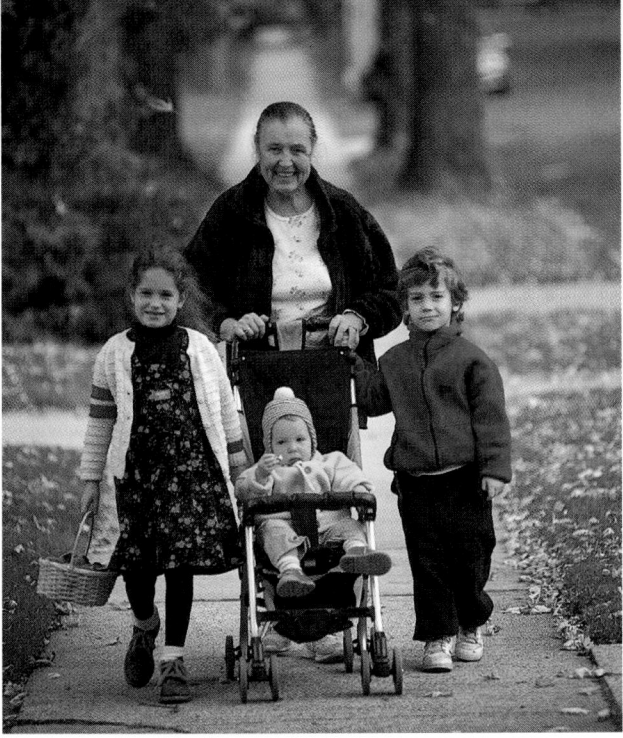

🔖 **Figure 18–4**
According to Erikson, a developmental task of older adulthood is generativity versus stagnation. A loving relationship with a spouse or grandchildren and active participation in community life (*e.g.*, shopping, socializing) are examples of positive influences during this stage of life.

The Dilemmas of the Second Half of Life

Abrahams (1983) identified a strong theme of "forgiveness seeking" in elderly people's attempts to master ego integrity and cope with guilt at the perceived failure in meeting their youthful grandiose expectations and omnipotent fantasies. It is important for nurses to recognize forgiveness seeking as a significant need.

Jung (1971) viewed the second half of life as having a purpose of its own. He believed that the tasks of the second half of life included reflective activity and inner discovery of other parts of the self previously left untapped. Jung's models are closely related to philosophical and spiritual aspects of aging.

Spiritual development is one aspect of adult development often overlooked in understanding how we age and the changes that occur. Because of its intangible nature, spiritual growth is not a well-researched dimension. However, if we are going to consider the whole human being, spirituality must be included. We can observe that more importance is placed on spirituality as people grow older. For example, more older adults than younger people support and attend religious institutions. Other creative outlets for spiritual growth are women's and men's circles, prayer groups, and religious services, which provide a center of activity for many senior groups.

Peck (cited in Carlsen, 1991) defined the tasks of the second half of life by building on Erikson's concepts (Table 18–6). Aging people must become actively engaged in the second half of life. Redefining the self, letting go of occupational identity, coping with bodily discomforts, and establishing personal meaning demand a shift from self-centeredness to

Table **18–6**	
PECK'S MODEL OF THE DILEMMAS OF THE SECOND HALF OF LIFE	
Midlife alternatives	Valuing wisdom vs. physical powers Socializing vs. sexualizing in human relationships Cathectic flexibility vs. cathectic impoverishment Mental flexibility vs. mental rigidity
Alternatives in later aging	Ego differentiation vs. work-role preoccupation Body transcendence vs. body preoccupation Ego transcendence vs. ego preoccupation

other-centeredness. Everyone may not be up to this task. Carlsen (1991), in her efforts to transform limiting patterns of thought and relationship, attempts to stimulate the following in her aging clients:

* Wisdom and integrity over stupidity, ignorance, and despair
* Generativity and care over self-aggrandizement and narcissistic preoccupation
* Open mindedness over rigid, closed thinking
* A willingness to entertain new ideas over opinionated self-righteousness
* Transcendent relationship over extremes of either self or other

Much of what happens during the second half of life is a recycling process. Old issues resurface and are recycled with a new perspective, and there is an opportunity to rework previous challenges. In this respect, the second half of life is a time of hope and renewal. The old adage applies: "We're not getting older, we're getting better."

Havighurst (1948) formulated a sequence of demands for successive periods of life that may be relevant today. His model is one of the few that breaks down in decades the tasks of the second half of life in a chronological manner. It is important not to view these tasks concretely but to remember that there is always movement across stages when one attempts to describe psychological development. Recently, developmental psychologists have reframed Havighurst's model as a sequence of thought questions useful in any period of transition.

The question to ask during this period is "How much and in what ways do I chose to engage?" The aging person possesses the freedom to decide what is possible rather than focusing on personal limitations or perhaps even to reframe personal limitations in light of what is possible.

Twelve percent of older Americans were in the labor force in 1992 (Gress & Bahr 1984) (Fig. 18–5). As we approach the end of the century, we will see many centenarians among our population. We hear examples of writers, artists, teachers all working well into the twilight of their life. Advances in medical science and technology have produced a shift in the definition of who is old and when work stops.

Nursing Process and the Older Adult

Assessment

The multiple theories that apply to the growth and development of the older adult require nurses to perform comprehensive, individualized, and multifactoral assessments. In some settings, the multidisciplinary team approach may be useful. Each team member reports from his or her area of expertise. Disciplines

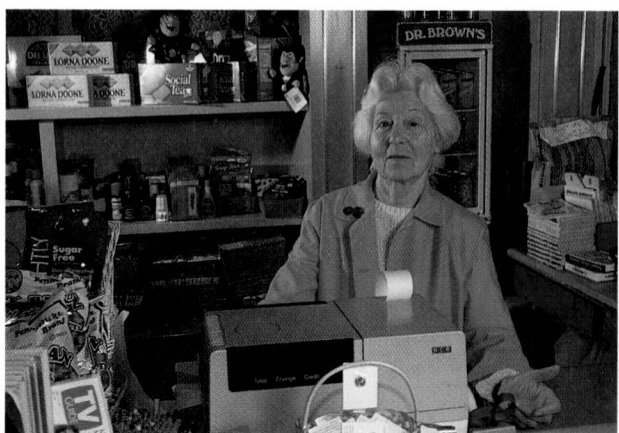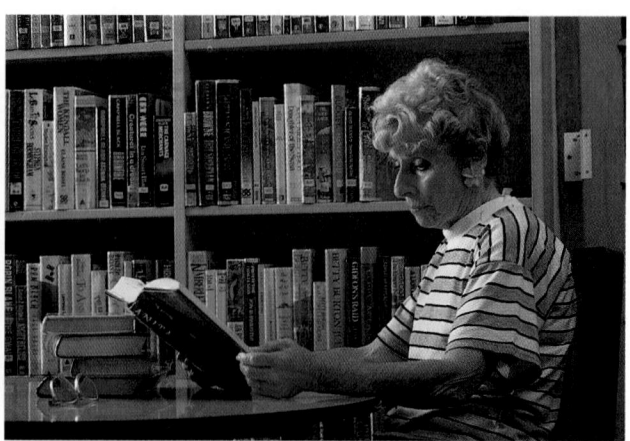

✦ **Figure 18–5**
Many older people continue to work and learn after the traditional retirement age. These activities provide intellectual stimulation and active engagement with others in the community.

represented on multidisciplinary teams include internal medicine, nursing, gerontology, psychiatry, nutrition, activity therapy, social services, clergy, and family members. The nurse's role in these settings is to coordinate all of this information into a holistic picture of the client. Sometimes special assessment forms are used.

Interviewing skills are among the most important tools that the nurse utilizes in assessing older adults. Listening actively and communicating clearly are fundamental when interviewing aging people. Other extremely important factors when interviewing older adults are

1. Sensitivity to perceptual losses.
2. An attitude of respect and caring. Adequate time must be set aside to make the experience pleasant. Elderly clients may require more time to answer questions, and if the nurse is rushed or pressured, clients may be inaccurately labeled as demented or noncooperative.

The setting should be quiet, private, and free of distractions. It may be necessary to reorient the client several times in the course of the interview. Verbal and nonverbal cues should be observed and integrated with cognitive and behavioral information. Emotional material may be harder to elicit in the older adult for a variety of reasons, including sensory losses, confusion, problems verbalizing feelings, shame and embarrassment, and fear of revealing too much of the self and thus becoming vulnerable to stigmatization. It is essential that the nurse establish a trusting, patient, and supportive attitude when interviewing elderly clients without becoming patronizing. The interview may need to take place in several short sessions if the client tires easily. When family members are present, they can provide invaluable assistance in providing the missing information or in assisting when information is contradictory.

Physical assessment skills utilized in assessment of the older adult include inspection, auscultation, palpation, percussion, and the ability to order the appropriate tests as needed. Initial data collection consists of subjective and objective data, including biological and psychological information, social support, financial aspects, spiritual beliefs, and ethnic differences. Comprehensive nursing assessments are required. For example, the Medical Data Set (MDS) 2.0 required for Medicare reimbursement insists on a systematic and thorough approach to data collection. The data are usually computerized, and analysis is necessary to make substantial nursing diagnoses. The nursing problems identified fuel the care planning process and often start with problems in cognition; move on to activities of daily living, such as dressing, grooming, and bathing; and include nutrition and toileting. There are scales to measure behavioral symptoms and degree of pain. The process is highly individualized and allows us to make objective and informed decisions as we plan nursing care for our aging population. In addition, it expands our thinking to include a global perspective so that we are making decisions based on objective data collection and analysis and not simply on our own assumptions or experience.

The expanding immigrant population in our country has significant implications for nursing. For instance, an Asian immigrant to this country may believe that Eastern remedies are the only methods that can cure an illness and may refuse to use "modern medicine." In addition, it is important to note strengths and previously useful coping mechanisms. Questions such as "How did you handle that the last time it happened to you?" are useful in eliciting this information.

The nursing assessment is usually completed on a form for this purpose. If the setting is a specialty center for the older adult, many of the modifications and adjustments necessary to conduct a comprehensive interview will be noted on the form.

The nursing assessment for the older client must be adapted to meet the unique problems associated with this age group. While basic nursing assessment tools provide baseline information, the following information should be added or included to produce a comprehensive view of the individual (Matteson and McConnell, 1988):

1. Activities of daily living: walking, transfer, bathing, dressing, continence, and eating
2. Instrumental activities of daily living: telephoning; household chores, including meal preparation, transportation, and shopping; and administering own medication
3. Mini-Mental Status Examination
4. Lifestyle, including exercise, diet, and use of social drugs including alcohol
5. Nutrition
6. Social support network
7. Family support
8. Recent life changes
9. Review of desire regarding living will and do not resuscitate orders
10. Sensory impairments, including hearing, vision, peripheral sensation
11. Immunization.
12. Cancer detection protocol: breast, colorectal, prostate, cervical, and oral
13. Fall-related injuries
14. Review of medications for possible adverse reactions

Nursing Diagnosis

Phase two of the nursing process begins when all the data have been collected and the team begins to formulate a plan of care for the client. Steps required in formulating nursing diagnosis are

- Analyzing data collected in the assessment phase
- Testing the diagnostic hypotheses
- Stating the nursing diagnosis

Nursing diagnoses frequently encountered with older persons include the following:

- Activity intolerance related to chronic inflamatory disease
- Risk for injury related to sensory dificit (vision or hearing)
- Self-care deficit related to reduced ability to perform ADL's
- Risk for impaired skin integrity related to thinning of skin tissue and lessened mobility
- Social isolation related to reduced mobility and/or economic hardship

Planning

The planning of care requires an ability to set goals, choose appropriate methods to achieve stated goals, and most importantly, being able to set priorities. Several factors must be considered when planning care for the older client (see Sample Nursing

---

SAMPLE NURSING CARE PLAN

THE CLIENT WITH ALZHEIMER'S DISEASE

Ms. W. is a 78-year-old woman admitted to the hospital for evaluation of Alzheimer's disease by her daughter, who is the primary caregiver. She is confused and disoriented, and her daughter feels burned out caring for her.

Nursing Diagnosis:
1. Alteration in thought process related to senile dementia, Alzheimer's type, as evidenced by impaired memory, judgment, and problem-solving ability.
2. Alteration in role relationships, secondary to extreme dependency needs, as evidenced by daughter's reports of feeling burned out.

Expected Outcomes:
1. Patient will function at highest possible level of independence and highest level of cognitive ability.
2. Family role relationships will return to preillness state. Daughter will no longer report feeling burned out.

Action	Rationale
1. Establish trust to perform assessments and ability to work with family caregivers by introducing self, modifying admission process to include patient as much as possible.	Provides role models for family members on how to interact with client post discharge and gives client some degree of control and mastery over hospital environment.
2. Teach caregivers communication techniques using simple patterns, reduce stimulation, and establish habits and routines.	Teaching family members new ways to communicate empowers them to enjoy a more satisfactory relationship with the patient and provides needed tools to use when they may be feeling helpless in coping with a progressive, chronic illness.
3. Assess mental status daily and record changes.	Changes in thought patterns may vary as environment changes and with medications and treatments prescribed. Mental status examinations provide a baseline.
4. Assess self-care deficits and provide assistance with hygiene and nutrition as needed.	Allows client to maintain as much independence as possible while decreasing dependency on caregivers.
5. Coordinate referral with social services for respite care post discharge.	Family members who are given breaks from caregiver roles return refreshed and able to maintain their equilibrium while caring for older parents.
6. Give daughter referral to counseling services, clergy, and/or support group.	The ability to verbalize stressful feelings strengthens coping skills.
7. Administer medications and treatments as ordered, while observing for untoward effects.	Biological therapies will stabilize a chronic illness; elderly persons may be more sensitive to medications and need frequent monitoring.
8. Document care provided, patient teaching, response to teaching, and outcome of referral process.	Documentation is crucial in maintaining clear communication among all disciplines and provides a picture of what actually happened to the client for future use.

Data from American Association of Retired Persons. (1986). *Truth about aging, guidelines for accurate communications.* Washington, DC: American Association of Retired Persons; Carlsen, M. B. (1991). *Creative aging: A meaning-making perspective.* New York: W. W. Norton; and *Aging America: Trends and projections.* (1991). Prepared by the US Senate Special Committee on Aging, the American Association of Retired Persons, the Federal Council on Aging, and the US Administration on Aging. Washington, DC.

Care Plan). First and foremost, the client of his or her advocate must be actively engaged and contribute to the care planning process. Choice of treatment is determined by the specific needs that the client presents. Many variations occur. Attention to individual differences is very important. For example, a 99-year-old female client who is a retired schoolteacher with sharp cognition will need a different level of activity and stimulation than an 83-year-old man who has had a stroke and has limited mobility.

Financing and availability of treatment are also important aspects of the planning process. For example, if the patient is not going to be in your care for more than a few days, it is unnecessary to develop an elaborate teaching plan requiring a week or more to implement. When financial limitations or probable transfer to another facility or program becomes evident, it is crucial that your goals are realistic and include available resources.

Discharge planning is an essential component of the nursing process. It should begin when the client enters a health care setting of any type.

Intervention

The following interventions may be modified in working with elderly clients to achieve stated goals: direct care interventions, such as further assessment, referral, caring, performing for another, teaching, exercising, creating and/or modifying the environment, and administering medications and treatments. Indirect skills such as coordinating, advocating, setting limits, lobbying, supervising, monitoring health status, and documentation are also important.

The 10 most prevalent health conditions for persons over age 65 are listed in Table 18–7. They are

useful touchstones when planning the type of care an elderly person may require.

Emotional support and teaching of new skills will allow the client to begin to incorporate new coping mechanisms into his or her daily routine and decrease dependency on the nurse. Older patients need to feel that they have some degree of control. Because of changes occurring on many levels, clients may feel out of control and express this feeling through noncompliance with recommended treatments. The nurse must always search for ways to give clients control and the reassurance and support needed to help them succeed in self-care. Often, the nurse is teaching significant others or family members how to provide nursing care. This is especially true in home care settings where family members and other caregivers assume responsibility for the elderly. Family caregivers must be treated with respect and tolerance. They require support and reassurance that they are doing a good job.

For some, this role reversal, may require an adjustment. To find yourself responsible for a parent who once cared for you can be a frightening experience.

Interventions with older clients often require creativity. Pets, plants, pictures, tape recorders, and videos are all tools nurses can use when intervening with the older adult. The presence of children can often provide stimulation and a sense of pleasure for older persons. Reminiscing groups and other socializing activities are a direct deterrent to the isolation and withdrawal that the elderly may experience due to a change in health status (Fig. 18–6).

Based on knowledge of changes that occur as the body, mind, and spirit grow and change, several principles emerge to help guide nursing interventions with the older adult:

				Table 18–7
TEN MOST PREVALENT HEALTH CONDITIONS FOR PERSONS 65 YEARS OF AGE AND OLDER, NUMBER PER 1000 PEOPLE, 1989				
CONDITION	**AGE 45–64 y**	**AGE 65+ y**	**AGE 65–74 y**	**AGE 75+ y**
Arthritis	253.8	483.0	437.3	554.5
Hypertension	229.1	380.6	383.8	375.6
Hearing Impairment	127.7	286.5	239.4	360.3
Heart Disease	118.9	278.9	231.6	353.0
Cataracts	16.1	156.8	107.4	234.3
Deformity or Orthopedic Impairment	155.5	115.2	141.4	177.0
Chronic Sinusitis	173.5	153.4	151.8	155.8
Diabetes	58.2	88.2	89.7	85.7
Visual Impairment	45.1	81.9	69.3	101.7
Varicose Veins	57.8	78.1	72.6	86.6

COMMUNITY BASED CARE

CHEMOTHERAPY AND RADIATION

The client undergoing cancer treatment, such as chemotherapy or radiation, is often referred for home nursing care. Chemotherapy administration may occur in the outpatient or home setting. Nursing interventions are critical and include assessment of coping and potential treatment complications, helping to alleviate anxiety and fear, and teaching side effect management. Nutrition is a major concern and challenge for these clients. Chemotherapy and radiation side effects include anorexia, nausea, vomiting, stomatitis, and diarrhea or constipation. Weakness and fatigue are common. Infection, along with bleeding, is a risk, especially during the nadir period, of the chemotherapy drugs. The nadir occurs when the blood count reaches its lowest point, usually between 7 to 21 days after chemotherapy, depending on the drugs administered.

Client education is essential. Many pamphlets and brochures are available from the American Cancer Society and the National Cancer Institute to use as teaching aids. Key teaching areas include

1. Dietary interventions: encouragement of foods and fluids rich in electrolytes, calories, and protein; using dietary supplements as needed; small, frequent meals

2. Preventative mouth care to reduce the risk and severity of stomatitis: good oral care, soft toothbrushes, saline rinsing

3. Setting realistic goals, pacing activities, getting adequate rest

4. Identification of early signs of infection or bleeding; monitoring temperature and reducing the risk of infection by avoiding crowds, individuals with contagious illness, and close contact with pets, especially during nadir

5. Signs and symptoms of dehydration, bowel impaction

6. Importance of good handwashing, general hygiene, and perineal care

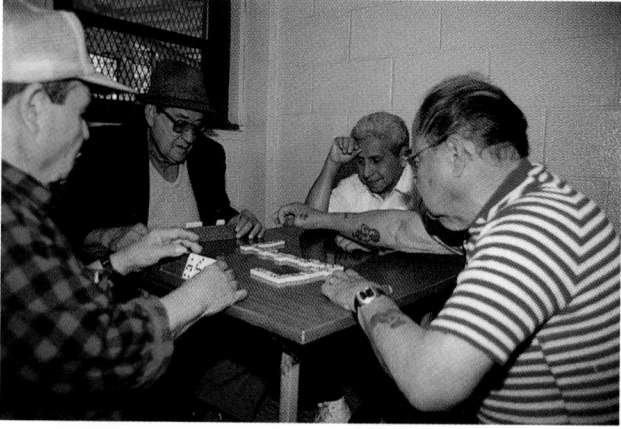

♦ **Figure 18–6**
Regularly scheduled socializing activities serve to combat isolation among older adults.

tivities that increase the older adult's sense of self-worth and self-esteem

• Establishing a safe, trusting, supportive environment in which honest expression of feelings such as loss, loneliness, and grief may be shared is essential

• Providing opportunities for life review is beneficial, as such opportunities assist individuals in resolving conflicts accrued over a lifetime to achieve a peaceful state of mind for the final stage of growth: death

• Health status and personality are important components of morale later in life and must be treated in a manner that enhances coping and reduces dysfunction and deterioration

• Americans are increasingly living longer and staying healthier, thus compressing the population of the frail elderly into a group that requires extensive services when they succumb to illness

Evaluation

As with the assessment and planning phases of the nursing process, evaluation is based on the client's appearance, behavior, and self-report. Outcome criteria guide the evaluation process. When evaluation is performed, reassessment data are compared with outcome criteria, and discrepancies are noted. If the nursing care plan is developed with realistic goals, objectives, and time frames, evaluation should reveal many achieved outcomes. Involving the elderly in outcome evaluation is important. This is another opportunity to give the client a sense of control and mastery over the environment.

As our society ages, we become increasingly dependent on our government and other groups to help meet health care needs. We will become increasingly accountable to those groups who pay some or all of the cost of care. Utilization review criteria demand that the nurse document carefully all nursing interventions and their outcomes. Thorough documentation presents a clear picture of what happened to the client while

• Sensitivity to differences among older clients requires a more thorough assessment, taking into consideration differences in psychological, cultural, spiritual, and sociological dimensions

• Ethnicity is a resource that must be treated sensitively and respectfully

• Perception and behavior are highly correlated with role changes and lack of social support in the individual's environment

• A focus on effective communication and social interactions with others through encouragement and positive reinforcement is necessary

• Behaving respectfully in all interactions helps promote ac-

under the care of the nurse. Remember, to a third party if it is not written down, it did not happen.

Aging as a Public Health Priority

As more Americans live longer lives, their impact on our health care system continues to spark intense debate. Some say that our health care system will struggle to provide fundamental services to a growing number of elderly and disabled. Others claim that as risk factors decrease and medical care improves, the onset of demanding, chronic disease will be postponed to ages even closer to death. This "compression" of morbidity will strain the health care system.

Some older persons warrant special medical attention. Two disciplines have evolved to address the specific problems of aging: **geriatrics** and **gerontology.** Geriatrics provides older persons specialized medical assistance. Gerontology studies the aging process. From the perspective of clinical care, older persons present a higher risk of frailty, a greater likelihood of having chronic disease, and a subsequent probability that their status will reflect the interaction of multiple problems rather than a single condition (Making Aging a Public Health Priority, 1994).

As we examine Table 18–5, we can readily see how illness coupled with lack of social support can create complex health care problems as one ages.

Policy Implications

The Baltimore Longitudinal Study seeks to determine what is attributable to normal aging and what is attributable to disease (National Institute on Aging, 1993). Public policy experts ask themselves questions such as "Should social security be reserved for the aged?" The aged have long been considered a separate group in our society. This group has enjoyed privileges and discounts and been favored in other ways. Now that it is no longer legal to discriminate on the basis of age and mandatory retirement is prohibited, we must ask ourselves some important questions, such as "Should social security benefits be assigned in response to need across all age groups?" Demographic trends and forecasts point to a need to study the epidemiology of aging as we consider the special needs that health care professionals will increasingly be called on to meet.

Aging represents a biological process and the accumulation of health insults over a period of time. As you begin to understand what constitutes normal aging at the individual level, you may begin to isolate environmental factors from intrinsic ones. Because older people are more sensitive to their environments, special attention needs to be paid to the threats the environment produces to optimize positive outcomes

and enhance the quality of life. Society faces enormous challenges in health care planning and public policy areas as we attempt to understand and address the challenges of an aging society.

Projections for the Future

A man is not old until regrets take the place of dreams
—John Barrymore

Emerging on the American scene is a healthier, wiser, and perhaps wealthier senior than the counterpart of only a generation ago. Characteristics of the new senior include

- Creativity and intellectual involvement: Available information in many media attract the interest of the senior, who is more likely to read books and newspapers than are younger, time-pressed adults. They travel widely and even return to college for course work and degrees. They investigate and analyze their purchases to a high degree.

- Experience and wisdom and the desire to share it: SCORE (Service Corps of Retired Executives), youth mentoring programs, and countless volunteer opportunities involve the active senior. Many find employment in settings with youthful workers, such as fast food franchises.

- Vitality and productivity: Most seniors want to remain productive members of society; they live on their own, drive themselves, and manage their affairs. Self-esteem generates from production rather than consumption. Therefore, look for seniors to be active in regular jobs and volunteer roles to a greater degree than in purely recreation pursuits.

- Compassion for others and concern for the world around them: This concern is well recognized in voting patterns and interest in political issues, particularly at the local level. Many older adults find meaning in their involvement in action programs of their religious institutions. Still others take on caring roles for relatives, grandchildren, or acquaintances.

Every decade in this century has been marked by significant tides of sociological changes. Given the upcoming increase in the older population, it is reasonable to expect the "invisible generation" to assume a stronger voice and a more visible presence in advertising, entertainment, and politics. Eldercare is likely to become a major issue and an important area of nursing care and research. Financing of care, housing the elderly, and caring for the caregivers present challenges for the nurse practicing in this rich and rewarding environment.

Summary

The fastest growing segment of the older population consists of those people 85 years of age and older. As they become frail and disabled, individual families and the health care system of the entire nation will feel the impact. There will be growing competition for resources as the senior boom and baby boom collide early in the next century, placing enormous pressures on programs that benefit the elderly. It becomes imperative that we find a solution to containing climbing health care costs before the senior boom begins.

Longitudinal research is being conducted to study the line between normal aging and the disease process, the relationship between health and disease, and the fundamental biology of aging. The findings can be studied from three perspectives: the aging body, the aging mind, and the aging spirit.

Multiple theories apply to the growth and development of the older adult. Assessments are conducted utilizing multidisciplinary teams. The actively engaged client is an important part of this process. Care planning and nursing diagnosis must be tailored to meet the individual needs of the older adult client. Care must be given based on the unique strengths and limitations of each individual. We all age differently. Greater numbers of active, productive older adults will demand increasing voice and focus by America's public policy makers as we move into the 21st century.

CHAPTER HIGHLIGHTS

✦

- ✦ We are an aging society with increasing numbers of women and minority groups represented. Compression of morbidity is a serious challenge for public policy.

- ✦ Ageism is a form of prejudice toward older persons similar to racism. Myths and stereotypes portray the elderly as invisible in our society.

- ✦ Longitudinal studies measure changes over time, the interface between health and disease, and the biology of aging. Personality remains stable over a lifetime.

- ✦ Nursing care of the elderly is much like nursing care of other populations with a sensitivity to diminished capacities in some specific areas.

Study Questions

Mrs. H. is a 62-year-old woman who lives in Sun City, Arizona. She arrives for her annual check-up at the doctor's office where you work as office nurse. She tells you that she has been staying at home a great deal and feels lonely and useless.

1. Which developmental stage is Mrs. H. currently experiencing?

   a. ego integrity versus despair

   b. generativity versus stagnation
   c. depression versus the normal aging process
   d. postmenopausal adaptation
   e. isolation versus socialization

2. The best nursing intervention you could design is to suggest that Mrs. H.

   a. go to the library, borrow some books on tape, and begin listening daily
   b. read the newspaper daily and keep up with current events
   c. volunteer her services at the local Meals-On-Wheels program
   d. recommend her husband take her to dinner and a movie weekly
   c. suggest she resume her interest in knitting

3. As you begin your physical assessment, you notice that Mrs. H. has a beautiful tan. She tells you that she takes daily walks on the golf course to stay fit. After you compliment on her exercise routine, you must further assess which of the following?

   a. the kind of walking shoes she wears to check for adequate support
   b. how long she walks and at what pace to determine cardiac fitness
   c. whether she walks alone or with friends
   d. what type of skin protection she uses
   e. whether she varies her routine with other fitness activities

4. While interviewing Mrs. H., you become impatient and feel a sense of urgency to move the interview along. The most likely reason for this is that

   a. Mrs. H. is lonely and enjoys talking to you
   b. sensory changes in aging include a slowing down of all sensory processes, including the ability to answer questions quickly
   c. Mrs. H. is not very intelligent and has difficulty answering the questions
   d. Mrs. H. is somatizing
   e. she is a new client and has lots to tell you

5. When Mrs. H. returns for a follow-up visit, she tells you that she recently was turned down for a job at a local fast food restaurant that "only hires kids." This is an example of

   a. sexism
   b. classism
   c. feminism
   d. rejection
   e. ageism

Critical Thinking Exercises

1. Ms. B. is a 60-year-old client with Alzheimer's disease who has been hospitalized for increasing confusion and disorientation. Discuss how role reversal may affect the developmental and psychosocial development of the client and her family of two daughters (ages 42 and 39). How would you begin to assess the client and her home situation? (What are the essential elements of the interview and assessment process for the aging client?)

2. New medical developments, economic security, and the ability to prolong life are contributing to an increasingly

aged population. What are some of the major medical, social, and political implications of this trend, and how might this phenomenon affect your career as a nurse?

References

Abrahams (1985). In Ebersole, H., *Towards healthy aging.* New York: C. V. Mosby.

Aging America: Trends and projections. (1991). Prepared by the US Senate Special Committee on Aging, the American Association of Retired Persons, the Federal Council on Aging, and the US Administration on Aging. Washington, DC.

American Association of Retired Persons. (1992). *Acronyms in aging.* Washington, DC: American Association of Retired Persons.

American Association of Retired Persons. (1993). *A profile of older Americans.* Washington, DC: American Association of Retired Persons.

American Association of Retired Persons. (1986). *Truth about aging, guidelines for accurate communications.* Washington, DC: American Association of Retired Persons.

Bureau of the Census, US Department of Commerce and National Institute on Aging, US Department of Health and Human Services. (1991). Growth of America's elderly in the 1980's. *Profiles of America's Elderly, 1.*

Bureau of the Census, US Department of Commerce and National Institute on Aging, US Department of Health and Human Services. (1993). Racial and ethnic diversity of America's elderly population. *Profiles of America's Elderly, 3.*

Carlsen, M. B. (1991). *Creative aging: A meaning-making perspective.* New York: W. W. Norton.

Congressional Clearinghouse on the Future. (1985). *Tomorrow's elderly: Issues for Congress.* Executive summary prepared for the House Select Committee on Aging. Washington, DC.

Erikson, E. (1963). *Childhood and society* (2nd ed.). New York: W. W. Norton.

Erikson, E. H., Erikson, J. M., & Kivnick, H. Q. (1986). *Vital involvement in old age.* New York: W. W. Norton.

Fowles, D. (1993). *A profile of older Americans.* Washington, DC: American Association of Retired Persons and the Administration on Aging, US Department of Health and Human Services.

Gress, L. D., & Bahr, R. T. Sr (1984). *The aging person: A holistic perspective.* New York: C. V. Mosby.

Havighurst, C. (1984). In L. D. Gress, & R. T. Bahr, Sr. *The aging person: A holistic perspective.* New York: C. V. Mosby.

Johnson, H. A. (Ed.). (1985). *Relation between normal aging and disease.* New York: Raven Press.

Jung, C. J. (1971). *The stages of life.* In J. Campbell (Ed.). *The portable Jung.* New York: Viking Press.

Making aging a public health priority. (1994). *American Journal of Public Health, 84,* August.

Martz, S. (Ed.) (1991). *When I am an old woman, I shall wear purple.* Watsonville, CA: Paper Mache Press.

Matteson, M. A., & McConnell, E. S. (1988). *Gerontological nursing.* Philadelphia: W. B. Saunders.

National Institute on Aging, National Institutes of Health. (1994). *Answers about: The aging man.* Bethesda, MD: National Institutes of Health.

National Institute on Aging, National Institutes of Health. (1994). *Answers about: The aging woman.* Bethesda, MD: National Institutes of Health.

National Institute on Aging, National Institutes of Health. (1993). *With the passage of time: The Baltimore Longitudinal Study of Aging.* NIH Publication No. 93-3685. Bethesda, MD: National Institutes of Health.

Peck (1988). In M. B. Carlsen, *Meaning-making perspective: Therapeutic processes in adult development.* New York: W. W. Norton.

Rogers, M. (1985). Change through environmental interaction makes aging exciting [Interview]. *Journal of Gerontological Nursing, 11,* 36.

Valliant, G. (1977). *Adaptation to life.* Boston: Little, Brown & Co.

Bibliography

Baressi, C. M., & Stull, D. E. (Eds.) (1992). *Ethnic elderly and long term care.* New York: Springer.

Birren, J. E., Bengston, V. L., & Deutchman, D. E. (Eds.) (1988). *Emergent theories of aging.* New York: Springer.

Carr, D. (1990). In D. Carr & C. A. Carr (Eds.), *Nursing care in an aging society.* New York: Springer.

Corlett, E. S., & Millner, N. B. (1993). *Navigating midlife: Using typology as a guide.* Palo Alto, CA: CPP Books.

Ebersole, H. (1985). *Towards healthy aging.* New York: C. V. Mosby.

Erikson, E. (1963). *Childhood and society* (2nd ed.). New York: W. W. Norton.

Heckheimer, E. F. (1989). *Health promotion of the elderly in the community.* Philadelphia: W. B. Saunders.

Johnson, H. A. (Ed.). (1985). *Relation between normal aging and disease.* New York: Raven Press.

Jung, C. J. (1971). *The stages of life.* In J. Campbell (Ed.). *The portable Jung.* New York: Viking Press.

Levinson, D. J., Darrow, C. N., Klein, E. B., Levinson, M. H., McKee, B. (1978). *The seasons of a man's life.* New York: A. Knopf.

Maddox, G. (1987). *The encyclopedia of aging.* New York: Springer.

Maslow, A. H. (1962). *Toward a psychology of being.* New York: Van Nostrand.

Rogers, M. (1985). Change through environmental interaction makes aging exciting [Interview]. *Journal of Gerontological Nursing, 11,* 36.

Chapter 19

THE FAMILY

SAUNDRA L. TURNER, EdD, RN, CS, FNP

KEY TERMS
◆

cultural norms
ecomap
family
family as client
family assessment

family theory
genogram
risk factors
roles
structure

LEARNING OBJECTIVES
◆

After studying this chapter, you should be able to

◆ Define terms related to family nursing

◆ Discuss theories such as developmental and systems theory

◆ Describe societal changes and their impact on family structure

◆ Define a variety of family units and inherent risk factors involved with each type

◆ Describe the nursing process in the context of the family

◆ Utilize a number of tools in the development of a family assessment and plan of care

Individual clients cope with the stressors of illness and crises in many ways. As nurses, we must make every attempt to understand which factors in clients' lives help to mediate and which increase their stress. To meet client needs effectively, the nurse must understand the environment from which the client has come. The values and beliefs, as well as cultural norms, originate from their family units. The main context within which a client defines his or her world is the family. The family unit is dynamic. As each member grows and changes, each other member is affected. The role each individual plays within the family unit is integral to the whole family system. Through increasing the understanding of the client's family, the nurse can learn how the client deals with his or her illness and what support mechanism he or she may have in moving to a higher level of wellness.

In this chapter, various types of family units are explored. Societal norms in the past and current trends are discussed. Theoretical approaches to understanding family dynamics also are outlined, and assessment tools for use in identifying strengths and needs in family support are explained.

In the delivery of nursing care to a client, the nurse must use all available resources to understand what issues are important, as well as how the client may cope with the stressors of illness. The best way in which to do this is to understand the client's context of living. The interaction patterns of the family unit and the role each individual plays in that group are of significance when trying to help both the client and the caregivers in dealing with the life crises of illness and the ensuing changes involved in recovery or lifestyle changes necessary for health promotion and illness prevention.

Not all families have positive interactions and behaviors with one another. Issues such as guilt, anger, and even fear can be identified by the astute nurse when performing a family assessment. Patterns of interaction that are normal in everyday life are often magnified in times of crisis, and health care providers must be alert to signs of both physical and emotional abuse.

The Family Defined

The Social Context

Family is a social term that is defined according to the era in which we live. It is the context of how an individual defines his or her past and present; his or her sense of belonging. In the 1950's, the family was a two-parent household with a minimum of one child. The mother was the homemaker, and the father was the breadwinner. Now as we prepare to enter a new century, a family is the group or persons with whom an individual identifies through bonds of responsibility and caring as he or she interacts with his

---

> **Box 19-1**
>
> ### FAMILY STRUCTURES
>
> Nuclear—two adults living in the home with one or more children
>
> Blended—families formed from members of previous marriages
>
> Single parent—one adult head of household with one or more children
>
> Communal—two or more family units living together
>
> Common law—two heterosexual adults living together without legal bonds
>
> Cohabiting—unmarried heterosexual or homosexual couples living together for a variety of reasons
>
> Single adult—adult living alone or with a pet
>
> Extended—family unit extended beyond the immediate boundaries of the nuclear unit, usually with parents or grandparents living in the household

or her world. As society has accepted new norms, other definitions have evolved, such as the dual-breadwinner, blended, single-parent, and single-sex family. Family members can be bound by blood, ceremony, location, or emotion. Any or all of these features can be involved in what someone calls family (see Box 19–1).

Nurses interact with clients, who also interact with their families as their caregivers, caretakers, and caring partners. Decisions that must be made about clients' worlds must be made with family members in mind.

The Family Unit

The American Family

In American society, the family norm takes many forms (Fig. 19–1). In 1970, 87% of family households consisted of married couples; in 1990, this percentage fell to 79%. In 1990, 17% of family households were female headed, up from 11% in 1970 (Haupt & Kane, 1991, p. 40). Although the traditional family unit may no longer be the actual norm in our society, it is still the ideal norm, and most adults spend at least a part of their lives in a nuclear household (Friedman, 1992). The traditions and expectations formed through time in a family are **cultural norms:** These are a family's ways of life that come from beliefs and traditions.

A family may consist of the *nuclear* family unit, or two adult family members, living in one household with dual careers. This can be a family from a first marriage or a *blended* family from previous marriages. Childless families and those with no children living at home are considered dyads. The single adult family has one adult head of household. This can result from

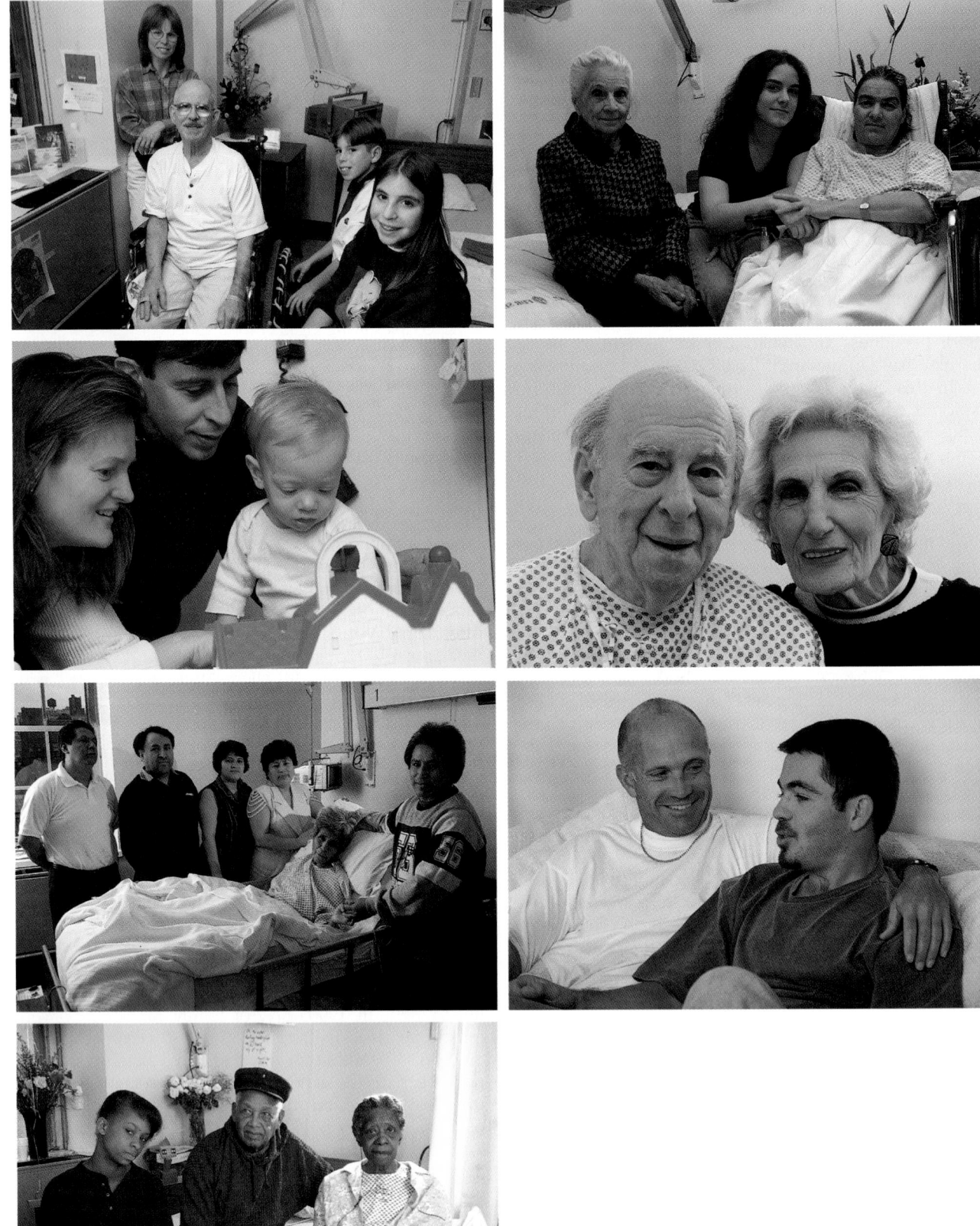

✦ **Figure 19–1**
Families have a variety of forms, and each one experiences its own strengths and stresses.

divorce, abandonment, separation, or death. A single adult can also live alone. An extended family comprises one or more family units living in the same household, often representing multiple generations.

An individual may be a member of many different families as he or she ages. One's family of origin is the family unit in which he or she was born or reared. When children mature and are launched into the world, they join with others in extended family units, as well as with other family units of their own.

Current Trends

One trend in our society is the dual-worker family, with both spouses working outside the home. Households with dual-career adults tend to have additional stressors related to the multiple demands of work and home life. Families need to have dual careers or occupations due to both economic demands and perceived survival needs, as well as personal growth needs to achieve competence through a career. When a family contains small children, the demands of child care and domestic tasks often still fall on the shoulders of the woman. The stress of feeling the need to become a "supermom," with expectations of being all things to everyone, becomes very real to many working mothers.

Another trend is the childless family. More and more women are choosing to remain childless or to delay childbearing so they can pursue educational and career opportunities denied to past generations of women. Women who delay childbearing have added stressors of balancing home, family, and career responsibilities.

Parents may find that they are in a position of caregiver to both aging parents and young children. Often it is the mother who finds herself "sandwiched" between giving care to and meeting expectations of multiple generations. Stressors, such as making a decision to move aging parents into their home or even into a tertiary care facility, can be a major burden to the family. Added concerns can involve end-of-life decisions that must be discussed with unemotional support persons to help the family determine the best route to take for the whole family while dealing with long-term issues that may be linked to the decision process.

A major demographic trend in the United States is the shift to single-parent families. Sole parents are usually mothers who are widowed, abandoned, divorced, separated, or never married. These single mothers may be fully involved with the care of their children or may have the support of the children's father living outside the home. Some single-parent families have a parental substitute or a parent in name only who abdicates the parental role to another member of the household, possibly a grandparent. A parental substitute may or may not be a relative. Even the child may take on the parenting role and the characteristics of a parent by being the decision-maker in the family. Parents who are in some way impaired, such as drug addicts, alcoholics, or mentally retarded people, may give up the parenting role.

Some mothers, such as teenage mothers, may in some way be unable to fulfill responsibilities of parenting; e.g., be unable to provide for the caring and financial needs of both themselves and their children. These parents may abdicate the parenting role altogether. A growing number of teenagers are becoming sexually active, and, as a result, births to teenage parents have increased dramatically. These teenage parents may remain in their family of origin and have their parents take on the responsibility of caring for their children. In this form of extended family, the teenager may never assume parental responsibility for his or her children.

Single-parent families experience more stressors than other forms of families. As a group, they usually experience greater poverty, are more mobile, and are more often female headed, with the parent being less educated and often from a minority background. Although the number of male-headed single-parent households is increasing, there are still relatively few. However, male-headed households are generally financially more secure than female-headed households.

Another growing segment of the society is the single adult living alone. This increase is seen in two age groups: elderly women and adults 20 to 30 years of age. Although solitary individuals may have extended family members somewhere in their environment, their social support is usually provided more by friends than by relatives. Pets also make up a vital part of their lives and are considered family members. Furthermore, some persons are truly loners and have no one they consider a part of their support system.

Blended families, those with a biological parent and a stepparent, have become increasingly common. These families involve multiple role changes and stresses as households merge. Problems such as identifying new expectations and roles among all members, disciplinary issues, and acceptance of change plague all members of the redefined household as they adjust to one another and work to develop a new group identity. Children of blended families may be a part of two households when their biological parent marries again and they become a part of a joint custody arrangement. Although the current trend is for the nonresidential parent to hold little or no responsibility for the child, societal norms indicate a growing intolerance for that practice. Terms such as *deadbeat dad* focus on the societal expectation that fathers will maintain responsibility for their children whether they have custody of them.

Other nontraditional family forms include unmarried couples or common law marriage couples with children, cohabiting unmarried couples, same-sex—gay or lesbian—partners, and communal families, with more than one monogamous couple with children living in the same household and sharing the same resources. These family units often experience additional stressors related to disapproval from extended family members and persons in their workplace or community. These strains can bring an extra burden on the family members, who may feel that they have little support, even in the health care community. Extended family members may also increase stressors and expectations on family members in times of crisis. Legal boundaries differ from state to state regarding rights and responsibilities in these nontraditional units.

As can be seen, there is now no "proper" or "right" form of family unit, but there are many varieties of households from which a client may draw his or her support and orientation. Each family must be understood in its uniqueness as it struggles with its own stressors in relating to the outside world. As health care professionals, we must be aware of the context of each family unit and be sensitive to the issues that each family may face in dealing with life. The nurse must take the time to understand whom the client needs for support and where they are. Furthermore, the interaction patterns of that group must be understood as the nurse helps the family members cope with additional stressors in their lives.

The family unit provides the environment for growth and maturation through the socialization process of each member. Major functions include the provision of safety and shelter, financial support, reproduction, and emotional support, as well as socialization and coping with the outside world (Friedman, 1992). As the basic unit of society, the family can provide the sense of belonging, love, and acceptance that is of major impact on the health and nurturing of each individual. The manner in which the unit is formed is called the family **structure.** Without the proper tools for cognitive and psychosocial growth, individuals have less protection from the outside world.

Family Roles

Specific **roles,** or tasks performed, such as those of parent and child, can be easily identifiable, but roles such as caretaker, breadwinner, or scapegoat may be less easily recognized. Also, roles that one normally maintains may have to be taken on by others in times of illness. For example, the father and breadwinner who becomes hospitalized for cancer may need to abdicate the role of minding the finances to his wife or even to an extended family member (Fig. 19–2). In the single-parent family, the child often takes on the role of caretaker of the parent, who must be concerned with the financial support of the unit. If one member becomes ill, stressors may become overwhelming for the other part of that unit.

Roles of childhood and position in the family (first, middle, or last child) may affect individuals for the rest of their lives. As people grow and move on to form another family unit, the roles that they held in their family of origin may resurface.

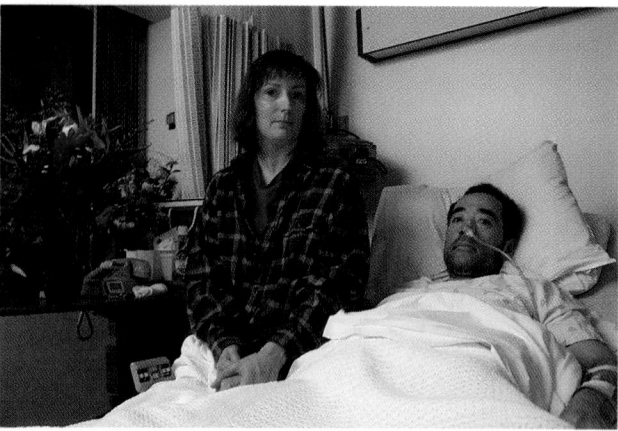

✦ **Figure 19–2**
Hospitalization can cause sudden shifts in roles and responsibilities.

✦ Theories of the Family System

A **family theory** is a framework used to understand how a family unit functions. The theories used when studying families include five major frameworks. The most commonly used framework (Bomar, 1989) is based on the general systems theory developed by Von Bertalanffy in 1968, which identifies a system as a functioning unit in the environment. Properties such as wholeness, openness, feedback, homeostasis, equifinality, boundaries, and environment are valid in relation to families. Therefore, the focus of this theory is more on the wholeness and complexity of the family unit and relationships within the system than on individual members. When relationships and interdependence in the family system are observed, the functional ability of the unit can be assessed. An open system has wholeness and relates to each part. Feedback that supports the functioning and equifinality occurs, which suggests that the system works toward a common goal. A closed system involves no exchange of energy with the environment. If the family is considered as an example of a social system, then the interactions with the environment are viewed as a process of adaptation and equilibrium seeking. Friedman (1992) believes that in the growth process, the family becomes more differentiated. During this process, the family becomes more discriminate, articulate, and complex. For example, a family in which the youngest child is leaving for college may experience stressors as the members remaining in the home redefine themselves in the context of the changed environment. The parents may find new experiences as they determine how to interact with each other without the third person in the household. The process of regaining equilibrium can be positive or negative for the system.

Another framework utilizes the structural-functional theory. The family is again considered a social system but is viewed in the context of its outcome rather than its process. The family structure is evaluated according to how well the family is able to fulfill its functions, both within and outside the unit. The goals of the family members and their ability to attain them are also determined. Family functions are the outcomes or consequences of the structure, or what the family does. Some examples of family function include meeting the psychological needs of members, socialization of the children as productive members of society, regeneration or reproduction, economic resource allocation, and maintenance of physical necessities, such as food, clothing, shelter, and health care. For example, parents traditionally function as the providers of shelter and security for the unit. A family in which the father is breadwinner and the mother is the social caregiver of the children may have to redefine itself if the mother determines that she needs to work outside the home. Structure and functional roles will need to be redefined to ensure that all needs are being met and that the desired outcomes are being attained.

The developmental theory (Duvall, 1977) analyzes the family as it progresses through the life cycle from inception to dissolution. Stages, as well as critical developmental tasks, are identified. Theories of Freud, Erikson, and Havighurst are used, and the concepts of role and interpersonal interactions are incorporated. Family members are viewed in the context of their growth and development stage, as well as the developmental stage of the family unit. For example, the beginning family is at a very different stage than one launching children into the world. Successful mastery of each developmental stage is important to move on to the next stage of growth. It is often helpful to identify the developmental stage of the family to determine situational crises that may be facing the family members, as well as the health care concerns. For example, the crisis of moving the children from the home, or "launching," can produce anxiety on the part of both the parents and the children. Children may return to their parents' home when they find that they are not able to live as comfortably on their own as they had with their parents. This phenomenon represents an unsuccessful launching. Conflict often results when children are unable to identify either with their former roles as children or their new ones as young adults. (See Table 19–1 for the developmental stages and tasks involved in each stage.) These stages occur in a linear process, or recur. For example, if a family has a child who grows up and leaves home, the parents can have another child, and the process can begin again. Also, in the blended family, individuals can move through the stages multiple times with each family unit.

A family with grown children who return to the home and with aging parents who return for care would exist in a multiple of stages. The core unit would be postparental, with an aging family and a beginning or childbearing family joining the home.

Table **19–1**

FAMILY DEVELOPMENTAL STAGES

THE EIGHT-STAGE FAMILY LIFE CYCLE	FAMILY DEVELOPMENTAL TASKS
I. Beginning family	To establish a mutually satisfying marriage To plan to have or not have children
II. Childbearing family	To have and adjust to infant To support needs of all three members To renegotiate marital relationship To expand relations with extended family
III. Family with preschool children	To adjust to costs of family life To socialize preschool children To cope with parental loss of energy and privacy
IV. Family with school-age children	To adjust to the activity of growing children To promote joint decision-making between children and parents To encourage and support children's educational achievements
V. Family with teenagers and young adults	To maintain open communication among members To support ethical and moral values within the family To balance freedom and responsibility for teenagers
VI. Family launching young adults	To release young adults with appropriate ritual and assistance To strengthen marital relationship To maintain supportive home base
VII. Postparental family	To prepare for retirement To maintain ties with older and younger generations
VIII. Aging family	To adjust to retirement To adjust to loss of spouse To close the family home

(Data from Friedman, M. M. (1992). *Family nursing: Theory and practice* (3rd ed.). Norwalk, CT: Appleton & Lange.)

Concepts used in this framework may be considered dated and difficult to adapt to nontraditional family units. Even traditional family units may not fit easily in the stages. Therefore, the nurse may need to use two stages or a variation of the developmental theory and explain reasoning used when making determinations.

The institutional historical theory examines a culture or society at some point in history and determines how the family unit mediates with the environment to accomplish the goals of the time. Social change and how societal institutions such as religious, educational, governmental, and economic systems affect and are affected by each other represent the main focus. One example of how this theory can be applied is to examine how a Catholic family deals with birth control decisions.

The nurse can assist the multigenerational family in reviewing their heritage by providing opportunities for the grandparents to discuss how they struggled through the Depression or preserved their religious beliefs through the Holocaust. A greater sense of tradition and family culture can be fostered through such a reflection and reminiscence process.

A final approach is to utilize multiple theories in an eclectic framework. All of the theories presented here can be drawn on when considered appropriate to the family under study. Also, theories such as conflict, stress, adaptation, and conflict can aid in understanding the dynamics and interactions involved in the functioning of the family system.

A specific issue in the family, such as bringing a new baby home, can be viewed by identifying the developmental stage — childbearing — and identifying how the system functions, the roles that each member plays, and how these roles will be altered by the new member of the group. Cultural considerations surrounding a new infant can be influenced by how well prepared each member was prior to the arrival. Positive and negative stressors and adaptation are often culturally determined. For example, a female infant may not be as desirable to families of Third World countries as a male child, and children with physical or emotional impairments may be more highly prized in these cultures than they are in ours. By utilizing multiple theoretical frameworks, the nurse can identify more possibilities in meeting the needs of complex family units.

See Chapter 2 for more information on theories and models of nursing practice.

The Family as Client

As nurses approach one or more members of a family unit, regarding the unit or **family as client** is the philosophical approach used in determination of and meeting health care needs. If the family is the main mechanism through which the individual interprets life, then to assist the individual client in attaining a

COMMUNITY BASED CARE

NURSE CASE MANAGER

Teamwork is critical in today's health care environment. Clients are discharged earlier than ever from the acute care hospital. They may spend time in a sub-acute care setting, return to outpatient clinics for care, or be referred for home care follow-up. In some cases, clients may experience *all* of these settings throughout the continuum of illness and recovery. In many cases, hospitalization is eliminated altogether, in favor of providing care safely, efficiently, and cost-effectively in other settings. Communication and case management are essential to ensure that health care resources are utilized appropriately and that no gaps occur in care.

When referred to a home care agency, the client is assigned a case manager. Although the case manager is usually a nurse, he or she could also be a physical therapist if only therapy services are being provided. The case manager visits the client at home and oversees and coordinates home care services. Specific responsibilities include

1. Physical assessment of the client. Communicating with the physician any problems or complications so that appropriate intervention can take place as needed. Assessment in the home setting may also include medical needs, psychosocial concerns, and financial concerns.

2. Coordinating care provided by all other disciplines involved in client care.

3. Arranging for medical supplies, equipment, and pharmaceutical needs as appropriate.

4. Ordering and monitoring laboratory work as ordered by the physician, with appropriate follow-up.

5. Updating and obtaining insurance authorization for home visits and payment.

6. Ensuring client follow-up (e.g., physician, outpatient) for ongoing health care needs after home care is discontinued.

higher level of wellness, the nurse must consider the context of the system from which he or she draws meaning. Therefore, the client is more than the individual, and the significant others are essential in care planning. In system theory terms, the individual is greater than the sum of his or her parts. Therefore, taking a part of the system without considering the whole is incomplete. The health care of the client's family should be a nursing focus in all interactions and a part of the planning of care.

When a member of a family is ill, each other family member is in some way affected, perhaps by having to take on the burden of that person's role or acting as caregiver. The added stress occurs as the roles shift and strain. The nurse must identify these stressors and help provide resources, as well as healthy means of coping, while the family members are in need of support. The overall health or stability of the family unit before illness strikes is an important factor in determining how effective coping strategies will be in the time of crisis. Maladaptive behaviors will have a negative impact on the family's ability to cope effectively with their problems. For example, a family member who is unable to communicate effectively or who will not talk at all when facing death can leave the remaining members guilt ridden and in need of counseling to deal effectively with the death.

Family members learn to deal with each other and sometimes to control one another through behaviors that would not be tolerated among individuals who do not have the bonds of responsibility and caring. Poor communication patterns are developed within the family unit. Withdrawing, or even verbal abuse, will be transmitted outside the family as the members transfer communication patterns to activities in the outside environment. Older family members can be taught that their relationships with each other and the support that they are able to show throughout each stage of growth are the main indicators of how their children will interact with the outside world and adjust to stressors.

Each family develops its own patterns of interaction and behavior among its members. The overall health or "hardiness" (Bigbee, 1992) of a family can be seen as the family's durability or ability to adjust to change and cope with stressors over time. The goal of the nurse is to help the family attain and maximize its health over time. To do that effectively, the nurse must become familiar with the family roles, structure, dynamics, strengths, and weaknesses.

The Process of Family Intervention in Family-Centered Nursing Care

Illness and crisis often precipitate stressors and behaviors that are not routinely seen within the family structure. Dynamics within the unit are magnified, and relationships may be compromised.

The nurse must identify the major person in that family unit who is the decision-maker and develop a trusting relationship. This cannot be done by pointing out negatives or needs for change immediately. The nurse must focus on strengths and the positives in the family unit to help the family trust enough to discuss the needs and concerns for change openly. Behaviors practiced sometimes over generations not only are difficult to change but also are difficult to recognize within the unit unless time is taken to discuss carefully and deal with multiple issues surrounding them. This may involve multiple interactions before discussion

can even begin on needs for changes and methods to attain them.

Chapter 13, "Communication," provides a helpful discussion on communication patterns and methods to support positive outcomes. Chapter 33, "Self-Esteem/Self-Concept," gives further information on ways to approach a client.

Nursing Process

Family Assessment

The *purpose* of a **family assessment** is to determine the strengths and needs of the family. In this process, the level of family functioning can be determined. Living patterns, interactions, coping strategies, as well as health status and practices, can be identified. The living environment should be assessed. This includes not only the home but also the surrounding community; safety and location in relation to groceries, schools, work, and health care should be assessed. The nurse and the family should perform the assessment together. If the family is a part of the assessment process and goal development, then the family and the health care team are likely to work together more cooperatively to accomplish the goals.

♦ **Cultural and Environmental Influences.** The cultural background is an important consideration. Cultural beliefs and values have a great impact on how the family views illness and copes with stress. By being sensitive to cultural differences, the nurse may be seen as more open to the family members. This supports communication and flexibility on the part of both the family and the health care provider.

Other considerations to be included in the assessment process are genetic background, or heredity, and environment. Diseases such as heart disease, cancer, diabetes, hypertension, mental illness, and genetic anomalies are important to identify. Environmental or lifestyle concerns would include the location or condition of the home, *e.g.*, urban or rural, high-crime or polluted area, and factors such as smoking or other modifiable behaviors that could affect health.

Identification of *support systems* available to family members is another important aspect of the assessment process. The mother may have consistent reliable child care or even an extended family member who helps with the child when needed. Friends and groups such as churches or other organizations are also valuable to identify. Families in crisis may turn inward and not seek the support of their friends, who may be very willing to offer assistance.

Several *tools can be used in assessing* the functioning of a family unit. The first, a **genogram,** much like a family tree, depicts the structure of the family system. The symbols utilized, such as the circle denoting female people and the box denoting male people, are generally accepted. Variable notations include the number of generations that should be identified, how the household should be described, and indicators such as divorce, death, and the index person or the focus client. Illnesses, surgeries, and birth and death dates can also be included. The genogram is a useful tool in identifying visually how each person in the unit is connected with each other. Especially with a blended family unit or multiple generations living in proximity, the genogram can become quite complex. Figure 19–3 gives an example of a three-generation genogram.

An **ecomap** is another valuable tool to utilize when looking at the function of the family. Family members are symbolized much like in the genogram, but environmental influences, such as school, work, church, and others, are also represented by hash marks across linking lines. Each member's interaction with the outside group is depicted by lines and ar-

rows. Conflict can also be noted; for example, one family member might have a problem with another's friends. An example of an ecomap is shown in Figure 19–4.

Concerns related to communication, support, economics, and health should be discussed. The assessment process involves data collection from a variety of resources, including the records from health services, the hospital, clinic, health department, or home health agency. Additional records can be obtained by speaking with school teachers and officials and employee health offices. Laboratory data, such as immunization records and past medical records from hospitalizations, may be helpful. With proper authorization from family members, data can be obtained for complete records.

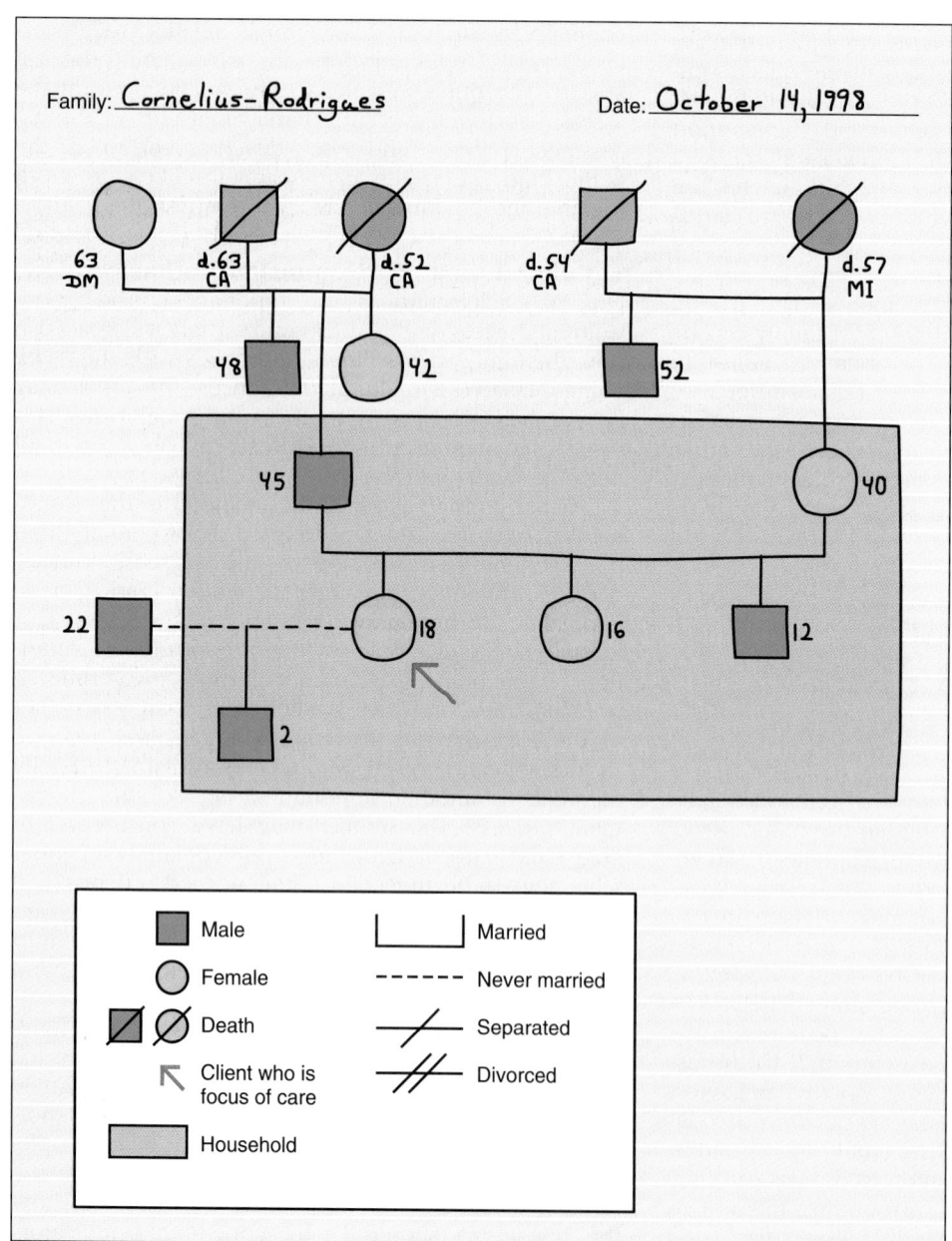

> ✦ **Figure 19–3**
> The genogram depicts relationships among family members. Many different symbols may be used in a genogram, and it is important to define each symbol when making the chart.

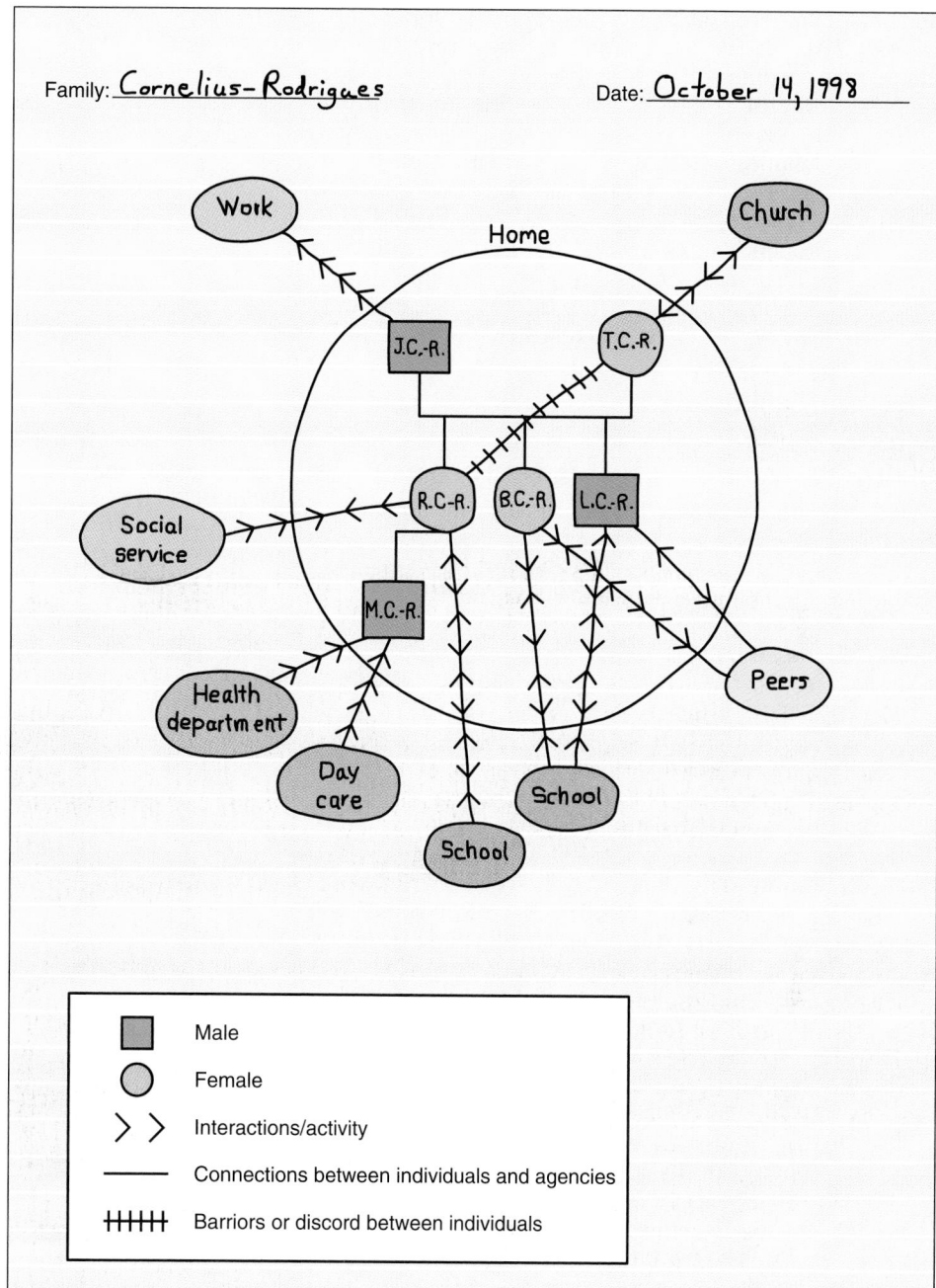

Family: _Cornelius-Rodrigues_   Date: _October 14, 1998_

Home

Work   Church

J.C.-R.   T.C.-R.

Social
service

R.C.-R.   B.C.-R.   L.C.-R.

M.C.-R.

Peers

Health
department

Day
care

School

School

■	Male
●	Female
＞ ＞	Interactions/activity
——	Connections between individuals and agencies
⊢⊢⊢⊢	Barriors or discord between individuals

✦ Figure 19–4
The ecomap shows interactions among family members and outside groups or activities, as well as areas of conflict or tension. The members of the household lie within the circle; the community, resources, and areas of interaction outside the home are placed outside the circle.

Discussions with the family can provide information regarding value systems, cultural norms from families of origin, and health belief systems. During discussions, information such as family interaction patterns and the role of each family member can be obtained. At these times, tools such as the genogram and ecomap can be used.

Nutritional information and meal patterns are also important to document for each family member. Medications prescribed are often different from those taken. A complete assessment of all medications taken by each family member is most helpful. The understanding of why each drug is taken is also needed. Clients often seek more than one health care provider.

Multiple providers rarely know that others are prescribing drugs to patients, so incomplete records are common. Clients may be taking multiple drugs for the same problem or sharing drugs with other family members or friends. Medications that clients may not view as drugs include birth control pills, vitamins, pain relievers, and many over-the-counter drugs that also need to be accounted for. The nurse should also inquire about use of illegal drugs and alcohol.

When assessing the client in the home setting, objective data can be obtained from records. However, the nurse may want to take blood pressures and do assessments of health status while in the home. Data such as limitations in function, wound healing, and adaptations made in the home are important to assess. As these data are compiled, the picture of the family unit becomes more complete.

A **risk factor** is anything that has the potential to decrease the strength or well-being of that family. Through identification of the family environment, genetic factors, sociocultural patterns, support systems within and outside the unit, and coping strategies, a needs assessment can be made. The nurse can determine overall strength or hardiness of the family, as well as areas in which support through community resources can be provided. Factors that may increase risk in families include

❧ Lifestyle
* Lack of knowledge or practice of safer sex related to teenage sexual activity or a newly divorced parent
* Altered nutritional status related to all family members eating outside the home
* Poor interpersonal communication patterns related to multiple individual activities outside the family unit

❧ Psychosocial
* Inadequate resources for appropriate child care related to age of children
* Lack of cultural identification with cultural group of origin due to living away from extended family
* Conflict or abusive behaviors between family members related to ineffective coping with stress

❧ Environmental
* Unsafe or violent neighborhood or living conditions related to inadequate housing for income group
* Environmentally unsafe work environment related to nature or place of employment of parent

❧ Developmental
* The addition or deletion of a family member from the unit related to the birth, death, or return of a family member to the home
* Limited resources and income related to retirement and fixed income status
* Ineffective coping with parenthood related to teenage motherhood without personal or financial resources

An example follows of a family assessment for a multigenerational family that is experiencing the stressors of change with added responsibilities as well as role changes within the family unit. The home health nurse comes into the Brown home to assess the situation and care needs of the elderly client, who has been newly diagnosed with Alzheimer's disease. Needs and concerns of the family unit are addressed as the assessment process unfolds.

CASE STUDY   **The Browns**
....

J. J., a home health nurse, has been notified that the Brown family is in need of a home evaluation visit. The family has just brought Mrs. Brown's mother into the home because she has become unable to care for herself with Alzheimer's disease. They also have their daughter and her young son in their home for an indefinite period. Mr. Brown has been diagnosed with hypertension and has just begun taking medication. Although the Browns have stated to their family doctor that they are experiencing a great deal of stress, they are anxious to look at ways that they can improve their lifestyle. Box 19–2 provides information about the Browns through use of a family assessment tool.

....

Nursing Diagnosis

The assessment data are used to develop a series of diagnoses to be used in determining the needs and plan for the family. Examples of diagnoses include Family Coping: Compromised, Ineffective; Family Process: Alcoholism, Altered. Examples of diagnoses with contributing factors are listed in the box. The nursing diagnoses help focus the concerns of both the family and the nurse to begin the process of planning to change the health status of the family unit. Nursing diagnoses that would apply to the Brown family described in the Case Study are as follows:

1. Family Process: Altered, related to structure change within home
2. Caregiver Role Strain: Related to ill parent and at-risk child
3. Communication, Impaired Verbal, related to altered mental status of MGM (maternal grandmother)

NURSING DIAGNOSES RELATED TO THE FAMILY

Family Process: Altered, related to
* Loss of mother
* Illness of father
* Birth of new family member

Family Coping: Compromised, related to
* Alcoholic parent
* Emotionally disturbed child
* Terminally ill grandparent

Caregiver Role Strain, related to
* Ill parent, spouse or child

At Risk for Emotional/Physical Exhaustion

Communication, Impaired Verbal, related to
* Lack of family interaction time
* Ineffective methods of dealing with anger

Parental Role Conflict, related to
* Single parent living with extended family
* Newly blended family

Box **19–2**

FAMILY ASSESSMENT TOOL—ASSESSMENT OF BROWN (FAMILY NAME)

Family Form: Multigenerational

Family Members

Initials	Sex	Position in Family	Birth Date	Role Outside Family
S. B.	M	Head of household	6/14/43	High school principal
J. B.	F	Wife, mother, daughter	10/5/45	Secretary
M. J.	F	Grandmother, mother-in-law	8/24/28	None identified
T. B.	F	Daughter, mother	4/3/72	College student
S. B.	M	Son, grandson	2/2/93	Preschooler

Address: _____

Home phone # _____ Work phone # _____

Cultural background: English-American, Polish (husband, third generation)

Spiritual/religious orientation: Catholic—strong religious beliefs

Formal roles of family members: S. B., father—breadwinner; J. B., mother—caregiver of parent and grandchild; T. B., daughter—support for mother, M. J., grandmother—ill person; S. B., child, grandchild—only child

Family development stage—Postparental with childbearing and aging units

Community resources currently in use by the family: Church, college counsellor, day care, Alzheimer's support group

Environmental Risks

Home characteristics and hazards: Single-family dwelling with three bedrooms; ample room for individual privacy; risks are throw rugs, walkways not cleared, small objects for child to break, cleaning products unlocked, electrical outlets open

Neighborhood characteristics (strengths and weaknesses): small neighborhood; longtime friends and support system for all members of unit; call frequently to assist; near busy intersection—noisy, crowded area

Health resources utilized (indicate by whom): Family physician cares for needs of all generations; T. B. uses family planning clinic and nurse practitioner; M. J. receives home health care by Visiting Nurses Association nurse; all use dental and eye care regularly.

Source of transportation: Cars (two) in home; daughter rides with friends

Social support (who offers support for the family and perceived adequacy): Church members offer support to mother and grandmother; they also receive support from neighborhood friends; mother goes to Alzheimer's support group for additional help; daughter has a close friend; father gets comfort from spending time with grandson; all seem positive about support systems

Ecomap for added documentation (see ecomap section)

Family structure and decision-making patterns: Mother and father are the main decision-makers who discuss issues about grandmother prior to making plans; daughter discusses concerns about herself and her son with her parents prior to making her own decisions

Genogram added for documentation (see genogram section)

Family Values With Highest Rank

1. A "good" future for daughter and her son
2. Security in retirement
3. Respect and care for elder parents
4. Health for each member

Value conflicts noted in family: Mother often feels torn between caring for her parent and meeting needs of other family members; daughter trying to be independent but remains in role of child to her parents; infant disciplined by all other family members and source of concern by his mother; grandmother seen as needing increasingly more care and source of guilt and bitterness on part of father and mother

Overall patterns of decision-making: Chaotic, authoritarian, democratic; rationale—family members discuss issues prior to making decisions; dependent members have little input; mother most influential in decision-making.

Communication patterns: Functional, dysfunctional; rationale—family members talk out concerns; anger is verbalized quickly, and care for each other is apparent

Goals Important to Family

Health of each member

Independence of daughter

Future of grandson

Care and safety of grandmother

Family health patterns: Members seek health care with signs of illness and practice preventive health care measures through exercise and healthful eating habits; screening measures taken for early detection of disease; medications are taken as directed

Member responsible for family health: Mother

Box continued on following page

Box 19–2

FAMILY ASSESSMENT TOOL—ASSESSMENT OF BROWN (FAMILY NAME)

(Continued)

Health History

Member Initials (Role)	Age, yr (Living or Dead)	Accidents/Illnesses	Year of Treatment (If Treated)	Amount of Tobacco, Drug, Alcohol Use
S. B., Sr. (paternal grandfather)	65 (dead)	Heart disease	None	Tobacco, 50 packs per year; alcohol 1 pt/wk
M. B. (paternal grandmother)	70 (dead)	Lung cancer	1980	None
S. B. (father)	54 (living)	Prostate cancer	1988	Alcohol, one or two drinks per day
M. J. (maternal grandmother)	69 (living)	Alzheimer's, breast cancer	1996, 1985	None
T. J. (maternal grandfather)	66 (dead)	Heart disease	None	Tobacco, 50 packs per year
J. B. (mother)	52 (living)	Breast cancer	1986	Alcohol, one or two drinks per night
T. B. (daughter)	25 (living)	No health problems	None	Alcohol, occasional use
D. B. (daughter)	10 (dead)	Motor vehicle accident	1980	None
S. B., III (grandson)	4 (living)	Asthma	1994	None

Family Illness History (Indicate Family Member; *e.g.,* Maternal Grandmother

a. Diabetes: Paternal grandmother

b. Heart disease: Paternal grandfather, maternal grandfather, father

c. Stroke

d. High blood pressure: Paternal grandfather, maternal grandfather

e. Seizure

f. Mental illness

g. Sickle cell

h. Allergies: Grandson

i. Cancer: Maternal grandmother, mother

j. Substance abuse

k. Communicable disease

l. See Genogram

Indicate family member's preference for health care resources: home remedies—none noted; clinic/physician —all family members prefer private family doctor; daughter also sees nurse practitioner at family planning clinic for gynecological needs; other resource for health information—physician's office records, home health nurse records; family perception of care—excellent, satisfied

Economic issues: Concerns of burden of added members to the family unit, maternal grandmother and future health care needs; also, daughter returning home with son will also give additional strain; family concerned about spending savings set aside for their retirement

Related to health: Stressors of maternal grandmother in home with inconsistent level of mental status; inability to leave unattended; infant in home with needs for care

Related to lifestyle: Mother, father, and daughter all experiencing decreased independence; maternal grandmother removed from own home and friends; grandson moved from home and friends

Box 19–2

FAMILY ASSESSMENT TOOL—ASSESSMENT OF BROWN (FAMILY NAME)
(Continued)

Current Health Status of Family Members

Member	Height	Weight, lb	Blood Pressure	Temperature, °F	Pulse	Respiration	Diagnosed Illness	Medications; Dosage frequency
S. B. (father)	6 ft	230	160/90	98	78	18	Hypertension, angina	Enalapril, 10 mg/d
J. B. (mother)	5 ft 6 in	170	140/80	98	72	18	Breast cancer	Tamoxifen, discontinued last year
T. B. (daughter)	5 ft 5 in	125	122/80	98	78	18	No illnesses	Triphasil 28
S. B., III (grandson)	3 ft 4 in	66		98	100	20	Asthma, allergies	Medication only with attacks, Loratadine syrup
M. J. (maternal grandmother)	5 ft 4 in	145	150/88	98	88	18	Alzheimer's, osteoporosis, non–insulin-dependent diabetes mellitus	Triazolam, Tums, five per day; Glipizide, 5 mg

Sources of stress for family and perceived ability to deal with stressors: Responsibilities related to the declining mental status of M. J.; a young child in the home and the daughter returning as an adult; new diagnosis of hypertension and angina for S. B.

Family strengths and resources: Financial stability with savings, strong social supports outside the home, good communication patterns within the home.

Assessment format for Brown family was adapted from Pender, N. J. (1987). *Health promotion in nursing practice* (2nd ed.). Norwalk, CT: Appleton & Lange.

4. Parental Role Conflict: related to single parent living with extended family

Planning

The planning of change begins with the identification of risks inherent in the assessment and the formation of diagnoses. The planning process needs to be mutually determined to ensure that the strategies are realistic from both the nurse's and the family's point of view. The goals of the strategies should be to improve the well-being or functioning level of the family.

A time frame for making those changes can then be made. For example, a family may determine that they need to decrease their debt. The goal would be that by the end of the year they would be able to manage their finances by being able to pay off all of their monthly bills on time. The nurse can help them by assisting with the budget process or locating a resource to assist them in social service. The nurse might also act as an advocate for the family by speaking with the utility companies and obtaining a planned payment system to allow a gradual payment of back bills and to prevent the loss of power and gas to the home.

Other possible examples of family goals and interventions follow:

Goal: Within 6 months, the family will be actively involved in school activities

Intervention: Mother and father will attend parent-teacher conferences and at least one school activity per child a month

Goal: Within 3 months, the family members will incorporate healthier behaviors

Intervention: The mother will take blood pressure medications regularly; the father will begin cutting down or stop smoking, especially in the home; all family members will work together to improve eating habits and eat at least one meal together daily

In this way, it can be seen that goals are both measurable and attainable. The nurse can assist with realistic goals as well as provide support for the development of an intervention plan. In family nursing care, plans may need to be developed for several different members or subgroups (Box 19–3).

Implementation

As the nurse identifies strengths and needs, the potential concerns or risks are outlined with the family. Mutual goals are then set to modify those risks and increase the level of wellness for all members of that family unit. For example, if adult family members are smoking in the home, there is not only immediate risk for cardiovascular disease for themselves but also long-term risk for damage to children in the home

---

Box 19–3

GENERAL PLAN FOR THE BROWN FAMILY

Number	Target Family Member	Intervention Strategy	Resolution Goal Date
1	Mother/father	Methods to obtain respite	2 mo
2	Mother	Support programs	2 wk
3	Mother, father, daughter	Support programs, respite	1 mo
4	Daughter	Friends, school	Indefinite

Intervention format for Brown family was adapted from Pender, N. J. (1987). *Health promotion in nursing practice* (2nd ed.). Norwalk, CT: Appleton & Lange.

---

who are breathing secondary smoke. Education and support could begin by having the smokers first change habits to protect the children (*e.g.,* only smoke outdoors) and later consider quitting smoking to support personal health care needs.

Addressing poor communication patterns is an important nursing intervention. When older family members are shown how their children will repeat destructive or unsupportive patterns outside the family, they are often more willing to evaluate their own responses to stress and to accept outside help in modifying those patterns. Nursing interventions to help the family members identify triggers that initiate negative communication and to help the family learn positive patterns will support a healthier environment for all members of the family.

Health beliefs and practices are learned and nurtured within the family unit. The nurse must be sensitive to those practices while maintaining concerns for the safety and health of the members. For example, female circumcision, while accepted widely in many African cultures, is considered mutilation in Western society and is punishable by law. Nurses must practice care and understanding when exploring cultures different from their own and should help the family understand the context of the society in which they are living and the standards by which they are judged.

Negative behaviors such as substance abuse and violence can be extremely detrimental to the family. Immediate dangers must be explored. The nurse may need to assist the mother with a plan to help move the children to safety if necessary. In an effort to support the desires of the family member of focus, the nurse must always maintain awareness that he or she has an obligation to protect the client from harm. Legal authorities, such as child protective services, social service, or even police, must always be kept apprised of dangers to vulnerable family members.

Resources and support systems can be mobilized

to aid the family in crisis to give its members the assistance they need to decrease immediate stressors and resolve issues effectively. The nurse can organize assistance in resolving family crises. The nurse can also teach the family members how to access resources themselves so that they can avert or diminish the impact of crises in the future and thereby increase their coping mechanisms for dealing with other events in their lives.

The intervention strategies used for the Brown family were developed by viewing the family members in the different roles they hold in the family group. The nurse and the family formulate the assessment together as the data are compiled. They discuss together concerns and goals for the health of the family members. Options are evaluated. For example, Mr. and Mrs. Brown have a need for time alone while being comfortable that the mother is safe. Therefore, day care and respite options can be suggested by the nurse, and Mrs. Brown can visit and evaluate the services for herself. Mr. Brown has a long-term goal of retirement. This dream can be discussed and dealt with productively by discussing healthful choices he can make to decrease his risk for heart disease through changing eating patterns, increasing exercise, and determining healthy ways to decrease stress.

By acknowledging the family's risk for disease, the nurse and family can work together to decrease risks and to detect early signs that problems might arise. For example, the child has asthma, and the home will need to be evaluated for possible allergens. The parents will need to reduce the allergen level in his bedroom. The grandmother will need to be given an area to live in which it is safe for her to "wander," where potential hazards for falls or injuries will need to be removed. Both she and Mr. Brown will need to be on an American Diabetes Association (ADA) diet to keep her blood sugar down and moderate his cholesterol and salt for his heart disease. Because both the mother and the grandmother have histories of breast cancer, the daughter is at very high risk. She should have instruction on breast self-examination and be examined each year for changes or lumps in her breasts. All members need to be able to discuss issues freely. Open communication will be essential with the added stressors that have come to this household.

The nurse would be particularly concerned about the wife, Mrs. Brown, who was identified as the key family member. She is the caregiver of her mother and the manager of the household. She carries the responsibility of monitoring the needs of all other family members and is at very high risk for problems due to the stress that she is experiencing.

Evaluation

Periodically, the nurse and the family members should discuss the plan of care that they have mutually established. They should determine if they have accomplished any of the goals that they have set or if

SAMPLE NURSING CARE PLAN

NURSING CARE PLAN FOR MRS. BROWN

Nursing Diagnosis: Caregiver Role Strain, related to ill parent and at-risk child

Expected Outcome: Family members will find acceptable programs to provide short-term care for relief and respite of caregivers

Action	Rationale
1. Assess the client (J. B.) and child (S. B., III) for level of wellness and determine health promotion needs.	1. Obtain baseline data on health status and determine whether level of wellness can be enhanced prior to exposing the child to community environments, *e.g.,* immunization updates
2. Assess cognitive level of client (J. B.)	2. Obtain baseline assessment for use in future comparison
3. Assess the strengths and needs of care providers (financial, social, emotional, psychological)	3. To determine when and if the care providers will need outside support and which resources would be needed
4. Evaluate the availability and appropriateness of adult day care facilities for Alzheimer's patients and child care facilities	4. Know facilities and program availability and assess "goodness of fit" as much as possible prior to utilization
5. Encourage family members' involvement in decision-making regarding choices of community resources for support in care	5. Increases acceptance and participation in use of resources
6. Establish a date for utilization of day care facilities	6. Provides a goal for family members to commit to utilization of outside services
7. Provide instruction to family members on coping and caregiver skills as needed	7. Care provision needs change continuously, and family members' ability to deal with those needs must be evaluated and addressed in an ongoing manner
8. Document care, progress, and needs as they change in the client record	8. Maintain an updated account of progress toward the accomplishment of the goal as well as changes and new goals as they occur; agency will have documentation requirements for utilization review and reimbursement

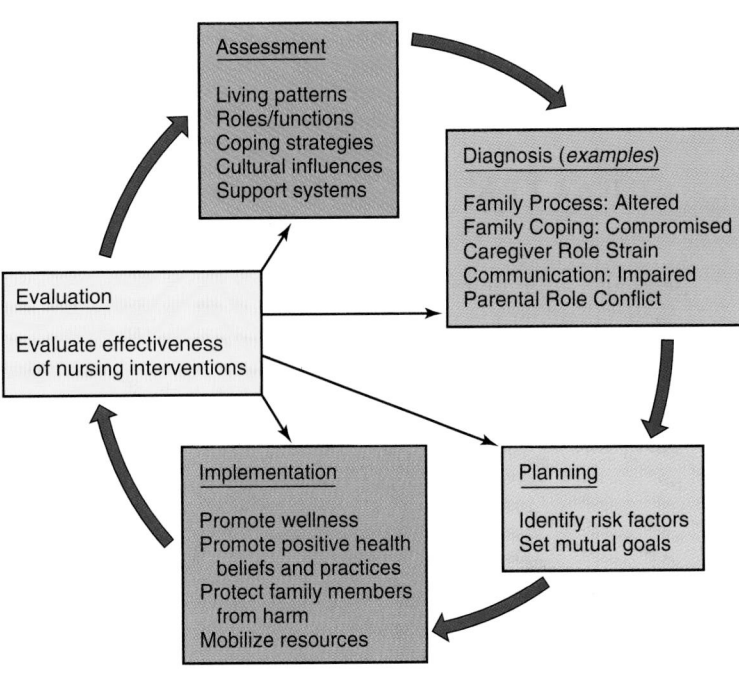

✦ **Figure 19–5**

Nursing approach to the family within the nursing process. Note that the fifth step of the nursing process—evaluation—is actually ongoing throughout the other four stages.

any need to be adjusted. In this manner, the progress toward those goals is evaluated throughout the time period of the caregiving. Evaluation is a continuous process that enables the nurse and the family members to revisit what they discussed when they initially developed the plan of care (Fig. 19–5). Lofty goals that may have been unrealistic can be adjusted when it becomes evident that they will not be attained, and new goals can be dealt with. Time frames are established when goals are discussed. As those deadlines near, the nurse and family members can discuss readjusting those dates forward or back, as appropriate. In this way, the nurse and the family work together to increase the level of wellness in the entire family, while the bonds of trust increase between the family and the nurse, promoting positive health outcomes.

Summary

Families are varied and complex. It is important for the nurse to assess the dynamics both within and outside the home to assist the family members in attaining a higher level of health. An appropriate tool for mutual use is the family assessment. This is used in data collection to compile information related to the strengths and stressors in the lives of family members, to diagnose the problems and needs of the family, and to plan interventions. The utility of the family assessment is limited to the willingness of the family members to communicate openly with the nurse and their ability to relate openly to one another as they mutually determine the needs for each member of the family. The nurse then is able to identify resources and to support the family through health education and advocacy to deal with their needs and to develop coping mechanisms for future concerns.

CHAPTER HIGHLIGHTS

✦

✦ The family is the unit of support with which the individual patient identifies as he or she deals with the stressors of life

✦ Families may be composed of the traditional unit of husband, wife, and child or of various combinations of groups bound by blood, law, or responsibility

✦ Various theories can be used to understand family functioning, such as general systems theory, structural-functional theory, developmental theory, institutional-historical theory, and eclectic theory

✦ Visual assessment tools used in family assessment

include the genogram and the ecomap, which are used to identify linear patterns in families and family dynamics, both internally and externally

✦ Assessments identify strengths as well as risks in health promotion; as the nurse works with the family members, needs and resources can be matched to increase the level of wellness of each family member and the health of the family unit as a whole

Study Questions

1. By viewing a family group in terms of how well it works together and performs its roles, the nurse is utilizing which family theory?

   a. systems
   b. structural-functional
   c. institutional-historical
   d. developmental

2. Family member roles

   a. are well defined and never change
   b. reflect the health of the family unit
   c. change as the family grows
   d. are specific and identifiable

3. Through completing a family assessment, the nurse is able to

   a. identify health issues of the family
   b. establish goals for the family
   c. evaluate the success of treatments done
   d. plan for future crises in the family

4. Cultural influences in a family are important to determine to assess differences in

   a. caring for each other
   b. physical responses to illness
   c. patterns of coping with stress
   d. ability to deal with change

5. A genogram is a useful tool to determine

   a. how family members interact with their external environment
   b. patterns of health problems through multiple generations
   c. friends and support systems
   d. community resources used by the family

Critical Thinking Exercises

1. Discuss how trends in the family and the increase of heart disease in women affect the health care needs of women.

2. How will the trend of persons becoming homeless affect health care needs of the family?

References

Bigbee, J. L. (1992). Family stress, hardiness, and illness: A pilot study. *Family Relations, 41*(2), 212.

Bomar, P. J. (1989). *Nurses and family health promotion: Concepts, assessment, and interventions.* Williams & Wilkins: Baltimore.

Duvall, E. (1977). *Marriage and family development* (5th ed.). Philadelphia: J. B. Lippincott.

Friedman, M. M. (1992). *Family nursing: Theory and practice* (3rd ed.). Norwalk, CT: Appleton & Lange.

Haupt, A., & Kane, T. T. (1991). *Population handbook* (3rd ed.). Washington, DC: Population Reference Bureau.

Pender, N. J. (1987). *Health promotion in nursing practice* (2nd ed.). Norwalk, CT: Appleton & Lange.

Bigbee, J. L. (1992). Family stress, hardiness, and illness: A pilot study. *Family Relations, 41*(2), 212.

Clark, M. J. (1996). *Nursing in the community* (2nd ed.). Norwalk, CT: Appleton & Lange.

North American Nursing Diagnosis Association. (1995–1996). *Nursing diagnoses: Definitions & classification.* Philadelphia: W. B. Saunders.

Stanhope, M., & Knollmueller, R. N. (1992). *Handbook for community and home health nursing: Tools for assessment, intervention, and education.* St. Louis: Mosby-Year Book.

Wright, L. M., & Leahey, M. (1994). *Nurses and families: A guide to family assessment and interventions* (2nd ed.). Philadelphia: F. A. Davis.

Bibliography

Aldous, J. (1975). *The developmental approach to family analysis.* Minneapolis: University of Minnesota Press.

Unit ✦ V

APPLICATION OF THE NURSING PROCESS TO SAFE AND PROTECTIVE ENVIRONMENT

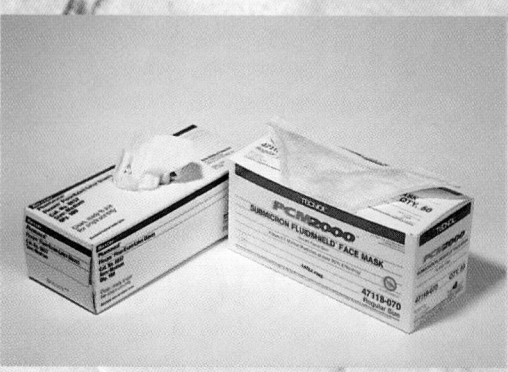

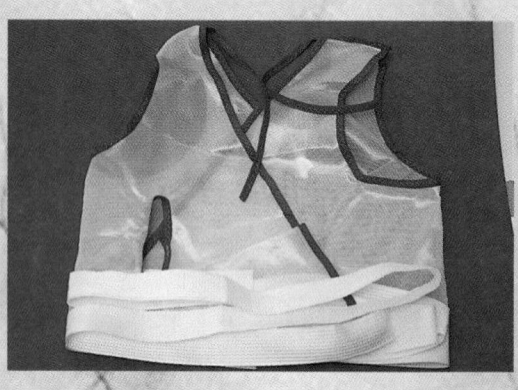

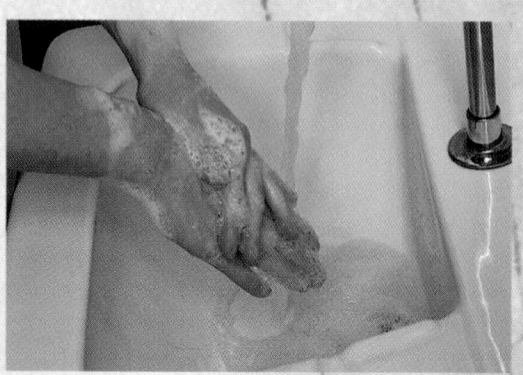

MATERIAL SAFETY DATA SHEETS

Would I miss providing direct, hands-on client care? Would I miss client-centered conferences and assisting in developing a specific plan of care for my clients? Would I miss client contact? Would I survive working independently— without a peer group within the Medical Center? Would I be self-motivated? Would I ever learn to spell and/or pronounce the names of bacteria and learn enough about microbes to teach others about them? Those were just some of the numerous concerns I had more than 24 years ago as I assumed the nurse epidemiologist role. As I quickly learned, there was much more to professional nursing and I had much more to offer than being a direct, hands-on care provider. This role would turn out to provide the most fulfilling years of my nursing career, and I would learn a lot about myself.

As the nurse epidemiologist I worked with everyone in the Medical Center, because infection prevention and control is an integral part of life in a health care setting. I facilitated and promoted the delivery of high-quality client care; coordinated the Infection Control Program; ensured a safe environment for clients, staff members, consultants, volunteers, and visitors; developed policies and procedures; served as a consultant, mentor, preceptor, and role model; participated in conferences and seminars; and planned, conducted, and evaluated continuing education programs in infection control. And that's only the short list. Infection control is risk management and quality assurance all rolled into one!

The most rewarding aspect of my role was teaching about infection control (and I seemed to always be doing just that) and seeing evidence that the staff members got the message. On the other hand, the most frustrating aspect of my role was also related to teaching. How do you make in-service infection control classes interesting and different year after year, knowing that some people will never get the message? Mark Twain probably said it best: "Never teach a pig to sing. . . . It wastes your time and annoys the pig!"

Ronnie E. Leibowitz, RN, MA, CIC
Ms. Leibowitz recently retired after working more than 35 years at the New York Department of Veterans Affairs Medical Center (New York City), where she served as the nurse epidemiologist for the past 24 years. She is a recognized national and international expert in infection control, HIV/AIDS, and tuberculosis, having published and presented widely in her areas of expertise. She has been a member of the New York State Bar Association Special Committee on AIDS and the Law since 1988 and serves as an HIV/AIDS advisor to the New York State Nurses Association.

Chapter 20

PHYSICAL AND BIOLOGICAL SAFETY

VICKI BRINSKO, BA, RN, CIC

JOHN D. BRINSKO, BS, IHIT

KEY TERMS
✦

aerosolization

antimicrobial agent

antiseptic

asepsis

bacteria

body substance isolation

CDC

colonization

communicable

community-acquired infections

contaminated

disinfectant

endogenous infection

EPA

epidemiology

exogenous infection

exotoxin

fungus

gram-negative bacteria

gram-positive bacteria

host

iatrogenic infections

immunity

incubation period

infection

isolation

JCAHO

medical asepsis

NIOSH

normal flora

nosocomial infections

opportunistic organisms

OSHA

pathogen

percutaneous injury

poison

pyuria

restraint

seroconversion

sterilization

sundowning

syrup of ipecac

transient flora

virulence

virus

LEARNING OBJECTIVES
✦

After studying this chapter, you should be able to

✦ List at least three safe practices to prevent home accidents

✦ List, in order, four actions the nurse should take in the event of a hospital fire

✦ Describe two ways to prevent falls in the elderly

✦ List two ways that restraints are used

✦ Describe the difference between medical waste and infectious waste

✦ State the difference between infection and colonization

✦ Describe the chain of infection

✦ List the types of isolation categories

✦ Identify communicable diseases that require special room ventilation

✦ State the easiest, most effective action anyone can take to prevent infections

✦ Describe medical asepsis

✦ Discuss OSHA's influence on health care workers in preventing needle sticks and hepatitis B

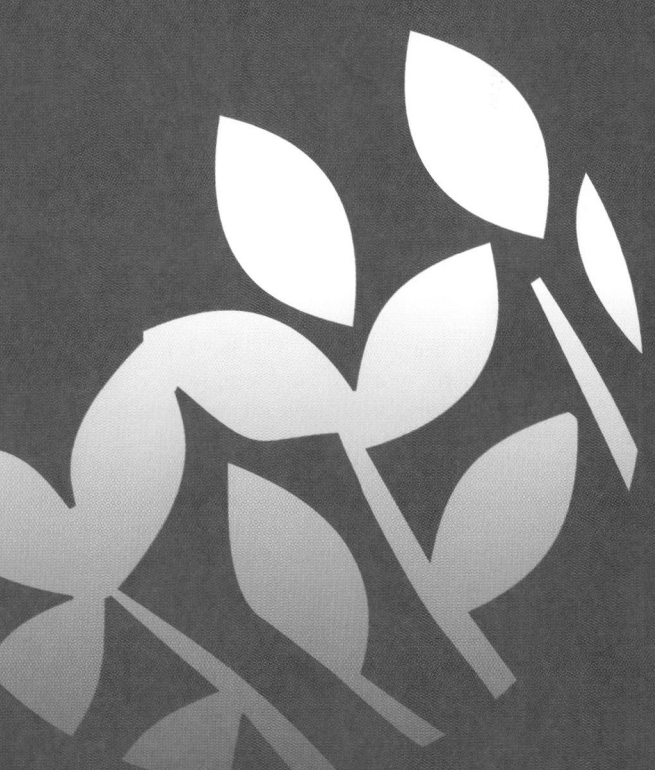

Safety is everyone's business. Each member of the health care team is a practicing safety officer and infection control practitioner. The health care worker who is at the client's bedside day in and day out can observe the safety and infection control issues that the client faces on a firsthand basis.

Safety, for both the client and the health care worker, has been addressed on a national level by such organizations as the Occupational Safety and Health Administration (OSHA) and the Centers for Disease Control and Prevention (CDC). Safety concerns for the client in the hospital and for the client discharged to a home setting are issues that nurses contend with on a daily basis. The nurse is the primary safety advocate and safety instructor for the client and the client's family. Thus, understanding how to provide a safe environment for the client is fundamental for nursing practice.

This chapter explores safety both in health care institutions, such as hospitals, clinics, and physicians' offices, and in clients' homes. This exploration includes aspects of physical and environmental safety, as well as biological safety.

Physical safety refers to the physical hazards a client may encounter while hospitalized or at home. The nurse can help prevent falls, poisonings, and other physical injuries by performing a home safety audit with the client and family.

Physical safety also refers to the environment the client inhabits and can involve such toxic hazards as radon, carbon monoxide, and lead. The nurse can assist the client at home by checking for smoke detectors, radon, and other environmental hazards. Diabetic clients and others who use needles at home can be instructed in safe needle disposal.

Biological safety refers to infection control, isolation, and disease transmission. The easiest and most effective method of preventing infection is handwashing—a simple act that often gets neglected.

Physical Safety

Safety begins at home. Home accidents injure or kill hundreds of men, women, and children each year. The majority of these accidents are preventable. Current health care trends are focusing on early discharge from hospitals and a greater reliance on home health care. Thus, many clients are encountered in home health care settings. Providing a safe home environment and advising the client on how that can be achieved are the keys to preventive health care.

Safety needs differ for each client. A nurse would assess a home with a toddler far differently from a home with an elderly client. For example, medication would require child safety locks in the home of the toddler but easy-open containers in the home of the elderly client.

Personal Risk Factors

The nurse must assess the client on various safety-related issues, including attitude toward safety, educational level, and developmental level. The safety needs of a client change as the client moves from hospitalized care to home care. Safety needs also change as clients and their families receive more health-related education from the nursing staff while hospitalized and as an ongoing process through the home health care agency. Thus, as the client's health improves, safety needs often change. This makes assessing risk factors for safety a dynamic process.

❥ **Age.** From infancy to senior citizenship, safety plays a key role in maintaining quality of life.

Infancy. Often, postpartum stays in the hospital are 24 hours. The nurse assumes the essential role of teacher for the new parents. When the nurse instructs new parents on infant care at home, the goal is to make the child's world safe, to allow the parents and child to bond, and to allow the child freedom to explore, learn, and grow. The nurse can help new parents safe-proof their home by conducting a safety audit (Table 20–1).

Infants explore their environment using their mouths as a key investigative tool for testing, tasting, and general exploration. Thus, choking hazards are an issue. The nurse can assist parents by pointing out the need to remove small items left on the floor, keep poisonous plants out of reach, lock cabinets containing cleaning agents, and keep all medications out of reach of children.

Burns and scalds result from placing infants in bathwater that is too hot or from feeding formula that has been overheated in the microwave. Consumer products are available to check the temperature of the bathwater. Parents can buy thermometers or heat-sensitive bath toys that change color when exposed to temperatures over 110°F (43.3°C). The nurse should advise parents to turn the thermostat of the water heater down to 120°F (48.8°C). Nurses can also instruct parents to test the temperature of heated infant formula by shaking some formula onto the inner aspect of the wrist. If the formula feels too hot to the parent, it is too hot for the delicate tissues of the infant's mouth. Microwaving infant formula is discouraged by most pediatricians because of the risk of burns. The bottle may feel cool to the touch or only slightly warm, but the liquid inside has hot spots that can burn the infant's mouth.

The crib should have slats that are spaced 2⅜ inches or less apart, have a mattress that fits snugly, and be painted with lead-free paint. Many parents want to use heirloom cribs and bassinets only to discover that they do not meet federal safety guidelines. Playpens should also meet federal safety guidelines.

Injuries from motor vehicle accidents are preventable by using federally approved rear-facing infant car seats. In cars equipped with passenger-side air bags,

Table 20–1

INFANT/TODDLER SAFE-PROOF CHECKS

CHECK	RATIONALE
Electrical wiring	
Replace worn, frayed cords	Prevent shock
Use safety guards/shorteners	Prevent hanging
Use outlet covers	Prevent shock
Floor	
Use fireplace screens	Prevent burns
Place gates at top and bottom of stairs	Prevent falls
Remove small objects	Prevent choking
Kitchen	
Turn pot handles toward back of stove	Prevent scalds/burns
Remove tablecloths	Prevent scalds
Use door lock on cleaning supplies	Prevent poisoning
Use drawer lock on sharp utensils	Prevent injury
Keep safe objects such as plastic bowls, pots, and pans in lower cabinets	Encourage exploration
Bathroom	
Lower hot water thermostat to below 130°F	Prevent scalds
Keep medication in locked cabinet out of reach	Prevent poisoning
Keep toilet lids closed or locked	Prevent drowning
Never leave child unattended in bathtub	Prevent drowning
Keep syrup of ipecac in medicine cabinet	To induce vomiting if instructed by physician or poison control center

these rear-facing seats should never be used in the front seat. During an accident, the force with which the air bag is deployed can severely injure the infant. Some hospitals give new parents an approved infant car seat as a promotional gift. These seats should also be used during air travel, but the parent may have to purchase an airline ticket for the infant. In cases of emergency landings, infants who were restrained in car seats survived and with few or no injuries.

Toddlerhood. The toddler often experiences physical trauma from falls in a test of newfound mobility. Nurses can advise parents to pad sharp-cornered furniture or purchase rounded corner protectors. Newfound mobility also poses drowning hazards from swimming pools or even the toilet bowl. Pool alarms are available, as well as toilet bowl locks. The swimming pool should be fenced with a secure gate. Parents can be instructed never to leave infants or children alone in or around the pool or the bathtub—not even for a moment. Drownings can occur in only a couple of inches of water.

Scalds and burns are also among the injuries that toddlers experience as they reach for that enticing cup of steaming coffee on the table edge. The nurse can instruct parents to keep hot liquids away from toddlers and to place all pots and pans on the back burners of the stove or turn the pot handles to an inward position. Control knob locks are available for both gas and electric ranges.

As the toddler becomes more adept at eating adult foods, his or her eagerness to try finger foods such as grapes, popcorn, and hot dogs often leads to choking. All medicines look like candy to toddlers. The nurse should advise parents never to refer to any medication as candy.

Syrup of ipecac is a nonprescription liquid that, when given orally, induces vomiting. All homes with children should have a bottle on hand in case the physician or poison control center instructs the parent to induce vomiting. Emergency phone numbers for the physician, hospital emergency room, or poison control center should be readily available.

Electrical outlets should be covered with safety plugs or covers. Toddlers enjoy sticking objects (such as knives, forks, or toys) into outlets or may bite on the electrical cord in an effort to relieve teething pain. Electrical cords, as well as miniblind and/or drapery cords, can be bound and tucked out of view.

Preschool. The preschooler wants to "do it myself." Playground injuries occur when the child tackles a toy that proves to be physically overwhelming. Poisoning, drowning, and burns are still concerns. Children can be taught to swim at very early ages, and parents should be encouraged to do so.

Animal bites are prevalent at this age. Earlier fears of dogs and other animals are replaced by the desire to befriend all animals. Preschoolers should be taught to avoid stray animals and never to tease or mistreat an animal.

Formal safety instruction begins at this age. The

preschooler is taught how to ride a tricycle or bicycle properly and with a safety helmet and that traffic signals and signs must be obeyed. The preschooler is instructed to cross the street only with an adult (that the child knows).

Fire safety includes warnings to preschoolers about the hazards of playing with matches or lighters. Parents can show the home smoke detector to the preschooler and give specific instructions about what to do (crawl on the floor) and where to meet once outside the house. Home fire drills may reinforce verbal instruction. Some local fire departments go to daycare centers and nursery schools to meet the children and do some hands-on teaching. Often in a fire situation, preschoolers panic and hide from rescuers. Meeting the firefighters before adverse circumstances occur reinforces that the firefighters are there to help.

School Age. Keen observance of traffic rules as they apply to bicycles, skates (including in-line skates), skateboards, and other recreational activities continues during the school-age years. The appropriate safety equipment (*e.g.,* helmets, knee pads) is essential.

"Never talk to strangers" is the advice most parents give their children. However, many child abductions and cases of molestation are at the hands of an individual the child knows, such as a neighbor, a relative, or a trusted friend (Wooden, 1995). According to Wooden, pedophiles prey on children at the brink of puberty. They are commonly found in occupations that give them close access to or authority over children, such as scout leaders or coaches. Many child molesters, pedophiles, and child abductors lure unsuspecting children with such tactics as:

- Name recognition—knows the child's name because it is on a personalized shirt, jacket, or backpack
- Emergency lure—claims that the child's parents have been involved in an accident and tells the child to "come with me" to the hospital
- Computer/on-line lure—offers to play computer games with the child at a designated location
- Assistance lure—claims to have a lost puppy (shows the child a collar and leash) and asks the child to help find the dog

For 15 years, Wooden interviewed pedophiles and collated the different child lures they used and possible prevention strategies. Prevention strategies include having continual open conversations with the child. Parents can practice lure scenarios and the specific actions that a child can take. Parents and health care professionals should encourage children to trust their instincts and to realize that they have a right to "basic body privacy" (Wooden, 1995).

Elementary schools often launch antidrug campaigns that include education about the harmful effects that drugs and alcohol can have on the body. Parents and all health care workers should join in this effort to stop drug use before it starts.

Adolescence. Adolescence is the age that knows no fear. Teens believe that they are immortal and thus are big risk takers. Experimentation with drugs, sex, and alcohol make the teen years particularly volatile. Although education on the ill effects of drug and alcohol use is best started at an earlier age, reinforcement of the basic message is always important. Parents and health care providers need to set good examples for teens.

Recreational thrill seeking such as drinking and driving, exceeding the speed limit, and unusual hobbies such as bungee jumping can be lethal. The teen years are indeed turbulent, and suicide is another safety risk. Parental authority, limit setting, and encouragement from health care providers never to drink and drive and to call for a ride home can offer options to the adolescent.

Adulthood. Adults who engage in smoking, excessive drinking, or continued drug abuse face long-term health and safety issues. Keeping home repairs current and mechanical equipment in working order is a major concern for busy career- and family-minded adults.

Food poisoning can occur when items such as raw chicken are cut and prepared on the same cutting board as salads and raw vegetables. Perishable food items should be promptly stored after purchase. Hands should be washed after preparing and handling all raw meats or eggs.

Always using a seat belt while driving and using life jackets while boating are fundamental safety principles.

Senior Adulthood. As the body ages, a number of physical changes occur that contribute to a decrease in coordination and mobility. Falls become an important safety issue with senior adults. The nurse can assist with fall prevention by anticipating some common causes of falls (see box).

Burn injuries are also a concern among senior adults. Hot water thermostats should be lowered to 120°F (48.8°C) or less to prevent scalding. Functioning smoke alarms with yearly battery changes and kitchen fire extinguishers are a must for every home, not just homes with senior adults.

❥ Lifestyle. More individuals are enjoying unusual hobbies such as hang gliding, bungee jumping, skydiving, and rock climbing. Along with the thrills that these hobbies bring come certain inevitable injuries. Smoking, heavy alcohol consumption, and drug abuse are lifestyle choices with both safety and health concerns. Smoking in bed is associated with home fires, lung cancer, and heart disease. Drinking alcohol and driving is associated with motor vehicle accidents. Drug abuse is associated with impaired judgment leading to numerous adverse consequences, including chronic illnesses such as hepatitis and acquired immunodeficiency syndrome (AIDS).

Workplace safety often depends on a choice that an individual makes. The employer may provide ear

COMMON CAUSES OF FALLS AMONG SENIOR ADULTS
• Poorly lit, cluttered stairs
• Stairs in poor repair
• Frayed or slippery rugs/carpets
• Slippery bathroom floors
• Slippery bathtubs
• Dark, poorly lit rooms
• Electric cords across floor

plugs or safety goggles, but without strict enforcement, employees often choose to avoid safety equipment, citing that it is too cumbersome, awkward, heavy, or hot. Safe work practices take time and effort. Many employers are interested in the bottom line, and safety is often an issue that gets ignored or low priority.

Where a client resides can affect safety, especially if the neighborhood is in a high crime area. As gang activity increases and drive-by killings become commonplace, where a client lives may be hazardous to the client's health and well-being.

✦ **Mobility.** Impaired mobility, whether from advancing age or physical handicaps, can compromise safety. A client who must use a cane or walker has an increased likelihood of injury.

Handicapped individuals may have difficulty navigating stairs or performing activities of daily living. Clients with debilitating diseases such as multiple sclerosis or advanced AIDS have difficulty performing even the most mundane tasks. Older clients may have difficulty getting into or out of the tub or shower because of unsteadiness.

✦ **Sensory Impairments.** The five senses—touch, sight, hearing, smell, and taste—are sometimes taken for granted. Safety can be affected for a client who is losing just one of these vital senses. Newly blind and deaf clients present particular challenges as they try to acclimate and often injure themselves. Older clients who are experiencing diminished sight, smell, taste, and tactile sensation are prone to falls, burns, and other injuries.

Loss of depth perception affects even a client who has lost vision in a single eye, impairing the ability to judge distances and to drive, especially at night.

✦ **Communication.** The inability to communicate with others or to understand the surrounding environment poses a safety hazard. Individuals who cannot read or understand English are likely to have difficulty with traffic signs and other written or spoken warnings. Deaf clients cannot hear sirens and other audible alarms. Clients recovering from stroke may have difficulty speaking (aphasia) or assimilating information in order to understand warning alarms or interpret safety information.

Environmental Factors

Promoting a safe environment in a world with limited resources is a concern of more and more individuals. Air, earth, and water pollution are topics that are receiving national recognition and political attention.

✦ **Radon.** Radon is a naturally occurring radioactive gas produced by the breakdown of uranium deposits in soil, rocks, and water. Radon can leak into homes from cracks in the foundation and other openings. With the emphasis on energy conservation, homes are being built with less fresh air supply to dilute potential indoor pollutants. Radon levels can build up over time and may contribute to certain cancers. It is estimated that radon causes 7000 to 30,000 cancer deaths each year (EPA, USHHS, & PHS, 1992). The Surgeon General has warned that radon exposure is the second leading cause of lung cancer in the United States (EPA, USHHS, & PHS, 1992). The nurse can obtain a radon detection kit from the local Environmental Protection Agency (EPA) office. The nurse must also counsel clients who smoke that if radon levels in the home are high, the risk of lung cancer is especially high.

✦ **Carbon Monoxide.** Carbon monoxide levels build up silently in homes that have fireplaces, kerosene heaters, gas water heaters, and wood-burning stoves that are not properly vented. This colorless, odorless gas can catch a family completely off guard, because its effects are insidious. By the time confusion and coma set in, it may be too late. Fireplace flues and woodstove pipes should be inspected annually for buildup and cleaned as needed. Carbon monoxide detectors can be placed in the home to detect unsafe levels. These detectors work much like smoke detectors and are similar in size and appearance.

✦ **Lead.** Lead is not a household toxin that most people think about. However, most homes built before 1950 contain leaded paint, and a few homes built in the 1970s may have it as well. Leaded paint actually tastes sweet, so the inquisitive toddler who notices the attractive, shiny flecks on the floor puts them in his or her mouth. The sweet flavor encourages the child to search for more. Windowsills frequently have peeling paint owing to sunlight and weather exposure. Even in modern-day America, 17% of all children have lead levels in the toxic range. Children absorb roughly half of the lead ingested, compared with adults, who absorb only one tenth. Prolonged high lead levels in blood lead to behavioral changes and decreased intellectual skills in these children. Reproductive disorders, including low sperm count and decreased fertility, can also be associated with high lead levels.

Paint is not the only source of lead in the home. Lead can leach into the water supply through old lead water pipes (especially pipes more than 40 years old), lead solder, ceramic dinnerware, or lead crystal. Many homes now have water-softening systems that may leach lead more easily than hard water. Water stands in the pipes overnight, and the lead-containing water is used to mix orange juice or make the morning coffee first thing the next day. Allowing tap water to run for approximately 1½ minutes should be enough time to purge the pipes. Additionally, hot water contains higher lead concentrations than cold water, so advise clients to cook with cold water.

Fire. Thousands of people are killed and tens of thousands of people are injured annually as the result of home fires. The U.S. Consumer Product Safety Commission has identified fires as the second leading cause of accidental death in the home. Smoke is the greatest threat.

Nurses can assist their clients in the home with fire safety tips (see box). Nurses and their clients must be familiar with fire extinguishers. Home fire extinguishers are usually located near or in the kitchen, where many home fires begin. An evacuation plan is essential both in the home and in the institution. Knowing at least two escape routes and practicing them can reassure the client during a difficult situation.

Hospitals are required by numerous agencies to conduct routine fire drills. Many of these agencies require annual fire safety training for the nursing staff and other health care workers. Most hospitals have specific protocols to follow in the event of a fire (see box). Nurses should know the exact location of the

nearest fire extinguisher and how to use it. A mnemonic for fire extinguisher use is PASS:

* Pull the pin
* Aim at the base of the fire
* Squeeze the handles
* Sweep from side to side

Pesticides. Busy families use lawn care companies to fertilize and "de-bug" their lawns. Many of the chemicals used to accomplish this task are toxic to children (who also happen to spend a great deal of time on those lawns) and to family pets. An insecticide known as chlordane was once used to treat homes for termites. However, it was found to linger in treated basements and foundations for a long time. It is now banned by the EPA. Although it has been linked to some forms of human cancer, some unscrupulous pest-control companies may still use it.

Tobacco Smoke. There has been much debate about whether secondhand, or passive, tobacco smoke is harmful to the nonsmoking occupants of a household. There is overwhelming medical evidence linking everything from cervical cancer, sudden infant death syndrome, tooth loss, osteoporosis, and head, neck, and lung cancer to smoking. Recently, passive smoking has been labeled as a serious pediatric health problem and linked to alterations in children's behavior and intelligence, as well as being a risk factor for developing lung cancer as adults (Committee on Atherosclerosis and Hypertension in Children, 1994).

The prevention of smoking in children and teens is a key determinant in preventing nicotine addiction. Those already hooked on nicotine are a tougher audience to address, especially because most teens engage in numerous risk-taking behaviors. Parental education can be helpful, because smoking parents are role models for their future smoking progeny.

Physical Safety and the Nursing Process

Assessment

Home Safety. The nurse must interview the client and the family members to determine the knowledge base and how to build on that knowledge base. Many times, the client and family are unaware that any safety problem exists until it is too late and the elderly client falls, breaking a hip, or the toddler is rushed to the local emergency room because of an accidental poisoning. A tour of the home with the client and family can help the nurse evaluate and identify the safety enhancements needed. Home safety guidelines are summarized in the accompanying box.

During the home assessment, the nurse may note particular safety challenges, such as cluttered stairs, which can be a safety hazard at any age. Other evalu-

HEALTH PROMOTION AND PREVENTION

FIRE SAFETY AT HOME

* Use smoke detectors.
* Replace batteries yearly.
* Plan and practice escape routes.
* Keep space heaters at least 3 feet from anything that can burn.
* Never smoke in bed or when drowsy.
* Never leave cooking food unattended.
* Keep matches and lighters away from children.
* Replace frayed electrical cords.
* If burned, place the area in cool water for 10–15 minutes. Contact a physician if the burn blisters or chars.
* If clothing catches fire, STOP, DROP, and ROLL.
* If in a smoked-filled room, crawl to the nearest safe exit.

HEALTH PROMOTION AND PREVENTION

HOSPITAL FIRE SAFETY

R—RESCUE patients in immediate danger.
A—ALARM, sound the alarm.
C—CONFINE the fire by closing all doors.
E—EXTINGUISH or EVACUATE.

Extinguish a fire by smothering it with a blanket, or use a fire extinguisher. To use the extinguisher:

P—PULL the pin.
A—AIM at the base of the fire.
S—SQUEEZE the handles.
S—SWEEP from side to side to coat the area evenly.

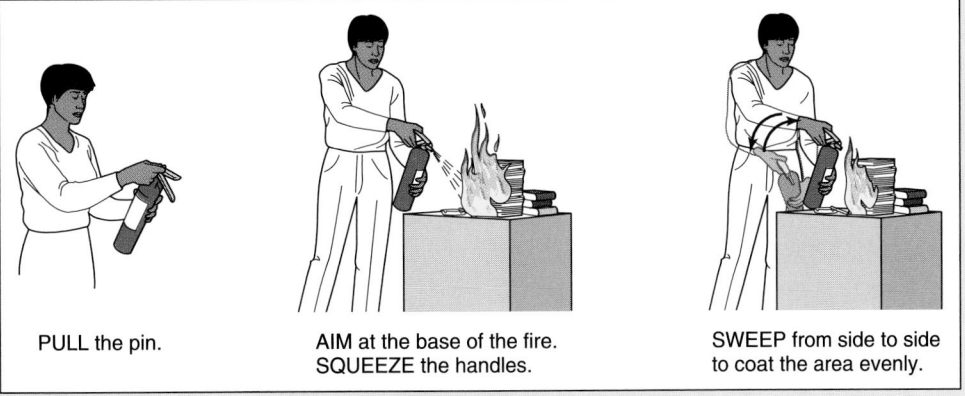

PULL the pin.

AIM at the base of the fire.
SQUEEZE the handles.

SWEEP from side to side
to coat the area evenly.

---

ations may be more client focused and age adjusted, such as when a nurse assists parents in performing toddler checks as they baby-proof their home.

✦ **Institutional Safety.** Just as the home can harbor many safety hazards, so can the hospital or clinic. Common safety practices with hospitalized clients include a thorough orientation to the room and instruction on how to use the nurse call-light system. Some institutions have policies and safe work practices that require the side rails of the hospital bed or crib to be left in the upright position at all times unless assisting the client into or out of bed. Needle disposal boxes located on pediatric floors or in exam rooms should be placed where it is inconvenient for little hands to explore. Hospitals and clinics with a pediatric clientele may opt for smaller needle disposal boxes that the nurse can bring into the room each time they are needed or for boxes that lock. Psychiatric facilities share the same concern.

✦ **Workplace Safety.** Hospitals, clinics, nursing homes, and home health care agencies are all part of a larger industry—the health care industry. This industry, like the auto industry or the chemical industry, has its share of occupational injuries. Injuries occur-

ring in the health care industry range from back strains and sprains to the occupational acquisition of infectious diseases such as tuberculosis through unprotected airborne exposure or HIV infection through needle-stick injuries. Nurses can strive to avoid these occupational injuries by safe work practices, as outlined in the accompanying box.

✦ **Workplace Violence.** Workplace violence can be defined as physical violence, verbal threats, or harassment occurring in a workplace situation. The nurse may experience physical violence in an attack by a chemically dependent client, verbal threats from disgruntled family members, or sexual harassment from a fellow employee. Coworkers, clients, and family members who are upset and demoralized are prime targets for workplace violence—both as victims and as perpetrators. Stress is usually the trigger in violent situations.

Nurses are under the constant stress of making life-and-death decisions that affect their clients. Along with these specific stressors is the job stress created by situations such as downsizing, terminations, and occupational accidents that could lead to long-term disability or even death. Outside stressors such as substance abuse, economic hardship, and marital dis-

HEALTH PROMOTION AND PREVENTION

BASIC HOME SAFETY GUIDELINES

Bathroom Safety

* Test bath water before placing client into water.
* Never leave client unattended in tub/shower.
* Use nonskid mats or strips on bathtub/shower floor.
* Use tub/shower grab bars for safety.

Medication Safety

* All medications must be clearly labeled.
* Keep all medications out of reach of children.
* If a medication reaction occurs, call a physician.

Oxygen Safety

* No smoking.
* Do not have oxygen in same room with fireplace; wood, gas, or kerosene stove/heater; or candles.
* Avoid sparks.

Fire and Burn Safety

* Use flame-resistant clothing/bedclothes whenever possible.
* Do not smoke while reclining or in bed.
* Turn handles of pots away from edge of stove.
* Lower hot water thermostat to below 130°F.
* Store flammable liquids, paints, and so forth in well-vented areas.
* Use smoke detectors; replace batteries yearly.
* Do not use electric blankets or heating pads on young children or older adults.
* Have a fire evacuation plan.

Miscellaneous Recommendations

* Remove clutter from stairs.
* Keep emergency phone numbers near phone.
* Wipe up all spills immediately.

HEALTH PROMOTION AND PREVENTION

SAFE WORK PRACTICES TO PREVENT OCCUPATIONAL INJURIES

To prevent back injuries:

* Wear low-heeled comfortable shoes.
* Keep object close to body.
* Bend at knees.

When lifting clients in bed:

* Get assistance whenever possible.
* Use a lifting blanket or draw sheet.
* Bend at knees.
* Raise the bed to a comfortable height.

When transferring client from bed to chair:

* Have chair close to bed.
* Keep knees bent.
* Pivot feet while using both arms to support client.

To prevent blood and body fluid exposures:

* Never recap a needle by hand.
* Use PPEs (mask, goggles, gowns, gloves).
* Clean up and disinfect all blood/body fluid spills.
* Dispose all sharps in sharps container.
* Use safety needles or needleless systems whenever possible.

* Risk for Suffocation
* Risk for Violence: Self-directed or directed at others

Risk for Poisoning

Poisoning results when substances that interfere with life functions are ingested, inhaled, injected, or absorbed. These interferences range in intensity from complete destruction of bodily functions, resulting in death, to partial impairment and reversal of the tissue damage. Home poisoning commonly results from ingestion of plants or household chemicals. Yet accidental or purposeful drug overdosage, poisonous insect bites (usually spider), and snakebites contribute to the total poisoning picture.

Small children, toddlers, and infants are frequently victims of accidental ingestion of common household products that resemble familiar edible products. A cleaning product may be the same color as a familiar juice. Other products such as milk and bleach come in containers that are the same shape. Adult medication may appear to be candy to some children.

Well-known poisonous plants include poison ivy, poison oak, and poison sumac. However, there are

cord often play an intrinsic role in the development of an acute decompensation. Certain behaviors by the nurse can deescalate a potentially violent situation (Table 20–2).

Nursing Diagnosis

The North American Nursing Diagnosis Association (NANDA)–approved nursing diagnoses for a client at risk for physical injury are the following:

* Risk for Poisoning
* Risk for Injury
* Risk for Trauma

Table **20–2**

NURSING ACTIONS TO MINIMIZE VIOLENCE

DO	DON'T
Move and speak slowly	Make sudden movements, which can be viewed as threatening
Project calmness	
Focus on the agitated person	
Validate the person's feelings; say, "I can see you are upset"	Criticize or judge the person
Use delay tactics—offer a drink, to sit down, or to move to a quieter location	Bargain with or make promises to the person
	Be impatient
Reflect back the person's feelings or requests	Try to make the situation seem less serious than it is
Maintain a position slightly to the side of the agitated person with clear access to an exit	Stand in front of the person with hands on hips in a challenging stance

many plants that are eaten by children that can cause impaired bodily functions. (These plants include, but are not limited to, those listed in Box 20–1.) Often, house plants purchased at the holidays have red berries or leaves that are enticing to toddlers. The effects of ingesting these common plants vary from mild stomach cramps to skin rash. Ingestion of dumb cane causes mouth swelling, impairing the ability to talk (thus the name).

Many large cities have poison control centers that can answer phone calls for panicky parents. A call to the poison control center can often avert an emergency room visit by directing the caller to simple, safe antidotes and/or home treatments. Certain cases are automatically referred to local emergency rooms for more advanced treatment.

Risk for Injury Related to Falls

Once the client moves from a home situation to the hospital, a whole array of new hazards is encountered. Fall hazards for elderly clients are a great nursing challenge.

Typically, some elderly individuals fall because, during the normal aging process, their eyesight becomes poor and their balance falters. The unfamiliarity of the hospital room, especially at night, can be especially disorienting.

"Sundowning" is a term used to describe the tendency for the elderly to become confused at the end of the day. As daylight diminishes, vision often fades with the light. The elderly client can bump into things and perhaps fall. To combat this, night-lights are used. Call lights are placed within easy reach, sturdy bed rails are used, and hand rails in the bathroom and along hallways decrease the possibility of a fall (Fig. 20–1).

Bed rails should be in the upright position and documented in the chart. If they are lowered, documentation should reflect the reason. Conservative use of vest restraints and mitten or wrist restraints can assist the nurse in preventing a wandering client from making nightly excursions. However, it must be ac-

knowledged that restraints often contribute to agitation in the elderly and can facilitate injury as the client endeavors to escape. A medical order is needed to restrain a client, even for the prevention of falls. These orders must be continually renewed as long as the client remains confused or is a potential fall risk.

Planning

Assisting the client and his or her family to set priorities and helping them plan for feasible interventions are two of the goals of the nursing process. Care plans or critical pathways are ways that the nurse can record these plans. Fall prevention is summarized in Nursing Care Plan 20–1.

Box **20–1**

COMMON GARDEN AND HOUSEHOLD POISONOUS PLANTS

Amaryllis	Hyacinth
Arrowhead	Hydrangea
Azalea	Iris
Bleeding heart	Jerusalem cherry
Boston ivy	Jonquil
Buttercup	Lily of the valley
Caladium	Mistletoe (berries)
Calla lily	Morning glory
Daffodil	Narcissus
Delphinium	Peony
Devil's ivy	Periwinkle
Dumb cane	Philodendron
Elephant ear	Poinsettia
English ivy	Sweet pea
Foxglove	Wisteria
Holly (berries)	

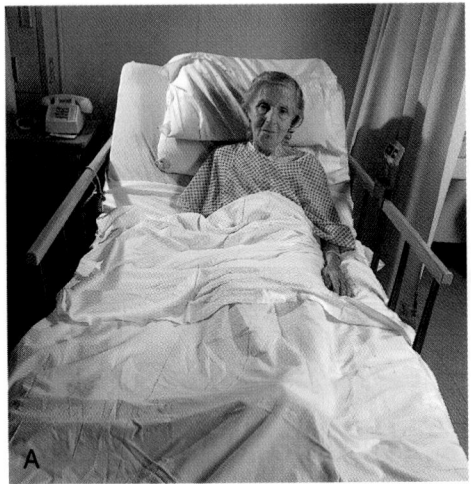
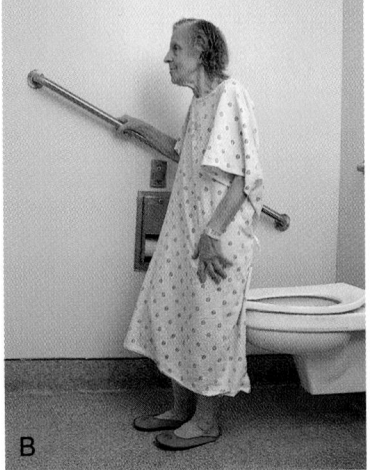
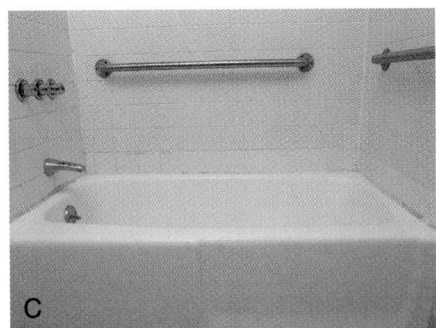

❧ **Figure 20–1**
Bed rails, hand rails, and other devices can help prevent falls in the elderly. *A*, bed rails in the upright position. *B*, Hand rails near the toilet and in the bathtub decrease the likelihood of a fall. *C*, Hand rails help the elderly or disabled client get into or out of the tub or shower.

Planning can also involve a team approach. This team approach involves all disciplines from the physician to the technician and all health care workers in between. Critical pathways outline goals, treatments, and other daily activities, as well as plan for discharge. A sample of a critical pathway for fall prevention is shown in Table 20–3. Family or primary caretaker involvement is crucial to the smooth functioning of the pathway.

Implementation

One of the roles the nurse assumes is that of educator. Some clients and their families are unaware

---

SAMPLE NURSING CARE PLAN

PREVENTING FALLS

Situation: A 90-year-old man lives with his daughter and her husband. The client has fallen several times during wandering episodes at night. The daughter states that the client seems more confused and disoriented at night. The daughter is seeking home health nursing advice on managing her father at night.

Nursing Diagnosis: Risk for injury related to wandering behavior and disorientation.

Expected Outcomes: Client will wander only while attended. Client is oriented to time, person, and place.

Action	Rationale
1. Encourage family member or sitter to stay with client at all times.	1. Client may wander if left alone.
2. Keep side rails up while client is in bed or asleep.	2. Side rails in the up position will prevent the client from rolling out of bed.
3. Use a night-light or keep the bathroom or hall light on.	3. A night-light may prevent "sundowning"—an increase in disorientation with approaching darkness.
4. For hospitalized clients or those in nursing homes, place the bed, table, and so forth in similar positions as they were at home.	4. Familiar surroundings or the illusion of familiar surroundings may decrease disorientation.
5. Place the bed in the lowest position with the call light nearby.	5. The low bed position will minimize injury if a fall should occur.
6. Walk with the client at the same time daily. Encourage family members to assist. Provide a walker or use hand rails for support.	6. Regular exercise as tolerated decreases restlessness and agitation and contributes to a sense of well-being.

CRITICAL PATHWAY FOR FALL PREVENTION

	DAY 1	DAY 2	DAY 3	DAY 4
Goals	Prevent injury while maximizing independence Family can list 5 home safety measures by the time the client is discharged Client will wander only when attended Client will perform daily exercises	Night-lights, call bell within reach Bed in low position Review teaching plan Begin walk around unit at same time every day		Family able to provide care
Treatments	Vital signs every shift Posey vest restraint when unattended			
Activity	As tolerated; encourage daily morning walk			
Diet	As tolerated			
Labs	Not applicable			
Meds/IVs	Not applicable			
Consults	Social work	Make arrangements for home health nurse, if needed	Check with family concerning "meals on wheels"	
Teaching/ discharge plan	Recommend the following home safety measures: Install tub side rails Use night-light Use bells, alarm system, secure door locks Safely store household chemicals Have family look for nonverbal injury cues such as grimacing, protecting injured part	Refer family to local medical supplier Ask family if they have one or suggest using a lamp with low wattage Ask family about door locks, bell on client's bedroom door Family understands that elderly clients may not recognize familiar objects		
Equipment	Posey vest restraint	Try to avoid use unless unattended		

of state and federal laws dealing with safety issues. It is the nurse's task to facilitate learning with an introduction to safety devices and literature.

Safety Devices

Many safety devices, especially car safety devices, are now regulated and/or mandated by federal law. Many states have enacted child restraint laws requiring parents to secure children in car seats while they are traveling in the vehicle (Fig. 20–2). These same states have also enacted legislation requiring adults to use car seat belts and fine drivers for not buckling up.

Other home safety devices focus on preventing injuries in infants and toddlers. Children are curious and love to stick items in holes or place loose objects in their mouths in an endless effort to investigate their surroundings. Thus, items such as electrical plug covers and door safety locks are essential.

Bathrooms are fascinating places for toddlers and

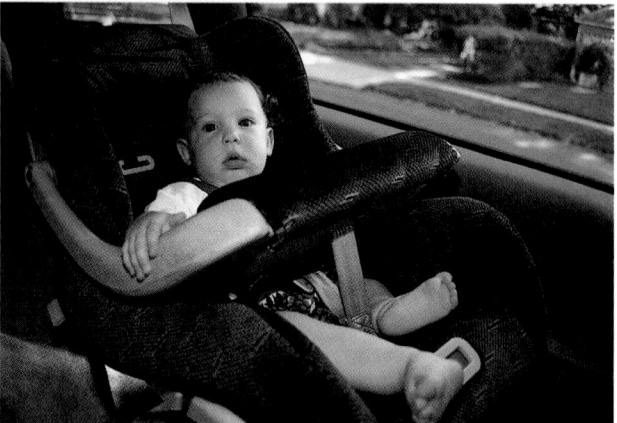

❧ **Figure 20–2**
Most states require parents to secure infants and young children in car seats while traveling in the vehicle. In cars equipped with passenger-side air bags, the car seat should never be placed in the front passenger seat because of the possibility of severe injury to the infant or child if the airbag deploys.

slippery places for older clients. Commode locks can prevent accidental drowning in toddlers, whose curiosity might prove deadly. Elderly clients can benefit by adding tub hand rails to facilitate getting into and out of the tub (see Fig. 20–1). Similarly, shower chairs with nonskid legs can help support older clients as they shower. Nonslip tub mats can prevent both infants and the elderly from slipping in the tub. Additionally, water spout covers prevent accidental head injuries in toddlers during bath time. Finally, lowering the thermostat on the hot water heater to 120°F can prevent scald burns in both age groups.

CASE STUDY **Ms. Satterfield Needs Safety Teaching**
....

Virginia Satterfield is a 17-year-old unwed mother who has delivered a small, premature, but healthy baby girl. She received no prenatal care. Ms. Satterfield expresses to her nurse that she wishes to breast-feed her baby but is not sure that she is doing it right. She plans to live with an older sister once she is discharged but has no baby care equipment. Her nurse offers to contact the hospital's social worker for assistance.

Ms. Satterfield has many learning needs. Her nurse is wise to involve the social worker to assist with locating baby care equipment from outside charitable institutions. The nurse should have the new mother demonstrate how to correctly use a car seat prior to discharge. The nurse can also explore the basics of early infant safety with the new mom, such as proper bathing, feeding, and even burping. Since Ms. Satterfield received no prenatal care, the nurse must emphasize the importance of well-baby checkups. The local health department can schedule appointments for exams and immunizations.

....

Restraints

A **restraint** is a physical or mechanical device used to limit or prevent a client's movement. The purpose of a restraint is to limit or prevent movement of the client's body as a means of controlling his or her activities, or to restrict the client's movement solely to stabilize the client's position or protect the client from a fall during the performance of a medical interventions or during transport.

The use of restraints has come under close scrutiny. In some states, strict regulations have been enacted regarding the use of restraints. The use of restraints has been associated with increased client confusion, agitation, pressure ulcers, nosocomial infection, incontinence, and death by strangulation (Sandler, 1995). The conditions for the use of restraints for protective/supportive reasons and restraining purposes are summarized in Table 20–4. Before deciding that restraints are necessary for the client, the nurse should explore other options such as moving the client closer

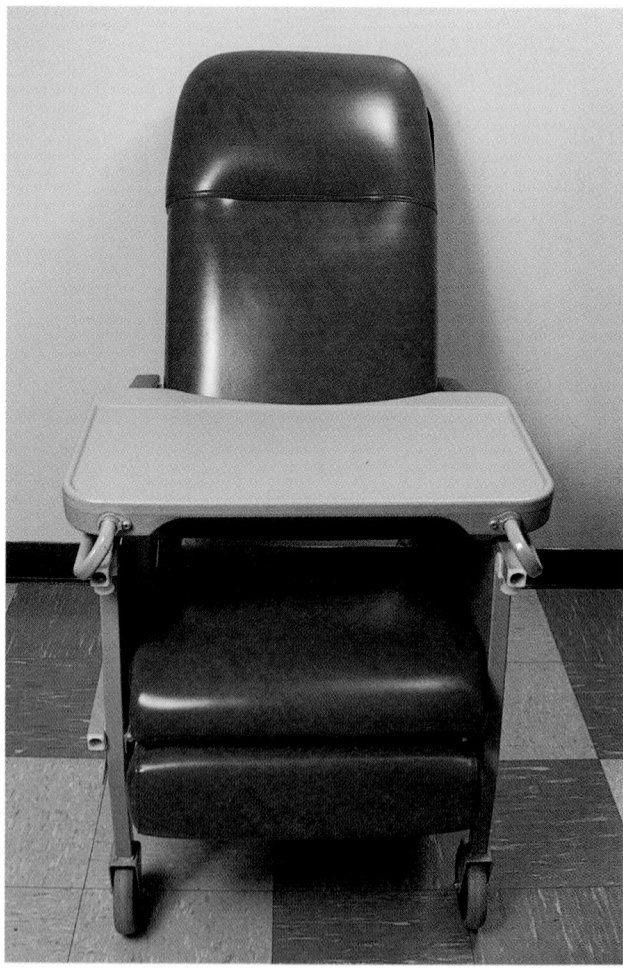

❧ **Figure 20–3**
A geriatric chair is an alternative to the use of restraints in the elderly. The use of restraints has come under close scrutiny and regulation because they have been associated with increased client confusion and agitation, pressure ulcers, nosocomial infection, incontinence, and even death by strangulation.

Table 20–4

CONDITIONS FOR USE OF RESTRAINTS

USE	EXAMPLES

Restraining purposes
   Prevention of falls
   Confused/disoriented clients
   Agitated/combative clients
	Posey vest to prevent unsupervised ambulation/falls in a confused client
	Soft limb restraints to prevent combative client from hurting self/others

Protective/supportive purposes
   Positioning/protecting during surgery
   Prevention of falls from stretcher, surgical table
   Protection/maintenance of ongoing care (endotracheal [ET] tube, nasogastric [NG] tube, IV)
	Side rails or belt on transport stretcher
	Draw sheet or posey vest used to support client in chair
	Soft limb restraints to prevent client from pulling out ET tube, NG tube, or IV
	IV arm boards
	Cast, splints, braces

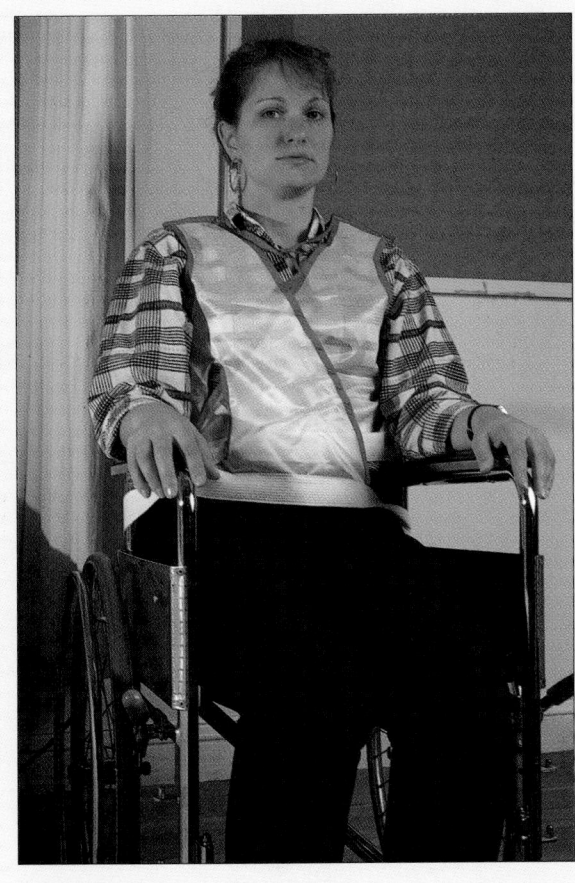

Posey vest

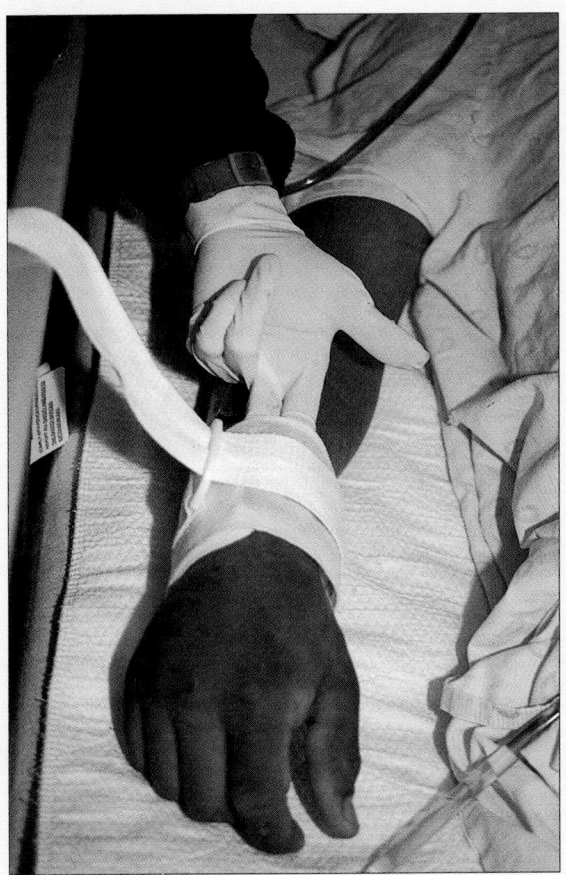

Wrist restraint

to the nurses station, using sitters, or using a geriatric chair (Fig. 20–3).

A physician's order must clearly define the type of restraint to be used, the purpose of the restraining device, and a time limit. The time limit may be 2 or 24 hours, depending on the situation and the events leading to the decision to use restraints. The nurse must document in the chart the client's behavior that led to the use of restraints. If less restrictive measures were tried and failed, these are documented. The nurse ex-

plains the purpose of using the restraint to the client and/or the client's family. If the client and/or family refuses the restraining device, the nurse documents this as well.

There are many restraining devices. Nurses must be familiar with each device and how it is used. The device is applied securely, but not tightly. Straps are secured to the bed or chair frame—*never* to side rails or other movable parts. A hitch knot or other knot that can be released quickly is used. Restraining devices are released and reevaluated every 2 hours (Sandler, 1995), at which time the nurse monitors skin integrity, circulation, and the continued need for restraints. Active or passive range-of-motion exercises are provided to the affected joints, as medically indicated. A temporary release from the restraints for up to 1 hour can be tried to evaluate whether the restraints need to be continued. The call light is placed in the client's hand for easy access.

Evaluation

A favorable client outcome—mainly, no physical injury—is an excellent measure of the effectiveness of a safety plan. If the client is injured, the nurse must reassess the plan of care and consider the following issues:

* Were there safety issues or concerns raised by the client or family that were not addressed?
* Did the client or family agree to the safety recommendations made by the nurse and follow through on implementation?

◆ Biological Safety

Infection Control

Infection control is a major responsibility of every health care worker, regardless of the setting. Nurses in

hospitals care for clients who have a variety of infections, such as tuberculosis or wound infections, on a day-to-day basis. A major resource for health care workers is the infection control practitioner, who should be used by the nursing staff as a valuable resource person knowledgeable about disease transmission, current isolation techniques, and the latest CDC guidelines.

Infection Control Terms

The world of infection is somewhat mysterious, in that the items we are trying to control are not usually visible to the naked eye. These invisible entities are called microorganisms and may be a simple one-celled animal, such as a protozoon *(Giardia),* or a virus that is so small that it can be seen only at magnifications provided by an electron microscope.

Microorganisms comprise bacteria, fungi, viruses, and protozoa. Some microorganisms produce disease and, as a result, are referred to as **pathogens.** In the strictest sense, the degree of pathogenicity is referred to as **virulence,** or the degree to which an organism produces disease. Some organisms require fewer numbers to produce disease than others. It may take a hundred shigellae to produce acute gastroenteritis, whereas it takes a million salmonellae to produce the same effect. A summary of these disease-causing microorganisms can be found in Table 20–5.

Microorganisms either always cause disease *(Bordetella pertussis)* or almost never cause disease *(Peni-*

Table 20–5

MICROBIAL AGENTS OF DISEASE

BACTERIA TYPE	ORGANISM	DISEASE
Spirochetes	*Treponema* *Borrelia* *Leptospira*	Syphilis Lyme disease Swimmer's itch
Gram-negative rods	*Legionella* *Bordetella* *Salmonella/Shigella* *Vibrio*	Legionnaire's disease Pertussis (whooping cough) Food poisoning/acute gastroenteritis Cholera
Gram-negative cocci	*Neisseria*	Meningitis Gonorrhea
Gram-positive rods	*Listeria* *Clostridium*	Listeriosis Gangrene
Gram-positive cocci	*Staphylococcus* *Streptococcus*	Wound/skin infections Toxic shock syndrome Scarlet fever "Strep throat"
Unusual bacteria	*Rickettsia* *Erlichia* *Bartonella* *Chlamydia* *Mycoplasma*	Rocky Mountain spotted fever Erlichiosis Cat scratch fever Atypical pneumonia
Mycobacterium	*Mycobacterium*	Tuberculosis Leprosy

cillium). Some microorganisms may cause disease in one area but not another. *Staphylococcus* is a bacterium commonly found on the skin. If it is somehow introduced to the bloodstream, it can cause a severe infection with multiorgan involvement, as in toxic shock syndrome. On the skin, *Staphylococcus* is benign and is referred to as **normal flora.**

Normal flora are the resident bacteria and other microorganisms that are regularly found in certain areas. **Transient flora** are the microorganisms that inhabit the skin or mucous membranes temporarily. These organisms can be pathogenic or nonpathogenic and can be removed by handwashing. Finally, some microorganisms take advantage of an opportunity. These organisms move in when the defense system of the body, the immune system, has been altered either through disease (human immunodeficiency virus [HIV]) or through drugs (chemotherapy for cancer or immune suppression for organ transplantation). These diseases or powerful drugs kill off the normal flora, weaken the body's immune system, and allow **opportunistic organisms** to flourish. To a certain extent, all infectious diseases are the result of opportunistic infections, because infectious diseases are not a normal state. Opportunistic organisms *(Aspergillus, Pneumocystis carinii)* do not usually cause disease in persons with normal immune systems. Often the client's own flora, such as *Candida,* produce infections once the immune system has been altered.

Bacteria come in many shapes and forms—from oblong rods to round cocci to corkscrew-shaped spirochetes. Typically, the microbiology laboratory stains the organisms with special dyes in order to see them under the magnification of a microscope. **Gram-negative bacteria** appear red after receiving the stain, and **gram-positive bacteria** appear blue after staining. The task of the microbiology laboratory is to identify the bacteria so that the physician can order the correct drugs to treat the client.

There are a variety of chemicals and biological agents that can destroy microorganisms. **Disinfectants** are chemicals that destroy microorganisms on inanimate surfaces such as floors, countertops, beds, and medical equipment. Examples of disinfectants include chlorine (bleach) and phenol (Lysol or other hospital-grade phenolics). **Antiseptics** are chemicals that destroy microorganisms but are used on living tissue. Examples include alcohol or iodine compounds. Antiseptics are used as handwashing agents, surgical scrubs, and skin preparation agents used before surgery or before inserting invasive devices (urinary catheters or intravenous lines). **Antimicrobial agents** are drugs that can stop a microorganism from growing or destroy it. Antibiotics (penicillin, gentamicin) are used against bacteria. Antiviral agents (ribavirin, acyclovir) are used against viruses. Antifungal agents (fluconazole, amphotericin) are used against fungi.

Sterilization is the process by which *all* microorganisms are absolutely destroyed. This process is accomplished by steam, gas, or certain chemical sterilizing processes. In the operating room, sterility is critical

COMMUNITY BASED CARE

TUBERCULOSIS

Clients who have tuberculosis are likely to remain at home, an environment that presents many challenges. The nurse's instructions must be clear and comprehensive; the client and caregivers must follow those instructions to prevent further spread of the disease. Because airborne droplets spread tuberculosis, teaching clients and caregivers to decrease contact with the droplets is imperative. If possible, the infectious client should stay in a separate room, keeping the doors closed and limiting the number of people who go into the room. The client should wear a surgical mask when leaving the room.

Other infection control measures the client and household members should follow include

1. Scrupulous handwashing

2. Keeping the client's window open when the physical structure of the home and weather permit

3. Before the nurse arrives, moving the client to another area of the home with increased ventilation, or even to an outside patio; the nurse should wear a particulate respirator until the client is no longer infectious

4. Client always covering mouth and nose with tissues when sneezing or coughing; if clients are unable to follow these protective measures, they should wear surgical masks; change the mask if it becomes moist or torn

5. Placing tissues and other infectious waste in a plastic-lined trash container in the client's room; wearing gloves to tie the plastic liner and to dispose of the trash

6. The client and all riders wearing surgical masks and keeping the windows open when riding in a car

for items that will be touching normally sterile tissues during an operative procedure. To maintain sterility, sterile items can touch only sterile items. If a sterile instrument (no organisms) is dropped on the floor, it becomes contaminated (acquires undesirable organisms). Infection can result if undesirable organisms gain access to normally sterile body sites.

The Disease Process

Infection is the result of an interaction between a susceptible host and an infectious agent (bacteria, viruses, and so forth). Infectious diseases follow a pattern of disease development in a susceptible host. This process can be divided into four major parts: incubation period, prodromal period, period of illness, and convalescent period.

The length of time between exposure to the agent and development of symptoms in the susceptible host is called the **incubation period.** Incubation periods may be short (staphylococcal food poisoning—30 minutes) or long (hepatitis B—6 months). A **prodromal period** begins at the end of the incubation period and can last 24 to 48 hours (as in chicken pox) or 1 week or more (as in pertussis). During the prodromal phase, the host may experience only vague complaints, if any at all. The host is able to transmit the infection (*i.e.,* the disease is contagious or communicable) but shows no outward signs or symptoms of the disease. Classic symptoms of the disease develop during the period of illness. The actual illness may last from days to months or years. As symptoms of the disease wane, the host begins to recover from the illness. This is referred to as the convalescent period.

Infection Versus Colonization

Infection is defined as a condition in which microorganisms are present in body tissues, resulting in tissue damage. An example is the classic streptococcal throat infection. The person has a fever and a sore throat and complains of not feeling well. The throat is inflamed and reddened, which makes swallowing difficult or painful. The surrounding lymph nodes in the neck are enlarged, and the white blood cell count is elevated.

Colonization is defined as a condition in which microorganisms are present in body tissues, but there is no damage to the tissues and no local signs and symptoms of infection. If a bacteriological culture is taken of the throat, for example, the laboratory report will be positive for some microorganisms that normally live there. These organisms are referred to as normal flora and are summarized in Table 20–6. The person is not ill, the body temperature is normal or near normal, and the white blood cell count is not elevated. The microorganisms are in the throat growing and multiplying but are not invading tissue and causing damage. In this case, a positive culture does not indicate that an infection is present.

Infections that occur during hospitalization or are the result of hospitalization are referred to as **nosocomial infections.** Nosocomial infections can occur up to 30 days after the person has been discharged. Examples are postoperative wound infections and central venous line–related sepsis. Some infections are acquired as a result of the medical treatment received. The person may become infected from normal flora—organisms that normally live in the mouth or bowel or on the skin. These types of infections are referred to as **iatrogenic infections.** Finally, the person may bring an infection, such as influenza or pneumonia, into the hospital on admission. The infections that a person is admitted with or is incubating on admission to the hospital are referred to as **community-acquired infections.**

Community-acquired infections are not preventable from an infection control standpoint. Iatrogenic infections can sometimes be prevented by giving the person oral antibiotics to clear the bowels of normal flora or an antibiotic mouth rinse to suppress the normal flora of the mouth. Of course, skin flora can be suppressed temporarily by adequate skin preparation before inserting an intravenous device, Foley catheter, or other invasive device. Most nosocomial infections can be prevented by handwashing before invasive procedures, between clients, and after removing gloves. Handwashing should become a reflex action.

The Chain of Infection

Few things in the world are actually sterile or absolutely devoid of microorganisms. A multitude of microorganisms lives on the skin, inside the mouth, and in the intestines to help the body function normally. For infections to occur, three conditions must be met: there must be a source of infection or microorganisms, a means or mode of transmission, and a susceptible host. Somehow, organisms must exit the source and invade another susceptible host. This process can be illustrated as a chain of infection (Fig. 20–4).

There are six links in the chain of infection: source, reservoir, portal of exit, mode of transmission, portal of entry, and susceptible host.

Table 20–6	
COMMON NORMAL FLORA BY BODY SITE	
BODY SITE	**NORMAL FLORA**
Upper respiratory tract	Staphylococci
	Alpha, beta, nonhemolytic streptococci
	Neisseria species
Mouth/upper gastrointestinal tract	Alpha, hemolytic streptococci
	Neisseria species
	Haemophilus species
	Candida albicans
Skin	Staphylococci
	Propionibacterium acnes
	Corynebacterium species
Lower gastrointestinal tract (stool/feces)	Assortment of gram-negative bacteria
	Enterococcus species
	Bacteroides species
	Clostridium species
	Staphylococcus species
Vagina/cervix	*Staphylococcus* species
	Lactobacillus
	Alpha, beta, nonhemolytic streptococci
	Anaerobic streptococci
	Escherichia coli
	Candida albicans
	Neisseria species
Eye	Nonhemolytic, alpha streptococci
	Coagulase-negative staphylococci

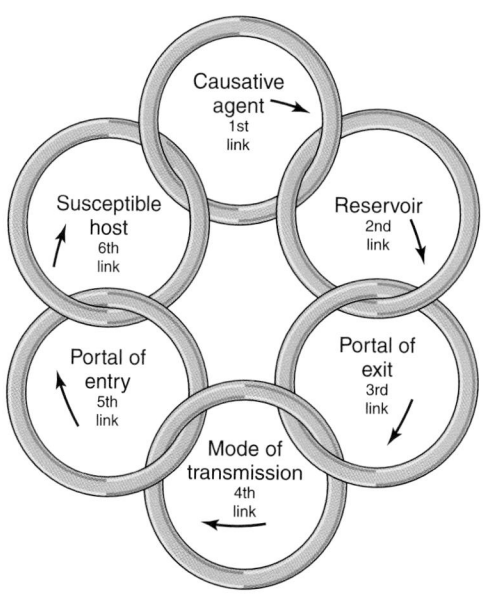

♪ Figure 20–4
The chain of infection.

Table 20–7	
EXAMPLES OF ANIMAL RESERVOIRS	
ANIMAL	**DISEASE**
Dog	Toxocariasis, ringworm, leptospirosis, rabies, giardiasis, leishmaniasis
Cat	Toxoplasmosis, cat scratch fever, rabies
Poultry	Salmonellosis
Cattle	*E. coli* 0157:H57, brucellosis, anthrax, rabies, toxoplasmosis
Pig	Trichinosis, toxoplasmosis
Sheep	Q fever, giardiasis, toxoplasmosis, anthrax
Wild carnivores (bats, skunks, raccoons)	Rabies, leishmaniasis
Wild rodents	Hantavirus infection, bubonic plague, giardiasis, leishmaniasis, tularemia

The source of an infection is often referred to as the causative agent. This is the first link of the chain of infection. These agents are usually bacteria, viruses, fungi, protozoa, or helminths (worms). Sources of infectious agents can be contaminated food, the hands of health care workers, or even the client's own flora. When the client's own throat, skin, or bowel organisms are the source of infection, these infections are referred to as **endogenous infections.** When the source of infection is outside the client's body—from health care workers, visitors, food, and so forth—the infections are referred to as **exogenous infections.**

Characteristics of infectious agents are summarized in Box 20–2. Characteristics such as virulence vary in different strains of the same agent or organism. For example, a nonvirulent strain of group A streptococci causes classic strep throat. A more virulent strain of group A streptococci causes a necrotizing pneumonia. Similarly, viability, or the ability to survive in the free state, varies with each organism. Respiratory syncytial virus and hepatitis B virus can linger for

hours on inanimate objects. *Neisseria gonorrhea,* in contrast, dies rapidly when exposed to environmental surfaces.

The second link in the chain of infection is the reservoir. Reservoirs are sources of infection where the organisms can live but do not necessarily multiply. There are three common reservoirs of infection: humans, animals and insects, and the environment.

Common reservoirs in a health care institution or clinic situation include health care workers, health care equipment, and other clients. Classic examples of animal reservoirs are summarized in Table 20–7. Diseases transmitted by various insects are summarized in Figure 20–5. The environment includes water, food sources, and soil—the inanimate environment.

Humans as reservoirs exist in two distinct states: cases and carriers. Humans with actual clinical disease are referred to as cases. Individuals without symptoms, but who are still shedding the disease-causing agent, are known as carriers. Reservoirs can be insects, as in the case of malaria, or inanimate objects such as tabletops, door knobs, and bed rails, as in the case of respiratory syncytial virus (RSV).

Next, the organism leaves the reservoir. This is referred to as a portal of exit, the third link. Organisms leave humans and animals by a variety of routes. Microorganisms in the respiratory tract may exit through coughing, sneezing, laughing, talking, or singing. Genitourinary release is generally through urine and genital secretions. Gastrointestinal exits can be through vomiting or in feces. Examples of portals of exit using skin or mucous membranes are touching the skin, as in holding hands, or touching mucous

Box 20–2	
CHARACTERISTICS OF INFECTIOUS AGENTS	

- Invasiveness
- Pathogenicity
- Virulence
- Infectious dose
- Viability
- Host specificity
- Ability to develop resistance

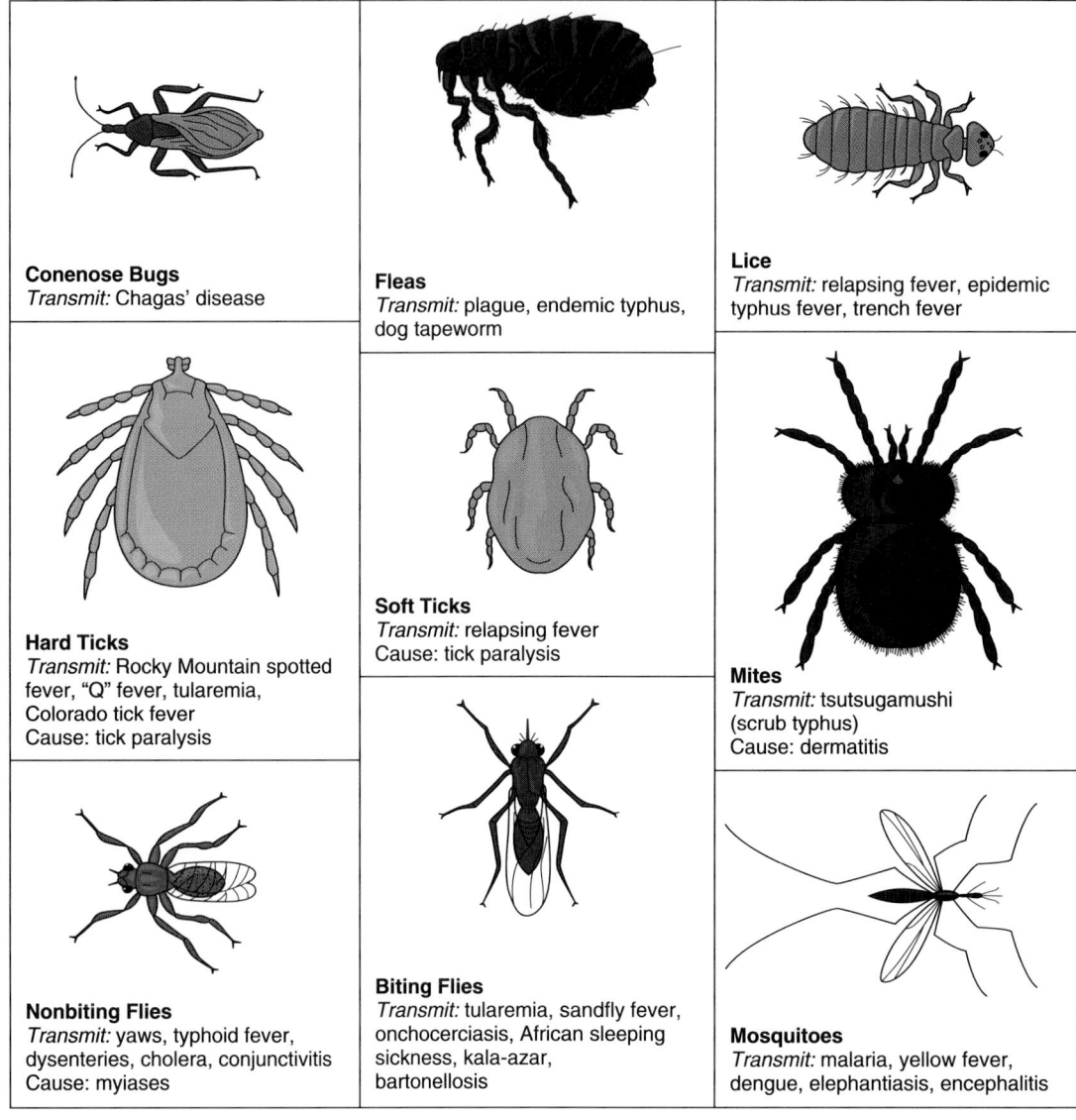

Conenose Bugs
Transmit: Chagas' disease

Fleas
Transmit: plague, endemic typhus, dog tapeworm

Lice
Transmit: relapsing fever, epidemic typhus fever, trench fever

Hard Ticks
Transmit: Rocky Mountain spotted fever, "Q" fever, tularemia, Colorado tick fever
Cause: tick paralysis

Soft Ticks
Transmit: relapsing fever
Cause: tick paralysis

Mites
Transmit: tsutsugamushi (scrub typhus)
Cause: dermatitis

Nonbiting Flies
Transmit: yaws, typhoid fever, dysenteries, cholera, conjunctivitis
Cause: myiases

Biting Flies
Transmit: tularemia, sandfly fever, onchocerciasis, African sleeping sickness, kala-azar, bartonellosis

Mosquitoes
Transmit: malaria, yellow fever, dengue, elephantiasis, encephalitis

❧ Figure 20–5
Insect vectors of disease. (Courtesy of the Centers for Disease Control and Prevention.)

membranes, as in kissing. Organisms can escape the mother's body and travel through the placenta to reach the fetus (transplacental exit). Organisms can also use blood to exit the body. If the organism cannot exit, the chain of infection can be broken.

Once the organism has left, it needs to get to a new susceptible host. This mechanism of transferring the newly exited organism to a new host is called mode of transmission, the fourth link. There are four major modes of transmission: contact, vehicular, airborne, and vector borne (Fig. 20–6).

The contact route of transmission is the most common route. It includes direct contact, indirect contact, and droplet spread. Direct contact, or person-to-person spread, is usually direct physical contact between the reservoir and the new host. Herpes simplex and most other venereal diseases, such as gonorrhea and syphilis, are spread in this manner. Indirect contact involves some intermediate object. Contaminated secretions containing RSV can be coughed or sneezed onto bed rails or tabletops. Because the virus can live on inanimate objects for an hour or longer, touching a table or bed rail contaminated with RSV can transfer the virus. In contrast, most organisms cannot survive outside of a cell, much less on inanimate objects, but those organisms that do survive use indirect contact as a mode of transmission.

Droplet spread is another form of the contact mode of transmission. Droplets are produced by coughing or sneezing. They are heavy and succumb to gravity at a very short distance, usually 3 feet. In order for droplets to infect a new source, the source must be relatively close, within a few feet of the source. The droplets are airborne for a short distance before gravity pulls them down to horizontal surfaces such as tables, beds, or floors. Many respiratory illnesses, in-

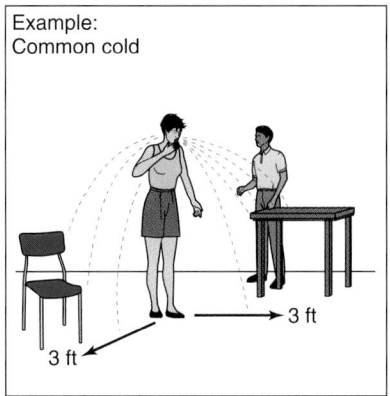

A Droplet mode (sneezing)

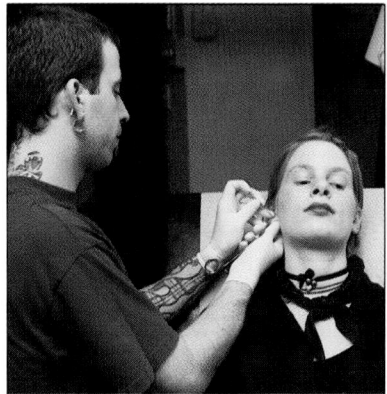

B Vehicular mode

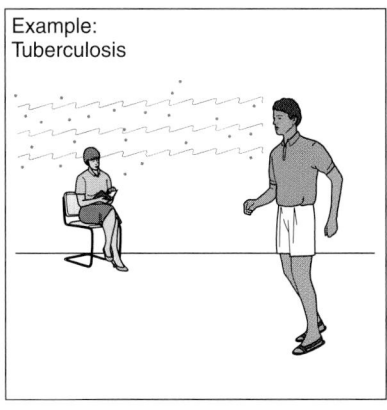

C Airborne mode

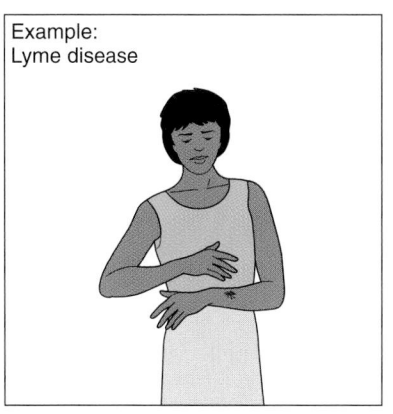

D Vector-borne mode

✦ **Figure 20–6**
Four major modes of transmission of an infectious agent. *A*, Contact mode; in this case, by droplets. *B*, Vehicular mode; in this case, piercing of an ear with a used needle. *C*, Airborne mode, with droplets wafting on an airstream. *D*, Vector-borne mode; in this case, via tick bite.

cluding the common cold, are spread by this type of contact. The most important factor here is proximity. Generally, 3 feet or less is needed for these airborne droplets to be inhaled.

In the vehicular mode of transmission, some common vehicle is used to transport the organisms to the new host. Food, blood, water, medicines, and intravenous (IV) fluids can become contaminated through various means. Once contaminated, the potential for infection occurs.

Food is often contaminated by such organisms as *Salmonella, Shigella, Campylobacter,* and hepatitis A virus. The food becomes contaminated when it is prepared by infected individuals who do not wash their hands after toileting. Improper refrigeration also allows organisms such as *Staphylococcus* to grow in food and contaminate it. Undercooking meats, especially ground beef, can transmit *Escherichia coli* 0157:H7. A well-documented outbreak of *E. coli* 0157:H7 plagued a fast-food chain, causing illness and several deaths (Griffin & Tauxe, 1991). Contamination of the meat typically occurs during butchering. The carcass of a properly butchered animal should have minimal surface contamination. However, if intestinal contents from the carcass are accidentally allowed to mingle

with the beef, gross contamination of all surfaces results. As the carcass is cut, each new cut surface adds new contamination. Ground beef is at the greatest risk for contamination because the non–prime choice cuts are combined and ground up together—contaminated and noncontaminated. *E. coli* 0157:H7 grows and flourishes in the ground beef and produces exotoxins that are heat tolerant; in other words, it takes very high heat to destroy these toxins. Individuals eat the undercooked beef and become ill.

Hepatitis B virus and HIV use blood as a vehicle of transmission. Although hepatitis B virus is responsible for a large percentage of the yearly morbidity and mortality, emphasis is placed on HIV. IV drug abusers often share needles, and any bloodborne infections on needles are passed from person to person. Tattooing and ear piercing at establishments with lax disinfection practices are other examples of bloodborne transmission. Occupational needle sticks, cuts during suturing, and scalpel injuries during surgery can also transmit bloodborne pathogens.

Water can become a vehicle of transmission when it becomes contaminated with raw sewage. This often occurs during disasters such as hurricanes and earthquakes. *Vibrio cholerae, Salmonella, Shigella, Cryp-*

Box 20–3

FACTORS CONTRIBUTING TO HOST SUSCEPTIBILITY

* Age (extremes—very young or very old)
* Underlying disease
* Ethnicity (ethnic or racial group)
* Heredity
* Immunization status
* Lifestyle (IV drug abuse, homelessness)
* Medications
* Nutritional status
* Occupation
* Pregnancy
* Sex
* Therapeutic procedures (surgery, chemotherapy)
* Trauma

---

tosporidium, and *Campylobacter* can contaminate municipal water supplies, rendering large numbers of people at risk for waterborne illness.

In the airborne route, the source sneezes, coughs, or talks, and the organism is expelled encapsulated in saliva. The saliva evaporates, leaving behind a smaller, lighter droplet nucleus. These droplet nuclei can be suspended in the air for long periods of time or drift on air currents traveling down the hall or into the ventilation system. Tuberculosis is a prime example of a disease with an airborne route of transmission.

Finally, vector-borne transmission usually involves insects (see Fig. 20–6). Flies and other insects can transfer organisms on the sticky pads of their feet. Some organisms actually use insects to transmit themselves to human and animal hosts. Certain species of mosquitoes transmit malaria, yellow fever, dengue fever, and several types of encephalitis. Different species of ticks can transmit Lyme disease, Rocky Mountain spotted fever, Colorado tick fever, and erlichiosis. Fleas can transmit plague and murine typhus.

Once the organisms have found a way out of the host, they must gain entry into a new host. The portal of entry, the fifth link, is the pathway the organism uses to gain entry into a susceptible host. These pathways are generally the same pathways used to exit a host, namely, respiratory tract, genitourinary tract, gastrointestinal tract, skin and mucous membranes, transplacentally, and percutaneously (via blood).

The new host that the organism enters must be a susceptible host, the sixth and final link. Being susceptible means that the individual is lacking immunity to the particular organism. Many extraneous factors can play a role in how susceptible a host is to disease (see Box 20–3). Extremes in age, for example, play an extraordinary role as predictors of infection. Premature infants, by nature of their immature immune systems,

are highly susceptible hosts, as are the very old with waning immune systems. Immunization status also plays an important role in disease susceptibility. Some parents elect not to immunize their children for certain vaccine-preventable diseases out of fear of side effects of the vaccine. Unfortunately, the actual severity of the disease far outweighs any potential side effects. Some lifestyle choices also influence susceptibility to disease, such as IV drug abuse and the risk of HIV and hepatitis B.

Medical Waste Disposal

Medical wastes are the end materials generated as a result of medical treatment. Medical waste can include paper waste such as letters and memos, soda cans, daily newspapers, old flowers, and wrapping paper, as well as bloody dressings and IV tubing. Medical waste can be produced at private physicians' offices, walk-in clinics, hospitals, extended care facilities, rehabilitation facilities, or client homes. Infectious waste is that portion of medical waste that could contain microorganisms capable of producing disease.

Hospitals and other health care institutions are heavily regulated by the EPA and state waste regulations as to exactly how medical and infectious waste must be managed. Most hospitals incinerate medical waste, but some use steam sterilization, and some disinfect prior to a grinding process that renders the waste unidentifiable.

The client and the home health care nurse will have to deal with medical waste generated at home (*e.g.,* insulin syringes, dressings, bandages). Box 20–4 summarizes acceptable ways to discard medical waste at home. A convenient and sturdy container that clients can use to dispose of needles is an empty liquid laundry detergent bottle. These plastic bottles are thicker than bleach bottles, thus decreasing the chance that needles could inadvertently poke through. After the bottle is filled with needles, syringes, lancets, and

---

Box 20–4

HOME MEDICAL WASTE DISPOSAL

1. **Use heavy plastic jugs** with screw-on caps (as from concentrated liquid laundry detergents) for syringe disposal. After reaching capacity, place 1 cup of chlorine bleach into the container. Fill the remainder of the container with water. Screw on cap. Discard with household waste.

2. **Place bloody dressings,** latex gloves, urinary catheters, and intravenous tubing (without needles attached) into a securely fastened plastic garbage bag.

3. **Do not use glass** or clear plastic containers for syringe disposal.

4. **Keep containers** with sharp objects out of the reach of young children.

so forth, 1 cup of bleach is added to the bottle, and then it is filled with water. This submerges the needles and syringes in a disinfecting solution of chlorine. The screw cap is reapplied, and the entire container is discarded with regular household waste. Some states have specific regulations that address home disposal of medical waste. The nurse should consult the infection control practitioner or hospital safety officer for local requirements.

Personal Safety

Employee Safety

The devastating consequences of HIV infection have changed the way nurses and other health care workers approach their clients. The emphasis of all hospital safety and infection control programs is *not* to have nurses think that all clients are infected, but rather that all blood and body fluids are universally hazardous substances. This is an industrial approach to client care. For example, when a chemical worker sees an unknown liquid on the floor, he or she approaches it as a hazardous liquid. The worker first dons appropriate personal protective gear to clean up the spill. Nurses and other health care workers should approach clients' blood and body fluids in a similar manner by wearing gloves, masks, gowns, and eye protection when needed.

Although strict adherence to universal precautions or standard precautions can reduce blood and body fluid exposures significantly, latex gloves cannot stop a needle stick. Eighty percent of occupationally acquired HIV infections were a direct result of accidental needle-stick injuries (Wugofski *et al.,* 1993). Consequently, much effort has been focused on the development and use of needleless devices, recessed needles, and shielded needles.

OSHA has focused attention on nurses and other health care workers as groups of relatively underprotected workers. Preventing blood and body fluid exposures was the driving force behind the 1991 OSHA bloodborne pathogen standard (Department of Labor, 1991). This standard also recognizes the importance of hepatitis B vaccine as an excellent preventive tool. The bloodborne pathogen standard, coupled with ever-increasing requirements from the Joint Commission on the Accreditation of Healthcare Organizations (JCAHO), has focused major regulatory attention on hospitals and health care workers. Major health care unions and nurses are increasingly concerned about safety and health issues.

Bloodborne Hazards

The driving force behind the implementation of universal precautions and standard precautions is the occupational transmission of HIV. Risk of HIV infection from an occupational injury is quite small, only 0.3%. The CDC reported 49 health care workers in the United States as having documented seroconversion: 18 laboratory technicians, 19 nurses, 6 physicians, 2 surgical technicians, 1 dialysis technician, 1 respiratory therapist, 1 health aide, and 1 housekeeping/maintenance worker. Forty-two of these workers had some sort of needle stick, puncture, or cut; several had splashes to eyes, nose, or mouth; and at least one experienced both a percutaneous injury and a splash. Those health care workers who were stuck by needles or experienced splashes or cuts with blood or body fluids immediately went for baseline HIV tests. In these 49 individuals, the baseline HIV test was negative. Over the next 3 months, all 49 health care workers eventually tested positive for HIV. An additional 102 health care workers who became HIV-positive had no documented exposure other than being a nurse or physician or working in the health care industry (Table 20–8).

In order to prevent these injuries and the devastating consequences, the 1991 OSHA bloodborne pathogen standard includes a hierarchy of control measures that hospitals are required by law to adhere to:

* Universal precautions
* Engineering controls
* Work practice controls
* Personal protective equipment

♦ **Universal Precautions/Standard Precautions.** Treating all body fluids from all clients as if they are contaminated and never recapping needles are principles that must be taught to nurses and other health care workers annually. Hospitals are also required to evaluate and adopt engineering controls that include the use of sharps disposal containers, safer needles, needleless systems, biosafety cabinets, and other specially designed containers. Work practice controls include such mandates as not eating or drinking at the client's bedside (which is very tempting in an intensive care situation). Finally, personal protective equipment has taken on new importance. Gloves, gowns, masks, and eye protection are designed to protect nurses and other health care workers as they perform their daily duties. However, to be effective, the protective gear must be worn every time a blood or body fluid exposure is anticipated.

♦ **Engineering Controls.** The CDC has issued universal precaution guidelines to decrease or eliminate needle sticks and blood and body fluid exposures to health care workers. A summary of the needle-stick guidelines can be found in Table 20–9. Many hospitals have adapted the suggested engineering controls and use at least one safety product. The nurse must be familiar with the basic premises of these safety products and how they are used.

Many of the safety syringes require that the nurse slide a shield over the syringe after use. The shield is then locked into place, and the entire safety syringe can be discarded in a needle box (Fig. 20–7). Intravenous delivery systems are more diverse. Some systems have specially made blunt-point syringes that slide into preslit IV tubing ports. Others have needleless valves that twist onto the tubing itself. Whatever sys-

Table 20–8

U.S. HEALTH CARE WORKERS WITH AIDS/HIV INFECTION BY OCCUPATION REPORTED THROUGH DECEMBER 1995

OCCUPATION	DOCUMENTED OCCUPATIONAL TRANSMISSION	UNDOCUMENTED OCCUPATIONAL TRANSMISSION
Dental worker/dentist	—	7
Embalmer/morgue technician	—	3
Emergency medical technician	—	9
Health aide/attendant	1	12
Housekeeper/maintenance worker	1	7
Laboratory technician, clinical	15	15
Laboratory technician, nonclinical	3	0
Nurse	19	24
Physician, nonsurgical	6	10
Physician, surgical	—	4
Respiratory therapist	1	2
Technician, dialysis	1	2
Technician, surgical	2	1
Technician, therapist (not listed above)	—	4
Other health care worker		2
Total	49	102

Adapted from HIV/AIDS Surveillance Report, Fourth Quarter Edition, December 1995, CDC.

tem the hospital has in place, the nurse must be familiar with the proper use of it.

Measures to prevent needle-stick injuries combine an emphasis on careful technique and universal precautions with safer needle devices. With needle designs, simple is generally best. Numerous blunted needles, retractable needles, and needleless systems have flooded the medical marketplace. Samples of just a few of these devices are shown in Figure 20–7(D).

With the mandates of universal precautions and the numerous safe needle devices that are available, needle-stick injuries should not be a problem. Yet needle-stick injuries still occur and, unfortunately, so does occupational seroconversion with HIV.

Activities among health care workers that can lead to HIV seroconversion include recapping needles,

Table 20–9

PREVENTING NEEDLE STICKS

Never recap needles by hand
Use needle guards, retractable needles
Use resheathing devices
Use needleless or blunt needle systems
Use the scoop method; place the cap on a tabletop and, with a sweeping motion, scoop it onto the needle
Use a specified sharps container
Keep the sharps container close to the point of use

splashing of blood or bloody fluids onto nonintact skin, suturing, and inflicting cuts with scalpels or other sharp instruments. The actual risk of HIV transmission after a needle-stick exposure depends on many different factors. High amounts of HIV circulating in the client (end-stage AIDS clients carry the highest risk), a deep injury to the health care worker, visible blood on the device, and a device that was previously placed in an HIV client's vein or artery increase the likelihood that HIV will be transmitted during an exposure (CDC, 1996b).

The CDC currently recommends three antiretroviral drugs as postexposure prophylaxis after an occupational exposure to HIV. These drugs are zidovudine (ZDV), lamivudine (3TC), and indinivir (IDV) (CDC, 1996b). These drugs are recommended for exposed workers at the highest risk for HIV transmission. Postexposure prophylaxis should be initiated within the first 1 to 2 hours after the injury. The CDC further recommends that the drug regimen be followed for at least 4 weeks to be protective.

Transmission of hepatitis B is much more likely. The risk of developing hepatitis B after a needle-stick injury from a client who is positive for hepatitis B surface antigen (has active hepatitis B) is approximately 30%. Comparing the same needle-stick injury involving a client who is HIV-positive, the risk to the health care worker is 0.3% (Robert & Bell, 1994). These data are summarized in Table 20–10. Conversely, the reported fatality rate is 80% for health care workers infected with HIV, compared with 1 to 2% for health care workers infected with hepatitis B.

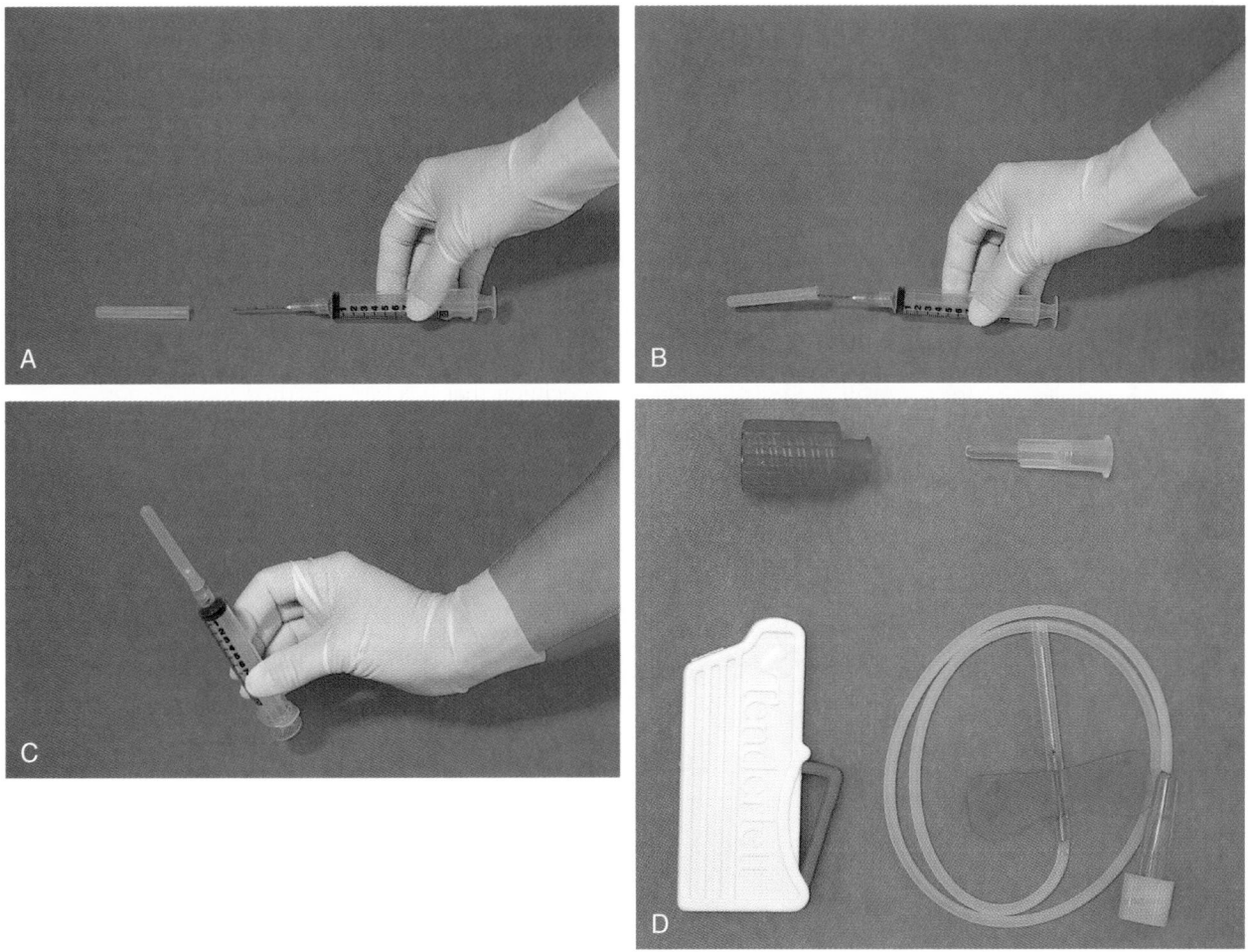

✦ **Figure 20–7**
Safer needle techniques and devices have been developed to help prevent needle sticks. *A–C,* Needle cap is placed on table and scooped up onto needle. The shield is then locked into place and the entire safety syringe discarded. *D,* Samples of safer needles: Blunt needle *(top left),* butterfly needle *(top right),* threaded lock cannula *(bottom left),* and retractable needle *(bottom right).*

Hepatitis B transmission among nurses and other health care workers can be avoided altogether with hepatitis B vaccine. The CDC estimates that approximately 8700 health care workers are infected with hepatitis B annually. Each year, 200 of those infected health care workers die from fulminant hepatitis B, a

vaccine-preventable disease (Department of Labor, 1991). OSHA estimates that approximately 2 to 2.5 million health care workers have declined the hepatitis B vaccine (Chiarello, 1995).

✦ **Work Practice Controls.** In addition to the engineering controls, nurses must be keenly aware of what constitutes good work practice. The bloodborne pathogen standard clearly states that eating, drinking, applying cosmetics such as lip balm, and even handling contact lenses are strictly prohibited at the workplace. Any food or drink brought on to the nursing unit for use by the nursing staff or ancillary staff must be stored in a refrigerator that is separate from the refrigerator used to store specimens or client nutrition. Food cannot be consumed at the client's bedside or anywhere there is a potential for blood or other possibly infectious material to splash or spill on the food items. Eating in areas designated for that purpose, such as the cafeteria or break room (lounge), is not only practical but is federal law.

All biohazardous materials, such as blood or body

Table **20–10**

RISK OF TRANSMISSION OF BLOODBORNE PATHOGENS AFTER PERCUTANEOUS INJURY

PATHOGEN	TRANSMISSION RISK
Hepatitis B	6–30%
Hepatitis C	2.7–10%
HIV	0.31%

Adapted from Chiarello, L. (1995). Sharps-related injuries in the health-care setting: Impact and prevention strategies. *Asepsis, 17,* 18–21.

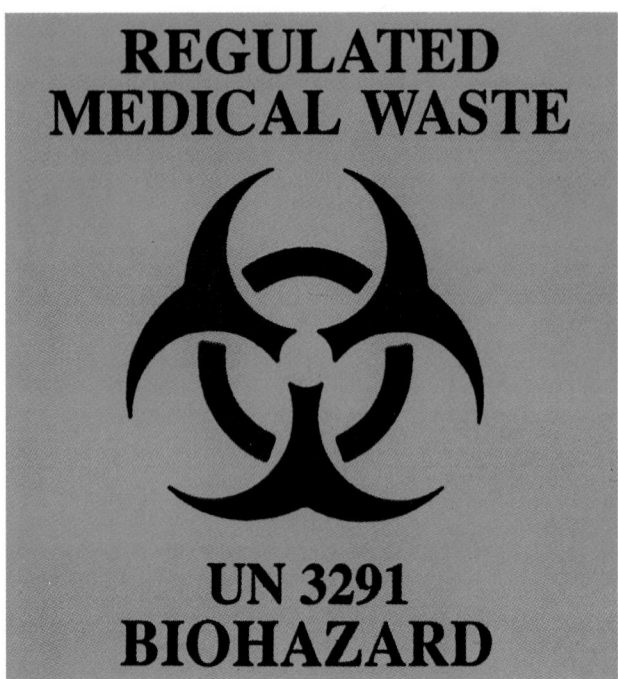

❧ **Figure 20–8**
All biohazardous materials must be appropriately labeled with the biohazard symbol on a bright orange background.

fluid specimens or items contaminated with blood or body fluids, must be labeled with appropriate signs. The nurse must be familiar with these signs and know exactly what they mean. The biohazard symbol (Fig. 20–8) is fluorescent orange or orange-red with lettering or symbols in a contrasting color (Department of Labor, 1991). Warning labels appear on refrigerators and freezers containing blood or body fluids, containers used to transport specimens to the laboratory, and containers used for infectious waste. Substitutes for the biohazard symbol are the red bags or boxes used for infectious waste and needle disposal. The nurse may be required to affix a biohazard symbol to a lab specimen that has been readied for transport.

Sometimes accidental spills of blood or other potentially contaminated body fluids occur. The health care worker who created the spill is responsible for making sure that the spill is cleaned up. Fluid on the floor is a slipping hazard as well as a biohazard. The appropriate action to take is outlined in Procedure 20–1.

❧ **Personal Protective Equipment.** Masks, gloves, gowns, and eye protection are the basic four when it comes to barrier precautions. Nurses must use the appropriate barrier for each activity. These barriers and the corresponding activities are summarized in Table

Table 20–11

PERSONAL PROTECTIVE EQUIPMENT AND SAMPLE NURSING CARE ACTIVITIES

NURSING ACTIVITY	GLOVES	GOWN	MASK	EYE PROTECTION
Taking vital signs				
Drawing blood	X			
Discontinuing IV	X			
Performing finger stick	X			
Emptying Foley bag	X		SP	SP
Changing visibly soiled bed	X	SO		
Performing postmortem care	X	SO		
Irrigating a wound	X	SO		
Suctioning, nasotracheal/endotracheal	X		SP	SP
Cleaning up blood spill	X			
Starting IV line	X			
Giving an enema	X	SO		
Removing fecal impaction	X	SO		
Providing ostomy care	X	SO		
Cleaning up incontinent client	X	SO		

X = routinely
SO = if soiling likely
SP = if splattering likely

HOW TO CLEAN UP A BLOOD OR BODY FLUID SPILL

Equipment: *Spill kit or gloves, absorbent disposable material such as paper towels, disposable tongs or brush and dustpan (to pick up broken glass), disinfectant.*

Action	Rationale
1. Apply gloves.	**1.** Protects hands from gross soilage by blood or body fluids.
2. Blot spill with absorbent disposable material such as paper towels or terry wipes. Use tongs or brush and dustpan to collect any broken glass.	**2.** Contains the spill and prevents it from spreading. Tongs, brushes, or other instruments are used to avoid touching broken glass to prevent getting cut.

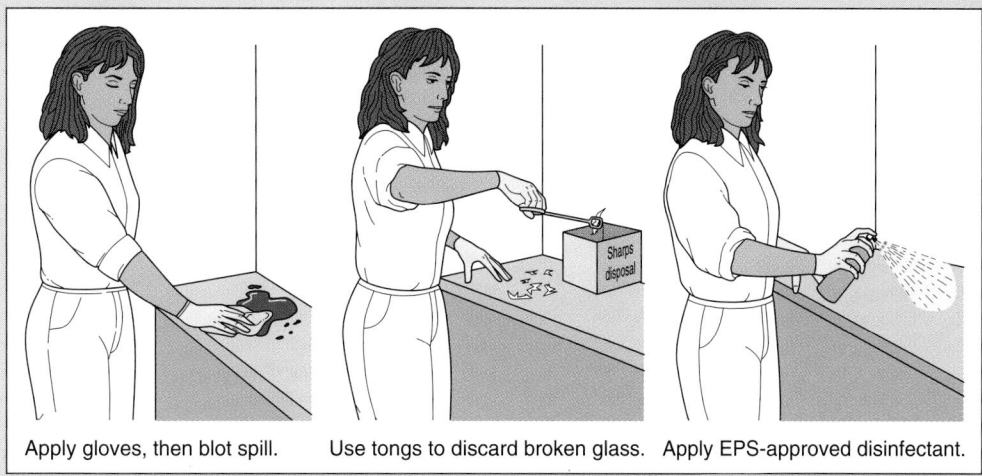

Apply gloves, then blot spill.   Use tongs to discard broken glass.   Apply EPS-approved disinfectant.

Step 2.

3. Discard blood/body fluid–soaked material in a biohazard bag. Discard broken glass in a sharps box.	**3.** Blood and other potentially contaminated body fluids are considered by OSHA to be a biohazard.
4. Use an EPA-approved disinfectant product (*e.g.,* phenol-based products, dilute bleach 1:10) to disinfect the area. Wipe with paper towels. Discard in a biohazard bag.	**4.** OSHA requires that disinfectants kill TB. Viruses, bacteria, spores, HIV, and hepatitis B, as well as TB, are easily killed by phenol products or dilute bleach.
5. Remove gloves. Discard in a biohazard bag. Wash hands.	**5.** Gloves have been contaminated by blood or other potentially infectious material and are considered a biohazard.

20–11. Housekeeping/maintenance workers should wear heavier gloves in comparison to the thin latex examination gloves. Nurses and other direct client caregivers should wear nonsterile latex or vinyl exam gloves when performing noninvasive procedures such as cleaning an incontinent client or performing mouth care. Often, health care workers develop either a true latex allergy or a hypersensitivity to the powder used on latex gloves to make them easy to don. In these cases, employers, whether they are hospitals, clinics, or home health care agencies, must provide an alternative product such as powder-free gloves or a nonlatex product. Invasive procedures, such as inserting an indwelling urinary catheter, should be performed using sterile gloves (usually provided in the Foley insertion kit).

Glove use soared after the 1991 OSHA bloodborne pathogen standard was enacted. However, nurses must pay particular attention to glove overuse. Some nurses get so engrossed in protecting themselves that they forget to remove the gloves between clients. They go from client to client without changing gloves. This phenomenon is identical to not washing hands between client care activities.

Tuberculosis Control Program

Respiratory protection for nurses and other health care workers has evolved from teaching clients to cough into tissues to using high-efficiency particulate air (HEPA) respirators that must be fit tested before being used. Because tuberculosis (TB) was a disease on the decline, many hospitals built in the early to mid-1980s gave little thought to its control. Then, in 1985, reported cases of tuberculosis increased by 20% (CDC, 1994).

From 1985 to 1992, there was a noted increase in the number of TB cases. Then, in 1992, there was an 8.7% decline in the number of TB cases reported to the CDC. The decline held true for 1993 and 1994. There were many deliberate actions taken by hospitals, public health departments, the CDC, and OSHA in an effort to stop the rising TB epidemic. Those efforts were apparently successful.

Nurses and other health care workers must wear respirators when rendering direct care to clients suspected of having or diagnosed with pulmonary tuberculosis. HEPA respirators are 99.97% efficient at screening out particles that are the size of the TB bacillus or smaller (Fig. 20–9). The higher efficiency of HEPA respirators makes them ideal for bronchoscopy or induction sputum procedures in which the client coughs profusely and respiratory secretions have a greater chance of becoming aerosolized. The N-95 respirator is 95% efficient at filtering particles that are the size of the TB bacillus. These masks are somewhat more comfortable to wear, which makes them more suited to bedside nursing care. Both of these respirators must be fit tested before use to ensure a tight, secure fit.

In addition to using respiratory protection, nurses must place clients suspected of having pulmonary tuberculosis into negative air pressure rooms. Some hospitals do not have negative air pressure rooms and cannot add airflow to the current ventilation system that the hospital uses. These hospitals use portable HEPA filter units. Some of the portable HEPA filters also have ultraviolet (UV) light capabilities. UV light can destroy the TB bacillus and many other bacteria and viruses. The HEPA filter filters the air as it passes through the unit. Thus, HEPA/UV systems are a "belt and suspenders" approach to air filtration. The nurses' responsibility is to order the HEPA unit for any client admitted with suspected or diagnosed pulmonary tuberculosis.

Finally, all nursing staff and other health care workers, including physicians, should receive a tuberculin skin test at least yearly. Some nurses who work on units that admit many clients with suspected or proven diagnoses of pulmonary tuberculosis or who assist in high-risk procedures such as bronchoscopy or induction sputum procedures may need more frequent skin testing (every 3 months).

Chemical Hazards

Nurses face a variety of chemical hazards, radiation exposures, and exposures to chemotherapeutic agents. In 1983, OSHA issued the hazard communication standard, which was later referred to as the right-to-know standard (Department of Labor, 1983). The purpose of the standard is to ensure that all employees have information about the chemicals they work with. Most people work with chemicals on a daily basis, and they are not necessarily employed in a chemical factory.

Hospitals and other health care institutions use many chemicals for cleaning and disinfecting that emit hazardous fumes. These chemicals must be handled carefully. Chemotherapeutic agents are drugs used to treat cancer. Some of these agents are radioactive, and some are cytotoxic, in that they target specific cells. The nursing staff and other health care workers have a right to know about these chemical hazards in the workplace. The nurse should be familiar with the chemical before using it, read the label, and follow warnings and instructions.

Chemical labels typically have the name of the chemical and the name, address, and emergency phone number of the manufacturer. A large signal word such as DANGER or CAUTION appears next, followed by the physical hazards (will it explode or catch fire?) and the health hazards (is it toxic? can it cause cancer?). This is followed by precautionary measures, which include whether gloves or other protec-

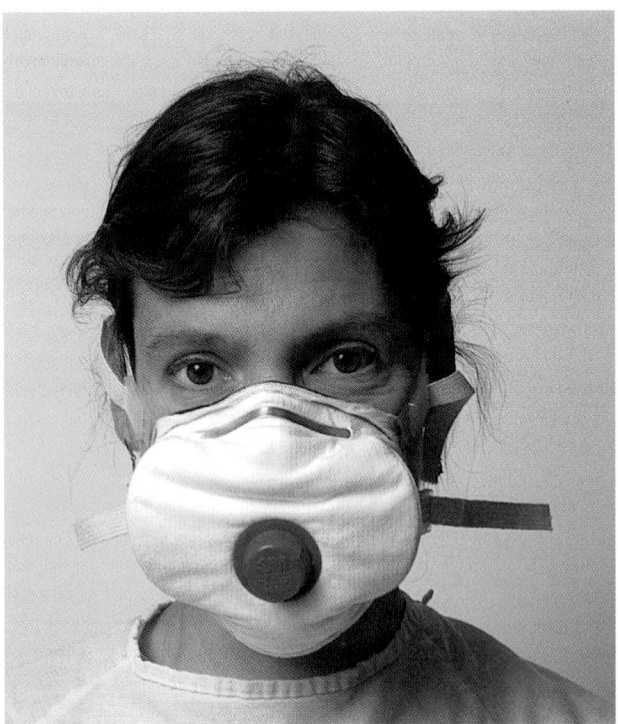

Figure 20–9

The HEPA respirator is 99.97% efficient in screening out particles the size of the TB bacillus and even smaller. A HEPA respirator should be worn for bronchoscopy or induction sputum procedures during which the patient coughs profusely. The respirator must be fit-tested prior to use to ensure a tight, secure fit.

tive equipment should be worn when working with the chemical. First-aid instructions are listed, as well as proper storage instructions. Finally, special instructions concerning children are given. A material safety data sheet should be available on the nursing unit to supply additional information not covered on the product label.

Biological Safety and the Nursing Process

Assessment

Clients who have or are prone to developing infections should be closely assessed and monitored. In order to classify a client as having a nosocomial infection, certain criteria must be met. Along with vital signs, laboratory tests such as microbiological cultures of body fluids, complete blood counts, and certain virological titers can be used to determine the presence or absence of infection.

✦ **Nursing History.** The nurse collects information from the client and/or family about:

* *Immunization history.* The immunization status of the client is recorded. Dates of vaccinations are documented as accurately as possible. Tests such as tuberculin skin tests are recorded.

* *Nutrition.* Record any fluctuations in diet, any weight loss the client has experienced, and over what period of time the weight loss has occurred. Clients with certain infectious diseases such as tuberculosis or HIV experience significant weight loss as part of the disease process.

✦ **Physical Assessment.** Accurately recorded vital signs and physical assessment tools can help sway the verdict of infection versus colonization. Fluctuations in vital signs occur as infection creeps in. For example, a temperature of 101.8°F (38.7°C) on admission to an institution may be indicative of a community-acquired infection. A temperature of 101.8°F (38.7°C) 2 days after surgery may indicate a postoperative wound infection. Is the temperature normal or elevated? Is the elevated temperature constant, or does it occur in cycles (*e.g.,* in malaria, temperature spikes occur in the evening)? How do the lungs sound to percussion and auscultation? Is the skin cold and clammy, or is the client diaphoretic? Are rashes present? A thorough physical assessment, including eyes, ears, nose, and throat examination, is warranted. Examine the neck and chest for palpable lymph nodes, check breath sounds, and look for the presence or absence of rashes or mottling.

Certain tick-borne diseases, such as Lyme disease, have a peculiar patterned rash that starts from the tick bite and extends outward in waves of erythema. It is described as alternating patterns of redness and clear zones in concentric circles. Another tick-borne disease, Rocky Mountain spotted fever, has a more diffuse rash pattern. Thus, it is essential that the characteristics of a rash, if present, be accurately recorded.

✦ **Diagnostic Testing.** Diagnostic tests play a key role in nursing assessment and infection detection. The most common diagnostic test is a culture, which involves determining what organisms are present in the specimen. Often it is the positive culture result that cues the nurse to the fact that an infection may be present.

Cultures. Specimen collection is performed using appropriate personal protective equipment (PPE), such as gloves. Masks and eye protection are worn when necessary. The specimen containers are sterile and leakproof and are transported to the laboratory in leakproof plastic bags. Nurses must ensure that the containers are properly sealed to prevent leakage while in transport. Syringes with needles still attached are inappropriate specimen containers. The specimen can be transferred to a sterile tube or the needle can be removed with a protective device and the specimen placed in a sealable plastic bag.

When collecting the specimen, the nurse avoids contamination by normal flora that resides on the skin and mucous membranes. The most common types of specimens that are collected are urine, sputum, blood, throat, and wound (see Procedures 20–2 through 20–7). As always, appropriate PPE is a must. An adequate volume of body fluids must be collected, so the nurse should check with the laboratory to ascertain the specific requirements and quantities. Insufficient volumes may give false-negative results. All specimens are labeled with the client's name, identification number, date of collection, and specimen source. Some laboratories require the time of collection and the client's attending physician's name.

Specimens should be transported to the laboratory promptly (within 2 hours). Specimens collected on evening or night shifts may be refrigerated for up to 24 hours. Some organisms have specific growth requirements and are very sensitive to temperature change. If the following organisms are suspected, the specimen should immediately be taken to the laboratory: *Neisseria gonorrhoeae, Neisseria meningitidis, Haemophilus influenzae,* and *Shigella.* Specimens from the eye, internal ear, or genital area and spinal fluid should also be sent to the laboratory immediately and should not be refrigerated.

Hematologic Studies. The complete blood counts (CBC) offers a wealth of data. It consists of a group of tests that includes:

* Hemoglobin
* Hematocrit
* Red blood cell count (RBC)
* White blood cell count (WBC)
* Differential white cell count

Text continued on page 418

COLLECTING A URINE SPECIMEN USING STRAIGHT CATHETERIZATION

Equipment: *Urinary straight catheterization kit (catheter, lubricating jelly, underpad, drapes, sterile gloves, forceps, povidone-iodine solution and prep balls or presoaked povidone-iodine swabs, sterile specimen container).*

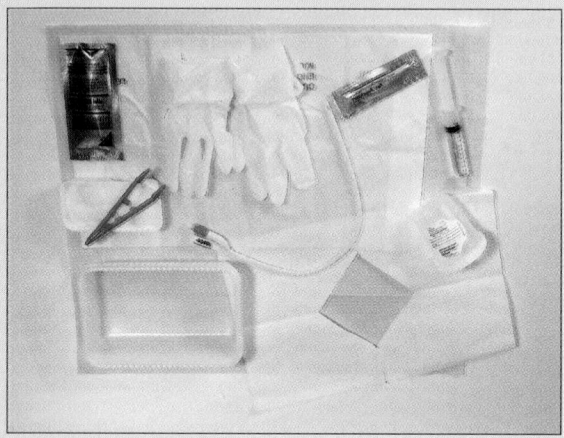

Action	Rationale
1. Wash hands. Open catheter kit to create a sterile field.	**1.** Removes transient flora.
2. Place underpad under client's buttocks.	**2.** Prevents soilage of the bed.
3. Don sterile gloves.	**3.** Sterile gloves are used at this point to prepare for the catheterization (opening sterile solutions and so forth).
4. Open povidone-iodine solution and pour onto prep balls, or open all presoaked povidone-iodine swabs and lay on sterile field.	**4.** Solution and equipment must be opened and prepared before touching the client (and thus contaminating the gloves).
5. Open lubricating jelly and pour into slot on the tray. Lubricate the tip of the catheter and the first 5 inches.	**5.** Lubrication is necessary to ease the catheter into the urethra without pain and irritation.
6. For women, with the nondominant hand, hold the labia apart. Grasp the povidone-iodine–soaked balls with forceps and cleanse the meatus using downward strokes and working from the outside toward the center. Use one ball per stroke and discard. For men, retract the foreskin.	**6.** Cleansing is accomplished from clean to dirty. The anus is contaminated with normal bacterial flora and is considered dirty compared with the sterile bladder.

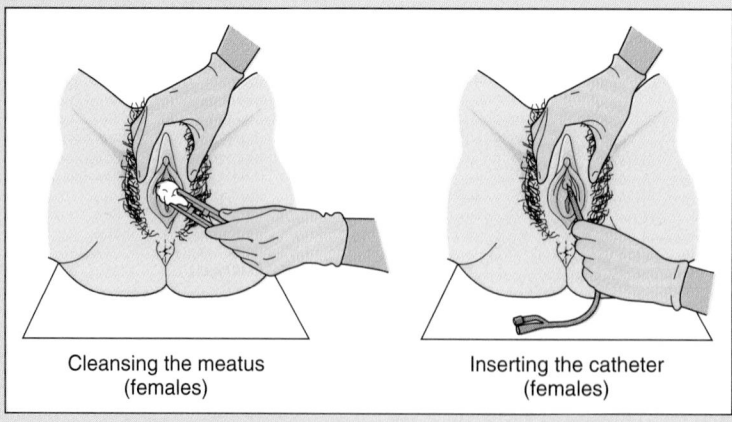

Cleansing the meatus (females)

Inserting the catheter (females)

Step 6.

Continued

20–2

COLLECTING A URINE SPECIMEN USING STRAIGHT CATHETERIZATION
(Continued)

Action	Rationale
7. While still holding the labia apart (or keeping the foreskin retracted on the penis), pick up the catheter (with the dominant hand) without touching the tip and gently insert it into the urethra.	**7.** The catheter tip must remain sterile. The gloved dominant hand may have accidentally touched tissue while cleansing the urethra.
8. If a preattached collection bag is not present, place the sterile cup at the end of the catheter after 15 ml of urine has passed.	**8.** The first 15 ml could be contaminated with ascending organisms from the perineal area.
9. Remove the catheter. Cap and label the specimen with the client's name, date, and so forth. Place it in a biohazard bag and send it to the lab.	**9.** The OSHA bloodborne pathogen standard requires the appropriate biohazard symbol on all lab specimens.

20–3

COLLECTING A URINE SPECIMEN USING A FOLEY CATHETER

Equipment: *20-ml syringe, antiseptic pad, sterile cup, nonsterile gloves.*

Action	Rationale
1. Wash hands and don gloves.	**1.** Removes transient flora on the hands. Gloves are used to protect the hands from gross soilage from the urine in case of spill or splatter.
2. Kink the tubing 3 inches from the sample port until urine becomes visible under the puncture site.	**2.** If tubing is not kinked, the urine will drain into the bag.
3. Swab the surface of the sample port with the antiseptic pad.	**3.** Removes transient bacteria on the port.
4. Insert the needle/syringe in the center of the sample port and withdraw the desired amount of urine (15 ml).	**4.** Sample from the appropriate port to obtain a sterile sample. Some Foley catheter systems do not need a needle to puncture the sample port (needleless systems).
5. Place the specimen in the sterile cup. Cap and label the specimen with the client's name, date, and so forth.	**5.** A sterile cup avoids environmental contamination. Label all lab specimens with the identity of the client to avoid specimen mix-up.
6. Place the specimen in a biohazard bag and send it to the lab.	**6.** The OSHA bloodborne pathogen standard requires the appropriate biohazard label on all lab specimens.

PROCEDURE

20–4

COLLECTING A MIDSTREAM (CLEAN CATCH) URINE SPECIMEN: FEMALES

Equipment: *Antiseptic pads, sterile collection cup.*

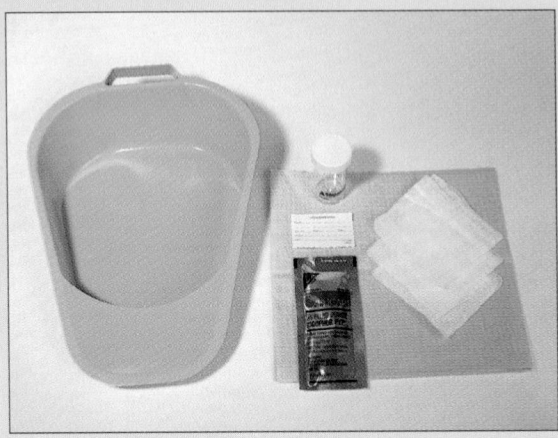

Action	Rationale
1. Instruct the client to clean the meatus with antiseptic pads. Use at least two pads per each labial side and clean using a downward stroke. Instruct the client to use a new pad with each stroke. The last pad should clean over the urethra (down the center).	1. Client instruction is crucial to obtaining this specimen. Cleansing is accomplished from clean to dirty. The anus is contaminated with normal bacteria.
2. Instruct the client to void while holding the labia apart.	2. Avoids the stream of urine touching the labial tissue (which is clean but not sterile).
3. After some urine has passed, instruct the client to collect urine in the sterile container. Make sure that her fingers do not touch the inside of the specimen cup.	3. The first 15 ml of urine could be contaminated with ascending bacteria from the urethra and must be discarded.
4. Cap and label the specimen with the client's name, date, and so forth. Place the container in a biohazard bag.	4. The OSHA bloodborne pathogen standard requires that all lab specimens be labeled as biohazards.

COLLECTING A MIDSTREAM (CLEAN CATCH) URINE SPECIMEN: MALES

Equipment: *Antiseptic pads, sterile specimen cup.*

Action	Rationale
1. Instruct the client to wash his hands and retract the foreskin. Instruct the client to clean the glans with antiseptic pads and to use a circular motion, cleaning from the urethra outward.	1. Cleansing is accomplished from clean to dirty. There are higher concentrations of bacteria at the edges of the glans as opposed to the urethra.
2. Instruct the client to void while retracting the foreskin.	2. Avoids the urine stream touching tissue.
3. After some urine has passed, collect the urine in a sterile container. Instruct the client not to touch the inside of the container with his fingers.	3. The first 15 ml may be contaminated with ascending bacteria from the urethra. If fingers touch the inside of the sterile container, the specimen will be contaminated.
4. Cap and label the specimen with the client's name, date, and so forth. Place the specimen in a biohazard bag.	4. The OSHA bloodborne pathogen standard requires that all lab specimens be labeled as biohazards.

COLLECTING EXPECTORATED SPUTUM

Equipment: *Sterile specimen cup.*

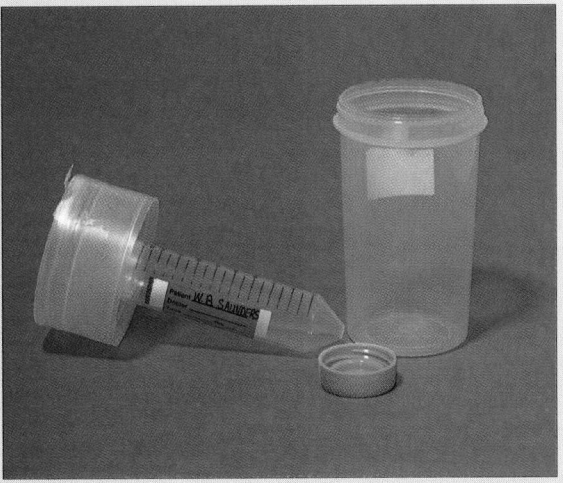

Action	**Rationale**
1. Instruct the client to rinse mouth with water. Collect early morning specimens for AFB (tuberculosis) as soon as the client awakes and before breakfast.	**1.** Rinsing decreases normal flora of the mouth. AFB (tuberculosis bacilli) are concentrated in the sputum in the morning. Three specimens on three consecutive mornings are necessary to conclusively demonstrate the pathogen's presence.
2. Instruct the client to cough deeply, producing a lower respiratory specimen.	**2.** Postnasal fluid is unacceptable.

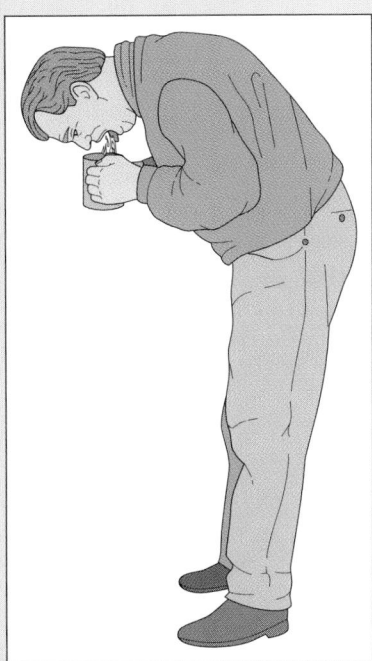

Step 2.

3. Collect the specimen in the sterile container. Cap and label the container with the client's name, date, and so forth. Place the specimen in a biohazard bag.	**3.** Minimizes contamination. The OSHA bloodborne pathogen standard requires the appropriate biohazard label on all lab specimens.

Continued

PROCEDURE

20–5

COLLECTING SPUTUM FROM AN INTUBATED CLIENT
(Continued)

Equipment: *Sputum specimen trap, suction kit (contains catheter, gloves, saline).*

Action	Rationale
1. Wash hands. Open suction kit. Pour saline into sterile compartment on the tray (kit). Open sputum specimen trap.	**1.** Washing hands removes transient flora. All necessary procedures, such as opening bottles, are performed before donning sterile gloves.
2. Don gloves. Attach suction catheter to latex tubing on sputum trap. Attach the suction tubing (which is connected to wall suction) to the male connector on top of the trap. Suction endotracheal tube.	**2.** Gloves prevent gross soilage. The sputum will collect in the trap.
3. Dip the tip of the suction catheter into saline. Disconnect the catheter from the trap and discard the catheter.	**3.** Flushes any remaining sputum into the trap.
4. Bend the latex tubing onto the male end of the connector at the top of the trap. Press firmly into place.	**4.** The latex tubing forms a sealed container.
5. Label the specimen with the client's name, date, and so forth. Place the specimen in a biohazard bag.	**5.** The OSHA bloodborne pathogen standard requires the appropriate biohazard label on all lab specimens.

• Red cell indices

• Stained red cell examination

In particular, levels of the white blood cells known as polymorphonuclear leukocytes (polys) above the norm (5000 to 10,000/cubic mm blood) are indicative of an infectious process. These polys, also known as neutrophils or PMNs, have a protective function that includes phagocytosis.

A differential white cell count is done to identify the five different types of normal white cells. The cells are counted and the results are expressed as percentages, the total equaling 100%. An increase in the number of neutrophils (normal range, 60 to 70%) indicates the presence of a bacterial or parasitic infection. With viral infections, usually the lymphocyte count is elevated.

Urinalysis. Urine studies are also helpful. When a urinary tract infection is present, the urine is positive for leukocyte esterase and/or nitrate. Pyuria is the presence of white blood cells in the urine. If an infection is present, there will be greater than 10 WBC/cubic mm of unspun urine per high-powered field (under the microscope). Sometimes laboratory technicians Gram stain unspun urine. If microorganisms are present, so is an infection.

Virologic Studies. The virology laboratory unleashes an entirely different set of tests that at first glance seem to be in a foreign language. Most of the specimens are from blood, but some could be from spinal fluid. These tests include the IgM and IgG antibody titers to determine immunity to such viral diseases as hepatitis A and varicella (chicken pox). *Proteus* XO titers are used to determine if a patient has a tickborne illness such as Rocky Mountain spotted fever. The enzyme-linked immunosorbent assay (ELISA) and Western blot are two virology tests that are quite well known and are used to determine if the client has HIV.

Any positive blood culture is worthy of scrutiny. However, an occasional false-positive blood culture results if the site was inadequately prepared or the specimen was subject to poor handling techniques in the lab. In general, positive blood culture results, particularly if the results indicate gram-negative rod bacteria or streptococci, are indicative of infection. Results with coagulase-negative staphylococci in one bottle out of four, for example, could indicate a skin contaminant from a poorly prepared site. This is especially true if the client does not have other signs or symptoms of infection.

Some body systems always have sterile body fluids (see Box 20–5). The presence of bacteria in these normally sterile body fluids indicates infection. Other body fluids and sites have organisms that are always present. Cultures of sputum, for example, always show growth of some kind of organism. Whether a culture is positive or not may not be an indication of infection. It is the combination of signs, symptoms, culture results, and overall patient well-being that determines whether infection is present.

Once laboratory data have been collected, it can be difficult to determine whether the results indicate

PROCEDURE

20–6

COLLECTING A BLOOD CULTURE

Equipment: *70% alcohol pads, 20-ml syringe with 20-gauge needle, blood culture bottles, gloves, povidone-iodine pads, labels.*

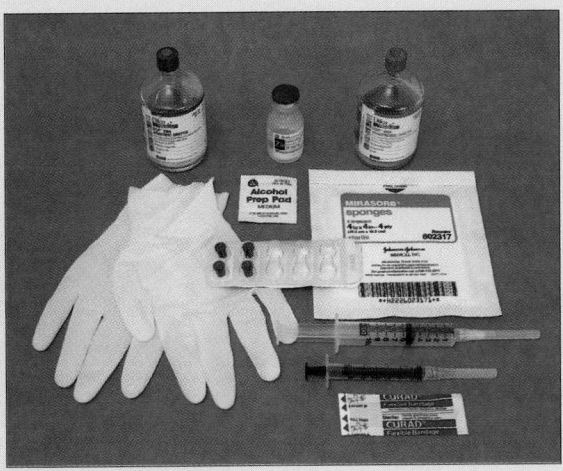

Action	**Rationale**
1. Wash hands and don gloves. Apply tourniquet and select venipuncture site.	1. Handwashing before the procedure removes transient bacterial flora. Wearing gloves prevents gross soilage of the hands with blood. Gloves are also mandated by OSHA for all venipuncture/IV starts.

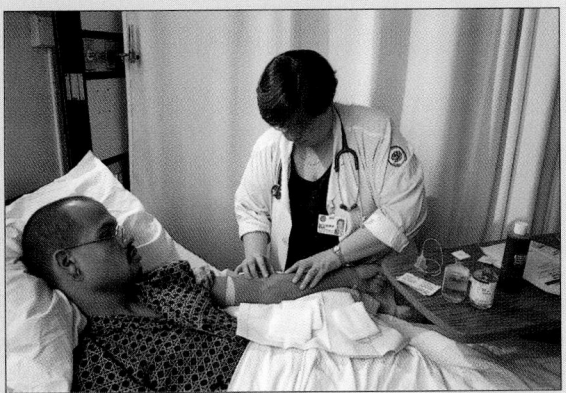

Step 1. *Looking for vein*

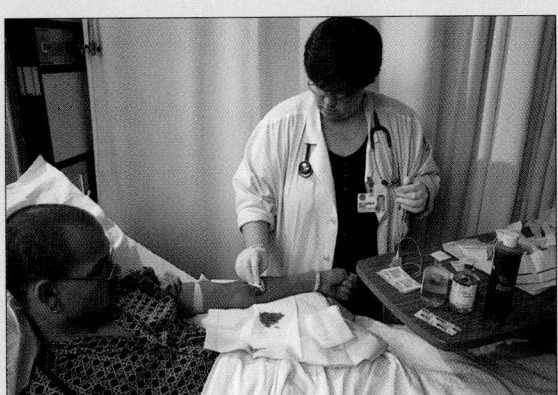

Step 2. *Skin preparation*

2. Cleanse skin thoroughly with alcohol pads. Allow the skin to dry.	2. Alcohol serves as an initial disinfectant and cleans the skin. Disinfectants are deactivated by organic material.
3. Swab the site with povidone-iodine pad in a circular action (from projected injection site outward.) Allow to dry.	3. Povidone-iodine serves as a disinfectant but needs time to kill bacteria. Allowing the antiseptic to dry provides this time.

Continued

PROCEDURE

20–6

COLLECTING A BLOOD CULTURE
(Continued)

Action	Rationale
4. Perform the venipuncture, withdrawing 20 ml of blood for adults, 6 ml for children, and 1 ml for neonates/infants/young children. Use smaller size syringe for children or neonates. Remove tourniquet.	**4.** Adequate blood volumes are essential for the automated blood culture analysis. Pediatric blood culture bottles are necessary for pediatric clients.

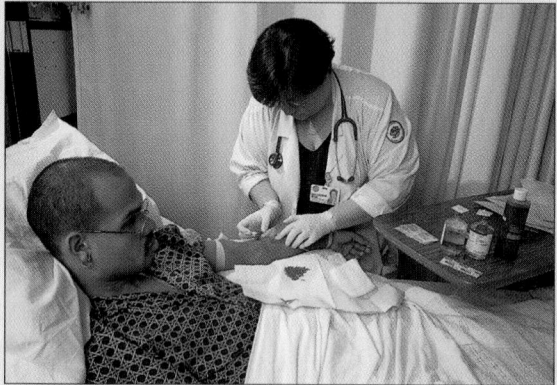

Step 4. *Puncture*

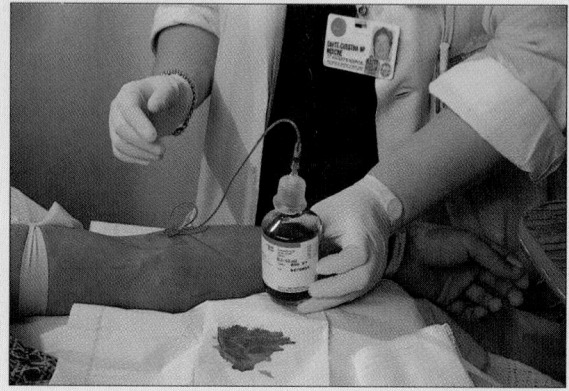

Step 4. *Filling bottle*

Action	Rationale
5. Swab the top of the blood culture with 70% alcohol pad and allow to dry.	**5.** Povidone-iodine interferes with the blood culture machine.
6. Transfer blood into culture bottle without changing needles. Instill half the sample into the aerobic bottle and half into the anaerobic bottle.	**6.** Changing needles increases the chances for contamination and a false reading of the blood culture. Blood transfer devices are available to ensure that this process is safe.
7. Label the bottles with the client's name, date, and so forth. Place the cultures in a biohazard bag and send them to the lab.	**7.** The OSHA bloodborne pathogen standard requires the appropriate biohazard label on all lab specimens.

an infection or represent colonization. The nurse can look for other clues to assist in making this determination. If the cultured organism is considered normal flora, it becomes even more difficult. Yet the overall clinical picture of the client is a valuable indicator.

Box 20–5

EXAMPLES OF STERILE BODY SITES

* Blood
* Cerebrospinal fluid (CSF)
* Urine (catheterized)
* Bronchoscopy washing (lower lung)
* Bronchi
* Sinuses
* Middle and inner ear

All tests play a part in the total picture of the disease process the client is experiencing. Data collected can then be assembled to form a nursing diagnosis and to develop an appropriate plan of care.

High-Risk Clients

Clients with severe trauma or burns, those admitted to intensive care units, and those at the extremes of age (premature infants and the extremely aged) often pose special infection risks. Usually these clients are the sickest and most fragile. Most have multiple lines, ventilators, and other invasive devices, providing many opportunities to bypass normal host defenses. Each intensive care unit or special care unit presents a unique challenge.

✦ **Neonatal Intensive Care Unit.** Infants born prematurely (before 37 weeks gestation) are low birth weight (weighing 1000 to 1500 grams) or very low birth weight (weighing less than 1000 grams) and can have a gestational age of 24 to 36 weeks. Prior to birth, the fetus is uniquely protected against many pathogens and acquires infections only as the result of transplacental transmission or passage through an infected birth canal. Once born, a normal newborn becomes colonized with the organisms from the mother, family members, and hospital personnel. A premature infant, however, has limited maternal contact, and many have antibiotics, invasive devices, delayed feeding, and more hospital personnel exposure.

Sources of infection for the premature infant include hands of hospital personnel; contact with inadequately decontaminated hospital equipment; water sources such as humidifiers, nebulizers, and ventilator tubing; manipulation of invasive lines; banked breast milk; and hospital-prepared formula. Many premature infants undergo surgery soon after birth and thus are at risk for surgical site infections.

The largest nosocomial risk for the premature infant is indwelling devices. Intravenous catheters, endotracheal tubes, central venous catheters, and umbilical catheters all bypass the body's main defenses. Many institutions require elaborate scrubs and donning of protective gowns before entering the neonatal intensive care unit. The rationale is to protect the nursery as a whole from outside organisms. Current infection control thought is to treat each infant as unique and as a potential source and recipient of infection. Handwashing becomes crucial to prevent the spread of microorganisms from infant to infant on the hands of personnel.

✦ **Immunocompromised Clients.** Transplantation has virtually revolutionized medicine in the twentieth century. Solid organ transplants and bone marrow transplants are increasing. Because of similarities in drug combinations and the shared immunosuppressive state, clients with neoplastic disease (cancer) are at the same risk for infection as clients receiving transplants. Associated with these modalities are high-dose chemotherapy and radiation therapy. The goal of these complex modalities is to suppress or destroy the body's immune system to allow the transplanted organ to graft. The radiation and chemotherapy serve to halt cancer growth or even destroy the rapidly metabolizing cancer cells.

In the early 1970s, the CDC recommended protective isolation. This involved the health care worker donning mask, gown, and gloves to protect the immune-suppressed client from outside contamination. In 1983, the CDC removed protective isolation as a category of isolation, calling it an expensive endeavor of little value in preventing infections (Garner & Simmons, 1983). Many severely immunocompromised clients develop infections from their own endogenous microflora. HEPA filters are used, along with topical antiseptics and oral antibiotics (to decrease intestinal flora), in an effort to control infections (Oniboni, 1990).

One of the major determinants of infection in this group of clients is the degree of immune suppression. High doses of steroids, such as prednisone, tend to predispose these clients to opportunistic fungal infections. The actual location of the transplant is also a

PROCEDURE 20–7

COLLECTING A THROAT CULTURE

Equipment: *Face shield or mask and goggles, culture swab, gloves, tongue depressors.*

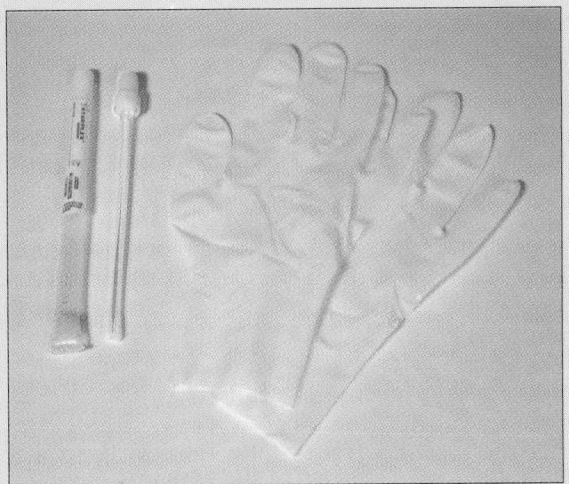

Continued

PROCEDURE

20–7

COLLECTING A THROAT CULTURE
(Continued)

Action	**Rationale**
1. Wash hands. Don face shield and gloves.	1. Handwashing removes transient flora. The face shield and gloves protect the health care worker's eyes, nose, and hands from gross soilage and possible coughing or splatter. This is an OSHA requirement.
2. Have the client open mouth. With the tongue depressor, depress the tongue. With the culture swab, swipe the back of the pharynx or exudate on the tonsils.	2. The tongue depressor prevents the tongue from touching the culture swab.

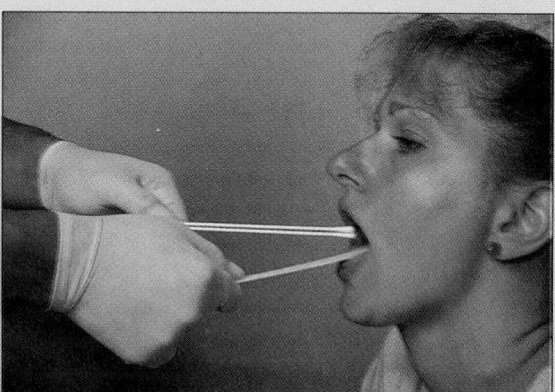

Step 2. *Collecting culture*

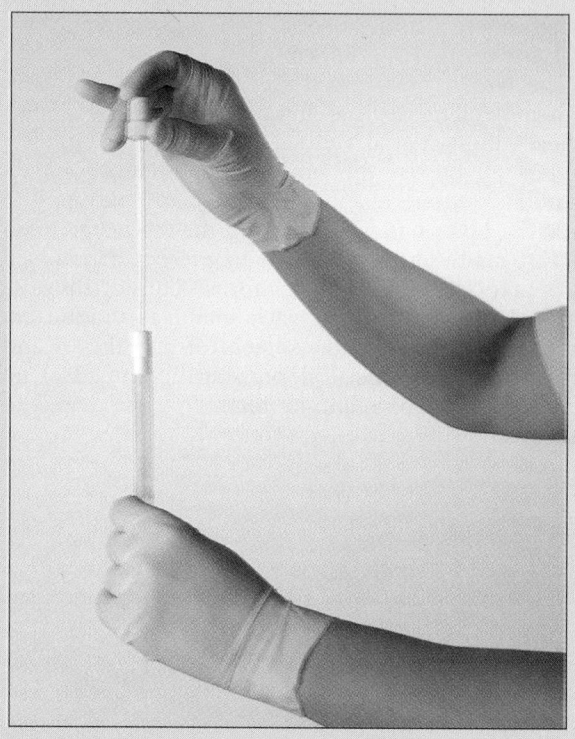

Step 3. *Replacing swab in holder*

3. Carefully reinsert the swab into its plastic holder and depress the capsule.	3. The capsule holds a transport liquid that keeps organisms viable during the trip to the lab.
4. Label the specimen with the client's name, date, and so forth. Place the specimen in a biohazard bag.	4. The OSHA bloodborne pathogen standard requires the appropriate biohazard label on all lab specimens.

factor in the risk of infection. For example, a cytomegalovirus pneumonia is much more severe in a lung transplant recipient than in a client with a renal transplant.

✦ **Critical Care Clients.** Because health care and managed care practices focus on early discharge and home-based care for many clients, the remainder are usually critically ill. These clients usually have multiple invasive devices: indwelling urinary catheters, central venous lines, pulmonary artery lines, arterial lines,

chest tubes, surgical drains, and intracranial monitors. Specialized trauma units and burn units have clients with multiple injuries and large areas of body surface involved (major burns, asphalt and road abrasions in multitrauma clients), placing these clients at particularly high risk for infection.

Critical care clients usually become colonized with the resident flora of that particular intensive care unit within the first 24 to 48 hours after admission to the unit. According to surveillance data from the CDC, nosocomial bloodstream infections and ventilator-associated pneumonia are frequently the most common cause of morbidity and mortality in intensive care units. Widespread use of mechanical ventilation and central venous lines has defined a high-risk population that is at increased risk for infection.

Nursing Diagnosis

Nursing diagnoses that typically reflect infection or infectious processes include the following:

Activity Intolerance related to weakness associated with many illnesses, including AIDS

Airway Clearance, Ineffective related to pneumonia

Body Temperature, Risk for Altered (fever)

Diarrhea related to intestinal infection with such organisms as *Salmonella, Shigella, Campylobacter,* and *Clostridium difficile*

Hyperthermia related to sepsis and other infections

Hypothermia related to sepsis

Infection, Risk for: all nosocomial infection types, especially when devices (*e.g.,* lines, ventilators) are present

Noncompliance with TB medications, leading to drug resistance

Skin Integrity, Impaired: clients with burns, decubitus ulcers

This list is not exclusive. Any aspect of any infection can easily lend itself to many of the NANDA-approved nursing diagnostic categories. One infectious disease, AIDS, covers most of the diagnoses in broad ranges of categories. Once a nursing diagnosis is established, implementing a plan of care is the next step.

Planning

The desired outcome is for the client to have no evidence of infection or resolution of the infection. The nursing plan of care carefully outlines the problems encountered, expected outcomes, and any nursing interventions. An example of a plan of care is given for a client diagnosed with respiratory syncytial virus (RSV) (see Nursing Care Plan 20–2).

Implementation

Resolution of the infection can be fostered by administering antibiotics, antifungal agents, or antiviral agents. Preventing the infection in the first place is the

PROCEDURE

20–8

HANDWASHING

Equipment: *Sink, soap, paper towels.*

Action	Rationale
1. Turn on water. Adjust temperature. Wet hands with warm water. Leave water running if no foot control, knee control, or automatic shutoff during all steps.	**1.** Warm water improves the sudsing action of the soap. The sink and the handles on the sink are considered dirty. The health care worker uses dirty hands to turn the water on. If the worker retouches the handles at any point during the handwashing procedure, the hands become recontaminated.

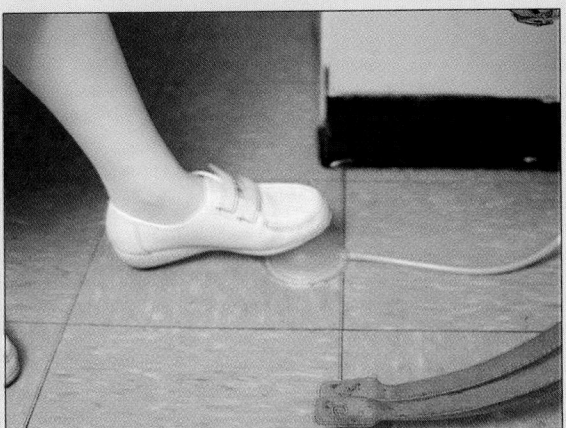

Using foot pedal to turn on water

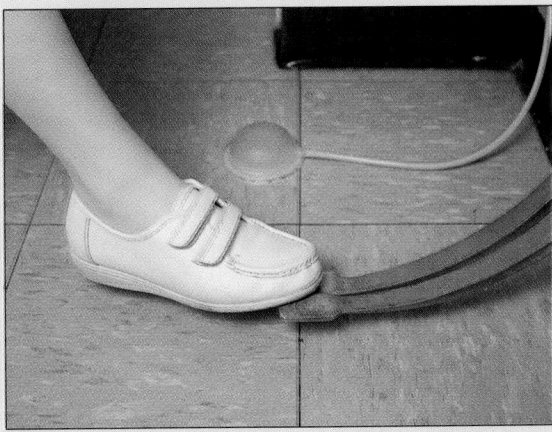

Soap dispenser pressed with foot

Continued

HANDWASHING
(Continued)

Action	**Rationale**

2. Apply liquid soap to hands. Vigorously rub all surfaces of hands, between fingers, and under nails for 10–15 seconds. Keep hands pointed downward.

2. Friction is important for removing dirt and microbial substances. Bacteria collect in crevices and under nails. Pointing hands downward allows contaminated material to drip off skin.

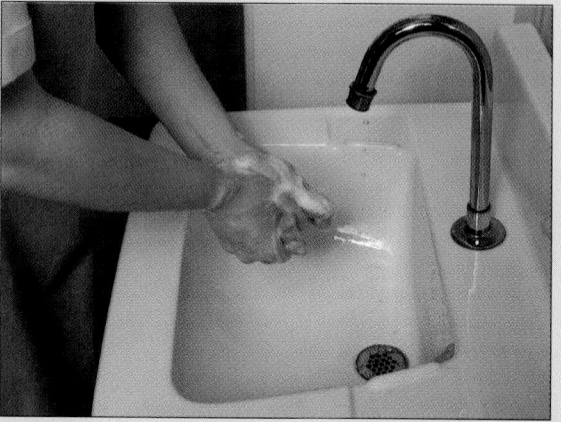

Step 2.

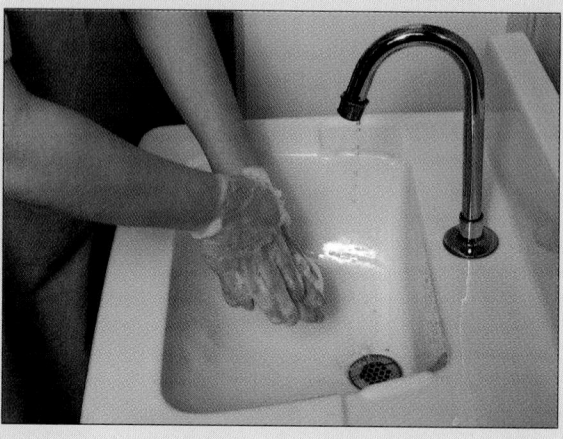

3. Rinse hands thoroughly.

3. Removes contaminated material from skin.

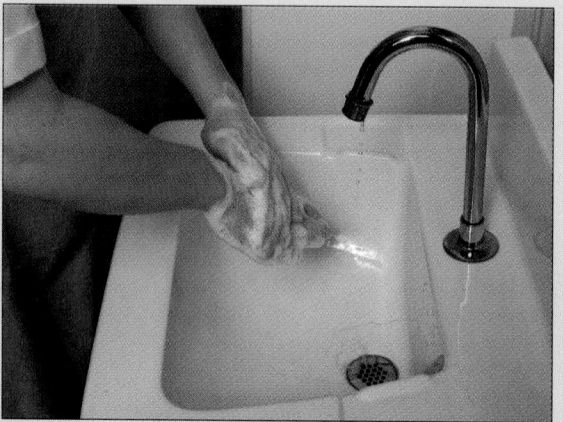

Step 3.

4. Dry hands with a paper towel. Use a paper towel to turn the water faucet off.

4. Touching dirty handles with clean hands would recontaminate hands. Paper towel acts as a barrier to prevent hands from becoming recontaminated.

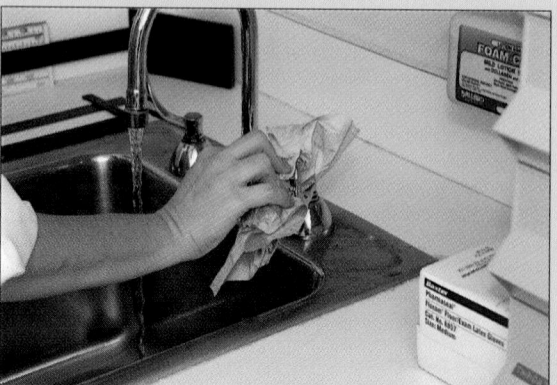

Step 4.

goal of infection control and can be accomplished by handwashing, use of aseptic technique, and isolation.

Handwashing

Handwashing is the single most important means of preventing infections in both the hospital and the home. Hands should be washed:

- Before beginning any client care activity
- Before exiting the room
- After removing gloves, in case there are microscopic holes or tears in the gloves
- Between clients

As simple as handwashing seems, there is a definite technique to good handwashing (see Procedure 20–8). The fingertips should always point downward to allow the water to drain from the least contaminated area (arms, elbows) to the most contaminated (fingertips). If knee or foot controls are not available, the nurse should always turn the water off using a paper towel to avoid recontaminating freshly cleaned hands.

For routine nursing care, any plain soap (bar, leaflets, liquid, or powder) is acceptable (Larson, 1995). The amount of soap used is irrelevant. It is the friction of rubbing the hands together during the act of handwashing that is important for removing surface organisms. Antimicrobial soaps are recommended for intensive care areas or areas where invasive procedures, such as central line placement or intracranial monitor placement, are done. Antimicrobial soap not only

eliminates transient flora on the hands but also reduces resident flora. These soaps bind to the skin's top layers, resulting in antimicrobial activity that lingers after the handwashing stops (Larson, 1995). Finally, the duration of handwashing stops (Larson, 1995). Finally, the duration of handwashing is important to allow antimicrobial soaps sufficient contact time with the skin to kill organisms.

Often, handwashing sinks and soap and water are not available or conveniently located. Alcohol-based handwashing agents, which are used without water, are an acceptable alternative, provided that hands are not visibly soiled (Larson, 1995).

Handwashing products can become contaminated with microorganisms, so it is important that dispensers and bar soap racks be kept clean. If bar soaps are used, slotted bar soap racks should be used to promote drainage, along with small bars of soap that encourage frequent changing. Liquid soaps are ideally dispensed from disposable containers, or the containers can be rinsed and thoroughly dried before being refilled (Larson, 1995). Some states require only liquid soaps in hospitals and other public places. Just like soap, hand lotion can support the growth of bacteria. Nurses should use small individual-sized hand lotion bottles rather than large refillable bottles that are shared among the nursing staff. Hand lotions should be water based, not petroleum based. Petroleum-based emollients may degrade latex gloves, causing them to rip or tear more easily or increasing their permeability (Larson, 1995).

Nurses should keep fingernails short. Long nails

SAMPLE NURSING CARE PLAN

THE CLIENT WITH BRONCHIOLITIS

Situation: A 9-month-old premature infant was discharged from the neonatal intensive care unit 2 weeks ago. The infant returned to the emergency department with signs and symptoms of RSV bronchiolitis. The child was admitted to the pediatric unit and placed on contact isolation. The parents are observed taking the infant to the playroom and being noncompliant with the isolation precautions.

Nursing Diagnosis: Knowledge deficit—RSV isolation procedures.

Expected Outcome: Family demonstrates compliance with isolation.

Action	Rationale
1. Use mask, gown, and gloves with each client encounter.	1. RSV can linger on inanimate objects such as bed rails for up to 1½ hours. The example the nurse sets demonstrates correct technique.
2. Instruct the family in isolation techniques. Apply gown, gloves, and mask and have parents demonstrate. Explain why each item is used.	2. A demonstration of correct technique coupled with an explanation will clarify hospital isolation procedures. Gowns and gloves protect hands and clothing from RSV, which can linger on inanimate objects for long periods. Masks are used to keep hands (gloved and ungloved) from touching the face to avoid autoinnoculation of RSV from the environment to the mouth or nose (from contaminated hands).

pierce latex gloves easily. The majority of the microorganisms found on hands are under and around the nails. If nail polish is worn at all, clear is preferred, because dark colors obscure the nail bed and prevent adequate cleaning. Artificial nails have been associated with high bacterial counts on the hands. Jewelry can increase the microbial load of the hands, as well as making glove application more difficult. At least one organization, the Association of Operating Room Nurses (AORN), prohibits nail polish, jewelry, and artificial nails. AORN publishes guidelines that cover dress codes for the operating room.

Asepsis

Asepsis is the absence of microorganisms that produce disease. Aseptic technique is the practice of reducing the total numbers of organisms to prevent the transmission of infection. **Medical asepsis** is often referred to as "clean technique." It includes handwashing, barrier precautions, and environmental concerns (see Box 20–6). It is important to note that with medical asepsis, the emphasis is on clean, not sterile. It is also important to clean from areas that are the cleanest to areas that are less clean. For example, when preparing the skin for a peripheral intravenous catheter insertion, cleaning of the skin with an antiseptic solution such as povidone-iodine (Betadine) begins at the potential injection site and moves outward in a circular fashion to the less clean area. Likewise,

when the client's room is being mopped, the health care worker mops from the corner most distal to the door. The hallway would be considered dirtier than the client's room, simply because there is more traffic and activity in the hallway than in the client's room. Finally, all hospital floors are to be considered dirty (even freshly mopped floors).

The main purpose of surgical asepsis is to render items maximally free from microorganisms, including spores, and to maintain this germ-free state. One procedure included in surgical asepsis is the surgical handwash scrub, or the surgical scrub. This is the special handwashing that surgeons and other operating room personnel engage in before donning the sterile operating room attire. Antimicrobial handwashing agents are used for a specified time. A sterile towel is used to dry the hands. A sterile cover gown is donned, along with sterile surgical gloves (Procedure 20–9).

Isolation Precautions

Isolation can also be used to control infection by isolating the client or, in some cases, the client's body fluids (body substance isolation) and following guidelines issued by the CDC commonly referred to as standard precautions (see box). The CDC has also issued guidelines to prevent the transmission of diseases in hospitals (CDC, 1996a). These guidelines break isolation down into standard precautions, which apply to all clients regardless of disease, and three transmission-based isolation categories: airborne precautions, which apply to those diseases contracted by the airborne route of transmission; droplet precautions, which apply to diseases in which the droplet route is used; and contact precautions, which apply to those diseases transmitted by contact.

PPE is required to be worn when entering isolation rooms. HEPA or N-95 masks should be worn when caring for clients with tuberculosis. How to don and remove PPE is addressed in Procedure 20–10.

✦ **Body Substance Isolation.** An alternative isolation system that some hospitals use is body substance isolation. It was developed at Harborview Medical Center as an alternative to the old category and disease-specific isolation systems (Lynch *et al.,* 1990). Body substance isolation focuses on moist body substances (liquid and solid) instead of disease processes.

All clients in this isolation system are considered to be isolated. Exceptions occur with clients who have airborne diseases such as pulmonary tuberculosis or varicella (chicken pox). A large red "STOP" sign is placed on the door of a client with an airborne communicable disease, instructing all who enter to check at the nurses' station for special instructions. Private rooms are used for clients with diseases transmitted by the airborne route.

Gloves are used before any contact with moist body substances on any client. Gloves are changed between each client and should also be changed be-

---

Box **20–6**

MEDICAL ASEPSIS (CLEAN TECHNIQUES)

Purpose: To reduce the number of organisms and prevent transmission from person to person (or person to object).

Handwashing: Use soap for routine care and antimicrobial soap for intensive care areas or special procedures.
- Duration: 10–15 seconds.
- Friction: The mechanical action of rubbing hands together increases the amount of soil removed.
- Clean from areas of clean to areas of less clean.

Barrier techniques: Interrupt transmission by use of physical barriers—mask, gown, gloves, eye protection.
- Change gloves and wash hands between clients.
- Use "no touch" dressing technique to avoid contamination of sterile supplies.
- Wear eye protection and mask or face shield to protect face.

Environmental controls
- Use monitored negative pressure rooms for diseases requiring airborne precautions (especially TB).
- Clean up blood spills promptly with spill kit or OSHA-approved disinfectant.

PROCEDURE

20–9

DONNING AND REMOVING STERILE GLOVES

Equipment: *Package of sterile gloves.*

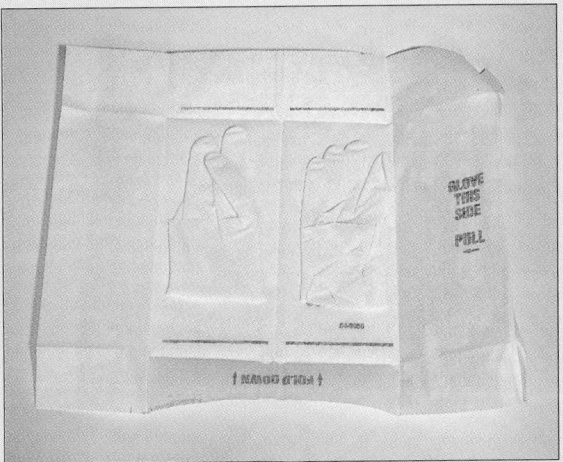

Action	**Rationale**
1. Wash hands. Open package of sterile gloves by pulling the package apart at the indicator tabs. Place opened package on a clean, dry surface.	1. Moisture can contaminate sterile gloves by striking through the outer paper wrap.
2. Fold open the inner wrapper of the glove packet like a book. With thumb and index finger, pull open the folded edges until they lie flat.	2. The inner wrapper serves as a sterile field.
3. Pick up the glove for the dominant hand by the cuff with the thumb and index finger of the nondominant hand, touching only the cuff. Slip the dominant hand into the glove.	3. The cuff is considered contaminated, because it will eventually touch the skin.

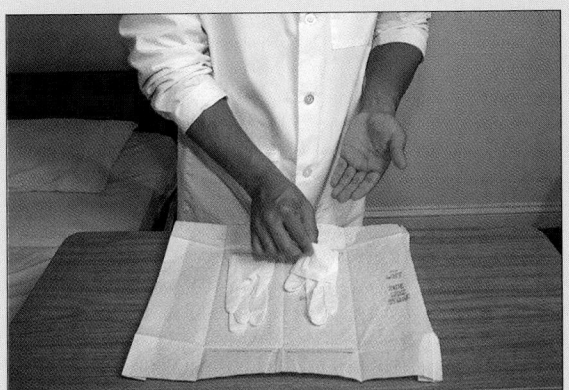

Step 3.

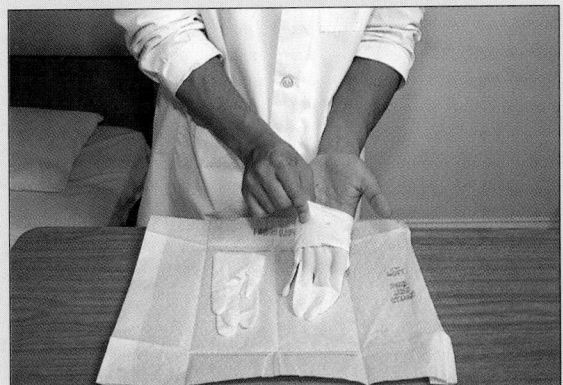

Step 3.

4. With the now gloved dominant hand, slip gloved fingers under the cuff of the second glove. Do not allow the sterile second glove to touch any nonsterile surfaces such as the tabletop. Slip the nondominant hand into the glove and push into place.	4. To maintain sterility, sterile items can touch only sterile items.

Continued

PROCEDURE

20–9

DONNING AND REMOVING STERILE GLOVES
(Continued)

Action	**Rationale**
5. Adjust each glove to fit by touching only the outside of the glove and gently pulling.	**5.** If the nurse sticks a gloved thumb under the cuff to pull the glove for adjustment, the glove will become contaminated.

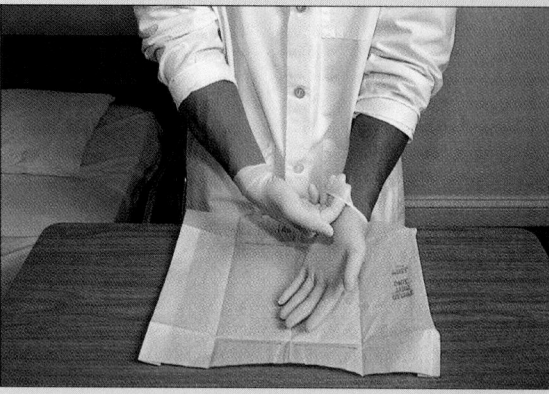

Step 5.

6. Use one hand to grasp other glove near cuff end and remove by inverting glove.	**6.** This keeps the contaminated area on the inside.
7. Hold removed glove in palm of gloved hand.	**7.** Contamination is contained.
8. Slide fingers of ungloved hand inside and remove other glove by turning inside out.	**8.** Prevents spread of contamination.
9. Discard gloves in Biohazard container or prepared baggie.	**9.** Institutions have special containers for contaminated materials; community health nurses pour disinfectant into contaminated bags.
10. Wash hands.	**10.** Reduces spread of microorganisms.

tween two different procedures on the same client. Handwashing is indicated after the gloves are removed (a point that the universal precautions do not emphasize). Thus, the purpose of body substance isolation is to decrease the chance of client-to-client and client–to–health care worker transmission of infection.

❧ **Standard Precautions.** Standard precautions combine universal precautions and body substance isolation. With universal precautions, all blood and bloody body fluids are handled with extreme caution, but handwashing is not necessarily emphasized. The body fluids of most concern are body fluids with visible blood present. With body substance isolation, all body fluids and moist body substances are handled with extreme caution and protective gear, regardless of the presence of blood. Clients with certain diseases transmitted by the airborne route, such as TB or varicella, are placed in private rooms with signs instructing all who wish to enter to report to the nurses' station. Thus, in this system, negative air pressure and special

masks are not indicated. Standard precautions combine the two forms, using the best aspects of each. The differences in the three systems are summarized in Table 20–12.

Airborne Precautions. Airborne precautions were designed to go one step further than standard precautions. These precautions apply to clients with known or suspected infections transmitted by the airborne route. These diseases are listed in Table 20–13. Diseases covered in this category center around three main diseases: varicella zoster (chicken pox), rubeola (measles), and pulmonary tuberculosis (TB).

Varicella zoster first occurs as chicken pox, a common childhood illness. However, because the varicella zoster virus is a member of the herpes family of viruses, it shares the characteristic of latency. This means that once one is infected with the virus, it never actually leaves the body. Infection can recur under the right set of circumstances, such as stress or chemotherapy, as zoster—otherwise known as shingles.

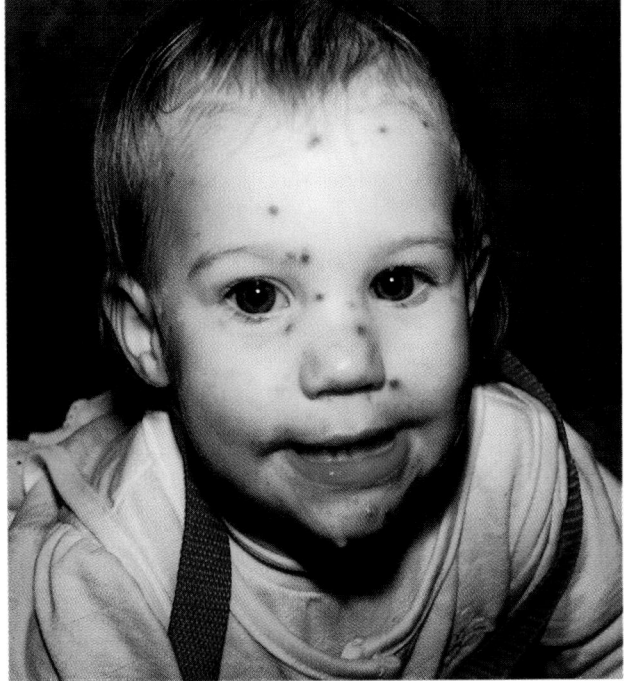

❧ Figure 20–10

Child with varicella (chickenpox) lesions in various stages of evolution.

coughs or speaks, the virus becomes airborne (Fig. 20–10). Since 95% of most adults have already had varicella, it is likely that these clients will be children. A private room is needed with negative air pressure. Negative air pressure rooms typically bring air into the room from the hallway and have a separate exhaust system (Fig. 20–11). A regular surgical mask, gown, and gloves should be worn to prevent cross-contamination. Unimmunized, susceptible health care workers should avoid caring for clients with varicella.

Varicella in the form of shingles is not very contagious. It usually recurs along a nerve grouping, such as the trigeminal nerves along the face or the thoracic nerves along the back and flank. The recurrence resembles chicken pox in that the lesions are vesicular on a reddened base. However, unlike the lesions of

Varicella in the form of chicken pox is extremely contagious by the airborne route. Lesions containing the virus appear on all skin surfaces, in the eyes, and inside the mouth and throat, so that as the person

Negative air pressure room

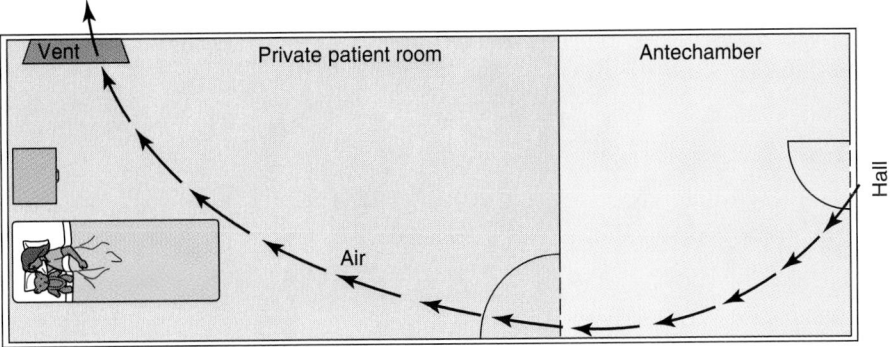

❧ Figure 20–11

A private negative air pressure room is used for clients with extremely contagious infections such as varicella.

DONNING AND REMOVING PERSONAL PROTECTIVE EQUIPMENT (PPE)

Equipment: *Gown, mask, gloves.*

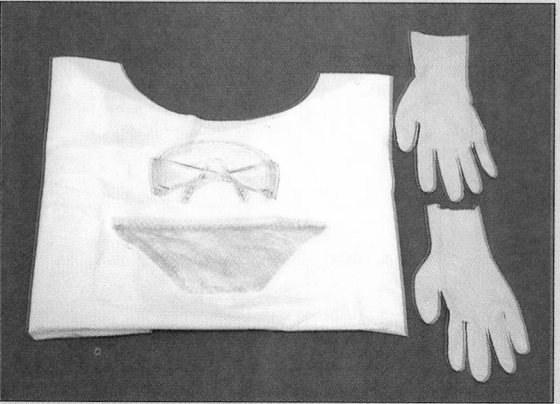

Action	**Rationale**
Gowning	
1. Slip hands between back of gown and shoulders. Hold arms high to allow sleeves to fall over arms.	1. Many disposable gowns are made from plastic-coated paperlike material that could tear if not donned correctly.
2. Secure neck ties or strings. Tie waistband, if present.	2. Loose-fitting gowns may impede nursing care.
Masking	
1. With one hand, grasp the face piece of the mask; with the other hand, grab the elastic. Pull it over the head. The elastic should rest at the crown of the head. If the mask has strings, secure the top set at the crown and the bottom set at the nape of the neck.	1. The mask should cover the nose and mouth with no gaps.

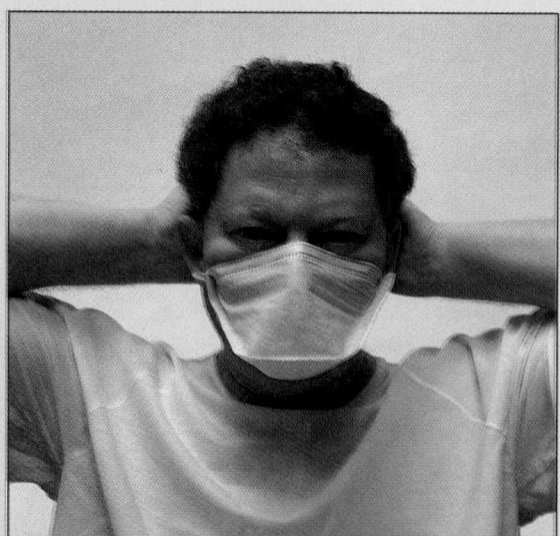

Step 1.

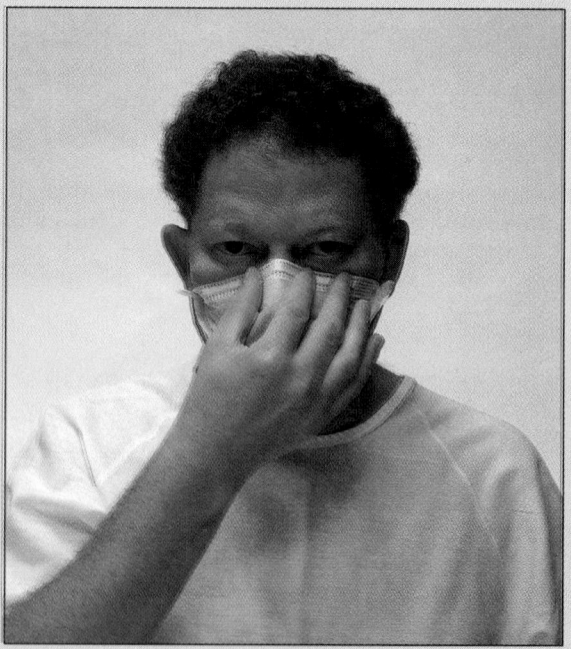

Step 1.

DONNING AND REMOVING PERSONAL PROTECTIVE EQUIPMENT (PPE)
(Continued)

Action	Rationale

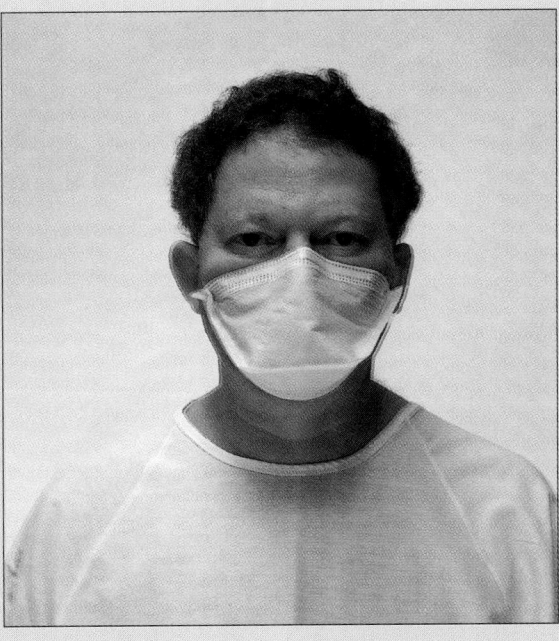

Step 1.

Action	Rationale
2. Adjust the nose piece by pressing the mask down along the bridge of the nose. Replace the mask if it becomes moist (usually after about 20 minutes) or soiled with blood or other body fluids.	**2.** Moisture decreases the effectiveness of the mask.
Gloves	
1. Wash hands.	**1.** Removes transient flora that might multiply on the skin surface.
2. Slip fingers between glove and pull onto hand. Bring cuff of glove over to cover the gown cuff.	**2.** Provides a complete protective barrier without exposed skin.

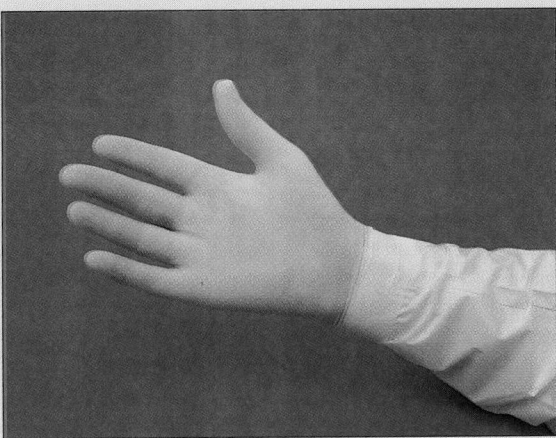

Step 2.

Continued

PROCEDURE

20–10

DONNING AND REMOVING PERSONAL PROTECTIVE EQUIPMENT (PPE)
(Continued)

Action	Rationale
Removing PPE	
1. Remove gloves first. Grasp edge of glove cuff and pull off hand until the inside is out. Slip ungloved fingers under cuff of remaining glove. Touch only the inside cuff. Pull inside out. Discard in biohazard bag.	**1.** Gloves are the most contaminated. The inside of the glove (next to the skin) is uncontaminated, but the glove surface is contaminated.
2. With ungloved hands, remove gown at the neck tapes or ties (some gowns have breakaway features). Roll the gown inside out. Discard in a biohazard bag.	**2.** The inside of the gown is uncontaminated. The back of the neck and upper back areas are also considered uncontaminated.

Step 2.

3. Remove mask or respirator at the ties or straps. Do not touch the face piece. Store respirators in appropriate bags. Discard surgical mask in biohazard bag.	**3.** The face piece may be contaminated with organisms.
4. Wash hands.	**4.** Removes any bacteria inadvertently acquired.

chicken pox, which appear all over the body, the lesions of zoster cluster along those nerve routes. Clients with zoster do not need isolation unless they are immunocompromised. In clients with suppressed immune function, shingles can disseminate or spread all over the body, similar to the first encounter as chicken pox. The virus again becomes airborne, owing to mouth and throat lesions.

Rubeola, or measles, is a disease that is seldom seen, except in underimmunized populations such as new immigrants or certain religious groups that forbid immunization. The disease is characterized by a fine red rash that occurs over the entire body. These clients should be placed in private negative air pressure rooms. Regular surgical masks, gowns, and gloves are indicated for all caregivers. Nonimmunized, susceptible health care workers should avoid caring for clients with rubeola.

Pulmonary TB is a disease that was predicted to be completely eradicated by the year 2010 by the CDC (CDC, 1994). In 1985, this downward trend reversed itself, much to the alarm of the CDC and other public health agencies. At the crest of this new wave of pulmonary TB cases were clients with AIDS. Clients with

Table 20-12

COMPARISON OF ISOLATION SYSTEMS

SYSTEM	DESCRIPTION	ADVANTAGES	DISADVANTAGES
Universal precautions	Barrier precautions for blood and certain bloody body fluids: blood cerebrospinal fluid synovial fluid pleural fluid peritoneal fluid pericardial fluid amniotic fluid fluids with visible blood	OSHA mandated Protects worker against bloodborne pathogens	Does not protect against communicable disease, so must be used in combination with another system Must determine what is "visibly bloody" Does not emphasize removing gloves between clients Does not emphasize handwashing
Body substance isolation	Barrier precautions for all moist body substances	Isolates body substances and not the client Used for bloodborne pathogens and communicable diseases	No recommendations for diseases transmitted by the respiratory route No recommendations for negative air pressure rooms Emphasizes gloves over handwashing
Two-tiered standard precautions (with three isolation categories)	Barrier precautions for all moist body substances	Transmission driven Protects worker and client from disease transmission	Some confusion over name—OSHA bloodborne pathogen standard

Table 20-13

DISEASES COVERED UNDER AIRBORNE PRECAUTIONS

DISEASE	DURATION OF PRECAUTIONS
Chicken pox (varicella) Exposure to varicella in susceptible people	Until all lesions crusted 8–21 days after exposure (28 days if varicella-zoster immune globulin given)
Measles (rubeola), all forms	Duration of illness
Tuberculosis, pulmonary (confirmed or suspected)	Until effective therapy is given, clinical improvement is seen, and sputum smears are negative for AFB on 3 consecutive days
Zoster, disseminated (in immunocompromised client)	Until lesions crusted
HIV/AIDS with cough (assume pulmonary TB)	Until 3 negative AFB smears or another disease is identified

HIV or AIDS are at great risk for acquiring TB because of their depressed immune status, their less than optimal nutritional status, and, for some, their lifestyle (IV drug abuse). Some groups are at increased risk for TB, including foreign immigrants from countries in Southeast Asia or Africa, where TB infects a great portion of the population; homeless people, because of crowded shelters or minimal nutritional status; and alcoholics, owing to poor nutrition (CDC, 1994).

A client with confirmed or suspected TB should be placed in a single negative air pressure room. A regular surgical mask must not be worn into these rooms. Instead, HEPA or N-95 respirators must be worn when providing care to these clients. These masks must be properly fitted to the face of the health care worker and then checked to ensure that the mask fits as securely as possible. This procedure is called fit testing and is performed by the hospital industrial hygienist or other trained individual. In one type of fit testing, the industrial hygienist sprays various concentrations of a sodium saccharin aerosol into a fit-testing hood.

Once the N-95 or HEPA respirator has been properly fitted, the health care worker should perform a fit check every time the mask is worn. For the N-95 respirator, a positive-pressure fit check is performed:

• Place both hands completely over the respirator and exhale forcefully.

- If air escapes around the nose piece, readjust the nose piece.
- If air leaks at the respirator edge, adjust the strap to obtain a better fit.

A negative fit check is performed on the HEPA respirator. The procedure is identical to the positive fit check outlined earlier, except that the wearer sharply inhales. If a good fit cannot be obtained, the health care worker should notify a supervisor and not enter the room.

CASE STUDY   Mr. Smith Needs Isolation

Charles Smith is a 33-year-old homeless man who is admitted from a homeless shelter with a tentative diagnosis of pneumonia. A thorough nursing history reveals that he has a history of alcohol and IV drug abuse. He appears quite thin and admits to the nurse that he has lost about 30 lb over the past month. He complains of coughing up thick tan sputum and waking at night with cold sweats.

Mr. Smith is in several risk groups for pulmonary TB. He is homeless and a former abuser of alcohol and IV drugs. These risk groups share poor nutrition and close physical contact with other individuals who may be infected with pulmonary TB. The nursing history also reveals information that should alert the nurse to possible TB (weight loss, productive cough, and night sweats). Based on his risk groups alone, Mr. Smith should be placed on airborne precautions in a negative air pressure room for possible pulmonary TB. Health care workers should wear respirators while in his room.

Medical orders may include a purified protein derivative (PPD) tuberculin skin test to be administered intradermally by the nurse and read within 48 hours of placement. Three sputum cultures with smears may be ordered by the physician to document a diagnosis of TB. The nurse should collect these specimens in the early morning, just after Mr. Smith awakes—one specimen daily for 3 days. Smear results are available in some laboratories as little as 4 to 6 hours after laboratory processing. The actual culture may take up to 6 weeks to become positive.

The ward dietitian may be contacted to lend nutritional teaching and advice to Mr. Smith. Social services can arrange for his postdischarge housing needs. The infection control practitioner will notify the local health department if Mr. Smith is diagnosed with pulmonary TB. Most local health departments will supply antituberculosis medication to clients. The health department will notify the homeless shelter and perform tuberculin skin tests on exposed individuals.

All clients on airborne precautions should wear surgical masks when leaving the negative air pressure room for x-rays, tests, or procedures. Clients who have confirmed or suspected TB should likewise wear surgical masks when leaving the negative air pressure room. A HEPA or N-95 respirator should not be placed on a client who has a suspected or confirmed diagnosis of TB, because these masks are too thick for someone with a compromised pulmonary system to breathe through. Two brands of HEPA respirators have nonfiltered expiratory ports (purple plastic round valve). If a client with TB wears a HEPA respirator with one of these ports, TB bacteria will escape from the port into the ambient air, possibly infecting susceptible persons.

Droplet Precautions. Droplet precautions were designed to prevent diseases transmitted by the droplet route. When an infected client coughs or sneezes and does not cover his or her mouth, large droplets of sputum are sprayed outward, up to about 3 feet. These large airborne droplets can be inhaled by health care workers or visitors.

Some droplets can fall into the eyes or even the mouths of persons occupying a 3-foot radius around the client. Diseases most often associated with droplet transmission are respiratory illnesses with adenovirus, influenza, mycoplasma, and group A streptococcus, along with meningitis involving *Haemophilus influenzae* or *Neisseria meningitidis*. The childhood diseases mumps, rubella, pertussis, and parvovirus B-19 are also included.

Single rooms are preferable, but clients with the same disease can share a room. Surgical masks are required for anyone coming within 3 feet of the client. Gowns should be worn if clothing or uniforms are likely to become contaminated with respiratory secretions. Whenever handling tissues or any items contaminated with respiratory secretions, gloves should be worn.

CASE STUDY   Lisa Malone Has Pertussis

The Admitting Office calls the pediatric floor for a room assignment for Lisa Malone, an 11-month-old child being admitted from the emergency room with possible pertussis (whooping cough). The charge nurse reminds the Admitting Office that the only two empty beds are in semiprivate rooms. Room 5243 has a 9-month-old girl with short bowel syndrome who is on total parenteral nutrition therapy. Room 5250 has a 3-year-old boy who has just left the floor for a cardiac catheterization.

The charge nurse realizes that admitting a child with a diagnosis of pertussis to either room is in conflict with sound infection control practices. Droplet precautions advise a single room unless two clients have the same disease. The charge nurse elects to move the child who is currently off the floor in the cardiac catheterization suite. This frees room 5250 for Lisa Malone to be admitted on droplet precautions. The other bed in the room is blocked by the charge nurse to further admissions, except for another pertussis case.

Contact Precautions. Contact precautions prevent the transmission of diseases that use the direct or indirect mode of transmission. Direct contact involves touching, bathing, or other activities with skin-to-skin contact. Indirect contact involves inanimate objects such as doorknobs, light switches, or tabletops in the transfer of organisms from one person to another. The diseases covered under contact precautions include RSV, congenital herpes, rubella, multiply drug-resistant organisms such as methicillin-resistant *Staphylococcus aureus* (MRSA) and vancomycin-resistant enterococci (VRE), and diarrhea in diapered infants or incontinent clients (namely, with hemorrhagic *E. coli,* rotavirus, *Shigella,* or hepatitis A virus). Major wound infections involving uncontrolled draining wounds, cellulitis, abscesses, or major burns and infections involving the skin such as lice, scabies, and zoster are also included.

Handwashing is the foundation of contact precautions. Gloves should be worn if the nurse will be touching the client or the client's body fluids. Gowns are worn to prevent contamination of the health care worker's clothing or uniform. Masks are generally not indicated, with a few exceptions. RSV can linger for long periods on bed rails, tabletops, call-light buttons, and other objects. Some researchers recommend wearing masks just to remind health care workers to keep their hands away from their noses and mouths (Filippell & Rearick, 1993). Caring for clients with pneumonia infections or upper respiratory colonization involving multiply resistent organisms such as VRE also requires a mask (CDC & HICPAC, 1995).

CASE STUDY Mr. Brown Has VRE

James Brown, a 47-year-old liver transplant recipient, has been hospitalized for over a month. He has been on numerous antibiotics and immunosuppressive drugs for his transplant. He has experienced a few infection complications, including pneumonia and a wound infection. His nurse now receives a phone call from the microbiology laboratory stating that Mr. Brown is growing vancomycin-resistant enterococci (VRE) from his sputum. The nurse notes his fever and cough. His morning chest x-ray reveals a new onset of pneumonia. The nurse promptly notifies infection control and the attending physician. Mr. Brown is promptly placed on strick contact precautions.

Fortunately, Mr. Brown is already in a private room and does not have to be moved. His nurse, along with the infection control practitioner, can explain to him why all the health care workers and his visitors must now wear masks, gowns, and gloves to enter his room. The nurse also serves as the client's advocate, reminding everyone, including physicians, of the strict adherence to isolation protocol.

Infection control is everyone's business. Meticulous handwashing protects not only the client but also the health care worker. Isolation is merely a small part of the overall care plan for most clients.

Evaluation

Once a plan of care has been devised, the nurse must carefully document the response. Whether it is a response to medication given to control fever or wet-to-dry dressing techniques to assist in wound débridement, each action must be recorded. Questions the nurse should consider when evaluating the effectiveness of the plan of care include the following:

* Were the family and other visitors informed of the purpose and importance of the isolation precautions?
* Was the disease contained (*i.e.,* not spread to other clients, personnel, or visitors)?
* Were the specific isolation recommendations for mask, gown, gloves, and so forth consistently followed?
* If negative air pressure rooms were used, were they monitored daily to ascertain that they were indeed maintaining negative pressure?

Careful recording and documentation of PPD skin tests, for example, could determine whether a client will receive preventive isoniazid (INH) therapy for tuberculosis infection. Accurate documentation of the appearance of the PPD as well as exact millimeters of induration is required by some local health departments when reporting new cases of pulmonary tuberculosis.

Summary

The ultimate outcome of all safety and infection control endeavors is the prevention of injuries and the prevention and control of infections. Safety takes time. Safe work practices and surveys of the client's environment can prevent injury and help ensure the client's well-being. Through adherence to isolation techniques, some diseases will be prevented. Outbreaks of seasonal infections, such as influenza and RSV, or epidemic outbreaks of multiple drug-resistant organisms, such as MRSA and VRE, can also be reduced by barrier techniques. However, in certain epidemic situations, constant feedback to the unit involved becomes critical. The nurses and the staff need to know how well they are doing or receive input from infection control on what else they could do to stop the spread of the particular infection in question.

When revision of safety measures or isolation precautions is necessary, a multidisciplinary task force can be helpful in assessing safety needs from all angles. Monitoring adherence to handwashing, standard precautions, and specialized isolation is sometimes necessary. Demonstrations and reeducation, especially when involved staff members participate, can expedite "buy-in" from all parties.

The ultimate goal is decreased injury and infection

rates or an end to the outbreak situation. Allowing the nurses, nursing aides, and orderlies to participate in the decision-making and planning can be paramount to a successful outcome.

Thus, safety involves providing a safe environment for the client, the family, and visitors, as well as hospital staff members. General safety, like infection control, usually requires nothing more than common sense. Yet sometimes in the day-to-day flurry of routine activities, personal protection issues take a back seat to other pressing needs. It is in these moments when clients fall, needle sticks occur, and exposures to infectious disease happen. We must teach ourselves to be more careful and more alert.

When compared with the high-tech equipment in most modern hospitals, the simple task of washing hands seems almost out of place. Yet it is usually the simplest things that the nurse does for the client that eventually become the most valuable. Things such as using a night-light and placing the call light within reach may prevent an elderly client from falling out of bed. Teaching a new mother about the importance of using an infant car seat every time the infant travels could save that infant's life. Finally, the simple act of handwashing could prevent a client with leukemia from acquiring a life-threatening MRSA infection and the nurse from becoming colonized as well.

CHAPTER HIGHLIGHTS

✦

+ Risk factors that impede safety include age, lifestyle, mobility, and sensory impairment.

+ Safe practices that prevent home accidents include lowering the water heater thermostat to 120°F and clearing the stairs of tripping hazards.

+ Actions a nurse should take in the event of a fire in a hospital are rescue clients in immediate danger, sound the alarm, confine the fire by closing all doors, and extinguish the fire or evacuate the clients.

+ Useful home safety devices include infant car seats, electrical outlet covers, commode locks, tub hand rails, and shower chairs.

+ Common household plants that could be poisonous if eaten are poinsettia, dumb cane, and mistletoe.

+ The use of sturdy bed rails and night-lights can prevent falls among the elderly.

+ Restraints are used for two purposes: to protect and support, and to restrain physical or combative activity.

+ Medical waste is any waste produced in a medical environment; infectious waste contains pathogens that could cause disease.

+ The difference between infection and colonization is that infection invades and damages tissue, whereas colonization does not.

+ The six links in the chain of infection are agent, reservoir, portal of exit, mode of transmission, portal of entry, and susceptible host.

+ Standard precautions and the three isolation categories (airborne precautions, droplet precautions, and contact precautions) serve as the major infection control components of isolation.

+ Three communicable diseases that require negative air pressure ventilation are measles, pulmonary tuberculosis, and varicella.

+ Handwashing is the easiest, most effective way to prevent infections.

+ Medical asepsis is the technique of preventing infection by using barriers, gloves, and handwashing.

+ OSHA's 1991 bloodborne pathogen standard highlights the need for free hepatitis B vaccine to all health care workers and encourages hospitals to explore safer needle options.

Study Questions

1. A nurse has just finished dressing the wound of a client with AIDS. The nurse should

   a. dispose of the dressing in the regular waste can
   b. double bag the dressing and dispose of it in the regular waste can
   c. dispose of the dressing in a biohazard bag that is placed in the infectious waste container
   d. none of the above

2. In the event of a fire in the client's room, the nurse should

   a. rescue the client, close all doors, and fight the fire
   b. close the client's door, rescue other clients, and pull the fire alarm
   c. close the client's door, sound the alarm, and extinguish the fire
   d. rescue the client, close all doors, sound the alarm, evacuate, or extinguish the fire

3. Standard precautions stress that

   a. all body fluids from the client are potentially infectious
   b. only bloody body fluids from the client are potentially infectious
   c. only body fluids from a client in isolation are infectious
   d. none of the above

4. The three communicable diseases that require a special private room with negative air flow are

   a. measles, AIDs, and meningitis
   b. measles, chickenpox, and TB
   c. measles, TB, and meningitis
   d. measles, mumps, and rubella

5. The easiest, most effective way to prevent transmission of infections is to

a. wash hands
b. administer antibiotics
c. isolate all clients with infections
d. use gloves, masks, gowns, goggles, and face shields for all clients

Critical Thinking Exercises

1. Ms. C., age 45 years, is diagnosed with retinitis pigmentosis and will be living alone in a two-story condominium. She is active in her church and community and works as a computer programmer. She has been advised to discontinue driving because of poor vision. She has a 2-year-old son and cares for her 90-year-old mother, who has Alzheimer's disease. Discuss the safety issues involved in this situation.

2. Mr. T. is admitted to the hospital with tuberculosis. Discuss mode of transmission and precautions needed for staff and visitors.

References

Centers for Disease Control and Prevention. (1994). Guidelines for preventing the transmissions of tuberculosis in health care facilities. *MMWR, 43*(RR-13), 1–132, and *Federal Register, 59*(208), 54242–54303.

Centers for Disease Control and Prevention. (1996a). Guideline for isolation precautions in hospitals. *American Journal of Infection Control, 24,* 24–52.

Centers for Disease Control and Prevention. (1996b). Update: Provisional public health service recommendations for chemoprophylaxis after occupational exposure to HIV. *MMWR, 45*(22), 468–472.

Centers for Disease Control and Prevention & Hospital Infection Control Practices Advisory Committee. (1995). Recommendation for preventing the spread of vancomycin resistance. *Infection Control and Hospital Epidemiology, 16,* 105–113.

Charney, W., Corkery, K. J., Kraemer, R., & Wugofski, L. (1993). Ribavirin aerosol. In W. Charney & J. Schirmer (Eds.), *Essentials of modern hospital safety* (Vol. 2, pp. 239–312). Boca Raton, FL: Lewis Publishers.

Chiarello, L. A. (1995). Selection of needlestick prevention devices: A conceptual framework for approaching product evaluation. *American Journal of Infection Control, 23*(6), 386–395.

Committee on Atherosclerosis and Hypertension in Children, Council on Cardiovascular Disease in the Young, American Heart Association. (1994). Active and passive tobacco exposure: A serious pediatric health problem. *Circulation, 90*(5), 2581–2590.

Department of Labor, Occupational Safety and Health Administration. (1983). Hazard communication. *Federal Register, 59,* 6126–6184.

Department of Labor, Occupational Safety and Health Administration. (1991). Occupational exposure to bloodborne pathogens: Final rule. *Federal Register, 56*(235), 64175–64182.

Filippell, M. B., & Rearick, T. (1993). Respiratory syncytial virus. In K. Saleh & V. Brinsko (Eds.), *The nursing clinics of North America* (pp. 651–671). Philadelphia: W. B. Saunders.

Finucane, E. (1993). Monitoring aldehydes in the hospital. In W. Charney & J. Schirmer (Eds.), *Essentials of modern hospital safety* (Vol. 2, pp. 191–211). Boca Raton, FL: Lewis Publishers.

Garner, J. S, & Simmons, B. P. (1983). Guideline for isolation precautions in hospitals. *Infection Control, 4(suppl),* 245–325.

Griffin, P. M., & Tauxe, R. V. (1991). The epidemiology of infections caused by *Escherichia coli 0157:H57,* other enterohemorrhagic *E. coli,* and the associated hemolytic uremic syndrome. *Epidemiologic Reviews, 13,* 60–98.

Larson, E. (1995). APIC guideline for handwashing and hand antisepsis in health care settings. *American Journal of Infection Control, 23*(4), 251–269.

Lynch, P., Cummings, M. J., Roberts, P. L., Herriott, M. J., Yates, B., & Stamm, W. E. (1990). Implementing and evaluating a system of generic infection precautions: Body substance isolation. *American Journal of Infection Control, 18*(1), 1–12.

Oniboni, A. (1990). Infections in the neutropenic patient. *Seminars in Oncology Nursing, 6*(1), 50–60.

Reich, A. (1990). Safe use of ethylene oxide in the hospital environment. In W. Charney & J. Schimer (Eds.), *Essentials of modern hospital safety* (Vol. 1, pp. 3–35). Boca Raton, FL: Lewis Publishers.

Robert, L., & Bell, D. M. (1994). HIV transmission in the health-care setting: Risks to health-care workers and patients. In A. E. Glatt (Ed.), *Infectious disease clinics of North America* (pp. 319–333). Philadelphia: W. B. Saunders.

Sandler, R. L. (1995). Clinical snapshot. Restraining devices. *American Journal of Nursing, 7,* 34–35.

US Environmental Protection Agency, US Department of Health and Human Services, US Public Health Service. (1992). *A citizen's guide to radon.* Washington, DC: US Government Printing Office.

Wooden, K. (1995). *Child lures.* Arlington, TX: Summit Publishing Group.

Wugofski, L., Makofsky, D., Cone, J. E., & Mehring, J. (1993). Occupational needlestick injuries. In W. Charney & J. Schirmer (Eds.), *Essentials of modern hospital safety* (Vol. 2, pp. 37–152). Boca Raton, FL: Lewis Publishers.

Bibliography

Boyce, J. M. (1995). Vancomycin resistant enterococci: Pervasive and persistent pathogens. *Infection Control and Hospital Epidemiology, 16*(12), 676–679.

Committee on Infectious Diseases, American Academy of Pediatrics. (1994). *The 1994 red book: Report of the Committee on Infectious Diseases,* (23rd ed.). Elk Grove Village, IL: American Academy of Pediatrics.

Hospital Infection Control Practices Advisory Committee & Centers for Disease Control and Prevention. (1995). Recommendations for preventing the spread of vancomycin resistance: Recommendations of the Hospital Infection Control Practices Advisory Committee. *American Journal of Infection Control, 23*(2), 87–94.

Mayhall, C. G. (ed.). (1996). *Hospital epidemiology and infection control.* Baltimore: Williams & Wilkins.

Rutala, W. A., & 1994, 1995, and 1996 APIC Guidelines Committee. (1996). APIC guideline for the selection and use of disinfectants. *American Journal of Infection Control, 24*(4), 313–342.

Wenzel, R. P. (1993). *Prevention and control of nosocomial infections* (2nd ed.). Baltimore: Williams & Wilkins.

Chapter 21

ADMINISTERING MEDICATIONS

✧

JULIA M. LEAHY, PhD, RN

PATRICIA NUTZ, RN, MSN, MEd

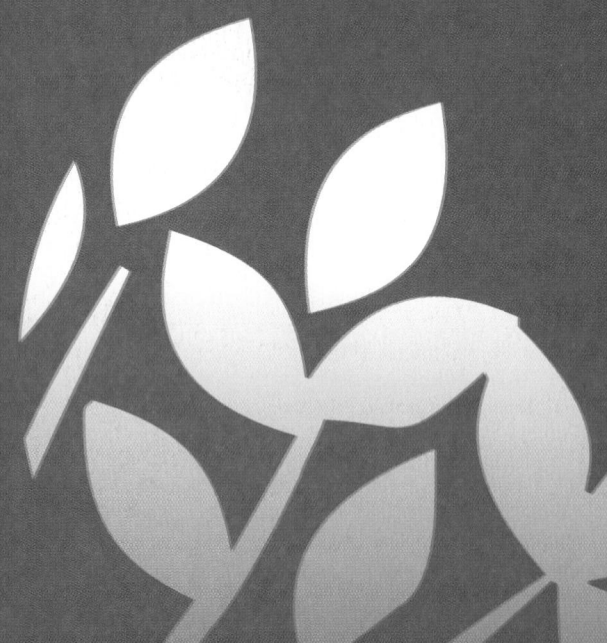

absorption	over-the-counter drugs
addiction	pharmacy
adverse effect	pharmacokinetics
bioavailability	pharmacology
biotransformation	poisons
distribution	prescriptions drugs
drug	substance abuse
drug action	teratogenicity
drug dose	therapeutic effect
drug effect	tolerance
excretion	toxicology
hypersensitivity	toxicity
idiosyncrasy	withdrawal

LEARNING OBJECTIVES

✦

After studying this chapter, you should be able to
- ✦ Define the terms drug and pharmacology
- ✦ Identify four types of drug names
- ✦ Describe sources of drugs
- ✦ Describe the concept and phases of pharmacokinetics
- ✦ Differentiate between drug effect and drug action
- ✦ Describe the concept of drug toxicity
- ✦ Differentiate between therapeutic and adverse drug effects
- ✦ Differentiate between predictable and unpredictable drug effects
- ✦ Discuss the concept of substance abuse
- ✦ Identify the components of a medication order
- ✦ Identify the "five rights" of medication administration
- ✦ Identify major drug classifications
- ✦ Describe three systems of measurement of drug therapy
- ✦ Discuss the development factors that affect drug actions
- ✦ Describe procedures for administration of drugs

Chemicals affect every aspect of human life. They surround us and help to make up our very existence, providing us with nutrients, creating our environment, and playing a vital role in the metabolic processes of the human body. Chemicals can be either helpful, such as drugs or medications that alter pathophysiological processes to restore homeostasis, or harmful, such as poisons that have a negative impact on the human organism. Even when chemicals are beneficial to humans, safety in the use of these chemicals is of utmost importance. Health care professionals must be continuously aware of safety considerations in relation to both the therapeutic and nontherapeutic chemicals that are used daily.

Chemical substances are often used to promote equilibrium and maintain homeostasis. A **drug,** or medication, is a chemical that is introduced into the body to act on body cells for an intended therapeutic effect. Drugs replace missing substances, protect bodily functions, and prevent, eliminate, and alleviate a variety of pathophysiological conditions. They maintain the biochemical processes that provide people with the energy to accomplish both simple activities and monumental achievements.

This chapter examines the concepts and principles related to chemical safety in the delivery of competent, quality health care to clients in a variety of clinical settings and the role of the nurse in administering medications safely. The role of the nurse is to assess the client, determine the appropriateness of prescribed drug therapy, implement procedures to ensure the client's safety when administering medications, and evaluate the client's response to the prescribed medication.

Basic Terms

There are some basic terms that the nurse should be aware of when administering medications.

Pharmacology: the study of the physical and chemical properties of drugs and their effects on the human body.

Pharmacy: the site where drugs are prepared, dispensed, and sold.

Pharmacokinetics: the study of movement of drugs in the body, including absorption, distribution, biotransformation, and excretion.

Toxicology: the study of poisons.

Prescription drugs: drugs, such as antibiotics, that can be dispensed only if they are legally prescribed by a physician or other duly authorized individual.

Over-the-counter drugs: drugs that can be sold without a prescription, such as aspirin, acetaminophen, and cough medications.

Drug Legislation and Standards

Chemical substances used in the United States and Canada must adhere to governmental standards to ensure purity and uniformity of strength. Health care providers depend on drug standards to determine the effectiveness and safety of a drug as well as its strength, purity, and bioavailability at the drug receptor site.

Drug Legislation

The first federal drug law in the United States was the Pure Food and Drug Act of 1906, which was enacted to ensure the strength and purity of marketed drugs and establish official drug standards. This act required that drugs be accurately labeled and meet standards regarding quality of chemical composition and potency of the dose. A number of laws related to drug use and control have since been enacted which further clarify the requirements for meeting federal standards. In Canada, the Proprietary or Patent Medicine Act of 1908 first set standards for the use of nonprescription medications. Table 21–1 provides a listing of significant US drug legislation.

Laws enacted in both the United States (Controlled Substance Act of 1970) and Canada (Canadian Narcotic Control Act of 1961) establish standards for the prescription and administration of controlled substances and for their labeling. Table 21–2 provides a description of the schedules for controlled substances in the United States. Institutions have strict protocols for control of narcotics, including storage in a locked, secure cabinet and maintenance of detailed inventory records. During a change of shift, a complete count of all controlled substances is performed by two nurses, one going off duty and one coming on duty.

In addition to federal legislation, state and local drug regulations exist. These laws govern the prescription of medications, the administration of medications including intravenous (IV) drug therapy, the control of mind-altering chemical substances, and the distribution of medications.

In addition, the nurse practice act of each state regulates specific aspects of drug administration, which pertain to the responsibilities of the nurse and may vary with the educational preparation of the nurse. For instance, in most states nurse practitioners with advanced educational preparation are granted prescription-writing privileges. Also, there may be specific restrictions on a nurse's practice; for instance, in some states, licensed practical nurses may not administer IV medications. Nurses need to become familiar with state practice acts when moving from state to state.

Health care and community-based institutions have administrative policies concerning administration of medications to clients. The nurse should be fully

Table 21–1

OVERVIEW OF DRUG LEGISLATION IN THE UNITED STATES

DATE	TITLE	PROVISIONS
1906	Pure Food and Drug Act	Established standards for strength and purity of drugs; protected public from mislabeled and adulterated drugs
1938	Food, Drug and Cosmetic Act	Established regulations for safety testing of all new drugs; set requirements for labeling of drugs
1952	Durham-Humphrey Amendment	Established guidelines for prescription (legend) drugs and refills and for over-the-counter drugs
1958	Kefauver-Harris Act	Established criteria for drug safety and efficacy
1970	Controlled Substance Act	Established schedules for controlled substances based on their potential for abuse

informed about these policies and procedures. Standing orders may exist that provide specific direction for the nurse in designated situations. In many emergency departments, for example, the nurse is permitted to administer nitroglycerin given verification of severe cardiac distress.

Workplace Legislation

Legislation exists for chemical safety in an occupational setting. The Occupational Safety and Health Act (OSHA) of 1991 outlines policies and regulations to ensure employee protection from hazards in the work environment. OSHA provides regulations governing such aspects of safety as needlesticks, exposure to sources of infection, use of protective equipment, and employee training related to the safe administration of chemical substances.

Substance Abuse

Throughout history, people have used chemical substances to change or modify behavior. When a specific chemical substance that is used on a regular basis to produce behavioral alterations impairs functioning, produces a lack of control over taking the substance, and brings about withdrawal symptoms after intake is stopped, **substance abuse** is said to occur. This pathological, maladaptive condition involves repetition of a harmful pattern that ultimately leads to impaired judgment, lack of control, and a significant decline in physiological and psychosocial functioning. Symptoms typically persist for a period of at least 1 month. Many factors have been implicated as causes of substance abuse, including poor self-esteem, inability to tolerate stress, and impaired coping ability. Chemical substances that are typically abused include

Table 21–2

SCHEDULE CATEGORIES OF CONTROLLED SUBSTANCES

SCHEDULE	DESCRIPTION	EXAMPLES
I	Drugs with high abuse potential Have no accepted medical indications	Heroin, hallucinogenics (LSD, marijuana, peyote)
II	Drugs with high potential for drug abuse Have acceptable medical uses Have strong potential for physical and psychological dependency	Morphine, meperidine (Demerol), codeine, methadone, oxycodone, amphetamines, secobarbital, phenobarbital
III	Drugs that are medically accepted Have less potential for drug abuse than schedule I or II drugs Have some tendency to cause dependence	Codeine preparations, nonnarcotic drugs (propoxyphene)
IV	Drugs that are medically accepted Have some tendency to cause dependence	Phenobarbital, benzodiazepines (diazepam, chloral hydrate, meprobamate)
V	Drugs that are medically accepted Have minimal potential for dependence	Opioid controlled substances found in cough and diarrhea medications

cocaine, hallucinogens, barbiturates, narcotic analgesics, and alcohol.

Any chemical substance that is capable of producing a heightened sense of well-being or euphoria has the ability to induce psychological dependence or **addiction.** When a person becomes physically dependent on the substance, tolerance and withdrawal are commonly seen. If **tolerance** occurs, the individual must increase the amount of the chemical substance taken over a period of time in order to achieve the same desired effect. If, on the other hand, the chemical substance is abruptly withheld, the person experiences unpleasant physiological changes that are characteristic of **withdrawal.**

Substance abuse seriously alters the user's interpersonal relationships, productivity, and status in society. It often leads to illegal activity in pursuit of the abused substance. And, despite the best of intentions, the recovery process from abuse of a chemical substance is a long and tedious one, which requires a considerable amount of physical and psychosocial support.

Health care professionals have been involved in abuse of chemical substances. Nurses need to be aware of behaviors that may indicate a colleague is abusing drugs and/or alcohol. Several factors, such as occupational and personal stress, along with the presence of addicting substances in the workplace, predispose a nurse to abuse medications and to become an impaired health professional. Because safety of clients may be affected, it is essential that incidences of abuse be reported according to the institution's and the state's policies. In many instances, the first line of action is to direct the health care professional into a recovery program through the institution's Employee Assistance Program, if available. Other programs may be offered by the state. The license of the health care professional could be suspended or revoked, depending on the extent of the problem and any resultant malpractice action.

✦ General Concepts of Pharmacology

Drug Names

Every drug is known by more than one name, and each name has particular significance to the client and the health team member. Drugs can be known by their chemical, trademark, generic, and official names. The *chemical* name is the first name given to a drug. It specifically describes the exact arrangement of the chemical components of the drug. This name is given to the drug by the chemist who formulates the substance to be used as a medication. The *trademark* or *brand* name is the name registered by the manufacturer who is the legal owner of this drug name. Because the manufacturer owns this drug, the brand name is often referred to as the proprietary name or trade name. The same drug can be sold under a number of different trade names. The *generic* name is often referred to as the nonproprietary name of the drug. It is the permanent drug name that is used in all countries and usually reflects the chemical makeup of the drug. A generic name is never capitalized and is always given to the new drug before it becomes "official" or listed in official drug publications. The *official* name is the name by which the drug is identified or appears in the official drug publications, the *United States Pharmacopeia (USP)* in the United States or the *British Pharmacopeia (BP)* in Canada. The official name is the same as the generic name. Table 21–3 provides an example of types of drug names.

Drug Classifications and Sources

Drugs are also classified according to their characteristics. Drugs within a specific classification have similar actions, are prescribed to treat similar conditions or symptoms, or target similar body systems or functions. Drugs within a classification do not necessarily have similar chemical composition. For example, one type of drug classification is antiinfectives; within this classification there are both natural substances and semisynthetic substances.

Drugs come from a variety of sources. Most drugs originate from natural sources, such as plants and animals. These natural product drugs all contain protein and are composed of the elements carbon, hydrogen, oxygen, and nitrogen. Because of these elements, natural product drugs are highly antigenic, that is, capable of producing a hypersensitivity reaction. Penicillin and other antibiotics are examples of drugs derived from natural, living sources, which explains why clients are prone to developing allergic responses to them.

Drugs also can be derived from chemicals and minerals found in the environment. Vitamin and mineral supplements are representative of these kinds of drugs. Some drugs are chemically synthesized in the laboratory and are distinctly foreign to the body's composition. Most recently, drugs such as human insulin have been synthesized from recombinant bacterial DNA, opening new avenues for pharmacological development in the field of molecular biology.

Mechanisms of Drug Actions

Drugs are capable of producing both therapeutic and adverse effects throughout the body. As chemicals, drugs are introduced into the body to act on body cells for an intended therapeutic effect. They are frequently used to promote equilibrium and maintain homeostasis in the body. Drugs replace missing substances such as insulin and other hormones; protect weakened bodily functions; prevent insult from for-

Table 21–3

THREE TYPES OF DRUG NAMES*

TYPE OF DRUG NAME	EXAMPLES
Chemical name	N-acetyl-para-aminophenol
Generic name (nonproprietary name)	Acetaminophen
Trade name (proprietary name)	Acephen
	Aceta
	Apacet
	Arthritis Pain Formula Aspirin-Free
	Aspirin Free Anacin
	Aspirin-Free Pain Relief
	Banesin
	Bromo-Seltzer
	Dapa
	Dolanex
	Dorcol Children's Fever & Pain Reducer
	Feverall
	Genapap
	Genebs
	Halenol
	Liquiprin
	Meda Tab
	Myapap
	Neopap
	Oraphen-PD
	Panadol
	Panex
	Panex 500
	St. Joseph Aspirin-Free for Children
	Suppap-325
	Tapanol
	Tempra
	Tylenol

*The chemical, generic, and trade names listed are all names for the drug whose structure is pictured. This drug is most familiar under its trade name of Tylenol.
From Lehne, R. A. (1994). *Pharmacology for Nursing Care* (2nd ed.). Philadelphia: W. B. Saunders.

eign substances such as bacteria; eliminate noxious chemicals within the body; promote cellular function (*e.g.,* cardiotonics); and alleviate symptoms such as fever.

Drugs are intended to act at specific receptors, or pharmacologically active sites, throughout the body to produce an effect. The mechanism of drug-receptor interaction resembles a lock and key. When the drug, or key, is attached to a specific receptor, or lock, a cascade of physiological events is "locked," altering a physiological response and producing a specific drug effect.

➤ **Pharmacokinetics.** The movement of drug molecules throughout the body is referred to as **pharmacokinetics.** This process encompasses everything that happens to the drug from the time that it is absorbed into the bloodstream and distributed throughout the body to the time it is metabolized and then eliminated. Four distinct processes are included in pharmacokinetics: absorption, distribution, biotransformation, and excretion (Fig. 21–1).

Absorption is the process by which the drug molecule is transferred from the site at which it enters the body to the circulating body fluids. Most drugs must enter the systemic circulation to exert their therapeutic effects.

Drugs are administered by various routes, and each route has its characteristic influence on the drug's absorption (Fig. 21–2). The extent to which the active ingredients of a drug are absorbed and transported to their sites of action is termed **bioavailability.** Typical routes for drug administration are topical (to the skin), inhalant, oral, and parenteral (including subcutaneous, intramuscular, and IV). Topical absorption is the slowest, and IV absorption is the fastest. Drugs that are inhaled are rapidly absorbed through the mucous membranes of the respiratory tract.

Oral administration, although safe, convenient, and inexpensive in comparison to parenteral administration, is affected by the presence or absence of food in the gastrointestinal tract and by the lipid solubility and ionization of the drug molecule. The presence of food usually delays absorption, which is why most medications are administered between meals. In some instances, the presence of food is required to protect the lining of the stomach from the harsh effects of the drug, as with aspirin or ibuprofen, or to promote absorption, as with orange juice for iron absorption. The form of the oral medication is also important; liquid medications are absorbed more readily than capsules. Enteric-coated medications are protected against gastric acid and do not disintegrate until they reach the small intestine, thus protecting the lining of the stomach. The small intestine is the primary site of oral drug absorption, because its vast number of villi provide an increased surface area for drug absorption.

Absorption rates for parenteral medications depend on many factors. The primary factor is the blood supply to the area. Poor blood supply that accompanies circulatory problems decreases the absorption rate of medications. The presence of edema, bruises, or scarring can severely affect absorption rates, thus limiting the effect of the drug. A drug administered into subcutaneous tissue is absorbed more slowly than one administered into a muscle. IV administration of a drug is the most rapid route; it provides an immediate effect because drugs admitted by this route bypass absorption.

Distribution refers to the process by which the drug molecule is transported by the circulating body fluids to various areas of the body (see Fig. 21–1). Transportation of the drug molecule is accomplished through attachment to plasma proteins, during which

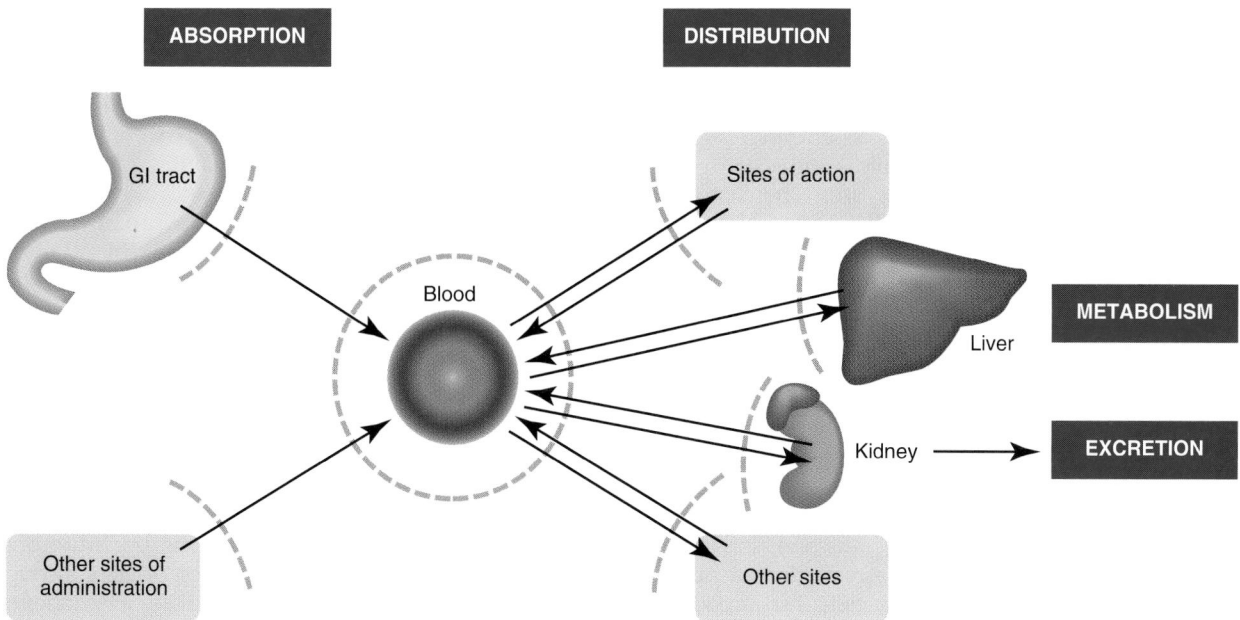

✦ **Figure 21–1**
The four basic pharmacokinetic processes. *Dotted lines* represent membranes that must be crossed as drugs move throughout the body. (GI = gastrointestinal.)

time the "bound" drug molecule remains inactive or incapable of producing a drug effect. Once the drug molecule is no longer bound to protein, it is capable of acting at tissue receptor sites and being metabolized and eliminated from the body. The blood is primarily responsible for drug distribution because of its intimate relation with all body tissues.

There are physiological barriers that prevent the distribution of certain drugs. The blood-brain barrier prevents entrance of drugs such as dopamine into the central nervous system because they are poorly soluble in lipids; drugs such as barbiturates pass readily into the brain. The placental barrier is not as selective

as the blood-brain barrier, but it is also highly sensitive to drugs soluble in lipids. Some drugs are prohibited for pregnant women because of their potential effect on the developing fetus.

Factors that affect distribution include body weight and composition, circulatory dynamics, and protein binding. The size of the client has a direct relation to the amount of drug that is needed to achieve a therapeutic effect. Infants and children require smaller doses of drugs, whereas obese adults require larger doses. Listings for average drug doses are based on an average-sized adult. Also, older adults have less body water, so drugs that are water soluble are distributed either slowly or unevenly, causing slower onset of drug action and longer duration of effect.

Distribution of a medication is highly dependent on the quality of the circulatory system and the ability to diffuse the medication from the intravascular to the interstitial layers. Vasodilation and vasoconstriction, which can occur normally with changes in temperature, affect the distribution rate of a drug. Clients with poor circulation to hands and feet tend to receive considerably less therapeutic benefit from drug therapy than clients with adequate tissue perfusion. For example, if tissue edema is present, diffusion from the vascular system to the interstitial tissue is hampered.

Most medications bind to serum albumin to some extent and are inactive when protein bound. Decreased levels of serum albumin result in higher levels of the active form of the drug. Clients who have liver disease or who are malnourished are at risk for drug toxicity because of decreased albumin levels. The same is true for infants and older adults. For these

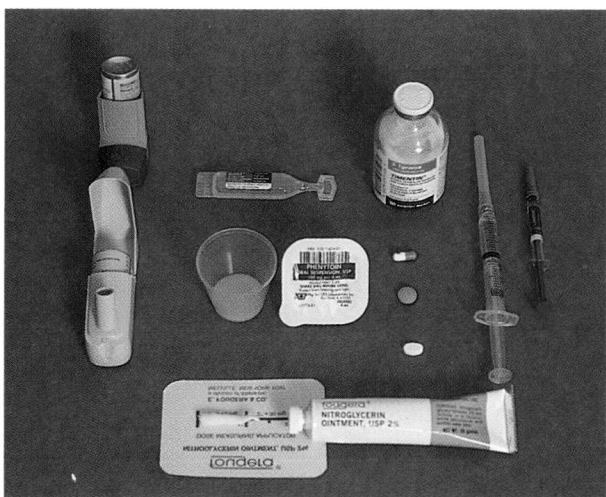

✦ **Figure 21–2**
Various forms of medications.

clients, smaller amounts of the drug are required to produce the desired drug effect.

Biotransformation, or metabolism, refers to the process by which a drug molecule becomes chemically altered through the action of enzymes and is converted to a less active, harmless substance. The enzymes function to detoxify the drug chemical, degrade or break it down into simpler components, and remove active components. This process is also referred to as drug metabolism or drug detoxification.

The liver is the primary site of drug transformation because the hepatic microsomes initiate enzymatic metabolic reactions. The liver is able to oxidize a chemical substance and transform it into a less toxic substance before it is distributed to other tissues. People with poor liver function are at high risk for development of toxic reactions to many drugs because the liver is unable or has an impaired ability to detoxify the drug. Clients who experience infection, inflammation, or fibrosis of the liver have a reduction of microsomal function, with a consequent negative impact on drug metabolism. In these clients, large amounts of the drug accumulate, and a toxic or adverse effect may occur. Metabolism of drugs also occurs in the lungs, kidneys, blood, and intestines.

Excretion refers to the process by which the less active, biotransformed drug molecule is removed from the body. Drugs may be eliminated from the body through urine, saliva, bile, milk and sweat gland secretions, and feces.

The kidney is the primary organ of drug excretion because of the large number of nephrons that promote tubular secretion of substances to be eliminated from the body. Some drugs are excreted in their original form, totally untransformed while in the body. Excretion of the drug through the kidney depends on an adequate glomerular filtration rate within the nephrons. In clients who have diminished kidney function, excretion of drugs is decreased. Acute or chronic renal failure significantly reduces urine output by the kidney and results in an accumulation of drug molecules to a level that is toxic and harmful to other bodily tissues. Older adults frequently have slowed kidney function and should be observed carefully for toxic drug reactions that may result from delayed excretion.

♦ **Effects of Drugs.** A **drug effect** is the observed manifestation of the actions of chemical substances on the body. The term *drug action* refers to the physiological and biochemical mechanisms that underlie how the drug responds in the body. Drug effects are produced by specific drug actions throughout the body. In other words, drug effects are what the drug does, and drug actions are how the drug does what it is supposed to do.

Every drug is capable of producing a desired or therapeutic effect. The **therapeutic effect** is the intended effect of the drug when it is introduced into the body. A drug may produce more than one therapeutic effect. For instance, digoxin acts to strengthen the force of cardiac contractions and to slow the heart rate by suppressing the sinoatrial node. Aspirin has many therapeutic effects: an analgesic effect that relieves pain; an antipyretic effect that reduces fever; an antiinflammatory effect that reduces swelling; and an anticoagulant effect that limits the ability of platelets to clump together.

The drug's *onset of action* is the point at which the level of the drug begins to rise in the blood after it is absorbed. *Peak effect* refers to the point at which maximal concentration of the drug is reached, whereas *duration of action* refers to the time from onset of action through the period of time that the drug is above minimal concentration levels. A drug's *half-life* is the time it takes for one-half of the drug to reduce its plasma concentration.

An **adverse effect,** or side effect, is a drug action that is not intended or is not a therapeutic effect. Each drug is capable of causing side effects by virtue of its ability to interact at a variety of receptor sites throughout the body. When drugs accumulate in concentrations that are too high within the body, as in overdoses, the phenomenon of drug **toxicity** occurs. Adverse effects are often relatively harmless. For example, a person who is taking an antibiotic may become nauseated; someone who takes a narcotic may experience constipation. However, many drugs cause severe adverse effects and require close monitoring. Clients receiving cancer chemotherapy are at high risk for many toxic effects, such as severe anemia, bleeding tendencies, and mouth ulcerations. The hematological studies of such clients must be monitored for possible toxic effects.

Some adverse effects are predictable; that is, the effect is an expected consequence associated with taking the drug. For example, a narcotic agent such as morphine or codeine produces the predictable side effects of nausea and vomiting resulting from stimulation of the medullary vomiting center, as well as constipation resulting from a decrease in peristalsis. Drugs may also produce unpredictable adverse effects that are not associated with a pharmacological drug effect. These unexpected results can be caused by a disease process, an interaction with another drug that is being taken, or the individual physiological makeup of the client. Types of unpredictable adverse effects are idiosyncrasy, hypersensitivity, and teratogenicity.

Idiosyncrasy is an unexplainable, unique reaction that occurs when a client takes a drug that typically does not produce this type of reaction. A client who develops a rapid heart rate after taking a drug intended to slow the heart rate is having an idiosyncratic reaction. **Hypersensitivity,** or an allergic reaction, may be slight with manifestations such as skin rash, hives, and itching, or it may be very severe, resulting in anaphylaxis or death. Antibiotics commonly cause allergic reactions, both mild and severe. Anaphylactic reactions are characterized by sudden constriction of the bronchioles, edema of the larynx, and severe shortness of breath. When anaphylaxis occurs, a client needs emergency treatment that usually includes administration of epinephrine. Nurses should carefully question clients about their history of drug allergies before administering any medications.

Teratogenicity occurs when a drug crosses the placenta and produces abnormalities in fetal development resulting in deformities. Drugs are currently classified by the US Food and Drug Administration (FDA) as Pregnancy Category A, B, C, D, or X to reflect their teratogenicity on the developing fetus. Category X drugs produce the most devastating effects (Table 21–4). It is important that nurses provide anticipatory guidance to clients about potential drug adverse effects in order to reduce anxiety associated with medication administration and increase compliance with drug therapy.

A *drug interaction* occurs when the action of one drug is altered by the simultaneous presence of another drug in the client's system. A drug's pharmacokinetics may be intensified, reduced, or negated by the interaction of two drugs or by a drug-food combination. On many occasions, two medications are prescribed together for a therapeutic effect, such as a narcotic and a nonnarcotic analgesic combination to enhance pain relief. A combination of medication and food can prevent an adverse effect, as when prednisone is administered with food or milk to prevent gastrointestinal irritation.

♣ **Poisons.** Chemical substances exist in the environment that can be very harmful to human life if they come in contact with the body through inhalation, digestion, or absorption. These substances, known as **poisons,** have the potential to produce effects that can impair the function of all essential bodily systems. Specific antidotes can be used to reverse the harmful effects of some poisons, such as naloxone to treat narcotic overdoses or ethylenediaminetetraacetic acid (EDTA) to treat lead poisoning. There are specific treatment protocols for most types of poisons. If a poisoning situation occurs, the local poison control center should be contacted immediately for appropriate treatment. Most poisonings occur in young children, because they are most likely to ingest household chemicals and plants. Poisoning situations involving older adults usually result from the accidental overdose of prescription medications. Regardless of the age of the client, poisoning presents a challenge for the nurse related to chemical safety and environmental influence.

Factors Affecting Drug Actions

A variety of factors other than the chemical structure of the drug affect the action of the drug in the body. Because of the unique characteristics of the individual, drug effects may vary from one client to another. These variations may include differences in the number or type of side effects; in some clients, effects may be severe or toxic.

Physiological Considerations

When determining the dose of a drug, the size of the client is a major consideration. Drugs are designed to cause certain physiological responses in an average-sized adult person. Infants and young children, as well as obese adults, may have altered responses because of their size. Doses for clients whose size varies significantly from the average should be calculated according to weight or body surface area.

The health status of the client has a major role in altering the metabolism and biotransformation of drugs. The presence of any illness or disease state affects the pharmacokinetics of drugs. Clients with metabolic disorders, such as liver cirrhosis or impaired renal function, respond to drugs differently than clients with normal health. As a result, absorption may be slowed, distribution altered and uneven, detoxification impaired, and excretion altered. When a drug's effectiveness is seriously affected, the client is at high risk for development of a toxic reaction.

Nutrition is an important component of normal cellular functioning. Deficient intake of important vitamins, minerals, and nutrients impairs body systems

---

Table 21–4

FDA PREGNANCY CATEGORIES

CATEGORY	DESCRIPTION
A	No risk to fetus. Studies have shown no evidence of fetal harm.
B	No risk in animal studies, but well-controlled studies in pregnant women are not available. It is assumed there is little or no risk in pregnant women.
C	Animal studies indicate a risk to the fetus. Controlled studies on pregnant women are not available. Risk versus benefit of the drug must be determined.
D	A risk to the human fetus has been proved. Risk versus benefit of the drug must be determined. It could be used in life-threatening conditions.
X	A risk to the human fetus has been proved. Risks outweigh the benefits, and the drug should be avoided during pregnancy.

Kee, J. L., & Hayes, E. R. (1997). *Pharmacology: A nursing process approach* (2nd ed., p. 136). Philadelphia: W. B. Saunders.

and interferes with normal metabolic activity. Clients with moderate to severe nutritional deficiencies are at higher risk for development of a toxic drug effect. Even clients with good nutritional habits may have ingested dietary substances that can alter the action of drugs. Orange juice has been shown to increase absorption of iron; milk and milk products alter the absorption of tetracycline; and green leafy vegetables with high amounts of vitamin K can alter the effects of warfarin sodium as an anticoagulant.

Another major physiological consideration is gender, because differences in the physiological processes of men and women affect drug actions. Varying levels of male and female hormones can affect the way a drug is absorbed, metabolized, and excreted. Also, there are distinct differences in body fat and fluid levels between men and women. The great majority of research on drug effects is done with male subjects, and, as a result, the effects of such drugs on women may be different from those expected.

Developmental Considerations

Age is a major factor affecting the action of drugs. Because of immature body systems, differences in the balance between fluid and body mass, and limited liver enzymes, the neonate and the infant require special consideration in drug dosage calculation. A slight increase in the dose administered to a young child may result in a significant overdose with toxic effects (Table 21–5).

Geriatric clients experience changes in normal physiological functioning that can place them at risk for alterations in drug pharmacokinetics (Table 21–6). The normal aging process affects liver and kidney function, which primarily influence biotransformation and excretion of drugs. As a result, the older client is more susceptible to drug overdose and toxicity. Older clients are more likely to experience multiple drug interactions from polypharmacy, because they may require medications for several conditions at once.

Psychological Considerations

The distribution and metabolism of drugs are highly affected by stress level. A person under severe emotional and physical stress tends to have heightened sympathetic responses, which increase blood pressure and circulation but tend to slow many metabolic functions. Under periods of great stress, drugs tend to be absorbed more slowly from the gastrointestinal tract, delaying the onset of drug action.

Table 21–5

PHARMACOKINETICS IN INFANTS AND CHILDREN

PHASES	BODILY EFFECTS AND POSSIBLE DRUG RESPONSES
Absorption	Reduced gastric acid production; gastric pH is higher than in adults. Drugs such as penicillin that are absorbed poorly with low gastric pH are absorbed faster in children. Smaller drug doses may be required.
	Slow gastric emptying time caused by slow or irregular peristalsis may delay drug absorption. Drugs given orally take longer to reach peak plasma levels. Adults and older children have a faster absorption rate.
	First-pass elimination by the liver is reduced. More drug is available for distribution, so a smaller drug dose is required. Topical drugs may be absorbed faster because infants have a proportionally larger body surface area.
Distribution	Infants and children have lower blood pressure, which affects blood flow to tissues. The liver and brain are proportionally larger and receive more blood flow; the kidneys receive less.
	Infants are composed of 65 to 75% water; premature infants are 85% water. Water-soluble drugs are diluted in the large volume of their body fluid; a larger drug dose may be needed.
	Since infants have fewer plasma protein-binding sites, lower doses are needed. With fewer available binding sites, there is more free drug.
	The blood-brain barrier is not completely developed in the infant, so more drug passes into the cerebral cells.
Biotransformation	There is a decreased activity of liver enzymes as a result of the immaturity of the infant liver. The half-life of a drug may be longer than it would be in an older child or adult; therefore, drug accumulation can occur.
	Drug half-life in the older child can be shorter because of the increased metabolic rate. Higher doses for the older child may be needed to offset the increased metabolic rate.
Excretion	Drug elimination via the kidneys is decreased until after the first year of life. Blood flow volume through the kidneys is less than in adults, and the glomerular filtration rate is approximately 30 to 40% of the adult rate. A decrease in drug excretion leads to a longer half-life and possible drug toxicity.

Kee, J. L., & Hayes, E. R. (1997). *Pharmacology: A nursing process approach* (2nd ed.). Philadelphia: W. B. Saunders.

Table **21–6**

PHARMACOKINETICS IN GERIATRIC CLIENTS

PHASES	BODILY EFFECTS AND POSSIBLE DRUG RESPONSES
Absorption	Decreased gastric acidity alters absorption of weak acid drugs, such as aspirin.
	Decreased blood flow to the gastrointestinal tract (40–50% less) is caused by decreased cardiac output. Because of the reduction in blood flow, absorption is slowed but not decreased.
	Reduced gastrointestinal motility rate (peristalsis) may delay onset of action.
Distribution	Because of decreased body water in the older adult, water-soluble drugs are more concentrated. There is an increase in the fat-to-water ratio in the older adult; fat-soluble drugs are stored and are likely to accumulate. Older adults have decreased serum protein and albumin levels; therefore, there are fewer protein-binding sites, resulting in more free drug. Drugs with a high affinity for protein compete for protein-binding sites with other drugs. Drug interactions result from the lack of protein sites and the increase in free drugs.
Biotransformation	In the older adult, there is decreased hepatic enzyme production, hepatic blood flow, and total liver function. These decreases cause a reduction in drug metabolism.
	With the reduction in metabolic rate, the half-life of drugs increases, and drug accumulation can result. Metabolism inactivates a drug and prepares it for elimination via the kidney. Drug toxicity may occur when the half-life is prolonged.
Excretion	The older adult has a decrease in renal blood flow and a decrease in glomerular filtration rate by 4–50%. With a decrease in renal function, there is a decrease in drug excretion, and drug accumulation results. Drug toxicity should be assessed continually while the client is taking the drug.

Kee, J. L., & Hayes, E. R. (1997). *Pharmacology: A nursing process approach* (2nd ed.). Philadelphia: W. B. Saunders.

Each client has a unique reaction to a drug, based on the client's past experience with medication administration, the client's personal health goals, and the beliefs of the client and his or her significant others about achieving the highest level of wellness. Thus, medication administration is influenced by a potential psychological effect that the client's environment brings to the situation. For example, the client may consciously or unconsciously desire to remain ill in order to receive compensation from an employer. In this situation, the psychological factors of power and security may influence the client's compliance with a medication regimen. Positive and negative influences, addiction, and the perception of drugs as dangerous are all psychological aspects that determine a client's reaction to drug therapy. The nurse must consider the psychological dynamics of the client's environment as it affects drug therapy and the client's capacity to get well.

Sociocultural Considerations

The client's sociocultural background and environment play a major role in the pharmacokinetics of drugs and the quality of the client's response to a drug's chemical actions. For instance, rural versus urban residency involves multiple factors that could affect the action of a drug, including air quality, living conditions, and job commuting. Economic conditions affect the extent to which clients seek medical care and have prescriptions filled. When a person has limited financial resources, his or her choices are restricted by the costs of available services. Frequently, health maintenance activities, such as making routine visits to a community health center, become luxuries. Minor health problems may be delayed until the situation becomes critical. Drug prescriptions are often expensive, and a client with limited resources may be unable to pay the costs.

The client's culture plays an important role in health beliefs and medication compliance. It is important to know how the client views the use of prescription medication. Two basic frameworks have been identified by anthropologists to classify views of health and illness: Western belief systems and non-Western belief systems (Edmisson, 1996). A person with a Western philosphy generally believes that the use of prescription medications will be effective, whereas an individual with a non-Western philosophy may prefer alternative modalities, such as herbs, spiritual solace, or special talismans. A client who believes that a drug is harmful will not follow a prescription given by a health care provider. It is important for the nurse to ascertain the client's cultural mores about pharmacological therapies in order to determine the likelihood of expected outcomes of therapy.

Types of Preparations

Drugs are available in many types of preparations depending on the route of administration, the action of the drug, the metabolism of the drug, and the therapeutic use of the drug. The form of the drug determines how it is administered. For instance, a supposi-

Table **21–7**

TYPES OF DRUG PREPARATIONS AND FORMS

ROUTE	TYPE	DESCRIPTION
Oral	Capsule	Medication in powder, liquid, or oil form encased in a gelatin shell
	Tablet	Medication in compressed disk or cylinder form that contains pure drug and inactive components
	Enteric-coated tablet	Tablet coated with substance that does not dissolve in stomach but does dissolve in intestines
	Suspension	Medication in finely divided particles dissolved in liquid; will separate if left standing
	Lozenge	Medication flavored with sugar and mucilage, compressed into a round form; dissolves in mouth
	Sustained-release spansule	Contains small drug-impregnated beads that slowly release the drug at different times
	Solution	Medication dissolved in at least one liquid substance, usually water (as in an aqueous solution)
Parenteral	Ampule	Medication contained in a molded glass container for single-use only
	Vial	Medication contained in a glass or plastic container, which may be either single or multiple dose
	Cartridge	Medication contained in a single-dose tube or cylinder for single-use only
Dermal	Transdermal disk	Medication contained in a semipermeable patch for absorption through skin
	Ointment	Medication that is semisolid in form for application to skin
	Lotion	Medication that is contained in an aqueous suspension, solution, or emulsion
	Cream	Medication that is a semisolid, nongreasy, water-soluble emulsion
	Suppository	Medication mixed with a solid base such as glycerin that melts at body temperature
Inhalant	Spray or mist	Hand-held inhaler disperses medication in an aerosol spray or mist, which the client inhales
	Gas	Gas is administered through an endotracheal or tracheal tube

tory is taken either rectally or vaginally; a patch is applied to the skin; a tablet is taken orally. Many drugs are available in multiple forms, allowing flexibility in relation to the client's situation and illness. For instance, if a client is unable to take an oral form of aspirin, rectal administration of a suppository may be used; if a client has difficulty swallowing pills or capsules, a liquid form may help; if rapid administration of digoxin is needed to decrease a client's heart rate, it may be administered intravenously. Table 21–7 lists several types of medication preparations.

Routes of Administration

Drugs can be administered through a variety of routes, the choice depending on the chemical properties of the drug, the intended effect of the drug, and the physical condition of the client. Administration routes are categorized as oral, parenteral, topical, or inhalant.

Oral Administration

The most common route of drug administration is the oral route (Fig. 21–3), which involves taking the medication by mouth and swallowing it, placing the medication under the tongue for it to be dissolved (sublingually), or placing a solid form of the medication against the mucous membrane of the mouth (buccally). Generally, the oral route is considered the least expensive. Drugs have a slower rate of onset when taken orally because of the time required for digestion and absorption in the intestinal tract. Some clients receive drugs that are directly instilled into the stomach through a tube, such as a nasogastric or gastrostomy tube. This is referred to as *enteral* drug administration.

Sublingual administration of a drug is designed to promote rapid absorption through the mucous membranes of the mouth. The client places the medication under the tongue for absorption. Nitroglycerin is administered sublingually to a client who is having chest pain to provide rapid pain relief. Buccal administration involves placing the drug against the surface of the mucous membranes of the cheek and is designed for a more local effect rather than the systemic effect that occurs if the drug is swallowed orally.

Parenteral Administration

Parenteral administration involves injection of a medication into a body tissue, such as subcutaneous tissue, muscles, or veins.

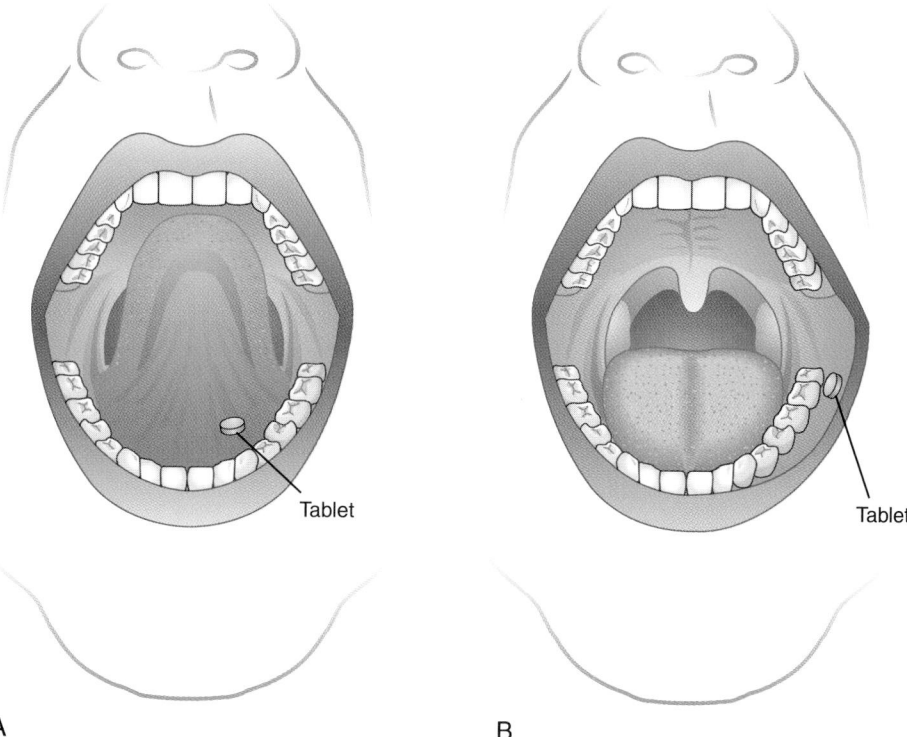

Tablet

Tablet

A   B

♦ **Figure 21–3**
A, Sublingual administration of a
tablet. *B*, Buccal administration of
a tablet.

Intradermal administration involves injection of a medication into the dermis layer of the skin; common examples are the administration of substances for allergy or tuberculin skin testing.

Subcutaneous administration involves injection of a medication into the subcutaneous tissue below the dermis; a common example is the administration of insulin.

Intramuscular administration involves injection of a medication into a muscle, such as the deltoid or the gluteus maximus; common examples are the administration of narcotic analgesics or penicillin.

Intravenous administration involves injection of a medication into a vein; common examples are antibiotics administered piggyback or narcotic analgesics administered via patient-controlled analgesia.

Intracavitary administration involves the injection of a medication into a body cavity. There are several types of intracavitary administration:

- *Epidural*—into the epidural space. The most common type is the administration of an analgesic, such as morphine sulfate, postoperatively through a catheter inserted into the epidural space.
- *Intrathecal*—into a subarachnoid space of the brain.
- *Intrapleural*—into the pleural space around the lungs, either through an injection or through a chest tube. A common type of intrapleural administration is the injection of a chemotherapeutic agent for treatment of a cancer.
- *Intraperitoneal*—into the peritoneal cavity. This method is used for administration of antibiotics or chemotherapy.
- *Intraosseus*—into the bone marrow.
- *Intraarterial*—into an artery.

Topical Administration

Topical administration involves application of a drug directly to the surface of the skin by spreading it over the skin surface, soaking the skin or body part in a solution, or applying a patch to the surface of the skin. The medication is absorbed through the skin and distributed systemically throughout the body.

A drug in the form of an ointment or cream is applied to the skin and smoothed over a designated area. Some of the topical medications dissolve into the skin, whereas others must be removed before a repeat dose is applied. Nitroglycerin ointment should be cleaned off the skin before a second dose is applied to prevent high levels of the medication circulating in the body. The patch form consists of a disk containing the medication; it provides for continuous administration over a prolonged period of time.

Instillations are another form of topical administration comprising those drugs that are placed into a body cavity or orifice. Included in this category are vaginal and rectal suppositories, body cavity irrigations (*e.g.*, eye, ear), and nasal or throat sprays. The drug effect of medications administered by instillation may be local or systemic.

Inhalatory Administration

Drugs can be inhaled through the nose or mouth into the respiratory tract for local or systemic effects. There are many bronchial inhalants that are targeted to exert a direct effect on the bronchial mucosa. Clients who have asthma commonly take inhalants such

ADMINISTRATION OF INHALED MEDICATIONS WITH A METERED-DOSE INHALER

Medications may be inhaled into the respiratory tract to provide rapid relief of symptoms caused by bronchospasm. Clients who receive inhalation therapy frequently suffer from chronic respiratory disease. Common medications delivered through the respiratory tract include bronchodilators, mucolytic agents, steroids, and antibiotics. Medications may also be inhaled to block local allergic reactions. The medications may be administered with a hand-held inhaler and dispersed through an aerosol spray, mist, or fine powder that penetrates lung airways.

The inhaled medications produce dilation of the bronchioles, relieving symptoms of bronchospasm by opening narrowed airways. Mucolytic agents and inhaled sterile saline help to liquefy thick secretions. The metered dose from an inhaler delivers a measured amount of medication with each depression of the canister.

Equipment:

Hand-held inhaler

Action	Rationale
1. Verify the physician's order for the client's name, drug name, dose, and time and route of administration.	**1.** This ensures that the client receives the correct medication by the proper route.
2. Assess the client's allergy history.	**2.** This alerts the nurse to potential reactions to observe during the drug administration.
3. Select the prescribed medication and verify against order on medication card or printout.	**3.** Verification of the order averts medication errors.
4. Ask the client to state his or her name, and check the client's identity by reading the wristband.	**4.** This verifies the identity of the client.
5. Explain the medication and review the procedure with the client.	**5.** This increases cooperation and reduces anxiety.
6. Shake the container well before each use.	**6.** This builds up aerosol pressure within the canister.
7. Have the client exhale slowly and as completely as possible through the mouth.	**7.** This increases the client's ability to inhale medication as deeply as possible for maximal penetration.
8. Instruct the client to place mouthpiece fully into mouth, holding inhaler upright, one to two finger-widths from mouth.	**8.** This allows inspired air to mix with medication.

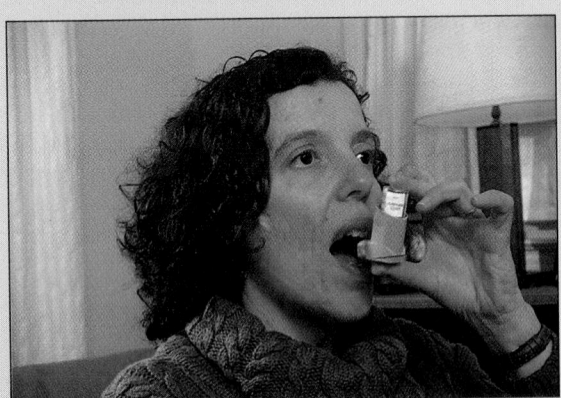

Step 8.

9. Have the client inhale deeply through the mouth while depressing the top of the canister with the middle finger so the medication is inhaled.

10. Tell the client to hold the breath for as long as possible before exhaling slowly and gently.

10. This allows time for the medication to penetrate the bronchioles, thereby producing bronchodilating effects.

ADMINISTRATION OF INHALED MEDICATIONS WITH A METERED-DOSE INHALER

(Continued)

Action	Rationale
11. When two puffs are prescribed, wait 2 minutes and shake the container again before administering a second puff.	**11.** This allows for deeper bronchial penetration.
12. Provide water to rinse mouth after inhalation.	**12.** This prevents mouth and throat dryness, or candidiasis if steroid inhalation is ordered.
13. Document the medication form, the time, and the client's response.	
14. Assess breath sounds for wheezing; record pulse.	

Example of Documentation

Date	Time	Notes
1/1/98	0800	c/o Shortness of breath. Bilateral wheezing noted with auscultation. Mary Smith, RN
1/1/98	0810	No wheezes auscultated. No c/o shortness of breath. Mary Smith, RN

as bronchodilators and steroids. Using hand-held inhalers that disperse the medication in an aerosol spray or mist, the client inhales while the medication is delivered from the inhaler. A metered-dose inhaler (MDI) is relatively easy to use when correct technique is applied (Procedure 21–1).

Anesthesia is commonly administered as an inhalant. Usually, an endotracheal or tracheal tube has been inserted, so the anesthetic gas is administered through the tube. Anesthesia is administered under controlled situations and by an anesthesiologist or nurse anesthetist. The nurse is responsible for monitoring clients as they come out of anesthesia. Medications may be administered through an endotracheal tube during an emergency situation. For clients who are in severe shock or cardiac arrest, endotracheal inhalation provides the most rapid onset of action.

Drug Measurement Systems

The amount of medication that is administered to a client is the *dose* of the medication. Calculation of dose requires accurate measurement of the drug. Inaccurate measurement can be dangerous or even fatal for the client. The nurse must be aware of the various measurement systems that are used to calculate drug doses. These are the metric, the apothecary, and the household systems. In the United States and Canada, the metric system is the primary measurement system,

but many drug doses are still calculated by the apothecary or household systems.

Metric System

The metric system is a decimal system based on units of ten; this allows for easy conversion by moving the decimal through multiplication and division. The basic units of measurement in the metric system are the liter (volume), the gram (weight), and the meter (length). Table 21–8 provides a description of the units for each measurement and their conversion equivalents. The prefix *kilo-* is used to describe a measurement of 1000 times the base measurement; for example, 1 kilometer is equal to 1000 meters. The prefix *milli-* is used to describe a measurement $\frac{1}{1000}$ or 0.001 times the base; for instance, 1 meter is equal to 1000 millimeters (or 0.001 meter). In the metric system, all units are written in decimals (e.g., 1.5, 0.05) and not in fractions.

Apothecary System

The apothecary system has been used for a long time in both the United States and Canada. Common units in the apothecary system are the pint and the quart (volume); the inch and the foot (length); and the ounce and pound (weight). For medications, the common unit of measurement is the grain for weight and the minim for volume. One minim of water weighs approximately 1 grain. See Table 21–8 for apothecary equivalents in weight and fluid volume.

Table 21–8

UNITS OF VARIOUS MEASUREMENT SYSTEMS

WEIGHT	LENGTH	VOLUME
Metric System 1 kilogram (kg) = 1000 gram (gm) 1 gram (g) = 1000 milligrams (mg)	1 kilometer (km) = 1000 meters (m) 1 meter (m) = 1000 millimeters (mm) 12 inches = 1 foot 3 feet = 1 yard	1 kiloliter (kl) = 1000 liters (L) 1 liter (L) = 1000 milliliters (ml)
Apothecary System 1 pound (lb) = 12 ounces (℥) 1 ounce (℥) = 8 drams (ℨ)		1 gallon (C.) = 8 pints (O.) 1 pint (O.) = 16 fluid ounces (fl. ℥) 1 fluid ounce (fl. ℥) = 8 fluid drams (f ℨ) 1 fluid dram (f ℨ) = 60 minims (♏)
Household System 1 pound (lb) = 16 ounces (oz)		1 gallon (gal) = 4 quarts (qt) 1 quart (qt) = 2 pints (pt) 1 pint (pt) = 2 cups (c) 1 cup (c) = 16 tablespoons (tbsp) 1 tablespoon (tbsp) = 3 teaspoons (tsp) 1 teaspoon (tsp) = 60 drops (gtt)

UNITS OF EXCHANGE AMONG SYSTEMS OF DRUG MEASUREMENT

Household	Apothecary	Metric	Avoirdupois
1 tsp	1 fluidram (f ℨ)	5 ml	
1 tbsp	½ fluidounce (f ℥)	15 ml	
2 tbsp	1 f ℥	30 ml	
1 measuring cupful	8 f ℥	240 ml	
1 pt	16 F ℥	473 ml	
1 qt	32 f ℥	946 ml (1 L)	
1 gal	128 f ℥	3785 ml	
15 gr		1.0 g (1000 mg)	
1 gr		0.6 g (60 mg) or 0.065 g (65 mg)	
$\frac{1}{120}$ gr		0.5 mg	
$\frac{1}{150}$ gr		0.4 mg	
	1 gr	0.065 g	1 gr
	15 gr	1.0 g	15.4 gr
	480 gr	28.35 g	1 oz
	1 oz	31 g	437.5 gr
	1.33 lb	454 g	1 lb
	1 lb	373 g	0.75 lb
		1 kg	2.2 lb

Household Measurements

Household measurements commonly used are the teaspoon, the tablespoon, and the cup for volume and the ounce and pound for weight. These measurements are convenient, and many household utensils use these scales. Recipes for baking and cooking use these measurements. Their major disadvantage is their inaccuracy compared with the metric or apothecary systems. They are not used with medications that require careful measurement. In less critical situations, where slight variations in measurement will not cause major harm, household measurements are used. Directions for taking most over-the-counter cough medicines and laxatives include measurements in teaspoons because these are the measurement scales that the client would have in the home. Table 21–8 presents a list of household equivalents in fluid volume.

Converting Different Measurement Units

There are times when it is necessary for the nurse to convert drug doses from one system to another. The nurse must be aware of the equivalents of measurement between systems and how to calculate the conversion. Table 21–8 provides a listing of common measurement equivalents between systems.

Calculating Prescribed Doses

Frequently, the nurse must calculate the prescribed dose because the dose available is in not the exact quantity needed. Several formulas are available. The following formula is a simple method for calculating doses:

$$\frac{\text{Dose ordered}}{\text{Dose on hand}} \times \text{Amount on hand} = \text{Prescribed dose}$$

Dose ordered is the amount of the drug prescribed by the physician. Dose on hand is the amount of the drug that is available. Amount on hand is the volume or weight of the drug that is available. This may be the number of tablets or capsules or the volume of the liquid that makes up the dose on hand. For instance, if the physician prescribes a dose of 650 mg of aspirin for a client and the drug is available in tablet form at 325 mg per tablet, the calculation of the prescribed dose is as follows:

$$\frac{650 \text{ mg}}{325 \text{ mg}} \times 1 \text{ tablet} = 2 \text{ tablets}$$

By dividing, the nurse determines that 650 is twice the amount of 325. Therefore, the nurse should administer two tablets to the client.

Another example is a prescription for 60 mg of Garamycin. On hand is a vial containing 80 mg in 2 ml. The calculation is as follows:

$$\frac{60 \text{ mg}}{80 \text{ mg}} \times 2 \text{ ml} = 1.5 \text{ ml}$$

By dividing 60 by 80, the nurse obtains a fraction of ¾. Multiplying ¾ by 2 equals a prescribed dose of 1.5 ml.

Another formula is the ratio method. This involves setting up a proportion.

Dose on hand : Quantity on hand :: Dose desired : Desired quantity (X)

When using a ratio formula, the nurse multiplies the dose on hand times the desired quantity (or X) and multiplies the quantity on hand times the dose desired, then solves for X. In the following example, Tylenol 650 mg is prescribed, and the drug on hand is 325 mg in 5 ml.

$$325 \text{ mg} : 5 \text{ ml} :: 650 \text{ mg} : X$$

Cross-multiplying gives 325X = 3250; solving for X yields a dose of 10 ml.

Pediatric Calculations

Doses for pediatric clients can be calculated by two methods. First, the dose may be calculated based on the client's body surface area (BSA). The BSA formula considers both the height and the weight of the child. To find the child's BSA, a nomogram (Fig. 21–4) is used. The height is found on the left column, and the weight on the right. A straight line is drawn between the two points, and the point at which it crosses the surface area column is the child's BSA. The formula then used is the following:

$$\frac{\text{BSA (child)}}{\text{BSA (adult)}} \times \text{adult's dose} = \text{child's dose}$$

The average BSA for adults is 1.7 square meters.

Types of Medication Distribution Systems

Institutions have medication distribution systems that are designed to coordinate activities among the various health team members. From the form that is used to prescribe the medication, to the dispensing of the medication by the pharmacy, to the administration of the medication to the client, each component of the system works in tandem with the others. The nurse is usually the person who coordinates all activities to ensure that the medication is available for the client when needed. There are three general types of systems: the stock supply system; the unit-dose system; and the computer-controlled dispensing system.

✦ **Stock Supply System.** In some situations, an institution may keep a stock supply of medications that are available in quantities for several clients. For instance, narcotics and barbiturates are frequently available as a stock supply; they are kept in a locked cabinet, and documentation of each dose administered is required. Many emergency departments keep a stock supply of medications for use in urgent situations. Most other units within an acute care or long-term care facility do not stock large quantities of medications because of the expense and errors associated with calculation of the dose.

✦ **Unit-Dose System.** More common than the stock supply system is the unit-dose system, which provides a supply of medications for a prescribed period, usually 24 hours. Each client has a drawer that is stocked daily by the pharmacist with the quantity of medication that will be required for that period. Each oral medication is individually wrapped, to be opened at the client's bedside and not ahead of time. The nurse should check the client's drawer after it has been stocked to verify that the correct amount of medication has been stocked. Any discrepancies should be reported immediately to the pharmacist. Usually, there are fewer medication errors with the unit-dose system because the amount of medication dispensed is the amount prescribed.

✦ **Computer-Controlled Dispensing System.** A computer-controlled dispensing system improves both accuracy and security of medication administration. The nurse is assigned an access code that must be entered into the system before a medication is dispensed. Once the system is accessed, the nurse enters

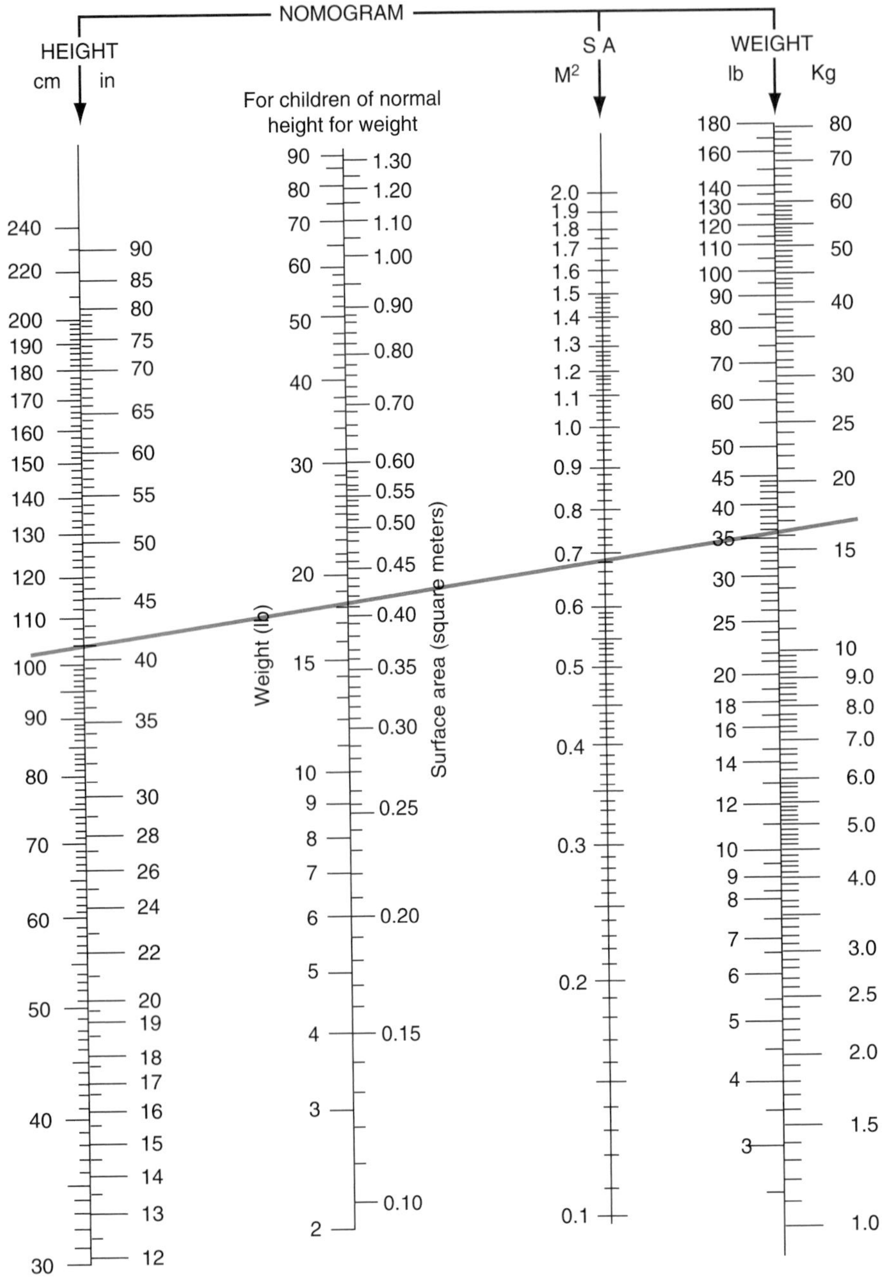

── NOMOGRAM ──

HEIGHT   SA   WEIGHT
cm   in   M²   lb   Kg

For children of normal
height for weight

HEIGHT
cm
240
220
200
190
180
170
160
150
140
130
120
110
100
90
80
70
60
50
40
30

in
90
85
80
75
70
65
60
55
50
45
40
35
30
28
26
24
22
20
19
18
17
16
15
14
13
12

Weight (lb)
90
80
70
60
50
40
30
20
15
10
9
8
7
6
5
4
3
2

Surface area (square meters)
1.30
1.20
1.10
1.00
0.90
0.80
0.70
0.60
0.55
0.50
0.45
0.40
0.35
0.30
0.25
0.20
0.15
0.10

SA
M²
2.0
1.9
1.8
1.7
1.6
1.5
1.4
1.3
1.2
1.1
1.0
0.9
0.8
0.7
0.6
0.5
0.4
0.3
0.2
0.1

WEIGHT
lb
180
160
140
130
120
110
100
90
80
70
60
50
45
40
35
30
25
20
18
16
14
12
10
9
8
7
6
5
4
3

Kg
80
70
60
50
40
30
25
20
15
10
9.0
8.0
7.0
6.0
5.0
4.0
3.0
2.5
2.0
1.5
1.0

❥ Figure 21–4
Nomogram for estimating body surface areas. The *straight line* is drawn between body weight and height. The point at which the line intersects the surface area (SA) column is the estimated body surface area.

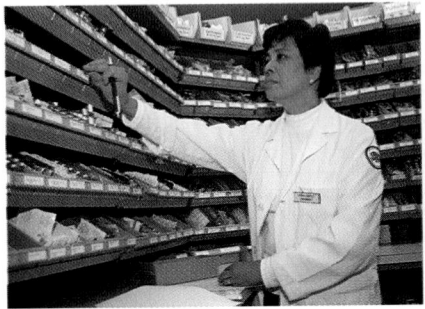
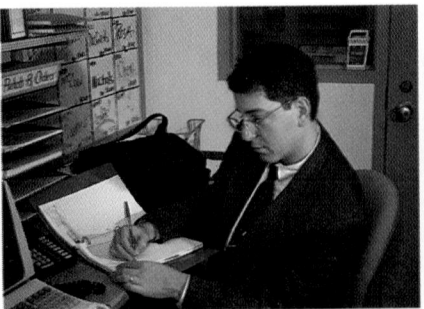
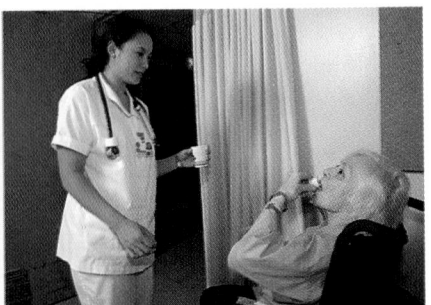

❥ Figure 21–5
Team responsible for safe drug administration: the pharmacist, physician, nurse, and client.

the client's name, the drug required, the dose, and the route of administration. Through the computer, the system verifies the request, dispenses the medication to the nurse, and records it on the client's record. This system is usually integrated with the client's record, so that maintenance and updating of the record is done automatically.

Principles in Administering Medications

A number of health team members play a vital role in drug therapy (Fig. 21–5). The primary team members that participate in ensuring safe, effective medication administration are the physician, the pharmacist, the nurse, and the client.

The Physician

The physician is the team member who prescribes the drug. In some states, advance practice nurses, such as nurse practitioners, may be granted prescriptive authority. When prescribing a medication, the prescriber considers the client's diagnosis, the need for the medication, the desired effect to be achieved, and the potential risks for the client. The prescription is written on the client's medical record according to the policies and procedures of the health care institution. In certain situations, the physician may be permitted to give an order for a medication verbally or over the telephone. When this occurs, the nurse should enter the verbal prescription on the client's record and obtain the physician's signature for the prescription within 24 hours.

A prescription should contain the following parts:

- *Client's full name.* It is imperative that the client be identified clearly to prevent administration of the medication to the wrong client. On inpatient units, the client's name is stamped on his or her chart.

- *Date the prescription was written.* The date of the prescription should include the day, month, and year. On inpatient units, the time that the prescription was written is also included. The date and time of the prescription are especially crucial if the medication is to be stopped automatically after a specified period.

- *Name of the drug.* The exact name of the medication should be identified clearly. In some situations, both the generic and the trade name should be given; in some clinical facilities, only generic names are used. For outpatient prescriptions, the prescriber should identify whether the generic or trade form of the drug should be used.

- *Dose of the drug.* The exact dose of the drug should be identified.

- *Frequency of the dose.* The prescription should include the number of times per day and the schedule for administering the drug. For instance, a drug that is to be taken three times a day may also need to be taken at 8-hour intervals.

- *Route of administration.* The specific route by which the drug should be administered must be identified clearly, because many drugs can be administered by more than one route.

- *Signature of the prescribing health care provider.* The prescription becomes a legally binding document only on evidence that the provider has signed it. The nurse should implement only prescriptions that include the signature of the prescribing person.

When a prescription is written, the nurse should follow institutional protocols for noting the order, transcribing the order onto the medication record, and submitting a copy of the prescription to the pharmacist who will dispense the drug. The medication record should be legible and should contain any special limitations that may exist. For instance, a medication may be prescribed to be withheld if the client's blood pressure is below a designated level.

There are several types of medication orders that

Table **21–9**

TYPES OF MEDICATION ORDERS

TYPE	DEFINITION	EXAMPLES
Standing order	Ongoing prescription to be administered until discontinued by physician; may be given only for a prescribed number of days	Digoxin (Lanoxin) 0.25 mg p.o. q.d.
p.r.n. order	A prescription to be administered when necessary for a specified problem/ condition	Aspirin 650 mg q 4h for temperature above 101°F; ibuprofen (Advil) 400 mg q 4h for complaints of pain
Stat order	A prescription to be administered immediately for an emergency situation	Morphine sulfate 10 mg IV stat for respiratory distress
One-time order	A prescription to be administered only once, not necessarily for an emergency situation	Diazepam (Valium) 10 mg IM on call to the operating room

Table 21–10

COMMONLY USED ABBREVIATIONS

ABBREVIATION	MEANING
a.c.	before meals
ad lib.	freely as desired
b.i.d.	twice a day
cc	cubic centimeter (same as a milliliter)
gtt.	drops
h.s.	at bedtime
I.M.	intramuscular
I.V.	intravenous
I.V.P.B	IV piggyback
mg	milligram
ml	milliliter
O.D.	right eye
O.S.	left eye
O.U.	each eye
p.c.	after meals
p.o.	by mouth
p.r.	by rectum
p.r.n.	when necessary
q.d.	every day
q. 1h.	every 1 hour
q. 4h.	every 4 hours
q. 6h.	every 6 hours
q.i.d.	four times a day
q.s.	quantity sufficient
S.C.	subcutaneously
S.L.	sublingual
stat	immediately
tbsp.	tablespoon
t.i.d.	three times a day
tsp.	teaspoonful

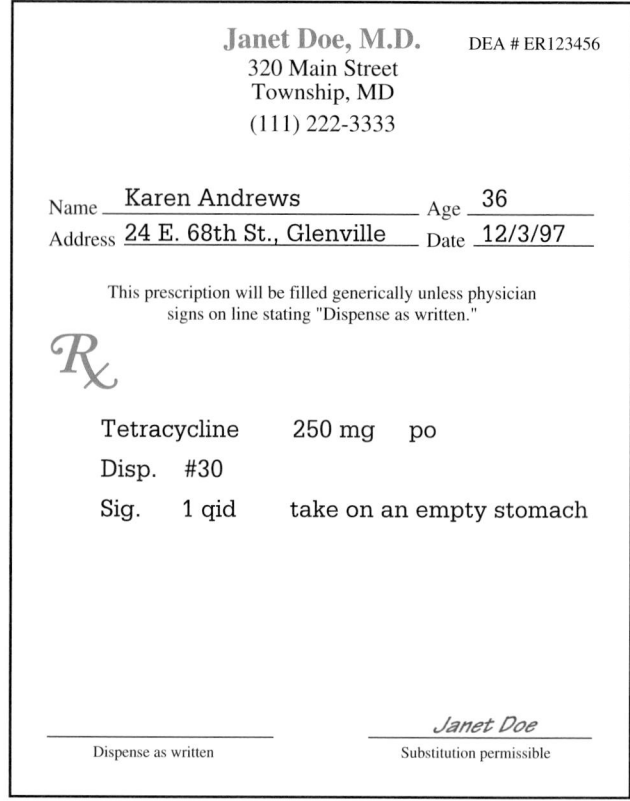

Figure 21–6
An example of a prescription filled out by a physician.

may be written (Table 21–9). The most common type is a standing order, which is to be implemented until such time as the physician discontinues the prescription. Usually, medication orders are canceled when a client undergoes surgery, transfers to another health care facility, or is discharged from a health care service or institution. When these events occur, the prescribing health care professional must either renew the previous prescription or write a new prescription. Each health care agency has specific policies for review and implementation of medication administration orders.

The written prescription should contain all the elements listed previously. The prescriber must sign the order and provide a registration number if the drug is a controlled substance.

When the prescription is written, it is common for approved abbreviations to be used to identify the dose of the medication, the route of administration, and the frequency with which the medication is to be administered. The nurse is responsible for recognizing appropriate abbreviations, for transcribing them accurately into the medication administration record (MAR), and for following their directions. Table 21–10 lists commonly used abbreviations.

The Pharmacist

The pharmacist is responsible for dispensing the medication as prescribed by the physician or health care provider. It is the pharmacist's responsibility to fill the prescription accurately and appropriately. If the prescription is incomplete, if it is thought to be inaccurate, or if it appears questionable for any reason, the pharmacist is obligated to refuse to fill the prescription until further clarification is obtained.

Pharmacists work within health care agencies and in the community. In an acute care institution, the pharmacist rarely sees the client; the nurse sends the prescription to the pharmacist, who fills it and returns it to the nurse for administration. In ambulatory settings such as community-based pharmacies, the pharmacist receives the prescription from the client (Fig. 21–6), who waits while the pharmacist fills it. In these situations, the pharmacist interacts with the client and provides direct instruction to the client about the purpose of the medication and how to take it properly.

The Nurse

The nurse is responsible for administering the medication as prescribed by the physician or health care provider. Inherent in this responsibility is the need to consider the client's physiological status, the predictable effects of the drug (both therapeutic and nontherapeutic), and the role that drug therapy plays in the client's total plan of care. In acute or extended care settings, the nurse is the health team member who is responsible 24 hours a day for assessing, monitoring, and evaluating the impact of the drug therapy on the client. In community health settings, the nurse is available for consultation to teach the client about the drug and to monitor the effects of the drug.

Nurses are responsible for their own actions when administering medications and are therefore accountable for implementing care that is deemed accurate and reasonable. The nurse is responsible for knowing about the medication that is being prescribed, how it should be administered, what the expected actions and side effects are, and when the medication should be withheld. If any part of a prescription seems unusual or incorrect, it is the nurse's responsibility to question the prescription and ask for clarification before administering the medication. The nurse should approach the prescriber in a professional manner and ask for the clarification. In most instances, the clarification is given and the prescription is implemented. In a few situations, the nurse may still not accept the clarification, and the nurse should approach the supervisor for further clarification and instructions. At no time should the nurse simply decide not to give the medication; appropriate follow-up with supervisory personnel is required, and documentation concerning the situation should follow institutional guidelines. The nurse needs to maintain a record of the situation while demonstrating appropriate professional accountability.

The Client

It is important to remember that the client is the person who is taking the drug and who is directly affected by the drug. The client is in the best position to evaluate the action and effects of the drug. The client provides valuable input that assists in identifying potentially problematic situations. The client, through communication with the other health team members, can give insight into therapeutic and nontherapeutic effects of the medication.

Maintaining Safety When Administering Medications: Five Rights

Administration of medications requires careful adherence to established principles. The nurse must adhere to the "five rights" of medication administration to ensure accuracy of administration and to maintain safety.

The five rights are: right drug, right dose, right client, right time, and right route.

Right Drug

Every drug is prescribed for a client because it has a specific therapeutic effect that is intended. The client is experiencing some pathophysiological change in body function and requires a specific drug to produce a change in physiological response and promote a higher level of wellness. With this in mind, the nurse must recognize that a drug is ordered for a client because there is a specific deviation from wellness and that it is imperative that the correct drug be administered. Table 21–11 summarizes the major categories of drugs used clinically, with definitions of their therapeutic effects and major prototype examples.

When administering the medication, the nurse should carefully compare the prescription with the MAR to ensure that the medication name has been correctly transcribed. Then the MAR should be carefully compared with the label of the medication before it is prepared. The nurse should check the name of the drug three times: when removing the drug container or unit-dose packet from the drawer or cabinet, when taking the drug out of the container, and when returning the container to the drawer or cabinet.

Once a medication is removed from its container, it should never be returned to the container if not used. Instead, it should be discarded. If it is a narcotic or controlled substance, another nurse must witness and sign that the medication was discarded. If a medication is in a unit-dose packet, the medication should be removed from the packet just before it is administered to the client.

Right Dose

Every drug is prescribed in a specific dose to produce a safe, therapeutic effect for the client. The dose of a drug is given in one of the three measurement systems described previously. Administering too small a dose, or underdosing the client, may result in decreased blood levels of the drug with a decline of therapeutic response for the client. On the other hand, administering too large a dose, or overdosing the client, may result in increased blood levels of the drug with a toxic or harmful effect on the client.

In unit-dose systems, many drugs come prepackaged in the dose prescribed. However, in some circumstances, the nurse must calculate the dose of the drug because the available amount is not the same as the prescribed amount. For instance, the prescription may read, "Lasix 80 mg, p.o." If only 40-mg tablets of Lasix are available, the nurse would have to calculate the dose and administer two tablets of Lasix (equal to 80 mg). The dose may be prescribed in a different system than that available. For example, the prescription may read, "Nitroglycerin gr 1/100 S.L.," but nitroglycerin 0.4 mg is available. The nurse must calculate the dose and administer one tablet.

Table 21-11

COMMON DRUG CLASSIFICATIONS, THERAPEUTIC EFFECTS, AND PROTOTYPES

DRUG CLASSIFICATION AND MAJOR THERAPEUTIC EFFECTS	PROTOTYPE
α-Adrenergic blocking agents Prevent vasoconstriction normally caused by the catecholamines epinephrine and norepinephrine	Phentolamine (Regitine)
Antacids Neutralize gastric acid	Magnesium hydroxide (Milk of Magnesia)
Antianginals Increase blood supply to myocardial tissue primarily through vasodilation	Isosorbide dinitrate (Sorbitrate)
Antiarrhythmics Promote normal cardiac rate and rhythm	Procainamide (Pronestyl)
Anticholinergics Block the effects of acetylcholine at muscarinic receptor sites in the autonomic nervous system	Atropine sulfate
Anticoagulants Prevent the formation and/or extension of clots	Heparin sodium
Anticonvulsants Control seizures	Phenytoin (Dilantin)
Antidepressants Elevate the mood by promoting accumulation of neurotransmitters (norepinephrine and serotonin) at CNS synapses	Amitriptyline (Elavil)
Antidiabetic agents Reduce blood sugar levels	Insulin (regular or NPH)
Antidiarrheals Promote defecation of normally formed stools	Loperamide (Imodium)
Antiemetics Prevent nausea and vomiting	Prochlorperazine (Compazine)
Antifungals Kill or inhibit growth of susceptible fungi	Fluconazole (Diflucan)
Antigout agents Control symptoms of gout	Allopurinol (Zyloprim)
Antihistamines Block the effects of histamine at H_1 receptors throughout the body	Diphenhydramine (Benadryl)
Antihyperlipidemic agents Decrease blood lipid levels	Clofibrate (Atromid-S)
Antihypertensive agents Reduce blood pressure	Enalapril (Vasotec)
Antiinfectives Kill or inhibit growth of susceptible bacteria	Penicillin
Antimanic agents Treat and prevent recurrence of manic episodes	Lithium
Antineoplastics Treat and control symptoms of malignant neoplasms	Cisplatin (Platinol)
Antiparkinson agents Treat symptoms of Parkinson's disease by restoring balance between acetylcholine and dopamine in the basal ganglia of the brain	Benztropine (Cogentin)
Antiplatelets Interfere with the ability of platelets to adhere to each other	Dipyridamole (Persantine)
Antipsychotics Alleviate psychotic symptoms by blocking dopamine receptors in the brain	Chlorpromazine (Thorazine)
Antipyretics Lower body temperature	Acetaminophen (Tylenol)
Antithyroid agents Inhibit thyroid hormone synthesis, thereby reducing basal metabolic rate	Propylthiouracil
Antituberculars Kill or inhibit growth of mycobacteria	Isoniazid (INH)
Antitussives Suppress cough reflex	Codeine
Antivirals Inhibit viral growth	Acyclovir (Zovirax)

Table 21–11

COMMON DRUG CLASSIFICATIONS, THERAPEUTIC EFFECTS, AND PROTOTYPES
(Continued)

DRUG CLASSIFICATION AND MAJOR THERAPEUTIC EFFECTS	PROTOTYPE
β-Adrenergic blocking agents Block the effects of the catecholamines epinephrine and norepinephrine on β-adrenergic receptors in the autonomic nervous system	Propranolol (Inderal)
Bronchodilators Relieve bronchospasm through bronchodilation	Theophylline
Calcium channel blockers Treat angina pectoris, hypertension, and coronary artery spasm by vasodilation	Verapamil (Calan)
Central nervous system stimulants Increase levels of catecholamines in the central nervous system	Amphetamine
Cholinergics Prolong the action of acetylcholine at receptor sites in the body	Bethanechol (Urecholine)
Diuretics Increase urine output by the kidney	Furosemide (Lasix)
Expectorants Decrease viscosity of bronchial secretions	Guaifenesin and alcohol (Robitussin)
Glucocorticoids Affect carbohydrate, fat, and protein metabolism; depress the immune response; exhibit antiinflammatory effects	Prednisone
Hematologic agents Increase blood-forming components of the circulatory system	Ferrous sulfate (Feosol)
Histamine (H_1) antagonists Inhibit gastric acid secretion by blocking H_1 receptors	Cimetidine (Tagamet)
Immunosuppressants Inhibit cell-mediated immune responses in the body	Cyclosporine (Sandimmune)
Inotropic agents Increase strength and force of myocardial contractility	Digoxin (Lanoxin)
Laxatives Promote defecation of normal, soft stool, thus relieving constipation	Psyllium (Metamucil)
Narcotic analgesics Relieve moderate or severe pain	Morphine
Neuromuscular blocking agents Block transmission of nerve impulses at the neuromuscular junction in the peripheral nervous system	Succinylcholine (Anectine)
Nonnarcotic analgesics Relieve mild to moderate pain	Aspirin
Nonsteroidal antiinflammatory drugs Relieve mild to moderate pain, fever, and inflammation through inhibition of prostaglandin synthesis	Ibuprofen (Motrin)
Sedatives/Hypnotics Reduce anxiety, promote sleep	Phenobarbital (Luminal)
Skeletal muscle relaxants Decrease skeletal muscle spasm	Baclofen (Lioresal)
Thrombolytic agents Dissolve existing blood clots	Alteplase (Activase)
Thyroid hormones Increase basal metabolic rate through replacement of deficient thyroid levels	Levothyroxine (Synthroid)
Vasopressors Increase blood pressure, cardiac output, and urinary output by affecting vasoconstriction	Dopamine (Intropin)

Right Client

The drug is prescribed for administration to a specific client. The nurse must properly identify each client before a medication is administered. This is extremely important because nurses are assigned many clients and must identify the correct client. Each client in an acute care or extended care facility has an identification band; this is the primary method for identifying clients. It is the nurse's responsibility to check the identification band and compare it with the name on the prescription. Extra care must be taken when clients have similar names.

Asking the client to state his or her name or asking the parent of a young child to state the child's name is another appropriate method of identifying clients. Do not ask the client, for example, "Are you Mr. Jones?" Some clients who are confused or disoriented may answer affirmatively when in fact they are not that person. The nurse should always have the client state his or her name. For a client who is unable to provide information, some method of ensuring that the drug is administered to the correct client must be instituted. A client whose identity is unknown may be identified as "John (or Jane) Doe" until accurate documentation of identity is obtained.

Clients who take medications at home should be instructed to refrain from sharing them with others. A medication is prescribed for a specific client and may be dangerous for others.

Right Time

Drugs are prescribed to be administered at designated times and at designated frequencies. The pharmacokinetics of a drug determine the time and frequency of medication administration. Some drugs require once-a-day dosing and should be administered consistently at the same time each day, for example, with breakfast. Other drugs are metabolized quickly

from the system and require administration at more frequent, equal intervals around the clock to maintain therapeutic blood levels.

Right Route

A drug prescription must specify the route that is to be used when administering the medication. If the route is not clearly identified, the nurse is responsible for consulting the physician to clarify the order.

◆
Medication Errors

At times, the nurse may not adhere to institutional policy and procedures governing the administration of medications. Usually, a medication error occurs when the nurse has not followed the "five rights" of medication administration (Fig. 21–7). A client may receive the wrong medication or the wrong amount of medication, or be given the medication at the wrong time or by the wrong route. When this occurs, the nurse is at risk for a charge of negligence for failing to follow the appropriate protocol for administering medications.

The multiple checks that are required when administering medications serve to prevent medication errors. The nurse plays an important role in administering medications correctly, including ensuring that the prescription is legible, is correctly transcribed, is correctly filled by the pharmacist, and is correctly administered to the client.

When a medication error does occur, it is the professional and ethical responsibility of the nurse to report the error to the physician and the nursing supervisor according to institutional policy. The well-being of the client should be of utmost concern to the nurse. The physician will determine what follow-up activities need to be done, from performing a diagnostic evaluation to prescribing an antidote. The client should be closely monitored for any adverse effects.

When the error is reported, the nurse must complete required documentation. In most institutions, an incident (or occurrence) report should be completed and the risk management department should be notified. This report does not become part of the client's medical record but is used by the institution for evaluation and follow-up to improve the quality of care. The client's record should have documentation concerning the drug that was erroneously administered (or not administered). Most institutions have guidelines about how this is recorded as part of their risk management initiatives. For instance, if a client receives twice the prescribed dose of furosemide, the record would reflect the actual dose given, instead of the prescribed dose. The nurse should document that the physician was notified, what follow-up care was instituted, and the client's status in response to the error. The completion of the incident report is not

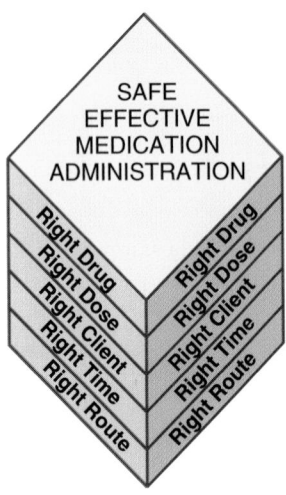

♦ **Figure 21–7**
Five "rights" of medication administration.

noted in the client's medical record, nor is the term "error" or similar terminology used to describe the incident. The nurse should be as objective as possible and report the facts of the incident only.

Application of the Nursing Process to Administration of Medications

Assessment

There are many variables that can affect safe, effective medication administration for the client. Before initiating drug therapy, the nurse must consider many client aspects that have an impact on the therapeutic effects of prescribed medications.

Nursing History

An initial review of the client's history is a major component of maintaining safety when administering medications to clients. A review of the client's medical history provides information about the client's past and current illnesses and previous surgical procedures, conditions that can have a serious impact on current medication regimens. Clients who have chronic illnesses may be taking medications on a long-term basis that would affect the actions of other drugs. The presence of liver disease should result in careful consideration of specific drugs and the amount of each drug that is prescribed. Clients with heart failure have impaired circulation, which limits or hampers distribution of drugs. Clients who take steroids are at risk for development of gastric ulcers; drugs that are irritating to the stomach mucosa should not be administered to such clients. It is important that the nurse know which illnesses or diseases the client has had and which medications he or she is taking on a regular basis. Clients should be questioned with regard to the over-the-counter drugs they may be taking. For example, the nurse should know whether a client takes aspirin frequently during the day for joint stiffness; such a client would be at risk for bleeding tendencies, especially if a gastric-irritating medication were prescribed.

A history of allergies to any medications or foods must be obtained from each client. Serious adverse hypersensitivity reactions could result if a medication is administered to a client who has an allergy. Knowledge of food allergies is critical because some food substances are chemically related to drug substances. For instance, certain contrast media used during many radiological procedures (*e.g.*, IV pyelography of the kidneys) are contraindicated in clients who have an allergy to shellfish. The presence of the allergy should be clearly noted in the client's record, and all members of the health team should be informed. In most institutions, a special note or tape is placed across the front of the client's record to indicate the allergy, and the client's identification band may also be marked with the allergy information.

A complete history of the client's previous and current use of medications should be obtained. Specific names of prescribed and over-the-counter drugs, the reasons for their use, and their frequency of administration are important components of the assessment. For current medications, information should be obtained about personal practices used by clients when taking the medication, as well as expected and actual responses to the medication.

Information about the client's lifestyle also should be obtained. The use of tobacco, alcohol, caffeine, and mind-altering drugs may alter the effectiveness of

NURSING DIAGNOSES FOR CLIENTS RECEIVING DRUG THERAPY

Knowledge Deficit

Clients who are receiving medications need to be informed about the actions of the drug, their purpose for the client, the expected frequency of administration, specific activities when taking the medication, and possible side effects. The nursing diagnosis of knowledge deficit may be related to lack of experience with the drug, cognitive limitations, or language barriers.

Noncompliance With Prescribed Regimen

Some clients fail to follow the prescribed regimen for taking the medication. A variety of reasons may exist for this. For instance, the client may have a lack of information, a different cultural perspective than the majority, a different health belief than expected, or limited financial resources. It is important for the nurse to identify the reason for noncompliance to provide the direction for subsequent interventions.

Risk for Injury

Drugs are necessary components of treatment for many illnesses. Yet, drugs have a potential for causing serious side effects and toxic reactions. The degree of risk for injury to the client depends on the type of drug, the dose, and the client's overall health status.

Risk for Aspiration

Some clients have difficulty swallowing, which leads to a possible risk for aspiration of the medication. Aspiration is a life-threatening situation.

Anxiety

Many clients may have anxious feelings about their health status and the need to take prescribed medications. Clients who need to take long-term insulin injections may be anxious about the parenteral injections. Clients who are receiving cancer chemotherapy may be anxious about whether the drugs will arrest the cancerous growth.

drug therapy. Cultural practices that are followed should be investigated. For instance, does the client use medicinal herbs or special potions to treat common ailments? Does the client wear crystals as part of a treatment modality? Does the client believe in the spiritual component of treatment as opposed to the use of drugs?

Physical Examination

A complete head-to-toe assessment should be performed and documented on the client's record. A baseline physical examination provides the guideline for evaluating the progress of the client's condition in response to the medication. Some of the important baseline assessments are pulse, blood pressure, temperature, respirations, height, and weight.

The nurse must be aware of physical conditions of the client that may have an impact on the effect of the drug. If the intended effect of an antibiotic is to treat an infected leg ulcer, the nurse needs to have objective physical data about the resolution of the infection and the healing of the ulcer. If the intended effect of a diuretic is to reduce edema of the lower extremities, then the nurse needs to document both the extent of the leg edema and the amount of urinary output.

Psychosocial Assessment

How a client perceives his or her own health and the importance of medical therapies greatly affects the client's compliance with the medical regimen. The nurse should assess the client's perceptions about health and illness and the client's attitude toward treatment. If the client believes that treatment is an important aspect of health promotion and maintenance, then he or she is likely to adhere to prescribed therapies.

Specifically, the nurse should determine the client's attitudes and beliefs about drugs and the client's previous experiences with taking prescriptions. How did the client perceive the effect that the drug had in the past? Did the drug achieve the desired outcome? Was the client satisfied with the prescribed drug? Did the client have any adverse side effects? How does the client react when describing past drug history? Is the client pleasant or angry?

Diagnostic Testing

Many drugs require preliminary screening before drug therapy is initiated. For instance, clients with suspected infections should have a culture from the infected area taken before any antibiotic is administered. An electrocardiogram should be obtained before administration of many cardiac medications. Checking renal function is important before administration of potassium chloride or aminoglycoside antibiotics.

Once drug administration is started, many diagnostic tests should be performed to monitor the effect of the drug on the client. Clients receiving cancer chemotherapy should have their hematological values monitored, because severe decreases in red blood cells, leukocytes, and platelets are common side effects. Clients receiving diurectics such as furosemide should have their serum potassium level monitored. Serum levels of antibiotics can be obtained to monitor their pharmacokinetics.

Diagnosis

Nursing diagnoses for clients receiving drug therapy may span the entire list of diagnoses because of the underlying medical conditions. For clients who are receiving prescription drugs, the nursing diagnoses shown in the Nursing Diagnoses box are quite common.

Planning

Planning is the interim step between formulating the nursing diagnosis and implementing activities to resolve the client's health problems. After the nursing diagnoses are identified, the nurse should determine which of them have priority over the others. A variety of nursing strategies are employed to assist the client who is taking prescribed medications. The nurse should engage both the client and significant others in the planning phase.

For clients who are taking prescribed medications, the following expected outcomes are applicable:

- Client will be able to describe the action and purpose of the prescribed drug
- Client will comply with the prescribed medication regimen by taking the correct dose of the correct drug on time
- Client will self-administer the medication by the prescribed route
- Client will achieve the intended therapeutic effect of the prescribed medication without developing any complications
- Client will report the development of side effects to the health team.

Implementation

General Measures When Administering Medications and Handling Related Equipment

The nurse must properly handle and dispose of drugs and drug-related equipment to maintain safety for both clients and health care workers. Medication administration may place the nurse in jeopardy from some of the effects of the drug. Special precautions must be taken to promote chemical safety in the delivery of health care to clients in a variety of clinical settings. Boxes 21–1 and 21–2 provide an outline of the procedure for medication administration and a listing of things to avoid when administering medications.

Before administering any medication, the nurse must use effective hand washing to decrease microbial

Box 21–1

GUIDELINES FOR CORRECT ADMINISTRATION OF MEDICATIONS

Preparation

- Wash hands before preparing medications
- Check for drug allergies: check the nursing history, chart, and kardex
- Check medication order with physician's orders, kardex, and MAR
- Check label on drug container three times
- Check expiration date on drug label; use only if date is current
- Recheck calculation of drug dose with another nurse
- Pour tablet or capsule into the cap of the drug container; with unit-dose packaging, open the packet at bedside after verifying client identification
- Pour liquid at eye level; base of meniscus should be at line of desired dose
- Dilute drugs that irritate gastric mucosa (e.g., potassium, aspirin) or give with meals

Administration

- Identify the client by examining the identification band
- Administer only those drugs that have been prepared
- Help the client get into an appropriate position depending on the route of administration
- Stay with the client when giving oral medications until the medications are taken

- When administering drugs to a group of clients, give drugs last to clients who need extra assistance
- Discard needles and syringes in appropriate containers
- Discard unused portions of drugs in the sink or toilet, never in a trash can; controlled substances are either returned to the pharmacy (pills) or discarded in the sink and witnessed by another nurse (solutions)
- Keep narcotics in a double-locked drawer or closet
- Keys to the narcotics drawer must be kept by the nurse and not stored in a drawer or closet

Recording

- Report drug error immediately to the client's physician and the nursing supervisor; complete an incident report in accordance with institutional policy
- Record administration of drugs promptly after they are given, especially stat doses
- Report and record drugs that were refused by the client with reason for refusal
- Record amount of fluid taken with medication on intake/output record; provide only liquids allowed on the client's diet

Adapted with permission from Kee, J. L. & Hayes, E. R. (1993). *Pharmacology: A nursing process approach*. Philadelphia: W. B. Saunders.

transfer. When preparing the medication for administration, the nurse should avoid touching or dropping the drug to prevent contamination of the medication. In some situations, touching the medication in any way can cause contact dermatitis if the skin reacts to physical exposure to the substance. In preparing parenteral medications for administration, ampules should not be allowed to stand open, and needles should not come into contact with any contaminated surface. Ampules are no longer commonly used. An alcohol prep or gauze pad should be used when breaking the ampule neck to protect the nurse's fingers from possible trauma due to broken glass. Disposable gloves should be used when administering parenteral medications to protect the nurse from exposure to body fluids.

The nurse is responsible for the safe-keeping of medications; with this in mind, the nurse must never leave medications unattended. Medications should never be left at the client's bedside because it is the nurse's responsibility to ensure that the client has taken the medication as prescribed by the physician. Gloves should be worn when administering most topical medications to protect the nurse from drug effects and contamination. Finally, the nurse should never return an unused medication or portion of a medication

to a container; rather, the unused medication should be discarded according to the institution's policy.

Safety in working with medications does not end with administration of the drug to the client. Proper disposal of unused portions of the drug and safe disposal of equipment used in medication administration are important aspects of chemical safety for the nurse (Fig. 21–8). Basic principles of infection control must be followed to prevent cross-contamination. Use of disposable, single-dose, prefilled syringes decreases the chance of accidental needlesticks. Excess fluid medications should be discarded in the sink. Used needles and syringes should be discarded unsheathed into appropriately labeled containers to prevent injury.

Administering Oral Medications

Oral administration, the most common method, is the safest and easiest route for the client (Procedure 21–2). Unless the client is unable to swallow, is to have nothing by mouth (NPO) in preparation for a procedure, or has a malabsorption syndrome, oral administration is the preferred method.

For adults, oral medications are usually tablets or capsules. The client should be able to swallow the

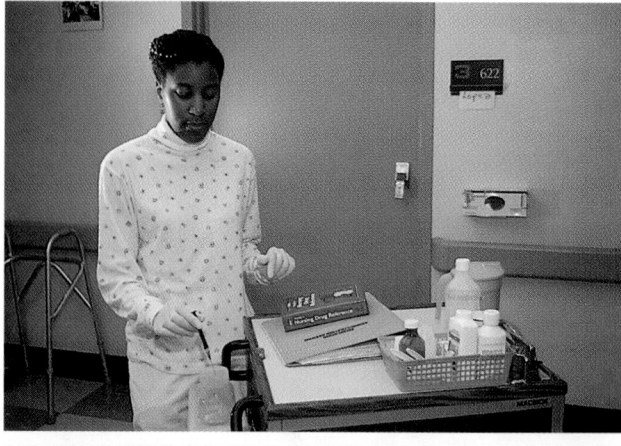

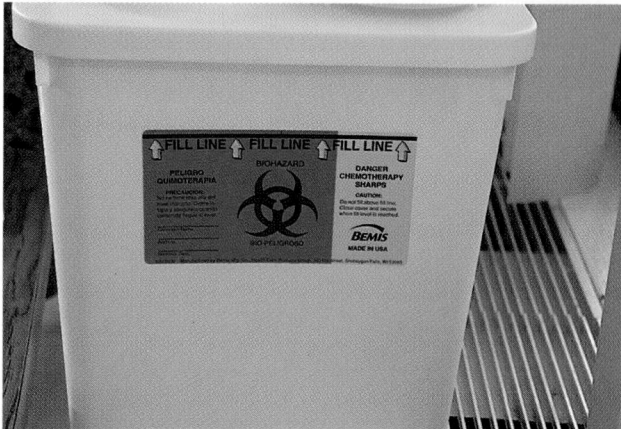

Box **21–2**

THE "DON'TS" OF ADMINISTERING MEDICATIONS

* Do not act distracted when preparing medications
* Do not give drugs poured by another staff member
* Do not pour drugs from containers with labels that are difficult to read or whose labels are partially removed or have fallen off
* Do not transfer drugs from one container to another
* Do not pour drugs onto your hand
* Do not give medications for which the expiration date has passed
* Do not guess about drugs and drug doses; ask when in doubt
* Do not use drugs that have sediment, are discolored, or are cloudy (and should not be)
* Do not leave medications by bedside or with visitors
* Do not leave prepared medications out of sight
* Do not give drugs if the client says he or she has allergies to the drug or drug group
* Do not call the client's name as the sole means of identification
* Do not give the drug if the client states it is different from the one he or she has been receiving
* Do not recap needles

Adapted with permission from Kee, J. L., & Hayes, E. R. (1993). *Pharmacology: A nursing process approach*. Philadelphia: W. B. Saunders.

❧ **Figure 21–8**
After administering injections, a nurse must properly dispose of used equipment in institutions and the home care settings.

medication and should take a sufficient amount of fluid with it. Liquid forms of the medication are used when the client has difficulty swallowing pills or when the medication is to be instilled through a nasogastric tube. Children usually prefer the liquid form, because they have difficulty swallowing pills. It is important for the nurse to make sure that the client can swallow without difficulty. When in doubt, always try water first; if the client has difficulty swallowing and begins to aspirate, water is easily absorbed by the body.

For many clients, oral medications are administered through an enteral feeding tube, either a nasogastric tube or a gastrostomy tube. When giving an oral medication through a feeding tube, medications that are in liquid form or can be crushed and mixed with liquids are preferred. Spansule medications should not be administered by this route because they will clump and clog the tube. Before administering the medication, the nurse should verify placement of the tube (see Chapter 27 for procedure to verify tube placement). If the client is receiving a feeding, the feeding should be stopped and the tube should be flushed with 15 to 30 ml of water before the medication is instilled. The tube should be flushed again after

each medication is administered. Usually the feeding is not restarted for about 15 minutes to allow for absorption of the medication. If the client has a tube connected to suction, the nurse should wait up to 30 minutes before reconnecting the tube to the suction apparatus. See the accompanying research box regarding client compliance with oral medication regimens.

Administering Parenteral Medications

There are several types of parenteral medication administrations requiring skill to ensure that client safety is maintained. All must be done under aseptic conditions, because parenteral administration is an invasive procedure. Equipment must be sterile to avoid introducing any organisms that could cause an infection.

❧ **Needles and Syringes.** Administration of a parenteral medication requires the use of a needle and syringe. There are a variety of needles and syringes, and the type chosen depends on the medication, the site to be used, and the method of administration. Syringes come in sizes from 1 to 50 ml (Fig. 21–9). Smaller-volume syringes are used for children, for insulin, or

PROCEDURE

21–2

ADMINISTRATION OF ORAL MEDICATIONS

Oral medications can be given either in liquid or in solid state for absorption from the gastrointestinal tract. The disadvantages of oral administration are that the medication may have an unpleasant taste, may be difficult to swallow, may irritate the gastric mucosa, may be absorbed irregularly from the gastrointestinal tract, or may be absorbed too slowly. Scored tablets may be crushed; enteric-coated tablets and capsules must not be broken.

Equipment:

Medication
Soufflé cup for tablet, capsule
Plastic cup for liquid
Cup of water or juice
For nasogastric administration:
60-ml catheter-tipped syringe
Glass of water
Disposable waterproof pad
Stethoscope
Clamp for nasogastric tube
Disposable gloves

Action	**Rationale**
1. Verify the physician's order for the client's name, drug name, dose, and time and route of administration.	1. This ensures that the client receives the correct medication by the proper route.
2. Assess the client's allergy history.	2. This alerts the nurse to potential reactions to observe after drug administration.
3. Select the prescribed medication and verify against order on medication card or printout.	3. Verification of the order averts medication errors.
4. Ask the client to state his or her name, and also check the client's identity by reading the wristband.	4. This verifies the client's identity.

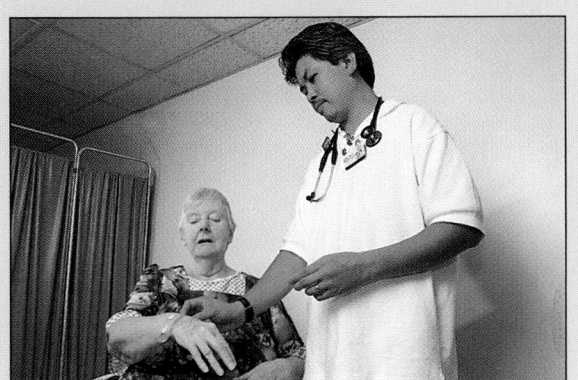

Step 4.

Continued

PROCEDURE

21–2

ADMINISTRATION OF ORAL MEDICATIONS
(Continued)

Action	Rationale
5. Explain the medication name and the intended therapeutic effect of the drug.	**5.** This increases cooperation and reduces anxiety.
6. Question the client regarding any difficulty swallowing pills.	**6.** Verify that the medication can be crushed before administration.
7. Prepare medication for one client.	**7.** Read the medication label three times to prevent medication errors.

Tablets, Capsules

8. Place the required number of tablets or capsules into the medication cup. Do not touch medication with fingers as you prepare it.	**8.** This maintains the cleanliness of the drug.

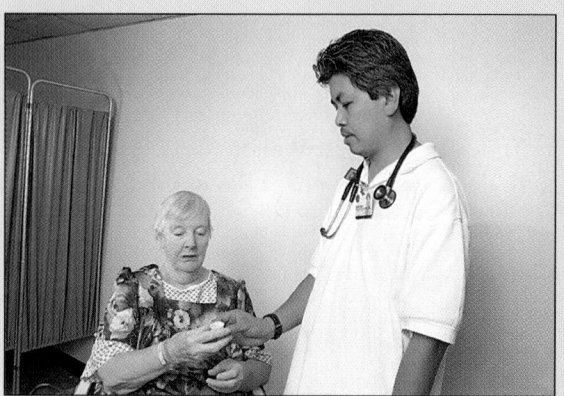

Step 8.

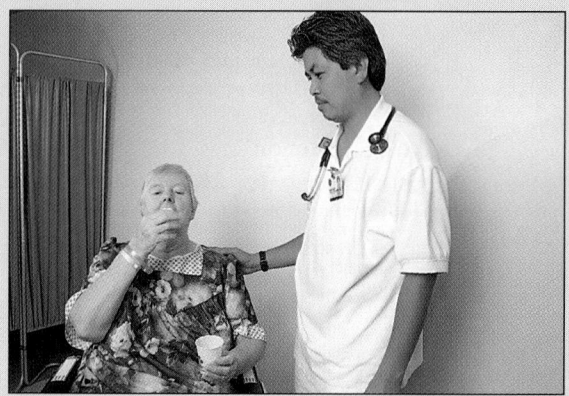

Step 8.

9. If necessary, crush tablets before administering. Some tablets may be dissolved in liquid or mixed with a small amount of custard or applesauce.

9. This makes swallowing easier.

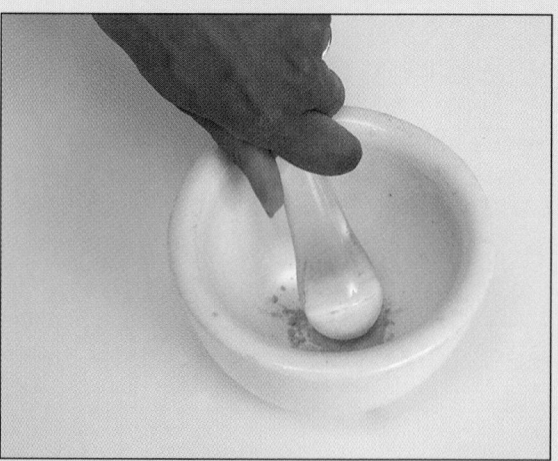

Step 9.

PROCEDURE

21–2

ADMINISTRATION OF ORAL MEDICATIONS
(Continued)

Action	Rationale
10. If giving enteric-coated medication, do not crush or break.	**10.** Gastric mucosa may be irritated or destroyed if the medication is released in the stomach.

Liquid—Normal Oral Route

Action	Rationale
11. Place medicine cup on a level surface.	**11.** This facilitates accuracy of measurement.
12. Remove the cap; hold the bottle with the label against the palm of your hand and pour the prescribed amount into the medicine cup.	**12.** This prevents the liquid from dripping down the label and rendering it illegible.
13. Measure the volume at the base of the meniscus.	**13.** Measures liquids precisely.

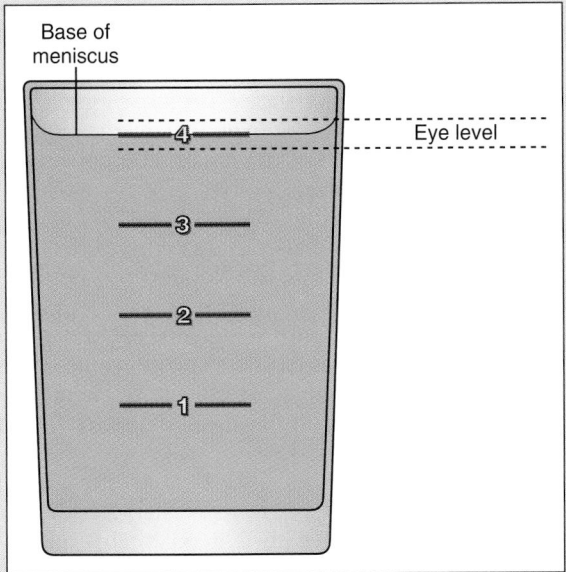

Step 13.

Action	Rationale
14. If preparing a narcotic, complete the narcotic signout form.	**14.** Controlled substance law requires monitoring of dispensed narcotics.

Liquid—Nasogastric Route

Action	Rationale
15. Elevate head of bed 30 to 45 degrees unless contraindicated.	**15.** This prevents aspiration.
16. Place waterproof pad between tube and bedding, and don gloves.	**16.** This protects linen and clothing of client, protects caregiver and client.
17. Check for proper positioning of nasogastric tube by (1) suctioning contents or (2) instilling small amount of air while auscultating with stethoscope.	**17.** This prevents aspiration: (1) gastric contents indicate correct positioning, (2) auscultation of air rushing into stomach indicates tip of tube is in stomach.
18. Draw up medication into syringe, clear syringe of air, and inject medication into tube.	**18.** Excess air may lead to flatus and abdominal discomfort.
19. Flush tube with 30 ml of water.	**19.** This ensures medication reaches stomach and clears tube.
20. Clamp tube for 30 minutes.	**20.** This allows time for medication to be absorbed.
21. Chart the medication given: time, route, and other pertinent information.	**21.** Prompt charting prevents errors such as repeated dosing and provides a legal record.

Continued

PROCEDURE

21–2

ADMINISTRATION OF ORAL MEDICATIONS
(Continued)

Action	Rationale
22. Return to client's room within 30 minutes to evaluate response.	**22.** Nurse is responsible for monitoring therapeutic effects, side effects, and allergic reactions.

Example of Documentation

Date	Time	Notes
1/1/98	0800	Acetaminophen, 1000 mg, P.O. for T. 100.5°
		M. Smith, RN
1/1/98	0900	T. 99.2°
		M. Smith, RN

RESEARCH BOX

Abstract

Factors affecting compliance with medication regimen and ability to self-medicate were investigated in relation to clients' health care beliefs. The sample consisted of 60 adult, English-speaking subjects who were able to read a medication label, were physically able to administer an oral medication, were receiving treatment for a chronic disease, and had been taking medications for at least 3 months. Findings indicated that a client's ability to perform those tasks required to self-administer medications was consistently 6 to 9% lower than his or her reading (or educational) level. Although 93% of the subjects took responsibility for their medication regimen, increasing complexity of medication instruction significantly affected their ability to read and perform the required tasks.

Nursing Implications

* Proper performance ability on the part of the client may not be evident regardless of educational expectations as the complexity of the medication instruction increases.

* Nurses need to be more vigilant with clients who have weak reading skills and lower levels of formal education.

* Clients will exercise their responsibility with self-medication but this may be different from what is actually prescribed.

* Clients will adapt their regimens to their lifestyles, requiring that nurses be aware of how the medication regimen may be affected by the client's lifestyle.

Bailey, A., Ferguson, E., & Voss, S. (1995). Factors affecting an individual's ability to administer medication. *Home Healthcare Nurse,* 13, 57–63.

for intradermal administrations. Larger-volume syringes are used to prepare intravenous medications. For adults, a 3-ml syringe is adequate for subcutaneous and intramuscular administrations.

Syringes are usually made of disposable plastic and designed for single use; glass syringes that can be sterilized and reused are no longer commonly employed. In some situations a syringe may be reused by a client. For instance, the American Diabetes Association has guidelines for home use of insulin syringes that cover the reuse of a syringe by a client who is self-administering insulin in the home. In hospitals, syringes are never reused.

Each syringe consists of a barrel with a plunger (Fig. 21–10). Many syringes are available with a Luer-lok tip for connection with a needle. This allows for the nurse to change the needle if it is contaminated or if a larger or smaller needle is required. Other syringes, such as an insulin syringe, have a needle attached and are provided as a complete unit.

Needles are measured in length and in diameter. They have three basic parts: the hub, the shaft, and the bevel (Fig. 21–11). Needles come in lengths from

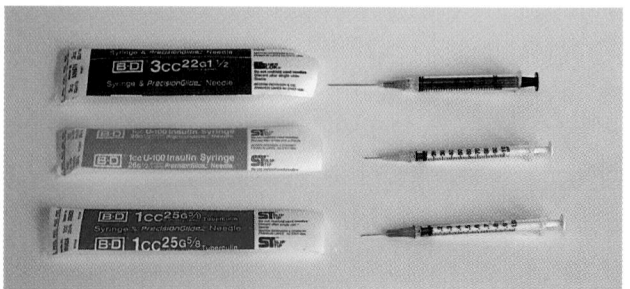

❧ **Figure 21–9**
A sampling of available syringe sizes and types: *top,* hypodermic; *middle,* insulin; *bottom,* tuberculin.

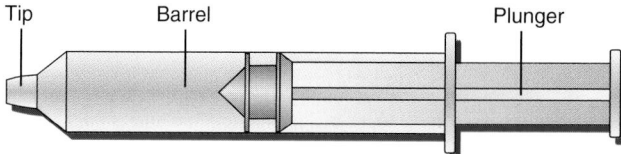

Figure 21–10
The parts of a syringe.

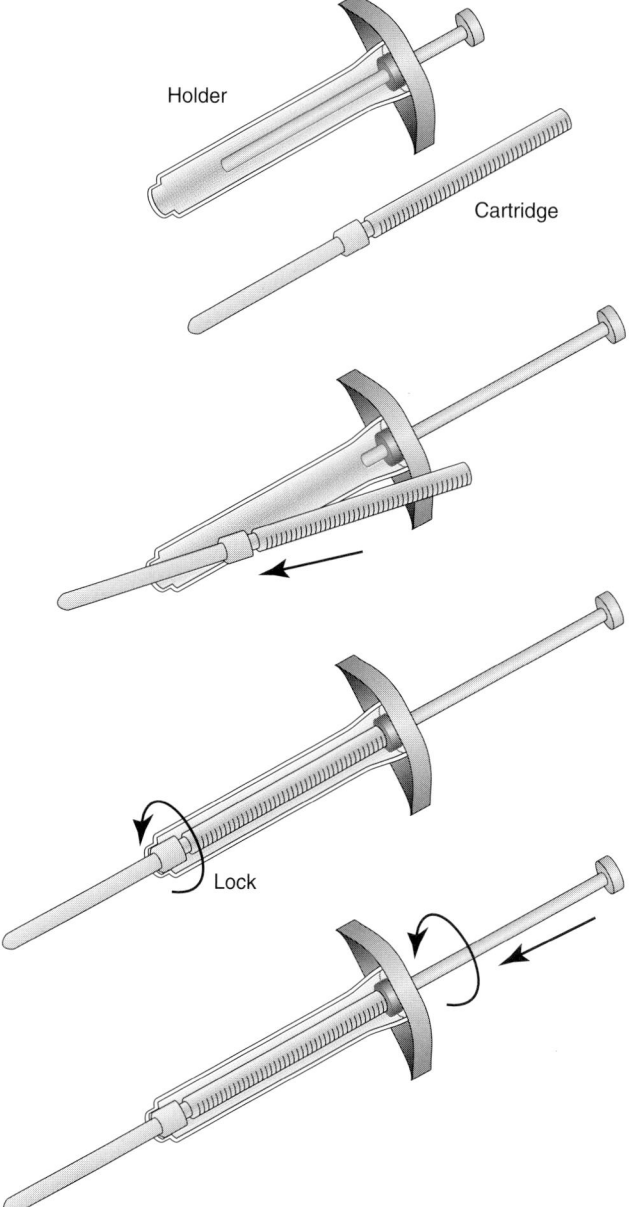

Figure 21–12
Cartridge-type syringe, Tubex.

0.375 in (⅜ in) to 1.5 in. A child or an underweight, slender adult requires a short needle, even for subcutaneous and intramuscular injections. A 1- to 1.5-in needle can be used on an average-sized adult for an intramuscular injection.

Gauge size describes the diameter of the needle: the smaller the gauge, the larger the diameter. An 18-gauge needle is larger, or fatter, than a 25-gauge needle. For adults, a 19- to 23-gauge needle is used for intramuscular injections, a 25-gauge needle is used for subcutaneous injections. For infants and young children, smaller gauges are used, usually a 23- or 25-gauge needle.

Another type of syringe is the cartridge syringe, which is prefilled with a medication and has a needle already attached. A commonly used cartridge-type syringe is the Tubex (Fig. 21–12). The cartridge is inserted into a metal or plastic holder and secured. The holder contains the plunger. Once the cartridge is secured into the holder, the plunger is manipulated to expel air from the cartridge. After the medication is administered, the cartridge is removed and discarded in the appropriate disposal container. The holder can then be reused.

A variety of systems are available on the market and fall generally into three categories (Gurevich, 1994):

- IV delivery systems that use no needle or a recessed needle in a protective housing—this type of system is suitable for connecting tubing to a piggyback setup.
- Needles that are used for percutaneous injections—either the needle is retracted into a guard or there is a protective shield that is slid forward over the needle.
- Blunt needles for blood collection and suturing—these needle systems have a blunt inner cannula, recessed slightly from the sharp tip, which slides forward over the needle as it is withdrawn from the client.

♦ **Preparing Medications.** Parenteral medications are available in single-dose ampules or vials, multiple-dose vials, or prefilled syringes. Ampules must be

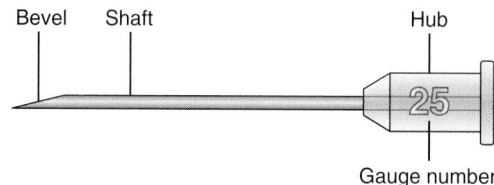

Figure 21–11
The parts of a needle.

snapped open in a direction away from the nurse, and the needle must be inserted into the ampule to be aspirated by the syringe (Fig. 21–13). A multiple-dose vial contains a glass container with a rubber seal at the top. Some vials contain powder medication and require that the nurse dissolve the powder before administering the medication. When a medication is in powder form, there are directions that indicate which solvent is to be used. Some medications can be dissolved only in distilled water or normal saline; others can be dissolved in either. Many medications have a larger volume after dilution than the volume of diluent used. It is important for the nurse to read the directions for dilution carefully. See Procedure 21–3 for a detailed description of how to prepare medications.

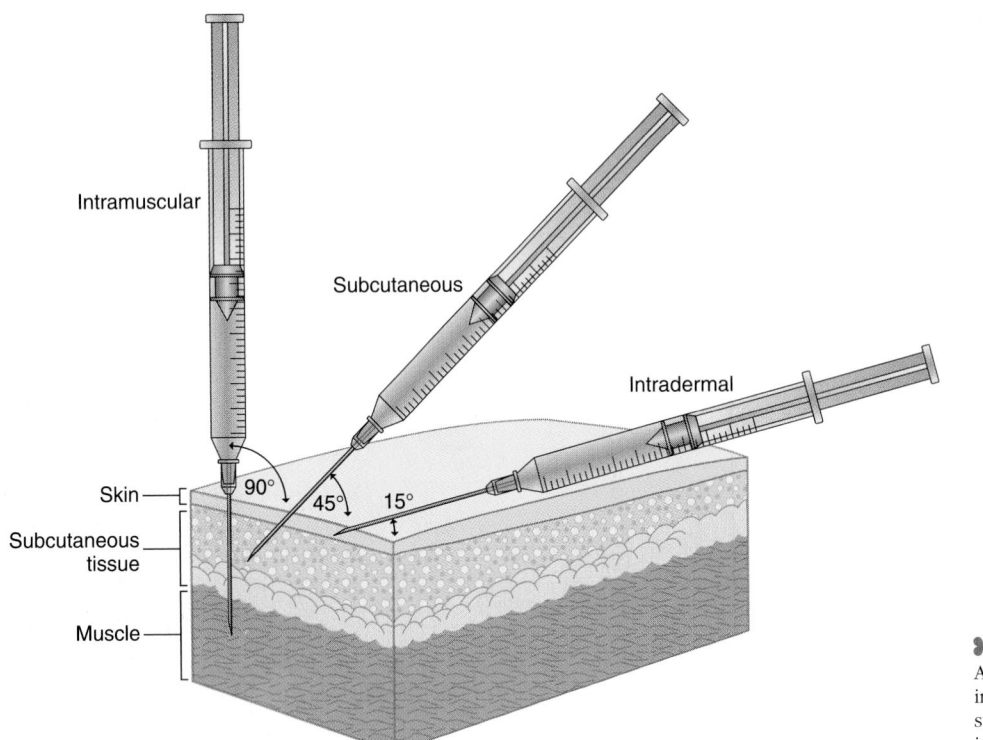

❧ Figure 21–13
A comparison of the angles of insertion for intramuscular, subcutaneous, and intradermal injections.

❧ **Subcutaneous Administration.** A subcutaneous injection involves insertion of a needle into the loose connective tissue under the dermis (Procedure 21–4). Absorption of a medication through the subcutaneous tissue is slower than absorption from a muscle because the subcutaneous tissue is not as richly supplied with blood vessels.

Common sites for subcutaneous drug administra-

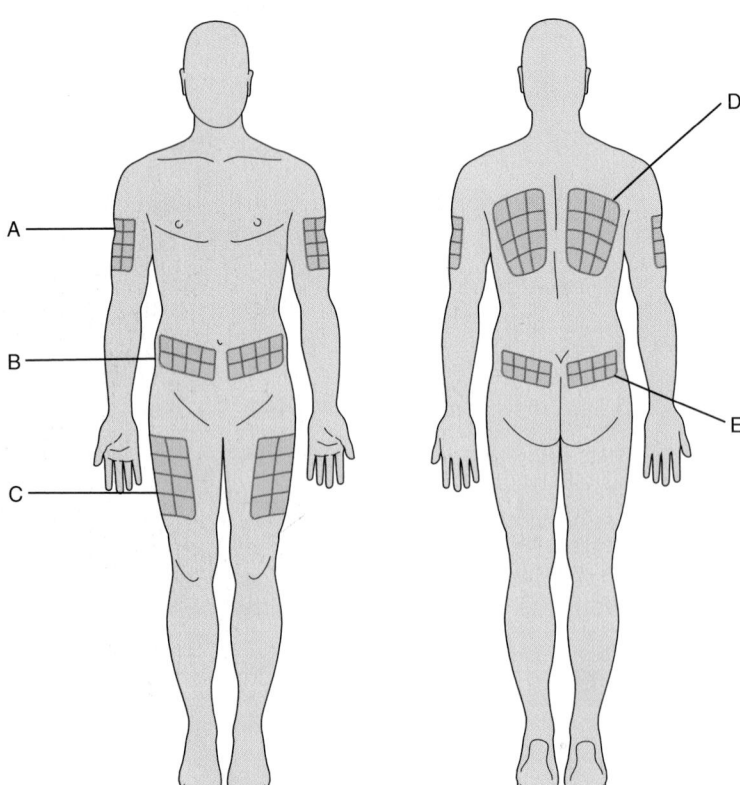

❧ Figure 21–14
Common sites for subcutaneous injections. *A*, Upper outer arm; *B*, lower abdomen; *C*, upper outer thigh; *D*, upper back; *E* flank region.

PROCEDURE

21–3

PREPARING MEDICATIONS WITH AN AMPULE AND A VIAL

Ampules contain single doses of liquid medication. The glass ampule has a constricted neck that must be snapped off manually to access the medication and aspirate the drug into a syringe.

Vials are either single-dose or multiple-dose glass containers and contain either liquid or powdered medication. The vial has a rubber top with a metal cap to protect the rubber until the vial is ready to use. Unlike ampules, air must be injected into the vial from the syringe to create a vacuum so that medication can be withdrawn. Vials containing a powdered form of medication must be mixed with a solution (usually normal saline) to dissolve the powdered drug.

Equipment:

Medication ampule or vial
Needle and syringe
Alcohol wipe or gauze pad
Disposable gloves

Action	Rationale
1. Verify the physician's order for the client's name, drug name, dose, and time and route of administration.	1. This ensures that the client receives the correct medication by the proper route.
2. Assess the client's allergy history.	2. This alerts the nurse to potential reactions to observe during the drug administration.
3. Select the prescribed medication and verify it against order on medication card or printout.	3. Verification of the order averts medication errors.
4. Ask the client to state his or her name.	4. Check the client's identity by reading the wristband.
5. Explain the medication and review the procedure with the client.	5. This increases cooperation and reduces anxiety.
6. Don gloves.	6. This protects both client and health care provider.

Ampule

7. To distribute medication from the top to the bottom of the ampule, tap the top lightly with fingers.	7. Solution trapped at the top will move into the lower chamber.

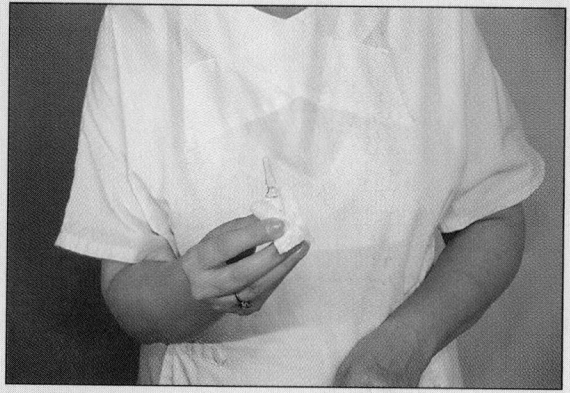

Step 7.

Continued

PROCEDURE

21–3

PREPARING MEDICATIONS WITH AN AMPULE AND A VIAL
(Continued)

Action	Rationale
8. Place alcohol wipe or gauze pad around the neck of the ampule and snap neck away from the body of the ampule.	8. This protects the fingers from injury as the tip is broken off.

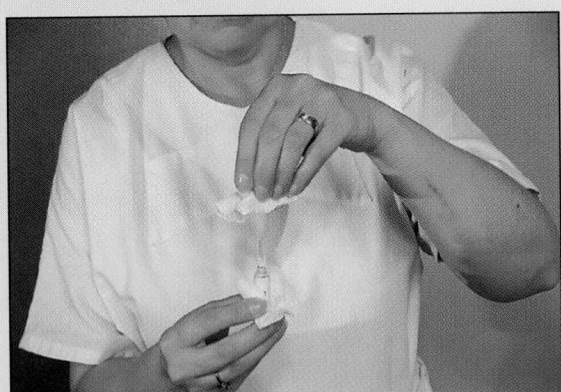

Step 8A.

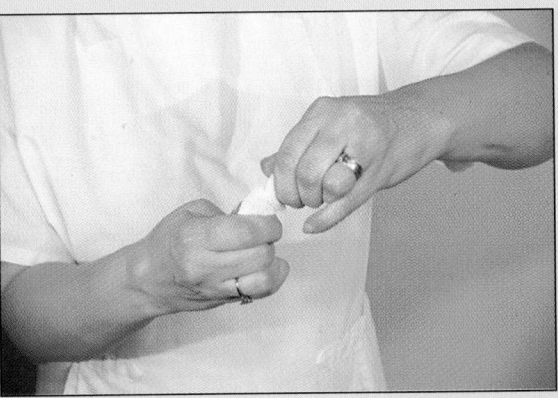

Step 8B.

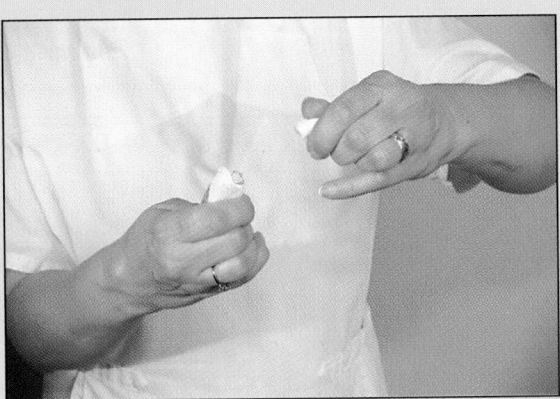

Step 8C.

9. Set the ampule on a flat surface or turn the ampule upside down and withdraw the medication.	9. So long as the needle does not touch the rim of the ampule, the medication will not spill out of container.

PROCEDURE

21–3

PREPARING MEDICATIONS WITH AN AMPULE AND A VIAL

(Continued)

Action	**Rationale**
10. Keep the tip of the needle within the surface of the solution and draw medication up with syringe.	**10.** This creates negative pressure within the syringe, pulling fluid from the ampule.

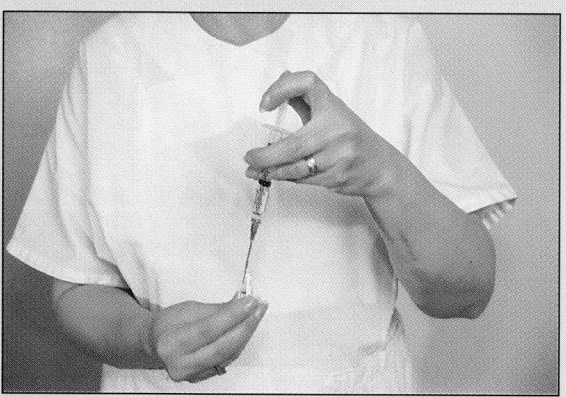

Step 10.

Vial

11. Remove metal cap from unused vial.	**11.** The metal cap prevents contamination of the rubber top of the vial.
12. Disinfect rubber top of vial with alcohol wipe.	**12.** This disinfects the top of the vial.
13. Fill the syringe with the same amount of air as the amount of medication to be aspirated from the vial.	**13.** Air must be injected into the vial in order for medication to be withdrawn from the vial.
14. Insert the tip of the needle into the center of the rubber top.	**14.** The center allows easiest access to the medication.
15. Inverting the vial, inject air into the vial and withdraw the medication, keeping the tip of the needle below fluid level.	**15.** This permits the medication to enter into the syringe because of positive pressure.
16. Remove needle from vial while holding plunger steady.	**16.** Not holding the plunger while removing needle from vial produces loss of medication.
17. Tap the syringe barrel lightly to dislodge air bubbles.	**17.** Air can displace volume of medication, allowing for medication error.
18. Change needle and cover.	**18.** This prevents tracking of medication through tissue.

tion are the outer aspects of the upper arm, the abdomen below the costal margins, and the outer aspects of the thigh (Figure 21–14*A*–*C*). Two common medications administered as a subcutaneous injection are heparin and insulin. Heparin is most commonly administered into the abdominal subcutaneous tissue, but reseach has shown that lower absorption rates and incidences of bruising did not occur significantly more often with injection in other sites (Fahs & Kinney, 1991). Insulin administration is discussed separately in the next section.

Subcutaneous administration involves small doses (0.5–1.0 ml) to avoid irritation of tissues and development of a sterile abscess, manifested as hard lumps under the skin. When administering a subcutaneous injection, the angle of insertion depends on the weight of the client. For an average-sized adult, a 25-gauge, 0.625-in needle is used, and it is inserted at a 45-degree angle. For an obese client, the needle may be inserted at a 90-degree angle. For a very thin client, an angle of less than 45 degrees may be best.

When administering heparin subcutaneously, the

ADMINISTRATION OF SUBCUTANEOUS MEDICATIONS

Subcutaneous injection allows medication to enter into the loose connective tissue between the skin and the muscle by inserting it at a 45-degree angle. The sites for subcutaneous injections include the outer aspect of the upper arms, the anterior aspect of the thighs, the abdominal area surrounding the umbilicus, and the back.

Equipment:

Syringe (1 to 2 ml)
Needle (27 to 25 gauge, 0.375 to 0.675 in)
Alcohol swabs
Medication ampule or vial
Disposable gloves

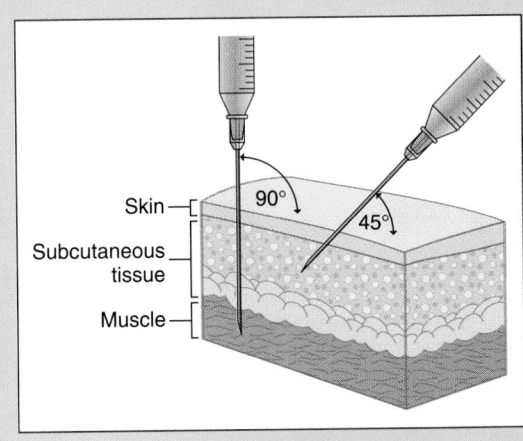

Action	**Rationale**
1. Verify the physician's order for the client's name, drug name, dose, and time and route of administration.	1. This ensures that the client receives the right medication by the right route.
2. Assess the client's allergy history.	2. This alerts the nurse to the potential for allergic reaction.
3. Select the prescribed medication and verify it against order on medication card or printout.	3. Verification of the order averts medication errors.
4. Check the expiration date and physical properties of the vial or ampule contents for color change, change in clarity, or precipitation.	4. Expired medications and medications that exhibit a change in physical properties may not produce the desired effect.
5. Select the appropriate syringe and needle for administration. The choice for an average-sized adult is a 25-gauge, 0.625-in needle.	5. The syringe and needle used for a subcutaneous injection depend on the medication to be given. An insulin syringe is used for insulin, and a tuberculin syringe is used for heparin. (Heparin is also supplied in a prefilled cartridge.)
6. Read the label a second time.	6. This prevents a medication error.
7. Draw up the correct dose of medication into the syringe, using sterile technique. Recap needle according to agency policy.	7. This ensures correct dose and ensures sterility.
8. Prepare medication for only one client. Do not discard ampule or vial until checking label (for the third time) to determine that you have the correct medication.	8. The label should be read three times to prevent errors in preparation or administration.
9. Check client's identification band and ask client to state his or her name.	9. This prevents administration of the medication to the wrong client. Wristbands are a reliable means of identification, and having the client state his or her name is a second means of proper identification.
10. Ask client about any drug allergies.	10. This serves as a final safety check.
11. Explain to the client the procedure, the purpose for giving the medication, and its mode of action; allow for questions.	11. The client has the right to be informed about the medication given.
12. Wash hands and put on clean gloves.	12. This decreases the transmission of microorganisms from person to person.

ADMINISTRATION OF SUBCUTANEOUS MEDICATIONS

(Continued)

Action	Rationale
13. Ask the client where the last subcutaneous injection was given. Inspect skin over proposed injection site for inflammation, edema, or hematoma, and palpate proposed site for masses or tenderness.	**13.** Rotation of injection sites avoids damage to tissue and maximizes the amount of drug absorbed.
14. Place client in a position in which the extremity or abdomen can be relaxed.	**14.** Relaxation minimizes injection discomfort.
15. Clean chosen site with alcohol swab, beginning at center and rotating outward; allow to air-dry. Continue to hold swab between two fingers.	**15.** Friction of the swab cleans the skin. Circular swabbing starting at the center ensures that injection site will be the cleanest area. Swab is readily accessible when needle is withdrawn.

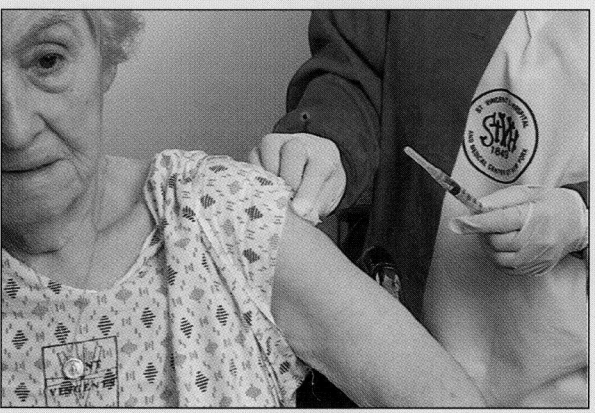

Step 15.

Action	Rationale
16. Remove cap from needle and hold barrel of syringe between thumb and forefinger of dominant hand, with palm facing down.	**16.** Contamination of the needle is prevented. Placement of fingers allows for deft manipulation of syringe.
17. Grasp the skin between thumb and forefinger, creating a roll of about ½ inch. For obese clients, grasp skin below a fold of tissue.	**17.** Well-nourished, well-hydrated clients have a good supply of subcutaneous tissue; emaciated, thin, or dehydrated clients have very little tissue. In the obese client, there is a layer of fat tissue above the layer of subcutaneous tissue.
18. Holding the barrel of the syringe like a dart and with a dart like motion, inject the needle quickly and firmly at a 45- to 90-degree angle, depending on whether the client has abundant or sparse subcutaneous tissue.	**18.** Dart like, firm insertion minimizes discomfort.

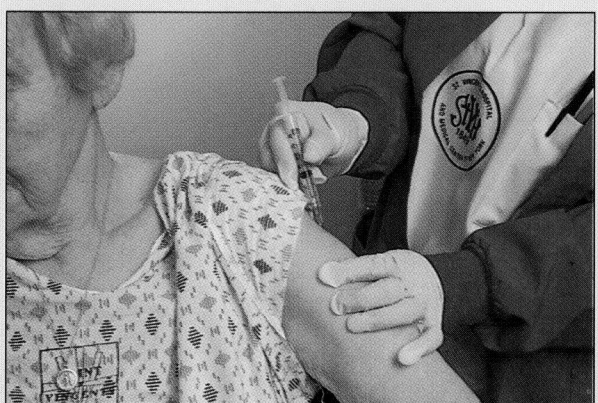

Step 18A.

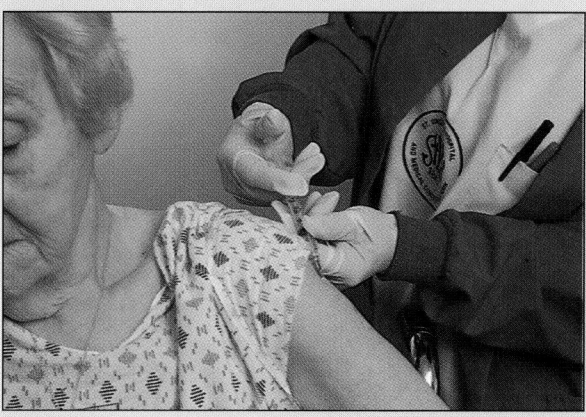

Step 18B.

Continued

PROCEDURE

21–4

ADMINISTRATION OF SUBCUTANEOUS MEDICATIONS

(Continued)

Action	Rationale
19. After the needle is in the subcutaneous tissue, release the skin and grasp the end of the syringe closest to the needle. Syringe is steadied for aspiration. Pull back on the plunger and observe for bloody aspirate. If blood is aspirated, remove the needle, discard the syringe, and repeat the procedure. *If injecting heparin, do not aspirate.*	**19.** Movement of syringe may cause the client discomfort. Bloody aspirate may indicate that the needle has entered a blood vessel. Avoids systemic injection.

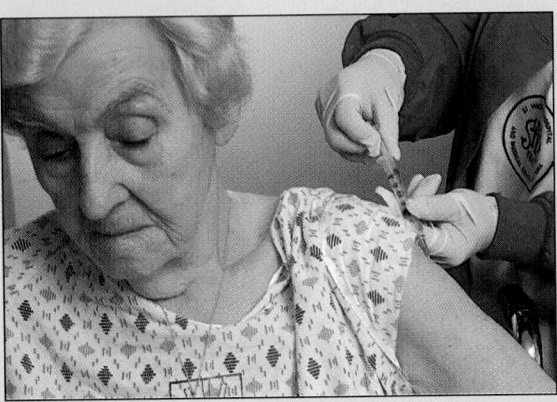

Step 19.

Action	Rationale
20. Inject the medication slowly.	**20.** This reduces pain and tissue to trauma.
21. Withdraw needle while applying the alcohol wipe over the injection site.	**21.** Maintaining the swab against the injection site minimizes discomfort during needle withdrawal.

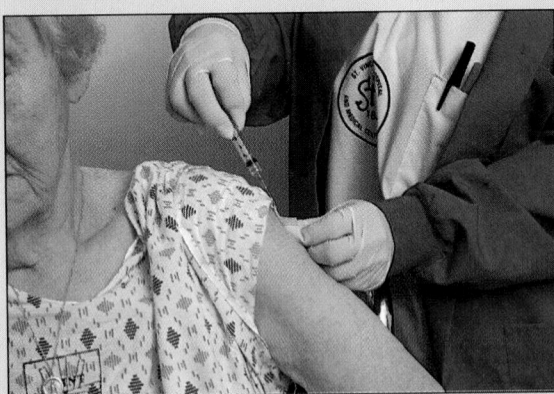

Step 21.

PROCEDURE

21–4

ADMINISTRATION OF SUBCUTANEOUS MEDICATIONS
(Continued)

Action	Rationale
22. Massage the injection site. *However, do not massage if you are injecting subcutaneous heparin or insulin.*	**22.** Massage stimulates blood circulation and absorption of the medication. With heparin, massage produces ecchymosis.
23. Discard uncapped needle and syringe in sharps receptacle.	**23.** This prevents needlestick injury to client and health care personnel.
24. Document immediately after administration. Chart medication dose, route, site, and time and date administered. Sign your full name.	**24.** This prevents repeated medication administration.

Example of Documentation

Date	Time	Notes
1/1/98	0800	Heparin, 5000 U, given SC in abdomen. Mary Smith, RN
1/1/98	1000	No ecchymosis, bleeding noted at site. Mary Smith, RN

nurse should use the anterior abdominal wall fold above the iliac crest and a site that is 2 in or more from the umbilicus to reduce the risk of bleeding. After inserting the needle, the nurse should not aspirate before injecting the heparin, and the nurse should avoid massaging the area after removal of the needle. Heparin should never be administered intramuscularly.

✦ **Administering Insulin.** Because insulin can be destroyed by gastrointestinal fluids, it is administered subcutaneously. Insulin is derived from either pork, beef, or human sources and comes in short-acting, intermediate-acting, and long-acting forms. The type of insulin used depends on the degree of severity of the client's diabetes and the client's response to the insulin. Many clients take both a short-acting form, such as regular insulin, and an intermediate form, such as NPH insulin.

Insulin dosages are expressed in USP units and generally are available in concentrations of 100 U/ml. This is commonly referred to as U100. Less common concentrations are U40, indicating a concentration of 40 U/ml, and U500, or 500 U/ml (Pinnell, 1996). Disposable plastic syringes for insulin administration that contain 1 ml and are scaled for insulin units are available.

Insulin can be stored unrefrigerated at room temperature (15–30°C, or 59–86°F) for long periods while it is being used. An open vial of insulin can be used safely for as long as 4 to 6 weeks before being replaced. Unused, unopened insulin vials should be stored in a refrigerator until opened. Ensure that any insulin is at room temperature before it is administered to a client. Use of cold insulin can cause lipodystrophy (atrophy of the tissue), reduced absorption rates, and local reactions (Pinnell, 1996).

Regular insulin is a clear solution; the other types of insulin are cloudy because they have been modified by the addition of a protein. When two insulin preparations are prescribed, the two insulins can be mixed together in the same syringe (Procedure 21–5). Regular insulin is the only type of insulin that can be administered intravenously, and, because it is clear and unmodified, it can be mixed with other intermediate- or long-acting insulins. When regular insulin is mixed with a modified insulin, the mixture should be administered within 5 minutes, because the action of the regular insulin is reduced when it binds with the modified form.

To prevent complications of lipodystrophy and hypertrophy (thickening of the skin), insulin administration sites should be rotated. The preferred rotation method is to remain at one location for about a week, separating the injections by at least 0.5 to 1 in within the site. After about 1 week, the injections should be switched to a new site (Pinnell, 1996).

Most insulin-dependent diabetics self-administer their insulin. Procedures for client administration of insulin are the same as when the nurse administers the insulin, with a few exceptions. The American Diabetes Association (1997) has published guidelines indicating that clients who self-administer insulin at home

MIXING INSULIN IN A SYRINGE

Diabetes mellitus occurs when the body does not produce enough insulin, a natural hormone, to meet the body's requirements. Because oral insulin is destroyed by digestive enzymes, it must be administered by the subcutaneous route. Insulin is given in a dosage strength called a unit (U). Most commonly, the outside of the insulin syringe shows a calibrated 100-U scale for use with U100 insulin.

Insulin is given according to the rate of action required by the client, that is, rapid-intermediate-, or long-acting. Some clients require more than one type of insulin for control of their diabetes. Rapid-acting insulin is presented as regular insulin, intermediate-acting insulin as NPH insulin. Regular insulin appears as a clear solution, whereas other (modified) insulins appear cloudy because of the protein that has been added to slow absorption. Unused, unopened insulin should be refrigerated until use but can be kept at room temperature for 4 weeks.

Equipment:

> 1-ml syringe
> Insulin vials
> Disposable gloves

Action	Rationale
1. Don gloves.	**1.** Protects both client and health care provider.
2. Before drawing up the drug, rotate each vial for at least 1 minute between both hands.	**2.** Helps warm the medication, and resuspends modified insulin.
3. Do not shake vials.	**3.** Shaking produces foaming and bubbles, thereby trapping insulin particles and altering the dose given.
4. With an insulin syringe and needle, inject an amount of air equal to the amount of insulin to be given into the vial of the modified insulin (cloudy vial) without touching the tip of the needle to the insulin, and remove the syringe from the vial.	**4.** Actions 3–7 are designed to prevent adding unmodified (regular) insulin into the modified (cloudy) insulin vial. This prevents the action of the regular insulin from being reduced.

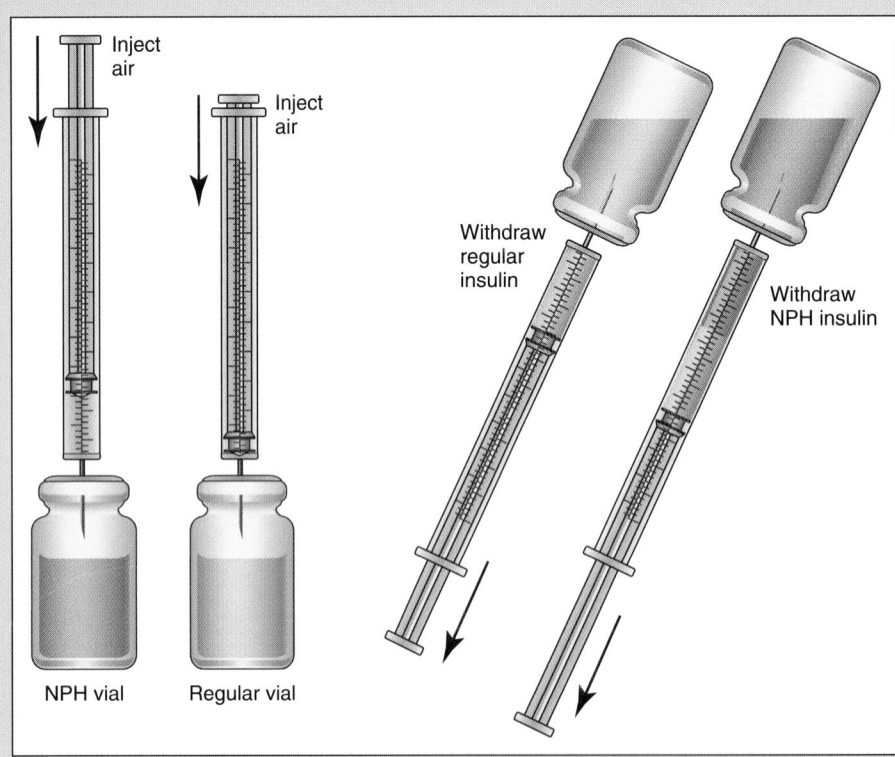

Step 5.

PROCEDURE

21–5

MIXING INSULIN IN A SYRINGE
(Continued)

Action	Rationale
5. With the same syringe, inject air equal to the amount of insulin to be given into the vial of regular insulin (clear vial), and then withdraw the correct dose.	
6. Remove the syringe from the regular insulin (clear vial) and remove air bubbles in the syringe.	
7. With the same syringe return to the vial of the modified insulin (cloudy vial) and withdraw the correct dose.	
8. It is common practice for one nurse to double check the type and dose to be given with another nurse.	**8.** An error in the type or dose of insulin can produce a life-threatening event.
9. Subcutaneous administration must be given within 5 minutes of drawing up the drug.	**9.** A longer wait may reduce the rate of action of the insulin.
10. Injection sites should be rotated consistently.	**10.** Tissue breakdown occurs depending on the frequency of insulin injection at the same site.

may reuse their syringes. For most clients, reusing a syringe is both safe and practical. Reuse should be cautioned in clients "with poor personal hygiene, an acute concurrent illness, open wounds on the hands, or decreased resistance to infection" (American Diabetes Association, 1997, p. S47). See Box 21–3 for points to review with clients who are self-administering insulin.

✦ **Intramuscular Administration.** An intramuscular injection involves the insertion of a needle deep into a

---

Box **21–3**

SELF-ADMINISTRATION OF INSULIN

- Vials of insulin do not need to be refrigerated after they are opened. Avoid extremes of temperature (below 59°F [15°C] or above 86°F [30°C]).
- Keep a spare bottle of insulin available; a slight loss in potency may occur after 30 days.
- Inspect vials before use; short-acting, regular insulin should be clear; other insulin types should be uniformly cloudy.
- If insulin types are mixed, they should be administered within 15 minutes.
- An insulin syringe may be reused if client is self-administering the insulin until needle becomes dull, becomes bent, or comes in contact with any surface other than the client's skin.
- Used syringes may be stored at room temperature.

---

muscle, where faster absorption of the drug will occur (Procedure 21–6). Muscles have a greater supply of blood vessels, which increases the absorption rate of the medication.

Because muscles lie deeper than the subcutaneous tissue, a longer needle is required to penetrate deeper into the tissue layers. Usually, a 1.5-in needle is used for an average-sized adult, and the needle is inserted at a 90-degree angle. The amount of medication that can be administered intramuscularly at one site into an adult is 3 ml, whereas children, older adults, and very thin adults may be able to tolerate only 2 ml or less.

Sites for intramuscular administration include the vastus lateralis muscle in the anterolateral, lateral aspect of the thigh; the ventrogluteal muscle along the outer aspect of the upper thigh near the hip; the dorsogluteal muscle in the upper outer aspect of the buttocks; and the deltoid muscle at the upper outer aspect of the upper arm (Fig. 21–15). The vastus lateralis is preferred for children, infants, and cachectic adults. Although the dorsogluteal site has long been preferred, use of this injection site can damage the sciatic nerve. The deltoid muscle is rarely used and should be avoided in infants and most children.

✦ **Z-Track Method.** Certain medications are very irritating to dermal and subcutaneous tissues when administered intramuscularly. To avoid tissue irritation, the Z-track method is employed. This method seals the medication in the muscle and prevents leakage into the tissues. For administration of an irritating medication, a large, well-developed muscle is selected.

PROCEDURE

21–6

ADMINISTRATION OF INTRAMUSCULAR MEDICATIONS

Intramuscular medications are administered past the subcutaneous tissue into deep muscle tissue. Because muscle has greater vascularity than subcutaneous tissue, intramuscular administration provides faster drug absorption. The angle of insertion is 90 degrees. Up to 3 ml of medication can be administered at one site in a well-developed client; elderly, thin clients and children can tolerate only 2 ml in one location. When selecting an intramuscular site, the dorsogluteal (upper outer quadrant), the ventrogluteal, the deltoid, and, in children the anterolateral thigh muscles are used.

Equipment:

> Syringe (2 to 3 ml for an adult, 1 to 2 ml for a child)
> Needle (19 to 23 gauge, 1 to 1.5 in for an adult; 25 to 27 gauge, 0.5 to 1 in for a child)
> Alcohol wipes
> Medication ampule or vial
> Disposable gloves

Action	**Rationale**
1. Verify the physician's order for the client's name, drug name, dose, and time and route of administration.	1. This ensures that the client receives the correct medication by the proper route.
2. Assess the client's allergy history.	2. This alerts the nurse to potential reactions to observe during drug administration.
3. Select the prescribed medication and verify it against order on medication card or printout.	3. Verification of the order averts medication errors.
4. Don gloves.	4. This protects both client and health care provider.
5. After drawing up the correct medication dose into the syringe, draw up 0.2 ml of air into the syringe.	5. This prevents tracking of drug through tissue after needle withdrawal.
6. Ask the client to state his or her name, and check the client's identity by reading the wristband.	6. This verifies the client's identity.
7. Explain the medication and review the procedure with the client.	7. This increases cooperation and reduces anxiety.
8. Assess the appropriate injection site for bruising, inflammation, edema; palpate for tenderness.	8. This allows you to note integrity of muscle to be injected to permit maximum drug absorption.
9. Assist the client into a comfortable position.	9. Relaxation of the site during administration produces less discomfort.

ADMINISTRATION OF INTRAMUSCULAR MEDICATIONS
(Continued)

Action	**Rationale**
10. Locate site for injection by using anatomical landmarks.	**10.** Accurate administration prevents injury to nerves, blood vessels, and bony prominences.

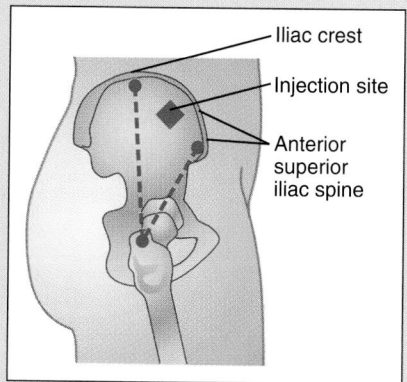

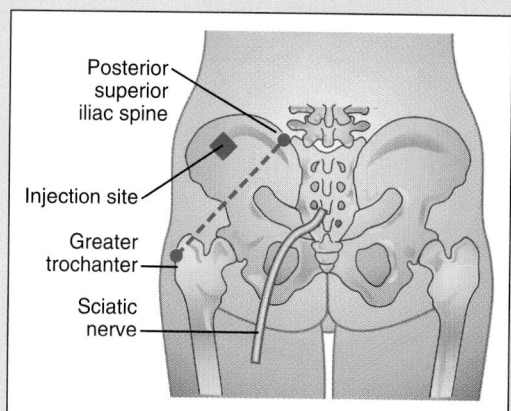

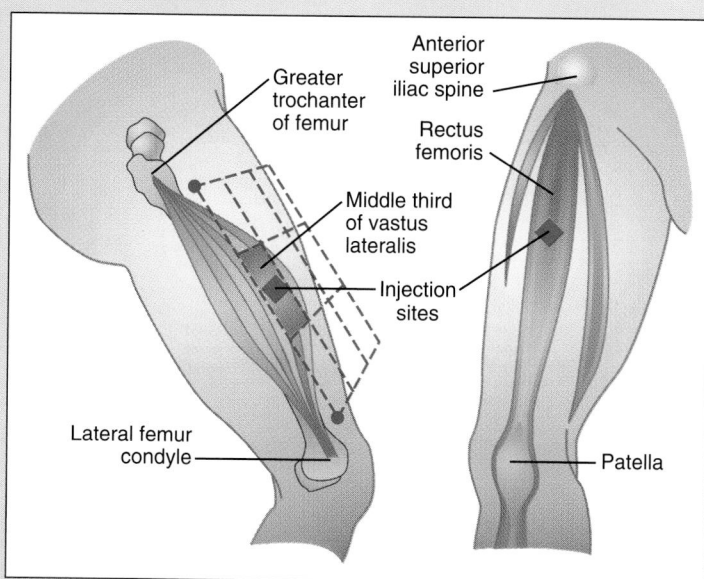

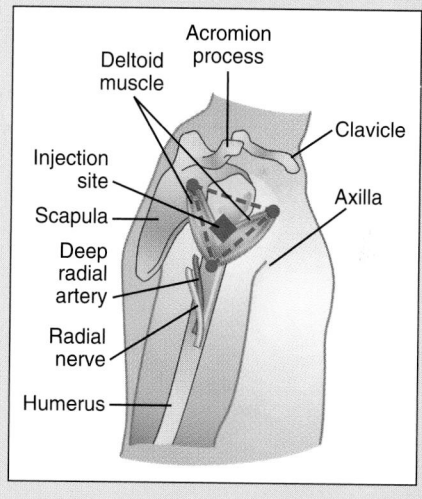

Step 10.

11. Clean the site with an alcohol swab by rotating from the center of the site outward in a circular motion.	**11.** This action removes microorganisms.
12. Select the appropriate injection site.	**12.** The dorsogluteal (upper outer quadrant), the ventrogluteal, the deltoid, and in children the anterolateral thigh muscles are used.
13. Holding syringe like a dart, palm down, between the thumb and forefinger, spread the skin tightly and inject the needle at a 90-degree angle. If the client has small muscle mass, grasp the muscle with the thumb and fingers before injection.	**13.** Proper manipulation permits quick, smooth technique with minimal discomfort. Grasping action allows medication to reach muscle mass rather than subcutaneous tissue.

Continued

PROCEDURE

21–6

ADMINISTRATION OF INTRAMUSCULAR MEDICATIONS
(Continued)

Action	Rationale
14. After the needle is inserted, pull back on the plunger to observe for blood aspirate. If bloody aspirate appears, withdraw the needle, discard it, and repeat the procedure.	**14.** Bloody aspirate indicates intravenous needle placement.
15. Inject the medication slowly and withdraw the needle while applying alcohol swab over injection site.	**15.** Slow injection minimizes discomfort.
16. Massage skin at injection site lightly.	**16.** This stimulates circulation, improving drug distribution.
17. Document the medication dose, route, site, time, and date.	**17.** This prevents potential repeated injection and medication errors.

Z-Track Method

Action	Rationale
18. Select an appropriate site.	**18.** The ventrogluteal site is preferred.
19. Apply a new needle to the syringe after drawing up the medication.	**19.** This prevents the solution from remaining on the outside of the needle shaft.
20. Draw up 0.2 ml air into the syringe after drawing up the medication.	**20.** This creates an air lock and prevents tissue "tracking."
21. Pull the overlying skin and subcutaneous tissue 1 to 1.5 in laterally away from the injection site and aspirate for bloody return.	**21.** This spreads tissues away from normal position.
22. Inject medication and air slowly, maintaining needle in place for 10 seconds after injecting the drug.	**22.** This allows the medication to disperse evenly.
23. Release the skin only after withdrawing the needle.	**23.** This leaves a zigzag path in the tissue, sealing the needle track, preventing the escape of the medication from muscle tissue.

Example of Documentation

Date	Time	Notes
1/1/98	0800	Demerol, 75 mg, IM right ventrogluteal M. Smith, RN

After the medication is drawn up into the syringe, the needle should be changed, because otherwise some of the irritating medication may remain on the outside of the needle. When administering the medication, the nurse pulls the skin and tissues approximately 2.5 to 3.5 cm (1–1.5 in) to the side. The needle is inserted while the skin is held. The medication is injected and the needle is held in place for about 10 seconds. Then the nurse withdraws the needle and releases the skin immediately. The result is that the medication is sealed within the muscle as the overlapping layers of skin and tissue move back to their original places (Fig. 21–16).

✦ **Intradermal Administration.** Intradermal administration of a medication is used primarily for skin testing, such as testing for tuberculosis and allergies (Procedure 21–7). A tuberculin or minim syringe is used to administer an intradermal medication. Typically, the medication is administered at a 5- to 15-degree angle into the layer just under the epidermis. A small bleb should appear as the medication is injected (Fig. 21–17). Because these solutions are generally very potent, it is important that they be administered into the correct layer and not into the subcutaneous tissues, where they would be absorbed more readily into the systemic circulation.

✦ **Intravenous Administration.** IV administration involves the infusion of a medication through an IV line or access site. The IV route is used when a more rapid onset of action is required or when a client's

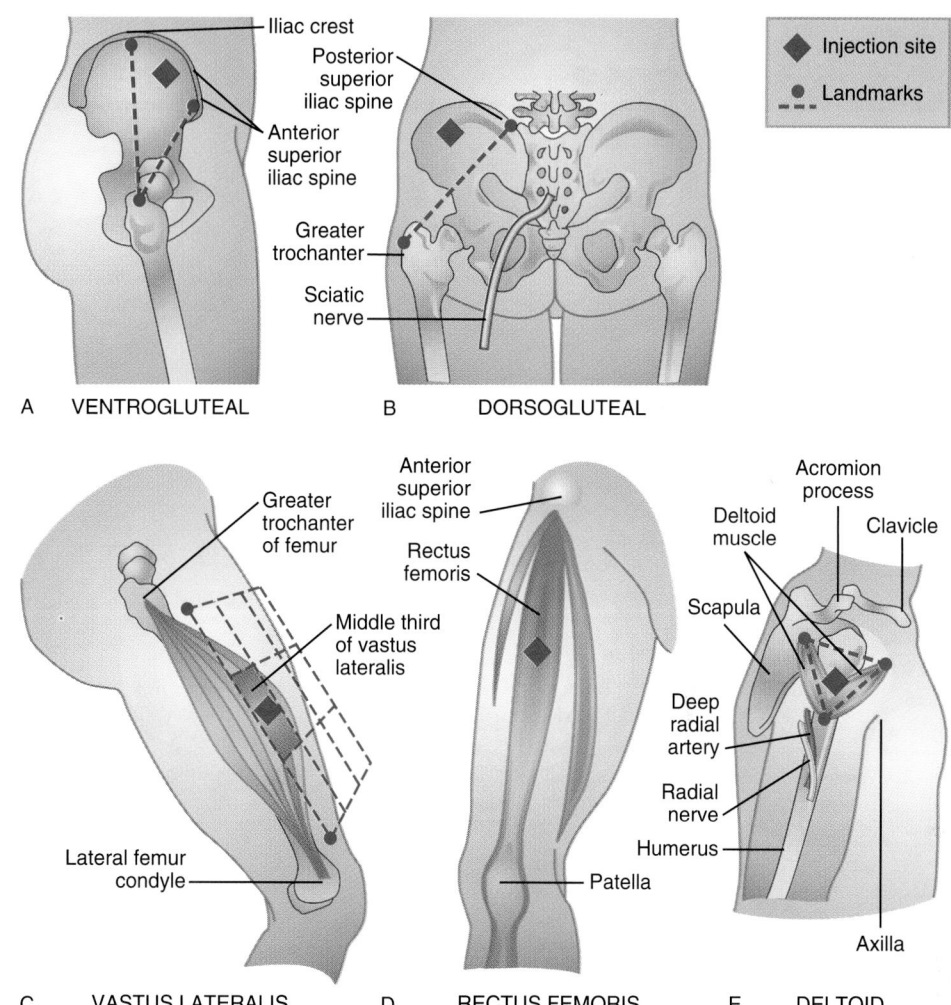

Injection site
Landmarks

A VENTROGLUTEAL   B DORSOGLUTEAL

C VASTUS LATERALIS   D RECTUS FEMORIS   E DELTOID

❥ **Figure 21–15**
Sites of intramuscular injections. **A,** Ventrogluteal muscle; **B,** dorsogluteal muscle; **C,** vastus lateralis muscle; **D,** rectus femoris muscle; and **E,** deltoid muscle.

physical status prevents oral or intramuscular administration. Yet this route has the potential for being the most dangerous. Clients are more at risk for developing an adverse reaction because the medication acts within a very short period of time, if not immediately. Once the medication is injected into a vein, there is no time to interrupt the distribution of the drug and its subsequent effect on the body. Close monitoring of

the client is necessary to identify onset of an adverse reaction and to implement available antidotes, if needed.

A medication can be administered as an admixture to an IV solution, as a bolus injection, or as an IV infusion piggybacked to an existing IV line. The method selected depends on the medication and its action and the client's health status. The procedures to

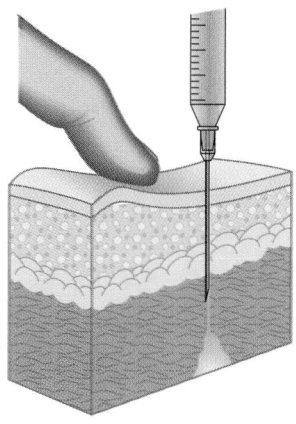

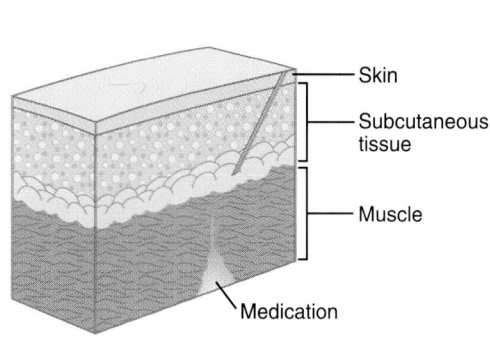

Skin
Subcutaneous tissue
Muscle
Medication

❥ **Figure 21–16**
The Z-track method of intramuscular injection. Skin is pulled to the side and then released. This prevents the deposit of medicine into sensitive tissue.

PROCEDURE

21–7

ADMINISTRATION OF INTRADERMAL MEDICATIONS

Intradermal injections are generally used for tuberculin screening, allergy testing, and vaccinations. They are administered into the dermal layer of the skin, just beneath the epidermis. The sites of intradermal injections are the medial and upper forearm, the back beneath the scapula, and the upper chest.

Equipment:

Tuberculin syringe (1 ml)
Needle (25 to 27 gauge, 0.25 to 0.625 in)
Alcohol swabs
Vial or ampule of test solution or vaccine
Disposable gloves

Action	Rationale
1. Verify the physician's order for the client's name, drug name, dose, and time and route of administration.	1. This ensures that the client receives the correct medication by the proper route. Incorrect doses of allergens can cause significant reactions.
2. Assess the client's medical and allergy history. When performing allergy testing, know the client's usual allergic reaction.	2. This alerts the nurse to potential reactions to observe during the drug administration.
3. Explain the procedure to the client. Inform the client that a slight stinging sensation will be felt as the needle enters the skin. The medication will produce a small bleb, resembling a mosquito bite, which will gradually disappear. Certain medications may produce redness and induration, which will need to be interpreted in 24 to 72 hours; this reaction will also disappear gradually. Instruct the client not to rub the injection site.	3. This encourages cooperation and reduces anxiety. The client will be knowledgeable about how to check for a reaction and when to follow up with the health care provider.
4. Wash hands and apply disposable gloves.	4. Hand washing prevents the spread of microorganisms. Gloves protect the nurse's hands from accidental exposure to blood during the procedure.
5. Withdraw the medication from the vial or ampule.	5. Medication should be withdrawn accurately and according to aseptic technique.
6. Select an appropriate injection site.	6. The forearm is a convenient location and can be monitored easily by the client. Select an area that is free of lesions, lightly pigmented, and free of hair. Measure three to four fingerwidths below the antecubital space and a handwidth above the wrist. The upper chest or upper back beneath the scapula may also be used.
7. Clean the site with alcohol using a firm, circular motion, moving outward from the injection site. Allow the skin to dry.	7. Mechanical action of the swab cleanses site.
8. Using the nondominant hand, pull the skin taut at the injection site.	8. Taut skin facilitates entrance of medication into the intradermal tissue.

ADMINISTRATION OF INTRADERMAL MEDICATIONS
(Continued)

Action	Rationale
9. Remove excess air from the syringe before beginning the injection into the dermis. Place the needle bevel side up at a 5- to 15-degree angle, until resistance is felt. Advance the needle through the epidermis approximately 0.125 in.	**9.** Holding the bevel side up helps keep medication from being injected into the tissue below the dermis.

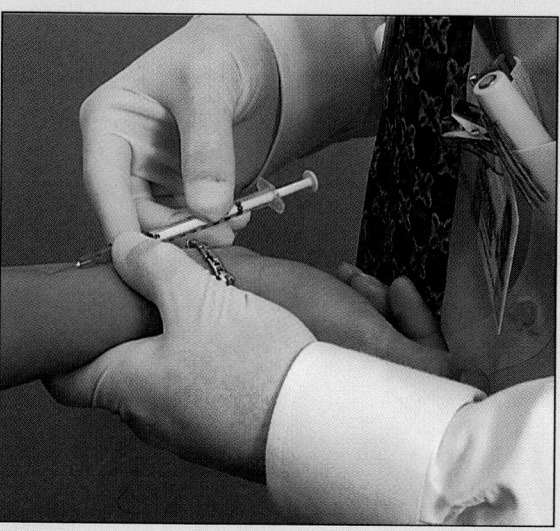

Step 9.

Action	Rationale
10. Slowly inject the medication so that a small bleb appears on the skin.	**10.** The presence of a bleb indicates that the medication is in the intradermal tissue.

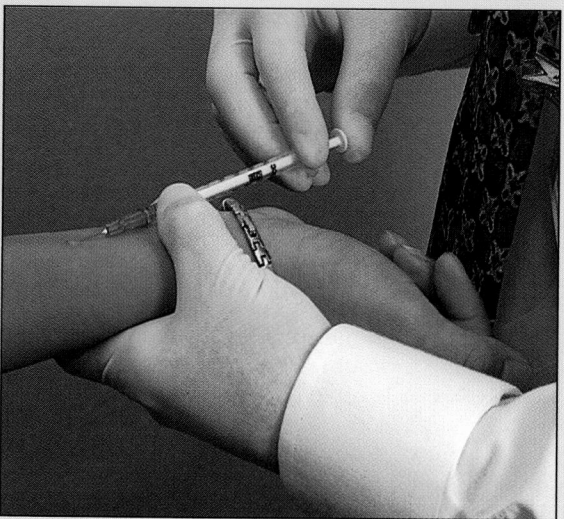

Step 10.

Continued

PROCEDURE

21-7

ADMINISTRATION OF INTRADERMAL MEDICATIONS

(Continued)

Action	Rationale
11. Withdraw the needle quickly at the same angle at which it was inserted, while applying an alcohol swab gently over the site. Do not massage the site.	**11.** Withdrawing the needle quickly and at the proper angle minimizes tissue damage and discomfort. Massaging the site may cause the medication to enter the subcutaneous tissue and may alter the test results.
12. Discard the needle and syringe in the appropriate receptable. Do not recap the used needle.	**12.** Proper needle disposal prevents accidental puncture wounds.
13. Remove gloves and properly dispose of them. Wash hands.	**13.** Hand washing prevents the spread of microorganisms.
14. Properly document medication administered, time, dose, route, site, and nursing assessments. Circle test sites in ink, according to agency policy.	**14.** Accurate documentation helps prevent medication errors and identifies the site for observation in 24 to 72 hours.
15. Assess the client's response to the substance administered. Observe for any evidence of an allergic reaction. Have antidote (epinephrine hydrochloride, a bronchodilator, and an antihistamine) available.	**15.** Anaphylactic reactions may occur with allergy testing. Dyspnea, wheezing, and circulatory collapse may occur and must be reported immediately.
16. Evaluate the intradermal injection site in 24 to 72 hours, depending on the test. Measure and record areas of induration at the largest diameter.	**16.** Careful observation of the area may reveal the presence of a positive reaction or sensitivity to an injected allergen.

Example of Documentation

Date	Time	Notes
1/1/98	0800	PPD (Mantoux), 0.1 ml, given intradermally in left medial forearm. No adverse reaction noted. M. Smith, RN
1/3/98	0800	5 mm area of induration noted. M. Smith, RN

be followed are guided by the institution's policies governing IV administration. There may be specific requirements for demonstrating competence in administering selected medications (*e.g.,* chemotherapy) as well as specific limitations on who may administer these medications. Many institutions have specific guidelines regarding personnel who are permitted to administer IV bolus medications and the drugs that may be administered by this method.

Administration of IV infusions is discussed in Chapter 28 (Procedure 28–1). In some situations, a medication is prescribed to be mixed with a large-volume IV solution and administered over a long period (Procedure 21–8). For instance, a common medication added to IV solutions is potassium chloride. This is a preferred method for administering potassium because of the potential negative effect on the body if potassium is delivered in too high a concentration. Other examples include emergency medications for controlling blood pressure, cardiac arrhythmias, or the progress of labor.

Regardless of the type of medication, admixtures to IV solutions usually are prepared by the pharmacist, although nurses usually are permitted to perform an admixture when needed. When a medication is added to an IV solution, a label must be clearly affixed to the container that indicates the name of the drug, the amount of drug added, the date and time that the drug was added, and the name of the person performing the admixture (Boxes 21–4 and 21–5).

Intermittent administration of medications may be done through a volume-controlled or piggyback setup or as a bolus. A volume-controlled setup is a container that can be attached either to the primary IV container or to a separate line that is then piggybacked to the primary infusion line (Procedure 21–9). These containers hold 100 to 150 ml of solution, which permits dilution of a medication into smaller amounts than a large IV solution; allows for control of the amount of IV fluid intake; and prevents the rapid-dose infusion that can occur with an IV bolus.

Another type of piggyback setup uses small, 50-

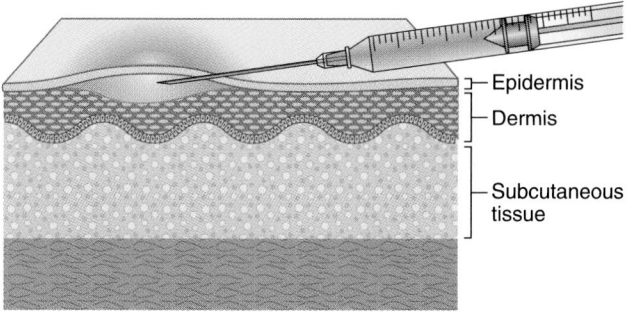

Epidermis
Dermis
Subcutaneous tissue

A

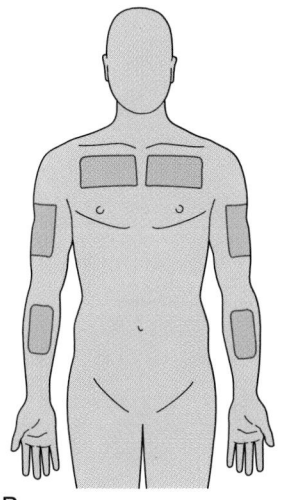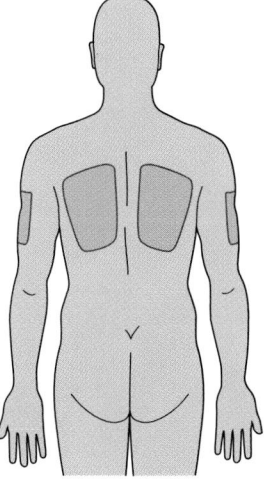

B

❧ **Figure 21–17**
A, For intradermal injection, the syringe is held almost parallel to the skin, and the medicine forms a small bleb under the epidermis. *B,* Commonly used body sites for intradermal injections.

or 100-ml solution bags that are connected through a port on the primary infusion line (Procedure 21–10). The tubing is smaller and has a microdrip or macrodrip chamber. The nurse connects the tubing to the primary line by use of a connector that retards needle-stick injuries or a needle.

Box 21–4

ADMINISTRATION OF INTRAVENOUS MEDICATIONS

* Carefully read the prescription
* Check the client's allergies
* Prepare medication adhering to the five rights of drug administration
* Explain the medication to the client
* Assess the intravenous site for patency
* Administer the dose within the prescribed time
* Observe the client for therapeutic response and adverse reactions
* Document the response to medication

Box 21–5

DOCUMENTATION OF THERAPEUTIC RESPONSE

Response to therapy can be documented as in this example using APIE (Assessment, Plan, Implementation, Evaluation) format.
5/5/97　#5 Fluid volume excess
　10 A.M.
　　A—Patient states "I feel SOB" and positioned self in high Fowler's
　　　BP 160/90, P 100, R 30
　　　Coarse rales auscultated in bilateral lung bases
　　P—Notify physician
　　　Decrease fluid intake
　　　Assess frequently
　　I—Lasix 60 mg IV bolus given via VAD right arm
　　E—Patient states, "I am breathing easier now."
　　　Voided 700 cc of urine
　　　BP 146/84, P 86, R 28

Bolus injection of a drug (Procedure 21–11) into an appropriate vein is a fast method for administering a medication in emergencies or whenever an immediate effect is desired. This method is the most hazardous, because adverse reactions can develop suddenly. Any known antidotes should be readily available in case of an adverse reaction. If there is no known antidote, support measures such as oxygen or suctioning equipment should be available. One major concern when administering a bolus medication is to prevent speed shock, which occurs when an IV bolus medication is given too quickly and causes a marked increase in plasma levels of the drug (Konick-McMahan, 1996). The nurse should carefully note the recommended administration rate and administer the medication accordingly.

Administering Topical Medications

❧ **Ophthalmic Instillations.** Common applications of ophthalmic instillations are eye drops and ointments. The most frequently used type of ophthalmic medication is eye drops for treatment of glaucoma. The client needs to be able to demonstrate adequate vision and dexterity to self-administer these drops safely. Many older clients take ophthalmic medications yet are at risk for problems with vision or manual dexterity, which can hamper their ability to self-administer the medications. The nurse must assist the client in learning the procedure to ensure accuracy and safety.

It is important that the client's cornea, which is very sensitive to irritants, be protected from injury when the medication is instilled. Therefore, the medication should be instilled into the lower conjunctival sac. Also, in cases of infection, cross-contamination from one eye to another should be avoided; medications should not be used in an unaffected eye. When

PROCEDURE

21–8

ADMINISTRATION OF CONTINUOUS INFUSION INTRAVENOUS MEDICATIONS

Medications are administered by the IV route through a variety of methods. If the IV catheter is patent, medications are administered by (1) continuous infusion, (2) piggyback (intermittent) infusion, (3) volume-controlled setup (with the medication contained in a chamber between the IV solution bag and the patient), or (4) bolus dose or "push" (a single dose of medication given through an infusion line or heparin lock).

Equipment:

Alcohol swabs
Syringe (3 to 20 ml)
Needle (19 to 21 gauge, 1 to
   1.5 in)
Ampule or vial of prescribed
   medication
Bag of IV fluid
Normal saline or sterile water
   to mix with the prescribed
   medications
IV label
Disposable gloves

Action	Rationale
1. Verify the physician's order for the client's name, drug name, dose, and time and route of administration.	1. This ensures that the client receives the correct medication by the proper route.
2. Assess the client's medical and allergy history.	2. This alerts the nurse to potential reactions to observe during the drug administration.
3. Select the prescribed medication and verify it against order on medication card or printout.	3. Verification of the order averts medication errors.
4. Explain the medication and review the procedure with the client.	4. This promotes patient cooperation and reduces anxiety.
5. Assess for evidence of infiltration or infection from previous intravenous administration.	5. Inspect the insertion site for redness, pallor, or swelling. Palpate the tissue for edema and coldness, which indicate the blockage of fluid into the tissues.
6. Check the physician's order for the type of IV solution, the medication additive, and the dose.	6. Verification of the order averts medication errors.
7. Verify the compatibility of the medication with the IV fluids. When more than one medication is ordered, review drug compatibility.	7. This prevents clouding, crystallization, and drug interactions.
8. Wash hands thoroughly and apply disposable gloves.	8. This decreases the transfer of microorganisms to supplies.

Adding Medication to a Newly Prescribed IV Bag

Action	Rationale
9. Remove the plastic cover of the IV bag.	9. This promotes sterility.
10. Clean rubber port with an alcohol swab.	10. This reduces microorganisms that can be introduced into a vial with a needle puncture.
11. Remove the needle cap from the syringe. Insert the needle into the center of the rubber port.	11. Injection into the side of the port can cause leakage.
12. Inject the medication.	12. This permits mixture of medication and solution.
13. Withdraw the syringe from the port.	13. This maintains a closed system.
14. Gently rotate the container to mix the solution.	14. This distributes the medication evenly.
15. Label the IV bag including the date, time, medication, and dose. It should be placed so it is easily read when hanging.	15. This promotes easy assessment of IV fluids being infused.

PROCEDURE

21-8

ADMINISTRATION OF CONTINUOUS INFUSION INTRAVENOUS MEDICATIONS
(Continued)

Action	Rationale
16. Spike the IV tubing and prime the tubing.	**16.** This removes air from the tubing to prevent an air embolism.
17. Attach a sterile needle to end of tubing.	**17.** A sterile needle is essential for connection.
18. Clean the port with an alcohol swab.	**18.** This reduces the concentration of microorganisms.
19. Connect the sterile needle adapter to the venous access device (VAD) or IV apparatus (Y port).	
20. If a sterile needle is used, secure it with tape.	**20.** Needle dislodgment can cause a needlestick injury, or the client may not receive the prescribed dose.
21. Verify that the prescribed solution is infusing.	

Adding Medication to an Infusing IV Bag

Action	Rationale
22. Perform steps 1 through 8.	
23. Assess the amount of fluid hanging.	**23.** Insufficient solution decreases the dilution of the medication.
24. Close the IV clamp before adding the medication. Reopen clamp after rotating container.	**24.** A closed clamp prevents medication from infusing into the client before it is properly diluted.
25. Verify that the prescribed solution is infusing.	**25.** This ensures that setup is connected.

PROCEDURE

21-9

ADMINISTRATION OF INTRAVENOUS MEDICATIONS THROUGH A VOLUME-CONTROLLED SETUP

Equipment:

> Alcohol swabs
> Syringe (3 to 20 ml)
> Needle (19 to 21 gauge, 1 to 1.5 in)
> Ampule or vial of prescribed medication
> Bag of IV fluid
> Normal saline or sterile water to mix with the prescribed medications
> IV label
> Disposable gloves

Action	Rationale
1. Perform steps 1 through 8 from Procedure 21–8.	**1.** This is correct procedure.
2. Insert the spike of the volume-controlled set (Buretrol, Soluset, Pediatrol) into the primary solution container.	**2.** Volume-controlled sets contain a maximum of 150 ml.

Continued

PROCEDURE

21–9

ADMINISTRATION OF INTRAVENOUS MEDICATIONS THROUGH A VOLUME-CONTROLLED SETUP
(Continued)

Action	Rationale
3. Open the air vent clamp on the volume-controlled-set.	**3.** An open air vent allows for fluid displacement.
4. Fill the volume-controlled-device with 30 ml of fluid by opening the clamp between the primary solution and the volume-controlled device.	**4.** This is an adequate amount of fluid to fill the drip chamber and prime the IV line.
5. Follow the directions of the manufacturer for filling the drip chamber. Sets have a stationary membrane filter or a floating valve filter.	**5.** It is necessary to create a vacuum so that the solution from the fluid chamber will flow into the drip chamber.

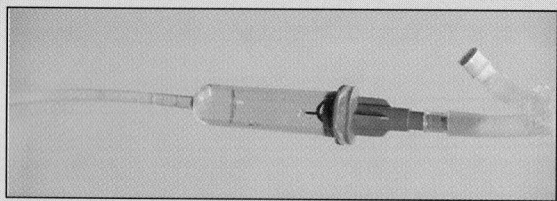

Step 5.

6. Attach a sterile needle or needleless adapter to the IV tubing.	**6.** A sterile needle/adapter is necessary for connections.
7. Open the upper clamp and allow sufficient fluid into volume-controlled chamber to dilute the medication. Usually 50 to 100 ml of IV fluid is used depending on the prescribed medication.	**7.** Insufficient solution decreases the dilution of the medication.
8. Use an alcohol wipe to clean the rubber port of the volume-controlled set.	**8.** This decreases the risk of introducing microorganisms into the container when the needle is inserted.
9. Inject the medication into the volume-controlled port using a sterile needle and syringe.	**9.** Medication is mixed with solution.
10. Label the volume-controlled chamber including the date, time, medication, and dosage.	**10.** This promotes easy assessment of IV fluids that are infusing.
11. Gently rotate the container to mix the solutions.	**11.** This distributes the medication evenly.

two or more medications are prescribed, a specific sequence of administration may be indicated. The nurse should carefully follow specific guidelines when administering eye drops to a client (Procedure 21–12).

Another type of ophthalmic application is administration of an ointment. Generally, an ointment is prescribed when a longer contact time with the external eye is indicated or when a lubricating effect is desired (Pinnell, 1996). Because ointments have a longer contact time, they are administered less frequently than eye drops. Yet, they have a higher tendency for causing blurred vision. When administering both an eye drop and an ointment, administer the eye drop first. See Procedure 21–12 for how to administer an ointment.

✦ **Otic Instillations.** Ear instillations, involving either drops or irrigations, should be done with the solution at room temperature to avoid vestibular stimulation, which may cause nausea or dizziness. Solutions that are warmed to body temperature are tolerated better (Pinnell, 1996). The nurse should use caution to avoid instilling medications into an ear canal with a punctured eardrum.

The client should be positioned lying on the side of the unaffected ear. To ensure proper administration of the medication, the pinna in an adult should be pulled up and back before administration; for a child, the pinna is pulled down, out, and back. After the drops have been instilled, the client should remain on the side for a short time to allow for the medication to be absorbed. The ear canal should never be occluded,

PROCEDURE

21–10

ADMINISTRATION OF INTRAVENOUS MEDICATIONS THROUGH A PIGGYBACK SETUP

Equipment:

Alcohol swabs
Syringe (3 to 20 ml)
Needle (19 to 21 gauge, 1 to 1.5 in)
Ampule or vial of prescribed medication
Bag of IV fluid
Normal saline or sterile water to mix with the prescribed medications
IV label
Disposable gloves

Action	Rationale
1. Perform steps 1 through 11 from Procedure 21–8 using either primary or secondary tubing as needed.	1. Primary set tubing is used to infuse medications into a venous access device (VAD). It is also used when the medication is not compatible with the primary intravenous solution. Secondary set tubing is used when a primary IV is infusing.
2. If the medication to be infused is not compatible with the primary intravenous fluid, turn the roller clamp off above the port closest to the intravenous site. Flush the port using a sterile needle and a syringe containing a few milliliters of normal saline to clear the intravenous line of the primary fluid.	2. This prevents mixing of solutions, which may cause crystallization or cloudiness in the tubing.

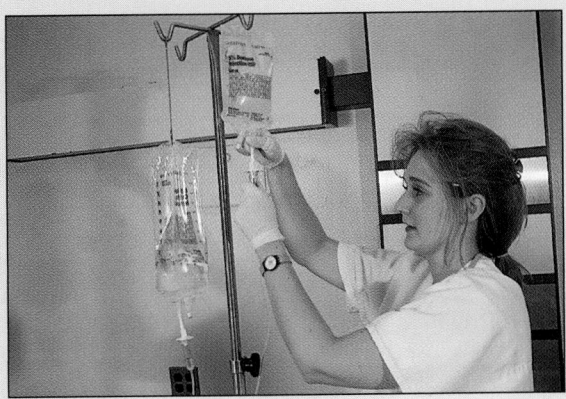

Step 2.

Continued

PROCEDURE

21–10

ADMINISTRATION OF INTRAVENOUS MEDICATIONS THROUGH A PIGGYBACK SETUP
(Continued)

Action	Rationale
3. Using the piggyback method, lower the primary bag 6 in below the secondary bag.	**3.** Secondary bag will empty first because of gravity.

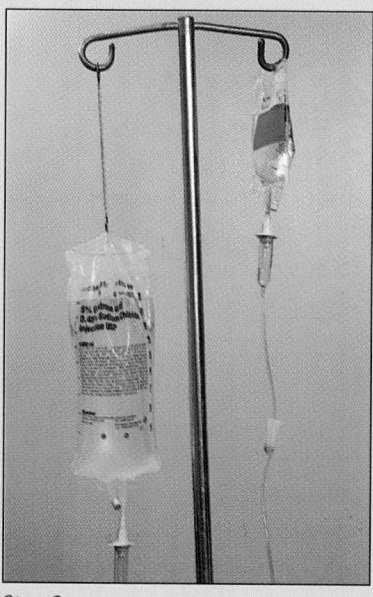

Step 3.

Action	Rationale
4. Regulate the piggyback medication by using the roller clamp.	**4.** Medications usually infuse over 20 to 60 minutes.

and the medication should never be forced into the canal (Procedure 21–13).

✦ **Nasal Instillations.** Instillation of nasal medications is usually done with the use of a nasal spray, for example, a nasal decongestant spray to relieve symptoms of a cold. Most nasal sprays are available over the counter. Clients should be instructed on their use and on how to avoid overuse. The client inserts the spray container into the nares and inhales through the nose as the container is compressed. Inspection of the nares should reveal any signs of irritation from the spray. Nasal drops are used to administer antibiotic medications to treat infections (Procedure 21–14).

✦ **Vaginal Irrigations and Instillations.** Medications may be administered into the vagina by several methods: suppositories, creams, jellies, or foams. Suppositories are kept refrigerated until used to prevent melting. Foams, jellies, and creams are administered

with an applicator. Once in the body, the medication melts or dissolves and may cause some drainage. Many of the medications are applied just before bedtime so that gravity drainage is avoided. In case of drainage, the client may prefer to wear a sanitary pad.

For irrigation of the vagina, a specially designed applicator is used that can easily be inserted into the vagina. The client is usually positioned on the toilet (or on a bedpan if in bed). Many vaginal douches are commercially available over the counter and come in an all-in-one kit. Clients should be cautioned about using these douches excessively. See Procedure 21–15 for a discussion of vaginal instillations.

Administering Inhalants

Inhalants are commonly prescribed for clients with respiratory problems to dilate air passages, reduce inflammation, or thin secretions. Clients with chronic respiratory diseases may take inhaled medications fre-

ADMINISTRATION OF INTRAVENOUS MEDICATIONS AS A BOLUS DOSE

Equipment:

Alcohol swabs
Syringe (3 to 20 ml)
Needle (19 to 21 gauge, 1 to 1.5 in)
Ampule or vial of prescribed medication
Normal saline or sterile water to mix with the prescribed medication
Disposable gloves

Action	Rationale
1. Perform steps 1 and 2 from Procedure 21–8.	
2. Prepare prescribed medication from a vial or ampule and normal saline flushes if indicated.	2. This allows you to prepare accurate dosage.
3. Explain the procedure to the client and examine the client's identification bracelet.	3. Identify the correct medication with the correct client.
4. Don gloves.	4. This protects both the client and the health care provider.
5. Clean the port with an alcohol swab.	5. This decreases microorganisms that can be introduced when the port is punctured with a needle.
6. If an existing IV is infusing, stop the infusion by pinching the tubing above the port.	6. If the IV is infusing properly with no signs of infiltration or inflammation, it should be patent.
7. Insert the needle into the port and aspirate to observe for a bloody return.	7. Blood indicates that the IV line is in the vein.
8. Inject the medication at the prescribed rate.	8. Side effects can occur from rapid IV administration.
9. Remove the needle and regulate the IV as prescribed.	9. The IV should infuse to maintain patency.

Using a Venous Access Device

Action	Rationale
10. Insert a needle connected to a syringe with saline.	10. Flush before and after giving IV medication through VAD to maintain patency.

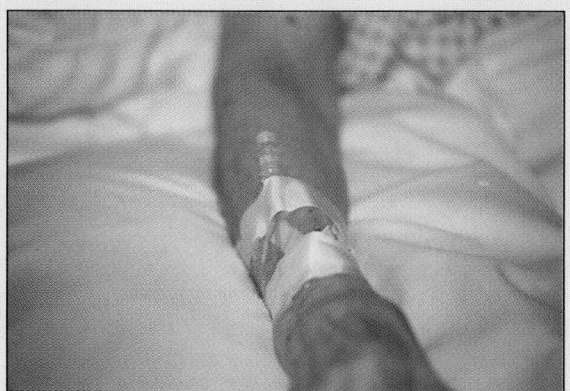

Step 10A.

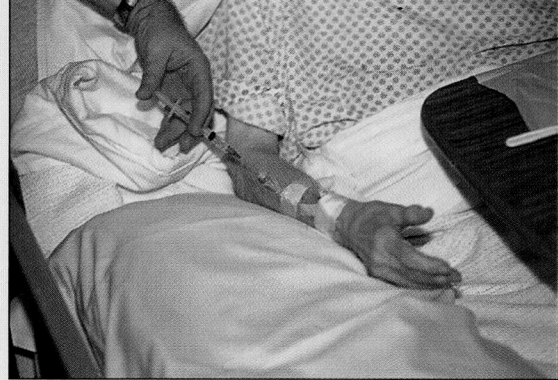

Step 10B.

Action	Rationale
11. Aspirate to observe for a bloody return. If none is observed, inject slowly 1 to 2 ml of normal saline while observing for signs of infiltration.	11. If a bloody return is not present, the saline flush can verify patency.

Continued

PROCEDURE

21–11

ADMINISTRATION OF INTRAVENOUS MEDICATIONS AS A BOLUS DOSE
(Continued)

Action	Rationale
12. Remove the needle with the normal saline.	**12.** Flushes VAD to ensure patency.
13. Attack a syringe with medication and inject medication slowly. Remove needle when finished.	**13.** Slowly administering medication reduces side effects.

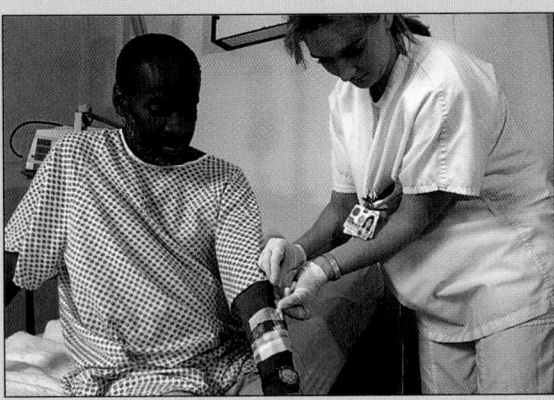

Step 13.

14. Attach the second syringe with saline and flush with 1 to 2 ml.	**14.** Flush the medication through the catheter line.
15. Remove the needle with the normal saline.	

Example of Documentation

Date	Time	Notes
1/1/98	0800	Lasix, 60 mg, IV bolus given via VAD right arm Mary Smith, RN
1/1/98	1200	Voided 700 cc clear, yellow urine Mary Smith, RN

quently at home. A typical apparatus for administration of inhaled medications is the metered dose inhaler (MDI). Nurses should instruct clients on the proper use of an MDI to avoid serious side effects. It is important that the MDI is shaken before use, held correctly in the mouth, and pressed down while the client breathes in. Medications commonly administered as inhalants are sympathomimetics, which cause bronchial smooth muscle relaxation; anticholinergics, which inhibit vagal reflexes that contribute to excessive vagal tone; and corticosteroids, which decrease inflammation of the airway passages (Rokosky, 1997). See Procedure 21–14 for steps in using a nasal inhalant.

Client Teaching

An important component of administering medications is providing the client with information about the medication. Clients need to be kept informed about their health status in relation to the medications that they are taking. In most situations, clients need to be given written information about the medication, its action, what to expect from the medication, when to take it, how to take it, what side effects to look for, and what should be reported to the health care provider. In many facilities, this information is preprinted; in others, there may be blank forms that are filled out for the specific medication. The nurse is responsible for ensuring that the client receives the appropriate

PROCEDURE

21–12

ADMINISTRATION OF OPHTHALMIC DROPS AND OINTMENTS

Ophthalmic medications are administered for treatment of infection, relief of inflammation, treatment of glaucoma, and diagnosis of foreign bodies and corneal abrasions. Eye irrigation is used to wash the conjunctival sac of the eye. The medications instilled are available in the form of ointments or liquids.

Equipment:

Medication
Tissue
Wash basin with warm water
Washcloth
Disposable gloves

Action	Rationale
1. Verify the physician's order for the client's name, drug name, dose, and time and route of administration.	1. This ensures that the client receives the correct medication by the proper route.
2. Assess the client's allergy history.	2. This alerts the nurse to potential reactions to observe during the drug administration.
3. Select the prescribed medication and verify against order on medication card or printout.	3. Verification of the order averts medication errors.
4. Ask the client to state his or her name.	4. Check the client's identity by reading the wristband.
5. Explain the medication and review the procedure with the client.	5. This promotes cooperation and reduces anxiety.
6. Assist the client into a comfortable sitting or lying position.	6. In a sitting position, the client's neck should be hyperextended.
7. Assess the eye. If exudate is noted, gently cleanse with warm water, wiping from inner to outer canthus.	7. Observe for redness, drainage, crusting, or lesions.
8. Draw the correct number of drops into the dropper. If ointment is used, discard the first bead.	8. The first bead of ointment is considered contaminated.
9. While holding the eye dropper in one hand 0.25 in above the conjunctival sac and resting your other hand on the client's forehead, instill the drops into the corner of the eye.	9. This prevents eye injury and possible dropper contamination.

Continued

21–12

ADMINISTRATION OF OPHTHALMIC DROPS AND OINTMENTS
(Continued)

Action	Rationale
10. If ointment is prescribed, apply a thin line from the inner canthus along the lower eyelid inside the conjunctival sac.	**10.** This spreads the medication evenly over the eye.

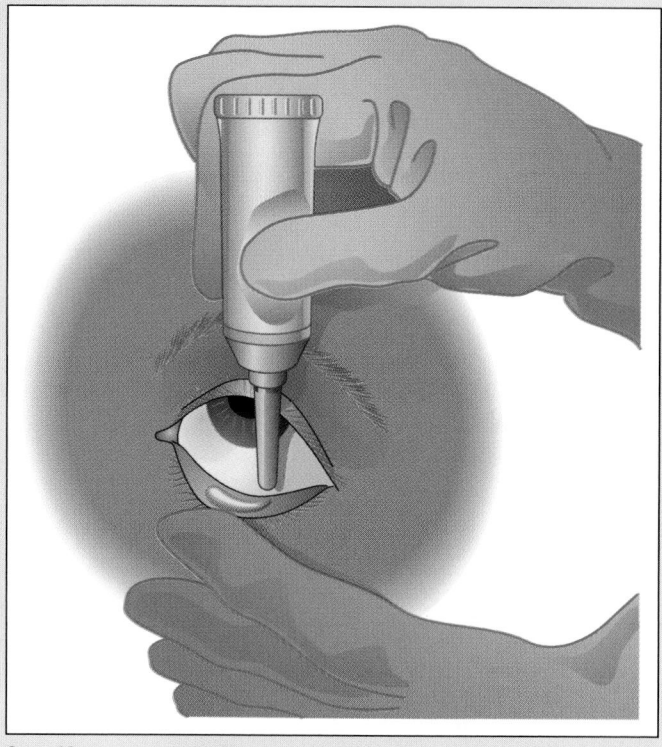

Step 10.

Action	Rationale
11. Allow the client to close both eyes gently.	**11.** This provides comfort for the client.
12. If administering dropper medication, apply gentle pressure to the nasolacrimal duct for 1 minute.	**12.** This prevents the medication from flowing into the tear duct and minimizes the risk of systemic effects.
13. Document the medication form, the time, and the client's response.	**13.** Chart O.D. (right eye), O.S. (left eye), or O.U. (each eye).

Example of Documentation

Date	Time	Notes
1/1/98	0800	Timoptic, 0.5%, 1 gtt OS Mary Smith, RN

information about the medication and has the opportunity to understand this information. The nurse should question the client about the medication to verify that learning has occurred.

Clients who will be self-administering parenteral medications need practice time to perform the designated skill. If instruction begins in an acute or subacute care facility but continues to the home environment, a referral for a home health nurse is required to follow up on the client's learning at home. The client should be given a phone number that can be called when he or she has a question about the procedure.

Text continued on page 501

PROCEDURE

21-13

ADMINISTRATION OF OTIC MEDICATIONS

Otic medications are administered to treat infection, relieve ear pain, or soften and remove cerumen (wax). The position of the external ear canal is variable with age.

Equipment:

Medication
Cotton ball
Cotton-tipped applicator
Examination gloves
Don gloves
Chart

Action	Rationale
1. Verify the physician's order for the client's name, drug name, dose, and time and route of administration.	**1.** This ensures that the client receives the correct medication by the proper route.
2. Assess the client's allergy history.	**2.** This alerts the nurse to potential reactions to observe during the drug administration.
3. Select the prescribed medication and verify it against order on medication card or printout.	**3.** Verification of the order averts medication errors.
4. Ask the client to state his or her name.	**4.** Check the client's identity by reading the wristband.
5. Explain the medication and review the procedure with the client.	**5.** This promotes cooperation and reduces anxiety.
6. Don gloves. Position the client in the side-lying position with the affected ear facing upward.	**6.** This facilitates the flow of the ear drops down the ear canal.
7. Assess the ear for drainage, pain, or inflammation.	**7.** Observe for redness, exudate, or tenderness.
8. If drainage or cerumen is seen in the outer ear, gently cleanse the outer ear with a cotton-tipped applicator. Do not push the applicator into the ear canal.	**8.** This removes the medium for bacterial growth and provides hygienic care.
9. Prepare medication for one client.	**9.** Read medication label three times to prevent medication errors.
10. Grasp the external ear and pull to straighten the ear canal. For adults, pull the ear up and back; for children, pull the ear down, back, and out.	**10.** This ensures correct placement of medication.

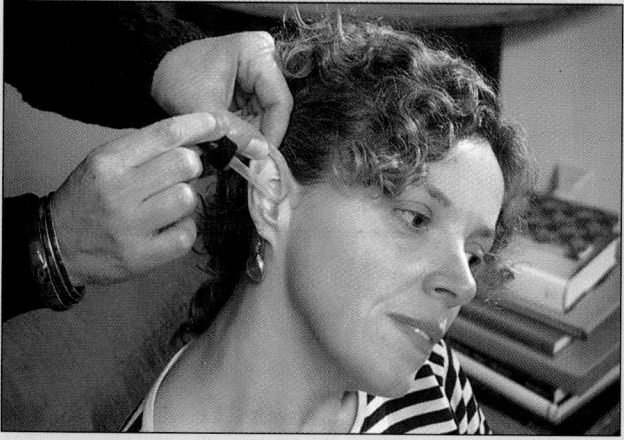 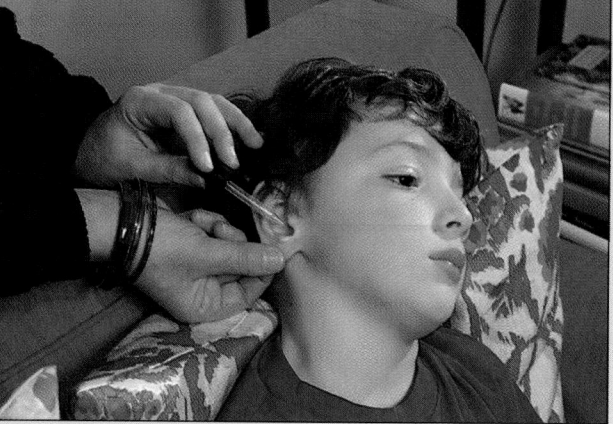

Step 10.

Continued

PROCEDURE

21-13

ADMINISTRATION OF OTIC MEDICATIONS
(Continued)

Action	**Rationale**
11. While holding the ear dropper in one hand 0.5 in above the ear and resting your other hand on the client's head, instill the prescribed number of drops into the ear.	**11.** Contamination of the ear dropper will occur if contact is made with the ear.
12. Instruct the client to continue to remain in side-lying position for 2 to 3 minutes.	**12.** This facilitates the spread of the medication evenly down the ear canal.
13. Apply gentle pressure on the tragus of the ear with your finger.	**13.** This facilitates the flow of the ear drops down the ear canal.
14. Apply an ear plug or a portion of a cotton ball into the client's external ear canal if physician ordered. Remove after 15 to 30 minutes.	**14.** This prevents the medication from draining out of the ear canal.
15. Document the medication given, the time, the route, and the client's response.	**15.** Prompt documentation prevents repeated-dose errors.
16. Return to client within 30 minutes to evaluate the response to the drug.	**16.** This monitors expected effect and side effects.

Example of Documentation

Date	Time	Notes
1/1/98	0800	Auralgan, 2 gg, left ear canal for c/o of pain Mary Smith, RN

PROCEDURE

21-14

ADMINISTRATION OF NASAL MEDICATIONS

Nasal medications are administered via drops or sprays. Nose drops may be prescribed to shrink swollen membranes or to treat infections of the sinuses or nasal cavity. Nasal instillation is usually treated as a clean procedure unless the client has had sinus or facial surgery.

The four sinuses are the frontal, ethmoid, sphenoid, and maxillary. If the ethmoid or sphenoid sinus is to be medicated, position the client with the head over the edge of the bed, or place a pillow under the shoulders with the head leaning backward. If the client is an infant, position the head in a football hold and allow the neck to hyperextend slightly. If the maxillary or frontal sinus requires treatment, the client should lie down with the head turned to the affected side.

Equipment:

> Nasal sprays or drops
> Dropper
> Tissue
> Chart
> Disposable gloves

PROCEDURE

21–14

ADMINISTRATION OF NASAL MEDICATIONS
(Continued)

Action	Rationale
1. Verify the physician's order for the client's name, drug name, dose, and time and route of administration.	1. This ensures that the client receives the correct medication by the proper route.
2. Assess the client's allergy history.	2. This alerts the nurse to potential reactions to observe during the drug administration.
3. Select the prescribed medication and verify it against order on medication card or printout.	3. Verification of the order averts medication errors.
4. Ask the client to state his or her name, and check the client's identity by reading the wristband.	4. This verifies the identity of the client.
5. Explain the medication and expected sensations (stinging, burning, or choking as the solution drips into the throat) to the client.	5. This promotes cooperation and reduces anxiety.
6. Don gloves. Assess the client for discharge, redness, or encrustation of the nares. A nasal speculum may be used to inspect the mucosa.	6. Observe for redness, exudate, or tenderness.
7. Prepare medication for one client.	7. Read medication label three times to prevent medication errors.
8. Instruct client to blow nose gently.	8. This clears the nasal passages and aids in absorption.
9. Inspect discharge on the tissue for color, odor, and consistency.	9. This provides objective documentation.
10. Assist the client to assume the correct position for instillation of medication and ask the client to breathe through the mouth.	10. This reduces the risk of aspiration.
11. Hold the dropper just above the nares and direct the tip toward the midline of the ethmoid bone. Do not touch the dropper to nose or nasal mucosa.	11. If the medication is directed toward the posterior wall, little absorption will occur and the solution will flow to the posterior nasal pharynx. Touching the dropper may produce contamination or damage the nasal mucosa.
12. Instill drops and ask client to remain in position for 5 minutes.	12. This facilitates absorption of the medication.

Instilling Sprays

Action	Rationale
13. Instruct the client to exhale and then close one nostril.	13. Closing one nostril facilitates installation of the spray into the other nostril.
14. Instruct the client to inhale while the spray is instilled into the first nostril.	14. This assists in distributing the spray.
15. Offer a clean tissue, but caution the client not to blow the nose.	15. Excess spray may be blotted, but blowing the nose expels the solution.
16. Document type of medication instilled, time, and route of administration.	16. Prompt documentation prevents repeated-dose errors.

Example of Documentation

Date	Time	Notes
1/1/98	0800	c/o fullness, pressure in right supraorbital region. Positioned with head lowered and turned to right. Nasal spray instilled M. Smith, RN
1/1/98	0815	States that nasal fullness, pressure decreased M. Smith, RN

PROCEDURE

21–15

ADMINISTRATION OF VAGINAL MEDICATIONS

Vaginal medications are administered in the form of suppository, foam, jelly, or cream in order to deliver medication to the vagina or cervix. Suppositories should be stored in the refrigerator to prevent melting.

Equipment:

Vaginal medication (cream, suppository, or foam)
Applicator
Water-soluble jelly
Perineal pad
Examination gloves

Action	Rationale
1. Verify the physician's order for the client's name, drug name, dose, and time and route of administration.	1. This ensures that the client receives the right medication by the right route.
2. Provide privacy. Ask client to void.	2. Discomfort is lessened if the bladder is empty.
3. Wash hands and arrange supplies.	3. This decreases risk of transmission.
4. Close the door and pull curtain around the bed.	4. This provides privacy and protects modesty.
5. Place client on her back with hips slightly higher than shoulders.	5. This promotes visibility and access to the vaginal area.
6. Drape the abdomen and lower extremities.	6. This provides the client with privacy.
7. Adjust the lighting and apply gloves.	7. This protects both client and health care provider.

Suppository

8. Remove suppository from wrapper and place in applicator if indicated.	8. Either an applicator or a gloved hand may be used to insert the medication.
9. Lubricate the rounded end of the suppository.	9. This promotes ease of insertion and provides patient comfort.
10. Separate the labia with the nondominant hand, and insert the suppository along the posterior wall of the vagina.	10. Complete insertion is necessary to dissolve and cover the entire vagina.

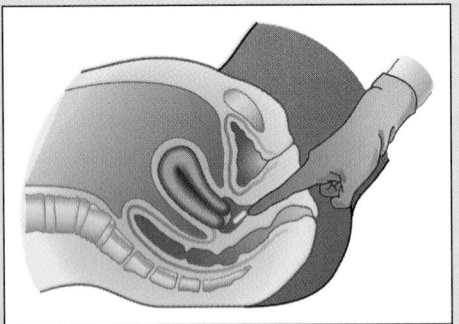

Step 10.

11. Apply a perineal pad.	11. This absorbs excess drainage.
12. Instruct the client to remain lying in supine position for 10 minutes.	12. This allows the medication to remain in the vagina while the drug is being absorbed.

Foam, Jelly, Cream

13. Fill applicator with the prescribed amount of medication.	13. The prescribed amount of the drug should be prepared.
14. Retract the labia with the nondominant hand.	14. This promotes ease of insertion.

21–15

ADMINISTRATION OF VAGINAL MEDICATIONS
(Continued)

Action	Rationale
15. Insert the plunger 2 to 3 in into the vagina toward the sacral area. Slowly push the applicator plunger until it is empty and remove the applicator from the vagina.	**15.** The medication spreads more evenly if insertion is midvaginal.

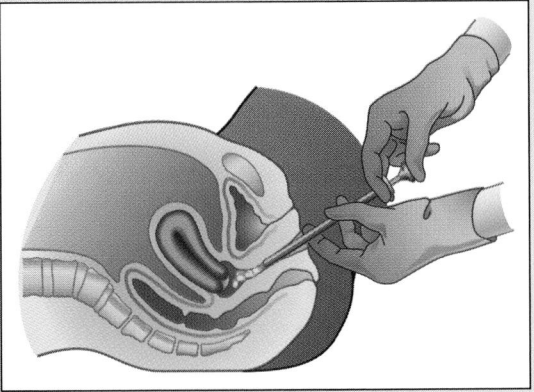

Step 15.

16. Apply a perineal pad.	**16.** This absorbs excess medication drainage.

Example of Documentation

Date	Time	Notes
1/1/98	0800	Vaginal cream administered. Tolerated procedure well with no c/o discomfort noted. Mary Smith, RN

It is also important that the client's family or significant other be given the information, as long as the client agrees. Having someone else in the home who is knowledgeable about the medication and the administration protocol helps to ensure that the prescription will be followed. Clients who have sensory deficits may need to be provided with devices to assist them in following the prescribed regimen. For instance, a client who is visually impaired may need a container that is divided into compartments, each compartment to be filled with one dose of a medication. This assists the client in taking only the prescribed amount of the correct medication.

Evaluation

During the evaluation step, the nurse should determine whether desired outcomes associated with the medications have been achieved. This requires that the nurse be knowledgeable about the actions and purposes of the prescribed medications and focus assessment on determining the presence of the desired physiological changes or behaviors. Sometimes, results of diagnostic laboratory tests may be needed to complete the evaluation. For a client who is receiving an antiarrhythmic medication to control ventricular arrhythmias, the nurse should obtain an electrocardiogram or a rhythm strip from a cardiac monitor to verify the abolition of the arrhythmia.

Evaluation of the effects of drugs is an essential component of safe administration of medications. Documentation in the client's medical record should include not only verification that the medication was administered but discussion of the client's understanding of the action and purpose of the medication, the client's acceptance of the medication regimen, the client's ability to self-medicate, and the presence of any side effects that may forewarn of potential toxic reactions. Any objective data (vital signs, cardiac rhythm strips, diagnostic laboratory results, intake/output monitoring) should be noted where applicable. Documentation of these data is an integral component of

MEDICATION MANAGEMENT

Medication management is a common reason for referral to a home health care agency. Many home care clients require teaching, especially older, chronically ill adults receiving multiple medications. Dose changes and introduction to new prescriptions can be very confusing. Compliance may be an issue. It is essential to assess reasons for noncompliance, such as lack of knowledge, unpleasant side effects, or forgetfulness. Assess the client for visual, auditory, cognitive, and physical impairments. Determine who will administer the medications and how the client will obtain the filled prescription. If the client is unable to successfully learn about or manage the medications, a caregiver must be identified. Teaching topics include name and purpose of the medication; prescribed dose and administration times; and side effects and what to do if they occur.

A number of tools can help with the teaching process, including a written list of medications, printed drug education cards, and medication organizers (*e.g.*, a 7-day pill box). Medication teaching usually takes several home visits. To be successful, keep the teaching simple. Use common drug names whenever possible. Focus on the most important information necessary. For some clients, the teaching goals may need to be *very* simple (*e.g.*, naming the drug and administration times); ability to verbalize medication purpose and side effects may not be realistic. If compliance is a concern, counting out remaining pills in the vial or pill box may be necessary. Medication management is a challenging area of home care practice that requires creativity and client individualization.

the ongoing monitoring process to provide continuity of care. As chemicals, drugs are a critical part of client care; evaluation of the client is crucial to maintain safety when using them. See the accompanying box for medication management in community-based care situations.

✦ Summary

Chemical substances, such as drugs, are prescribed to promote equilibrium and maintain homeostasis in clients who for some reason require intervention. Although drugs can be helpful in altering a physiological process or replacing a missing substance, they can become toxic if administered incorrectly. An essential component of safe nursing practice is to administer drugs in a safe manner using the "five rights" as a guideline.

The client is an integral member of the health care team and, as such, needs to be fully informed about the purpose and actions of the prescribed medication. The nurse should provide detailed instructions to the client both verbally and in writing. With more clients self-medicating, the potential for problems associated with medication administration will increase. A large number of clients take multiple prescriptions, creating interaction effects among the different medications.

The nurse's role in safe administration of medications, whether in an inpatient setting or in a community-based environment, is to safeguard the client's welfare. The changing roles of the nurse with the rise of managed care affect the way in which nurses interact with clients who are receiving prescription medications. Instead of close supervision in a structured environment, clients now require intermittent monitoring and assistance as they function within their usual living conditions. It is essential that the nurse's assessment skills be focused on evaluating clients in the home or at work.

■   ■

CHAPTER HIGHLIGHTS
✦

✦ Federal legislation regulates the prescription and administration of drugs and establishes standards for the prescription and administration of controlled substances and for their labeling.

✦ The nurse practice act of each state regulates specific aspects of drug administration that pertain to the individual responsibilities of the nurse and that may vary with the education preparation of the nurse.

✦ Every drug is known by more than one name, with each name having particular significance to the client and the health team member. Drugs can be known by the following names: chemical, trademark, generic, and official. Drugs are also classified according to their similar characteristics.

✦ Drugs are capable of producing both therapeutic and adverse effects throughout the body. Drugs replace missing substances such as insulin and other hormones; protect weakened bodily functions; prevent insult from foreign substances such as bacteria; eliminate noxious chemicals within the body; promote cellular function (*e.g.*, cardiotonics); and alleviate symptoms such as fever.

✦ A drug effect is the observed manifestation of the action of a chemical substance on the body. The therapeutic effect of a drug is the intended effect of the drug when it is introduced into the body. A drug may produce more than one therapeutic effect in the body.

◆ Adverse effects (side effects) are those drug actions that occur and are not the intended or therapeutic effect.

◆ A variety of factors other than the chemical structure of the drug affect the action of the drug in the body. Because of the unique characteristics of clients, drugs can cause different types of effects from one client to another.

◆ Drugs are available in many types of preparations depending on the route of administration, the action of the drug, the metabolism of the drug, and the therapeutic use of the drug. The form of the drug determines how it is administered.

◆ Drugs can be administered through a variety of routes, with the choice depending on the chemical properties of the drug and the intended effect of the drug. Administration routes are categorized as oral, parenteral, topical, or inhalant.

◆ The amount of medication that is administered to a client is described as the dose of the medication. Calculation of the dose requires accurate measurement of the drug.

◆ The major measurement systems for calculating drug dosages are the metric, the apothecary, and the household systems.

◆ The physician is the team member who prescribes the drug. The pharmacist is responsible for dispensing the medication as prescribed by the physician or health care provider.

◆ Administration of medications requires careful adherence to established principles. The nurse must adhere to the "five rights" of medication administration to ensure accuracy of administration and to maintain safety. The five rights are right drug, right dose, right client, right time, and right route.

◆ There are times when an incorrect medication is administered to a client. If a medication error does occur, it is the professional and ethical responsibility of the nurse to report the error to the physician and to the nursing supervisor according to institutional policy. When the error is reported, the nurse should complete the required documentation.

◆ The nursing process should serve as a guideline for the nurse when administering medications.

◆ The nurse should follow accurately the procedures for administering medications.

◆ Documentation of medication administration, the client's knowledge of the action and purposes of the medication, the client's ability to self-medicate, the achievement of the intended effect of the drug, and the presence or absence of side effects are crucial components of the nurse's role in administering medications safely.

Study Questions

1. The name of a drug that is considered the permanent drug name and reflects the chemical name is

   a. trade name
   b. chemical name
   c. scientific name
   d. generic name

2. The process by which a drug is transported by the circulating body fluids to various areas of the body is called

   a. bioavailability
   b. distribution
   c. absorption
   d. metabolism

3. Which of the following is a unit of weight measurement in the metric system?

   a. milliliter
   b. kilogram
   c. decimeter
   d. minim

4. Which of the following persons is legally permitted to dispense drugs?

   a. physician
   b. nurse practitioner
   c. pharmacist
   d. nurse

5. For an average-sized adult, which of the following needle sizes would be appropriate to use when administering a subcutaneous injection?

   a. 0.5 in
   b. 0.625 in
   c. 0.75 in
   d. 1 in

Critical Thinking Exercises

1. You are ordered to give Demerol, 75 mg I.M. Discuss how to give the injection and safety measures you would implement regarding drug administration.

2. Ms. M. is 82 years old. She is 5 ft 2 in tall and weighs 90 lb. She lives in a personal care home and has slightly altered mental status and mild renal failure. Discuss the pharmacokinetics involved in giving her Lanoxin and Lasix.

References

American Diabetic Association (1997). Clinical practice guidelines. *Diabetic Care, 20*(1).

Bailey, A., Ferguson, E., & Voss, S. (1995). Factors affecting an individual's ability to administer medication. *Home Healthcare Nurse, 13,* 57–63.

Edmisson, K. W. (1996). Psychosocial dimensions of medical-surgical nursing. In J. M. Black & E. Mattassarin-Jacobs (Eds.), *Medical Surgical Nursing* (5th ed.). Philadelphia: W. B. Saunders.

Fahs, P. S., & Kinney, M. (1991). The abdomen, thigh, and arm sites for subcutaneous sodium heparin injections. *Nursing Research, 40,* 204–207.

Gurevich, I. (1994). Preventing needlesticks: A market survey. *RN, 57,* 44–49.

Kee, J. L., & Hayes, E. R. (1997). *Pharmacology: A nursing process approach* (2nd ed.). Philadelphia: W. B. Saunders.

Konick-McMahan, J. (1996). Full speed ahead—with caution. *Nursing 96, 26,* 26–31.

Lehne, R. A. (1994). *Pharmacology for nursing care* (2nd ed.). Philadelphia: W. B. Saunders.

Pinnell, N. L. (1996). *Nursing pharmacology.* Philadelphia: W. B. Saunders.

Rokosky, J. M. (1997). Misuse of metered-dose inhalers: Helping patients get it right. *Home Healthcare Nurse, 15,* 13–21.

Bibliography

Beyea, S. C., & Nicoll, L. H. (1996). Back to basics: Administering IM injections the right way. *AJN, 96,* 34–35.

Blodget, J. B. (1995). Managing injection reactions. *Nursing 95, 25,* 46–47.

Covington, B. P., & Trattler, M. R. (1997). Bull's eye: Finding the right target for IM injections. *Nursing 97, 27,* 62–63.

Hussar, D. A. (1995). Helping your patient follow his drug regimen. *Nursing 95, 25,* 62–64.

Kee, J. L., & Marshall, S. M. (1996). *Clinical calculations* (3rd ed.). Philadelphia: W. B. Saunders.

Levins, T. T. (1996). Central IV lines: Your role. *Nursing 96, 26,* 48–49.

Segbefia, I. L., & Mallet, L. (1997). Are your patients taking their medications correctly? *Nursing 97, 27,* 58–60.

Whitman, M. (1995). The push is on: Delivering medications safely by IV bolus. *Nursing 95, 25,* 52–54.

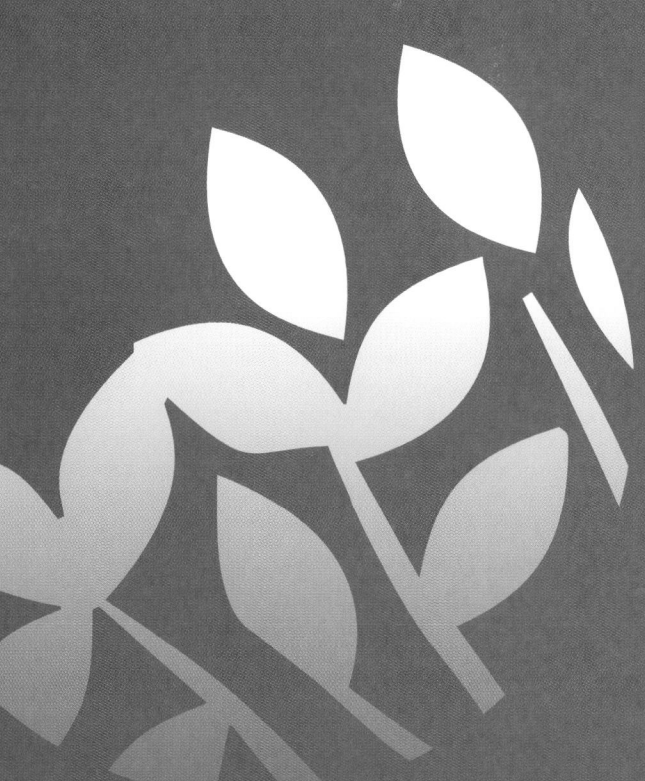

Chapter **22**

HYGIENE

LISA K. ANDERSON SHAW,
RNC, MSN, MA

KEY TERMS

◆

acne
alopecia
A.M. care
caries
cerumen
ceruminal gland
complete bed bath
dandruff
dermis
epidermis
gingiva
gingivitis
halitosis
hirsutism
H.S. care
integument
integumentary system

morning care
necrosis
oral care
partial bed bath
perineal care
periodontal (gum) disease
personal hygiene
plaque
P.M. care
pressure ulcer
P.R.N. care
pyorrhea
sebaceous glands
self-care
subcutaneous layer
tartar

LEARNING OBJECTIVES

◆

After studying this chapter, you should be able to

◆ Define key terms
◆ Relate the history of hygiene to current nursing practice
◆ Identify functions of the skin
◆ Explain the need for comprehensive hygiene
◆ Identify factors that may alter self-care
◆ Identify appropriate hygiene practices for various age groups
◆ Describe methods to encompass cultural and personal hygiene preferences
◆ Perform a complete bed bath, skin assessment, and back rub in acute and home settings
◆ Perform complete oral care in various settings according to client needs
◆ Provide specific hygiene measures regarding hair, nail, eyes, ears, nose, and foot care, including such aids such as glasses, dentures, contacts, and hearing aids
◆ Identify important environmental hygiene measures
◆ Develop nursing process for nursing diagnosis related to client-specific hygiene needs
◆ Utilize proper body mechanics and ancillary equipment
◆ Make unoccupied and occupied beds (and surgical bed)
◆ Demonstrate or explain use of specialty beds and mattresses
◆ Incorporate client and family teaching throughout interactions
◆ Identify potential community health and discharge needs of clients

505

Many of the aids and practices used for personal hygiene today have their origins in ancient times. However, the importance of hygiene and health was brought to modern attention when Florence Nightingale instituted basic hygienic and sanitation measures at the battlefront during the Crimean war.

The practice of personal hygiene measures is a health-promoting behavior. The word *hygiene* refers to the science of health and its maintenance, the prevention of disease, and sanitary practices. **Personal hygiene** is the activity of self-care, including bathing and grooming. Hygiene includes care of the skin, hair, nails, mouth, teeth, eyes, ears, nasal cavities, and perineal and genital areas. The activities by which hygiene is achieved are influenced by many factors, of which cultural and developmental variables are often the most influential (Box 22–1).

Because hygiene practices are often of a personal nature, the manner in which a nurse provides hygiene measures can foster trust and comfort between the client and the nurse and can provide opportunities for communication and teaching. Assessing client hygiene needs is very important to implementing appropriate hygiene activities. Nurses must also be aware of the type of assistance required by their clients for hygiene measures to be effective. It is very important that the nurse allows the client to perform as much of his or her own care as possible independently and to allow the client privacy while doing so. Maintaining and encouraging independence is extremely important, especially in debilitated or older clients, so they do not lose whatever self-care abilities they have. Respecting independence is not always easy, especially when the nurse could perform certain activities much faster than the client can. However, it is always of benefit to the client if independence is respected and fostered.

Hygienic Practices and Nursing Care

Assisting the client with hygiene measures provides the nurse with an excellent opportunity to learn more about the client while making skilled observations about the person's condition. The nurse must first assess what hygiene procedures can be done independently by the client and which ones will require assistance. While the client is performing hygiene measures or while the nurse is assisting with such measures, ongoing nursing assessments of many body regions may be done. Assessments during this time may be convenient for both the client and the nurse. For example, a full skin assessment is more convenient for a client if done while bathing rather than at another time when clothing might have to be removed simply for this purpose. The oral mucosa and teeth may also be better assessed after proper oral hygiene procedures have been completed.

The development of therapeutic relationships may also be enhanced while providing a client's hygiene care. During this time, the nurse may speak to the client about specific assessment concerns or may teach the client important hygienic techniques that would be of benefit. For example, if the nurse notices that the client has dry, cracking skin, the nurse may educate him or her about the use of lotions to decrease the possibility of further skin breakdown while providing such skin care.

Hygiene measures often provide comfort to clients who are hospitalized. Hygienic measures such as applying lotion to dry itchy skin or performing soothing oral care to a client with stomatitis may relieve discomfort. Clients may be embarrassed if they are not able to perform personal hygiene measures that they may routinely perform at home, such as shaving or washing hair on a daily basis. The nurse may be able to assist with specific needs and may also offer understanding and support to clients who may not be able to perform their routine hygiene measures.

Box **22–1**

FACTORS INFLUENCING PERSONAL HYGIENE PRACTICES

1. Developmental level: Children learn most of their hygiene practices at home and in their personal environment. They model their behavior after other family members, and many of these behaviors stick with them throughout life. With advancing age, hormonal levels and changes in the integumentary system often require hygiene measures to be altered.

2. Cultural background: Norms related to hygiene practices differ from culture to culture. For example, North American culture places a high value on personal cleanliness, and people tend to bathe daily, whereas people from other cultures may consider bathing once a week to be the norm. Privacy practices vary from culture to culture. The use of deodorants, perfumes, and lotions may also vary from culture to culture.

3. Socioeconomic status: Financial status often affects a person's ability to purchase hygiene products. Living arrangements may also affect hygiene practices, such as frequency of bathing, and perhaps the assistive needs of a person (especially those living in nursing homes). Socially, people tend to conform to the hygiene expectations of those around them.

4. Religion: Some religions observe specific rules related to personal hygiene, especially regarding the opposite sex.

5. Personal habits: Some people have specific preferences about their hygiene practices; *i.e.,* preferring a shower to a tub bath.

6. Health status: Persons who are ill are often unable to attend to personal hygiene activities, either because they have a low energy supply or because of a specific physical deficit.

Bathing may offer clients a sense of normalcy in otherwise uncontrolled hospital situations. Allowing a client to make some decisions regarding hygiene activities may also enhance his or her sense of control. Allowing clients to perform as many procedures as they can independently and, if possible, to choose the time they wish to do such activity can foster this sense of control.

Although the client may request that personal hygiene measures be done at specific times, there are some routine scheduled times for hygienic care practiced in most institutions. Such scheduled times are usually individualized to clients according to their personal and cultural preferences. The following is a list of most common scheduled hygiene care times:

* Early morning care (**A.M. care**): After the client awakens, the nurse assists with toileting if needed and then provides comfort measures to refresh the client and prepare him or her for breakfast (or diagnostic or therapeutic procedures). Such hygiene and comfort measures include washing the face and hands and providing oral hygiene. This activity may be facilitated by the night shift staff or by the day shift staff, depending on the institution policy for such care.

* **Morning care:** Such care is usually performed after the client has had breakfast or prior to diagnostic or therapeutic procedures if the client's breakfast has been held. Morning care measures include assisting with toileting as needed; providing a bath or shower; oral care; foot, nail, and hair care (including shaving, if indicated); giving a back rub and providing appropriate skin care; changing the client's gown or pajamas; changing bed linens; and providing environmental hygiene measures. The client is assessed for comfort, and the client's room is assessed for safety. The call bell should be placed within the client's reach, and protective measures should be in place as needed (*e.g.,* bed rails). Morning care is often described in terms of how much assistance a client will need from the

nursing staff. See Box 22–2 for a description of the levels of hygiene care.

* Afternoon care (**P.M. care**): Hospitalized clients are often very busy in the mornings with tests, procedures, and therapies. Often, simple hygiene measures offered in the afternoon may refresh and comfort clients. Such measures include washing of hands and face; assisting with oral care; assisting with toileting as needed; and providing environmental hygiene. For those clients who are immobile, positioning for comfort is also very important.

* Evening care (**H.S. care**): Personal hygiene care before bedtime often helps the client relax and promotes sleep. The nurse again offers assistance with toileting, handwashing, and oral care. Clients may find a back massage relaxing. The call light should always be placed within the client's reach, and protective devices should be secured as needed.

* As-needed care (**P.R.N. care**): Some clients might require hygiene measures in addition to the previously noted scheduled ones. Clients who are on a routine toileting schedule may require assistance every 2 hours. Clients who are incontinent of bowel or bladder should be assessed frequently for hygiene needs. Clients who are very diaphoretic (sweat profusely) may need assistance with clothes and bed linen changes at frequent intervals. The nursing staff should assess each individual client for special hygienic needs so that such needs may be met.

Functions of Skin

The skin, or **integument,** is considered the largest organ system of the human body (Fig. 22–1). The **integumentary system** includes the skin, hair, glands located in the skin, and the nails. This integumentary system is extremely important in the maintenance of good health and provides the following functions (see Chapter 23):

1. Protection:

   The skin is the body's first line of defense against many types of injury. The **epidermis** (the skin's outer layer) is fairly waterproof, which prevents entrance of microorganisms into the body's system. The **dermis** (or corium) is the layer under the epidermis. It is composed of connective tissue containing blood vessels, nerves, and sweat and sebaceous glands. The inner layer of skin is the **subcutaneous layer,** which helps insulate the body and absorb shock. The skin is usually dry, thus inhibiting the growth of bacteria that normally reside on the skin's surface. When intact, the skin also shields the body from certain effects of slight trauma. Mucous membranes also serve to protect the body. For example, nasal hair assists in stopping small particles from entering the respiratory tract, and irritating substances sensed in the respiratory system cause a person to sneeze or cough as a warning.

2. Temperature regulation:

   Sebaceous glands and sweat glands assist the body in temperature control through the secretion of fluids from the body, which then evaporate outside the body's surface. Heat is also lost through radiation and conduction through vasodilation. Lack of perspiration and vasoconstriction assist the body in heat retention.

Box 22–2

LEVELS OF HYGIENE CARE NEEDS

I. Self-care: Self-care describes when clients can perform all hygiene activities independently. The nurse only needs to offer supplies and to perform specific assessments as needed (*e.g.,* skin or oral assessments).

II. Partial care: Partial care describes when clients need hygiene care supplies set up for them, most often at the bedside or near the sink in the bathroom. These clients may only be able to perform part of their hygiene measures due to weakness or immobility. The nurse should assist these clients in being as independent as possible while performing measures that cannot be done by the client.

III. Complete care: Complete care describes when clients cannot perform any hygienic measures without the assistance of the nursing staff. The nurse must provide a complete bed bath and perform all other measures indicated by the client's condition.

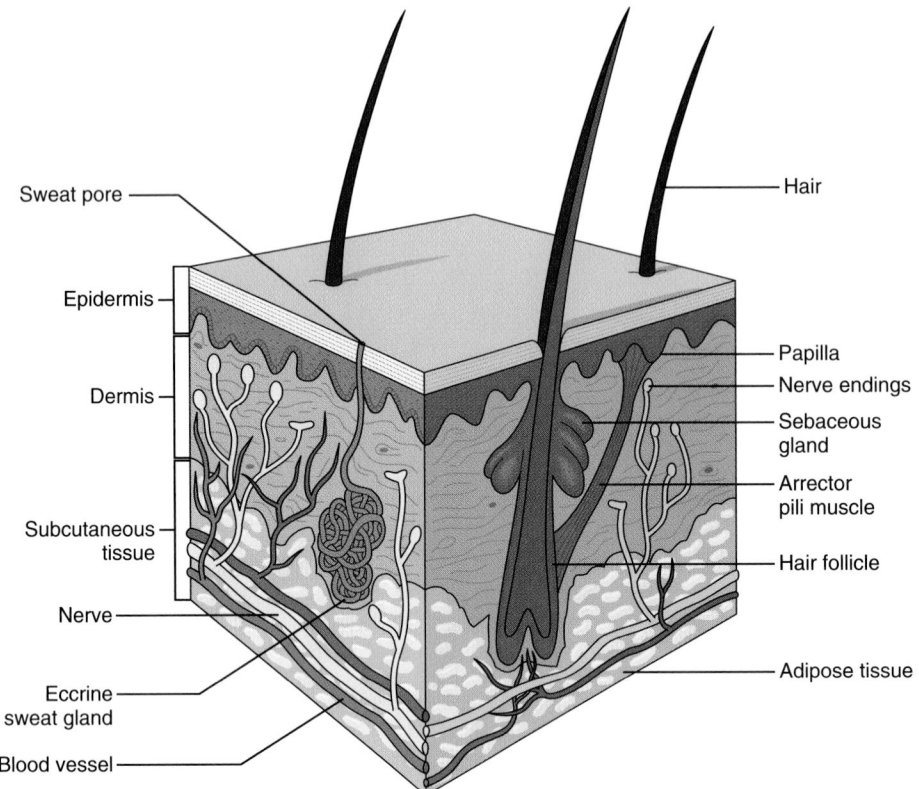

Sweat pore

Epidermis

Dermis

Subcutaneous tissue

Nerve

Eccrine sweat gland

Blood vessel

Hair

Papilla

Nerve endings

Sebaceous gland

Arrector pili muscle

Hair follicle

Adipose tissue

❧ **Figure 22–1**
Cross-section of normal skin.

3. Sensation:

The skin contains sensory nerve receptors, which transmit sensations of touch, pressure, pain, and temperature.

4. Secretion and excretion:

Sebaceous glands and **ceruminal glands** secrete materials that assist in lubricating the skin and in trapping foreign substances. Water, salts, and nitrogenous wastes are excreted through the skin.

5. Production and absorption of vitamin D:

The skin produces needed vitamin D through exposure to sunlight (a precursor for vitamin D is contained in the skin and becomes activated when exposed to the sun's ultraviolet rays).

Principles of Skin Care

The skin often is a reflection of underlying disease processes; thus, the assessment of this system is extremely important in the management of illness. The normal integumentary system has the following characteristics:

* Skin should be smooth, soft, and intact
* Skin should be warm and dry to touch
* Skin turgor should be good (feels firm and has elastic quality)
* Skin color may vary in different body areas
* Skin temperature may vary to touch across the skin's surface

* Hair should be evenly distributed
* Nail beds should be pink and blanch well
* Nails should be smooth and strong
* Mucous membranes should be moist and of normal color for skin type
* Mucous membranes should be intact

Because the skin is the body's first line of defense against microorganisms and infection entering the body, it is very important to assist clients in keeping their skin intact and healthy. While caring for clients, it is important to provide client education regarding the importance of good skin care (see Health Promotion and Prevention Box).

Developmental and Cultural Factors Affecting Hygiene

Personal hygiene practices are often learned from the family and community in which one is raised. These practices are learned in the early years of one's life and are modeled after family members, friends, and other community members (*e.g.,* caretakers, teachers, neighbors). Hygiene preferences may vary significantly from person to person and from culture to culture. The environment one is exposed to also has a great influence on hygiene practices. This also includes one's socioeconomic status. Financial resources may influence the amount and type of hygiene products one has, as well as the availability of a well-balanced diet, which promotes a healthy body.

In addition to cultural factors, normal growth and development factors play an important part in hygiene self-care practices. The nurse must consider the client's age and developmental stage when planning hygiene interventions for assigned clients.

Newborns and Infants

The basic needs of a newborn must be supplied by a caregiver. Newborns can communicate certain needs through crying, such as when they need a diaper change. Infants are totally dependent on caregivers for toileting. Bowel and bladder activity can be frequent. Keeping the skin clean and dry is important in preventing skin irritation and possible skin breakdown. During diaper changes and feeding activity, in-

fants should never be left unattended, as falls or choking could result.

Bathing infants and newborns is important for comfort and assessment reasons, as well as for basic hygiene. Skin should be assessed for rashes or other irritations. Bathing should be done with slightly tepid water so as not to burn the baby, and babies should never be left unattended during bathing. Newborns and younger infants may lose a lot of heat when unclothed, so it is important to complete bathing care as efficiently as possible and to clothe them soon after the bath. The frequency of bathing depends on the individual baby, but daily bathing of newborns and infants is usually not needed. Skin lotions applied after bathing may be comforting to the infant and may help to keep skin from drying out.

Toddlers and Preschool-Age Children

Self-care abilities regarding hygiene care, toileting, and feeding increase rapidly in toddlers and preschool-age children, who begin to show mastery of their environment and a desire to be more independent. Most children at this age achieve daytime bowel and bladder control (between ages 2 and 3 y). Nighttime control comes later and depends on the individual child. Most children at this stage can feed themselves and drink from a cup with a moderate amount of independence. They often ask for assistance from their caregivers to meet the needs they are not independent with.

Bathing continues to require assistance and supervision at this stage. Toddlers and preschoolers often want to help bathe themselves or do it themselves, and most can perform some simple hygiene measures with minimal assistance. Children in this stage need supervision to make sure activities are thoroughly completed, but allowing them some independence is important for their development.

During hospitalization, it is common for toddlers and preschoolers to regress in their toileting and feeding habits. This behavior allows the child to cope with the stress of change and illness and to try to regain some control of his or her environment. This is a common coping mechanism and should be recognized and permitted by the nursing staff.

Children and Adolescents

Children and adolescents are typically independent in their hygiene practices. However, they may require reminders to complete such practices. They are independent in eating but may need direction in maintaining a well-balanced diet. As their bodies mature, hygiene practices should be implemented to meet these body changes.

In adolescence, hormonal changes occur, resulting in the growth of pubic and axillary hair. Boys begin to grow facial hair and may even begin shaving. Skin changes occur as the sebaceous glands begin to produce more oil on the skin, which may result in **acne,** an inflammation of the sebaceous glands, on the face, chest, and back. Acne can negatively affect an adolescent's self-image as he or she becomes more sensitive to his or her physical appearance. Bathing and shampooing become very important at this time because the sweat glands fully develop. The use of deodorants usually begins at this time to control body odor.

When caring for children and adolescents, it is important to allow independence and privacy when possible. Adolescents are often very sensitive about their physical development and their physical appearance.

Adults and Older Adults

Young and middle-aged adults are usually very independent in their hygiene care practices and preferences. Although they may have specific needs related to their health status, most young and middle-aged adults require little assistance from caregivers.

Older adults begin to see changes in their skin that may predispose them to injury or complications (Fig. 22–2). As skin ages, it becomes thinner and less elastic. The structural attachments between epidermis and dermis break down, so that the epidermis can actually tear away with slight trauma, such as when a person is pulled across a bed or when adhesive tape is removed abruptly. Older adults also tend to bruise easily because their dermal circulation becomes less efficient and the vascular walls become thinner (Fenske *et al.,* 1992). Both men and women may experience thinning hair and hair color changes. Many older adults wear dentures because of gradual deterioration of teeth from periodontal disease or caries.

Physically, older adults experience a loss of muscle mass and joint flexibility. This results in motor weakness and agility. They may require more time to perform tasks. They also experience a decrease in bone mass, which may predispose them to injury or fracture when falls occur. Some older adults also suffer from chronic and disabling diseases, which greatly affect their self-care abilities (see the box entitled "Skin Care Needs of the Elderly").

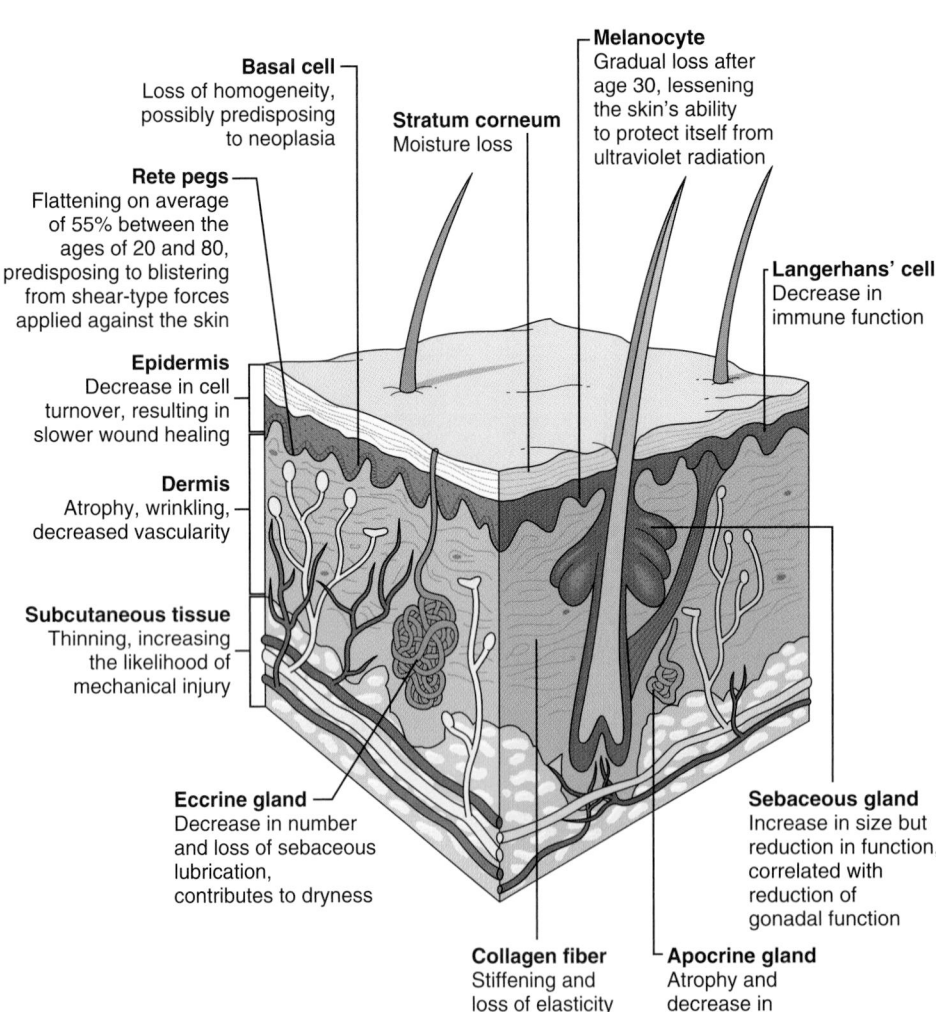

Basal cell
Loss of homogeneity, possibly predisposing to neoplasia

Rete pegs
Flattening on average of 55% between the ages of 20 and 80, predisposing to blistering from shear-type forces applied against the skin

Epidermis
Decrease in cell turnover, resulting in slower wound healing

Dermis
Atrophy, wrinkling, decreased vascularity

Subcutaneous tissue
Thinning, increasing the likelihood of mechanical injury

Stratum corneum
Moisture loss

Melanocyte
Gradual loss after age 30, lessening the skin's ability to protect itself from ultraviolet radiation

Langerhans' cell
Decrease in immune function

Eccrine gland
Decrease in number and loss of sebaceous lubrication, contributes to dryness

Collagen fiber
Stiffening and loss of elasticity

Apocrine gland
Atrophy and decrease in function

Sebaceous gland
Increase in size but reduction in function, correlated with reduction of gonadal function

❥ **Figure 22–2**
The skin undergoes many changes over time.

SKIN CARE NEEDS OF THE ELDERLY

Nutrition

Poor eating habits and possible dental problems may contribute to the malnutrition of the older adult. Because a healthy diet is important for adequate skin integrity, assessment and education are very important for the older adult.

Teaching should include

* Reviewing simple healthy menu plans
* Encouraging clients to drink six to eight glasses of water per day
* Encouraging self-assessment of skin and weight on a routine basis
* Encouraging the use of liquid dietary supplements to enhance caloric and vitamin intake

Bathing and Skin Care

Older adults need not bathe as frequently because of a decrease in glandular secretions. Skin care is very important to avoid breaks in skin integrity and other skin problems.

Client teaching should include

* Encouraging clients to take a full bath two or three times per week and wash up in between
* Encourage the use of a lotion soap to avoid drying out of skin
* Encourage the use of moisturizers after bathing
* Tell clients to increase the humidity in the house to decrease effects of dry skin—especially during winter months
* Warn against direct sun exposure; tell clients to wear a sunscreen with a sun protection factor (SPF) of 15 or greater
* Encourage clients to perform skin self-assessments during bathing, noting any spots or lesions or changes in moles

Oral Hygiene

Daily oral hygiene procedures are essential components of total health care. Nurses have a very important role in assisting clients to maintain an acceptable level of oral health (Miller & Rubinstein, 1992). Mouth care is not only an essential part of overall good health, but it is also a comfort measure for clients of all ages, which is why oral hygiene should be offered frequently during the day. Comfort may come from the aesthetic value of clean teeth and gums or from the therapeutic value of comfort from pain for a client with stomatitis or gum disease.

Common Oral Problems

Problems within the oral cavity can affect any system within the body. If the oral mucosa is interrupted by sores, or the teeth and gums are in poor condition, bacteria can enter the body's system and can cause infection. Problems within the oral cavity may also lead to poor nutritional intake, especially for persons who have inadequately fitting dentures or have pain within the oral cavity while eating. Clients who are immunosuppressed due to illness or medications are also more susceptible to oral cavity problems, such as opportunistic infections. Although oral hygiene is extremely important to hospitalized clients, such measures are often overlooked by the clients as well as by the nursing staff.

Dental **caries** (decay) and **periodontal (gum) disease** are the most frequent sources of tooth loss. Dental caries is a progressive erosion and destruction of the outer enamel of the tooth. If caries is not effectively treated, damage to the tooth's pulp can occur (Fig. 22–3). Other dental problems include:

> **Plaque,** a buildup of bacteria, Saliva, and epithelial cells which adheres to teeth and gums
>
> **Tartar,** a hardened buildup of plaque that must be removed by a dental professional
>
> **Pyorrhea,** an infection of the gums located between the roots of the teeth and their surrounding tissue—may lead to loss of teeth

The prevalence of dental disorders is quite high in the United States, and the major risk factor for dental caries is poor dental care. Other risk factors for dental caries include (Tinanoff, 1995):

* High consumption of sucrose
* Exposure to high levels of cariogenic microorganisms
* Previous caries exposure
* Poor oral hygiene practices
* Lack of fluoride exposure
* Low socioeconomic status
* Poor familial patterns

Primary prevention of dental caries includes daily brushing and flossing, routine dental visits with cleaning, maintaining a healthy diet, and, in children, the application of fluoride (Black & Matassarin-Jacobs, 1993).

Special oral hygiene measures should be implemented for clients who are being treated for cancer or other conditions that can result in immunosuppression. Two conditions that are common in immunosuppressed clients are stomatitis and candidiasis (moniliasis). Stomatitis is simply an inflammation of the oral cavity that can be caused when the client's resistance is lowered and an opportunistic infection results. Such infections may be caused by viruses, bacteria, yeast, or fungus. All clients with disease processes that cause immunosuppression should have frequent, thorough oral examinations for stomatitis so that prompt treat-

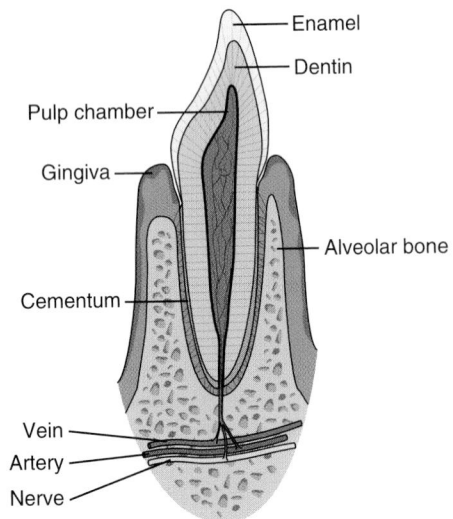

A

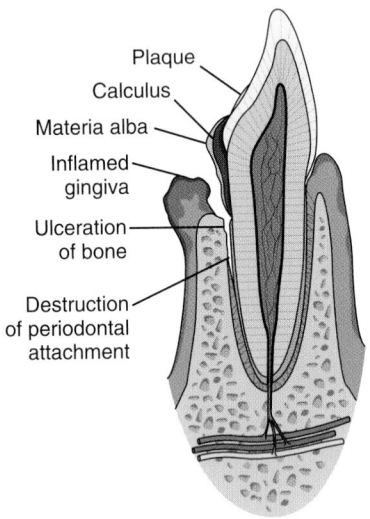

B

✦ **Figure 22–3**
Cross-section of a normal tooth.

ment may be initiated. Stomatitis can be very painful and may include one lesion or many lesions within the oral cavity.

Candidiasis (moniliasis), commonly called thrush, is also a common oral problem of clients who are immunosuppressed. The organism, *Candida albicans,* is part of the normal flora of the oral cavity; however, when clients are immunosuppressed, an overgrowth of normal flora candida may occur. Clinical assessment of a client with candidiasis usually reveals white patches on the tongue, palate, and buccal mucosa. These patches may be irritating or painful. Inspection of the oral cavity should, again, be routine care for the client with immunosuppression. Treatments for both stomatitis and candidiasis include good oral hygiene measures, along with prescribed treatments from the client's physician.

The elderly experience changes in the oral cavity. These changes, mainly caused by atrophy of the mucosa and a decrease in salivation, often predispose the elderly to oral problems. Older clients often experience dental caries and may lose some or all of their teeth. Oral cavity problems also predispose them to nutritional deficits. Elderly clients often experience an inability to perform adequate oral hygiene measures because of a decrease in manual dexterity and strength. The goal of dental care in the elderly is to maintain a healthy oral cavity and to decrease tooth decay, tooth loss, and gum disease.

Brushing, flossing, denture care, and care of unconscious or debilitated clients are discussed in the implementation section of this chapter.

Providing Oral Care

It is very important for the nurse to obtain a detailed dental history from each client, which includes any existing dental problems, routine dental care information and current routine oral hygiene practices. The nurse should also note the client's overall nutritional status and ability to chew, including the use of dentures. After a complete history, the oral cavity should be assessed. The nurse should perform this inspection wearing nonsterile gloves and with the use of a tongue blade and a light source (penlight or flashlight). The nurse should note the overall appearance of the oral cavity, teeth, and gingiva. Missing teeth, oral lesions, dental caries, hydration status, and mucosa color should be noted. Normal **gingiva** should be smooth, shiny, and an uneven red color. Any areas of edema or tenderness should be noted, and the client should be asked about their presence for further information (Black & Matassarin-Jacobs, 1993) (see Box 22–3).

Education is extremely important for clients with oral hygiene problems as studies have shown that compliance with oral hygiene measures can be increased by 30 to 50% with a combination of written information and verbal counseling (Crosby, 1989). Nurses should reinforce good oral hygiene as they provide such care to their clients. **Oral care** should include reinforcement of healthy practices such as

- Brushing teeth at least in the morning and at night (and after each meal if possible)
- Using a small-headed, soft-bristled tooth brush, stroking horizontally across the tooth to protect gingival tissue (even immunosuppressed clients benefit from the same oral care routine, including very gentle toothbrushing) (Crosby, 1989)
- Obtaining routine dental care from a dentist for fluoride treatments, radiographs, professional cleaning, and treatment of dental caries
- Assessing the oral cavity routinely for lesions, growths, tenderness, and edema and seeking prompt professional care for such abnormal findings
- Flossing teeth daily

Box 22–3

COMMON ORAL CAVITY PROBLEMS

Dental plaque: Soft mass of bacteria, leukocytes, macrophages, and epithelial cells that adheres to the teeth. Plaque can be removed only by mechanical cleaning.

Dental caries: Tooth decay. Causes progressive demineralization and destruction of outer enamel of tooth. Plaque buildup is the most important cause of tooth decay. Such decay can be decreased by removal of plaque through good oral hygiene practices.

Periodontal Disease

Gingivitis: Bacterial colonization from plaque buildup on or around the gingiva (gums). Pockets of inflammation may develop and deepen, causing separation of the gingiva from the tooth. Gingivitis may be avoided by plaque removal through brushing and flossing.

Periodontitis: Includes gingivitis, but destruction extends to the alveolar bone and periodontal ligament, destroying supporting structures of the teeth. Tooth loss may occur. Good oral hygiene, including brushing and flossing, may decrease risk of developing periodontitis.

Other problems

Stomatitis: Inflammation of the oral cavity.
Candidiasis: "Thrush," caused by the organism *Candida albicans.*
Glossitis: Inflammation of the tongue.
Halitosis: Bad breath.
Cheilosis: Cracked lips.

From Black, J., & Matassarin-Jacobs, E. (Eds.). (1993). *Luckmann and Sorensen's Medical-Surgical Nursing* (4th ed.). Philadelphia: W. B. Saunders.

- Using commercially prepared mouthwashes or rinses, as needed for desired effects (decrease bacteria and **halitosis** [bad breath])
- Maintaining a healthy, well-balanced diet
- Obtaining adequate denture care and assessment of dentures (make sure dentures fit well, are not broken, and do not cause pain); seeking prompt assistance if denture problems are noted

Care of Eyes, Ears, and Nose

Eye Care

Routine eye care is usually very basic and mostly involves assessment skills. The normal eye is self-contained and protected by the eyelids and eyelashes. The eyes are also continuously cleansed by natural tear activity (Fig. 22–4). The eyes should be carefully assessed for any abnormal anatomy or lesions, abnormal discharge or tearing, the presence of any infec-

tions such as conjunctivitis (inflammation of the conjunctiva), and the use of any visual aids (glasses, contact lenses). An ocular history should also be obtained from the client regarding previous eye injuries, infections, surgeries, visual limitations (*i.e.,* night or color blindness), decrease in visual perception, history of cataracts, glaucoma or other eye conditions, and the use of any ocular medications. If any visual aids, such as glasses or contact lenses, are worn, then the nurse should ask the client when he or she needs such devices (*e.g.,* just for reading) and the normal care routine (*e.g.,* with contact lens care). Does the client have an artificial eye? If so, how does he or she care for it?

A normal eye assessment would show the following:

- Both eyes are centered on the face
- Eyelids (upper and lower) open in close approximation with the eyeball
- The sclera are clear
- There is no redness, edema, lesions, or drainage noted on the eyelids or lid margins
- Upper and lower lid lashes are turned outward
- Pupils are round and not dilated
- No excess tearing is noted from the eyes
- Gross eye movements are symmetrical

Routine eye care includes simply washing around the eyes with a warm, moist washcloth. Soap or astringents should not be used around the eyes, as they may be irritating. Special attention should be made to the medial canthus area, where normal secretions may pool or crust. Such secretions should be gently removed with a warm, moist washcloth. If a client has conjunctivitis, then it is important for the nurse and the client to observe meticulous handwashing after contact with eye secretions to prevent the spread of infection to other persons.

Clients who are unconscious have special eye care needs. Because they are unconscious, they do not blink frequently enough to produce adequate tearing to cleanse the eyes naturally. These clients require frequent eye care to remove accumulated secretions and also may require the use of artificial tears or a similar lubricant, as ordered by a physician to keep the eyes moist. Dry eyes are more prone to infection and injury. If the unconscious client is unable to keep his or her eyelids closed, a light patch may be applied to keep the eyes closed protecting the cornea from becoming dry or irritated (see the box entitled "Effects of Aging on the Eye").

Ear Care

Routine ear care usually involves simple cleansing and inspection of the outer ear (Fig. 22–5). However, when **cerumen** (wax) production is visible in the external ear canal or when clients complain of hearing deficits due to cerumen buildup, hygiene procedures should include the removal of such cerumen. Ceru-

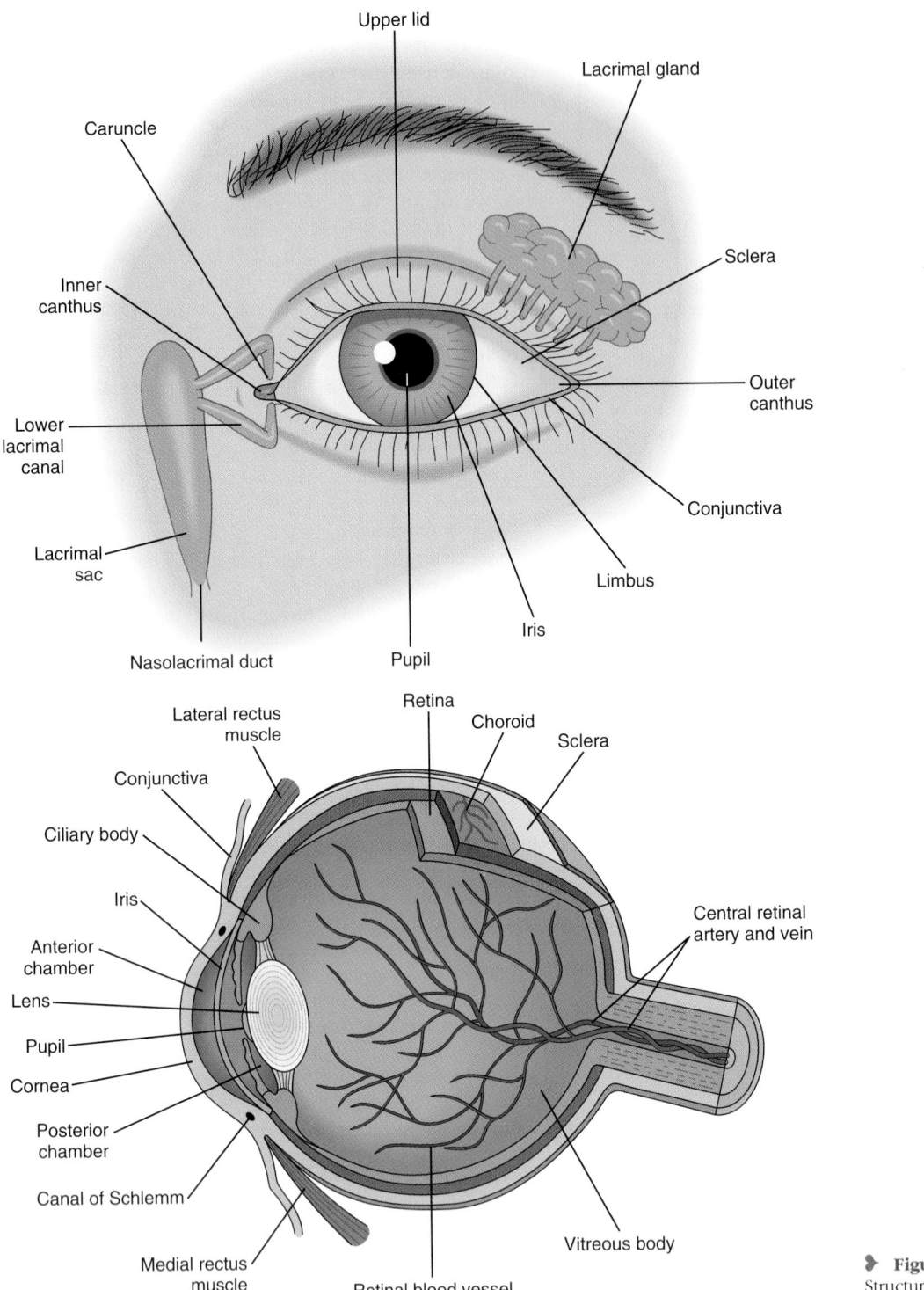

❧ **Figure 22–4**
Structures of the normal eye.

men can affect hearing because it interferes with sound conduction through the external ear canal. Obvious cerumen does not necessarily indicate poor hygiene; it may indicate that the client simply produces more cerumen than is usually seen. Those clients who know they produce more cerumen than usual should have their ears checked by a health care provider frequently to avoid a cerumen impaction.

For most clients, gently cleansing the ear canal with a clean, moistened washcloth is all that is needed as part of daily routine hygiene care. If visible cerumen is noted, a gentle downward motion with the washcloth may remove it. However, if impacted cerumen is noted, the client will need to have the impaction removed by irrigation (usually done by a physician or nurse practitioner). Prior to irrigation, the

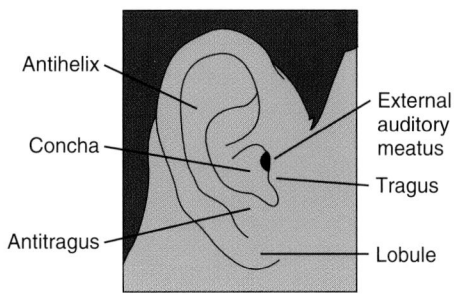

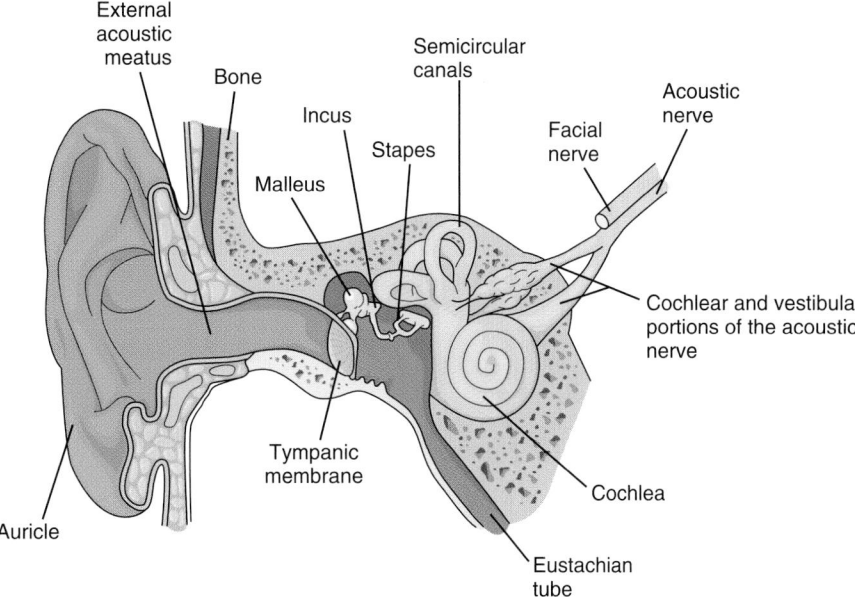

 Figure 22–5
Structures of the normal ear.

---

client should use softening agent drops, such as Debrox, in the impacted ear canal for several days. Irrigation can then be done easily with about 250 ml of warm water. Clients should be instructed *never* to cleanse ears with cotton-tipped applicators or sharp objects. These objects often push the cerumen against the tympanic membrane, making the impaction worse.

A short history should be obtained from the client regarding any ear problems. Such a history should include information about injuries, surgical procedures, infections, medications, hearing deficits, the use of hearing assistive devices, and any inner ear troubles that might affect balance. A normal assessment of the ear would provide the following observations:

* The auricles, or pinna, are well developed and easily visualized
* The auricle is attached to the side of the head at approximately a 10-degree angle
* The auricle is flexible
* No lesions, drainage, or growths are noted
* The ears are symmetrically located
* The client does not exhibit any signs of a hearing deficit (Black & Matassarin-Jacobs, 1993)

Older people have changes in the external auditory canal that may affect the production and movement of cerumen, which may cause some conductive hearing loss. These people need to pay special attention to ear hygiene practices (Ney, 1993) (see Box).

Hearing impairments occur in about 25 to 40% of people older than 65 years, and the figure increases to more than 90% of people in their ninth decade of life (Ney, 1993). (Hearing aids and their care are discussed in the implementation section of the nursing process.) Because hearing difficulties are so prevalent, nurses need to be aware of how they communicate with hearing-impaired clients so that effective communication may be accomplished (Box 22–4).

Nose Care

The nose allows a person to smell and also protects the respiratory tract from the entrance of foreign bodies. The nose controls temperature and humidity of inhaled air. Problems within the nasal passages, such as crusting of secretions or swelling of tissue, can impede normal breathing and cause distress. Careful assessment of the nose and nasal passages, as well as the employment of simple hygiene measures, such as removing secretions with a soft tissue or moist washcloth, is important. Clients who experience dry, crusting secretions may need to increase the humidity in their environment or may use topical lubricants, such as petroleum jelly, to moisten secretions for removal. Picking of crusted secretions should be discouraged, as this can lead to trauma of the membranes.

Assessment of the nose should reveal placement in midface; no swelling, lesions, or growths; moist, pink nasal mucosa; and no active secretions. The client should be able to breathe freely through both nares. A client history should include information about any previous trauma, surgical procedures, problems with breathing or smelling, medications, abnormal bleeding or secretions, or history of sinus prob-

EFFECTS OF AGING ON THE EAR

* The hairs in the ear become coarser, resulting in less movement and a potential for retaining cerumen
* Presbycusis (hearing loss in the elderly) is a result of changes in the labyrinthine structures that produce loss of sounds, predominantly at higher frequencies
* Presbycusis may also be associated with stiffening of the tissues of the cochlea
* Presbycusis is mainly treated with the use of hearing aids, as it cannot be treated medically or with surgery

---

Box **22–4**

IMPROVING COMMUNICATION WITH HEARING-IMPAIRED CLIENTS

* Get the client's attention by raising an arm or hand.
* Stand with a light on your face; this will help the client speech read.
* Talk directly to the client while facing him or her.
* Speak clearly, but do not overaccentuate words.
* Speak in a normal tone; do not shout. Shouting overuses normal speaking movements and may cause distortion and be too loud for the client with sensorineural damage. If the client has conductive loss only, sometimes making the voice louder without shouting is helpful.
* If the client does not seem to understand what is said, express it differently. Some words are difficult to "see" in speech reading, such as "white" and "red."
* Move closer to the client and toward the better ear.
* Write out proper names or any statement that you are not sure was understood.
* Do not smile, chew gum, or cover the mouth when talking.
* Inattention may indicate tiredness or lack of understanding.
* Use phrases to convey meaning rather than one-word answers. State the major topic of the discussion first and then give details.
* Do not show annoyance by careless facial expression. Clients who are hard of hearing depend more on visual clues for understanding
* Encourage the use of a hearing aid if it is available; allow the client to adjust it before speaking.
* In a group, repeat important statements and avoid asides to others in the group.
* Avoid the use of the intercommunication system because this may distort sound and cause poor communication.
* Do not avoid conversation with a client who has hearing loss. It has been said that to live in a silent world is much more devastating than to live in darkness, and clients with hearing loss appear to have more emotional difficulties than do those who are blind.

From Black, J., & Matassarin-Jacobs, E. (Eds.). (1993). *Luckmann and Sorensen's Medical-Surgical Nursing* (4th ed.; p. 891). Philadelphia: W. B. Saunders.

---

lems and allergies. Client education includes teaching about routine nasal assessments, prompt treatment for abnormal findings, the use of humidifiers as needed, not picking at nares, and not blowing the nose with excessive force.

Clients who have special hygiene needs regarding

the nasal area include those who have nasogastric tubes in their nares. Such tubes should be secured comfortably with tape. The nares with the tube should be assessed frequently for possible skin breakdown, redness, swelling, or discomfort. Secretions around the tube should be cleansed frequently. A cotton-tipped applicator may be used to cleanse debris from around the tube.

♦ Foot Care and Nail Care

The care of a person's feet and nails can be very important, especially for those clients with diabetes or poor circulation to their lower extremities. In these clients, incidental problems, such as a small wound or an ingrown toenail, may become serious sites for infection. Age may be a factor in the care of feet and nails (Box 22–5). As a person ages, his or her nails become thicker and harder, which may make it difficult for the client to trim his or her own nails. Because the back of an older client may not be flexible, he or she may be unable to assess the feet and nails on a routine basis. Thus he or she may not notice problems with his or her feet until they become quite serious.

The feet also support total body weight, and if these are problems with the feet, then there are usually problems with mobility. It is very important that nurses assess feet and nails carefully while providing or assisting with hygiene measures to clients. If problems are noted, prompt interventions prevent more serious problems from developing. Common foot and nail problems include the following:

Bunions (hallux valgus)—a swelling of the bursa of the foot, usually of the metatarsophalangeal joint to the great toe, appearing as a lateral deviation of the great toe

Hammer toes—abnormal flexion of the proximal interphalangeal joint of one of the lesser four toes

Plantar warts—warts that usually appear on the sole of the foot; they are caused by the virus *Papovavirus hominis* and can be painful during walking; they are usually removed by a physician; the virus is moderately contagious

Corns—painful circular thickening of skin over a bone; corns commonly occur on a toe at a joint; sometimes corns can be so deep that they attach to the bone and are generally removed surgically

Calluses—thickened portions of epidermis, usually caused by pressure from shoes; they are usually located on the bottom or sides of the foot over a bony prominence; calluses are usually painless and flat

Ingrown toenails—inward growth of the nail into soft tissues around the nail; it is caused most often by improper nail trimming; ingrown toenails can be painful when pressure is applied over the area or if they become infected (Gregory, 1994)

First, a careful nursing assessment must be done. Assessment of the feet would require the nurse to:

Box 22–5

AGE-RELATED NAIL CARE NEEDS

Infants and Toddlers

1. Infants should have their nails trimmed straight across with blunt scissors or blunt baby nail clippers

2. Infants often scratch their face (especially while sleeping), so it is important to keep nail edges smooth

3. It is best to trim infants' nails while they are sleeping to prevent injury

4. Toddlers may enjoy having their nails trimmed as part of their clean-up rituals

School-Age Children

1. School-age children should have their nails trimmed routinely, as long, jagged nails may injure other children during group play activities

2. Nails should be assessed for nail biting habits, which may form during this age

3. Over-the-counter preparations are available to assist children to stop biting nails, as severe nail biting can often lead to infections

Adults and Older Adults

1. Normal physiologic changes in older adults may affect their nails by making them hard, thick, and brittle; such changes may predispose the older client to breaks in skin integrity and infection

2. Older clients may need to soak their nails in warm, soapy water before trimming

3. Nails should be trimmed straight across and filed smooth

- Ask client about his or her normal foot care routine
- Observe client walking around the room—note any trouble with gait or complaints of foot discomfort
- Observe condition of client's shoes and socks, noting cleanliness and areas of wear to shoes
- Assess client's feet and toes and nails for cleanliness, sores, lesions, hydration status, fungal growths, cracks, and other problems
- Assess lower legs and ankles for edema, skin temperature changes, and peripheral vascular problems (purple discoloration, weak pedal or post tibial pulses)
- Inspect toenails for any problems (*e.g.*, ingrown nails; thickened, overgrown, or discolored nails)
- Check point sensation of lower legs and feet with blunt point
- Inspect sides and bottom of feet for problems such as corns, calluses, bunions

Clients may also require care of their fingernails. If fingernails are jagged and have sharp borders, they

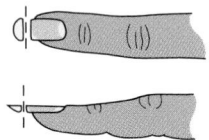

Figure 22–6
When the client is unable to trim his or her own nails, cut the nail straight across and file the edges.

need to be filed straight across and smoothed with a fingernail file (Fig. 22–6). Jagged nails may scratch skin or cause interruption in skin integrity, which could lead to infection.

Care of the toenails is often difficult for clients, especially older adults, to perform. Special care must be used when providing toenail care:

* Always trim or cut toenails after a bath or shower or after soaking in warm soapy water for 15 to 20 minutes
* Avoid clipping or cutting entire nail at once, clip or cut small areas of nail at a time
* Clip or cut nail straight across; do not clip or cut nails at the corners. Short, rounded edges may expose some of the toe tissue that the toenail is meant to protect
* Refer clients with extremely thick nails or other nail problems to a podiatrist or foot clinic for follow-up care
* Dry feet and nails well after procedure before putting on socks or shoes

Clients often enjoy receiving foot and nail care, and this provides a very good opportunity for client teaching. Teaching the basic care skills, as have already been discussed, should include information about:

1. Purchasing shoes that fit well and are made well
2. The importance of good nutrition
3. Walking slowly and using a heel-to-toe motion to avoid injury
4. Wearing clean socks that fit comfortably in shoes
5. Seeking medical attention when alterations in feet and nails are noticed
6. Performing routine foot and nail assessments; if self-assessment cannot be easily performed, then the client should have someone else assess or use a mirror

Special Diabetic Foot Care

The client with diabetes mellitus requires special attention in caring for his or her feet. The disease process of diabetes seriously affects the nerve fibers in the body—especially those in the extremities. This condition is called diabetic neuropathy and is usually caused by vascular insufficiency, chronic elevations in blood glucose levels, hypertension, cigarette smoking, and increasing age. Neuropathy in the lower extremities may cause the client to have an inability to per-

ceive pain, which is a very dangerous condition. Because the client cannot feel pain in his or her feet or toes, he or she may be totally unaware that an injury has occurred.

Such injuries can be very serious because of the decreased ability to fight infection, especially in the lower extremities. There is usually a reduced blood supply to the feet with diabetes, which causes delayed healing of foot lesions. Delayed healing can lead to serious complications such as ulcerations and even gangrene. For these reasons, meticulous foot care principles should be reviewed with all diabetic clients (see Box).

HEALTH PROMOTION AND PREVENTION

CLIENT EDUCATION FOR SPECIAL DIABETIC FOOT CARE

Daily Foot Care

1. Assess feet daily. Use good lighting and a mirror to see bottom of feet. If needed, have significant other, or family member assist with assessment.
2. Do not wash feet with harsh soaps or chemicals or use hot water. Wash feet daily.
3. Dry feet well after cleansing.
4. Do not use lotions between toes.
5. Lotions may be used on bottoms of feet if feet are dry.
6. Never use a razor, knives, or corn remedies to remove calluses or corns.
7. Do not use heating pads, hot water bottles, or electric blankets on feet.
8. Never go barefoot; wear shoes or slippers at all times.
9. Always wear comfortable shoes that fit well.
10. Break in new shoes gradually.
11. Change socks daily and check socks for any signs of infections, such as bleeding or pus.

Nail Care

1. Cut toenails straight across, and file rough edges as needed.
2. Trim nails after a shower, bath, or foot soak.

Injuries

1. Assess feet daily for signs of injury or infection (*i.e.,* redness, swelling, drainage, odor).
2. If injury is noted, cleanse area with soap and water and cover with a dry gauze dressing.
3. Notify physician immediately if signs of infection are noted.

Hair Care

The appearance of one's hair is often a very important part of one's sense of well-being. This sense of well-being is interrupted when a client is sick and unable to tend to his or her hair as he or she might otherwise. The appearance of one's hair can also reflect one's health status. For example, many people undergoing chemotherapy experience hair loss. Hair loss and color changes may also be associated with the aging process.

People tend to have a hair care routine that is included in their overall hygiene routine. Some people wash their hair daily, while others might do so less frequently. Adolescents tend to spend a great deal of time grooming their hair, partly because hormonal changes increase the oil content in their hair and partly because experimenting with their sense of personal identity is a characteristic of this developmental stage. Hair care routines are also often influenced by cultural factors that influence the hair. For example, people of African descent often have very dry hair, which requires that they apply oil to their scalp on a daily basis. For these people, washing hair once a week is sufficient because their hair tends to be very dry.

Developmental changes influence hair care needs. Many newborns have little, if any, hair on their scalp. By the end of their first year, hair is usually noticeable. Infants, toddlers, and school-age children require hair care (most do not require daily shampooing). As mentioned previously, during adolescence, hormonal changes may cause hair to be more oily. Changes in routine hair care must follow to meet their body's changing needs. In older age, hair may become thinner, grow more slowly, and begin to gray. Some older people lose their scalp hair and become completely bald. Axillary and pubic hair also becomes finer and thinner with advancing age.

Assessment of the hair is a routine part of the nursing assessment. It is important to have a good look at the client's hair in relation to his or her age, physical condition, and cultural background. It is also important to ask the client how he or she usually cares for his or her hair, if he or she has any deficits with self-care, and if he or she has a history of hair or scalp problems.

Common hair and scalp problems are as follows:

Alopecia
　Acute hair loss
　Chemotherapy, hypothyroidism, and radiation of the head may cause this acute hair loss

Dandruff
　Diffuse scaling of the epidermis of the scalp
　Usually is accompanied by itching and flaking, whitish scales

Hair loss
　Natural hair loss associated with age and heredity

Pediculosis (lice)
　Pediculus capitis (head louse)
　Pediculus pubis (crab louse)
　Lice are parasitic insects that can infect humans
　Head and pubic lice lay their eggs, which look like white oval particles, on the hairs
　Can be contracted from infested clothes or direct contact with an infected person
　Often seen in school-age children
　Often treated with gamma benzene hexachloride shampoo

Scabies
　Skin infestation by the itch mite
　Contagious
　Mite penetrates upper layers of skin, commonly between the webs of the fingers and folds of wrists and elbows
　Produces very intense itching, which is more pronounced at night

Hirsutism
　Excessive growth of body hair

Such information would be noted in the client's record. Hair care would be maintained as close to the normal routine as possible to fasten a sense of well-being. Hair should be brushed or combed daily. The hair should be arranged so it is out of the way of the client's face and does not interfere with any therapeutic procedures.

Environmental Hygiene

The environment where care is provided should always be safe and clean. Although housekeeping services are provided, especially in hospital settings, it is the nursing staff who must assess the client's environment on an ongoing basis and implement environmental hygiene measures as needed.

Safety is very important within a client's living space, whether that be in an institution or at home (see Community Based Care Box). Beds should always be in the low position, and the wheels should be locked. Walking paths should always be free of clutter and unnecessary furniture. Floors should be dry, and carpets secured to prevent slipping or tripping. Garbage containers should not be overflowing onto the floor and should be placed out of the way. Furniture such as bedside tables or bedside cabinets should be free of clutter, garbage, or unnecessary items. Opened containers of food should never be left at the client's bedside unless they will be consumed in a reasonable amount of time. Such containers may accidentally get spilled, and the client may slip on the spill. Open containers may also attract unwanted pests.

Extra linens and client care supplies should be placed in a closet or drawer to avoid stacking items on a window sill or air duct. Only approved room equipment should be in a client's room, such as:

COMMUNITY BASED CARE

HYGIENE AND THE PHYSICAL ENVIRONMENT

Factors in the physical environment can potentially affect the client's recovery, as well as his or her safety, his or her family, and you. Simultaneously, your behavior and attitudes must always indicate that you are the *guest* and the client is the *host*. Modifying the physical environment is the client's responsibility, not yours; develop a partnership with the client and his or her family so they will make needed modifications. You may be asked to leave or not be invited to return if you are impatient and not sensitive to the values of clients and their families.

A comprehensive nursing assessment includes:

1. The neighborhood: Observe for evidence of pollution, physical hazards, crime, uncontrolled animals, and unsafe play areas when approaching the home.

2. Outside the home: Observe for inadequate lighting, unsafe entrances, lack of structural soundness, and evidence of lead-based paint when approaching the door.

3. Inside the home: Observe for inadequate supplies and equipment, inadequate water supply, inadequate sewage disposal, soiled living areas, insects or rodents, inadequate heating or cooling, steep stairs, unsafe mats or throw rugs, inadequate safety devices, and crowded living space.

Document the presence or absence of problems in the physical environment on the client's record and share pertinent information with colleagues. It is important to use these data to develop the plan of care and to schedule the date, time of day, and length of future visits. Follow the same process for collecting, analyzing, and using data about the client's physiological and psychosocial problems to provide the best possible nursing care.

Bed—the bed should always be in proper working condition with safety devices intact and client call bell in working condition and within client reach at all times

Over-bed table—the over-bed table should be in working condition and should be free of clutter at all times

Bedside chest of drawers—the bedside chest of drawers should be free of clutter at all times and should be placed near the bed for easy client access; client items, such as hygiene accessories or personal belongings, may be stored here; *note:* money or other valuable client belongings should never be kept in the client's room but should be taken home by the client's family or secured through the institution per policy

Bedside chair—the bedside chair should be clean and easy to access at all times; avoid using chairs to store equipment or linens, as this can be a safety hazard for the client

Bedside commodes—bedside commodes are used for clients who may not be able to ambulate to the bathroom; the commode should always be cleaned after client use and should also be easily accessible at all times

A client's bathroom should also be kept free of clutter to prevent injury when a client needs to use it. Keeping the client's environment clean and free of clutter provides the client with a sense of safety and also with a sense of security with his or her caregivers. These are important aspects of care and should not be overlooked.

Some clients' charts list special orders for the position of the hospital bed (Box 22–6). Many clients benefit from the use of special beds, which are different from the usual hospital bed and are used according to the special needs of the client. A major reason special beds are used is to reduce pressure over a client's bony prominences to prevent **pressure ulcers** from developing or getting worse. Pressure ulcers occur when damage or **necrosis** (morphological changes indicative of cell death) of underlying tissue occurs due to unrelieved pressure or from tissue shearing. Treating pressure ulcers can be a long and expensive process; thus, it is better to prevent such ulcers from developing in the first place. Nurses play a major role in preventing these ulcers by assessing clients at risk and then providing proper skin care and special assistive resources, such as pressure-reducing beds, mattresses, and overlays. Client risk factors for skin breakdown that must be assessed include immobility, tissue friability, poor nutrition, incontinence, impaired cognitive ability, and a decreased ability to respond to the environment (Kresevic & Naylor, 1995).

Clients who are identified at risk for skin breakdown should be assessed on an ongoing basis (see Fig. 23–1). Several rating scales are identified in the literature and are used in various institutions (see Tables 23–3 and 23–4). These rating scales assist nurses in identifying clients who need to be using a special bed, mattress, or overlay to prevent pressure ulcer formation. Getting a specialty bed, mattress, or overlay for a client usually requires a physician's order (see Box 23–9). Some clients do not require the use of special beds, mattresses, or overlays but do require a special device to protect a specific part of the body. These include the following:

Foot board—foot boards are used to prevent foot drop in certain patients; the foot board is a flat piece of wood or plastic placed vertically against the mattress at the foot of the bed

Bunny boots—bunny boots are plastic boots lined with soft sheepskin or foam, used to prevent foot drop and also to take pressure off the heel while the client is in bed

Bed cradle—a bed cradle is a curved, bridge-shaped device most often made of metal and placed over the body part that needs protection; the cradle keeps the pressure of bed linens off the affected area

Box 22–6

COMMON BED POSITIONS

Flat: The entire bed is flat, parallel with the floor

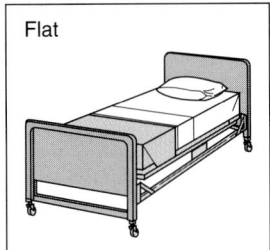

Flat

Semi-Fowler's: The head of bed is raised 30 degrees, with the foot of the bed flat; this position promotes expansion of the lungs

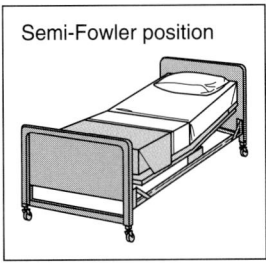

Semi-Fowler position

Fowler's: The head of the bed is raised 45 degrees or more; this position also promotes lung expansion and is most comfortable for clients while eating

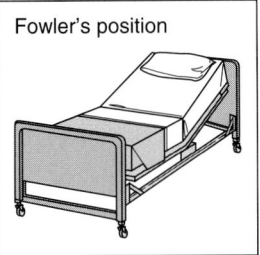

Fowler's position

Trendelenburg: The head of the bed is at an incline lower than the foot of the bed; often used when clients experience hypotension

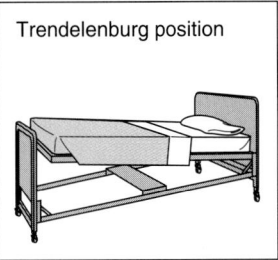

Trendelenburg position

Reverse Trendelenburg: The foot of the bed is at an incline lower than the head of the bed; often used to relieve esophageal reflux

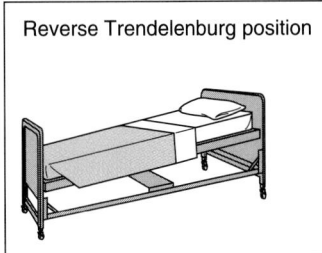

Reverse Trendelenburg position

Trapeze—a bed trapeze is a special hardware device placed on the bed frame to allow a client to move more independently in bed; most often this is used for clients with lower extremity weakness

An important part of environmental hygiene is bed-making. A clean, well-made bed provides comfort to the client. Beds are prepared in different ways for specific purposes. Most of the time, beds are made unoccupied while the client is out of the room or is sitting up in a chair. If a client cannot get out of bed, the bed must be made while the client is still in the bed. A surgical bed is made ready to receive the client after surgery (see Procedures 22–1 and 22–2).

Application of the Nursing Process Related to Hygiene

The nursing process is the process by which nurses perform their work. This process is extremely important in providing the best overall plan of care for each client. The process includes assessment, diagnosis, planning, implementation, and evaluation and plan adjustment. Each step is very important on its own but becomes essential when looking at a client's overall treatment plan. Personal hygiene can be easily

Text continued on page 529

PROCEDURE

22–1

MAKING AN UNOCCUPIED BED

Preparation: Linens are usually changed after the client's bath so that all soiled linens may be discarded together. Assess whether client can safely get out of bed and comfortably stay out of bed while bed is being made. (If client is unable to tolerate being out of bed, the nurse must make an occupied bed; see Procedure 22–2.) Assist client to a comfortable position in the bedside chair. (Note whether client is going out of the room for a test or procedure; it might be more convenient to change linens while client is absent.)

Tips and Precautions:

Do not use another client's area to place fresh linen, as this could cause cross-contamination

When holding soiled linens, always hold away from your body to avoid self-contamination

Never shake soiled linen; this could disseminate secretions and microorganisms into the air

Always work from one side of the bed to the other to conserve time and energy

Equipment:

Bottom sheet
Top sheet
Draw sheet (optional)
Blanket
Bedspread (change only if soiled)
Mattress pad (change only if soiled)
Pillow slips (for each pillow used by the client)
Waterproof pads (as needed)
Linen bag or hamper

Action	Rationale
1. Wash hands well. Wear gloves if linens are visibly soiled.	1. To avoid self-contamination.
2. Raise bed to comfortable working level.	2. To avoid joint and back strain.
3. Remove soiled linen, keeping watch for any personal items the client might have placed in the bed. Personal items can be placed in bedside cabinet.	3. To avoid loss of personal items.
4. Place pillows on bedside chair or table after removing soiled pillow slips.	4. To avoid contamination.
5. If bedspread is not visibly soiled, fold and place with pillows.	5. To avoid contamination.
6. Discard any soiled disposable pads into the appropriate trash receptacle.	6. To avoid contamination.
7. Assess mattress for any dysfunction. Pull mattress up to the head of the bed.	7. This position is most comfortable for clients.

PROCEDURE

22–1

MAKING AN UNOCCUPIED BED
(Continued)

Action	Rationale
8. Place clean bottom sheet and clean draw sheet (if needed).	**8.** Decreases chance of shearing.

    a. Some institutions use fitted bottom sheets.

    b. If a flat sheet is used, unfold sheet on bed with the hem side down. Place sheet with its center fold in the center of the bed and high enough to have a sufficient amount to tuck under the head.

    c. Unfold sheet over entire bed.

    d. Place waterproof pad or protective barrier (if needed) in the areas needed.

    e. Place draw sheet (if needed) over waterproof pad/barrier.

    f. Tuck the bottom sheet and the draw sheet under the bed on the side you are working on. A mitered corner is preferable if a flat sheet is used. The bottom sheet should be tucked under at the head of the bed. The sheet should be placed along the edge at the foot of the bed without being tucked in.

    g. Repeat steps on the other side of the bed. Remember to pull sheets smooth and tight.

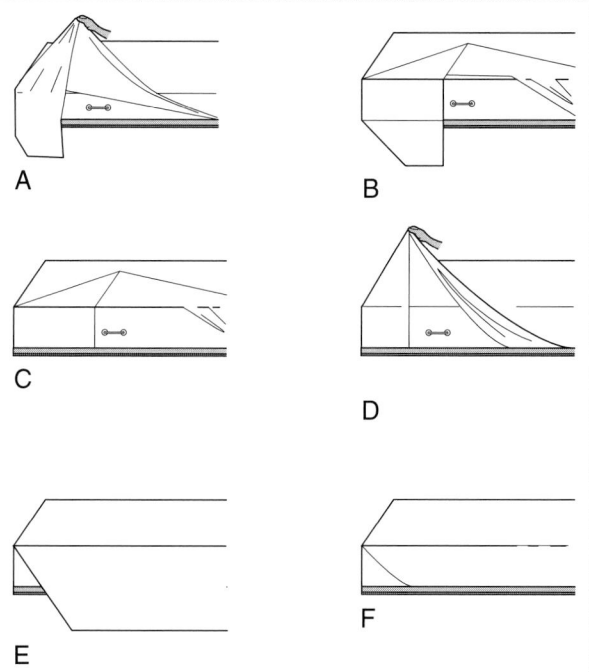

A   B

C   D

E   F

Step 8.

Continued

MAKING AN UNOCCUPIED BED
(Continued)

Action	**Rationale**
9. Place the top sheet, blanket, and bedspread:	**9.** Makes clean bed neat and tidy.

9. Place the top sheet, blanket, and bedspread:

  a. Open the top sheet on the bed, hem side up, with the center fold in the center of the bed. The top edge of the sheet should be parallel with the top edge of the mattress.

  b. Open the sheet up over the head.

  c. Allow the bottom edge of sheet the to hang over the foot of the bed.

  d. Repeat the same steps for the blanket and the spread. Allow enough space at the head of the bed for a cuff to be made with the sheet cuffed over the blanket and spread.

  e. Allow bottom edges of blanket and spread to hang over foot of bed on top of sheet.

  f. Tuck in the top sheet, blanket, and spread at the foot of the bed, using mitered corners. Leave the sides of the top sheet, blanket, and spread untucked.

  g. Cuff the top sheet over the blanket and spread at the head of the bed.

  h. Fold down the top sheet, blanket, and spread in a fanlike fashion to make the bed ready to receive the client.

9. Makes clean bed neat and tidy.

10. Place clean pillow slips on pillows:

  a. Place hand inside clean pillow slip and grasp bottom center.

10. This makes the slips go on easier and also decreases the chance of disseminating microorganisms.

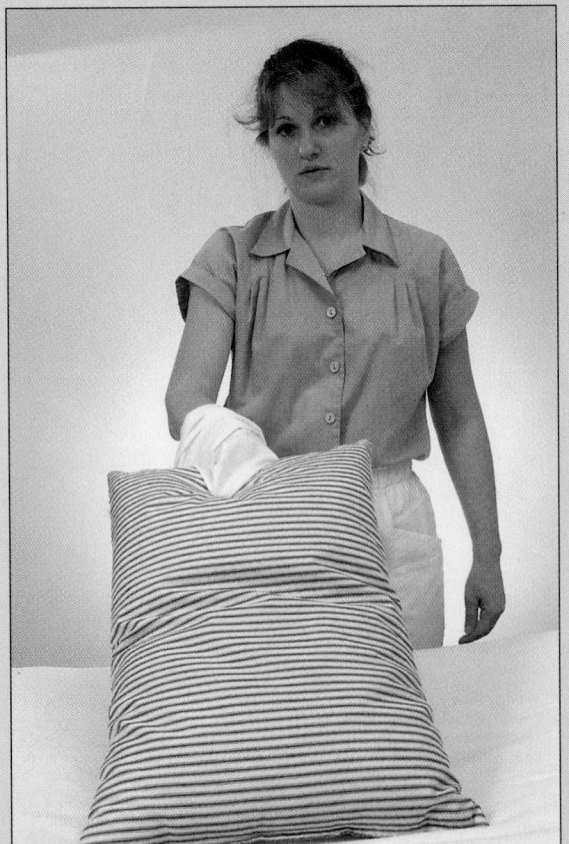

Step 10A.

MAKING AN UNOCCUPIED BED
(Continued)

Action	Rationale
b. Pull slip up over hand. c. With same hand, grasp center of one end of the pillow. d. Pull pillow slip over pillow with free hand.	

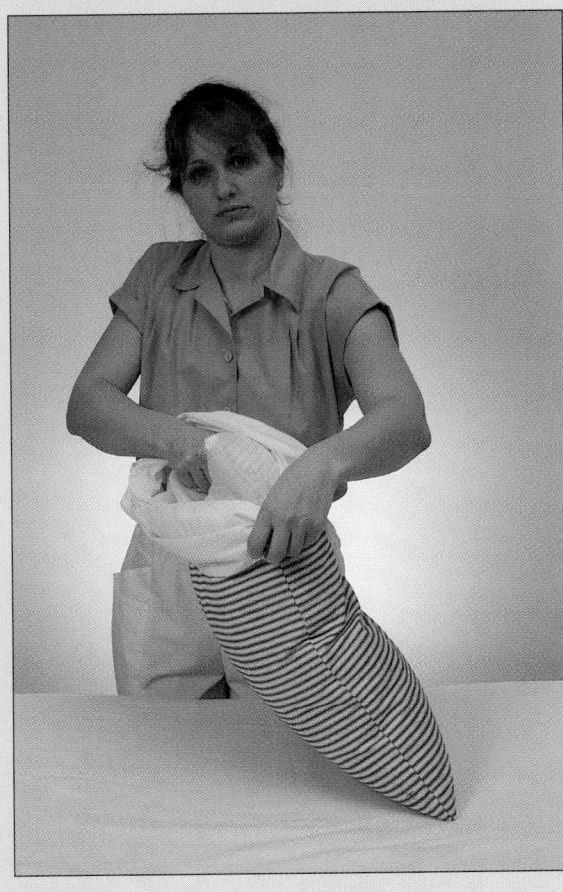

Step 10D.

Continued

PROCEDURE

22–1

MAKING AN UNOCCUPIED BED
(Continued)

Action	Rationale
e. Smooth pillow slip over pillow, especially in the corners.	

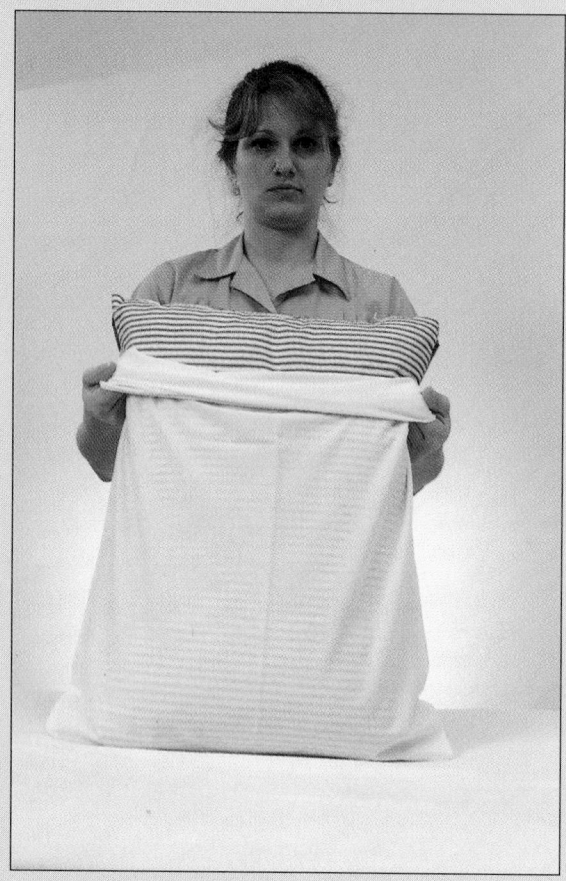

Step 10E.

f. Repeat steps for additional pillows if needed.

g. Place one pillow in center of head of bed. Additional pillows may be laced at the foot of the bed.

11. Prepare bed to receive client:
    a. Lower bed to low position and lock wheels.
    b. For a surgical bed, leave bed in high position and fan back the top sheet and bedspread.
    c. Raise side rails on one side of bed (opposite to the side of bed where the client will get in).
    d. Secure call light so client can easily reach it.
    e. Place bedside table or overbed table in convenient place for client use.
    f. Discard soiled linen.
    g. Wash hands.
    h. Assist client back into bed, if needed.

11. a. Client can safely get into bed.
    b. Client can safely transfer from the surgical cart into bed.
    c. To ensure client safety.
    d. Client can easily call for assistance.

PROCEDURE

22–2

MAKING AN OCCUPIED BED

There are occasions when a client is on strict bed rest and is unable to get out of bed while the linens are being changed. For example, a client may be too weak or may be in traction or have several monitors placed on him or her that cause him or her to be immobile. In such cases, the nurse must change soiled linens with the client remaining in the bed.

When changing an occupied bed, it is very important to keep the client in proper body alignment while changing the linen. To do so often requires the assistance of another person. It is during this time that a total skin assessment and bed bath may be done also. It is important that safety issues are noted and assistance is obtained, not only for the safety of the client, but also for the safety of the nurse. The nurse must be careful to avoid back strain when working with clients in bed and to explain procedures before implementing them.

Preparation: Assess the client's condition and activity level. Assess need for assistance with procedure and get assistance if needed. Explain the procedure to the client. If bathing is to be done, perform bathing procedure first (see Procedure 22–3). Talk to client and explain activity as it is being done, allowing client to rest as needed.

Tips and Precautions:

Do not use another client's area to place fresh linen, as this could cause cross-contamination

When holding soiled linens, always hold away from your body to avoid self-contamination

Never shake soiled linen; this could disseminate secretions and microorganisms into the air

Always work from one side of the bed to the other, to conserve time and energy

Equipment:

Bottom sheet (fitted or flat)
Top sheet
Draw sheet (optional)
Blanket
Bedspread (change only if soiled)
Mattress pad (change only if soiled)
Pillow slips (for each pillow used by the client)
Waterproof pads (as needed)
Linen bag or hamper

Action	Rationale
1. Wash hands well. Wear gloves if linens are visibly soiled.	1. To avoid self-contamination.
2. Raise bed up to comfortable level.	2. To avoid joint/back strain.
3. Secure safety devices on side of bed opposite of where you are working, even if assistance is present.	3. For client safety.
4. Remove any equipment attached to bed that can be removed.	4. To ensure client safety and ease of activity.

Continued

PROCEDURE

22–2

MAKING AN OCCUPIED BED
(Continued)

Action	Rationale
5. Remove blanket and bedspread and loosen sheet. Client may remain covered with sheet for comfort.	**5.** Do not need bulky linens when performing bath.
6. Place bed in as flat a position as the client can tolerate.	**6.** Making bed is easier with bed flat.
7. Change bottom sheet and draw sheet: 　a. Ask client to roll onto his or her side away from the side you are changing. The side rail on the side to which he or she is turning should be raised for safety. An assistant may help client stay on side while work is being done. 　b. Loosen up the linens on the side you are changing. 　c. Remove any soiled protective pads and discard appropriately. 　d. Fan fold bottom sheet toward the center of the bed and place as near to the client as possible. 　e. Place clean bottom sheet on bed with center fold in center of bed. Edge of sheet at bottom should be parallel to bottom edge of mattress. Open up sheet at center and fan fold to center, placing under the soiled linen.	**7.** a–c. Working from one side to another conserves energy. d–h. Decreases effects of shearing.

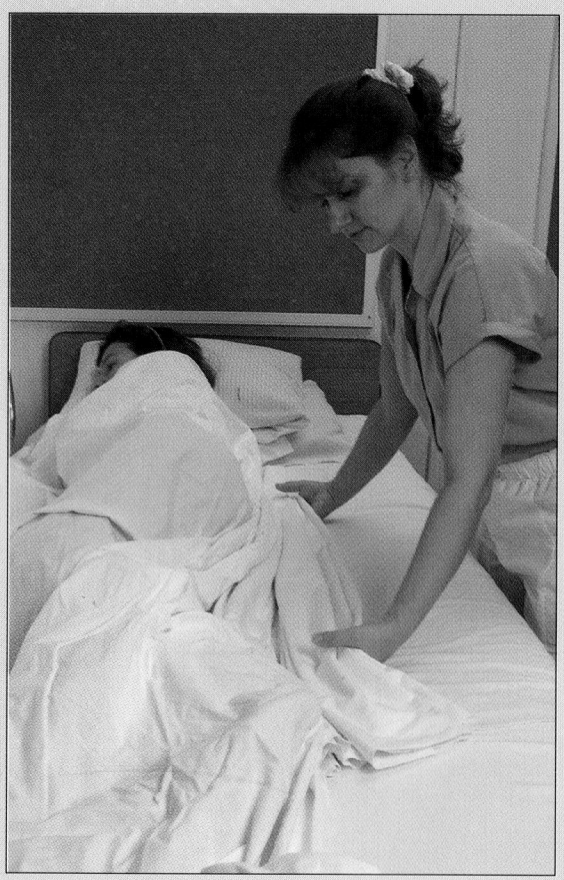

Step 7.

PROCEDURE

22–2

MAKING AN OCCUPIED BED
(Continued)

Action	Rationale
7. f. Tuck in the head and miter corner unless fitted sheet is used.	
g. Place draw sheet on bed with center fold at center of bed. Open up draw sheet and fan fold to center, placing under the clean untucked portion of the bottom sheet.	
h. Tuck in draw sheet under the side of the mattress.	
i. Raise side rails on finished side and ask client to roll over onto his or her other side. Assist client as needed. Explain that he or she will be rolling over a small "bump" where the linens have been rolled up under him or her.	
j. When client is safe and comfortable, move to other side of bed and lower side rails.	
k. Remove soiled linen and place in soiled linen bag or hamper.	
l. Unfold and smooth out fan-folded clean linens under client.	
m. Tuck in linens as done on opposite side.	
8. Reposition client and position for comfort (get assistance with this as needed).	**8.** To make client comfortable.
9. Change pillow slips as described in Procedure 22–1.	**9.** To avoid disseminating secretions and microorganisms.
10. Place pillows for client comfort.	**10.** To make client comfortable.
11. Place sheet, blanket, and bedspread over client.	**11.** To keep client warm.
12. Loosely tuck sheet, blanket, and bedspread at the foot of the bed, allowing room for client's feet.	**12.** Avoids pressure over toes—allows for comfort.
13. Assist client in safety and comfort measures; *e.g.,* secure call light within client reach, raise head of bed for comfort, raise side rails for safety, position overbed table and bedside chest of drawers for convenient client use.	**13.** Allows for safety and comfort.
14. Discard soiled linens.	**14.** Avoids cross-contamination.
15. Wash hands.	**15.** Prevents cross-contamination.

mapped out in the nursing process format, which begins with assessment.

Assessment

The hygiene assessment begins with a basic history of the client's current routine hygiene practices, current deficits that hinder him or her from performing routine hygiene care, and any additional cultural or developmental information that may assist in his or her overall hygiene history.

Next, a head-to-toe assessment must be performed by the nurse so that a baseline hygiene level might be noted. Expected findings for each hygiene area have already been explored in this chapter. Assessment findings should be compared with expected findings, and any and all deficits should be noted in the client's record.

Subjective, as well as objective, findings should be noted. It is not uncommon for the nurse to note an objective deficit, such as poor dental hygiene. The client may not subjectively be aware of such a deficit. These subjective findings should be used as a basis for initial and ongoing client education. It is extremely important that both the client and the nurse identify any self-care deficits and any knowledge deficits that may exist. The client and the nurse must both agree that certain deficits exist for the implementation phase of the treatment plan to be successful. If a client does not acknowledge the need for a specific treatment or educative process, the process will most likely not be successful.

It is important for the nurse to follow up with the identification of any special equipment needs of the client. Assistive devices, such as bedside commodes, walkers, and special beds, are usually easy to secure for clients who need them. Assistive devices might also need to be secured for the client when he or she goes home; thus, meticulous nursing assessment skills are extremely important so that the client receives the care that he or she needs.

Community Health and Discharge Planning

Currently, people do not stay in the hospital for their illnesses as long as they used to. There is great pressure on health care institutions to discharge people sooner than ever before. Clients are frequently discharged to home, often in need of follow-up nursing care in their homes. Therefore, it is essential that nurses truly begin their discharge planning on admission of the client to the institution.

On admission, nurses must evaluate all of the client's resources that might be of importance at the time of discharge. These resources include identifying any and all family members who will be available to assist the client with home care needs. These family members may need to be taught certain skills while the client is hospitalized, so it is important to identify them early so that teaching may begin as soon as possible. Economic resources need to be assessed. For example, if the client needs assistance that requires durable medical equipment, arrangements need to be made so that the client receives the equipment at discharge. Most companies that supply equipment (*e.g.,* special beds, oxygen, dressing supplies) require financial information up front, and the nurse usually arranges for this equipment while the client is still in the hospital. Other economic issues may include the client's ability to purchase nutritious food, medications, or personal hygiene items. Nurses must also assess the environment to which clients are to be discharged. Questions about the home environment might include how many steps clients must walk in their home, and whether the home environment is safe and free from clutter.

Discharge planning is very much an interdisciplinary activity. It is often the nurses who first assess the client's potential discharge needs. However, nurses may use other disciplines to assist clients in meeting these potential needs. For example, social workers may assist clients with certain economic needs and may assist clients in signing up for specific social services, such as Meals on Wheels. Dietitians may be consulted to review specific diets, such as a diabetic diet, with clients. Physicians must also be aware of potential client needs, as most home care nursing agencies require physician orders to render their services.

Many services may be required of clients on discharge, which is why prompt discharge planning is essential in coordinating a smooth transition from hospital to home care.

Nursing Diagnosis

The second phase of the nursing process is diagnosis. Examples of hygiene-related nursing diagnoses are listed in the Nursing Diagnoses box.

Activity Intolerance

Activity intolerance is a decrease in one's physiological ability to endure activities to the level desired or required. Related factors include any activity that compromises oxygen transport or lead to physical deconditioning. Such related factors may be classified as pathophysiological (*e.g.,* obesity, malnourishment), treatment related (*e.g.,* surgery, diagnostic studies), situational (*e.g.,* depression, pain), or maturational (*e.g.,* elderly with decreased muscle strength). Outcome criteria include identifying all factors that may reduce activity intolerance and allow progress toward meeting the hygiene activity goal.

Impaired Skin Integrity and Tissue Integrity

Impaired skin integrity is the actual or potential damage to epidermal and dermal tissue. Impaired tissue integrity is the actual or potential damage to the integumentary, corneal, or mucous membrane tissues. These two nursing diagnoses are closely related. Such impairment is related to pathophysiological factors (*e.g.,* diabetes, peripheral vascular alterations, cancer), treatment-related factors (*e.g.,* surgery, mechanical irritants such as dressings or tape), situational factors (*e.g.,* radiation, secretions, immobility), and maturational factors (*e.g.,* dry skin associated with advanced age). Outcome criteria should include the avoidance or resolution of impaired skin or tissue integrity.

Risk for Infection

Risk for infection is the potential invasion by an opportunistic or pathogenic agent. Related factors include pathophysiological (*e.g.,* chronic disease, diabetes, immunosuppression), treatment-related (*e.g.,* surgery, chemotherapy), situational (*e.g.,* immobility, poor hygiene, stress), and maturational (*e.g.,* open wounds, debilitated condition) factors. Outcome criteria should stress that the client will demonstrate knowledge of his or her personal risk factors associated with a risk for infection and demonstrate appropriate precautions to prevent infections.

then the ability of the client to demonstrate correction of the deficit (*e.g.*, proper care of dentures, contact lens care, foot care).

Health Maintenance, Altered

Health maintenance, altered, is a disruption of health because of an unhealthy lifestyle or lack of knowledge to manage a condition. Related factors include situational (*e.g.*, lack of motivation, lack of education or readiness to learn) and maturational factors (*e.g.*, for a child or adolescent, nutrition or substance abuse; for an adult, parenthood and safety practices; for the elderly, sensory deficits). The outcome criteria should include that the client will be able to demonstrate knowledge of lifestyles that promote health and describe signs and symptoms that would need to be reported to a health care provider (*e.g.*, diabetic foot ulcer, changing skin condition, broken dentures).

Self-Care Deficit

Self-care deficit describes a decreased ability to care for oneself due to impaired motor or cognitive function. **Self-care** includes all activities needed to meet daily needs. Related factors include pathophysiological (*e.g.*, muscle weakness, visual disturbance), treatment-related (*e.g.*, external devices, pain or fatigue), situational (*e.g.*, cognitive deficits, anxiety), and maturational factors (*e.g.*, elderly often experience a decrease in visual and motor activity). Outcome criteria should include that the client will be able to perform certain self-care activities at his or her highest possible level of function.

Sensory-Perceptual Alteration

Sensory-perceptual alteration describes altered perception and cognition influenced by physiological factors. Such alterations result when barriers or factors interfere with a client's ability to interpret stimuli accurately, such as when experiencing visual, auditory, tactile, or olfactory deficits. Related factors include pathophysiological (*e.g.*, sensory organ alterations, neurological alterations), treatment-related (*e.g.*, medications, surgery), and situational factors (*e.g.*, pain, excessive noise, loss of socialization). Outcome criteria should stress that the client can acknowledge sensory perception alterations and can identify safe compensatory activities to meet activities of daily living.

Planning

Once a nursing diagnosis has been made and outcome criteria (expected outcomes) related to the diagnosis have begun to be identified, the planning of specific care activities is addressed. The planning phase consists of setting goals, identifying priorities, selecting nursing interventions, and noting available resources to assist in reaching the expected outcomes. All activities should be planned to meet the desired

---

POTENTIAL NURSING DIAGNOSES CONCERNING HYGIENE

Activity Intolerance (Actual or at Risk For) Related To
* Obesity or malnutrition
* Surgery
* Diagnostic studies
* Depression or pain
* Decreased muscle strength

Skin Integrity, Impaired (Actual or at Risk For)

Tissue Integrity, Impaired (Actual or at Risk For) Related To
* Diabetes, peripheral vascular alterations, cancer
* Surgery, mechanical irritants (*e.g.*, dressings and tapes)
* Radiation, secretions
* Immobility
* Dry skin associated with advanced age

Knowledge Deficit Related To
* Anxiety

Health Maintenance, Altered, Related To
* Lack of motivation
* Lack of education
* Developmental stage

Self-Care Deficit Related To
* Muscle weakness, visual disturbance
* External devices
* Pain, fatigue
* Cognitive problems, anxiety
* Maturational factors

Sensory/Perceptual Alteration (Actual or at Risk For) Related To
* Sensory organ alterations, neurological alterations
* Medications, surgery
* Pain
* Excessive noise
* Loss of socialization

Knowledge Deficit

Knowledge deficit describes a deficiency in knowledge or psychomotor skills concerning the condition or treatment plan. Related factors may include anxiety, which hinders the learning process. Knowledge deficits can be detected when a client verbalizes a deficiency in knowledge or skill or expresses an inaccurate perception of health status or care procedures. Outcome criteria should include the identification and acknowledgment of a specific deficit and

SAMPLE NURSING CARE PLAN

FOOT CARE

A 75-year-old person is admitted to your medical surgical unit. During your admission history, you note that the client has been a diabetic for over 40 years. You also note that the client's feet are very dry and scaly. The client states there is little feeling in the toes or feet.

Nursing Diagnosis: Risk for Impaired Skin Integrity
Expected Outcome: Client will perform foot care correctly.

Action	**Rationale**
1. Instruct client about importance of daily assessment of feet.	**1.** Because diabetic neuropathy may decrease sensation to feet and toes, daily assessment is needed to note any lesions, bruises, or other problems that could lead to infection.
2. Discuss with client proper foot care measures.	**2.** Wound healing is often impaired with diabetics. Because of this, proper foot care may help prevent complications that go along with diabetic wounds.
3. While instructing client, observe client demonstrate proper foot care measures	
a. Carefully inspect all areas of both feet and of all toes. Make sure lighting is good. It may be helpful to have a mirror available.	a. Inspection can help identify problems with feet that may not be felt by the client. Good lighting helps to view all areas of toes and feet. A mirror can assist in viewing bottoms of toes and feet.
b. Use warm water to soak feet.	b. Because sensation is impaired, clients may not feel that the water is too hot, and burning may result.
c. Cleanse feet and toes with mild cleanser.	c. Harsh soaps may dry skin and predispose skin to cracking.
d. Dry feet and toes well after cleansing.	d. Moist areas, especially between toes, may predispose skin to breakdown.
e. Apply lotion to tops and bottoms of feet and toes as needed.	e. Softens skin and may help prevent skin from cracking.
f. Document care, instructions, and client demonstration on the client record.	f. Provides information and accountability.

outcomes for the client, as they relate to the nursing diagnosis (see Sample Nursing Care Plan).

Priorities are set according to the most prevalent needs of the client. Once these needs are prioritized, realistic goals that will serve as guides toward the attainment of expected outcomes should be written. It is important to write the goals and expected outcomes in the client's record so they can be easily evaluated for effectiveness. Once goals are identified, nursing interventions can be chosen so that the goals may be met. Expected outcomes related to hygiene must be formulated in ways in which such outcomes can be measured or evaluated.

The following are examples of expected outcomes that can be measured either by direct observation, return demonstration, or verbal acknowledgement:

1. The client will verbally acknowledge effective hygiene practices
2. The client will actively participate in specific hygiene or self-care measures at his or her optimal level of function
3. Skin will remain intact, supple, warm, and odor free
4. The client will maintain appropriate personal hygiene
5. The client will not develop problems related to total personal hygiene (skin, nails, hair, feet, eyes, ears, nose, oral cavity)
6. Oral hygiene will be maintained or enhanced
7. The client will not experience alteration in skin integrity related to foot and nail care
8. The client will verbally acknowledge actions that will enhance personal hygiene and that will decrease risks of impaired skin integrity
9. The client will not experience any sensory or perceptual alterations

Once the expected outcomes have been noted, a time frame should be identified for each outcome. The time frame may be short term, which means that the outcome will be expected on a daily basis or at the time of the client's discharge. The time frame may be long term, such as within 6 months. After expected outcomes and time frames are noted, the next step is to plan interventions that will work toward completing the expected outcomes within the time frames noted.

Sometimes the time frame will need to be changed to suit the needs of the client.

CASE STUDY Clients Have a Right to Refuse Activities
....

A 62-year-old woman has suffered a stroke, which has left her speech garbled and her left side flaccid. Otherwise, she appears in no apparent distress. When the nurse asks her if she would like her bath, she refuses. What should be the revised plan of care?

First, it is always important to allow clients as much independence as possible while still meeting their health care objectives. It is also very important to allow clients with physical deficits to maintain a sense of control.

Clients have a right to refuse activities, but often their initial refusal does not mean that they never want to perform the activity. Keeping all this in mind, when the client refuses her bath, the nurse should respond, "We don't have to do your bath now. I will come back in 30 minutes and I can assist you then." This lets the client know her bath is important and that she will be allowed to assist as much as she can. It also gives the client a sense of control over her environment, which is very important.

Implementation

Planning interventions must be personalized to each client according to his or her nursing diagnosis, expected outcomes and goals, and current state of health. Hygiene interventions within a hospital setting are often different than if the client were in a home environment. However, as much as possible, hygiene interventions should be arranged as close to the client's normal routine as possible. The hygiene interventions should also be planned to meet expected outcomes. Examples of planned hygiene interventions may include

1. Assisting with a bed bath, allowing the client to perform as much of the bath as he or she can
2. Observing the client do a skin assessment and reinforcing skin assessment technique
3. Observing the client perform oral hygiene (brushing teeth, flossing teeth, denture care) and reinforcing proper technique
4. Assisting the client with foot care and reinforcing proper skin care of the feet
5. Listening to the client as he or she describes safety measures related to sun exposure

Again, it is very important to document the effect of your nursing interventions in the client record so that adequate evaluation and possible plan modifications may be made, all of which will ultimately be of benefit to the client.

The following is a step-by-step guide to specific identified hygiene interventions.

Bathing

Most clients in the hospital receive one of several types of baths on a daily basis. The type of bath depends on the client's ability to assist in the bathing activity, his or her health status, and his or her planned therapeutic activities. If a client is independent with bathing, the nurse usually gives him or her the supplies and clean linens and gowns and allows the client to wash up independently, either at the sink, at the bedside, or in a tub or shower. If the client requires assistance, the nurse usually stays with him or her during the activity and assists as needed; this is termed a partial assist bath, or **partial bed bath.** The client may require the nurse to perform the entire bath in bed; this is termed a **complete bed bath.**

During bathing procedures, care must be taken to provide the client with privacy, safety, and warmth. The temperature of the water used should be checked on the inside of the nurse's wrist before it is used on the client's skin (Fig. 22–7). The water temperature should be comfortable and safe. Safety devices are available for use in tubs and showers. Always make sure the nursing call light is available to clients during bathing. When bathing infants and children, never leave them alone. Wash basins should be rinsed and dried well after use to prevent contamination with bacteria (Skewes, 1994). (See Procedure 22–3).

Another type of bath recently used is called a "bag bath." This method uses prepacked washcloths that are soaked in a mixture of water and nonrinsable cleanser and are packaged in individual plastic bags. A different cloth is used to cleanse each part of the client's body, and the skin is allowed to air dry. The bag bath is useful for clients with dry skin, as the drying effects of soap are avoided. The use of poten-

Text continued on page 537

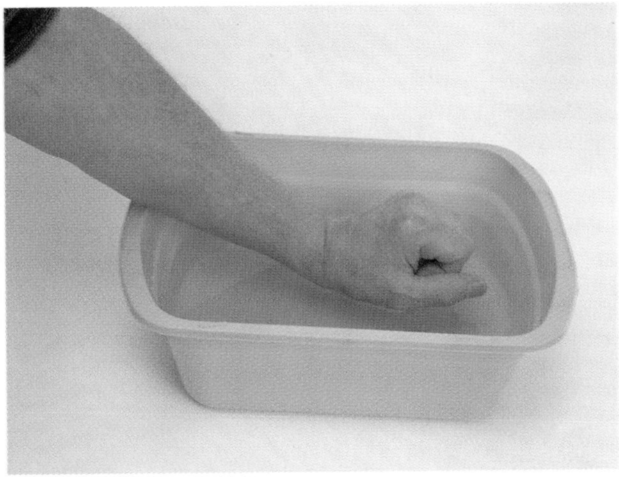

Figure 22–7
Water temperature for a bath should be comfortable against the inner wrist.

PROCEDURE

22–3

PERFORMING A BED BATH

Preparation: Assist client with use of bedpan, urinal, or commode if needed. Position client for comfort. Provide safety measures (side rails). Place water basin, towels, wash cloths, and personal hygiene products within reach. If client is not able to bathe at present time, postpone activity until client is physically and mentally able to do so.

Tips and Precautions:

Ensure privacy (close curtains and door)

Keep temperature of room comfortable

Remove clutter from overbed table

Assess client's health status and readiness to bathe

Assess client's knowledge and routine hygiene practices

Include range of motion exercises in bathing routine

Use proper body mechanics at all times during bathing activities

Perform comprehensive skin and body assessment with bathing activities

Equipment:

Wash cloth (at least two)

Towels (at least two)

Cleanser

Personal hygiene products (*e.g.,* deodorant, powder, lotion)

Bath blanket (if needed)

Clean pajamas or gown

Laundry bag or hamper

Wash basin with warm water (test temperature by placing drops of water on inner forearm)

Action	Rationale
1. Wash hands well. Wear disposable gloves.	1. To avoid cross-contamination.
2. Provide for privacy.	2. To decrease client anxiety.
3. Raise bed to comfortable level.	3. Prevents joint/back strain.
4. Fold down top sheet, blanket, and bedspread and place bath blanket over client.	4. For client comfort.
5. Remove client gown or pajamas under blanket.	5. Makes skin easily accessible.
6. Keep linens to be reused clean and dry during procedure (if client has an intravenous line, place intravenous container through arm hole of gown, unless snap gowns are used).	6. To avoid contamination or getting wet.

PROCEDURE

22–3

PERFORMING A BED BATH
(Continued)

Action	Rationale
7. Place dry towel under client's chin.	**7.** Keeps lower skin warm and dry.
8. Fold a wash cloth to make a bath mitt.	**8.** Makes cleaning skin easier.

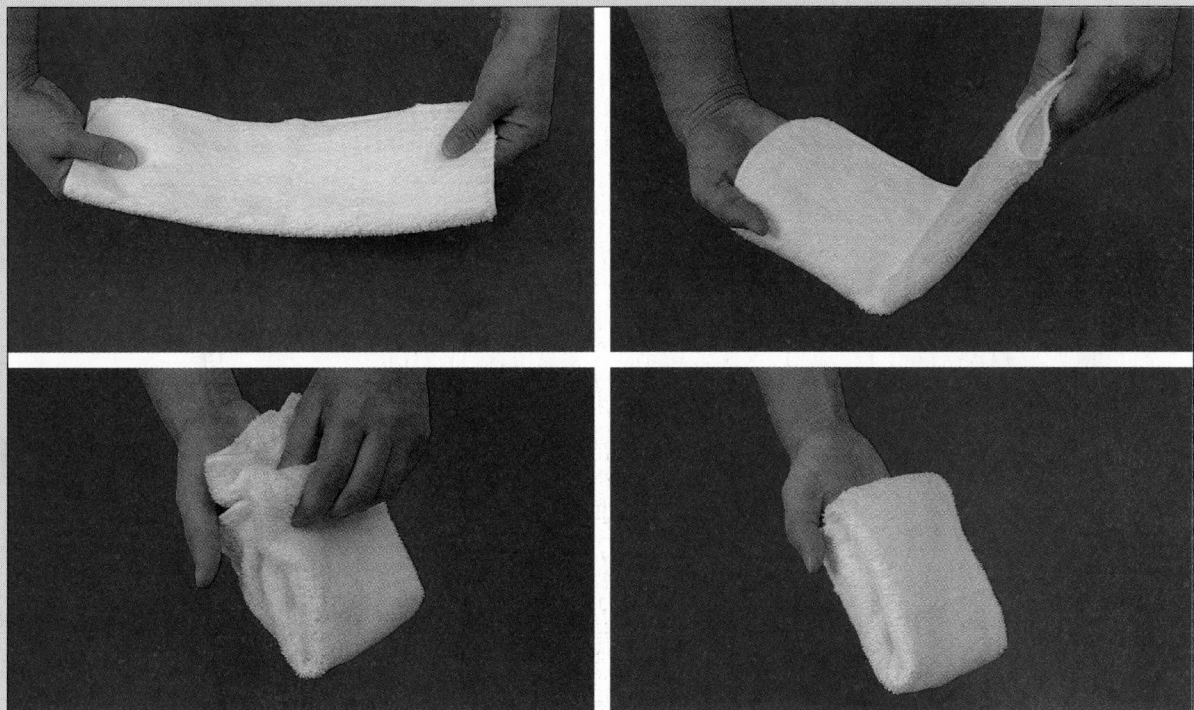

Step 8. *Rectangular fold.*

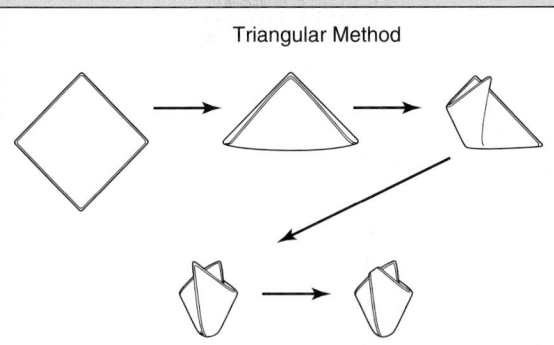

Step 8. *Triangular fold.*

Continued

PROCEDURE

22–3

PERFORMING A BED BATH

(Continued)

Action	**Rationale**
9. Wash eyes with water only. Cleanse from inner to outer canthus, using different corner of wash cloth for each eye.	**9.** Soap can be irritating to eye.

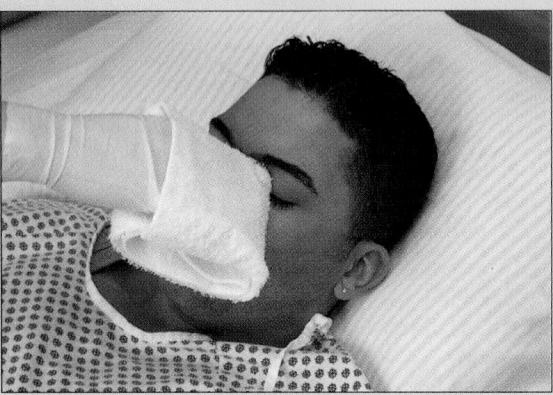

Step 9.

Action	**Rationale**
10. Wash face, neck, and ears with water only and dry with towel. Do not forget to wash back of neck.	**10.** Soap can be irritating or drying to the face, neck, and ears.
11. Cover the right side of the client while washing the left side and vice versa.	**11.** Keeps client warm.
12. Wash, rinse, and dry hands, fingers, arms, and axilla. Stroke from distal to proximal to stimulate circulation. (Remember to do range of motion to all joints while giving bath.)	**12.** Stimulates circulation and exercises joints.

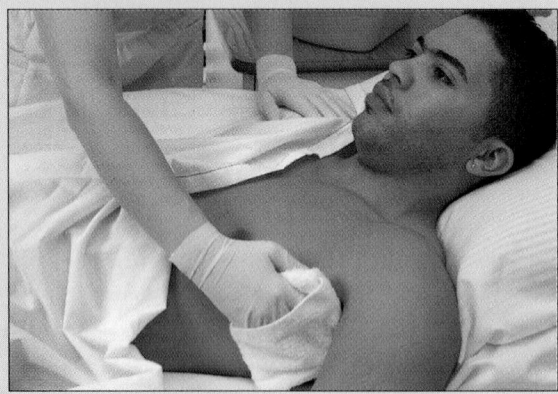

Step 12.

Action	**Rationale**
13. Apply lotion, powder, and deodorant as needed.	**13.** For client comfort.
14. Wash, rinse, and dry chest. Lower bath blanket to waist and cover one side of chest with towel while washing the opposite side.	**14.** To ensure client comfort.
15. Apply lotion as needed. Cover chest with towel.	**15.** For client comfort.

PROCEDURE

22–3

PERFORMING A BED BATH
(Continued)

Action	Rationale
16. Wash, rinse, and dry abdomen.	**16.** To provide comfort.

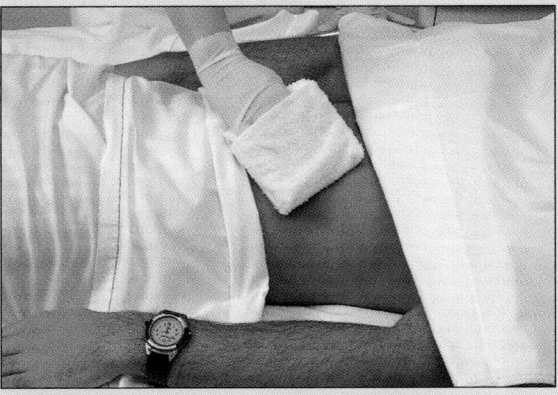

Step 16.

Action	Rationale
17. Apply lotion as needed.	**17.** To ensure comfort.
18. Place clean gown over client's arms, chest, and abdomen.	**18.** For client comfort.
19. Place bath blanket over one leg/foot while you wash, rinse, and dry opposite leg/foot. Use long strokes to clean leg and foot.	**19.** For comfort.
20. Apply lotion as needed.	**20.** To ensure client comfort.
21. Assist client to roll to one side, and wash, rinse, and dry back. Back massage may be done now (see Procedure 22–5).	**21.** For comfort.
22. Discard dirty water, rinse basin, and obtain clean basin of water for perineal care.	**22.** Avoids cross-contamination.
23. Wash, rinse, and dry genitalia and anal area (see Procedure 22–4).	**23.** Comfort.
24. Discard dirty water and linens.	**23.** Avoids cross-contamination.
25. Assist with hair and oral care.	**29.** To provide client comfort.
26. Change bed linen.	**26.** For client comfort and avoids cross-contamination.
27. Position client for comfort.	**27.** To ensure client safety and client comfort.
28. Return bed to low position.	**28.** To ensure client safety.
29. Wash hands.	**29.** Avoids cross-contamination.
30. Document procedure and assessment findings.	**30.** Provides information and accountability.

tially contaminated basins is also avoided (Skewes, 1994).

Perineal Care

Perineal care involves those hygienic measures related to care of the perineum and is an important part of personal hygiene but can often be embarrassing for the nurse and the client. If the client can perform his or her own perineal care, then he or she should do so. However, the nurse needs to assess for certain perineal problems, such as vaginal or urethral discharge, and for skin irritations. If a client has an indwelling bladder catheter, perineal assessment is also important. (See Procedure 22–4.)

Text continued on page 540

PROCEDURE

22–4

PERFORMING PERINEAL CARE

Preparation: Place supplies in convenient location for easy access.

Tips and Precautions:

Ensure privacy (close curtains and door)
Explain procedure to client
Assess if client has an indwelling bladder catheter
Assess if client has incontinence of bowel or bladder
Assess client for complaints of vaginal or urethral discharge, irritations, or other problems

Equipment:

Wash basin
Towels (two)
Wash cloths (two)
Cleanser
Powder
Disposable gloves
Laundry bag or hamper

Action	Rationale
1. Provide for safety (*e.g.,* side rails).	**1.** To ensure client safety.
2. Provide for privacy (close curtains, close door)	**2.** Decreases client anxiety.
3. Assist client with bed pan, urinal, or bedside commode if needed.	**3.** For client comfort. Best to clean area after urination/bowel movement.
4. Raise bed to comfortable position.	**4.** Prevents joint/back pain.
5. Don disposable gloves.	**5.** To prevent cross-contamination.
6. Assist female clients into dorsal recumbent position and males into supine position.	**6.** Allows for easier access to area.
7. Place waterproof pad under client.	**7.** Keeps linens dry.
8. Remove gown/pajamas/linen to expose only area to be cleansed. Clients may be draped as shown.	**8.** Decreases client anxiety.

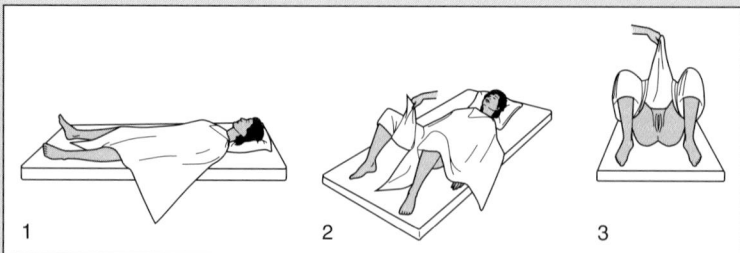

Step 8. *Providing comfort.*

PERFORMING PERINEAL CARE
(Continued)

Action	Rationale
9. Female genital care:	**9.** a–d. Cleansing from least contaminated areas to most contaminated areas helps to avoid cross-contamination.
a. Wash, rinse, and dry upper inner thighs.	
b. Wash labia majora by retracting labia with non-dominant hand and washing skin fold with dominant hand.	
c. Always wash from cleanest area to dirtiest area (from perineum to rectum).	
d. Wash urethral meatus and vaginal orifice in the same manner as in step B. Always use separate section of washcloth for each stroke. Carefully cleanse labia minora, clitoris, and vaginal orifice.	
e. Dry areas well and apply powder if needed.	

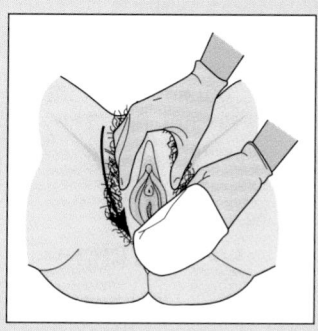

Step 9.

Action	Rationale
10. Male genital care:	**10.** a–d. Cleansing from least contaminated areas to most contaminated areas helps to avoid cross-contamination.
a. Gently cleanse tip of penis and urethral meatus first. (If client is not circumcised, the foreskin must be retracted; if client has an erection, provide care at later time.)	
b. Cleanse shaft of penis and scrotum with clean washcloth.	
c. Rinse and dry areas well.	
d. Apply powder if needed.	

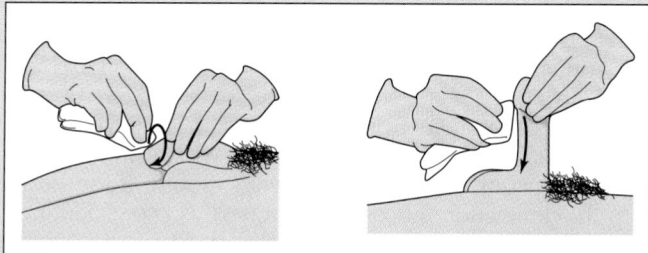

Step 10.

Action	Rationale
11. Rectal care:	**11.** a–b. Most comfortable position for activity also exposes area well.
a. Assist client to side-lying position.	
b. Cleanse, rinse, and dry rectal area with a clean washcloth.	c. Such areas need intervention.
c. Note any reddened areas or irritations on coccyx area.	d. To avoid skin breakdown.
d. Apply moisture barrier products if needed (if client is incontinent).	

Continued

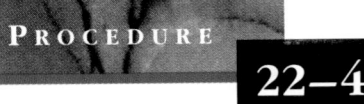

PERFORMING PERINEAL CARE
(Continued)

Action	Rationale
12. Position client for comfort.	**12.** For client comfort.
13. Place bed in low position.	**13.** To provide client safety.
14. Discard soiled linens.	**14.** To avoid cross-contamination.
15. Discard gloves and wash hands.	**15.** To avoid cross-contamination.
16. Document procedure and any abnormal assessment findings.	**16.** For ongoing client record.

Back Rub

Back rubs are often comforting to clients. Back rubs can also stimulate circulation and assist in relation. Furthermore, providing a back rub allows the nurse the opportunity to assess the skin on the back and look for any pressure points that may have developed along the spine. The back rub usually follows the client's bath and can take from 3 to 5 minutes to complete. (See Procedure 22–5.)

Antiembolism Stockings

Antiembolism stockings and devices, such as sequential compression devices are worn on the lower extremities to enhance venous blood flow and avoid venous stasis, which could lead to deep vein thrombosis or pulmonary embolus, both of which are serious conditions. Clients who have decreased mobility or are immobile are at greater risk for developing such conditions. When these stockings or devices are in place, they may be removed for a short time so that the lower extremities and feet may be washed.

Elimination Hygiene

Clients who use bedpans, urinals, and bedside commodes often need perineal hygiene after each elimination activity and often require assistance from the nurse with this. These clients often have impaired mobility. It can be embarrassing or uncomfortable for clients to ask for assistance with elimination needs. Therefore, it is important to assist clients with their needs in a kind and gentle fashion. Clients should be assisted for comfort, especially when using a bedpan. They should be allowed privacy and enough time so that they do not feel hurried (see Chapter 31).

Clients who can should be encouraged to use a bedside commode if they cannot ambulate into the bathroom. A bedside commode, which looks like a bathroom commode, is a portable chair with an opening in the center. Under the opening is a pail that can easily be removed and cleansed after each use. Clients usually prefer to use a bedside commode rather than a bedpan if the activity is allowed. Toilet tissue should be easily available to clients, and they should be instructed to call for nursing assistance when using the commode so they do not fall. They may also require assistance with washing of hands and perineal hygiene measures.

Oral Hygiene

Proper oral hygiene includes at least daily brushing and flossing of the teeth and stimulation of the gums. Brushing of teeth not only removes particles that may be trapped in the teeth but also comforts the client by making his or her mouth taste fresh and clean. Brushing also can help in preventing dental caries by removing bacteria from the teeth and gums. Children as well as adults need reinforcement by the nurse on the proper technique of brushing and flossing the teeth. (See Procedure 22–6.)

Denture Care

Clients often present with artificial dentures. They may have a few false teeth, an upper plate, a lower plate, or a full set of artificial teeth. If the client has only a few artificial teeth, they may be connected to a bridge, which may or may not be removable from the client's mouth. If the bridge can be removed, it can be cleansed as other dentures are, and the client's natural teeth can be brushed and flossed as usual also. Clients should be encouraged to use their dentures while in the hospital. However, if they choose not to, it may be safer for the client's family to take the dentures home to prevent loss or breakage of the dentures.

Although artificial teeth cannot decay, they can harbor microorganisms that can then contribute to oral cavity problems. Thus, dentures need to be removed and cleaned at least once each day. Clients often prefer privacy when performing denture care, as they

Text continued on page 545

PROCEDURE

22–5

PERFORMING A BACK RUB

Preparation: Ask client if he or she would like a back rub. Provide for safety (*e.g.,* side rails). Provide for privacy (close curtains, close door).

Tips and Precautions:

Ensure privacy (close curtains/
  door)
Explain procedure to client
Assess skin and spinal areas
  for lesions or reddened
  pressure points

Equipment:

Powder and/or lotion

Action	Rationale
1. Provide for privacy.	**1.** To decrease client anxiety.
2. Assist client to a side-lying position.	**2.** Most comfortable position for activity.
3. Adjust bed to high position.	**3.** To prevent joint/back strain.
4. Expose client's back, shoulders, and upper arms. Cover rest of body with towel, blanket, or pajamas.	**4.** To ensure privacy.
5. Apply moderate amount of lotion in hands and warm lotion.	**5.** Lubricates skin for back rub.
6. Explain to client that lotion may feel a little cool.	**6.** Decreases client anxiety.
7. Begin massaging at lower back and move upward toward shoulders.	**7.** Helps relax client, as shoulders and upper back are usually the most tight.
8. Using both hands—one on the right side and one on the left side of the back—massage in a circular motion.	**8.** Increases circulation to back.

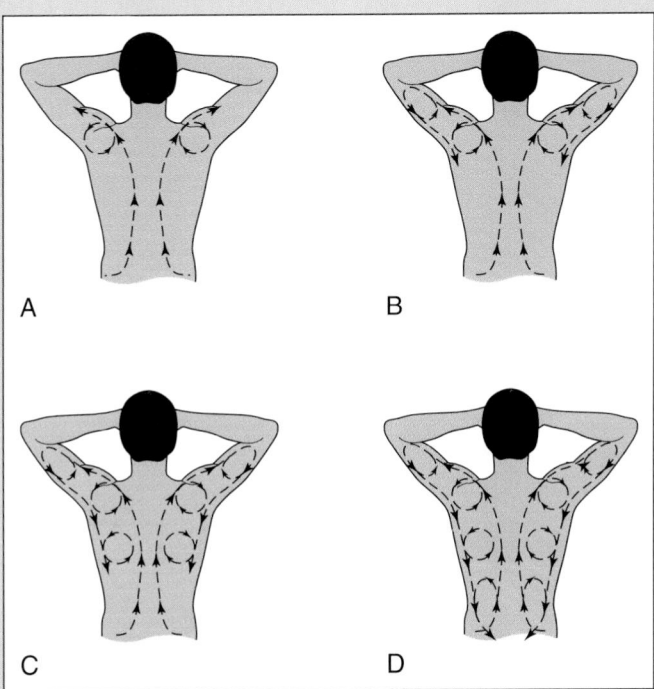

A   B

C   D

Method of giving a backrub.

Continued

PROCEDURE

22–5

PERFORMING A BACK RUB
(Continued)

Action	Rationale
9. Keep hands on client during entire massage (3–5 min).	9. Allows for comfort and reassurance.
10. Pat dry any excess lotion left on client's back.	10. To ensure client comfort.
11. Assist client to a comfortable position.	11. To provide client comfort.
12. Lower bed to low position.	12. To ensure client safety.
13. Wash hands.	13. Avoids cross-contamination.

PROCEDURE

22–6

BRUSHING AND FLOSSING TEETH

Preparation: Collect supplies and place them in convenient location at client bedside for easy access.

Equipment:

Toothbrush
Toothpaste
Dental floss
Mouth rinse
Cup of tepid water
Towel
Curved basin (emesis basin)
Disposable gloves

Action	Rationale
1. Provide for safety (*e.g.,* side rails).	1. To ensure client safety.
2. Explain procedure to client.	2. Decreases client anxiety.
3. Assist positioning client for comfort.	3. For client comfort.
4. Raise head of bed as much as possible.	4. Helps prevent aspiration of fluids.
5. Wash hands.	5. Prevents cross-contamination.
6. Don disposable gloves.	6. Prevents cross-contamination.
7. Place towel under client's chin.	7. Keep client's chin and neck dry.
8. Moisten toothbrush in cup of water.	8. Softens brush bristles.
9. Apply toothpaste to brush.	9. Acts as a cleansing agent.
10. Place the emesis basin under client's chin.	10. To keep client's chin and neck dry.
11. Inspect the mouth, gums, and teeth.	11. While oral cavity is exposed is the best time to perform assessment.

PROCEDURE

22–6

BRUSHING AND FLOSSING TEETH
(Continued)

Action	Rationale

Brushing

12. Brush the client's teeth, holding the bristles at a 45-degree angle.

12. Removes plaque buildup and food particles.

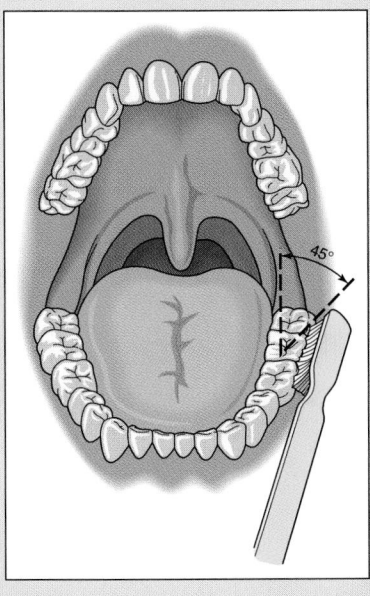

Step 12.

Brush from the gum line to the crown of the tooth in a semicircular motion.

13. Brush the biting surfaces of the teeth by moving the brush back and forth on top of the tooth's surface.

13. Removes food particles.

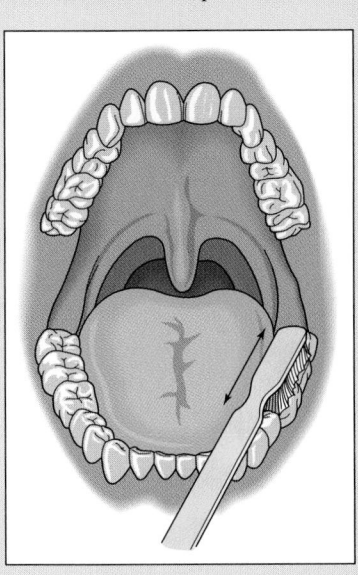

Step 13.

Continued

PROCEDURE

22–6

BRUSHING AND FLOSSING TEETH

(Continued)

Action	Rationale
14. Brush the sides of the teeth by gently brushing the sides back and forth.	**14.** Removes plaque buildup and food particles.

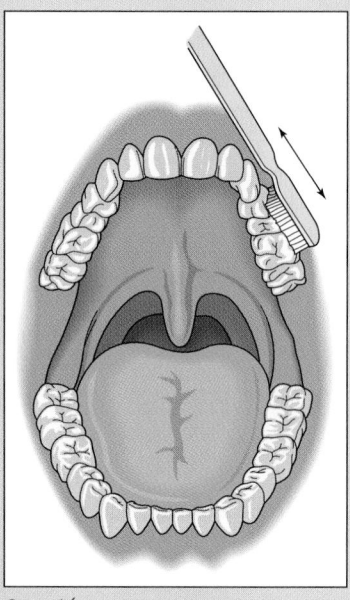

Step 14.

15. Assist client in rinsing of mouth with cup of water. The client may spit excess water into emesis basin.	**15.** Removes waste contents from oral cavity.
16. If a mouthwash is used, follow step 15.	**16.** Prevents cross-contamination.

Flossing

17. Hold about 1.5 in of floss tightly between fingers, with enough floss wrapped around the fingers to prevent slipping.	**17.** Such tension is needed.

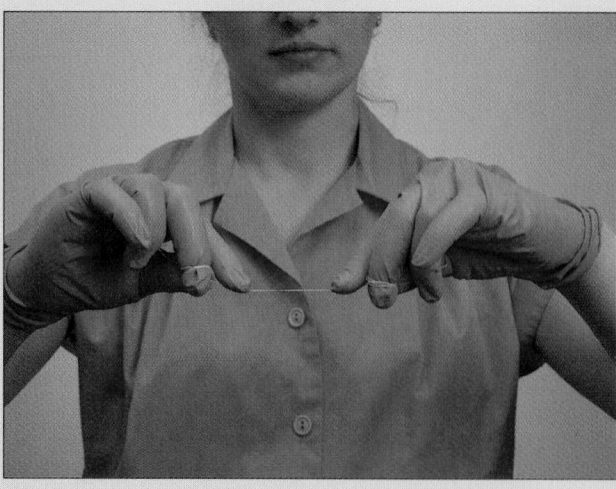

Step 17.

PROCEDURE

22–6

BRUSHING AND FLOSSING TEETH
(Continued)

Action	Rationale
18. Ask client to open mouth and smile to reveal teeth.	**18.** Easy access to areas between the teeth.
19. Gently insert floss between teeth and move it back and forth between the teeth and gums.	**19.** To remove plaque and food particles.

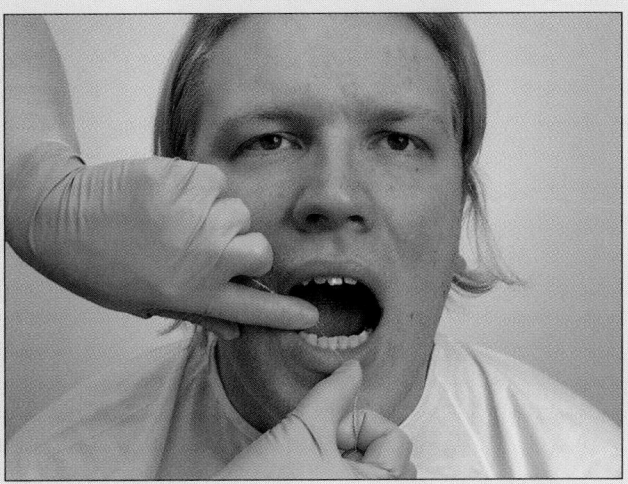

Step 19.

20. Move floss up and down until the sides of both teeth are clean.	**20.** Removes plaque buildup.
21. Repeat steps so all teeth are flossed.	**21.** Removes plaque buildup.
22. Assist client to rinse mouth as in step 15 of brushing procedure. Flossing may induce a small amount of bleeding—this is normal.	**22.** Removes waste contents from oral cavity.
23. Clean up emesis basin and supplies.	**23.** Prevents cross-contamination.
24. Apply lubricant to client lips as needed.	**24.** For client comfort. Prevents cracking of lips.
25. Discard gloves.	**25.** Prevents cross-contamination.
26. Wash hands.	**26.** Prevents cross-contamination.
27. Document procedure and any pertinent assessment findings.	**27.** For ongoing client record.

may be embarrassed to be seen without their "teeth in." If the client can perform denture care independently, he or she should be encouraged to do so. Dentures should be assessed by the nurse for effectiveness of cleansing, and teaching should be done with the client if a deficit is noted. Most dentures can be removed, brushed, rinsed and then reinserted. Clients may have special products they use for cleansing their dentures and may even bring such products to the hospital with them. If a client removes his or her dentures at night, they should be stored in a denture case, and the client's name should be clearly marked on the denture case. The dentures should be placed in a drawer in the client's bedside table so they will not be knocked on the floor, broken, or lost.

Some clients may require assistance with their denture care (see Procedure 22–7). While performing denture care, the nurse may take the opportunity to demonstrate and teach the client proper care technique.

Mouth Care of the Unconscious or Debilitated Client

Clients who are unconscious have special mouth care needs. Because they are unconscious, they are

PROCEDURE

22–7

DENTURE CARE

Preparation: Collect supplies and place them in convenient location at client bedside for easy access.

Equipment:

Toothbrush
Toothpaste
Denture cup
Mouth rinse
Small basin of tepid water
(unless sink is used)
Towel
Disposable gloves

Action	Rationale
1. Provide for safety (*e.g.,* side rails).	1. To ensure client safety.
2. Explain procedure to client.	2. Decreases client anxiety.
3. Assist client in removing dentures.	3. Client may need help with this.
4. Place dentures in denture cup.	4. To avoid breakage.
5. Carefully inspect the client's oral mucosa and gums (wearing gloves and using a tongue blade and light source).	5. While doing dental care, oral mucosa is exposed, and assessment is easily done.
6. Assist client in rinsing mouth.	6. Provides comfort.
7. Wash hands.	7. Prevents cross-contamination.
8. Don disposable gloves.	8. Prevents cross-contamination.
9. Place dentures in basin of tepid water (if sink is used, place paper towels in sink to pad sink and prevent denture breakage).	9. Extreme water temperatures may harm dentures.
10. Hold dentures in nondominant hand.	10. Dominant hand needed for brushing dentures.
11. Brush the dentures with the dominant hand using toothpaste in the same manner as described in Procedure 22–5.	11. Dominant hand will provide safer and more efficient brushing activity.
12. Brush all denture surfaces well.	12. To clean entire denture surface.
13. Rinse out denture cup.	13. To discard contaminated water.
14. Rinse clean dentures in cold water and place in denture cup with a small amount of water.	14. For clean storage.
15. Assist client in inserting dentures if needed.	15. Many clients like to wear dentures at all times.
16. Assess fit of dentures and ask client if dentures are comfortable.	16. Ill-fitting dentures can cause pain.
17. Discard gloves.	17. Prevents cross-contamination.
18. Document procedure and any pertinent assessment.	18. Provides information and accountability.

unable to report any dryness, sores, or irritations in the mouth. Unconscious clients may breathe more from their mouth, making the mouth very dry; this may predispose them to infection. Their oral mucosa also becomes dry because they are not taking fluids by mouth.

Mouth care should be performed on the unconscious client at least every 4 hours and more fre-quently if needed. Commercially prepared swabs may be used in the mouth to decrease dryness. The oral mucosa should be assessed every 8 hours for sores, lesions, and irritations. The lips should be lubricated with petroleum jelly or a similar lubricant to prevent them from cracking. Some clients who are very ill and debilitated may require the same oral care as the unconscious client. (See Procedure 22–8.)

22–8

MOUTH CARE FOR THE UNCONSCIOUS OR DEBILITATED CLIENT

Preparation: Collect and place supplies in convenient location at client bedside for easy access.

Tips and Precautions:
Never place fingers in an unconscious client's mouth.

Equipment:
Toothbrush
Toothpaste
Pretreated foam toothettes
Towel
Curved basin (emesis basin)
Disposable gloves
Bite block (optional)
Cup of tepid water
Mouthwash
Petroleum jelly or similar lubricant

Action	Rationale
1. Position client in a side-lying position with the head of the bed as flat as possible.	1. Prevents aspiration of fluids.
2. Provide for safety (*e.g.,* side rails)	2. Provides client safety.
3. Provide for privacy.	3. Decreases client anxiety.
4. Place towel under client's head.	4. Keeps neck dry.
5. Place curved basin under client's chin.	5. Catches fluids and keeps chin and neck dry.
6. Place bite block in client's mouth—*never* place fingers in an unconscious client's mouth.	6. Bite block helps keep mouth open so care may be provided. Fingers should never be placed in client's mouth, as biting may occur.
7. Inspect client's oral cavity wearing gloves and using a tongue blade and light source.	7. Inspection is best done while providing mouth care.
8. Brush teeth as much as possible, as described in Procedure 22–6.	8. Removes plaque.
9. If brushing is too difficult, swab teeth, oral mucosa, and gums with moistened foam toothette.	9. Such mouth care is better than doing none at all.
10. Allow fluid to run out of client mouth into basin.	10. Prevents aspiration.
11. If needed, suction may be used to remove excess fluid from the mouth.	11. Prevents aspiration.
12. Swab roof of mouth and tongue with foam toothette as well.	12. Cleans areas and provides moisture.
13. Apply lubricant to lips as needed.	13. Provides client comfort and helps to prevent cracking of lips.
14. Inspect oral cavity again.	14. Cleaning of oral cavity may allow for closer inspection of mucosa.
15. Clean up supplies and client.	15. Prevents cross-contamination.
16. Position client for comfort.	16. Provides client comfort.
17. Discard gloves.	17. Prevents cross-contamination.
18. Wash hands.	18. Prevents cross-contamination.
19. Document procedure and any pertinent assessment findings.	19. Provides information and accountability.

Shampooing Hair

Hair care in a hospital or home environment can be very difficult for a person who is ill. If he or she is dependent, it is difficult for a caregiver to provide such care, and if he or she is independent, the client may not feel well enough to wash his or her hair as usual.

The independent client may perform hair care in the shower or tub. The nurse need only provide the client with needed supplies and linen. The use of a shower chair may be helpful for ambulatory clients who may become fatigued or lightheaded with such activity. For the dependent client, the caregiver must perform the cleansing and grooming of hair. When it is not possible to shampoo a client's hair in bed with water, dry shampoos (or no-rinse shampoos) are available. Dry shampoos are not as good as wet shampoos, but they are helpful in removing some of the dirt, oils, and odors from the hair until a wet shampoo can be performed. The dry shampoo is simply applied to the client's hair and scalp and is combed or brushed through the client's hair until the shampoo is entirely combed through. Dry shampoos are not rec-

ommended for persons with very dry hair, as the dry shampoo tends to dry the hair out even more.

Some clients may tolerate being transferred from a bed to a stretcher, on which they can be bathed, and have their hair washed over a sink or shower. To shampoo hair using this method, the sink should be equipped with a hand-held shower nozzle to make the procedure comfortable for both client and caregiver. Special attention must be given to the client's neck and shoulders—pillows or towels may be placed under the neck and shoulders for positioning and comfort. The stretcher wheels should be locked, and a waterproof pad should be placed over the end of the stretcher.

If a client can tolerate a wet shampoo in bed, the nurse should provide such care as needed. (Note, some institutions may require a physician's order for shampooing a client's hair.) (See Procedure 22–9.)

Shaving a Male Patient

Male clients who do not usually have a beard or moustache may feel uncomfortable as their facial hair grows. Clients who are independent with care can

Text continued on page 551

PROCEDURE

22–9

WET SHAMPOOING OF A CLIENT ON BED REST

Preparation: Collect and place supplies in convenient location at head of client's bed. Review physician's order (if needed). Assess client for ability to tolerate procedure. If client is unable to tolerate the procedure, postpone it until another time.

Equipment:

Shampoo and conditioner
Towels (at least two)
Face cloth (wash cloth)
Plastic shampoo basin
Garbage can or basin to collect rinse water
Water pitcher
Clean comb and brush
Waterproof pad
Hair dryer
Disposable gloves

Action	Rationale
1. Provide safety measures.	**1.** Ensures client safety.
2. Explain procedure to client.	**2.** Decreases client anxiety.
3. Provide for privacy.	**3.** Decreases client anxiety.
4. Raise bed to convenient height for procedure.	**4.** To avoid joint/back strain.
5. Place waterproof pad under client's head, neck, and shoulders.	**5.** Keeps bed linens dry.
6. Wash hands.	**6.** Prevents cross-contamination.
7. Don disposable gloves.	**7.** Prevents cross-contamination.

PROCEDURE

22–9

WET SHAMPOOING OF A CLIENT ON BED REST
(Continued)

Action	Rationale
8. Place client in supine position and place plastic shampoo basin under client's head. Make sure shampoo basin spout empties into a catch basin or garbage can.	**8.** Prevents linens from getting wet and provides exit for water.

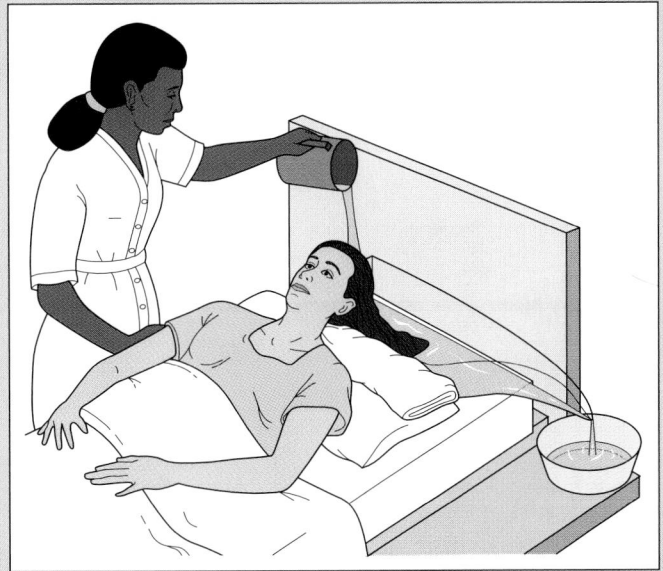

Step 8.

Action	Rationale
9. Place a towel roll under client's neck for comfort and support.	**9.** Provides client comfort and support.
10. Wet hair using water pitcher (temperature should be warm—between 109°F [42.7°C] and 111°F [43.8°C]). Check temperature by placing drops of water on forearm.	**10.** To avoid injury and to provide comfort.
11. Place face towel/washcloth over client's face or ask him or her to close his or her eyes.	**11.** To prevent fluids from going into client's eyes.
12. Place small amount of shampoo on client's hair and work into lather, starting at hairline and working toward the posterior neck—massage all areas of the scalp while shampooing.	**12.** Increases circulation to the scalp.
13. Assess scalp and hair.	**13.** To provide interventions according to assessment.
14. Rinse shampoo thoroughly, and repeat as needed.	**14.** To remove dirty water.
15. Condition as needed and rinse thoroughly.	**15.** To make combing out hair easier.
16. Wrap wet hair in towel.	**16.** To dry hair.
17. Remove shampoo basin.	**17.** For client comfort.
18. Complete drying hair and neck with dry towel.	**18.** To provide client comfort.
19. Position client for comfort.	**19.** For client comfort.
20. Raise head of bed to 30 degrees.	**20.** Easier to comb hair at this position.
21. Comb hair and dry with dryer.	**21.** For client comfort.

Continued

PROCEDURE

22–9

WET SHAMPOOING OF A CLIENT ON BED REST
(Continued)

Action	Rationale
22. Style hair.	**22.** To provide client comfort.
23. Discard soiled linen and clean up area.	**23.** Prevents cross-contamination.
24. Assess client for positioning and comfort.	**24.** To ensure client safety.
25. Lower bed to low position.	**25.** For client safety and comfort.
26. Document procedure and pertinent assessment findings.	**26.** Provides information and accountability.

PROCEDURE

22–10

SHAVING A MALE CLIENT

Preparation: Collect and place supplies in convenient location at client bedside. Assess client for ability to tolerate procedure. If client is unable to tolerate, postpone activity until later. Explain procedure to client.

Equipment:

Washcloth
Towel
Water basin
Safety razor
Shaving cream
Shaving lotion (optional)
Electric razor (if safety razor is
    contraindicated)

Action	Rationale
1. Provide safety measures.	**1.** Ensures client safety.
2. Assist with positioning client for comfort (usually head of bed is raised at least 30 degrees).	**2.** For client comfort.
3. Provide for privacy.	**3.** Decreases client anxiety.
4. Raise bed to comfortable working level.	**4.** Prevents joint/back strain.
5. Wash hands.	**5.** Prevents cross-contamination.
6. Don disposable gloves.	**6.** Prevents cross-contamination.
7. Fill water basin with warm water.	**7.** Extreme water temperatures may be uncomfortable for client.
8. Moisten face with warm washcloth.	**8.** Moisture softens facial hair and allows for easier removal.
9. Apply shaving cream to facial areas to be shaved.	**9.** Lubricates face for easier and less painful hair removal.
10. With nondominant hand, pull facial area taut.	**10.** Smooths out facial surface area.

SHAVING A MALE CLIENT
(Continued)

Action	Rationale
11. Shave facial area with dominant hand using short, firm strokes in the direction of hair growth.	**11.** Removes hair more efficiently.

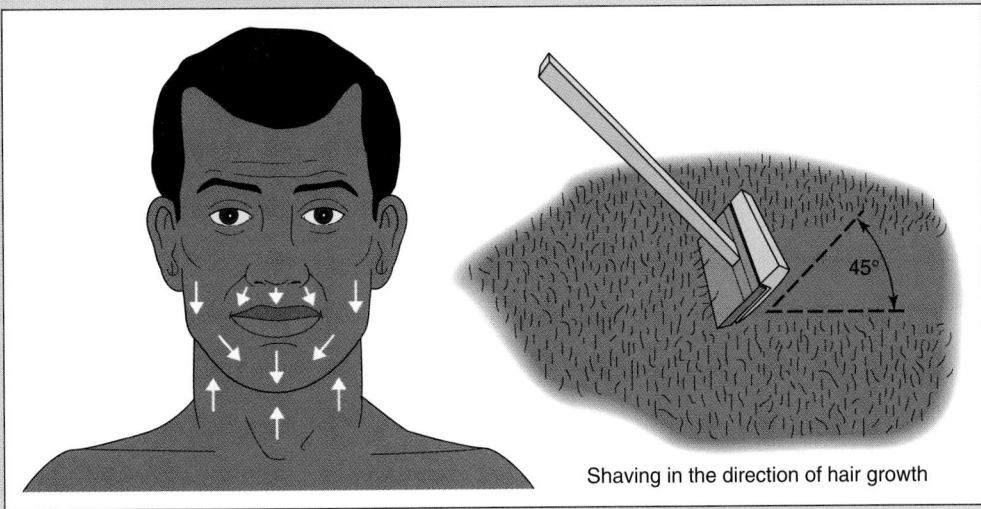

Shaving in the direction of hair growth

Step 11.

Action	Rationale
12. Repeat steps 8 and 9 as necessary.	**12.** Removes unwanted hair.
13. Wash client's face with warm washcloth.	**13.** Rinses off excess shaving cream.
14. Apply facial lotion.	**14.** Moisturizes face.
15. Position client for comfort.	**15.** To provide client comfort.
16. Lower bed to low position.	**16.** Ensures client safety.
17. Clean up supplies and linen.	**17.** Prevents cross-contamination.
18. Discard gloves and wash hands.	**18.** Prevents cross-contamination.
19. Document procedure and pertinent assessment findings.	**19.** Provides information and accountability.

usually shave themselves with a disposable razor or an electric razor. Before a client uses an electric razor, however, it should be checked by the nurse or bioinstrument department for any electrical hazards. Electric razors are usually recommended for clients receiving anticoagulant therapy or who have any type of bleeding disorders.

Some clients are dependent on the nursing staff to have their shaving needs met. Shaving of the client should be planned to follow the bath. (See Procedure 22–10.)

Contact Lens Care and Removal

Many people wear corrective contact lenses. These lenses are worn directly on the eyeball and can either be hard or soft. Hard lenses are usually made of a rigid plastic that is not gas or liquid permeable. Soft lenses are made of a gas- and liquid-permeable plastic material. Most hard lenses must be removed after 14 hours of wear because they restrict the oxygen supply to the cornea. Soft contact lenses may be worn for extended periods, some as long as 30 days (depending on the manufacturer's recommendations). Most soft lenses should be cleansed at least weekly, using the appropriate manufacturer's recommended method. Eye damage may result if contact lenses of any kind are left in for too long.

Most clients who wear contact lenses can provide independent care or choose to wear eyeglasses when hospitalized or ill. However, there may be times when the nurse must remove and care for a client's contact

Text continued on page 554

PROCEDURE

22–11

CARE OF CONTACT LENSES AND CONTACT LENS REMOVAL

Preparation: Prepare supplies in convenient location near client's head. Assess if client has glasses to wear while contact lenses are removed. Assess client for ability to tolerate procedure. If client is unable to tolerate, postpone until a later time.

Equipment:

> Sterile saline solution
> Contact lens solution (often supplied by client)
> Contact lens cleaning solution (often supplied by client)
> Contact lens storage case (often supplied by client)
> Towel

Action	**Rationale**
1. Raise bed to convenient height for procedure.	**1.** Prevents joint/back strain.
2. Provide for safety and privacy.	**2.** Ensures client safety and privacy.
3. Wash hands.	**3.** Prevents cross-contamination.
4. Assist client to supine position.	**4.** Most efficient position for procedure.
5. Place towel near client's face.	**5.** To dry tearing if needed.
6. Instill a few drops of sterile saline into client's eye.	**6.** To lubricate lens and make removal easier.
7. Using nondominant index finger and thumb, open eye by pulling up on upper lid and down on lower lid.	**7.** To make removal of lens easier.

Removing Soft Lenses

8. With dominant index finger and thumb, gently pinch contact lens and lift it out of eye.	**8.** For comfortable lens removal.

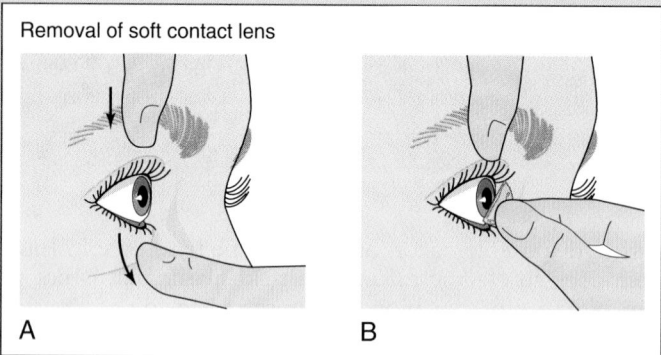

Removal of soft contact lens

A   B

Step 8. *Removing soft contact lenses.*

Removing Rigid (Hard) Lenses:

Note: This procedure is for a nurse to remove a lens from a client's eye, not the client removing the lens. Observe all steps in preparation and client assessments as with soft lens care. Observe steps 3–7 of soft lens care and removal.

a. Position lens into center of cornea (have client close eye and gently massage lens to center).	a. Efficient location for lens removal.
b. Method 1: With nondominant index finger and thumb, gently pull outer corner of eye.	b. Places pressure on lens.

PROCEDURE

22–11

CARE OF CONTACT LENSES AND CONTACT LENS REMOVAL

(Continued)

Action	**Rationale**
c. With dominant hand remove lens as client blinks and pops lens out.	c. Safely removes lens without scratching lens on eye surface.

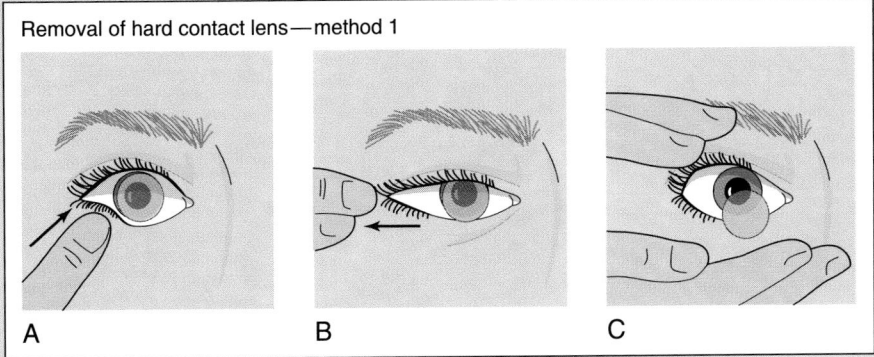

Step 8C.

Action	**Rationale**
d. Method 2: Separate the eyelids to expose edges of lens. Hold the eyelid above the eye.	d. Stabilizes the lens for removal.
e. Gently press the bottom of the lens to lift it away from the eye; then move lids together to slide out lens.	e. Removes lens safely.

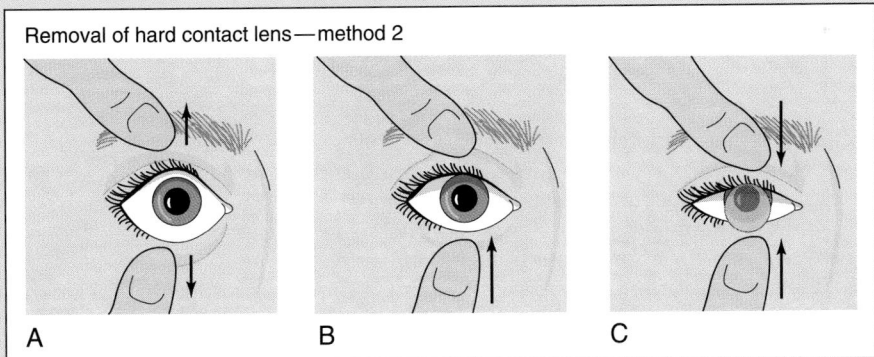

Step 8E.

Action	**Rationale**
f. Observe steps 9 through 18 of soft lens care and removal.	f. Provides for cleanliness and safety.
9. Gently cleanse lens with contact lens cleaning solution by placing lens in nondominant palm and gently rubbing lens with dominant index finger.	9. To cleanse lens before storage.
10. Rinse lens with sterile saline solution.	10. To cleanse lens before storage.

Continued

PROCEDURE

22–11

CARE OF CONTACT LENSES AND CONTACT LENS REMOVAL

(Continued)

Action	Rationale
11. Place lens in appropriate side of storage container (right or left).	**11.** Keeps lenses in correct order.

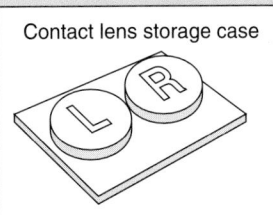

Step 11. *Place contact lenses in correct side of case.*

Action	Rationale
12. Repeat steps 6 through 11 to remove and care for other lens.	**12.** See steps 6 through 11.
13. Place contact lens in safe area.	**13.** To avoid losing contact lens.
14. Assess eyes.	**14.** To see if irritated from lens.
15. Assist client for comfort and positioning.	**15.** For client comfort.
16. Lower bed to low position.	**16.** To ensure client safety.
17. Clean up area.	**17.** Ensures client safety and prevents cross-contamination.
18. Wash hands.	**18.** To provide for client safety and prevent cross-contamination.
19. Document procedure.	**19.** Provides information and accountability.

lenses (*e.g.,* if the client is unconscious). If an eye injury is present, the nurse should not try to remove a contact lens because of the danger of further injury. A client with an eye injury wearing contact lenses should be referred to a physician for appropriate treatment. (See Procedure 22–11.)

Care of the Artificial Eye

Clients who have had an entire eye enucleated (removed) as a result of illness or injury often wear an artificial eye (prosthesis). Clients who wear an artificial eye usually have a routine of eye care and should be encouraged to continue such care when hospitalized or ill.

If the client is unconscious or is dependent for care, the nurse must provide hygiene measures to the artificial eye. The artificial eye can be removed by retracting the lower eyelid and applying gentle pressure just below the eye. The prosthesis is usually made of glass or plastic and can therefore be easily cleaned with normal saline. The eye socket should be cleansed with warm water and a washcloth and the tissue assessed. The prosthesis can be reinserted by retracting the lower lid and gently placing the eye into the socket. The nurse should document the procedure and any pertinent findings in the client's record. Clients who wear artificial eyes often require the use of eye lubricants to keep the eye and inner lids moist. Ask the client if he or she uses such lubricants and secure a physician's order for the lubricant if needed. Remember that the client cannot see out of an artificial eye, so direct all activity toward the client's good eye.

Hearing Aids

Between 25 and 40% of people over the age of 65 are hearing impaired, and many of them require the use of hearing aids. Advances in hearing aid technology have made modern hearing aids more efficient and more compact than ever before. Most modern devices are digital and can be programmed for up to eight quiet or noisy situations, according to the client's preferences (see Chapter 34). Hearing devices can be very expensive (from $500–2000), so it is very important that clients' hearing aids be taken care of during hospitalization. Care must be taken that hearing aids do not get lost or broken. Nurses may need to review hearing aid care with clients.

Evaluation

The evaluation and plan modification phase is the final activity of the nursing process. Although it is a final step, evaluation and plan modification is really an ongoing process until full resolution of expected outcomes is attained. First, the nurse must look at the planned interventions and decide if the interventions were effective in meeting the outcomes expected. If the client responded to the interventions as planned and attained the expected outcomes, then no additional modification needs to be made to the plan. Such interventions are then either reinforced through their continuance or are stopped if they are no longer needed. If the expected outcome was not met through the planned interventions, then the interventions must be modified and tested again for their effectiveness. Reevaluation of interventions must then continue. If evaluation of the implemented interventions results in the identification of a new problem, then the nursing process must be used on the new problem.

The evaluation step is essential in measuring the effectiveness of the nursing process as it relates to specific client problems. Documentation of such evaluations is also essential so that all those who care for a particular client may assist in providing continuity of care through the communication of planned nursing interventions.

Summary

A person's state of personal hygiene often tells a lot about his or her current state of health. It is at this basic level where much of a nurse's work is done. Providing hygiene measures allows the nurse to learn much about clients through skilled observation and assessment and also allows the nurse to provide comfort to clients while at the same time developing therapeutic relationships with them.

Although hygiene measures are often basic, the opportunities to educate clients about the importance of specific activities are extremely valuable. For example, teaching proper foot care is essential for diabetic clients. Proper oral hygiene is also important to teach, as the prevalence of gum disease is so high and can be prevented by simple hygiene measures. By providing appropriate hygiene and educative interventions, nurses not only gain valuable information from their clients but also provide valuable care to them.

The role of the professional nurse is rapidly changing. Managed care and budget cuts are forcing health care institutions and other providers of health care services to look closely at how they utilize nurses in client care activities. In many cases, nurses are now delegating specific client care tasks to nonlicensed caregivers. These nonlicensed caregivers work under the direction of the professional nurse. The nurse may not actually be carrying out all the steps in such care, but he or she is still responsible for the overall management of client care and the outcomes of care.

The changing roles are forcing nurses to learn management skills that in the past were reserved for nurse managers. These management skills include the assessment of their provider skills mix, the appropriate delegation of tasks to the appropriately trained provider, and the overall assessment of their clients related to their multidisciplinary care.

CHAPTER HIGHLIGHTS

♦

- ♦ Personal hygiene refers to the activity of self-care, including bathing and grooming
- ♦ Hygiene includes care of the skin, hair, nails, mouth, teeth, eyes, ears, nasal cavities, and perineal and genital areas
- ♦ Proper personal hygiene is essential for overall good health
- ♦ Hygiene practices are influenced by many factors, including developmental level, cultural background, socioeconomic status, religion, personal preferences, and overall status of health
- ♦ Performing or assisting in the performance of hygiene measures allows the nurse to do a total skin assessment of the client and allows the opportunity for teaching; such activity can also help foster trust and a therapeutic relationship between the nurse and the client
- ♦ Special hygiene needs are noted for clients who might be diabetic or suffer from immunosuppressive diseases
- ♦ Hospitalized clients usually receive scheduled hygiene-related care; however, it is important to allow clients as much privacy and independence as possible when planning their care
- ♦ The nursing process is important to follow when addressing hygiene problems; this process allows for modification of plans so that expected outcomes might be achieved
- ♦ Discharge planning should always begin as soon as possible so that client needs are taken care of in an organized and timely fashion

Study Questions

1. During a bath, the nurse observes that a diabetic client's feet are very dry and cracking. The nurse should plan to

   a. wash feet daily with an astringent soap
   b. assess feet three times a week and bathe as needed
   c. assess feet daily and apply lotion to feet
   d. wash feet daily in hot water

2. Performing hygiene measures allows the nurse to do the following:

   a. perform a thorough skin assessment of the client
   b. develop a therapeutic relationship with the client
   c. provide comfort to the client
   d. all of the above

3. The layer of the skin that contains blood vessels, nerves, connective tissue, and glands is the

   a. integument
   b. dermis
   c. subcutaneous
   d. adipose

4. Tartar on the teeth can

   a. only be removed by a dental professional
   b. be easily removed by brushing
   c. only be removed by brushing and flossing
   d. be removed with the use of an oral water pic

5. When performing hygiene measures, the first thing the nurse should do is

   a. explain the procedure to the client
   b. assess the independence of the client
   c. provide for the client's safety and privacy
   d. perform an assessment of the client's skin

Critical Thinking Exercises

1. Mr. T. is homeless and falls on the ice. He is admitted to your floor with a fractured hip. He is adentulous and dirty. Discuss hygiene needs and considerations for teaching.

2. Ms. Y. is unconscious. Discuss the skin and hygiene needs of Ms. Y.

References

Black, J., & Matassarin-Jacobs, E. (Eds.). (1993). *Luckmann and Sorensen's medical-surgical nursing* (4th ed; pp. 829–940, 1572–1583.) Philadelphia: W. B. Saunders.

Carpenito, L. (1995). *Handbook of nursing diagnosis* (6th ed.). Philadelphia: J. B. Lippincott.

Carroll, P. (1995). Bed selection helps patients rest easy. *RN, May,* 44–50.

Christensen, M., Funnell, M., Ehrlich, M., Fellows, E., & Floyd, J. (1991). How to care for the diabetic foot. *American Journal of Nursing, March,* 50–56.

Crosby, C. (1989). Method in mouth care. *Nursing Times, 85* (35), 38–41.

Fenske, N., Grayson, L., & Newcomer, V. (1992). Tips for treating aging skin. *Patient Care, March,* 61–72.

Gregory, B. (1994). *Orthopaedic surgery* (pp. 135–140). Philadelphia: Mosby.

Kresevic, D., & Naylor, M. (1995). Preventing pressure ulcers through use of protocols in a mentored nursing model. *Geriatric Nursing, 16*(5), 225–229.

Miller, R., & Rubinstein, L. (1992). Oral health care for hospitalized patients: The nurse's role. *Journal of Nursing Education, 26*(9), 362–366.

Ney, D. (1993). Cerumen impaction, ear hygiene practices, and hearing acuity. *Geriatric Nursing, March/April,* 70–85.

Pascucci, M. (1992). Measuring incentives to health promotion in older adults. *Journal of Gerontological Nursing, March,* 16–23.

Skewes, S. (1994). No more bed baths. *RN, January,* 34.

Tinanoff, J. (1995). Dental caries risk assessment and prevention. *Dental Clinics of North America, 39*(4), 709–719.

Bibliography

Braden, B., & Bergstrom, N. (1994). Predictive validity of the Braden scale for pressure sore risk in a nursing home population. *Research in Nursing & Health, 17,* 459–470.

Bryant, R. (1992). *Acute and chronic wounds—nursing management.* Chicago: Mosby.

Burgess, R. (1995). Assessment of caries risk factors and preventive practices. *Journal of Dental Education, 59*(10), 962–971.

Carroll, P. (1995). Bed selection helps patients rest easy. *RN, May,* 44–50.

Easton, K. (1993). Defining the concept of self-care. *Rehabilitation Nursing, 18*(6), 383–387.

Erwin-Toth, P. (1995). Cost effectiveness of pressure ulcer care in the United States. *Advances in Wound Care, Sept/Oct,* 59–61.

Esernio-Jenssen, D. (1995). Teaching and reinforcing hygienic practices in child care centers. *American Journal of Public Health, 85*(12), 1710.

Futrell, A., Forst, S., Harrell, J., Adams, L. (1991). Effects of occupied and unoccupied bed making on myocardial work in healthy subjects. *Heart and Lung, 20*(2), 161–167.

Gould, D. (1994). Infection control—helping the patient with personal hygiene. *Nurs Standards, 8*(34); 30–32.

Griffiths, G. M., Wieman, T. (1992). Meticulous attention to foot care improves the prognosis in diabetic ulceration of the foot. *Surg Gynecol Obstet, 174*(1), 49–51.

Hunter, S., Langemo, D., Olson, B., *et al.* (1995). The effectiveness of skin care protocols for pressure ulcers. *Rehabilitation Nursing, 20*(5), 250–255.

Jagger, D., Harrison, A. (1995). Denture cleansing—the best approach. *British Dental Journal, 178*(11), 413–417.

Kresevic, D., & Naylor, M. (1995). Preventing pressure ulcers through use of protocols in a mentored nursing model. *Geriatric Nursing, 16*(5), 225–229.

Lovell, H., & Anderson, C. (1990). Put your patient on the right bed. *RN, 53*(5), 66–72.

Maklebust, J. (1995). Pressure ulcers: What works. *RN, 58*(9), 46–50.

Maklebust, J., & Sieggreen, M. (1996). *Pressure ulcers: Guidelines for prevention and nursing management* (2nd ed.), Springhouse, PA: Springhouse Corporation.

Mcdermott, J. (1992). Dentures and denture care. *North Carolina Medical Journal. 53*(2), 93–95.

Meintz, S. (1995). Whatever became of the back rub? *RN, 58*(4), 49–50, 53, 56.

Miller, K. (1978). Assessing peripheral perfusion. *American Journal of Nursing, October,* 1673–1674.

Miller, R., & Rubinstein, L. (1987). Oral health care for hospitalized patients: The nurse's role. *Journal of Nursing Education, 26*(9), 362–366.

Nosek, M. (1993). Personal assistance: Its effect on the long-term health of a rehabilitation hospital population. *Archives of Physical Medicine and Rehabilitation, 74*(2), 127–132.

Pase, M. (1994). Pressure relief devices, risk factors, and development of pressure ulcers in elderly patients with limited mobility. *Advances in Wound Care, 7*(2), 38–42.

Pieper, B., & Mott, M. (1995). Nurse's knowledge of pressure ulcer prevention, staging, and description. *Advances in Wound Care, 8*(3), 34–46.

Ransier, A., Epstein, J., Lunn, R., & Spinelli, J. (1995). A combined analysis of a toothbrush, foam brush, and a chlorhexidine-soaked foam brush in maintaining oral hygiene. *Cancer Nursing, 18*(5), 393–396.

Rieber, G. (1992). Diabetic foot care—financial implications and practice guidelines. *Diabetes Care, 15 (suppl 1),* 29–31.

Renn, N. (1989). Oral health and hygiene for the elderly. *Home Health Care Nurse, 7*(3), 37–39.

Salvadalena, G., Snyder, M., & Brogdon, K., (1992). Clinical trial of the Braden scale on an acute care medical unit. *Journal of ET Nurse, 19*(5), 160–165.

Santen, S., & Scott, J. (1995). Ophthalmic procedures. *Emergency Treatment of the Eye, 13*(3), 681–695.

Specht, J., Bergquist, S., & Frantz, R. (1995). Adoption of a research-based practice for treatment of pressure ulcers. *Nursing Clinics of North America, 30*(3), 553–563.

Stillman, M. (1978). Territoriality and personal space. *American Journal of Nursing, Oct,* 1670–1672.

Suarez, C., & Reynolds, A. (1995). Pressure reduction with a hospitalized population using a mattress overlay. *Ostomy Wound Management, 41*(1), 58–60.

Tinanoff, N. (1995). Dental caries risk assessment and prevention. *Dental Clinics of North America, 39*(4), 709–719.

Tombes, M., & Gallucci, B. (1993). The effects of hydrogen peroxide rinses on the normal oral mucosa. *Nursing Research, Nov/Dec,* 332–336.

Treloar, D., & Stechmiller, J. (1995). Use of a clinical assessment tool for orally intubated patients. *American Journal of Critical Care, 4*(5), 355–360.

Chapter 23

SKIN
INTEGRITY

PATRICIA ALBANO SLACHTA,
PhD, RN, CS, CETN

KEY TERMS
✦

clean wound	pressure ulcer
dirty wound	purulent
granulation	reactive hyperemia
infected wound	sanguineous
ischemia	serosanguineous
necrosis	serous

LEARNING OBJECTIVES
✦

After studying this chapter you should be able to

✦ List the four causal factors of pressure ulcer development

✦ Identify the contributing factors to pressure ulcer development

✦ Describe the four stages of pressure ulcers

✦ Assess clients at risk for skin breakdown

✦ Discuss the pathology of pressure ulcer development

✦ Identify the role of the nurse in the prevention and management of pressure ulcers

✦ Discuss the standards of care for clients with causal factors for pressure ulcer development

✦ Identify individualized plans of care related to causal/contributing factors of skin breakdown

✦ List the phases of wound healing

✦ Explain the concept of a moist wound healing environment

✦ Identify wound care treatments based on research

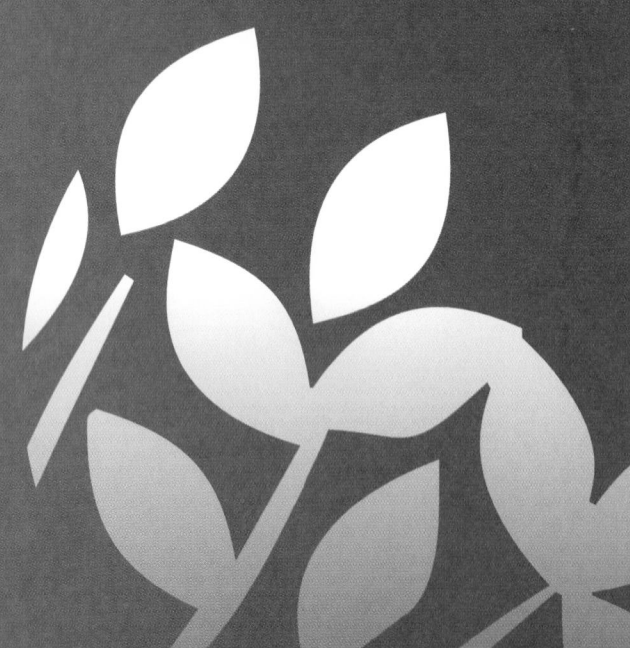

During the past decade, the importance of maintaining a client's skin integrity has gained nationwide recognition. Nursing has been at the forefront of this movement and has clearly identified maintaining skin integrity as one of the autonomous roles of the nurse. Much research has been done during this period related to wound healing and interventions for prevention of skin breakdown. To function within the scope of nursing practice, even the novice nurse needs to know the basics about prevention and management of skin integrity problems.

One of the main purposes of this chapter is to provide the nurse with the essential knowledge and standards for caring for clients at risk for or who have developed skin integrity problems. The chapter addresses two major areas: the first is pressure ulcers, and the second is acute wounds.

The environment in which the nurse is practicing (*e.g.,* home care, acute care, long-term care) does not change the principles of the nursing process. However, dressing selection and topical treatments may be affected by practice area because reimbursement may be relevant in determining the most cost-effective plan of care for the client.

Physiology of Skin

The integumentary system is the largest organ in the body and functions as an organ of protection, temperature regulation, sensation, excretion, and absorption. The skin is the body's first line of defense.

The three predominant layers of the skin are epidermis, dermis, and subcutaneous. The epidermal layer is dry, stratified, squamous epithelium that is thin over most of the body. This layer consists of four or five layers of avascular cells, with regeneration occurring from the basal cell layer approximately every 28 days. The outermost layer is the stratum corneum. The epidermal layer is primarily responsible for preventing mechanical, chemical, or bacterial injury and preventing underlying tissues from suffering water loss.

The dermal layer is the connective tissue layer of the skin and supports the epidermis with collagen bundles and elastic fibers. It separates the epidermis from the cutaneous adipose tissue and acts as a nutritional source for the epidermis. The dermal layer also contains blood vessels, nerve fibers, sebaceous glands, sweat glands, and hair follicles. The sebaceous glands secrete sebum which contains fats, soaps, cholesterol, and other materials. Sebum forms a thin protective layer on the skin to prevent undue absorption or evaporation of water from the skin and keeps the skin and hair soft and pliable. Sweat glands are either eccrine, which are found on the surface of the skin and regulate body temperature by evaporative cooling, or apocrine, whose ducts open into hair follicles and are found in the axilla, anogenital areas, nipples, and areolae. The bacterial decomposition that occurs in these areas is responsible for body odor.

The subcutaneous layer is of dense cellular composition and anchors, insulates, and supports the dermis. Fatty tissue is present in the loose connective tissue that is in the subcutaneous layer, along with blood vessels, lymph, and nerve fibers. Below the subcutaneous tissue is the muscle layer and then the bone.

Factors That Alter Skin Condition

The major function of the skin is that of protection. Skin is our first line of defense against chemical and ultraviolet exposures, bacterial and viral organisms, mechanical trauma, and temperature changes. Five predominant factors alter skin condition: age, ultraviolet radiation, hydration, nutrition, and medication.

As aging occurs, the epidermis and dermis decrease in thickness; epidermal turnover time increases, causing slower wound healing; and barrier function and sensory perception are decreased, leading to greater potential for injury (Box 23–1). The young child has skin tissues that are the most elastic and resistant to injury and, if injured, heal readily.

Adolescence creates different effects in girls and boys, as hormonal influence is a large factor. Eccrine and apocrine sweat glands become active during this period, and hygienic measures for the adolescent become more significant. Use of antiperspirants and face astringents and more frequent bathing and hair shampooing may be needed.

The thermoregulatory function of the skin is affected throughout aging as the number of sweat

---

Box **23–1**

SKIN CHANGES WITH AGING

Factors That Decrease With Age

Epidermis/dermis in thickness

Barrier function of skin

Sensory perception

Number of sweat glands

Sebum production

Vascularity of tissues

Hydration of skin

Subcutaneous fat

Skin turgor

Elasticity of dermis and collagen

Slower growing nails

Factors That Increase With Age

Turnover time for epidermal regeneration

Thickness and brittleness of nails

glands, vascularity of the tissues, and subcutaneous fat are decreased (Wysocki & Bryant, 1992). Skin turgor also decreases, as does elasticity of the dermis as collagen and elastic fibers are lost. Because of the smaller dermal underbase, the epidermis begins to fold and appear wrinkled. Gravity also pulls the skin downward so that drooping eyelids, earlobes, and jowls occur. Nails grow slower because of decreased peripheral circulation and also change color to yellowish or grayish and become thicker and more brittle.

The ultraviolet radiation from the sun is a second factor that alters skin characteristics. The aging of the skin is accelerated with this exposure, and if excessive exposure occurs, there is an increased risk of developing skin cancers due to DNA damage.

Hydration, a third factor, is supplied by sebum secretion and the intact stratum corneum's keratinized cells. Aging decreases hydration of the skin, as does the humidity of the environment and the removal of sebum. Soaps also affect the skin's protective ability, as alkaline soap diminishes the thickness and numbers of cell layers in the stratum corneum. Soap also emulsifies the lipid coating of the skin; therefore, excessive use of soap and detergents may interfere with the ability of the skin to hold water and to resist bacterial invasion, as alkaline soaps increase the skin pH (normal pH is 5.5). This is especially significant for the elderly person, as the skin is already losing some of its hydration from decreased sebum production.

Adequate nutrition is also important for maintaining skin integrity; however, increased nutrition is not necessarily beneficial under normal circumstances (Wysocki & Bryant, 1992). Vitamin A and protein are the main constituents of skin cells. Vitamin C supports the capillary beds supplying the skin cells. Clients who have a disease process that impairs adequate digestion and/or absorption and those who are not permitted to eat or drink preceding surgery are more susceptible to skin integrity impairments.

The fifth factor noted by Ehrlich and Hunt (1968) is the effect of medication on the skin. Interference with epidermal regeneration and collagen synthesis has been identified as a result of corticosteroid ingestion. There are many other categories of drugs that can affect the skin, so if any skin reactions occur, medications should be examined (Wysocki & Bryant, 1992).

✦ Nursing Process and Skin Integrity

Before assessing the client in relation to skin integrity, the nurse must identify the type of wound: acute or chronic. Acute wounds are wounds that have been present for less than 1 month. Chronic wounds have usually been present for longer than 1 month and are usually colonized with bacteria. (See Nursing Diagnosis box for a list of nursing diagnoses related to skin integrity. Note that nursing diagnoses do not relate to surgically created, acute wounds.)

The specific assessment of clients at risk for or with chronic wounds such as pressure ulcers is presented in more detail in the chapter, as pressure ulcer care is a significant independent practice domain for the professional nurse.

Assessment
Nursing History

Obtaining an accurate clinical picture of the client is important in determining the risk that the client has for developing impairments in skin integrity or for the healing of those impairments that are present.

NURSING DIAGNOSES RELATED TO IMPAIRED SKIN INTEGRITY

Impaired Tissue Integrity Related To

- Effects of mechanical destruction
- Effects of chemical destruction

Defining characteristics that are specific should be noted. This diagnosis should be used for all impairments that are deeper than the dermis.

Impaired Skin Integrity, Actual or Risk Related To

- Pressure from immobility, decreased activity, or altered mental status
- Moisture from incontinence, excessive perspiration, excessive wound drainage
- Friction and shear from sensory deficits, or immobility/inactivity

Skin integrity should be used as a diagnosis only for those injuries that are stage I or II.

Impaired Physical Mobility Related To

- Musculoskeletal impairment
- Mental status deficit

Risk for Infection Related To

- Open wound
- Surgical incision

Anxiety Related To

- Perceived threat to self-concept, health status, socioeconomic status, role functioning, interaction patterns, or environment

Pain

BOX 23-2

TYPES OF SKIN LESIONS

Macule: Flat, nonpalpable skin lesion, noticeable only because it differs in color from the surrounding skin.

Papule: Small, raised, solid skin lesion usually under 0.5 cm in diameter.

Nodule: A raised lesion greater than 0.5 cm in both width and depth.

Plaque: A raised, plateaulike lesion greater in diameter than in depth. Surface may or may not have secondary changes such as scale or crusting.

Vesicle: A small lesion (0.5 cm in diameter) filled with serous fluid.

Bulla: A large lesion (> 0.5 cm in diameter) filled with serous fluid. In both vesicles and bullae, clear fluid accumulates within the epidermis or at the dermal-epidermal junction. Both vesicles and bullae can develop into pustules.

Pustule: A sack or blister filled with cloudy or purulent material (lymph, pus).

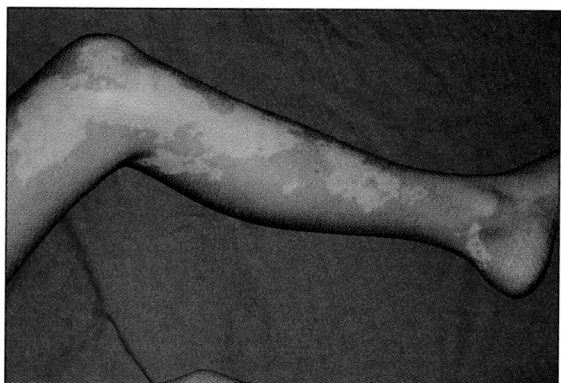

Macules (vitiligo)

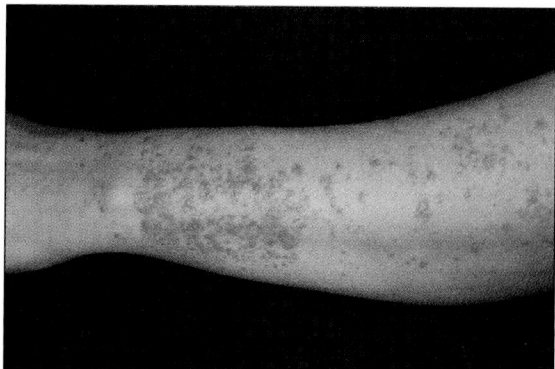

Papules

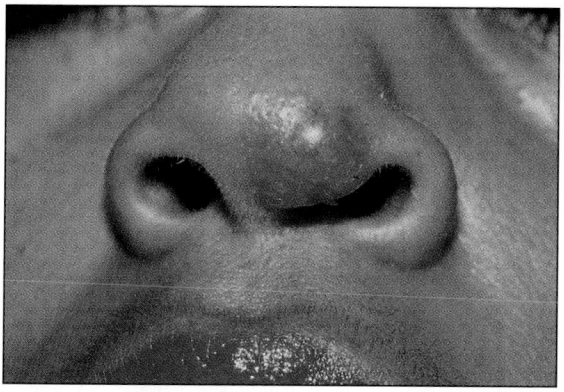

Nodule (sarcoidosis)

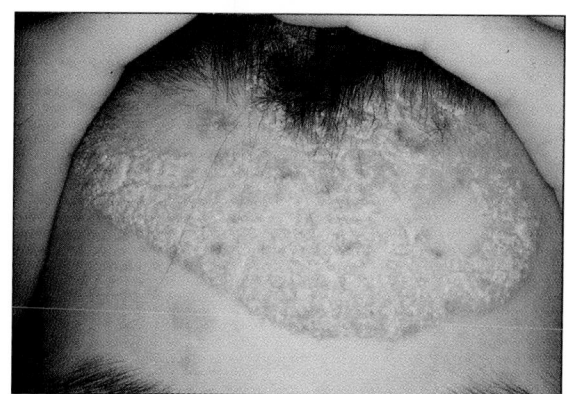

Plaque (psoriasis)

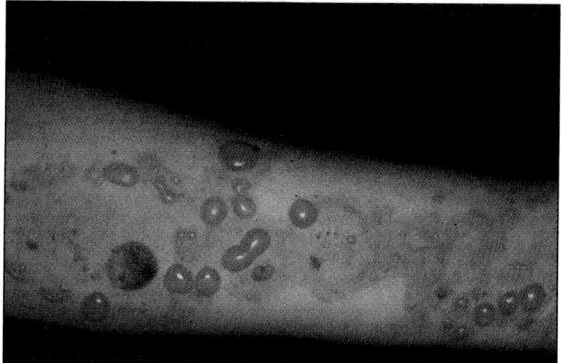

Vesicles and bullae

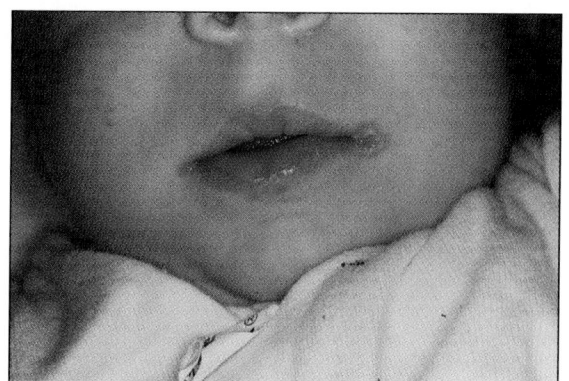

Pustules

Photos from Callen, J. P., Greer, K. E., Hood, A. F., Paller, A. S., & Swinyer, L. J. (1993). *Color atlas of dermatology.* Philadelphia: W. B. Saunders.

Nutrition

The following nutritional questions should be reviewed with all clients on admission to any agency. Deficits that are determined will need further follow-up with either the nurse or dietitian.

Describe and Examine the Pattern of Food and Fluid Intake Relative to Body Needs

1. Typical daily food and fluid intake: Determining the typical intake of the client will assist the nurse in determining his or her likes and dislikes as well as the general caloric and nutritional intake of the client. Gaps in the food pyramid should be discussed to determine if there is a knowledge deficit, a narrow range of likes and dislikes, cultural issues, or social issues such as finances that are preventing the client from eating a nutritionally adequate diet. Nursing interventions should address identified problems, and a consult to social services should be done for clients with social issues.

2. Appetite and changes in appetite: Determining whether the client has had any appetite changes may assist the nurse in planning the nutritional intake of the client. Reporting changes in appetite to the physician is a collaborative function of the nurse, as there may be an unidentified medical problem contributing to the appetite change.

3. Dental problems: Clients who cannot chew because of pain from dental caries or ill-fitting or missing dentures may not be receiving adequate nutrition. Many clients, regardless of age, may not have healthy teeth. Referral to a dentist for tooth inspection and repair or to a social worker for financial issues may be necessary.

4. Consults: Consulting with a dietitian is also imperative if nutritional deficits are noted or suspected. The dietitian will examine the client in relation to fat and muscle stores by determining the anthropometric assessments. These noninvasive assessments consist of weight, midarm circumference, triceps skinfold, and arm muscle circumference.

History of Skin Lesions, Difficulty With Wound Healing, General Skin Condition

1. Any skin lesions? When a client reports the presence of skin lesions, the nurse needs to obtain more information about the lesions, what, if anything, precipitates the lesions, and whether there is pain. The location, number, and appearance of the lesions also need to be assessed (Box 23–2).

2. Skin dryness? During aging, the dermis becomes dehydrated because of the decreased production of sebum. Drinking adequate amounts of fluid, not bathing excessively with hot water, and applying lotions may relieve some of the dryness. Dehydrated skin loses strength and elasticity; therefore, the skin is more fragile and tears more easily.

Physical Examination and Diagnostics

Limited equipment is needed for skin inspection. A strong, direct light and a measurement device for lesions and wounds are necessary. The light should be halogen or natural instead of fluorescent, as fluorescent light produces a blue tone to dark skin, which impedes accurate assessment (Bennett, 1995).

General Physical Appearance

1. Height, weight, and weight loss or gain: The client's height and weight are reported on admission. *This should be an actual measurement and not ascertained by client report.* Subsequent management of nutrition, as well as selected pharmacological therapy, may depend on accurate measurements of height and weight.

   Clients who have experienced weight loss or gain will have additional factors involved in their illness. Adequate nutrition is essential for maintaining wellness as well as for enhancing wound healing. (See Box 23–3 for pertinent laboratory tests.)

   The client who gains weight may not have an adequate nutritional intake, although the caloric intake may be increased. Heavy clients are also susceptible to skin breakdown because the blood flow to the tissues is decreased due to the obesity. Weight loss predisposes the client to nutritional inadequacies as well as susceptibility to skin breakdown related to pressure. Unintentional weight loss of 10% or more within a 6-week period is considered significant (Konstantinides & Lehmann, 1993).

   Anthropomorphic measurements complete the somatic protein picture and are usually done by the dietitian. Somatic (muscle) protein status is assessed by determining the client's ideal weight in relation to his or her actual height and weight. Adult ideal body weight can be ascertained by using the Metropolitan Life Insurance chart or by calculating the ideal weight. In 1986, Blazey and coworkers noted the formula for women as follows: allow 100 lb for the first 5 ft, and then add 5 lb/in. For men, 106 pounds is allowed for the first 5 ft, with an additional 6 lb/in added. Body frame type may reveal a 10% variation in either direction. In addition to the somatic protein measurement, the visceral proteins (all other proteins) can also be assessed.

2. Color: Skin color is consistent with genetic background. If erythema is noted, especially on one of the pressure points (Fig. 23–1), examine this area carefully for nonblanching erythema, which heralds a stage I skin breakdown. Darkly pigmented skin does not show the typical erythema, but an area in jeopardy may appear darker than surrounding skin, taut, shiny, or indurated or have a purplish/bluish hue (Bennett, 1995). The recommended period of time between turning that is needed for a client can be calculated by examining the duration of redness (see Health Promotion and Prevention box).

3. Texture: Normal skin has an even surface and feels smooth and firm.

4. Turgor: *Turgor* reflects the elasticity of the dermis. When the skin is gently pinched in a large fold (use skin on the anterior chest under the clavicle), it should return to place immediately when released instead of standing by itself or "tenting" (Jarvis, 1992). Poor skin turgor is found in clients with dehydration and in the elderly, as the skin elasticity is decreased.

5. Temperature: Using the back of the hand, feel the skin. The temperature should be warm and equal bilaterally, indicating normal circulatory status. Areas of increased warmth are indicative of possible infection or compromised circulation. An area of increased warmth or coolness in a dark-skinned person may be an indication of a stage I pressure ulcer (Bennett, 1995).

Box 23–3

NUTRITIONAL DIAGNOSTICS

Creatinine height index (CHI) is a laboratory test that also assesses the somatic muscle. The CHI measures lean body mass and is a percentage as expressed by the milligrams of creatinine excreted in 24 hours by a normal subject of the same height and sex as the client (Blazey et al., 1986). A CHI (the ratio of actual creatinine excretion versus the ideal creatinine excretion) of less than 40% of the standard is interpreted as severe nutritional depletion and a 40 to 60% of the standard is interpreted as a marginal depletion.

Serum albumin is a visceral protein that decreases slowly in malnutrition (the half-life of albumin is approximately 18 to 20 days); therefore, a low serum albumin level is a late manifestation of protein deficiency (Blazey et al., 1986; Charney, 1995). Serum albumin levels of less than 3.0 g/dl usually indicate hypoalbuminemic tissue edema.

Prealbumin contains a high level of tryptophan content, which is an amino acid thought to be crucial for protein synthesis control. The advantage of prealbumin over albumin is its significantly shorter half-life (2 days). Changes in prealbumin status can be noted within 72 hours of protein restriction (Charney, 1995), and the normal range is 10 to 40 mg/dl.

Total protein—Hypoproteinemia results in interstitial edema because the fluid between the cells reduces the ability of the body to oxygenate the tissues. Therefore, maintaining a total protein level high enough to keep the client's colloid osmotic pressures higher than his or her hydrostatic pressures eliminates the possibility of edematous tissues (Kaminski et al., 1989).

Serum transferrin is more indicative of nutritional status, as transferrin has small extravascular stores (half-life, 7 days), and low levels reflect the present state of nutrition. Using serum transferrin levels remains controversial in terms of diagnosing malnutrition because the concentrations vary widely, even in the diagnosed malnourished client. Concentrations of less than 100 mg/dl are indicative of severe protein depletion, and those concentrations between 100 and 200 mg/dl are indicative of a marginal protein depletion and need for further assessment.

Total lymphocyte counts (TLCs) that are depressed have been associated with increased morbidity and mortality, as these cells are major constituents of the immune system. Protein is a component of various immune system structures, such as lymphocytes and antibodies; therefore, malnutrition and TLC of less than 1500 cells per millimeter are related. This low count indicates the need for further nutritional evaluation (Konstantinides & Lehmann, 1993). A TLC of less than 1000 cells per millimeter is a significant lymphocytopenia.

Leukocyte counts are increased in a chronic or acute infection, and this blood test (a component of the white blood cell [WBC] count) is done with the complete blood cell (CBC) count. The leukocyte count can also be done alone.

---

6. Intactness: If the skin is not intact, the wound can be described as a *partial-thickness wound* or as a *full-thickness wound* or by a *four-stage system.* Partial-thickness wounds are those limited to skin layers and not penetrating below the dermis, with reepithelialization usually occurring to heal these partial-thickness wounds. Abrasions, lacerations, and blisters are partial-thickness wounds. Full-thickness wounds have tissue loss below the dermis. All types of wounds may be described as partial-thickness or full-thickness wounds.

Pressure ulcers are also categorized using a four-stage description (Fig. 23–2):

Stage I: Nonblanching erythema of intact skin is the heralding lesion of skin ulceration. An area of nonblanching erythema *does not* turn white when finger pressure is applied. Reactive hyperemia, on the other hand, is a normal response in tissues subjected to pressure. After the pressure is released, oxygen floods the tissues that were previously starved for oxygen; therefore reactive hyperemia is a bright flush of the skin. Irreparable damage does not occur if the pressure is of short duration. Note that reactive hyperemia can normally be expected to be present for one half to three fourths as long as the pressure occluded blood flow to the area; it should not be confused with a stage I pressure ulcer (Berecek, 1981). Remember that reactive hyperemia and nonblanching erythema are not indicators of stage I areas in dark-skinned people. Bennett (1995) stated that the National Pressure Ulcer Advisory Panel suggested the following addition to the definition of stage I: "For persons with darkly pigmented intact skin, assess for erythema and/or inflammation with localized changes in skin temperature in comparison to the surrounding tissue, edema, and/or induration" (p. 35).

Stage II: Partial-thickness skin loss involving epidermis and/or dermis. The ulcer is superficial and presents clinically as an abrasion, blister, or shallow crater.

Stage III: Full-thickness skin loss involving damage to or necrosis of subcutaneous tissue that may extend down to, but not through, underlying fascia. The ulcer presents clinically as a deep crater with or without undermining of adjacent tissue.

Stage IV: Full-thickness skin loss with extensive destruction, tissue necrosis, or damage to muscle, bone, or supporting structures (*e.g.*, tendon or joint capsule). Note: Undermining and sinus tracts may also be associated with stage IV pressure ulcers (Panel for the Prediction and Prevention of Pressure Ulcers in Adults, 1992).

The effectiveness of this staging system, as first described

Pressure ulcer sites

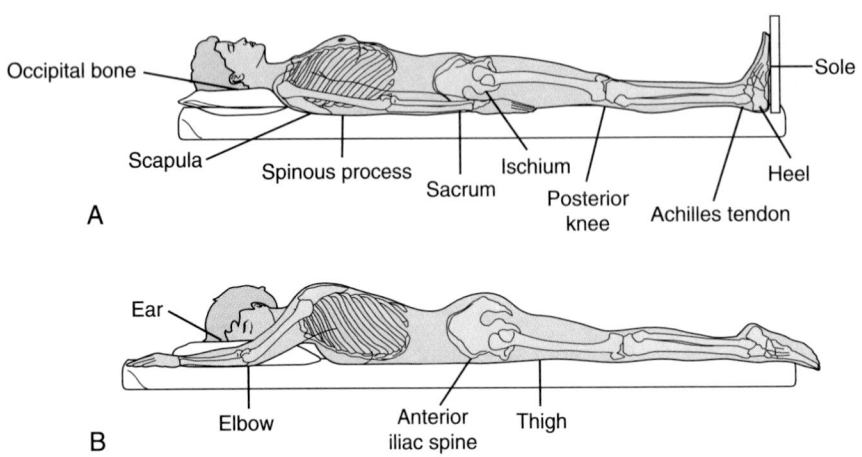

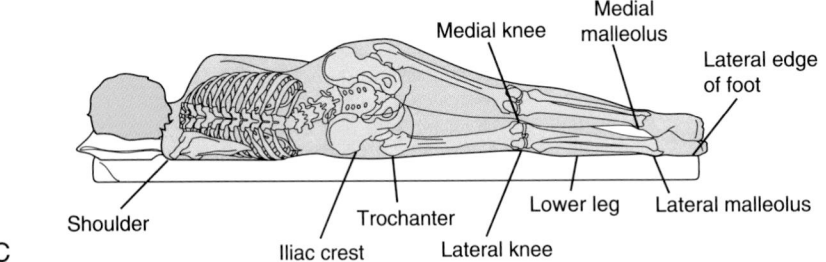

✦ **Figure 23–1**
Pressure points are areas of the skin overlying bony prominences where pressure ulcers are most likely to occur. Careful examination of the skin in these areas and turning of the client at regular intervals are necessary to prevent pressure ulcers. (See Box 23–1.)

by Shea (1975), depends on the knowledge of the examiner of anatomy of skin and deeper tissue and the ability of the examiner to differentiate between these.

In addition to staging an area of skin breakdown, other data need to be collected. Staging of any kind *cannot* be done if the wound bed contains necrotic or scar tissue.

7. Wound assessment: Accurate wound assessments are hard to obtain, as wounds are irregular and change over short periods of time. In addition, more than one caregiver is often involved with the client, thereby making wound assessment subject to caregiver judgments. The following areas need to be addressed when assessing wounds (Box 23–4).

Anatomic Wound Location

Because accurate communication is important when documenting wounds, the exact anatomical location of the wound should be noted. Upper body wounds heal more easily than those on the lower body.

Size — Circumference, Depth, and Stage

Paper or plastic measuring devices are available for the clinician to use for measuring in centimeters or millimeters. To obtain consistent measurements from day to day and/or from clinician to clinician, reference points for the measurements need to be determined. One method for doing this is to identify the wound in relation to the client's head and feet, using the face of

a clock: The client's head is 12 o'clock, and the feet are 6 o'clock. The length and width of the wound are measured, and then the depth is measured. Wound area is obtained by multiplying the length by the width. Depth may need to be identified in several areas, as many wound beds are irregular. Although linear measurements are imprecise, when repeated over time they do provide gross information in relation to the wound healing (Cooper, 1992).

Because many wound care products are packaged in transparent wrappings, a tracing of the wound using this transparent paper and permanent ink marker can also be made. Precision should be used when tracing, and the tracing should be dated.

Photography is a third method for documenting wound size and shape. Permission must be received from the client prior to taking photographs. The use of measuring devices placed next to the wound assist in sizing. Date each picture if the camera does not automatically provide this information on the photograph.

Appearance of Surrounding Skin

In addition to actually measuring the wound opening itself, the surrounding tissue must be evaluated. Any erythema, edema, and/or ecchymosis within 4 cm of the wound edges is noted and measured. For an area that is erythematous, remember to reevaluate the erythema on two consecutive observations or more than 48 hours apart for the chronic wound. The

HEALTH PROMOTION AND PREVENTION

GOALS OF THE AGENCY FOR HEALTH CARE POLICY AND RESEARCH PREVENTION GUIDELINES*

Risk Assessment Tools and Risk Factors

Identify at-risk individuals needing prevention and the specific factors placing them at risk

Pressure ulcer risk should be reassessed periodically (A)

All assessments of risk should be documented (C)

Skin Care and Early Treatment

Maintain and improve tissue tolerance to pressure to prevent injury

At-risk individuals need systematic skin inspection at least daily, with special attention to bony prominences (C)

Skin cleansing should occur at the time of soiling, avoiding hot water and using mild cleansing agent (C)

Minimize environmental factors leading to skin drying (low humidity and exposure to cold) (C)

Avoid massage over bony prominences (B)

Minimize skin exposure to moisture due to incontinence, perspiration, or wound drainage (C)

Minimize skin injury due to friction and shear by proper positioning, transferring, and turning techniques (C)

Discover factors compromising appropriate dietary intake, and offer nutritional support if needed (C)

For nutritionally compromised individuals, implement a plan for adequate supplementation to meet individual needs (C)

Institute rehabilitation efforts if potential for improving mobility and activity status exists (C)

Monitor interventions and outcomes (C)

Mechanical Loading and Support Surfaces

Protect against the adverse effects of external mechanical forces: pressure, friction, and shear

Reposition any individual in bed at risk for pressure ulcers every 2 hours according to a written schedule (B)

Keep bony prominences from direct contact with one another by using positioning devices (C)

Immobile individuals in bed should have care plan that includes total relief of pressure on the heels (C)

Avoid direct positioning on trochanter when the client is side-lying (C)

Maintain head of bed at lowest degree of elevation (C)

Use lifting devices for individuals who cannot assist during transfers and position changes (C)

Use pressure-reducing device in bed for any individual assessed to be at risk for developing pressure ulcers (B)

At-risk individual should avoid uninterrupted sitting in chair or wheelchair (C)

Use pressure-reducing device for chair-bound individual (C)

Position chair-bound individual in chairs and wheelchairs considering postural alignment, distribution of weight, balance and stability, and pressure relief (C)

A written plan for the use of positioning devices and schedules will be helpful (C)

Education

Reduce the incidence of pressure ulcers through educational programs

Educational programs should be structured, organized, and comprehensive and directed at all levels of health care providers, clients, family, or caregivers (A)

The program for the prevention of pressure ulcers should include all aspects of these guidelines (B)

The educational program should identify those responsible for pressure ulcer prevention and should be updated on a regular basis (C)

Principles of adult learning should be used when developing the educational program (C)

* Strength of evidence: A = there is good research-based evidence to support the recommendation; B = there is fair research-based evidence to support the recommendation; C = the recommendation is based on expert opinion and panel consensus.

From Panel for the Prediction and Prevention of Pressure Ulcers in Adults. (1992). *Pressure ulcers in adults: Prediction and prevention. Clinical practice guideline, number 3.* AHCPR Pub. No. 92-0047. Rockville, MD: Agency for Health Care Policy and Research, Public Health Service, US Department of Health and Human Services.

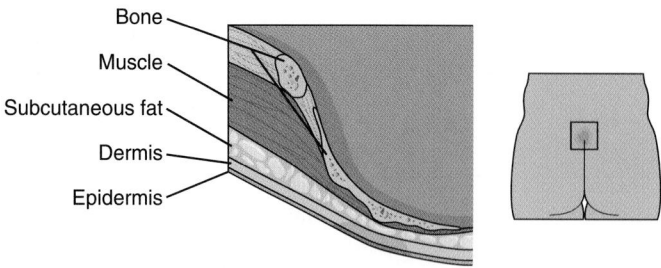

Stage I: Reddened intact epidermis does not blanch under light pressure—a sign of future skin ulceration

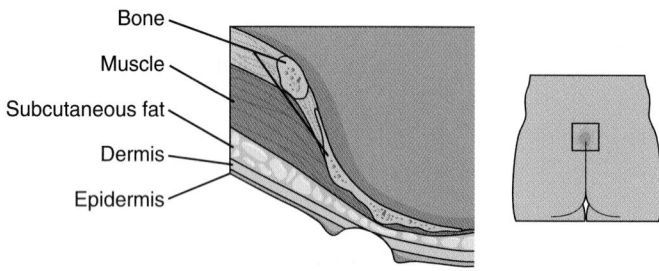

Stage II: Partial-thickness skin loss; epidermis and/or dermis affected; superficial ulcer resembles a shallow crater, blister, or abrasion

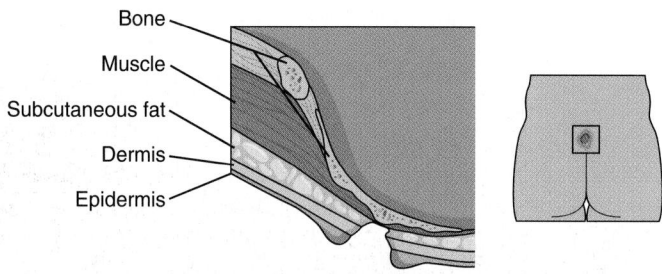

Stage III: Full-thickness skin loss with damage to subcutaneous tissue that may extend to the underlying fascia; resembles a deep crater

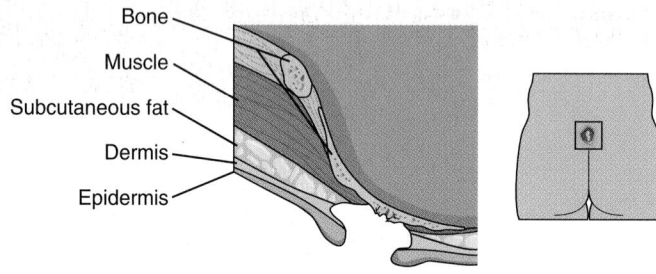

Stage IV: Full-thickness skin loss; extensive damage that may involve muscle, bone, or supporting structures

❧ **Figure 23–2**
Stages of pressure ulcers. The effectiveness of this staging system depends on the ability of the examiner to differentiate the stages.

acute wound needs to be evaluated daily (Bergstrom & Braden, 1992).

Tissue Appearance in Wound Bed

Viable tissue in the wound bed is categorized as granulation, epithelialization, muscle, or subcutaneous tissue. Granulation tissue is connective tissue containing multiple small blood vessels to assist in rapid healing of the wound bed. Granulation tissue is red or pink. Epithelialization is the regeneration of epidermal cells across the wound bed.

Nonviable tissue, also known as necrotic or slough tissue, is associated with impeded wound healing. This nonviable tissue can be many colors, such as black, yellow, or tan, and may also be firmly or loosely adherent to the wound bed. Although describing color is important, the range of colors in a wound may be extensive (Cooper, 1992).

Drainage or Exudate

The amount, consistency, and color of exudate in the wound are assessed. Wound drainage is often

DOCUMENTATION OF WOUNDS

The following items are documented:

- Wound location—anatomical
- Wound size—circumference, depth, stage
- Appearance of surrounding skin, including measurement of affected tissue
- Tissue appearance in wound bed
- Drainage or exudate
- Presence of undermining and/or tracts

Example of Documentation

Mr. Smith has a pressure sore located on the right ischium. The area measurements are as follows: width = 1 cm; length = 2 cm; depth = 0.5 cm; irregular shape with no undermining edges or tracts noted. The ulcer is stage 2 and has minimal drainage with no odor or color. Tissue in the wound bed is light pink with no necrotic areas or slough. There is nonblanching erythema for 2 cm around the wound.

serous—clear, watery plasma. **Serosanguineous** drainage is also watery but is pink tinged, indicating some bleeding. **Sanguineous** drainage is bloody and indicates active bleeding. Extremely odorous, **purulent** exudate may suggest an anaerobic infection (Cooper, 1992). Purulent exudate may be a variety of colors from yellow to green to brown or tan. Green drainage may indicate infection with *Pseudomonas aeruginosa*. Assessing wound drainage from a wound covered by an occlusive dressing should be done *after* cleansing the wound.

Presence of Undermining and/or Tracts

Gentle probing around the edges of the wound and in the wound bed will usually evidence undermining or tracts if they are present. The location of the undermined area or tract is noted, again by identifying it in relation to the face of a clock, and the depth is documented. Insert the applicator as far as it will go without using force, and then mark the skin on the outside where the tip can be seen or felt. Undermining often occurs as a result of shear forces in addition to pressure (Cooper, 1992).

Documentation of Healing Wounds and Pressure Ulcers

The parameters for wound and pressure ulcer description in the previous sections are the same parameters that the nurse documents as the wound heals, *with the exception of stage*. A stage 4 ulcer does not become a stage 3 or stage 2 as it heals, as this presumes that the tissue structure of the healing ulcer is the same as the normal skin. Previously lost muscle, fat, and dermis are not replaced during healing, but this ulcer is filled instead with granulation tissue, fibroblasts, collagen, and an extracellular matrix. Therefore, *reverse staging* does not follow the anatomical and structural layers of the skin and tissues (National Pressure Ulcer Advisory Panel [NPUAP], 1995).

Wound Classification

Wound classification can be done in a variety of ways. In addition to the acute versus chronic classification discussed earlier, wounds may be open (when there is a break in the skin) or closed (a wound with traumatized tissue that occurs without a skin break). Intentional wounds are those that are caused by surgery, radiation, or other therapies. An unintentional wound is accidental. Wounds can also be classified as **clean wounds** (no pathogens are present) or **dirty wounds** (microorganisms are present), also identified as contaminated or colonized. The contaminated wound may be **infected,** which is determined by the number of microorganisms present, usually greater than 10^5 organisms per gram of tissue. A colonized or contaminated wound is one in which there are multiple microorganisms but not the number required to classify it as an infection (Crow, 1997). This is an important distinction, as the colonized wound may still be susceptible to the natural defenses of the body. In colonization, there is no tissue invasion or immune response to the organisms.

One of the major issues related to skin integrity is the development of pressure ulcers, classified after a few weeks as a chronic wound. The independent, autonomous role of the nurse in pressure ulcer prevention and management has been well documented in the literature (Mundinger, 1980; Singleton & Nail, 1984; Willey, 1992). Pressure ulcers are defined as areas of localized tissue necrosis. This tissue **necrosis** develops when soft tissue is compressed between a bony prominence and an external surface (NPUAP, 1992). As the tissue is compressed, blood flow to that area decreases, and death of the cells begins. Time is also a factor, as the longer the pressure is exerted, the greater the likelihood of breakdown (Kosiak, 1961).

Nationally, two organizations have developed statements on and guidelines for prevention and treatment of pressure ulcers. The NPUAP (1992) and the Agency for Health Care Policy and Research (AHCPR) (Panel for the Prediction and Prevention of Pressure Ulcers, 1992) have published several booklets on pressure ulcers that are available to health care professionals and the public. The goals of the AHCPR guidelines for the prediction and prevention of pressure ulcers in adults are listed in the box. Pressure ulcer development occurs in clients in hospitals, nursing homes, and the home. In addition to the assessment done with the client admitted to an agency, there are several other parameters that need to be addressed in relation to pressure ulcers.

HEALTH PROMOTION AND PREVENTION

PREVENTING PRESSURE ULCERS

Check skin color over pressure points (see Fig. 23–1) to determine how often a client needs to be turned. Non-blanching erythema is a danger sign that heralds a stage I skin breakdown (see Box 23–2). In dark skin, check for areas darker than the surrounding skin and areas that are taut, shiny, indurated, or with a purplish/bluish hue. Redness or darkness usually persists for 50% of the time hypoxia to the tissues actually occurred. Therefore, if the redness lasts for 30 minutes, the hypoxia time for that tissue was 1 hour. To calculate the recommended turning interval, use the following formula:

Recommended turning interval
$$= \text{Previous turning interval} - \text{hypoxia time}$$

In the example given earlier, if the previous turning time was 2 hours, then the recommended turning interval is

$$2 \text{ hours} - 1 \text{ hour} = \text{turn every 1 hour}$$

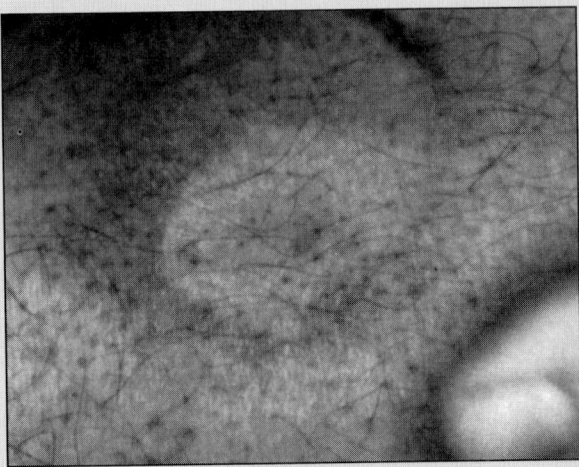

Normal blanching erythema: Erythema blanches completely on digital compression. Earliest stage of decubitus ulcer development. (From Moschella, S. L., & Hurley, H. J. [1992]. Dermatology [3rd ed., pp. 2240–2241]. Philadelphia: W. B. Saunders.)

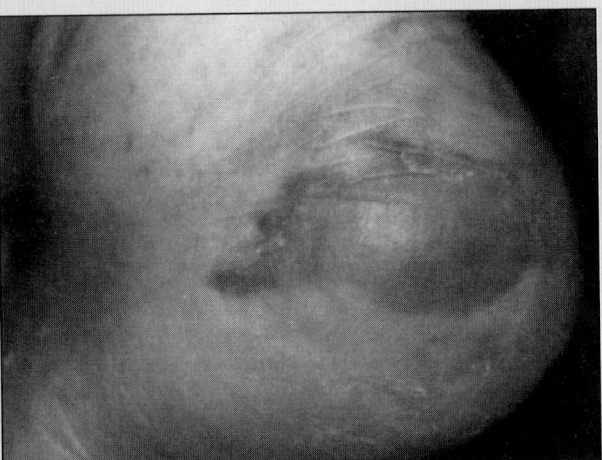

Abnormal nonblanching erythema: Does not blanch on digital depression. Heralds a stage I skin breakdown. (From Moschella, S. L., & Hurley, H. J. [1992]. Dermatology [3rd ed., pp. 2240–2241]. Philadelphia: W. B. Saunders.)

Assessing for Pressure Ulcer Risk

Pressure ulcers have received significant attention during the past 10 years, especially since the AHCPR selected this topic for two of their guideline publications.

Pressure ulcers are being tracked in all areas of health care. Prevalence, which is determined by assessing all clients in a facility or setting for the presence of pressure ulcers during a specified period, is now reported frequently in the literature. This statistic looks at both old and new cases at one point in time. Incidence, which refers to the number of new cases that develop over a period of time, is then monitored as part of the total quality assurance program in most agencies (NPUAP, 1992).

The increase in prevalence is a critical factor in today's economic environment, and nurses must be prepared to take a leading role in the prevention and treatment aspects of pressure ulcers, regardless of the setting.

Risk Factors, Scores, and Instruments

There are multiple risk factors related to skin breakdown, and these can be classified into causal factors and contributing factors.

Causal Factors

✦ **Pressure.** Most pressure ulcers are caused by occlusion of capillaries, veins, and lymphatics. If skin does not receive adequate oxygenation, the tissue becomes ischemic and eventually begins to die, because the skin needs to receive nutrients and eliminate metabolites and carbon dioxide. Because the circulating peripheral blood aids in this process of normal cell metabolism, it is imperative that there not be any prolonged interference with the peripheral circulation. Several classic studies related to vascular hemodynamics are highlighted in the Clinical Insight box.

✦ **Moisture.** In 1969, Adams and Hunter observed that friction in the paws of a cat increased 51% with mild or moderate sweating. It is known that constant moisture on intact skin increases the potential for skin breakdown. In addition, the alkalinity of the urine affects the acid mantle of the skin, which contributes to the potential for impairments in skin integrity.

✦ **Friction and Shear.** In 1958, Reichel identified shear as a cause of pressure sores in semirecumbent paraplegic clients. Since that time, it has been a recognized factor in skin breakdown. Shear occurs when

forces act parallel to skin surfaces. The blood supply in the area is stretched and compromised, and, over time, extensive venous thrombosis of the deep superficial fascia occurs. The classic example of shear occurs when the head of the client's bed is elevated. The skin and sheets remain in contact and stationary due to friction, the deep superficial fascia slides between the skin (which is in a fixed position) and the deep fascia, and the shearing force causes stretching and angulation of the blood vessels. Friction and shear are significant forces in the immobile client, as the client is moved by the nurse (Fig. 23–3). In practice, nurses often move clients by pulling them from side to side or up in bed, and this increases friction on the client's skin. Friction injuries usually affect the epidermis and not the deeper tissues.

Contributing Factors

✦ **Nutritional and Hydration Status.** See the previous discussion under "Assessment."

✦ **Immobility—Sensory and Motor Impairments.** Mobility and activity are not synonymous. Changing, maintaining, or sustaining a body position is related to a person's mobility, while standing and walking reflect the activity of the client. Sensory perception of pain and/or discomfort is a part of mobility and activity—when a client responds purposefully to pain or discomfort by seeking assistance to change position or changing position himself or herself, this is a reflection

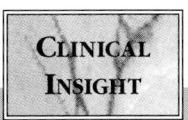

CLINICAL INSIGHT

Pressure Ulcers: Prevalence, Incidence, and Causal Factors

Two research studies noted that persons in skilled care and nursing homes had a pressure ulcer prevalence of 23% (Langemo *et al.,* 1989; Young, 1989). Meehan (1994) looked at the prevalence of pressure ulcers in acute care hospitals and found that the prevalence in 1989 was 9.2% and in 1993, 11.1% in the 177 hospitals surveyed. In 1994, Gawron noted a 12% prevalence rate in a large midwestern hospital. Oot-Giromini (1993) noted the prevalence rate in a community setting was 29%, with an incidence rate of 16.5%.

Nichol (1951) found that capillaries have some instability at low perfusion pressures, which may actually cause cessation of or temporary reversal of blood flow. Landis (1930) found the average pressure in the arteriolar limb to be 32 mmHg. Kosiak (1959) postulated that "because the hydrostatic pressures in capillaries are relatively low, and because cessation of flow occurs even in the presence of positive arterial pressure, it would seem logical that complete tissue ischemia might be present when pressures of the order or capillary blood pressure are applied to the body" (p. 63). Therefore, unevenly distributed, localized pressure on a part of the body that is greater than 32 mmHg may cause tissue damage.

In studies on dogs, Kosiak (1959) also found that intense pressures of a short duration were as significant in injuring tissue as low pressures for long duration.

Data from Langemo, D. K., Olson, B., Hunter, S., Burd, C., Hanson, D., & Cathcart-Silberberg, T. (1989). Incidence of pressure sores in acute care, rehabilitation, extended care, home health, and hospice in one locale. *Decubitus, 2*(2), 42; Meehan, M. (1994). National pressure ulcer prevalence survey. *Advances in Wound Care, 7,* 27–38; Nichol J. (1951). Fundamental instability of the small blood vessels and critical closing pressures in vascular beds. *American Journal of Physiology, 64,* 330.

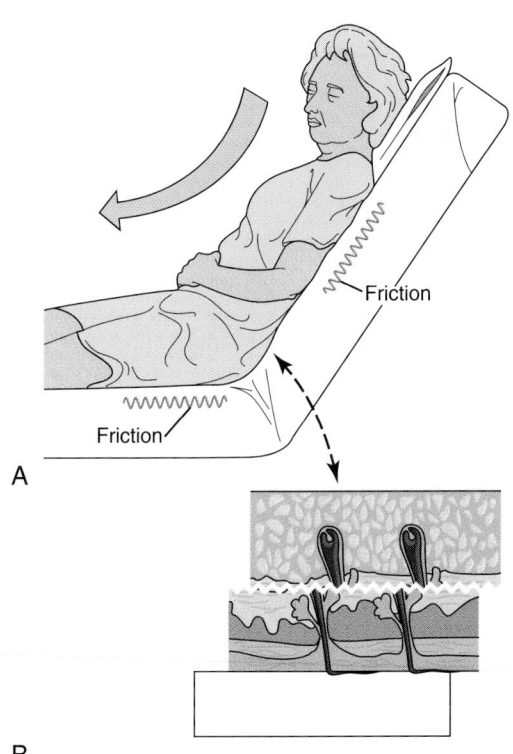

✦ **Figure 23–3**
A and *B,* Friction and shear can cause skin breakdown.

of this perception (Bergstrom *et al.*, 1987a). Documentation of these aspects of mobility is part of the baseline assessment.

✦ **Mental Status.** The client who is semiconscious or unconscious is frequently unable to move voluntarily or sufficiently to change pressure points adequately and is therefore at risk for developing pressure ulcers.

✦ **Altered Peripheral Vascular Circulation.** Peripheral vascular disease (PVD) involves the arteries, veins, and lymph vessels of the lower extremities. There is no cure—just palliative measures. Blood flow is compromised, and even benign trauma can cause an impairment in skin integrity.

Risk Scores

In addition to the initial client history and physical assessment, determining the client's risk for skin breakdown is important. Several at-risk scales have been developed to determine which clients are at high risk for developing skin breakdown. Although nurses often have an idea of clients who are at risk, determining this risk in an objective manner is more scientific. The risk instrument should also lead the nurse to the development of an appropriate nursing plan of care based on the causal and contributing factors noted during the assessment.

As early as 1962 in London, England, Norton developed a scale designed to reflect five areas of assessment: physical condition, mental condition, activity, mobility, and incontinence. A total score of 14 or less indicated that the client was likely to develop pressure ulcers, and a score lower than 12 indicated a very great risk (Norton, 1975).

The Knoll scale, developed in 1975, is an instrument that incorporates those factors found to be related to pressure ulcer formation into either the variables or the descriptors of the variables (Abruzzese, 1981). The instrument includes the variables of general health, predisposing diseases, mental status, activity, mobility, incontinence, oral nutrition intake, and oral fluid intake (Table 23–1). This instrument has some demonstrated reliability and validity in the prediction of pressure ulcer development (Towey & Erland, 1988). A total score of 12 is purported to discriminate between those clients who will be more likely to develop pressure ulcers and those who will not (Towey & Erland, 1988).

The Braden scale measures six characteristics: sensory perception, moisture, activity, mobility, nutrition, and friction and shear. Each of these characteristics or subscales is designed to be mutually exclusive and to reflect the critical determinants of pressure and other factors that influence the tolerance of the skin (Bergstrom *et al.*, 1987b). The Braden scale is used frequently in institutions to determine risk for breakdown (Table 23–2). A score of 16 or less, or a score of 18 or less for the client over 75 years of age, indicates risk for breakdown.

Psychosocial Assessment

Clients with pressure ulcer formation may have an altered body image. The young, immobile adult who develops pressure ulcers from sitting in the wheelchair may be concerned about the reactions of friends or loved ones. The family of a client in a long-term care facility who develops an impairment in skin or tissue integrity may believe that the client is not receiving adequate care and may feel guilty about their decision in placing the client in the home. Guilt sometimes leads to avoidance and less frequent visits.

If the client is being cared for in the home, the caretaker may exhibit guilt over the development of skin breakdown. Baharestani conducted a qualitative study on wife caregivers of totally dependent husbands who had stage IV pressure ulcers and concluded that the wife had ". . . grossly limited finances, physical abilities, knowledge sources, and support systems" in the home environment (1994, p. 52). Supporting the client who is at high risk for developing impairments in skin and tissue integrity and his or her family is a major role for the nurse. Informing and educating clients and families about the prevention of impaired skin integrity is essential. The AHCPR guidelines for both prevention and treatment of pressure ulcers are available for the clients and families to assist them in identifying their role in prevention and management.

Wound Healing

Another part of assessment is the determination of the healing of an existing wound (see Community Based Care box, p. 574). Wounds heal by primary, secondary, or delayed primary intention. Although all wounds heal by the same orderly sequence of events, we can affect the healing rate by our treatment methods.

Primary Intention

Tissue edges are approximated, and there is minimal tissue loss and scar formation in first intention healing. A surgical incision is an example of primary intention healing.

Secondary Intention

This wound healing occurs when the wound is extensive and there is considerable tissue loss. Wound healing by secondary intention takes longer, has a greater incidence of scarring, and tends to have an increased chance for infection.

Delayed Primary

The wound is left open for a period of time to monitor the healing process and assess for infection. This third intention closure actually has facets of both primary and secondary closure. When the open wound is determined to be healing adequately without infection, the wound may be sutured and allowed to heal as a primary closure.

Text continued on page 574

Table 23–1

KNOLL SCALE

PARAMETERS	0	1	2	3	DATE/ SCORE	DATE/ SCORE	DATE/ SCORE
General state of health	Good	Fair	Poor	Moribund			
Predisposing diseases	Absent	Slight	Moderate	Severe			
Mental status	Alert	Lethargic	Semicomatose	Comatose			
Oral nutrition intake	Good	Fair	Poor	None			
Oral fluid intake	Good	Fair	Poor	None			
Activity	Ambulatory	Assist	Chairfast*	Bedfast*			
Mobility	Full	Limited	Very limited*	Immobile*			
Incontinence	None	Occasional	Frequent*	Totally*			
				TOTAL SCORE =			

General State of Health

0   GOOD: Injury limited to one area; usually free of major health problem
1   FAIR: Minor surgery; major health problems but controlled
2   POOR: Chronic, serious health problems; major surgery
3   MORIBUND: Prognosis fatal; death expected within 3 months

Predisposing Diseases

0   ABSENT: Has no vascular disease, neuropathies, diabetes, anemia, steroid use, acquired immunodeficiency syndrome or human immunodeficiency virus present; skin breakdown
1   SLIGHT: Controlled diabetes or anemias; incipient vascular disease; incipient skin disease
2   MODERATE: Brittle diabetes; advanced vascular disease evidenced by frequent unhealed areas on skin; absent pedal pulses
3   SEVERE: Uncontrolled diabetes/anemias; well-advanced disease manifested by lack of sensation in extremities, constant unhealed areas of skin, edema of ankles and feet, thin pallid atrophic skin, brown pigmentation around ankles with stasis dermatitis

Mental Status

0   ALERT: Aware of time and place; communicates appropriately
1   LETHARGIC OR CONFUSED: Listless conversation; sleeps for long periods; sleeps most of day and night
2   SEMICOMATOSE: Responds only to painful stimuli; does not cooperate in pressure relief
3   COMATOSE: Does not respond verbally or to painful stimuli

Nutrition Intake

0   GOOD: Eats adequate amounts for age and size; weight within normal limits; gets sufficient intake from tube feedings
1   FAIR: Eats smaller than usual portions (¾); snacks between meals; under weight or over weight; tolerates diluted tube feedings; meets minimal recommended dietary allowance with feedings or total parenteral nutrition
2   POOR: Seldom eats half of served portions; snacks very little; losing weight slowly; obese; tolerates tube feedings poorly;
3   NONE: unable to eat/refuses to eat; losing weight rapidly; emaciated; nothing by mouth; no nutritional support

Fluid Intake

0   GOOD: Drinks sufficient fluids; good skin turgor (warm and resilient); sufficient intake of fluid via feeding tube or intravenously, at least 1500 ml
1   FAIR: Must be encouraged to drink fluids; skin dry and flaccid; concentration urine; 1000–1500 ml/d
2   POOR: Drinks <1000 ml/d; lips parched, mouth dry, scanty urine with no renal disease; skin dry and flaking
3   NONE: Refuses oral fluids; incapable of swallowing

Activity

0   AMBULATORY: Walks freely without help
1   NEEDS HELP: Requires assistance to walk; uses crutches or walker
4   CHAIRFAST: Cannot ambulate; confined to chair or wheelchair
6   BEDFAST: Cannot sit in chair; remains constantly in bed

Mobility

0   FULL: Can move all extremities at will; voluntarily changes position
1   LIMITED: Cannot voluntarily move all extremities; cast on arm or leg; pain on joint movement
4   VERY LIMITED: Moves extremities only with assistance; severe pain on joint movement; body cast; paraplegic or hemiparesis
5   IMMOBILE: Never voluntarily changes position; contractures prevent movement; all extremities paralyzed

Incontinence

0   NONE: Has control of bowel and bladder
1   OCCASIONAL: Stress incontinence; occasional diarrhea
4   FREQUENT: Usually incontinent of urine; frequently incontinent of stool
6   TOTAL: No control over bowel or bladder

*Count as double.

Table 23–2

BRADEN RISK SCALE

					Date	Date	Date	Date
SENSORY PERCEPTION								
Ability to respond meaningfully to pressure-related discomfort	**1. Completely limited:** Unresponsive (does not moan, flinch, or grasp) to painful stimuli due to diminished level of consciousness or sedation OR Limited ability to feel pain over most of body surface	**2. Very limited:** Responds only to painful stimuli; cannot communicate discomfort except by moaning or restlessness OR Has a sensory impairment that limits the ability to feel pain or discomfort over half of body	**3. Slightly limited:** Responds to verbal commands but cannot always communicate discomfort or need to be turned OR Has some sensory impairment that limits ability to feel pain or discomfort in one or two extremities	**4. No impairment:** Responds to verbal commands; has no sensory deficit that would limit ability to feel or voice pain or discomfort				
MOISTURE								
Degree to which skin is exposed to moisture	**1. Constantly moist:** Skin is kept moist almost constantly by perspiration, urine, etc; dampness is detected every time patient is moved or turned	**2. Moist:** Skin is often but not always moist; linen must be changed at least once a shift	**3. Occasionally moist:** Skin is occasionally moist, requiring an extra linen change approximately once a day	**4. Rarely moist:** Skin is usually dry; linen requires changing only at routine intervals				
ACTIVITY								
Degree of physical activity	**1. Bedfast:** Confined to bed	**2. Chairfast:** Ability to walk severely limited or nonexistent; cannot bear own weight and/or must be assisted into chair or wheelchair	**3. Walks occasionally:** Walks occasionally during day but for very short distances, with or without assistance; spends majority of each shift in bed or chair	**4. Walks frequently:** Walks outside the room at least twice a day and inside room at least once every 2 h during waking hours				
MOBILITY								
Ability to change and control body position	**1. Completely immobile:** Does not make even slight changes in body or extremity position without assistance	**2. Very limited:** Makes occasional slight changes in body or extremity position, but unable to make frequent or significant changes independently	**3. Slightly limited:** Makes frequent, though slight, changes in body or extremity position independently	**4. No limitations:** Makes major and frequent changes in position without assistance				

NUTRITION

Usual food intake pattern

1. Very poor:
Never eats a complete meal; rarely eats more than a third of any food offered; eats two servings or less of protein (meat or dairy products) per day; takes fluids poorly; does not take a liquid dietary supplement
OR
Is on nothing by mouth diet and/or maintained on clear liquids or intravenous feeding for more than 5 d

2. Probably inadequate:
Rarely eats a complete meal and generally eats only about half of any food offered; protein intake includes only three servings of meat or dairy products per day; occasionally will take a dietary supplement
OR
Receives less than optimal amount of liquid diet or tube feeding

3. Adequate:
Eats over half of most meals; eats a total of four servings of protein (meat, dairy products) each day; occasionally will refuse a meal, but will usually take a supplement if offered
OR
Is on a tube feeding or total parenteral nutrition regimen, which probably meets most of nutritional needs

4. Excellent:
Eats most of every meal; never refuses a meal; usually eats a total of four or more servings of meat and dairy products; occasionally eats between meals; does not require supplementation

FRICTION AND SHEAR

1. Problem:
Requires moderate to maximum assistance in moving; complete lifting without sliding against sheets is impossible; frequently slides down in bed or chair, requiring frequent repositioning with maximum assistance; spasticity, contractures, or agitation leads to almost constant friction

2. Potential problem:
Moves feebly or requires minimum assistance; during a move, skin probably slides to some extent against sheets, chair, restraints, or other devices; maintains relatively good position in chair or bed most of the time, but occasionally slides down

3. No apparent problem:
Moves in bed and in chair independently and has sufficient muscle strength to lift up completely during move; maintains good position in bed or chair at all times

Bergstrom, N., Braden, B. J., Laguzza, A., & Holman, V. (1989). Clinical utility of The Braden Scale for predicting pressure sore risk. *Decubitus, 2,* 44–51.

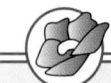

COMMUNITY BASED CARE

WOUNDS

Clients are frequently discharged from the hospital with open wounds resulting from surgery, venous/arterial disease, pressure ulcers, burns, injuries, skin infections, or other dermatological conditions. The goals of the home care nurse are to promote wound healing, prevent further breakdown, and teach the client or caregiver to care for the wound independently. Most wounds are cleansed with saline or a wound cleansing solution to remove exudate. Hydrogels are very useful to keep the wound bed moist; deep wounds may need packing with moist gauze or a calcium alginate product to absorb heavy drainage. Dressing changes are usually done daily, unless drainage is heavy, significant infection is present, or frequent soilage of the dressings occurs. Most wounds are managed using clean technique, except for open surgical wounds.

The nurse documents a wound assessment with each dressing change, including amount and character of drainage, wound bed, and periwound appearance. Wound dimensions are measured regularly—usually weekly. A wound care flow sheet can facilitate documentation.

Additional teaching topics for home wound care include

1. Promoting wound healing by encouraging nutrition and hydration, adequate rest, and moderate exercise as tolerated

2. Recognizing the signs and symptoms of wound infection and knowing when to call the nurse or physician

3. Preventing further skin breakdown by frequent repositioning and weight shifting, meticulous skin care, pressure-relieving devices or special mattresses, proper lifting and turning techniques, and good nutrition and hydration

4. Proper disposal of soiled dressings—generally double bagging before putting into the trash

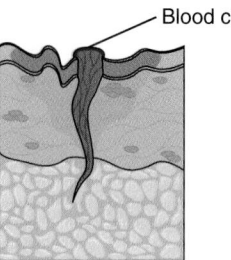

Phase 1: Inflammation
  Lasts up to 4 days
  Vasoconstriction occurs; clot forms to control bleeding
  Histamine released
  Redness, edema, warmth, and pain with damage
    to the microcirculation

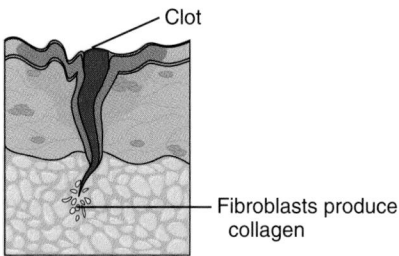

Phase 2: Granulation
  Lasts for 5–20 days
  Collagen synthesized
  Granulation tissue forms

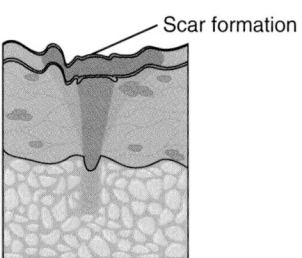

Phase 3: Remodeling
  Lasts for > 20 days
  Wound contracts due to collagen fiber
    reorganization

❥ **Figure 23–4**
Three phases of wound healing.

Phases of Wound Healing

There are three generally recognized phases of wound healing that do not occur discretely but have some overlap (Fig. 23–4). Understanding the phases is helpful in making informed wound treatment decisions.

Phase I — Inflammation

This first phase is a defensive phase or an exudative phase and begins as soon as the body is injured (Bryant, 1987). During this phase, bleeding is controlled by the formation of a fibrin clot and hemostasis, and bacterial invasion is fought by inflammation.

Because of the tissue injury, histamine is released at the injury site, allowing the surrounding vessels to dilate and become more permeable, leading to vasocongestion. These phenomena lead to the clinical observations of erythema, warmth, edema, and pain. Leukocytes are attracted to the wound to protect the wound from bacterial invasion. Approximately 4 days later, macrophages enter the wound. Macrophages continue the débridement and attraction of growth factors throughout the healing process (Doughty, 1992).

Phase II — Proliferative

During this second phase, **granulation** and epithelialization occur in the wound bed. *Granulation* refers to the formation of the new connective tissue by collagen synthesis and angiogenesis. *Epithelialization* is the resurfacing of the wound bed by the migration of epithelial cells. This cell proliferation phase has also been known as the fibroblastic phase and lasts for 4 to 20 days after the injury. The events during this phase occur as follows: macrophage entry; fibroblast production, which yields the secretion of collagen; and lastly, the development of new capillary networks to support the new tissue development (angiogenesis). Collagen provides tensile strength to the body tissue. This tensile strength refers to the amount of pressure that can be applied to the wound without the wound rupturing. This new wound bed, filled with granulation tissue, has a unique appearance: moist, beefy red, shiny, and fragile. Epithelialization occurs over this surface as the epithelial cells migrate across a wound bed free of devitalized tissue such as eschar (thick, leathery or woody, necrotic tissue), necrotic tissue, and blood clots (Bryant, 1987). Epithelial tissue appears as a silvery layer (Eaglstein, 1990) and then gradually matches the skin tone of the person.

Phase III—Remodeling

Also known as the maturation or matrix formation phase, remodeling actually begins as soon as granulation tissue forms. This final phase may continue for up to 2 years, with the macrophages playing an important role as they mediate collagen lysis and collagen synthesis. The final result is a reorganization of the collagen-formed scar tissue, hopefully to a scar with the most tensile strength. Tensile strength is sufficient at 15 to 20 days postoperatively to resist normal stress. The remodeling continues, and wound strength increases so that 70 to 80% of the original intact skin strength is reached within 3 to 6 months.

Factors Affecting Wound Healing

Local and systemic factors may be present that negatively affect wound healing. The presence of microorganisms, necrotic tissue, edema, poor nutrition, certain disease entities, selected medications, and aging are a few examples of impediments to wound healing.

Infection

Wound infections prolong the inflammatory phase of wound healing and delay the synthesis of collagen and, subsequently, the granulation and epithelialization of the wound.

Tissue Perfusion and Oxygenation

Necrotic tissue and edema are negative factors in wound beds. Wound repair is contingent on the cells receiving enough oxygen to fuel their repair functions. The rate of collagen synthesis and epithelial proliferation and migration is dependent on adequate levels of oxygen in the tissues. Edematous tissues decrease the flow of oxygen to the area and affect the wound

healing. The phagocytotic activity occurs in both hypoxic and oxygenated tissue, but the ability of phagocytes to kill bacteria is predominantly oxygen dependent (Bryant, 1992). Necrotic tissue, therefore, increases the need for phagocytosis and, subsequently, oxygen. The body works harder to heal the wound.

Nutrition

As discussed earlier in the chapter, adequate nutrition is important for collagen synthesis (protein, vitamin C, zinc, iron), collagen fiber cross-linking (copper, B complex), and energy needed to do repairs (calories).

Diseases

Diabetes mellitus is a disease that has significant negative effects on wound healing. Because of the angiopathic changes in vessels, oxygenation to the wound bed is impaired. Decreased collagen synthesis and increased infections are two results of this decreased tissue perfusion. Clients with malignancies or renal or hepatic diseases also demonstrate a decreased ability to heal wounds.

Medications

Corticosteroids are known for their antiinflammatory actions. The movement of neutrophils and macrophages into the wound is affected, and the wound is susceptible to infection and retarded healing because the macrophages attract the growth factors that stimulate the collagen synthesis. Immunosuppressive medications also affect the inflammatory response and delay wound healing.

Aging

Cells are less proliferative as age progresses, leading to decreased wound contraction rates, impaired wound remodeling, and decreased ability to reepithelialize. (See previous discussion on aging at beginning of chapter.)

Drainage

Excessive drainage in a wound area may impede healing, as it places pressure on granulating tissue, and the drainage may harbor bacterial growth. The physician may insert a drain into the incision or into a wound area to minimize the pooling fluid. Penrose drains are most commonly used and work on the principle of gravity and a path of least resistance to aid in drainage from an area. A pin is often placed in the Penrose to prevent it from going into the wound, and the pin can be seen on x-ray if the drain does slide into the wound. The T-tube used for clients who have had common bile duct surgery is another example of a gravity drain.

Suction drains are also frequently used for clients. Hemovacs and Jackson-Pratt tubes are closed-suction drains that exert only low pressure on the wound area as long as the bladder of the drain is compressed. If the vacuum is unable to be maintained, the surgeon may use larger drains such as sump drains that are connected to a secondary vacuum source, such as wall suction.

Complications of Wound Healing
Infection

A major complication of wound healing is the development of an infection. Débriding, wound cleansing, and appropriate dressing technique assist in keeping a wound clean. Wound infections are a major nosocomial problem in the hospitalized client but occur in clients in all settings.

Hemorrhage

A profuse amount of bloody drainage is abnormal in a wound. Hemorrhage may be caused by a ruptured blood vessel, loose suture, or dislodged blood clot. The hemorrhage may be external or internal. The external hemorrhage is more easily noted, as the wound dressing becomes wet. Initially, the nurse may mark the extent of the saturation, but a saturated or leaking dressing needs attention. The physician should be notified, and the dressing should usually be changed, not reinforced, as the wet dressing macerates the good skin and is an excellent medium for bacterial growth. A pressure dressing that is saturated should be reinforced until the physician arrives. Risk of hemorrhage is the greatest during the first 24 to 48 hours after surgery. Internal hemorrhage can be more subtle, and the nurse must assess the wound for distention or swelling, and assess the client for signs of hypovolemic shock.

Dehiscence

Dehiscence is a total or partial separation of the wound edges and tissue layers and usually occurs before the second phase of wound healing when collagen formation is beginning. Abdominal surgical wounds are the most susceptible to dehiscence, which may occur after some type of strain such as sneezing, coughing, or vomiting. Obese and malnourished clients are more susceptible to dehiscence because they have increased fat tissue and therefore a decreased blood supply to the surgical area. On assessment, a noted increase in serosanguineous drainage or a client's comment about feeling as if the wound is separating may be an indication of impending dehiscence.

Evisceration

This is a phenomenon predominantly of abdominal wounds and is characterized by the total separation of the wound edges with protrusion of the visceral organs through the opening. It is a medical emergency and requires surgical repair. The nurse should soak sterile dressings or towels in saline solution and place them over the wound and organs until the physician arrives. The sterile saline soaks keep the organs moist and may decrease the chances of infection. Do not force the organs back into the cavity and do not move the client until the client returns to the operating room.

Fistulas

A fistula is an abnormal tract between an internal organ and the skin or between internal organs. Fistulas may be surgically created for gastrostomy or tracheostomy tubes, but many occur because of poor wound healing. This tract may result in fluid and electrolyte imbalances, infection risks, or skin breakdown from the drainage.

Traumatic Wounds

Persons who have suffered trauma from any cause and have a wound should be assessed for bleeding and broken bones. If the wound is bleeding profusely, applying pressure with a clean cloth to decrease or stop the bleeding is important. If there is an opportunity to rinse the wound of any debris, the nurse may do so; however, most traumatic wounds occur in a location that precludes any but the basic first aid measures.

Diagnostic Studies
Collecting a Wound Culture

A client with a wound that is erythematous, painful, indurated, and/or edematous should be observed for a possible wound infection. The physician should be notified of this finding, and a culture may be ordered. Cultures are aerobic or anaerobic.

Aerobic cultures are usually obtained as swab cultures, which are often done with a "culturette" tube that contains a cotton-tipped applicator. After the culture is obtained, the applicator is returned to the tube, and the bottom of the tube is crushed to activate the medium.

Anaerobic cultures are obtained without exposing the culture sample to air during the collection and transport or laboratory procedure. This is usually accomplished by aspirating fluid with a needle and syringe, changing the needle after expelling any extra air from the syringe, and injecting the aspirant into a special anaerobic culture medium in a vial.

There is some controversy regarding the necessity of wound cultures and the techniques that should be used to complete these cultures. Swab cultures are the most common and may demonstrate infection, especially in the acute wound versus the chronic wound. The chronic wound, however, is known to be contaminated with bacteria, and generally swabbing is not productive to determine organisms responsible for infection. It is suggested that wound aspiration or bi-

OBTAINING A WOUND CULTURE

Equipment:

Irrigation set
Sterile gloves or clean gloves
Sterile or clean gauze
Wound culture bottle or culturette tube

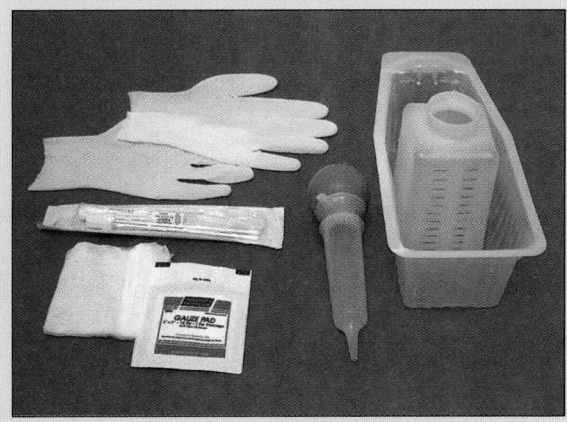

Action	Rationale
1. Gently irrigate wound with normal saline solution to remove all visible debris, topical ointments or creams, and/or excessive drainage.	**1.** DO NOT use an antiseptic solution, as causative organisms might be killed.
2. Open gauze pads and wound culture kit. For sterile procedure, apply sterile gloves.	**2.** Reduces possibility of contamination.
3. Absorb excess saline with appropriate gauze pad.	**3.** Excess fluid may impede culture results.
4. Separate margins of deep wounds.	**4.** Do not touch skin edges with swab, as this area contains natural microorganisms.
5. Insert swab into granulating, viable tissue. Press and rotate swab over wound surface for at least 30 seconds in ziz-zag pattern.	**5.** Microorganisms live in viable tissue; do not swab necrotic tissue.

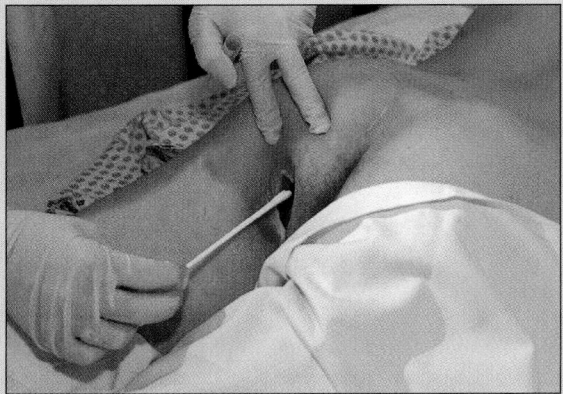

Step 5

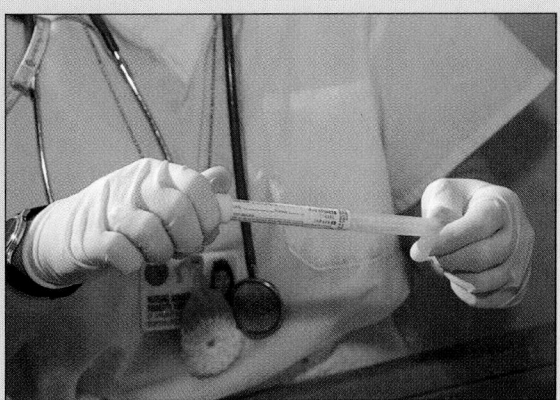

Step 6

6. Place swab in sterile culture tube with medium immediately.	**6.** Do not touch swab end to any other surface, or contamination may occur.
7. Label specimen with client name, date, time, anatomical site, type of specimen, and laboratory test to be performed. List any topical therapy the client is receiving.	**7.** Proper labeling is required to ensure accuracy.
8. Send specimen to laboratory immediately.	**8.** Cultures need to be implanted on correct medium as soon as possible.

Documentation: Document appearance of wound and that culture was sent.

opsy is more accurate for cultures, especially of the chronic wound (Cuzzell, 1993).

A wound aspiration for culture should be done by cleansing the wound with normal saline solution after dressing removal, then instilling approximately 10 ml of normal saline solution into the wound bed, allowing it to interact with the wound tissue for approximately 10 minutes, and then aspirating the saline solution from the wound and transferring it to the appropriate container. (See Procedure 23–1, Obtaining a Wound Culture.)

Nursing Diagnosis

Nursing diagnosis for the client with wounds relates only to those clients with pressure sores or other impairments of skin integrity as a result of moisture, pressure, friction, or shear. Surgical wounds should not be reclassified into a nursing diagnosis of skin or tissue integrity impairment.

The most common North American Nursing Diagnosis Association (NANDA) nursing diagnoses for clients with wounds are

* Impaired Tissue Integrity, which Gordon (1993) describes as "a state in which an individual experiences damage to mucous membrane or to corneal, integumentary, or subcutaneous tissue."
* Risk for Infection should also be considered for clients with Impaired Tissue Integrity as these clients are subject to infection due to the damaged skin.
* Impaired Skin Integrity is a third nursing diagnosis to consider if the wound is superficial. There are other issues that a client may face because of a wound; see the Nursing Diagnoses box, which also notes those diagnoses and contributing factors.

Assessment reveals data that determine whether there is an actual or potential risk for impaired skin or tissue integrity. The diagnosis should include the defining characteristics that support the diagnostic label (Gordon, 1993). Many physiological alterations may affect skin integrity. By analyzing the causal and contributing factors, the nurse can determine the focus of the plan. Also, the outcome objectives for the plan of care should reflect the factors that may create a problem for the client. For instance, if mobility is a factor, then the plan should address the decrease of pressure for the client. Time frames should be as realistic as possible.

Planning

Preventing skin breakdown is much more cost-effective than treating breakdown once it has occurred (see Sample Nursing Care Plan for the Client with Anginal Pain). The goals for preventing skin breakdown are that

1. The skin will remain clean and dry
2. The skin will not be subjected to pressure, friction, and/or shear forces

All wounds, whether acute or chronic, are subject to pressure from dressings or the body, depending on the location of the wound; moisture breakdown if the wound is draining; and friction and shear injury from tape and dressings. Therefore, if the nurse is caring for existing skin breakdown, a pressure ulcer, or a surgical wound, the goals for skin care are maintained for the periwound area. Additional goals for existing wounds are that

1. The skin will maintain a moist and protected wound environment that promotes healing and inhibits infection
2. The client will report decreased pain related to the wound
3. The client will maintain adequate nutrition to enhance wound healing
4. The client will be able to discuss the signs and symptoms of wound complications

To determine the best treatment, the wound should be assessed and cleansed before dressing. Assessment of any wound, whether surgically or traumatically created, requires the same assessment data.

Methods for prevention of skin breakdown for clients with moisture, pressure, friction, and/or shear problems is well documented in the literature, should follow the AHCPR guidelines (Panel for the Prediction and Prevention of Pressure Ulcers, 1992), and can be classified as standards of care. These standards of care are independent nursing functions and apply to the chronic pressure ulcer as well as the acute surgical wound.

Implementation

Developing the individualized plan of care from the following standards is the role of the professional nurse. Based on the assessment of the causal and contributing factors related to skin breakdown, specific interventions may be identified and implemented.

Providing Measures to Control Moisture

To meet the first outcome goal, the standard of care for moisture is reviewed. Clients must be assessed daily for skin breakdown. Effectiveness of the specific plan based on the standard should be monitored and changed if not effective in preventing skin breakdown. Unless detrimental effects are noted, the plan of care should remain in effect for at least 3 days. (See Box 23–5, Standards of Care, concerning the three steps in preventing skin breakdown from moisture.)

Cleanse

1. Keeping skin clean and dry by using mild soap and water or specially formulated bath cleanser is important, as moisture macerates skin over time.

SAMPLE NURSING CARE PLAN

THE CLIENT WITH ANGINAL PAIN

A 78-year-old client, Mr. B., is admitted to your medical unit for anginal pain to rule out myocardial infarction. The client lives at home with his wife and is not active, as he also has severe arthritis. Based on the nursing history, his risk score on the Knoll scale is

General state of health—1

Mental status—0

Activity—4

Mobility—4

Incontinence—4

Oral nutrition—2

Oral fluid—2

Predisposing diseases—1

Total score of 18

Mr. B. has antiembolic stockings ordered for each leg, is on bedrest with bathroom privileges, and has a low-fat, low-sodium diet ordered.

Nursing Diagnosis: Risk for skin breakdown related to (1) pressure, (2) friction and shear related to immobility and inactivity, and (3) moisture from occasional urine incontinence.

Expected Outcome: Client will not develop any skin breakdown during hospitalization.

Action	Rationale
1. Assess the client for the presence of any skin breakdown every day.	**1.** Obtain a baseline assessment for purposes of comparison.
2. Change every client's position in bed at least every 2 hours—turning schedule on bedside table—right side; back; left side; back; right side. Assess effectiveness of turning by skin examination 30 minutes after each turn, and change schedule as needed.	**2.** Changing position relieves pressure to allow blood flow to tissue over bony prominences. Development of a turning schedule will assist other staff members in following prescribed plan. Reddened areas should blanch when pressed; if not, more frequent turning is needed (nonblanching erythema is a hallmark of tissue ischemia) (Maklebust, 1991).
3. Place client on pressure-reducing surface of *brand name* alternating-pressure mattress.	**3.** Client's risk score on mobility and activity warrants focus on pressure as causal factor.
4. Remove elastic stockings each shift for 30 minutes @ 0600, 1400, 2200 and check heels.	**4.** Standard of care recommends removal every shift. Standard of care for pressure recommends checking pressure points on removal of special equipment.
5. Move client with cotton underpad. DO NOT use extra sheets/blankets, paper/plastic pads under this client.	**5.** Standard of care for friction/shear recommends lifting versus dragging/sliding clients. Standard of care for pressure suggests minimal layers between client and pressure reduction device.
6. When head of bed is elevated to 30 degrees, gatch knees slightly.	**6.** Standard of care for friction/shear recommends this to prevent sliding of client in bed.
7. Wash client's skin as soon as possible after each incontinent episode with *brand name* balanced wash. Protect client's skin from moisture with *brand name* protectant ointment.	**7.** Standard of care for moisture notes that washing with pH-balanced wash is important to avoid changing the pH mantle of the skin. Protecting the skin from wetness is accomplished with selected protectant ointments that impede the moisture from attacking the skin.
8. Educate client and family about pressure relief, friction and shear, and moisture effects on skin integrity.	**8.** Client/family education is important to development of and participation in the plan of care.
9. Document turning, inspection of pressure points and perineal area, and client/family education on flow sheet at bedside.	**9.** Documentation of these factors is needed to ascertain the progress toward the outcome goal.

Box **23–5**

SKIN INTEGRITY STANDARD OF CARE: MOISTURE

Goal

Protect intact or impaired skin from further breakdown due to moisture from incontinence of urine or stool, from perspiration, or from draining wounds.

Nursing Interventions

Step 1: Cleanse

* Wash with mild soap and water and rinse well

OR

* Use no rinse—pH wash to cleanse skin

Step 2: Protect

Choose one:

* Apply skin protectant ointment only; apply liberally
* Apply occlusive ointment
* Apply transparent polyurethane dressing
* Apply hydrocolloid wafer

Remember to "picture frame" edges of transparent and hydrocolloid dressings. Avoid powders, ointments (especially zinc oxide–based ointments) to radiation fields without physician order.

Step 3: Contain

Choose appropriate containment method based on person's activity and needs.

* Condom catheter for incontinent males
* Fecal incontinence collector for bed-bound person with diarrhea or constant oozing
* Pouch draining wounds
* *One* underpad to absorb wetness
* *Selective* diapering for ambulatory client or client who is restless—Consider diaper with gel formation

Avoid rectal tubes, as they may break down bowel mucosa.

---

2. In acute care settings, use a pH-balanced cleanser for incontinent clients to minimize changing the acid mantle of the skin, which acts as a protectant. The cleanser may also be used *around* a wound when cleansing caustic wound drainage. For clients in long-term care facilities or in the home, if the client is developing increased redness with the usual washing and protecting standard for the agency, a pH-balanced cleanser should be the next plan.

3. Pat skin while washing and drying. Rubbing or massaging is not indicated, as fragile tissues may be torn.

Protect

1. Moisturizing creams keep skin from becoming dry and cracked. Cracked skin is more susceptible to bacterial invasion.

2. Moisture-repellent ointments protect skin from wetness. These are especially useful in the perineal and perianal areas, but consider other options for periwound areas, as ointments may "migrate" into the wound.

3. Apply protective barrier spray or wipes for protecting skin from incontinence, draining wounds, or moist dressings, as these products act as a water repellent. Barrier sprays or wipes do not migrate into wounds, as they dry on the skin.

4. Selected dressings that do not allow moisture to penetrate the skin, such as polyurethane films, hydrocolloids, or pectin wafers are useful. These dressings are placed on the skin that may come in contact with wound drainage, stool, or urine.

5. Protect skin from moisture with products that are easily removed with pH-balanced washes. Avoid talcum powder (it produces grit that acts like sandpaper), cornstarch (it breaks down into a sugar, which promotes yeast development), and zinc oxide products that are not manufactured for easy removal.

Contain

Because decreasing exposure of skin to moisture is more effective than healing macerated and denuded skin, containment of drainage is a significant nursing care measure.

1. Apply a fecal incontinence collector to the anal opening for the client who has diarrhea and is bedridden. The collector is not usually effective for the ambulatory client. These collectors are very advantageous, but the nurse may need assistance with the application to position the device correctly. Careful removal of this adhesive-backed product from the skin is a factor in preventing unnecessary skin tears from the adhesive.

2. Do not diaper bedridden clients unless absolutely necessary, as the diaper traps wetness next to the skin, and the plastic increases surface temperature, which increases susceptibility of skin to effects of pressure and moisture. (There are some diapers that trap moisture and turn into a gel, which may decrease effects of moisture next to the skin.) Consider the psychological effects of a diaper on an adult, and use this method as a last resort.

3. Pouch draining wounds to minimize moisture on skin. A variety of wound pouches or ostomy pouches are available. The product lines that may be used in the standards listed here are varied and extensive. Consult the policies and procedures of the agency and the clinical nurse specialist for wound and skin care or the enterostomal therapy nurse for additional information.

Minimizing Pressure

Education is a key factor for prevention of pressure ulcers (Box 23–6).

1. Research has noted that frequent small body shifts change pressure points enough so that the length of time for remaining in one general position can be tolerated for a longer period of time. The nurse needs to develop a plan for moving various parts of the client's body on each visit to the room because within a 2-hour time period, slight pressure changes will have taken place. For the client at home, the caregiver needs to participate in the moving of the client with the nurse so he or she will understand the

Box 23–6

STANDARD OF CARE FOR PRESSURE, FRICTION, AND SHEAR

Assessment for Pressure Risk

- Assess scores on risk form for significant causal and/or contributing factors for this protocol. Nursing care plan should reflect actions to alleviate the *causal* factors.

- Remove all elastic stockings, immobilizers, splints, restraints at least every 8 hours. **EXCEPTION:** Check with physician before removing any orthopedic equipment.

Nursing Interventions

Education

Teach client/caregiver the following:

Positioning/Activity

- Make small changes in position to alter pressure points every 30 to 60 minutes (develop schedule)

- Turn to side, back, side, abdomen every 2 hours or more frequently as needed (develop schedule)

- Conduct active or passive ROM to involved extremities every 4 hours while client is awake, unless contraindicated (develop schedule)

- Maintain activity as tolerated

Get client out of bed whenever possible (develop schedule)

Do not allow client to sit in chair for more than 1 hour without significant change in position. (Stand client and sit client down in a different position or change position of recliner or put client back to bed; develop schedule)

Pressure Reduction/Relief

- Separate all pressure points (*e.g.,* knees, ankles) with pillows or other padding (identify what is to be used and where)

- Elevate reddened heels off of bed with pillow under calves or use selected foot splints/heel pressure-relief devices ("sheepskin" booties and padded socks DO NOT provide pressure relief)

- Mattress replacements to reduce pressure (identify product)

- Use *minimal number* of sheets, diapers, underpads, as thick layers decrease effectiveness of pressure-reduction products

- Evaluate patients for specialty pressure-relief beds as necessary

Friction and Shear

- Lift versus slide client (use underpad or draw sheet)

- Elevate the head of the client's bed no more than 30 degrees unless tube fed

- Gatch bed to raise knees slightly to decrease down-sliding if in hospital bed

techniques that may be used to facilitate repositioning without injuring themselves or the client.

2. Removal of stockings and other tight items is important, as all devices place pressure on the skin, and this pressure needs to be relieved on a regular basis. After removal of items, check possible pressure points for non-blanchable erythema.

Positioning/Activity

1. Schedules serve as reminders for nursing staff or family and ensure that the client has been positioned on a regular basis. These schedules need to be developed by the client with the caregiver or nurse and should include small body shifts as well as turning and out-of-bed plans.

2. Active and passive range of motion (ROM) exercises decrease the development of contractures and pressure points. The ROM plan needs to highlight the extremities and actual exercises that are to be done for the client, and the family and client should be involved in these plans.

3. The heels are very susceptible to pressure, and breakdown has been documented even in pressure relief specialty beds. Elevating the heels off of the bed with special products may be an effective method for relieving heel pressure. However, heel protection research is limited and inconclusive at this time. A partial list of products that have received attention in the literature includes Span-aid foot-drop stop, Span-aid cradle boot, Lunax foam boot, L'Nard Multi-Podus splint, Stryker Air-Shu, and Spenco Silicore Foot Pillow. Accurate placement of the foot in the device and correct sizing are important facets of protecting heels (Fig. 23–5). Elevating the heel with pillows or blankets may not be reliable, as the pillows or blankets may move or may elevate the leg so that proper body alignment is not maintained. Pressure is also exerted by immobilizers; they should be removed at least once per shift. The condition of the skin on the heels should be checked and documented each time a device is removed.

Teaching the family or caregiver of the client who will be at home is of paramount importance. Not only does the plan need to be developed *with* this person to ensure that it is realistic but also the nurse needs to

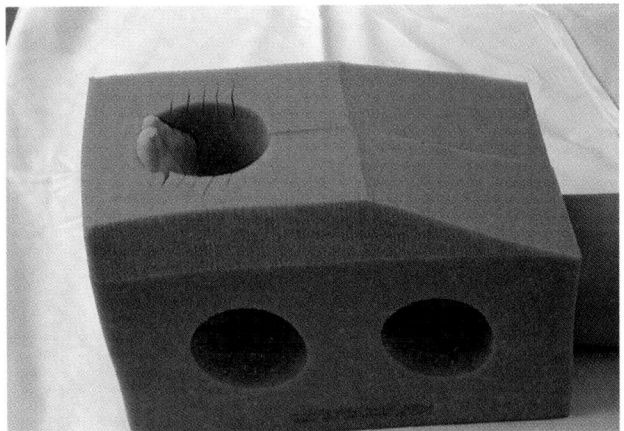

❧ **Figure 23–5**
A heel protector device can relieve heel pressure, preventing skin breakdown in that area.

ensure that the plan and its implementation are understood and can be physically and emotionally accomplished.

Pressure reduction and relief for the immobilized client is a significant business in today's health care market. Preventing pressure ulcers by reducing or eliminating pressure is a goal of nurses, and the number of products available to attempt to meet this goal is extensive. Pressure reduction is used for clients who may be able to reposition themselves or need minimal

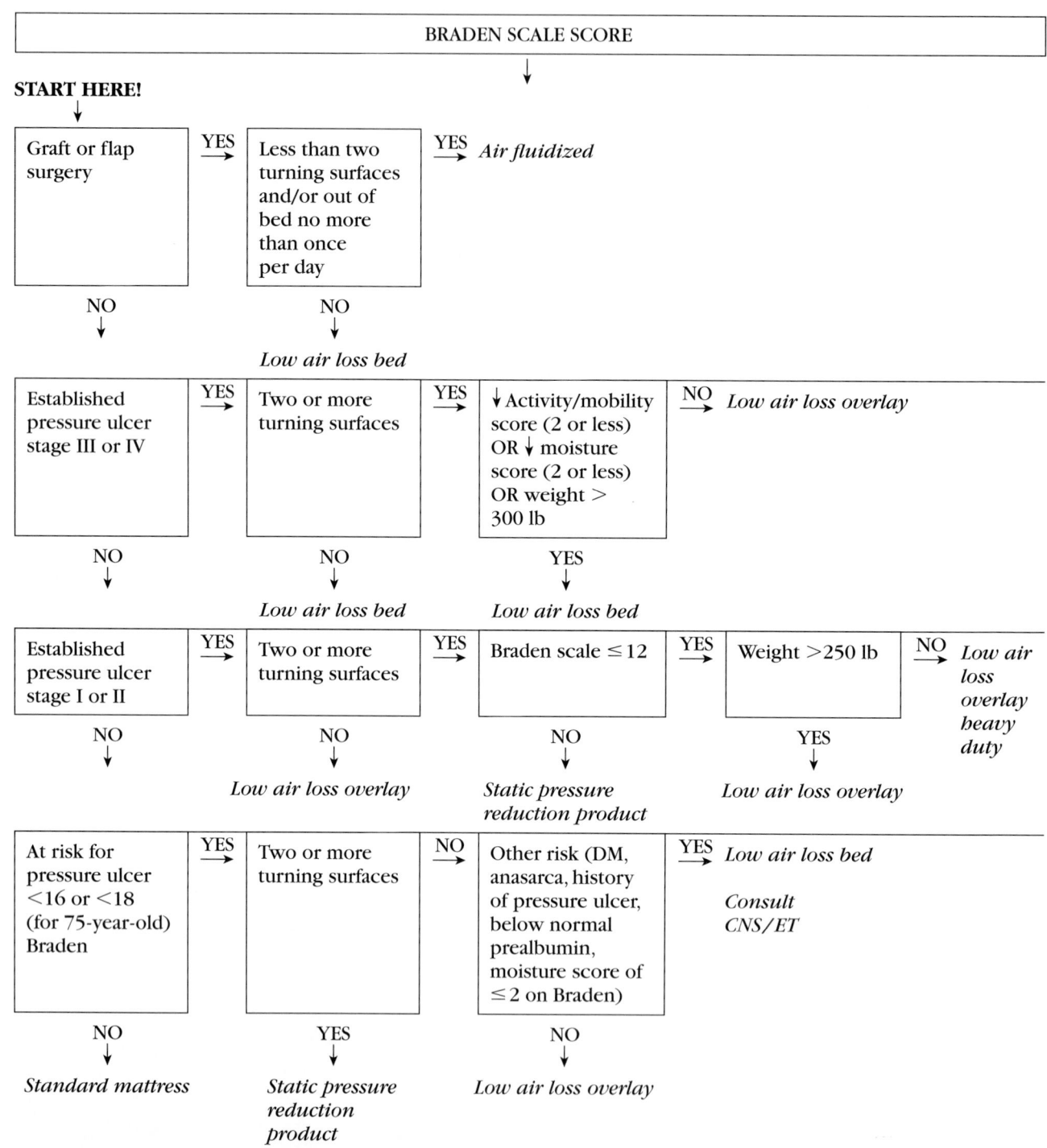

Consult CNS/ET as needed for treatment plans
Consult CNS/ET for any patient who has a pressure ulcer that is not healing

✦ Figure 23–6
Flow chart for selecting a pressure-relieving device based on client needs. (CNS/ET = clinical nurse specialist/enterostomal therapist; DM = diabetes mellitus; OOB = out of bed; prn = as needed.)

assistance. These devices are usually overlays of foam, water, or air. Pressure-relieving devices consistently maintain interface pressures that are below arterial capillary closing pressure. These products subsequently reduce the risk of cell hypoxia, which causes cell necrosis. This type of product is helpful for the client who is unable to move or shift position without assistance or who is limited to positioning on one skin surface (Johnson *et al.*, 1991). Specialty mattress and bed products for reduction or relief of pressure *do not* negate the need for turning clients on a regular schedule.

Pressure-Reduction and Pressure-Relief Devices

There is a difference between pressure relief and pressure reduction. "Pressure reduction devices are defined as a mattress that reduces pressure as compared with the standard hospital mattress surface yet does not keep interface pressure consistently below capillary closing pressure" (Petrie & Hummel, 1990).

1. Pressure-reducing mattresses (*e.g.*, foam, gel, water, alternating pressure) should be used with all clients who are at low to moderate risk for pressure as determined by the risk instrument.
2. Pressure-relieving devices (*e.g.*, selected dynamic mattresses and beds) may be necessary for the high-risk client as determined by the risk instrument score and other variables. (See Fig. 23–6 for sample selection process.)
3. Utilizing multiple layers of sheets, pads, and blankets decreases the effectiveness of pressure-reducing or pressure-relieving devices.

Reducing Friction and Shear

1. Sliding or dragging clients across sheets creates shearing.
2. The client's plan of care should be based on the standards of care and developed with the client so that the specifics of the plan will reflect the client's particular problems as well as preferences.
3. Timely implementation of the individualized plan of care based on the causal and contributing factors placing the client at risk is imperative.

The development of specific nursing interventions for clients with moisture and friction and shear follows the example of nursing interventions for pressure. General statements as noted in the standards of care are not complete enough for other nurses to implement. Therefore, for the individualized plan of care, the categories in the standards need to be elaborated on in terms of time frames, specific products, and other factors. Prevention and/or treatment of skin integrity problems should be planned, directed, and assessed by the professional nurse. (See Sample Nursing Care Plan box for the plan of care.)

Treatment of pressure ulcers in particular has been highlighted in the AHCPR guidelines (Panel for the Prediction and Prevention of Pressure Ulcers in Adults, 1994) (Box 23–7). Although these guidelines were written for pressure ulcers in particular, there are facets that are applicable to all wounds.

Wound Cleansing

Cleansing wounds serves the purpose of providing a moist wound environment and removing bacteria and slough on the surface of the wound, which impede healing.

When planning what to use for wound cleansing, the nurse decides what type of wound is present: clean or dirty. Clean wounds do not have excessive, odorous drainage or necrotic or slough tissue that characterizes a dirty wound.

Clean Wounds

Gentle cleansing with a noncytotoxic agent (normal saline irrigating solution and some of the manufactured cleansing agents available) should be done prior to applying any dressing. Noncytotoxic agents decrease the amount of disruption to the wound bed of proliferating cells that otherwise occurs with antiseptic solutions (*e.g.*, povidone-iodine, hypochlorite, hydrogen peroxide, or acetic acid). The nurse selects one of these solutions, depending on the products that the agency uses. Table 23–3 lists common wound cleansing solutions.

Gentle irrigation is accomplished by pouring solution over the wound bed or gently flushing the wound with a 60-ml catheter tip syringe until the drainage is clear. Pressurized irrigation techniques and whirlpool therapy are *not* indicated for clean wounds, as these methods disturb cell proliferation in the wound bed (Doughty, 1992).

Text continued on page 587

Table 23–3

WOUND CLEANSING SOLUTIONS*

SOLUTIONS	"SAFE" CONCENTRATIONS
Povidone-iodine solution	1% (1 : 10 dilution) or 0.001% (1 : 1000)
Sodium hypochlorite (Dakin's)	0.025% (1 : 10 dilution) or 0.005% (1 : 200)
Acetic acid	No "safe" concentration with bactericidal activity
Hydrogen peroxide	No "safe" concentration with bactericidal activity
Normal saline solution	0.9%

*Universal precautions should be used as necessary when wound cleansing is needed. Vigorous cleansing or cleansing that may result in splashing drainage will require gown, mask, goggles, and gloves as appropriate.
Doughty, D., (1994). A rational approach to the use of topical antiseptics. *JWOCN, 21*(6), 224–231.

Box 23-7

AGENCY FOR HEALTH CARE POLICY AND RESEARCH TREATMENT OF PRESSURE ULCER GUIDELINES

Assessment*

Assessing the Pressure Ulcer

- Assess the pressure ulcer(s) initially for location, stage (NPUAP, 1992), size, sinus tracts, undermining, tunneling, exudate, necrotic tissue, and the presence or absence of granulation tissue and epithelialization. (C)

- Reassess pressure ulcers at least weekly. If the condition of the client or of the wound deteriorates, reevaluate the treatment plan as soon as any evidence of deterioration is noted. (C)

- A clean pressure ulcer should show evidence of some healing within 2 to 4 weeks. If no progress can be demonstrated, reevaluate the adequacy of the overall treatment plan as well as adherence to this plan, making modifications as necessary. (C)

Assessing the Individual With a Pressure Ulcer

- Perform a complete history and physical examination, because a pressure ulcer should be assessed in the context of the client's overall physical and psychosocial health. (C)

- Clinicians should be alert to the potential complications associated with pressure ulcers. (C)

- Perform an abbreviated nutritional assessment, as defined by the Nutrition Screening Initiative, at least every 3 months for individuals at risk for malnutrition. These include individuals who are unable to take food by mouth or who experience an involuntary change in weight. (C) (See AHCPR Guidelines for more in-depth information on nutrition, supplements, and pain management for clients with pressure ulcers.)

- All individuals being treated for pressure ulcers should undergo a psychosocial assessment to determine their ability and motivation to comprehend and adhere to the treatment program. The assessment should include, but not be limited to, the following: mental status, learning ability, depression; social support; polypharmacy or overmedication; alcohol and/or drug abuse; goals, values, lifestyles; culture and ethnicity; stressors. Periodic reassessment is recommended. (C)

- Assess resources (e.g., availability and skill of caregivers, finances, equipment) of individuals being treated for pressure ulcers in the home. (C)

- Set treatment goals consistent with the values and lifestyle of the individual, family, and caregiver. (C)

- Arrange interventions to meet identified psychosocial needs and goals. Follow-up should be planned in cooperation with the individual and caregiver. (C)

Managing Tissue Loads

While in Bed

Positioning Techniques

- Avoid positioning a client on a pressure ulcer. (C) (See Guidelines for more information on positioning devices, schedules, assessment of pressure problems, and positioning of immobile individuals.)

- Assess all clients with existing pressure ulcers to determine their risk for developing additional pressure ulcers. For those individuals who remain at risk, institute the measures recommended in Panel for the Prediction and Prevention of Pressure Ulcers in Adults, 1992.

Support Surfaces

- Assess all clients with existing pressure ulcers to determine their risk for developing additional pressure ulcers. If the client remains at risk, use a pressure-reducing surface. (C) (See Guidelines for suggestions on static and dynamic surfaces and surfaces for clients with stage III or IV pressure ulcers or excess moisture exposure.)

While Sitting

Positioning Techniques

- A client who has a pressure ulcer on a sitting surface should avoid sitting. If pressure on the ulcer can be relieved, limited sitting may be allowed. (C)

Support surfaces

See Guidelines for more information regarding positioning techniques and support surfaces.

Ulcer Care

Débridement

- Remove devitalized tissue in pressure ulcers when appropriate for the client's condition and consistent with client goals. (C)

---

* Strength of evidence: A = results of two or more randomized controlled clinical trials on pressure ulcers in humans provide support; B = results of two or more randomized controlled clinical trials on pressure ulcers in humans provide support, or when appropriate, results of two or more controlled trials in an animal model provide indirect support; C = this rating requires one or more of the following: (1) results of one controlled trial; (2) results of at least two case series/descriptive studies on pressure ulcers in humans; or (3) expert opinion.

Adapted from Bergstrom, N., Bennett, M. A., Carlson, C. E., et al. (1994). *Treatment of pressure ulcers. Clinical practice guideline. Number 15.* AHCPR Publication No. 95-0652. Rockville, MD: US Department of Health and Human Services. Public Health Service, Agency for Health Care Policy and Research.

Box 23–7

AGENCY FOR HEALTH CARE POLICY AND RESEARCH TREATMENT OF PRESSURE ULCER GUIDELINES
(Continued)

- Select the method of débridement most appropriate to the client's condition and goals. Sharp, mechanical, enzymatic, and/or autolytic débridement techniques may be used when there is no urgent clinical need for drainage or removal of devitalized tissue. If there is urgent need for débridement, as with advancing cellulitis or sepsis, sharp débridement should be used. (C) Sharp débridement is urgently indicated when there are signs of advancing cellulitis or sepsis.

- Use clean, dry dressings for 8 to 24 hours after sharp débridement associated with bleeding; then reinstitute moist dressings. Clean dressings may be used in conjunction with mechanical or enzymatic débridement techniques. (C)

- Heel ulcers with dry eschar need not be débrided if they do not have edema, erythema, fluctuance, or drainage. Assess these wounds daily to monitor for pressure ulcer complications that would require débridement (*e.g.,* edema, erythema, fluctuance, drainage). (C)

- Prevent or manage pain associated with débridement as needed. (C)

Wound Cleansing

- Cleanse wounds initially and at each dressing change. (C)

- Use minimal mechanical force when cleansing the ulcer with gauze, cloth, or sponges. (C)

- Do not clean ulcer wounds with skin cleansers or antiseptic agents (*e.g.,* povidone-iodine, iodophor, sodium hypochlorite solution [Dakin's® solution], hydrogen peroxide, acetic acid). (B)

- Use normal saline for cleansing most pressure ulcers. (C)

- Use enough irrigation pressure to enhance wound cleansing without causing trauma to the wound bed. Safe and effective ulcer irrigation pressures range from 4 to 15 psi. (B)

- Consider whirlpool treatment for cleansing pressure ulcers that contain thick exudate, slough, or necrotic tissue. Discontinue whirlpool when the ulcer is clean. (C)

Dressings

- Use a dressing that will keep the ulcer bed continuously moist. Wet-to-dry dressings should be used only for débridement and should not be considered when continuously moist saline dressings are required. (B)

- Use clinical judgment to select a type of moist wound dressing suitable for the ulcer. Studies of different types of moist wound dressings showed no difference in pressure ulcer healing outcomes. (B)

- Choose a dressing that keeps the surrounding intact (periulcer) skin dry while keeping the ulcer bed moist. (C)

- Choose a dressing that controls exudate but does not desiccate the ulcer bed. (C)

- Consider caregiver time when selecting a dressing. (B)

- Eliminate wound dead space by loosely filling all cavities with dressing material. Avoid overpacking the wound. (C)

- Monitor dressings applied near the anus, because they are difficult to keep intact. (C)

Adjunctive Therapies

See Guidelines for different adjunctive therapy options.

Managing Bacterial Colonization and Infection

Pressure Ulcer Colonization and Infection

- Minimize pressure ulcer colonization and enhance wound healing by effective wound cleansing and débridement. (A)

- If purulence or foul odor is present, more frequent cleansing and possibly débridement are required. (C)

- Do not use swab cultures to diagnose wound infection, because all pressure ulcers are colonized. (C)

- Consider initiating a 2-week trial of topical antibiotics for clean pressure ulcers that are not healing or are continuing to produce exudate after 2 to 4 weeks of optimal patient care (as defined in this guideline). The antibiotic should be effective against gram-negative, gram-positive, and anaerobic organisms (*e.g.,* silver sulfadiazine, triple antibiotic). (A)

- Perform quantitative bacterial cultures of the soft tissue and evaluate the patient for osteomyelitis when the ulcer does not respond to topical antibiotic therapy. (C)

- Do not use topical antiseptics (*e.g.,* povidone-iodine, iodophor, sodium hypochlorite [Dakin's® solution], hydrogen peroxide, acetic acid) to reduce bacteria in wound tissue. (B)

- Institute appropriate systemic antibiotic therapy for clients with bacteremia, sepsis, advancing cellulitis, or osteomyelitis. (A)

- Systemic antibiotics are not required for pressure ulcers with only clinical signs of local infection. (C)

- Protect pressure ulcers from exogenous sources of contamination (*e.g.,* feces). (C)

Continued

Box 23–7

AGENCY FOR HEALTH CARE POLICY AND RESEARCH TREATMENT OF PRESSURE ULCER GUIDELINES

(Continued)

Infection Control

* Follow body substance isolation (BSI) precautions or an equivalent system appropriate for the health care setting and the client's condition. (C)

* Use clean gloves for each patient. When treating multiple ulcers on the same patient, attend to the most contaminated ulcer last (*e.g.,* the perianal region). Remove gloves and wash hands between patients. (C)

* Use sterile instruments to débride pressure ulcers. (C)

* Use clean dressings, rather than sterile ones, to treat pressure ulcers, as long as dressing procedures comply with institutional infection control guidelines. (C)

* Clean dressings may also be used in the home setting. Disposal of contaminated dressings in the home should be done in a manner consistent with local regulations. (C)

Operative Repair of Pressure Ulcers

Patient Selection

See AHCPR Guidelines for more detailed information.

Controlling Factors That Impair Healing

See AHCPR Guidelines for more detailed information.

Operative Procedures

See AHCPR Guidelines for more detailed information.

Postoperative Care

* Minimize pressure to the operative site by use of an air-fluidized bed, a low-air-loss bed, or a Stryker frame for a minimum of 2 weeks. Assess postoperative viability of the surgical site as clinically indicated. Have the client slowly increase periods of time sitting or lying on the flap to increase its tolerance to pressure. To determine the degree of tolerance, monitor the flap for pallor, redness, or both not resolving after 10 minutes of pressure relief. Ongoing client education is imperative to reduce the risk of recurrence. (C)

* Assess for recurrence of pressure ulcers as an ongoing component of care. Caregivers should provide education and encourage adherence to measures for pressure reduction, daily skin examination, and intermittent relief techniques. (A)

Education and Quality Improvement

Education

Prevention and Treatment: A Continuum

* Design, develop, and implement educational programs for patients, caregivers, and health care providers that reflect a continuum of care. The program should begin with a structured, comprehensive, and organized approach to prevention and should culminate in effective treatment protocols that promote healing as well as prevent recurrence. (C) (See AHCPR Guidelines for information regarding target populations, information to be covered, involvement of client and caregiver, and roles.)

Assessing Tissue Damage

* Educational programs should emphasize the need for accurate, consistent, and uniform assessment; description; and documentation of the extent of tissue damage. (C)

* Update educational programs on an ongoing and regular basis to integrate new knowledge, techniques, or technologies. (C) (See AHCPR Guidelines for information to be included in educational programs.)

Monitoring Outcomes

See Guidelines for information to be monitored.

Quality Improvement

* Obtain intradepartmental and interdepartmental quality improvement support for pressure ulcer management as a major aspect of care. (C)

* Convene an interdisciplinary committee of interested and knowledgeable persons to address quality improvement in pressure ulcer management. (C)

* Identify and monitor the occurrence of pressure ulcers to determine their incidence and prevalence. This information will serve as a baseline to the development, implementation, and evaluation of treatment protocols. (C)

* Monitor the incidence and prevalence of pressure ulcers on a regular basis. (C)

* Develop, implement, and evaluate educational programs based on the data obtained from quality improvement monitoring. (C)

Dirty Wounds

Wound healing is more likely to occur when necrotic tissue and exudate are removed from the wound bed. Cleansing should be done gently with the correct solution to maximize the wound environment without causing trauma to the granulating wound bed (Panel for the Prediction and Prevention of Pressure Ulcers in Adults, 1994).

Although the application of antiseptic solutions as irrigations or dressings for wounds is controversial, nurses will find these products in use. The antiseptic solutions, if used, should be in dilute concentrations, as they are toxic to fibroblasts and other wound repair cells (Glugla & Mulder, 1990). If the nurse is managing a wound, the nursing order for cleansing should be normal saline solution.

Removing slough and necrotic debris is imperative for wounds to heal, and this procedure is called débridement. *Selective* débridement is the removal of necrotic tissue only, whereas *nonselective* débridement is the removal of any type of tissue within the wound bed. Wound débridement may be accomplished by mechanical, chemical, or autolytic techniques.

Mechanical Débridement

Surgical débridement, the use of wet-to-dry dressings, hydrotherapy, and irrigation are examples of mechanical débridement. Surgical débridement is done by a physician and may require local or general anesthesia. This option may be used for clients with extensive necrotic tissue who are surgical candidates. Avascular, loose tissue may be débrided by a surgeon or

---

PROCEDURE

23–2

WOUND IRRIGATION

Equipment:

> Underpad, graduated container, catheter-tipped syringe, basin (may be available as an irrigation set)
> OR
> 30-ml syringe and 19-gauge angiocatheter or needle
> OR
> Catheter tipped syringe and red rubber catheter
> Solution
> Sterile or clean gloves
> Dressing material as ordered by nurse or physician

Action	Rationale
1. Explain procedure to client and provide privacy.	1. Decreases client anxiety.
2. Wash hands and dry.	2. Reduces spread of microorganisms.
3. Assemble equipment as needed per nursing or physician orders. Pour estimated or ordered volume of solution into graduated container.	3. Prepares irrigation solution.
4. Position client comfortably and cover to expose only wound site.	4. Enhances client privacy and decreases unnecessary exposure.
5. Apply clean, disposable gloves.	5. Dressing is considered contaminated and needs to be disposed of in appropriate container.
6. Place absorbent pad under area to be irrigated.	6. Collects drainage and/or spills.
7. Remove tape gently pulling parallel to skin.	7. Tape removal can tear skin and/or place stress on suture line or wound.
8. Gently remove old dressing, taking care not to dislodge tubes or drains in wound bed.	8. Dislodgement can disrupt wound healing.

Continued

PROCEDURE

23–2

WOUND IRRIGATION
(Continued)

Action	Rationale
9. Observe and assess wound.	**9.** Facilitates documentation of wound appearance after procedure.
10. a. Wide open wounds: Fill syringe with irrigating solution. Hold syringe close to wound and flush wound using gentle, continuous pressure. Continue this until solution returned is clear or without residue.	**10a.** Decreases trauma to wound bed. Ensures adequate cleansing of wound.
b. Narrow and/or deep wounds: Fill 30-ml syringe with catheter/needle with irrigating solution (fill catheter-tipped syringe and then attach to red rubber). Gently insert syringe/catheter into wound until resistance felt, pull syringe/catheter out slightly. Flush wound using gentle, continuous pressure. Continue this until solution returned is clear or without residue.	**10b.** Decreases possibility of trauma to inner wall of wound.

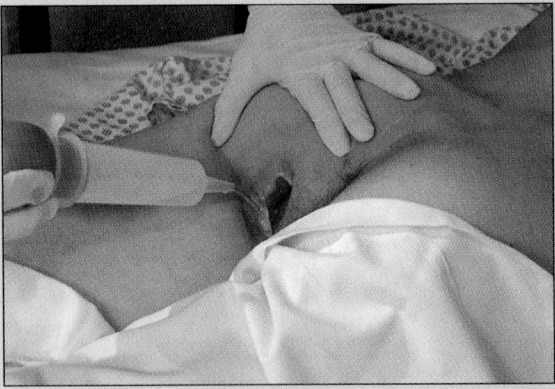

Step 10. *Irrigating wound.*

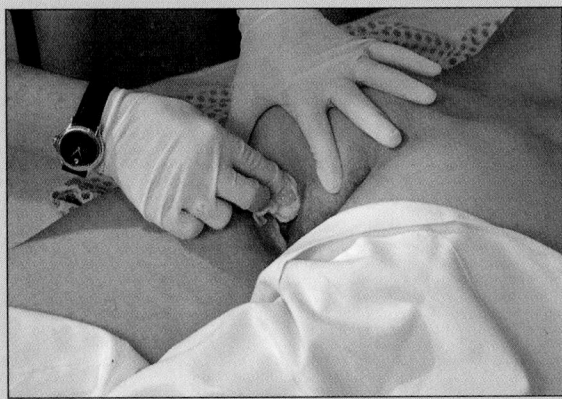

Step 11. *Cleaning and drying wound.*

11. Dry peri wound edges with gauze.	**11.** Prevents maceration of skin surrounding wound.
12. Apply dressing as ordered by nurse or physician	**12.** Protects wound.

Documentation: Document appearance of wound and describe procedure.

---

nurse experienced in the procedure and is done with sterile instruments in the client's room. Surgical débridement is generally selective.

Moist-to-damp dressings (usually ordered and referred to as wet-to-dry dressings), another method of mechanical débridement, should be done every 4 to 6 hours, as the devitalized tissue adheres to the drying gauze and is partially removed when the dressing is removed. However, moist-to-damp dressings also adhere to granulating tissue; therefore, this is a nonselective technique that may traumatize new epithelial tissue (Alterescu, 1983).

Hydrotherapy and wound irrigation are also nonselective, mechanical methods of débridement. Irrigation of a dirty wound surface with pressure is recommended to remove debris and bacteria. Whirlpool

therapy is often used for cleansing large infected wounds. At the bedside or in the home, a forceful irrigation can be done with a 35-ml syringe and a 19-gauge needle (Procedure 23–2).

Chemical Débridement

Débridement accomplished with enzyme ointments is chemical. Enzymes are physician ordered, and product guidelines must be followed. Enzymatic agents may not work over dry eschar, and a moist environment may also be necessary for the action. Enzymatic débridement may be selective or nonselective, depending on the enzyme agent.

Text continued on page 598

Table 23–4

DRESSING CLASSIFICATIONS

This table contains dressing classifications with some actions, indications, contraindications, and application tips for the classifications. The following companies have products that are listed in the table.

Acme United—LYOfoam™
Bard—Bard Absorption Dressing™
Biocore—Kollagen™ (SkinTemp™ and Medifil™)
Carrington—Carrasyn™ V Gel
Convatec—Kaltostat™, DuoDERM®
DeRoyal—Multidex®™
Dow Hickam—Sorbsan™
Hollister—Restore™

Johnson & Johnson—Sof-Wick, Mirasorb, Bioclusive®, Algosteril®, Fibracol
Kendall—Kerlix™, Versalon™, Exilon™, Curaderm™, Curasorb™, Curafil™, Curafoam™
Knoll—Collagenase Santyl®
NDM—ClearSite®
Smith & Nephew—RepliCare™, Allevyn®, SoloSite™, OpSite®
Sween—WounDres™, Triad™
3M—Tegasorb™, Tegaderm™

DRESSING CLASSIFICATIONS	ACTIONS	INDICATIONS	CONTRAINDICATIONS	APPLICATION TIPS
Gauze (Johnson & Johnson, Kendall); "gauze" dressings were traditionally woven cotton, nonfilled, sponges that are loosely (Kerlix™) woven or a fine mesh; 2 × 2 and 4 × 4 are most common sizes; synthetic gauze is now available in several combinations—polyester and/or rayon	**Kerlix and woven gauze** Absorbs exudate and allows fluid to transfer to secondary dressing; nonselective débridement of wound bed; fills dead space of wound, sinus tract, or undermining edges. Gauze dressings will Keep wound bed moist Débride Absorb exudate **Noncotton, nonwoven** (Mirasorb, Sof-Wick by Johnson & Johnson; Versalon, Excilon by Kendall) More absorbent than woven, but does not transfer drainage to secondary dressing Less adherent—not for débriding Good for cleaning and prepping	Gauze dressings are used on all wound stages, and gauze is often the outer or secondary dressing layer. Most effective on stages 3 and 4, but needs to be changed every 4–6 h to maintain moisture or every 6–8 h if used for débriding (gauze dressings are usually ordered wet to dry, but in practice they should *never* be allowed to dry out, as this is contrary to moist wound healing) Exudative wound—nonwoven sponges may be more absorbent	Packed in dry wounds unless moistened. Woven gauze (Kerlix) should not be used as a secondary dressing. For some draining wounds, use cotton gauze to "wick" drainage into cover dressing	Fine mesh gauze to decrease damage to wound bed on removal (do not use cotton-filled sponges such as "Toppers" by Johnson & Johnson) Pack lightly to avoid compromised blood flow or delay wound closure Protect surrounding skin with a skin protector when moist gauze used Change every 4–8 h, depending on purpose, amount of drainage Gauze should be applied moist to damp to prevent "drowning" wound or "drying" wound bed too much
Transparent, polyurethane adhesive (OpSite®, Tegaderm™, Bioclusive®, Polyskin®)	Semipermeable membrane that permits water vapor and oxygen to pass between wound bed and environment but keeps bacteria from coming in because of pore size Maintains moist wound environment so that resurfacing of the wound is enhanced Occlusion reduces local wound pain Autolytic débridement enhanced by moist, warm environment Does not require secondary dressing	Indicated for nondraining wounds; promotes autolytic débridement of dry eschar and fibrin slough Maintains moist, nonadherent surface next to wound Protects blisters and superficial wounds easily Wound can be monitored through transparent dressing Stages 1 and 2 May be used as secondary dressing for selected wound (but is not Medicare part B reimbursed as secondary dressing)	Exudating wounds Clinically infected wounds Wounds with sinus tracts or undermining edges, unless this "dead space" is packed	1.5–2 in of intact skin around wound allows for better seal Use skin protector around wound to defat area and protect skin from adhesive Shave or clip excessive hair to decrease bacterial invasion of wound and increase adhesion Change when dressing is leaking or no longer intact or every 3–5 d Exudate is usually cloudy and foul smelling until wound cleansed with normal saline solution; therefore, do not assess wound drainage until wound cleansed

Continued

Table 23–4

DRESSING CLASSIFICATIONS
(Continued)

DRESSING CLASSIFICATIONS	ACTIONS	INDICATIONS	CONTRAINDICATIONS	APPLICATION TIPS
Hydrocolloid (DuoDERM®, Restore™, Tegasorb™, RepliCare™, [Comfeel Plus, Curderm™])	Contains hydroactive particles Occlusive and adhesive Some products react with wound exudate to form gel-like covering to maintain moist wound environment Absorbs low to moderate amount of exudate	Assists with autolytic débridement by keeping wound bed moist Absorbs light to moderate wound drainage Insulates wound and, because of occlusion, provides some protection against secondary infection Used with compression dressings for venous ulcers for protection against infection and/or autolysis Stages 1, 2, and 3 noninfected wounds	Highly exudating wounds Clinically infected wounds Wounds with sinus tracts or undermining edges, unless this "dead space" is packed Wear time <24 h	1.5–2 in of intact skin around wound allows for better adherence May use skin protector around wound to defat area and protect skin from adhesive if fragile skin Shave or clip excessive hair to decrease bacterial invasion of wound and increase adhesion "Picture frame" edges with tape if dressing not prepackaged with this feature (especially on sacral or coccyx wounds) Change every 3 d or when dressing is no longer occlusive, is leaking, or is wrinkled Exudate is usually yellowish and odorous—assess wound *after* cleaning
Polyurethane foam (LYOfoam™, Allevyn®, Curafoam™)	Absorbs exudate with nonstick surface and holds exudate away from wound bed to permit moist environment without maceration	Absorbs moderate to heavy exudate while maintaining moist wound bed Insulates wound surface Provides nontraumatic removal Stage 2 and stages 3 and 4 if dead space is packed (space may be packed with selected foam products or gauze or other products) May be used as a secondary dressing for additional absorption	Wounds with no exudate Wounds with dry eschar Wounds with undermining edges or sinus tracts unless areas are packed	Does not require secondary dressing Foam needs to be secured if it is nonadhesive (tape, gauze wrap, mesh net wrap, elastic bandage) May be cut to fit Use skin protectant around wound to protect periwound skin from drainage Change when drainage strikes through to outer edges of foam every 1–4 d
Absorption dressing (Bard Absorption Dressing™, Debrisan®, Multidex™), available as copolymer starches and dextranomer bead dressings	Absorbs moderate to heavy amounts of exudate while maintaining a moist wound bed	Clean or dirty Wounds with large amounts of exudate that need to be packed Wounds with necrosis and exudate Stages 3 and 4 Clean or dirty	Wounds with minimal exudate Wounds covered with dry eschar	Absorptive dressings require a secondary or cover dressing Copolymer starches should be thoroughly rinsed from wound bed before assessment of wound and reapplication of dressing Change when strike through to outer dressing occurs

Alginates (Kaltostat™, Sorbsan, Curasorb™)	Absorb moderate to heavy amounts of exudate while maintaining a moist wound bed Alginates are derived from seaweed and absorb many times their own weight Exchange Ca^+ and Na^+ ions between dressing and wound bed	Wounds with large amounts of exudate that need to be packed Wounds with necrosis and exudate Selected wounds with sinus tracts and undermining edges, depending on ability to *remove all of dressing material* at each dressing change Stages 3 and 4 Clean or dirty	Wounds with minimal exudate—DO NOT moisten dressing Wounds covered with dry eschar Burns	Alginates come in ropes or sheets Alginates may change to a tan color—assess wound *after* cleansing DO NOT pack with torn pieces of alginate Change when strike through to outer dressing occurs Always rinse wound during dressing change, as some alginates dissolve in wound while others can be removed in one piece
Hydrogel dressings **Sheets** (Vigilon®, Geliperm®, ClearSite®) **Amorphous** (Carrasyn V™, SoloSite, DuoDERM® gel, WounDres™, Curafil™, Restore™) **Gauze impregnated** (Curafil™, Resore™)	Maintain a moist wound surface, as they are composed of mostly water or glycerin (promote granulation and reepithelialization) Nonadherent Minimal absorption Autolytic débridement because of eschar hydration (sheets are not the best for this action) Act like second layer of skin and decrease pain Gels have different hydrophilic properties and therefore have different wound-hydrating capacities—check product information	Maintain moist wound environment in clean wounds Promote autolytic débridement in wounds with thin fibrin cover Provide comfort to wound Clean or dirty Create a moist wound surface by hydrating Stages 3 and 4 if used on gauze and "dead space" lightly packed Skin tears (sheets especially useful here)	Moderate to heavily exudating wounds Wounds with gelatinous fibrin	Secondary dressings may be needed Change dressings when strike through occurs for amorphous and gauze impregnated; may be once or twice a day to every other day Change sheet dressings when drainage has pooled under dressing Cut to fit wound, as moist dressing can macerate intact skin around the wound Skin prep periwound skin
Collagen dressings (Kollagen™ [Medifil particles, paste, pad, or SkinTemp pad], Triad™)	Help body stabilize the wound and optimize the environment for wound healing, as they lay a collagen base in the wound bed	Kollagen™ can be used on all types of wounds; selection of Kollagen™ form depends on which is easiest to apply, change, and/or secure and the frequency with which the dressing must be changed	Patients allergic to bovine material, as Kollagen™ is derived from bovine hide	Medifil particles, pad, and SkinTemp pad are used on wet wounds Particles good on nonresponding wounds Medifil paste is used on dry wounds—changed daily Medifil pad good for heavily draining wounds and when nonadherent surface is required SkinTemp pad good for multiday application and partial-thickness wounds Use cover dressings as needed (e.g., for absorbency, protection) Remove by rinsing wound with normal saline solution and reapplying dressing material
Enzymatic agents (Collagenase Santyl®, Elase® Granulex®, Travase®, Panafil®)	Selective enzyme activity to dissolve necrotic tissue without injuring healthy tissue (check each product for selectivity of tissues)	Necrotic tissue in wound bed	Adverse reactions of periulcer area, such as burning, stinging, bleeding, transient dermatitis	*Dressing change frequently:* Collagenase Santyl® every day; Travase® three or four times a day; Elase® is two to three times a day; Granulex® is at least twice a day Score (cross-hatch) hard eschar or soften by autolysis before applying enzyme to increase penetration
Combination dressings (Fibracol®, Curaderm™, Comfeel Plus)	These dressings are a combination of products	Curaderm™ and Comfeel Plus are a combination of *hydrocolloid* and *alginate*, and Fibracol® is *collagen* and *alginate*	Follow contraindications of each component of product	

Copyright Nursing Educational Programs and Services, Inc., Longmeadow, MA, May 30, 1996.

Table 23–5

DRESSING OPTIONS BASED ON STAGE, DRAINAGE, WOUND BED

WOUND CARE GOAL: Maintain a *moist* and *protected* wound environment that promotes healing and inhibits infection*

1. Cleanse wounds with normal saline solution or other noncytotoxic solutions before dressing
2. Select ONE of the following dressing options based on the above goal: stage, amount of exudate, presence of necrotic tissue (any tissue that is nonviable, including fibrinous and eschar), presence of infection, client's ability, and/or caregiver support
3. **Always** protect skin around draining wounds with a spray or wipe skin protector
4. Infected wounds should be treated in consultation with a clinical nurse specialist, enterostomal therapy nurse, and physician; patients with infected wounds may be on systemic antibiotics, and the wound and wound dressings are monitored closely
5. When wounds have granulation and nonviable tissue in the wound bed, usually treat the wound in relation to the largest portion of tissue present

STAGE II

Clean, Minimal Drainage	Clean, Moderate Drainage
A. Protectant spray or barrier ointment Re-apply as needed, per package directions	
B. Polyurethane transparent dressing (adhesive film) Maintains moist wound bed Apply skin protector around wound Change every 2–4 d or if leaking or no longer occlusive Extend 1.5–2 in beyond wound edges Tape edges of dressing to prevent lifting	
C. Hydrocolloid Maintains moist wound bed Change every 2–5 d or if leaking/nonocclusive Extend dressing 1 in beyond wound Tape edges to prevent rolling if product requires	**C. Hydrocolloid** Maintains moist wound bed Change every 2–5 d or if leaking/nonocclusive Extend dressing 1 in beyond wound Tape edges to prevent rolling if product requires
D. Amorphous wound gel/impregnated gauze Maintains moist wound bed Apply thin layer over entire wound bed Skin protector around wound Cut impregnated gauze to fit wound Change every day to every 72 h (check with manufacturer) Cover with gauze or polyurethane film	**D. Amorphous wound gel/impregnated gauze** Maintains moist wound bed Apply thin layer over entire wound bed Skin protector around wound Cut impregnated gauze to fit wound Change every day to every 72 h (check with manufacturer) Cover with gauze or polyurethane film

E. Hydrogen sheet dressing
Maintains moist wound bed
Skin protector around wound
Cut to fit wound
Remove plastic film from side next to wound if product requires
Cover with surginet or gauze to keep in place as needed
Change when dry (1–2 d) or for drainage strike through to outer dressing

F. Moist normal saline solution gauze
Skin protector around wound
Cut dressing to fit inside wound (synthetic gauze)
Cover with dry gauze dressing
Change every 4–6 hours and as needed—do not allow to dry out completely

G. Absorption Dressings
Alginate
  Cover with sheet dressing
  Apply gauze as secondary dressing
  Change when strike through to outer dressing occurs or every 3 d
Polyurethane foam
  Check package directions for application
  Nonadherent
  Cover with surginet or gauze to keep in place
  Change when strike through occurs

H. Collagen gels, pastes, pad
Maintains moist wound bed; provides collagen base
Change gels and pastes daily
Cover collagen dressings as needed for absorbency and protection

E. Hydrogen sheet dressing
Maintains moist wound bed
Skin protector around wound
Cut to fit wound
Remove plastic film from side next to wound if product requires
Cover with surginet or gauze to keep in place as needed
Change when dry (1–2 d) or for drainage strike through to outer dressing

F. Moist normal saline solution gauze
Skin protector around wound
Cut dressing to fit inside wound (synthetic gauze)
Cover with dry gauze dressing
Change every 4–6 hours and as needed—do not allow to dry out completely

H. Collagen gels, pastes, pad
Maintain moist wound bed; provide collagen base
Change gels and pastes daily
Cover collagen dressings as needed for absorbency and protection

Continued

Table 23–5

DRESSING OPTIONS BASED ON STAGE, DRAINAGE, WOUND BED

(Continued)

STAGE II

Necrotic, Minimal Drainage	Necrotic, Moderate Drainage	Necrotic, Heavy Drainage
B. Polyurethane transparent dressing Maintains moist wound bed Provides autolytic débridement Apply skin protector around wound Change every 2–3 d or if leaking or no longer occlusive Extend 1.5–2 in beyond wound edges Tape edges of dressing to prevent lifting		
C. Hydrocolloid Maintains moist wound bed Provides autolytic débridement Change every 2–5 d or if leaking/nonocclusive Extend dressing 1 in beyond wound Tape edges to prevent rolling if product requires	**C. Hydrocolloid** Maintains moist wound bed Provides autolytic débridement Change when leaking/nonocclusive Extend dressing 1 in beyond wound Tape edges to prevent rolling if product requires	
D. Amorphous wound gel/impregnated gauze Soften eschar/enhance autolytic débridement Apply thin layer over entire wound bed Skin protector around wound Cut impregnated gauze to fit wound Change every day to every 72 h (check with manufacturer) Cover with gauze or polyurethane film		
E. Hydrogel sheet dressing Soften eschar/enhance autolytic débridement Skin protector around wound Cut to fit wound Remove plastic film from side next to wound if product requires Cover with surginet or gauze to keep in place as needed Change when dry (1–2 d) or for drainage strike through to outer dressing **Not all sheet dressings provide enough moisture to assist with autolytic débridement**		

F. Moist-to-damp normal saline solution gauze
Skin protector around wound
Cut dressing to fit inside wound
Cover with dry gauze dressing
Change every 6 h and as needed—do not allow to dry out completely

G. Absorption Dressings
Alginate
Cover with sheet dressing
Apply gauze as secondary dressing
Change when strike through to outer dressing occurs or every 3 d
Polyurethane foam
Check package directions for application
Nonadherent
Cover with surginet or gauze to keep in place
Change when strike through occurs

H. Collagen particles, pad
Maintains moist wound bed; provides collagen base
Change particles every 48 h or as needed
Cover collagen dressings as needed for absorbency and protection

Continued

F. Moist-to-damp normal saline solution gauze
Skin protector around wound
Cut dressing to fit inside wound
Cover with dry gauze dressing
Change every 6 h and as needed—do not allow to dry out completely

G. Absorption dressings
Alginate
Cover with sheet dressing
Apply gauze as secondary dressing
Change when strike through to outer dressing occurs or every 3 d
Polyurethane foam
Check package directions for application
Nonadherent
Cover with surginet or gauze to keep in place
Change when strike through occurs

H. Collagen gels, pastes, pad
Maintains moist wound bed; provides collagen base
Change gels and pastes daily
Cover collagen dressings as needed for absorbency and protection

I. Enzymes
Apply to necrotic tissue in wound bed
Change dressings every 8 h or every day, depending on product instructions
Use requires physician's order
May use selected antibiotic preparations with physician's order
Check manufacturer; some require moist wound environment

Table 23–5

DRESSING OPTIONS BASED ON STAGE, DRAINAGE, WOUND BED
(Continued)

STAGES III AND IV

Clean, Minimal Drainage	Clean, Moderate Drainage	Clean, Heavy Drainage

C. Hydrocolloid
Maintains moist wound bed
Fill/pack dead space lightly
Change when leaking/nonocclusive
Extend dressing 1 in beyond wound
Tape edges to prevent rolling if product requires
 	
D. Amorphous wound gel/impregnated gauze
Maintains moist wound bed
Select wound gel with appropriate properties
Apply thin layer over entire wound bed (fill dead space with fluffed gauze)
Skin protector around wound
Cut impregnated gauze to fit wound
Change every day to every 72 h (check with manufacturer)
Cover with gauze or polyurethane film
 	
F. Moist normal saline solution gauze
Skin protector around wound
Cut dressing to fit inside wound
Cover with dry gauze dressing
Change every 4–6 h and as needed—do not allow to dry out
 	
H. Collagen gels, pastes, pad
Maintains moist wound bed; provides collagen base
Change gels and pastes daily
Cover collagen dressings as needed for absorbency and protection
	C. Hydrocolloid
	Maintains moist wound bed
	Fill/pack dead space lightly
	Change when leaking/nonocclusive
	Extend dressing 1 in beyond wound
	Tape edges to prevent rolling if product requires
	
	F. Moist normal saline solution gauze
	Skin protector around wound
	Cut dressing to fit inside wound
	Cover with dry gauze dressing
	Change every 6 h and as needed—do not allow to dry out
	
	G. Absorption dressings
	  Alginate
	  Pack lightly with rope or sheet dressing
	  Cover with gauze or polyurethane transparent dressing
	  Change when strike through to outer dressing occurs or every 3 d
	  Polyurethane foam sheets or cavity dressings
	  Check package directions for application
	  Nonadherent
	  Cover with surginet or gauze to keep in place
	  Change when strike through occurs to outer edges
	
	H. Collagen gels, pastes, pad
	Maintains moist wound bed; provides collagen base
	Change gels and pastes daily
	Cover collagen dressings as needed for absorbency and protection
		F. Moist normal saline solution gauze
		Skin protector around wound
		Cut dressing to fit inside wound
		Cover with dry gauze dressing
		Change every 6 h and as needed—do not allow to dry out
		
		G. Absorption dressings
		  Alginate
		  Pack lightly with rope or sheet dressing
		  Cover with gauze or polyurethane transparent dressing
		  Change when strike through to outer dressing occurs or every 3 d
		  Polyurethane foam sheets or cavity dressings
		  Check package directions for application
		  Nonadherent
		  Cover with surginet or gauze to keep in place
		  Change when strike through occurs to outer edges
		
		H. Collagen particles, pad
		Maintains moist wound bed; provides collagen base
		Change particles every 48 h or as needed
		Cover collagen dressings as needed for absorbency and protection

Necrotic, Minimal Drainage	Necrotic, Moderate Drainage	Necrotic, Heavy Drainage
C. Hydrocolloid Maintains moist wound bed Provides autolytic débridement Fill/pack dead space lightly Change when leaking/nonocclusive Extend dressing 1 in beyond wound Tape edges to prevent rolling if product requires **D. Amorphous wound gel/impregnated gauze** Softens necrotic tissue/enhances autolytic débridement Select wound gel with appropriate properties Apply thin layer over entire wound bed (fill dead space with fluffed gauze) Skin protector around wound Cut impregnated gauze to fit wound Change every day to every 72 h (check with manufacturer) Cover with gauze or polyurethane film **F. Moist to damp normal saline solution gauze** Skin protector around wound Cut dressing to fit inside wound Cover with dry gauze dressing Change every 6 h and as needed—do not allow to dry out completely **G. Absorption dressings** **Alginate** Pack lightly with rope or sheet dressing Cover with gauze or polyurethane foam Change when strike through to outer dressing occurs or every 3 d **Polyurethane foam sheets or cavity dressings** Check package directions for application Nonadherent Cover with surginet or gauze to keep in place Change when strike through occurs to outer edges **H. Collagen gels, pastes, pad** Maintains moist wound bed; provides collagen base Change gels and pastes daily Cover collagen dressings as needed for absorbency and protection **I. Enzymes** Apply to necrotic tissue in wound bed Change dressings every 8 h or every day, depending on product instructions Use requires physician's order May use selected antibiotic preparations with physician's order Check manufacturer; some require moist wound environment	**C. Hydrocolloid** Maintains moist wound bed Provides autolytic débridement Fill/pack dead space lightly Change when leaking/nonocclusive Extend dressing 1 in beyond wound Tape edges to prevent rolling if product requires **F. Moist to damp normal saline solution gauze** Skin protector around wound Cut dressing to fit inside wound Cover with dry gauze dressing Change every 6 h and as needed—do not allow to dry out completely **G. Absorption dressings** **Alginate** Pack lightly with rope or sheet dressing Cover with gauze or polyurethane foam Change when strike through to outer dressing occurs or every 3 d **Polyurethane foam sheets or cavity dressings** Check package directions for application Nonadherent Cover with surginet or gauze to keep in place Change when strike through occurs to outer edges **H. Collagen gels, pastes, pad** Maintains moist wound bed; provides collagen base Change gels and pastes daily Cover collagen dressings as needed for absorbency and protection **I. Enzymes** Apply to necrotic tissue in wound bed Change dressings every 8 h or everyday, depending on product instructions Use requires physician's order May use selected antibiotic preparations with physician's order Check manufacturer; some require moist wound environment	**F. Moist to damp normal saline solution gauze** Skin protector around wound Cut dressing to fit inside wound Cover with dry gauze dressing Change every 6 h and as needed—do not allow to dry out completely **G. Absorption dressings** **Alginate** Pack lightly with rope or sheet dressing Cover with gauze or polyurethane foam Change when strike through to outer dressing occurs or every 3 d **Polyurethane foam sheets or cavity dressings** Check package directions for application Nonadherent Cover with surginet or gauze to keep in place Change when strike through occurs to outer edges **H. Collagen particles, pad** Maintains moist wound bed; provides collagen base Change particles every 48 h or as needed Cover collagen dressings as needed for absorbency and protection	

*Remember, pouch with heavily draining wounds. Question the need for surgical débridement if wound bed continues to be covered with fibrous tissue or necrotic tissue after enzymatic or autolytic débridement has been in place for over 2 weeks.

Autolytic

The last method of débridement is autolytic. The body's own white blood cells break down the necrotic tissue under the correct conditions. Occlusive or transparent dressings, hydrogels, and alginate dressings assist the body in autolytic débridement. These dressings promote rehydration of the wound bed, as they are moisture retentive and attract phagocytic cells to the wound.

Dressing Materials

Determining the type of wound dressings to use has become a major decision in today's health care environment. There are a myriad of dressing categories with multiple products within each category. Each category has specific actions with advantages and disadvantages. For the nurse, the decision as to which dressing is best for the client becomes multifaceted.

Wounds have historically been covered to protect them from further injury and/or infection. Between the 1600s and the 1960s, little was done to change the wound coverings that were used. We now know that a moist wound bed heals more rapidly than a wound bed that is dried out or has necrotic tissue of any type (*e.g.*, eschar, slough) (Alvarez *et al.*, 1989). In addition, dressings are also used for hemostasis (to stop bleeding) in the form of a pressure dressing. Elastic adhesive bandages are usually used with a pressure dressing, and the application technique creates pressure over an actual or potential bleeding site (see Fig. 23–7). Ascertaining the adequacy of circulation in the area of the pressure dressing is done as ordered or at least every 4 hours.

Traditional dressing techniques use gauze and are done in layers. The initial layer that is in contact with the wound bed absorbs drainage and wicks it to the next layer. Woven cotton gauze or synthetic gauze is most commonly used. The dressing should be removed gently, as the initial layer (especially if cotton gauze) may be stuck to the wound or incision. Moistening the dressing with normal saline solution will loosen the dressing for easier removal (unless it is a moist-to-damp dressing for débriding).

The dressing that is used for the cover layer or secondary dressing (often called an abdominal pad) has a barrier on the top of the dressing to prevent strike-through of drainage and is larger (often 5 × 8 in) to cover the inner layers of dressings and protect the wound from outside contamination. Dressings need to be taped into place to prevent them from falling off the site as the client ambulates or moves in bed.

To prepare for a dressing change, the nurse needs to know the type of wound, presence of drains or tubing, and types of dressings that would be appropriate for the wound. If the physician has ordered a certain dressing, then that procedure is followed unless the nurse obtains a new order.

Drains or tubes are used in a variety of surgical wounds to facilitate drainage from an organ, cavity, or surrounding anatomical space. See "Complications of Wound Healing" earlier in the chapter for further discussion of drains.

Table 23–4 lists dressings by category with information regarding indications. Table 23–5 lists stages of wounds and dressings that can be used for those stages. Table 23–5 may be used to assist the nurse in making dressing decisions.

Before changing any dressing, the nurse informs the client of the procedure to take place and medicates the client for discomfort so that the peak effect of the analgesia will occur during the dressing change. Procedures 23–3 and 23–4 outline two different dressing application techniques. Traditional gauze dressings that are moistened with normal saline are still used frequently. Although these dressings provide a positive environment for wound healing, they require frequent changing, as they dry out and do not keep the wound bed moist (usually within 4–6 hours).

Moist wound healing is supported by polyurethane film and hydrocolloid dressings that may remain in place for up to several days. These dressings are easily used on partial-thickness wounds. If the wound is full thickness, the use of the dressings requires astute decision making by the nurse. Is the wound draining profusely? Is it infected? Does the cavity (dead space) of the wound need to be lightly packed to promote healing from the base of the wound bed? If the nurse is unsure of the correct dressing option for the client, the clinical nurse specialist in wound and skin care or the enterostomal therapy nurse should be consulted.

Tapes and Binders

Dressings need to be secured to remain in place unless they have their own adhesive. The choice of bandage depends on the size and location of the wound, purpose of dressing, and frequency of dressing changes.

Tape is available in various widths (*e.g.*, ½, ¾, 1, 2, 3, 4 in) and different types. The nurse chooses the size of the tape based on the size of the dressing to be affixed. Tape should extend at least 2 in on either side of the dressing to remain in place as the client moves.

Tape should be removed gently, with the outer end being pulled toward the wound and with traction being applied to the skin away from the wound as the tape is peeled away. Adhesive removers may be used if the client has fragile skin, but the remover must be kept out of the client's wound, and any traces need to be removed from the skin so the tape will adhere. Use a spray or wipe skin protector if necessary to protect the client's skin from the tape.

Binders are pieces of material that have various configurations. Their purpose is to secure dressings or secure an incisional area. The most common binder is

Text continued on page 604

PROCEDURE

23–3

APPLYING STERILE GAUZE DRESSING—DRY AND MOIST

Equipment: *Required*

Disposable gloves
Sterile gloves
Swabs
Sterile solution
Tape or Montgomery straps
Cleansing solution
Gauze pads for cleaning
Gauze dressing of appropriate
  size

As needed

Skin protector
Sterile tongue blades
Medication as ordered
Face mask
Gown

Action	Rationale
1. Explain procedure to client and provide privacy.	1. Decreases client's anxiety.
2. Assemble equipment as needed per nursing or physician orders.	2. Maintains standards.
3. Wash hands and dry.	3. Reduces spread of microorganisms.
4. Position client comfortably and cover to expose only wound site.	4. Enhances client privacy and decreases unnecessary exposure.
5. Apply clean, disposable gloves.	5. Dressing is considered contaminated and needs to be disposed of in appropriate container.
6. Remove tape gently pulling parallel to skin.	6. Tape removal can tear skin and/or place stress on suture line or wound.
7. Gently remove old dressing, taking care not to dislodge tubes or drains in wound bed.	7. Dislodgement can disrupt wound healing.

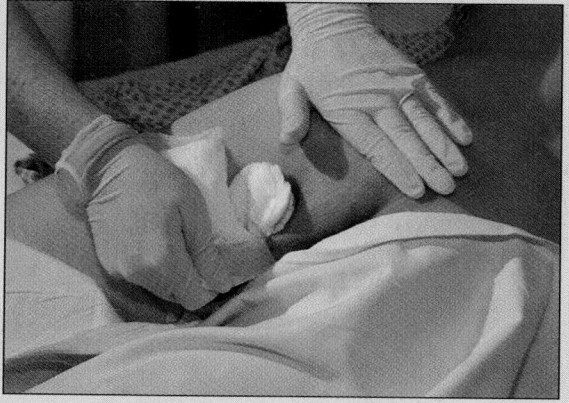

Step 7

8. A dressing that was ordered wet to dry and is stuck to the wound bed should not be moistened. Continue to remove, and warn client of discomfort. Dispose of dressings in appropriate container.	8. An ordered wet-to-dry dressing is to débride wound by gauze clinging to necrotic tissue and, as it dries, shrinking slightly to have necrotic tissue cling to dressing. It also absorbs moisture and wicks it from base of the wound to the outer dressing. All agencies have protocols for disposing of contaminated material.

Continued

PROCEDURE

23–3

APPLYING STERILE GAUZE DRESSING—DRY AND MOIST

(Continued)

Action	**Rationale**
9. Observe type and amount of drainage on dressing.	**9.** Assessment data need to be collected.
10. Remove soiled gloves and dispose of in appropriate container.	**10.** All agencies have protocols for disposing of contaminated material.

11. Open sterile supplies and arrange on sterile field.
    Pour cleansing solution onto gauze pads for cleansing of wound (use plastic wrapper of gauze if available or use a sterile barrier or container for solution and drop sterile gauze onto barrier or into container).
    Apply medication to sterile tongue blade or applicator with squeeze technique or open top to container.
	11. Sterile field reduces contamination of sterile supplies.
	    Moisture can strike through paper packages and bacteria migrate through wet.
	
	    Tongue blades and swabs are sterile and cannot be touched until sterile gloves are on.

12. Apply sterile gloves.	**12.** Allows handling of sterile supplies without contaminating the supplies.
13. Clean the wound from top to bottom or from the center of the wound to the outside in a circular motion.	**13.** Wounds are cleaned from the least to the most contaminated area (drainage collects at the bottom of the wound, and the outer area of the incision/wound is most contaminated).
14. Assess the wound bed or incision now that the area is clean.	**14.** Assessing an area before cleansing does not give a valid picture of wound bed appearance, drainage color, odor, and other factors.
15. Apply any ordered medicine.	**15.** Creams and ointments can be applied with a sterile tongue blade or swab.

16. Apply sterile dressings as ordered.
    If dry dressing, apply gauze singly over wound, starting at center and moving outward. Use only a few gauze sponges.
    If wet-to-dry dressings ordered, wring out each dressing and open each gauze before applying. Pack wounds lightly until all dead space is filled.
	16. Excessive use of pads does not provide any benefits to wound. Purpose of dressing is to protect wound.
	    Wet-to-dry dressings should actually be damp, as they will not begin to dry if too wet. Although moisture is needed for the wound to heal, excessive moisture does not speed the process. Opening the gauze and packing lightly allows the cells to migrate easily across the wound bed and does not impede blood flow to the wound.

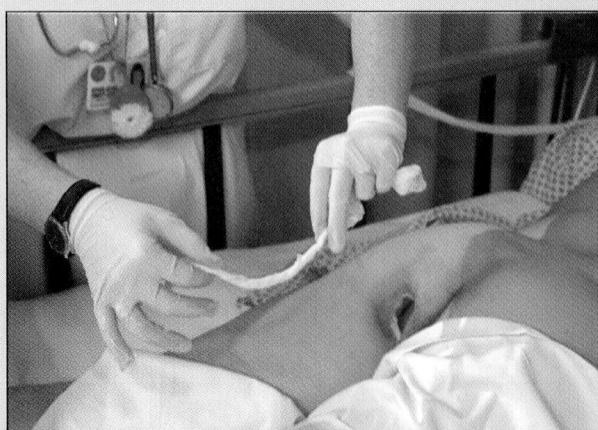

Step 16. *Wringing out moist dressing.*

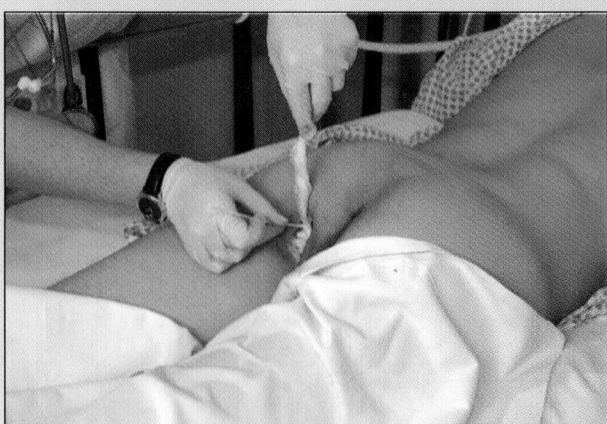

Step 16. *Packing wound*

APPLYING STERILE GAUZE DRESSING—DRY AND MOIST

(Continued)

Action	Rationale
17. If moist dressings are used, apply a skin protector to area around wound.	**17.** Standard of care for moisture notes the need to protect skin from moisture.
18. Cover moist dressings with dry dressing—surgical or abdominal pad.	**18.** Outer dressing is needed to protect the wound from external contaminants and to protect client's clothing from damp dressings. These outer pads have a top liner layer to prevent wetness from striking through.

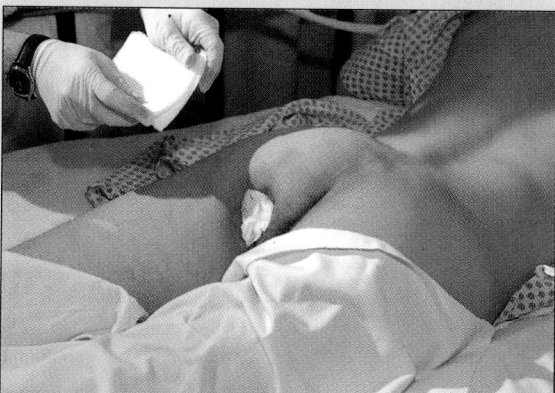

Step 18

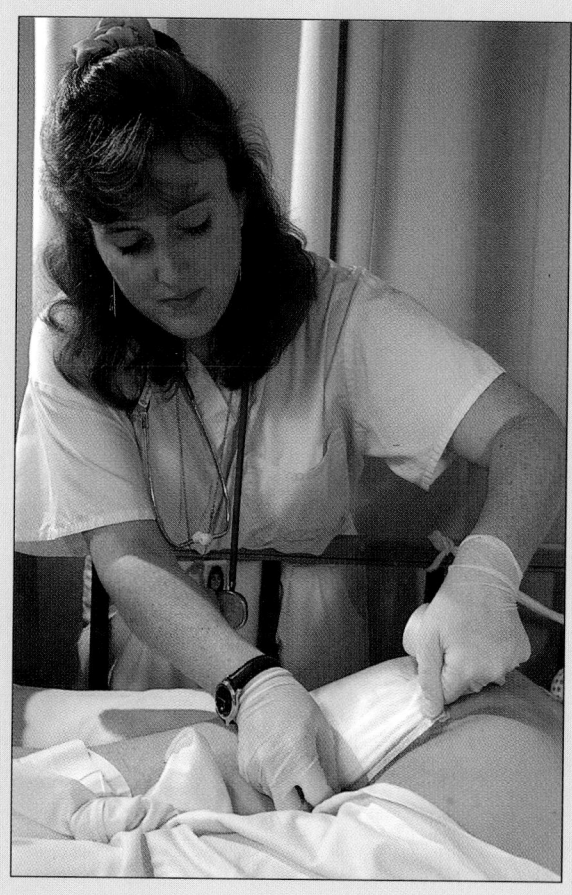

Step 19

19. Secure dressings with minimal amount of tape.	**19.** Consider using Montgomery straps and skin protectors for any tape applications if dressing change is very frequent or large amounts of tape are used. Consult clinical nurse specialist or enterostomal therapy nurse for assistance with wounds that are complicated or heavily draining or require frequent dressing changes.
20. Dispose of equipment in appropriate container and remove gloves.	**20.** Prevents spread of contamination.
21. Position client for comfort.	**21.** Promotes rest.
22. Wash hands.	**22.** Reduces spread of microorganisms.

Documentation: Document wound appearance and dressing application. Evaluate/update plan of care for dressing change.

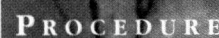

PROCEDURE

23–4

APPLYING TRANSPARENT OR HYDROCOLLOID DRESSING

Equipment:

Clean gloves
Gauze, nonwoven, synthetic
Selected transparent/hydrocol-
    loid dressing
Skin protector
Normal saline

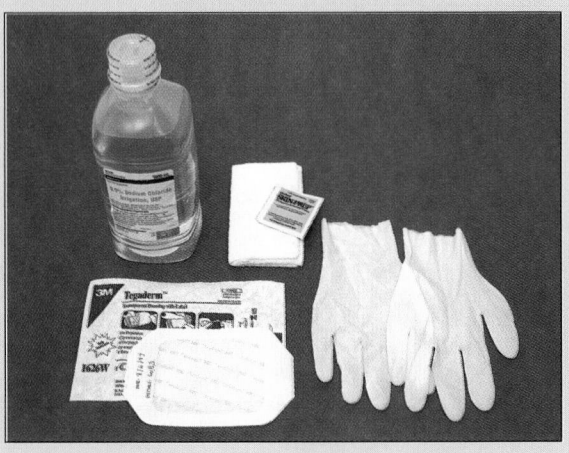

Action	Rationale
1. Protect client's privacy.	
2. Wash hands.	
3. Apply clean gloves.	
4. Remove old dressing. Gently peel adhesive dressings from skin. Use moist gauze or an adhesive remover to assist release of adhesive.	4. Peeling skin away with adhesive is possible if care is not taken.
5. Open gauze and pour saline onto pads for cleansing wound. Absorb excess irrigant with gauze.	5. Use synthetic gauze, as this is more cost-effective and also does not leave lint inside the wound.
6. Select dressing size that is appropriate for the wound (usually 1.5 to 2 in larger than wound size). Cut dressings as needed.	6. Wound healing may increase wound drainage, especially if autolytic débridement is occurring. A dressing that is too small will allow drainage to leak too quickly.

7. If using transparent dressing, apply a skin protector around edges of wound to area covered by adhesive.
    Allow skin protector to dry thoroughly before applying dressing.
	7. Skin protectors defat (or remove oil from skin surface) the area and provide a base to protect the skin from the adhesive.
	    Wet skin protector does not allow the dressing to adhere well, and if alcohol based, the alcohol can be trapped underneath and cause skin rash or breakdown.

8. Apply dressing evenly without tension.	8. Stretching the dressing during application may cause skin to wrinkle underneath and lead to irritation.
9. Tape edges of either dressing as needed.	9. Taping edges of those dressings that are not manufactured with edging is helpful in preventing the dressing from "rolling." This is especially important in the sacral area or other areas of high friction.

Documentation: Document wound appearance and dressing application. Evaluate/update plan of care for dressing change.

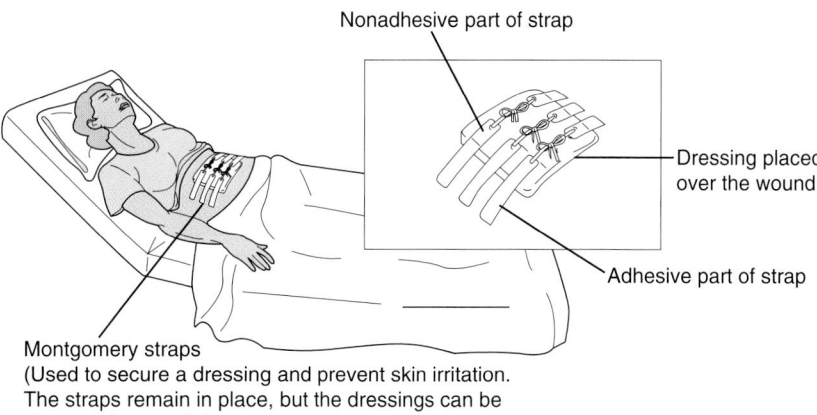

❥ **Figure 23–7**
Montgomery straps are used for dressings that need to be changed frequently. Skin protector should be applied to the skin where the adhesive will adhere to protect against skin tearing when the Montgomery straps are removed.

Nonadhesive part of strap

Dressing placed over the wound

Adhesive part of strap

Montgomery straps
(Used to secure a dressing and prevent skin irritation. The straps remain in place, but the dressings can be changed frequently.)

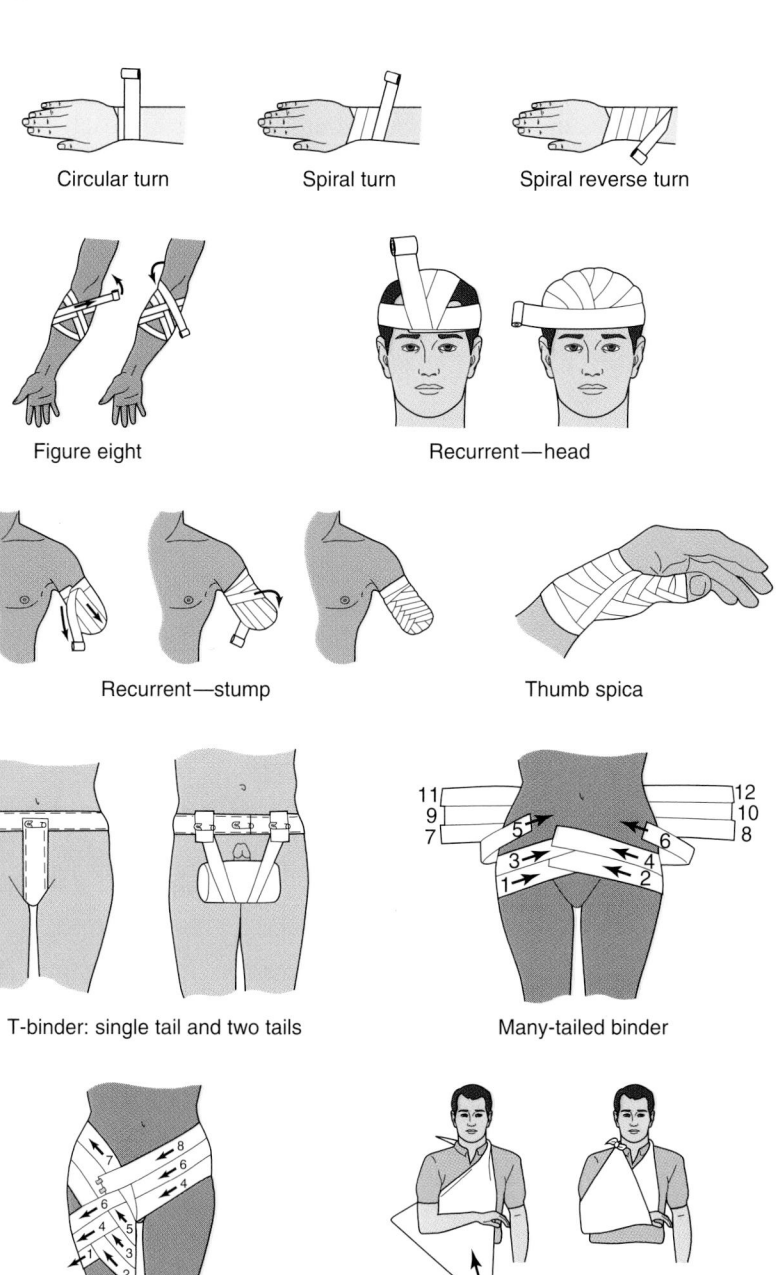

Circular turn

Spiral turn

Spiral reverse turn

Figure eight

Recurrent—head

Recurrent—stump

Thumb spica

T-binder: single tail and two tails

Many-tailed binder

Spica

Sling

❥ **Figure 23–8**
Application techniques for elastic bandages, used to keep dressings in place.

the abdominal binder, which is elastic, applied around the abdomen, and attaches to itself with Velcro strips.

If dressings are to be changed frequently, Montgomery straps should be used (Fig. 23–7). This tape is available in large pieces and can be cut to fit body contours and dressing sizes. Approximately three fourths of the strap is adhesive-backed tape, with about 1 in of one side a nonadhesive, reinforced area with holes to attach ties available with the Montgomery straps. Montgomery straps are placed on either side of the wound, and the dressing is "tied" into place, with the ties being laced like a shoe. The Montgomery straps need to be changed when they are wet or soiled. The nurse should always apply a spray or wipe skin protector on the skin to be exposed to the Montgomery straps, as they are predominantly adhesive and could tear the skin when removed. For the client with very sensitive skin, place the Montgomery straps over pectin wafers (such as Stomahesive by Convatec), which are applied to either side of the wound first.

Elastic Bandages and Gauze Wrap Bandages

Elastic bandages (the most well-known brand of which is the Ace bandage) vary in width (*e.g.*, 2, 3, 4 in). They are wrapped predominantly around extremities to apply pressure or to keep bandages in place (Fig. 23–8).

Gauze wrap bandages are used as a primary or secondary dressing on extremities. These wraps are approximately 4 yards in length and vary from 2 to 4 in in width.

Evaluation

The evaluation of the plan of care is based on the specific outcome goals established in the plan. These goals should be reassessed daily by a professional nurse to determine the effectiveness of the nursing actions and orders. For pressure ulcers or skin or tissue integrity impairments from moisture, the causal factor needs to be considered. If the cause is not addressed, healing cannot occur. Unless the situation is deteriorating, the nursing orders in the plan of care should be in effect for approximately 3 days to 1 week to determine effectiveness.

When evaluating wounds that are managed by the physician, the role of the nurse continues to be to monitor and assess the progress of wound healing. Dressing orders for clients with such wounds may be changed only as directed by the physician.

Documentation

The documentation of the wound assessment is of the utmost importance and assists clinicians in determining whether the wound or skin integrity impairment is progressing toward healing. Flow sheets for documenting the size, depth, and other wound char-

acteristics are succinct and guide the clinician in the measurements and assessments to be made. However, if a wound flow sheet is not used by the agency, the nurse needs to write detailed narrative notes that describe those aspects of a wound or skin impairment as discussed under "Assessment" earlier in the chapter.

◆ Summary

Skin integrity issues have a major role in today's health care economics. Clients in hospitals, nursing homes, and at home are susceptible to skin breakdown for a variety of reasons. The nurse has the opportunity to diagnose the client at risk and to institute preventive measures quickly. Astute nursing care in the skin and wound arenas will save health care dollars by preventing and/or treating problems in a timely and cost-effective manner.

In addition to instituting prevention measures to prevent skin breakdown, nurses need to be able to make decisions about different dressing materials and their appropriate use in different types of wounds.

CHAPTER HIGHLIGHTS
◆

◆ Maintaining skin integrity remains a challenge in all arenas of nursing, acute, long-term, and community care.

◆ There are five factors that alter skin condition.

◆ The causal factors of skin breakdown are pressure, moisture, friction, and shear.

◆ Nurses must be able to assess a client's risk for breakdown and develop a plan of care to prevent breakdown based on the predominant causal and risk factors.

◆ The contributing risk factors to breakdown are nutrition, mental status changes, immobility and inactivity, and peripheral vascular problems.

◆ There are four stages of pressure ulcer development.

◆ Wound description is important in determining cause, treatment, and progress of healing.

◆ The AHCPR has developed a guideline for the prediction and prevention of pressure ulcers (Panel for the Prediction and Prevention of Pressure Ulcers in Adults, 1992) in adults and a guideline for treatment of pressure ulcers (Panel for the Prediction and Prevention of Pressure Ulcers, 1994).

- Treating wounds based on scientific research is the basis for nursing practice.
- Moist wound healing has been identified as the best method of allowing wounds to heal at their optimal rate.
- Dressing selection entails consideration of a variety of wound characteristics.
- Documentation of wounds and treatments assists the health care team in evaluating the success of the plan of care.

Study Questions

1. When turning a client after 60 minutes, the nurse notices a reddened area on the coccyx that remains for 15 seconds after the client was turned. Which of the following should the nurse do after measuring the reddened area?

   a. apply nonalcohol body lotion
   b. turn the client every 30 minutes
   c. apply a transparent dressing
   d. turn the client every 2 hours

2. The most appropriate nursing intervention for a preulcer is to

   a. vigorously massage the skin
   b. determine cause and alleviate
   c. apply an occlusive dressing
   d. provide ROM to the affected extremity

3. The nurse notes a client's skin is reddened, with a small abrasion and serous fluid present. The nurse classifies this stage of ulcer formation as

   a. stage I
   b. stage II
   c. stage III
   d. stage IV

4. The thick, black, leatherlike crust of dead tissue that covers the ulcer is called

   a. eschar
   b. slough
   c. undermining
   d. stage 3

5. In assessing wound drainage on a dressing from an abdominal incision, the nurse notes the drainage to be yellow, thick, and with a foul odor. The nurse would describe the drainage as

   a. purulent
   b. serosanguineous
   c. sanguineous
   d. serous

Critical Thinking Exercises

1. Ms. Z., age 42 years, has a history of spinal cord injury 20 years ago. She is paralyzed from the waist down. She is admitted to your facility with a stage 3 pressure ulcer. Wet-to-dry dressings are ordered. As you are changing Ms. Z's dressing, the gauze begins to stick to the wound. Discuss the implications of wetting the gauze to allow for easier removal of it from the wound base.

2. Ms. P., age 82 years, is admitted with a new diagnosis of cerebrovascular accident (stroke). She is having difficulty swallowing, is now bedridden, and weighs 90 lb. Discuss the nursing care needed for Ms. P. to maintain skin integrity.

References

Abruzzese, R. (1981). The effectiveness of an assessment tool in specifying nursing care to prevent decubitus ulcers. *Adelphi PRN*, 43–62.

Alterescu, V. (1983). Toward a physiologic approach to the topical treatment of wounds. *Journal of Enterostomal Therapy, 10* (3), 101–107.

Alvarez, O., Rozint, J., & Wiseman, D. (1989). Moist environment for healing: Matching the dressing to the wound. *Wounds, April*, 35–51.

Baharestani, M. M. (1994). The lived experience of wives caring for their frail, homebound, elderly husbands with pressure ulcers. *Advances in Wound Care, 7*, 40–52.

Bennett, M. A. (1995). Report of the task force on the implications for darkly pigmented intact skin in the prediction and prevention of pressure ulcers. *Advances in Wound Care, 8*(6), 34–35.

Berecek, K. (1981). The etiology of decubitus ulcers. In *Preventing decubitus ulcers*. New York: Grune & Stratton.

Bergstrom, N., Bennett, M. A., Carlson, C. E., *et al.* (1994). *Treatment of pressure ulcers*. Clinical Practice Guideline, No. 15. AHCPR Publication No. 95-0652. Rockville, MD: US Department of Health and Human Services. Public Health Service, Agency for Health Care Policy and Research.

Bergstrom, N., & Braden, B. (1992). A prospective study of pressure sore risk among institutionalized elderly. *Journal of the American Geriatrics Society, 40*, 747–758.

Bergstrom, N., Braden, B. J., Laguzza, A., & Holman, V. (1987a). The Braden Scale for predicting pressure sore risk. *Nursing Research, 36*(4), 205–210.

Bergstrom, N., Demuth, P. J., & Braden, B. J. (1987b). A clinical trial of the Braden Scale for predicting pressure sore risk. *Nursing Clinics of North America, 22*(2), 417–428.

Blazey, M. E., Brewer, E. M., Hudson, M. A., & Wilson, M. F. (1986). Nutritional assessment of protein status. *Dimensions of Critical Care Nursing, 5*(6), 328–332.

Braden, B. J. (1997). Risk assessment in pressure ulcer prevention. In D. Krasner & D. Kane (Eds.), *Chronic wound care: A clinical source book for healthcare professionals* (pp. 29–36). Wayne, PA: Health Management Publications.

Breslow, R. A., Hallfrisch, D. G., Guy, D. G., Crawley, B., & Goldberg, A. P. (1993). The importance of dietary protein in healing pressure ulcers. *Journal of the American Geriatric Society, 41,* 357–362.

Bryant, R. A. (Ed.). (1992). *Acute and chronic wounds: Nursing management*. St. Louis: Mosby-Year Book.

Bryant, R. A. (1987). Wound repair: A review. *Journal of Enterostomal Therapy, 14*, 262–266.

Burd, C., Langemo, D. K., Olson, B., Hanson, D., Hunter, S., & Sauvage, T. R. (1992). Skin problems: Epidemiology of pressure ulcers in a skilled care facility. *Journal of Gerontological Nursing, 18*(9), 29–39.

Caroll, P. (1995). Bed selection: Help patients rest easy. *RN, May, 44–51.*

Charney, P. (1995). Nutrition assessment in the 1990s: Where are we now? *Nutrition in Clinical Practice, 10, 131–139.*

Cheneworth, C. C., Hagglund, K. H., Valmassoi, B., & Brannon, C. (1994). Portrait of practice: Healing heel ulcers. *Advances in Wound Care, 7*(2), 44–48.

Cheney, A. M. (1993). Portrait of practice: A successful approach to preventing heel pressure ulcers after surgery. *Decubitus, 6*(4), 39–40.

Cooper, D. M. (1992). Wound assessment and evaluation of healing. In R. A. Bryant (Ed.), *Acute and chronic wounds: Nursing management* (pp. 69–90). St. Louis: Mosby-Year Book.

Crow, S. (1997). Infection control perspectives. In D. Krasner (Ed.), *Chronic wound care: A clinical source book for healthcare professionals* (pp. 367–377). King of Prussia, PA: Health Management Publications.

Cuzzell, J. Z. (1993). The right way to culture a wound. *American Journal of Nursing, 5,* 48–50.

Doughty, D. B. (1992). Principles of wound healing and wound management. In R. A. Bryant (Ed.), *Acute and chronic wounds: Nursing management* (pp. 31–68). St. Louis: Mosby-Year Book.

Doughty, D. B. (1994). A rational approach to the use of topical antiseptics. *JWOCN, 21*(6), 224–231.

Edlich, R. F., Morgan, R. F., Edlich, H. S., & Rodeheaver, G. T. (1987). Puncture wounds. *Current Concepts in Wound Care, Winter,* 11–18.

Ehrlich, H. P., & Hunt, T. L. (1968). Effects of cortisone and vitamin A on wound healing. *Annals of Surgery,* 167: 324.

Gawron, C. L. (1994). Risk factors for and prevalence of pressure ulcers among hospitalized patients. *JWOCN, 21* (6), 232–240.

Glugla, M., & Mulder, G. D. (1990). The diabetic foot: Medical management of foot ulcers. In D. Krasner (Ed.), *Chronic wound care: A clinical source book for healthcare professionals* (pp. 223–239). King of Prussia, PA: Health Management Publications.

Gordon, M. (1993). *Manual of nursing diagnosis.* St. Louis: C. V. Mosby.

Guin, P., Hudson, A., & Gallo, J. (1991). The efficacy of six heel pressure reducing devices. *Decubitus, 4,* 15–23.

Jarvis, C. (1992). *Physical examination and health assessment.* Philadelphia: W. B. Saunders.

Johnson, G., Daily, C., & Franciscus, V. (1991). A clinical study of hospital replacement mattresses. *Journal of Enterostomal Therapy, 18*(5), 153–157.

Kaminski, M. V., Pinchcofsky-Devin, G., & Williams, S. D. (1989). Nutritional management of decubitus ulcers in the elderly. *Decubitus, 2,* 20–30.

Konstantinides, N. N., Lehmann, S. (1993). The impact of nutrition on wound healing. *Critical Care Nurse, October,* 25–33.

Kosiak, M. (1959). Etiology and pathology of ischemic ulcers. *Archives of Physical Medicine and Rehabilitation, 40,* 62.

Kosiak, M. (1961). Etiology of decubitus ulcers. *Archives of Physical Medicine and Rehabilitation, 42,* 19–29.

Krasner, D. (1992). The 12 commandments. *Nursing, 12,* 34–41.

Landis, E. M. (1930). Micro-injection studies of capillary blood pressure in human skin. *Heart, 15,* 209.

Langemo, D. K., Olson, B., Hunter, S., Burd, C., Hanson, D.,

& Cathcart-Silberberg, T. (1989). Incidence of pressure sores in acute care, rehabilitation, extended care, home health, and hospice in one locale. *Decubitus, 2*(2), 42.

Langemo, D. K., Olson, B., Hunter, S., Hanson, D., Burd, C., & Cathcart-Silberberg, T. (1991). Incidence and prediction of pressure ulcers in five patient care settings. *Decubitus, 4*(3), 25–36.

Lyder, C. H. (1991). Conceptualization of the stage 1 pressure ulcer. *Journal of Enterostomal Therapy, 18*(5), 162–165.

Maklebust, J. (1991). Pressure ulcer update. *RN, 12,* 56–63.

Meehan, M. (1994). National pressure ulcer prevalence survey. *Advances in Wound Care, 7,* 27–38.

Mundinger, M. (1980). *Autonomy in nursing.* Germantown, MD: Aspen Systems.

National Pressure Ulcer Advisory Panel (1995). *NPUAP Report, 4* (2). Reported in *Advances in Wound Care, 8* (6), 32–33.

National Pressure Ulcer Advisory Panel. (1992). Statement on pressure ulcer prevention. Buffalo, NY: State University of New York at Buffalo.

Nichol, J. (1951). Fundamental instability of the small blood vessels and critical closing pressures in vascular beds. *American Journal of Physiology, 64,* 330.

Norton, D. (1975). Research and the problem of pressure sores. *Nursing Mirror, February,* 65–67.

Oot-Giromini, B. A. (1993). Pressure ulcer prevalence, incidence and associated risk factors in the community. *Decubitus, 6*(5), 24–32.

Panel for the Prediction and Prevention of Pressure Ulcers in Adults. (1992). *Pressure ulcers in adults: Prediction and prevention. Clinical practice guideline, number 3.* AHCPR Pub. No. 92-0047. Rockville, MD: Agency for Health Care Policy and Research, Public Health Service, US Department of Health and Human Services.

Panel for the Prediction and Prevention of Pressure Ulcers in Adults. (1994). *Treatment of pressure ulcers. Clinical practice guideline, number 15.* AHCPR Pub. No. 95-0652. Rockville, MD: Agency for Health Care Policy and Research, Public Health Service, US Department of Health and Human Services.

Petrie, L. A., & Hummel, R. S. (1990). A study of interface pressure for pressure reduction and relief mattresses. *Journal of Enterostomal Therapy, 17*(5), 212–216.

Shea, T. D. (1975). Pressure sores: Classification and management. *Clinical Orthopedics, 112,* 89–100.

Singleton, E. K., & Nail, F. C. (1984). Autonomy in nursing. *Nursing Forum, 21*(3), 123–130.

Strauss, M. B. (1987). Improving host factors: Hyperbaric oxygen, secondary mechanisms. *Current Concepts in Wound Care, Winter,* 7–10.

Towey, A. P., & Erland, S. M. (1988). Validity and reliability of an assessment tool for pressure ulcer risk. *Decubitus, 1*(2), 40–48.

Willey, T. (1992). Use a decision tree to choose wound dressings. *American Journal of Nursing, 92*(2), 43–46.

Williams, A. (1972). A study of factors contributing to skin breakdown. *Nursing Research, 21,* 238–243.

Wolf, J. G. (1995). Selection of appropriate support surfaces. *JWOCN, 22*(6), 259–262.

Wysocki, A. B., & Bryant, R. A. (1992). Skin. In R. A. Bryant (Ed.), *Acute and chronic wounds: Nursing management* (pp. 1–30). St. Louis: Mosby-Year Book.

Young, L. (1989). Pressure ulcer prevalence and associated patient characteristics in one long-term care facility. *Decubitus, 2*(2), 52.

Bibliography

Braun, J. L., Silvetti, A. N., & Xakellis, G. C. (1992). What really works for pressure sores. *Patient Care, January,* 63–83.

Brylinsky, D. M. (1995). Nutrition and wound healing: An overview. *Ostomy/Wound Management, 41*(10), 14–24.

Carpenito, L. J. (1992). *Nursing diagnosis: Application to clinical practice.* Philadelphia: J. B. Lippincott.

Colwell, J. C., Foreman, M. D., & Trotter, J. P. (1993). A comparison of the efficacy and cost-effectiveness of two methods of managing pressure ulcers. *Decubitus, 6,* 28–36.

Day, A., & Leonard, F. (1993). Seeking quality care for patients with pressure ulcers. *Decubitus, 6,* 32–43.

Ferrell, B. A., Osterweil, D., & Christenson, P. (1993). A randomized trial of low-air-loss beds for treatment of pressure ulcers. *JAMA, 269,* 494–497.

Flynn, M. E., & Rovee, D. T. (1982). CE: Wound healing mechanisms. *American Journal of Nursing, 82,* 1543–1553.

Goodridge, D. (1993). Pressure ulcer risk assessment tools: What's new for gerontological nurses. *Journal of Gerontological Nursing, 19,* 23–27.

Hanson, D., Langemo, D. K., Olson, B., Hunter, S., Burd, C., & Cathcart-Silberberg, T. (1993). The prevalence and incidence of pressure ulcers in home care: Are patients at risk? *Journal of Home Health Care Practice, 5,* 25–32.

Holmes, R., Macchiano, K., Jhangiani, S. S., Agarwal, N. R., & Savino, J. A. (1987). Combating pressure sores nutritionally. *AJN, 87*(10), 1301–1303.

International Association of Enterostomal Therapy. (1987). *Standards of care: Dermal wound and pressure sores.* Irvine, CA: International Association of Enterostomal Therapy.

Kaminski, M. V., Pinchcofsky-Devin, G., & Williams, S. D. (1989). Nutritional management of decubitus ulcers in the elderly. *Decubitus, 2,* 20–30.

Kerr, J. C., Stinson, S. M., Bay K., Thurston, N. E., Leatt, P. (1980). *Pressure sores: Nurses' knowledge, attitudes and clinical judgment—A preliminary investigation.* Edmonton, Alberta: The University of Alberta.

Kravitz, R. (1993). Development and implementation of a nursing skin care protocol. *Journal of Enterostomal Therapy, 20*(1), 4–8.

Kuhn, B. A., & Coulter, S. J. (1992). Balancing the pressure ulcer cost and quality equation. *Nursing Economics, 10*(5), 353–359.

Maklebust, J. (1991). Pressure ulcer update. *RN, 12,* 56–63.

Martinez, J. A., & Burns, C. R. (1987). Wound management. *Current Concepts in Wound Care, Summer,* 9–16.

Olshansky, K. (1994). Essay on knowledge, caring, and psychological factors in prevention and treatment of pressure ulcers. *Advances in Wound Care, 7,* 64–68.

Ratra, I. (1990). Nutritional care plan for pressure ulcers. *Decubitus, 3,* 36–37.

Richelson, C. N. (1990). Leg ulcers. *Journal of Enterostomal Therapy, 17*(5), 217–220.

Russell, M. (1995). Serum proteins and nitrogen balance: Evaluating response to nutrition support. *Support Line, February,* 3–6.

Shannon, M. L., Skorga, P. (1989). Pressure ulcer prevalence in two general hospitals. *Decubitus, 2*(4), 38–43.

Taylor, K. J. (1988). Assessment tools for the identification of patients at risk for the development of pressure sores: A review. *Journal of Enterostomal Therapy, 15*(5), 201–205.

Thomas, A. C., & Wysocki, A. B. (1990). The healing wound: A comparison of three clinically useful methods of measurement. *Decubitus, 3,* 18–25.

Thomas, C. (1988). Wound healing halted with the use of povidone-iodine. *Ostomy and Wound Management, Spring,* 30–33.

Timberlake, G. A. (1986). Wound healing: The physiology of scar formation. *Current Concepts in Wound Care, Summer,* 4–14.

Wallace, D. M., Archer, P., Roznos, K., Peters, S., & Strauss, M. B. (1989). Use of directional irrigation (Ingress-egress tubes for complex wound care management). *Ostomy/Wound Management, Spring,* 34–40.

Chapter ✦ 24

THERMO-REGULATION

JUNE BURGESS LEWIS, RN, BSN, MSN, ACCE

KEY TERMS
✦

antipyretic	heat exhaustion
basal metabolic rate	homeotherm
body temperature	hyperthermia
conduction	hypothermia
convection	pyrexia
core temperature	pyrogen
diurnal rhythm	radiation
evaporation	set point
fever	surface temperature
heat cramps	

LEARNING OBJECTIVES
✦

After studying this chapter, you should be able to

✦ Describe the difference between core temperature and surface temperature

✦ Describe four factors that affect heat production by altering the basal metabolism

✦ Compare physiological effects of heat production with physiological effects of heat loss

✦ Describe eight factors affecting thermoregulation

✦ Explain the effects of pyrexia and hypothermia and identify appropriate nursing assessments of pyrexic and hypothermic clients

✦ State appropriate nursing diagnoses for pyrexic and hypothermic clients

✦ Describe implementation of appropriate nursing care for pyrexic and hypothermic clients

✦ Compare electronic, mercury-in-glass, and tympanic thermometers

✦ Compare axillary, bladder, oral, pulmonary artery, tympanic, and rectal temperature assessment sites

✦ Discuss the therapeutic use of heat and cold

✦ Identify appropriate nursing assessment of the client receiving thermal therapy

✦ Discuss the implementation of the various types of thermal therapy

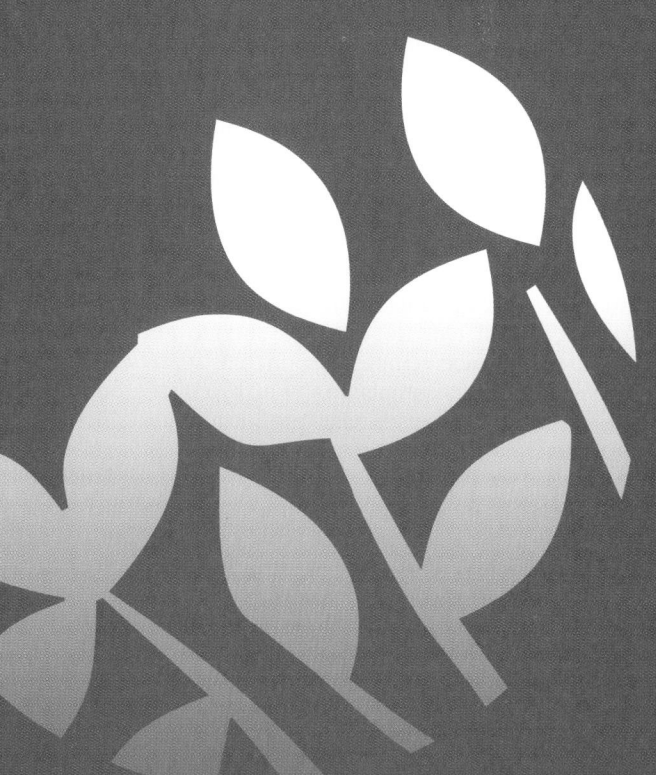

In a healthy state, the human body's temperature is maintained within a narrow range under a wide variety of environmental conditions or physical activities. The body continuously produces heat as a byproduct of metabolism and loses heat to the surroundings. The body is in heat balance when the amount lost is equal to the amount gained. An organism with this ability to maintain a steady body temperature under a variety of conditions is defined by the term *homeotherm.* Deviations above or below the normal range may be indicative of a disease process, deterioration in physical condition, or a disorder in the thermoregulatory function. The most common temperature alteration is fever, which frequently indicates the presence of disease, often an infection. Therefore, assessment of body by thermometry is one of the most common clinical procedures.

✦ Physiology of Thermoregulation

Normal Body Temperature

Body temperature is the balance of body heat produced and heat lost. The average body temperature is generally considered to be 37°C (98.6°F) but may vary between 36 and 37.2°C (97–99°F). When measured rectally, the values are approximately 0.6°C (1.0°F) greater than when measured orally (Guyton, 1992).

Normal variations in body temperature occur during hard work, exercise, and heightened emotional responses, as well as during varying times of the day. These short-term changes are not a reflection of disease or body dysfunction but rather reflect the body's ability to adapt to changing needs through heat production or heat loss.

Temperature balance is maintained by receptors located in the hypothalamus. The anterior hypothalamus controls heat dissipation, and the posterior hypothalamus controls heat conservation. The hypothalamus acts as a central thermostat, receiving input from sensors that detect hot or cold surface temperatures. When the surface temperature increases, a message is relayed to the hypothalamus, which initiates body responses that decrease heat production and increase heat loss.

There are two types of body temperature. **Surface temperature** relates to the temperature of the skin, subcutaneous tissue, and fat. Two thirds of the body mass is maintained at **core temperature,** which is the temperature of the deep tissues, such as the abdominal cavity, cranium, and thoracic cavity. Changes in body core temperature are detected by temposensors present in the abdominal viscera, spinal cord, and around large arteries. These sensors seem to be more sensitive to cold than heat. The remaining third of the body mass (the body surface) regulates core temperature by either gaining or losing heat (Fulbrook, 1993). The assessment of body core temperature may be made by oral, rectal, tympanic, or axillary measurement.

Heat Production

Heat is produced by the metabolism of food and the expenditure of energy by the body. Essentially all the energy expended by the body is eventually converted into heat. The rate of energy usage by the body is referred to as the metabolic rate. The **basal metabolic rate** is the amount of energy necessary for the body to function at its minimum level of productivity. The average basal metabolic rate is 70 calories per hour but will vary with age, sex, and body size.

Heat production may be altered with a change in the basal metabolic rate, which may be caused by an increase in exercise, a change in thyroid function, altered sympathetic nervous system functioning, and increased muscular activity (Box 24–1).

Heat Loss

Body heat is lost through four routes: (1) the skin by radiation, conduction, and convection; (2) humidification and warming of inspired air; (3) sweat evaporation and insensible perspiration; and (4) urine and feces (Brobeck, 1991). The majority of heat loss (65%) occurs from the skin through radiation, convection, and conduction (Fig. 24–1). Heat loss through **radiation** occurs in the form of infrared heat rays that move from a warmer object to a cooler object without actual physical contact. In an unheated cold room where walls and furniture are colder than body temperature, there will be a transfer of heat from the body through infrared rays to the colder objects in the room without actual contact. Sixty percent of body heat lost by a nude person will be by radiation (Guyton, 1992). If the body is overheated, the excess heat can be removed through radiation facilitated by an increased cardiac output. This results in rapid blood flow through dilated blood vessels, which allows for increased amounts of body heat to be moved to the body surface and lost through radiation.

Conduction refers to heat loss that occurs by actual physical contact between the body and substances or objects touching the skin. These substances or objects might include furniture, walls, clothing, air, water, or anything that comes into direct contact with the skin. For example, if a person sits on a cold chair, body heat would transfer to that chair. Heat loss varies with the amount of exposure; for example, the amount of heat lost by a person immersed in a cold tub of water depends on the water temperature and the amount of time exposed to the cold water. Normally, heat loss through conduction accounts for only 3% of total body heat loss. Heat loss through **convection** is closely related to that of conduction. Convection is the loss of heat through air currents. Body heat

FACTORS AFFECTING METABOLIC RATE

Exercise: The metabolic rate increases with muscle activity. Short bursts of maximal contraction in a single muscle can increase heat production for a few seconds at a time by as much as 100 times its normal resting state. In the entire body, maximal muscle exercise in a well-trained athlete can increase heat production to 20 times normal and sustain it for several minutes (Guyton, 1992).

Thyroid Hormone: Thyroxine, a hormone secreted by the thyroid gland, increases cellular mitochondrial activity. Maximal secretion of thyroxine by the thyroid gland may increase the metabolic rate by as much as 60 to 100% above normal. This increased metabolic activity results in increased energy expenditure and heat production. On the other hand, total loss of thyroid secretion decreases the metabolic rate to as little as 50 to 60% of normal (Guyton, 1992). Temperature changes due to thyroid function occur gradually over a period of weeks or months.

Sympathetic Nervous System: Epinephrine and norepinephrine, mediators in the sympathetic nervous system, affect the basal metabolic rate by increasing cellular metabolism. This effect is called chemical thermogenesis. In the adult, thermogenesis increases body heat production only 10 to 15%, but in newborns, this increase may be as high as 100%, which helps the newborn adapt to extrauterine life.

Muscular Activity: The body can also regulate heat production by increasing muscular activity according to the degree of heat production needed. The most common muscular activity related to thermoregulation is shivering. When chilled to 23°C (73.4°F), the body automatically begins to shiver. Shivering consists of small increases and decreases of nerve impulses to a muscle, causing inapparent tensing and relaxing. This results in considerable muscle activity, which increases the metabolic rate and causes heat production. During maximal shivering, body heat production can rise to as high as four to five times normal (West, 1991).

Data in part from Guyton, A. (1992). *Human physiology and mechanisms of disease* (5th ed.; p. 533). Philadelphia: W. B. Saunders; and West, J. B. (Ed.). (1991). *Best and Taylor's physiological basis of medical practice* (p. 1064). Baltimore: Williams & Wilkins.

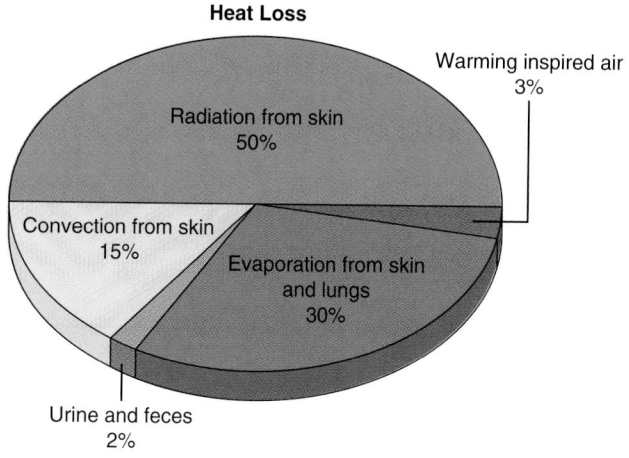

Figure 24–1
How body heat is lost.

which is the loss of body heat when body liquids are converted to a vapor. The majority of evaporation occurs through insensible water loss through the skin and lungs. Water loss by evaporation accounts for a total of 600 ml of fluid per day. This loss is not controlled by environmental temperatures; however, if the body overheats, an increased amount of evaporation can be instigated by an increase in sweat production. In cold temperature, there is little sweat production, but as environmental temperatures rise, so does the amount of sweat produced. A maximum rate of sweat production is thought to be 1.5 to 2 L/hour for a climatized athlete. A climatized athlete has gradually worked to adjust the body's response to hot weather training. The climatized body has an increased level of efficiency to dissipate or lose heat. It is interesting to note that a climatized person will have an increased amount of sweating but a decreased amount of electrolyte loss (Jacobson, 1992).

The amount of heat loss is affected by the humidity of the air. When the humidity increases, the amount of heat lost from sweat decreases.

Factors That Affect Thermoregulation

The nursing assessment of the client with problems of thermoregulation would include vital signs and physical assessment, but it is important to assess for preexisting factors as well. When obtaining a nursing history the identification of factors affecting thermoregulation is an important step in providing care. Preexisting factors that could affect thermoregulation include size, age, exercise, hormones, environmental exposure, stress, diurnal variations, and behavioral controls (Box 24–2).

is first conducted to the air in contact with the skin surface and is then removed by air currents. This could be demonstrated by setting a person in a warm room in front of an electric fan. Heat loss by convection would be that heat removed by the moving air current.

Heat loss from the body can occur when the environmental temperature is very close to the normal body temperature. This occurs through **evaporation,**

Body Size

Stability of body temperature is affected by the size of the person. An infant or toddler has a greater amount of body surface exposed to environmental conditions and is therefore more easily affected by environmental temperatures than is an adult.

Internal tissues of the body are insulated by the skin, subcutaneous tissues, and fat. The amount of body fat present affects the body temperature because fat conducts heat only one third as readily as the rest of the tissues and therefore serves as an insulating layer. Women usually have better insulation because of the higher percent of body fat than men (Guyton, 1992). The obese client would lose less body heat than a thin client in a cool environment. Body weight has a great impact on the elderly client: A thin, frail elderly person would have a low metabolic rate.

Age

The metabolic rate is affected a great deal by the age of the client. An infant's metabolic rate is very high, which works to compensate for a greater body surface area (Table 24–1). In the elderly, however, a decreased rate of metabolism results in a decreased amount of heat production and makes them more vulnerable to cold temperatures (Fig. 24–2). Other factors that alter the elderly client's response to temperature changes are listed in the accompanying box.

Exercise

Body heat production is greatly affected by the amount of energy used. Energy utilization varies greatly with activity. For example, a person climbing stairs uses 17 times the amount of energy as a person asleep in bed (Guyton, 1992). The postoperative client often experiences low body temperature, caused by decreased muscle activity, and a suppressed shivering response, caused by the anesthesia (Heidenreich & Giuffre, 1990). High amounts of extreme exercise or prolonged exercise may produce high body temperatures. An example of this is the marathon runner who may experience temperatures of 39.5 to 41°C (103.2–105.8°F) (Braunwald, 1987). The heat balance that is disrupted by exercise when a greater heat production than loss occurs is restored by rest and activation of heat loss mechanisms.

Hormones

Body temperature is affected by the endocrine system. This is especially true for women; the endocrine influence on temperature is seen throughout the menstrual cycle. During the second half of the menstrual cycle, the mean body temperature of a woman is higher than it is between the onset of menstruation and the time of ovulation (Braunwald, 1987). Ovulation may be tracked by monitoring the basal body temperature daily. During menopause, the sudden "hot flashes" that produce a sensation of intense heat followed by profuse sweating are caused by an endocrine disbalance.

Environment

Overheating or heat loss can easily occur from exposure to the environmental temperatures when

Table **24–1**

DEVELOPMENTAL FACTORS THAT AFFECT TEMPERATURE REGULATION

AGE	FACTORS	TEMPERATURE RANGE
Infant	Increased body surface area Increased metabolism rate	36.1–37.7°C (97–100°F)
Child	Increased activity Increased metabolism rate	37–37.6°C (98.6–99.6°F)
Adult	Increased physical work increases temperature Alcohol intake increases body heat loss	37–37.6°C (98.6–99.6°F)
Elderly Person	Decreased metabolism Decreased body fat Decreased activity	36.0–36.9°C (96.9–98.3°F)

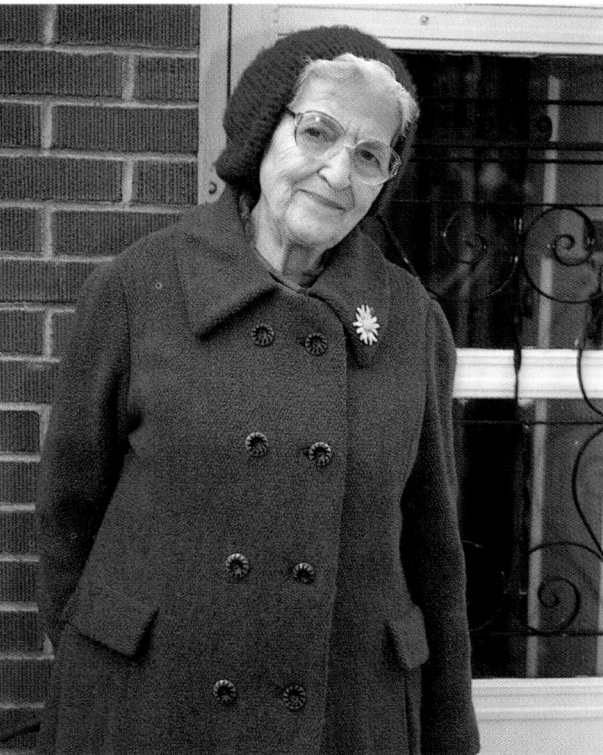

FACTORS THAT ALTER THE ELDER CLIENT'S RESPONSE TO TEMPERATURE CHANGES

Factors increasing hypothermia

* Decreased body fat
* Decreased metabolism
* Endocrine dysfunction
    Hypoglycemia
    Hypothyroidism
    Hypopituitarism
* Infections
    Pneumonia and sepsis
* Neurological impairment
* Inactivity
* Fatigue and hypoxia suppress shivering

Factors increasing hyperthermia

* Decreased sensation of thirst
* Decreased efficiency of kidney to concentrate urine, causing dehydration
* Impaired sweating
    Higher threshold for onset
* Decreased cardiac output
* Decreased conscious awareness

Data from Miller, C. (1995). *Nursing care of older adults* (2nd ed.). Philadelphia: J. B. Lippincott.

> **Figure 24–2**
Elderly people are more vulnerable to cold temperatures because of decreased metabolism, decreased body fat, and a lower level of physical activity.

they are excessively warm or cold. For example, a summer hike in the mountains when the hiker is lightly clad, perspiring heavily, and buffeted by wind can lower the body's core temperature to below 35°C (95°F) (Walhout, 1992). Frostbite and decreased body temperature are often experienced with snow and freezing temperatures when the exposed person is inadequately dressed or exposed for prolonged periods. Exposure to high temperatures also is a very serious problem and is compounded when the humidity is high. In dry air, a person can withstand several hours of temperatures as high as 54°C (130°F), whereas the person exposed to a temperature of 34.3°C (94°F) at 100% humidity will begin to overheat (Guyton, 1992).

Stress

An increased level of stress results in the activation of the sympathetic nervous system, which in turn increases the production of epinephrine and norepinephrine, causing an increased metabolic rate. The emergency room client who is highly stressed may experience a slightly increased temperature level, which may return to normal once he or she has calmed down.

Diurnal Effects

Diurnal temperature variations occur in most people. The variations usually result in a lowered body temperature in the early morning hours and a higher body temperature in the afternoon and most likely relate to the circadian cycle. Plasma cortisol levels are thought to influence these normal 24-hour circadian fluctuations in temperature by 0.2 to 0.3°C (1°F) (Osguthorpe, 1993). The circadian cycle remains fairly stable throughout life but can be affected by emotional strain, pain, trauma, and changes in the sleep pattern.

Behavioral Control

An important factor affecting the body heat regulation is that of behavioral control. This is both a psychological and a neurological function. Behavioral control involves the conscious recognition that the body is either too hot or too cold. The mechanism can be explained in this way: When the body becomes too cold, neuroreceptors evoke the sensation of cold discomfort. The person then makes a conscious effort to adjust the environmental temperature by putting on more clothing, adjusting the thermostat, moving to a warmer place, or moving the extremities to increase muscle activity. Unfortunately, the judgment needed for behavioral control may be limited because of drug or alcohol use, illness, brain impairment, or unconsciousness.

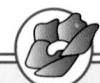

Spinal Cord Impairment

Damage to the spinal cord may interrupt nerve pathways, resulting in an abnormal response to temperature changes. Injury to the hypothalamus disrupts the body's ability to adapt to temperature alterations and may be life threatening.

Temperature Assessment Techniques

Types of Thermometers

A wide variety of mercury-in-glass thermometers, electronic probes, liquid crystal thermometers, tympanic membrane thermometers, and pulmonary artery catheter thermistors are available. The most commonly used in the clinical setting are the mercury-in-glass thermometer, electronic probe, and tympanic thermometer.

The body temperature is measured in degrees, using either a Fahrenheit (°F) or a Celsius (°C) scale. On a mercury-in-glass thermometer, the scale for Celsius usually runs between 34.0 to 42°C, and the scale for Fahrenheit runs from 94 to 108°F.

To convert a temperature from one scale to another, the following formulas are used:

To change Celsius to Fahrenheit: F = (Celsius temperature × 9/5) + 32

To change Fahrenheit to Celsius: C = (Fahrenheit − 32) × 5/9

Mercury-in-Glass Thermometer

The most commonly used thermometer is the mercury-in-glass thermometer, which was first developed in 1867 and continues to be used to this day. This thermometer is a glass rod that measures temperature by the movement of mercury, seen as a sliver line through the calibrated glass (Procedure 24–1). The tip of the thermometer may be short and rounded, pear shaped, or long. The short rounded tip is used for rectal temperatures most commonly but may also be used for oral or axillary measurement. The long tip and the pear-shaped tip are used for oral or axillary temperature measurement. The thermometer may be calibrated in either the Fahrenheit or the Celsius scale.

The mercury in the glass thermometer must be shaken down until it is below 35°C (95°F) before a reading can be taken. This is done by holding the thermometer at the opposite end from the bulb with the thumb and forefinger. The hand is then snapped in a downward movement from the wrist (see Procedure 24–1).

Electronic Thermometer

The electronic thermometer is a battery-operated portable unit with an attached probe and disposable probe cover (Procedure 24–2). This thermometer offers a more rapid reading of the body temperature. The time needed to get an accurate reading varies from between 2 seconds to 1 minute, depending on

PROCEDURE

24–1

ORAL TEMPERATURE ASSESSMENT

Gather equipment and explain procedure to client.

Equipment:

Mercury-in-glass thermometer
and disposable cover
Clean, dry gauze or tissue
OR
Electronic thermometer and
disposable cover

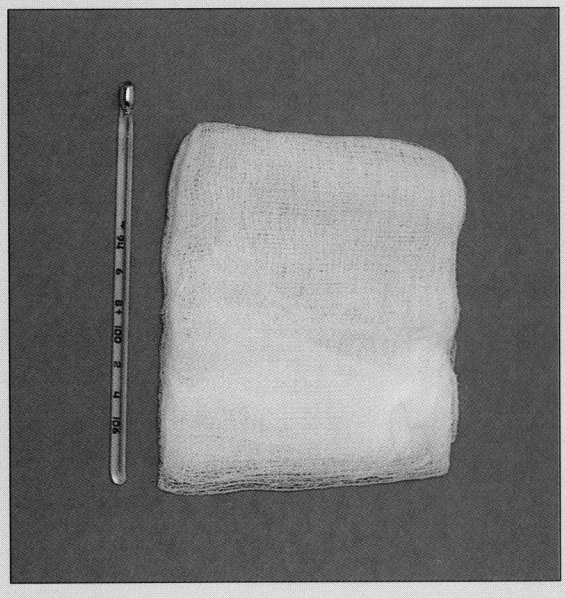

Equipment

Action	**Rationale**
1. Wash hands	1. Infection control
2. *Glass thermometer:* Dry thermometer with dry tissue or gauze if it has been stored in a chemical solution *Electronic thermometer:* Remove temperature probe from the unit	2. To prepare for thermometer insertion
3. *Glass thermometer:* Grasp thermometer (at opposite end from bulb) between thumb and forefinger and shake with a snapping motion of the wrist; continue shaking until mercury reaches at least 95°F (36°C) *Electronic thermometer:* Probe is ready for use	3. Mercury must be shaken down in glass thermometer to obtain an accurate reading

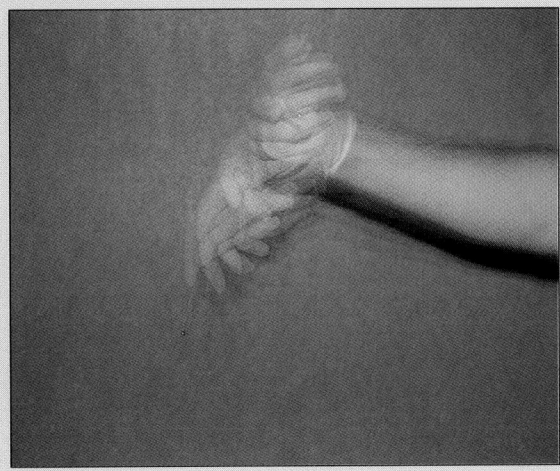

Step 3. *Shaking glass thermometer*

4. Cover thermometer or probe with a disposable cover	4. Disposable cover is important for infection control

Continued

PROCEDURE

24–1

ORAL TEMPERATURE ASSESSMENT
(Continued)

Action	Rationale
5. Place thermometer or probe at the base of the tongue on the left or right side of the frenulum; have client close lips around thermometer or probe and instruct client not to talk	**5.** For accurate measurement of an oral temperature, placement must be near blood vessels in posterior sublingual pocket
6. A glass thermometer should remain in place for at least 3 minutes; the probe of an electronic thermometer should remain in place until the unit records a reading	**6.** Adequate time must be allowed for an accurate reading

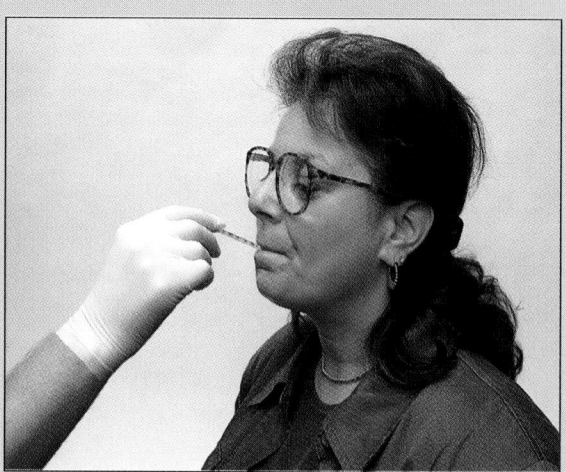

Step 4. *Glass thermometer in place*

Action	Rationale
7. Remove thermometer or probe; remove disposable cover with a gloved hand	**7.** Hand is gloved for infection control
8. *Glass thermometer:* Read the point at which the mercury marks to the nearest tenth *Electronic thermometer:* Unit records reading	**8.** To obtain accurate reading
9. *Glass thermometer:* Place in storage container *Electronic thermometer:* Return to charging unit	**9.** Returning glass thermometer promptly to storage container prevents breakage Returning electronic thermometer to charging unit ensures recharging of thermometer

Documentation: *Record reading in client's record/chart.*

---

the type of unit used. An electronic thermometer may be used to obtain oral, rectal, or axillary temperatures. However, research findings question the accuracy of the axillary measurement (Heidenreich & Giuffre, 1990). The probe placement for temperature measurement is the same as that used with the mercury-in-glass thermometer.

Tympanic Thermometer

The tympanic thermometer is a relatively new form of electronic thermometer. The most recent one, the infrared light reflectance thermometer, determines the temperature of the tympanic membrane by mea-

suring heat radiated as infrared energy from that site (Holtzclaw, 1993). Because the hypothalamus and the tympanic membrane share the same vasculature, the temperature measured reflects the core temperature at the hypothalamus. The accuracy of the tympanic thermometer depends a great deal on the correct placement of the probe, which should be placed in the ear canal, directed toward the tympanic membrane. Researchers have compared the pulmonary artery blood temperature to that of the tympanic membrane temperature and have found no significant difference between the two (Ferrara-Love, 1991).

The thermometers generally have the appearance of a small otoscope and either have an attached porta-

RECTAL TEMPERATURE ASSESSMENT

Gather equipment and explain procedure to client.

Equipment:

Glass thermometer or electronic unit
Disposable cover or probe cover
Lubricant
Disposable gloves

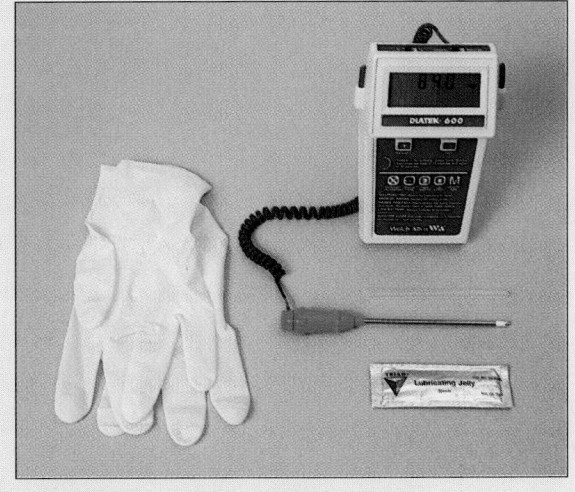

Equipment

Action	Rationale
1. Wash your hands and put on disposable gloves	1. Infection control
2. *Glass thermometer:* Dry thermometer off with dry tissue if it has been stored in a chemical solution *Electronic thermometer:* Remove temperature probe from the unit	2. To prepare for thermometer insertion
3. *Glass thermometer:* Grasp thermometer (at opposite end from bulb) between thumb and forefinger and shake with a snapping motion of the wrist; continue shaking until the mercury reaches at least 95°F, then cover thermometer with a disposable cover and lubricate *Electronic thermometer:* Remove electronic unit from the charging unit; securely attach a disposable cover over temperature probe and lubricate	3. The mercury in glass thermometer must be shaken down to obtain an accurate reading

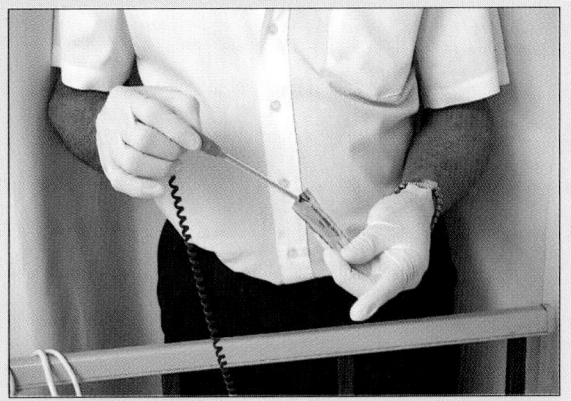

Step 3. *Lubricating probe*

Continued

ble module with a digital readout or the module is contained in the probe unit itself (Procedure 24–3).

Temperature-Sensitive Tape

The use of temperature-sensitive tape provides a generalization of body temperature and is not an ac-curate measurement of temperature. This method is used often with well children or infants as a screening mechanism. If a temperature elevation is noted, a more accurate measurement can then be obtained using a more reliable instrument.

Temperature-sensitive tape, which is adhesive, is
Text continued on page 620

RECTAL TEMPERATURE ASSESSMENT
(Continued)

Action	Rationale
4. Turn client to lateral position and separate buttocks until you can see the anus	**4.** For comfort and ease of insertion

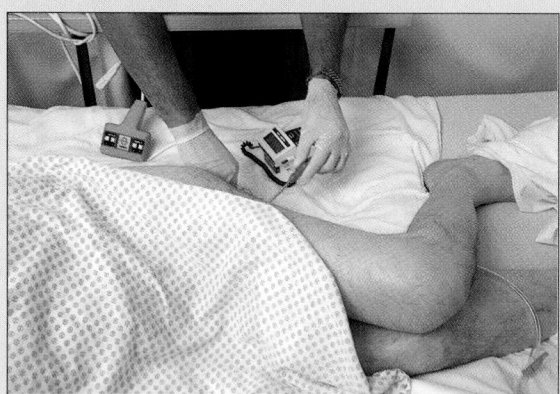

Step 4. *Client in position (adult)*

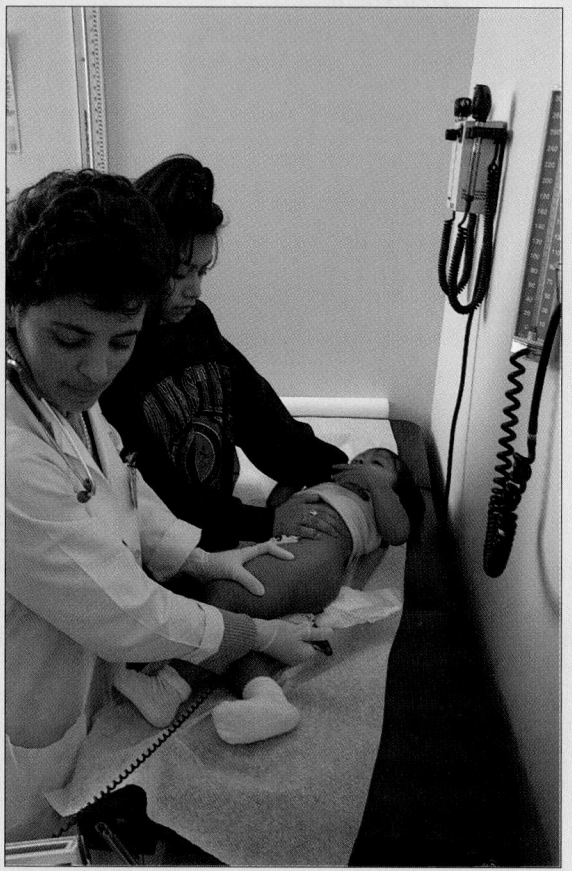

Step 4. *Inserting probe (infant)*

Action	Rationale
5. Insert the thermometer or probe gently into the rectum 1.5 in (3.7 cm) in an adult, 1 in (2.5 cm) in a child, and 0.5 in (1.5 cm) in an infant	**5.** To prevent trauma or puncture of rectal mucosa
6. *Glass thermometer:* Hold securely in place for 2 minutes or more *Electronic thermometer:* Hold probe securely in place until electronic alarm sounds	**6.** To prevent displacement or complete insertion of thermometer
7. *Glass thermometer:* Remove thermometer and remove disposable cover; read temperature *Electronic thermometer:* Remove probe and note temperature registered on display	**7.** To obtain temperature reading
8. Remove gloves *Electronic thermometer:* Remove probe cover without touching by pressing release button while probe is held pointing down into a waste basket	**8.** Infection control
9. *Glass thermometer:* Store thermometer in container *Electronic thermometer:* Return thermometer to its charging unit	**9.** To prevent breakage or to recharge electronic thermometer

Documentation: *Record reading in client's record/chart.*

24–3

TYMPANIC TEMPERATURE ASSESSMENT

Gather equipment and explain procedure to client.

Equipment:

Tympanic thermometer
Disposable probe cover

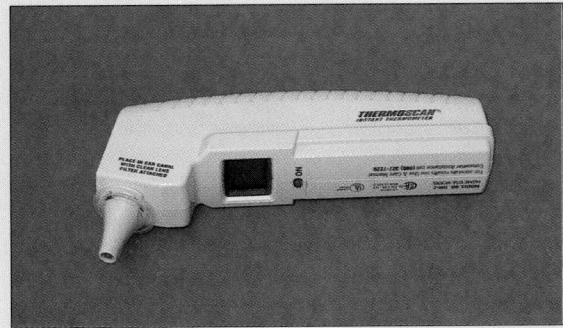

Equipment

Action	**Rationale**
1. Remove tympanic thermometer from charger; check to see if disposable probe covers are available for use	1. Tympanic thermometers should be kept stored in the charger to prevent the battery from running down; disposable probe covers are for infection control
2. Some thermometers will not immediately function and require a 15-second time period; the thermometer should read "ready"	2. Some thermometers require several seconds to recalibrate and be ready for use
3. Apply a disposable cover to probe (read directions on your thermometer)	3. This is done differently with some thermometers
4. Explain the procedure to the client	4. This decreases anxiety and increases cooperation
5. Place the probe in the ear canal, pointed toward the tympanic member (the same way you would view the tympanic membrane with an otoscope)	5. The temperature will only be accurate if it can measure the infrared rays from the tympanic membrane

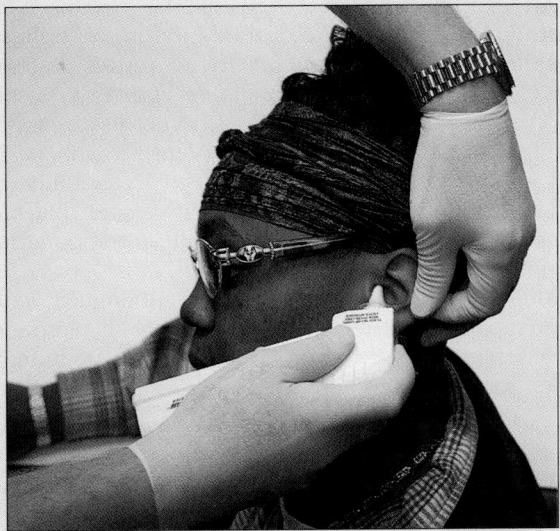

Step 5. *Tympanic temperature assessment*

6. Press "scan" button; this must be done with some thermometers within 25 or 30 seconds after it is removed from the cradle (review directions on your thermometer)	6. This activates the thermometer

Continued

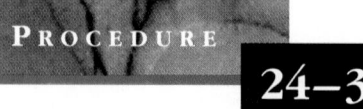

TYMPANIC TEMPERATURE ASSESSMENT
(Continued)

Action	Rationale
7. Hold the probe gently in place until alarm goes off (either beeper or light)	**7.** Thermometer usually registers temperature within 2 or 3 seconds
8. Correct thermometer reading should be displayed at that time	**8.** Read temperature
9. Remove from ear and discard disposable cover into trash can	**9.** For infection control
10. Return thermometer to recharger	**10.** To keep unit charged
11. Record temperature	**11.** To monitor changes in temperature

Documentation: *Record reading in client's record/chart.*
Note: *If this is the first time the thermometer is used on a shift, it is recommended that a second reading be taken. The second reading is the most accurate and should be the one that is recorded.*

applied to dry skin and left in place for 15 to 60 seconds. The most frequently used site is the forehead. A color change occurs on the tape to indicate the approximate body temperature.

Body Temperature Assessment Sites

An exact core temperature can be obtained by measuring the temperature of the blood in the pulmonary artery. Only in the pulmonary artery does a convective mixture of blood from all over the body occur. However, in most cases this site is rarely used except with the surgical or critically ill client (Bligh, 1973, cited in Fulbrook, 1993). The lack of accessibility of this site presents the need for alternative sites that are both easy to access and fairly accurate in temperature measurement.

Multiple sites, including oral or sublingual, axillary, tympanic, and rectal, are used daily in temperature assessment. The route of assessment is frequently chosen for safety and convenience.

Oral Temperatures

The oral or sublingual temperature is the most commonly used temperature assessment site because of its convenient location and vascular blood supply. At the base of the tongue lies the sublingual pocket, which receives its blood supply from branches of the external artery, which is close to the internal carotid artery (Clemente, 1985, cited in Erickson and Yount, 1991). Because of its location next to these arteries, the sublingual pocket responds very quickly to changes in the core temperature. The thermometer is

inserted into the mouth at the base of the tongue beside the frenulum. The client is instructed to close his or her lips around the thermometer but to avoid biting down on the thermometer because of the possibility of breaking it. The thermometer should be left in place, with the client keeping his or her mouth closed and not talking for at least 3 minutes (Holtzclaw, 1993; Togawa, 1985, cited in Fulbrook, 1993). However, some researchers believe that up to 12 minutes are required to obtain a fully accurate reading on a mercury-in-glass thermometer. An electronic probe is used in the same way but is left in place only until a reading is obtained, usually approximately 30 seconds.

Researchers found that, compared with rectal temperatures, the oral or sublingual temperatures were 0.2 to 0.5°F lower (Fulbrook, 1993; Holtzclaw, 1993). Oral temperatures, however, may be influenced by external factors, including mouth breathing, talking, gum chewing, eating, and smoking. For example, ingestion of liquids that are either hot or cold can alter the temperature for as long as 9 minutes (Terndrup, 1987, cited in Holtzclaw, 1993). Because of this alteration, it is recommended that 30 minutes should pass between the ingestion of iced drinks and temperature assessment.

The oral temperature site, although easily accessible and convenient, is not always the best method. Cross-infection is considered a risk of oral temperature measurement. Dry storage of thermometers allows for bacterial colonization to occur (Litsdky, cited in Fulbrook, 1993). With either mercury thermometers or electronic probes, disposable covers are now used to cover the thermometer to prevent this problem. The disposable cover should be discarded after each use, and a new one used for the next temperature measurement.

Oral thermometers are not considered safe for use in infants, small children, or the elderly, or in demented, epileptic, or unconscious clients. A risk occurs because of the possibility of a mercury thermometer breaking, with ingestion of the mercury or injury to the client. Oral measurements should not be taken in the client with recent oral surgery or current oral infection because the accuracy would be impaired by the increased heat production caused by local inflammation (Fulbrook, 1993).

See Procedure 24–1 for steps in taking oral temperature.

Rectal Temperatures

The rectum, which is supplied by the hemorrhoidal artery, serves as a good site for temperature measurement. The rectum is well insulated and does not vary with outside environmental temperature influences. The rectal temperature is 0.2 to 0.3°C (1°F) higher than that of the pulmonary artery (Holtzclaw, 1993), possibly as a result of the increased metabolic activity of fecal bacteria (Benzinger, 1969, cited in Fulbrook, 1991). To take a rectal temperature, a disposable covering is first placed over the thermometer, and water soluble lubricant is then applied to the bulb end of the thermometer. About 1 in of the thermometer should be coated with lubricant to ease insertion of the thermometer into the rectum and to avoid trauma to the rectal mucosa. To insert the thermometer, the client is placed in a lateral position with the anterior leg flexed. The client should be carefully draped to avoid exposure, as most clients are uncomfortable or embarrassed when having a rectal temperature taken. The nurse should always wear disposable gloves when taking a rectal temperature. An accurate measurement of rectal temperature requires correct positioning of the rectal thermometer. The thermometer is inserted 1.5 in (3.7 cm) in an adult, almost 1 in (2.5 cm) in a child, and 0.5 in (1.5 cm) in an infant. *The mercury thermometer or temperature probe should always be held firmly in place for 2 minutes or more and never left unattended because of the risk of breakage or complete insertion of the thermometer into the rectum* (Nichols, 1972, cited in Holtzclaw, 1993).

Disadvantages of rectal temperature measurement include client embarrassment and discomfort and the necessity of repositioning the client to gain access to the site. The possibility of bradycardia due to parasympathetic stimulation was thought to be a potential problem, but recent research does not support that theory (Fulbrook, 1991). However, many critical care units do not take rectal temperatures due to possible vagal stimulation.

Another disadvantage is that the rectal temperature response to core temperature changes is slower than the oral site. Inaccuracies in the rectal temperature may also occur due to the presence of stool, regional inflammation, or ischemia.

See Procedure 24–2 for steps in taking rectal temperatures.

Axillary Temperatures

The axillary site is frequently chosen because it is safe and easily accessed; however, it is known to be the least consistent and accurate in measurement of core temperature and more likely to be influenced by environmental changes. The axillary temperature is 0.6 to 0.8°C lower than the rectal temperature (Holtzclaw, 1993). However, Fulbrook (1993) found that the difference was 0.19°C below the temperature of the pulmonary artery when measured for 10 minutes.

The measurement of the axillary temperature is actually a measurement of two body surfaces. To take an axillary temperature, insert the thermometer probe in the middle of the arm pit (Fig. 24–3). The arm is then pulled close to the body, which traps air into the axillary pocket between skin surfaces and decreases some of the environmental effects. The mercury thermometer should be held in place for 10 minutes (Fulbrook, 1993). It is known, however, that when the client is chilled, hypothermic, or experiencing some form of vasoconstriction, the temperature measurement does not reflect core body temperature (Holtzclaw, 1993). Axillary measurement may have a greater accuracy in children because of the decreased amount of subcutaneous tissue and skin depth. One study of elderly women found a temperature variation of 0.2 to 1.4°C between the left and right axilla, with the left axilla usually having a higher temperature (Howell, 1972, cited in Fulbrook, 1993). Therefore, when using the axillary site, documentation of site and side and repeatedly using the same site would increase accuracy in determining changes in temperature.

Accuracy of the temperature measurement depends on the correct placement of the thermometer, the length of time used for measurement, and the type of thermometer used. The use of mercury-in-glass

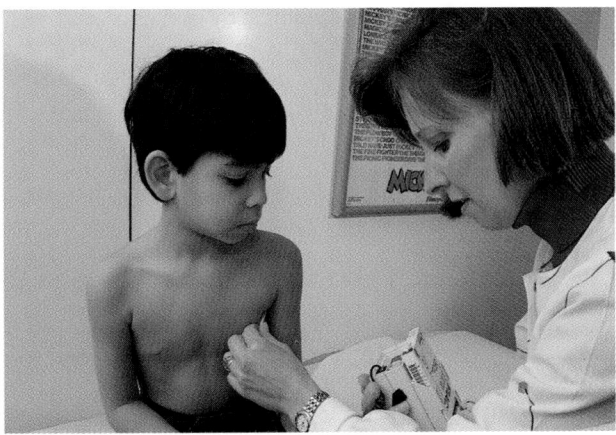

♦ **Figure 24–3**
The axillary site provides easy access for temperature assessment, but it is the least accurate way to measure temperature. A mercury-in-glass thermometer placed correctly for 10 minutes will give the most accurate reading at this site.

thermometers gives a more consistent and accurate reading of axillary temperatures than those obtained with an electronic thermometer (Giuffre *et al.,* 1990).

Disadvantages with the axillary site include the necessity of using a glass thermometer, the duration of thermometer placement, and the possibility of thermometer displacement during that time.

Tympanic Temperatures

The measurement of body temperature using a tympanic thermometer has become common and is frequently used in the clinical setting. The ability to measure body temperature through the external auditory canal has proven to have several advantages. Its easy accessibility and minimal discomfort make this method very useful for children and confused adults. It is even possible to take the temperature without awakening the client.

The tympanic temperature has been found to be 0.05 to .25°C lower than rectal temperatures.

The steps followed when assessing the temperature are to (1) place a disposable cover over the scope, (2) straighten the auditory canal by slightly retracting the external ear, (3) gently direct the scope into the ear canal (holding the thermometer as you would hold an otoscope), and (4) direct the scope toward the tympanic membrane. The reading will be produced within a few seconds. A recent study found that the first tympanic thermometer reading on a thermometer that had been in the recharging mode was slightly higher than later measurements (Baird *et al.,* 1992). Therefore, when using a freshly recharged thermometer, take two readings on the first client and record the second reading.

An advantage of the tympanic thermometer is that the auditory canal itself has a much lower bacterial count than the mucous membranes of the mouth or rectum (Ferrara-Love, 1991). Disposable covers are also made for the tympanic thermometer to prevent any risk of cross-contamination.

A disadvantage of the tympanic thermometer is a reported inaccuracy of readings by nursing staff. Researchers have found that the greatest cause of this inaccuracy is the incorrect positioning of the instrument (Holtzclaw, 1993). The probe should be directed toward the tympanic membrane to get the most accurate reading.

See Procedure 24–3 for steps in taking tympanic temperatures.

Pulmonary Artery Temperatures

The temperature of the blood in the pulmonary artery may now be measured as a result of the advancement of hemodynamic instrumentation and technology. This is done in a critical care setting because it requires the insertion of a pulmonary artery catheter and would not be justified for temperature verification alone.

The thermistor-tipped quadruple-lumen catheter is used in major vascular surgery. Most clinicians consider the pulmonary artery temperature reading to be the gold standard of temperature measurement. The thermistors used in these devices are known to be exceptionally sensitive and accurate (Holtzclaw, 1993). Their use and availability would only be for critically ill clients.

Bladder Temperatures

Measuring the bladder temperature has only recently become possible through the development of Foley catheters that have a thermistor tip. The calibration of the bladder thermistor, however, requires skilled intervention. Because the technique is relatively new, the future usefulness and accuracy of bladder temperatures will become more evident as the use of the catheter increases.

Therapeutic Use of Heat and Cold

The daily care of clients frequently involves the use of heat or cold as therapeutic treatment for injuries and infectious processes. The use of therapeutic heat and cold ranges from an ice pack for a sports injury, to warm whirlpool treatment for joint immobility, to a cool sponge bath for the hyperthermic client.

Heat Therapy

The application of heat improves blood flow to the involved area by causing vasodilation. This in turn results in the delivery of increased oxygen and nutrients, as well as an increased removal of wastes. Heat therapy facilitates soft tissue repair through accelerated cellular metabolism. Heat also results in decreased blood viscosity and increased capillary permeability, thereby aiding in the rebuilding and recovery process.

Muscle spasm and secondary muscle pain are decreased by the application of heat, which interferes with the pain reception of the nerve fiber. This in turn results in increased range of motion because of increased extensibility of collagen and the reduced spasm (Halvorson, 1990).

Heat therapy could be used for inflammation of an edematous body part; joint pain, such as arthritis; muscle strain; menstrual cramping; perianal and vaginal inflammation; hemorrhoids; and local abscesses.

Cold Therapy

Cold has almost the opposite effect of heat on the body tissues. It causes vasoconstriction and therefore decreases blood flow to the involved area. Cooling of the tissue decreases the cell metabolism, increases the blood viscosity, decreases muscle tension, and results in anesthetic effects by numbing the tissue.

When treating an acute injury, it is important to

control soft tissue swelling. Swelling results in cellular damage because of hypoxia and indirect release of chemical mediators. Cold applied to an acute injury decreases swelling and bleeding as a result of vasoconstriction. Inflammation is decreased because of slowed cellular metabolism. The pain is decreased because of its effect on nerve fiber transmission and indirectly through the reduced amount of swelling (Halvorson, 1990).

Assessment for Thermal Therapy

Therapeutic application of heat and cold is frequently used to treat acute and chronic injuries. However, the proper selection and application of heat or cold require an understanding of cellular and neuromuscular responses. The application of heat or cold for therapeutic use requires a physician's order.

When implementing the physician's order, the nurse should assess the area to which the thermotherapy is to be applied. The risk of damage from thermotherapy is greater if the area has impaired circulation, impaired skin integrity, or edema.

Assessment for circulation in the area would include color, warmth, and sensation. Skin integrity assessment includes open lesions, blisters, amount of drainage, and bleeding. The presence of edema and the amount of involvement should be noted. Tissue that is impaired in any of these ways will be at greater risk for trauma from cold therapy, although it is frequently necessary to aid in recovery. The nurse must therefore assess at the time of application and then repeatedly reassess the skin for changes once the thermotherapy is initiated. If any negative change should occur, reevaluation of the therapy with the physician is necessary.

Implementation of Thermal Therapy

Heat therapy is divided into moist heat, such as a warm wet dressing or sitz bath, and dry heat, such as electric heating pads or hot water bottles. The advantage of warm moist heat is the dissipation or conduction into superficial tissues. Moist applications may be used to soften wound exudate and do not result in insensible fluid loss.

Warm Moist Heat

Warm moist heat may be as simple as the application of a wet towel that has been warmed in the microwave to a tolerable level (the nurse should be able to hold the warmed towel in his or her bare hand). A nonsterile, warm wet towel can be used if the skin is intact. If the skin is broken, sterile dressings and sterile water would be used to prevent contamination of the wound. The top side of the wet towel or sterile dressing should be covered with plastic or a dry towel to prevent saturating the bed linens.

Whirlpool Therapy

A whirlpool bath applies warm moist heat by the immersion of the involved part or most of the body in warm water (Fig. 24–4). Hubbard tanks are frequently used for this type of therapy. In a Hubbard tank, water jets force air and water into the tub, circulating the water in a whirlpool-type motion. Immersion in a Hubbard tank is frequently used to obtain pain relief, increase range of motion, stimulate circulation, and débride wounds or burns. The use of Hubbard tanks and whirlpools is most commonly found in physical therapy, although some health care facilities, especially those for rehabilitation, have them available on the health care unit.

Sitz Bath

A sitz bath is used to apply warm moist heat to the pelvic area. It is most frequently used with the postpartum client who is recovering from a vaginal delivery. It applies heat and warmth to the perianal, vaginal, and perineal areas. The whirlpool effect of the sitz bath aids in cleansing the area as well.

To decrease cross-contamination, a plastic disposable sitz bath (a round basin designed to fit into the base of the commode) is usually used. The basin and the bag are filled with fresh warm water. The client sits with the buttocks and perineal area in the basin for approximately 10 to 20 minutes while the water from the bag is allowed to circulate through the basin. This process is usually repeated three to four times a day. The use and frequency of use of the sitz bath is ordered by the physician.

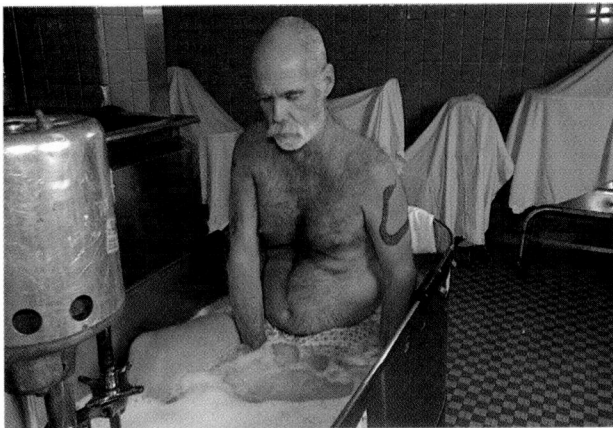

❧ **Figure 24–4**
The warm, moist heat of a whirlpool bath may be used to relieve pain, increase range of motion, stimulate circulation, or débride wounds or burns.

Dry Heat

Dry heat can be applied through conduction (aquathermia pad, electric heating pad, or hot water bottle) or radiation (heat lamp or heat cradle). The method of heat application would depend on the part of the body involved, the presence of open lesions, and the physical condition of the client.

Electric Heating Pad

An electric heating pad can be relatively safe if used correctly. The area on which the electric pad is used should be assessed frequently to avoid overheating the tissue. The electric heating pad should always be set on a low setting. It should never be placed under the client but should be laid lightly against or on top of the involved area. Burns to the skin can occur when the client lies on the pad (Lindsey, 1990). Bed linens should never be wet or damp when the electric pad is in use because of the risk of electrical shock. The possibility of equipment malfunction by the electric heating pad should always be considered; therefore, the pad should be periodically checked for proper electrical function.

Hot Water Bottle

The hot water bottle is still occasionally used, but its use has decreased. The risks with a hot water bottle include leakage of the hot water and burns from too high a temperature or improper placement of the bottle under a body part. The hot water bottle should always be covered with a pillowcase or towel to prevent direct contact with skin surfaces. It should lie against or on top of the involved area. Frequent assessment of the involved site should be done to prevent increased tissue damage from excessive heat.

Aquathermia Pad

The aquathermia pad is used to supply heat to a localized area. This pad is a rubber or plastic pad connected to a heating unit, which supplies it with warmed water in the 43.3 to 46°C (110–115°F) range. The water circulates through rubber hoses in the pad. The plastic pad must be covered with a pillowcase or towel to prevent direct contact with the skin. Nursing assessment would be the same as with an electric heating pad.

Disposable Chemically Activated Hot Pack

Use of disposable chemically activated hot packs has replaced electric heating pads and hot water bottles when short-term use is desired. The heat pack is chemically activated by twisting the pad. This breaks an internal container that holds chemicals that produce heat when mixed. The limitations of the pad are the short length of heat production and the need to replace it once it cools.

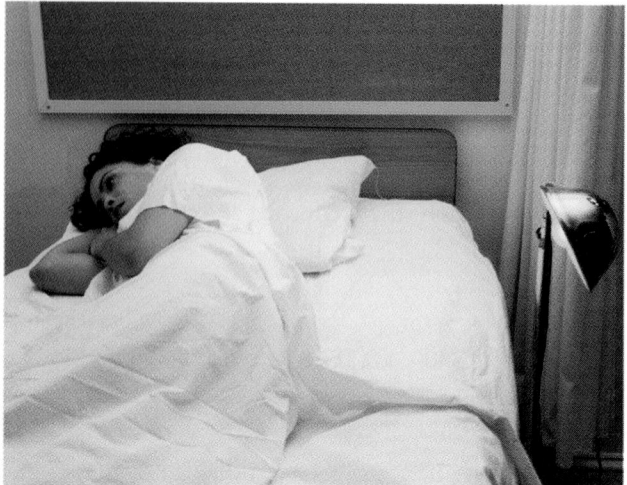

✦ **Figure 24–5**
A heat lamp is used to apply heat to a localized area. Note that the lamp should be placed no closer than 24 to 30 in, depending on the wattage of the bulb.

Heat Lamp and Cradles

A heat lamp consists of a small adjustable lamp with a 40- to 75-watt infrared or regular household bulb (Fig. 24–5). The lamp is used to apply heat to small localized areas; for example, a decubitus. The lamp should be placed no closer than 24 in (with a 40-watt–60-watt bulb) or 30 in (with a 75-watt bulb) from the involved area (Perry & Potter, 1986). It is usually left in place for approximately 20 minutes, with frequent assessment of the involved area during this period.

The heat cradle provides heat to a broader area than a heat lamp. A heat cradle consists of a half-circle frame that fits over the bed and lifts the bed linens up off the involved area. The heat cradle has a 25-watt bulb attached to it, which releases heat down over the exposed area. It is generally safer than a heat lamp since the wattage is lower and is less likely to cause tissue damage.

Implementation of Cold Therapy

Therapeutic cold is best used in the first 24 to 72 hours after acute tissue injury (Halvorson, 1990). Cold therapy may be applied in the form of an ice pack, disposable cold packs, cold compresses, or a cool sponge bath.

Ice Packs

An ice pack, which is similar to a hot water bottle, is filled with small chunks of ice. If it is placed directly against the skin or left in place for an extended amount of time, it carries a risk of tissue damage similar to that of the hot water bottle.

An ice pack may consist of a commercially prepared ice bag, an ice collar, a plastic bag filled with ice, or a disposable glove filled with ice. It should never be placed directly against the skin but should be covered with a pillowcase or towel. To prevent tissue damage from excessive cold exposure, the ice pack should be removed in most cases after 30 minutes and after a short time may be reapplied.

Disposable Cold Packs

Disposable cold packs are frequently used in the clinical setting (Fig. 24–6). These are commercially produced cold packs that contain a nontoxic frozen solution. The advantage of these packs is their ability to bend or fold over the involved part. The cold gel inside makes the bag very pliable. These nonreuseable bags are kept frozen until needed.

Disposable chemically activated cold packs are also available. These do not require refrigeration and are activated by twisting the bag to activate the chemicals inside.

Cold Compresses

A cold compress may consist of a cold wash cloth or surgical gauze saturated with cold water. The most frequent uses of cold compresses are for eye injuries, following mouth surgery or tooth extraction, or for postpartum edema and hemorrhoids.

A cold compress should be saturated in ice-cold water. It is important to remove excess water from the compress to prevent dripping. The compress is left in place at the involved site for 15 to 20 minutes and may be replaced several times during the day, per physician's order.

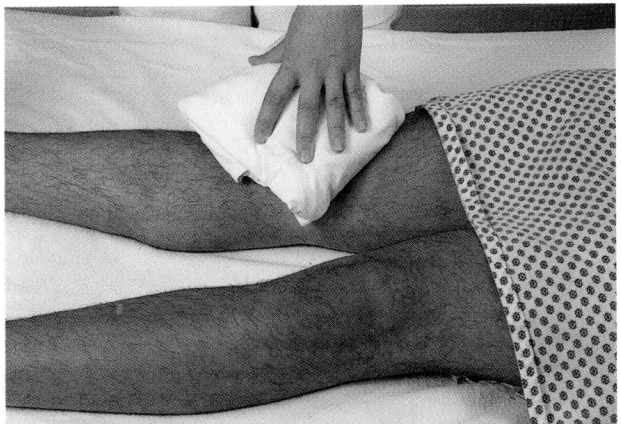

♦ **Figure 24–6**
A folded, disposable cold pack applied to a client's leg. Cold therapy is most useful in the first 24 to 72 hours after acute tissue injury.

Cool Sponge Bath

Cool sponge baths are used to cool the hyperthermic client. The cause of the hyperthermia may be fever or overheating, such as heat stroke. The purpose of the cool sponge bath is to lower the body temperature.

The sponge bath is started by placing ice packs at the armpit, groin, and throat areas, where major blood vessels come in close contact with the skin.

The client should be draped, and skin areas not being bathed should remain covered to prevent excessive shivering. The skin of the extremities, face, and neck is then bathed with water that is initially 29 to 35°C (85–95°F). Alcohol is frequently added to the water to facilitate evaporation for rapid cooling of the skin. Bathing should continue for approximately 30 minutes to ensure benefit from the cooling process. Vital signs should be monitored during the bathing process.

Application of the Nursing Process to the Pyrexic Client

The provision of care to the client with pyrexia requires a full understanding of the disorder. **Pyrexia,** a body temperature above the normal range, may be caused by bacterial infections, dehydration, brain abnormalities, toxins, or brain tumors. Two types of pyrexia most commonly seen in the health care system are hyperthermia and fever. Hyperthermia occurs when there is damage to the hypothalamus. It is frequently a critical condition in which dysfunction of the thermoregulatory system increases the body temperature but fails to activate compensatory cooling mechanisms (Osguthorp 1993). This might be seen in a client with a basal brain injury or a cerebral infarction (stroke).

Fever occurs when the body temperature is above the client's normal body temperature range. Fever most frequently is caused by the action of exogenous and endogenous **pyrogens.** The exogenous pyrogens include bacteria and their endotoxins, protozoa, spirochetes, viruses, yeast, and progestational hormones and drugs. Endogenous pyrogens are produced by the cell interacting with the exogenous pyrogens (Wilson *et al.,* 1991). The pyrogens affect the thermostatic set point of the hypothalamus, causing the normal set point (37°C, 98.6°F) in the hypothalamus to be moved to a higher setting. For example, a client with an infection may have a thermostat set point of 38.8°C (102°F). The body in this febrile state recognizes that it is cooler than the set point and goes into action to increase body heat. This results in vasoconstriction and shivering, which increases muscle work. The client may add an additional blanket or clothing because he or she feels cool. Once this new thermostatic set point is reached, the normal heat-dissipating mechanisms will resume, and the temperature will remain at this elevated level. When the temperature goes higher than the set point or when the pyrogen is no longer present, a temperature crisis will occur. What actually happens is that the thermostatic set point has been moved back down to a lower setting. The body suddenly recognizes its overheated state, and heat-dissipating mechanisms go into action. These include intense sweating and sudden development of hot skin (flushing) caused by vasodilation. The client may respond to this crisis by feeling "very hot" and removing additional clothing or bed coverings. Before the use of antibiotics, doctors always awaited the crisis as an indication that the temperature would soon drop.

The main concern with a fever is the temperature of the brain. Hypothalamic temperatures higher than 42°C (107.6°F) can result in impaired thermoregulation and may cause permanent brain damage. Therefore, frequent assessment of body core temperature is important in identifying and preventing high temperatures.

Assessment

Nursing History

The nursing assessment should start with a complete nursing history to identify preexisting factors, the onset of pyrexia, and accompanying symptoms. An accurate record of temperature onset and duration is important. Recording activity and environmental exposure is also necessary to identify types of heat disorders (Box 24–3).

Several types of fever patterns are experienced by clients. A constant fever or sustained fever is one in which the temperature remains elevated, with variations of no more than 1 to 2°C throughout the day. Low-grade constant fever is often seen in a client having a malignant disease. An intermittent fever rises, then drops to normal, and then elevates again during a 24-hour period. A remittent fever, which rises and falls throughout the day but never drops to a normal level, is seen with tuberculosis and influenza. A re-

---

Box **24–3**

HEAT SYNDROMES

High environmental temperatures frequently result in heat overload. Four syndromes that are caused by high environmental temperatures are heat cramps, heat exhaustion, heat stroke, and exertional heat injury. Heat syndromes most frequently occur at elevated ambient temperatures (>32°C or >90°F) and at high relative humidities (>60%). These syndromes occur more frequently in the elderly population, particularly those who are mentally impaired or alcohol abusers or those who receive antipsychotic drugs, diuretics, and anticholinergics (Wilson *et al.,* 1991). Poorly ventilated homes without air conditioning compound the problem. An increase of heat syndromes is seen during the first few days of a heat wave. The best prevention of a heat syndrome is increased hydration, light clothing, frequent cool baths, decreased activity, and resting in a cool place.

Heat Cramps

Heat cramps are a fairly mild complication of heat exposure. This syndrome results in muscular cramping after strenuous exercise. The muscle cramps may be extremely painful but usually only last a short time. The body temperature remains at a normal level. Treatment involves resting in a cool place and replacement of sodium, potassium, and fluid.

Heat Exhaustion

Heat exhaustion is the most common of the heat syndromes. It is often call heat prostration or heat collapse. The onset is fairly rapid, and the duration is relatively brief. The client experiences weakness, fatigue, dizziness, anxiety, thirst, headache, and often nausea and vomiting. The skin is cool and clammy, the eyes dilated, and the pulse rapid. The care required for this client is a cool

environment, increased hydration, and resting in a recumbent position. Recovery is fairly rapid.

Heat Stroke

Heat stroke occurs most frequently with the elderly and is epidemic during heat waves. In classic case of heat stroke, the client is pyrexic, often with a core temperature as high as 40.7°C (106°F), but does not sweat. The client may complain of a headache, dizziness, faintness, abdominal discomfort, and hyperpnea. He or she may experience confusion, delirium, or loss of consciousness. Heat stroke is a critical situation that requires immediate care. The most common treatment is rapid cooling by placing the client in a tub of iced water or sponging the client with cold water. Other emergency procedures are often needed for this critically ill client.

Exertional Heat Injury

This syndrome is seen frequently with runners who enter races without adequate acclimatization or with poor hydration. Risk factors for this syndrome include age; obesity; hypertension; and use of anticholinergics, antihistamines, beta-blockers, diuretics, sedatives, tranquilizers, and vasodilators. This client will experience sweating and an elevated temperature, but the temperature will only be in the 38.5 to 39.6°C (102–104°F) range. Headache, chills, hyperventilation, nausea and vomiting, muscle cramps, weakness, an unsteady gait, and loss of consciousness may occur. The treatment is rapid cooling by sponging the client with cool water or a cool shower. Muscle massage increases blood flow and increases cooling of body core temperature. The client should remain in the hospital for observation (Wilson *et al.,* 1991).

lapsing fever occurs with the malaria client and is characterized by prolonged periods of fever followed by periods of several weeks or months without fever and then recurring bouts of fever (Osguthorpe, 1993).

Physical Assessment

When assessing the pyrexic client, frequent monitoring of the body temperature and its alterations is important. The temperature should be assessed using the same site, method, and times during the day to avoid recording fluctuations in the temperature that do not relate to the disease process.

The nurse should assess the client not only for an alteration in the temperature range but also for other clinical signs of pyrexia. The vital signs should reflect an increased pulse and respiratory rate, caused by sympathetic nervous system stimulation. An accentuated cardiac S_1 often occurs in the hyperkinetic state experienced with hyperthermia. At the onset of hyperthermia, a client's skin may actually feel cold, and nails may appear cyanotic. This may be caused by the vasoconstriction that occurs with the onset of fever. A "gooseflesh" appearance of the skin and shivering may also be evident as the body increases muscular activity for heat production. The client may complain of feeling cold. As increased heat production occurs, the skin becomes warm or hot to touch, and shivering ceases. The temperature should be monitored frequently throughout the 24-hour period. Malaise, generalized discomfort, and fatigue accompanied by a headache frequently occur with the temperature elevation. The level of consciousness should be monitored with extreme hyperthermia. Simple drowsiness and restlessness may progress to delirium and convulsions due to nerve cell irritation. This is frequently seen in small children and the elderly when they experience high temperatures. The client may also experience photophobia.

The hyperthermic client may have anorexia and may have to be encouraged to adequately meet nutrient and fluid needs. Monitoring fluid intake and output is also important because of the potential for dehydration from excessive sweating. A decreased urine output or urine that is more concentrated in appearance is common if adequate fluid replacement is not made. Careful assessment of the elderly client experiencing hyperthermia is important—particularly those with cardiac or cerebrovascular disease—because these conditions may limit the client's ability to sense or dissipate heat.

Diagnostic Tests

Diagnostic tests ordered for the pyrexic client often depend on the nature of the physical disorder that he or she is experiencing. The most common diagnostic test done is the complete blood count. This gives an overall picture of the response to hyperthermia. The white blood cell count elevates as a normal re-

sponse to infection. A rapid erythrocyte sedimentation rate reflects the response to tissue injury. If an infection is obvious, for example, the wound should be drained and then a culture and sensitivity test should be done prior to antibiotic therapy. This would identify the specific organism causing the infection and its resistance to antibiotics. An elevated hematocrit level would indicate the presence of dehydration due to loss of fluids through excessive sweating. The sodium and potassium levels may be decreased because of excess loss, which also occurs with sweating. Arterial blood gases may be drawn to monitor oxygen, carbon dioxide, and pH levels because of the increased oxygen utilization and the risk of acid-base disbalance that occur with hyperthermia.

Other diagnostic tests are performed, depending on the cause of the hyperthermia. For example, the client with a respiratory infection or pneumonia would have chest x-rays and pulmonary function studies done. The choice for diagnostic testing would also reflect the epidemiological setting. The college student's hyperthermia may result from mononucleosis or some viral infection, whereas the client from Asia or Africa may have malaria, and the appropriate testing for these diseases should be performed.

Nursing Diagnosis

The appropriate nursing diagnosis for the client with pyrexia would be related to the reason for the elevated temperature. The diagnosis would be Risk for Altered Body Temperature if the client has not been experiencing a temperature elevation but has a medical or surgical reason that would increase his or her chances of developing an elevated temperature. The client who is already experiencing a temperature elevation would have a nursing diagnosis of Hyperthermia. For a client who has bacterial pneumonia, the nursing diagnosis would be Hyperthermia related to Bacterial Infection of the Lungs as evidenced by Temperature Elevation (see Nursing Diagnosis box).

Planning

In planning the care of the pyrexic client, the projected outcome would be the return of the temperature to a normal range. The outcomes would vary with the cause of the temperature elevation. (See Sample Nursing Care Plan: The Client With Pyrexia.)

Implementation

The nursing care of the pyrexic client is directed toward providing comfort, preventing complications, and supporting the body's physiological response to fever. This may include providing the client with extra blankets during the onset of a fever or giving a tepid sponge bath during the height or crisis of a fever. Replacing wet bed clothes and sheets is necessary when profuse sweating occurs. By monitoring fluid intake and output and maintaining adequate hydration, the nurse can prevent possible dehydration. Providing for adequate oral hygiene is also necessary with the pyrexic client, because increased respiration and dehydration often result in dry mucosal membranes. Should the fever last several days, it would be important for the nurse to monitor the white blood cell count and hematocrit.

Nursing implementations should include the administration of **antipyretics,** drugs that reduce fever, as ordered by the physician. These drugs act by lowering the thermostatic set point of the pyrexic client but do not affect normal body temperature. Examples of these drugs are aspirin, acetaminophen, and ibuprofen. These drugs also offer relief some for the discomforts associated with fever. Antipyretics are frequently ordered to be given every 3 to 4 hours and should be accompanied by liberal amounts of fluids.

For the client with a bacterial infection, antibiotic drug therapy would also be expected.

Care of the client in the community setting should be directed toward the prevention of the hyperthermia (see box).

Evaluation

When evaluating the hyperthermic client and whether the temperature has returned to normal, other factors should be considered. With the hyperthermic client, it would be necessary to determine if the return of the temperature to the normal range is a long-term change or the result of diurnal effects. For example, the client's temperature may be 37.1°C (99°F) at 4:00 A.M., when diurnal effects naturally lower body temperature, but at noon and at 4:00 P.M., the client's temperature may be 39.4°C (103°F).

Continuous reevaluation for temperature stability

NURSING DIAGNOSES USED WITH IMBALANCES IN TEMPERATURE REGULATION

Ineffective Thermoregulation
Related to

Disease or injury
Age (newborn infant or elderly)

Examples

Physical trauma to the hypothalamus
Thyroid dysfunction
Newborn with immature thermoregulation function
Emaciated elderly

Hypothermia
Related to

Extended exposure to cold
Inadequate home heating or clothing
Poor physical condition caused by debilitating illness

Examples

Accidentally trapped in cold environment (immersion in cold water, automobile accident)
Homeless, elderly person in an unheated house, hiker poorly dressed for cold weather
Client with tuberculosis

Hyperthermia
Related to

Overexposure to hot, humid climate
Dehydration or poor fluid intake in relationship to heat exposure
Illness or disease

Examples

Homeless, elderly person in home without adequate cooling
Tennis player or marathon runner in excessive humidity
Patient with pneumonia, influenza, Rocky Mountain spotted fever

Potential Altered Body Temperature
Related to

Disease, trauma, or surgery altering thermoregulation
Drugs or medications that cause sedation, decreased muscle activity, or blood vessel changes (dilation or constriction)

Examples

Postoperative client exposed to cold surgical room environment
Anesthesia resulting in decreased muscle activity
Antihypertensive drugs and exposure to excessive heat
Antipsychotic drugs, which also decrease sweat production

SAMPLE NURSING CARE PLAN

THE CLIENT WITH PYREXIA

A 56-year-old female client is admitted to your clinical care center with a diagnosis of an acute respiratory infection. She appears very flushed and is complaining of being hot. She states that she has had chills and fever for the past 4 days.

Nursing Diagnosis: Hyperthermia related to an upper respiratory infection

Expected Outcome: Client's body temperature will return to the 36.3 to 36.9°C (98–99°F) range following treatment

Action	Rationale
1. Assess the client's vital signs. Take the temperature either by the oral or tympanic method.	1. Cardiac and respiratory functions increase with hyperthermia, as the body tries to remove excess heat by conduction, radiation, and convection.
2. Assess the skin for color, temperature, gooseflesh appearance, and sweating.	2. The presence of gooseflesh or piloerection is evidence that the body is trying to produce heat and would be present during a chill. The presence of sweating would indicate that the body was attempting to cool down.
3. Monitor laboratory values (white blood cell count, sedimentation rate, hematocrit, and urinalysis).	3. An elevated white blood cell and sedimentation rate would be suggestive of an infectious process, whereas an elevated hematocrit level would suggest dehydration. A temperature elevation occurs with most urinary tract infections.
4. Keep client comfortable. Cover lightly with blankets when cold, and remove blankets when hot. Replace wet linens if client is sweating.	4. When excessive chilling occurs, increased amounts of body energy are needed to supply warmth. Applying a blanket will decrease the amount of heat needed. When the client is sweating, excessive blankets will only slow the cooling process.
5. Encourage rest and energy conservation.	5. Heat production by shivering, piloerection, and increased metabolic rate utilizes a great deal of the body's energy.
6. Encourage fluid and nutrient intake.	6. Dehydration frequently occurs due to excessive fluid loss with sweating. Additional nutrient needs are present due to increased metabolic rate.
7. Administer antipyretics as ordered by physician.	7. Antipyretics assist the hypothalamus in resetting the thermostat and lower the temperature experienced with fever.
8. Administer an antibiotic as ordered by the physician.	8. Antibiotics treat the infectious disorder, which is the cause of the hyperthermia.
9. Give the client a sponge bath using tepid or cool water if the temperature elevates above 38.5°C (102°F).	9. A cool sponge bath increases the conduction of heat from the hyperthermic client and speeds the cooling process. Convection by air movement over the damp skin also removes heat.
10. Evaluate client's response to therapy. Reassess temperature using same sites.	10. Continued evaluation of the client's response to antipyretics, antibiotics, comfort techniques, and their temperature range is necessary to determine the client's response to therapy.
11. Document care given.	11. A continuous documentation of the temperature is necessary to determine if the client has an intermittent, continuous, or remitting fever. Documentation of temperature site is also important because of variation of temperatures depending on the site at which it is taken. Documentation of treatment and care given is also important in reevaluating the client's response during the disease process.

HEALTH PROMOTION AND PREVENTION

PREVENTION OF HYPERTHERMIA

• Participants in hot weather sports events should be adequately acclimatized. At least a 5- to 6-week training period with a slow increase of activity should be followed.

• Sports activity should be avoided during the hottest part of the day.

• Increased fluid intake is essential before and during strenuous activity. Thirst is not a reliable indicator of body need. Long-distance runners should drink 100 to 200 ml for every 2 to 3 km.

• Alcoholic beverages should be avoided in high temperatures because they cause dehydration. Sugary beverages should also be omitted, as they decrease gastric emptying.

• Children and pets should never be left in closed automobiles on hot days, as the temperature within the vehicle will soar rapidly, inducing hyperthermia within a few minutes.

• Elderly adults are prone to develop hyperthermia due to non–air conditioned homes. The gradual heat increase in the home is not recognized by the elderly person as life threatening.

Data from Jacobson, S. (1992). The ill effects of heat. *Emergency Medicine. 24*(7), 313–314, 317–316, 321–324.

is necessary for revision of the plan of care. For example, the client whose temperature spikes to 40°C (104.6°F) is going to require an immediate change in action, as compared to a client experiencing a temperature of 37.4°C (100°F).

Nursing Care of the Hypothermic Client

Hypothermia means a body temperature lowered to 35°C (95°F) or lower (Wilson *et al.,* 1991). It most commonly occurs as a result of an overexposure to cold environmental temperatures. However, physical problems, disease, and some medications also may alter the regulatory ability of the hypothalamus to maintain a normal body temperature. The care of the hypothermic client requires an understanding of the body's reaction to cold, as well as the different types of cold disorders.

A body temperature of 37°C (98.6°F) results in the activation of heat-conserving mechanisms. These include intense vasoconstriction, piloerection, abolition of sweating, and increased body heat production. The

posterior hypothalamus activates the sympathetic nervous system, and signals are sent to the superficial blood vessels in the skin, causing constriction. Therefore, decreased amounts of blood will be exposed to the cold temperature, and a warmer core temperature will be maintained.

Piloerection simply means that the hairs stand on end, which does not do a great deal to increase the human core temperature. However, in animals, piloerection increases the thickness of the fur and results in an increased amount of insulating air being trapped in the fur.

The abolition of sweating occurs once the body temperature starts to drop below the 37°C (98.6°F) normal temperature. This results in decreased evaporative cooling of the body and therefore conserves body heat.

Increased heat production occurs in the following three ways. The posterior hypothalamus activates the motor center for shivering. Sympathetic stimulation also results in an increased amount of epinephrine in the blood, which increases cellular metabolism and, therefore, heat production. The third occurrence is the release of increased amounts of thyroxin.

Hypothermia may be categorized by type. The types include accidental hypothermia, inadvertent hypothermia, and intentional hypothermia (Table 24–2).

Accidental hypothermia is classified as a body temperature of 35°C (95°F) that occurs from exposure to cold. The causes of accidental hypothermia may be exposure to snow, wind, or rain during participation in winter sports or in poorly clothed children or the elderly exposed to a cold environment. The drowning victim may be exposed to cold water temperatures. The homeless and those who lack heat in their homes are at risk for hypothermia. The alcoholic is at risk because of vasodilation and increased heat loss, along with impaired judgment.

Inadvertent hypothermia may occur when surgical clients are exposed to a cold operating room environ-

Table 24–2	
TYPES OF HYPOTHERMIA	
TYPE	**CAUSE**
Accidental hypothermia	Cold water drowning, extended exposure to cold weather without adequate clothing
Inadvertent hypothermia	Exposure to cool surgical room temperature and medications that alter body temperature–regulating mechanism
Intentional hypothermia	Purposeful cooling of the body temperature for cardiac and transplant surgical procedures

ment. This is an unintentional hypothermia that must be anticipated with surgical clients. It occurs for several reasons: The temperature of most operating rooms is set between 15.5 and 16.6°C (60 and 64°F), because low humidity and low temperatures are thought to decrease bacterial growth (Summers, 1992). Furthermore, surgical clients are frequently medicated with drugs that inadvertently affect the body temperature by decreasing the hypothalamic regulation mechanisms or increasing vasodilation.

Intentional hypothermia is the purposeful cooling of a client's body core temperature for surgical reasons, such as for cardiac bypass grafts and heart transplants. The body temperature is decreased to 26 to 32°C (80–90°F) during the surgical process (Summers, 1992).

Assessment

Nursing History

An accurate and complete nursing history is necessary to determine the type of heat loss that has occurred. The cause, the type of exposure, the length of time exposed to low temperatures, and socioeconomic factors all help identify possible problems that may be experienced with hypothermia. For example, an elderly lady admitted with a temperature of 35°C (95°F) may be experiencing gradual hypothermia due to a lack of heat in her home.

Hypothermia may be categorized by the rate at which it occurs. Nursing care must be individualized to the type and extent of hypothermia present.

1. Acute heat loss most frequently refers to heat loss that has occurred by conduction through immersion in water. In acute heat loss, the body temperature drops from normal to a hypothermic level within 1 hour.
2. Subacute heat loss occurs over several hours, most frequently as a result of conduction, convection, radiation, and evaporation. A good example would be the hiker who has dressed lightly and is exposed to lower environmental temperatures than expected.
3. Gradual hypothermia occurs over several days or weeks and is most frequently seen in the elderly (Summers, 1992).

Physical Assessment

The assessment of a client who is experiencing hypothermia will have findings that differ depending on the degree of hypothermia experienced. If the client is only mildly hypothermic, which is most frequently seen in the postoperative client, body temperature would be in the range of 32 to 35°C (90–95°F). Symptoms of mild hypothermia would include shivering, cool skin, piloerection, slow capillary refill, and altered nail bed color. There is usually a loss of dexterity. Tachycardia and hypertension may also be noted.

In newborn infants, the assessment would also include oxygen saturation. This is important because newborn infants do not shiver when temperatures

drop but generate additional heat by burning brown fat, which is stored around abdominal organs. This heat generation requires an increased use of oxygen so infants with mild hypothermia may become hypoxic as well (Walhout, 1992).

Moderate hypothermia occurs when the body core temperature has dropped to 30 to 32°C (86–90°F). Shivering is usually not present because of impaired hypothalamic function. The client is confused and often stuporous. Other symptoms include decreased recognition, decreased respiratory rate, and decreased cardiac rate and output.

Severe hypothermia occurs when the body core temperature drops below 30°C (86°F). The client may be unconscious and in fact may appear dead. The client's pupils are dilated and often do not react to light. The functioning of the vital organs will be greatly impaired, and respiration may decrease or completely cease. Cardiac function is depressed to the point that the client is extremely hypotensive, or the client may experience a complete cardiac arrest.

Nursing Diagnosis

The nursing diagnosis of Hypothermia is used for the client who has a body temperature below 35.6°C (96°F) in an adult or 36.4°C (97.5°F) in infants. The surgical client who has a normal temperature preoperatively would have a nursing diagnosis of Risk for Ineffective Thermoregulation. The newborn with a subnormal temperature would have the diagnosis of Ineffective Thermoregulation (see Nursing Diagnoses box, p. 628).

Planning

In planning the care of the hypothermic client, the major objective or outcome would be the return of the body temperature to a normal range. However, the severity of the hypothermic condition would affect the overall care of the client. If the client were severely hypothermic and had no cardiac or respiratory function, then the outcomes would also include the return of cardiac and respiratory function. (See Sample Nursing Care Plan: The Client with Hypothermia.)

Implementation

The primary intervention in the care of the hypothermic client is to increase body core temperature. When caring for the immediately postoperative client, as seen in a recovery setting, warmed blankets are placed over the client immediately. These may be replaced several times with additional warmed blankets. This facilitates the client's rewarming process. A warmed towel may also be placed around the head to increase body temperature. These warming methods are referred to as passive rewarming and work rather slowly. Temperature probes (an electronic temperature monitoring device) that were attached in the operating room may be left in place through the recovery pro-

SAMPLE NURSING CARE PLAN

THE CLIENT WITH HYPOTHERMIA

A 20-year-old man is admitted to the emergency department following an automobile accident in which he lost control of his car and went down a deep embankment. He was trapped in his car for several hours and was exposed to temperatures in the 30 to 40°F range. He will respond to pain and forced arousal but is very lethargic. His respiration rate is very slow, and he has a very slow, weak pulse.

Nursing Diagnosis: Hypothermia related to extended exposure to cold temperatures

Expected Outcome: Client's body temperature will return to the 98 to 99°F range following emergency treatment

Action	Rationale
1. Assess the client's vital signs. Monitor temperature with a rectal probe.	1. Obtain a baseline assessment. Implementations of care will differ with severity of hypothermia.
2. Assess the client's level of consciousness, response to commands, and alertness.	2. The level of consciousness determines the severity of the hypothermia. The mental state also affects the type of care chosen.
3. Assess the client's skin for color, capillary refill, piloerection, and response to stimuli.	3. The presence of shivering and piloerection occurs with mild to moderate hypothermia but is absent in severe cases. These symptoms indicate proper functioning of the hypothalamus in trying to reheat the body.
4. Assess the client for neurological impairment.	4. Continued poor response to stimuli would suggest neurological damage, either of the involved body part or of the central nervous system.
5. Warm the client with electric or rewarming blankets or hot water bottles or by immersion if the client is responsive and alert.	5. External or passive rewarming is used with mild to moderate hypothermia to aid the body's effort to reheat itself to a normal core temperature.
6. Administer warmed intravenous fluids.	6. Warm intravenous fluids increase the blood temperature and aid in rewarming.
7. Massage extremities to aid in rewarming.	7. Massage increases circulation and muscle tone, therefore increasing the return of warmth to the extremity.
8. Encourage client to move extremities.	8. Movement of extremities increases muscle tone and circulation.
9. Evaluate client's response to rewarming. Inspect extremities for tissue damage.	9. Only after rewarming does frostbite and tissue damage become apparent.
10. Document care given on the client's record.	10. Documentation is important for legal reasons and for follow-up care.

cess to further monitor the body core temperature and its return to normal.

In the moderately hypothermic client, maintaining an airway and increasing oxygenation if bradypnea is occurring is important. The oxygen administered should be warmed to aid rewarming of the client. External rewarming devices such as electric or rewarming blankets, which work by heating the surface of the body, would most likely be necessary. Placing the client in a warm bath or Hubbard tank at 40 to 42°C (104–108°F) would be beneficial. Caution should be taken in case the client should develop an arrhythmia, because time would be lost getting the client out of the tub and dried prior to starting cardiopulmonary resuscitation. The client's electrolytes should be moni-

tored, and, if necessary, blood volume should be expanded with warmed glucose and saline. In the severely hypothermic client, rewarming may necessitate the use of extracorporeal circulation, in which the blood is removed from the body and warmed by an external device.

In the intentional hypothermic client, rewarming is frequently accomplished through reoxygenation and rewarming of the blood through a cardiac bypass machine. Because a cardiac bypass machine is used with the cardiac bypass client and the cardiac transplant client during surgery, it is the easiest tool to use for rewarming. The severely hypothermic client may be rewarmed in surgery by attaching the femoral vessels to the cardiac bypass machine (Walhout, 1992).

Box 24-4

COLD INJURIES

The term *frostnip* refers to cold injury of earlobes, nose, cheeks, fingers, toes, hands, and feet. Frostnip is reversible damage characterized by blanching of the skin and numbness. It can be reversed simply by re-warming the extremity. *Frostbite* is a cold injury that results in damage to tissue and blood vessels. This injury may be severe and sometimes irreparable. Warming of the involved limb should occur once the core temperature of the patient is returned to normal. The warming process starts slowly with the immersion of the limb in water at 10 to 15°C (50–59°F) and is increased by 5° (9°F) every 5 minutes until a maximum temperature of 40°C (104°F) is reached. Once the limb is warmed, therapy usually includes bed rest, elevation of the limb, antibiotic therapy, tetanus toxoid, and daily washes with chorhexidine or an iodophor and physiotherapy.

Data from Wilson, J. *et al.* (Eds.). (1991). *Harrison's principles of internal medicine* (11th ed.; p. 2199). New York: McGraw-Hill.

Evaluation

The evaluation of the hypothermic client's response to care is important when revising the plan of care. For example, the temperature of the client who is severely hypothermic may have returned to the normal range, but he or she may still be maintained on life support because of neurologic damage. In another client, the body core temperature may be normal but the client has frostbite in the fingers and toes (Box 24–4). An ongoing reevaluation of the applicability of outcomes or needed revisions is important in providing care.

Summary

Thermoregulation remains a complex process affected by both external and internal factors that require immediate physiological responses from the hypothalamus. An alternation of this regulatory balance is evidenced by either hypothermia or hyperthermia. The state of hypothermia or hyperthermia may be resolved normally by the human body or may remain unresolved and require medical intervention.

The nurse plays a major role in the medical care of clients who experience a disbalance in thermoregulation through assessment, nursing diagnosis, intervention, and evaluation.

CHAPTER HIGHLIGHTS

♦

♦ Body temperature is controlled by the hypothalamus, with the average body core temperature set at 37°C (98.6°F).

♦ Basal metabolism is affected by exercise, thyroid hormone, sympathetic nervous system, and muscular activity. The basal metabolism level directly affects heat production.

♦ Heat production is produced by the metabolism of food and the expenditure of energy, whereas heat loss occurs by radiation, conduction, convection, and evaporation.

♦ Thermoregulation is affected by body size, age, exercise, hormones, environment, stress, diurnal effects, and behavioral control.

♦ Pyrexia, an increased body temperature, is a common symptom of disease. It is most frequently referred to as fever and is most commonly caused by pyrogens. Pyrexia may also result from damage to or dysfunction of the hypothalamus.

♦ Fever may occur in several patterns. These include constant, intermittent, remittent, and relapsing.

♦ Hypothermia is a decrease in body temperature, most frequently caused by overexposure to a cold environment. It may also be caused by disease, dysfunction of the hypothalamus, or medications.

♦ The nursing diagnoses for problems with thermoregulation may include Ineffective Thermoregulation, Hypothermia, Hyperthermia, and Risk for Altered Body Temperature.

♦ Assessment of the pyrexic client includes complete history, vital signs, skin color and temperature, sweat production, and neurological functioning. Symptoms related to a possible infection should be noted.

♦ Care planning and implementation for hyperthermia should be directed at cooling the body core temperature as well as treating the disorder that caused the temperature alteration.

♦ Assessment of the hypothermic client should include complete history, vital signs, skin color, presence of piloerection or shivering, capillary refill, and neurological functioning.

♦ Care planning and implementation for the hypothermic client should be directed at maintenance of cardiopulmonary function as well as body core temperature rewarming.

♦ The body temperature may be measured using the mercury-in-glass. electronic, or tympanic thermometer.

✦ Body temperature is most commonly measured at the axillary, oral, rectal, or tympanic sites, but it is also possible to measure the pulmonary artery and bladder temperature using special devices.

✦ Therapeutic heat may be used to treat pain, discomfort, soft tissue damage, impaired mobility, and decreased circulation. Moist heat includes the use of whirlpools, sitz baths, and heat applications. Dry heat involves the use of electric heating pads, hot water bottles, aquathermia pads, hot packs, and heat lamp and cradles.

✦ Cold therapy is frequently used to prevent swelling and inflammation with injuries and surgery. Cold therapy includes the use of ice packs, cold compresses, and cool sponge baths.

Study Questions

1. In normal everyday experiences, the regulation of body temperature to changing environmental temperatures is controlled by

   a. the density of body fat and piloerection
   b. the anterior and posterior hypothalamus
   c. the liver's utilization of fat
   d. hormone levels

2. Heat loss in the operating room where the air temperature is considerably lower than the body's temperature, would primarily result from

   a. conduction
   b. convection
   c. radiation
   d. evaporation

3. Norma Johnson, an 80-year-old client, was discovered in her unheated home during freezing weather. She is admitted for suspected moderate hypothermia. Which of the following symptoms support this?

   a. decreased respiratory and cardiac rate
   b. an unconscious state
   c. extreme shivering
   d. a body temperature of 85°F

4. When taking a rectal temperature in an infant, the thermometer should be inserted into the rectum

   a. 1.5 in
   b. 1 in
   c. 0.5 in
   d. with the bulb only placed inside the anus

5. Nancy Thomas injured her foot while riding a bike. She was seen in the emergency department and had multiple sutures for a large laceration and was also told she had a severe sprain of her ankle. She was instructed to use cold therapy during the next 24 hours. What is the reason for the use of cold?

   a. muscle spasms are relaxed with the use of cold applications
   b. blood viscosity is increased, but a decrease of cellular metabolism occurs

   c. an increase of the extensibility of collagen results
   d. increased capillary permeability occurs

Critical Thinking Exercises

1. Ms. C., age 84 years, fell on the ice while going to her mailbox. She was discovered after 2 hours of lying in the snow while it was 20°F outside. She arrived at the emergency department with a body temperature of 94°F. Discuss the implications of trying to rewarm Ms. C. physiologically and the nursing implications. She begins to shiver during the rewarming process. Discuss the physiological implications of shivering.

2. Mr. D. is in the hospital with pneumonia. You take his temperature and discover an oral temperature of 103°F. Discuss the nursing care of the patient with hyperthermia.

References

Baird, S. C., White, N. E., & Basinger, M. (1992). Can you rely on tympanic thermometers? *RN, 55*(8), 48–51.

Braunwald, E. *et al.* (Eds.). (1993). *Harrison's principles of internal medicine* (11th ed.). New York: McGraw-Hill.

Brobeck, J.R., (1991). In *Best and Taylor's basis of medical practice* (9th ed.). Baltimore: Williams & Wilkins.

Erickson, R. S., & Yount, S. T. (1991). Comparison of tympanic and oral temperatures in surgical patients. *Nursing Research, 40*(2), 90–93.

Ferrara-Love, R. (1991). A comparison of tympanic and pulmonary artery measures of core temperatures. *Journal of Post Anesthesia Nursing, 6*(3), 161–164.

Fulbrook, P. (1993). Core temperature measurement in adults. *Journal of Advanced Nursing, 18,* 1451–1460.

Giuffre, M., Heidenreich, T., Carney-Gerston, F., *et al.* (1990). The relationship between axillary and core body temperature measurements. *Applied Nursing Research. 3*(2), 52–55.

Guyton, A. (1992). *Human physiology and mechanisms of disease.* Philadelphia: W. B. Saunders.

Halvorson, G. (1990). Therapeutic heat and cold for athletic injuries. *The Physician and Sportsmedicine, 18*(5), 87–94.

Heidenreich, T., & Giuffre, M. (1990). Postoperative temperature measurement. *Nursing Research, 39*(3), 153–155.

Holtzclaw, B. J. (1993). Monitoring body temperature. *AACN Clinical Issues in Critical Care Nursing, 4*(1), 44–55.

Jacobson, S. (1992). The ill effects of heat. *Emergency Medicine, 24*(7), 313–314, 317–318, 321–324.

Lindsey, B. (1990). Cold and heat application in musculoskeletal injury. *Journal of Emergency Nursing, 16,* 54–7.

Miller, C. (1995). *Nursing care of older adults* (2nd ed.). Philadelphia: J. B. Lippincott.

Osguthorpe, S. (1993). Monitoring body temperature. *AACN Clinical Issues in Critical Care Nursing, 4*(1), 44–55.

Perry, A. G., & Potter, P. A. (1986). *Clinical nursing skills and techniques.* St. Louis: C. V. Mosby.

Summers, S. (1992). Hypothermia: One nursing diagnosis or three? *Nursing Diagnosis, 3*(1), 2–11.

Walhout, M. F. (1992). Treatment for hypothermia. *RN, 55*(4), 50–55.

West, J. B. (Ed.). (1991). In *Best and Taylor's physiological basis of medical practice.* Baltimore: Williams & Wilkins.

Wilson, J. *et al.* (Eds.). (1991). *Harrison's principles of internal medicine* (11th ed.). New York: McGraw-Hill.

Bibliography

Barhydt, S. J., & Berkowita, C. (Eds.). (1988). *Nursing and the aged.* New York: McGraw-Hill.

Berne, R., & Levy, M. (Eds.). (1993). *Physiology* (3rd ed.). St. Louis: C. V. Mosby.

Birrer, R. B. (1988). Heat stroke: Don't wait for the classic signs. *Emergency Medicine, 20*(12), 8–10, 12–13, 16.

Darowski, A., Weinberg, J. R., & Guz, A. (1991). Normal rectal, auditory canal, sublingual and axillary temperatures in elderly febrile patients in a warm environment. *Age and Aging, 20,* 113–119.

Erickson, R. S., & Yount, S. T. (1991). Comparison of tympanic and oral temperatures in surgical patients. *Nursing Research, 40*(2), 90–93.

Fuller, J., & Schaller-Avers, J. (1994). *Health assessment: A nursing approach* (2nd ed.). Philadelphia: J. B. Lippincott.

Jarvis, C. (1996). *Physical examination and health assessment* (2nd ed.). Philadelphia: W. B. Saunders.

McConnel, E. (1991). Using an aquathermia pad safely. *Nursing, 21*(12), 72.

Memmier, R. L., Cohen, B. J., & Wood, D. L. (1992). *Structure and function of the human* (5th ed.). Philadelphia: J. B. Lippincott.

Samples, J. F., Van Cott, M. L., Long, C., King, I. M., & Kersenbrock, A. (1985). Circadian rhythms: Basis for screening for fever. *Nursing Research, 34*(6), 377–379.

Suddarth, D. S. (1991). *Lippincott manual of nursing practice* (5th ed.). Philadelphia: J. B. Lippincott.

Tortora, G. J., & Grabowski, S. R. (1993). *Principles of anatomy and physiology.* New York: Harper Collins.

Walhout, M. F. (1992). Treatment for hypothermia. *RN, 55*(4), 50–55.

Unit ◆ VI

APPLICATION OF THE NURSING PROCESS TO PHYSIOLOGICAL NEEDS

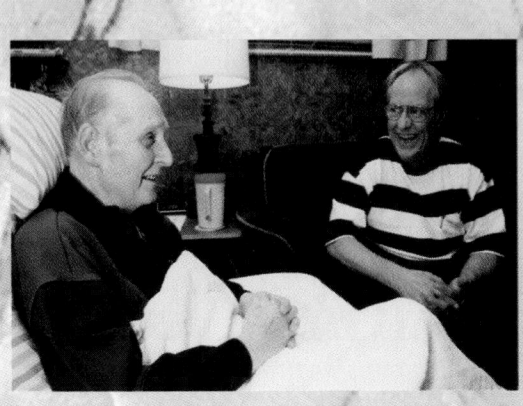

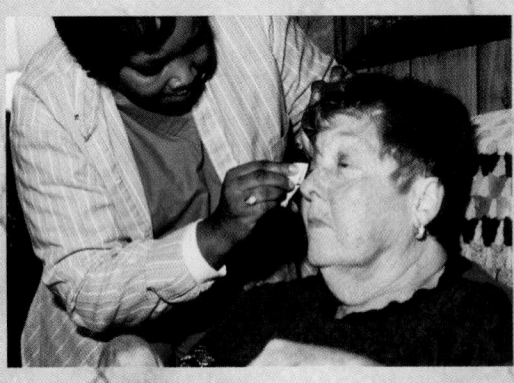

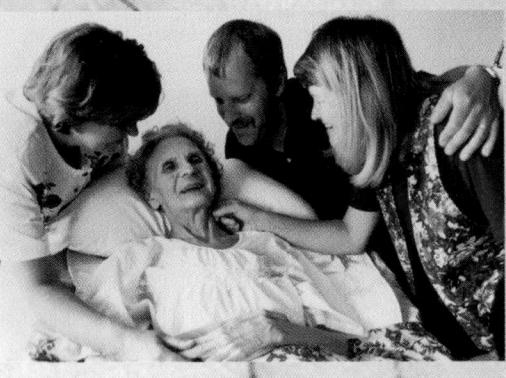

"Death and dying: Isn't it depressing to work with these every day? How do you cope?" I've answered these questions many times over my 10 years of hospice nursing: No, it isn't depressing. And I cope knowing that although I can't prevent death, I make a difference in the lives of my clients and their families. Symptom management, or addressing the client's physiological needs, is an important aspect of enhancing the client's total well-being. As clients decline, they can develop multiple symptoms such as dyspnea, nausea, constipation, agitation, insomnia, and pain, just to name a few. It is important as a nurse to listen attentively to the client's complaints and aggressively treat these symptoms, not only to provide physical comfort but also to give the client a sense of being cared for and valued and to dispel any fears of abandonment.

I can't imagine work more personally satisfying than that of a hospice nurse, which is to be part of a supportive team while practicing my nursing skills independently; to exercise and be recognized for expertise in symptom management; to prioritize client/family needs into a plan of care; to help clients and families do what they thought they couldn't do and take charge of their own care; to ease their emotional pain and enable them to spend this time at home sharing peaceful moments, reliving special memories, laughing, crying, and just being together; to be there as the client is dying and to truly experience that moment, which is just as emotionally powerful as assisting in a birth; to increase comfort and quality of life; and to help people live during the last days and moments of their lives.

This is what hospice care does. In return for my work as a hospice nurse, I receive the extraordinary gift of understanding better what it means to live each day to its fullest.

Mary Ann Coletta, RN, CRNH, Director of Nursing at Hospice of Naples, Inc., Naples, Florida

Mary Ann has been a nurse for 32 years. In 1987 she joined the new Hospice of Naples. At the time, the staff consisted of one-full time and one part-time nurse, with a case load of 10. Currently, there are 36 nurses, a six-bed residence, and an average daily case load of 100. As the program has grown, Mary Ann has moved to administrative positions but still takes calls and fills in with visits on weekends and regards this as one of the most rewarding aspects of her work. In 1996, she was named Hospice Nurses Association Certified Hospice Nurse of the year.

MOBILITY

JENNIFER M. LOEPER, RN, MS

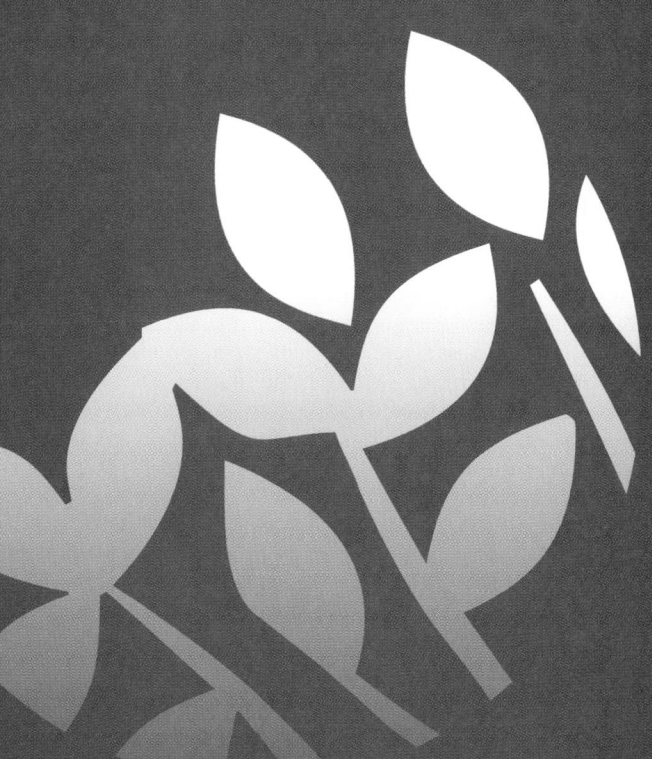

LEARNING OBJECTIVES
✦

After studying this chapter, you should be able to

✦ Describe the purpose of mobility

✦ Discuss the physiology of movement

✦ Describe the effects of immobility on the client

✦ Incorporate the client's socioeconomic factors into the plan of care

✦ Identify the key factors that must be considered when developing a plan of care

✦ Discuss the factors that put a client into a high-risk category

✦ Accurately diagnose a client with impaired mobility

✦ Incorporate turning and positioning schedules into a client's plan of care

✦ Perform range of motion and passive range of motion exercises on a client

✦ Position a client appropriately, based on the medical and nursing diagnoses

✦ Help a client with impaired mobility ambulate

✦ Discuss the client and caregiver safety needs

✦ Evaluate a client against stated outcomes and revise the plan

✦ Describe the special home care needs of a client with impaired mobility

✦ Discuss the role of the members of the health care team with the client and family

It is hard to imagine life without motion. In fact, without motion, we would not exist. Even at rest, the human body is in a state of continuous motion. Being mobile gets an individual from one place to another with relative ease. It supports our need to interact with each other; allows us to attend to our basic human needs for food, clothing, and shelter; and enables us to defend ourselves when necessary.

At some point in life, everyone has been confined to bed for a time. The first few hours or days may be therapeutic. Soon, however, restlessness and boredom begin. A child will begin to plead with his or her parents to be allowed to get up, go outside, and play, and nothing will divert the child's attention. Bed rest has accomplished the goal of healing. A decreased sense of awareness develops, and a generalized state of fatigue and weakness occurs if bed rest continues. These responses to decreased mobility have a physiological basis and in relatively healthy persons are quickly reversed once the need for bed rest is diminished. In an individual who is chronically ill, has multiple health problems, or is elderly, the negative outcomes can take weeks or months to reverse and, in fact, may not be reversible to the prior level of functioning.

Mobility is the state of movement or the facility of movement. Being mobile enables a person to interact with the environment, defines self-concept, and promotes a general sense of well-being. Challenges to the ease of mobility in a healthy individual occur at all stages of life. However, the response to mobility impairments or limitations changes as aging occurs. A cast on the leg of a 2-year-old child will evoke a much different response than one on an 80-year-old person.

A sedentary lifestyle creates and supports negative changes within the body. Research shows that movement on a routine basis improves the level of cardiovascular functioning, muscle tone, and a sense of well-being; at the same time, it decreases levels of cholesterol, excess weight, and the side effects of immobility. In the elderly, mobility, range of motion (ROM), and cognitive functioning have been shown to improve when a routine program of movement and exercise is added to the daily routine (Mobily and Kelley, 1991).

It is the nurse's responsibility as a member of the health care team to address the issues surrounding decreased or impaired mobility, to participate in the process of developing and implementing a mobility plan while the client is in the hospital, and to plan for home care following discharge.

The purpose of this chapter is to describe the importance of maintaining mobility in a client, minimizing the effects of impaired mobility on the client, and maximizing client outcomes. Mobility is incorporated into all phases of the client care plan because the effects of decreased mobility and immobility are profound and far reaching. The goals of assisting with mobility are threefold: prevention of disabilities or problems, maintenance of the present level of function, and the restoration of function to the highest degree possible. This chapter focuses on mobility, positioning, ambulation, and transferring clients. It also explores the effects of immobility on the client, the impact of injury on mobility, and the role of the nurse in minimizing these effects.

Physiology of Movement

Mobility at the microscopic or cellular level supports the transportation of the cell nutrients in the living organism. At the macroscopic level, mobility is evident in all daily activities (*e.g.*, walking, sitting, lifting). When mobility is impaired, negative consequences begin to occur within the individual. It becomes extremely important to minimize these problems and begin addressing mobility as early as possible. Maintaining the current level of functioning not only preserves the self-esteem of the individual but also reduces the risk of further problems. Finally, the goal of restoration allows the individual to maintain control over as much of the daily routine as possible during a stressful time of life when much of the control in the hospital setting is eliminated.

Joint Classification

Movement occurs through the interaction of muscle with bones or a joint. It involves the structures of skeletal muscle, bone, and the nervous system. The **joints** in the body are junctions between two bony surfaces surrounded by ligaments, muscles, and a joint capsule. The joint allows movement between the two bony surfaces.

The joints are classified according to the amount of movement permitted and by the shape that the two surfaces assume. Joints classified by movement are synarthrodial, amphiarthrodial, and diarthrodial (Table 25–1). The synarthrodial joint allows no movement

Table 25-1

JOINT CLASSIFICATION		
TYPE OF JOINT	**EXAMPLE**	**LIMITATIONS OF MOVEMENT**
Synarthrodial	Suture lines of skull	Permits no movement
Amphiarthrodial	Vertebrae of the spine	Permits limited motion
Diarthrodial	Intercarpal joints of hand	Allows the most movement

between the surfaces. An example of such a joint would be the suture lines of the skull. An amphiarthrodial joint, on the other hand, permits limited motion between the joint surfaces and has a membrane or ligament between the bony surfaces. A vertebra in the spine is an example of such a joint. The type of joint that permits the most movement is the diarthrodial joint. To support movement in many directions, the bone ends in diarthrodial joints are covered by cartilaginous sheets and connected by ligaments. The joint itself is lined with a synovial membrane, which secretes a liquid to lubricate the joint. The ligaments around a joint reinforce and stabilize the joint capsule as well as direct movement and limit excessive motion. Muscles stabilize the joint, permitting the firm contact between the joint surfaces and allowing movement.

Diarthrodial Joints

The diarthrodial joints are further defined by the shape of the articulating surfaces. These include the ball and socket, hinge, pivot, condyloid, saddle, and gliding joint.

The ball-and-socket joint consists of a ball-shaped head fitting into a concave socket and allows the most movement. The joint is located in the shoulder and the hip.

The hinge joint has a concave surface fitting into a convex shape. The motion in this joint is limited to flexion and extension. The knee is a hinge joint.

The pivot joint consists of a rounded, pointed, or concave surface fitting into a depression. Motion is limited to rotation. An example of a pivot joint is the radius, which articulates with the notch of the ulna.

Condyloid joints, found in the wrist between the radius and carpal bone, are similar to ball-and-socket joints. They contain an oval-shaped head fitting into an elliptical surface. This joint does not permit rotation to occur.

The saddle joint has a concave surface moving in one direction and convex surface moving in the other. Movement is allowed in most directions, but rotation is limited. The thumb joint, between the first metacarpal and the trapezium of the thumb is an example of such a joint.

The intercarpal joints of the hand are examples of a gliding joint. The surfaces in this type of joint are slightly convex, articulating with a slightly concave surface. The possible motions are abduction, adduction, flexion, and extension.

✦ Muscle Function

Muscle tissue comprises 40 to 50% of the body. This tissue is classified as skeletal, smooth, or cardiac. In this chapter, skeletal muscle tissue is addressed.

Skeletal muscle is made up of numerous fibers that extend, in most muscles, the entire length of the muscle. Because of these fibers, muscle can be stretched or shortened, depending on the stimuli. There are certain points in the muscle fiber, called neuromuscular junctions, where the muscles are more easily stimulated. These areas, called motor points, can be used in therapy to stimulate contraction of the muscle more easily.

✦ Muscle Contractions

Skeletal muscle consists of bands of actin and myosin filament. When stretched, these filaments pull apart to allow the muscle to contract or relax. Muscles shorten to perform the work of lifting or to move objects against force, and they lengthen to relax or stretch. During this work, the muscles consume large quantities of oxygen and other nutrients.

Muscles contract either isometrically or isotonically. During the isometric contraction, muscles do not shorten; in an isotonic contraction, muscles shorten, and tension remains constant. An isotonic contraction causes work to occur, i.e., a load is moved. Momentum, caused by the movement, continues even after the muscle contraction is over, and more energy is used. In an isometric contraction, the fibrils in the muscle do not slide among each other, and less energy is consumed. The isotonic contraction, therefore, lasts longer. During the daily activity of the body, the muscle contractions usually are a mixture of the two types. A weightlifter uses isotonic contractions when lifting arm weights and at the same time uses isometric contractions in the legs while standing.

Muscles, which come in different sizes, are attached to bones, connective tissue, soft tissue, skin, and other muscles. Muscles initiate movement, produce heat, and maintain posture. Some contract slowly, whereas others contract rapidly; the duration is related to the function of the muscle. The force of the contraction depends on the state of the muscle. If the fibers are lacking certain nutrients or are fatigued, the contraction may be weak. A muscle that is warm and highly contractible may contract more strongly than usual. Athletes use this concept when preparing for participation in an event. Warm muscles are more flexible and ready to respond to the rigors of exercise and less likely to become injured.

The contraction of a muscle is initiated in the central nervous system by a motor neuron from the spinal cord. The motor neuron affects many muscle fibers or motor units in the same area, causing a reaction. Muscles that react rapidly have few muscle fibers in each motor unit. The slower-acting muscles, such as those that maintain posture, have many fibers that support each other.

If certain nerve fibers are lost to a muscle, the remaining fibers can grow and take over the lost function. This can account for the regaining of function when nerve damage occurs, even though the degree of the control may be compromised.

Skeletal System

The skeleton is the framework for the body. Because of its rigidity, it provides shape and form, protects internal vital organs, acts as a storage system for nutrients, affects the hemoregulatory system, and participates in movement. Muscles and ligaments attach to the bones of the skeleton at various points. The contraction of the muscle, along with motion in the joint, facilitates movement.

Bone formation and reabsorption is kept in balance by the hormonal system, along with certain vitamins and the stress that muscles place on the bones. Stress or weight bearing stimulates the bone into formation and reabsorption. The long thick bones are the weight-bearing bones and are affected by activity or inactivity quickly.

Body Alignment

Normal movement and posture are not conscious but rather are automatic responses that develop early in infancy. This development involves integration of early primitive reflexes, which at first are automatic. As higher brain centers are more developed and refined, they exhibit control over movement. Normal movement occurs in all directions when the center of gravity is kept over the base of support.

Muscle tone is a prerequisite for normal movement. **Tone** is the state of muscle readiness; it occurs on a continuum from low to high. Normal tone is high enough to resist gravity's effect yet low enough to allow movement. The trunk of the body is the stabilizer, and the extremities move about the trunk. The stabilization of the trunk develops from infancy on, and it is a gradual process; *i.e.,* the infant progresses from lying to sitting to standing postures. An injury or insult to the central nervous system can affect the trunk's stability and cause a return to primitive styles of movement. When this occurs, the goal of the therapist is to inhibit these styles and to encourage as normal movement as possible.

The head is centered over the trunk, usually oriented to midline and the horizon. If the trunk shifts away from the midline, readjustment occurs to bring the head back to midline. This orientation to midline defines the amount of the body's rotation. An example of this is seen when a person shifts balance or is spinning. The head stays near midline to maintain stability even though the trunk rotates, such as in a spinning dancer.

The spine centers over a stable pelvis with an anterior lordosis (curvature). This allows the head to remain in a midline position. If a shift occurs, the spine can compensate. For example, while sitting, try bearing weight on one hip and notice what happens to the spine. This is an example of functional scoliosis.

Truncal balance reactions are an automatic response to changes in posture. The reactions are bilateral, *i.e.,* change on one side produces a change on the other. These reactions are important components in normal movement because they maintain stability while allowing independent extremity movement. The extremities will assist in maintaining balance by broadening the base of support. Notice what happens with the arms when standing on one foot—the arms automatically extend in an attempt to maintain balance.

Posture

Both the client and the caregiver (who may be either the nurse or a family member) must consider **posture** and body alignment when moving. Attempts should be made to maintain or achieve as normal a body position as possible.

The line of gravity, the center of gravity, and the base of support are important when someone is moving and lifting either an object or a client. When these factors are ignored, inefficiency in energy expenditure causes fatigue in the person lifting and may result in injury.

The line of gravity is an imaginary line that runs down the center of the body, passing through the center of gravity and exiting the body through the base of support (Fig. 25–1). The goal of posture is to arrange the segments of the body in a vertical column so that the line of gravity is within the base of sup-

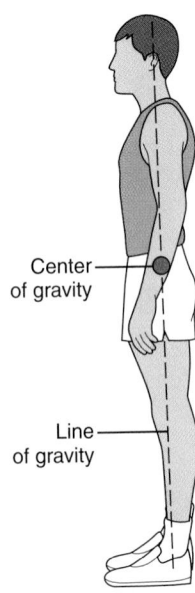

Center of gravity

Line of gravity

❧ **Figure 25–1**

Proper body alignment. The segments of the body are in a vertical column.

port. This alignment gives the musculoskeletal system the most stability when a person is standing and minimizes the expenditure of energy when he or she attempts to stand upright.

The center of gravity is that part of the body where the center of its mass is located. For the adult in a standing position, the center is located in the pelvic region about 55% of the total height from the floor. As long as the line of gravity falls through the center of gravity and within the base of support, the person will maintain a stable posture with minimal exertion.

The base of support is that area defined by the person's feet. The closer the feet are to each other, the narrower the base of support. Again, the line of gravity should fall through the center of the base of support.

Sitting Posture

The normal **sitting posture** is mostly dynamic rather than static (Fig. 25–2). In other words, one cannot sit still. In the sitting posture, the hips are level and flexed at a 90-degree angle, and the pelvis is tilted forward to create a lumbar curve (lordosis). The trunk is centered over the pelvis and shoulders at an equal height, with the shoulder blades parallel to the chair back without retraction of the shoulder blades. The head is held in midline, the neck neutral, and the chin centered under the forehead. The hips, knees, and ankles are flexed at 90 degrees without any rotation. The hip and knee should be in line with one another. There is no normal position for the upper extremities, but if they are left to hang or are unsupported, they may cause a downward pull of the spine and shoulders.

Standing Posture

In a standing posture (Fig. 25–3), the feet are shoulder width apart, with the toes pointing forward and the knees straight but not locked. Weight is distributed evenly over both feet, and the shoulders are equal in height. The pelvis is in a neutral position, with the lumbar spine extended over the pelvis and the head centered over the spine in a midline position. The chin in centered under the forehead, with the face forward.

Lying Posture

In the lying position, increased neck and upper back flexion should be avoided. Otherwise, there is no one correct lying position.

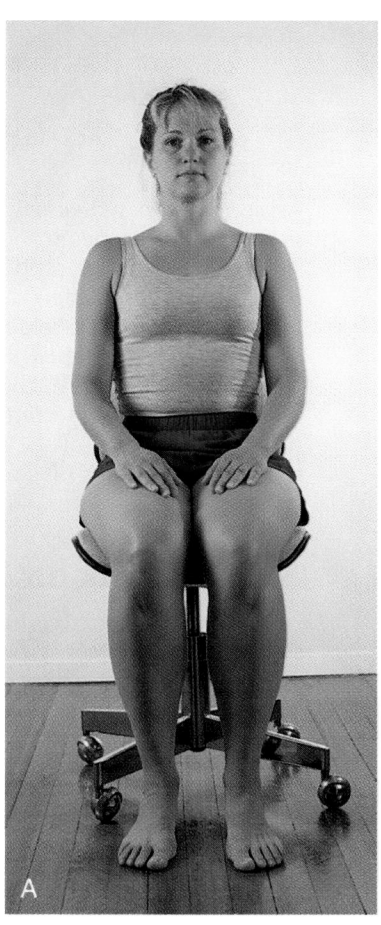
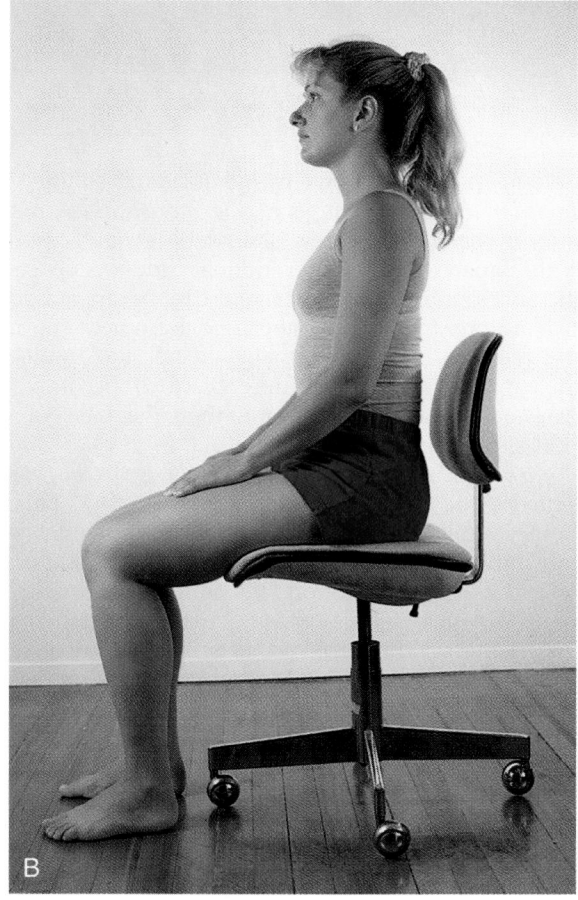

✦ **Figure 25–2**
Normal sitting posture. *A,* Front view. *B,* Side view.

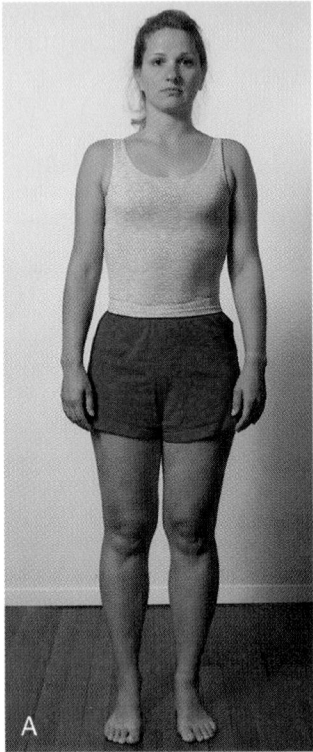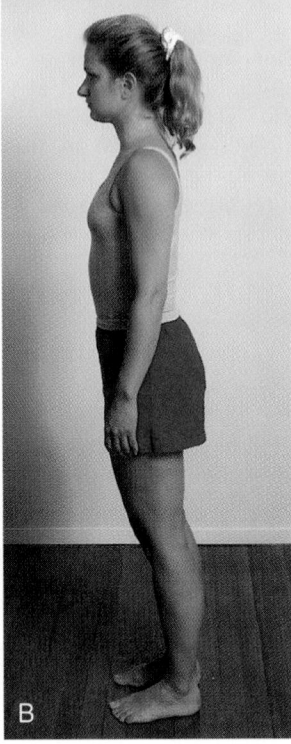

❧ **Figure 25–3**
Normal standing posture. *A,* Front view. *B,* Side view.

lifting. However, when caring for the client, it is important to remember the effects of shearing and friction on the skin that can occur from sliding. Tissue damage can occur and becomes an especially critical factor for a client with thin skin or a fragile health status. (Refer to Chapter 23 for further information on skin care.)

More muscular effort is needed as the body shifts away from the center of the supporting base. The human body was designed in such a way as to provide a means to move and lift. The large muscles in the legs are designed to provide force, speed, and balance. The upper extremities are designed to produce fine coordination and rest on a flexible base of support. *For a nurse to work as an efficient machine, it is extremely important that the body be maintained in prime working order.* Any excess weight carried adds to the work required to maintain stability and function efficiently. Muscles must be toned and flexibility supported. If excess weight is carried in the abdominal area, the low back curve increases in an attempt to maintain an upright posture. The increased curve causes back pain and is especially evident in the advanced stages of pregnancy. The cardiovascular system must function efficiently to provide the nutrients to the muscles and support the body when stress of any nature is added. If a conscious effort is made, then the body will serve the individual well throughout the years of moving and lifting and client care.

Moving and Lifting Principles

Certain principles govern moving and lifting. *The broader the base of support, the more stable an individual becomes.* The feet should be at least shoulder width apart to allow for normal side-to-side movement. Front-to-back movement can be increased by placing one foot slightly ahead of the other. The more the feet are moved apart, the greater the stability in the upright position. If the object to be moved is extremely heavy or awkward, then the base of support should be widened.

The lower the center of gravity is to the base of support, the more stable the object becomes. This can be accomplished by bending the knees slightly when moving or lifting. When the line of gravity shifts outside the base of support, the amount of energy required to maintain stability is considerably increased. To counteract this problem, it is necessary to use the large muscle groups within the body, such as the legs and arms. Getting as close to the object also reduces the problem of maintaining good body alignment.

Changing positions frequently reduces the fatigue of the body's muscles. In addition, using mechanical devices, such as lifts, to accomplish the tasks preserves muscle tone and efficiency. When appropriate, moving or sliding an object or a client requires less force than

Pathophysiology of Immobility

As soon as an individual becomes ill and is confined in bed, changes begin, both internally and externally. Although rest is prescribed as a means to a cure, 2 days of rest can affect the client adversely (Kottke, 1966). If the client is elderly, the result can be devastating and sometimes irreversible. The following changes occur in all clients, but the extent of the effects depends on a number of factors, including (but not limited to) age of the client, comorbidities present, extent and length of immobilization, and treatment plan.

Effects on Body System
Musculoskeletal System

Studies have been done on healthy men who were immobilized for different lengths of time. In the absence of any involuntary muscle contraction, muscle strength decreased by 5% per day. In individuals who remained in bed for one week, muscle strength decreased by 1 to 1.5% per day (Creditor, 1993). The changes in muscle strength were seen most noticeably in the lower extremities. Contractures and atrophy resulted.

Bone density changes dramatically with immobilization. Bones need the wear and tear of muscles and weight bearing to retain calcium and phosphorus salts. Vertebral bone loss accelerates with bed rest. In one study, loss that occurred with 10 days of bed rest took 4 months to restore (Kottke, 1966). The effects of bed rest on the skeletal system can cause osteoporosis, leading to fractures, urinary tract stone formation, bone deformity, and osteoarthropathy due to calcium salt deposits in the joints.

Gastrointestinal System

Immobility affects all body systems, and the initial effects may be unnoticeable, especially in the digestive system. Changes in the gastrointestinal system are often subtle and undiagnosed. The most prominent effect is on the functions of digestion and elimination. Digestion slows and results in a negative nitrogen balance due to an increase in catabolism, or the breakdown of tissue, and the decrease in anabolism, or the buildup of tissue. Marked protein deficiency, which can lead to anorexia, malnutrition, and decreased tissue healing and repair, can occur. The increased level of nitrogen in the blood causes a decrease in appetite, escalating the problems. The client needs to maintain the basal metabolism and compensate for protein loss. This is difficult to do during immobility or when the body is attempting to repair tissue in a state of decreased protein supply.

Muscle activity is reduced, and atrophy occurs in the muscles needed in elimination (abdominal muscle, diaphragm, and levator ani). Constipation occurs because of changes in the environment, the patterns of living, and the manner of defecation, as well as neglect of the urge to defecate. Constipation can eventually lead to fecal impaction and/or obstruction.

Integumentary System

The integumentary system, or skin, is affected by immobility. The response is rapid and visible. Redness, edema, and eventual tissue breakdown occur in areas where pressure occurs. Direct pressure greater than 32 mmHg for 2 hours results in tissue necrosis. Normally, a person changes positions approximately 50 times per hour. Studies show that if someone changes position less than 25 times per day, pressure ulcers will develop (Kottke, 1966).

An ulcer does not appear initially, but edema and redness are early signs of tissue damage. If the pressure is removed, no further tissue breakdown will occur. Pressure that is unrelieved will cause damage in a short time, depending on the condition of the patient. (Refer to Chapter 23.)

Genitourinary System

The genitourinary system is adversely affected by the lack of mobility. Gravity encourages the flow of urine from the kidneys to the bladder. When the client lies down for long periods, urine pools in the kidney and can produce infection and permanent damage. Urinary retention can lead to bladder distention, a decreased or absent bladder muscle tone and strength, kidney and bladder stones, and urinary tract infections. Failure to empty the bladder can also result in dribbling, leaking, and voiding in small amounts. The stasis of urine in the bladder, as well as the presence of indwelling catheters, provide an ideal medium for bacterial growth that leads to infection (Fig. 25–4).

As a result of tissue breakdown and the body's response to being immobile, renal stones form from minerals, crystals, or other particles in the kidney. Stones form in approximately 30% of immobilized clients 14 to 21 days after being put on bed rest. If a client is losing large amounts of calcium, stones form from around these salts. Excretion of minerals from tissue breakdown into the urine has been found in clients as little as 2 days after confinement to bed, an indication of the speed with which complication can occur (Kottke, 1966).

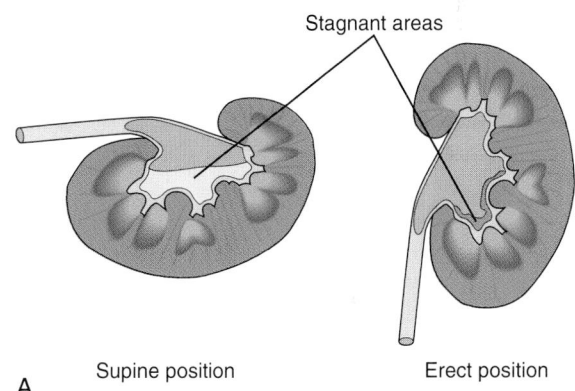

Stasis of urine in bladder

Stagnant areas

Supine position   Erect position

A

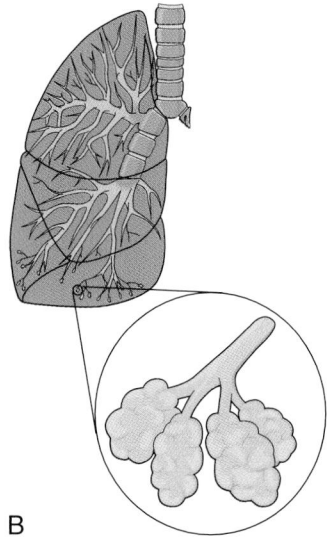

Hypostatic pneumonia

B

❧ **Figure 25–4**
Bacterial growth due to stasis of urine leads to an infection. *A,* Urinary stasis. *B,* Hypostatic pneumonia.

Cardiovascular System

The cardiovascular system begins to decompensate shortly after immobilization begins. Three major problems have the potential to develop: orthostatic hypotension, venous stasis and thrombus formation, and cardiovascular deconditioning.

Orthostatic hypotension is the rapid falling of the blood pressure that occurs when an individual goes from a lying to a sitting or standing position. Dizziness or vertigo, pedal and leg edema, weakness, giddiness, and fainting can occur. The individual can also experience an increase in the pulse rate, pallor, and sweating of the palms of the hands. These symptoms are related to venous stasis in the lower limbs, a decrease in muscle tone, and dilation of blood vessels in the abdomen and legs, allowing the blood to pool. The muscles are not able to pump blood from these areas to the brain when positions are shifted.

Venous stasis and thrombus formation result from a lack of muscular contraction, especially in the lower extremities. Blood pools and edema develops. The pooling of the blood, along with the external pressure of the bed on the blood vessels and the dehydration that occurs from being immobile, causes the blood to become thicker and prone to thrombus formation. The increased level of calcium in the blood contributes to clot formation, because calcium plays a role in the development of thrombi. Edema, redness, warmth, and a positive Homans' sign are all possible indications of venous thrombosis.

Cardiovascular deconditioning is a result of immobility. The heart works harder in the resting supine position than in the sitting position to offset the effects of gravity. Vascular resistance and hydrostatic pressure in the blood vessels change when the person is lying down. The heart must deal with an increase in blood volume when gravity is overcome, and pulse rates increase as does blood pressure. When an individual begins to increase the level of activity, the heart must work harder to handle the increased volume of blood and a decreased recovery time.

Valsalva's maneuver also increases the workload of the heart. This maneuver occurs as an individual holds the breath during strenuous activity, moving in bed, or having a bowel movement. The breath is pushed against a closed glottis, and the intrathoracic pressure is raised. As a result, blood flow to the heart is temporarily diminished. When the breath is released, blood rushes to the heart, causing an increased workload, rapid pulse, and possible cardiac arrest.

Respiratory System

Respiratory infections, a pulmonary embolus, pneumonia, atelectasis, and respiratory acidosis are effects of immobility. These occur because there is either a decreased movement of the lungs or an imbalance of oxygen–carbon dioxide exchange.

Decreased expansion of the lungs can be a result of external pressure from the bed or chair or from the lying or sitting posture on the chest. Medication, abdominal distention, or binders, as well as pain, can decrease the rate and depth of the respirations. Normal respirations cause the lungs to remove 100 cc (or ml) of mucus in a 24-hour period. If the lungs are limited in their movement, removal of this fluid becomes difficult, pooling of secretions occurs, and pneumonia develops. Muscle weakness from immobility directly affects the individual's ability to cough up secretions from the lower lobes of the lungs. Secretions become thick and difficult to move—the perfect medium for bacterial growth, leading to respiratory infections and further immobility. Hypostatic pneumonia, an inflammation of the alveoli and buildup of secretions in the alveoli, develops as a result of the decreased mobility, a weakened cough, and the pooling of secretions (see Fig. 24–4B).

Atelectasis, a collapse of alveoli caused by external pressure of fluid accumulation, blocks the bronchial tree, preventing air exchange. The collapse of the alveoli causes dyspnea and cyanosis.

Respiratory acidosis occurs because of the inadequate exchange of oxygen and carbon dioxide. Normal gas exchange is impaired by the pooling of the secretions and the decreased respiratory movement. Acidosis produces drowsiness, irritability, confusion, headaches, and cardiac arrhythmias. If left untreated, death will occur.

Pulmonary emboli (blood clots) are another common problem due to immobility. A clot forms in the lower part of the leg. When movement is initiated, the thrombus can break loose and form an embolus that travels to the lungs. Death can occur rapidly if emboli are not treated.

Metabolic System

Metabolic changes occur rapidly, although they are less visible than other changes. Included among the changes are a reduced metabolic rate, tissue atrophy and protein catabolism, bone demineralization, fluid and electrolyte imbalance, and gastrointestinal hypermobility or hypomotility. The supine position decreases adrenocortical hormone production, affecting the metabolism of carbohydrates, protein, fat, and minerals. This position also increases circulation to the kidney, increasing urinary output. The impact on metabolism is closely intertwined with the other changes occurring in all body systems and illustrates how closely related and dependent all systems are within the body.

Psychological System

The mind and spirit are adversely affected by immobility. An individual adapts to the surroundings, and if a situation is present that does not challenge independence and intellectual needs, the person becomes more dependent. Disorientation occurs because of the lack of interaction with and stimulation from the environment. A person takes cues from the activity around, and if isolation occurs, disorientation and possible regression in behavior are seen. Often the immobilized individual is isolated from the environment and experiences minimal stimulation. Immobility fosters a decreased level of motivation and ability to learn. Studies show difficulty with problem solving and retention of new material and a decrease in the ability to discriminate (Kottke, 1966).

Immobility can also cause an individual to have exaggerated reactions to incidents. Anger, depression, or sudden outbursts are not uncommon and may be related to changes in body image brought on by the illness or disease producing the immobility. Insomnia is often present with immobilization. Those on bed rest take frequent naps and expend little energy and, as a result, have difficulty sleeping at night.

Effect on the Elderly

Immobility presents a significant challenge to the elderly—especially the hospitalized elderly. The elderly client often has very little reserved energy, has one or more chronic illnesses, and views the hospitalization as a threat to his or her current level of independence. Illness induced by medical diagnosis or the medical treatment prescribed (**iatrogenesis**) is one result of immobility in the elderly and is a serious health hazard (see Box). The hospital, although a place to receive treatment, is very dangerous for the elderly.

The effects of immobility in the elderly can be seen as soon as 24 hours after bed rest has begun

Organ Systems	**Clinical Effect**
• Cardiovascular	• Blood pressure drops
	• Diminished physical work tolerance
	• Atelectasis
• Pulmonary	• Decreases muscle strength, contraction
• Dermatological	• Pressure ulcers
• Neurological	• Compression neuropathy leading to decreased sensation
	• Increased body sway leading to falls
• Gastrointestinal	• Constipation
• Genitourinary	• Hypercalcemia
	• Urinary incontinence leading to infection
• Psychological	• Depression, anxiety, delirium

IMMOBILITY IN THE ELDERLY: NEGATIVE EFFECTS OF BED REST ON SELECTED BODY SYSTEMS

(Gorbien, 1992). Most immobility in the elderly is the result of problems with the musculoskeletal, neurological, or cardiovascular system. Within these systems, the most common diagnoses are degenerative joint disease, fractures of the hip, advanced osteoporosis, stroke, congestive heart failure, coronary disease, and peripheral vascular disease. These diseases require frequent contact with the health care system and complex care, increasing the risk of iatrogenesis.

Hospital practices often debilitate an elderly person more than the physical problems or primary reason for admission. The routines often keep the older person in bed for long periods of time in uncomfortable or prolonged positions, promoting the development of contractures, skin breakdown, and deconditioning. Staff are unable to ambulate clients frequently, and the halls are often cluttered and busy. Restraints, which may be applied if the client is confused or combative, contribute further to immobilization. If medications are used to sedate or quiet an elderly person, they often cause an unsteady gait, increased confusion, and orthostatic hypotension, affecting the ability to ambulate. Often the client is confined to the bed just by the various tubes being used, such as a catheter, intravenous line, or nasogastric tube.

Changes that normally occur with aging are similar to those that occur in a younger person who is immobilized for a period. Because these changes take place gradually, the elderly person's body adjusts to these changes and continues to function adequately, provided no further incidences stress the fragile systems. Thus, when an elderly person enters the hospital, he or she is at risk of developing complications quickly if the special needs are not addressed in the plan of care.

The skin of the elderly is thin and dry and has little fat to pad the areas over the bony prominences. As a result, being in bed can cause friction and shearing when the client moves. Tearing of the skin and the formation of pressure ulcers can occur in a matter of a few days.

The nutritional status of the elderly is often less than ideal. Adequate intake of fluids and needed nutrients is often absent and can be a result of the inability to prepare food or buy food, poorly fitting dentures, loss of appetite, and decreased sensation of thirst. Once a person is hospitalized, the need for good nutrition becomes even more important to promote wound and tissue healing. However, fluids may not be accessible, the food may be difficult to eat, and insufficient time may be allowed for meals. The elderly may need help with food preparation, and appetite may be poor due to inactivity or medications.

Elimination quickly becomes an issue with the elderly client. Constipation may result from the lack of activity, medications, poor food and fluid intake, lack of privacy, and disruption in routine. Urinary incontinence can become an issue, especially if the client is unable to get to the bathroom easily. Incontinence may also contribute to skin breakdown.

Newly admitted clients are at a high risk for falls.

Falls are common because of environmental barriers and the client's attempt to overcome them. For example, crawling over the bed's side rails to get to the bathroom is prompted by the client's attempt to address the urgency need or the desire to maintain independence. Calling for the nurse when the call light is out of reach is not a possibility. The bathroom is the place where falls are most likely to occur. Transfers off and onto the toilet can cause a fall, especially if the client is in a hurry. A poorly lit bathroom at night presents an added hazard and contributes to incontinence. Even when the nurse has taken the time to orient the client to the room, sometimes the client cannot learn new things because he or she is under stress or has impaired cognition. Often the client becomes more confused.

Hospital-acquired (nosocomial) infections continue to be a major complication of hospital care. Studies show that in the general population, the risk of acquiring an infection during a hospital admission is about 5%. The elderly client's chance of getting an infection, however, increases fivefold for a urinary tract infection, threefold for pneumonia, fivefold for bacteremia, and twofold for a wound infection (Creditor, 1993). These same statistics are seen in residents of nursing homes.

Muscle strength decreases at a rate of 1 to 2% per day (Kottke, 1966). This and increased weakness often lead to falls and fractures. Minimal contractions of the muscles are needed to maintain the strength and mass. Immobility produces contractures in the elderly. The contractures are due to both the loss of energy reserve that occurs with aging and the muscle shortening from inactivity. Contractures and limited motion occur most rapidly in the lower extremities—especially the ankles (Creditor, 1993). It is no wonder, then that bed rest prescribed for the purpose of healing can actually cause harm to the client—more specifically, the elderly client.

CASE STUDY **Mrs. Bridges Falls**

Mrs. Bridges, a relatively healthy woman, is admitted to the emergency department after a fall at home. She is complaining of pain in her hip, and after an examination and x-ray, it is determined that she has broken her hip. She is admitted to the orthopedic unit for preparation for surgery. She is accompanied by her husband, who seems somewhat bewildered by the incident and who expresses great concern over what is happening to his wife.

After surgery and hip replacement, Mrs. Bridges is confused, is unable to participate in the ambulation program, and is not eating well. Her husband is worried about caring for her after discharge because he is unable to drive and has a cardiac condition that limits his activity. The physician orders Mrs. Bridges' discharge in 4 days.

This elderly couple has suffered a tremendous blow to their lifestyle. The challenges seem insurmountable to them and require a team conference. It is decided that it is most appropriate for Mrs. Bridges to be transferred to a skilled nursing facility before going home. Her confusion was a result of both the surgery and the pain medication she was receiving, as well as the isolation she was experiencing in her room. She is moved nearer to the nurse's station and put in a room with a roommate. As her confusion clears, she begins to eat, and an attempt is made to serve her the foods that she likes.

It also is determined that Mrs. Bridges is the caregiver in the home, and her husband depends on her for transportation, decision-making, and meal preparation. The social service department arranges transportation to and from the hospital and the skilled nursing facility. In addition, Mr. Bridges is able to eat his meals at the hospital with his wife. Arrangements are made for home services in the form of a home-delivered meal service and a homemaker when Mrs. Bridges is discharged home. Nursing care at home will be provided by a nurse and the home health aide. With these arrangements, the couple is able to continue living at home and strive toward the independence they had prior to Mrs. Bridges' fall.

Nervous System Impairment

Interference with the central nervous system often leads to mobility problems. When blood flow to the brain is impaired, the continuous flow of needed oxygen is disrupted. This can be caused by a hemorrhage, occlusion of a vessel, vasospasm, or a lesion. The resulting immediate and residual impairment depends on where the incident occurred in the brain. If hemorrhage occurs in the brainstem or the internal capsule, weakness on one side of the body (hemiplegia) results. Hemiplegia also results from interruption of the blood supply to the middle cerebral artery or anterior cerebral artery. Occlusion of the posterior cerebral artery causes uncoordinated voluntary movement. Deficits within the sensory areas of the brain make it difficult to process information and understand where and what information that relates to mobility and body position is being received.

Diseases that interfere with the pathways within the brain, such as cerebral palsy and Parkinson's disease, affect movement. Cerebral palsy, which is caused by trauma at birth or shortly after birth by central nervous system damage, involves lack of muscle control. Symptoms include a clumsy walk, lack of balance, shaking, jerky movements, and unclear speech. The long-term results are spasticity, ataxia, or athetoid, involuntary movements depending on the affected area of the brain. Movement is difficult, and lifelong interventions are needed.

Parkinson's disease is another example of neural

pathway interference. The disease is characterized by a resting tremor, muscle rigidity, difficulty initiating movement, and gait disturbances. Slow in onset, it usually occurs later in life and causes increasing problems with movement.

Multiple sclerosis is an example of a disease that interferes with the spinal cord pathways. The disease involves destruction of the nerve sheaths in the white matter of the brain and spinal cord and produces mobility problems, as messages along the nerves are interrupted. It is characterized by a series of remissions and exacerbations over a long time. Symptoms, often vague initially, include weakness, incoordination, numbness, and difficulty with movement. These symptoms are made worse by heat and stress.

Quadriplegia (paralysis of all extremities) and paraplegia (paralysis of two extremities) result from an injury to or lesion of the spinal cord. The degree of paralysis depends on the level of the injury and its severity. Transmission of impulses to the brain are interrupted, and movement is impaired or absent. The effects of immobility can be severe, and measures need to be taken to minimize the effects.

Usually paralysis is a result of trauma to the spinal cord. However, inflammation or viruses can attack the spinal cord and cause varying degrees of paralysis or paresis (muscle weakness). In addition to the impairments to the central nervous system, interferences with peripheral motor and sensory pathways also occur. Guillain-Barré syndrome is a degeneration of the myelin in the peripheral motor and sensory nerves. Paraesthesia, motor weakness, respiratory paralysis, and pain are common symptoms, and flaccid paralysis occurs. The syndrome does terminate, and recovery occurs with little or no residual effects.

Muscular dystrophy is an example of an inherited disorder that involves degeneration of muscle fibers in skeletal muscle. Degeneration occurs slowly over time and affects the amount and type of movement left in an individual. Because the disease is progressive and impairs movement, a long-term plan is needed to minimize the effects of immobility.

Factors other than nervous system problems that interfere with skeletal functioning are hip fractures, joint replacement, stroke, and degenerative and juvenile arthritis. Clients must be provided with the necessary information to deal with the challenges they face and to maintain independent functioning.

Application of the Nursing Process to Mobility

Assessment

Nursing History

The nurse begins to develop a nursing history when the client enters the health care system. All cli-

ents should be assessed for any mobility problems regardless of the reason for admission. This process can be initiated either in the physician's office, in the emergency department, or during the admission to the hospital. The history should include the degree of mobility at home, the daily routine, any accommodations made to address the mobility needs, and available caregivers and equipment. If possible, interview both the client and family. This is especially significant if the client has a cognitive impairment and is unable to give an accurate history. Include questions that will elicit information about precipitating factors for this admission or visit and whether the problem has occurred before; if so, determine the course of events, any problem resolution, and the methods used. It is appropriate at this time to begin planning for discharge, especially if the client is going to need assistance then.

The elderly client who is hospitalized and immobile experiences sensory deprivation. Isolation occurs, and the client begins to lose contact with the world. If the client has some degree of cognitive impairment, delirium results. The elderly are often on many medications (polypharmacy), and the combinations can contribute to delirium or even be lethal. Some clients never recover from delirium and may in fact be misdiagnosed. As a result, more medications may be added to treat the delirium, and a cascade of events leads the client to more dependency and the inability to return to the previous living situation.

Physical Assessment

Because all body systems are affected by movement or immobility, a baseline physical assessment is done. The cardiac status, respiratory function, elimination patterns, cognitive and psychosocial functioning, condition of the skin, and the mobility status should be established on admission. Information is retrieved from the physician's history and physical, along with other team members' notes, impressions, and an interview with the client and family.

The physical assessment can be done on both a formal and an informal basis. On initial contact with the client, be aware of how independently he or she moves. Is there a need for assistive devices to aid with mobility? If the client has a cane or walker and is independent, the aid should be brought to the hospital and placed within easy reach. As the client changes into hospital clothing or pajamas, observe the amount of assistance needed, as well as signs of restricted movement or any indication of pain (*e.g.,* facial expressions, the willingness or hesitation to participate in the process, and the guarding of any joint motion). The level of pain can also be evaluated through a formal process by having the client rate the level, intensity, and duration of pain on a scale or merely by asking the client to describe the pain. Pain in various joints of the body may make certain positions difficult to achieve or impossible to maintain for any length of time.

Note whether the client is able to understand and complete the task of getting ready for and into bed. Also note whether he or she can move and change positions in bed. This information can give the nurse clues as to the level of cognition present and can be used to formulate the methods needed for client education.

A thorough inspection of the skin should be done to establish a baseline for comparison if any skin problems arise due to decreased mobility. Note the texture of the skin, the condition (whether oily or dry), and the amount of subcutaneous tissue. Chart any bruises or breaks in the skin and how these were acquired, as well as any reddened areas—especially over the bony prominences and in places that are prone to continuous pressure or shearing. Redness should disappear within 30 minutes of pressure relief. Palpation of the pressure area will also tell whether edema—another sign of tissue damage—has begun. For the frail elderly person, 2 hours in one position may be too long and may cause damage to the skin. Pressure-relieving devices are needed, and skin creams should be used to increase skin tolerance (see Chapter 23).

Determine the level of continence. Continual drainage from either the bladder or the bowel onto the skin is extremely irritating and debilitating. It can also make it socially unacceptable for the client to ambulate or be out in the community and difficult for him or her to maintain any one position for a period of time. In addition, excess moisture on the skin can increase the risk of skin breakdown.

Perform **passive range of motion** (PROM; range of motion in which the nurse moves the extremities through full range) to determine which, if any, of the joints have restricted movement. The plan, when developed, will focus on those areas that have restricted motion and maintain the function in the joints and extremities so that they are functioning at the maximum level. Note the presence of any spasticity when the extremities are moved. This is characterized by muscle spasm, jerky movements, or a tightening of the limb into a position. If spasticity is a problem, it can affect skin care and positioning as well as ambulation techniques.

When a client has experienced immobility for a time, contractures may be present on admission to the hospital. These contractures alter the way in which a client is positioned, affect whether ambulation is possible, and determine how much ROM can be performed on an extremity. As the contracture is released, changing the positioning program will inhibit further development of contractures and skin breakdown.

Define the baseline neurological status. As was mentioned previously, the neurological system has a significant role in mobility. The level of consciousness is established as a baseline reference. The Glasgow Coma Scale, which defines consciousness at four levels—alert, lethargic, stuporous, or coma—can be used. If the client is not alert, then determine whether he or she is easily arousable (lethargic), difficult to arouse (stuporous), or comatose (does not respond to even painful stimuli). Check the orientation of the awake client to person, place, and time. Test whether the client can follow one-part, two-part, and multipart commands.

Assess the color, sensation, and movement of each extremity and compare the findings to identify any type of bilateral deviation. The color can be tested by visualization of the hands and feet and observation of the filling of the nail beds after pressure is applied. To test for sensation, poke the extremities with a blunt object and a sharp object while the client closes his or her eyes, and ask the client to verbalize when and what is being felt and where. Movement is tested by asking the client to wiggle the fingers and toes and the other extremities.

Stability, position sense, and coordination are also part of the neurological assessment. Stability can be assessed by asking the client to stand if possible with the eyes closed and watching for any signs of swaying or loss of balance. If the client cannot stand, having him or her sit on the side of the bed with the eyes closed also tests for stability. Ask the client to hold his or her arms out in front with eyes closed to determine position sense. Coordination assessment involves asking the client to touch his or her nose. The client should also be asked to place the heel on the opposite knee and then slide the heel up and down the shin. Ask the client to touch his or her nose and then the nurse's finger. Have the client repeat the task as the nurse's finger moves right and left.

Finally, the grasp and strength in the extremities should be noted. The client should squeeze the nurse's hands (right to right and left to left) at the same time to compare grasp strength. The client should push against the hand of the nurse with the feet to test for lower extremity strength. Note any variation on either side. Consult a physical examination text for further information or a more detailed explanation.

Assess the client's psychological state. A positive attitude can influence motivation toward independence and commitment to a program. A client and family who are cooperative and involved initially with the client's care will make a successful plan easier to achieve.

Diagnostic Testing

Diagnostic testing is aimed at two distinct areas of concern: the reason for the mobility impairment and the impact of immobility on the general welfare of the client. Tests to determine the cause of the immobility include x-rays of the limb or joint to rule out or identify a fracture. More extensive radiographic tests, such as computed tomographic scanning or magnetic resonance imaging, or diagnostic tests, such as a myelogram or angiogram, may be used if a condition more serious than a fracture is suspected or if the client fails to respond to initial treatment. Any test preparation is completed by the nurse. This includes not only administration of any preparations such as sedatives but also client education about the examination itself. Once the tests are completed, results should be noted and communicated to the physician.

Chest x-rays may be ordered to rule out pneumonia, a common problem with immobilized clients—especially the elderly. Auscultation of the chest may find lung sounds of rales, rhonchi, or wheezing. A productive cough also warrants further testing, including sputum cultures.

Physical and occupational therapists are often asked to evaluate the extent of immobility. This is especially true if a permanent or long-term problem, such as a stroke, head injury, or fracture of the lower limb, is diagnosed. Instruments to assess physical function, such as the Barthel Index and the Functional Independence Measure, are available.

Diagnostic laboratory tests should be used to monitor the client for reactions to immobility. Laboratory tests on blood, urine, and other body fluids can identify areas of concern. Because changes caused by bed rest occur rapidly, a systematic process for client monitoring should be initiated by the physician. Testing electrolytes, hematocrit, and hemoglobin and blood urea nitrogen will identify the client's status in terms of tissue breakdown, level of nutrition, the status of tissue repair, and the body's ability to cope with the illness. A urine culture should be done if there is reason to suspect an infection. The client may be experiencing fever, chills, passage of blood, or burning and frequency of urination. The level of calcium salts and the acidity or alkalinity of the urine could indicate the potential for stone formation. Increased serum calcium causes higher coagulability of the blood, promoting thrombus formation along with venous stasis. Low hemoglobin and hematocrit levels signal problems with oxygen transportation and tissue healing, as well as with the client's energy level. As a result, participation in a mobility program may be compromised. The albumin level of a client identifies the nutritional status and the potential for malnutrition. This is especially significant in the elderly, whose status may be very fragile on admission. A poor nutritional status delays healing and could delay discharge from the acute setting.

The immobilized client is at risk for developing thromboemboli, especially in the lower extremities. If the client complains of a dull ache, tight feeling, or frank pain in the calf, then a thrombus should be suspected. On palpation in about half of the cases, slight swelling, increased warmth or redness, fever, or tachycardia may be present. The Doppler ultrasound is an inexpensive and easy test for detecting thrombosis.

Safety and Risk Factors

An issue to consider when caring for a client with a mobility problem is client safety. The client's degree of steadiness, independence, cognition, and mobility affects how he or she moves around the environment

COMMON SAFETY OR RISK FACTORS IN THE ELDERLY

- Impaired postural control
- Changes in gait
- Presence of chronic pathological conditions associated with instability (*e.g.,* Parkinson's disease)
- Visual impairment
- Nocturia
- Increased presence of dementia
- Medications and alcohol use

and defines the level of risk for falling. As part of the initial assessment, all clients with impaired mobility should be screened for their risk of falling. Screening tools are often developed by various institutions and incorporate identified risk factors. Intrinsic and extrinsic risk factors include clinical factors that impair sensory input or judgment. Blood pressure regulation, reaction time, and balance and gait are some of the items included in the tools. See the box Common Safety or Risk Factors in the Elderly for common age-related factors.

For a hospitalized client, there are many environmental hazards that place him or her at risk for falls. These include

Furniture

Inadequate grab bars

High beds and bedrails

Restraints

Inadequate lighting and glare

Inaccessible nurse call devices

Nursing Diagnosis

After assessment, it is necessary to determine a nursing diagnosis. The diagnosis may be made on admission or any time during hospitalization. The most common diagnoses are (1) Impaired Physical Mobility, related to insufficient knowledge of techniques to either increase lower limb or upper limb function; (2) Risk for Injury related to lack of awareness of environmental hazards; (3) Disuse Syndrome; and (4) Self Care Deficit (see Nursing Diagnosis box).

A diagnosis of Risk for Injury is made for those clients whose level of cognition is impaired, such as those with head trauma or a central nervous system deficit or the frail elderly, who may have some visual impairment or failing eyesight.

The diagnosis of Impaired Physical Mobility describes an individual with limited use of either the arms or legs. It is not appropriate to use this diagnosis to describe total immobility: It should be used for the client who, for example, has a cast for a fracture, has

Impaired Physical Mobility

Examples of related factors include inability to transfer, limited ability to participate in activities of daily living, decreased exercise, fatigue, sleep disturbance

Risk for Injury

Examples of related factors include unsteadiness, poor balance, gait impairment, impaired vision, decreased mobility due to cast

Disuse Syndrome

Examples of related factors include muscle tissue atrophy, disorientation, deconditioning, kidney stones, urine stasis, sleep disturbance, depression

Self Care Deficit

Examples of related factors include inability to bathe self, difficulty with dressing, poor nutritional intake

Knowledge Deficit

Examples of related factors include lack of understanding of positioning needs, inability to participate in exercises, lack of understanding of transfer techniques, lack of understanding of skin care regimen

Pain

Examples of related factors include infrequent change of position, surgical incision, joint stiffness

Activity Intolerance

Examples of related factors include fatigue, dizziness, shortness of breath, weakness

Altered Health Maintenance

Examples of related factors include activities of daily living, inability to perform decreased nutritional intake, activity intolerance, decreased exercise

Impaired Skin Integrity

Examples of related factors include inability to shift weight, inability to change positions frequently, poor nutrition, inadequate protein intake

Sleep Pattern Disturbance

Examples of related factors include interruption of day-night cycle, interaction of medications, environmental noise and activity, lack of social stimulation

Anxiety

Examples of related factors include loss of control over independent mobility, uncertainty of future, inconsistent caregivers, limited financial resources

---

an individual is at risk for deterioration of body systems or altered functioning as the result of prescribed or unavoidable musculoskeletal inactivity (Carpenito, 1993). It describes a situation in which a person is experiencing or is at risk for the adverse effects of immobility. This diagnosis now includes 11 high-risk or actual diagnoses. It identifies an individual as vulnerable to certain complications or as experiencing altered functioning in a health pattern. Disuse Syndrome should be used even if the individual manifests the signs and symptoms of another diagnosis. In such a situation, the nurse should identify and use the specific diagnosis but continue to use Disuse Syndrome so that further deterioration of other body systems does not occur.

Self Care Deficit is another diagnosis used for the client with impaired mobility. It is manifested by the client who has upper and/or lower limb impairments. The level of deficit depends on the prior activity level, the severity of the impairment, and the aids available to the client. As the level of deficit changes, the client's activity level increases and the healing process improves his or her ability to participate in self-care. This diagnosis is also made when the client does not have the ability to cognitively understand the directions of the caregiver.

Additionally, a diagnosis of Knowledge Deficit can be used with mobility problems if the primary cause of the diagnosis is a lack of knowledge. An immobilized client with a cast may experience problems because of a lack of information and understanding about cast care. In this case, the diagnosis could be related to anxiety from unfamiliarity with a cast. Remember, however, that most people have a knowledge deficit about something, and it is only when this deficit affects the course of treatment that this diagnosis should be made.

The diagnosis of Pain must be specifically defined in terms of what the pain is related to. The immobilized client may be experiencing pain from contractures, postoperative procedures, or the underlying pathology that is producing the impaired mobility. Be specific when making this diagnosis, and identify the location and intensity of the pain; e.g., Pain in the abdomen related to a surgical incision.

Activity Intolerance is a nursing diagnosis that can be used if the client's physiological capacity to endure activities to the degree required is reduced (Carpenito, 1993). This particular diagnosis often is seen in the elderly individual who is deconditioned from bed rest and must participate in a rehabilitation program. Currently, Medicare requires 3 hours of therapy per day, 6 days a week, which is often too rigorous, fatiguing the client. The diagnosis is made throughout the process of activity by measuring the client's vital signs before, during, and after activity, as well as asking the client about his or her tolerance level. If fatigue is and continues to be a factor or physiological problems occur, a diagnosis should be made and interventions initiated to address the problem. Nursing diagnoses are made over the course of the hospitalization and resolve or

---

had a joint replaced, or has a paresis in a limb. The interventions are focused on strengthening and restoring function and preventing any deterioration.

The diagnosis of Disuse Syndrome is used when

change, depending on the medical diagnoses and subsequent treatment.

Planning

The purpose of developing a plan of care is to define systematically what is to be done, to provide consistency and continuity, to minimize the negative effects of hospitalization and immobility, and to establish a means of communication among caregivers, client, and family. It is essential that the client and family be involved in the plan to identify the process and agree on the outcomes. When their participation is obtained, the chances of compliance are much greater.

The plan includes turning and positioning schedules, periodic skin assessment and management, ROM exercises, and an ambulation plan. Client and family education and planning for discharge are key components of any plan of care, but these are often the two factors that are omitted or given superficial consideration by the nursing staff.

The overall goal for the client is to maximize the level of independence. For some clients, the goal is stated in terms of returning to the level of functioning prior to the admission to the hospital. This level may not be total independence—especially in the elderly population. The elderly client may need some assistance at home to allow him or her to remain in the home. Other groups of clients may have a temporary mobility impairment, and time for healing is all that is needed. Still others are faced with a permanent impairment, and the long-term level of independence is not known. This is especially true for someone with a central nervous system impairment or a stroke. Goals for these clients would be short-term ones that are achievable. For example, a goal for a paraplegic client might be transfers in and out of the wheelchair independently. The short-term goals could be

1. Demonstrates ability to do push-ups while in wheelchair
2. Transfers into wheelchair from bed with minimal assistance
3. Uses sliding board for transferring out of bed independently
4. Transfers into chair without the use of the sliding board

The evaluation of the client's functional abilities and limitations occurs on admission. Usually, these are compared against a set of standards—either internal or national. If nationally established standards are used, the outcomes are usually based on a database that is sound and recognized by third-party payers as valid and reliable. The Barthel Index is an example of a tool used to measure functional abilities. Those instruments developed internally (*e.g.*, within a hospital) have a small data sample and may be of questionable validity. An example of this kind of instrument may be a screening tool for risk of falls.

The long-term outcomes for the client with Impaired Physical Mobility include, but are not limited to, the following:

1. Increases mobility with the use of adaptive equipment
2. Increases or maintains muscle strength in the extremities
3. Demonstrates safe methods of transfers
4. Incorporates positioning plan into daily routine where appropriate
5. Ambulates with minimal assistance
6. Articulates safety measures instituted in hospital and home

Outcomes for the diagnosis of Disuse Syndrome include

1. Improves or maintains ROM
2. Maintains skin integrity
3. Describes understanding of treatment
4. Participates in ROM plan
5. Maintains or improves circulatory blood flow
6. Maximizes pulmonary status and minimizes pulmonary complications
7. Maintains or improves bowel, bladder, and kidney function
8. Maximizes nutritional status

Outcomes for a diagnosis of Knowledge Deficit may include

1. Increases understanding of physical impairment by verbalizing limitations
2. Identifies high-risk behavior
3. Participates in self-care through return demonstration
4. Lists symptoms and signs of skin care problems (*e.g.*, with cast)
5. Verbalizes emergent situations and appropriate action

Possible outcomes for a diagnosis of Pain include

1. Identifies possible source of pain
2. Describes appropriate treatment for pain
3. Manages pain adequately
4. Seeks help when pain control measures fail
5. Achieves pain control

Each goal identified by the client needs to be measurable, and the criteria indicating achievement must be agreed on by the health care team.

Implementation

The client with mobility problems benefits from a team approach to the plan of care. The nurse often assumes the role of coordinator of the care in addition to the role of direct caregiver. The approach to the plan warrants consistency, repetition, and active involvement through education of the client and family. This facilitates recovery, minimizes stress for the family and client, and offers a sound base from which to evaluate the client's response to care.

The primary means of communication between team members is the client's medical record. Hospitals are required by external regulatory agencies to provide some form of documentation. The plan of care is the means of informing colleagues what is important to maintain continuity of care. The format varies between hospitals and may include charting by exception through the use of flow sheets, clinical progressions, multidisciplinary action plans, or computerized documentation.

Document the client's response to the positioning schedule. Note the condition of the skin, the tolerance level, the presence or absence of pain, and the teaching done. Monitor the ambulation program through charting, noting the variations in progression toward or regression away from the goals. When performing ROM exercises, chart any improvement in the joint range or tightening, any signs of pain, as well as the client's level of participation.

Continually monitor the client for the risk of developing any iatrogenic complications. The risk factors for falling should also be noted in the chart, and the client should be continually screened for any added factors that might increase the risk of falling. Examples to watch for are changes in the level of consciousness, cognition, and level of mobility impairment. Noting any changes in the client's chart helps to provide the continuity of care and foster a proactive response to potential complications.

Range of Motion Exercises

Range of motion exercises begin as soon as the client is admitted. The client's current condition determines which joint motions are of the highest priority. Preference is given to those movements that are weak or limited due to the position that the client frequently assumes; *e.g.*, knee extension is emphasized in a client who sits for long periods. It is the nurse's responsibility to perform ROM exercises within the pain-free range. It is outside the realm of nursing practice to stretch tight joints and attempt to release contractures unless supervised by a therapist. As the range increases, the exercises can be modified to increase the joint range.

Before beginning the exercises, consider the amount of pain the client is experiencing along with the activity or exercise. Fatigue will always be a factor as the level of activity is increased. The exercise should be stopped or modified before the point of exhaustion. Pain medications should be given routinely—especially before the client is scheduled for any therapy or increase in activity. Other methods of pain control should also be explored with the client and physician to eliminate reliance on drugs.

Under normal circumstances, joint motion is an active process; *i.e.*, motion is produced by the individual independently without assistance or resistance from an outside force. Joint motions also may be performed passively or with some help, depending on the client's level of immobility. Emphasize the motions that are limited when performing the exercises; for example, it is not necessary to spend time flexing the knee if the client is able to walk. Use the client's ability to assist whenever possible.

COMMUNITY-BASED CARE

MOBILITY, ADAPTIVE EQUIPMENT, AND TRANSPORTATION

Illnesses such as strokes and Parkinson's disease often produce long-term or permanent mobility problems, hindering clients' independence and quality of living. Frequently, nurses, social workers, and physical and occupational therapists work collaboratively with these clients to increase their mobility and endurance. Although services need to be tailored to the client's needs and disease, interventions involve adaptive equipment, transportation, exercise programs, skin care, and other physiological and emotional issues.

If the client or family purchases or rents equipment from a medical equipment company, that company is responsible for installation. However, if the equipment is obtained from a home care agency's loan closet or from a retail outlet, installation may not be provided. In those situations, staff from local agencies on aging or volunteers from churches may be willing to install the equipment.

Clients may require assistance with transportation to obtain medical care, go grocery shopping, and attend church or events that others take for granted. Although services for those who cannot drive or have special transportation needs are increasing, barriers to using those services include expense and scheduling. In many communities, the public transportation system and private cab and van services operate handicapped-accessible vehicles; the Area Agency on Aging, the Salvation Army, and other volunteer organizations may also offer transportation services. Senior centers provide numerous services to center participants, such as weekly grocery shopping assistance on a designated day. Some health care systems offer transportation as a value-added service to attract and keep clients, providing rides for appointments with physicians or other outpatient services.

Clients may perform PROM, active ROM exercises (AROM), or active assistive ROM exercises (AAROM). PROM exercises are those that clients cannot do themselves and are performed by a caregiver, AROM exercises are those that clients can do alone, and AAROM exercises are performed with some assistance from a caregiver or a device.

Excessive stretching of joints in clients who have tight joints or spasticity or who actively resist movement may cause bleeding into the joint. This can lead to a condition known as myositis ossificans. The joint becomes stiff and difficult to move, causing further immobility. Excessive stretching can also cause edema and overstretching or tearing of the tendons, muscles, or ligaments around the joint.

Notice the client's facial expression and "body language" as the exercise is performed. If the client grimaces in pain, verify that the movement is causing the pain. Withdrawal of the limb or tensing of the body is another sign that pain or discomfort is occurring. Remember that some immobilized clients are unable to verbalize their level of pain because of communication difficulties, such as aphasia.

The movement of the joint is determined by the classification of the joint. The location of joint motions can be seen in Figure 25–5.

Before beginning ROM exercises, position the client properly. A smooth surface that is at the nurse's waist level is ideal. This keeps the activity near the nurse's center of gravity, facilitates movement with the least of amount of energy expended because the nurse does not have to work outside the base of support, and reduces the friction and shearing of the client's skin. In the supine position, the client should be placed on his or her back without a pillow under the head. Heels should be close together, and arms

should be at the side. When a client is unable to be placed in the prone position, use a side-lying position. Support the client's back with pillows to prevent his or her rolling away from the nurse. An alternative for upper extremity ROM is to place the client in a seated position. Place both of the client's feet on the floor or on footrests of a wheelchair and firmly support the client's back.

Usually ROM exercises are performed in a sequence from head to toe. They should involve the client as much as possible. Inform the client before beginning what is happening, as explaining the purpose of the exercise ensures cooperation and alleviates any fear. Support the limb that is being exercised to avoid overextension or flexion of the joint. Perform each set of exercises three times slowly. Most nurses incorporate the exercises with the morning care or bath. During the sets, notice the joints' response to the

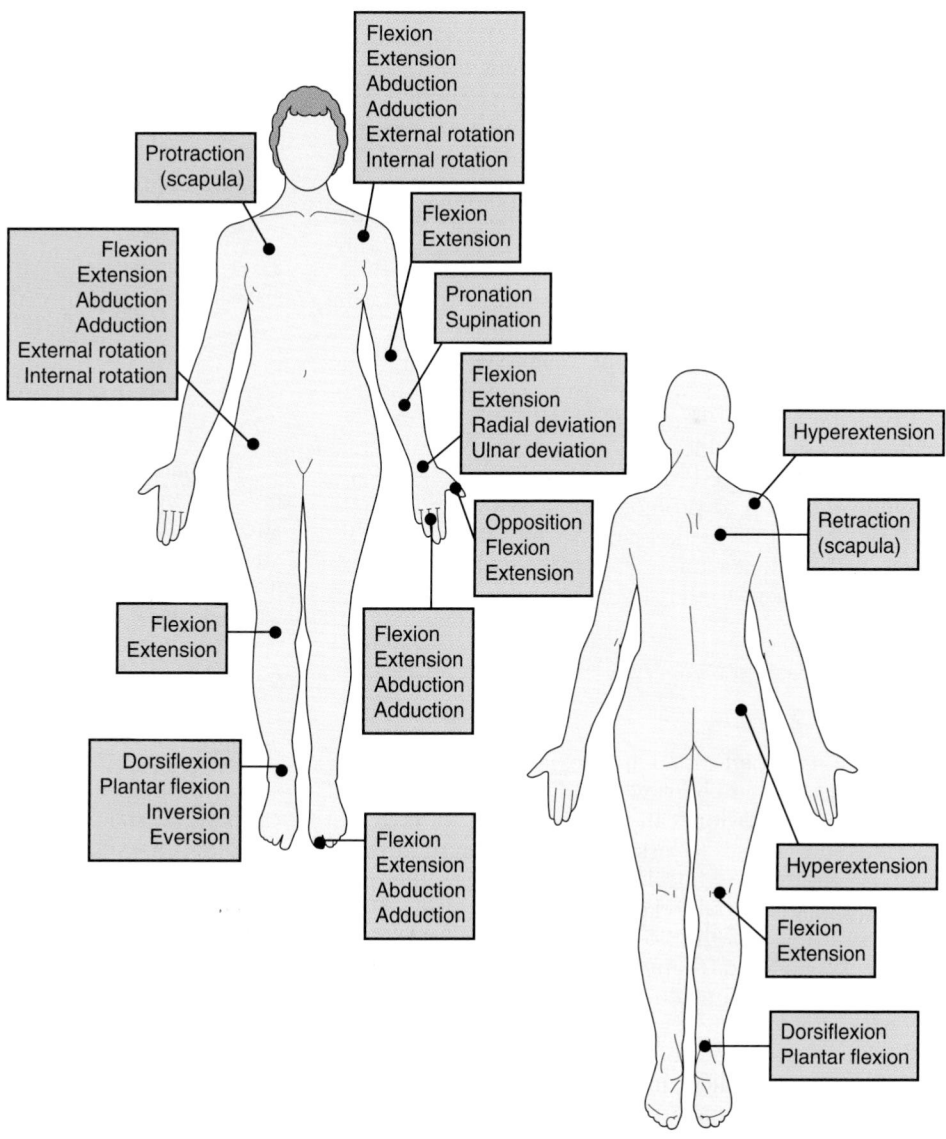

❥ **Figure 25–5**
Location of joint motions.

Anterior or supine   Posterior or prone

movement. If increased resistance or more pain occurs, make note and have the physician or therapist perform a more formal evaluation. Procedure 25–1 details ROM exercises.

Upper and Lower Extremity Exercise Variations

The client should be encouraged to participate in the exercises as much as possible. Some of the exercises do not need to be done if the client performs them as part of the daily routine and joint motion seems to be adequate. The client with a weakened upper extremity can be taught to exercise this extremity with the stronger arm. This can be accomplished either while in bed or when sitting in the chair.

Upper extremity ROM generally requires less effort than lower extremity ROM. In the case of an upper extremity with decreased sensation, a full-length mirror placed in front of the client will assist with position sense.

As the client's ability to participate in self-care increases, ROM exercises to the extremities can be done by him or her. These motions can be continued in a formal exercise program, as well as incorporated into activities of daily living. Clients maintain some ROM through walking, self-care activities such as dressing and bathing, daily tasks such as cleaning, mowing the lawn, and participation in crafts and hobbies of various kinds. It is only necessary to focus on those movements that are impaired—not those that occur naturally in everyday activities.

The client should grasp the uninvolved arm at the wrist and raise and lower the arm, as well as moving it from side to side. The client should follow the same pattern for the shoulder as is done with PROM. While the hands are clasped, the thumb of the weaker hand should be on top to promote abduction of the thumb. Do not assist the weaker arm to more than 100 degrees if the client cannot externally rotate the shoulder. Impingement to the shoulder could result.

Upper Extremity Exercises

Shoulder

Flexion is performed in the sitting position, and the stability of the client while in this position should be evaluated. Flexion can be frightening at first and requires the nurse to assist the client and possibly stabilize the trunk while he or she performs the exercise. The client should clasp the hands and reach forward and down to the floor, straightening the elbows. He or she should then raise the hands above the shoulders and return them to his or her lap. This exercise should be repeated 10 times (Fig. 25–6).

Abduction is initiated with the arms folded on the chest, with the weaker arm placed on top for support. The client should move the arms up and away from the chest and then move them from one side to another. This exercise should be repeated 10 times.

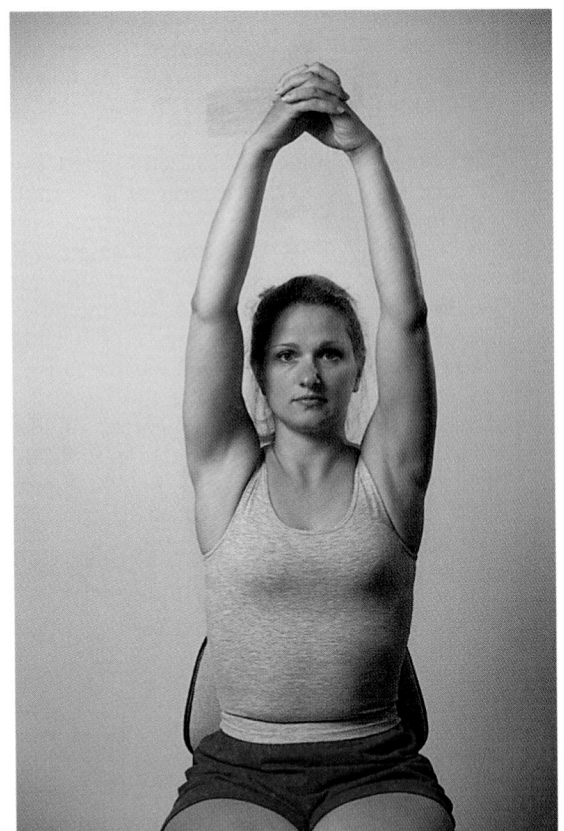

✤ **Figure 25–6**
Shoulder exercise.

Forearm

Pronation and supination are achieved by the client grasping the wrist of the weaker hand with the stronger hand while bending the elbows. He or she should turn the palm of the hand toward the ceiling and then toward the floor or table. It may be necessary for the client to sit at a table or use a lapboard in a wheelchair to facilitate this exercise (Fig. 25–7). The exercise should be repeated 10 times.

Elbow

The elbow's flexion and extension can be accomplished by the client clasping the hands in the lap, keeping the weaker thumb on top of the hand. He or she should bring the hands toward the chest, bending the elbows and then return the hands toward the lap and touch the knees, straightening the elbows as much as possible (Fig. 25–8). The exercise should be repeated 10 times.

Wrist and Finger

These exercises should also be repeated at least 10 times and can be done more than once a day if the client desires. The client clasps the hands, interlacing

Text continued on page 668

PROCEDURE

25–1

RANGE OF MOTION EXERCISES

Equipment:

Hospital bed
Pillows (small and large)
Wheelchair

Steps	Rationale

Head and Neck

1. Ask the client to "roll" the head gently down, to the right, around to the back, to the left, and then return it to the erect position. Have the client turn the head as far as possible to the left and then to the right.

1. Movements of the head and neck are active motions. They are seldom done passively because of the danger of causing an injury to the cervical spine.

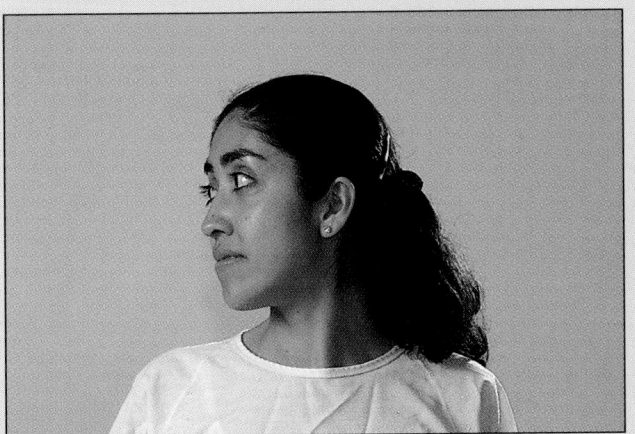

Step 1. *Neck pivot to right.*

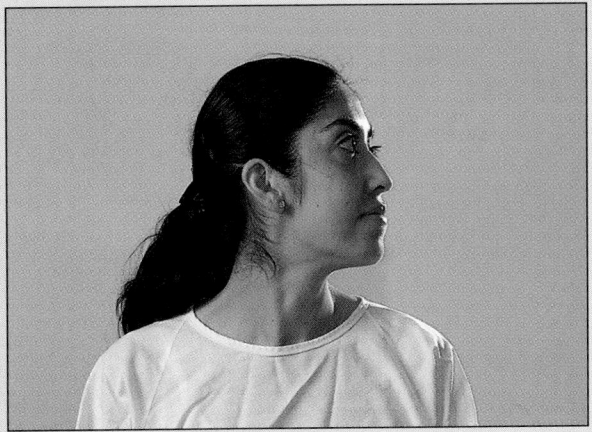

Step 1. *Neck pivot to left.*

2. Ask the client to bring the chin to the chest, return to the erect position, tilt head back as far as possible, and return to the erect position.

3. Have the client tilt the head toward each shoulder and then return to the erect position.

2, 3. The joints in the neck and head are amphiarthrodial and pivot joints. They allow rotation, side bending, flexion, extension, and limited movement between the bodies of the vertebrae.

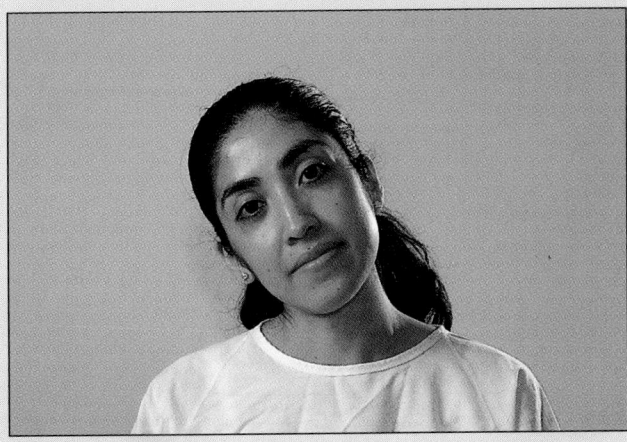

Step 3. *Neck tilt to right.*

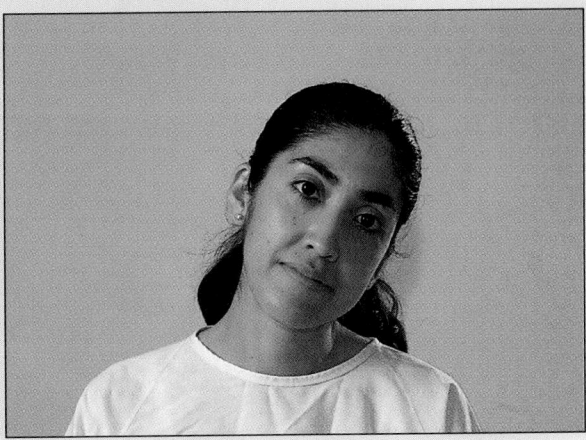

Step 3. *Neck tilt to left.*

Continued

RANGE OF MOTION EXERCISES
(Continued)

Steps	Rationale
Trunk	
4. Support the client as he or she leans forward from the waist, returns to erect standing position, arches back as far as possible, and returns to neutral standing position.	**4.** The joints in the trunk are amphiarthrodial and gliding, permitting slight movement; joints glide on each other between the arches of the vertebrae.
5. Assist the client to lean to either side and then return to neutral standing position.	**5.** These activities are done when transferring and positioning a client. They can be harmful to the lower back of the nurse and therefore require the use of good body mechanics.
Shoulder	
6. Flexion and extension—cup the client's elbow with the hand and grasp the client's wrist. Lift the arm, "reaching" toward the ceiling, keeping the client's arm to the side of the body. Keep the elbow as close to the client's head as possible. Then return the arm to the resting position while continuing to support it.	**6.** It may be necessary to bend the elbow as the arm is brought over the head to avoid hitting the head.

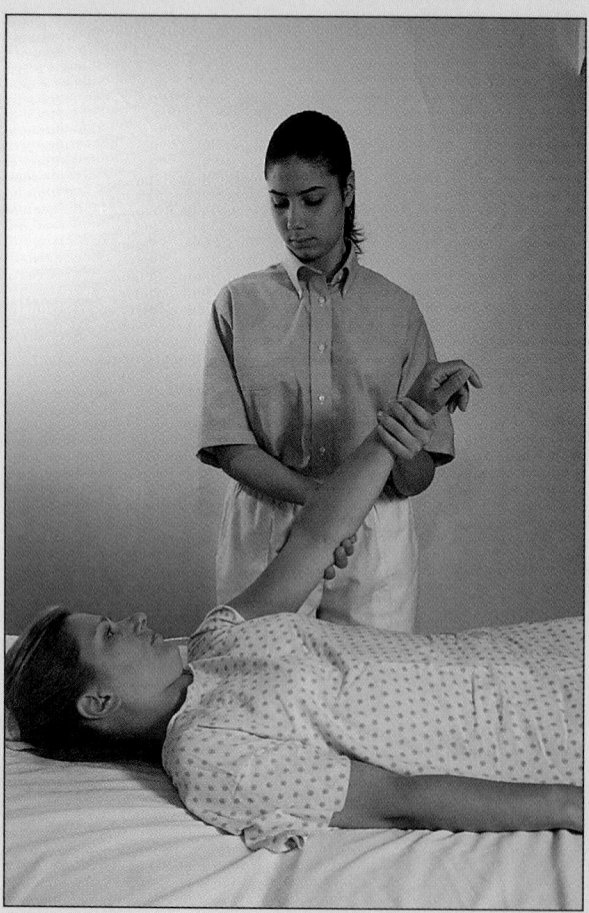

Step 6. *Shoulder flexion.*

RANGE OF MOTION EXERCISES
(Continued)

Steps	Rationale
7. Externally rotate the shoulder to 90 degrees.	**7.** The shoulder is a ball-and-socket joint that allows the maximal amount of movement possible. The potential also exists for causing further damage to the shoulder if care is not taken. The exercises for the shoulder should be performed in the sequence indicated.
8. Protraction—place one hand under the client's scapula and lift the shoulder off the bed, bringing the shoulder forward.	**8.** Pay special attention to the scapula. Evaluate the mobility of the joint by placing a hand over the scapula. A forward glide of the scapula is necessary to reduce the possibility of injury. If any question arises, check with the physician before beginning the exercise.

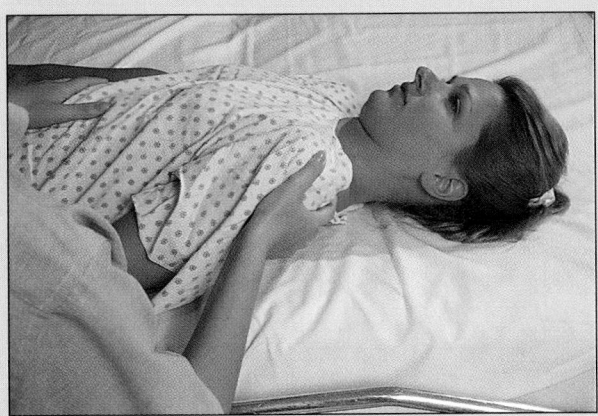

Step 8. *Shoulder protraction.*

9. Abduction and adduction—place your hand under the client's elbow and support the client's forearm with your own arm. Bring the arm out to the side and move it away from the body until it reaches a 90-degree angle. Continue to move the client's arm toward the head while grasping the client's arm at the wrist. Flex the elbow as the arm is moved overhead. Keep the elbow as close to the bed as possible and keep the shoulder in external rotation. Return to starting position.	**9.** Flexing the elbow when the arm is overhead increases the range.

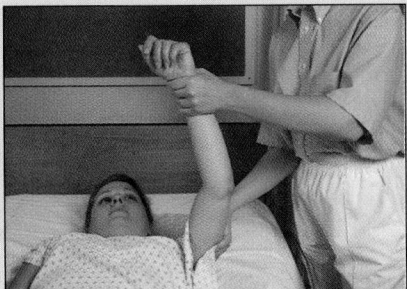

Step 9. *Shoulder abduction.*

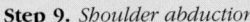

Step 9. *Shoulder abduction.*

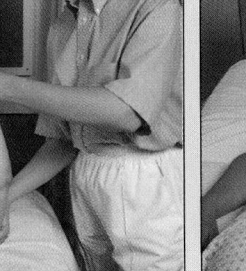

Step 9. *Shoulder adduction.*

Continued

PROCEDURE

25–1

RANGE OF MOTION EXERCISES
(Continued)

Steps

Rationale

10. Hyperextension—place one hand on the client's shoulder and grasp the arm at the wrist with the other hand. While standing slightly behind the client, bring the arm straight back, keeping the trunk from bending forward.

10. Hyperextension can be done while the client is in the prone position. Perform all exercises that require the prone position at one time to conserve the client's energy.

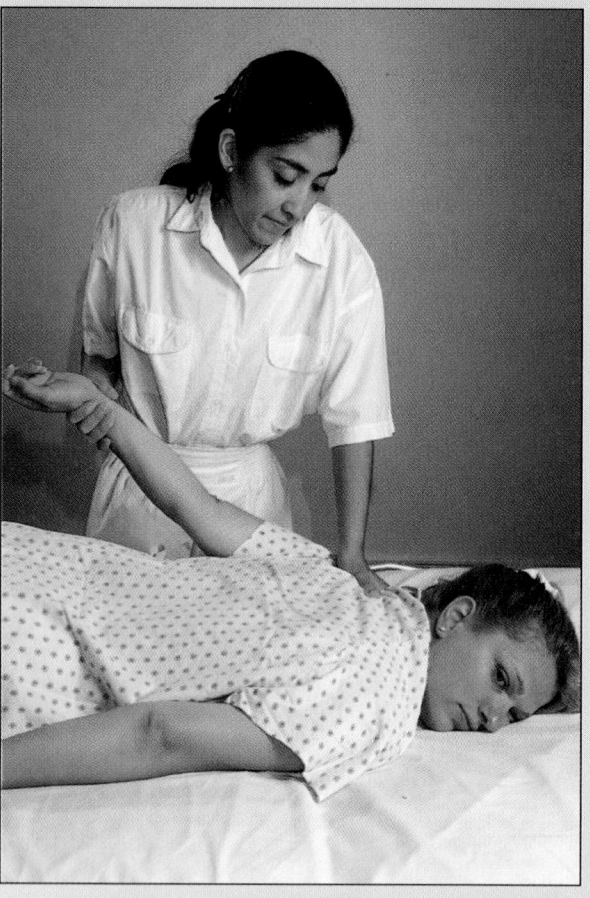

Step 10. *Shoulder hyperextension—prone position.*

11. Rotation—support the elbow with one hand and grasp the palmar surface of the client's hand with the other. Place your thumb on the back of the client's hand. Bring the arm out to the side at shoulder level and bend the elbow to achieve a right angle with the forearm. Roll the forearm down so that the palm touches the bed and then rotate it so the back of the hand touches the bed.

11. Full ROM.

RANGE OF MOTION EXERCISES
(Continued)

Steps	Rationale
12. Retraction—with the client in prone position, cup one hand over the client's shoulder. Lift the shoulder off the bed as if bringing the shoulder blades together.	**12.** See rationale for Step 8.

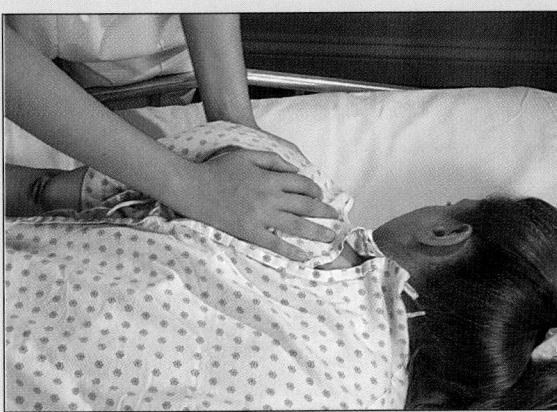

Step 12. *Shoulder retraction.*

Elbow and Forearm

13. Flexion and extension—grasp the client's hand and place the thumb over the back of the client's hand and fingers. Bend the elbow. Return the arm to starting position.	**13.** The elbow is a hinge joint whose ROM is limited to flexion and extension.

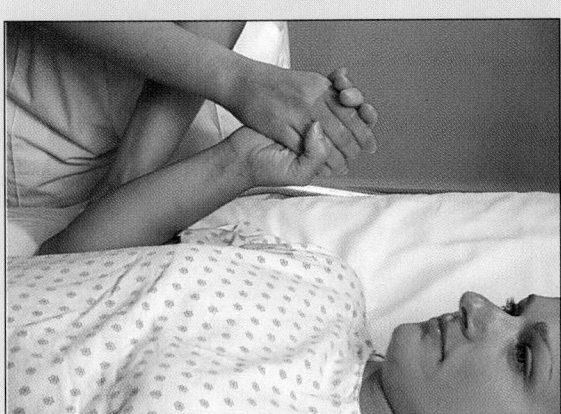

Step 13. *Elbow flexion.*

14. Pronation and supination—secure the client's hand close to the wrist. Place your index finger over the wrist to keep it straight and avoid movement in the wrist joint. Turn the palm downward and then upward.	**14.** The forearm is a pivot joint whose motion is limited to rotation. Motions should take place in the forearm, not the wrist or shoulder.

Continued

RANGE OF MOTION EXERCISES
(Continued)

Steps	Rationale

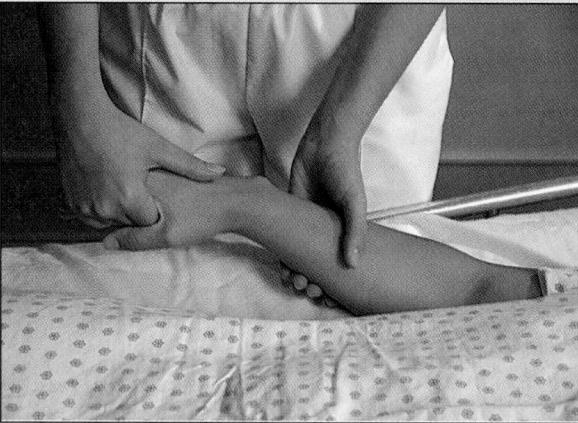

Step 14. *Forearm pronation.*

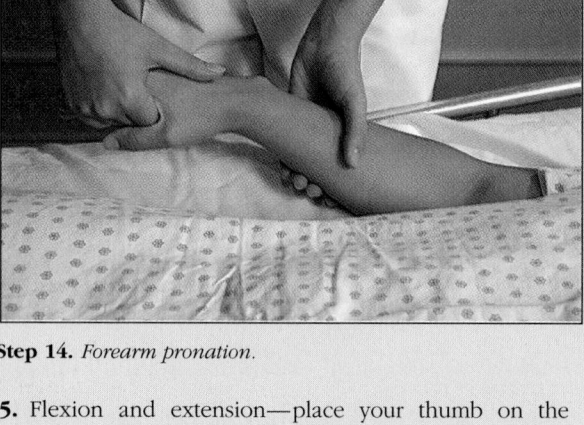

Step 14. *Forearm supination.*

15. Flexion and extension—place your thumb on the back of the client's wrist. While supporting the forearm with the other hand, bend the wrist forward, return to neutral, and then bend wrist backward, monitoring the client at all times for any sign of pain.

15, 16. The wrist joint is a condyloid joint that permits a wide range of motion, excluding rotation.

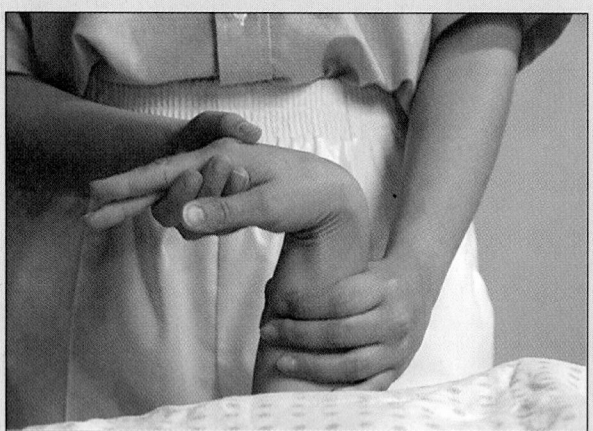

Step 15. *Passive range of motion—wrist flexion.*

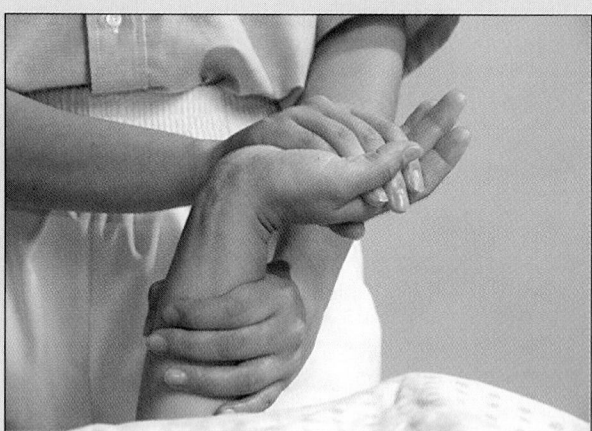

Step 15. *Passive range of motion—wrist extension.*

25–1

RANGE OF MOTION EXERCISES
(Continued)

Steps	**Rationale**
16. Radial and ulnar deviation—while supporting the wrist, move the hand first toward the thumb and then toward the little finger side.	

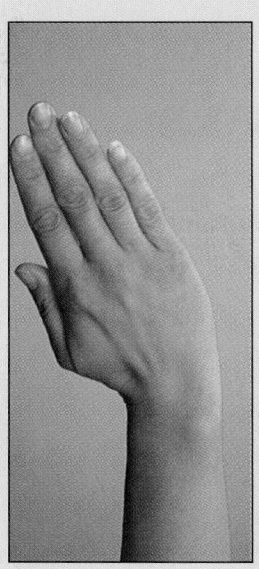 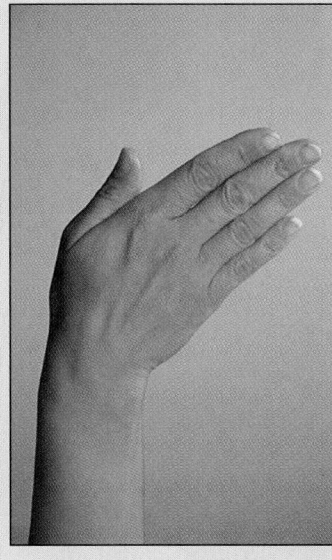

Step 16. *Radial deviation.*   **Step 16.** *Ulnar deviation.*

Fingers

17. Flexion and extension—flex the client's elbow and cup your hand over the back of the client's hand. Support the forearm and wrist with the other hand. Curl the fingers down to make a fist and then straighten out the fingers.	**17.** Support the wrist in the neutral position.

Continued

PROCEDURE

25–1

RANGE OF MOTION EXERCISES
(Continued)

Steps	Rationale

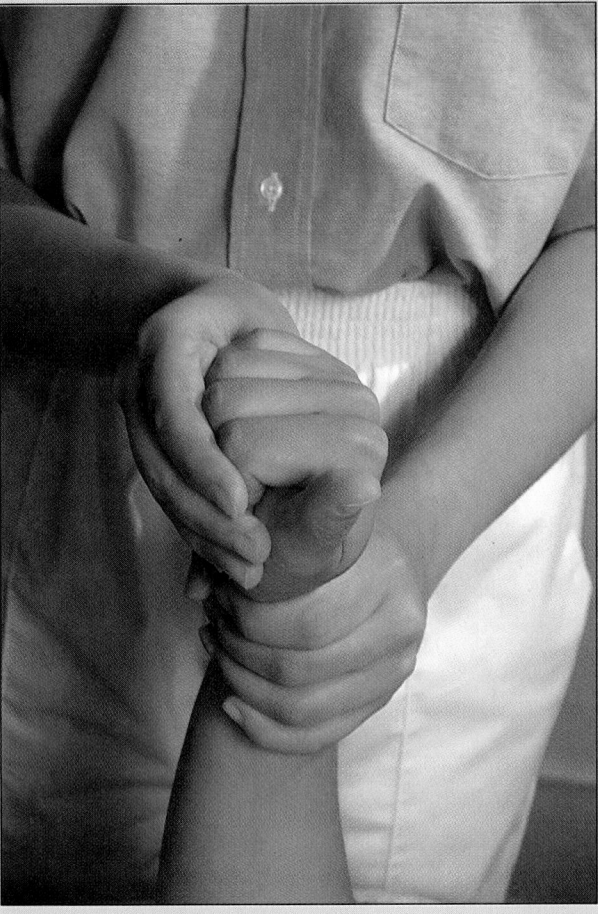

Step 17. *Passive range of motion—finger flexion.*

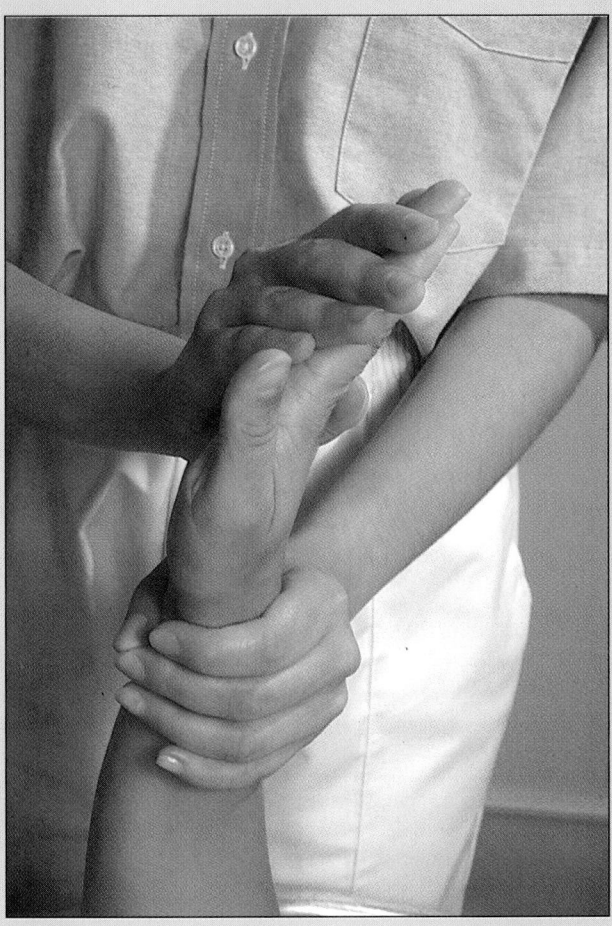

Step 17. *Passive range of motion—finger extension.*

18. Abduction and adduction—move the fingers one at a time away from the adjacent fingers and then back. This exercise can be done with the client's hand on the bed or with the elbow flexed.

Thumb

19. Opposition—move the client's thumb in an outward circling motion.

Hip

20. Flexion and extension—while supporting the knee with one hand and the heel with the other, raise the leg and bring the knee up toward the client's chest but not beyond a 90-degree angle unless the therapist or physician has written an order to do so; return to starting position.

18. The fingers are condyloid and hinge joints, whose movement is limited to flexion and extension, as well as motion similar to that of the ball-and-socket joint, excluding rotation.

19. The thumb is a saddle joint, which allows motion in all directions but has limited rotation. Abduction and adduction were included in exercises for fingers.

20. The hip joint is a ball-and-socket joint that allows the widest ROM. If increased motion is desired at the hip, bend the knee and move it toward the client's chin.

RANGE OF MOTION EXERCISES
(Continued)

Steps	**Rationale**
21. Hyperextension—with the client in the prone position, place one hand on the buttock and move the leg up to achieve optimal mobility.	**21.** The hand prevents the hip from lifting off the bed.
22. Abduction and adduction—support the knee and heel while keeping the client's leg close to, but not on, the bed. Move the leg away from midline, return to midline, and then move across the opposite leg; return the leg to midline.	**22.** Avoid dragging the leg on the bed.

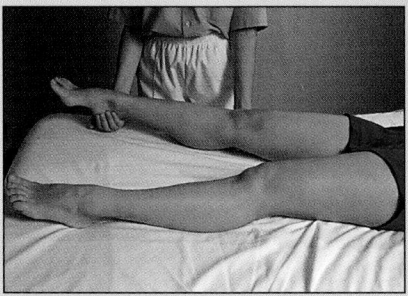

Step 22. *Passive range of motion— abduction of hip.*

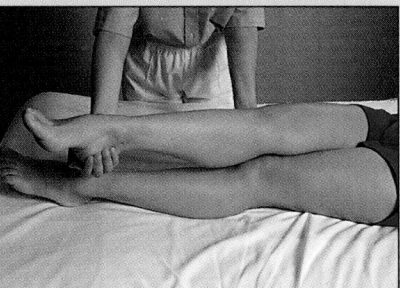

Step 22. *Adduction of hip—across opposite leg.*

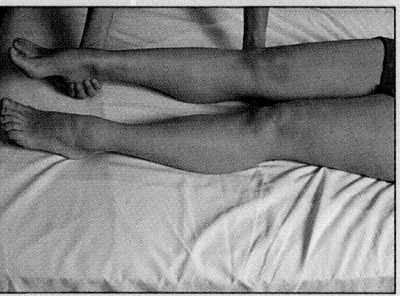

Step 22. *Adduction of hip—return to midline.*

23. Internal and external rotation—roll the leg inward and then outward.	**23.** Note that outward motion may not be needed if you find the leg naturally moving into this position when the client is lying down.

Step 23. *Internal rotation.*

Knee

24. Place one hand under the client's knee and hold the heel with the other hand. Bend the hip to a 90-degree angle, then bend the knee by bringing the ankle toward the buttocks without forcing. Support the leg at all times and avoid dropping the leg when straightening. Return to starting position.	**24.** The knee is a hinge joint, with motion limited to flexion and extension. The exercise can be done with the client in the prone position, but knee flexion will be less because of secondary muscles crossing both hip and knee.

Continued

PROCEDURE

25–1

RANGE OF MOTION EXERCISES
(Continued)

Steps	Rationale

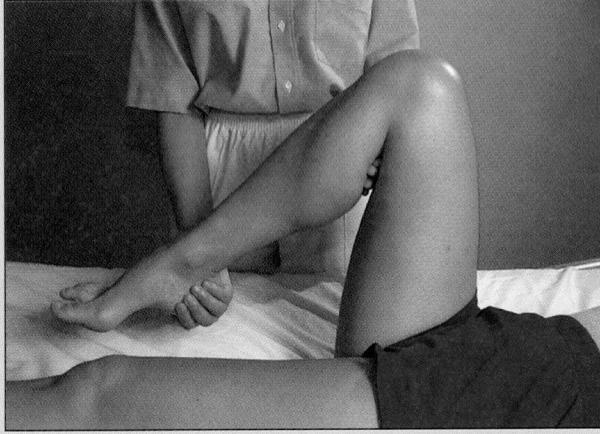

Step 24. *Knee flexion—supine.*

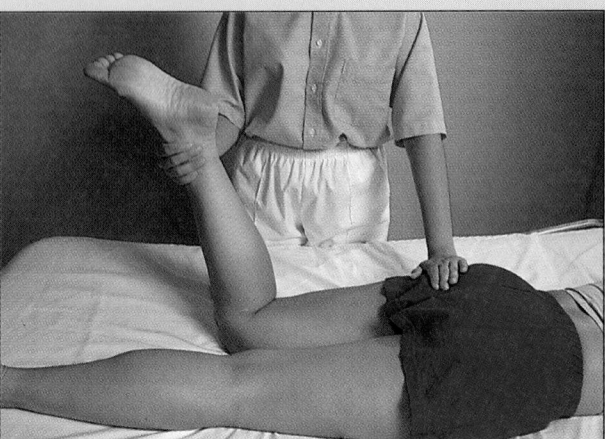

Step 24. *Knee flexion—prone position.*

Ankle

25. Flexion and extension—grasp the ankle with one hand while holding the foot with the other. Bend the foot toward the toes and then bend the foot down.

25. The ankle is a hinge joint, with motion limited to flexion and extension. The ankle needs only to achieve a 90-degree angle to support the standing position and slightly more to aid walking.

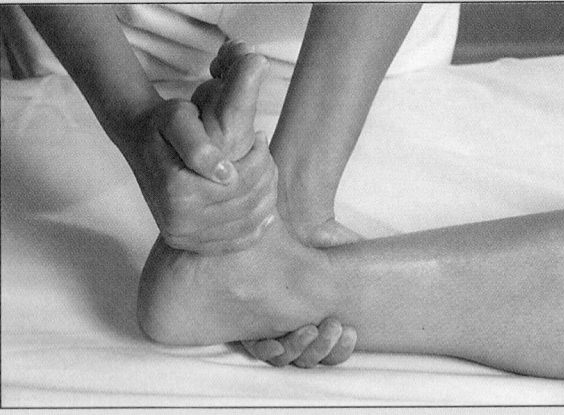

Step 25. *Ankle flexion.*

RANGE OF MOTION EXERCISES
(Continued)

Steps	Rationale
26. Inversion and eversion—turn the foot toward the outside and then the inside.	**26.** This helps tone the muscles supporting the foot.

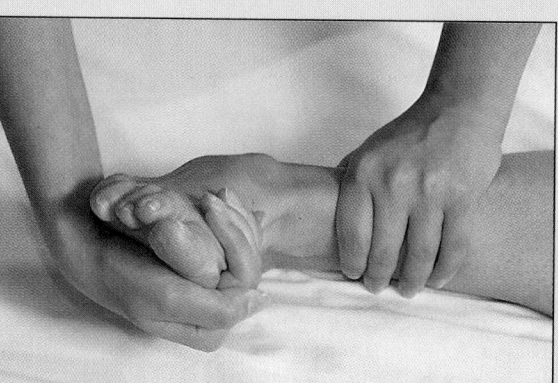

Step 26. *Ankle inversion.*

Toes

27. Flexion and extension—cup the hands over the toes and curl them toward the sole of the foot, then straighten them.	**27, 28.** The toes consist of a modified ball-and-socket joint and a condyloid joint. These joints allow the widest ROM, except for the condyloid joint, which does not permit rotation.
28. Abduction and adduction—move the toes apart and then bring them together.	

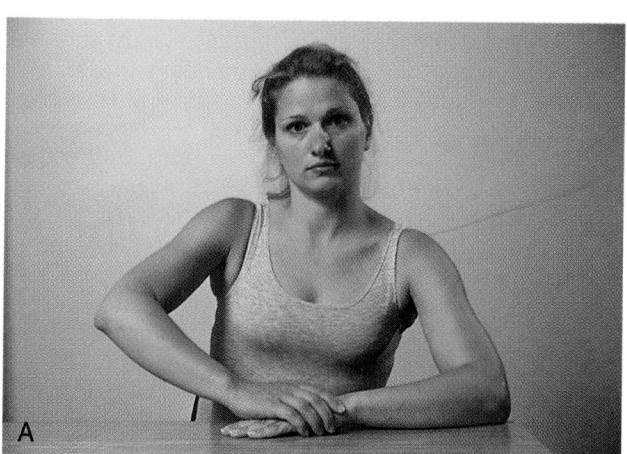
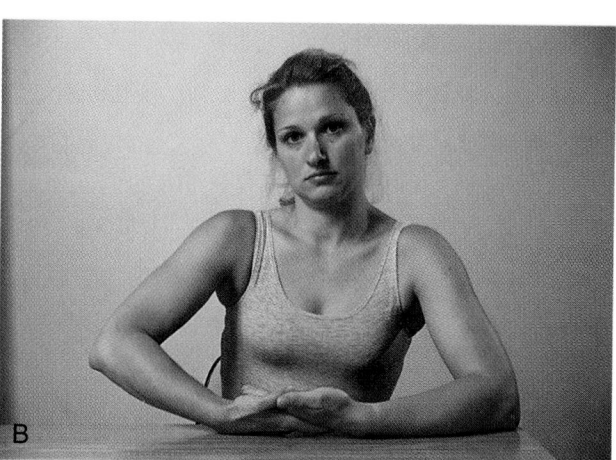

🔖 **Figure 25–7**
Forearm exercise. *A,* Pronation. *B,* Supination.

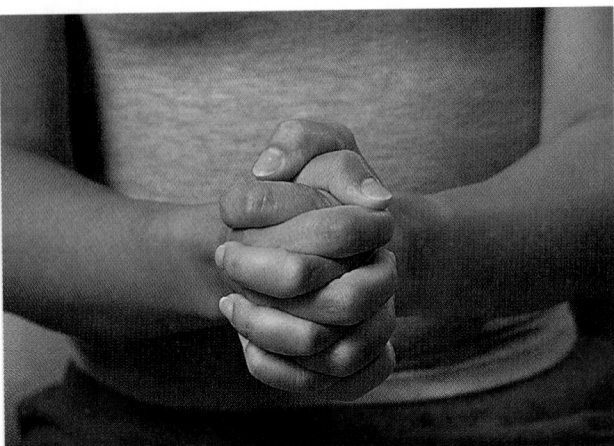

❧ **Figure 25–8**
Wrist exercise—clasped hands.

the fingers, with the weaker thumb on top. He or she should then extend and flex the wrist by bending the wrist first to one side and then the other (Fig. 25–9). The client should bend the wrist toward the ceiling and then the floor to accomplish radial and ulnar deviation. With the stronger hand, he or she grasps the thumb of the weaker hand and rotates in a circle to promote thumb extension. Using the stronger hand, the client should grasp the fingers of the weaker hand and curl them into a fist to facilitate finger extension and flexion.

The weaker hand often assumes the position of having the wrist bent forward and the fingers curled over the thumb into a fist. If the hand is left in this position, it will develop contractures and be nonfunctional. The flexor muscles are much stronger than the extensors and must be overridden. A splint may be needed to inhibit flexor muscle strength, and exercises should be done to promote extensor activity.

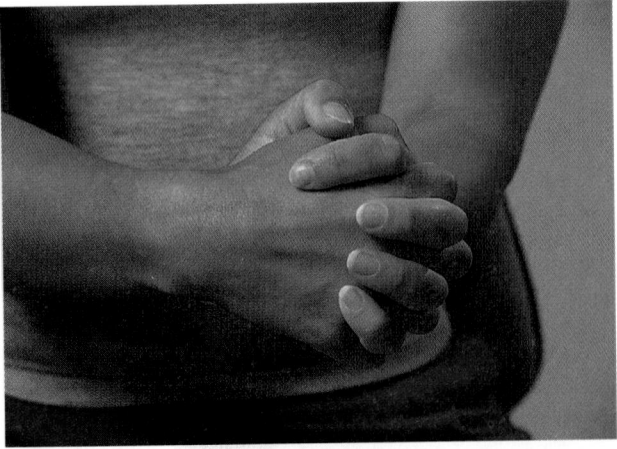

❧ **Figure 25–9**
Wrist exercise—flexion and extension of wrist.

Lower Extremity Exercises

The following exercises can be done either in the sitting or the lying position. The safety of the client should be considered, and the trunk stability and sitting balance should be evaluated before the exercises are recommended. These exercises should be repeated 10 times.

While lying in bed in the supine position, the client should slide the foot of the stronger leg under the knee of the weaker leg and down the leg to the ankle. He or she should bend the stronger leg, causing the weaker one to bend at the knee and the hip. As the leg is brought up toward the body, the client grasps the weaker leg and pulls the knee toward the chest (Fig. 25–10) and then reverses the procedure. Initially, this exercise will need to be demonstrated and supported. Less help will be needed as the client progresses. Clients who have paralyzed or very weak lower extremities can perform exercises on their lower extremities after they have learned to maintain upper body stability. The client can achieve stability by resting against the wall or the headboard of the bed.

The client can perform hip and knee flexion by placing one hand under the knee and pulling it toward the chest. He or she should then place one hand on the shin and the other on the knee, pulling the leg as close to the chest as possible. The client repeats this procedure with the other leg (Fig. 25–11).

Rotation, abduction, and adduction of the hip are accomplished when the client places one foot against the opposite leg, holding it and gently pushing down the knee of the bent leg with the other hand to achieve hip rotation and abduction (Fig. 25–12). Toe flexion and extension can be done in this position (Fig. 25–13). The client should then balance on one arm while bringing the knee toward the chest and placing the foot flat on the floor. He or she then gently presses the bent knee over the straight leg as far as possible, rotating and adducting the hip (Fig. 25–14).

The client can perform straight leg raising while lying down. He or she grasps one leg and pulls toward the chest until he or she is able to grasp the ankle. The client then pulls the leg toward the chest with the hand and begins to straighten the knee by pushing on it with one hand. He or she should not pull the leg so far as to lift the other leg off the bed or floor; doing this causes a stretch to the low back rather than to the hamstrings (Fig. 25–15).

At all times, continue to teach the client what to do to achieve maximal independence. Encourage the client to use either the uninvolved extremities (self-assistive) or other devices. AAROM exercises are so called because the client is actively doing part of the motion. Use of devices often makes the exercise easier and more interesting for the client.

PROM machines are often used with clients who have undergone joint replacement because they eliminate the fatigue factor for the client. However, consul-

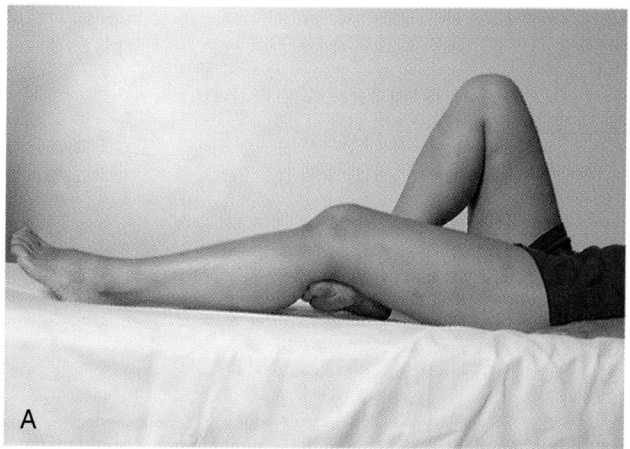

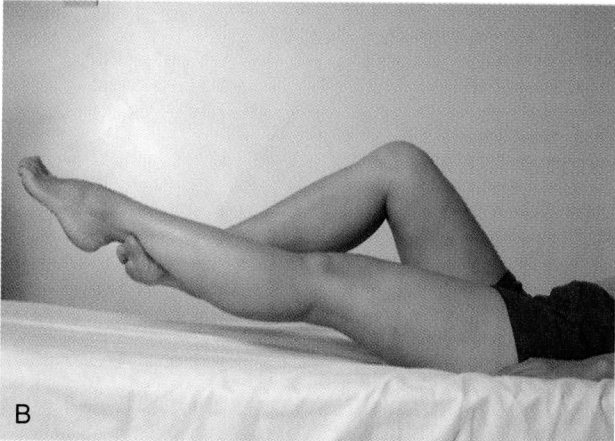

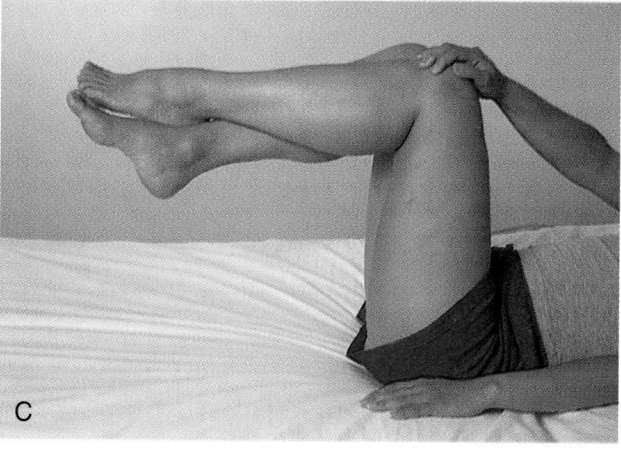

♪ Figure 25–10
Lower extremity exercise. *A,* Foot under knee. *B,* Foot under ankle.
C, Leg and hand pulling leg up.

tation with a therapist is essential before any program is started—especially if pulleys or other mechanical devices are to be used. It is very easy to cause more damage if aids are used that are not familiar to the nurse.

Incorporating exercises into daily activities can achieve several client goals simultaneously. Increased joint ROM, increased participation in self-care, and a variation in the ROM program are a few of these goals. For example, sweeping involves several upper and lower extremity and trunk motions. Dressing accomplishes gross motions of the joints when the client puts on the larger articles of clothing. Encouraging these activities gives a client a sense of control and increases self-worth, which is important for quick recovery.

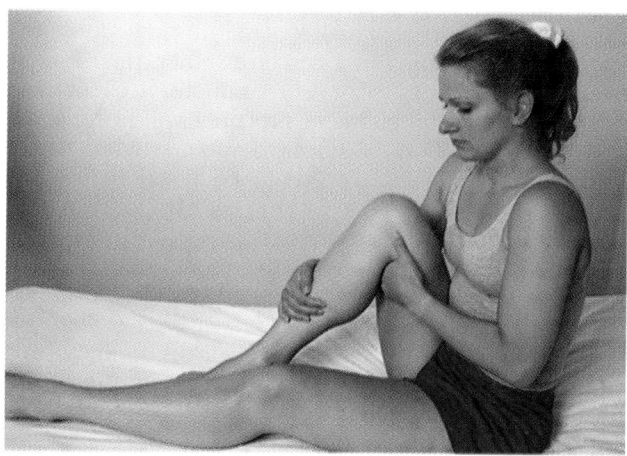

♪ Figure 25–11
Hip and knee flexion.

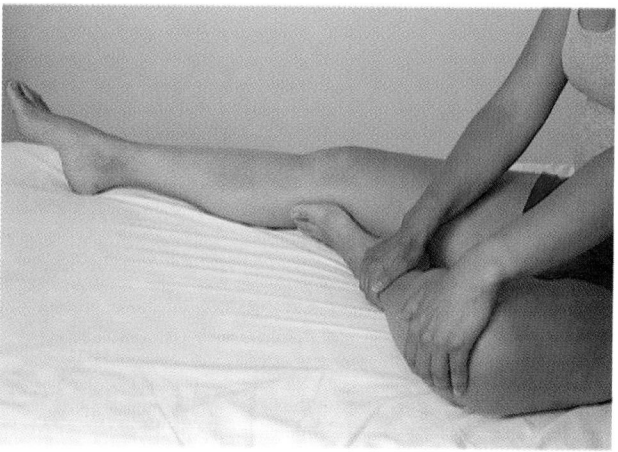

♪ Figure 25–12
Rotation and abduction of hip—knee toward chest.

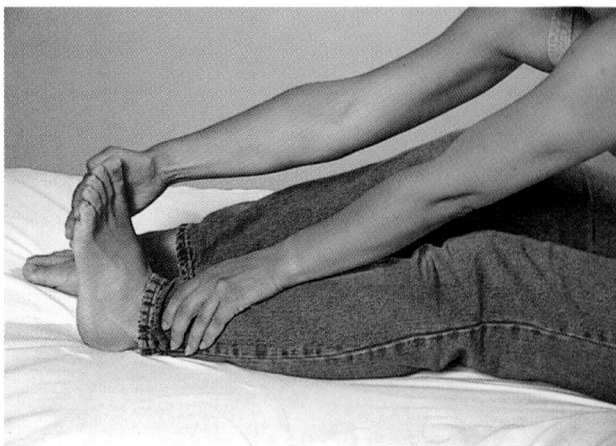

❯ **Figure 25–13**
Toe flexion.

Table **25–2**		
POSITIONING SCHEDULE		
TIME	**POSITION**	**COMMENTS**
6:00–8:00 A.M.	Left side lying	8:00 A.M. breakfast, followed by bowel program
8:00–10:00 A.M.	Supine	Bed bath, including ROM to lower extremities
10:00–11:00 A.M.	Prone	Back care; work up tolerance—now at 40 min
11:00–1:00 P.M.	Sitting	Lunch—feeds self
1:00–3:00 P.M.	Left side lying	Visiting with family
3:00–4:00 P.M.	Prone	Back; ROM—tolerates 35 min; need to increase
4:00–6:00 P.M.	Supine	Dinner—feeds self
6:00–8:00 P.M.	Right side lying	Visiting
8:00–11:00 P.M.	Left side lying	HS care
11:00–3:00 A.M.	Supine	Sleeping
3:00–6:00 A.M.	Right side lying	Sleeping; skin intact with no red areas

Positioning

Positioning Schedule

A **positioning schedule** is developed to achieve the goals of preventing skin breakdown and contractures and promoting adequate ventilation of the lungs. It is necessary for clients who have a mobility impairment who are usually confined to bed or are in a wheelchair for the majority of the day. The frequency of position change depends on a number variables, including comfort, amount of self-movement, edema in the extremities, sensation, pain, and physical status. The standard rule has been that the schedule should cover the entire day and the position should be changed every 2 hours. See Table 25–2 for an example of a positioning schedule. However, for some clients, 2 hours is too long a time to maintain one position. Some individuals become extremely uncomfortable after 30 minutes, whereas others can tolerate the same position for up to 4 hours. If an individual either can shift weight or has some movement, he or

she should be encouraged to change positions frequently independently. For a paralyzed person or someone who has lost sensation, especially in the lower limbs, 2 hours may be too long to wait. These clients usually are unaware of the problems associated with sitting too long because they do not feel the discomfort. Therefore, the nurse must intervene. Edematous tissue, coupled with decreased sensation, is much more susceptible to the development of pressure ulcers and bears close inspection in a positioning program.

The plan is developed based on the following considerations. Do any specific medical or surgical conditions affect the client's positioning needs? Certain conditions determine what the client can and cannot do. If the client has had a surgical procedure that precludes positioning in a certain manner, then it must be factored into the plan. For example, a client who has a respiratory impairment probably will not tolerate the prone position, whereas someone who has a lower limb amputation needs to be positioned prone at least once during the 24-hour shift to prevent hip and knee flexion contractures.

The client's pulse should be monitored to determine the tolerance level. If he or she has been on bed rest for a time, the pulse will increase as activity increases, and dizziness, lightheadedness, and nausea can result. This is the cardiovascular system's response to being deconditioned.

The time of day is an important factor to consider when developing a plan. If the client is able to tolerate a longer period between position changes, the nurse should plan to use this extended period for

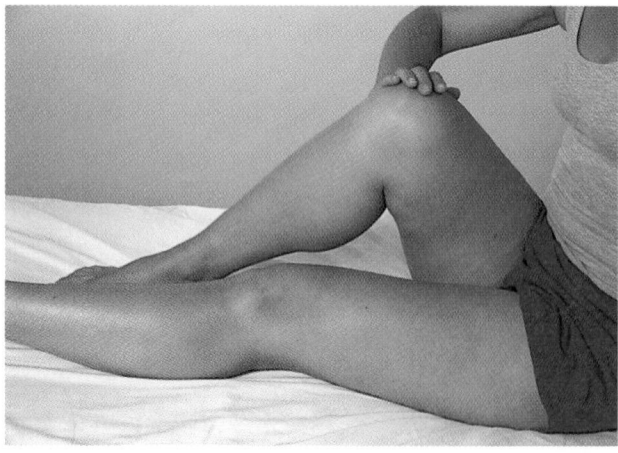

❯ **Figure 25–14**
Rotation and abduction of the hip—press bent knee over straight leg.

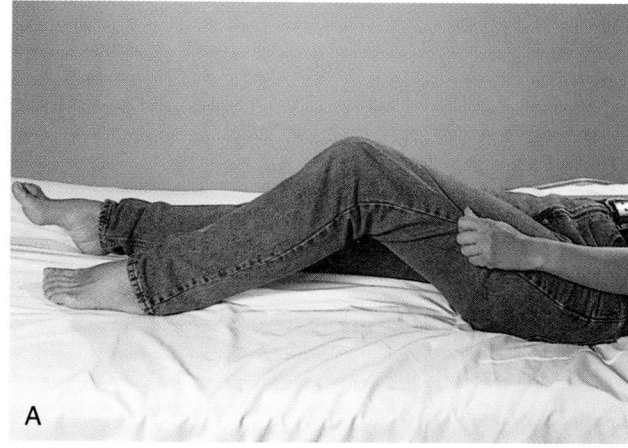
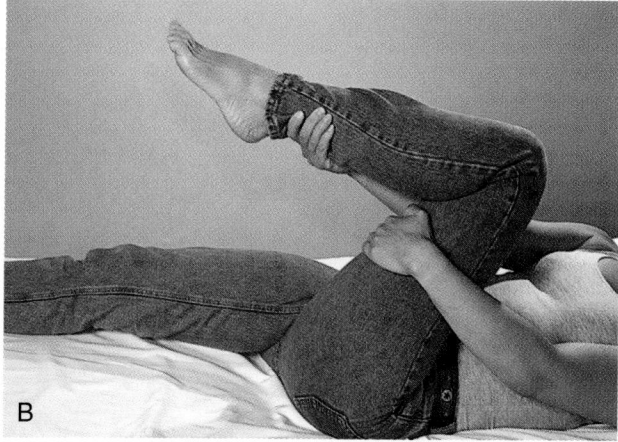
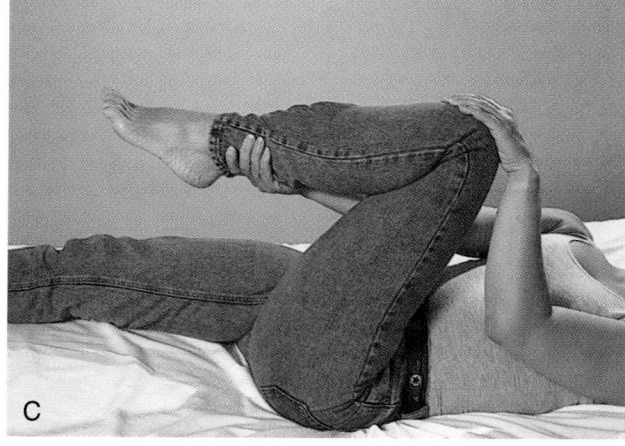
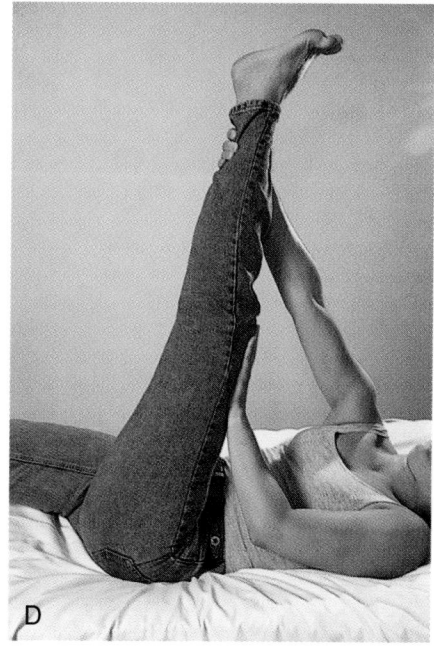

❧ **Figure 25–15**
Straight leg raising. *A*, Grasp leg. *B*, Pull leg toward chest. *C*, Prepare for straightening. *D*, Leg straight.

sleep at night. This will help to reduce the amount of fatigue the client is experiencing due to constant disruption of the sleep cycle. If the client participates in therapies, he or she should sit between position changes.

Posting the positioning and **turning schedule** (a planned schedule for turning to minimize contractures and to relieve skin pressure) at the bedside allows communication among the nursing staff and the client and family. Knowledge of the schedule gives the client the ability to control part of the care and supports the goal of independence. The schedule also facilitates the education of the family and client about positioning, allows the family to participate in the care of the client, and affords the nurse the time to evaluate the effects of the education.

A client who has a central nervous system insult or injury, such as a stroke or head injury, will experience either muscle weakness or paralysis in some part of the body. Noting how the client compensates for the deficits is a part of the basic care plan and is

included in the positioning plan by identifying the impact of these deficits. For example, if a client has a weak or paralyzed side and tends to ignore it because of sensory loss, spatial problems, or a cognitive deficit, the nurse and the therapists must build into the plan interventions to focus on that side. The Sample Nursing Care Plan describes care for a client who has had a stroke.

An injury to the brain causes the muscle reflexes to become exaggerated. A lesion, such as a tumor in the brain, interferes with the normal postural reflexes of activities such as standing, sitting, and lying. A pattern of muscle spasm develops, in which most commonly, the affected shoulder is retracted, the forearm is pronated, the wrist and hand are flexed, the pelvis is retracted, and the leg is internally rotated. The hip, knee, and ankle are extended on the affected side, while the ankle inverts and shows plantar flexion. The trunk is flexed toward the side that has been affected. This position is often seen in a client who has had a stroke when he or she is lying in bed without any

SAMPLE NURSING CARE PLAN

CLIENT WHO HAS HAD A STROKE

A 55-year-old man, Mr. Bigelow, is admitted to the nursing unit from another hospital. His wife was unable to arouse him in the morning 2 days ago. There is weakness on the left side of the body, and he is unable to move about in bed. A diagnosis of cerebral vascular accident (stroke) has been made. The left side of his body has flaccid muscle tone. As his nurse, you must begin to teach him to turn in bed, especially onto his left side, as part of his plan of care.

Nursing Diagnosis: Impaired Physical Mobility related to paralysis of the left side of the body, secondary to the cerebral vascular accident.

Expected Outcome: Client will be able to turn onto the left side with minimal assistance.

Action	Rationale
1. Assess the level of understanding.	1. Clients often have communication impairments after a stroke.
2. Develop, in writing, a teaching plan.	2. Writing down the plan will help with consistency of approach.
3. Explain plan to the client through the use of demonstration, pictures, touch, and verbal cues.	3. The client will participate more when he or she understands the plan. Stimulating multiple senses will assist with comprehension.
4. Instruct the client to lift leg with the right hand while demonstrating action.	4. Lifting the leg off bed reduces friction.
5. Instruct the client to grasp side rail with right hand	5. This action uses the client's own muscle strength and promotes a feeling of independence.
6. Roll the client onto the left side.	6. Initially, assistance from the nurse conserves the client's strength.
7. Evaluate the client's response.	7. Evaluation guides the nurse in determining what changes must be made.
8. Document care given and the response in the client's medical record.	8. Documentation provides the consistency that is needed between caregivers.

positioning. The tendency when there is no voluntary control of the muscles is for the body to develop synergistic patterns; **synergy** involves combined contractions of muscles working together as a unit with cortical control of the brain. The goal of a positioning program with such a client is to position "out of synergy" and reeducate the limbs to achieve maximal recovery. Another goal is to reduce the amount of **spasticity** (an involuntary movement of the muscle to a stimulus) that may develop. For this reason, restraints are not used with clients who have muscle spasticity. The stimulus of the restraint against movement causes further spasticity in the restrained limb and negates the impact of the positioning program.

Occasionally, a client's preexisting condition may prevent the ideal positioning plan from being used. Fractures or a pressure ulcer may preclude the ideal, and adjustments must be made. For example, positioning the client on an ulcer is not an option. Casts, splints, and other devices affect the plan, as well as pain or contractures from arthritis or prolonged immobility, and they should be accommodated. Procedure 25–2 describes positioning.

Sitting Positions

During sitting, the pelvis assumes an anterior tilt and a normal lumbar lordosis and an upright spine are present, with the head centered. The average chair supports the trunk and thigh at an angle of 100 to 105 degrees, with a seat height 16 in from the floor. The back of the chair supports the scapula and promotes lumbar lordosis when it has a support in the low back region.

A wheelchair that is not modified does not provide these features or support the seated position. The wheelchair seat is a sling designed for ease of storage and not for a stable base of support. These seats promote internal rotation and adduction of the legs and a posterior pelvic tilt. Often, clients who sit in wheelchairs develop uneven hip heights, and the weaker hip retracts. The results are often seen as an angular orientation in the chair. Because of the sling seat and back of a wheelchair, it is difficult for the client to maintain an anterior tilt. As a result, the client tends to slide forward in the chair, the foot often falls off the footrest, and the client has a difficult time maintaining any kind of correct sitting posture (Fig. 25–16).

Text continued on page 677

PROCEDURE

25-2

POSITIONING

Equipment:

Hospital bed
Small and large pillows
Footboard
Trochanter roll
Transfer belt

Steps	Rationale
Bed Positioning: Supine	
1. Place a small pillow under the scapula, which extends to the arm and supports it in an abducted and slightly elevated position. Position this pillow between the arm and the side.	**1.** When positioning the client supine, the affected upper extremity should be placed in the abducted position; the shoulder is protracted and rotated externally, the wrist is extended, and the elbow and the forearm are supinated.
2. If the hand is held in a fist, a splint may be needed.	**2.** Avoid soft rolls, such as a rolled washcloth or sponge. These only increase the flexor tone of the muscle in the hand and promote the clenched fist position.
3. The hip is protracted, slightly flexed, and held in a neutral position. Slight flexion of the knee is supported with a flat pillow that can also support the hip. Also, a trochanter roll can be used to hold the hip in position.	**3.** A trochanter roll prevents excessive external rotation of hip.
4. A footboard may be used to keep linen off the feet. If the client has spasticity in the foot, a footboard should be avoided.	**4.** A footboard increases muscle tone, as the foot presses against the board.
Bed Positioning: Side-Lying—Stronger Side	
1. Protract the shoulder and the weaker arm forward on a pillow. Extend the elbow and wrist, keeping the forearm in a neutral position or slightly pronated.	**1.** If the hand tends to remain in a fist, use a hard splint. If edema is present, elevate the hand.
2. Protract the lower extremity and flex it slightly at the hip. Place the top or weaker knee in a slight flexion and support it with pillows between the lower extremities. Extend the lower leg and position slightly behind the top leg.	**2.** Pillows help maintain good spinal alignment.
3. Place a small pillow or rolled up bath sheet under the stronger side between the crest of the pelvis and the rib cage. Use a small pillow under the head to flex the neck laterally.	**3.** The bed mattress tends to sag and encourages shortening of the trunk on the weaker side. A pillow near the rib cage offsets this. A pillow under head stretches the muscles on the weaker side.
Bed Positioning: Side-Lying—Weaker Side	
1. The shoulder is protracted, and the arm is in a neutral position. The elbow and wrist are extended, and the hand is positioned as before.	**1.** An alternative to a hard splint in the hand is a cone with the large end on the little finger side.
2. The lower extremities should have the hip and knee of the weaker side protracted and slightly flexed, along with the knee. The top leg is extended in a line with the trunk.	**2.** The top leg is stronger.

Continued

PROCEDURE

25–2

POSITIONING
(Continued)

Steps

Rationale

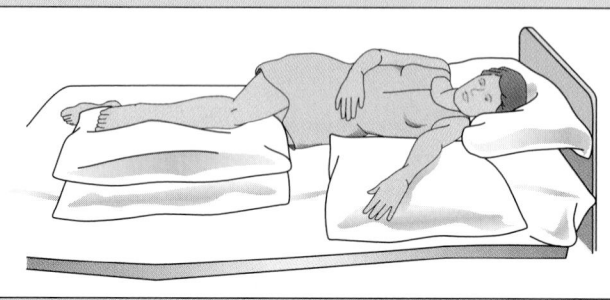

Step 2. *Side-lying position—weaker side.*

3. Place pillows between the legs. A pillow under the waist area is not needed in the position.

3. If the client cannot tolerate a full side-lying position, place pillows behind the back and allow the client to roll back against them. A pillow under the waist is not needed because the goal is to lengthen the affected side of the trunk, and this occurs naturally.

4. Assist the client to roll on the affected side.

4. The nurse helps the client to protract the scapula while avoiding pain and trauma to the shoulder joint.

Bed Positioning: Fowler's and Semi-Fowler's

1. The client is positioned on the back with the head of the bed elevated and legs extended (Fowler's) or legs slightly flexed (semi-Fowler's).

1. This position is often used for clients with respiratory problems. Semi-Fowler's helps prevent the client from sliding down in the bed. It is most often used when the client is eating, reading; or participating in hygienic activities. The client who stays in this position too long may have a tendency to develop contractures of the knee and pressure on the heels and sacrum.

2. Use a small pillow, no pillow, or the large pillow under the shoulders and under the head.

2. There is a danger of using too large a pillow behind the head, which could cause an increase in neck flexion.

3. Place a trochanter roll lateral to the femur.

3. A trochanter roll counteracts the tendency of the hips to rotate externally.

Bed Positioning: Prone

1. Place the client in the center of the bed, with the feet positioned between the mattress and the foot of the bed. Align the shoulders and hips with each other.

1. This position is highly desirable for clients who have had lower limb amputations, spinal cord injuries, or pressure ulcers over the coccyx. If breathing is a problem, a pillow can be placed under the chest to allow for chest expansion.

POSITIONING
(Continued)

Steps	**Rationale**
2. Place the arms in an alternating position, with one over the head and the other along the side. The head usually faces the overhead arm. Small pillows can be placed under the shoulders.	**2.** This is often the position of choice for sleeping at night.

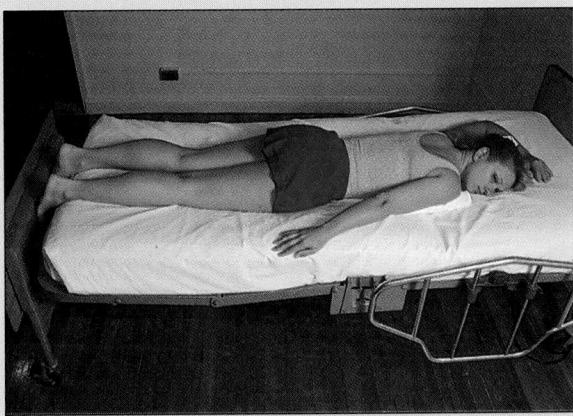

Step 2. *Prone position—chest expansion.*

Bed Positioning: Spinal Cord Injury

1. When supine, the client should have a lumbar roll placed in the lumbar region.	**1.** The lumbar musculature of the paralyzed client will assume a kyphotic, or flexed, posture when in the supine position.
2. During side-lying, a pillow should be placed between the pelvic crest and the axilla. The shoulder of the bottom arm is protracted, and the upper arm is supported on a pillow alongside the trunk. The bottom hip is protracted, and the leg is slightly flexed at the hip and knee. The upper leg can rest on pillows and should be fully extended in direct alignment with the trunk. Place pillows behind the back.	**2.** The trunk sags into the bed in the side-lying position. Pillows behind the back help maintain balance.

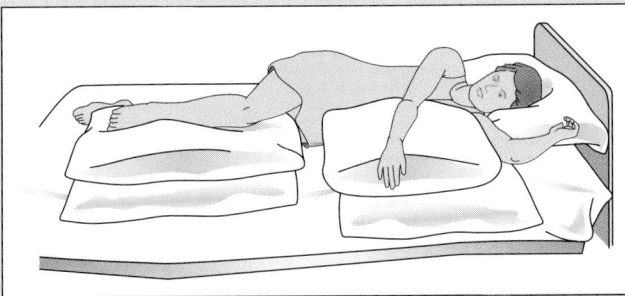

Step 2. *Spinal cord injury—side-lying position.*

3. When the head of the bed is elevated, the knees should be slightly flexed.	**3.** This prevents the client from sliding down in bed, and it also increases the curve in the low back area.

Continued

Procedure

25–2

POSITIONING
(Continued)

Steps	Rationale
4. Inspect the client's position visually to identify any misalignment.	**4.** Clients with spinal cord injury may not automatically turn in bed or sense discomfort because of decreased sensation. If the injury is high enough in the spinal cord, position sense may also be affected.

Sitting

1. Position the client with the hips against the backrest of chair. A belt should cross the hip at a 45-degree angle.

1. A hip belt keeps the hips in place but should not cut across the waist or the top of the pelvis.

2. Hips should be at a 90- to 95-degree angle; knees and ankles should also be at 90 degrees. Support the feet on footrests or on the floor.

2. This is the most functional sitting position.

3. A pad can be added behind the scapula or pelvis; a lapboard and armrests should be at elbow height. A lumbar roll should be placed behind the back.

3. Pads can discourage retraction on the weaker side. Armrests can keep the client from leaning to one side for support. A lumbar roll supports proper lumbar lordosis.

Standing

1. Your feet should be parallel and shoulder width apart. Place your foot on the outside of the weaker foot and assist the client to a standing position. Protract (bring forward) the client's hip, and brace the client's knee with your knee.

1. The client with hemiplegia often experiences pelvic retraction and knee hyperextension when standing. The nurse's knee stabilizes the client's weaker knee.

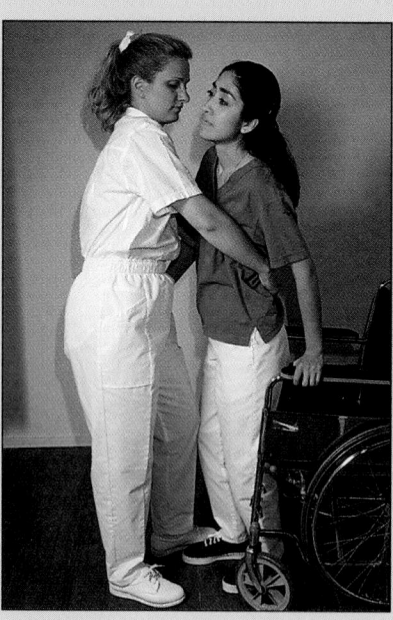

Step 1. *Standing position with nurse support.*

2. Once the client is standing, encourage him or her to shift weight toward the weaker side. Ask the client to stand as straight as possible with eyes forward.

2. This is proper body position. The nurse can assist the client at the waist by holding on to a transfer belt.

Before beginning any sitting program, the wheelchair deficiencies should be addressed. A consultation may need to be held with an occupational therapist to determine the modifications needed. A firm seat and back are necessities. A seat cushion may be needed to support proper positioning (Fig. 25–17). The need should be evaluated early in the course of hospitalization with the help of the physical and occupational therapists.

Ambulation

As a client begins an ambulation program, safety is of primary concern. The nurse should remain close by and allow the client ample rest when fatigue becomes apparent. When ambulation (or walking) begins, the nurse should make certain that the floor is dry and clear of any objects. If the floor is waxed, a nonslip wax should be used to prevent falls. Handrails are suggested to provide a secure feeling, especially for going up and down stairs. A safety belt is worn around the client's waist and is secured firmly to provide additional support. The client's own belt is less than ideal because of the possibility of it slipping or tearing. Sturdy shoes with soles that do not skid on the floor are worn.

When the client is standing, the nurse should

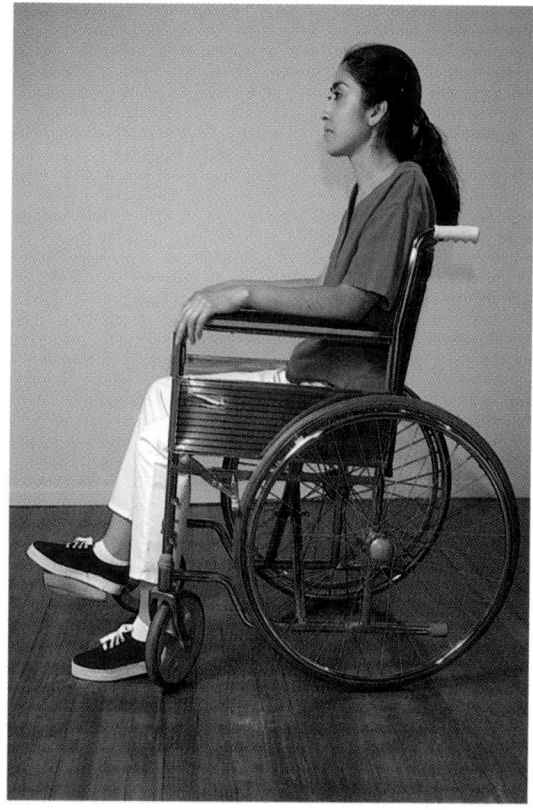

✦ **Figure 25–17**
Correct sitting position in a wheelchair.

stand to the side and slightly behind the client, grasping the safety or transfer belt and placing the other hand on his or her shoulder. If the client has extensive weakness, an assistant may be needed. One person should sit or stand in front of the client, and the other should stand behind and to one side. If the weakness is in one extremity, such as in the person with hemiplegia or hemiparesis, the nurse either sits or stands in front of the client and puts the hands on the hips to keep the client positioned forward. When standing to the side of the client, the nurse would stand on the weaker side to assist the client should he or she be unsteady. If the client will be going up and down stairs, the nurse should stand behind the client when he or she goes up and should stand in front when he or she goes down the steps, grasping the safety belt at all times.

Fatigue is always a factor when the client begins to ambulate. Allow for this when developing a plan and schedule rest periods during the day. Begin with short periods of ambulation and gradually increase the time and distance as the client develops more tolerance.

The client who uses a cane or crutch can use these devices to come to a standing position. He or she holds the cane or crutches on the weaker side, placing the tips on the floor slightly to the side and ahead of the feet. The client should place one hand

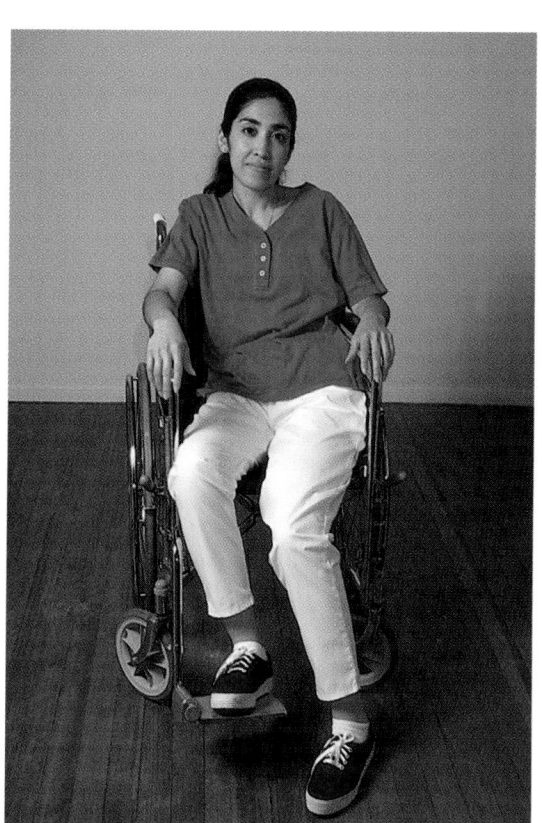

✦ **Figure 25–16**
Incorrect sitting position in a wheelchair.

on the armrest or seat of the chair and the other one on the handgrips of the crutches, pushing to a standing position. Once in the standing position, the client should put the crutches under his or her arms. If a cane is used, he or she should hold it in the weaker hand, using the armrests to push off the chair and coming to a standing position. The client reverses the procedure when sitting down, removing the crutches from under the arms before sitting.

The proper crutch stance is standing erect with the crutches 4 to 6 in in front and slightly to the side of either foot. The body weight should be on the palms of the hands—not on the axilla. The axillary bar should be approximately 2 in below and resting against the chest to promote stability.

The nurse is usually concerned with ambulation only for the less severely or temporarily disabled client. For this group of clients, the nurse may be responsible for providing crutches, a walker, or a cane of the proper length and for showing the client the gait needed to use the equipment. If the client has learned a gait pattern in physical therapy with orders to ambulate on the unit, it will be the nurse who supervises and evaluates this activity.

Patience and understanding are required throughout this period of early ambulation. The nurse must encourage the client to continue through periods of frustration and notify the physician or therapist when positive or negative changes occur.

A gait training program is usually needed for anyone using ambulation aids and should always be done under supervision of the physical therapist or physician. In consultation with the health care team, the appropriate program, aids, and gait can be prescribed. As progress occurs, changes should be made to maximize the abilities of the client. Less assistance is needed, and the assistive devices are changed or eliminated as the stability and independence of the client increase.

At the beginning of an ambulation program, the client assumes the correct standing posture. The body is aligned vertically, with the center of gravity of the head, arms, and trunk in a plane slightly behind the hip joints and in front of the knee joints. Check that the feet are slightly apart and parallel, knees flexed, and head held high, eyes forward. Some clients may deviate from the ideal, but they should try to move as close to normal as possible. Encourage the client to tuck in the abdomen and buttocks, hold the shoulders level, and achieve as tall a posture as possible. The nurse should also assume this posture when helping the client ambulate.

Clients are often resistant to using assistive devices for a variety of reasons, including fear of falling, fear of using equipment that may indicate to the world that they have a disability, and concern that dependence on the aids may be permanent. To help the client overcome these concerns, familiarize him or her with the equipment. Allowing the client to handle the aids and providing a demonstration of use will lessen the concerns. It may also help to have the client watch others use the equipment successfully. Sufficient help must be available initially to alleviate the fear of falling. Assure the client that someone will be present to help until he or she appears stable and confident in the use of the equipment. Listen to the client so that any expression of fear or concern can be heard and resolved to his or her satisfaction. Use a liberal amount of praise and positive feedback as progress is made. Allow for negative comments, but try not to reinforce them. At all times, convey a positive attitude that the client will succeed and will find the aids a means to increased mobility and independence.

Proper use of crutches, walker, and cane is best learned through a step-by-step program of regular practice. A client experiencing mobility problems uses the following sequence to lead to ambulation:

1. Maintain muscle strength and ROM
2. Develop sitting balance
3. Develop standing balance
4. Learn to shift body weight
5. Learn a specific gait

It is not necessary to go through every step in the sequence if that activity has already been achieved. Start at the level of the client and progress from that point on to the final goal.

The client's ability to bear weight also affects the ambulation program. Non–weight-bearing activity refers to the fact that no weight is put on the affected extremity and it is kept off the floor at times. Partial weight bearing allows the client to bear up to half of the weight on the affected extremity during stance. Tolerance weight bearing is defined as bearing weight on the affected extremity to pain tolerance. Full weight bearing is normal weight bearing on the affected extremity during stance.

Muscle Strength

Muscle strength is maintained by instituting ROM exercises early in the hospitalization or as soon as the client is stable. The nurse can initiate a maintenance program and refer the client to physical therapy for a strengthening program. The physician may order muscle strengthening exercises to maintain the use of extremities and joint mobility.

Balance and strength are often more of a problem for the elderly. The older client does not have much reserve to draw on, and if a situation occurs in which ambulation aids are required, it may push the client into a greater degree of dependence.

Muscles used for crutch walking extend the elbow and depress the shoulders. Use of a trapeze on the bed does not exercise these muscles. Once the client is in the seated position, encourage pushing down with the arms to make to transfer and doing seated push-ups when possible to strengthen the upper extremities (Fig. 25–18).

It is recommended that the client participate in isometric resistive exercises to increase strength, be-

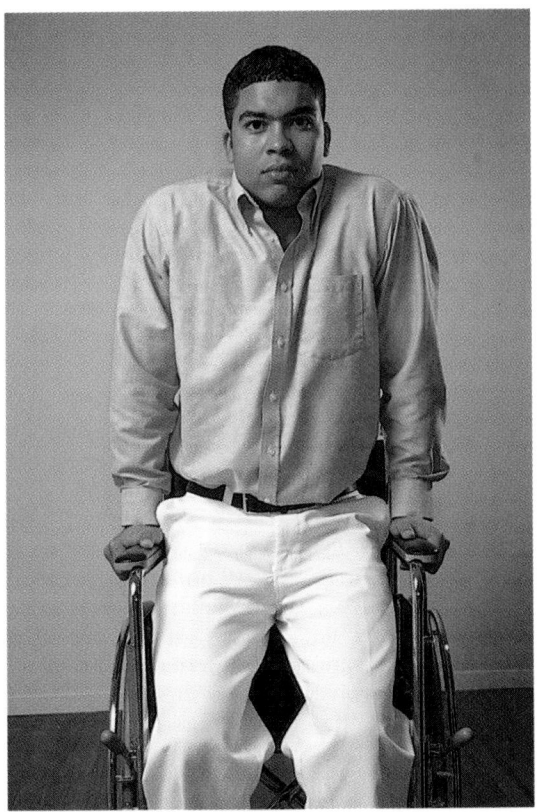

> **Figure 25–18**
Sitting push-ups.

cause they require little time and no special equipment. The muscle should exert as much effort as possible against resistance for a set time, usually 5 to 15 seconds.

Resistance in the following exercises is provided either by the bed, by the client pushing against the body, or by the nurse. Again, check with the physician or therapist before starting such a program. While the client is lying in bed, instruct him or her to place the arms at the side and push down on the bed with the head and back of the arms as if trying to raise the chest off the bed. With the arms straight at the side, thumbs up, have the client pull the arms as tightly into the side of the body as possible. While the client's legs are extended, have him or her push the heels into the mattress as if trying to raise the buttocks off the bed. Ask the client to push hard against the foot of the bed with the balls of the feet while grasping the edge of the mattress to keep from sliding up in bed (Fig. 25–19). If a high degree of arm strength is needed, such as with crutch walking, it may be necessary to do sitting push-ups. The client does these by keeping the elbows straight and shoulders fully depressed. Instruct the client to slowly lift the body off the chair. He or she should slowly flex the elbows to lower the body while refraining from using the feet or legs to assist with the push-up. It is obvious that the client will need full use of the arms.

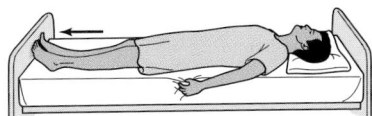

> **Figure 25–19**
Resistance exercises.

Sitting Balance

Sitting balance is addressed by the nursing staff as soon as the client is medically stable. Begin by elevating the head of the bed and dangling the client's legs at the edge of the bed. Remain with the client to promote safety and monitor the client. Many clients feel dizzy initially, but this should cease over time. If dizziness continues, an underlying cause should be suspected and evaluated. Monitor the blood pressure during the initial phases.

The client must have good sitting balance before coming to a standing position. Instruct the client to practice sitting by coming to the edge of the bed and placing the feet firmly on the floor or a footstool. The nurse should stand in front of the client and offer a steadying hand on the client's shoulder if it is needed. When the client can raise the arms over the head without losing balance, then this exercise is no longer needed.

Standing Balance

Some clients lose the physical or mental ability to come to a standing position. To relearn this motion, while the client is in a seated position, he or she should slide forward to the edge of the bed or a chair with arms, keeping the feet back under the body. Instruct the client to lean forward with the trunk while pushing down with the arms and legs to come to a standing position. The client should push rather than pull up to a standing position (Fig. 25–20). This helps strengthen the muscles of the upper extremities that are used most for cane and crutch walking.

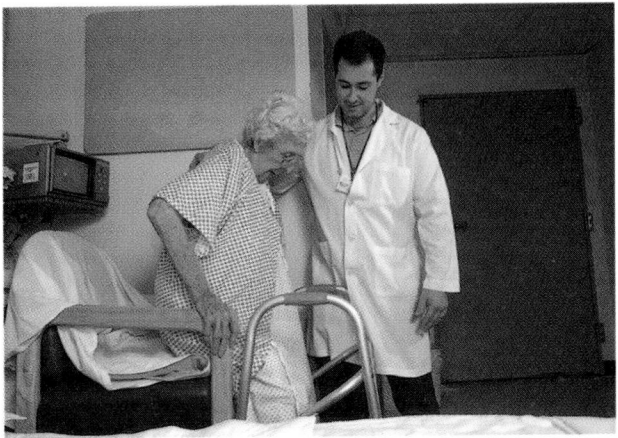

> **Figure 25–20**
Mobilizing an elderly client.

The client may be able to come to a standing position without assistance. If assistance is needed, use a safety or transfer belt around the waist of the client. The nurse is nearer the client's center of gravity and should not pull on the client's arms or shoulders. If the client needs minimal assistance, then the nurse should stand at the side and grab the belt to offer a secure feeling.

Standing balance is essential for walking to occur. The client should practice standing next to a stable support that is at about wrist level while standing erect. He or she should keep the trunk in balance while moving the extremities. When the client is able to do this without swaying, then he or she is ready to walk.

Some clients have a greater degree of immobility and less trunk stability and may need some assistance with standing in the form of a passive standing device—either a standing frame or a tilt table. These devices are used outside the realm of nursing, but this does not preclude the nurse from being aware of their existence or use. Clients with spinal cord injuries, brain damage, cerebral vascular accidents, arthritis, and fractures are among those who may benefit from these devices. The goal for this activity varies. Eventual ambulation is a possibility for some, and for others, the goal may be improved body functioning. The weight-bearing activity of standing helps the bones

retain the calcium salts and delays the onset of severity of osteoporosis (Kottke, 1966).

Tilt tables are used for clients who are extremely deconditioned or have poor endurance or poor balance. The table is tilted vertically at a gradual angle while the client is secured to the top. The table is elevated 15 to 20 degrees initially, and the client's tolerance is monitored through blood pressure readings and the client's verbal response. Gradually the table is elevated more and more until a 70-degree angle is reached (Fig. 25–21). At this angle, the client may initially feel like he or she is falling forward. The tolerance and blood pressure are monitored until the client can tolerate this position for 20 to 30 minutes. Once the client can tolerate this elevation without difficulty, the standing position becomes more of an option, and the client is ready to try ambulating.

The nurse's role during use of these devices is limited by some problems that do occur that require a nursing intervention. Passive standing can cause postural hypotension that is detrimental to the client and, in a severe case, could produce fatal results. Careful and constant observation of the client must be maintained until all involved parties are certain that the position can be tolerated. The nurse should take the blood pressure at frequent intervals and observe for dizziness, sweating, blurred vision, fainting, or a drop in blood pressure. Abdominal binders or supportive stockings are used to promote venous return and maintain a constant flow of blood to the brain.

Weight Shifting

The client must also be able to shift weight while sitting and while ambulating. This is accomplished through exercises learned in therapy and practiced on the client units. Clients must be able to shift their weight while sitting to relieve pressure on the buttocks and sacrum and to reposition themselves in the chair. Push-ups (described previously) help accomplish the weight shifting. Stand-ups are another form of exercise that improve standing balance and facilitate weight shifting. The client is in a seated position with both feet firmly on the floor, facing a table. The client is instructed to place the hands on the table, slide to the edge of the chair, and lean forward slightly while pushing down with the hands. Instruct the client to straighten the knees and back while coming to a standing position. The work should be done by the legs and not the arms. Once this is accomplished, the client can shift the weight of the body as he or she will need to do when walking or climbing stairs.

Gait

Gait patterns that are developed for clients should be individualized, differing in speed, safety, and the amount of energy required. Various patterns are taught to accommodate the different needs of the client, especially if crutches will be used for a long time. If the client will be going home with the aids, the

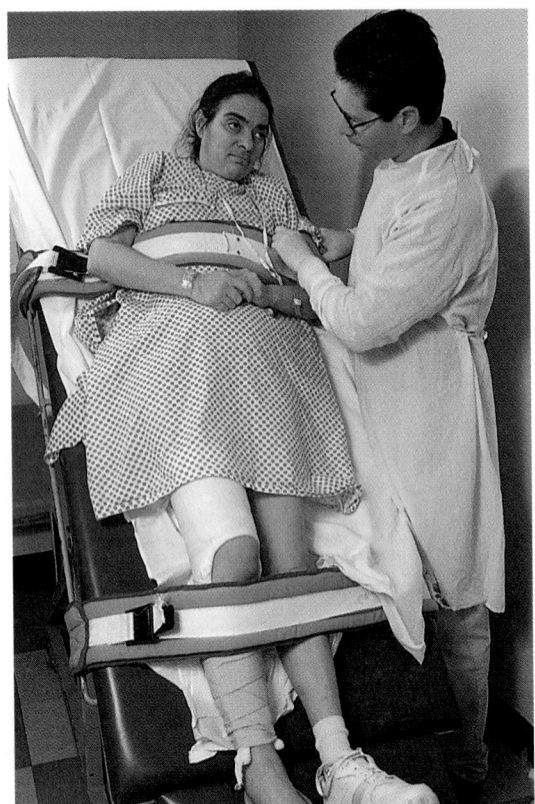

⇥ Figure 25–21
Tilt table.

family members should also be taught how to facilitate ambulation, and their abilities should be evaluated based on the instructions given them by the staff.

Normal gait patterns for walking consist of two phases: the stance phase and the swing phase, when the leg is advanced. The stance begins when the heel strikes the floor and does not end until the foot is plantar flexed and the weight has shifted up over the opposite extended leg. The swing phase begins when the weight is shifted off the leg and the hip and knee are flexed. As the leg is brought forward, the knee is gradually extended so it is close to full extension as the heel strikes the floor. During walking, one leg is always in the stance phase while the other is in the swing phase (Fig. 25–22). This is the ideal pattern that the gait training program is trying to promote through retraining.

Gaits are classified as two point, three point, step through, three point and one, or four point. The nurse does not have the responsibility of deciding which is the most appropriate gait pattern. That decision is left to the therapist or physician. The nurse's responsibility is to reinforce those things taught in therapy and make note of any changes when the client is ambulating on the unit.

The two-point gait is a faster way of walking than the four-point gait but requires that the client have more stability because there only two points of contact with the ground at any one time. The client be-

gins with a weight shift to the left leg and the right crutch, followed with the movement of the right leg forward along with the left crutch. The client then shifts the weight to the right leg and the left crutch and finally moves the left leg with the right crutch (Fig. 25–23A). In this gait, the client would start out with the stronger leg (if one is stronger)—not necessarily the right leg. The pattern is a leg with the opposite crutch and then the other leg with the opposite crutch.

The three-point gait is a non–weight-bearing gait and is often seen in the client who has had an orthopedic procedure done on one lower extremity. The client may be restricted to partial weight bearing or may use full weight bearing. The three-point gait requires upper body strength, trunk stability, and balance because the client bears the entire body weight on the arms. The client begins by supporting the weight on the strong leg while moving the crutches forward about 4 in. He or she shifts the weight to the crutches and steps ahead, with the strong leg landing just behind the crutches. He or she then shifts the weight to the strong leg and moves the crutches ahead again (Fig. 25–23B). Instruct the client to avoid moving the crutches so far forward that it becomes necessary to overreach and lose balance. The pattern is both crutches, step with the strong leg, and then both crutches.

As the client becomes more confident and comfortable with this gait, the step-through gait can be shown. This is a more efficient and faster gait, but it requires more space to maneuver. The client must swing the leg in front of the crutches because the crutches offer no help in maintaining balance. The client should be instructed to keep the hips forward while the body is ahead of the crutches. Caution the client not to step too far forward or balance will become a problem. Instruct the client to shift the weight to the strong leg and then move the crutches ahead about 4 in and shift the weight onto the crutches. He or she then steps through, with the strong leg landing in front of the crutches and shifts the weight to the strong leg and moves the crutches ahead again (Fig. 25–23C). The pattern is both crutches, step through, and then both crutches.

The three-point-and-one gait is prescribed for a client who has had an orthopedic procedure and is instructed to begin a partial–weight-bearing program. The weight bearing will stimulate the healing of the bone and help offset the development of osteoporosis that occurs as a result of no weight bearing. If a cast is on the limb, the physician may put a rubber caliper on the bottom of the cast to support the partial weight bearing.

The client begins the gait by standing with crutches, bearing full weight on the strong leg and partial weight on the weaker leg. He or she shifts weight to the stronger leg and then moves both crutches and the weaker leg ahead, shifting weight onto the crutches and partially bearing weight on the weaker leg. The client should then step ahead with

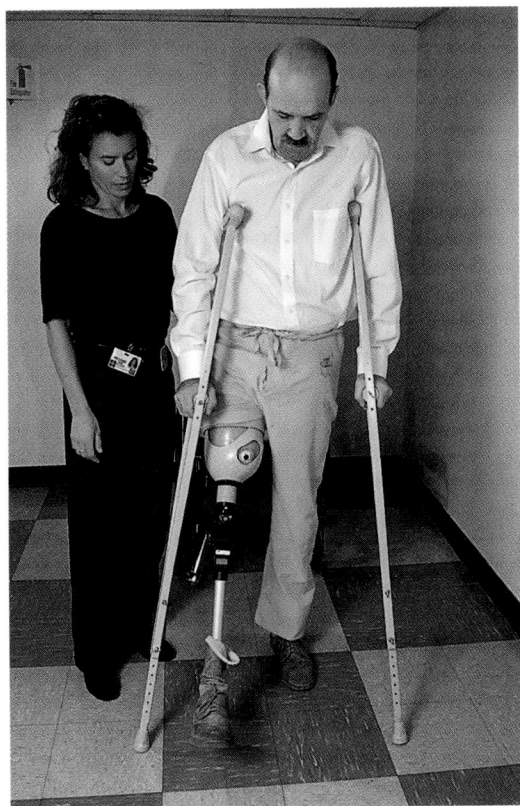

❧ **Figure 25–22**
Learning to walk with prosthesis.

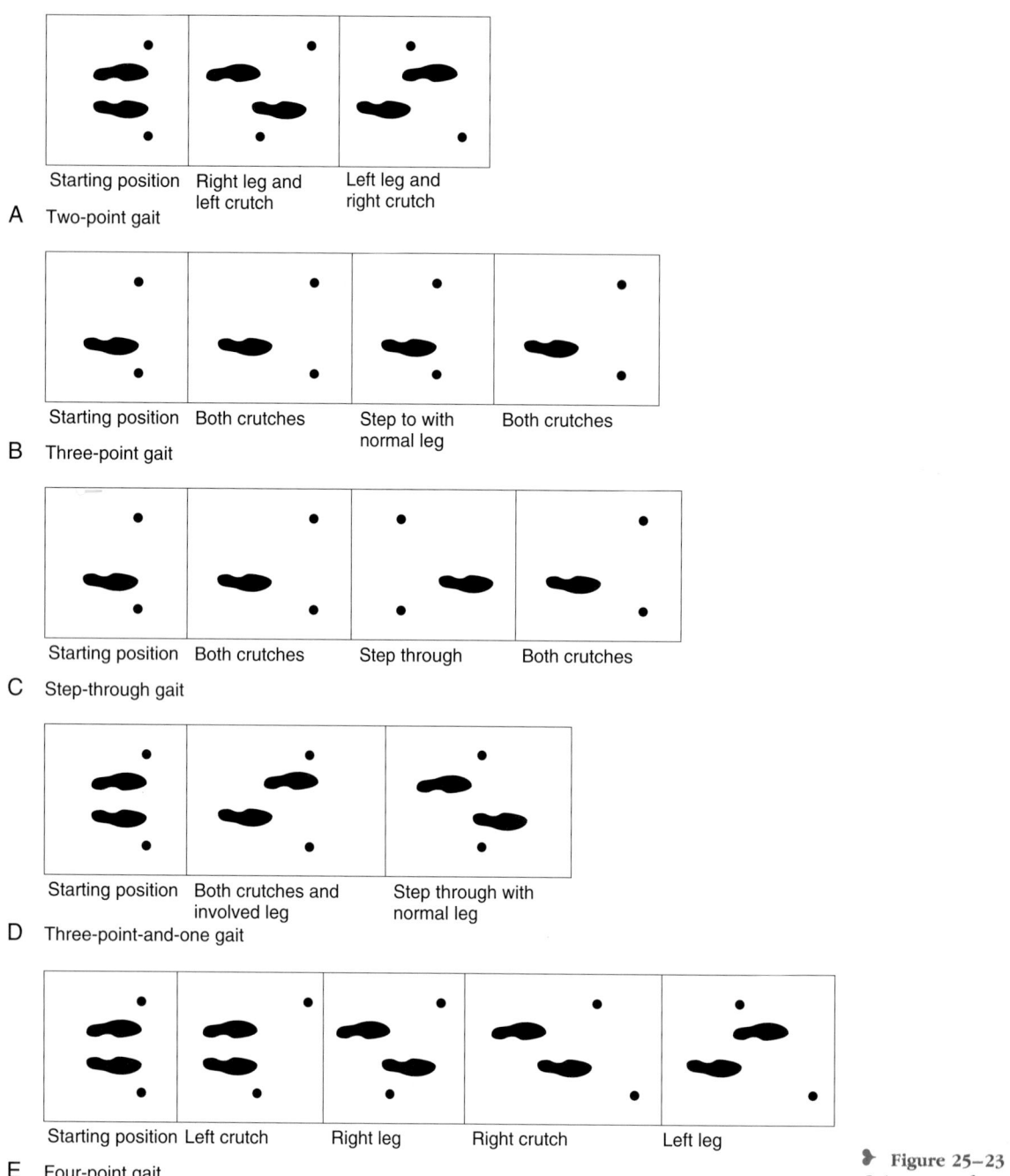

A   Two-point gait

Starting position | Right leg and left crutch | Left leg and right crutch

B   Three-point gait

Starting position | Both crutches | Step to with normal leg | Both crutches

C   Step-through gait

Starting position | Both crutches | Step through | Both crutches

D   Three-point-and-one gait

Starting position | Both crutches and involved leg | Step through with normal leg

E   Four-point gait

Starting position | Left crutch | Right leg | Right crutch | Left leg

Figure 25–23
Gait patterns for crutch use.

the stronger leg (Fig. 25–23D). The pattern is both crutches and weaker leg and then step through with the stronger leg. When the client changes to a cane, the cane should be held on the side opposite the weaker leg. The client must be able to bear full weight to use a cane.

The four-point gait is used for clients who have lower extremity weakness or lack of coordination or balance or for the elderly person who is afraid of falling. The client with lower limb amputations also uses this gait once the prostheses have been fitted. This gait requires that the client have enough muscle

power in the arms to hold the handgrips and lift the crutches as well as enough leg power to move the foot forward and straighten the knee. This gait is the safest and most stable of all gaits because there are four points touching the floor at all times.

The client begins this gait by bearing weight on both legs and both crutches. The nurse stands at the side with one hand on the safety belt and the other on the front of the client's shoulder. Instruct the client to shift the weight to both legs and one crutch. It is suggested that the client begin with the weaker leg (if one is weaker) and thus shift to the crutch on the weaker side first. He or she should move the other crutch forward and shift the weight to that leg and the opposite crutch. The pattern becomes one of left crutch, right leg, right crutch, and left leg (Fig. 25–23E).

Navigating the stairs is a challenge for clients using a four-point gait. Once a comfort level has been achieved, the client can be taught to use the stairs. The nurse should stand behind the client with one hand on the safety belt and the other on the railing. Instruct the client to step onto the first step with the strong leg, making sure that the heel of the foot is fully on the step before transferring the weight. The client should press on the crutch and the handrail and use the strong leg to pull the weight forward, positioning over the leg until stable. Finally, he or she should lift the crutch onto the step. The client repeats the sequence until the top stair is reached.

When a client is going down the stairs, the nurse should stand in front of him or her. Instruct the client to lift the crutch down along with the weak lower extremity onto the first step and step down with the strong leg. The temptation when going up or down the stairs is to lean onto the railing with the forearm. This is awkward and fatiguing and should be discouraged.

Ambulation Aids

Physical therapists, in conjunction with the physician, are responsible for prescribing the type of equipment that the client should use. As the client's condition improves, the team should discuss the need for continued use of equipment or the possibility of a change in equipment. The usual progression is from a walker to underarm crutches, to elbow-length crutches, to broad-based canes, and, finally, to regular canes, which are mostly used for balance. For the client with a progressive disease, such as multiple sclerosis, the progression may be reversed, requiring more support rather than less.

Usually the client who has a fractured leg or has had a joint replaced uses a pick-up walker or underarm crutches until full weight bearing is achieved. At this point, the client may have a walking cast or a cane. An elderly person may use a cane for a longer time—more for assurance than for balance. A client who has had an amputation of the lower extremity and is using a prosthesis may learn to walk with a walker or an underarm or elbow-length crutches but can rapidly progress to a cane. Eliminating the cane is a possibility, but canes are often kept for balance. The client who has undergone bilateral amputations and has prostheses may learn to walk indoors without any aids but usually needs two canes or crutches when walking outside or up any elevation to promote stability and safety on uneven surfaces or slippery ground. If the client is elderly and somewhat unsteady, continuous use of the aids may be needed because of an ongoing problem with poor balance and a need for reassurance.

Clients who have spinal cord injuries that result in paraplegia may use underarm crutches because the pressure of the bar on the axillae helps compensate for lack of position sense and provides stability. A younger person with paraplegia, especially one with good balance and some muscle function, may prefer elbow-length crutches. Walking is probably not functional for any distance, but walking does provide some weight bearing on the long bones and changes the client's perspective from constantly sitting to standing.

When walkers are used, it is often because other aids are not an option. Elderly clients often prefer the walker. A client who has hemiplegia and good function in one arm may use a pick-up walker. However, a client may become too dependent on the walker and reluctant to advance to any other aid. The wheeled walker stays on the floor and does not have to be picked up but is not usually recommended because this type of walker may roll away from the client, causing a loss of balance. The client should advance the walker, making sure that all four legs contact the floor simultaneously; take a step with the weaker leg and then the stronger leg; and advance the walker again. This kind of walker provides a more normal gait because it allows for continuous steps.

One of the most necessary pieces of equipment and one that is often neglected is a properly fitting pair of shoes. Shoes protect the feet, give the client position sense, and provide adequate support. Consider the following features when looking at the shoes a client wears. A steel shank may be needed—especially if a brace is to be attached. The shoe needs a leather sole, rubber heels, and a hard counter to give form to the shoe around the heel. The oxford shoe is the shoe of choice and should have at least four eyelets on each side to ensure adequate support if a brace is needed. The physical therapist serves as an excellent resource for help with selecting a shoe.

Measuring Equipment

Clients who need to use crutches must have crutches of the correct length if they are to be useful. The client should be measured while standing (Fig. 25–24). It may be necessary to assist the client during the measurement process. Nurses are not usually responsible for this process and should seek the advice of the physical therapist if needed.

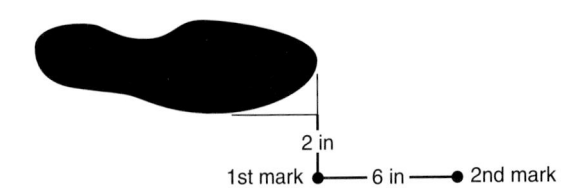

♪ Figure 25–24
Marks used for measuring correct crutch length.

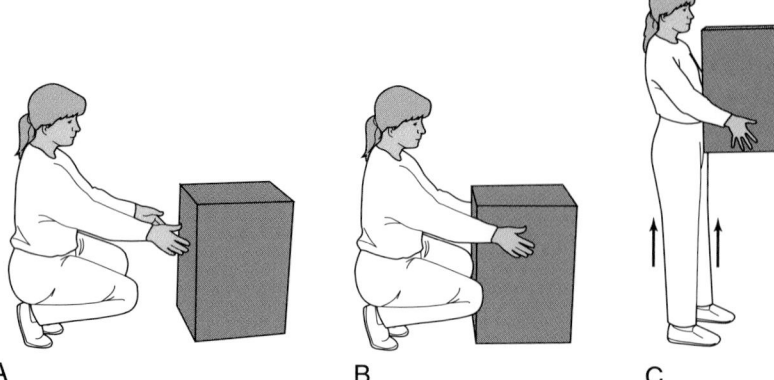

A   B   C

Figure 25–25
Proper lifting techniques.

Principles of Body Mechanics

Transferring clients from one surface to another is a process that affects both the client and the nurse. This activity is one that requires a significant amount of patience, client education and goal setting, and consistency and creativity in the approach. In addition, nurses often must carry heavy supplies, move awkward objects, or work in a less than ideal environment for back safety.

When the body is used as a lifting machine, it takes considerable muscular effort to keep the body stable, lift the object against gravity, and lift the upper body weight. Test the weight of the object to be lifted. Lift one side of the object slightly or, in the case of a patient, know the body weight and the amount of assistance that the client can provide. If the object is too heavy or awkward to handle, then it is necessary to get help or find an alternative method to move the object.

The nurse should keep the client or object as close to the body as possible. If moving an object, try to position it between the knees when moving from a low surface. This action helps get the object closer to the center of gravity. (More stress and strain is exerted on the low back when the object is farther away from the center of gravity.) It also helps if you can grip the object with the whole hand and not just the fingers. Tighten the abdominal muscles and raise straight up, using the legs to lift (Fig. 25–25). Strong contractions of the abdominal muscles increase the pressure within the abdomen. This pressure lifts the chest and helps counteract the downward forces on the low back area.

Weak abdominal muscles cause the loss of this important uplifting effect. They also cause the small back muscles to bear more of the strain from lifting. One of the initial effects of gaining weight in the abdominal region is the thinning of the muscles and the increasing of the curve in the lower back because of the effect of gravity on the protruding abdomen. This is often seen as the stages of pregnancy advance in women and the abdomen becomes larger. The woman must lean farther back to prevent falling forward, and the curve in the back also increases.

Strengthening the stomach muscles along with losing weight spares the back.

Turn the feet, not the back, if a change of direction is required when carrying the object or client. Twisting the back causes a shift in balance and can strain the structures in the low back area. When turning, keep the back straight and take small steps with your feet.

Not all objects that need to be lifted can conveniently fit within the base of support, and some weigh too much. If an object is too heavy or awkward, some alternative lifting methods can be used.

Certain considerations must be made when working at various height levels. One of the areas that often threatens the back is lifting or working above the head. As the arms begin to raise, the arch in the low back increases. The higher the arms are raised, the farther down the back the arch travels. The legs

---

HEALTH PROMOTION AND PREVENTION

HANDLING HEAVY OR AWKWARD WEIGHTS

1. **Get help.** Staff know their own abilities and limitations when lifting a heavy object.

2. **Push or pull an object.** This is most efficiently done by applying force in the direction of the move. Place the hand in line with the object's center of gravity. If there is friction or resistance between the object and the floor or the client and the bed, place the hands below the center of gravity of the object or person. Use the legs and lean toward the weight being pushed, away from weight being pulled. Pushing is easier than pulling if possible.

3. **Avoid twisting.**

4. When moving an awkward object, try turning the object end over end, rotating the object as if "walking" the object, rolling the object as when rolling a barrel, using a mechanical device such as a dolly or cart, or moving the object in sections.

provide some support but do not add to the lifting power. The abdominal muscles are also less effective as protectors of the low back. It is much more efficient to use a stool or stepladder. Tightening the abdominal muscles while lifting also protects the back. Whenever possible, store lightweight or infrequently used items overhead. Try lifting the object in sections and avoid twisting or overreaching. Take frequent short breaks if the task is to take a long time.

Many activities require constant bending at the waist or working at lower levels for long periods. Often, the nurse fails to raise the level of the bed to waist height when administering client care and bends over the client. If the nurse's thigh muscles are weak or the heel cords are tight, squatting is difficult for any length of time. The natural tendency is to bend at the waist with the legs straight. Instead, squat slowly and keep the back straight when getting closer to the lower level. Tighten the abdominal and buttock muscles and, if necessary, kneel on one or both knees. If bending at the waist cannot be avoided, place one foot in front of the other. This reduces stress on the lower back.

There are also situations in which lifting an object from a difficult position or location is required. In these instances, people have a tendency to lean forward while keeping the knees straight and bending at the waist. Examples of this are the nurse reaching across the litter to move a client from the bed to the litter or reaching for a child in a crib or playpen. Ideally, the nurse should get as close to the object as possible, using the body as counterweight. Then he or she should use the lifting rules: (1) broaden the base of support by placing the feet farther apart, (2) bend the knees to lower the body to the object, (3) keep the object as close to the body as possible, (4) tighten the abdominal and buttock muscles and breathe normally, and (5) shift the position of the feet rather than twisting the back if a change in direction is required (Fig. 25–26). Sometimes the nurse will climb into the bed to move the client. However, the problem then exists of using the back and arms rather than the legs to lift and move.

Carry the object as close to the body as possible, ideally in front. Many nurses carry a child on their hip and tend to always carry the child on the same hip. If this is the only option available, change sides frequently and take short breaks.

Often, a simple modification in the way the task is performed increases the nurse's safety. On the job or at home, continual awareness of how the task is performed is essential. *Remember to assess each situation to minimize risk, minimize exertion, and maximize effectiveness.* Keep in mind that the guidelines presented can easily be adapted to everyday situations. The prevention of future back problems is usually possible through the correct use of body mechanics. Even if the task is awkward, using these principles minimizes the strain on the low back and serves the nurse well in the daily moving and lifting of objects and clients.

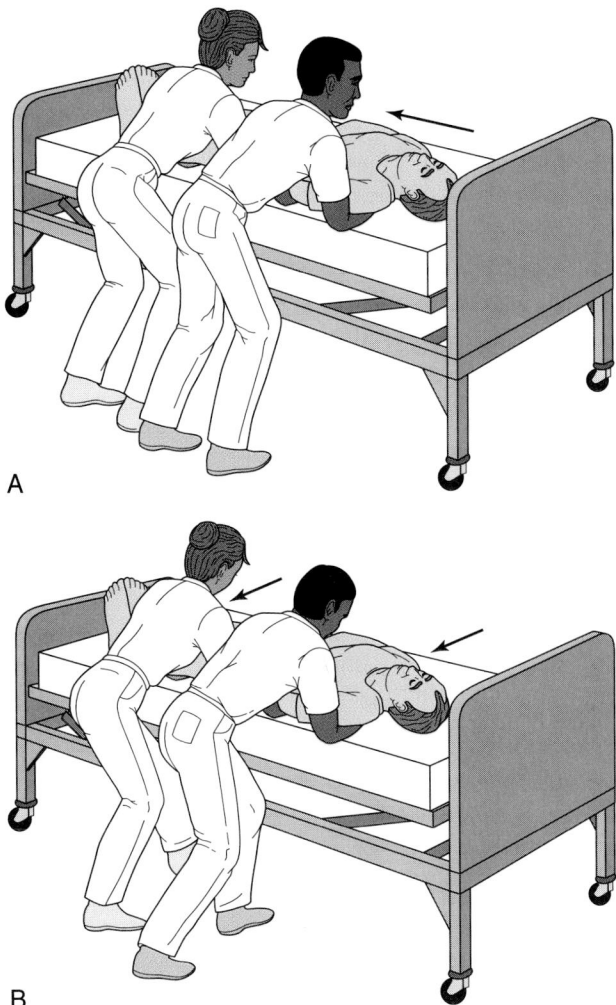

A

B

✦ **Figure 25–26**
Lifting a client from a difficult position.

Moving and Lifting Clients

Once a client is stable and able to move around, steps for developing a transfer plan begin. A **transfer** refers to moving the client from one surface to another; *e.g.,* bed to chair, wheelchair to toilet or car, or litter to bed. It is essential that the nurse involve the client in the plan from the very beginning, because the goal is to enable the client to become as independent as possible.

Transfers are classified as either active or passive and as requiring minimal, moderate, or maximal assistance. The transfer is considered to be active if the client contributes to the procedure, even if some assistance is needed. If the client is unable to help or needs mechanical assistance, the transfer is considered passive or dependent. In either case, supervision and verbal cues are necessary for a safe technique.

As soon as the client is medically able, the opportunity must be provided for him or her to get out of bed. Increasing the client's activity level improves the recovery process, shortens the time in the hospital, and achieves better outcomes. Selecting a method of transfer, at the very least, is the responsibility of the nurse. However, it can be a collaborative effort of the interdisciplinary team. It is essential that the nurse select a method in which the client can participate and that follows a consistent approach to teach the client.

Minimizing the negative effects of prolonged bedrest prepares the client for transfer out of the bed. This is accomplished by gradually elevating the head of the bed while assessing the client's response to the upright position. Maintain joint ROM to prepare the client for assisting with the transfer process. Transfers are easier if the client's strength and endurance are supported through daily activity. Any self-care activities in which a client can participate should be encouraged, along with daily upper extremity strengthening. If the client's endurance is poor, plan to provide a high degree of assistance initially until adequate strength is achieved. Include periods of rest in between activities to minimize fatigue.

The client needs to have a good degree of balance while sitting. If he or she tends to lean or fall to one side while sitting, this will probably become more obvious when he or she is transferred. The nurse places a hand on the client's shoulder to compensate for the imbalance. Provide assistance at the client's waist with a belt. Suggest that the client use the bed rail or the arm of a chair for support. Observe the client's response during the transfers. If pain seems to be interfering with the process, it may be helpful to administer pain medication at least a half hour before the activity begins. If fear is an issue, explore it with the client and take the measures previously identified to reduce his or her fear.

A client who has difficulty comprehending what is being said presents a challenge when being taught the transfer techniques. The nurse should plan thoroughly not only what needs to be taught but also when it should be taught. Fatigue plays a major role in the client's ability to participate in the process and understand and retain what is being said. It may be helpful at this point to break the task into several short steps, repeat them as often as needed, be consistent in the approach, use demonstration when appropriate, be patient, and use praise to encourage the client.

Equipment

Particular attention is paid to the environment and to the pieces of equipment that are needed when determining the type of transfer to be used. Environmental concerns include adequate lighting, transfer surfaces of equal height, and space to accommodate equipment needed and movement by the client and nurse. Equipment needs range from walking aids to a wheelchair. Wheelchairs should have brakes, swing-away or removable footrests, and removable armrests and should be collapsible. A sliding board bridges the distance between transfer surfaces but needs removable arm rests to function properly (see "Sitting Transfers"). Carts or litters ideally need to be positioned

near the bed. If a mechanical lift is used, it must have enough space in which to maneuver properly.

Transfer surfaces should be fairly firm. It is much easier to transfer out of a firm bed than one with a soft mattress. The client's energy is transferred to the soft surface rather than being used for the movement required. Stabilize the surfaces by applying the brakes, not only on a wheelchair or litter but also on the bed.

Short or half side rails stabilize the client and are used when the client turns in bed or comes to a sitting position. Some clients use a trapeze, but those with weak upper extremities or pain when lifting the arm will find this option unsatisfactory. Grab bars strategically placed in the bathroom assist with a sitting transfer. It is important for the client to avoid becoming dependent on equipment that will not be available at home.

Types of Transfers

There are basically two different types of transfers: sitting and standing. The client's physical and cognitive abilities direct which of these two types is most appropriate.

Sitting Transfers

A sitting transfer is used when the client has weakness or paralysis in the lower extremities, has had lower limb amputations, or has weak upper extremities. The client can use a long sitting or a short sitting position. The long sitting position is used by paraplegic or quadriplegic clients because it requires little effort and provides good sitting balance. The hips and knees must be flexible because the client needs to lean forward to maintain an upright, balanced position. The short sitting position is used by clients who have weakness in the lower extremities and good sitting balance. This method is used by someone whose degree of disability is not severe. Transfers can be made laterally or, on occasion, backward or forward. Procedure 25–3 describes the different types of transfers.

If assistance is needed, it can be either maximal, moderate, or minimal. Maximal assistance implies that the client is completely dependent and participates minimally; the nurse does all the work. Moderate assistance means that a client participates to some degree; however, the nurse still does more than 50% of the work. With minimal assistance, the client does the majority of the work, with guidance and stabilizing assistance provided by the nurse. Contact assistance (contact guard, stand-by assistance, or supervision) means that the client does all of the work; however, the nurse holds or stands next to the client for safety and very minimal guidance. The client is independent when he or she transfers safely with no guidance or contact from the nurse.

The bathroom presents some challenges to the client's ability to do a sitting transfer. Often, the area is cramped, and the doorway is too narrow to accommo-

Text continued on page 694

PROCEDURE

25–3

TRANSFERS

Equipment:

Hospital bed
Wheelchair
Transfer belt
Transfer board
Side rails
Nonslip footwear
Cart
Sheet for lifting
Car
Tub rails
Toilet rails

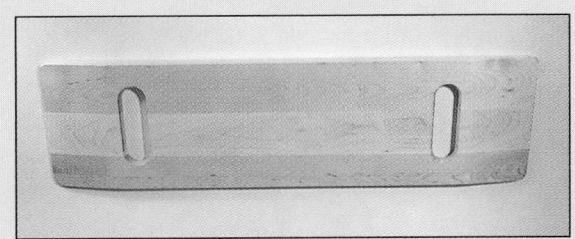

Steps	Rationale

Unassisted Sitting Transfer

1. Place the wheelchair at a 45-degree angle to the bed, remove the armrests, make sure surfaces are level, and apply brakes.

2. Instruct the client to come to a sitting position in the bed and to swing the legs over the side of the bed onto the floor.

3. Have the client move to the edge of the bed and lean forward, with the feet well under the client and in a wide base of support. Then instruct the client to place one hand on the farthest armrest of the chair and swing the hips onto the seat of the chair.

1. Prepares the environment to ensure client safety and minimal energy expenditure.

2. Bringing legs to the floor is advised for the short sitting transfer.

3. The client must have fairly good upper body and extremity strength and balance to change position safely and efficiently without assistance.

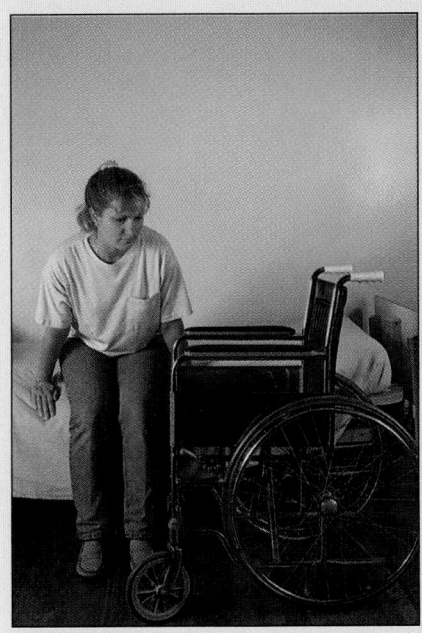
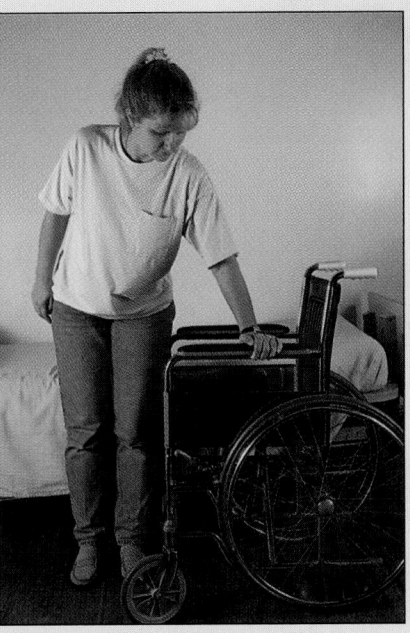
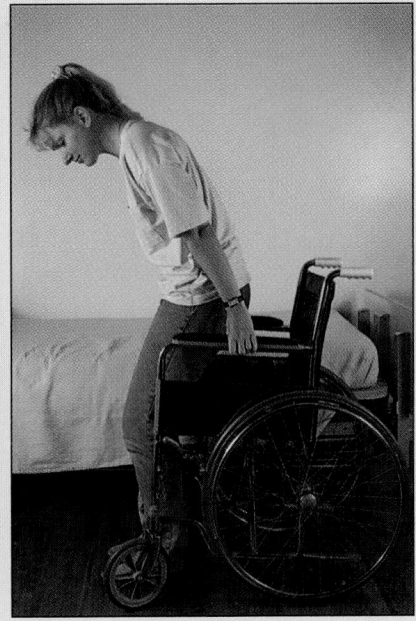

Step 3. *Independent transfer—bed to chair.*   **Step 3.** *Independent transfer—bed to chair.*   **Step 3.** *Independent transfer—bed to chair.*

Continued

PROCEDURE

25-3

TRANSFERS
(Continued)

Steps	Rationale
4. The final step is to arrange the feet on the footrests of the chair and replace the armrests.	**4.** Provides safety and comfort.

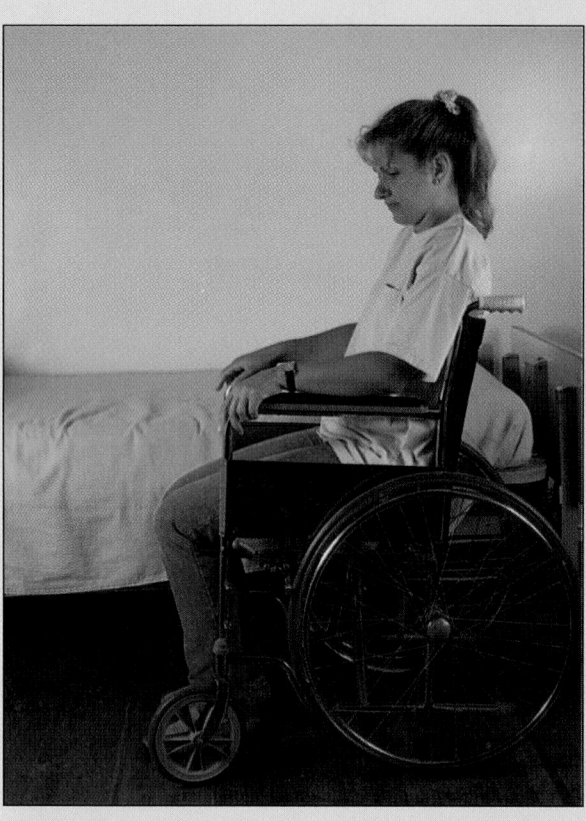

Step 4. *Independent transfer—bed to chair.*

Long Sitting Transfer

1. Wheelchair is positioned at a right angle to the bed, and brakes are locked.	**1.** The wheelchair must be stable before the transfer is begun.

TRANSFERS
(Continued)

Steps	**Rationale**
2. The client does push-ups to position his or her back to the wheelchair, then reaches back, grabs the armrests, and pulls the body into the chair.	**2.** Clients with no use of the lower extremities but good sitting balance can do this transfer.

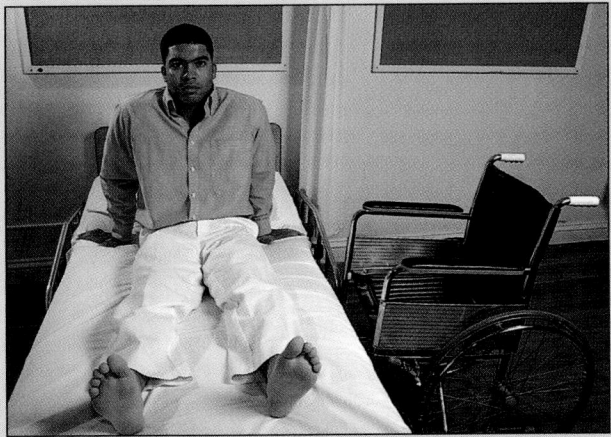

Step 2. *Long sitting transfer—facing forward.*

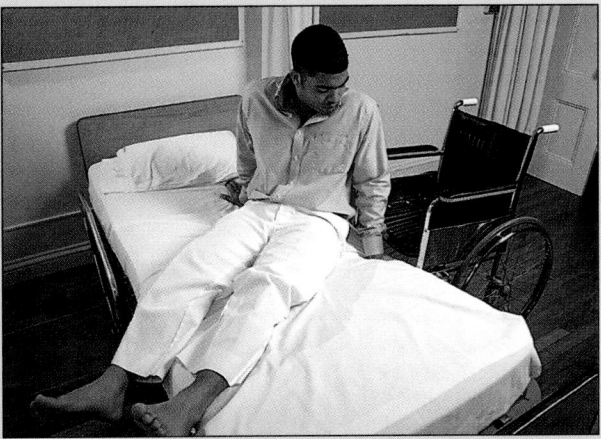

Step 2. *Long sitting transfer—diagonal on bed.*

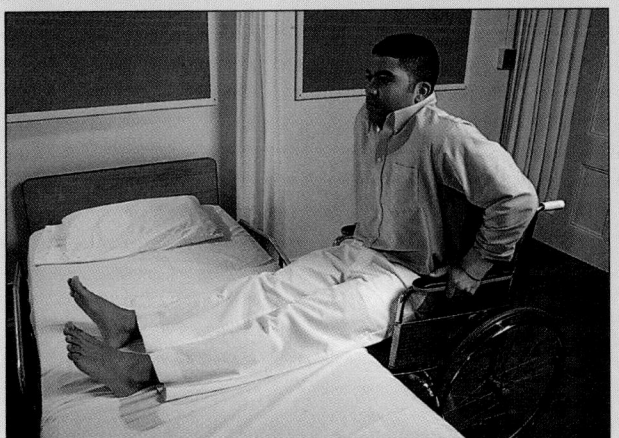

Step 2. *Long sitting transfer—moving into chair.*

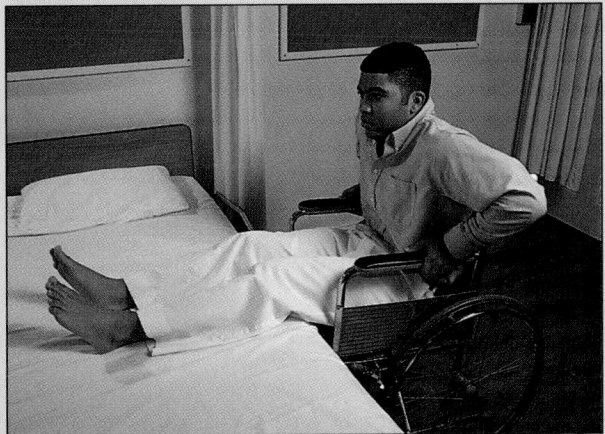

Step 2. *Long sitting transfer—sitting in chair.*

Maximum Assistance Sitting Transfer

1. Two nurses move the client. The client is instructed to cross the arms in front of the body.

2. One nurse reaches around the client from behind and grasps the client around the waist or ribcage. The other nurse lifts the lower extremities off the bed. In a coordinated movement, the nurses shift the client to the chair.

1. The client is unable to help in the transfer; the client's arms when crossed will not impede transfer.

2. Smooth shifting of weight creates the least strain and discomfort and helps ensure safety.

Moderate Assistance Sitting Transfer

1. With help, the client comes forward on the sitting surface, either by doing push-ups or by sliding one hip and then the other forward. The nurse may assist by grasping the hip as the client comes forward.

1. The client participates, but the nurse still does more than 50% of the work. It is easier for a client to move toward the stronger side.

Continued

TRANSFERS
(Continued)

Steps	Rationale
2. The nurse assists the client at the waist with the transfer belt, helping the client to bear as much weight as possible while shifting the hips onto the chair surface.	**2.** The nurse helps to carry the client's weight across to the chair. Proper footwear prevents sudden loss of balance.
3. The nurse's knees brace the client's knees while the client scoots back into the chair.	**3.** This provides for correct posture and comfort.

Transfer Board

1. Place one end of the board under the client's hip and the other end securely on the surface to which he or she will be transferred.	**1.** It is sometimes difficult to get two transferring surfaces close to each other.
2. Assist the client to slide along the board to the new location; then remove the board.	**2.** The client can be taught to use the board independently by doing push-ups while moving across the board.

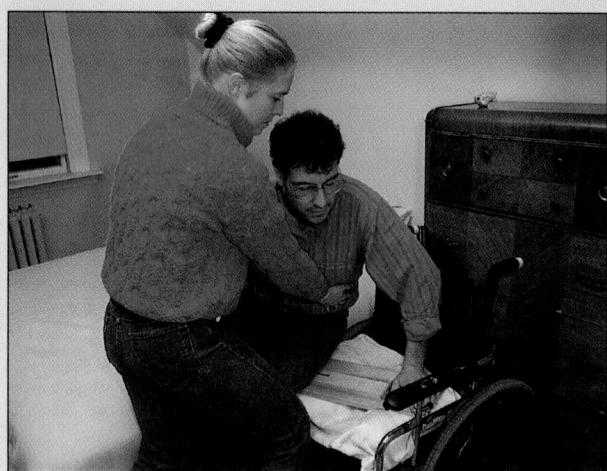

Step 2. *Assisting with sliding board transfer.*

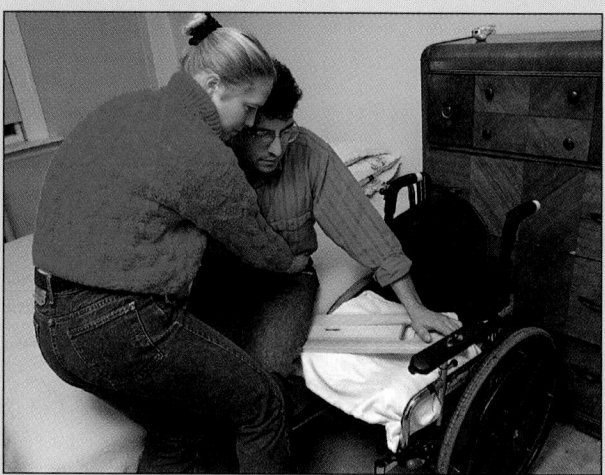

Step 2. *Assisting with sliding board transfer.*

Toilet Transfer

1. Position the chair at a 45-degree angle to the toilet and lock the brakes. Instruct the client to remove his or her feet from the footrests, and, if necessary, shift the chair closer to the toilet.	**1.** The client should be as close as possible to the toilet.
2. Have the client shift the hips so that they are sideways to the seat, remove the armrest, and reach for the opposite side of the toilet seat. The client uses the upper extremities to swing the hips onto the toilet seat.	**2.** Toilet rails or grab bars are an alternative to the toilet seat.
3. Reverse the process to return to chair.	**3.** Employing the same steps ensures safe transfer.

Tub Transfer

1. Position the wheelchair as close to the tub as possible and transfer the client to the edge of the tub.	**1.** The client should be as close as possible to the tub bottom or the tub chair. Upper body strength and good balance are needed to get into and out of the bottom of the tub.

PROCEDURE

25–3

TRANSFERS
(Continued)

Steps	**Rationale**
2. Lift the client's legs into the tub one at a time. Then have the client reach for the tub or for grab bars on the far side of the tub. Keeping the knees extended and the head and trunk forward, the client lowers into the tub, gradually bending the elbows to lower the body. The process is reversed to get out.	**2.** The client with a weaker extremity will probably want to transfer into the tub toward the weaker side and go to the stronger side when getting out. Legs will need to be tucked under the body as much as possible.
3. Draw the water into the tub after the client is in the tub; drain it before the client gets out.	**3.** Water makes the body buoyant and can cause instability.

Car Transfer—Standing

1. Position the wheelchair near the open front car door, remove the feet from the footrests, and swing the rests away. Lock the brakes. Instruct the client to move forward in the chair, placing the feet firmly on the ground with one foot slightly behind the other.	**1.** The wheelchair must be stable. Position of the feet helps in weight bearing. The nurse can assist the client by holding the transfer belt.
2. Have the client use the armrests of the wheelchair to come to a standing position and then reach for the seat or doorframe of the car. The client pivots and lowers the body to the seat, leaning forward to maintain stability and avoid hitting the head. Once seated, the client swing the legs into the car and fastens the seat belt. The process is reversed to exit.	**2.** It is usually easier for the client to ride in the front seat because of the accessibility of the seat. Make sure the door is open as far as it can go to avoid movement of the door as the client stands.

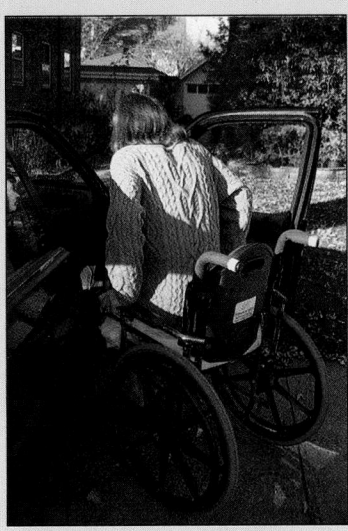 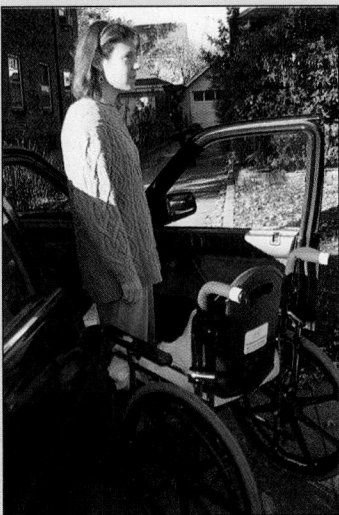

Step 2. *Car standing transfer—standing.*   **Step 2.** *Car standing transfer—turning.*

Continued

PROCEDURE

25-3

TRANSFERS
(Continued)

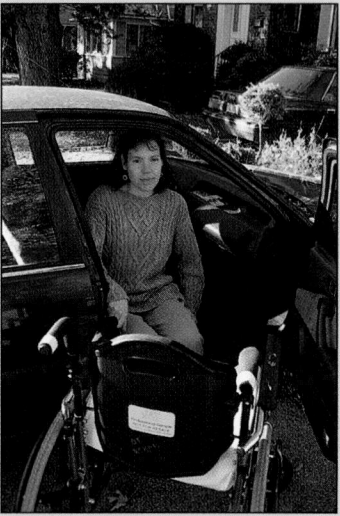 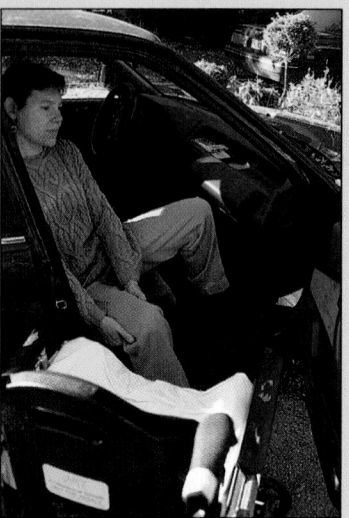

Step 2. *Car standing transfer—sitting.*   **Step 2.** *Car standing transfer—bringing in right leg.*

Steps	Rationale
Car Transfer—Sitting	
1. Instruct the client to position the chair, lock the brakes, and remove the footrests or lift the footpedal.	1. Maintains stability and promotes ease of transfer.
2. The client places one hand on the seat of the car and the other on the armrest of the chair. Using the upper extremities, he or she lifts the hips off the chair and swings them into the car. The client then places the legs into the car and buckles the seatbelt.	2. If the distance between the chair and the car seat is too far, a sliding board may be used to bridge the gap.
3. If the client is the driver, the pieces of the chair must be placed in the car, not in the trunk.	3. Some clients may prefer to transfer into the passenger side and then slide over to the driver's side; others transfer into the driver's seat and place the equipment in the back seat. This maneuver requires that the client be independent.
Three-Person Transfer	
1. If possible, discuss this maneuver with the client before beginning. Lock the brakes of the hospital cart or chair. Move any bottles or drainage bags to the transfer site before beginning.	1. This maneuver can be very frightening for the client. It requires coordination and should be discussed by all before it is begun. The bed and cart should be stable and in the high position to avoid injury to the caregivers' backs.
2. Move the client to the side of the bed in a coordinated manner. Place the client's arms across the chest. Position one caregiver at the client's shoulders, one at the waist, and one at the knees.	2. The client's arms should not interfere with the transfer. Weight should be distributed among the caregivers.
3. Caregivers bend at the knees and hips and slide arms under the client until the hands have grasped the opposite side of the client's body. Using the elbows as a lever on the mattress, the caregivers roll the client into their chests.	3. Care with this step ensures a firm hold. Leverage reduces muscle strain.

PROCEDURE

25–3

TRANSFERS
(Continued)

Steps	**Rationale**
4. Lift the client by straightening the knees and hips on the count of three, then pivot to the transferring surface and lower the client to the chair or cart.	4. All steps must be coordinated carefully. The client should be encouraged and supported to eliminate fear.
5. If moving the client from a stretcher back to the bed, one nurse holds the client's head and shoulders, while two others kneel on or stand at the far side of the client's bed. At the count of three, they lift the client onto the bed, then move the client again into the center of the bed. A doubled sheet placed under the client from head to foot can also be used to assist in transfer.	5. The caregivers across the bed must operate outside their base of support; caregivers on the bed must operate outside their center of gravity. Neither position is ideal. The nurse who is standing across the bed should place one leg behind the other, brace the front leg against the bed, and shift the weight as the move is made from the front leg to the back leg, using the momentum of the move and large muscle strength to facilitate the transfer.

Standing Transfer

1. Have the client wear a good pair of shoes and a brace if one has been prescribed.	1. This provides the client with as much stability and strength as possible.

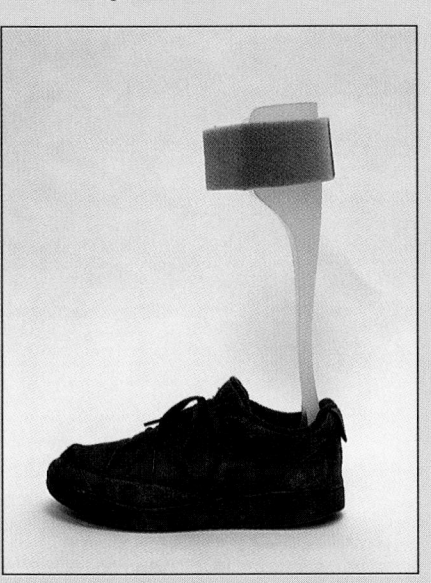

Step 1. *Ankle splint as used during standing.*

2. Stand as close to the client as possible. This can be in front for maximum assistance, or to the weaker side by the person's waist for partial assistance. Stand with a broad base of support, with feet shoulder width apart and one foot slightly ahead of the other.	2. Proper body mechanics prevent injury. Holding the client at the waist is nearer to both the client's and nurse's center of gravity. Use large muscles for lifting by bending at the knees and hips while keeping the back straight.
3. Instruct the client to look in the direction of the transfer to see the transfer surface.	3. Affords the client a sense of security and encourages participation in the process.

Continued

PROCEDURE

25-3

TRANSFERS
(Continued)

Steps	Rationale
4. Assist the client at the waist rather than under the arms. Use a transfer belt if possible. Move your body in the direction of the transfer.	**4.** Position provides enough support for the client but encourages client independence.

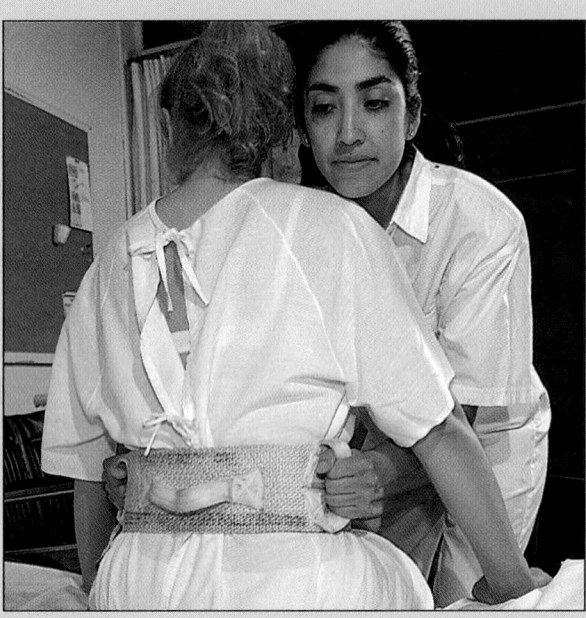

Step 4. Nurse-assisted ambulation with transfer belt.

Steps	Rationale
5. Be consistent when doing a transfer. Teach the client the same sequence of steps and communicate them to other health care team members.	**5.** Reinforces teaching that needs to occur for the client to become independent.

date a wheelchair. The surfaces are difficult to get close to, and the presence of water imposes an added safety hazard. Steps must be taken and adaptations installed to reduce or eliminate the problems. Safety strips can be applied to the bottom of the tub or shower. Grab bars can be added to the area around the toilet and tub. An elevated toilet seat is available to level the transfer surfaces. Shower and tub chairs facilitate the client's ability to get into and out of the bathroom.

A shower chair can be used to enable the client to bathe independently. A chair is desirable when the client is unable to transfer to the bottom of the tub. If a client does not have adequate upper body strength, it is difficult for him or her to get into and out of the bottom of the tub. The chair is the ideal alternative and should be used with a hand-held shower head. The chair is placed in the tub, or the client can trans-

fer to a shower chair and then be wheeled into the shower.

Standing Transfers

Standing transfers require that the client be able to bear some weight or pivot on one or both legs. Clients who have hemiplegia, a fractured hip or leg, unilateral amputation, or any type of weakened extremity usually are able to bear some weight and can perform a standing transfer. Standing transfers produce weight bearing on the long bones and help retain some of the calcium salts that are lost with immobility.

Standing transfers also require that the client has some upper extremity strength. Give the client only the assistance that is needed. Keep in mind the idea of safety and protection for both the nurse and the client.

Client Education

Teaching can occur both formally and informally. The goal for a client with impaired mobility is to maximize the level of independence. The implications for client teaching are significant because the client must learn self-care if independence is to be achieved. Family members are also heavily involved in the care of the client and must also be taught. A formal teaching plan is identified by the nurse shortly after admission. The plan identifies the content to be taught, when, by whom, the method used, and the outcome of the teaching. Specific content includes ROM exercises, ambulation techniques, positioning schedules, self-care activities, management of medication or treatments, hygiene techniques for the skin, as well as any management of the disease process.

The setting in which the teaching occurs can be the client's room or a formal classroom setting. It may be more efficient to have the client and family involved in classes held on the unit. The dynamics of a group interaction can be invaluable and reinforce what the nurse has been trying to teach. If time is a factor, one-to-one teaching may be necessary. Schedule a session when the client is not too tired to learn and when family members are present. The cognitively impaired client will need the material to be presented in a simple manner, consistent in content, and repeated many times. A return demonstration is very helpful, because most of the skills taught are best learned by demonstration and return demonstration. Use of print media and visual aids increases the chances of success with the client.

Caregivers also need education. Involve them in the classes with the client. Allow for many questions and time to assimilate the information. A referral to a home care agency or a public health nurse to reinforce teaching and evaluate the client at home is appropriate. Some hospitals have separate classes for the caregivers. Encourage attendance if this is an option.

Evaluation

The goals for the client are the criteria to measure his or her activity and whether the outcomes have been achieved. The goals developed for mobility are specific to the client and factor in the diagnosis, prognosis, and treatment plan. Outcomes are defined in terms of client behavior and not in terms of nursing interventions (see "Planning").

Client learning, a change in behavior, movement toward independence, and readiness for discharge need to be evaluated and noted in the client record. The nurse must maintain objectivity when evaluating the client, basing the evaluation on where the client currently is in the process of returning to health and not where he or she should be or is hoped to be.

Clients involved in a rehabilitation environment have the added advantage of the interdisciplinary team formally evaluating his or her progress on a planned schedule. Goals that are set by the whole team, including the client and family, are evaluated, and adjustments are made, depending on the response. Open discussion and problem solving, in the spirit of collaboration among team members, provides the optimal environment for the client and ensures that he or she is getting the best care possible. Clients covered by Medicare must show progress toward the outcomes or they become ineligible to continue in a formal rehabilitation program.

Discharge Planning

Discharge planning is a form of evaluation that begins on the day of admission. All members of the team anticipate the needs of the client after discharge. Clients with impaired mobility usually have multiple needs once they leave the hospital and therefore benefit from discharge planning. Mobilizing the forces needed takes careful coordination of the energy and resources available in the community. That is why it is ideal if all members of the team agree on a plan, articulate it, and identify the outcomes that will indicate success. A client may need some environmental modifications that will take time to implement. Performing a home evaluation and then making any necessary changes, such as building ramps or making changes to the bathroom, are some of the factors involved in the discharge plan.

For some families, the options are limited. Geographical distance or financial limitations may make it unrealistic for family members to be able to support the client at home. Alternatives should be explored early in the hospitalization. It may be necessary for the client to move into an extended care unit or nursing home on a temporary basis.

Home Care

Evaluation of the home is essential for the client with a mobility impairment. The first step is an interview with the client and family. Questions should focus on the floor plan, the ease of movement in the house, the anticipated problems the client can identify through the nurse's prompting, and the financial resources available to provide any changes needed. A home visit may be needed and can be done by the nurse or therapists.

The entrance into the home may need to be modified to accommodate a wheelchair. If stairs lead into the house, a ramp with a gradual incline may be needed to make it easier to enter the home. A ramp can be constructed with a 1-in rise for every 12 in of elevation. The incline cannot be too great, or the person will be unable to navigate the ramp. Railings are provided to steady the client when he or she is moving up or down a ramp. If the client resides in a residence that cannot be modified with ramps, temporary or permanent changes in living arrangements may be necessary.

The flooring in the home can make it difficult to ambulate. Carpeting is difficult to roll a wheelchair over, and scatter rugs are especially dangerous because they slip and slide easily and can get caught on a walker or crutch base. Remove the rugs that are unsafe and offer assistance with moving the wheelchair. A wet floor is dangerous for both the able bodied and the disabled. Wipe up spills and make sure the floor in the bathroom is dry. Apply safety strips to the bottom of the bathtub or shower to provide sure footing.

Grab bars near the toilet and tub can be installed either permanently or temporarily to support safe transfers. The occupational or physical therapist or social service worker can be a valuable resource in recommending and securing these items for the client. Lists of the vendors in the area can be obtained from social service or home care.

Standard doorways are often too narrow to allow the passage of a wheelchair. A commode may be needed if the client is unable to get into the bathroom. Often, the client will have to attend to hygiene needs at the bedside or in the kitchen. Every attempt should be made to provide the client with privacy. Commodes or bedpans may negatively affect the client's elimination habits. Develop a routine as close as possible to the one the client had prior to the mobility problems. A raised toilet seat may be all that is needed to modify the bathroom.

Adaptive equipment is available to assist the client. Equipment ranges from grooming and bathing aids to eating utensils and devices that enable a client to return to work. If an occupational therapist is available, a consultation can prove invaluable. Not only do occupational therapists have numerous items available, but they also can modify items that the client has in the home. If a therapist is not available, medical supply companies can be of assistance and have access to supply catalogues.

Adaptations can be made to the client's automobile to allow him or her to continue to drive. Special steering wheels are available if the client is unable to grasp the standard wheel. A thicker rim is sometimes all that is needed. Hand controls are available for those who are unable to use the lower extremities. The client must take lessons to learn to use the devices. Modifications to the client's car allow him or her the ability to continue with the mobility enjoyed before the impairment occurred.

Safety issues are also of concern to the client and caregiver, who may be a family member. If the client requires a high degree of assistance to move about, the safety of the caregiver should be addressed. If the caregiver is a healthy individual, then instructions on body mechanics and moving and lifting can spare the back. Often—especially with an older client—the caregiver is elderly and experiencing some limitations of activities. An elderly caregiver may only be able to assist in lighter interventions. In such cases, it is necessary to secure the services of home health aides or a personal attendant.

To protect the client and caregiver from further injury, education is essential. Actively involve the client and those concerned from the beginning. Use every situation to teach the care required. Demonstration and return demonstration are extremely effective. This allows the nurse the opportunity to evaluate the interaction that is occurring between the client and caregiver. Watch for signs such as follow-through or initiation of activity that indicate an understanding of the instructions given. A change in behavior also indicates that people involved in the process are learning. Evaluate the interpersonal dynamics between client and caregiver and watch for signs of support, tension, or misunderstanding. This may be the time to promote a discussion of the issues surrounding the hospitalization, the potential changing of roles within the family, and the goals that the client and family hope to achieve.

◆ Summary

This chapter has focused on the concept of mobility as it relates to both the client and the nurse. Mobility impairments affect not only the client's ability to move around but also his or her physiological and social needs. The nurse must consider the mobility needs when the client first enters the health care system. A plan is initiated and revised as the client's status changes. The ultimate goal is to return the client to the level of independence before the incident occurred. Client care is shifting from the acute care setting to the home and requires adaptations that support the family and caregivers in the home.

The actions of moving and lifting the client affect the caregivers because they require that the nurse use good body mechanics to prevent an injury from occurring. If the client is going to require assistance at home, it is imperative that the family or caregiver be instructed in the techniques of client assistance. The caregiver also needs guidance in monitoring the client's progress and reporting changes to the appropriate people. It is the responsibility of the nurse and the other members of the health care team to provide this information in the form of instruction, handouts, and demonstration so that the care of the client is safe, consistent, and appropriate. The client and family are seen as key members of the team and must be included in the process that guides the decisions.

The population most vulnerable to immobility or impaired mobility is the elderly. Changes that can often spell the difference between independence and dependence occur quickly. Chronic diseases and co-morbidities affect the reserve that the elderly client maintains, and often hospitalization initiates the cascade to dependency. The nurse's role with the elderly client is to minimize the impact of hospitalization, mobilize the client early, and facilitate discharge to home or an intermediate facility.

CHAPTER HIGHLIGHTS

◆

◆ Every living organism requires mobility as part of its function.

◆ Movement transports objects from one point to another.

◆ Immobility creates negative effects on the body. The extent is determined by the length of time the client is immobile, any chronic diseases present, and the age of the client.

◆ Factors to be considered when developing a plan of care include strength of the client, mobility impairments, nature of the impairment, cognitive level of functioning, any complicating factors, and the resources available to the client after discharge.

◆ Risk factors that affect the level of immobility are age of the client, mental status, functional status, chronic diseases, visual impairments, medications, and environmental barriers or hazards.

◆ The most frequently used nursing diagnoses concerning mobility are Disuse Syndrome; Physical Mobility, Impaired; High Risk for Injury; and Self Care Deficit Syndrome.

◆ Positioning and turning schedules are incorporated into the plan of care to minimize complications, maximize results, and promote a timely discharge from the hospital.

◆ Nurses and caregivers are at high risk for back injuries because of the amount of moving and lifting required when caring for an immobilized client. To offset this risk, they must incorporate good body mechanics into their activities.

◆ The nursing staff and other members of the health care team must evaluate the client's home setting. Environmental barriers should be modified and special equipment made available prior to discharge to maximize the independence of the client.

Study Questions

1. The hip joint is an example of a

    a. pivot joint
    b. ball-and-socket joint
    c. condyloid joint
    d. hinge joint

2. The center of gravity is

    a. located in the pelvic region
    b. the point at which the body's mass is located
    c. outside the base of support in a side-to-side motion
    d. a key component of body mechanics

3. Risk factors for the immobilized elderly client include

    a. decreased cognition
    b. incontinence of the bladder
    c. incontinence of the bowel
    d. visual impairment
    e. multiple chronic diseases
        1. a, b
        2. b only
        3. all of the above
        4. d, e

4. Which of the following statements are true?

    a. abduction of a limb means moving toward midline
    b. flexion of a joint is possible with a hinge joint
    c. the prone position is a face-up position
    d. the joints in the fingers and toes are primarily gliding joints
        1. a, d
        2. b, d
        3. b, c
        4. a, c, d

5. Mr. Smith is going home after having a hip joint replaced. He is able to partially bear weight and needs to use crutches. Which gait pattern is most appropriate for him?

    a. four-point gait
    b. three-point-and-one gait
    c. three-point gait
    d. two-point gait

Critical Thinking Exercises

1. You are preparing to transfer Ms. T., who has a right hemiparalysis, from the bed to a wheelchair. Discuss how you would transfer her.

2. Amy, 18 years old, is a new quadraplegic patient following a motor vehicle accident. Discuss the important principles of positioning and early mobility for Amy.

References

Carpenito, L. J. (1993). *Nursing diagnosis: Application to clinical practice* (3rd. ed.). Philadelphia: J. B. Lippincott.

Creditor, M. C. (1993). Hazards of hospitalization of the elderly. *Annals of Internal Medicine, 118* (3), 221.

Gorbien, M., Bishop, J., Beers, M., *et al.* (1992). Iatrogenic illness in hospitalized people. *Journal of American Geriatric Society, 40* (10), 103.

Kottke, F. (1966). The effects of limitation of activity upon the human body. *Journal of American Medical Association, 196*, 835–840.

Mobily, P., & Skemp Kelley, L. (1991). Iatrogenesis in the elderly: Factors of immobility. *Journal of Gerontological Nursing, 17* (9), 9.

Bibliography

Carpenito, L. J. (1993). *Nursing diagnosis: Application to clinical practice* (3rd ed.). New York: J. B. Lippincott.

Chenitz, W. C., Stone, J. T., & Salisbury, S. A. (1991). *Clinical gerontological nursing: A guide to advanced practice.* Philadelphia: W. B. Saunders.

Christian, B. J. (1982). Immobilization: Psychosocial aspects. In C. Nomis (Ed.), *Concept clarification in nursing,* Rockville, MD: Aspen Publications.

Creditor, M. C. (1993). Hazards of hospitalization of the elderly. *Annals of Internal Medicine, 118* (3), 219–223.

Curry, K., & Casady, L. (1992). The relationship between extended periods of immobility and decubitus ulcer formation in the acutely spinal cord–injured individual, *Journal of Neuroscience Nursing, 24* (4), 185–189.

Dean, E. (1985). Effect of body position on pulmonary function. *Physical Therapy, 65* (5), 613–618.

Dittmar, S. (1989). *Rehabilitation nursing: Process and application.* St. Louis: C. V. Mosby.

Ferris, F., & Fretwell, M. (1992). *Practical guide to the care of the geriatric patient.* St. Louis: Mosby-Year Book.

Flinn, N., Loeper, J., Irrgang, S., *et al.* (1986). *Therapeutic positioning and skin care.* Minneapolis: Sister Kenny Institute.

Gee, Z. L., & Passarella, P. M. (1985). *Nursing care of the stroke patient: A therapeutic approach.* Pittsburgh: AREN Publications.

Gorbien, M., *et al.* (1992). Iatrogenic illness in hospitalized people. *Journal of American Geriatric Society, 40* (10), 103.

Hersberg, S. R. (1993). Positioning the nursing home resident. An issue of quality of life. *American Journal of Occupational Therapy, 47* (1), 75–77.

Hinderer, S. R., & Steinberg, F. U. (1990). Physicatric therapeutics. 4, Transfers and mobility/community reentry. *Archives of Physical Medicine & Rehabilitation, 71* (4-S), S267–S270.

Hirsch, C. H., *et al.* (1990). The natural history of functional morbidity in hospitalized older patients. *Journal of American Geriatric Society, 38* (12), 1296–1303.

Kane, R. L., Sommers, L., Olsen, A., & Mullen, L. (1994). *Essentials of clinical geriatrics* (3rd ed.). New York: McGraw-Hill.

Kottke, F. (1965). Deterioration of the bedfast patient. *Public Health Reports, 80,* 437.

Kottke, F. (1966). The effects of limitation of activity upon the human body. *Journal of American Medical Association, 196,* 835–840.

Loeper, J. (1985). *Range of motion exercise.* Minneapolis: Sister Kenny Institute.

Miller, C. A. (1990). *Nursing care of older adults.* Glenview, IL: Scott-Foresman.

Quellet, L. L., & Rush, K. (1992). A synthesis of selected literature on mobility. A basis for studying impaired mobility. *Nursing Diagnosis, 3* (2), 72–80.

Rush, K. L. & Quellet, L. L. (1993). Mobility: A concept analysis. *Journal of Advanced Nursing, 18* (3), 486–492.

Steel, K., *et al.* (1981). Iatrogenic illness on a general medicine service at a university hospital. *New England Journal of Medicine, 304,* 638–642.

Whaley, L. F., & Wong, D. L. (1989). *Essentials of pediatric nursing* (3rd ed.). St. Louis: C. V. Mosby.

York, J. (1989). Mobility methods selected for use in home and community environments. *Physical Therapy, 69* (9), 736–744.

Chapter 26

REST AND COMFORT

CHRISTINE MIASKOWSKI, RN, PHD, FAAN

LEARNING OBJECTIVES

✦

After studying this chapter, you should be able to
✦ Define sleep
✦ Describe the physiology of sleep
✦ Explain the differences between REM and non-REM
  sleep
✦ Describe developmental changes in the physiology
  of sleep and the need for sleep
✦ List six problems that can alter an individual's
  sleep-rest cycle
✦ Define insomnia, narcolepsy, sleep apnea, and
  sleep deprivation
✦ Perform a sleep assessment
✦ Develop a nursing care plan for a client experienc-
  ing an alteration in the sleep-wake cycle
✦ Define pain
✦ Describe the four physiological processes involved
  in pain physiology
✦ Describe the developmental changes in pain pro-
  cessing that occur in neonates and the elderly
✦ Differentiate among acute pain, chronic pain of
  nonmalignant origin, and chronic pain of malignant
  origin
✦ Differentiate among somatic, visceral, and neuro-
  pathic pain
✦ Perform a pain assessment
✦ Develop a nursing care plan for a client in acute
  pain
✦ Develop a nursing care plan for a client in chronic
  pain

Rest and comfort are two fundamental human needs that contribute to the physical well-being and quality of life of every individual. When illness or injury results in pain or sleep disruption, an individual often requires pharmacological or nonpharmacological interventions to promote rest and comfort. This chapter describes the physiological mechanisms underlying sleep and pain. In addition, the most common sleep disorders and pain problems are described. The nursing assessment of these two clinical problems is addressed, and developmental considerations are stressed. Emphasis is placed on understanding both the pharmacological and nonpharmacological management of these two clinical conditions.

Rest

Rest can be defined as a state of mental relaxation and decreased physical activity. Adequate rest leaves an individual feeling refreshed and rejuvenated. Every person has his or her own ways of attaining adequate rest. Rest may be obtained by watching television, reading a book, or taking a walk. Many clients need to be encouraged to obtain adequate rest to meet the physiological and psychological demands placed on the body by illness or physiological changes such as pregnancy. Nurses can help clients recognize the importance of rest and learn how to promote it at home or in a health care facility.

Sleep is a common human experience. Humans spend approximately one third of their lives asleep. Sleep can be defined as a regular, recurrent, easily reversible state of an organism, characterized by relative quiescence and by a great increase in the threshold of response to external stimuli (Turpin, 1986). However, as noted by Turpin (1986, p. 313), "sleep is not a period of mere physiological quiescence, but a complex phenomenon which results from numerous different physiological processes."

Sleep has been shown to be an essential component of health, affecting the well-being and quality of life of individuals (Jensen & Herr, 1993). It is estimated that over 100 million people in the United States have sleep disorders (Manfredi, Vgontzas, & Kales, 1989). Sleep disorders may result in an occasional "bad day" or completely disrupt an individual's normal work and social activities. Disruptions in the normal sleep-wake cycle may have profound physiological as well as psychological and socioeconomic consequences (Robinson, 1993).

Normal Physiology of Sleep and Wakefulness

Sleep is a state of reduced responsiveness to external stimuli, an altered state of consciousness from which a person can be aroused only if a stimulus is of sufficient magnitude. Sleep is the physically inactive part of the circadian sleep-wake-activity cycle and is characterized by cyclical changes in the electroencephalogram (EEG) and other physiological parameters (Hodgson, 1991).

The circadian sleep-wake-activity cycle refers to one type of cyclical rhythm that regulates a variety of physiological functions. The most familiar rhythm is the 24-hour day-night cycle, known as a circadian or diurnal rhythm. The circadian sleep-wake-activity cycle is affected by light and temperature. Light and darkness provide environmental cues to when a person should sleep or awaken. However, circadian cycles are also influenced by work schedules and social activities. For example, individuals who work nights adjust their sleep-wake-activity cycles to accommodate their work schedules. When individuals enter health care facilities, they often experience disruptions in their sleep-wake-activity cycles that can lead to inadequate sleep and rest.

Anatomy and Physiology of Sleep

The exact anatomical and physiological mechanisms of sleep are not completely understood. Two interrelated cerebral mechanisms—the reticular activating system (RAS) and the bulbar synchronizing region (BSR)—are involved in controlling the sleep-wake cycle.

The RAS appears to be responsible for maintaining arousal and wakefulness. The RAS receives visual, auditory, gustatory, olfactory, tactile, visceral, kinesthetic, somatic, and cognitive input. As illustrated in Figure 26–1, the RAS has numerous connections between higher and lower brain centers (Lee, 1991). The BSR is located in the brain stem and contains specialized cells that release a neurotransmitter (i.e., serotonin) that is involved in promoting sleep. A reduction in sensory input to the RAS (e.g., closing one's eyes, being in a quiet room) and enhanced activity in the BSR cause sleep. However, increased sensory input to the RAS (e.g., disturbing thoughts, heightened emotions, loud noises, bright lights) at bedtime results in increased activity in the RAS and decreased activity in the BSR, promoting wakefulness rather than sleep.

Sleep occurs when there is decreased input into the RAS and serotonin is released from the BSR. As people prepare to fall asleep, they close their eyes and assume relaxed positions. These activities reduce input to the RAS. Being in a darkened and quiet room further decreases the environmental inputs into the RAS and lets the BSR take over, producing sleep.

States and Stages of Sleep

Two states of sleep can be recognized using EEG recordings. The first state, called non–rapid eye movement (NREM) sleep, is characterized by a sleeping posture, with the eyes closed and the pupils myotic. However, a certain degree of tone remains in all mus-

Functions of Sleep

The exact functions of sleep are unknown. Most of the theories about the functions of human sleep come from observations of individuals who have been deprived of sleep. For example, sleep deprivation is associated with irritability, decreased mental functioning, and, in some cases, psychotic behavior. Therefore, sleep has been viewed as a time of restoration for the body (Guyton, 1991). NREM sleep appears to be necessary for a person to be restored physiologically and to feel well rested. REM sleep appears to be necessary for psychological restoration and for learning and memory to occur (Lee, 1991).

Developmental Changes in the Need for Rest and Sleep

The amount of sleep that individuals require varies a great deal. However, distinct changes in the amount of sleep required during different developmental stages have been documented and are summarized in Table 26–2.

✦ **Neonates.** Neonates sleep for approximately 16 hours per day (range, 10–23 h). Part of their sleep-rest activity involves recovering from the stress of the birth process. Approximately 50% of a neonate's sleep is REM. The states of a neonate's sleep-wake pattern are summarized in Table 26–2.

✦ **Infants.** Infants vary in the amount of sleep they require. Most infant sleep is characterized as REM sleep and occurs for about 10 to 15 hours per day. Usually by 4 months of age, an infant sleeps through the night. It should be noted that breast-fed infants exhibit more nighttime awakenings than bottle-fed infants.

✦ **Toddlers.** The sleep-wake cycle in toddlers begins to mature, and the amount of time spent in REM sleep decreases. Napping is a common experience for toddlers. The need for two or three naps per day decreases as the toddler approaches the preschool years. Toddlers often awake during the night (two or three times each night) because of separation anxiety, teething pain, or nightmares and sometimes require parental attention to return to sleep.

✦ **Preschoolers.** Preschoolers average about 12 hours of sleep per night. Preschoolers need to develop a nighttime routine and an established bedtime ritual. Nightmares are common in preschoolers, and children need to be comforted by parents in their own beds.

✦ **School-Age Children.** School-age children have variable sleep needs, depending on the activity level and the physical growth needs of the child. School-age children require encouragement to go to sleep on a schedule and develop a normal sleep routine.

✦ **Adolescents.** Increasing social demands and a desire to be part of a peer group affect the sleep patterns of adolescents. The sleep needs of adolescents vary widely. For example, adolescents may enjoy social activities that continue into the night. These late-night hours may result in adolescents sleeping late in the morning.

✦ **Young Adults.** Sleep in healthy young adults begins to establish adult routines. Various factors (e.g., stress, work, recreational activities, social relationships) can influence young adults' need for sleep and their ability to fall asleep. In young adults, 80% of an individual's total sleep is NREM and 20% is REM.

✦ **Middle-Aged Adults.** Middle-aged adults experience a total decrease in sleep time and an increase in the amount of time spent in bed awake. The total amount of time in stage 4 NREM sleep decreases. Sleep disturbances, particularly insomnia, become more common. Women may experience sleep disturbances as they go through menopause.

✦ **Older Adults.** Changes in the sleep patterns of older adults may be caused by changes in the central nervous system (CNS) that affect sleep regulation. In addition, chronic illnesses in older adults may alter their sleep-wake cycles. Therefore, the quality of sleep as one ages markedly deteriorates. The elderly experience a significant decrease in the amount of time spent in stages 3 and 4 of NREM. In addition, older adults tend to awaken repeatedly during the night and spend more time awake before falling asleep. Another change in the sleep-activity pattern in the elderly is the need for frequent naps and rest periods during the day.

Common Problems That Alter Sleep and Rest

Numerous factors can enhance or detract from an individual's ability to sleep, as well as the amount of time an individual spends in sleep. These factors include illness, drugs, activity, diet, stress, and the environment (Lee, 1991).

✦ **Illness.** Physical and psychological illnesses can cause disruptions in the sleep-wake cycle. Certain illnesses (e.g., respiratory disease, cardiac disease, hypertension, gastrointestinal disorders, restless leg syndrome) can result in sleep disturbances. For example, asthma, bronchitis, or the common cold may interrupt normal breathing and disrupt sleep. With regard to cardiac disease, it is known that myocardial infarctions occur more often during REM sleep, and deaths from cardiac disease occur most frequently between 5 and 6 A.M., when REM sleep lasts the longest. In addition, clients with chronic medical illnesses may experience pain that can interfere with their ability to sleep and rest.

Table **26–2**

AGE-RELATED CHANGES IN SLEEP-WAKE CYCLE

AGE GROUP	DURATION OF SLEEP, HOURS	BEHAVIORAL CHARACTERISTICS
Neonates	10–23	Six distinct levels of arousal: **1.** Regular sleep—eyes are closed, no muscle jerks, regular respiratory pattern **2.** Irregular sleep—eyes are closed, irregular respiratory pattern, involuntary muscle activity **3.** Periodic sleep—periodic respiratory pattern (*e.g.,* tachypnea to Cheyne-Stokes) **4.** Drowsiness—eyes open or closed; irregular breathing pattern; neonate may squeal **5.** Alert inactivity—eyes open, infant responds to environmental stimuli, irregular respiratory pattern **6.** Crying—open or closed eyes, vocalization associated with gross motor movements
Infants	10–15	REM sleep predominates Circadian (day-night) sleep cycle develops By 4 mo of age, infants sleep through the night
Toddlers	10–15	Amount of REM sleep decreases Naps needed up to 3 y of age Two or three nighttime awakenings
Preschoolers	9–16	REM sleep pattern resembles that of adults Nightmares are common Need for a consistent bedtime routine
School-age children	8–10	Sleep needs are highly individualized Nap not required Sleep needs increase during periods of physical growth
Adolescents	8–9	Sleep needs vary widely Sleeping late in the morning is common
Young adults	6–8.5	REM sleep accounts for 20% of sleep time Sleep-wake cycle establishes adult routines
Middle-aged adults	6–8.5	Total sleep time decreases Stage 4 sleep decreases Number of sleep arousals increases Time spent awake in bed increases
Older adults	6–8.5	Deep sleep is decreased Difficulty falling asleep is common Awakening easily is common Decrease in the total number of hours of sleep Stages 3 and 4 of NREM sleep decrease No stage 4 NREM sleep Nap time increases

✦ **Drugs.** Many different types of medications, including sedatives and hypnotics, can affect sleep stage cycles and the sleep-wake cycle. Sedatives and hypnotics produce a more rapid sleep onset by reducing the amount of sensory input to the RAS. Many drugs (*e.g.,* opioids, alcohol, barbiturates, tricyclic antidepressants, antihypertensives) suppress REM sleep regardless of the time of day the drugs are administered.

Short-acting benzodiazepines (*e.g.,* triazolam) are used to initiate and maintain sleep. These drugs may act by stimulating an inhibitory neurotransmitter called gamma-aminobutyric acid (GABA). These drugs induce the rapid onset of sleep, but they suppress deep sleep as well as REM sleep.

Central nervous system stimulants (*e.g.,* caffeine) have been shown to delay the time of sleep onset and decrease the total amount of sleep time. CNS stimulants that contain caffeine include coffee, tea, and chocolate. Even decaffeinated coffee contains small amounts of caffeine.

❧ **Activity.** Exercise associated with moderate fatigue enhances sleep. Research has demonstrated that physical exercise during the early part of the day increases the amount of deep sleep during the night and reduces the amount of REM sleep. It should be noted that excessive fatigue may result in difficulty falling asleep. In addition, individuals who are placed on bed rest or are immobile demonstrate a need for more deep sleep.

❧ **Diet.** Individuals experiencing sudden weight changes have an increased need for sleep. Clients experiencing malnutrition or hyperthyroidism have increases in the deep stages of sleep, most likely because they are in an increased catabolic state.

❧ **Stress.** Individuals who experience physical stress (*e.g.*, intense physical labor or exercise) appear to require less total sleep time, have fewer episodes of light sleep, and have fewer interruptions in all stages of sleep. In contrast, when an individual experiences psychological stress, the amount of deep sleep and total sleep time appear to increase. However, high levels of anxiety produce disruptions in the sleep-wake cycle by activating the RAS and preventing the onset of sleep.

❧ **Environment.** The environment is a critical component in initiating the sleep cycle. The environment and environmental clues (*e.g.*, darkness, nightclothes, bed, pillows) are often part of an individual's sleep rituals that promote sleep onset and sleep efficiency. Alterations in the environment (*e.g.*, being admitted to a hospital, attempting to sleep in a noisy hotel room) often disrupt the initiation and maintenance of the sleep cycle.

Sleep Disorders

Impaired sleep is a global and nonspecific term used to describe an alteration in sleep cycles and daytime functioning (Robinson, 1993). Originally, sleep disorders were divided into four major categories, based on an individual's symptoms (Sleep Disorders Classification Committee, 1979). Gradually, this classification system became unsatisfactory, because individuals reported sleep-related symptoms that fell into more than one category. In 1990, a new classification system, with more discrete categories, was published (American Sleep Disorders Association, 1990). The major diagnostic categories are listed in Box 26–1. Several of the more common sleep disorders are discussed here.

Insomnia

Insomnia is a perception of inadequate sleep and includes difficulty in initiating sleep, frequent awakenings from sleep, and a perception of a nonrestorative sleep. It is the most common sleep disorder. Insomnia may be classified as idiopathic or psychophysiological.

Idiopathic insomnia usually begins in childhood. It may be caused by a neurochemical imbalance of the arousal system, the sleep-onset mechanisms, or the sleep-maintenance system. The syndrome is usually associated with a decreased feeling of well-being during the day, a deterioration of mood and motivation, decreased attention span, low levels of energy and concentration, and increased fatigue (American Sleep Disorders Association, 1990).

Psychophysiological insomnia can occur from a variety of causes, including stress and tension. Individuals with this disorder are usually not sleepy during the day but function poorly in terms of cognitive skills and also report fatigue (Robinson, 1993).

Narcolepsy

Narcolepsy is a disorder characterized by a set of clinical symptoms including abnormal sleep, overwhelming episodes of sleep that may occur at inappropriate times, excessive daytime sleepiness, hallucinations, disturbances in nighttime sleep, paroxysmal muscle weakness, cataplexy (a sudden loss of muscle tone involving specific small muscle groups or generalized muscle weakness that may cause a person to slump to the floor), and sleep paralysis (a generalized flaccidity of muscles with full consciousness in the transitional period between sleep and waking) (American Sleep Disorders Association, 1990). The cause of narcolepsy is unknown, but there is a strong genetic component to this disorder (Billard, 1985). The disorder begins in early adult life and occurs equally in men and women. Individuals with this disorder may fall asleep while totally engaged in a stimulating activity. An abrupt and reversible decrease in or loss of voluntary muscle tone (cataplexy) can occur during an attack. Attacks generally last from a few seconds to 30 minutes and begin with REM sleep.

Sleep Apnea

Sleep apnea syndrome can be classified as obstructive or central; more commonly, it has characteristics of both. Obstructive sleep apnea (OSA) is characterized by cessation of breathing for at least 10 seconds that occurs at least 30 times during sleep. The syndrome is associated with loud snores or gasps followed by a period of apnea that lasts 20 to 30 seconds. The total number of apneic episodes may be in the hundreds.

Obstructive sleep apnea is associated with nasopharyngeal abnormalities, neurological abnormalities of the airway muscles, and/or obesity. The typical client is an overweight male. Most clients, as well as their sleep partners, are aware of the sleep disorder. Clients may experience a variety of physiological and psychological consequences associated with OSA, including depression, anxiety, irritability, loss of libido,

Box **26–1**

DIAGNOSTIC CLASSIFICATION OF SLEEP-WAKE DISORDERS

I. Dyssomnias
  A. Intrinsic sleep disorders
    1. Psychophysiological insomnia
    2. Sleep-state misperception
    3. Idiopathic insomnia
    4. Narcolepsy
    5. Recurrent hypersomnia
    6. Idiopathic hypersomnia
    7. Posttraumatic hypersomnia
    8. Obstructive sleep apnea syndrome
    9. Central sleep apnea syndrome
    10. Central alveolar hypoventilation
    11. Periodic limb movement disorder
    12. Restless legs syndrome
  B. Extrinsic sleep disorders
    1. Inadequate sleep hygiene
    2. Environmental sleep disorder
    3. Altitude insomnia
    4. Adjustment sleep disorder
    5. Insufficient sleep syndrome
    6. Limit-setting sleep disorder
    7. Sleep-onset association disorder
    8. Food allergy insomnia
    9. Nocturnal eating (drinking) syndrome
    10. Hypnotic-dependent sleep disorder
    11. Stimulant-dependent sleep disorder
    12. Alcohol-dependent sleep disorder
    13. Toxin-induced sleep disorder
  C. Circadian rhythm sleep disorders
    1. Time zone change (jet lag) syndrome
    2. Shift work sleep disorder
    3. Irregular sleep-wake pattern
    4. Delayed sleep phase syndrome
    5. Advanced sleep phase syndrome
    6. Non-24-hour sleep-wake disorder
II. Parasomnias
  A. Arousal disorders
    1. Confusional arousals
    2. Sleepwalking
    3. Sleep terrors
  B. Sleep-wake transition disorders
    1. Rhythmic movement disorder
    2. Sleep starts
    3. Sleep talking
    4. Nocturnal leg cramps
  C. Parasomnias usually associated with REM sleep
    1. Nightmares
    2. Sleep paralysis
    3. Impaired sleep-related penile erections
    4. Sleep-related painful erections
    5. REM sleep-related sinus arrest
    6. REM sleep behavior disorder

  D. Other parasomnias
    1. Sleep bruxism
    2. Sleep enuresis
    3. Sleep-related abnormal swallowing syndrome
    4. Nocturnal paroxysmal dystonia
    5. Sudden unexplained nocturnal death syndrome
    6. Primary snoring
    7. Infant sleep apnea
    8. Congenital central hypoventilation syndrome
    9. Sudden infant death syndrome
    10. Benign neonatal sleep myoclonus
III. Medical/psychiatric sleep disorders
  A. Associated with mental disorders
    1. Psychoses
    2. Mood disorders
    3. Anxiety disorders
    4. Panic disorder
    5. Alcoholism
  B. Associated with neurological disorders
    1. Cerebral degenerative disorders
    2. Dementia
    3. Parkinsonism
    4. Fatal familial insomnia
    5. Sleep-related epilepsy
    6. Electrical status epilepticus of sleep
    7. Sleep-related headaches
  C. Associated with other medical disorders
    1. Sleeping sickness
    2. Nocturnal cardiac ischemia
    3. Chronic obstructive pulmonary disease
    4. Fragmentary myoclonus
    5. Sleep hyperhidrosis
    6. Peptic ulcer disease
    7. Fibrositis syndrome
IV. Proposed sleep disorders
    1. Short sleeper
    2. Long sleeper
    3. Subwakefulness syndrome
    4. Fragmentary myoclonus
    5. Sleep hyperhidrosis
    6. Menstrual-associated sleep disorder
    7. Pregnancy-associated sleep disorder
    8. Terrifying hypnagogic hallucinations
    9. Sleep-related neurogenic tachypnea
    10. Sleep-related laryngospasm
    11. Sleep choking syndrome

From American Sleep Disorders Association. (1997). *International classification of sleep disorders, revised: Diagnostic and coding manual.* Rochester, MN: American Sleep Disorders Association.

cardiac arrhythmias, premature ventricular contractions, hypertension, decreased oxygenation, polycythemia, and gastroesophageal reflux. Individuals with this disorder typically awaken feeling groggy, experience mental dullness and incoordination, complain of a

morning headache, and are excessively sleepy during the day.

Central sleep apnea (CSA) occurs because the normal respiratory drive mechanism fails during sleep. The condition is associated with a decrease in or cessation of respirations, usually accompanied by a decrease in arterial oxygen levels. These individuals often complain of insomnia and sometimes are sleepy during normal waking hours. Clients with CSA may also have hypertension, cardiac arrhythmias, pulmonary hypertension, and cardiac failure.

Sleep Deprivation

Sleep deprivation is a common problem when individuals are hospitalized or placed in an intensive care unit. The problem can also occur when an individual is in other unfamiliar surroundings, such as a hotel room. Disruption of the normal sleep-wake cycle occurs because of overstimulation and disruption of the normal bedtime routines. Disruption of the normal sleep-wake cycle can have profound physiological (e.g., tremors, cardiac arrhythmias, altered level of consciousness) and psychological (e.g., depression, irritability, agitation) consequences, because people are deprived of the restorative functions that occur during sleep.

Application of the Nursing Process

Assessment

Sleep is a subjective human experience. Therefore, an accurate assessment of an individual's sleep-wake cycle and the adequacy of the sleep experience must rely on self-reporting. With individuals who cannot self-report (e.g., children or cognitively impaired elderly), one needs to rely on reports from family caregivers (e.g., parents or significant others).

Nursing History

The purpose of the nursing history is to determine the usual sleep behavior of an individual and any factors that may influence the person's ability to maintain a normal sleep-wake cycle. A detailed sleep assessment is provided in Box 26–2.

The nurse needs to obtain a complete picture of the individual's normal sleep pattern and sleep behavior. Assessment questions focus on sleep time, sleep onset, number of nighttime awakenings, total hours of sleep time, and the individual's appraisal of sleep efficiency and satisfaction with the current sleep routine. In addition, the assessment includes questions about normal sleep routines (e.g., does a child need to have a bedtime story read to him or her prior to falling asleep?) and whether the individual needs to take sleeping medication. Finally, the assessment process gathers data on whether the person has any concurrent problems or is currently taking any medications (e.g., diuretics) that may be disrupting the normal sleep-wake cycle. Nurses need to remember that when conducting sleep assessments with shift workers,

COMMUNITY-BASED CARE

FATIGUE

One of the most common and overlooked barriers to successful recovery after hospitalization is the lack of adequate rest and sleep for both client and caregiver. During hospitalization, many clients do not get adequate sleep. The hospital activity, noises, and frequent interruptions when staff check vital signs or perform other assessments can be very disrupting. Even for the most healthy caregiver, frequent trips to the hospital for visits followed by tending to client care needs at home can be very stressful and fatiguing.

Once at home, lack of sleep causes or exacerbates symptoms, including increased pain, irritability, and decreased appetite and activity. If left unchecked, these symptoms can become so severe that psychoses and hallucinations may develop. The home care nurse must thoroughly assess each client for potential rest and sleep disturbances. It is also important to assess who will be the primary caregiver and identify the amount of caregiving and support required. Promote client recovery while reducing caregiver stress by

1. Controlling and managing all symptoms influencing client comfort, such as nausea, vomiting, anxiety, constipation, and pain

2. Providing additional home care services, such as therapy or a nursing assistant for bathing and personal care to allow for respite from the caregiver role, especially when caregiving needs are extensive

3. Involving the social worker in assisting in exploring available community resources, such as home-delivered meals, housekeeping assistance, and transportation for necessary appointments

4. Involving family members and/or neighbors in care if possible and appropriate

the questions in Box 26–2 need to be modified to reflect individual variations in bedtime and time of awakening.

Physical Examination

If an individual has an adequate sleep-wake cycle and is experiencing sufficient rest, physical findings will be absent and the individual will describe a normal pattern of physical and social activities. Individuals with sleep problems may exhibit a variety of physical and behavioral characteristics that provide evidence of the sleep problem (see Box 26–3).

If the nurse or sleep partner can evaluate the client's sleeping, other characteristics that should be assessed include restlessness, snoring, position changes during sleep, and jerking leg movements. Snoring is caused by an obstruction to airflow through the nose and mouth. Normally, snoring is not considered to be

Box 26-2

SLEEP ASSESSMENT

Normal Sleep Pattern and Sleep Behavior

1. What time do you go to sleep at night?
2. How long (minutes) does it take you to fall asleep?
3. How many times are you awakened during the night?
4. Do you experience any thoughts that keep you from falling asleep or awaken you during the night?
5. How many hours do you usually sleep during the night?
6. What time do you awaken from sleep?
7. How satisfied are you with your current sleep-wake cycle?
8. How rested do you feel after a night's sleep?
9. Do you take naps during the day? If yes, how many, for what period of time, and when during the day?
10. Do you dream during sleep?

Use of Sleep Aids

1. Describe your normal routine before going to sleep (*e.g.,* read, watch television, drink a glass of warm milk).
2. Do you take any medication to help you fall asleep? If yes, then determine
   a. name of the drug(s)
   b. dosage of the drug(s)
   c. frequency of use
   d. length of time used
   e. effectiveness of the medications
   f. side effects

Aggravating Factors

1. Do you have any of the following symptoms that may affect sleep (*e.g.,* pain, respiratory distress, tension, anxiety, depression)?
2. Do you routinely take any of the following substances before you go to sleep (*e.g.,* corticosteroids, caffeine, amphetamines)?

Box 26-3

PHYSICAL AND BEHAVIORAL CHARACTERISTICS OF A SLEEP DISORDER

Physical Characteristics

Narrowing of the eyes

Swelling of the eyelids

Obesity

Snoring

Deviated nasal septum

Behavioral Characteristics

Yawning

Rubbing eyes

Head bobbing

Dozing

Decreased attention span

---

ficient amounts of rest. Clients at particularly high risk for sleep disorders are those who are admitted to a hospital or require care in an intensive care unit. The new environment and hospital routines may disrupt their normal sleep activities and schedules. Nurses need to alter the hospital's routine as much as possible so that clients can continue to observe their sleep routines and obtain a sufficient amount of rest.

If an individual is suspected of having a chronic sleep disorder, the person should be evaluated by a sleep specialist. Individuals may be referred to a sleep disorders clinic, where they will spend several nights in a sleep laboratory. In this setting, individuals are monitored using an EEG, electro-oculogram, and electromyogram to evaluate brain waves, eye movements, and muscle activity, respectively, during sleep. With these procedures, a specific sleep disorder may be diagnosed.

Nursing Diagnosis

A careful and detailed assessment of an individual's normal sleep-wake cycle determines whether the person is experiencing a sleep problem or any other associated nursing problems. Several common nursing diagnoses associated with a disruption in an individual's sleep-wake cycle are listed in the accompanying box. By defining the etiology of the diagnosis, the nurse is better able to design specific interventions for an individual experiencing a sleep problem. Although the sleep problem may be the primary nursing diagnosis, associated diagnoses must be listed so that all of the individual's problems can be managed effectively. For example, a person with a sleep disorder may be experiencing difficulty coping with work activities because he or she is falling asleep on the

---

a sleep disorder. However, snoring accompanied by periods of apnea may indicate that the client is experiencing obstructive sleep apnea.

Jerking leg movements or nocturnal myoclonus is observed in 10 to 20% of chronic insomniacs. Nocturnal myoclonus results from marked involuntary muscle contractions that cause one or both legs to jerk during sleep. The jerking arouses the sleeper and causes daytime sleepiness, anxiety, depression, and cognitive impairments.

Specific Diagnostic Evaluation for a Sleep Disorder

Nurses need to evaluate all their clients for sleep disorders and determine whether they are getting suf-

NURSING DIAGNOSES RELATED TO SLEEP DISORDERS

Sleep pattern disturbance (long time to sleep onset) related to:

* Noisy environment
* Loss of normal bedtime routine
* Changes in the environment
* Pain

Sleep pattern disturbance (numerous awakenings) related to:

* Shift work
* Anxiety
* Depression

Fatigue related to:

* Sleep pattern disturbance

Ineffective individual coping related to:

* Sleep pattern disturbance

job. Poor job performance can lead to anxiety, particularly if supervisors are criticizing the individual's lack of productivity. Worrying about losing one's job could result in a further disruption of the normal sleep-wake cycle.

Planning

After identifying the specific nursing diagnoses, the nurse develops an individualized plan of care for the person experiencing a specific sleep disorder. The nursing plan of care involves the identification of specific client outcomes and nursing interventions that include pharmacological as well as nonpharmacological approaches.

Client Outcomes

Client outcomes need to be developed with the client and the family caregiver. The outcomes should be as specific as possible. Specific nursing interventions should be designed to help the client achieve the mutually established outcomes. Examples of specific outcomes for an individual with a sleep pattern disturbance might include: (1) Client manifests the absence of a sleep pattern disturbance, as evidenced by reports of an uninterrupted night's sleep and reports of feeling rested. (2) Client implements specific sleep hygiene measures as part of his or her bedtime routine. (3) Client takes sleep medications as prescribed. (4) Client identifies specific factors that interfere with the normal sleep-wake cycle.

Nursing Care Plan

When the nurse develops a plan of care for a client with a sleep pattern disturbance, consideration should be given to several specific interventions: bedtime rituals, environmental preparation, pharmacological management, scheduling of client care activities, and promotion of rest and relaxation (see Sample Nursing Care Plan). Each of these interventions is summarized in the implementation section (Page, 1991).

Implementation

Implementation of the plan of care for a client with a sleep pattern disturbance requires the active participation and cooperation of the client.

Bedtime Rituals

As part of the assessment process, the nurse ascertains the client's normal bedtime routine. Adults often describe specific rituals such as putting on bedclothes, brushing their teeth, reading or watching television, and/or praying prior to sleep. Children may describe going to bed with a favorite toy or blanket, having a story read to them, or saying their prayers with their parents (Fig. 26–3). These ritual practices provide the brain with the clues that sleep time is approaching.

Nurses must make careful notes of an individual's bedtime rituals, particularly when the person is hospitalized. These rituals should be adhered to as closely as possible to promote the optimal sleep-wake cycle for the client.

Environmental Preparation

Attention should be paid to the sleep environment. Minimizing noises, particularly strange noises, promotes sleep onset and prevents disruptions in the sleep cycle. In addition, sleep is promoted if the room is dark, as well as quiet. Shades or blinds should be

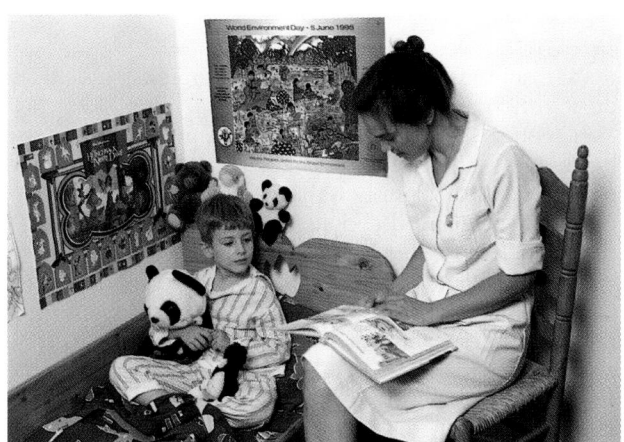

✦ **Figure 26–3**
A favorite blanket, a stuffed animal, saying prayers, and a bedtime story are examples of common bedtime rituals that help children make the transition to sleep.

SAMPLE NURSING CARE PLAN

THE CLIENT WITH A SLEEP PATTERN DISTURBANCE

Situation: A 60-year-old client is admitted to the hospital with a pathological fracture from metastatic bone cancer. The client complains of difficulty falling asleep and frequent nighttime awakenings because of pain and difficulty turning in bed.

Nursing Diagnosis: Sleep pattern disturbance related to pain and decreased mobility.

Expected Outcome: Client will report an intact and restful night's sleep.

Action	Rationale
1. Assess the client's normal sleep-wake cycle, including bedtime rituals and use of pharmacological agents for sleep and pain.	1. Baseline assessment assists in the development of an individualized plan for promoting sleep.
2. Institute an effective pain management plan.	2. A reduction in the client's pain will enhance sleep.
3. Establish a bedtime ritual, including: a. Maintain a routine exercise schedule during the day. b. Maintain a regular retirement time and arousal time. c. Provide a bedtime snack of a high-protein food or beverage (*e.g.,* milk).	3. Following a routine procedure before sleep facilitates the establishment of the normal sleep cycle. a. Moderate daytime exercise promotes sleep. b. A routine schedule facilitates the establishment of a sleep-wake cycle. c. Milk and high-protein foods contain the dietary amino acid L-tryptophan, which helps promote sleep.
4. Decrease environmental stimuli and adjust room temperature before sleep.	4. Loud noises interrupt sleep; excessive heat fragments sleep, and excessive cold prevents sleep.
5. Schedule nursing care before sleep and after awakening.	5. Coordination of nursing care prevents frequent awakenings.
6. Use diversional activities (*e.g.,* music, massage, reading, watching TV) to promote sleep.	6. Diversional activity before sleep helps the client relax and fall asleep more easily.
7. Administer sleep medication if nonpharmacological interventions are not effective.	7. Sleep medications promote an earlier sleep onset.
8. Evaluate the client's response to pharmacological and nonpharmacological interventions.	8. An evaluation of the effectiveness of the interventions determines whether the treatment plan needs to be revised.
9. Document care given on the client's record.	9. Documentation provides a record of nursing actions and a means of communication with other members of the health care team.

drawn shut. Individuals who work nights and sleep during the day and who are experiencing a sleep pattern disturbance should be encouraged to purchase blackout shades. These shades create a darkened room during daylight hours.

The client's bed should be as comfortable as possible. The client should select the firmness of the mattress to promote optimal back support and comfort. Particularly in the hospital setting, fresh linen promotes comfort and relaxation. To assist children to sleep, particularly in the hospital, parents should be encouraged to bring in the child's favorite toy or pillow.

Finally, environmental temperature should be optimized. An extremely cold environment prevents the onset of sleep. In contrast, an excessively warm environment tends to fragment sleep.

Pharmacological Management

Sleep medications include benzodiazepines, sedative-hypnotic drugs, and antianxiety medications. These drugs do *not* produce a normal sleep cycle but in some way disturb either REM or NREM sleep. Common sleep medications and associated side effects are listed in Table 26–3 (Becker & Jamieson, 1992). All the sedative-hypnotic drugs provide one or two nights of excellent sleep, and then their beneficial effects no longer occur. The decrease in effectiveness of these drugs tends to result in an escalation of the dose with no improvement in the client's sleep.

Clients need to be taught that they *cannot* abruptly stop taking sleep medications. Abrupt cessation of these drugs can result in withdrawal, which is manifested as weakness, tremulousness, restlessness,

Table 26–3
COMMON SLEEP MEDICATIONS

SLEEP PROBLEM	DRUG AND DOSE	SIDE EFFECTS
Sleep onset	Triazolam (Halcion), 0.125 mg	Early waking, daytime anxiety, memory change
Sleep maintenance	Estazolam (ProSom), 1 mg Temazepam (Restoril), 15 mg	Morning sedation
Daytime anxiety	Flurazepam (Dalmane), 15 mg	Sedation, poor coordination

insomnia, tachycardia, anxiety, seizures, and psychotic behavior.

Pharmacological agents used for sleep disorders are meant for short-term use. Clients should be encouraged to use nonpharmacological strategies to optimize their sleep-wake cycles.

Scheduling of Client Care Activities

When clients are admitted to a hospital, they are often required to adapt to hospital routines rather than having clinicians respect their normal routines. Nurses, particularly those who work evenings and nights, need to establish a schedule for client care activities that promotes sleep and rest. For example, medication administration and vital sign measurements need to be coordinated so that clients are not awakened to have their temperature and blood pressure checked shortly after receiving sleep medication.

Promotion of Rest and Relaxation

All types of nonpharmacological interventions can be used to promote rest and relaxation. Clients can listen to music or watch television as a way of promoting sleep and rest. In addition, massage is often relaxing and serves to enhance client comfort. Clients can also be taught specific relaxation exercises to promote a restful sleep.

The establishment of a specific bedtime ritual may be particularly beneficial. Clients should be encouraged to retire and awaken at a regular time each day. In addition, a routine exercise schedule during the day may help improve a client's sleep. Clients should be encouraged to have a bedtime snack that is high in protein (*e.g.*, a glass of warm milk). These high-protein foods contain the dietary amino acid L-tryptophan, which helps promote sleep.

Evaluation

The plan of care needs to be evaluated on the basis of the client's progress in achieving the specific outcomes that were mutually established by the client and the nurse. Failure to achieve the desired outcomes necessitates more data collection and revision of the plan of care.

Comfort

Pain, the disruption of comfort, is a universal human experience, but no one can experience another person's pain. Therefore, pain must be viewed as a subjective sensation, and nurses must obtain information about an individual's pain experience directly from the client.

Pain is defined as "an unpleasant sensory and emotional experience associated with actual or potential tissue damage, or described in terms of such damage" (International Association for the Study of Pain, 1979, p. 249). This definition considers two essential elements of pain: sensory perception of actual or potential tissue damage, and the emotional component of the pain experience. A second definition of pain emphasizes the importance of the individual's experience by stating that "pain is whatever the experiencing person says it is existing whenever he says it does" (McCaffery, 1979, p. 11). Both of these definitions emphasize the importance of understanding the individual's personal experience with pain and believing the client's self-report of pain.

Pain Mechanisms

Pain is a protective mechanism for the body. The physiology of pain is a question that has plagued scientists since the time of Aristotle. However, most of the progress in understanding pain physiology has occurred in the past 30 years. Pain physiology is often discussed in terms of four processes: transduction, transmission, perception, and modulation. These four processes are not totally distinct but overlap and interact to allow noxious stimuli to be processed by the peripheral and central nervous systems and to be interpreted as painful.

Transduction

Transduction is the process by which a noxious stimulus is changed into an electrical stimulus on a cell membrane (Fields, 1987). Transduction occurs within the peripheral nervous system. Specialized pain neurons, called primary afferent nociceptors, can be activated by thermal, mechanical, or chemical stimuli. Any type of tissue injury produced by chemical (*e.g.*, extravasation of chemotherapy into the skin), thermal (*e.g.*, a burn), or mechanical (*e.g.*, a surgical incision) stimuli results in the activation of an inflammatory response. Biochemical substances (*i.e.*, prostaglandins, bradykinin, histamine, hydrogen ions, potassium ions, substance P) are released or produced as part of the inflammatory response. These biochemical substances activate primary afferent nociceptors and initiate an action potential in the neuron. The action potential travels along the primary afferent nociceptor from the painful site to the spinal cord.

Transmission

Painful stimuli are transmitted from primary afferent nociceptors in the peripheral nervous system to the dorsal horn of the spinal cord. Pain impulses are transmitted from the primary afferent nociceptor to a second neuron through a synaptic connection in the dorsal horn of the spinal cord. Several neurotransmitters (*e.g.*, substance P, calcitonin gene-related peptide, glutamate, aspartate) are involved in transmitting the pain impulse across the synapse between the primary afferent nociceptor and the second neuron. The pain impulse crosses the spinal cord and ascends to multiple brain sites through the spinothalamic tract. It is in the cerebral cortex where the cognitive, perceptive, evaluative, and emotional responses to pain occur (Puntillo & Tesler, 1993).

Perception

A noxious stimulus becomes pain when it reaches conscious awareness. The perception of pain and an evaluation of its meaning are believed to occur in the cerebral cortex. Many areas of the somatosensory cortex are believed to be involved in the perception and response to noxious stimuli (Fields, 1987).

Modulation

Pain modulation can occur in many areas within the CNS. The gate control theory of pain helps explain pain modulation (Melzack & Wall, 1965, 1983). In addition, pain modulation occurs through endogenous opioid and nonopioid analgesic systems.

➤ **Gate Control Theory of Pain.** The gate control theory was developed to help explain some common pain experiences and why certain nonpharmacological interventions (*e.g.*, massage, transelectrical nerve stimulation) are effective in the treatment of pain (Hoffert, 1986). Controversy exists as to whether a "real" gating mechanism exists in the dorsal horn of the spinal cord. Research has shown that there are numerous neurotransmitters in the dorsal horn of the spinal cord that can enhance or inhibit the transmission of painful stimuli. These neurotransmitters may be thought of as controlling the gating mechanism for pain transmission and modulation within the spinal cord (Fig. 26–4).

According to the gate control theory, the dorsal horn of the spinal cord is an extremely important site for pain modulation (Melzack & Wall, 1965, 1983). The theory hypothesizes that in the dorsal horn of the spinal cord, a balance exists between large-diameter nonpain fibers and smaller-diameter pain fibers that synapse on central transmission cells. Stimulation of smaller-diameter, primary afferent nociceptors results in pain transmission (*i.e.*, the "gate is open"), whereas stimulation of large-diameter nonpain fibers inhibits transmission cell activity and "closes the gate." In addition, Melzack and Wall (1965) speculate that higher cortical centers within the CNS can influence the gate control system by delivering descending inhibitory messages to the dorsal horn of the spinal cord.

➤ **Endogenous Opioid System.** The CNS has its own internal system for producing analgesia called the endogenous opioid system. Endogenous opioids (*e.g.*, beta-endorphin, enkephalin, dynorphin) are substances that act like morphine. At the present time, we do not know how to control the release of these endogenous morphinelike substances to produce analgesia in humans. It is known that the endogenous opioid system is involved in the placebo response.

Developmental Changes in Pain Physiology

Neonates

A careful examination of the anatomical and physiological development of nociceptive pathways reveals that the neural elements involved in nociceptive processing are in place early in fetal life and continue to mature during postnatal development (Fitzgerald & Anand, 1993). In fact, there is ample evidence that the fetal nervous system is sufficiently mature at 20 weeks' gestation to experience painful stimuli. Furthermore, it appears that the neurotransmitters involved in pain processing are produced earlier than the endogenous opioids (*e.g.*, beta-endorphin), which would decrease painful stimuli (Anand & Hickey, 1987; Johnston & Stevens, 1992). Therefore, despite arguments to the contrary, newborn infants do experience pain. Unrelieved pain activates a stress response and can produce numerous deleterious consequences in neonates, including hypoxemia, increases in heart rate and blood pressure, and increased metabolic demands. The pain and stress responses can result in intraventricular hemorrhages, impaired wound healing, and resultant developmental delays, particularly in critically ill newborns or premature infants (Franck & Gregory, 1993).

Elderly

Studies of age-related changes in pain perception have produced inconclusive results. The majority of these studies have been done using "normal" elderly volunteers who were subjected to noxious thermal, mechanical, or electrical stimuli. In an excellent review, Harkins, Kwentus, and Price (1984) conclude that because of differences in methodology and participant selection, no consensus exists in the literature about how aging influences pain sensations or perception.

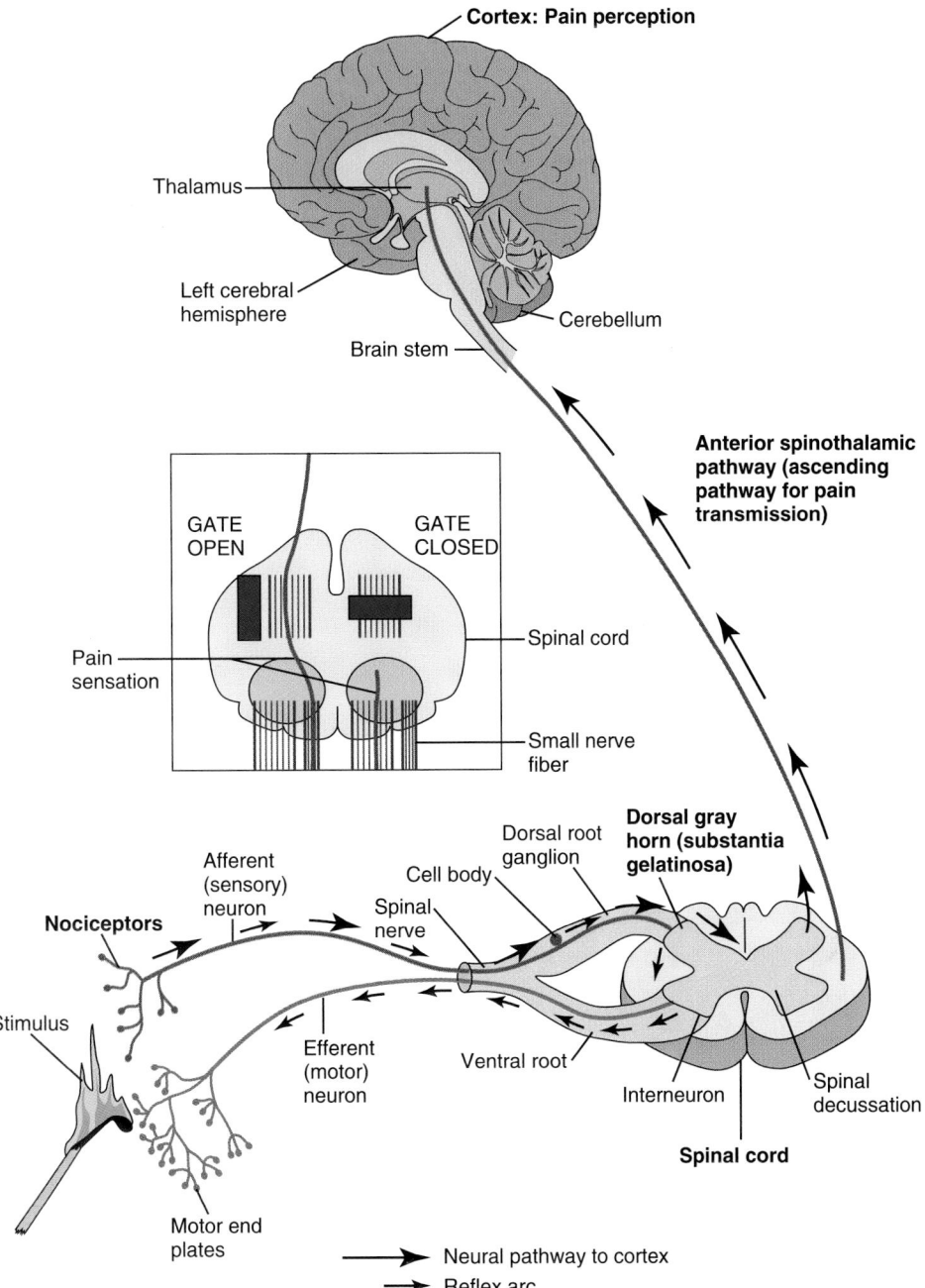

Figure 26–4

Transmission of pain. Receptive fibers in the sensory neuron carry messages to the dorsal column of the spinal cord, where the sensory neurons form synapses with the interneuron. The interneurons form synapses with motor neurons in the anterior horn to form a reflex arc. Also in the posterior horn, sensory neurons form synapses with fibers leading to the spinothalamic pathway, which allows incoming messages to be sent to the brain, where they are perceived as pain. *Inset,* According to the gate control theory of pain, a balance exists in the dorsal horn of the spinal cord between large-diameter nonpain fibers and smaller-diameter pain fibers that synapse on central transmission cells. Theoretically, stimulation of the smaller fibers results in pain ("open gate"), whereas stimulation of the larger fibers inhibits transmission from the smaller fibers, "closing the gate" to pain transmission. In addition, higher cortical centers can deliver descending inhibitory messages to the dorsal horn, also blocking pain. (Adapted from Bolander, V. B. [1994]. *Sorensen and Luckmann's basic nursing: A psychophysiologic approach* [3rd ed.]. Philadelphia: W. B. Saunders; and Ignatavicius, D. D., Workman, M. L., & Mishler, M. A. [1995]. *Medical-surgical nursing: A nursing process approach* [2nd ed.]. Philadelphia: W. B. Saunders.)

Pain Assessment

Pain assessment is the cornerstone of effective pain management. Recently, two clinical practice guidelines have been published by the Agency for Health Care Policy and Research (AHCPR) on the management of acute postoperative pain (Acute Pain Management Guideline Panel, 1992) and the management of cancer pain (Jacox *et al.*, 1994). These two federal guidelines emphasize the importance of a detailed initial assessment, as well as an ongoing assessment of a pain complaint. The initial pain assessment provides data for formulating an accurate diagnosis of the pain complaint, and the ongoing assessment provides data for evaluating the effectiveness of the pain management plan. Prior to discussing how a nurse should conduct a comprehensive pain assessment, the characteristics of acute and chronic pain are reviewed, and the major types of pain are described.

Classification of Pain

Pain is classified as either acute or chronic in nature. Acute pain serves as a warning signal for the body, indicating that something is wrong. Table 26–4 summarizes the differences in the characteristics of acute and chronic pain. Examples of acute pain include pain following surgery, pain following trauma, procedure-related pain, and acute pain associated with a medical condition (*e.g.*, cholecystitis, angina). In contrast, chronic pain can be divided into two distinct categories: chronic pain of nonmalignant origin (*e.g.*, pain associated with rheumatoid arthritis, low back pain), and chronic pain of malignant origin (*e.g.*, pain related to cancer or cancer treatment).

✦ **Acute Pain.** Acute pain serves as a protective mechanism for the body. The pain is of limited dura-

tion (usually less than 3 mo). In general, when the condition producing the acute pain is corrected or controlled, the pain abates. However, until the cause of the pain is identified, acute pain usually requires some type of intervention. Box 26–4 lists some common causes of acute pain. Acute pain typically results in activation of the sympathetic nervous system and produces a variety of physiological effects, including increased heart rate, increased respiratory rate, increased blood pressure, decreased gastrointestinal motility, increased rate of oxygen consumption, increased muscle tension, pupillary dilation, palmar and plantar sweating, and increased anxiety (Sternbach, 1990).

Recent evidence from studies of postoperative pain suggests that unrelieved acute pain may have negative physiological consequences on the individual. Unrelieved pain is believed to contribute to the overall stress response following surgery. These stress responses can promote tissue breakdown; produce increases in metabolic rate, blood clotting, and water retention; impair immune function; and trigger the "fight or flight" response (Kehlet, 1982; Kehlet, Brandt, & Rem, 1980). In addition, unrelieved acute pain, particularly following surgery, can result in shallow breathing and cough suppression, followed by retention of secretions and postoperative pulmonary complications (*e.g.*, atelectasis, pneumonia) (Marshall & Wycke, 1972; Sydow, 1989). Unrelieved acute pain may delay the return of normal gastrointestinal functioning (Wattwill, 1989). These unwanted complications, particularly in postoperative clients, may delay wound healing, impair mobility, and lengthen the period of recovery (Miaskowski, 1993a).

✦ **Chronic Pain of Nonmalignant Origin.** Chronic pain is defined as a pain problem of greater than 3 months' duration and is often associated with significant changes in the client's mood and quality of life. Examples of chronic pain of nonmalignant origin include headaches, low back pain, irritable bowel syndrome, and reflex sympathetic dystrophy. The pathophysiological causes of the pain may not be completely understood. Clients with chronic pain problems do not exhibit the same signs and symptoms of sympathetic nervous system activation as do those

Table 26–4

CHARACTERISTICS OF ACUTE AND CHRONIC PAIN

ACUTE PAIN	CHRONIC PAIN
Serves as a warning signal for the body, indicates something is wrong	Persistent pain, often meaningless
Time limited (<3 mo)	Indefinite duration (>3 mo)
Pathophysiological mechanisms causing the pain are well understood	Pathophysiological mechanisms causing the pain may not be understood
Sensory aspects of the pain are typically consistent with the pathophysiology	Sensory aspects of the pain are not consistent with the pathophysiology
Treatment is usually well defined, with a high probability of success	Multimodal treatment is often required, and the results of treatment are variable
Socioeconomic impact of the pain is often minimal	Socioeconomic impact of the pain is often substantial

Box 26–4

CAUSES OF ACUTE PAIN

Chemical injury (*e.g.*, chemotherapy-induced mucositis)

Infection

Medical procedures

Surgery

Thermal injury (*e.g.*, burns)

Traumatic injury

in acute pain. In fact, clients with chronic pain do not exhibit any physiological changes in heart rate, blood pressure, or respiratory rate. However, chronic pain sufferers may report significant changes in mood, ability to sleep, and ability to function. Because these pain problems can have a profound impact on client and family functioning, they often require intense multimodal management using the services provided in a chronic pain clinic.

♦ **Chronic Pain of Malignant Origin.** Pain related to cancer or cancer treatment is typically classified as chronic pain of malignant origin. However, individuals with cancer can also experience acute pain from a variety of causes. A classification system for cancer-related pain that can be used to determine whether clients with cancer are experiencing acute and/or chronic pain related to cancer or cancer treatment is depicted in Box 26–5 (Foley, 1985). Clients may experience acute pain, as discussed previously, as an initial symptom of cancer. In addition, clients with cancer may undergo diagnostic procedures or surgery that is painful. The nature of acute cancer-related pain is that it is time limited and is usually effectively managed with analgesic medications (Miaskowski, 1993b).

Clients with cancer can also experience chronic pain as a result of their disease or treatment. Tumor progression or metastasis to bone, nerves, or soft tissues can produce chronic pain. In addition, cancer treatment can cause chronic pain. Chronic pain can occur following surgery, chemotherapy, or radiation therapy. Chronic pain following a mastectomy, thora-cotomy, nephrectomy, or radical neck dissection is the result of nerve damage, with the development of a traumatic neuroma. Certain cancer chemotherapy drugs (*e.g.*, the vinca alkaloids) can produce a painful peripheral neuropathy in some people. Finally, radiation therapy can sometimes produce nerve injury and a resulting neuropathic-type pain (see later) in the injured area. Common causes of cancer-related pain, descriptions of the pain, and management options are listed in Table 26–5. The chronic nature of cancer pain is associated with sleep disturbances, a reduction in appetite, changes in mood, and a decrease in overall quality of life.

It should be noted that clients with cancer may experience chronic pain unrelated to their cancer. For example, a client with cancer may continue to suffer from low back pain or migraine headaches that began prior to the cancer diagnosis. If these clients develop a chronic cancer pain problem, treatment of both types of chronic pain must be initiated (Miaskowski, 1993b).

Types of Pain

Pain can be classified into three major types based on its underlying pathophysiological mechanisms: somatic, visceral, or neuropathic (also referred to as deafferentation). Each type of pain can occur in either an acute or a chronic form.

♦ **Somatic Pain.** Somatic pain occurs as a result of activation of nociceptors in cutaneous and deep tissues. This type of pain is caused by tissue injury. Somatic pain is typically described as constant, sharp, aching, or throbbing (Patt, 1993). In addition, clients can point to the site of their pain. Examples of acute pain of somatic origin include a toothache, a traumatic fracture, a burn, postoperative pain, or pain associated with chemotherapy-induced mucositis. Examples of chronic pain of somatic origin include pain caused by rheumatoid arthritis, bone metastasis, or fibromyalgia. Somatic pain usually responds well to opioid (*e.g.*, morphine) and nonopioid (*e.g.*, aspirin) analgesics. Sometimes a surgical intervention is required to correct the underlying cause of the pain.

♦ **Visceral Pain.** Visceral pain originates from injury to internal organs. When pain is caused by involvement of the abdominal or pelvic viscera, the pain is often difficult to localize and is characteristically described as deep, dull, aching, or pressurelike. When acute, the pain may occur in shooting paroxysms and may be associated with other symptoms (*e.g.*, nausea, vomiting, diaphoresis). Several mechanisms are involved in producing visceral pain, including distention or contraction of smooth muscle walls, rapid stretching of a capsule surrounding a solid visceral organ (*e.g.*, the liver), ischemia of a visceral muscle, or chemical irritation of the viscera (*e.g.*, peritonitis) (Patt, 1993). Examples of acute visceral pain include peritonitis, renal colic, and acute appendicitis. Chronic visceral pain is associated with such conditions as chronic pancreatitis or Crohn's disease. Visceral pain

---

Box 26–5

TYPES OF CANCER-RELATED PAIN

I. Acute cancer-related pain
  A. Tumor-associated pain
  B. Pain associated with cancer therapy (*e.g.*, mucositis, procedure-related pain, postoperative pain, radiation-induced skin desquamation)
II. Chronic cancer-related pain
  A. Chronic pain from tumor progression (*e.g.*, bone metastasis, spinal cord compression, lymphatic obstruction)
  B. Chronic pain associated with cancer therapy (*e.g.*, postsurgical pain syndromes, chemotherapy or radiation-induced peripheral neuropathies)
III. Preexisting chronic pain of nonmalignant origin associated with acute or chronic cancer-related pain
IV. Cancer-related pain accompanied by a history of substance abuse
V. Pain associated with the terminal phase of an illness

Adapted from Foley, K. M. (1985). The treatment of cancer pain. *New England Journal of Medicine, 313,* 84–95.

Table **26–5**

ASSESSMENT AND MANAGEMENT OF COMMON TYPES OF CANCER-RELATED PAIN

CAUSE	DESCRIPTION	TREATMENT OPTIONS
Bone metastases	Constant, aching, gnawing, deep, intense pain	Administer opioid analgesics Add a nonsteroidal antiinflammatory drug to the analgesic regimen
Spinal cord compression (SCC)	Intense, sharp, well-localized back pain If SCC is in the thoracic area, client may complain of pain like a "tight band" around the chest that worsens with defecation, sneezing, or bending forward; if SCC is located in the lumbosacral area, client may complain of back pain that radiates down one or both legs	Evaluate client for the most appropriate type of treatment (*i.e.,* surgery and/or radiation therapy) Administer corticosteroids Administer opioid analgesics with or without a nonsteroidal antiinflammatory drug
Postsurgical pain syndrome (following mastectomy, thoracotomy, nephrectomy, radical head and neck dissection)	Paroxysms of "shooting" or "shock-like" pain accompanied by a burning, dysesthetic sensation May be accompanied by a feeling of tightness at the site of the incision May be associated with decreased activity or range of motion	Administer tricyclic antidepressants (*e.g.,* amitriptyline) and/or an anticonvulsant (*e.g.,* phenytoin) May require an opioid analgesic
Postherpetic neuralgia	Paroxysms of "shooting" or "shock-like" pain accompanied by a burning, dysesthetic sensation	Administer tricyclic antidepressants (*e.g.,* amitriptyline) and/or an anticonvulsant (*e.g.,* phenytoin) May require an opioid analgesic
Obstruction of a hollow viscus	Constant aching, poorly localized pain or colicky-type pain that is poorly localized	Attempt to relieve the obstruction (*e.g.,* place a nasogastric tube or ureteral stints) Administer opioid analgesics

From Miaskowski, C. (1993). Current concepts in the assessment and management of cancer-related pain. *MEDSURG Nursing, 2*(2), 113–118. Reprinted with permission of the publisher, Jannetti Publications, Inc.

usually responds well to opioid and nonopioid analgesics. Sometimes a surgical procedure is required to correct the cause of the pain.

❦ **Neuropathic Pain.** Neuropathic (or deafferentation) pain refers to pain syndromes associated with damage to some part of the nervous system. Neuropathic pain is a dysesthetic-type pain. Dysesthesia refers to discomfort and altered sensations that are distinct from the ordinary sensations of pain. Typically, clients describe dysesthetic pain as burning, tingling, numbing, pressing, or squeezing. The pain is described as extremely unpleasant and unbearable (Patt, 1993).

The dysesthetic component of neuropathic pain is usually constant. In addition to the continuous pain, an intermittent, shocklike pain—often described as shooting or lancinating or like a jolt of electricity—may occur. This shocklike component is often superimposed on the burning, dysesthetic-type pain (Patt, 1993). Neuropathic pain is typically chronic in nature. Examples of neuropathic pain include trigeminal neuralgia, postherpetic neuralgia, and postthoracotomy pain. Neuropathic pain tends to respond to a combination of pharmacological (*e.g.,* tricyclic antidepressants) and nonpharmacological (*e.g.,* nerve blocks) interventions.

Application of the Nursing Process

Assessment

Initial Pain Assessment

A carefully collected pain history can facilitate the development of an effective pain management plan. An interview guide for conducting an initial pain assessment is outlined in Box 26–6. Asking these questions should provide the needed information about how the client reacted to past experiences of pain, the

Box 26–6

INITIAL PAIN ASSESSMENT

Previous Pain Experience. Would you please describe any previous instances of pain and the effect the painful experience had on you?

Previous Methods of Pain Control. What treatments have you used in the past to control pain? How effective were those treatments in relieving your pain?

Attitude About Taking Pain Medication. Do you have any concerns about taking pain medication?

Behavioral Responses to Pain. Please describe your typical behaviors when you are in pain.

Client Knowledge of, Expectations About, and Preferences for Pain Management Methods. Do you have a particular preference for a certain type of pain management (*e.g.,* intramuscular injections, patient-controlled analgesia)?

Family Expectations or Concerns About Pain Management. Does your family have any expectations or concerns about your pain management?

If the client is experiencing pain, also ask the following questions:

Description of the Pain. What does the pain feel like?

Location and Radiation. Show me where it hurts. Does the pain go anywhere else?

Severity/Intensity. On a scale of 0 to 10, with 0 being no pain and 10 being the worst pain you can imagine, how much does it hurt right now?

Aggravating and Relieving Factors. What makes your pain worse? Better?

Previous Treatment Modalities. What types of treatments have you tried to relieve your pain? Were they and/or are they effective?

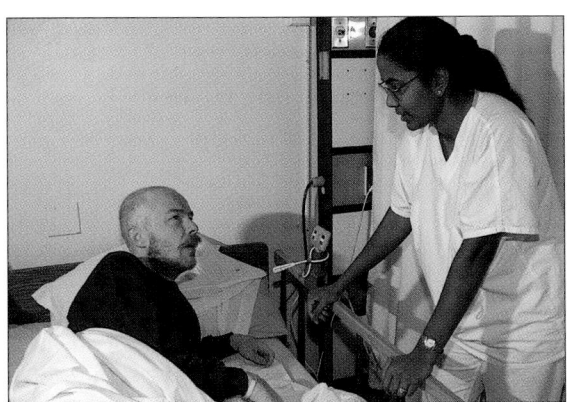

Patient describing his pain to nurse

client's current fears and concerns about pain management, and the client's preferences for particular pain management strategies (Miaskowski, 1993a, 1993b).

If the client is experiencing pain at the time of the interview, several additional questions must be asked (see Box 26–6) to obtain specific information about the pain complaint. This information often aids in diagnosing the cause of the pain. The first step in the assessment of the pain complaint is to have the client describe the character of the pain. Clients may need to be provided with words or phrases such as burning, tingling, heavy, sharp, or dull if they are having difficulty putting the pain sensation into words.

The second part of the pain assessment involves ascertaining the exact location of the pain and whether or not the pain radiates or goes anyplace else. The easiest way to obtain this information is to have the client indicate on his or her body the exact location of the pain or point to the location of the pain on the nurse. The nurse should carefully examine the painful area to determine whether movement or pressure exacerbates the pain.

The severity or integrity of the pain is the third assessment parameter. It is important to remember that a severity rating is a subjective report. What one person describes as a 9 on a pain-severity scale may be described as a 4 by another individual. Figure 26–5 provides examples of several different types of pain rating scales. The one that is the easiest to use in clinical practice is the verbal numerical rating scale. The reason for asking a client to rate his or her pain using a numerical rating scale is that, over time, the nurse can determine whether the pain management plan is effective or requires modification (*i.e.,* if the pain rating increases or decreases).

The fourth assessment parameter involves obtaining information on aggravating and relieving factors. This portion of the assessment is critical; by knowing what makes the pain better and worse, the nurse can modify the pain management plan to include interventions to enhance the client's level of comfort and, when possible, avoid painful activities. Finally, the nurse must assess the client's previous use and effectiveness of various pharmacological and non-pharmacological interventions and whether the present pain management plan is providing adequate pain control.

Physical Examination

The physical examination should be conducted in an organized and systematic fashion. Vital signs are obtained to determine whether the client is experiencing any of the physiological effects associated with activation of the sympathetic nervous system (*e.g.,* increases in heart rate, blood pressure, or respiratory rate). These physiological responses are more commonly associated with acute pain and are not seen in clients with chronic pain problems.

Careful attention is paid to examining the painful area and adjacent areas to determine whether the pain is referred to any other sites. Certain types of pain problems show characteristic patterns of referral (*e.g.,* pain associated with a herniated disk may radiate

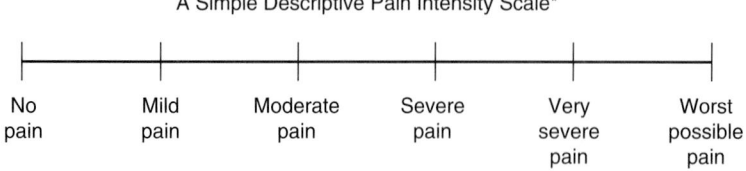

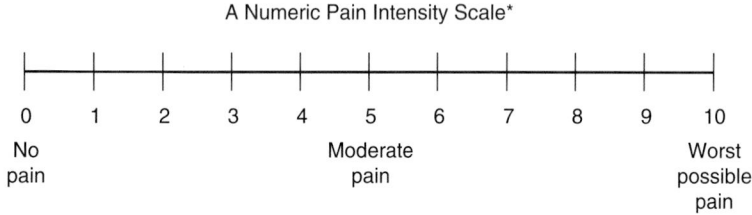

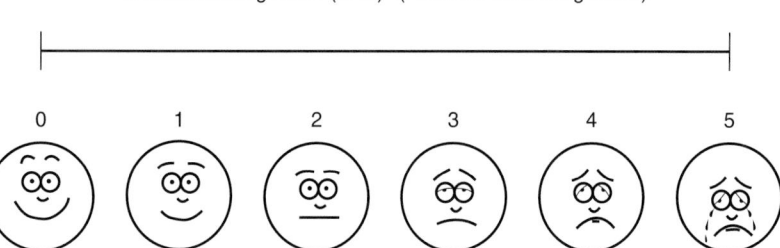

> ✦ **Figure 26–5**
> Several different pain intensity scales. (FACES Pain Rating Scale from Wong, D. L. [1997]. *Whaley & Wong's essentials of pediatric nursing* [5th ed.; p. 624]. St. Louis: Mosby-Year Book.)

down one or both legs). Particular attention is paid to whether palpation of the painful site produces pain and whether movement of a painful site exacerbates the pain. Detailed musculoskeletal and neurological examinations are part of the physical examination of a client complaining of acute or chronic pain, because many pain problems produce changes in the client's strength, ability to move, or ability to perform normal activities of daily living.

The neurological exam focuses on the client's pain problem to determine whether the pain problem is causing any neurological deficits. For example, a complaint of headache or neck pain requires careful evaluation of the cranial nerves. Back pain requires careful motor, sensory, and reflex evaluation in the arms and legs. In addition, the client should be evaluated for cues that indicate pain (*e.g.*, distorted posture, guarding of a painful site, impaired mobility, restricted movement of an extremity, anxiety, depression) (Jacox *et al.*, 1994).

Diagnostic Tests

There is no standardized group of tests to perform when a client presents with a pain complaint. The specific diagnostic tests that are used depend on the nature of the pain complaint. For example, a client presenting with acute abdominal pain may undergo a series of gastrointestinal radiological procedures. In contrast, a client complaining of low back pain may undergo a computerized axial tomography scan or a magnetic resonance imaging scan. Diagnostic tests are ordered to facilitate the accurate diagnosis of the cause of the client's pain.

Psychosocial Assessment

As part of a comprehensive assessment of a pain complaint, an evaluation of the impact of the pain on a client's psychosocial functioning is important. A psychosocial assessment is particularly useful with clients who are experiencing chronic pain of malignant or nonmalignant origin. Specific content areas for a focused assessment are listed in Box 26–7.

The psychosocial assessment provides data that are critical to the development of an individualized plan of care. An assessment of changes in the client's mood may lead to a recommendation for pharmacological therapy to relieve depression or anxiety or a referral to a psychiatrist or psychologist. An assessment of the client's understanding of the cause of the pain in relation to his or her specific clinical condition, as well as an understanding of the meaning of the pain to the individual (*e.g.*, some clients view pain as a punishment from God that must be endured), provides useful information to guide nursing interventions. A critical component of the psychosocial assessment is to evaluate the impact of the client's pain on family functioning. Part of the assessment must focus on the economic burden that the pain problem places on the family in terms of the financial cost of treatment, the number of days lost from work for caregiving activities, and role changes caused by the pain.

Developmental Assessment

Two distinct populations of clients require special consideration in terms of pain assessment: children and the elderly. Specific recommendations for assessing pain in these two populations are summarized.

✦ **Neonates, Children, and Adolescents.** An assessment of pain in the pediatric population is largely determined by the developmental age of the client and whether he or she is preverbal. Behavioral observation is the primary assessment approach for preverbal and nonverbal children and is an adjunct to pain assessment in verbal children. Behavioral observations include vocalizations (*e.g.*, crying, whining, groaning), facial expressions, muscle tension and rigidity, ability to be consoled, guarding of body parts, temperament, activity, and general appearance (Fig. 26–6) (Acute Pain Management Guideline Panel, 1992; Jacox *et al.*, 1994). Behaviors must be interpreted with caution in children, because other types of stimuli (*e.g.*, fear) may produce similar behaviors. In addition, behavioral indicators may be absent when they elicit more pain.

In a verbal child, careful attention must be paid to the language the child uses to communicate pain (*e.g.*, hurt, owie, boo-boo) and how and to whom the child communicates pain. An example of a pain history for a pediatric client is found in Box 26–8. In addition, several different types of pain intensity rating scales have been developed for pediatric clients. These tools are summarized in Table 26–6.

✦ **Elderly.** Pain assessment in the elderly should be done using the assessment tools described previously. In addition, careful attention must be paid to concurrent medical conditions that occur quite frequently in the elderly and produce pain. Elderly clients should be evaluated for such conditions as musculoskeletal problems, rheumatoid arthritis, osteoarthritis, postherpetic neuralgia, temporal arteritis, peripheral vascular disease, traumatic injuries, and vertebral compression fractures. Because of the elderly's hesitancy to report pain problems (see box), nurses should make pain assessment a routine part of every elderly person's health history.

Nursing Diagnosis

Initially, the nurse must determine whether the client is at risk for acute pain or is experiencing acute and/or chronic pain. Because of the nature and cause of the pain, there may be a number of different nursing diagnoses for the client. Following a detailed pain assessment and diagnostic work-up, the nurse should

---

Box **26–7**

COMPONENTS OF A PSYCHOSOCIAL PAIN ASSESSMENT

1. Have you noticed any changes in your mood (*e.g.*, depression, anxiety) as a result of the pain?

2. How has your pain affected your health and your family members' health?

3. Describe what your pain means to you.

4. How does the pain affect your functional abilities, work activities, social activities, and recreational activities.

5. How do you cope with the pain?

6. Do you have any preferences for pain medications?

7. Do you have any concerns about taking pain medication?

Adapted from Jacox, A., Carr, D. G., Payne, R., *et al.* (1994). *Management of cancer pain.* Clinical Practice Guideline No. 9 (AHCPR Publication No. 94-0592). Rockville, MD: Agency for Health Care Policy and Research, Public Health Service, U.S. Department of Health and Human Services.

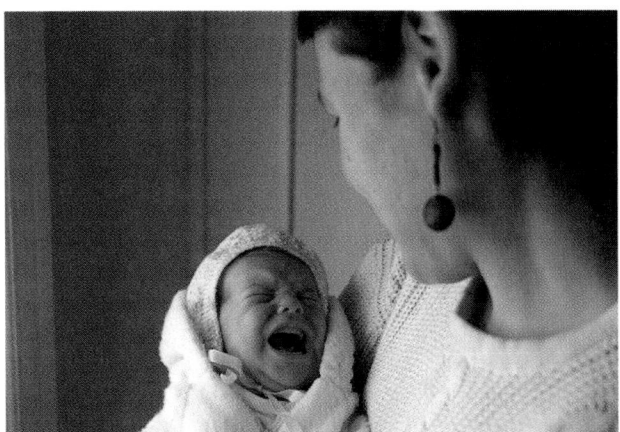

✦ **Figure 26–6**
Crying, muscle tension, and rigidity can be signs of pain in a neonate. Pain is assessed in preverbal children primarily through behavioral observation.

Box **26–8**

PEDIATRIC PAIN ASSESSMENT

1. Tell me what pain is.
2. Tell me about the hurt you have had before.
3. Do you tell others when you hurt? If yes, who?
4. What do you do for yourself when you hurt?
5. What do you want others to do for you when you hurt?
6. What helps the most to take your hurt away?
7. Is there anything special that you want me to know about you when you hurt?
8. What words would you use to describe your hurt?
9. Show me where it hurts.
10. What makes the hurt better?
11. What makes the hurt worse?

From Hester, N. O., & Barcus, C. S. (1986). Assessment and management of pain in children. *Pediatric Nursing Update, 1,* 1–8.

---

is often involved in coordinating the plan of care with the client, the family, and other members of the health care team.

Clients experiencing chronic pain may require the services of a multidisciplinary pain team, which typically consists of neurologists, anesthesiologists, psychiatrists, nurses, psychologists, physical therapists, pharmacists, social workers, and pastoral care counselors. Because of the variety of disciplines represented, a comprehensive pain management plan can be developed for a client with chronic pain.

Planning

The nursing care plan for a client experiencing acute or chronic pain must incorporate specific outcomes for each nursing diagnosis and should incorporate, based on client preferences, both pharmacological and nonpharmacological interventions. See Sample Nursing Care Plans for clients with chronic and acute pain.

Client Outcomes

Client outcomes need to be developed with the client and the family caregiver. The outcomes should be as specific as possible. Specific nursing interventions should be designed to facilitate the client's achievement of the mutually established outcomes. Examples of specific client outcomes for an individual with an acute pain problem might include: (1) Client manifests a significant reduction in acute postoperative pain, as evidenced by reports of pain intensity scores of less than 2 on a 0 to 10 scale. (2) Client uses the patient-controlled analgesia (PCA) pump with sufficient frequency to be able to ambulate without pain. (3) Client manifests a significant reduction in acute postoperative pain, as evidenced by being able to ambulate without pain and perform coughing and deep

be able to identify specific nursing diagnoses for the client. The etiology of the nursing diagnosis should accompany the diagnostic statement. By defining the etiology of the nursing diagnosis, the nurse is better able to design specific interventions for a client experiencing an acute or chronic pain problem and related nursing problems. See the accompanying box for a list of nursing diagnoses for clients experiencing acute and chronic pain.

An individualized plan of care must be developed for each client experiencing acute or chronic pain. The nurse, who spends the most time with the client,

---

Table **26–6**

PEDIATRIC PAIN ASSESSMENT TOOLS

TOOL	DESCRIPTION	AGE RANGE, YEARS	REFERENCE
Eland color assessment tool	Four of eight colored felt squares are selected to represent the most hurt, not quite as much hurt, just a little hurt, and no hurt	4–10	Eland, 1981
Oucher	Six photographs of a child in increasing levels of distress; 0 to 100 numerical scale for older children	3–12	Beyer, 1984
Poker chip tool	Four red poker chips representing pieces of hurt	4–12	Hester, 1979
Adolescent pediatric pain tool (APPT)	Multidimensional tool with word descriptors, body outline, and a word graphic rating scale	8–17	Savedra *et al.,* 1989

ELDERLY CLIENTS MAY UNDERREPORT PAIN

Elderly clients tend to underreport pain for a number of reasons. They may see pain as a normal part of the aging process and ignore the problem or bear it as a part of life. Some clients may strive to play the role of the "good patient" and are reluctant to report pain problems for fear of being labeled a "complainer." In addition, elderly clients may refrain from reporting pain complaints because they perceive that nurses are too busy and they do not want to bother them. Finally, elderly clients may refrain from reporting pain problems because they worry about the financial expenses associated with additional diagnostic tests (Dull & Stratton, 1991; Leech-Hofland, 1992). Because of the elderly's hesitancy to report pain problems, nurses should make pain assessment a routine part of every elderly person's health history.

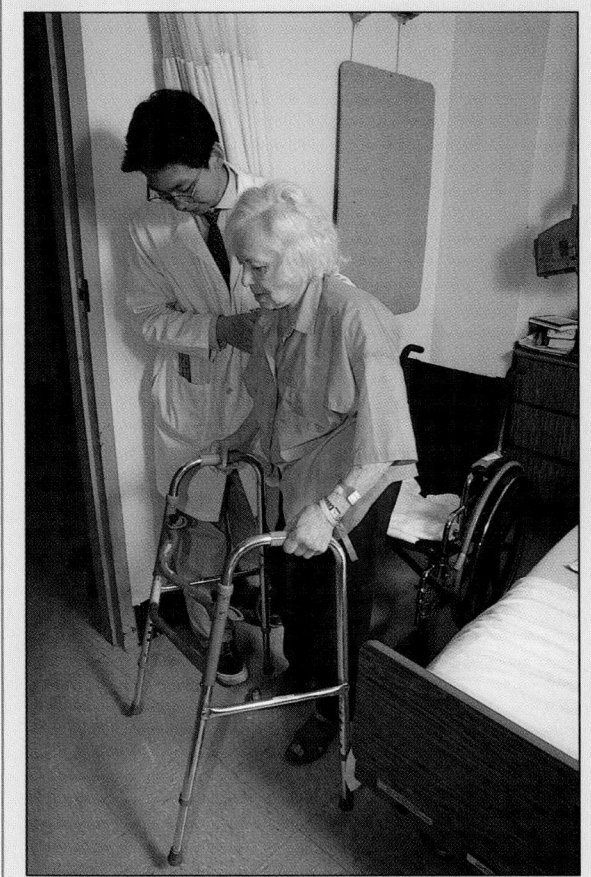

Arthritis is a common cause of pain in the elderly.

NURSING
DIAGNOSES
FOR ACUTE
AND
CHRONIC
PAIN

Nursing Diagnoses Related to Acute Pain

Pain related to myocardial ischemia

Anxiety related to unexplained abdominal pain

Activity intolerance related to pain from an abdominal incision

Ineffective breathing pattern related to incisional pain

Nursing Diagnoses Related to Chronic Pain

Chronic pain related to joint inflammation

Chronic pain related to metastatic bone cancer

Depression related to chronic pain

Fatigue related to chronic pain

Ineffective family coping related to chronic pain

chronic pain, as evidenced by an increase in functional status, an improvement in mood, and an improvement in quality of life.

Nursing Care Plan

Two clinical practice guidelines—one on the assessment and management of acute postoperative pain (Acute Pain Management Guideline Panel, 1992), and the other on the assessment and management of cancer pain (Jacox *et al.*, 1994)—have recently been published by the Federal Agency for Health Care Policy and Research. The two guidelines provide detailed information on the management of acute and cancer pain using pharmacological and nonpharmacological interventions. Much of the information presented in this section is from these two publications.

✦ **Pain Management Principles.** The management of pain should be governed by some fundamental principles. These principles are listed in Box 26–9. The fundamental principle underlying effective pain management is ascertaining the cause of the client's pain. A detailed assessment and diagnostic work-up provide the needed information to formulate an etiology for the pain complaint. The need to determine the etiology of the pain is linked to establishing an effective treatment plan. For example, a client presenting with abdominal pain may have acute appendicitis, which would require surgery. In contrast, abdominal pain could also indicate food poisoning, which would require a completely different set of interventions.

Once the cause of the pain has been established, the plan of care needs to be individualized to meet the unique needs of the client. Clients should be part of the pain management team and assist in formulat-

breathing exercises effectively. Examples of specific client outcomes for an individual with a chronic pain problem might include: (1) Client manifests a significant reduction in chronic pain, as evidenced by reports of pain intensity scores of less than 2 on a 0 to 10 scale. (2) Client takes analgesics on a routine schedule. (3) Client manifests a significant reduction in

SAMPLE NURSING CARE PLAN

THE CLIENT IN CHRONIC PAIN

Situation: A 75-year-old client with lung cancer is admitted in excruciating pain. A bone scan reveals disseminated bone metastases.

Nursing Diagnosis: Chronic pain related to bone metastases.

Expected Outcome: Client will state that pain is controlled to tolerable levels that permit ambulation.

Action	Rationale
1. Assess character, location, and intensity of the pain. Determine aggravating and relieving factors and previous pain treatment modalities.	1. A baseline assessment provides data for making comparisons over time.
2. Administer analgesics on an around-the-clock schedule.	2. Around-the-clock administration of analgesics maintains a constant blood level of the drug.
3. Treat constipation prophylactically using a stool softener and a laxative.	3. Constipation occurs with chronic administration of opioid analgesics and must be treated prophylactically.
4. Discuss different nonpharmacological options for pain control (*e.g.,* distraction, relaxation, imagery) with the client and, if client desires, teach the chosen option.	4. Nonpharmacological measures can temporarily decrease awareness of pain.
5. Evaluate the effectiveness of the pain management plan.	5. Reassessment is a critical part of the nursing process to determine whether the pain management plan needs to be revised.
6. Document care and instructions on the client's record.	6. Documentation provides a method for communicating with other members of the health care team.

SAMPLE NURSING CARE PLAN

THE CLIENT IN ACUTE PAIN

Situation: A 40-year-old client is admitted to the hospital for an emergency cholecystectomy. The client is complaining of severe pain at the site of the incision and will not move or cough and deep breathe.

Nursing Diagnosis: Acute pain related to surgery.

Expected Outcome: Client will report a pain intensity score of less than 2 and increase activity following the administration of pain medication.

Action	Rationale
1. Ask the client to rate the pain using a 0 to 10 scale.	1. Client self-report of pain intensity is the gold standard for assessment and provides data to evaluate the effectiveness of the pain management intervention.
2. Examine the incision for swelling, excessive draining, or bleeding.	2. Provides baseline data for comparison should the client's condition change.
3. Administer pain medication as prescribed.	3. The client should be given pain medication on a routine basis for the first 24–48 hours postoperatively.
4. Teach the client to use a pillow against the incision before coughing and deep breathing.	4. Placing a pillow over the incision splints it, providing support to make respiratory exercises easier.
5. Reassess the effectiveness of the analgesic in relieving the client's pain.	5. Reassessment is a critical component of the nursing care plan that allows the nurse to determine whether the analgesic medication is effective or whether the medication order requires modification.
6. Document care and instructions given on the client's record.	6. Documentation provides a method of communicating with other members of the health care team.

final component of an effective pain management plan is the evaluation of the effectiveness of the specific interventions being used. If the pain management plan is not working, additional data are often needed to make appropriate modifications in the therapeutic regimen. Clients may need to undergo additional diagnostic tests or be provided with different types of pain medications or other types of interventions to get their pain under control.

Implementation
Pharmacological Management

The pharmacological agents used to manage acute and chronic pain can be categorized as nonopioid analgesics, opioid analgesics, and adjuvant analgesics. The mechanism of action, therapeutic uses, and side effects of each of these groups of analgesics are reviewed here.

✦ **Nonopioid Analgesics.** Nonopioid analgesics (*i.e.*, aspirin, acetaminophen, and the nonsteroidal antiinflammatory drugs [NSAIDs]) are indicated for mild to moderate pain. These drugs produce their analgesic effects in the peripheral nervous system by interfering with the synthesis of prostaglandins (chemical substances that are irritating to primary afferent nociceptors). The different types of nonopioid analgesics and their recommended starting doses are listed in Table 26–8.

The NSAIDs and acetaminophen exhibit the pharmacological property of a ceiling effect, which means that beyond a certain dose, these drugs do not produce any greater analgesia, and with higher doses, the number and severity of side effects markedly increase. Clients receiving nonopioid analgesics, particularly NSAIDs, need to be monitored for the following side effects: gastrointestinal upset, gastrointestinal ulceration, bleeding, renal failure, and CNS toxicity (*e.g.*, confusion).

✦ **Opioid Analgesics.** Opioid analgesics are the medications of choice for moderate to severe pain. These drugs work in the CNS at the level of the spinal cord and midbrain to produce analgesia. The dose equivalents of the various opioids and the recommended starting doses for adults and children greater than and less than 50 kg who are in moderate to severe pain are listed in Tables 26–9 and 26–10, respectively. The recommended starting doses should be reduced by 30 to 50% in the elderly. Doses should be increased slowly until adequate analgesia is achieved with minimal side effects.

Morphine sulfate is the analgesic of choice for acute and cancer pain. If morphine cannot be used because of an unusual reaction or allergy, another opioid (*e.g.*, hydromorphone) can be substituted. Meperidine should be reserved only for brief courses of acute pain therapy in clients who have a demonstrated allergy or intolerance to morphine or hydromorphone.

ing the plan of care. They should be informed about the variety of pain treatment options that are available. Besides providing a list of options, nurses need to indicate the potential risks and benefits of each of the different pain management interventions. An example of such a teaching tool is found in Table 26–7. In addition, clients need to be taught the importance of notifying the nurse when they are experiencing pain and to take their pain medication *before* the pain becomes severe, thus necessitating less pain medication to get the pain under control.

Consideration needs to be given to using both pharmacological and nonpharmacological interventions. In most instances, the effective management of pain requires the use of analgesic drugs (Fig. 26–7). Nonpharmacological pain management strategies often serve as supplements to the analgesic regimen. The

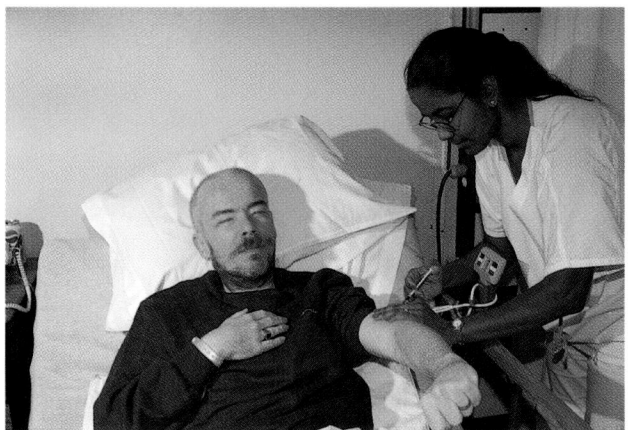

✦ **Figure 26–7**
Most clients in pain require drugs for effective pain management. Nonpharmacological pain management strategies can serve as supplements. Pain medications are administered initially on a regular schedule; the client is encouraged to request medication before the pain becomes severe. Later, when the pain is less acute, medications can be taken on an as-needed basis.

Table **26–7**

CLIENT TEACHING TOOL: RISKS AND BENEFITS OF PAIN MANAGEMENT INTERVENTIONS

PAIN RELIEF MEDICINES		
Description	Benefits	Risks
Nonsteroidal antiinflammatory drugs: acetaminophen (*e.g.,* Tylenol), aspirin, ibuprofen (*e.g.,* Motrin), and other NSAIDs reduce swelling and soreness and relieve mild to moderate pain	There is no risk of addiction to these medicines Depending on the amount of pain, these medicines can lessen or eliminate the need for stronger medicines (*e.g.,* morphine or another opioid)	Most NSAIDs interfere with blood clotting They may cause nausea, stomach bleeding, or kidney problems For severe pain, an opioid usually must be added
Opioids: morphine, codeine, and other opioids are most often used for acute pain, such as short-term pain after surgery	These medicines are effective for severe pain, and they do not cause bleeding in the stomach or elsewhere It is rare for a client to become addicted as a result of taking opioids for postoperative pain	Opioids may cause drowsiness, nausea, constipation, or itching or interfere with breathing or urination
NONDRUG PAIN RELIEF METHODS		
Description	Benefits	Risks
Client teaching: learning about the operation and the pain expected afterward (*e.g.,* when coughing or getting out of bed or a chair)	These techniques can reduce anxiety; they are simple to learn, and no equipment is needed	There are no risks; however, client attention and cooperation with staff are required
Relaxation: simple techniques, such as abdominal breathing and jaw relaxation, can help increase comfort after surgery	Relaxation techniques are easy to learn, and they can help reduce anxiety After instruction, the client can use relaxation at any time No equipment is needed	There are no risks, but instruction from a nurse or doctor is necessary
Physical agents: cold packs, massage, rest, and TENS therapy are some of the nondrug pain relief methods that might be used following surgery	In general, physical agents are safe and have no side effects TENS (transcutaneous electrical nerve stimulation) is often helpful; it is quick to act and can be controlled by the client	There are no risks related to the use of physical techniques for managing pain If TENS is used, there is some cost and staff time involved for purchasing the machine and instructing clients in its use There is only limited evidence to support the effectiveness of TENS for pain relief in certain situations

From Acute Pain Management Guideline Panel. (1992). *Pain control after surgery: A patient's guide* (AHCPR Publication No. 92-0021). Rockville, MD: Agency for Health Care Policy and Research, Public Health Service, U.S. Department of Health and Human Services.

Meperidine should not be administered chronically for the management of cancer pain. Meperidine is contraindicated in clients with impaired renal function or in those who are receiving monoamine oxidase inhibitors, because normeperidene, the first active metabolite of meperidine, is a cerebral irritant. Accumulation of normeperidene can cause effects ranging from dysphoria and irritable mood to seizures (Miaskowski, 1993a). Additional recommendations for the dosing, scheduling, and route of administration for opioid analgesics in the management of acute pain are listed in Box 26–10.

The dose of an opioid analgesic needed to control acute pain varies greatly among clients. Those in moderate to severe pain should be started on a dose of opioid analgesic (see Tables 26–9 and 26–10) and assessed to determine whether they are experiencing adequate pain relief. The dose of pain medication should be adjusted to achieve optimal analgesia with minimal side effects. If a client was taking opioid analgesics before the onset of the acute pain problem, he or she may require higher initial and maintenance doses of opioid analgesics.

Medications for acute pain should be administered

Text continued on page 727

Table 26–8

DOSING DATA FOR ACETAMINOPHEN AND NSAIDS

DRUG	USUAL DOSE FOR ADULTS AND CHILDREN ≥50 KG BODY WEIGHT	USUAL DOSE FOR CHILDREN* AND ADULTS† ≤50 KG BODY WEIGHT
Acetaminophen and over-the-counter NSAIDs		
Acetaminophen‡	650 mg q 4 h 975 mg q 6 h	10–15 mg/kg q 4 h 15–20 mg/kg q 4 h (rectal)
Aspirin§	650 mg q 4 h 975 mg q 6 h	10–15 mg/kg q 4 h 15–20 mg/kg q 4 h (rectal)
Ibuprofen (Motrin, others)	400–600 mg q 6 h	10 mg/kg q 6–8 h‖
Prescription NSAIDs		
Carprofen (Rimadyl)	100 mg tid	
Choline magnesium trisalicylate (Trilisate)¶	1000–1500 mg tid	25 mg/kg tid
Choline salicylate (Arthropan)¶	870 mg q 3–4 h	
Diflunisal (Dolobid)*	500 mg q 12 h	
Etodolac (Lodine)	200–400 mg q 6–8 h	
Fenoprofen calcium (Nalfon)	300–600 mg q 6 h	
Ketoprofen (Orudis)	25–60 mg q 6–8 h	
Ketorolac tromethamine (Toradol)**	10 mg q 4–6 h to a maximum of 40 mg/day	
Magnesium salicylate (Doan's, Magan, Mobidin, others)	650 mg q 4 h	
Meclofenamate sodium (Meclomen)‡	50–100 mg q 6 h	
Mefenamic acid (Ponstel)	250 mg q 6 h	
Naproxen (Naprosyn)	250–275 mg q 6–8 h	5 mg/kg q 8 h
Naproxen sodium (Anaprox)	275 mg q 6–8 h	
Sodium salicylate (generic)	325–650 mg q 3–4 h	
Parenteral NSAIDs		
Ketorolac tromethamine (Toradol)**,‡‡	60 mg initially, then 30 mg q 6 h; intramuscular dose not to exceed 5 days	

Note: Only the NSAIDs listed have FDA approval for use as simple analgesics, but clinical experience has been gained with other drugs as well.

*Only drugs that are FDA approved as an analgesic for use in children are included.

†Acetaminophen and NSAID dosages for adults weighing less than 50 kg should be adjusted for weight.

‡Acetaminophen lacks the peripheral antiinflammatory and antiplatelet activities of the other NSAIDs.

§The standard against which other NSAIDs are compared. May inhibit platelet aggregation for ≥1 wk and may cause bleeding. Aspirin is contraindicated in children with fever or other viral disease because of its association with Reye syndrome.

‖ Not FDA approved for use in children as an over-the-counter drug; has FDA approval for use in children as a prescription drug for fever, but clinicians have experience in prescribing ibuprofen for pain in children.

¶May have minimal antiplatelet activity.

#Administration with antacids may decrease absorption.

**For short-term use only.

††Coombs-positive autoimmune hemolytic anemia has been associated with prolonged use.

‡‡Has the same gastrointestinal toxicities as oral NSAIDs.

Table **26–9**

DOSE EQUIVALENTS FOR OPIOID ANALGESICS IN OPIOID-NAIVE ADULTS AND CHILDREN ≥ 50 KG BODY WEIGHT*

DRUG	APPROXIMATE EQUIANALGESIC DOSE		USUAL STARTING DOSE FOR MODERATE TO SEVERE PAIN	
	Oral	Parenteral	Oral	Parenteral
Opioid agonist[†]				
Morphine[‡]	30 mg q 3–4 h (repeat around-the-clock dosing) 60 mg q 3–4 h (single dose or intermittent dosing)	10 mg q 3–4 h	30 mg q 3–4 h	10 mg q 3–4 h
Morphine, controlled-release (MS Contin, Oramorph)[‡,§]	90–120 mg q 12 h	N/A	90–120 mg q 12 h	N/A
Hydromorphone (Dilaudid)[‡]	7.5 mg q 3–4 h	1.5 mg q 3–4 h	6 mg q 3–4 h	1.5 mg q 3–4 h
Levorphanol (Levo-Dromoran)	4 mg q 6–8 h	2 mg q 6–8 h	4 mg q 6–8 h	2 mg q 6–8 h
Meperidine (Demerol)	300 mg q 2–3 h	100 mg q 3 h	N/R	100 mg q 3 h
Methadone (Dolophine, others)	20 mg q 6–8 h	10 mg q 6–8 h	20 mg q 6–8 h	10 mg q 6–8 h
Oxymorphone (Numorphan)[‡]	N/A	1 mg q 3–4 h	N/A	1 mg q 3–4 h
Combination Opioid/NSAID Preparations[‖]				
Codeine (with aspirin or acetaminophen)[¶]	180–200 mg q 3–4 h	130 mg q 3–4 h	60 mg q 3–4 h	60 mg q 2 h (IM/SC)
Hydrocodone (in Lorcet, Lortab, Vicodin, others)	30 mg q 3–4 h	N/A	10 mg q 3–4 h	N/A
Oxycodone (Roxicodone; also in Percocet, Percodan, Tylox, others)	30 mg q 3–4 h	N/A	10 mg q 3–4 h	N/A

Note: Published tables vary in the suggested doses that are equianalgesic to morphine. Clinical response is the criterion that must be applied for each client; titration to clinical responses is necessary. Because there is not complete cross-tolerance among these drugs, it is usually necessary to use a lower than equianalgesic dose when changing drugs and to retitrate to response.

*Caution: Recommended doses do not apply for adults weighing less than 50 kg. For recommended starting doses for children and adults <50 kg body weight, see Table 26–10.

†Caution: Recommended doses do not apply to clients with renal or hepatic insufficiency or other conditions affecting drug metabolism and kinetics.

‡Caution: For morphine, hydromorphone, and oxymorphone, rectal administration is an alternative route for clients unable to take oral medications. Equianalgesic doses may differ between oral and parenteral doses because of pharmacokinetic differences.

*§Transdermal fentanyl (Duragesic) is an alternative option. The transdermal fentanyl dosage is not calculated as equianalgesic to a single morphine dose. See the package insert for dosing calculations. Doses above 25 µg/h should not be used in opioid-naive clients.

‖ Caution: Doses of aspirin and acetaminophen in combination opioid/NSAID preparations must also be adjusted to the client's body weight. Aspirin is contraindicated in children in the presence of fever or other viral disease because of its association with Reye syndrome.

¶Caution: Codeine doses above 65 mg are often inappropriate because of diminishing incremental analgesia with increasing doses but continually increasing nausea, constipation, and other side effects.

N/A = not available; N/R = not recommended; IM = intramuscular; SC = subcutaneous.

Table 26–10

DOSE EQUIVALENTS FOR OPIOID ANALGESICS IN OPIOID-NAIVE CHILDREN
AND ADULTS <50 KG BODY WEIGHT*

DRUG	APPROXIMATE EQUIANALGESIC DOSE		USUAL STARTING DOSE FOR MODERATE TO SEVERE PAIN	
	Oral	Parenteral	Oral	Parenteral
Opioid agonist†				
Morphine‡	30 mg q 3–4 h (repeat around-the-clock dosing) 60 mg q 3–4 h (single dose or intermittent dosing)	10 mg q 3–4 h	0.3 mg/kg q 3–4 h	0.1 mg q 3–4 h
Morphine, controlled-release (MS Contin, Oramorph)‡,§	90–120 mg q 12 h	N/A	N/A	N/A
Hydromorphone (Dilaudid)‡	7.5 mg q 3–4 h	1.5 mg q 3–4 h	0.06 mg/kg q 3–4 h	0.015 mg/kg q 3–4 h
Levorphanol (Levo-Dromo-ran)	4 mg q 6–8 h	2 mg q 6–8 h	0.04 mg/kg q 6–8 h	0.02 mg/kg q 6–8 h
Meperidine (Demerol)	300 mg q 2–3 h	100 mg q 3 h	N/R	0.75 mg/kg q 2–3 h
Methadone (Dolophine, others)	20 mg q 6–8 h	10 mg q 6–8 h	0.2 mg/kg q 6–8 h	0.1 mg/kg q 6–8 h
Combination Opioid/NSAID Preparations‖				
Codeine (with aspirin or acetaminophen)¶	180–200 mg q 3–4 h	130 mg q 3–4 h	0.5–1 mg/kg q 3–4 h	N/R
Hydrocodone (in Lorcet, Lortab, Vicodin, others)	30 mg q 3–4 h	N/A	0.2 mg/kg q 3–4 h	N/A
Oxycodone (Roxicodone; also in Percocet, Percodan, Tylox, others)	30 mg q 3–4 h	N/A	0.2 mg/kg q 3–4 h	N/A

Note: Published tables vary in the suggested doses that are equianalgesic to morphine. Clinical response is the criterion that must be applied for each client; titration to clinical responses is necessary. Because there is not complete cross-tolerance among these drugs, it is usually necessary to use a lower than equianalgesic dose when changing drugs and to retitrate to response.

*Caution: Doses listed for clients weighing less than 50 kg cannot be used as initial starting doses in babies less than 6 mo of age.

†Caution: Recommended doses do not apply to clients with renal or hepatic insufficiency or other conditions affecting drug metabolism and kinetics.

‡Caution: For morphine, hydromorphone, and oxymorphone, rectal administration is an alternative route for clients unable to take oral medications. Equianalgesic doses may differ between oral and parenteral doses because of pharmacokinetic differences.

§Transdermal fentanyl (Duragesic) is an alternative option. The transdermal fentanyl dosage is not calculated as equianalgesic to a single morphine dose. See the package insert for dosing calculations. Doses above 25 μg/h should not be used in opioid-naive clients.

‖ Caution: Doses of aspirin and acetaminophen in combination opioid/NSAID preparations must also be adjusted to the client's body weight. Aspirin is contraindicated in children in the presence of fever or other viral disease because of its association with Reye syndrome.

¶Caution: Some clinicians recommend not exceeding 1.5 mg/kg of codeine because of an increased incidence of side effects with higher doses.

N/A = not available; N/R = not recommended.

on a regular schedule. This maintains a steady concentration of the analgesic in the client's blood and prevents the recurrence of pain. Later, when the condition producing the acute pain problem is corrected and the pain is decreasing, pain medications can be administered on an as-needed basis.

If the client can take pain medication orally, this route is preferred. If the client needs to receive pain medication parenterally, the intravenous route is preferred. Clients, particularly children, should not receive pain medication by intramuscular injection, because the injections are painful and may deter clients from requesting pain medication.

Nurses need to assess clients at regular intervals to

Box **26–10**

RECOMMENDATIONS FOR DOSING, SCHEDULING, AND ROUTE OF ADMINISTRATION OF OPIOIDS FOR THE MANAGEMENT OF ACUTE PAIN

Dosages of Opioid Analgesics

- Clients vary greatly in their analgesic dose requirements and responses to opioid analgesics.
- Doses of opioids should be titrated to achieve optimal analgesia with minimal side effects.
- Relative potencies of opioid analgesics need to be considered when switching from one opioid to another or when changing the route of administration.
- Clients who have been receiving opioid analgesics prior to the episode of acute pain may require higher starting and maintenance doses of opioids.

Scheduling of Opioid Analgesics

- Unless contraindicated, analgesics for acute pain should initially be administered on a regular basis.
- Later, as the condition producing the acute pain is corrected, it may be acceptable to give analgesic agents on an as-needed basis.
- Nurses should assess clients at regular intervals to determine the efficacy of the intervention, the presence of side effects, the need for adjustments in dosage and/or interval, and the need for supplemental doses of medication for breakthrough pain.

Routes of Administration

- Intravenous administration is the parenteral route of choice.
- Repeated intramuscular injections can themselves cause pain and may deter clients from requesting pain medication.
- Oral administration of pain medications is convenient and inexpensive. It is appropriate as soon as a client can tolerate oral intake.

Adapted from Acute Pain Management Guideline Panel. (1992). *Acute pain management: Operative or medical procedures and trauma.* Clinical Practice Guideline (AHCPR Publication No. 92-0032). Rockville, MD: Agency for Health Care Policy and Research, Public Health Service, U.S. Department of Health and Human Services.

determine how well the pain medication is working and to determine whether adjustments need to be made in the dosage or in the frequency of drug administration.

The most common side effects associated with acute administration of opioid analgesics are sedation, hypotension, and respiratory depression. The actual incidence and severity of these side effects are unknown. Nurses should monitor clients for the develop-

ment of these side effects, as well as for the efficacy of the analgesics.

✦ **Adjuvant Analgesics.** Adjuvant analgesics are most commonly used in the management of cancer and chronic nonmalignant pain. In most cases, the primary indication for these agents is not pain relief. However, all the drugs used as adjuvant analgesics have pain-relieving properties or help counteract some of the side effects associated with the chronic administration of opioid analgesics. These drugs may be administered in combination with nonopioid or opioid analgesics. The adjuvant drugs that are most commonly used are the tricyclic antidepressants, antihistamines, dextroamphetamine, steroids, phenothiazines, and anticonvulsants.

The tricyclic antidepressants include amitriptyline, imipramine, desipramine, and doxepin. These drugs provide direct analgesic effects and may potentiate opioid analgesia by blocking the reuptake of serotonin. In addition, these drugs may enhance the client's ability to sleep. However, the tricyclic antidepressants have potent anticholinergic side effects (*e.g.*, dry mouth, urinary retention, blurred vision). Clients must be taught strategies to relieve dry mouth (*e.g.*, sucking on sugarless candy) and the importance of reporting symptoms of urinary retention and blurred vision (Miaskowski, 1993b).

Certain antihistamines (*e.g.*, hydroxyzine) may be useful in treating the anxiety or nausea associated with chronic or cancer pain. Dextroamphetamine, a psychostimulant, may be a useful adjuvant drug in helping to counteract the sedative effects associated with the chronic administration of opioid analgesics. Steroids may provide euphoria as well as relieve cancer pain associated with bone metastasis or spinal cord compression. The phenothiazines may be useful adjuncts in treating the nausea associated with the administration of opioid analgesics. It should be noted, however, that this group of drugs can enhance the sedative effects of opioid analgesics. Finally, anticonvulsants (*e.g.*, phenytoin, carbamazepine, sodium valproate, clonazepam) may be used to treat the lancinating pain associated with neuropathic pain.

Management of Cancer Pain

The management of cancer pain often requires a combination of nonopioid, opioid, and adjuvant analgesics. Work by several individuals, including clinicians who care for clients in hospice settings, has identified basic principles for the management of pain associated with cancer and/or cancer treatment (see Box 26–11) (American Pain Society, 1992).

Several of these principles are worth highlighting. First, opioid and nonopioid analgesics are the mainstay of cancer pain management. However, these pharmacological agents must be administered in the right dose, through the correct route, and with the right frequency. In addition, analgesics are more effec-

CANCER PAIN MANAGEMENT PRINCIPLES

1. Ascertain the cause of the pain.
2. Individualize the dose, route, and schedule of administration of nonopioid and opioid analgesics.
3. Use appropriate combinations of nonopioid and opioid analgesics.
4. Administer analgesics regularly (not as needed) if pain is present most of the day.
5. Understand the pharmacology, including the time course of effect, of several strong opioids (*e.g.,* morphine sulfate, hydromorphone, methadone).
6. Monitor clients closely, particularly when beginning or changing an analgesic regimen.
7. Monitor for and treat nonopioid- and opioid-induced side effects early.
8. Use adjuvant medications (*e.g.,* tricyclic antidepressants, steroids, anticonvulsants).
9. Monitor for signs and symptoms of tolerance, and initiate treatment when it occurs.
10. Be aware of the development of physical dependence, and prevent withdrawal.
11. Use nonpharmacologic strategies for pain control.

From Miaskowski, C. (1993). Current concepts in the assessment and management of cancer-related pain. *MEDSURG Nursing, 2*(1), 28–33. Reprinted with permission of the publisher, Jannetti Publications, Inc.

tive if they are administered in combinations based on their pharmacological mechanisms of action. For example, the addition of an NSAID, which acts on the peripheral nervous system, to an opioid analgesic, which acts on the central nervous system, results in enhanced analgesic efficacy.

Route of administration and frequency of administration must be considered when planning the client's pharmacological regimen. In general, the oral route is the most convenient; it is the method of choice and should be used for as long as possible. One must remember, however, that drugs administered orally have a slower onset of action (in most cases, at least 30 minutes) and a longer duration of effect. Drugs administered parenterally have a more rapid onset of action, with intravenous administration being the most rapid, but have a shorter duration of effect. If rapid pain relief is required, the medication should be administered intravenously and then followed by oral preparations of the drug.

Opioid and nonopioid analgesics should be administered around the clock, not on an as-needed basis, to clients with chronic cancer pain. Nurses are often hesitant to administer opioids to clients who do not request them or who do not "look like" they are in pain. It is important to remember that clients with cancer, particularly those in chronic pain, require around-the-clock administration of analgesics to maintain an adequate serum blood level of the opioid and to maintain adequate pain control.

Because clients with cancer receive opioids on a chronic basis, a major principle in their management is to anticipate opioid-induced side effects and treat them promptly or, in some cases, prophylactically. The major side effects associated with the chronic administration of opioid analgesics are constipation, respiratory depression, sedation, and nausea and vomiting. Nursing interventions for alleviating these side effects are provided in Box 26–12 (Miaskowski, 1993b).

Tolerance, Physical Dependence, and Addiction

All health care professionals need to be aware that tolerance and physical dependence occur in clients who receive opioids over a period of time. Tolerance

MANAGEMENT OF THE COMMON SIDE EFFECTS ASSOCIATED WITH CHRONIC ADMINISTRATION OF OPIOIDS

Constipation

- Start the client on a bowel regimen containing docusate sodium 100–200 mg two or three times a day and senna 1–2 tablets at bedtime.
- Maintain adequate fluid intake.
- Provide increased roughage in the diet, if the client can tolerate this.

Respiratory Depression

- Not a major problem in clients who are taking opioids chronically.
- If respiratory depression occurs, withhold a dose of the opioid and stimulate the client.
- If an opioid antagonist is required, dilute 1 ampule (0.4 mg) of naloxone in 10 ml of normal saline and administer *slowly* (*i.e.,* 0.5 ml every 1–2 min) until respiratory rate improves.

Sedation

- Sometimes this side effect is difficult to avoid.
- Dextroamphetamine in doses of 2.5–5 mg twice a day may be helpful.

Nausea and Vomiting

- Administer antiemetics as needed.

From Miaskowski, C. (1993). Current concepts in the assessment and management of cancer-related pain. *MEDSURG Nursing, 2*(1), 28–33. Reprinted with permission of the publisher, Jannetti Publications, Inc.

means that, over time, larger doses of opioids are required to maintain the original analgesic effect. One of the first signs that a client is becoming tolerant to an opioid is that the duration of action of the drug shortens.

Physical dependence is a condition that occurs in clients taking opioids chronically when the drugs are abruptly discontinued or an opioid antagonist, such as naloxone, is administered. The result is the production of an abstinence syndrome characterized by anxiety, irritability, chills alternating with hot flashes, salivation, lacrimation, nausea, vomiting, abdominal cramps, and insomnia.

Psychological dependence or addiction is defined as a pattern of compulsive drug use characterized by a continued craving for an opioid and the need to use the opioid for effects other than pain relief (American Pain Society, 1992). Psychological dependence should never be an issue in treating opioid-naive clients with acute or cancer-related pain. It must be made clear to nurses and physicians, as well as to clients and their family caregivers, that tolerance and physical dependence are *not* the equivalent of psychological dependence or addiction. In reality, the incidence of psychological dependence following either acute or chronic administration of opioids to clients with cancer is extremely small.

Nonpharmacological Management

Nonpharmacological approaches to managing pain can be divided into physical interventions and psychological interventions. Physical interventions may include any or all of the following: positioning, massage, use of heat or cold, and transelectrical nerve stimulation (TENS). Psychological interventions may include such techniques as distraction, relaxation, hypnosis, guided imagery, biofeedback, and music therapy. Each of these interventions is reviewed in this section.

Nonpharmacological interventions are appropriate for the client who (1) finds such interventions appealing; (2) expresses anxiety or fear, as long as the anxiety is not incapacitating or the result of a medical or psychiatric condition that requires specific interventions; (3) may benefit from avoiding or reducing drug therapy; (4) is likely to experience and need to cope with a prolonged interval of pain; or (5) has incomplete pain relief following pharmacological interventions (Acute Pain Management Guideline Panel, 1992).

When considering nonpharmacological interventions, the nurse should consider several factors, including the intensity of the client's pain, the expected duration of the pain, the client's cognitive/mental status, the client's previous experience with the technique and its efficacy, the client's physical ability, and the client's desire to use such techniques. Family caregivers may be involved in the process of selecting nonpharmacological interventions, as well as in implementing them.

◗ **Positioning.** Maintaining proper body alignment and positioning can facilitate a client's comfort. The use of pillows and wedges can provide additional support, particularly in those experiencing incisional pain or pain associated with bone fractures.

◗ **Massage.** Massage, a form of cutaneous stimulation, provides both physical and mental comfort and relaxation. Massage may produce pain relief mainly by relaxing muscles and improving circulation (Fig. 26–8).

◗ **Use of Heat and Cold.** The use of heat induces vasodilation, which increases the delivery of oxygen and nutrients to damaged tissues. Heat also decreases joint stiffness by increasing the elastic properties of muscles (Vasudevan *et al.*, 1992).

A variety of methods can be used to apply superficial heat, including hot packs, hot water bottles, hot/moist compresses, heating pads (see Fig. 26–8), and immersion in a bathtub or whirlpool. Care should be taken with all applications of heat to prevent burns. Clients with decreased sensation should be monitored closely when heat is applied to the skin to prevent tissue injury (Jacox *et al.*, 1994).

The use of cold causes vasoconstriction and hyperesthesia. Cold therapy is often effective in reducing swelling and inflammation following tissue injury. Safety precautions should be implemented when using cold to prevent skin irritation. The duration of ice application should be no longer than 15 minutes. The use of cold packs is contraindicated in any condition in which vasoconstriction increases symptoms, such as peripheral vascular disease, Raynaud syndrome, or other vascular or connective tissue disorders (Whitney, 1989). In addition, cold packs should not be applied to tissue that has been damaged by radiation therapy.

◗ **Transelectrical Nerve Stimulation (TENS).** TENS is a method of applying controlled, low-voltage electrical stimulation to large, myelinated peripheral nerve fibers through skin electrodes for the purpose of modulating stimulus transmission and relieving pain (see Fig. 26–8). TENS has been used to treat a variety of acute and chronic pain problems.

◗ **Distraction.** Distraction is the strategy of focusing the client's attention on stimuli other than pain or the accompanying negative emotions (see Fig. 26–8). Various forms of distraction can be implemented, including singing, praying, watching television, talking with family and friends, or reading. Distraction may be particularly useful as a pain-reducing strategy with children. Distraction can be used alone to manage mild pain or as an adjunct to analgesic drugs to manage brief episodes of severe pain, such as procedure-related pain (Jacox *et al.*, 1994).

◗ **Relaxation/Guided Imagery.** Relaxation techniques and imagery are used to achieve a state of mental and physical relaxation. Mental relaxation re-

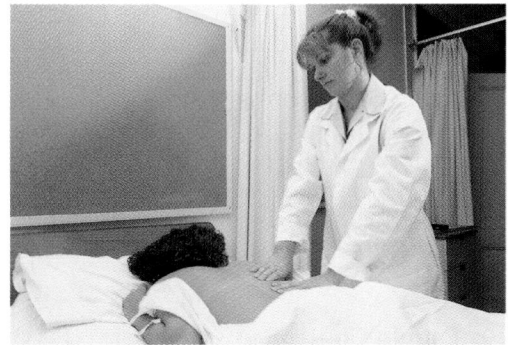

Massage *may relieve pain by relaxing muscles and improving circulation.*

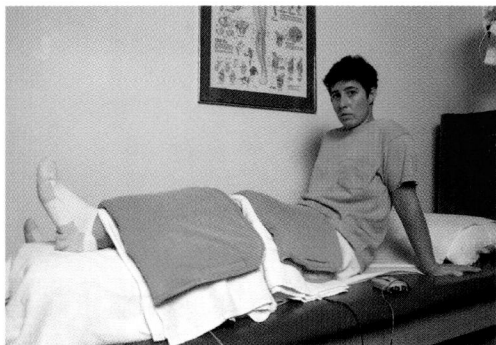

Heat application *can help control pain. Towels under these heat pads prevent burns..*

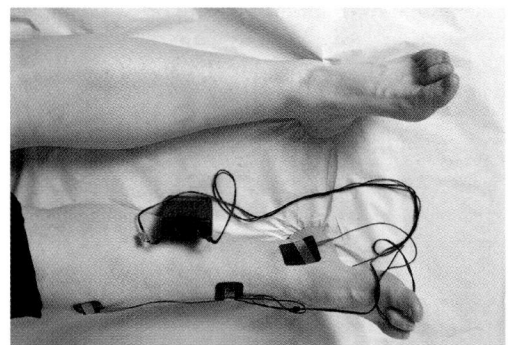

Transelectrical nerve stimulation (TENS) *unit in place.*

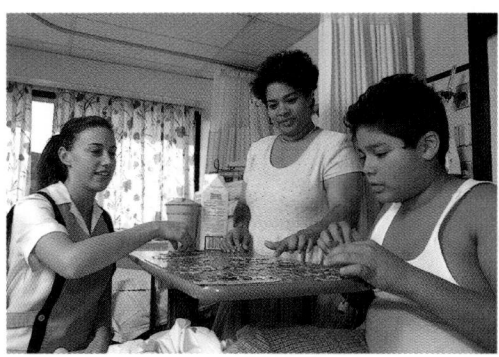

Distraction: *Nurse and mother help child with puzzle.*

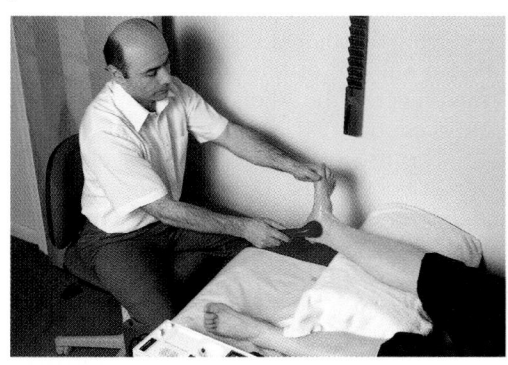

Ultrasound *to relieve pain.*

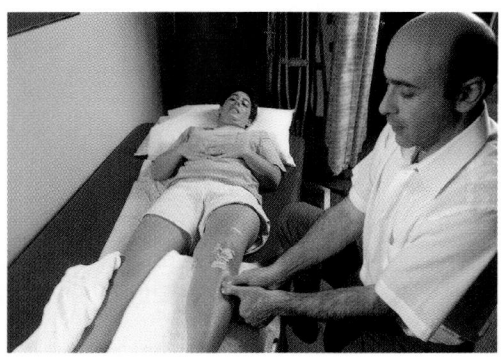

Stimulation of pressure points *for pain relief.*

✦ **Figure 26–8**
Nonpharmacological methods of pain management.

sults from an alleviation of anxiety. Physical relaxation results from a reduction in skeletal muscle tension. Relaxation techniques can focus on breathing exercises, progressive muscle relaxation, or meditation. An example of a relaxation exercise that can be used with a client in acute or chronic pain is found in Box 26–13.

Imagery can be used to aid relaxation. Clients should be encouraged to share pleasant images with the nurse. The nurse can then incorporate these pleasant images (*e.g.*, a walk on a beach, a picnic, a sunset, going skiing) into the relaxation exercise. Both pleasant imagery and progressive muscle relaxation have

been shown to decrease pain intensity and pain distress (Graffam & Johnson, 1987). Nurses can make tapes of relaxation exercises for clients to use when it is convenient for them.

✦ **Hypnosis.** Hypnosis is a state of heightened awareness and focused concentration that can be used to manipulate the perception of pain and has been found to be effective in the treatment of acute and cancer-related pain (Spiegel & Bloom, 1983; Syrjala, Cummings, & Donaldson, 1992). Hypnosis should be administered only by specially trained professionals (Jacox *et al.*, 1994).

Box 26–13

RELAXATION EXERCISE

Client Preparation: Have the client empty his or her bladder and remove glasses or contact lenses. Have the client assume a comfortable position, either sitting or lying down.

Exercise Steps

1. Close your eyes and slowly take in a deep breath.

2. Now slowly exhale. Feel your body begin to relax, feel the tension leaving your body.

3. Now take in another deep breath. Exhale slowly, feeling more relaxed and more comfortable.

4. Now take in a third deep breath, let the breath out slowly, and feel as relaxed and comfortable as you are ready to feel.

5. Continue to repeat this procedure, breathing in and out slowly, and let yourself feel more and more comfortable with each breath.

6. When you are ready, exhale slowly and tell yourself, "I feel very alert and relaxed."

Other Pain Management Procedures

A variety of pharmacological preparations (*e.g.*, sustained-release morphine, transdermal fentanyl) and technological advances (*e.g.*, patient-controlled analgesia [PCA] devices, spinal administration of opioids) have provided more options to improve the management of pain.

❧ **Sustained-Release Morphine Preparations.** Sustained-release or controlled-release morphine tablets are specially formulated pills in which morphine is contained in a resin matrix that slowly dissolves in the gastrointestinal tract, releasing the morphine over a 12-hour interval. This preparation (in contrast to immediate-release morphine, which must be administered every 3 to 4 hours) can be given every 8 to 12 hours. For clients experiencing chronic pain, an 8- or 12-hour dosing regimen allows an uninterrupted night's sleep.

Clients with chronic pain may experience "breakthrough" pain, or pain that occurs between regularly scheduled doses of sustained-release morphine. Clients should be provided with an immediate-release, short-acting opioid (*e.g.*, morphine, hydromorphone, oxycodone) to take in between doses of sustained-release morphine should breakthrough pain occur.

❧ **Transdermal Fentanyl.** Fentanyl is the only drug currently available in a transdermal delivery system. Fentanyl is readily absorbed through the skin, and the drug delivery system allows a continuous opioid infusion without the use of needles. Transdermal fentanyl (Duragesic) is approved by the Food and Drug Administration for use in chronic cancer pain.

Four doses of transdermal fentanyl are available: 25, 50, 75, and 100 μg/hour patches. Once the patch is applied to the skin, it takes approximately 12 to 16 hours for the drug to start working and approximately 48 hours to achieve steady-state blood concentrations. Clients should be given a short-acting opioid to take if breakthrough pain occurs.

❧ **Patient-Controlled Analgesia (PCA).** PCA is a regimen that allows the client to self-administer predetermined doses of an analgesic drug in sufficient amounts to maintain relatively constant plasma concentrations of the pain medication and a relatively constant amount of analgesia (Wasylak *et al.*, 1990). The major advantages of PCA are that it is an individualized approach to pain control, clients are given some control over their pain management, and pain management is improved. PCA delivery systems have been used in the management of acute postoperative pain and cancer pain.

Most PCA devices allow the client to self-administer a predetermined dose of medication by pressing a button (see Procedure 26–1). PCA devices can be attached to an intravenous line or an epidural catheter. Once the medication is delivered to the client, there is a preset lockout interval that prevents the client from receiving another dose of pain medication until a sufficient amount of time has elapsed. This lockout interval prevents the client from overdosing on the pain medication (Wasylak *et al.*, 1990).

The use of PCA requires adequate client preparation. Clients must be taught how to use the device and be instructed to administer the pain medication *before* the pain becomes severe, so that their pain is better controlled.

❧ **Spinal Analgesia.** Since the discovery of opioid receptors in the spinal cord, analgesics have been administered into the epidural or intrathecal space to treat acute postoperative pain, labor pain, and cancer-related pain. Spinal analgesia requires the placement of a temporary (for acute administration) or permanent (for chronic administration) catheter into the epidural or intrathecal space. The administration of opioids into the epidural or intrathecal space leads to binding of the analgesic to opioid receptors in the spinal cord (Fig. 26–9), thereby blocking the transmission of painful stimuli.

Nursing care of clients receiving spinal analgesia requires careful monitoring of catheter-related complications, including infection, leakage, hematoma formation, and catheter migration. In addition, clients must be monitored for the side effects of spinal analgesia: nausea and vomiting, pruritus, urinary retention, and respiratory depression. Explicit policies and procedures should be in place that specify how frequently

PROCEDURE

26–1

PATIENT-CONTROLLED ANALGESIA

Equipment:

PCA device
Prefilled syringe or intravenous solution with pain medication
Intravenous tubing
Client identification label
18- or 20-gauge needle
Alcohol swab
Adhesive tape
Disposable gloves

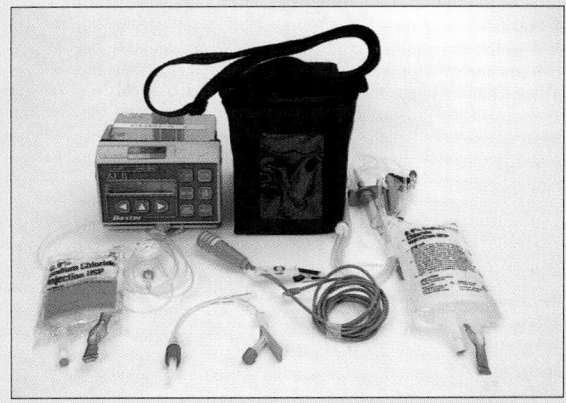

PCA device

Action	Rationale
1. Wash hands.	1. Reduces the risk of nosocomial infections and the spread of infections.
2. Check the settings on the PCA device to ensure that it is programmed to deliver specific physician-prescribed doses of pain medication at predetermined interval doses, bolus doses, a continuous infusion, or a combination of the three. In addition, check that the lockout interval has been programmed correctly.	2. Checking the programming of the PCA device ensures that the client is given the correct dose of pain medication over a specific period of time. The lockout interval prevents the client from inadvertently overdosing on pain medication; a preprogrammed delay time (usually set at 5 to 10 minutes) occurs between client-initiated doses of pain medication.
3. Check the client's identification band and call the client by name to ensure that the correct client is receiving the correct medication.	3. Minimizes the risk of a medication error.
4. Apply gloves.	4. Potential contact with blood can occur when initiating PCA.
5. Assess the patency of the existing IV line.	5. The IV line must be patent for pain medication to reach the venous circulation.
6. Attach an 18- or a 20-gauge needle to the intravenous tubing connected to the PCA device.	6. PCA-delivered medication is usually administered in a piggyback fashion through an existing IV line.
7. Wipe the injection port of the IV line with the alcohol swab.	7. Alcohol is a topical antiseptic that minimizes entry of surface microorganisms during needle insertion.
8. Insert the needle into the injection port nearest the IV insertion site.	8. PCA solution can enter the main IV line.
9. Secure the connection with a piece of adhesive tape.	9. Prevents dislodging of the needle from the IV tubing.
10. Discard the gloves and supplies in an appropriate container.	10. Reduces the transmission of infection.
11. Turn on PCA device.	11. Ensures that PCA device is working properly.
12. Demonstrate the use of the PCA device to the client.	12. Repeating instructions reinforces learning.
13. Wash hands.	13. Reduces the transmission of infection.
14. Document the initiation of PCA in the client's medical record.	14. Timely documentation prevents error and enhances communication among clinicians.

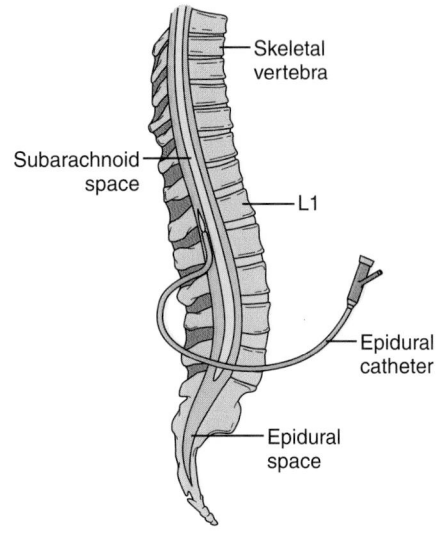

Skeletal
vertebra

Subarachnoid
space

L1

Epidural
catheter

Epidural
space

❧ **Figure 26–9**
Spinal analgesia.

clients with epidural catheters require monitoring of their vital signs.

Evaluation

An evaluation of the effectiveness of a pain management plan involves ongoing assessment of the pain complaint. The AHCPR pain management guidelines (Acute Pain Guideline Panel, 1992; Jacox *et al.*, 1994) recommend that frequent evaluations of the client's pain be done, using a simple measurement tool. Clients' self-reporting of pain intensity using a numerical rating scale is a simple and effective way to determine changes in their levels of pain, as well as to evaluate the effectiveness of pain management plans.

Ongoing evaluation should be done at regular intervals, depending on the nature of the pain; with each new report of pain; and at a suitable time interval after an analgesic intervention (for example, 1 hour after the administration of an oral analgesic).

Summary

All human beings, at various points in their development, experience alterations in rest and comfort. These alterations can occur as part of the normal growth and development processes or as a result of some type of pathophysiological process. Nurses are in a unique position to assess clients for alterations in rest and comfort. Numerous pharmacological and nonpharmacological interventions can be used to enhance an individual's ability to rest and to be comfortable.

CHAPTER HIGHLIGHTS
✦

✦ Sleep is an essential component of health and affects the well-being and quality of life of an individual.

✦ Sleep is divided into two distinct stages: NREM and REM.

✦ The amount of sleep that individuals require varies a great deal. In addition, distinct changes occur in the amount of sleep required during different developmental stages.

✦ Numerous factors can enhance or detract from an individual's ability to sleep and affect the amount of time an individual spends sleeping, including illness, drugs, activity, diet, stress, and the environment.

✦ Common sleep disorders include insomnia, narcolepsy, sleep apnea, and sleep deprivation.

✦ An accurate assessment of an individual's sleep-wake cycle and the adequacy of an individual's sleep must rely on self-reporting.

✦ When a nurse develops a plan of care for a client with a sleep pattern disturbance, consideration should be given to specific interventions related to bedtime rituals, environmental preparation, pharmacological management, scheduling client care activities, and the promotion of rest and relaxation.

✦ Pain is a universal human experience that is felt by the individual.

✦ Neonates and infants do experience pain.

✦ Pain assessment is the cornerstone of effective pain management.

✦ The initial pain history should focus on having the client provide the following information: a description of the pain, the location of the pain, the severity of the pain, aggravating and relieving factors, previous pain treatments and effectiveness, and any associated symptoms.

✦ Pharmacological and nonpharmacological interventions should be part of a pain management plan.

✦ The pharmacological agents used to manage acute and chronic pain can be categorized into nonopioid, opioid, and adjuvant analgesics.

✦ Doses of pain medication should be adjusted to provide optimal analgesia with minimal side effects.

✦ Pain medications should be administered around the clock or on a regular schedule.

✦ Clients need to be reassessed at appropriate intervals to determine the effectiveness of the pain management plan.

Study Questions

1. The stage of sleep that is necessary for psychological restoration and for learning and memory to occur is

   a. stage 2 NREM
   b. stage 3 NREM
   c. stage 4 NREM
   d. REM

2. A client reports that he is having difficulty falling asleep, is experiencing frequent awakenings, and feels that his sleep is totally inadequate. The sleep disorder the client is describing is

   a. narcolepsy
   b. insomnia
   c. sleep apnea
   d. sleep deprivation

3. Nursing interventions for a client with a sleep pattern disturbance include all of the following *except*

   a. maintaining bedtime rituals
   b. drinking a glass of warm milk
   c. increasing environmental stimuli
   d. reading a book

4. If a client is on 10 mg of intravenous morphine every 4 hours, what would be the 24-hour dose of hydromorphone to provide the same analgesic effect?

   a. 1.5 mg
   b. 3 mg
   c. 7.5 mg
   d. 9 mg

5. Nurses who are caring for clients with cancer who are taking opioids on a chronic basis need to assess them for all of the following *except*

   a. tolerance
   b. constipation
   c. sedation
   d. addiction

Critical Thinking Exercises

1. Ms. S. is an 80-year-old woman on the first day after hip replacement surgery. Discuss the effects of her age and surgery on your assessment of her pain.

2. Mr. W. is a 52-year-old man admitted to an eight-bed intensive care unit following coronary artery bypass grafting. Develop a plan of care to address the diagnosis of "sleep deprivation" for Mr. W.

References

Acute Pain Management Guideline Panel. (1992). *Acute pain management: Operative or medical procedures and trauma.* Clinical Practice Guideline (AHCPR Publication No. 92-0032). Rockville, MD: Agency for Health Care Policy and Research, Public Health Service, U.S. Department of Health and Human Services.

American Pain Society. (1992). *Principles of analgesic use in the treatment of acute pain and cancer pain.* Skokie, IL: American Pain Society.

American Sleep Disorders Association. (1990). *The international classification of sleep disorders: Diagnostic and coding manual.* Lawrence, KS: Allen Press.

Anand, K. J. S., & Hickey, P. R. (1987). Pain and its effects in the human neonate and fetus. *New England Journal of Medicine, 317,* 1321–1347.

Becker, P. M., & Jamieson, A. O. (1992). Common sleep disorders in the elderly: Diagnosis and treatment. *Geriatrics, 47,* 41–52.

Beyer, J. E. (1984). *The Oucher: A user's manual and technical report.* Charlottesville, VA: University of Virginia Alumni Patient Foundation.

Billard, M. (1985). Narcolepsy. *Annals of Clinical Research, 17,* 220–226.

Browne, R. (1996). Accepting the challenges of pain management. *British Journal of Nursing Care, 5*(9), 552–555.

Dull, W. B., & Stratton, M. (1991). Current approaches to chronic cancer pain in older adults. *Geriatrics, 46,* 47–52.

Eland, J. M. (1981). Minimizing pain associated with prekindergarten intramuscular injections. *Issues in Comprehensive Pediatric Nursing, 5,* 361–372.

Fields, H. L. (1987). *Pain: Mechanisms and management.* New York: McGraw-Hill.

Fitzgerald, M., & Anand, K. J. S. (1993). Developmental neuroanatomy and neurophysiology of pain. In N. L. Schecter, C. B. Berde, & M. Yaster (Eds.), *Pain in infants, children, and adolescents* (pp. 11–31). Baltimore: Williams & Wilkins.

Foley, K. M. (1985). The treatment of cancer pain. *New England Journal of Medicine, 313,* 84–95.

Foreman, M. D., & Wykle, M. (1995). Nursing standard-of-practice protocol: Sleep disturbances in elderly patients. *Geriatric Nursing, 16*(5), 238–243.

Franck, L. S., & Gregory, G. A. (1993). Clinical evaluation and treatment of infant pain in the neonatal intensive care unit. In N. L. Schecter, C. B. Berde, & M. Yaster (Eds.), *Pain in infants, children and adolescents* (pp. 519–535). Baltimore: Williams & Wilkins.

Graffam, S., & Johnson, A. (1987). A comparison of two relaxation strategies for the relief of pain and its distress. *Journal of Pain and Symptom Management, 2*(4), 229–231.

Guyton, A. C. (1991). States of brain activity—sleep; brain waves; epilepsy; psychoses. In A. C. Guyton, *Textbook of medical physiology* (8th ed., pp. 659–666). Philadelphia: W. B. Saunders.

Harkins, S. W., Kwentus, J., & Price, D. D. (1984). Pain in the elderly. In C. Benedetti (Ed.), *Advances in pain research and therapy* (Vol. 7). New York: Raven Press.

Hester, N. O. (1979). The preoperational child's reaction to immunization. *Nursing Research, 28*(4), 250–254.

Hester, N. O., & Barcus, C. S. (1986). Assessment and management of pain in children. *Pediatric Nursing Update, 1,* 1–8.

Hodgson, L. A. (1991). Why do we need sleep? Relating theory to nursing practice. *Journal of Advanced Nursing, 16,* 1503–1510.

Hoffert, M. (1986). The gate control theory revisited. *Journal of Pain and Symptom Management, 1,* 39–41.

International Association for the Study of Pain. (1979). Pain terms: A list with definitions and notes on usage. *Pain, 6,* 249–252.

Jacox, A., Carr, D. G., Payne, R., *et al.* (1994). *Management of cancer pain.* Clinical Practice Guideline No. 9 (AHCPR Publication No. 94-0592). Rockville, MD:

Agency for Health Care Policy and Research, Public Health Service, U.S. Department of Health and Human Services.

Jensen, D. P., & Herr, K. A. (1993). Sleeplessness. *Nursing Clinics of North America, 28*(2), 385–405.

Johnston, C., & Stevens, B. (1992). Pain in infants. In J. H. Watt-Watson & M. I. Donovan (Eds.), *Pain management: Nursing perspective* (pp. 203–235). St. Louis: C. V. Mosby.

Kehlet, H. (1982). The endocrine-metabolic response to postoperative pain. *Acta Anaesthesiologica Scandinavica, 74*(Suppl.), 173–175.

Kehlet, H., Brandt, M. R., & Rem, J. (1980). Role of neurogenic stimuli in mediating the endocrine-metabolic response to surgery. *Journal of Parenteral & Enteral Nutrition, 4,* 152–156.

Lee, K. A. (1991). Nursing care of patients with disturbances in arousal and sleep patterns. In M. C. Patrick, S. L. Woods, R. F. Craven, J. S. Rokosky, & P. M. Bruno (Eds.), *Medical-surgical nursing—Pathophysiological concepts* (2nd ed., pp. 79–91). Philadelphia: J. B. Lippincott.

Leech-Hofland, S. (1992). Elder beliefs: Blocks to pain management. *Journal of Gerontological Nursing, 18,* 19–24.

Manfredi, R. L., Vgontzas, A., & Kales, A. (1989). An update on sleep disorders. *Bulletin of the Menninger Clinics, 53,* 250–273.

Marshall, B. E., & Wycke, M. Q., Jr. (1972). Hypoxemia during and after anesthesia. *Anesthesiology, 37,* 178–209.

McCaffery, M. (1979). *Nursing management of the patient with pain.* Philadelphia: J. B. Lippincott.

Melzack, R., & Wall, P. D. (1965). Pain mechanisms: A new theory. *Science, 150,* 971–977.

Melzack, R., & Wall, P. D. (1983). *The challenge of pain.* New York: Basic Books.

Miaskowski, C. (1993a). Current concepts in the assessment and management of acute pain. *MEDSURG Nursing, 2*(1), 28–33.

Miaskowski, C. (1993b). Current concepts in the assessment and management of cancer-related pain. *MEDSURG Nursing, 2*(2), 113–118.

Page, M. A. (1991). Alteration in comfort: Sleep pattern disturbance. In J. C. McNally, E. T. Somerville, C. Miaskowski, & M. Rostad (Eds.), *Guidelines for oncology nursing practice* (2nd ed., pp. 148–154). Philadelphia: W. B. Saunders.

Patt, R. B. (1993). Classification of cancer pain and cancer pain syndromes. In R. B. Patt (Ed.), *Cancer pain* (pp. 3–22). Philadelphia: J. B. Lippincott.

Puntillo, K., & Tesler, M. D. (1993). Pain. In V. Carrieri-Kohlman, A. M. Lindsey, & C. M. West (Eds.), *Pathophysiological phenomenon in nursing: Human responses to illness* (2nd ed., pp. 303–339). Philadelphia: W. B. Saunders.

Richards, K. C. (1996). Sleep promotion. *Critical Care Nursing Clinics of North America, 8*(1), 39–52.

Robinson, C. R. (1993). Impaired sleep. In V. Carrieri-Kohlman, A. M. Lindsey, & C. M. West (Eds.), *Pathophysiological phenomenon in nursing: Human responses to illness* (2nd ed.). Philadelphia: W. B. Saunders. pp. 490–528.

Savedra, M. C., Tesler, M. D., Holzemer, W. L., & Ward, J. A. (1989). *Adolescent pediatric pain tool (APPT) preliminary user's manual.* San Francisco: University of California.

Sleep Disorders Classification Committee, Association of Sleep Disorders Centers. (1979). Diagnostic classification of sleep and arousal disorders. *Sleep, 2,* 137–150.

Spiegel, D., & Bloom, J. R. (1983). Group therapy and hypnosis reduce metastatic breast carcinoma pain. *Psychosomatic Medicine, 45*(4), 333–339.

Sternbach, R. A. (1990). Acute versus chronic pain. In R. Melzack & P. Wall (Eds.), *Textbook of pain* (pp. 242–246). New York: Churchill Livingstone.

Sydow, F. W. (1989). The influence of anesthesia and postoperative analgesic management on lung function. *Acta Chiurgica Scandinavica, 550*(Suppl.), 159–165.

Syrjala, K. L., Cummings, C., & Donaldson, G. W. (1992). Hypnosis or cognitive behavioral training for reduction of pain and nausea during cancer treatment: A controlled clinical trial. *Pain, 48*(2), 137–146.

Turpin, G. (1986). Psychophysiology of sleep. *Nursing, 3*(9), 313–320.

Vasudevan, S., Hegmann, K., Moore, A., & Cerletty, S. (1992). Physical methods of pain management. In P. P. Raj (Ed.), *Practical management of pain* (2nd ed., pp. 669–679). Baltimore: Mosby-Year Book.

Wasylak, T. J., Abbott, F. V., English, M. J., & Jeans, M. E. (1990). Reduction of postoperative morbidity following patient controlled morphine. *Canadian Journal of Anaesthesia, 37,* 726–731.

Wattwill, M. (1989). Postoperative pain relief and gastrointestinal motility. *Acta Chiurgica Scandinavica, 550* (Suppl.), 140–145.

Whitney, S. L. (1989). Physical agents: Heat and cold modalities. In R. Scully & M. Barnes (Eds.), *Physical therapy* (pp. 844–875). Philadelphia: J. B. Lippincott.

Bibliography

Ancoli-Israel, S. (1996). Sleep problems in older adults: Putting myths to bed. Geriatrics *52*(1), 20–30.

Chokroverty, S. (1996). Sleep and degenerative neurological disorders. Neurologic Clinics *14*(4), 807–826.

Magrum, L. C., Bentzen, C., & Landmark, S. (1996). Pain management in the home. *Seminars in Oncology Nursing, 12*(3), 202–218.

Marchiondo, K., & Thompson, A. (1996). Pain management in sickle cell disease. *Medsurg Nursing, 5*(1), 29–33.

Parkinson, D. (1994). Overcoming sleep problems in infants and toddlers. *Professional Care of Mother and Child, 4*(7), 215–217.

Simpson, T., Lee, E. R., & Cameron, C. (1996). Patient's perceptions of environmental factors that disturb sleep after cardiac surgery. *American Journal of Critical Care, 5*(3), 173–181.

NUTRITION

KIM SHERER, RN, MN

KEY TERMS

✦

absorption
anabolism
anorexia nervosa
anthropometric
  measurements
basal metabolic rate
bulimia
catabolism
daily reference values
dietitian
dysphagia
enteral nutrition

kilocalorie
malnutrition
metabolism
NPO (nothing by
  mouth)
nutrients
peristalsis
RDAs (recommended
  dietary allowances)
reference daily intakes
total parenteral
  nutrition

LEARNING OBJECTIVES

✦

After studying this chapter you should be able to

✦ Describe the roles, sources, and deficiencies
  of the six classes of nutrients

✦ Describe the processes of digestion, absorption, metabolism, anabolism, and catabolism

✦ Describe how nurses can help clients plan
  healthy diets

✦ Identify factors affecting nutrition

✦ Describe common problems in nutrition and
  how nursing care can assist in resolving these
  problems

✦ Apply the nursing process to meet various nutritional needs of clients

urses must have a basic understanding of nutrition to educate and care for healthy clients as well as clients with nutritional needs or problems. This chapter prepares nurses to provide optimal nutritional care by presenting a general review of basic nutrition and factors that affect nutrition. Applying the nursing process to meet the nutritional needs of clients is emphasized. After reading this chapter, the student will have acquired the necessary knowledge to assess nutrient intake, develop nutritional nursing diagnoses, make goals, suggest methods to improve food choices, and evaluate whether these suggestions were effective or ineffective.

Nutrition, a basic need that must be met for clients to live, is becoming more prominent in the health care field daily. What person has not heard about or read about the effects that nutrition can have on health? People are bombarded with nutritional information regarding cholesterol and how to lower it, saturated fat intake and how this promotes cardiac disease, and antioxidants and how they affect the development of cancer. In other words, nutrition can be a two-edged sword: it can either improve or adversely affect the health status of clients. Thus, nurses must be prepared to assist clients in meeting nutritional needs in a healthy, safe manner.

✦ Nutrients

The process of nutrition utilizes food for energy, growth, development, and maintenance of the human body. Nutrients, obtained from foods, must be supplied in adequate amounts for this process to be performed effectively. The six classes of nutrients are (1) carbohydrates, (2) fats/lipids, (3) proteins, (4) vitamins, (5) minerals, and (6) water.

Carbohydrates

Carbohydrates are the preferred source of energy for the body. Monosaccharides, disaccharides, and polysaccharides are classified as carbohydrates. Monosaccharides, also called simple sugars, can be absorbed without further digestion. Glucose is the major monosaccharide because it is the carbohydrate that provides energy to the body's cells. Other monosaccharides are galactose and fructose.

Disaccharides are two simple sugars joined together. Sucrose and lactose are disaccharides.

Polysaccharides are complex carbohydrates composed of numerous (over 1500) monosaccharides joined together. Examples of polysaccharides are starch, cellulose, and pectin. Starches, also called complex carbohydrates, are digestible and provide energy. Cellulose and pectin are types of fiber, which the body does not digest; no energy or kilocalories are produced. Cellulose increases stool bulk, which maintains digestive muscle tone, thereby decreasing chance of diverticulosis (bulging of the gastrointestinal [GI] tract into pouches). Pectin has gel-forming abilities and can bind bile acids and lower cholesterol levels (Bell *et al.*, 1991).

Functions

The major functions of carbohydrates include

1. Providing a source of energy. The body uses carbohydrates like a car uses gas. Carbohydrates are the fuel that runs the body, providing 4 kcal/g. The body's cells prefer glucose for cellular energy.
2. Promoting normal fat metabolism. Carbohydrates, when eaten in sufficient quantities, facilitate proper fat metabolism. Carbohydrates are required by the body to metabolize fats. If carbohydrate intake is low, fats will be incompletely metabolized, producing ketone bodies, which can be harmful to the body.
3. Sparing protein. With adequate carbohydrate intake, protein can be allowed to do its job of building and repairing tissues. If carbohydrate intake is inadequate, protein will be used as fuel to provide energy.
4. Enhancing lower GI functioning. Some complex carbohydrates provide fiber, which prevents constipation.

Sources

Milk, grains, fruits, and vegetables supply the major amount of dietary carbohydrates. Glucose is found in grapes, oranges, dates, corn, and carrots. Honey and fruits provide fructose. The most abundant form of sucrose is granulated table sugar. It is also found in molasses, apricots, peaches, plums, honeydew, cantaloupe, peas, and corn. Lactose is mainly found in milk. Starch is supplied by grain products such as wheat, corn, oats, rye, and barley. Potatoes, pasta, beets, carrots, and peas are also excellent starch sources. Cellulose (fiber) is found in bran, apples, beans, and cabbage. Fruits such as apples, citrus fruits, and strawberries contain pectin.

Deficiency

An insufficient amount of fiber can lead to constipation and possible colon cancer. Consuming fiber and cruciferous vegetables (*e.g.*, broccoli, cauliflower) can decrease the risk of colon cancer.

Inadequate carbohydrate intake has metabolic consequences: either energy intake will be too low, leading to body fat and muscles being used for energy, or too much fat will be consumed, possibly causing heart disease or other chronic diseases.

Fats/Lipids

Fats are an essential nutrient for healthy physical functioning and should not be totally eliminated from the diet. Clients mistakenly assume that because fat provides twice the amount of kilocalories as protein or carbohydrates, fats are forbidden. Linoleic acid, the only essential fatty acid, must be supplied in the diet because the body cannot make this fat. Thus, if fat is not consumed, linoleic acid deficiency would develop. Some authorities classify arachidonic and linolenic acids as essential fatty acids, but children and adults can make these fatty acids if sufficient quantities of linoleic acid are present in the body. Nonessential fatty acids can be manufactured by the body and include lecithin and omega 3.

Inside the body, fats exist as triglycerides or compound lipids. A compound lipid comprises a lipid and another substance such as protein (lipoproteins) or phosphate (phospholipids). Lipoproteins have been implicated in cardiac disease and strokes. Low-density lipoproteins (LDLs) are considered "bad," because high levels of LDL, the main transporter of cholesterol, increase the incidence of heart disease and strokes. High-density lipoproteins (HDLs) are classified as "good," because HDL tends to lower the cholesterol level by transporting cholesterol to the liver, where it is excreted as bile salts. An easy way to remember this is to think of the following phrase: clients want their *L*DL level to be *l*ow; if it is not low they will feel *l*ousy. Conversely, clients want their *H*DL level *h*igh to feel *h*ealthy.

There are several classifications of fats, based on their degree of saturation: saturated (hydrogen is attached to all carbon rings), monounsaturated (one carbon ring is not attached to hydrogen [*i.e.*, one double bond]), and polyunsaturated (many carbon rings are not attached to hydrogen [*i.e.*, many double bonds]). Most saturated fats are solid at room temperature, while monounsaturated and polyunsaturated fats are liquid at room temperature. High saturated fat intake has been linked to heart disease, strokes, and high cholesterol levels.

Cholesterol is another type of lipid. It is made by the body as well as ingested and is used to make hormones and bile.

Functions

The functions of fats include

1. Providing a concentrated source of energy and a stored form of energy. Fats furnish 9 kcal/g and form adipose tissue.
2. Sparing protein. With adequate fat intake, proteins can be spared to build and repair tissues rather than be used to provide energy.
3. Improving satiety (feeling of fullness) and palatability. Fats delay gastric emptying, inhibiting hunger and promoting a sense of satiety. Fats also add flavor to food, which enhances palatability.
4. Protecting internal organs. Adipose tissue provides a cushion for internal organs.
5. Maintaining body temperature. Subcutaneous fat acts as an insulator to preserve body heat.
6. Enhancing absorption of fat-soluble vitamins. Fats facilitate absorption of vitamins A, D, E, and K.
7. Providing the essential fatty acid.

Sources

Saturated fat is supplied by beef, luncheon meats, hard yellow cheeses, and butter; oils that contain saturated fat are palm and coconut. Monounsaturated fats are found in duck, goose, eggs, and olive and peanut oils. Polyunsaturated fats and linoleic acid are provided by safflower, corn, and sunflower oils. Cholesterol is only found in animal products, with the highest concentrations in egg yolks, liver, and organ meats.

Deficiency

If the client's intake of fat is inadequate, then the nurse may observe a thin appearance, sensitivity to cold temperatures, skin lesions, increased chance of infection, and amenorrhea in women. Continued inadequate fat intake could also lead to secondary fat-soluble vitamin deficiencies. Although most clients are not likely to experience a fat deficiency, chronically ill clients with a prolonged decreased food intake are most prone.

Conversely, diets high in fat have been linked to breast and colon cancer. Willet and associates (1990) found that colon cancer is strongly associated with a high intake of red meat and animal fat. Controversy still surrounds this issue, but encouraging clients to consume low-fat meats such as chicken and fish and to decrease, but not eliminate, consumption of high-fat meats is prudent advice.

Proteins

Protein is the second most plentiful substance in the body. (Water is the most plentiful.) Proteins are made from amino acids, which are classified as either essential or nonessential. The basic difference is that essential amino acids (EAAs) are required in the diet from foods because the body cannot manufacture these amino acids, and the nonessential amino acids are not required in the diet from foods because the body can produce them.

When a food contains adequate amounts of EAAs to support growth in the body, it is said to have high-quality proteins, also known as proteins of high biological value or complete proteins. Eggs, dairy products, meat, fish, and poultry are foods of high biological value, containing high-quality proteins. As one can see, animal products contain high-quality proteins. Foods that do not contain the EAAs in sufficient amounts are called lower-quality proteins or incomplete proteins. Example of these foods include legumes, nuts, and grains. However, incomplete proteins can be combined in a meal to complement one another and meet nutritional protein needs.

Functions

The major functions of protein include

1. Building and repairing body tissues. Protein is a component of all body cells.

2. Regulating fluid balance. Proteins such as albumin attract water, holding this fluid in the blood vessels.

3. Producing antibodies. Protein is needed to manufacture antibodies.

4. Providing energy. Protein supplies the body with 4 kcal/g.

5. Maintaining acid-base balance. Plasma proteins act as buffers to maintain the body's blood pH at 7.4.

6. Producing enzymes and hormones. Proteins are constituents of many enzymes and hormones in the body.

Sources

Meats (*e.g.,* chicken, beef, and pork) and dairy products (*e.g.,* milk, cottage cheese, and cheeses) provide most of the protein in US diets. Cereal products such as bread, cereal, rice, pasta, and dried beans can also contribute significantly to protein intake. Fruits and vegetables provide little, if any, protein.

Deficiency

Some clients are more prone to protein deficiency. These include clients who are elderly, homeless, unable to prepare nutritious meals, anorexic, on low incomes, strict vegetarians, uneducated about nutritional information, unwise shoppers, chronically ill and hospitalized, or have large, open draining wounds. Protein-deficient clients experience increased chance for infections, increased risk for pressure ulcers, and increased time for healing, resulting in a slower recovery period.

When clients have protein deficiency, it can cause protein-energy malnutrition (PEM). Kwashiorkor and marasmus are two forms of PEM. Kwashiorkor is most common in acute, severe deficiency, whereas, marasmus is more common in chronic long-term deficiency. There can be some overlap too.

Kwashiorkor primarily occurs in third world countries when a child is weaned from breast milk. Kwashiorkor is seen when the child receives adequate kilocalories but not enough high-quality protein. Aggressive treatment is indicated and may be in the form of enteral or parenteral feedings.

When both protein and kilocalories are deficient, marasmus develops, characterized by severe wasting of fat and muscle tissue. Slow increase of protein and kilocaloric intake is the preferred treatment.

The major physical difference between kwashiorkor and marasmus is edema. When protein (albumin) is severely low, as in kwashiorkor, fluid is not held in the blood vessels and leaks out into the tissue, causing edema. Thus, edema is seen with kwashiorkor (usually the feet and legs) but not with marasmus. The nurse can use this physical finding to distinguish between the two diseases.

Vitamins

Vitamins are organic substances found in foods that the body must have to function normally but that do not provide energy (kilocalories). Only protein, carbohydrates, and fats provide energy.

Fat-Soluble Versus Water-Soluble Vitamins

Vitamins are divided into two groups: fat-soluble and water-soluble vitamins. Vitamins A, D, K, and E are fat-soluble vitamins, whereas the B vitamins and vitamin C are water-soluble vitamins. Differences exist between these two types of vitamins. Fat-soluble vitamins can be stored in the body, so an excess of these can cause toxicities. Water-soluble vitamins are not stored in the body, and excess amounts are excreted in the urine; thus, daily intake is important. As the name indicates, fat-soluble vitamins are absorbed with fats and bile, while water-soluble vitamins are readily absorbed from the liquid intestinal contents in the small intestine.

Functions

The functions of vitamins include

1. Facilitating metabolism of proteins, fats, and carbohydrates. Vitamins such as riboflavin, pantothenic acid, and thiamine are required for proper metabolism of proteins, fats, and carbohydrates, respectively.

2. Acting as catalysts for metabolic functions. Vitamin K acts as a catalyst for facilitating blood clotting factors, especially prothrombin.

3. Promoting life and growth processes. Vitamin C produces collagen, a vital component in wound healing.

4. Maintaining and regulating body functions. Vitamin A maintains eyesight and epithelial linings.

Specific roles of vitamins are summarized in Table 27–1.

Sources

The main sources of vitamins are fruits, vegetables, grains, dairy products, and lean meats. A balanced, varied diet will supply the needed vitamins; supplements are not necessary for healthy clients. (See Table 27–1 for sources of each vitamin.)

Deficiency

Nurses need to be adept at performing physical assessment and analyzing findings, because fat-soluble and water-soluble vitamin deficiencies are more readily detected from physical assessment than from diagnostic tests. However, because fat-soluble vitamins are stored in the body, deficiencies may take months or years to develop. For ease of reading, refer to Table 27–1 for a synopsis of vitamin deficiencies. Generally, vitamin supplements are necessary to replenish the body's depleted stores.

Minerals

Minerals are inorganic elements that are subdivided into major, or macronutrients (minerals required in large amounts), and micronutrients, or trace elements (those required in small amounts). Even though

Table **27-1**

SUMMARY OF FAT-SOLUBLE AND WATER-SOLUBLE VITAMINS

VITAMIN	FUNCTIONS	SOURCES	DEFICIENCY
Fat Soluble			
Vitamin A	Maintains skin and mucous membranes, promotes eyesight	Yellow, green, or orange vegetables and fruits (*e.g.,* apricots, cantaloupes, carrots, spinach, sweet potatoes); whole milk; liver; egg yolk	Night blindness; dry, scaly skin
Vitamin D	Hardens bones and teeth, regulates serum calcium and phosphorus levels, helps body absorb calcium	Sunshine, fortified milk and cereals	Rickets (weak bones) (called osteomalacia with skeletal pain and muscle weakness in adults)
Vitamin E	Protects the integrity of normal cell membranes, prevents breakdown of red blood cells, acts as an antioxidant	Vegetable oils, margarines made with vegetable oils; whole-grain or fortified cereals; nuts; green leafy vegetables; apples; apricots; peaches	Deficiency is unlikely
Vitamin K	Involved in manufacture of prothrombin, which allows the blood to clot properly	Green leafy vegetables, cauliflower, cabbage; intestinal bacteria can also synthesize this vitamin in the body	Hemorrhage, clotting problems
Water Soluble			
Vitamin C **Ascorbic acid**	Helps to form collagen, enhances healing of wounds, increases iron absorption, acts as antioxidant	Strawberries, orange juice, grapefruit, cantaloupe, tomatoes, citrus fruits, broccoli	Scurvy, with easy bruising, bleeding gums, sore mouth, slow healing
Thiamine **Vitamin B_1**	Enhances carbohydrate metabolism	Whole or enriched grains, pork, nuts, legumes	Beriberi, with damage to the nervous and cardiovascular systems, depression, irritability, anorexia
Riboflavin **Vitamin B_2**	Enhances protein metabolism	Milk, milk products, enriched cereals, meat, fish	Cracked lips (cheilosis), scaly skin with red lesions, tongue inflammation (glossitis)
Niacin	Helps metabolize protein, carbohydrates, and fats	Meats, poultry, beef, fish, whole and enriched grains, legumes, seeds, nuts	Pellagra with the "three Ds": dermatitis, diarrhea, and depression or dementia; bilaterally reddish skin rash
Pyridoxine **Vitamin B_6**	Enhances protein metabolism, converts tryptophan to niacin, produces hemoglobin	Beef, poultry, fish, pork, legumes, nuts, green beans	Central nervous system abnormalities, convulsions, dermatitis, cheilosis, glossitis, anemia
Pantothenic acid	Enhances metabolism of carbohydrates, fats, and proteins	Legumes, whole-grain cereals, all meats	Deficiency is unlikely

Table continued on following page

Table 27–1

SUMMARY OF FAT-SOLUBLE AND WATER-SOLUBLE VITAMINS (Continued)			
Biotin	Enhances metabolism of carbohydrates, fats, and proteins	GI microflora synthesize this vitamin; liver, egg yolk	Anorexia; nausea; vomiting; glossitis; paleness; dry, scaly skin
Folate **Folacin or folic acid**	Maintains normal levels of mature red blood cells	Liver, green leafy vegetables, legumes, grapefruit, oranges, beef, fish	Megaloblastic (large fragile red blood cells) anemia, glossitis, diarrhea, poor growth
Cyanocobalamin **Vitamin B_{12}**	Helps red blood cells mature; produces myelin, a covering for nerve cells	Microorganisms can produce this vitamin in the body; meats and all animal foods	Pernicious anemia (lack of intrinsic factor) or megaloblastic anemia (lack of vitamin B_{12} intake)

trace elements are needed in smaller amounts, they are just as important for normal body function as the major minerals. See Table 27–2 for examples of macronutrients and micronutrients.

Functions

Minerals are

1. Components of hormones, cells, tissues, and bones. Calcium is a component of bone, and iron is a constituent of hemoglobin. Iodine is a part of thyroxine, a hormone that regulates basal metabolic rate.
2. Catalysts for chemical reactions. Copper stimulates production of dopamine, a neurotransmitter, and zinc is a component of 120 enzymes that the body needs for growth and physical development.
3. Enhancers of cell function. Sulfur can combine with harmful substances, rendering them harmless in the body; chromium enhances carbohydrate metabolism.

Sources

Almost all foods contain some form of minerals. A variety of foods is encouraged to obtain proper amounts of needed minerals. For a listing of foods that are high in certain minerals, see Table 27–2.

Deficiency

A deficiency of minerals can occur in chronically ill or hospitalized clients. For a summary of deficiencies, refer to Table 27–2. Mineral supplements are often needed to correct the imbalance, because increasing intake of foods that contain the mineral may not provide sufficient amounts.

Water

Water is the most important nutrient and the most abundant component in the body, representing 50 to 60% of the total adult body weight. Infants have a larger percentage (75–80%) of water content. Men have higher concentrations of water than women, because women have larger fat stores than men. (Adipose tissue contains less water than does lean muscle tissue.) Fat stores in women are usually about 25 to 30% of body weight, as compared to men's, which are only approximately 14%.

Functions

The functions of water include

1. Acting as a solvent for chemical reactions to occur. Water provides a medium for all of the body's chemical reactions.
2. Maintaining body fluid balance. Water is the principal component of fluids, secretions, and excretions within the body.
3. Transporting substances in the body. Water allows nutrients and waste products to be transported to various sites in the body.
4. Lubricating cells. Water between cells decreases friction.
5. Regulating body temperature. Water can evaporate through the skin to regulate body temperature.

Sources

Obviously, sources of water include liquids, but surprisingly, solid foods also provide water. Meats are more than half water. Other good sources are fruits and vegetables. The body itself also makes water through the process of metabolism; approximately 300 to 350 ml of water are supplied daily through metabolism.

Deficiency

A deficiency of water leads to dehydration or fluid volume deficit. Clients prone to a deficiency include those who sweat profusely; urinate large, frequent volumes; experience nausea, vomiting, hemorrhage, diar-

Table 27-2

SUMMARY OF MINERALS

MINERAL	FUNCTIONS	SOURCES	DEFICIENCY
Macronutrients			
Calcium	Component of bones and teeth; enhances muscle contractions and blood clotting	Milk and dairy products, dark green leafy vegetables, sardines, fortified orange juice	Rickets, osteoporosis (decreased bone mass), and tetany (uncontrolled muscle cramps, tremors, and convulsions)
Chloride	Major ion of extracellular fluid, regulates osmotic pressure and acid-base balance; constituent of gastric acid	Salt	Too much base in the blood (alkalosis)
Magnesium	Constituent of bones and heart muscle	Whole-grain products, nuts, beans, bananas, green leafy vegetables	Neuromuscular dysfunction (muscle spasms, convulsions, tremors, decreased reflexes), personality changes, heart irregularities
Phosphorus	Component of bones and teeth; enhances carbohydrate metabolism	Milk and dairy products, meats, whole grains, legumes, nuts	Muscle weakness, bone loss
Potassium	Conducts nerve impulses, helps muscles contract, facilitates heart contractions, regulates acid-base balance; major ion of intracellular fluid	Dried fruits, baked potato, cantaloupe, bananas, spinach, milk, steak, beans	Hypokalemia (low blood levels of potassium), anorexia, absence of bowel sounds, muscle weakness, leg cramps, heart abnormalities, even cardiac arrest
Sodium	Major ion of extracellular fluid; maintains fluid balance, regulates acid-base balance, facilitates nerve and muscle fiber impulses	Canned vegetables, soups, and meats; cheeses (especially processed); ham; pork; sausages; luncheon meat; frankfurters; soy sauce; salt	Hyponatremia (low blood levels of sodium), nausea, abdominal cramps, headache, confusion
Sulfur	Part of cartilage, tendons, bone, hair, nails; components of amino acids and vitamins; maintains acid-base balance, neutralizes toxins	All protein foods	Deficiency is unlikely
Micronutrients			
Chromium	Enhances glucose metabolism	Meats, whole-grain products	Deficiency is unlikely
Copper	Needed for red blood cell formation, produces dopamine and other neurotransmitters	Oysters, crabs, nuts, shellfish, sunflower seeds	Anemia, stunted growth, infections, mental retardation, impaired bone development
Fluoride	Deposits calcium into bone, prevents dental caries	Seafood, fluoridated water	Increased chance of dental caries

Table continued on following page

Table **27-2**

SUMMARY OF MINERALS
(Continued)

MINERAL	FUNCTIONS	SOURCES	DEFICIENCY
Iodine	Component of the thyroid hormone (thyroxine); regulates basal metabolic rate	Iodized salt, seafood	Goiter (enlarged thyroid gland, dry skin, depression), poor growth, cretinism (an infant disorder from a lack of iodine during pregnancy, which causes mental retardation and deaf mutism), stillbirths
Iron	Component of hemoglobin; helps in antibody formation	Liver, meats, egg yolk, dark green vegetables, enriched breads and cereals	Microcytic (small red blood cells) anemia, fatigue
Molybdenum	Helps produce uric acid	Legumes, whole grains, organ meats	Deficiency is unlikely
Selenium	Helps protect red blood cells, acts as an antioxidant	Seafood, liver, meats, dairy products	Heart damage, with possible heart attack
Zinc	Helps produce insulin and cell proteins; enhances normal growth, immune function, reproduction, night vision, taste and appetite	Meats, eggs, leafy vegetables, protein-rich foods	Growth failure; decreased wound healing; impaired taste; infections; dry, scaly skin with blisters containing pus

rhea, anorexia, or swallowing difficulties; and/or participate actively in sports.

A deficiency is most readily detected through physical assessment findings rather than through laboratory findings. The client may exhibit weight loss, hypotension, and on standing experience dizziness and a drop in blood pressure (orthostatic hypotension). Classic signs include poor skin turgor, dry tongue with longitudinal furrows, sunken eyes, decreased urinary output, and dry skin and mucous membranes. Fluids should be replaced either orally or intravenously.

✦ Digestion

The foods that clients eat must be broken down into useable forms. The digestive system is designed to do just that. It has three major functions: (1) to ingest food; (2) to break down carbohydrates, fats, and proteins into monosaccharides, fatty acids, and amino acids; and (3) to dispose of undigested substances. Vitamins, minerals, and water usually do not need to be digested; they are absorbed as eaten.

The GI tract extends from the mouth to the anus and comprises the mouth, pharynx, esophagus, stomach, small intestine, and large intestine (Fig. 27–1). Other organs that assist with digestion but are not in the GI tract are called accessory organs and include the salivary glands, liver, gallbladder, and pancreas.

Digestion is initiated in the mouth, with teeth chewing the food into smaller pieces and salivary glands secreting ptyalin, a starch-splitting enzyme. The mass of chewed food (bolus) is swallowed, enters the esophagus, and is carried to the stomach by gravity and peristalsis. In the stomach, the bolus is mixed with gastric juices to form a substance called chyme. This semifluid mass enters the small intestines by peristalsis. Here, the chyme is mixed with bile, pancreatic juices, and intestinal juices. The liver secretes bile, which is stored in the gallbladder and aids in fat digestion. Pancreatic juice is secreted by the pancreas to digest proteins, carbohydrates, and fats. Intestinal juices further digest carbohydrates, fats, and proteins.

Whatever has not been digested and absorbed is propelled by peristalsis into the large intestine, where water is absorbed. The resulting product (feces) is formed and stored in the large intestines until defecation.

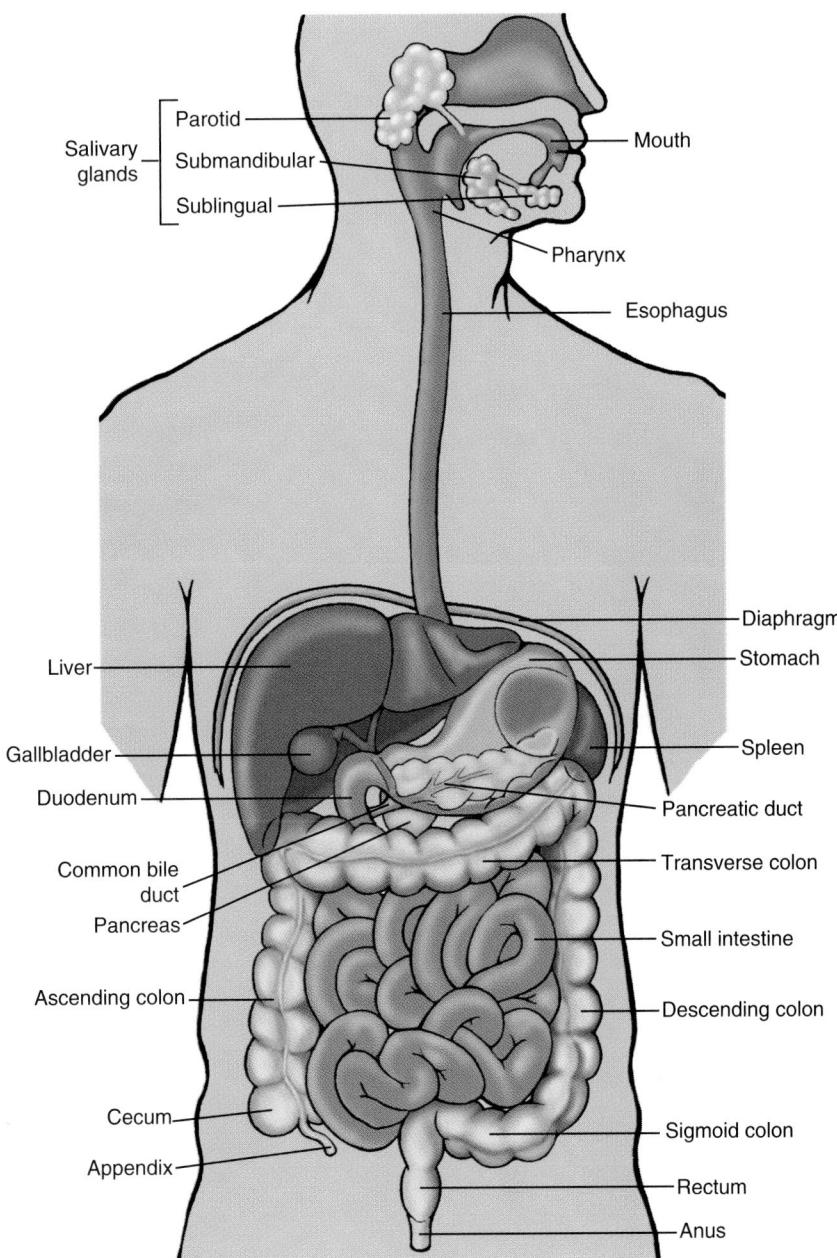

❥ Figure 27–1
The digestive system. (From Monahan, F. D.,
& Neighbors, M. [1998]. *Medical-surgical
nursing: Foundations for clinical practice*
[2nd ed.]. Philadelphia: W. B. Saunders.)

In the figure, the following labels appear:

Salivary glands
- Parotid
- Submandibular
- Sublingual

Mouth
Pharynx
Esophagus
Diaphragm
Stomach
Spleen
Pancreatic duct
Transverse colon
Small intestine
Descending colon
Sigmoid colon
Rectum
Anus

Liver
Gallbladder
Duodenum
Common bile duct
Pancreas
Ascending colon
Cecum
Appendix

✦ Absorption

Absorption is the passage of digested nutrients
through the stomach's or small intestine's wall into the
blood or lymph systems. Water, alcohol, potassium,
sodium, and glucose are absorbed in the stomach,
whereas all other nutrients, including vitamins and
minerals, are absorbed in the small intestine. Villi, fin-
gerlike projections arising from the intestinal lining,
vastly increase the small intestine's ability to absorb
nutrients.

Water-soluble nutrients enter the portal circulation,
whereas fat-soluble nutrients enter the lymphatic circulation. In portal circulation, the nutrients are transported through the portal vein directly to the liver.
Fat-soluble nutrients enter the lymphatic system, then
enter the left subclavian and left internal jugular veins,
travel to the heart, and finally enter the liver.

✦ Metabolism

Metabolism is an ongoing chemical process within
the body that converts digested nutrients into energy,
body structures, and waste (elimination). The principal
site for nutrient metabolism is the liver, which regulates the kinds and quantities of nutrients distributed

in the blood. Several functions that the liver performs include (1) maintaining blood glucose levels within a certain range; (2) storing excess glucose as glycogen or fat; (3) providing energy from metabolism of carbohydrates, fats, and proteins; (4) releasing nutrients as needed by the cells; and (5) promoting anabolism.

Anabolism

Anabolism, the conversion of simple substances into complex substances, is occurring continually in the body. This process allows the body to grow, build, and rebuild body tissue, muscles, bones, and other cells. The end products of digestion and metabolism (glucose, amino acids, fatty acids) are involved during anabolism to build the numerous substances that make up the body itself and the other substances necessary for the body to function. During growth spurts, recovery from disease or injury, or pregnancy, anabolism occurs at a faster rate than catabolism; normally, anabolism occurs at the same rate as catabolism.

Catabolism

Catabolism is the tearing down of body tissue, muscles, bones, and other cells. During illness or chronic physical stress, catabolism exceeds anabolism. If the body does not receive the nutrients and kilocalories it requires from food, the body itself will initiate processes to provide what is needed. In other words, the body takes what it needs to live from itself. Thus, body tissue, bone, muscle, and cells are destroyed to provide the needed nutrients and energy. If decreased intake is prolonged, death will occur. However, some catabolism is necessary for the body to function properly; dead, diseased, or abnormal body cells must be catabolized.

Basal Metabolic Rate

Basal metabolic rate (BMR) is the minimal amount of energy that the body requires to maintain life. A simple method to figure BMR is 10 or 11 times ideal body weight in pounds equals kilocalories for BMR daily. In general, for healthy men, 1500 to 1800 kilocalories is needed daily to maintain BMR, while healthy women need 1200 to 1350 kilocalories. Of course, several factors can alter the amount of energy used, which affects the amount of kilocalories needed. If BMR is high, kilocaloric needs will be increased; if BMR is low, kilocaloric requirements will be decreased.

Factors that lower the BMR include sleeping; aging; fasting; or decreasing food intake due to various disease processes, such as anorexia, malnourishment, hypothyroidism, or starvation. Conversely, BMR is elevated during growth spurts, pregnancy, lactation, stress, fever, and hyperthyroidism. Hyperthyroidism, in which excess thyroxine is secreted, can double the BMR. Nurses must be aware of these factors, because

kilocaloric intake will need to be adjusted accordingly for clients to regain their health.

◆ Healthy Diet

A healthy diet, consisting of 55 to 58% energy from carbohydrates, 12 to 15% energy from protein, and 30% energy from fat (10% saturated, 10% monunsaturated, and 10% polyunsaturated), provides the essential nutrients needed throughout life. Nurses should promote healthy dietary aspects and reduce unhealthy factors (see Box: Health Promotion for Nutrition).

Because clients eat foods, not nutrients, nurses must present nutrient requirements and information in a language that clients can understand. The Food Guide Pyramid, recommended dietary allowances (RDAs), and dietary guidelines are tools designed to help the patient and nurse communicate on the same level.

Food Guide Pyramid

The Food Guide Pyramid groups six broad families of foods with similar kinds of nutrients together (Fig. 27–2). Remember that this is based on like nutrients, not kilocalories or serving sizes; thus, within

HEALTH PROMOTION AND PREVENTION

HEALTH PROMOTION FOR NUTRITION

Primary Prevention: Health Promotion and Specific Protection Before Any Abnormal Condition Occurs

• Offer general nutritional teaching about the Food Guide Pyramid and Dietary Guidelines for Americans

• Offer specific instructions about how to lower fat intake and avoid problems with increased cholesterol in people at risk due to morbidity statistics

Secondary Prevention: Early Diagnosis and Prompt Treatment

• Suggest blood screening for cholesterol, LDL, and HDL levels scheduled with referrals, as needed

• Suggest the use of diet therapy, exercise, and medication, as needed, to people with an identified problem (elevated cholesterol levels)

Tertiary Prevention: Rehabilitation

• Provide active in-depth dietary planning with dietitian

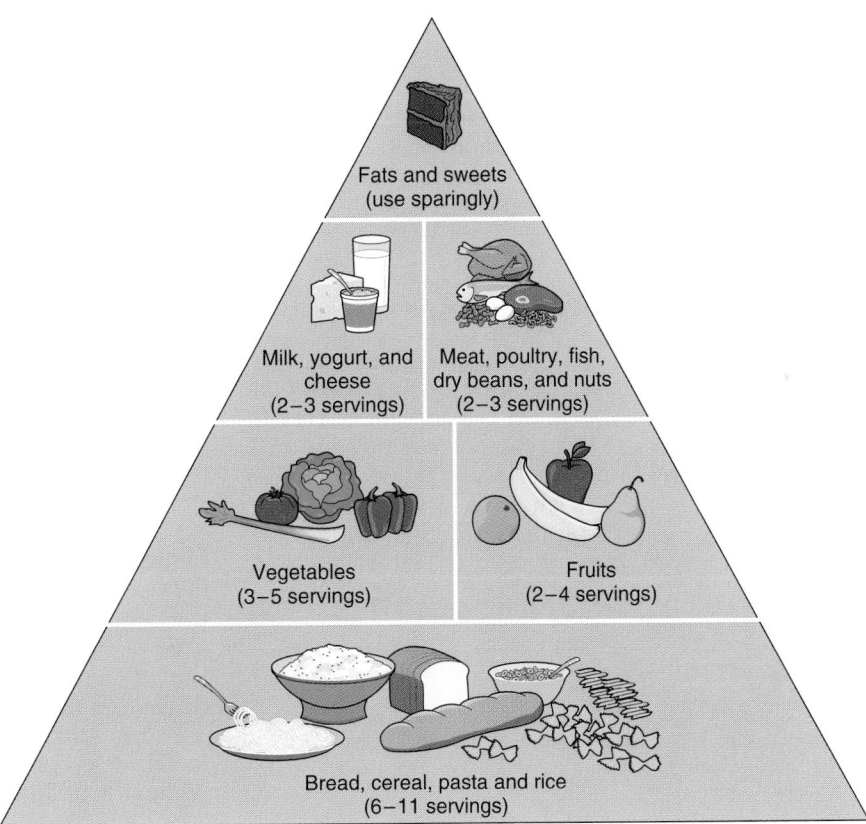

❥ **Figure 27–2**
The Food Guide Pyramid. (Adapted from the US Department of Agriculture and the US Department of Health and Human Services. Washington, DC, US Department of Agriculture and US Department of Health and Human Services, 1992.)

each food group, foods will vary widely in kilocalorie content, and serving sizes can differ.

The base of the pyramid is the bread, cereal, rice, and pasta group; 6 to 11 servings are recommended daily. Included in this group are all of the grain products (whole grain, refined, enriched, or fortified). Whole-grain products provide more fiber in comparison to enriched products. Enriched products replace the nutrients (iron, thiamin, riboflavin, and niacin) removed during processing. Fortified products, especially cereals, add nutrients not present or at a higher level than those occurring naturally.

The next level of the pyramid is divided into the vegetable and fruit groups. Three to five servings for the vegetable group and two to four servings for the fruit group are recommended. The only way for clients to consume vitamin C naturally is from eating foods in the fruit and vegetable groups; therefore, a good source of vitamin C should be eaten daily. Additionally, vitamin A–rich foods should be eaten three to four times a week.

The next pyramid level is also divided into two groups: the milk, yogurt, and cheese group and the meats, poultry, fish, dry beans and peas, eggs, and nuts group. Recommended servings for each group are two to three. The milk group is further defined according to various life stages: children 9 to 12 years of age need three or more servings, and teenagers, young adults, and pregnant or breast-feeding women need four or more servings. Calcium and vitamin D

are provided from the milk group, whereas meats supply protein and iron.

The tip of the pyramid is the fats and sweets group. These foods are to be eaten sparingly because they are kilocalorie-dense, nutrient-sparse foods that are high in fats, sugar, or alcohol.

Recommended Dietary Allowances

The **RDAs** are guidelines developed by the US government, based on findings from scientists and nutritionists, to delineate specific requirements for certain nutrients. Not all nutrients are addressed, because if people consume the recommended amounts of the listed nutrients, these other nutrients will also be furnished. Estimated safe and adequate daily dietary intake (ESADDI) for two vitamins and five minerals is included in the RDAs. If a healthy client consumes two thirds of the RDAs, the diet is adequate; below two thirds is considered poor or inadequate. The nurse must remember that this is a general guideline for healthy clients only.

Nurses must also be cognizant of the fact that there are terms used for food labeling that should not be confused with the RDAs. The **reference daily intakes** (RDIs) and the **daily reference values** (DRVs) are used to make labels more readable by the layperson. RDIs are percentages of daily values for protein, vitamins, and minerals depending on five various life cycles: infants, children under 4 years of age, children over 4 years and adults, women who are pregnant, and women who are breast-feeding. DRVs identify ranges considered healthy for carbohydrates, fats, protein, saturated fat, cholesterol, sodium, and fiber. These ranges are listed as guidelines, not as specific requirements.

Dietary Guidelines

To promote healthy food choices, the government established seven dietary guidelines for Americans (US Department of Agriculture & US Department of Health and Human Services, 1990). These guidelines are designed for healthy Americans and for people who want to decrease their chance of developing nutritional deficiencies or chronic diseases that are associated with diet, such as heart disease, certain types of cancer, high blood pressure, obesity, stroke, and atherosclerosis. The seven guidelines are

1. Eat a variety of foods from each of the food groups.
2. Maintain a healthy weight for height.
3. Choose a diet low in fat, saturated fat, and cholesterol to decrease chance of heart disease, obesity, and certain types of cancer.
4. Choose a diet with plenty of vegetables, fruits, and grain products to reduce the chance of developing chronic constipation, diverticular disease, hemorrhoids, and some cancers.
5. Use sugars only in moderation because they only furnish kilocalories; no other nutrients are provided.
6. Use table salt and other sodium only in moderation to protect against or possibly lower hypertension in sodium-sensitive individuals.
7. If one drinks alcoholic beverages, do so in moderation. One drink a day for women and no more than two drinks a day for men is considered moderate consumption. Alcohol is high in kilocalories (7 kcal/g) and low in nutrients, and its potential to cause serious health problems has been well documented.

Vegetarian Diets

Some clients choose to follow a vegetarian diet based on religious, cultural, or health beliefs, and/or other personal beliefs stemming from a desire to promote proper use of land for food production (it takes more land and grain to produce meat or animal food than it does to produce vegetarian food).

A vegetarian diet can be healthy, but careful planning is essential. Depending on the types of foods included in the diet, there are four types of vegetarian diets: (1) vegan or strict, (2) lactovegetarian, (3) ovolactovegetarian, and (4) ovovegetarian (Table 27–3).

A vegan, or strict, vegetarian diet eliminates all foods of animal origin, including meat, milk, cheese, eggs, and butter. Therefore, soups need to be made with vegetable-based stock, foods should not be cooked with lard or butter, and gelatin is avoided

because it is an animal product. However, all vegetables, fruits, and grains may be eaten. Because all animal products are eliminated, combinations of plant foods that provide the essential amounts of amino acids must be paramount. To provide these necessary proteins, nurses should encourage clients to combine the following groups: (1) grains and legumes (*e.g.*, rice and black-eyed peas, cornbread and brown beans, or corn tortillas and beans); (2) legumes and nuts or seeds (*e.g.*, peanuts and sunflower seed trail mix, stir fried tofu with cashews, or seed bread with split-pea soup); (3) grains and nuts or seeds (*e.g.*, rice and sesame seeds, rice and slivered almonds, or a peanut butter sandwich); and (4) vegetables and legumes, grains, corn, or potatoes (*e.g.*, stir-fried vegetables over brown rice, steamed vegetables with kidney beans, or corn and potato casserole).

To ensure an adequate intake of vitamin B_{12} (which only comes from animal products) encourage the use of foods fortified with vitamin B_{12} (*e.g.*, breakfast cereals, some soy milk, some fermented soy products) or B_{12} supplements. A vitamin B_{12} deficiency may lead to anemia, resulting in serious and irreversible damage to the central nervous system (Dwyer, 1991).

In a lactovegetarian diet, in addition to plant foods, dairy products can be eaten. However, meat, poultry, fish, and eggs are eliminated. The addition of

		Table 27–3
VEGETARIAN DIETS		
TYPE	**FOODS ALLOWED**	**FOODS OMITTED**
Vegan/strict	Vegetables Fruits Grains	Meats Poultry Fish Milk Dairy products Cheese Butter Eggs
Lactovegetarian	Vegetables Fruits Grains Dairy products Milk	Meat Poultry Fish Eggs
Ovolactovegetarian	Vegetables Fruits Grains Dairy products Milk Eggs	Meat Poultry Fish
Ovovegetarian	Vegetables Fruits Grains Eggs	Meat Poultry Fish Milk Dairy products

dairy products enhances the protein content of the diet. A lactovegetarian can use the combinations listed under strict vegetarian diet but can also include the following combinations: grains and milk products, such as cottage-cheese salad with sunflower seeds; milk in legume soups; or beans in cheese sauce.

Ovolactovegetarian diet is the same as the lactovegetarian diet, but eggs are added. Meat, poultry, and fish are excluded. All essential nutrients can be provided by this diet in sufficient amounts with not as much cautious planning as is required in the strict vegetarian diet.

When meat, poultry, fish, and dairy products are eliminated from the diet and only plant foods and eggs are eaten, this diet is called the ovovegetarian diet. Eggs provide a source of protein and vitamin B_{12}.

Factors Affecting Nutrition

Factors affecting nutritional status can be categorized into physiological, psychological, sociological, and economical aspects.

Physiological Factors

Physiological conditions that affect nutritional status include activity level, disease states, ability to purchase and prepare foods, and procedures or treatments performed. Depending on activity level, nutrients and kilocalories may need to be increased, as when activity level is high, or decreased, as when a client is sedentary. Smoking can be classified as a physiological factor. Physiologically, smoking increases most nutrient requirements, especially for vitamin C, which often is doubled (Schectman et al., 1991). Disease states and procedures or treatments performed have an impact on intake, digestion, absorption, metabolism, and excretion of nutrients.

Some physiological conditions may cause a decrease in certain nutrients, whereas some may cause an increase. Kidney diseases can decrease the requirements for protein because protein is excreted by the kidneys. However, numerous physical conditions increase nutrient requirements. Physical illnesses usually increase nutrient requirements at a time when the client feels least like eating. This is especially evident in any illness that involves the GI tract.

Physical disorders can strike all along the GI tract, resulting in decreased nutrient intake, impaired absorption, altered transportation, or improper utilization. Mouth ulcerations can cause a decrease in intake because of the pain associated with eating. Diarrhea can cause decreased absorption because the nutrients are propelled too quickly from the GI tract. In gallbladder disease, the gallbladder does not function properly; the bile, which is needed for fat digestion, is insufficient or ineffective. Thus, when the client eats fatty foods, pain occurs. Additionally, fat-soluble vita-

mins need fat and bile to be transported through the small intestines into the lymph system; fat-soluble vitamin deficiencies may develop. Some people do not have the enzyme to break down the lactose in milk, a condition called lactose intolerance. Instead of the body utilizing this nutrient, the lactose is fermented in the intestines, causing bloating and diarrhea.

Other specific physical conditions that affect nutritional needs and status are discussed separately.

Alcohol

Excessive alcohol consumption can affect every nutrient in the body, because alcohol dependency accelerates nutrient metabolism, increasing nutrient requirements. However, most alcohol-dependent patients would rather drink than eat.

Alcohol requires no digestion but is rapidly absorbed in the stomach; however, all of the alcohol drunk must be metabolized by the liver. Therefore, metabolism, transport, and utilization of every nutrient can be adversely affected. Uric acid and fat are elevated in the blood; fat accumulates in the liver; low blood sugar develops; appetite is poor; and the need for vitamins, especially the B complex vitamins, and minerals is increased. All of these factors combined can lead to malnutrition. A well-balanced diet, high in B complex vitamins and complex carbohydrates, is suggested.

Two syndromes that occur in chronic alcoholism are Wernicke-Korsakoff syndrome (the symptoms of which are confusion, hallucinations, loss of memory) and night blindness, each resulting from a lack of a vital nutrient, thiamin and vitamin A, respectively. Hepatitis and cirrhosis, which further affect nutritional requirements, may also develop.

Immobility

Clients who are immobile frequently have poor appetites, which can lead to an inadequate intake and malnutrition. This poor appetite is thought to result from decreased basal metabolism and decreased activity.

Decreased activity or decreased weight bearing can cause a loss of calcium from the bones. Even though calcium is lost, it is not advisable to increase calcium intake in clients who are bedfast. For the calcium to be deposited into the bone, weight bearing must occur; otherwise, the calcium is elevated in the blood, predisposing patients to kidney stones. The best intervention is early ambulation.

If immobile clients are not turned while in bed, pressure ulcers or decubiti may develop. Malnutrition and low blood protein levels have been associated with increased risk of pressure ulcers. A well-balanced diet, high in kilocalories and high-quality protein, is suggested. When kilocaloric and protein amounts are not adequate, attempt to discover factors compromising intake and offer assistance with eating (Bergstrom et al., 1992). If oral intake is still poor, nutritional supplements or enteral feeding may be required. Vitamin C, zinc, and iron are also recommended—vitamin C and zinc for proper wound healing and iron for hemoglobin synthesis, as adequate oxygen is essential for wound healing.

Human Immunodeficiency Virus and Acquired Immunodeficiency Syndrome

The human immunodeficiency virus (HIV) destroys the body's immune system. When the virus is present in the blood, the client is diagnosed as being HIV positive. Being HIV positive does not mean that the client has acquired immunodeficiency syndrome (AIDS). AIDS is diagnosed when infections occur that normally would not because the body is unable to protect itself.

Nutritional care should begin as soon as the client has been diagnosed as being HIV positive. Promoting an adequate, balanced diet is suggested. Healthy eating habits can maintain body strength and level of functioning.

Weight loss and malnutrition are often present because of anorexia, diarrhea, malabsorption, increased metabolism, and dementia. With dementia, some clients do not remember eating, do not remember how to prepare food, do not remember how to feed themselves, or do not realize that food is to be eaten. Clients with AIDS may develop depression and apathy, which adversely affect food intake.

Depending on whether a patient is HIV positive or has AIDS, nutritional needs will differ. However, prescribing a diet high in kilocalories and high-quality protein and avoiding self-prescribed unorthodox diets is recommended (Merrill, 1994). Enteral or parenteral feedings or both may be instituted when the client has AIDS.

Cancer

Nutritional care for cancer is similar to that of HIV and AIDS. Because rapidly growing cancer cells compete with the host's body needs, the host's body is deprived of needed nutrients. Therefore, all nutrient requirements are increased. Even the treatments for cancer (radiation, surgery, and chemotherapy) cause additional nutrient requirements. A high-kilocalorie, high-protein diet is often ordered.

The challenge is getting clients who have cancer to eat even when they do not feel like eating. Thus, individualizing diets is essential. The appetite of most clients with cancer is strongest in the morning, so a filling breakfast is advised, with small meals and snacks offered during the rest of the day.

Burns

Proper nutritional care can decrease healing time and length of hospital stay for burned clients. The severity of the burn will determine energy needs. Usually a high-kilocalorie (3000), high-protein (125 g) diet

is recommended. Nutritional supplements are often needed. Fluids must be provided in amounts of 2.5 to 4 L/day. If the burn covers more than 20% of total body surface, tube feedings are necessary. Parenteral feedings may also be required.

Surgery

Certain physical disorders require surgery. A light dinner with fluids allowed until midnight is the usual procedure preoperatively. Then, after midnight, clients are to have **nothing by mouth (NPO).** In the majority of clients, undergoing an NPO diet for this short amount of time is not detrimental.

After surgery, some clients are reluctant to eat or drink because of nausea and vomiting or presence of pain. Following minor or outpatient surgery, a client's regular diet is usually resumed as soon as possible. After major or involved surgery, especially of the GI tract, intravenous feedings may be necessary to allow the bowels to rest and heal. When peristalsis returns, clear liquids are provided, advancing to a regular diet as tolerated. Generally a high-kilocalorie, high-protein diet is recommended. Supplements or enteral feedings may be needed if oral intake is prohibited or poor. Vitamin C, iron, and zinc are also necessary for wound healing. Offering foods high in these nutrients is beneficial.

Psychological Factors

Almost everybody at one time or another has used food as a reward or punishment. What mother or father has not said to a child that good behavior will be rewarded with a cookie or an ice cream cone? Because emotional significance is placed on mealtimes and foods, food has often been associated with strong feelings. Some clients think they are being punished when familiar foods are not allowed on a special diet. Others may feel isolated and depressed because they cannot eat with their families or friends. Some may feel embarrassed, angry, or dependent if they must be fed by another or eat blenderized foods. On the other hand, some foods may cause feelings of acceptance and support. Familiar foods may be comforting during an illness and may be the only food that the client wants to eat or can tolerate. Remembering these emotional responses when planning nutritional care can alert the nurse to possible problems and solutions.

When clients are depressed, lonely, apathetic, fearful, grieving, or feeling hopeless, intake usually decreases. Of course, a small minority of clients may increase intake to cope with these feelings. Stress or anxiety may cause clients to increase or decrease intake.

Sociological Factors

Mealtimes are not only to nourish the body physically but also to nourish the body socially by providing interaction and conversation with others. Eating is a social experience, as most social gatherings involve food. People living alone usually do not eat as much as people who eat with family members or others.

Personal preferences are influenced by foods served at home or during the childhood years. If meat was served at every meal, this practice will more than likely continue into adulthood. Some people will not even consider adding tofu to their diet if it was never eaten during childhood. However, others, if trying new foods was encouraged in their family, may be very willing to eat this different food item.

Economic Factors

Income can influence intake. Employment or unemployment of a client can determine whether funds are available for providing a healthy nutrient intake. If funds are low, people tend to buy foods poor in nutrition, such as old food or food in dented cans. Or, if a client does not have enough money to buy food, meals may be confiscated from garbage bins or missed completely. A fixed income can also adversely affect food purchases. If a client cannot pay the electric or gas bill, the stove cannot be used to prepare meals. Continually missing meals can lead to malnutrition from the decreased intake.

Developmental Factors

Nutrition needs vary dramatically through the life span. The nurse must pay close attention to how developmental stages can affect adequate nutritional intake. (See "Assessment," "Developmental Aspects," in "Nursing Process.")

....✦..
Common Problems in Nutrition
....

Nurses must become familiar not only with factors that affect nutrition but also with nutritional problems that may occur when caring for clients. Some common problems and required nutritional care are addressed.

Malnutrition

Malnutrition not only indicates a lack of nutrient intake but can also reflect an excessive intake. (Remember in nursing that when *malnutrition* is used, the term generally refers to when nutrients are deficient.) Malnutrition from increased intake of fat, sodium, and kilocalories can lead to heart disease, high blood pressure, and obesity, respectively. Most people consume more kilocalories than are required, leading to excess fat storage, weight gain, and, eventually, obesity. *Obesity* is the term used when body weight is 15 to 20% above ideal body weight for height, gender, and age.

Nutritional care for obesity consists of balancing kilocaloric intake with the amount of energy needed for body processes and physical activities. If the client is consuming a diet high in fat, sodium, or another nutrient, nutritional care involves teaching the client about decreasing intake of that nutrient, not eliminating it from the diet.

Conversely, a decreased food intake can result in malnutrition (a lack of kilocalories or a decrease in several or one specific nutrient) or excessive catabolism. As one becomes malnourished, appetite decreases, which worsens malnutrition. If intake can be improved and malnutrition reversed, appetite also improves.

Clients at risk for malnutrition are those who are elderly, institutionalized, homeless, or immobile; other clients at risk include those living alone or those with injury, surgery, trauma or chronic illnesses that deplete appetite (Wells, 1994).

Decreased food intake may result from psychological as well as physical needs. Physical problems such as nausea and vomiting may also contribute to a decreased food intake, increasing the likelihood of malnutrition.

Nausea and Vomiting

Nausea and vomiting are common symptoms that nurses observe in clients. Nausea and vomiting may result from emotional problems (*e.g.*, bulimia, stress), physical problems (*e.g.*, chemotherapy, infection), or a combination of both. When the vomiting center in the medulla is stimulated, vomiting (reverse peristalsis) occurs. Projectile vomiting, when the stomach contents are forcefully ejected several feet, is typically a sign of severe GI problems, such as a bowel obstruction in infants. Nausea, a subjective feeling, usually precedes vomiting. Just the thought, site, or smell of food can intensify nausea.

Nutritional care for nausea and vomiting depends on the severity of the vomiting. If severe, liquids and foods are withheld; then clear liquids or crushed ice is offered, advancing to a regular diet. Apple juice, iced tea, dry crackers, dry toast, or gelatin is usually tolerated well (Fig. 27–3). Cold foods or foods at room temperature are also suggested. Hot foods seem to aggravate nausea from the aromas emitted. Avoiding fried, greasy, spicy, or fatty foods is also recommended. Offering oral care after vomiting can increase a patient's sense of well-being. Intravenous fluids and antiemetics (medicines that decrease vomiting) may be necessary. Nausea and vomiting can lead to anorexia.

Anorexia

Anorexia is a lack of appetite with no desire to eat; oral intake is decreased. Many diseases cause anorexia. In fact, anorexia is commonly the first sign of illness. Fever, altered taste sensations, and early satiety can also intensify anorexia. Disorders in the GI tract

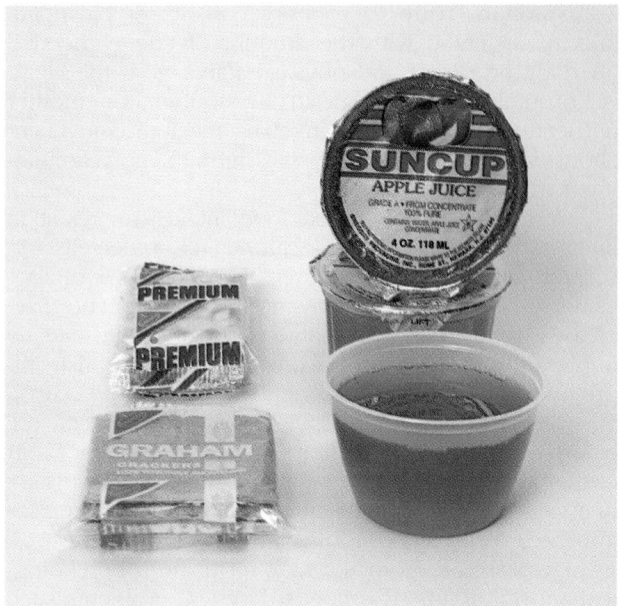

✦ Figure 27–3
Foods usually tolerated by the client with nausea include apple juice, dry crackers, and gelatin.

can lead to feelings of fullness after eating just a few bites of food (early satiety), which only worsens anorexia. Any condition that will decrease digestive juices, cause GI mucosal atrophy, or impair gastric emptying can contribute to anorexia. Adverse side effects of drugs may also cause anorexia. Not only physical but emotional conditions can result in anorexia and/or exacerbate anorectic behaviors.

Nutritional care involves stimulating the client's appetite. Encouraging oral intake of foods is preferred, but enteral and parenteral feedings may be advised.

Heartburn

Heartburn, called gastroesophageal reflux, is a very common GI disorder, especially in the elderly. This reflux typically occurs approximately 30 minutes to 1 hour after eating. Pregnancy, vigorous exercise, hiatal hernia (partial stomach protrusion through the diaphragm), and large, fatty meals can cause heartburn.

A change in some lifestyle habits is recommended. Waiting at least 2 hours after meals before lying down will allow the increased level of stomach acid to decrease and thereby lessen heartburn. Clients should not overeat; more food in the stomach means production of more acid and more stomach pressure. Chocolate, peppermint, acidic beverages (*e.g.*, fruit juices and soda), alcohol, and nicotine may stimulate acid production and weaken the stomach valve, allowing food to back up into the esophagus. Elevating the head of the bed about 4 to 6 in uses gravity to keep the acids in the stomach. A low-fat, high-protein diet is recommended; fat can aggravate heartburn by open-

ing the stomach valve, while protein closes the stomach valve. Antacids may also be ordered to neutralize stomach acidity.

Application of the Nursing Process to a Client's Nutritional Needs

The nursing process is an excellent method to assess nutritional status, monitor eating habits, and evaluate whether nutritional needs are met. The first and most important step in determining nutritional adequacy is assessment.

Assessment

Since nurses spend more time with the client than any other health care team member, nurses are in a unique position to assess nutritional status. As Kathleen Cope (1994) states, "Since illness starts at the cellular level, and the food we eat nourishes the body at the cellular level, the 'nutritional status' must be considered a vital sign as important and necessary as 'blood pressure' or 'pulse' or the seven warning signs of cancer" (p. 29). Therefore, nutritional assessment should be performed on every client, just as vital signs are performed on every client.

If any of the following conditions are identified on assessment, the physician or dietitian should be notified:

1. A greater than 10% unintended weight loss or gain within the past 6 months
2. A weight less than 80% or greater than 120% of ideal body weight
3. Less than 3.5 g/dl for serum albumin
4. A greater than 5% weight loss or gain within the last month.

Nursing History—Dietary

A thorough diet history (Box 27–1) will reveal food preferences, usual and actual nutrient intake, weight changes, kilocaloric needs, fluid intake, medications taken, and physiological and psychological aspects affecting nutrition.

Direct and indirect questioning of the client and/or family or significant others can be utilized to obtain this information. The information collected can be compared with the RDAs, Food Guide Pyramid, or dietary guidelines to determine whether diet is adequate.

Other techniques for assessing intake can be incorporated into the dietary history. The 24-hour dietary recall allows the client to state or write down a record of all foods and amounts eaten within the last 24 hours. Food models and examples of serving sizes may stimulate the client's memory.

Box 27–1

COMPONENTS OF A DIET HISTORY

Name

Age

Sex

Medical diagnosis/surgeries

Medical history

Exercise history

Emotional/mental health status

Food/drug allergies

Weight changes (present, usual, ideal)

Appetite or taste changes

Conditions of teeth and mouth

Dentures

Chewing, swallowing, choking problems

Favorite foods/fluids

Disliked foods/fluids

Personal or religious restrictions

Location and number of meals

Who purchases and prepares the food; finances for food

Eating and snacking habits

Nutritional supplements taken

Medications taken (prescribed and over the counter)

Fluid intake; alcohol intake

Cultural dietary beliefs

Any special diet; any problems with this diet

Problems with heartburn, indigestion, nausea, vomiting, diarrhea, constipation, laxative use

---

A food diary is a more precise record but is time consuming for the client. A client maintains a food diary for 3 to 7 days that includes all foods consumed with amounts, method of preparation, and location and time of meals. To provide a more realistic picture of usual foods eaten, at least one weekend day should be included in the diary.

A quick method to assess intake is the food frequency form. This is a food checklist that lists approximately 40 to 80 types of foods to determine the number of times per day, week, or month that each food is eaten. Portion sizes are not necessarily included. All of the three techniques require that the information obtained be compared with a standard to determine adequacy of diet.

Kilocalorie counts, usually done over a period of 3 days, can be used for hospitalized clients. Accuracy is of utmost importance. Usually, nurses are the ones responsible for charting the amounts and percentages of what clients ingest. Nurses must remember to include food provided by significant others and snacks.

After completion of this count, a dietitian evaluates the findings to determine whether more or fewer kilocalories are needed.

Physical Assessment

Nurses can also incorporate physical assessment findings to determine nutritional adequacy and detect possible nutritional deficiencies. Alerting the physician to abnormal findings could shorten a client's hospital stay or meet a client's nutritional need so that deficiencies could be averted.

Findings from a head-to-toe inspection that can alert the nurse to possible nutritional problems are listed in Box 27–2.

Mouth Assessment

The techniques required during a physical assessment include inspection, palpation, percussion, and auscultation. Inspection of the mouth is the first step. Inspection can indicate an obvious problem, such as wounds or ulcers in the mouth. Areas that would give some clues as to a client's nutritional status include the gums (bleeding may indicate a vitamin C deficiency), color of the mucous membranes (pallor could indicate poor nutrition as well as poor circulation), teeth (loose or no teeth could indicate lack of calcium and vitamin D), and number of caries (numerous caries could indicate poor hygiene practice, excessive intake of sugars, or excessive vomiting). While inspecting the mouth, have the client lift up the tongue; white, irregular patches under the tongue or on the sides of the mouth or tongue could indicate oral cancer. Report the findings to the physician. Dentures are removed after the nurse has assessed them for proper

Box 27–2

FINDINGS THAT MAY INDICATE NUTRITIONAL PROBLEMS

General appearance: Thin, "skin and bones"

Hair: Dull, sparse

Eyes: Pale conjunctivae, dry eye membranes, night blindness

Lips: Cheilosis (cracks and sores located by the corners of the mouth), cracked, chapped

Tongue: Glossitis, deep furrows

Teeth: Cavities, discolored

Gums: Bleeding, swollen, receding

Skin: Scaly, bruising, poor wound healing, pressure ulcers

Nails: Ridged, brittle

Muscles: Weak, flaccid, atrophied

Bones: Beading of ribs, bowlegs

Neurological: Depression, depressed reflexes

Cardiovascular: Tachycardia, hypertension

fit. Palpate the mouth with gloved hands to detect lumps or masses that may interfere, interrupt, or alter nutritional intake.

Auscultation and percussion are not performed during a mouth assessment. For the mouth assessment, the nurse asks about the last dental check-up, sore throats, and swallowing and chewing problems.

Abdominal Assessment

Mentally divide the client's abdomen into four quadrants by drawing a vertical line through the umbilicus and then a horizontal line through the umbilicus. These areas are called right upper quadrant, right lower quadrant, left lower quadrant, and left upper quadrant.

Inspection of the abdomen is the first step in the physical assessment. A rounded abdomen could indicate weight gain or edema, whereas a scaphoid (concave appearance when supine) abdomen could indicate malnutrition. Wounds, sores, and scars can also be observed.

Auscultating for bowel sounds is the next step of an abdominal assessment. Warm the diaphragm side of the stethoscope before auscultating all four quadrants of the client's abdomen in a clockwise manner. If the client has gastric suctioning, clamp tubing when auscultating abdomen. The nurse may mistakenly confuse the suction sound with bowel sounds.

Active bowel sounds indicate that peristalsis is occurring; nutrients will be able to be digested. If no bowel sounds are heard after listening for 2 to 5 minutes, alert the physician and do not let the client eat or drink. An ileus (absence of peristalsis) has occurred, and digestion is interrupted. When peristalsis is occurring slowly, as in constipation or after surgery, hypoactive bowel sounds result. Hyperactive bowel sounds may indicate that nutrients will not be absorbed properly, as transit time in the GI tract is accelerated, as in diarrhea.

Abdominal palpation is performed after auscultation to avoid interrupting or increasing bowel sounds. Before palpating all four quadrants in a clockwise manner, ask the client if abdominal pain is present, if so, palpate that area last. A midline pulsating mass should not be palpated, because it could be an aneurysm that could rupture if palpated. Palpate all areas of the abdomen for temperature, distention, lumps, masses, tenderness, and guarding. Guarding is present when the client tenses, indicating that pain or tenderness is present. Palpate with fingertips first and then follow with deep palpation by pressing about 3 in into the abdomen. Deep palpation on infants should be performed cautiously to avoid liver laceration. Rebound tenderness is checked by pressing the abdomen in and releasing very quickly. If the client feels pain on release, rebound tenderness is present, which may indicate appendicitis or peritonitis.

Percussion helps the nurse to estimate the location and size of abdominal organs. Because x-rays can de-tect organ sizes and locations accurately, percussion may or may not be performed.

During the abdominal assessment, the nurse inquires about problems with nausea, vomiting, diet, or intake.

Because physical findings by themselves are inconclusive for determining malnutrition, several findings must be correlated: physical assessment findings, anthropometric measures, diagnostic tests, and laboratory information.

Anthropometric Measures

Height, weight, lean body mass, and fat stores are anthropometric measures assessed to determine nutritional status. In fact, height and weight should be measured for every client on admission or during the admission assessment.

◆ **Height/Weight.** Direct measurements of height and weight are more accurate than information obtained from the client or family. However, when height and weight cannot be directly measured because of the client's medical condition, information from the client or family is better than none. To measure height, the client stands as straight as possible with legs together and shoes removed. A measuring rod, attached to either a wall or platform scale, is used to actually measure height.

Because the most quick and helpful indicator of nutritional status is body weight, an accurate weight is essential (Fig. 27–4). Weighing a client at the same time of day, in the same amount of clothing, and with the same scale will produce valid results. The best time of day is before breakfast and after urinating. Depending on the client's activity level, a platform, chair, or bed scale may be used.

The findings from height and weight measurements are compared with standard values. Height and weight tables may be used. The nurse can then compare the actual weight with the weight listed on the chart.

◆ **Skinfold Measurements.** To determine the amount of subcutaneous fat or energy reserves, skinfold measurements are obtained. Using special skinfold calipers, two sites can be measured: triceps or subscapular. In most facilities, triceps is the preferred site. The nondominant side or arm is measured three times and averaged. A normal finding for men is about 13 mm, and for women, about 17 mm. Low levels may indicate PEM.

◆ **Circumferences.** Kilocalorie and protein stores are determined by measuring midarm circumference. As the name indicates, the midpoint of the arm is measured with a tape measure. A normal finding for both men and women is about 29 cm.

Midarm muscle circumference estimates the amount of lean body mass. The skinfold measurement finding is subtracted from the midarm circumference

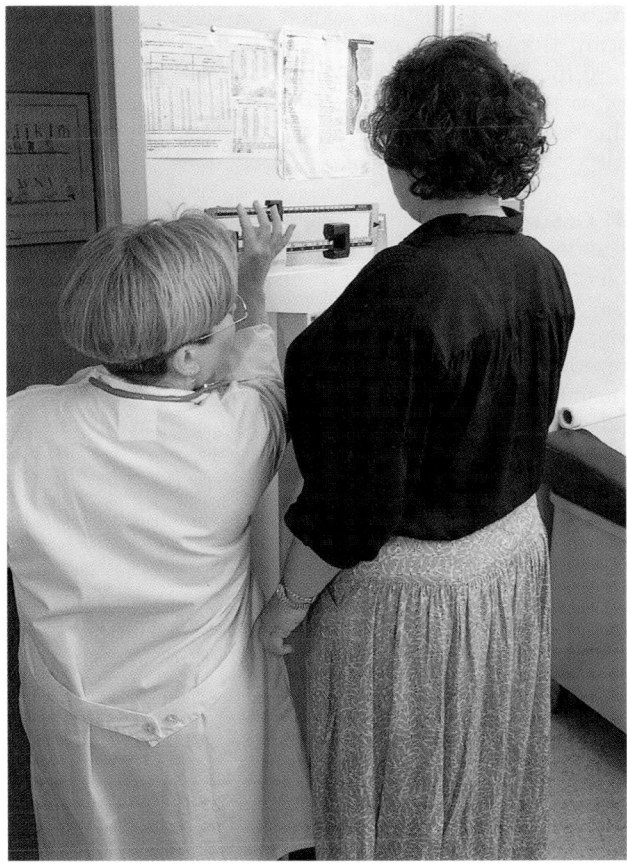

✦ **Figure 27–4**
Accurate weight measurement is an important means of assessing nutritional status. The client's weight can then be compared with the recommended weight on the chart for her height and body frame type.

amount to obtain the midarm muscle mass circumference. An average finding for men is approximately 25 cm, and for women, 23 cm. Malnutrition is usually severe if lower values are obtained. A nurse can also inspect the client's scapular, pelvic, and calf areas for muscle wasting to confirm midarm measurements.

Diagnostic Tests

Diagnostic tests are usually performed to detect GI masses, strictures (narrowing), tumors, or ulcers.

✦ **Barium Swallow and Upper GI Series.** Barium swallow and upper GI series are tests in which the client drinks barium that coats the GI lining to enhance findings from x-rays (Fig. 27–5). The evening before the test, the client eats a light supper and is then NPO at midnight or at least 8 hours before the test. The nurse informs the client that the barium tastes chalky, the room is dark to enhance fluoroscopy, and the x-ray table is tilted to assist the barium to flow. This test lasts about 45 minutes. Medications are not given to the client before the test unless ordered by the physician. After the test, nurses inform clients that their stools will be light colored (barium is being excreted) and not to be alarmed. Barium is constipating, so fluids are encouraged. Enemas or laxatives may be needed.

✦ **Computerized Axial Tomography.** Computerized axial tomography (CAT) makes a three-dimensional cross-section of the body being scanned. During an abdominal CAT scan, the client lies still as the CAT scan machine circles the body. This procedure causes no pain and can last from 15 to 60 minutes. Preparation before this test varies; therefore careful consultation with the radiology department is vital. An iodine contrast medium can be used during CAT scans. If

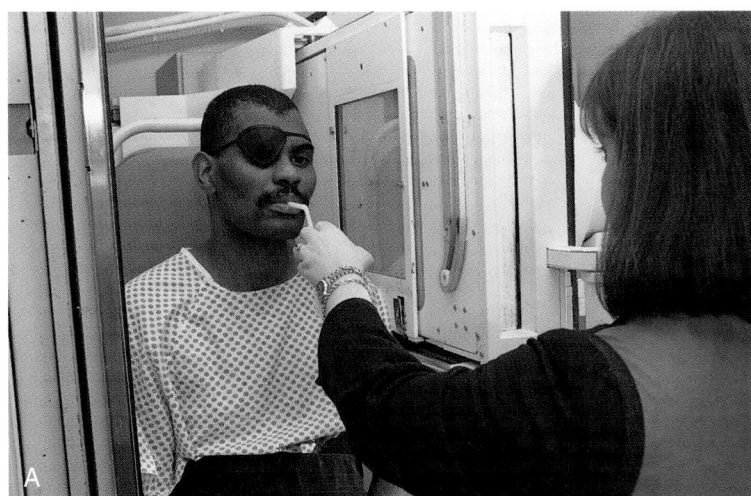
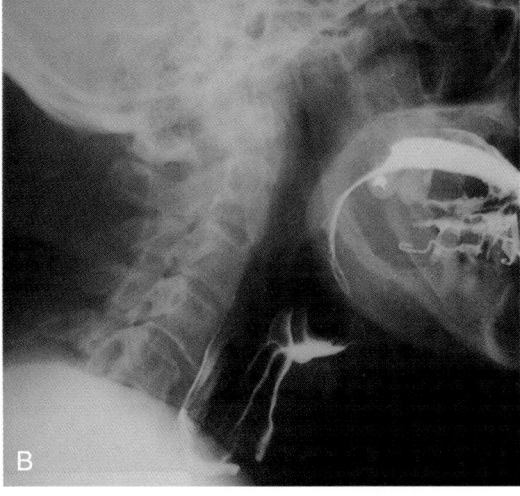

✦ **Figure 27–5**
A barium swallow and upper GI series may be ordered for a client with digestive problems. *A*, The client swallows a contrast substance, both in liquid and purée form, which coats the GI lining. *B*, The client is observed under fluoroscopy to determine the path of the swallowed substances. The x-ray shows that this client is aspirating.

iodine is used, ask clients if they are allergic to sea-food or iodine. Nurses should notify the radiology department if clients are allergic to the contrast medium. Nurses should also inform the client that a warm, flushing sensation will be experienced when the dye is injected. Following the procedure with contrast dye, the nurse should encourage the intake of fluids and monitor the injection site for redness, swelling, or warmth. If redness, swelling, or warmth is present, the nurse should apply a warm, moist pack to the site.

✦ **Magnetic Resonance Imaging.** Magnetic resonance imaging (MRI) uses no contrast medium or radiation to visualize internal organs for tumors. A client is placed on a sliding hard pallet and pushed into the large cylinder-like MRI machine. Because the machine works by magnetic fields, this test is contraindicated for clients with metal surgical clips, metal heart valves, pacemakers, or metal joint replacements. Nurses inform clients that clicking, drum beat, or muffled jack-hammer sounds may be heard during the test; food and fluids do not need to be restricted; a tingling sensation in teeth fillings is normal; and all metal items must be removed, including hair clips, credit cards, watches, and jewelry. If the nurse accompanies the client to the testing site, stethoscopes must be removed. There is no special care after the test.

✦ **Abdominal Ultrasound.** Abdominal ultrasound is a noninvasive, painless procedure that is becoming more popular. A lubricant is placed on the abdomen, and a transducer is then positioned on the abdomen. This transducer is moved to various parts of the abdomen, and a picture of internal structures is projected into a monitor much like a television screen (Fig. 27–6). This picture is obtained because the transducer emits sound waves, which the monitor converts into images. Depending on the reason for the abdominal ultrasound, the client is usually allowed fluids. Coordinating with the ultrasound department is essential. To

prevent gas formation, which can interfere with the scan, smoking and gum chewing are not allowed before the test, and simethicone (Mylicon) may be given prior to the test. If abdominal dressings are present, these must be removed before the test. Following the ultrasound, no special care is needed.

✦ **Gastroscopy.** Gastroscopy is used for direct visualization of the stomach (Fig. 27–7). Ulcers and active bleeding can be identified. Six to eight hours before the test, the client is NPO. A consent form must be signed by the client prior to the test. Dentures are removed prior to the procedure to reduce the risk of pushing the dentures into the trachea while the tube is passed or swallowed, leading to aspiration. A special procedure room or operating room is used to perform this test. While the client is lying on the left side, a flexible tube is swallowed. To prevent gagging, certain medications that promote relaxation are administered. After the test, the client is placed in a semi-Fowler's or side-lying position to prevent aspiration. Vital signs are taken every 30 minutes for 2 hours. If a local anesthetic was used to numb the throat during the procedure, liquids are not allowed until the gag reflex returns. A nurse checks this by stroking the back of the client's throat with a tongue depressor; if the client gags, the reflex is present. When the gag reflex is present, warm saline gargles or throat lozenges can be used if the client has a sore throat.

✦ **Gallbladder Tests.** Several tests can be performed to assess the functioning of the gallbladder. An oral cholecystogram can determine concentrating abilities of the gallbladder and can detect gallstones or an obstruction. The client must consume a high-fat diet and take medication to help visualize the gallbladder. The night before the test, the client eats a low-fat meal and takes more medication. The client is then given

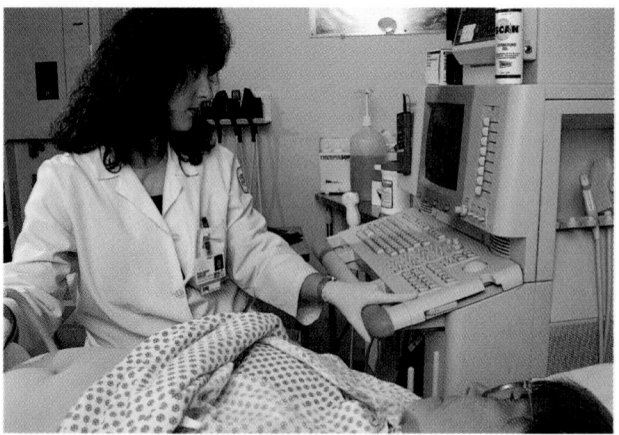

✦ **Figure 27–6**
Abdominal ultrasound is an increasingly popular diagnostic test for digestive problems. In this noninvasive, painless procedure, a transducer is moved across the abdomen, and a picture of the internal structures is projected via sound waves onto a monitor.

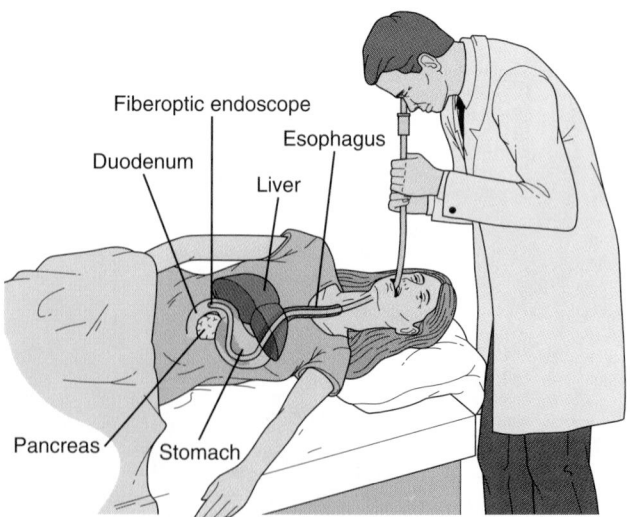

✦ **Figure 27–7**
A gastroscopy procedure is undertaken to directly visualize the stomach. The client is placed in a side-lying position on the left side to prevent aspiration and for ease of access.

an NPO order. Question the client about allergies to iodine, because these medications contain iodine compounds. If the client is allergic to iodine or shellfish, notify the physician before administering the tablets. Enemas or laxatives may be ordered before the test to clear the bowels. No special care is required after the test unless more films are planned. If so, a high-fat meal will be served to the client.

A more popular method to detect gallbladder anomalies such as gallstones, obstructions, or tumors is ultrasound of the gallbladder. This test resembles the abdominal ultrasound test, except that for this test, the client must be NPO 12 hours before the test and is fed a fat-free diet the night before the test. Eating before the test is contraindicated because the gallbladder will not be easily visualized if food is in the stomach. No special care is required after the test. However, in some cases, a client will be asked to eat a high-fat substance during the test to determine how the gallbladder contracts.

An intravenous cholangiogram allows an iodine-based contrast medium to be given intravenously, which assesses the condition of the gallbladder ducts to determine if stones, obstructions, or tumors are present. This can be performed in the radiology department or in surgery (Fig. 27–8). If this test is done in surgery, two methods may be employed: (1) inject- ing the dye through a tube into the ducts or (2) injecting the dye directly into the ducts. Because this is an invasive procedure, consent forms must be signed. The client is NPO 6 to 8 hours before the test. Enemas or laxatives are ordered to clean out the GI tract. Questioning the client for allergies to iodine is necessary. Tell the client that when the dye is injected, a warm, flushing feeling may be felt; this is normal. Following the test, nursing care consists of monitoring vital signs, offering fluids, and resuming diet.

Laboratory Tests

Results of blood and urine laboratory tests provide objective data to determine a client's nutritional status (Table 27–4). Urine results are an indication of recent, rather than usual, nutrient intake. Vitamin levels are usually not routinely obtained because of the expense.

For the findings to be meaningful, the nurse must know the purpose of each test, normal values, and proper client preparation. The laboratory tests described do not require special preparation, unless specified in the text.

✦ **Red Blood Cells.** Red blood cell (RBC) levels are an indication of iron, vitamin B_{12}, and folate status. If the RBC level is normal ($3.6-6.2$ million/mm³), iron, vitamin B_{12}, and folate intake is probably good.

✦ **Hemoglobin.** Normal levels of hemoglobin ($11-18$ g/dl) indicate that protein and iron intake is adequate. Conversely, if the hemoglobin level is low, the nurse should suspect a lack of protein and iron intake. However, bleeding can also cause the hemoglobin to be low.

✦ **Albumin.** Serum albumin levels can reflect protein stores. Normal levels ($3.5-5.5$ g/dl) indicate adequate protein intake. A client's protein status is compromised when levels fall below 3.5 g/dl. Also, hospital stays are longer and death is more likely in clients with albumin levels less than 3.4 g/dl (Herrmann *et al.*, 1992). The nurse must remember that dehydration may falsely elevate albumin levels.

✦ **Transferrin.** A more sensitive measure for current protein intake is serum transferrin, an iron-carrying protein. A level of 200 to 370 μg/dl indicates that protein intake is adequate.

✦ **Blood Urea Nitrogen.** When protein is catabolized, nitrogen and urea are produced. A normal level of blood urea nitrogen (BUN) ($8-23$ mg/dl) depicts good protein intake. Less than 8 mg/dl indicates poor protein intake.

✦ **Creatinine.** Muscle mass or lean tissue changes are reflected in creatinine levels. Normal creatinine levels ($0.6-1.6$ mg/dl) are desired. If kilocaloric intake is low, muscles atrophy. This atrophy results in a low

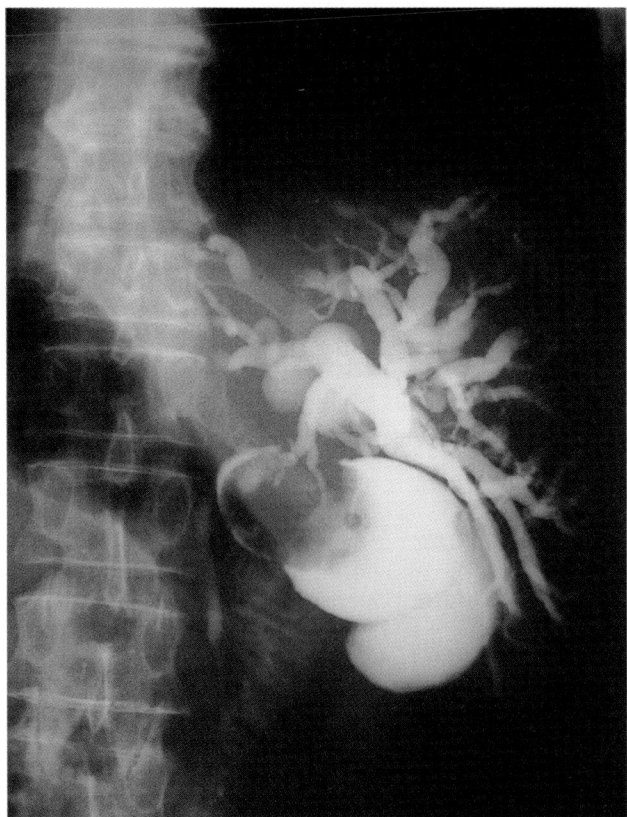

✦ **Figure 27–8**
An intravenous cholangiogram is used to assess the gallbladder ducts for stones, obstructions, and tumors. Iodine-based contrast medium is given to the client intravenously, and an x-ray is taken.

Table 27–4

LABORATORY TESTS

TEST	NORMAL	MALNOURISHED
Red blood cells	Male: 4.2–6.2 million/mm³ Female: 3.6–5.4 million/mm³ Children: 4.5–4.8 million/mm³	Depressed if iron, folate, or vitamin B_{12} intake is low
Hemoglobin	Male: 14–18 g/dl Female: 12–16 g/dl Children: 11–13 g/dl	Low values if iron intake is low
Albumin	3.5–5.5 g/dl	If 2.8–3.5, protein status compromised Less than 2.8, suspect kwashiorkor
Transferrin	200–370 μg/dl	If 180–200, mild malnutrition If 160–180, moderate malnutrition Lower than 160, severe malnutrition
Blood urea nitrogen	8–23 mg/dl	Lower than 8, protein intake inadequate
Serum creatinine	0.6–1.6 mg/dl	Below 0.5, muscle wasting secondary to decreased kilocaloric intake
Nitrogen balance	0 or above	Negative number, negative nitrogen balance or catabolism exceeding anabolism, which is common in malnutrition

creatinine level. Elevated creatinine and BUN levels indicate kidney problems, not a nutritional problem.

✦ **Nitrogen Balance.** Nitrogen balance reflects the extent of protein catabolism and protein intake. When protein catabolism and protein anabolism are equal, nitrogen is in balance. Determining nitrogen balance is an involved process that requires teamwork among laboratory, dietary, and nursing personnel. Nitrogen balance of a client is determined by measuring urinary urea nitrogen and comparing this result with the protein that the client consumes. The urine specimen is collected for a 24-hour period. No urine is discarded; it is placed in a special container. If all of the urine is not collected, the process must begin again for another 24 hours. Additionally, the nurse records all food intake, while the dietitian assesses the protein intake. Sometimes an estimate of a 3-day intake of protein is used rather than recording all food intake. A value below 0, such as − 2, indicates that protein catabolism is exceeding protein intake and the client is in negative nitrogen balance. Therefore, more protein and kilocalories are required.

Psychosocial

The assessment of both physical factors and psychosocial factors, such as culture, religion, and personal preferences, is necessary to recognize a high risk of or an actual problem with nutrient intake. Feelings that a client expresses or displays about ordered diet are also assessed. As nurses are assessing these areas, a nonjudgmental attitude is needed to obtain useful nutritional data.

Assessing personal preferences can also avert possible problems. Many likes and dislikes are influenced by cultural and religious beliefs.

Culture

Think of a favorite food. For some (e.g., people from the midwestern United States), this would be steak and potatoes. For others (e.g., Mexicans) it would be tacos and rice; several (e.g., Vietnamese) may think of tea and pho (a delicate beef and noodle soup). Still others, (e.g., Koreans) might think of toasted seaweed and kimchi (a combination of chopped vegetables that are highly seasoned, salted, and fermented). Cultural food preferences are as distinctly different as the cultures themselves. When people relocate, their favorite cultural food may not be available or may be too expensive to purchase.

In some cultures, foods are classified into certain categories, such as "hot" and "cold" or "yin" and "yang." Depending on the culture, some foods may be considered "hot" by one group and "cold" by another. Thus, it is very important to ask clients about their nutritional beliefs to determine in which category the food belongs. Generally, the intake of "hot" and "cold" or "yin" and "yang" foods should be balanced. Also, the disease can determine what foods are eaten to keep the body in balance. In some cultures, diseases are also classified as "hot" or "cold." Therefore, if the disease is "cold," "hot" foods should be consumed, and vice versa.

Because a nurse is assessing an individual client, cultural stereotypes are to be avoided. The nurse should use cultural food patterns as a guideline but also recognize that not all individuals will follow these guidelines explicitly. Nurses should be cautious about assuming that all patients from the same culture will eat the same foods.

It is not the focus of this chapter to address every culture's food preferences, but an overview is presented in the special box "Nursing Tips for Cultural Nutritional Care." If the nurse uses the dietary history discussed previously, valuable cultural and religious beliefs about food will be obtained.

Religion

Some people in the United States give no thought to eating beef, whereas for Hindu people in India, eating beef is taboo because of their religious beliefs. Seventh-Day Adventists are usually vegetarians who drink no alcoholic or caffeine-containing beverages. For Christians, usually no restrictions are placed on diets, but some may choose to eliminate a food item during Lent. Muslims eat no pork or pork products. Jewish people, depending on their degree of observance of dietary laws, may only eat kosher foods. A specific Jewish dietary custom is to avoid eating dairy products and meat at the same meal. Shellfish, catfish, shrimp, escargot, and lobster are not allowed in a traditional Jewish diet. When religious beliefs and dietary restrictions conflict, referrals to the dietitian are beneficial.

Developmental Aspects

When nurses are assessing the amount of basic nutrients that clients need, nurses should take into account the client's age. Age influences the quantities of nutrients that are required.

Infants

Height, weight, and head circumference are measured to determine adequacy of diet and appropriate weight gain. Height is measured with the infant recumbent. To gauge whether height is increasing as intended, use growth charts.

Tremendous growth occurs during the 1st year of life. At 4 months of age, an infant has doubled its birth weight; by 1 year, birth weight has tripled. By 2 years of age, an additional 4 to 6 pounds should be gained. Growth charts can be used to determine if weight gain is appropriate.

The brain is developing continuously in the womb and for another 2 years after the infant is born. To develop actual brain cells and increase head size, normally optimum nutrition is essential. The head circumference is measured and compared with measurements on a head circumference chart. If head circumference is normal, the number will correspond to the number on the head circumference chart. Conversely, if growth is not occurring properly, the head circumference finding will be lower than what is on the chart.

High energy requirements are necessary for the rapid growth rate that infants experience. Approximately 90 to 120 kcal/kg/day are needed. Fat requirements are high—50% of the kilocalories. Because infants do not have the ability to make vitamin K, a vitamin K injection is required after birth to prevent bleeding. Both breast-fed and bottle-fed infants can receive adequate amounts of nutrients for growth (Fig 27–9).

♦ **Breast-Fed Infants.** Breast-feeding is encouraged for full-term, premature, and low–birth-weight infants; breast-feeding is preferable to bottle-feeding. Evidence is accumulating that breast-feeding encourages optimal development and reduces lifetime problems with allergies and other chronic diseases. An early benefit of breast-feeding is the colostrum that the infant receives. Colostrum, a thick, yellowish fluid that is a precursor to mature milk, provides immunity from some diseases. Between the 3rd and 6th day after delivery, colostrum will change into mature milk.

When assessing an infant who is breast-fed, several factors are taken into consideration. A breast-fed infant will gain weight slower than a bottle-fed infant because of less milk intake. Breast-fed infants may also eat more often than bottle-fed infants. This is not an abnormal finding, and neither the mother nor the nurse should be alarmed. An infant's sucking stimulates milk production. Thus, the more an infant feeds, the more milk is produced.

Breast milk can meet nutritional needs for 4 to 6 months. Supplemental foods, such as cereal or juices, are not necessary during this time.

♦ **Bottle-Fed Infants.** When assessing bottle-fed infants, focus on the type of formula used, how formula is prepared, if overfeeding is present, and condition of the mouth.

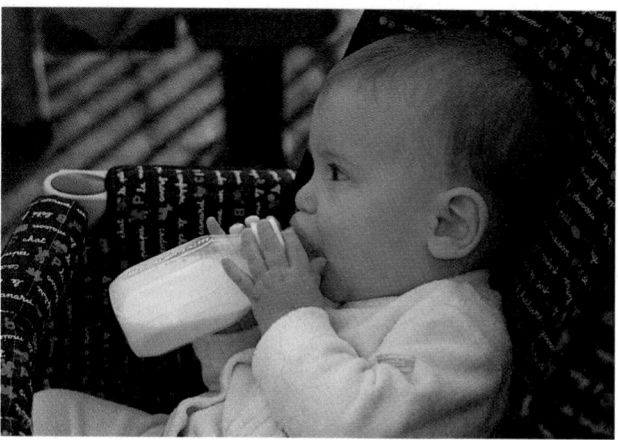

♦ **Figure 27–9**
Although breast milk is ideal for babies, commercial formulas also provide adequate nutrients for growth. Cow's milk is not recommended before 10 to 12 months of age. The fat in cow's milk is poorly digested. Also, cow's milk is higher in protein than formula or human milk, and the infant's kidneys are not developed enough to excrete the extra waste products of protein breakdown.

NURSING TIPS FOR CULTURAL NUTRITIONAL CARE

Culture	Traditional Foods	Nursing Tips
African-American	Fried and barbecued pork or chicken Sweet potatoes Black-eyed peas Yellow and dark green leafy vegetables	Encourage the use of yellow and dark green leafy vegetables
Mexican-American	Tortillas Refried beans Tacos Enchiladas Chili peppers	Incorporate the "hot/cold" beliefs of food into care plan as much as possible Encourage the use of beans, a good source of protein Suggest using unsaturated fat rather than lard to fry Encourage the use of cheese to increase calcium intake Encourage using chili peppers, which are good sources of vitamins A and C
Puerto Rican	Rice Safrito—spicy relish to season foods Viandas—starchy vegetables and fruit, *i.e.,* sweet potatoes and green bananas Bacalao—salted dried codfish	Refer to Mexican American
Cuban	Chicken, fish or meat soup Salad Fried fish, poultry, and eggs Rice and beans	Refer to Mexican American
Native American	Corn Beans Squash Chili peppers	Remember that each tribe has different customs and beliefs about food; incorporate these customs and beliefs as much as possible Include the extended family, especially grandparents and uncles, when relaying nutritional information, since communal decisions may be necessary When teaching, explain how information will help now in the present—not the future, *i.e.,* "eating calcium will help the bones be strong," not "eating calcium will help prevent osteoporosis when you are older."
Chinese	Rice Pork Soybeans Bean sprouts Bamboo shoots Soy sauce Snow peas	Incorporate the "yin-yang" concept into dietary needs as much as possible Encourage the use of foods high in calcium Ask if ice is wanted in beverages; some Chinese people believe this practice to be harmful because ice may shock the body
Japanese	Fish, sometimes eaten raw Tofu Rice or noodles Bean paste Soy sauce Green tea Sake—rice wine Many vegetables and fruit	Instruct that rinsing rice diminishes its nutrient value Encourage the use of tofu, which is high in protein and iron Suggest not eating or decreasing the intake of raw fish, since this poses many health hazards (e.g. cancer, gastroenteritis)

NURSING TIPS FOR CULTURAL NUTRITIONAL CARE		
Vietnamese	Rice Nuoc mam—liquid from fermenting fish and salt Pho—beef and noodle soup Tea Many vegetables	Encourage the use of vegetables When hospitalized, monitor for constipation, since the fiber content in hospital diets is not as high as in Vietnamese diets
Korean	Rice Barley Red beans Seaweed Fish Beef Ginseng Kimchi—spicy fermented combination of many chopped vegetables Fresh fruit Soybean products Barley water	Suggest using whole-grain or enriched rice If seaweed is unavailable, suggest using turnip greens, kale, or mustard greens, which are similar in taste If kimchi is unavailable, suggest using a Mexican salsa, which is similar in taste
Italian	Pastas Parmesan cheese Salads Bread Veal Fish Salami Pepperoni Garlic Wine Black coffee	Suggest using whole-grain or enriched breads Encourage the consumption of various pastas

Although they are not quite identical to breast milk, commercial formulas are used to bottle feed. Cow's milk is not recommended because of its high protein and mineral levels: An infant's kidneys are not fully developed and cannot excrete the extra waste products of protein breakdown. Additionally, the fat in cow's milk is poorly digested and absorbed.

Commercial formulas can provide adequate nutrition. These formulas are constituted to supply an appropriate amount of kilocalories (about 20 kcal/oz). Protein, fats, and carbohydrates are provided in forms that the infant can easily digest. Vitamins and minerals are also supplied. However, iron deficiency is possible if the formula does not contain iron. Iron-fortified formulas or supplements are recommended. Special formulas for premature and low–birth-weight infants are also available. It is essential to follow package directions to prepare formula from powder.

Overfeeding of the infant is more likely with bottle feeding than with breast-feeding because the amount of formula left in the bottle is visibly evident. Infants do not have to drink the bottle dry to be full. If an infant turns his or her head away or becomes interested in another activity, he or she is satisfied.

Overfeeding could result in weight gain, possibly leading to obesity.

Assessment of the infant's mouth is essential to determine if baby bottle tooth decay is present. An infant's gums may be swollen and red, and caries may be evident if baby bottle tooth decay has developed. This process occurs when the infant is put to bed with a bottle in his or her mouth. Teaching the caregiver to discontinue this behavior is necessary to prevent other health and nutritional problems. A pacifier can be substituted for the bottle.

✦ **Initiating Solids.** Observance of the child's physical growth and feeding methods are required to determine adequacy of intake when solids are started. Height, weight, and head circumference are measured to assess physical growth. The caretaker should be asked to list methods of feeding and foods given to the infant. The following are guidelines for initiating solid foods:

Four to six months of age is the suggested time for introducing solids. Some may start this process sooner, but this is unnecessary; no nutritional advantage is observed. In fact, this can be detrimental because introducing solids before 4 months can increase the risk of allergies and can dilute nutrient content of the diet.

The sequence for initiating solids is iron-fortified rice cereal, other types of cereal, strained vegetables and fruits, and then thin strained meats. However, this sequence may vary, depending on the pediatrician's philosophy. Rice cereal is chosen first because it is less allergy producing than other foods. The cereal is fortified with iron because the infant's own iron stores will be depleted by this time. Adding one food at a time is suggested to observe whether an allergic reaction occurs. Food is offered from a spoon—never a bottle. Formula or breast milk is still used but is usually offered after the solids. Offering solids first allows the infant to try new foods when he or she is most hungry.

At 6 to 9 months of age, finger foods are offered (Fig. 27–10). After 10 months to 1 year, homogenized whole milk can be taken from a cup, and foods that adhere to the spoon, such as applesauce, cottage cheese, and mashed potatoes, can be offered. Commercial baby food does not have to be purchased; foods that other family members eat may be utilized. Meats may be chopped or ground, and raw fruits and vegetables may be mashed and served. A well-balanced, varied diet is preferred.

Toddlers

When assessing toddlers, observe for physical ability to feed self, appetite changes, and food jags. Toddlers, aged 1 to 3 years, start learning to feed themselves. Bright-colored, crisp finger foods such as carrots or peeled apples are generally preferred. However, nuts, popcorn, whole grapes, and hot dogs are avoided because of the possibility of aspiration.

During this time, appetites are ever-changing—one way in which toddlers assert independence. Also, when growth rates are high, intake is high. At age 2 when toddlers are active and growth is still occurring, the child is always hungry. However, at age 3, the

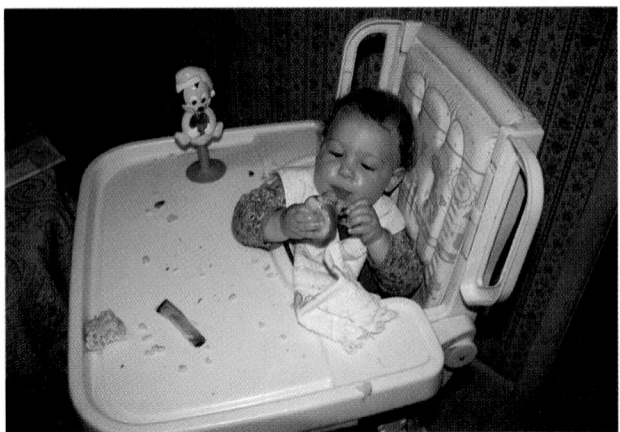

Figure 27–10
Finger foods are offered between 6 and 9 months of age to encourage self-feeding and allow older babies and young toddlers the independence they often crave. Care must be taken to observe the baby at all times for choking, and certain foods that are easily aspirated, such as nuts, popcorn, whole grapes, and hot dogs, should be avoided.

growth rate slows and appetite decreases, causing the child to appear to be a "picky" eater. The child should not be forced to eat if not hungry. Preparing parents for this change in appetite can avert power struggles regarding foods and prevent overfeeding, which can predispose toddlers to weight problems later in life.

When toddlers refuse to eat anything except one food item for several days, they are on a "food jag." Food jags are common but temporary if the caregiver does not display undue concern. The caregiver should serve the desired food along with other foods and should not comment if the added foods are not eaten. It is best simply to ignore the behavior.

Preschool and School-Age Children

For a preschooler or school-age child, the nurse assesses eating habits, food choices, presence of lead poisoning, and parental attitudes about nutrition. Meals and snacks are the usual eating habits. Fruits, yogurt, and low-fat cheeses are healthy snacks that can provide the needed nutrients and kilocalories. In school-age children, eating habits can be adversely affected by schoolwork concerns or emotional difficulties with friends, family, or school.

Food choices will vary. Most preschoolers prefer their foods fixed separately. Mixed foods, such as casseroles and stews, may be avoided. In the school-age child, almost all foods except vegetables are eaten.

Lead poisoning can occur in children who ingest dirt, lead-contaminated objects, lead-containing paint chips, or water from lead pipes. If the child lives in an old house and has eaten paint or dirt and displays vomiting, irritability, weight loss, malaise, headache, and insomnia, suspect lead poisoning. Lead levels above 25 μg/dl confirm the diagnosis. This blood test must be ordered by the physician. Chronic lead poisoning can seriously delay development. To decrease a child's chance of experiencing lead poisoning, encourage a well-balanced diet, with 4 cups of milk daily. Calcium in the milk decreases lead absorption.

Parental food likes or dislikes will affect children's intake. Foods that are not liked by parents will not be served. Children who eat meals together with the family will have a greater nutrient intake than children who do not eat meals with the family. Allowing children to prepare meals and snacks alongside a parent can be one of the best methods to enhance healthy eating. Providing a variety of foods, following the dietary guidelines for Americans, and allowing the child to eat without coercion can lead to healthy lifelong eating habits.

Adolescents

Nurses assess adolescents' nutritional intake and eating practices. Because of the growth spurt that occurs during adolescence, many teenagers are susceptible to nutrient deficiencies. About 3000 kilocalories are needed for adolescent boys, whereas, 2200 kilocalories are needed for girls.

Ensuring that foods high in calcium and iron are eaten is necessary during the assessment phase. Calcium and iron are minerals that are often deficient in a teenager's diet. A rapid increase in height and skeletal mass causes an increased need for calcium. Research also indicates that a lifelong high intake of calcium, especially for women, can protect against the development of osteoporosis later in life. Iron is required for the increase in blood volume and muscle mass in boys and for the onset of menses in girls.

Peer pressure is very great during adolescence and can affect eating practices and food choices. How many teenagers would eat tofu when the rest of the group is eating pizza? Eating times may be before, during, or after group events. For some teenagers, this practice may be easily tolerated, but for other teenagers with nutritional problems, this could cause adverse effects. For example, if a diabetic teenager does not eat food at regular intervals, hypoglycemia, which is life threatening, could result.

In some cases, because drugs and alcohol are part of the peer group activities, the nurse should assess the teenager's intake of these substances. Drugs and alcohol increase nutrient requirements. Couple this with the rapid growth requirements of adolescence and one can see how detrimental drug or alcohol use could be for normal growth and development. Money may not be spent on food purchases but rather on drugs and alcohol, resulting in a decreased intake, causing possible malnutrition and impaired growth.

Eating practices that are common during this time include ingesting excessive sodium, sugar, and fat because of eating fast foods or vending machine food; skipping meals or eating meals on the go because of busy schedules; and trying fad diets because of perceived weight problems. Additionally, carbonated beverages are often consumed rather than milk. Assessing eating practices may identify possible eating disorders (*e.g.*, anorexia nervosa and bulimia) common during this stage of life. For both disorders, the underlying cause of the problem must be investigated; psychiatric as well as medical follow-up care is usually necessary. Therapy, counseling, and/or support groups for the family as well as for the client are necessary and helpful. Inpatient and outpatient care settings are available for various levels of treatment.

❧ **Anorexia Nervosa. Anorexia nervosa** (AN) develops most often in adolescent girls, but adolescent boys and middle-aged adults can also be affected. When assessing these clients, use a structured, not open-ended, interview. Clients with AN have a distorted body image and a deep-seated fear of becoming fat. Ask clients how they view their body and then ask if other people see them in the same way to detect a distorted body image (Love & Seaton, 1991).

If a client exhibits the following, suspect AN: weight loss equal to or exceeding 15% below ideal body weight, lack of menstruation in girls, desiring thinness, being achievement oriented, eating little or

nothing, excessive dieting, excessive physical activity, or indepth knowledge of kilocaloric content of food. Clients with AN may also look like "skin and bones" (Fig 27–11). Clients with AN often want to weigh less than 100 pounds; this is a major achievement for them. Inquire about how much the client would like to weigh. Anorexics may check their weight up to 20 times a day to determine if this goal has been met (Edelstein *et al.*, 1989); ask how often clients weigh themselves.

Treatment for AN involves all the members of the health care team. Promoting intake and increasing weight are common goals. Promoting intake may be in the form of a regular diet, diet supplements, tube feedings, or intravenous feedings. Weight gain is usually set at 1 lb/week. Foods to offer include cereals, low-fat dairy products, yogurt, bagels, fish, poultry, and pudding. Mealtimes are limited to 30 minutes, and prolonged discussions about the kilocaloric content of foods are avoided.

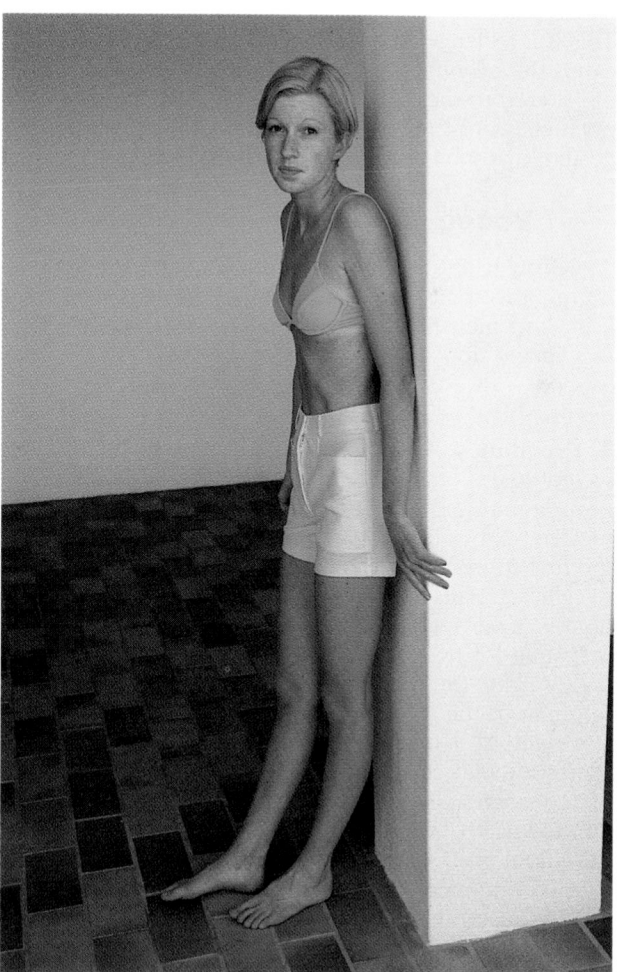

❧ **Figure 27–11**
A client who weighs 15% or more below ideal body weight should be carefully assessed for anorexia nervosa. Excess dieting, a stated desire for thinness or distorted perception of being overweight, and excessive physical activity in a client who is "skin and bones" are danger signs.

❧ **Bulimia. Bulimia** affects all ages and both male and female clients. However, adolescent girls are the most often affected. Bulimics also fear becoming fat, but they control this fear by at times overeating (binging) and then using laxatives, enemas, vomiting, diuretics, or exercise (purging) to undo their binging. Alcohol intake and prior sexual and/or physical abuse have been associated with bulimia.

A nurse should suspect bulimia when a client demonstrates the following: normal or slightly above-normal weight, kilocalorie intake above 10,000 at one meal, evident caries, swollen parotid glands, heavy laxative use (over 100 laxatives per day) (Edelstein *et al.*, 1989), or self-induced vomiting after the binge. Compulsive stealing or spending ($8–50) for food items is common, as is binging on high-carbohydrate, easily digested junk food (Plehn, 1990). When assessing the mouth, do not assume caries or swollen glands are from poor dental hygiene habits, but assume they may be secondary to the frequent vomiting of bulimia (Hofland & Dardis, 1992).

Treatment involves a multidisciplinary approach. Nurses monitor clients after meals to prevent purging. This surveillance may last up to 1 hour. Foods that cause the client to purge are excluded but then gradually added to the diet. Tell the client that purging does not necessarily reduce the number of kilocalories ingested; many bulimics have this misconception.

Young and Middle-Aged Adults

Growth and nutrient requirements have stabilized during this phase of life. Women need about 1900 kcal, and men need approximately 2500 kcal. Assessing intake for a well-balanced, varied diet is performed.

❧ **Pregnancy.** Kilocaloric intake, nutrient intake, and weight gain trends are assessed. An additional 300 kcal/day are required during the second and third trimesters. No additional kilocalories are needed during the first trimester unless the woman is severely underweight. Nurses should inform the woman that doubling her intake is not necessary, even though she is "eating for two."

Weight gain should be steady and gradual throughout the second and third trimesters. Normally, a weight gain of 2 to 4 lb is suggested for the first trimester, with a weight gain of 1 lb/week for the rest of the pregnancy. The overall weight gain should be approximately 25 to 35 lb. If the nurse detects major deviations in the weight changes, notifying the physician is warranted.

Because pregnancy is a time for increased growth, most nutrient needs are increased. Protein requirements are increased to provide amino acids to build the new tissues. An additional 10 to 14 g of protein is suggested: Drinking 2 cups of milk, eating 2 oz of extra meat, or drinking 1 cup of milk and eating 1 oz of additional meat will provide the needed protein.

Vitamin D and calcium intake are also assessed. These are increased to form the skeletal tissue of the fetus. An extra 400 mg of calcium is required. Drinking three or four glasses of milk per day will meet this recommendation. Other dairy products, such as cheeses, ice cream, and yogurt, can also be incorporated into the diet.

Folate requirements are established at 400 µg/day, more than double the allowance for nonpregnant women. Most women need to take a vitamin supplement to meet this requirement. Otherwise, women must consume raw fruits and green leafy vegetables, whole-grain cereals, or folate-enriched cereals to supply enough folate from the diet. If the daily requirement of folate is met, spinal cord defects usually do not occur. On the other hand, if folate intake is low, especially prior to conception, spinal cord defects may result.

Iron recommendations are raised from 15 mg to 30 mg/day during pregnancy to meet the increased demand for hemoglobin synthesis. Most women will need a mineral supplement to meet this need. Ask the woman what type of vitamin and mineral supplement is being taken. If the answer is none, refer to physician or dietitian.

Nutrient intake can affect the weight of the baby. If the mother's intake is adequate, then the baby's weight is usually normal; if intake is low, then the baby's weight is low. Improvement of the women's diet before pregnancy has produced better results than waiting to improve the women's diet once she becomes pregnant. However, increasing intake when needed after conception is prudent. In a study by Doyle and associates (1991), mothers who had poor nutrition delivered babies with low birth weight. These mothers were found to have a diet low in fruits, vegetables, dairy products, breakfast cereals, and whole-grain breads. If the pregnant woman's weight is 10% below ideal or 20% above the norm weight for height, she is more prone to deliver a low–birth-weight, premature infant (Naeye, 1990).

❧ **Lactation.** Fluid intake, kilocalories consumed, and weight are assessed. Fluid needs are increased to an additional 1000 ml/day or an extra 4 cups/day to replace the fluid secreted in the milk. An additional 500 kcal/day is recommended for women who are breast-feeding, making the total kilocaloric intake approximately 2000 to 2500. Prepregnancy weight may be achieved more quickly for the woman breast-feeding as compared to the woman who chooses to bottle feed. Producing the milk requires energy (kilocalories); the extra fat stores from pregnancy are used to meet this requirement, as the recommended 500 additional kilocalories do not fully meet this energy need.

Usual food intake is also assessed. The main emphasis is on a well-balanced, varied diet. If deficiencies are identified, the nurse teaches the woman about foods high in missing nutrients. If more than one nutrient is lacking, nutrient supplementation may be necessary, and a dietary consult is advised.

Elderly Clients

Kilocaloric intake, eating patterns, weight, medication history, and physical and mental functioning are parameters to be assessed in the elderly. Because of lowered BMR and physical activity levels, the kilocaloric requirement for the elderly is 2300 for men and 1900 for women. Even though kilocaloric intake is decreased, the elderly are still prone to nutrient deficiencies because of the many age-related changes occurring in the GI tract: Enzyme secretions, hydrochloric acid secretions, peristalsis, and GI muscle tone are all decreased. Other age-related changes and nursing care are addressed in the special box "Nutritional Care of the Elderly."

Eating patterns of the elderly reflect a decrease in foods consumed, making them prone to nutritional deficiencies and malnutrition. Malnutrition in the elderly may be related to physiological, psychological, and/or economic factors. The major factor is income.

NUTRITIONAL CARE OF THE ELDERLY

Below are nursing tips for age-related changes that may affect nutritional status in the elderly client:

Decreased Hydrochloric Acid Secretions

* Encourage chewing foods thoroughly
* Assess intake of calcium and vitamin D, because absorption of calcium may be decreased; offer foods high in calcium (*e.g.,* milk, cheese, yogurt) and vitamin D (*e.g.,* fortified milk or supplements).

Decreased Peristalsis and Gastrointestinal Muscle Tone

* Encourage a diet high in fiber
* Suggest chopped fresh or canned fruit for dessert instead of soft, chewable high-sugar desserts like cookies or cakes
* If not contraindicated, offer at least 2000 ml of fluid per day
* Encourage regular physical activity
* Teach not to abuse laxatives, especially mineral oil, since mineral oil can decrease the absorption of fat-soluble vitamins
* Plan largest meal at noon rather than at supper

Decreased Thirst Sensation

* Monitor for dehydration
* Monitor intake and output
* Offer favorite beverage frequently

Decreased Chewing Ability

* Encourage easily chewed foods, such as fish or chicken, beans, and eggs, rather than red or hard-to-chew meats
* Chop, shred, or grind food as needed

Decreased Sense of Smell and Taste

* Suggest using different spices such as lemon, garlic, pepper
* Avoid using salt, since cardiac problems are prevalent in the elderly
* Serve foods at proper temperature
* Alternate food textures, *i.e.,* offer a bite of meat, then vegetable, then fruit

Decreased Social Contacts or Support

* Eat with the client when possible
* Converse with the client while eating, unless contraindicated
* Let the client eat with other people if possible
* Suggest eating outside, if possible
* Refer to Meals on Wheels or other food programs
* Monitor for depression or loneliness, which could decrease intake

Decreased Funds for Food

* Refer to social worker
* Suggest the use of food stamps
* Teach ways to shop efficiently for food; *e.g.,* buy dry beans, eggs, peanut butter, and cheeses rather than meats; purchase foods on sale; buy store or generic brands; avoid impulse buying; purchase larger sizes; avoid buying highly processed foods or convenience items

Decreased Intake

* Monitor for malnutrition
* Monitor intake
* Offer foods that are high in needed nutrients
* Offer favorite foods

Decreased Physical Mobility

* Offer adaptive feeding devices (*e.g.,* larger utensils, specially designed cups or plates) when indicated
* Assist with serving, preparing (*e.g.,* cutting meats, opening cartons), and feeding of meals, as needed
* Refer to social worker or dietitian for programs such as Meals on Wheels
* Suggest having someone drive client to and from grocery store if needed

Most elderly people are on a fixed income, which may limit the amount of money available for food purchases. A lack of transportation also hinders ability to obtain food items, and decreased space and quality of food storage prevent proper storage of these food items. Remember to ask about these factors during assessment.

Also, assess for psychological factors such as loneliness, depression, withdrawal, and despair, which can lead to malnutrition. Congregate meal sites and elderly nutrition programs are helpful. A simple intervention that may avert a decreased intake is described in the Clinical Insight research box, "Increasing Intake in the Elderly."

Physical aspects to assess include disease processes; reduction in ability to perform activities of daily living, such as shopping or cooking; and cognitive impairment. Many elderly people may have numerous disease processes, making eating a chore rather than a pleasure. Sometimes these disease processes may cause a change in the elderly person's familiar diet to an unfamiliar diet.

Ability to perform activities of daily living (physical) and cognitive (mental) impairment can be assessed by observing the client getting out of bed, walking, and maneuvering a fork to place food in the mouth. If the client is unsteady while getting out of bed or walking, physical functioning may be impaired, which could affect ability to purchase and prepare foods. Furthermore, if the client cannot bring the fork to the mouth, it could be a physical or mental impairment. For example, the client may not be able to place the food in the mouth because of a weakness in the hand (physical) or because he or she does not realize that a fork is used to place food in the mouth (mental). Regardless of the reason for altered physical or mental functioning, nutritional intake may be affected.

Weight in the elderly tends to decrease with age. Weight measurements several days in a row, called serial weights, are indicated. For the elderly client, a desirable weight is one that corresponds to height or is slightly above ideal weight. If the client is underweight, mortality risk becomes greater. On the other hand, if the client is obese, heart disease is increased, disabilities occur, and mobility is impaired.

Another factor to consider is prescribed and over-the-counter medication use by the elderly. Many of the elderly take multiple drugs that can interfere with nutrient intake, absorption, or usage. Laxatives, antacids, blood cholesterol–lowering drugs, hypoglycemics, and cancer drugs are the main culprits. If a client is taking any of these drugs, assess nutrient intake thoroughly. If the client is taking two or more of these drugs, a dietary consult may be needed.

Additionally, some drugs are to be taken with food, before meals, on an empty stomach, or with large amounts of water. The client's knowledge of how to take the drug is assessed to determine if the medication is being taken appropriately according to time, route, and method.

To recognize possible nutritional deficits earlier, the nutrition screening initiative for the elderly was instituted. A checklist with 10 statements is completed by the client or significant other. The checklist assigns points to various risk factors. For example, 4 points are given if a client indicates that he or she does not have enough money to buy needed food; 3 points are given if fewer than two meals are eaten per day. Depending on the score, nutritional habits are good and do not need to be changed (a score of 0–2), nutritional habits are placing the client at moderate risk and need to be rechecked in 3 months (a score of 3–5), or nutritional habits are placing the client at high nutritional risk and need to be checked by a nurse practitioner, dietitian, or doctor (a score of 6 or greater). If the client needs to see the health care worker, there are two levels of screening: screen I and screen II. Screen I involves weighing the client, assessing nutrient intake, and determining whether physical, psychological, sociological, and economic factors are causing a problem. If weight and intake are low and factors that can cause a nutritional problem are present, referrals are made to appropriate agencies, *i.e.*, physicians, dietitians, or social workers. Preventive measures (*e.g.*, providing economic, shopping, or transportation assistance) are also instituted as needed. Screen II, which includes laboratory work and a physician or dietitian consult, is implemented when findings from assessment indicate actual nutritional problems like obesity, malnutrition, or osteoporosis.

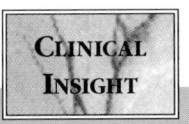

CLINICAL INSIGHT

Increasing Intake in the Elderly

A study by Lange-Alberts and Shott (1994) was undertaken to determine whether touching, verbal cuing, or a combination of the two could significantly increase the mean kilocaloric intake of hospitalized, elderly, oriented clients. In this study, elderly clients were touched on the forearm, verbally encouraged to eat, or received both touch and verbal encouragement.

All three types of contact increased kilocaloric intake. Based on these findings, nurses can provide touch during meals by touching the client's forearm; can perform verbal cuing by encouraging the client to eat during mealtimes; or can carry out both techniques.

These methods are inexpensive, practical, require no special equipment, take minimal time to perform, and can easily be done in any facility to improve the elderlys' nutritional status. Since the elderly people are prone to decreased intake and malnutrition, these simple techniques may avert nutritional complications.

Data from Lange-Alberts, M. E., & Shott, S. (1994). Nutritional intake: Use of touch and verbal cuing. *Journal of Gerontological Nursing, 20*(2), 36–40.

Nursing Diagnosis

After gathering data from the assessment, the nurse interprets and analyzes this information to form a nursing diagnosis. For the diagnosis to be appropriate for the client, an accurate and thorough assessment is essential. Possible nursing diagnoses related to nutrition are listed in the box.

The two main nursing diagnoses are (1) Altered Nutrition: More Than Body Requirements and (2) Altered Nutrition: Less Than Body Requirements. These diagnoses are used when an actual problem exists. If the client is at risk for these diagnoses (*i.e.*, does not have this diagnosis at the moment but could more than likely develop it), "risk" is used (*e.g.*, Risk for Altered Nutrition: Risk for More Than Body Requirements).

Altered Nutrition: More Than Body Requirements

A diagnosis of Altered Nutrition: More Than Body Requirements is applicable when the client weighs 10 to 20% more than the ideal weight for height, age, or sex; intake exceeds need for age, height, sex, and activity level; and triceps skinfold is greater than 15 mm in men or 25 mm in women. Basically, excessive intake is occurring in relation to physical needs.

Altered Nutrition: Less Than Body Requirements

As would be expected, a diagnosis of Altered Nutrition: Less Than Body Requirements is used when the intake of nutrients is insufficient to meet physical needs. A client's weight is 10 to 20% less than the ideal weight for height, age, or sex; intake does not meet requirements for age, height, sex, and activity level; and physical assessment findings suggesting malnutrition (*i.e.*, weakness; poor muscle tone; dull hair; low blood levels of albumin, transferrin, RBCs, hemoglobin, and creatinine; and negative nitrogen balance) are present. Any disorder that causes a problem with ingestion, digestion, or absorption can make a client prone to receive the diagnosis of Less Than Body Requirements.

Other Diagnoses

If a client's gag reflex is absent, coughing and choking occur while eating, or swallowing difficulties exist while eating or drinking, two diagnoses may be used: (1) Impaired Swallowing or (2) Risk for Aspiration. A client with mouth ulcerations, lesions, or inflammation could have the diagnosis of Altered Oral Mucous Membrane. For a breast-feeding mother, if the baby's weight is within normal limits for age and the mother has no concerns or problems about breast-feeding, then Effective Breast-Feeding is appropriate. Conversely, if the baby's weight is below normal limits for age and the mother has concerns or problems about breast-feeding, then the diagnosis of Ineffective

Breast-Feeding is chosen. For a client who is unable to bring food from a plate, dish, cup, or other utensil to the mouth because of weakness, poor coordination, or neurologic deficits, the diagnosis of choice is Self-Care Deficit: Feeding. For nursing diagnoses related to nutrition, see the special box "Nursing Diagnoses Related to Nutrition."

Planning

A nurse must set priorities based on identified nursing diagnoses before determining expected outcomes (goals). Nursing diagnoses for conditions that are life threatening need to be addressed first. If intake is severely limited, as in AN, then addressing the diagnosis of Altered Nutrition: Less Than Body Requirements would be the first priority. However, the main priority will depend on the client's condition. If none of the conditions are life threatening, choose the one that is causing the most problems from the client's point of view. Ask clients what one nutritional problem they would like resolved. Also consider which condition, if resolved, would improve other conditions that the client is experiencing. Suppose a client has pain and is not eating: The pain must be resolved before the client will eat. Another client might have mouth ulcerations (Oral Mucous Membrane, Altered) and decreased intake (Altered Nutrition: Less Than Body Requirements). Mouth ulcerations could be from ill-fitting dentures: The dentures would have to be replaced or removed and the ulcerations begun to heal before intake would improve.

Outcomes

General nutritional goals include preventing or correcting nutritional deficiencies or excesses, maintaining body weight for normal-weight clients, achieving normal body weight for overweight or underweight clients, promoting anabolism, and slowing or eliminating catabolism.

Specific goals would depend on the client's nursing diagnosis. Typical client outcomes may include "client will gain 1 to 2 lb a week until desired weight is achieved," or "client will consume 75% of each meal within 3 days" for a client with a diagnosis of Altered Nutrition: Less Than Body Requirements. For a client with a diagnosis of Altered Nutrition: More Than Body Requirements, the goal could be "client will lose 1 to 2 lb a week until desired weight is achieved." See the special box "Nursing Diagnoses Related to Nutrition" for other specific client outcomes.

Planning with the client and family is crucial for goals to be met. Goals need to be mutually attained. This method will most likely ensure compliance; addressing clients' concerns initially will indicate to clients that their own needs rather than the needs of the nurses, are being met. This also indicates to the client and family that they are active participants in their care and the nurse really cares about them as people, not just as clients.

Altered Nutrition: More Than Body Requirements Related to

- Imbalance of intake versus physical activity
- Sedentary lifestyle
- Self-prescribed doses of megavitamins and minerals
- Dysfunctional eating patterns

Outcome

- Client will lose 1 to 2 lb in 1 week until desired weight is attained
- Client will state methods to decrease kilocaloric intake by 500 kcal/day within 3 days
- Client will verbalize eating patterns that led to weight gain by end of 48 hours
- Client will demonstrate lifestyle and/or behavior changes that will help maintain weight loss by 3 days

Altered Nutrition: Less Than Body Requirements Related to

- Anorexia
- Impaired peristalsis
- Lack of funds
- Lack of information for adequate nutritional needs
- Misinformation concerning normal nutritional needs

Outcome

- Client will gain 1 to 2 lb/week until desired weight is obtained
- Client will state factors that led to weight loss within 3 days
- Client will plan 3 meals a day that reflect a 500-kcal increase
- Client will identify three foods that are high in kilocalories by the end of the shift
- Client's albumin will return to normal (3.5–5.5 g/dl) within 4 days

Self-Care Deficit: Feeding Related to

- Activity intolerance
- Weakness
- Pain
- Neuromuscular impairment
- Poor eyesight
- Impaired mobility

Outcome

- Client will eat 75% of meals within 3 days
- Client will independently feed self before discharge
- Client will use assistive feeding devices, as needed, to help feed self within 5 days

Risk for Aspiration Related to

- Decreased level of consciousness
- Tube feedings
- Wired jaws
- Depressed/absent gag reflex
- Regurgitation

Outcome

- Client will not aspirate
- Client will not choke on food
- Client will maintain patent airway

Effective Breast-Feeding Related to

- Prior proper breast-feeding information
- Normal breast structure
- Good sources of support
- Confidence of mother

Outcome

- Mother will state that she enjoys breast-feeding
- Baby will void six times a day
- Mother will state that she is glad she chose to breast-feed
- Baby wets diaper six times a day

Ineffective Breast-Feeding Related to

- Prior history of breast-feeding failure
- Abnormal breast structure
- Lack of support sources
- Interruption in breast-feeding
- Severe anxiety of the mother

Outcome

- Mother will verbalize satisfaction with breast-feeding within 3 days
- Baby will not require supplemental feeding by 3 days
- Mother will state pleasure in breast-feeding within 4 days
- Baby will void six times a day

Impaired Swallowing Related to

- Fatigue
- Depressed/absent gag reflex
- Neuromuscular impairment

Outcome

- Client will swallow food/fluids freely within 3 days
- Client will perform jaw exercises as prescribed every day
- Client will name foods that cause choking and avoid eating these foods within 4 days

Altered Oral Mucous Membrane Related to

- Dehydration
- Effects of radiation or cancer drugs
- Acidic foods
- Poisoning (specify)
- Nasogastric tubes

Outcome

- Client's affected area will not increase in size, and within 7 days, healing will be evident
- Client's oral mucous membrane will be moist and intact with no lesions by the end of 2 weeks

Care Plans

After the nurse has collaborated with the client, the nurse must write down this information for the plan to be implemented by all health care team members. Consistency is enhanced if the care plan is communicated to others via the written word. Suppose a client is allergic to nuts. If this were written and communicated not only to the nurses but also to the dietary department, hassles and misunderstandings could be avoided. The client would not have to continually repeat this information to every nurse who provided care. If the client wanted a quick snack, the nurse would know not to serve nuts, averting a possible life-threatening situation.

While writing the plan of care, interventions must be devised that are workable for the client; therefore, input must be obtained from the client and/or family. When diet needs to be altered because of health reasons, remembering early family influences and personal preferences is beneficial. Many clients are much more willing to comply with the modified diet when their likes and dislikes are incorporated into the new meal plan. Because most nutritional needs are related to excessive or deficient intake, specific interventions that correct these excesses or deficits are instituted.

✦ **Altered Nutrition: More Than Body Requirements.** Begin by asking if the client wants to lose weight to determine motivation. Client noncompliance and failure rates are high for obesity treatments. If motivation is low, compliance will possibly be low. If motivation is low, ascertain the reason; it could be a lack of knowledge or desire. Lack of knowledge would indicate to the nurse that teaching is needed, whereas a lack of desire could mean that motivational techniques are required. Highlighting how weight loss would improve health status may be the motivating factor. Weight loss lowers cholesterol levels, decreases blood pressure, increases energy level, enhances interest in sex, lessens joint pain, and eases shortness of breath.

The overall goal is to balance kilocaloric intake with the amount of energy needed for body processes and physical activities. Nutritional care is generally a combination of decreasing the number of kilocalories ingested and increasing activity levels. Interventions will focus on decreasing intake and increasing physical activity to decrease weight (Fig. 27–12).

One pound of fat is equal to 3500 kcal. For 1 lb of weight loss to occur, 3500 kcal must be eliminated from the diet. This is usually accomplished by decreasing the intake 500 kcal a day for a week to sustain a 1-lb weight loss in 1 week. However, clients may be more enthusiastic when the weight loss is 2 lb per week. For the other pound of weight loss, an additional energy expenditure of 500 kcal a day is recommended. Weight loss that is slow and gradual is more apt to "stay off" than rapid weight loss, which typically causes the lost weight plus extra pounds to be regained.

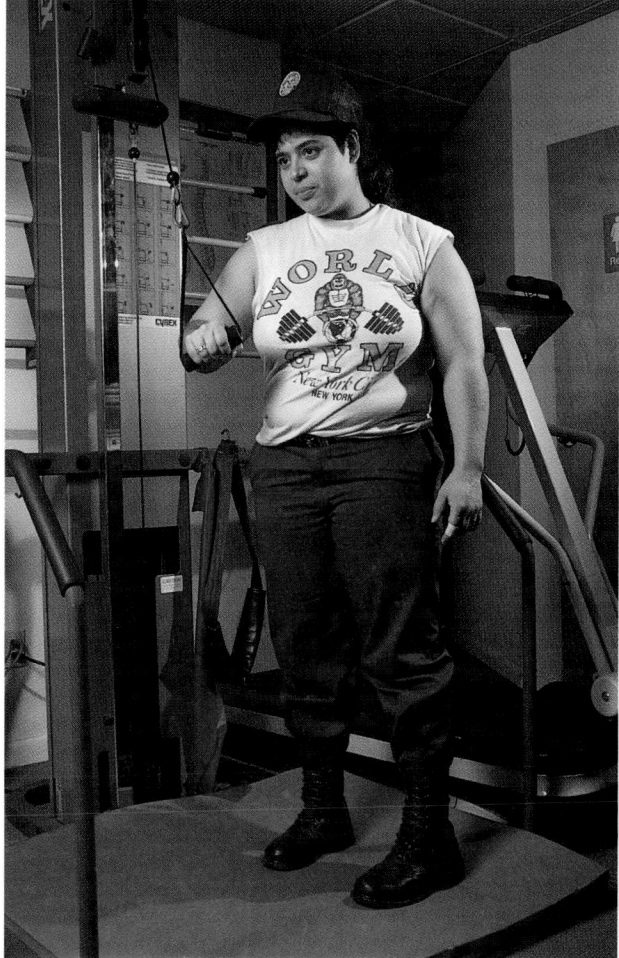

✦ **Figure 27–12**
Encourage the overweight client to increase physical activity, as well as decrease caloric intake, to accomplish a steady loss of weight. An additional energy expenditure of 500 kcal/day, along with a decreased consumption of 500 kcal/day, should result in the loss of 2 lb/week.

Behavior modification practices that increase energy expenditure, which will burn kilocalories and tone muscles, include using the stairs instead of the elevator or parking the car further away than normal. Exercising 20 minutes three times a week is recommended. Devising exercise plans that fit into the client's lifestyle rather than recommending a formal exercise program will increase the likelihood of this behavior being repeated. Swimming, walking, and bicycling are activities that could be incorporated. Playing with children and housekeeping chores can also burn kilocalories.

Other behavior modification practices that will decrease kilocaloric intake include using a smaller plate, chewing food 20 times before swallowing, putting the fork down after each bite, eating from plates or dishes rather than from the box, eating while sitting rather than standing, and shopping for food with a grocery list or after eating.

Avoid using terms like *loss* and *diet;* instead use

reduction or *meal plan* to enhance positive ideas about nutrition. A diet that totally eliminates one food group (*e.g.*, dairy products) or nutrient (*e.g.*, fat, carbohydrate) and fad diets are to be avoided, as deficiencies could develop. Meals are eaten three or more times a day; clients who only eat one or two meals a day may increase fat deposits, cholesterol levels, and snacking habits.

Involving the client in support groups or obtaining support from family and significant others is crucial. Clients with support maintain weight loss better than those with no support. More weight is also lost when spouses or significant others are involved with the process. (See the Sample Nursing Care Plan for the overweight client.)

❥ **Altered Nurtition: Less Than Body Requirements.** Overall, the goal is to promote food intake. Interventions may be as simple as increasing the frequency of feedings to 4 to 6 times a day, assisting with menu selections by completing the menu when the client is unable, or providing a pleasant environment by removing noxious odors and bedpans from sight. Offering the client's favorite food can be beneficial in providing the needed nutrients and energy. Unpleasant procedures, such as dressing changes, can depress the appetite; performing these procedures 2 hours before or after meals is recommended. Suggesting the use of food banks, food pantries, food stamps, or school lunch programs may positively affect a client's or child's nutritional status.

Nuts, some sauces, homogenized milk, sour cream, and ice cream are kilocaloric-dense foods that are offered to increase kilocaloric and protein intake. Snacking before bedtime can also be beneficial.

Exercise is also important for clients with this diagnosis. Exercise can stimulate the appetite and prevent nervous tension, which can cause an excessive use of kilocalories. (See the Sample Nursing Care Plan for the underweight client.)

SAMPLE NURSING CARE PLAN

THE OVERWEIGHT CLIENT

A client is 5 ft, 4 in tall, weighs 150 lbs and has triceps skinfold measurement of 30 mm. During the dietary assessment, the client states, "Food is my life" and "I can't stand those exercise programs.'" Her favorite food is chips and dip.

Nursing Diagnosis: Altered Nutrition: More Than Body Requirements related to excessive intake in relation to physical expenditure.

Expected Outcome: Client will lose 1 to 2 lb/week until desired body weight is obtained.
Client will verbalize three lifestyle changes that will help maintain weight loss within 2 days.

Action	Rationale
1. Discuss eating habits, low-kilocaloric, low-fat foods; provide written material as needed.	1. Client should receive written instructions to have as a resource to indicate which foods are allowed. This also focuses on positive aspects—not on foods that should be avoided.
2. Suggest activities such as walking, swimming, or playing golf or tennis with a partner.	2. Client states she hates exercise programs. These suggestions are more simple activities and sports that the client may be more willing to try and continue, especially if someone else is also involved.
3. Teach relationship among intake, exercise, and weight gain.	3. Knowledge can increase compliance and sense of control.
4. Weigh weekly.	4. Weighing weekly will determine if goal is being met.
5. Devise method of how to include chips and dip in the diet, such as eating baked chips and low-fat dip once a week, only eating 10 chips per day, or suggesting salsa and nonfat sour cream dips rather than fatty dips like sour cream or mayonnaise-based ones.	5. Client says favorite food is chips and dip. This will incorporate favorite food into meal plan, which will increase compliance and sense of ownership with plan. Salsa is a less fattening dip. Baked chips are less fattening than fried chips.
6. Encourage enrollment in a self-help or support group.	6. Client is more likely to follow through with the regimen if support is provided.
7. Document weight and instructions given on the patient record.	7. Documentation is a legal and ethical requirement to indicate that nursing care was individualized and properly implemented.

SAMPLE NURSING CARE PLAN

THE UNDERWEIGHT CLIENT

A client is 5 ft, 6 in tall, weighs 102 lb, and is only eating 20% of ordered diet. During the dietary assessment, the client states, "Food doesn't taste right, and I get full after a few bites." Favorite food is baked potato.

Nursing Diagnosis: Altered Nutrition: Less Than Body Requirements related to anorexia and taste changes.

Expected Outcome: Client will gain 1 to 2 lb/week until desired body weight is obtained.
Client will verbalize two foods that are high in kilocalories within 24 hours.
Client will consume supplements as ordered.

Action	Rationale
1. Offer baked potato with sour cream, butter, and cheese.	1. Favorite food is more likely to be consumed. Adding these kilocaloric-dense toppings can greatly increase intake, and they are likely to be eaten.
2. Weigh weekly.	2. Weighing will determine if goal is being met or if modifications are required.
3. Suggest food high in zinc, such as meats and milk.	3. A deficiency in zinc can cause taste alterations, a symptom the client is experiencing.
4. Encourage milkshakes, custards, dried fruits.	4. Foods that are kilocaloric-dense do not have to be eaten in large amounts to provide needed nutrients and energy.
5. Ask physician for supplements between meals.	5. Because client is not consuming diet, additional intake is required to provide adequate intake of nutrients and kilocalories. Also, client becomes full quickly, so this provides more opportunities to eat.
6. Document weight, percent of diet eaten, and supplements consumed; *i.e.,* "Weight 104 lb, eating 50% of diet, and drinking Ensure between meals."	6. Documentation is a legal and ethical standard that must be followed to indicate proper, safe care was rendered.

Implementation

Flexibility is the key to successful implementation of nutritional interventions. The client's status can change rapidly. One day the client is ready to eat, but the next day he or she refuses. Including the family or significant others at mealtime, especially with elderly clients, is important. Ordering trays for the spouse or family members helps to make mealtime more enjoyable, and many hospitals allow family members to order trays. Changing the routine hospital mealtimes to suit the client's routine may be necessary, especially with the elderly who may like to eat dinner earlier.

Most clients prefer to feed themselves, and, if possible, this should be encouraged, for it enhances self-esteem and feelings of independence; all clients should be allowed to do as much as they are able. Blind clients can usually feed themselves if the nurse describes the food's location in clock terms; *e.g.,* "the meat is at 3 o'clock, and the mashed potatoes are at 12 o'clock." Feeding clients when it is unnecessary can be offensive to some clients and foster dependence in others. Therefore, assess physical ability and nutri-

tional needs before feeding a client. If not sure, the nurse may ask the client in what way assistance is needed.

Several types of clients may need assistance with eating. These are clients with muscle weakness, casts on either arm, fatigue, handicaps, tubes in the dominant arm, joint pain, or tubes in the GI tract. Procedure 27–1 provides detailed steps for assisting clients with eating.

Providing Assistance

Whether the nursing diagnosis is Altered Nutrition: More Than Body Requirements or Less Than Body Requirements, nurses should monitor intake and weight, serve ordered diet or suggest change if indicated, and provide physical (*e.g.,* buttering bread) and emotional support of diet therapy. Emotional support can be as simple as conversing with the client during mealtimes or as complex as dealing with a client with AN who is beginning to put on weight.

For a client with a diagnosis of Less Than Body Requirements, the physician may have to be reminded

PROCEDURE

27–1

ASSISTING THE CLIENT WITH EATING

Action	Rationale
1. Compare client's name band to the name on the tray.	1. To ensure that the right client receives the right meal.
2. Compare the food on the tray to the diet ordered.	2. This ensures that the correct diet is being served.
3. Check to make sure the client does not have an NPO order.	3. No food is given to a patient who is on an NPO order; giving food could prolong the hospital stay or cause rescheduling of needed tests.
4. Place tray on overbed table with plate nearest the client.	4. This allows for easy access to food.
5. Raise head of bed, if permitted, to at least 30 degrees—preferably 90 degress; place client in chair if possible, or place client in side-lying position if raising head is not allowed.	5. Sitting is the preferred position for eating. Raising the head of the bed or placing the client in side-lying position reduces the chance of aspiration.
6. Sit down while feeding the client.	6. Displays to the client that nurse is unhurried and at ease, which will promote intake.
7. Assist as necessary, with, opening food containers, pouring beverages, cutting meat into bite-sized pieces.	7. Accessible food is more likely to be eaten.

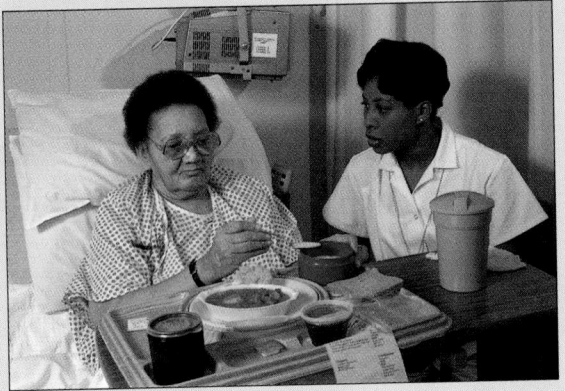

Step 6.

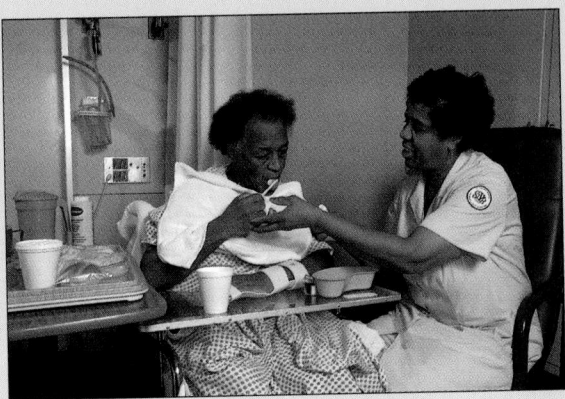

Step 9.

8. Place naking or towel over client's gown.	8. Protects gown and maintains dignity if spills occur.
9. Wipe client's mouth with a napkin as needed.	9. This also maintains a client's dignity.
10. Ask the client if all of one food should be served first, or if he or she prefers to alternate one food with another.	10. Adhering to the client's normal routine of eating will enhance nutrient intake.
11. If client has weak side, place food on good side of mouth.	11. Placing food on the good side enhances swallowing, decreasing the chance of aspiration and pocketing.
12. Converse with the client.	12. Socializing is a natural component of mealtimes and may help the client feel at ease.

how many meals the client has missed because of tests or surgeries or how many days the client has received nutritionally inadequate intake because of the diet ordered or from poor intake. Stimulating the client's appetite is required. This is sometimes easier said than done, because the client may not want to eat because of physical, psychological, cultural, or economic reasons. Nursing tips for stimulating appetite are listed in Table 27–5.

Nursing Measures to Stimulate Appetite

If a diagnosis of More Than Body Requirements is used for the client who is consuming a diet high in

PROCEDURE

27–1

ASSISTING THE CLIENT WITH EATING
(Continued)

Action	Rationale
13. Offer assistive devices as indicated; consult with physical therapy.	**13.** Large-handled eating utensils, plate guard, and special drinking glasses can promote intake and independence.

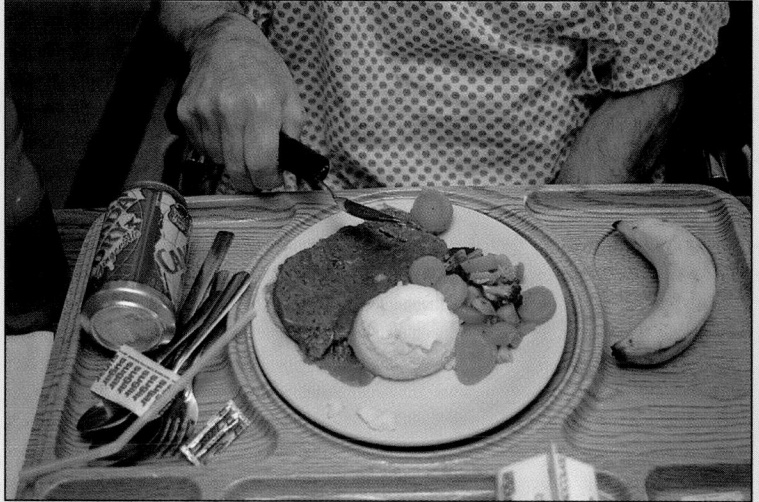
Step 13. *Large-handled utensil*

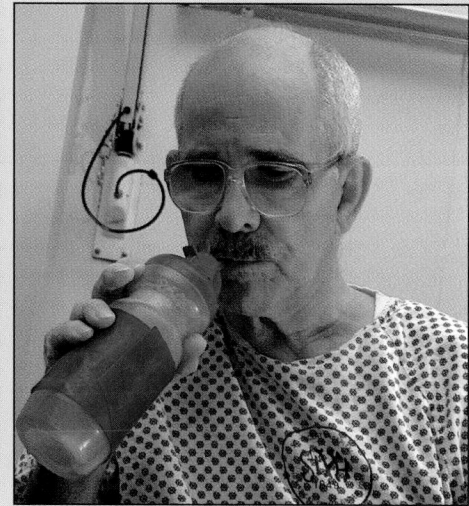
Step 13. *Drinking utensil with special grip*

14. Offer mouth care after meal.	**14.** Oral hygiene decreases the risk of caries and infection.

Documentation: *Document if assistance is needed;* i.e., *"Needed help with eating soup and meat but could handle finger foods on own."*

---

fat, sodium, and/or kilocalories, nursing care involves decreasing intake of the particular nutrients or kilocalories, not eliminating them. Collaboration and time are required for these changes in diet to be accomplished and continued. For example, suppose a client who uses large amounts of salt and consumes excess kilocalories is placed on a low-sodium, kilocalorie-restricted diet. This client is likely to be noncompliant unless the nurse takes time to listen to his or her concerns, feelings, and attitudes about the diet. The client needs to know why the diet is ordered, how sodium and kilocalories affect health or the disease process, and which foods are high and low in sodium and kilocalories. Then, collaboration between the nurse and client facilitates the decision as to which spices or seasonings (such as lemon juice, garlic, or pepper) can be used to help with the sodium restriction and which low-kilocalorie foods can be eaten (*i.e.,* broth soups, lettuce, or skim milk), based on the client's input (Fig. 27–13).

Involving the client in deciding which behavior modification practices to implement may be beneficial. A change in usual habits is needed to keep weight off. Anyone can go on a diet, but long-term weight maintenance requires lifelong behavior change. List several examples and then let the client decide which behavior modification to try.

Diet Modifications

The oral route is the preferred method of providing nutrients, as long as nutrients can be provided in adequate amounts and the GI tract is functional (bowel sounds normal). However, some disease processes require a special or modified diet.

The American Dietetic Association has published the *Handbook of Clinical Dietetics* (1992) and the *Manual of Clinical Dietetics* (1992). The manual is very comprehensive, and the handbook describes the scientific basis for diet therapy and lists foods and

Table 27–5

NURSING MEASURES TO STIMULATE APPETITE

NURSING ACTION	RATIONALE
If needed, give pain medication 30 minutes before meals	Pain can cause a decrease in intake
Plan a 30-minute rest period before meals	This allows the client to conserve energy for eating and digesting food
Offer mouth care before meals	This stimulates saliva production, moistening and freshening the mouth, which promotes eating
Insert dentures as indicated	Dentures provide mechanical means for adequate chewing, which facilitates digestion
Offer to wash client's hands and face before meals	Appetite is enhanced if personal comfort is experienced
Keep the food at proper temperature (use microwave as needed) or make arrangements for client to receive tray at a later time if the tray cannot be served because of factors such as tests, surgeries	Foods that are at proper temperature are more easily consumed
Remove tray cover outside of client's room	If the cover is removed in the client's room, the combined odors may be offensive to the client and cause nausea
Limit fluid intake during meals; offer fluid between meals	Fluids can occupy more space in the stomach, thus creating a "full" feeling and decreasing intake
Encourage eating with family, friend, or other clients	Socializing at mealtimes is the custom in this culture and will enhance intake
Praise for any intake but do not be harsh if intake is low	Praised behavior is repeated

sample menus for specific diets. If questions arise as to what foods may be eaten, these books can serve as reference material for both the nurse and client. Familiarity with these diets will allow the nurse to suggest substitutes when indicated, choose allowable foods when the client wants to snack, and determine whether food brought in by family, friends, or significant others is appropriate. Consultation with the dietitian is also helpful.

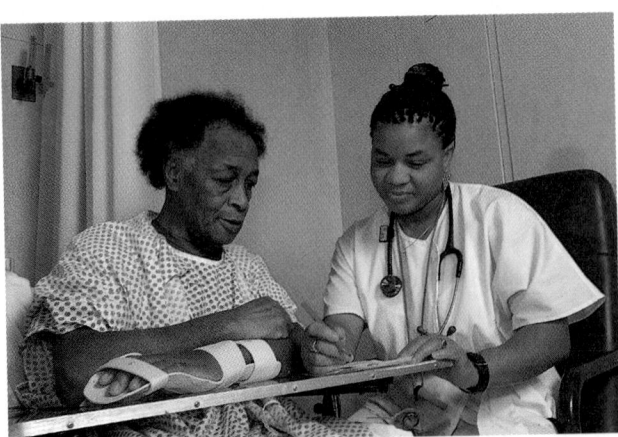

❧ **Figure 27–13**
Collaboration between the nurse and client in the selection of foods will help the client understand the reason for any dietary restrictions. Choice also encourages eating in clients with poor intake.

Since the diet is on the orders, no documentation is necessary in the nurse's notes unless modifications and/or teaching is indicated. For example, say the client is on a regular diet, but the nurse discovers that the client has no teeth and no dentures. The nurse documents the following: "Doctor called to see if diet could be changed because of having no teeth or dentures. New orders received (mechanical soft)."

❧ **Regular.** This diet has no restrictions; the client can eat whatever is desired. In some facilities, this is called a general diet. Usually there are no problems with this diet. However, feeding times, preparation, and foods offered are different from the client's normal routine, so criticisms may occur.

❧ **Soft or Mechanical Soft.** When a client cannot tolerate a regular diet, a soft diet may be ordered. Soft diets may be designed to be easily chewed or provide minimal fiber. The reason for the diet affects the specific foods included. Broiled and baked foods are served, but fried foods, rich pastries, highly spiced foods, and raw vegetables are avoided to minimize gas, distention, and nausea. Because fiber is limited, the nurse should monitor the client for constipation. Fluids, activity, and small, frequent feedings can be implemented on a soft diet if constipation develops.

For a client who has no teeth or has chewing or

swallowing difficulties, a mechanical soft diet is recommended. In some facilities, this is termed a dental soft diet. This resembles the regular diet in the food that is offered, but if the food is too tough to chew, the food is chopped, ground, or puréed. Usually no problems are encountered with this diet.

♦ **Puréed.** Soft, smooth, easily swallowed foods that require no chewing are offered on a puréed diet. This diet is indicated for the following clients: those learning to swallow again, as after a stroke; those experiencing head and neck abnormalities, such as in cancer; or those having their jaws wired for a jaw fracture. A puréed diet resembles a soft diet that is blenderized. Many clients do not like this diet because it reminds them of baby food. Careful observance of the client's intake is essential to ensure that food intake is optimal. Nurses can increase intake if they make comments positive, not negative (*e.g.*, "Here is your meal; which would you like to eat first, the meat or the vegetable?" rather than "This stuff looks awful; I'm glad you're eating it and not me"). A technique that is gaining popularity with puréed diets is component puréeing, which adds an instant food thickener to the puréed food to add consistency and allow the foods to be shaped back into their original form.

♦ **Dysphagia.** When the client is prone to aspiration because of swallowing difficulties, a dysphagia diet is ordered. Careful coordinating with the dietary and speech-language personnel is essential, because this diet varies widely from institution to institution and from client to client. The thickness of liquids will be specified: thin liquids (*e.g.*, water, apple juice, milk, tea, coffee, sherbet), medium thick (*e.g.*, vegetable juice, nectars, eggnog, cream soups, ice cream) or spoon thick (*e.g.*, yogurt, pudding). This specification must be followed, even when fluids are offered with medications. Liquids, especially thin, are easily aspirated, because liquids are more difficult to manipulate in the mouth. Special powders are available to thicken even thin liquids to desired thickness to reduce chance of aspiration.

Depending on the severity of the swallowing problems, clients may be NPO or have puréed, soft, or finely chopped foods. Raw vegetables (*e.g.*, carrots, apple), tough foods (*e.g.*, celery, melba toast), chewy foods (*e.g.*, raisins), and small-kernel foods (*e.g.*, peas, corn, nuts, popcorn) are to be avoided. Generally, frequent, small meals are served to prevent overtiring of the client. Frequent, small meals can decrease chance of aspiration and maintain nutrient intake.

With the dysphagia diet, the nurse observes for pocketing of food, especially on the weak or affected side, by inspecting the inside of the mouth. Clients may not be aware that food is still in their mouth, making them prone to aspiration. Manual removal of food may be necessary. Oral suction equipment should be nearby. If on tracheal suctioning, the secretions are green or are the same color as the food eaten, the nurse should suspect aspiration. With aspiration, clients may also exhibit bluish, dusky skin color, increased respiratory rate, and abnormal breath sounds on auscultation. Because talking increases the risk of choking or aspirating, the nurse should limit conversation during meals with the client who is dysphagic. With the threat of aspiration ever present, teaching the client and family the Heimlich maneuver can be a life-saving technique.

♦ **Clear Liquids.** As the name indicates, only clear liquids or foods that liquify at room temperature, such as gelatin, are allowed. This diet is ordered when the client experiences vomiting, diarrhea, or surgery. Because this diet is inadequate in all nutrients, the nurse must remind the physician after 48 hours that the client is still on this diet. Some facilities have eliminated this diet because of the nutrient inadequacies. Supplements such as high-protein, high-kilocalorie broth mixes are being added to supply the missing nutrients.

♦ **Full Liquids.** This diet is served to postoperative clients, especially after dental (*e.g.*, wired jaws), facial (*e.g.*, cancer), or neck (*e.g.*, tonsillectomy) surgeries. This diet is also utilized for clients unable to tolerate solid foods. All items on the clear liquid diet plus milk and milk-containing products that liquefy at room temperature are allowed. If the client requires more protein, then adding nonfat dry milk or puréed meats to liquids is advisable. If the client develops diarrhea, bloating, and flatus, notify the dietitian or physician; lactose intolerance may be occurring. Using lactose-free supplements may be required. Another factor to consider is that this diet is high in cholesterol. If the client's fat or lipid level is high or if he or she has heart disease, notify the dietary department to substitute skim milk for whole milk.

♦ **Low Fat or Low Cholesterol.** A low-fat and/or low-cholesterol diet is desirable to help reduce the incidence of heart disease by preventing atherosclerosis. Fat and cholesterol can cause plaque to form on the inside of vessels, accelerating the process of atherosclerosis. Substituting foods that contain monounsaturated or polyunsaturated fat for those containing saturated fats is recommended. Therefore, foods that are low in saturated fat and cholesterol are offered. Thus, some foods to avoid are gravies, lard, whole milk, egg yolks, fried foods, organ meats, and butter.

♦ **Sodium Restricted.** As the name implies, sodium is restricted to 2 to 3 g (mild), 1 g (moderate), 0.5 g (strict), or 0.25 g (severe). This diet is usually used when the client has high blood pressure, a heart attack, or heart disorders. Since water goes where sodium goes, when sodium is reduced, total fluid volume is decreased, which lowers blood pressure, heart workload, and excess fluid levels. Depending on the level of restriction, foods containing high amounts of sodium, such as potato chips, bacon, ham, canned goods, some frozen foods, and soy sauce, are reduced or eliminated from the diet.

Diabetic. When a client who has diabetes mellitus follows the "exchange system" diet, it is frequently referred to as the ADA diet. These exchange lists were developed by the American Diabetes Association, the American Dietetic Association, and the US Public Health Service to provide flexibility in meal planning and constancy of carbohydrate, protein, fat, and kilocaloric intake. There are six exchange lists. Within each list, the foods listed are approximately equal in kilocalories, carbohydrate, fat, and protein content. However, the lists are not quite the same as the Food Guide Pyramid food groups. In the ADA diet, cheese is in the meat group because of its high protein content, and starchy vegetables (*e.g.*, potatoes, corn, peas) are placed in the bread/starch list.

The standard ADA diet is three meals with a bedtime snack. The overall dietary goal is to keep the blood glucose level stable—not elevated or depressed; the glucose level must be stable for the body to function properly. Because this diet is followed for a lifetime and is such a change for the client, a dietary

consult is advised; a consult with the diabetic educator, if available, is also recommended.

Diet as Tolerated. Usually abbreviated as DAT, a diet as tolerated requires collaboration between the nurse and client. The client's preferences determine the diet ordered. For example, if the client wants a soft diet, a soft diet is ordered. After some surgeries, DAT is ordered. Discretion on the nurse's part may be needed. For example, if the client wants chicken noodle soup, this should be given to the client. However, if the client wants steak and potatoes immediately after surgery, the nurse may have to discourage this type of intake and suggest an alternative meal.

Overall, regardless of whether the client is on a regular diet, modified diet, or special diet, "food should be enjoyed for its taste and texture and the social opportunities it affords rather than be seen as a medicine which must be eaten in the prescribed amounts" (Halliday, 1991, p. 27).

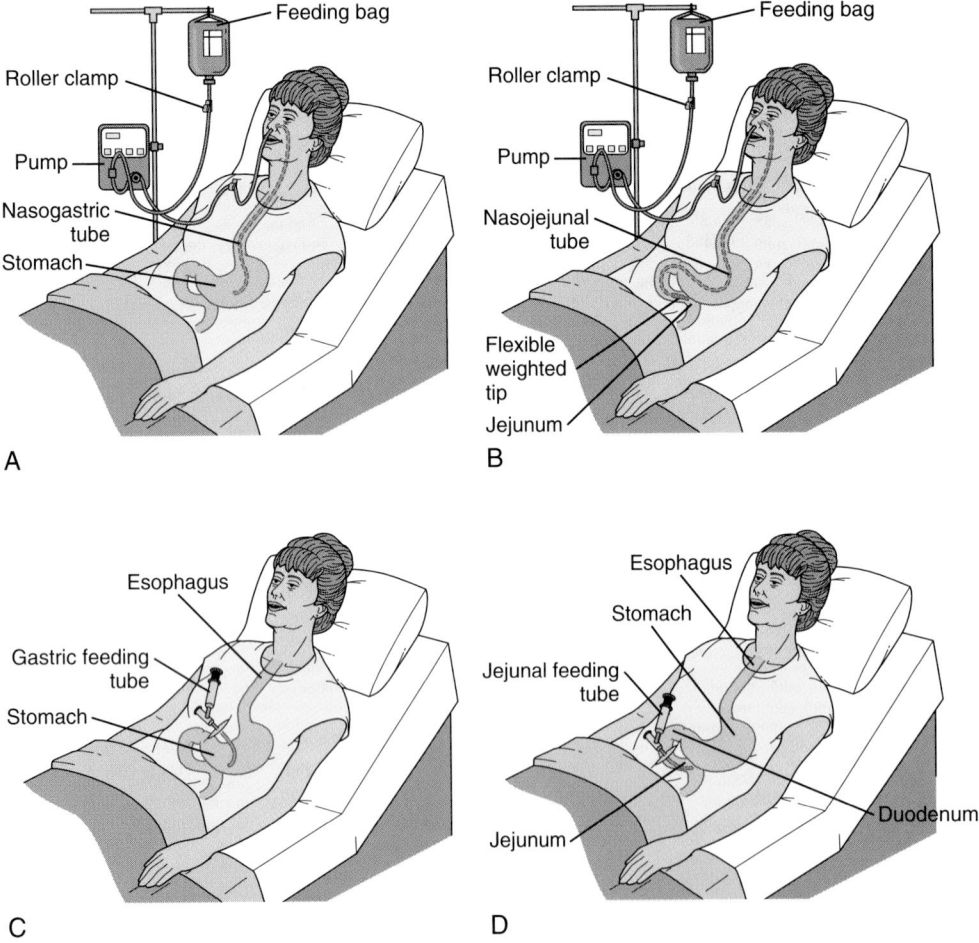

Figure 27–14
The client who has a functional GI tract but is unable to eat can be given enteral nutrition via the nose to the stomach *(panel A)* or directly into the stomach *(panel C)* if there is no danger of aspiration. If there is a risk of aspiration, enteral nutrition can be given via the nose to the duodenum or proximal jejunum *(panel B)* or directly into the jejunum *(panel D)*. Note that if the client is unable to eat and has a nonfunctional GI tract, total parenteral nutrition must be given via a central venous line (see Fig. 27–15).

✦ **Enteral Nutrition.** If the GI tract is not stimulated, the small and large bowel will atrophy. When the GI tract is functional but oral intake is not feasible, enteral nutrition is the treatment of choice. Clients with swallowing problems, burns, major trauma, liver failure, or severe malnutrition warrant enteral nutrition.

Enteral nutrition provides liquified foods into the GI tract via a tube; this type of feeding is commonly called tube feeding or enteral feeding. The tube can enter the GI tract via the nose to stomach (nasogastric), nose to duodenum or jejunum (nasoduodenal/nasojejunal), or directly into stomach (gastrostomy) or jejunum (jejunostomy) (Fig. 27–14). Most tubes are small in diameter for ease of passage and lessening of tissue irritation. Nurses can insert nasogastric, nasoduodenal, and nasojejunal tubes, but the other tubes must be placed during surgery. Another technique called the percutaneous endoscopic gastrostomy al- lows the stomach tube to be inserted by the physician at the bedside. When nurses insert the feeding tube, it is also performed at the bedside (see Procedure 27–2).

Tube feedings can be administered in three ways: by bolus, continuously, or cyclically. Cyclic feedings are given either in the daytime or nighttime for 8 to 16 hours. Feedings at night allow for more freedom during the day. As the name implies, continuous feedings are given continually for 24 hours a day. An infusion pump regulates the flow. Continuous feedings are the preferred method in a hospital setting. Bolus feedings resemble normal meal-feeding patterns. About every 3 to 6 hours, approximately 300 to 400 ml of ordered formula are administered over a 30- to 60-minute period. Enteral feeding bags are connected to a gravity drip system, in which a manually controlled mechanism regulates flow rate of the feeding, or an infusion

---

PROCEDURE

27–2

INSERTING A SMALL-BORE FEEDING TUBE

Equipment:

Clean gloves
8- to 12-French feeding tube
    with stylet or guidewire
30-ml Syringe
pH test strips
Tape
Straw in glass of water
Emesis basin
Tongue blade
Towel

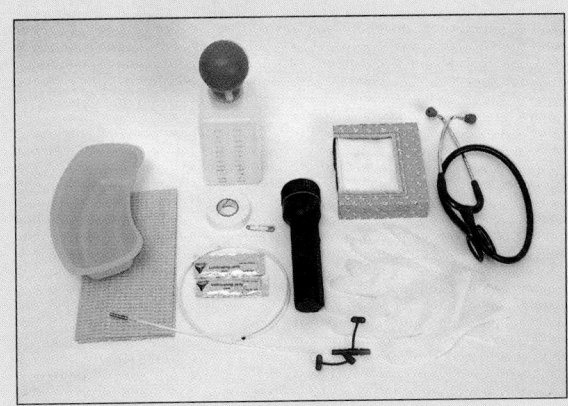

Action	**Rationale**
1. Check physician's order	1. Inserting a tube feeding requires a doctor's order.
2. Explain procedure to client.	2. Knowledge increases compliance and cooperation and decreases fear of the unknown.
3. Wash hands.	3. Washing hands decreases chance of infection by decreasing the number of microorganisms.
4. Stand on right side of bed if right handed; if left handed, stand on left side of bed.	4. This allows the nurse to easily use the dominant hand for insertion.
5. Elevate head of bed to 90 degrees if possible; if not, elevate to a 30- to 45-degree angle.	5. This position decreases chance of aspiration and facilitates insertion of tube.
6. Place towel over client's chest.	6. If vomiting occurs, the client's gown will be protected.
7. Ask client to breathe normally and occlude one nare at a time to determine which nostril has the greater air flow.	7. This helps determine which nostril to use (the one with the greatest air flow).

Continued

PROCEDURE

27–2

INSERTING A SMALL-BORE FEEDING TUBE
(Continued)

Action	Rationale

8. Measure length of tube and mark with tape. Choose one of the following methods:
  a. Using the distal end of the feeding tube, measure from tip of nose to earlobe to xiphoid process.
      OR
  b. Measure 20 in from distal tip of tube and mark, then measure from tip of nose to earlobe to xiphoid process; the midpoint between these two measurements is the length.
	8. These methods ensure tube is inserted into stomach.

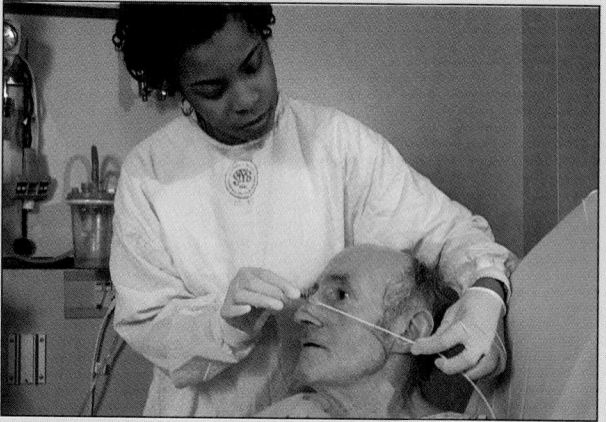

Step 8A.

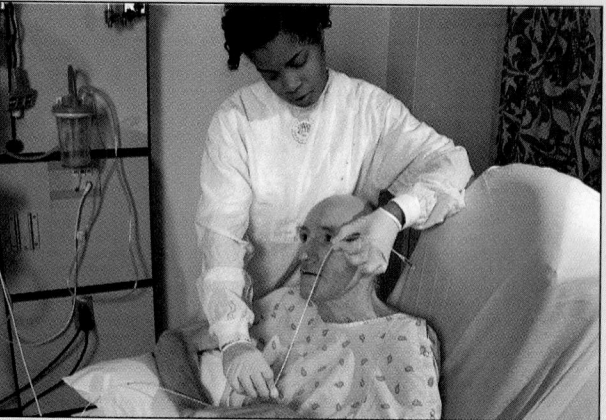

Step 8B.

9. Insert 10 ml of water into feeding tube; then insert guidewire into feeding tube, checking to make sure guidewire does not protrude through tube.	9. Water helps guidewire insert easier, and insertion of guidewire enhances passage of tube. Since the tube is so small and flexible, some stiffness is required to aid the passage of the tube into the stomach without coiling.
10. Insert distal tip of tube into a glass of water.	10. This activates lubricant, making insertion easier.
11. Prepare tape by splitting one end lengthwise and leaving the other end intact.	11. Preparing tape early can enhance proper anchoring of the tube in a timely manner.
12. Don clean gloves.	12. Gloves protect the nurse, since contact with body fluids is likely.

pump, which automatically controls flow rate. The nurse is responsible for initiating, maintaining, and regulating feedings (see Procedure 27–3, "Giving Enteral Feedings").

The nurse is also responsible for recognizing complications that can occur with tube feedings (Box 27–3). Most complications can be averted or lessened if the nurse is knowledgeable and observant.

Diarrhea is a common complication and develops for many reasons: (1) a too-concentrated feeding is given, (2) the feeding is contaminated with bacteria, (3) the feeding is too cold, (4) the feeding lacks fiber, (5) medications ordered cause a side effect of diarrhea, or (6) the client is malnourished. Treatment with an isotonic feeding may be beneficial. Before adding fresh feeding formula to the enteral bag, rinse it with water (Kohn & Keithley, 1989) to decrease the chance of infection, which can cause diarrhea. Follow institutional policies for hanging and changing a feeding delivery system to decrease the chance of contamination, thereby reducing infection. Before administering feedings, nurses should check the feeding to make sure that it is at room temperature. Extremes in temperatures can irritate the GI tract. During normal meal

PROCEDURE

27–2

INSERTING A SMALL-BORE FEEDING TUBE
(Continued)

Action	Rationale
13. Insert tube through nostril to back of throat by directing tube back and down.	**13.** This follows the natural curves of the body.

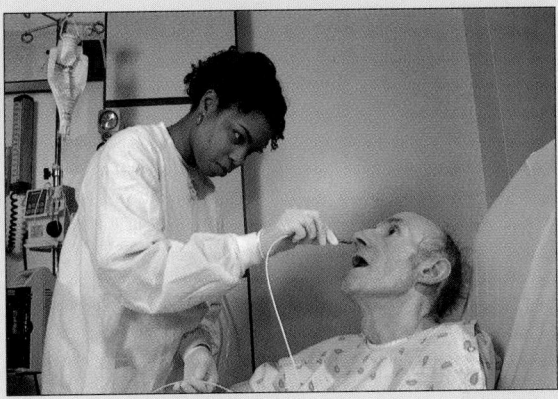

Step 13.

Action	Rationale
14. When tube reaches back of the throat, ask client to flex head forward and swallow.	**14.** Leaning the head forward decreases chance of tube entering the trachea by closing the glottis. Swallowing enhances insertion of the tube.
15. Have client swallow, using straw placed in the glass of water.	**15.** This facilitates the swallowing reflex.
16. Advance and rotate the tube 180 degrees while the client is swallowing.	**16.** All of these techniques decrease friction and enhance tube insertion.
17. Advance tube to predetermined measurement.	**17.** This ensures tube is in stomach.
18. Wait several seconds before advancing tube if client gags.	**18.** This allows client to rest. Some gagging is expected, since the gag reflex is stimulated by the passage of the tube.
19. Do not force the tube if it meets resistance.	**19.** This could cause trauma to the throat and esophagus.
20. Pull back on the tube (do not pull the tube completely out of the nostril, just to the back of the throat) if client experiences severe gagging, coughing, choking, or cyanosis.	**20.** The tube has entered the trachea rather than the esophagus, or the tube could be kinked or coiled.
21. Verify tube placement by at least one of the following methods: (1) aspirate gastric contents with syringe and measure pH with test strips (should be 4 or less) or (2) obtain x-rays.	**21.** This verifies that tube is in stomach and not the lungs.

Continued

ingestion, food moves from the mouth to the stomach, allowing for changes in the food's temperature. However, during tube feedings, this process is interrupted.

Aspiration, another complication of tube feedings, can be life threatening. An incorrectly placed tube can result in aspiration. Confirmation of tube placement is necessary before tube feedings are initiated. The best method to check placement is by x-ray. Nurses can aspirate gastric contents with a syringe or listen with a stethoscope over the epigastric region of the upper abdomen for a "swishing" sound while air is injected via syringe into the tube. However, if a small-diameter tube is inserted, aspiration of stomach contents may not be possible (Metheny *et al.*, 1988), and auscultation with a stethoscope may be inaccurate (Metheny *et al.*, 1990). If clients have frequent coughing spells, a decreased level of consciousness, an absent or depressed gag reflex, frequent suctioning, or upper airway tubes, they are prone to tube displacement, in-

PROCEDURE

27–2

INSERTING A SMALL-BORE FEEDING TUBE
(Continued)

Action	Rationale
22. Tape tube in place by placing intact end of tape on the bridge of the nose and wrapping the two split ends around the tube.	**22.** This holds the tube in place so it does not dislodge. Placing the tape as described also decreases pressure on the nares, so trauma and possible skin breakdown are lessened.

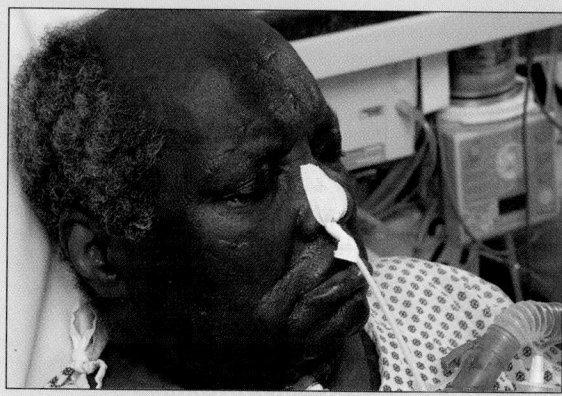

Step 22.

23. Slowly remove guidewire. Do not try to partially or fully reinsert guidewire once removed.	**23.** Guidewire needs to be removed so feedings may be initiated. If you try to partially or fully reinsert guidewire, trauma or perforation of the GI tract, especially of the esophagus, may occur.
24. Dispose of, clean, or store equipment as needed; remove gloves, and wash hands.	**24.** Ensures that nurse follows universal precautions to decrease spread of microorganisms.

Documentation: *Chart "10-French feeding tube placed with minimal gagging, aspirated greenish, yellowish fluid with a pH of 3."*

---

creasing the chance of aspiration (Metheny *et al.*, 1987).

Obstructed or clogged tubes can be problematic for the nurse and the client. Water, not normal saline, is the best irrigant for clogged tubes. Clogged tubes can mean missed feedings (Petrosino *et al.*, 1989), causing an inadequate intake of needed nutrients. Prevention is the best treatment. For bolus and continuous feedings, flush the tube with 20 to 50 ml of water after checking residuals, before and after administering drugs, and anytime the feeding is stopped (Bockus, 1991).

Whenever possible, use liquid forms of medicines. If this is not feasible, crush the medication and dissolve it in 10 ml of warm water before administering. Crushing time-released capsules is contraindicated. Spansules (*i.e.*, Theo-Dur [theophylline]) should not be crushed, because they do not dissolve and clog tubes easily.

Vomiting can result when the feeding is too large or given too fast. When the bolus feeding is quickly forced into the stomach, excessive pressure is likely to cause vomiting. If air enters the tube during feeding, gastric distention or reflux could occur, resulting in vomiting. Abdominal cramping and reflux can be avoided if the temperature of the feeding is at room temperature. Taking one's time lessens the chance of causing vomiting.

Numerous clients are discharged with enteral feedings. Many nursing interventions are the same as if the client was in the hospital, but there are some differences (see Box 27–4).

✦ **Total Parenteral Nutrition.** When the GI tract is severely dysfunctional or nonfunctional, total parenteral nutrition (TPN) is required to prevent subcutaneous fat and muscle protein from being catabolized by the body for energy. TPN solutions are provided and prepared by the pharmacy. Typical clients who receive TPN include those with multiple GI surgeries, GI

PROCEDURE

27–3

GIVING ENTERAL FEEDINGS

Equipment:

Feeding formula
Feeding pump
Clean examination gloves
Stethoscope
Feeding bag with tubing
50-ml Syringe
Catheter-tipped syringe

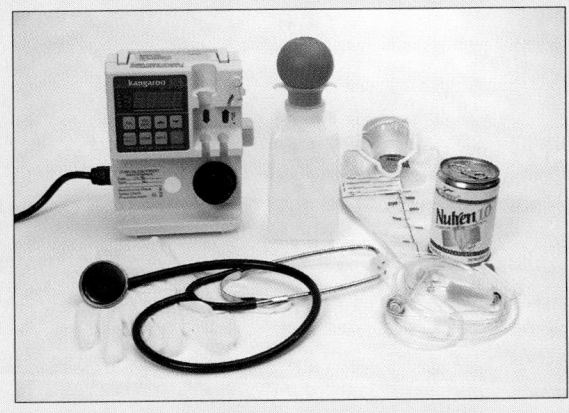

Action	**Rationale**
1. Check orders.	1. Enteral feeding requires an order.
2. Explain to client.	2. Knowledge increases compliance and cooperation and decreases fear of the unknown.
3. Position client in high Fowler's and on right side if comatose.	3. This helps prevent aspiration by gravity, and lying on right side enhances passage of formula to stomach, which is located on the right side.
4. Wash hands and don clean gloves.	4. This provides protection by following universal precautions.
5. Warm feeding to room temperature.	5. Cold feedings can cause diarrhea and cramps.
6. Verify placement of tube.	6. This confirms that the tube is in the stomach and not the lungs.
7. Aspirate all stomach contents (residual), measure amount, and return contents to stomach.	7. The amount of residual determines whether the feeding should be given. Usually if residual is less than 100 to 150 ml, give the feeding; if more than 150 ml, hold the feeding. Replacing the contents into the stomach prevents electrolyte imbalances.

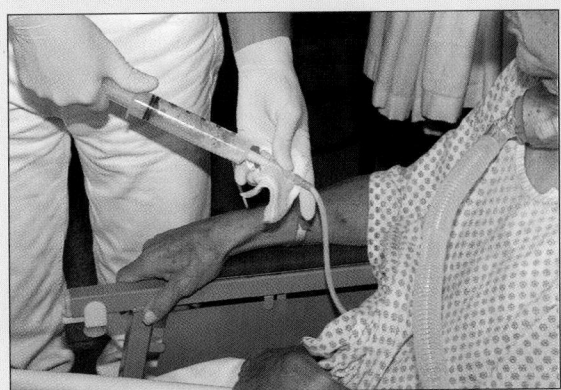

Step 7.

Continued

PROCEDURE

27–3

GIVING ENTERAL FEEDINGS
(Continued)

Action	Rationale
8. Assess bowel sounds.	**8.** Bowel sounds indicate peristalsis is occurring. Peristalsis is necessary for proper digestion of formula.
9. For bolus feedings: pinch the feeding tube; remove plunger from barrel of syringe; attach syringe to feeding tube and fill with prescribed amount of formula; elevate syringe to 18 in or less above client; unpinch tube; infuse formula between 30 and 60 minutes; do not let the syringe run dry; follow with water; clamp end of tube.	**9.** Following these procedures will decrease chance of complications and provide needed nutrients safely.

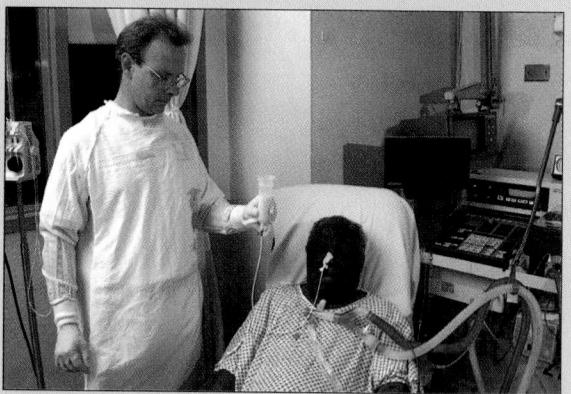

Step 9.

10. For continuous or cyclic feedings: attach feeding bag and tubing to intravenous pole; attach feeding bag and tubing to distal end of feeding tube; thread tubing through pump; set rate.	**10.** Following these procedures will decrease chance of complications and provide needed nutrients safely.

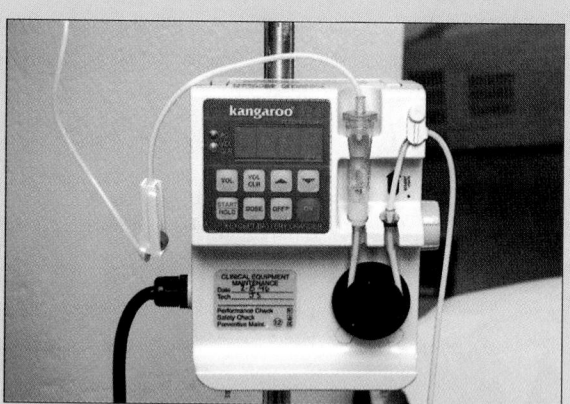

Step 10. *Kangaroo feeding pump for continuous feedings*

11. Flush tubing with prescribed amount of water.	**11.** Water helps maintain fluid balance and patency of tube.
12. For bolus feeding, leave client in a high Fowler's or at least elevated to 30 degrees for 30 minutes after feeding. If continuous, keep client in a 30-degree position at all times.	**12.** This helps reduce the incidence of aspiration.
13. Remove gloves and wash hands.	**13.** Following universal precautions decreases chance of contamination.

Documentation: *Active bowel sounds in all four quadrants. Returned residual of 50 ml into stomach. 250 ml of formula administered over 30 minutes in a high Fowler's position. Feeding followed with 30 ml of water. No nausea or vomiting.*

Box 27–3

NURSING CARE FOR COMPLICATIONS OF ENTERAL FEEDINGS

Diarrhea

- Suggest using fiber-containing feedings
- Administer feedings slowly and at room temperature

Aspiration

- Verify tube placement as needed
- Do not give feeding if residual is greater than 150 ml
- Keep head of bed elevated to 30 degrees at all times if on continuous feedings
- If on bolus feedings, elevate head of bed to at least 30 degrees, preferably 60 to 90, and keep in that position for 30 minutes after the feeding.
- If aspiration has occurred, suction as needed; monitor for temperature increase, since aspiration pneumonia may occur; auscultate lung sounds; assess respiratory rate; and obtain chest x-ray if necessary

Clogged Tube

- Avoid adding medication directly into formula
- Use liquid forms of medication whenever possible
- Flush tube with water before and after medication administration
- Flush tube with 20 to 50 ml water before and after bolus feedings
- For continuous feedings, flush tube with water every 4 hours

Vomiting

- Administer feedings slowly; for continuous feedings, use a slow rate; for bolus feedings, make feeding last for at least 30 minutes
- Measure abdominal girth
- Do not let the feeding run dry
- Do not let air enter the tubing
- Administer feeding at room temperature
- Elevate head of bed at least 30 degrees
- Administer antiemetic as ordered
- If client has vomited, place in side-lying position with head lowered to decrease chance of aspiration; suction if needed; offer oral care; if vomiting continues, tube may have to be discontinued

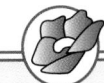

COMMUNITY-BASED CARE

ENTERAL FEEDINGS

Home enteral feedings may be initiated as a continuation of hospital care or may be initiated in the home setting. Careful planning, client and caregiver education, and support are essential components for successful enteral therapy. Some planning issues are as follows:

1. Reimbursement must be assessed; if limited, the client must understand any financial responsibility.

2. Enteral therapy must be medically necessary to sustain nutrition; common indications include neurological disorders with inability to swallow or suck (infants) and head or neck malignancy.

3. The client or caregiver must be capable of learning to administer the feedings; in many cases, enteral therapy may be a permanent form of nutrition and thus lifestyle.

4. If tube feedings are initiated in the home setting, the dietitian is consulted for nutritional assessment and recommendations regarding appropriate calories and feeding administration plan.

Education by the home care nurse includes

1. Feeding tube care

2. Feeding administration method—pump, gravity

3. Potential complications

4. Storage, management, and reordering of supplies

5. Handwashing and maintaining clean supplies, equipment, and environment

6. Resources and telephone numbers for questions and troubleshooting

Tube feeding dependence is difficult for many clients. They must adjust to the inability to enjoy food. They may avoid the kitchen and sitting down at the dinner table, where much socialization occurs. This is also difficult for the family. It is important to encourage both client and family to verbalize their concerns and feelings. A national support and information group for these clients exists; local support groups may also be available.

---

trauma, severe intolerance to enteral feedings, intestinal obstructions, and cancer. Clients with acquired immunodeficiency syndrome and malnourished clients who require surgery have become more frequent candidates for TPN. In some clients, the bowels must be rested for healing to occur; TPN is the method of choice for providing these clients with the needed nutrients.

Total parenteral nutrition is a feeding method that supplies necessary nutrients via veins; carbohydrates in the form of dextrose, fats in special emulsified form, proteins in the form of amino acids, vitamins, minerals, and water can all be provided. Two routes may be utilized: peripheral veins or central veins. Peripheral veins are used for short periods (5–7 days) and when the client only needs small concentrations of carbohydrate, fats, and proteins. Central veins (sub-

HOME ENTERAL NUTRITION

Intensive training while the client and family is in the hospital is essential to avert complications at home and to enhance compliance. A multidisciplinary team addresses physical, emotional, psychological, social, and financial aspects of home enteral nutrition. Providing written instructions is a must.

Bolus and cyclic feedings are the preferred method at home to facilitate normal activities of daily living. To decrease costs, the delivery system can be reused when bolus and cyclic feedings are chosen. Rinsing the set-up daily with either soapy water or diluted vinegar and then rinsing again with tap water allows the set-up to be used for 7 days without contamination (Grunow *et al.*, 1989).

Findings that suggest that the client is having trouble adjusting to home enteral feedings are frequent tube complications, weight loss despite adequate levels of protein and kilocalories provided in the feedings, and missing or overstocking pieces of equipment (Gulledge *et al.*, 1987). The nurse assesses the situation to determine if physical, psychological, economical, and/or social factors are interfering with adaptation. Goals and interventions are devised based on the information obtained.

can insert the catheter for peripheral lines, but the physician or intern places central lines, with the nurse assisting.

Methods to deliver TPN resemble those for enteral feedings: continuous or cyclic. Continuous infusion with the use of an infusion pump is the preferred method in the hospital setting.

A nurse's responsibility during TPN involves assessing, cleansing, and maintaining the intravenous line, educating the client and family about TPN, and detecting or preventing complications. The intravenous site is assessed for redness, swelling, tenderness, or drainage. Any of these signs could indicate that the line must be moved to another site. Cleansing the site, especially for central lines, with aseptic technique is crucial.

Teach the client and family the rationale for TPN: For peripheral route, the rationale is to prevent further deterioration of nutritional status, whereas central lines are used to promote cell growth and repair. The protein in the feeding enhances growth and repair; dextrose supplies the body's main source of energy (glucose) and allows protein to do its job; and fat emulsions provide a source of concentrated kilocalories and help prevent a deficiency of linoleic acid. Assuring the client or family that the body's nutritional needs are being met even though food is not ingested is helpful. Sometimes clients experience hunger pains and food cravings: Because the stomach is receiving no food, it sends messages to the brain that food is needed (Rodriguez, 1992). This is normal and not a cause for alarm; the body is receiving nutrients in a different manner that bypasses the stomach.

Nurses also monitor for infection, hyperglycemia, fluid overload, and air embolism, complications of TPN (Box 27–5). Infection, either at the intravenous site or in the bloodstream, is a common problem of

clavian or internal jugular) are chosen when the feedings must last for longer than 7 days and when the client requires a large concentration of carbohydrate (greater than 10% dextrose) (Fig. 27–15). The high rates of blood flow through the larger veins dilute the large concentration of dextrose rapidly. (If this large concentration is given in the peripheral veins, inflammation and scarring of the vessels will result.) Nurses

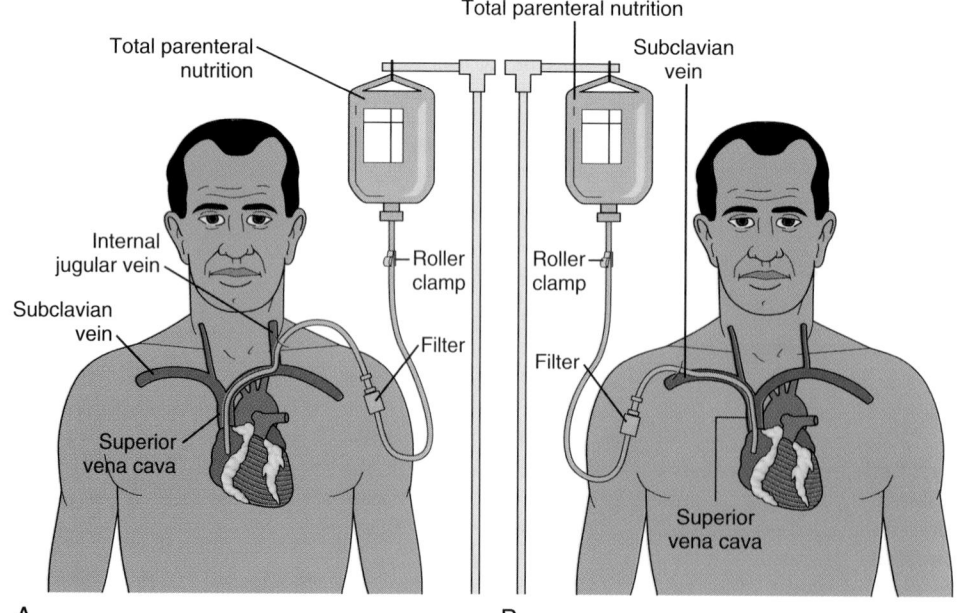

Total parenteral nutrition

Total parenteral nutrition

Subclavian vein

Internal jugular vein

Subclavian vein

Roller clamp

Roller clamp

Filter

Filter

Superior vena cava

Superior vena cava

A   B

🍝 **Figure 27–15**
Total parenteral nutrition is a type of nutritional support given to the client with a severely dysfunctional GI tract. TPN can be infused through a central venous line through the internal jugular vein *(panel A)* or the subclavian vein *(panel B)*.

NURSING CARE FOR COMPLICATIONS OF TOTAL PARENTERAL NUTRITION

Infection

- Monitor site for redness, swelling, warmth, tenderness, and increased body temperature and white blood cells—all are signs of infection
- Discontinue intravenous line if infection is present
- Maintain strict asepsis while preparing, cleansing, and administering intravenous fluid

Hyperglycemia

- Monitor for deep, rapid breathing, excessive urinary output, and malaise—all signs of hyperglycemia
- Place fluid on pump and monitor hourly
- Never "speed up" parenteral feeding
- Monitor glucose and ketone levels as ordered
- Give insulin if needed

Fluid Overload

- Monitor for bounding pulse, jugular vein distention, increased blood pressure, headache, and crackles on lung auscultation—all signs of fluid overload
- Maintain intravenous fluid on pump and monitor hourly
- Monitor intake and output
- Weigh daily

Air Embolism

- Teach client to use the Valsalva maneuver whenever the line is opened
- Tape tubing connections so that they cannot come apart accidentally
- Place in left side-lying position with head lower than feet if air embolism is suspected
- Contact physician

TPN. The high concentration of glucose is an ideal medium for bacteria growth. Strict asepsis while preparing and administering the fluid is paramount to prevent contamination. Cleaning and tubing or fluid change procedures must be strictly followed.

Because large amounts of glucose are being infused into the body, hyperglycemia is common. Never "speed up" the intravenous rate if the rate of infusion falls behind; this could lead to extremely high levels of glucose, predisposing clients to hyperglycemia. Blood or urine levels should be monitored for glucose. If the glucose levels are high, insulin may be given to return the blood glucose to normal. Clients and families are informed that the client has not developed diabetes, but that the high glucose levels are a result of the glucose in the feedings. When feedings are discontinued, insulin will no longer be required.

"Speeding up" the intravenous rate or administering the feeding at a too-rapid rate could lead to fluid overload, placing undue stress on the cardiac and respiratory systems. TPN is always administered using an infusion pump that automatically controls the flow rate. Checking the flow rate and settings on the pump hourly can avert this complication.

Another complication that could be fatal is air embolism. If air gets into the tubing, it enters the bloodstream and travels to the heart, causing life-threatening heart and lung problems. To prevent air embolism, the client is taught to perform the Valsalva maneuver whenever the line must be opened for tubing or bag changes.

Home TPN can be effective, safe, and economical for clients who do not require acute or long-term physical care. A multidisciplinary team approach is used to prepare the client and family for home TPN. Training may last from to 2 to 3 weeks with follow-up visits. Although these techniques are technical, motivated laypeople, with appropriate training, are very capable of performing these tasks (Bissett et al., 1992). For specific aspects related to home TPN, see Box 27–6.

Enteral and parenteral feedings require a more in-depth charting procedure than do modified diets. Charting varies from institution to institution, but generally a flow sheet limited to one or two pages to document feedings, times, amounts, fluid intake, weight, physical assessment findings, and possible complications with treatment is utilized.

Client Teaching

Health promotion for nutritional needs will become a major teaching issue for nurses. Knowing ba-

HOME PARENTERAL NUTRITION

As in enteral feeding, the preferred method of delivery for parenteral feedings at home is either daytime or nighttime cyclic schedules. Most clients feel that home TPN enhances quality of life by allowing a return to a more normal, familiar routine and allowing more time spent with family or significant others. However, psychosocial issues are present. Of 172 participants, over half indicated that they had problems with depression, control and independence issues, altered body image, sexual concerns, and relating problems with spouse or significant others (Rodriquez, 1992). Nurses initiate conversations with clients about these aspects nonjudgementally by stating, "Most clients when they go home with TPN have concerns about (specify which issue, such as body image or relationship). I was wondering if you had any questions or concerns?"

The most common cause for rehospitalization is catheter infections. Nurses must stress proper care for intravenous site and have patients demonstrate intravenous site care before discharge.

sic nutrition principles, the dietary guidelines for Americans, and foods high and low in certain nutrients (especially fats, sodium, and calcium) will be prerequisites for effective health promotion. A referral to a dietitian may be necessary. For example, if a client cannot tolerate milk but consumes cheeses, sardines, and green leafy vegetables, this is a healthy adaptation, promoting health. The nurse should praise and positively reinforce the client for choosing healthy alternatives. However, if a client cannot tolerate milk and makes no effort to eat good sources of calcium, rickets or osteoporosis or osteomalacia could develop. For this client, teaching is of utmost importance. The nurse could converse with the client to determine level of understanding. This client may not recognize the correlation between calcium intake and healthy bones or may not know food sources of calcium. Teaching the client about calcium's role in the body, foods high in calcium, and possible complications from a lack of calcium may be all that is required to correct this unhealthy behavior.

Interpreting principles of nutrition into practical terms that a client can understand is essential for the client's effective learning. Learning is enhanced when the client is actively involved. An optimal time to assess knowledge and initiate teaching is when the client is completing the menu selections.

For teaching to be effective, the client's knowledge level is assessed. It will be quite different teaching a client who has never heard of LDL how to decrease fat intake than teaching a client who knows desired LDL blood levels and foods to decrease LDL levels. Ask what the client would like to learn first and begin with that subject.

Telling a client to decrease fat intake is not sufficient. The nurse must identify specific foods that are low in fat, liked by the client, affordable, and readily available to promote compliance. Suppose that decreasing fat in the diet is a major change for the client. Start the change process gradually; if goals (outcomes) are set too high, failure is likely. If the client drinks whole milk, then suggesting that he or she switch to skim milk will probably cause no change in behavior. However, suggesting that 2% milk be drunk for a few weeks and then 1% milk for a few weeks is much more beneficial. Realistic changes can enhance successful, permanent lifestyle behaviors.

Explaining the health risk as it relates to nutrition can result in changes for the adult; decreasing fat intake can help prevent heart disease, strokes, and atherosclerosis. For teenagers, emphasizing how the change is beneficial for their physical appearance, acceptance among peers, and sports activities can motivate change, as can emphasizing that decreasing fat in the diet can cause weight loss, enhance endurance for sporting events, and reduce the size of a body part that the adolescent perceives is too big.

When teaching clients about diet modifications, if the nurse notes that the client says that he or she will comply, but the nurse observes that the food is un-touched, a change in plan is needed. Uneaten food does not provide the nutrients that clients require to heal or stay healthy. Commenting to the client about the lack of intake and then listening to the client's response is necessary. It may be that one item on the food tray is disliked, so no food is eaten, or it may be that the client does not understand why the diet is ordered. Finding out the client's reasons for not eating can allow the nurse to adjust the plan to the client's needs.

When discussing the diet modifications, focus on the positive, not the negative. For example, say "You like potatoes and they are allowed" rather than "This food and this food and this food will have to be eliminated from your diet."

Documentation should include not only what is taught or done but how the client responds. When the client refuses any nutritional interventions, this is documented in his or her chart, and possible complications that could result are communicated to the client and written in the chart. Suppose that the nurse taught the client about behavior modification techniques to decrease intake. The chart would read "Taught about behavior modification techniques to decrease intake while at home. States that she will chew her food 20 times; use a smaller plate, and eat while sitting rather than standing. Positive reinforcement given." Conversely, if the client does not comply, this would also be charted: "Taught about behavior modification techniques to decrease intake while at home. States that this is a 'waste of time' and 'don't expect me to use them when I go home'. Another example is as follows: "Reinforced benefits of weight loss, such as decreased blood pressure and cholesterol level and complications from weight gain; *i.e.,* increased blood pressure, heart and mobility problems, but still stated, 'I don't care what you say. I'm not doing them'.

Charting must be objective—not subjective. Facts, not opinions, are charted. Words such as "belligerent," "obnoxious," and "hateful" are avoided; rather, describe the behavior.

Working With the Health Team

A nurse coordinates care with other ancillary departments when indicated. For example, the client receives respiratory treatments right before meals. On assessing the situation, the nurse discovers that the treatments make the client nauseated, and meals are not eaten. Collaborating with the respiratory department to perform treatments 2 hours before or after meals may increase intake. Other departments that the nurse may have to coordinate with include radiology, nuclear medicine, and physical therapy.

Coordinating nutritional care also involves the use of referrals. Nurses must be knowledgeable about the various agencies available for nutrition support, because most clients require some type of special assistance, be it financial, educational, or emotional.

Clients with a diagnosis of Altered Nutrition: Less

Than Body Requirements may benefit from nutrition support services. City or county health departments are often the best sources. Well-baby clinics and family health centers can also provide nutrition services. Food stamps are available for the low-income family through welfare offices. The women, infants, and children program is designed to prevent nutritional problems in pregnant women, breast-feeding women, infants, and children up to 5 years of age. School breakfast and lunch programs provide nutritious meals for school-aged children. Headstart programs are available for qualified preschoolers. Some community agencies or churches have food banks or food pantries. Elderly meal programs and home-delivered meals are also available.

Numerous groups that facilitate weight loss for clients with a diagnosis of Altered Nutrition: More Than Body Requirements include Weight Watchers, Thin Within, TOPS, and Overeaters Anonymous. Depending on the community, other resources may be available.

People to contact if available include the dietitian, social worker, metabolic specialist, and nutrition support team. These specialists could then direct the nurse and client to various community resources. Any referrals are noted in the client's chart. For example, suppose a low-income mother is prescribed a high-protein diet but feels she cannot follow this diet because funds are low and high-protein foods are expensive.

Documentation would include: "States is afraid cannot follow diet when home because of lack of funds to purchase high-protein foods. Dietitian and social worker notified about patient's concerns." (In some areas, the physician is notified before referrals can be made.) The nurse could also begin teaching about economical protein foods such as beans, milk, cheese, and eggs.

Evaluation

During this step, the nurse determines whether nutritional goals (outcomes) were achieved. Client's responses are compared with the outcome. For example, weighing the client would be indicated because the primary nutritional goals are to increase or decrease weight by 1 to 2 lb/week. If the weight has been gained or lost, goals were met, indicating that interventions were successful; only periodic monitoring of nutritional status is required. Document that the client has gained or lost weight in the chart. However, if the weight was not lost or gained, then the nurse should begin with an assessment to determine why the goals were not met, following up with diagnosing, planning, implementing, and evaluating to modify or revise the care plan. Suppose the client did not lose 1 to 2 lb within a week. The first action that the nurse should perform is to ask the client, "What do you suppose happened that prevented the specified weight loss?" This will open up lines of communication to gather needed information. Several factors may be discovered.

1. The client states that the diet plan is being followed and can verbalize treatments and rationale. Based on this information, the client and nurse can decide that the plan just needs to be continued.

2. The client states that there is no motivation to change, he or she hoarded candy bars in the nightstand, felt depressed so he or she ate a whole bag of chips in one sitting, or thinks that low-kilocaloric food tastes "bland and flat." Depending on the data collected, the client and nurse can revise the care plan. Maybe the diagnosis needs to be changed to noncompliance, or the goal should be revised to say that weight loss of 1 lb over 2 weeks or other interventions, such as having the client keep a food diary to recognize vulnerable times for overeating and a chart to visually track food eaten and subsequent weight can be tried.

This process is implemented any time goals are not achieved. Unsuccessful goal achievement does not imply failure; it just means that other strategies need to be considered.

To evaluate nutritional care, refer to goals (outcomes) listed in the Nursing Diagnoses box on p. 768. If the client's behavior is congruent with the goal, nutritional needs have been met. Other methods to evaluate attainment of goals are to

1. Monitor intake: 75% or more of meals should be consumed
2. Recognize or prevent physical complications (*e.g.*, malnutrition, nausea, vomiting, PEM, noncompliance) from modified diets
3. Recognize or prevent physical complications (*e.g.*, diarrhea, aspiration, clogging) from tube feedings
4. Recognize or prevent physical complications (*e.g.*, infection, hyperglycemia, fluid overload, air embolism) from TPN
5. Recognize or prevent psychosocial complications (*e.g.*, depression, grieving, apathy, helplessness, irritability, withdrawal) from dietary changes
6. Identify changes in eating patterns, such as decreasing salt and cholesterol or increasing protein and kilocalories, when indicated
7. Ask clients to describe dietary modifications (*i.e.*, the client should be able to state the dietary changes made and reasons for them)
8. Ask clients what was learned or gained by using referrals, such as clients actually using nutritional resources (*e.g.*, low-income mother participates in the women, infants, and children program).

Dietary changes take time; lifelong patterns have to be altered. Sometimes a change in a client's behavior is more desirable than a change on the scales. Healthy dietary changes that will be used for a lifetime can lay a solid basis for enhancing, maintaining, and/or restoring optimal nutritional status.

Summary

Providing effective nutritional care can improve clients' physical and mental functioning, which will in turn enhance quality and productivity of life. To assist nurses in providing effective nutritional care, basic nutrition and factors that affect nutrition were reviewed. Common nutritional problems, with suggested interventions, were also addressed. Using the nursing process to meet clients' nutritional needs, especially in the assessment phase, was highly emphasized. Assessment of dietary habits, mouth, abdomen, anthropometric measures, diagnostic and laboratory tests, psychosocial factors, and developmental aspects is necessary to determine appropriate nutritional nursing diagnoses. Several nutritional diagnoses were discussed. Nutritional goals and interventions were also presented, as well as how to evaluate effectiveness of nutritional care.

CHAPTER HIGHLIGHTS

✦ The six classes of nutrients are carbohydrates, fats, proteins, vitamins, minerals, and water.

✦ Carbohydrates provide the body's preferred source of energy (glucose) and are supplied by grains. A decreased intake can cause constipation and utilization of protein for energy.

✦ Fats form adipose tissue and are supplied by meats and oils. A deficiency can cause inadequate energy intake.

✦ Proteins build and repair tissues and are supplied by meats. A decreased intake leads to PEM (marasmus or kwashiorkor).

✦ Vitamins and minerals enhance body processes and are supplied by most foods. Deficiencies can result in numerous disorders, depending on the specific substance lacking.

✦ Water maintains fluid balance and is provided by liquids and solid foods. A decreased intake results in dehydration.

✦ Digestion, absorption, and metabolism work together to provide the body with needed nutrients.

✦ Anabolism and catabolism are occurring simultaneously in the body.

✦ Nurses can use the Food Guide Pyramid, Dietary Guidelines for Americans, and the RDAs to help clients plan a healthy diet consisting of 55 to 58% of energy from carbohydrates, 12 to 15% from protein, and 30% from fat.

✦ Physiological, psychological, sociological, and economical factors can affect nutrition.

✦ Alcohol, immobility, human immunodeficiency virus or acquired immunodeficiency syndrome, cancer, burns, and surgery affect nutrition by increasing nutrient requirements.

✦ Malnutrition can be an increase or decrease in nutrient(s) or kilocalories.

✦ Obesity is a form of malnutrition. Nursing care focuses on balancing intake with energy expenditure.

✦ Nausea and vomiting can be eased with small, frequent, bland foods.

✦ Anorexia is a nutritional problem. Nursing care involves stimulating the client's appetite.

✦ Heartburn is another common nutritional problem. Changing lifestyle habits and avoiding some foods are recommended.

✦ Parameters assessed to determine nutritional status include a dietary nursing history, physical assessment findings, anthropometric measures, diagnostic tests, laboratory results, psychosocial factors, and developmental aspects.

✦ The two main nutritional diagnoses are Nutrition, Altered: More Than Body Requirements and Nutrition, Altered: Less Than Body Requirements.

✦ Depending on the nursing diagnosis, goals emphasize losing or gaining weight and promoting anabolism and decreasing catabolism.

✦ Nutritional interventions focus on stimulating appetite, facilitating weight loss, or enhancing healthy eating habits.

✦ Depending on the disease process, regular, modified, or special diets may be ordered.

✦ Enteral nutrition is ordered when the GI tract is functioning but intake is poor or prohibited. Nurses monitor clients to prevent complications.

✦ Parenteral nutrition is implemented when the GI tract is severely dysfunctional or nonfunctional. Complications are avoided by thorough nursing assessment and care.

✦ Teaching is of utmost importance in nutritional care.

✦ Nurses use referrals as needed to improve the nutritional status of clients.

✦ Clients' behaviors are compared with goals to evaluate nutritional care. Depending on data collected, nutritional care may be continued, modified, revised, or completed.

✦ Documentation of nutritional care is required to demonstrate that care was individualized, properly implemented, and coordinated.

Study Questions

1. A community health nurse is evaluating possible malnutrition in the elderly. Which of the following parameters should the nurse investigate?

    a. food jags
    b. lead levels
    c. support systems
    d. hemoglobin status

2. For a nurse to perform a nutritional assessment, which of the following is necessary?

    a. gather anthropometric data
    b. write dietary goals (objectives)
    c. develop a nutritional nursing diagnosis
    d. collaborate with client to determine interventions

3. Upon performing a nutritional assessment, which of the following findings would warrant notifying the doctor?

    a. weight decreased from 100 lb to 93 lb in 1 month
    b. hypoactive bowel sounds in all four quadrants
    c. transferrin levels 250 mg/dl
    d. albumin is 3.8 g/dl

4. A nurse writes a nutritional goal as follows: "Client will eat 95% of meals within 3 days." After 1 day, the nurse observes that the client ate 45% of meals. Which of the following should the nurse do?

    a. make the client eat the rest of the food
    b. continue to observe the client's intake
    c. revise the nutritional interventions
    d. change the nursing diagnosis

5. Which of the following interventions should the nurse perform for a client with a diagnosis of Altered Nutrition: Less Than Body Requirements?

    a. suggest three large meals a day
    b. offer favorite beverage with meals
    c. teach how to avoid kilocaloric-dense foods
    d. encourage exercising on a regular basis

Critical Thinking Exercises

1. Ms. H., age 33 years, comes to the community center for her children's check-up. She has a 6-month-old daughter and a 3.5-year-old son. She also cares for her 68-year-old mother with Alzheimer's disease. Discuss the implications for dietary teaching with Ms. H. regarding her children and mother.

2. Mr. G., age 29 years, has acquired immunodeficiency syndrome and is being evaluated by your home health care agency for malnutrition. It is determined that peripheral TPN is the best route for Mr. G. Discuss the nursing implications for the client receiving TPN.

References

American Dietetic Association. (1992). *Handbook of clinical dietetics* (2nd ed.). Chicago: American Dietetic Association.

American Dietetic Association. (1992). *Manual of clinical dietetics* (4th ed.). Chicago: American Dietetic Association.

Bell, L. P., *et al.* (1991). Cholesterol-lowering effects of soluble-fiber cereals as a part of a prudent diet for patients with mild to moderate hypercholesterolemia. *American Journal of Clinical Nutrition, 52*(6), 1020–1026.

Bergstrom, N., Carlson, C. E., Frantz, R. A., *et al.* (1992). How to predict and prevent pressure ulcers. *American Journal of Nursing, 92*(7), 52–54.

Bissett, W. M., *et al.* (1992). Home parenteral nutrition in chronic intestinal failure. *Archives of the Disabled Child, 67*(1), 109–114.

Bockus, S. (1991). Troubleshooting your tube feedings. *American Journal of Nursing, 19*(5), 24–30.

Burnes, J. U., *et al.* (1992). Home parenteral nutrition—A 3-year analysis of clinical laboratory monitoring. *Journal of Parenteral and Enteral Nutrition, 16*(4), 327–332.

Cope, K. A. (1994). Nutritional status: A basic "vital sign." *Home Healthcare Nurse, 12*(2), 29–34.

Davis, J. R., & Sherer, K. L. (1994). *Applied nutrition and diet therapy for nurses* (2nd ed.). Philadelphia: W. B. Saunders.

Doyle, W., *et al.* (1991). Low birth weight and maternal diet. *Midwife Health Visitor and Community Nurse, 27*(2), 44, 46.

Dwyer, J. T. (1991). Nutritional consequences of vegetarianism. *Annual Review Nutrition, 11,* 61–92.

Edelstein, C. K., Haskew, P., & Kramer, J. P. (1989). Early clues to anorexia and bulimia. *Patient Care, 23*(13), 155–175.

Grunow, J., *et al.* (1989). Contamination of enteral nutrition systems during prolonged intermittent use. *Journal of Parenteral and Enteral Nutrition, 13*(1), 23–25.

Gulledge, J., *et al.* (1987). Psychosocial issues of home parenteral and enteral nutrition. *Nutritional Clinical Practice, 2*(5), 183–194.

Halliday, A. (1991). Nutrition and the healthy adult. *Nursing Standard, 5*(21), 25–27.

Herrmann, F. R., *et al.* (1992). Serum albumin level on admission as a predictor of death, length of stay, and readmission. *Archives of Internal Medicine, 152*(1), 125–130.

Hofland, S. L., & Dardis, P. O. (1992). Bulimia nervosa: Associated physical problems. *Journal of Psychosocial Nursing, 30*(2), 23–27.

Kohn, C. L., & Keithley, J. K. (1989). Enteral nutrition: Potential complications and patient monitoring. *Nursing Clinics of North America, 24*(2), 339–352.

Lange-Alberts, M. E., & Shott, S. (1994). Nutritional intake: Use of touch and verbal cuing. *Journal of Gerontological Nursing, 20*(2), 36–40.

Love, C. C., Seaton, H. (1991). Eating disorders: Highlights of nursing assessment and therapeutics. *Nursing Clinics of North America, 26*(3), 677–697.

Merrill, A. (1994). Nutrition interventions for the HIV-positive client. *Home Healthcare Nurse, 12*(2), 35–38.

Metheny, N., *et al.* (1990). Effectiveness of the auscultatory method in predicting feeding tube location. *Nursing Research, 39*(5), 263–267.

Metheny, N., *et al.* (1987). Frequency of nasoenteral tube displacement and associated risk factors. *Research in Nursing Health, 9,* 241–247.

Metheny, N. A., Spies, M. A., & Eisenberg, P., *et al.* (1988). Measures to test placement of nasoenteral feeding tubes. *Western Journal of Nursing Research, 10*(4), 367–383.

Naeye, R. L. (1990). Maternal body weight and pregnancy outcome. *American Journal of Clinical Nutrition, 52*(2), 273–279.

Nutrition interventions manual for professionals: Caring for older Americans. (1992). Nutrition Screening Initiative, A

Joint Effort of the American Academy of Family Physicians, the American Dietetic Association, and the National Council on Aging, Inc., Washington, D.C.

Petrosino, B. M., et al. (1989). Implications of selected problems with nasoenteral tube feedings. *Critical Care Nursing Quarterly, 12*(3), 1–18.

Plehn, K. W. (1990). Anorexia nervosa and bulimia: Incidence and diagnosis. *Nurse Practitioner, 15*(4), 22–31.

Rodriquez, M. (1992). Effect of TPN on appetite. *Support Line, 14*(3), 11–12.

Schectman, G., et al. (1991). Ascorbic acid requirements for smokers: Analysis of a population survey. *American Journal of Clinical Nutrition, 53*(6), 1466–1470.

US Department of Agriculture, & US Department of Health and Human Services. (1990). *Nutrition and your health: Dietary guidelines for Americans* (3rd ed.). Home and Garden Bull. No. 232. Washington, DC: Government Printing Office.

US Department of Agriculture, & US Department of Health and Human Services. (1992). *The food guide pyramid.* Home and Garden Bull. No. 252. Washington, DC: Government Printing Office.

Wells, L. (1994). At the front line of care: The importance of nutrition in wound management. *Professional Nurse, 9*(8), 525–530.

Willett, W. C., Stampfer, M. J., Colditz, G. A., et al. (1990). Relation of meat, fat and fiber intake to the risk of colon cancer in a prospective study among women. *New England Journal of Medicine, 323*(24), 1664–1670.

Bibliography

American Institute for Cancer Research. (1992). *Diet and cancer . . . What's the link?* Washington, DC: American Institute for Cancer Research.

Grant, J. A., & Kennedy-Caldwell, C. (1988). *Nutritional support in nursing.* Philadelphia: W. B. Saunders.

Lin, E. M. (1991). Nutrition support: Making the difficult decision. *Cancer Nursing, 14*(5), 261–269.

Mahan, L. K., & Arlin, M. T. (1992). *Krause's food, nutrition, and diet therapy* (8th ed.). Philadelphia: W. B. Saunders.

Poleman, C. M., & Peckenpaugh, N. J. (1991). *Nutrition essentials and diet therapy* (6th ed.). Philadelphia: W. B. Saunders.

Saal, N. M., & Douglas, P. D. (1992). Teaching nutrition survival skills. *Journal of American Dietetic Association, 92*(5), 547.

Worthington, P. A., & Wagner, B. A. (1989). Total parenteral nutrition. *Nursing Clinics of North America, 24*(2), 355–370.

Young, C. K., & White, S. (1992). Preparing patients for tube feedings at home. *American Journal of Nursing, 24*(2), 46–53.

HYDRATION: PRINCIPLES OF FLUID-GAS TRANSPORT

KEETA P. WILBORN, MS, RN

KEY TERMS

✦

acid	electrolytes
acidosis	filtration
active transport	homeostasis
alkalosis	homologous blood
anions	hypertonic
autologous blood	hypotonic
base	isotonic
cations	osmolality
colloids	osmolarity
crystalloids	osmosis
designated blood	pH
diffusion	tetany
edema	

LEARNING OBJECTIVES

✦

After studying this chapter, you should be able to

✦ Describe the distribution and composition of body fluids
✦ Identify the various functions of sodium, potassium, calcium, phosphorus, and magnesium
✦ Discuss regulation mechanisms for body fluids and electrolytes
✦ Describe transport mechanisms for fluids and electrolytes
✦ Define edema
✦ Describe disturbances in hydration, including fluid volume deficit and fluid volume excess
✦ Identify electrolyte imbalances caused by either an increase or decrease in serum concentration of an electrolyte
✦ Describe three mechanisms within the human body to maintain acid-base balance
✦ Identify disturbances in acid-base balance
✦ Apply the nursing process to the nursing care of clients experiencing disturbances in hydration, electrolyte, or acid-base balance
✦ Administer intravenous fluids safely and accurately
✦ Administer blood products safely and accurately

Homeostasis, the maintenance of a stable or constant internal environment, depends on the regulation of oxygen, carbon dioxide, organic nutrients and wastes, inorganic ions, and temperature within the human body. Virtually every body system contributes to homeostasis to maintain normal cellular function (Chenevey, 1987).

This chapter explores hydration, as well as fluid, electrolyte, and acid-base balance necessary for homeostasis. Nursing care of people experiencing fluid, electrolyte, or acid-base imbalance is also presented, as well as a sample nursing care plan.

Hydration—Fluid and Electrolyte Balance

Distribution of Body Fluids

Body water constitutes approximately 50 to 55% of total body weight in adult women, 60% in young adult men, and 77% in newborn infants (Fig. 28–1*A*). However, the percentage of total body water (TBW) varies considerably depending on the amount of body fat, because fat tissue contains little water. In addition, TBW progressively decreases with age (Brown, 1993; Chenevey, 1987; Jones, 1991).

Total body water is distributed between two compartments, the intracellular fluid (ICF) compartment and the extracellular fluid (ECF) compartment (see Fig. 28–1*B*). Most body water is intracellular, accounting for 55 to 75% of TBW. The remaining 25 to 45% of TBW is distributed in the ECF compartment (Brown, 1993).

The ECF compartment is further divided into intravascular (plasma) and interstitial compartments. Eighty percent of the ECF is interstitial (the fluid that surrounds the cells), and the other 20% is plasma, the fluid portion of blood. Whereas a dynamic exchange of fluid continuously occurs among the intracellular, interstitial, and intravascular compartments, only the intravascular (plasma) compartment is directly affected by intake or elimination of fluid from the body (Kee & Paulanka, 1994).

Composition of Body Fluids

Body fluids contain water, nonelectrolytes, and electrolytes. Water has several functions in the body, including transportation of oxygen, electrolytes, and nutrients to the cells; regulation of body temperature; excretion of waste products; lubrication of joints and membranes; and a medium for food digestion (Kee & Paulanka, 1994).

Nonelectrolytes are solutes, such as glucose and urea, that do not break apart into electrically charged particles when placed into a solution. **Electrolytes** are chemical substances that dissociate into electrically charged particles called ions when placed into a solution (Weldy, 1992).

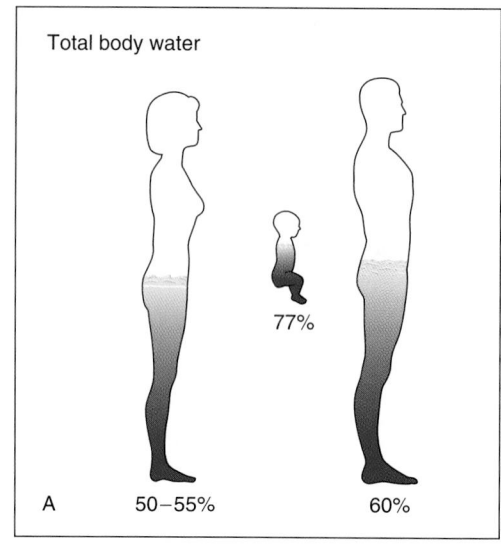

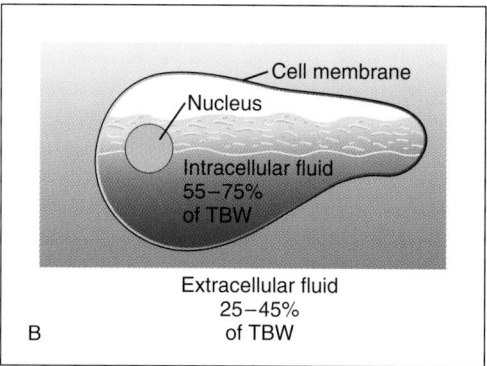

✦ **Figure 28–1**
Percentage of total body water (TBW) **(A)** and distribution of TBW in compartments **(B)**.

Electrolytes

Electrolytes are necessary for the maintenance of life. Four physiological processes for which electrolytes are essential include promotion of neuromuscular irritability, maintenance of body fluid osmolality, regulation of acid-base balance, and distribution of body fluids between the fluid compartments (Weldy, 1992).

Electrolytes are either positively or negatively charged ions. The positively charged electrolytes are called **cations** and include sodium (Na^+), calcium (Ca^{++}), potassium (K^+), and magnesium (Mg^{++}). The negatively charged electrolytes are called **anions** and include bicarbonate (HCO_3^-), chloride (Cl^-), phosphate (HPO_4^-), and sulfate (SO_4^-).

The concentration of electrolytes in the ECF differs from the concentration of electrolytes in the ICF (Table 28–1). Sodium, calcium, bicarbonate, and chloride are the major electrolytes found in the ECF; potassium, magnesium, phosphate, and sulfate are the major electrolytes found in the ICF.

Cellular function, as well as distribution of water in the various fluid spaces, is dependent on electrolyte

Table **28−1**

ELECTROLYTE CONCENTRATIONS IN BODY FLUIDS

ELECTROLYTE	EXTRACELLULAR CONCENTRATION, mEq/L	INTRACELLULAR CONCENTRATION, mEq/L
Cations		
Sodium (Na$^+$)	145	10
Potassium (K$^+$)	5	150
Calcium (Ca^{++})	5	2
Magnesium (Mg^{++})	2	27
Anions		
Chloride (Cl$^-$)	116	1
Bicarbonate (HCO$_3^-$)	26	10
Phosphate (HPO$_4^{--}$)	2	100

concentration. As electrolyte concentration changes in either the ECF or ICF, water shifts from an area of higher concentration of solutes to an area of lower concentration. Likewise, each compartment replaces and exchanges ions to maintain electrical stability of the fluids. This constant interchange of water and electrolytes between the ICF and ECF occurs through the semipermeable cell membrane (Chenevey, 1987).

Sodium

Sodium is the primary cation in the ECF and, as such, is the major determinant of plasma osmolality. Because water follows the osmotic gradients created by changes in salt concentration, sodium helps to regulate ECF fluid volume. Sodium also works with potassium and calcium in the transmission and conduction of nerve impulses and assists in the regulation of acid-base balance. The serum sodium concentration is usually 135 to 145 mEq/L (Isley, 1990; McCance & Huether, 1994).

Potassium

Potassium is the primary cation in the ICF, with a serum concentration of 3.5 to 5.3 mEq/L (Kee & Hayes, 1990). Potassium is essential for a variety of biochemical reactions, such as glycogen deposition in the liver and skeletal muscle cells and regulation of ICF osmolality. It also affects resting membrane potentials and plays a major role in nerve conduction, muscle contraction, and myocardial membrane responsiveness (Perez, 1995a).

Calcium

Calcium provides structural support to bone and teeth, and as an ion, it participates in neuromuscular

excitability, enzymatic and secretory activity, and blood coagulation. In plasma, approximately 50% of calcium is bound to serum protein, and the other half is unbound or ionized calcium (Graves, 1990). The serum concentration of calcium is 4.5 to 5.5 mEq/L or 9 to 11 mg/dL (Kee & Hayes, 1990).

Phosphorus

Phosphorus is more abundant in ICF and is important in tissue oxygenation, central nervous system function, carbohydrate utilization, and leukocyte function (Graves, 1990). The usual serum concentration of phosphorus is 2.5 to 4.5 mg/dL (Kee & Hayes, 1990).

Magnesium

Magnesium is primarily an intracellular cation that is important in numerous biochemical reactions—most notably those involved in the production and use of adenosine triphosphate (ATP). Only 1% of the body's magnesium is found in the serum, with the remainder being present in bone and soft tissues (Friday & Reinhart, 1991). The usual serum concentration of Mg^{++} is 1.5 to 2.5 mEq/L (Weldy, 1992).

Regulation of Body Fluids and Electrolytes

Water and Sodium

The intake and output of fluids must remain relatively equal to maintain homeostasis. In the healthy adult, between 1500 and 3000 ml of fluid per day are taken in and eliminated. Normal sources of water include ingestion of liquids and foods containing water, as well as water produced during metabolic activities (Chenevey, 1987).

Regulation of body water is maintained by control

of water intake and elimination. Volitional intake of water is regulated by thirst, which, in turn, is regulated by plasma osmolality. ***Osmolality*** refers to the total number of osmotically active particles in a solution (Chenevey, 1987). Osmoreceptors located in the hypothalamus stimulate thirst when the serum osmolality increases above normal (280–294 mOsm/kg). Thirst then increases the rate of water intake sufficiently to offset water loss (Brown, 1993).

Water elimination occurs through loss from skin, lungs, and kidneys. Insensible water loss, or loss from the skin and lungs, varies with temperature, humidity, activity, and respiratory rate and may account for approximately 500 to 1000 ml/day. The kidneys excrete excess body fluid as urine (Brown, 1993; Chenevey, 1987).

The rate at which the kidneys excrete urine is regulated primarily by the antidiuretic hormone (ADH), vasopressin. ADH is produced by the hypothalamus and stored in the posterior pituitary. Under the influence of ADH, the kidneys reabsorb water from the urine into the ECF compartment and excrete a low volume of concentrated urine (Brown, 1993).

Antidiuretic hormone is secreted in response to several different variables, including decreased blood pressure, decreased blood volume, nausea, acute hypoglycemia, increased ambient temperature, acute hypoxia, and hypercapnia. As plasma osmolality increases, osmoreceptors in the hypothalamus are stimulated, and ADH is released. In contrast, an acute rise in blood pressure or blood volume or a normal or low plasma osmolality inhibits the secretion of ADH (Brown, 1993).

In addition, renal conservation of sodium and water is affected by the secretion of aldosterone by the adrenal cortex. A decrease in arterial blood pressure results in a diminished renal perfusion pressure, which stimulates the kidneys to release renin. Renin in turn stimulates the conversion of angiotensin I to angiotensin II, which stimulates the release of aldosterone. Aldosterone increases sodium reabsorption from the distal tubule of the nephron and thus increases water retention by the kidneys (McCance & Huether, 1994).

Potassium

The serum potassium level is usually regulated by the kidney, which excretes excess potassium in the urine. However, the serum potassium level is also influenced by movement of potassium between the ICF and ECF compartments. The sodium-potassium pump moves sodium out of the cell and potassium back into the cell. Acidosis, increased plasma osmolality, and vigorous exercise can shift potassium from ICF to ECF. In contrast, alkalosis and insulin tend to shift potassium from ECF to ICF (Calhoun, 1990).

Calcium and Phosphorus

The serum concentration of calcium is regulated primarily by parathyroid hormone (PTH), vitamin D,

and calcitonin. The parathyroid glands release PTH in response to a low serum calcium level. PTH, along with vitamin D, increases absorption of calcium from bone and the intestines, as well as conservation of calcium by the kidneys. In contrast, a high serum calcium level results in a decreased release of PTH and an increased release of calcitonin by the thyroid gland. Calcium is then reabsorbed by bone and excreted in the urine and feces (Graves, 1990).

Phosphorus concentrations are in an inverse relationship with calcium; as serum calcium levels increase, serum phosphorus levels decrease. Excretion of excess phosphorus is regulated by the kidneys (Graves, 1990).

Magnesium

Serum magnesium concentration is regulated primarily by the kidney through increased or decreased reabsorption from the ascending limb of the loop of Henle (Graves, 1990).

Transport Mechanisms for Fluids and Electrolytes

Movement of water and particles through the semipermeable cell membrane occurs via diffusion, osmosis, active transport, and filtration.

Diffusion

Diffusion is the movement of particles from an area of greater concentration to an area of lesser concentration of solutes (Fig. 28–2*A*). Substances diffuse across the semipermeable cell membrane by passing through the pores or dissolving in the lipid matrix of the membrane wall. However, certain molecules, such as glucose, are too large to pass through the membrane pores and instead enter the cell via a carrier transport system called facilitated diffusion. The net diffusion of a molecule is primarily determined by the concentration difference of the substance crossing the cell membrane (Chenevey, 1987).

Osmosis

Osmosis is the net movement of water across the cell membrane in response to a concentration difference. Water moves from an area of lesser concentration of solute to an area of greater concentration of solute until equilibrium is achieved (see Fig. 28–2*B*).

Two terms often used interchangeably when describing osmosis are *osmolality* and *osmolarity*. Osmolality, the total number of osmotically active particles in a volume of solution, and **osmolarity,** the concentration of solute in a volume of solution, regulate the movement of water. Water diffuses from an area of low osmolality to an area of high osmolality until equilibrium is reached (Chenevey, 1987).

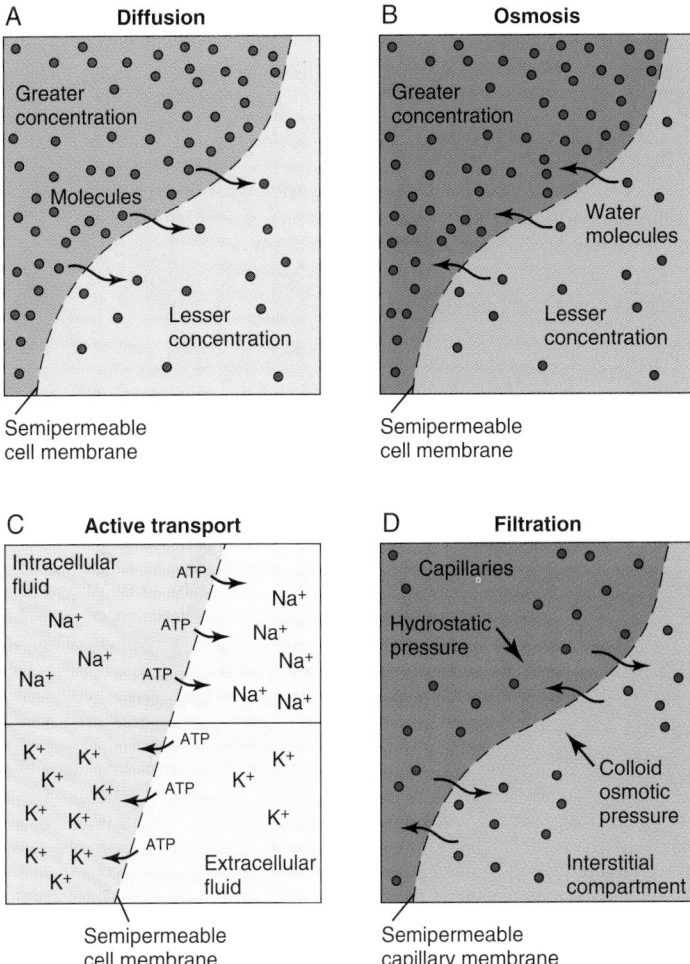

❧ **Figure 28–2**
Transport mechanisms for fluid and electrolytes.

Active Transport

Movement of substances against a concentration gradient, *i.e.,* from an area of lower concentration to an area of higher concentration, is called **active transport** and requires energy in the form of ATP, as well as a carrier substance. The sodium-potassium pump is an example of active transport, which is needed to maintain a greater concentration of sodium outside the cell and potassium inside the cell (see Fig. 28–2C).

Sodium inside the cell combines with a carrier and moves to the outer surface of the cell, where it is released. Potassium combines with a carrier outside the cell and moves to the interior of the cell, where it is released. Release of sodium and potassium from the carrier substances is facilitated by ATP, and this process continues indefinitely to maintain the concentration of sodium and potassium (Chenevey, 1987).

Filtration

Filtration is the transfer of water and dissolved substances through a semipermeable membrane in response to pressure. Hydrostatic pressure or blood pressure tends to force fluid and electrolytes out of capillaries into the interstitial compartment. Colloid osmotic pressure or the pressure created by plasma proteins tends to prevent the movement of fluid out of capillaries into the interstitial compartment (see Fig. 28–2D). The balance between hydrostatic and colloid osmotic pressure maintains fluid balance in the intravascular system (Chenevey, 1987).

Disturbances in Hydration and Electrolyte Balance

Hydration

Hydration status is closely tied to serum sodium. In fact, disorders affecting hydration and water balance are usually reflected by changes in the sodium concentration, and disorders affecting sodium balance are often reflected by changes in hydration and the volume of ECF (Brown, 1993). In determining hydration status, both the fluid volume status and serum sodium are assessed. Disorders of hydration may be the result of fluid distribution, fluid volume excess, or fluid volume depletion.

Disturbances in hydration status are more likely to occur and be severe in infants and in the elderly than in children and younger adults. Infants have a greater need for fluid due to their larger body surface area relative to their size and their higher metabolic rate, with greater heat production and insensible fluid loss. In addition, kidney function is immature at birth, with a limited capacity to concentrate or dilute urine. The elderly have a decrease in TBW, and with increasing age, the sensation of thirst decreases. In addition, urine-concentrating ability declines with age. Thus, hydration status in infants and the elderly should be carefully assessed (Weldy, 1992).

Edema

Edema is an accumulation of fluid in the interstitial spaces and is a problem of fluid distribution. Edema does not necessarily indicate a fluid excess and, in some cases, may occur with a fluid deficit. Edema may occur with an increase in forces that increase fluid filtration from the capillaries or lymphatic channels into the interstitial tissues. These forces include increased hydrostatic pressure, decreased plasma oncotic pressure, increased capillary membrane permeability, and lymphatic obstruction.

Edema may be localized or limited to a site of trauma or within a particular organ system. Cerebral edema, pulmonary edema, pleural effusion, and ascites are examples of localized edema. Dependent edema (Fig. 28–3) is an example of generalized edema, in which fluid accumulates in gravity-dependent areas of the body such as the feet and legs during standing or in the sacrum and buttocks during lying down. Edema may be associated with weight gain, swelling and puffiness, tight-fitting clothes and shoes, and limited movement of the affected area.

Whereas edema is associated with an accumulation of excessive fluid, this fluid is trapped within a "third space" and is not available for metabolic processes. Thus, a state of dehydration may develop as fluid leaves the vascular compartment and moves into interstitial tissues (McCance & Huether, 1994).

Fluid Volume Excess

An excess of extracellular fluid volume is usually associated with hypoosmolality and hyponatremia. The excess ECF volume decreases the concentration of solutes, resulting in a decrease in serum osmolality and a decrease in serum sodium (Brown, 1993). The overall effect is dilution of the ECF, causing movement of water into the intracellular space. Manifestations of water excess may include confusion, convulsions, weakness, nausea, muscle twitching, headache, and weight gain (McCance & Huether, 1994). If severe, fluid volume excess may lead to heart failure and pulmonary edema, especially in the individual with cardiovascular dysfunction (Horne *et al.*, 1991).

Fluid Volume Deficit

There are three types of fluid volume deficit:

1. **Isotonic**—the most common type, in which a loss of

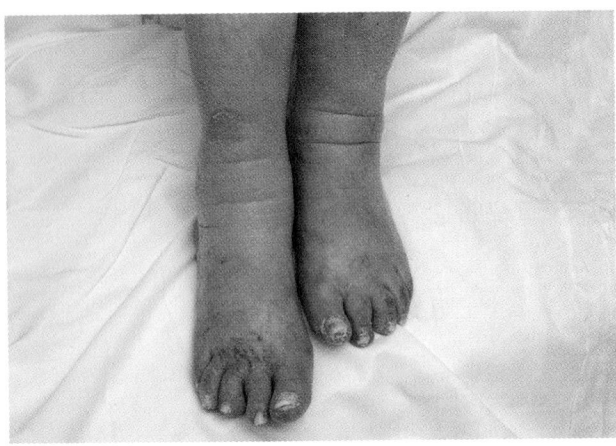

❥ Figure 28–3
In dependent edema, fluid accumulates in gravity-dependent areas of the body, such as the feet and legs.

fluid and electrolytes in approximately balanced proportion occurs.
2. **Hypotonic**—the electrolyte deficit is greater than the fluid deficit. With this type of fluid deficit, the ECF is hypotonic, and fluid moves from the ECF compartment into the ICF compartment.
3. **Hypertonic**—the loss of fluid is greater than the loss of electrolytes (Weldy, 1992). This type of fluid deficit is usually associated with hyperosmolality and hypernatremia. The decreased ECF volume increases the concentration of solutes, resulting in an increase in serum osmolality and an increase in serum sodium (Brown, 1993). This type of deficit is rare and is most often associated with diabetes insipidus.

Manifestations of fluid volume deficit may include thirst, dry skin and mucous membranes, elevated temperature, weight loss, and concentrated urine. Symptoms of hypovolemia may also be present and include increased heart rate, weak pulses, and postural hypotension (McCance & Huether, 1994).

Electrolyte Imbalances

Electrolyte imbalances may be due to either an increase or decrease in serum concentration of an electrolyte, and these imbalances may also affect the hydration status of the client. Electrolyte imbalances may occur with many disorders. Table 28–2 summarizes electrolyte imbalances, including possible etiological factors and signs and symptoms of each imbalance.

Sodium Imbalances

Hyponatremia

Hyponatremia, or a decrease in serum sodium, usually occurs in conjunction with a fluid imbalance, most commonly an excess fluid loss that results in loss of sodium. Hyponatremia may also occur as a result of dilution of serum sodium, as water is retained in excess of sodium. Sodium may be lost through diuresis,

Table 28–2

ELECTROLYTE IMBALANCES

IMBALANCE	CAUSATIVE FACTORS	MANIFESTATIONS
Hyponatremia	Loss of Na^+ by diuresis, vomiting, diarrhea, third spacing, diaphoresis Dilution of Na^+	Serum Na^+ <135 mEq/L, thirst, weakness, anorexia, nausea, muscle cramps, stupor, coma
Hypernatremia	Fluid loss in excess of Na^+ by osmotic diuresis, profuse sweating, vomiting, diarrhea	Serum Na^+ >145 mEq/L, altered mental status, coma, neuromuscular irritability, seizures, anorexia, nausea, vomiting
Hypokalemia	Loss of K^+ by diuretic therapy, nasogastric suction, vomiting, diarrhea, diaphoresis Shift of K^+ into the cells with alkalemia, insulin excess	Serum K^+ <3.5 mEq/L, electrocardiogram changes, cardiac arrhythmias, muscle weakness, fatigue, slurred speech, paralytic ileus
Hyperkalemia	Renal failure, aldosterone deficiency, burns, trauma Shift of K^+ out of cells with acidosis	Serum K^+ >5.3 mEq/L, ventricular arrhythmias, cardiac arrest, nausea, diarrhea, hypotension, irritability, restlessness, paresthesias, slurred speech, hyperreflexia
Hypocalcemia	Malnutrition, vitamin D deficiency, chronic diarrhea, malabsorption syndrome, alkalosis, acute pancreatitis, hypoparathyroidism	Serum Ca^{++} <8.8 mg/dl, anxiety, irritability, numbness and tingling of lips, twitching, cramps, increased deep tendon reflexes, positive Trousseau's and Chvostek's signs Serum Ca^{++} <7.4 mg/dl, impaired coagulation, tetany, convulsions, cardiac arrhythmias
Hypercalcemia	Overuse of calcium antacids, immobilization, malignancy, hyperparathyroidism, thiazide diuretic use	Serum Ca^{++} >11 mg/dl, constipation, anorexia, lethargy, fatigue, depression, confusion, coma, cardiac arrhythmias, renal lithiasis
Hypophosphatemia	Increased loss from diuretic therapy, osmotic diuresis Hyperparathyroidism, malabsorption syndromes, chronic antacid use Shift into cells with alkalosis	Serum phosphorus <2.5 mEq/L, weakness, mental confusion, anemia, bone brittleness, respiratory arrest
Hyperphosphatemia	Renal failure, hypocalcemia, phosphate laxative use, excess vitamin D intake	Serum phosphorus >4.5 mEq/L, and symptoms of low Ca^{++}, including fatigue and tetany
Hypomagnesemia	Starvation, chronic diarrhea, malabsorption syndromes, diuretic therapy, chronic alcohol use, hyperparathyroidism acute myocardial infarction, congestive heart failure, diaphoreses	Normal serum Mg^{++} levels or Mg^{++} <1.5 mEq/L, cardiac arrhythmias, coronary artery spasm, muscle weakness, muscle twitching, tremor, delirium, hyperreflexia, convulsions, coma, refractory hypokalemia, hypocalcemia
Hypermagnesemia	Renal failure, adrenal insufficiency, overuse of magnesium-containing medication or enemas	Serum Mg^{++} >2.5 mEq/L, weakness, hypotension, weak deep tendon reflexes, slurred speech, drowsiness, lethargy, cardiac arrhythmias With higher Mg^{++} levels, flaccid muscle paralysis, respiratory depression, apnea, coma, heart block, cardiac arrest

vomiting, diarrhea, diaphoresis, or movement of fluid into a third space. Sodium may be diluted as a result of congestive heart failure, cirrhosis, hypoalbuminemia, excess fluid intake, or a syndrome of inappropriate secretion of ADH. As sodium levels decrease, fluid moves from the vascular compartment into the cells or intracellular compartment. Symptoms associated with hyponatremia are nonspecific and include thirst, weakness, anorexia, nausea, muscle cramps, stupor, coma, and focal neurological signs. These symptoms are more likely to develop as the serum sodium concentration decreases below 125 mEq/L (Bove, 1996b; Isley, 1990).

Hypernatremia

Hypernatremia, or an increase in serum sodium, results in an increase in serum osmolality. Fluid then moves from the cells into the extracellular space, resulting in dehydration of the intracellular compartment. Hypernatremia usually occurs as a result of excess fluid loss from such disorders as osmotic diuresis, profuse sweating, vomiting, or diarrhea. The elderly are more prone to develop hypernatremia because they dehydrate more easily. Nonspecific symptoms of hypernatremia include fatigue, muscle weakness, restlessness, flushed skin, and a low-grade fever. Symptoms associated with hypernatremia as a result of cellular dehydration, particularly dehydration of brain cells, include altered mental status, coma, neuromuscular irritability, seizures, anorexia, nausea, and vomiting (Bove, 1996b; Isley, 1990).

Potassium Imbalances

Hypokalemia

Hypokalemia, or a decrease in serum potassium level below 3.5 mEq/L, may occur as a result of excessive loss of potassium from the body or a shift of potassium from the ECF into the ICF. Potassium loss may occur as a result of diuretic therapy, nasogastric suction, vomiting, diarrhea, or severe sweating. Potassium shift into the cells may occur with alkalemia or insulin excess. Symptoms of hypokalemia include changes in the electrocardiogram, cardiac arrhythmias, muscle weakness and fatigue, slurred speech, and paralytic ileus (Calhoun, 1990; DeAngelis & Lessig, 1991; Perez, 1995b).

Hyperkalemia

Hyperkalemia, or an excess of potassium, is a potentially life-threatening electrolyte disorder due to the risk of cardiac arrest as the potassium level exceeds 6.5 mEq/L. The primary cause of hyperkalemia is renal failure. It is also associated with aldosterone deficiency, burns, and trauma. Potassium levels may also increase when potassium shifts from the cells into the ECF. This shift may occur with acidosis, such as diabetic ketoacidosis. Symptoms of hyperkalemia include ventricular arrhythmias, cardiac arrest, nausea, diarrhea, hypotension, irritability, restlessness, paresthesias, slurred speech, and hyperreflexia (Calhoun, 1990; DeAngelis & Lessig, 1992; Innerarity, 1992).

Calcium Imbalances

Hypocalcemia

Hypocalcemia, or a low serum calcium level, may occur with malnutrition, vitamin D deficiency, chronic diarrhea, malabsorption syndrome, rapid or massive transfusion of citrated blood, alkalosis, acute pancreatitis, and hypoparathyroidism. Also, as the phosphorus level increases, the serum calcium level decreases. The first symptoms of hypocalcemia may appear when the serum level falls below 8.8 mg/dl and include anxiety, irritability, numbness and tingling of the lips, twitching, cramps, grimacing, and increased deep tendon reflexes. Trousseau's and Chvostek's signs may also be positive (Fig. 28–4). Trousseau's sign is contraction of the hand and fingers when the arterial blood flow in the arm is occluded for 5 minutes. Chvostek's sign is twitching of the nose or lip when the facial nerve is tapped just below the temple. As the calcium level falls below 7.4 mg/dl, impaired coagulation, generalized muscle spasms, tetany, convulsions, and cardiac arrhythmias may develop (Bove, 1996a; McCance & Huether, 1994).

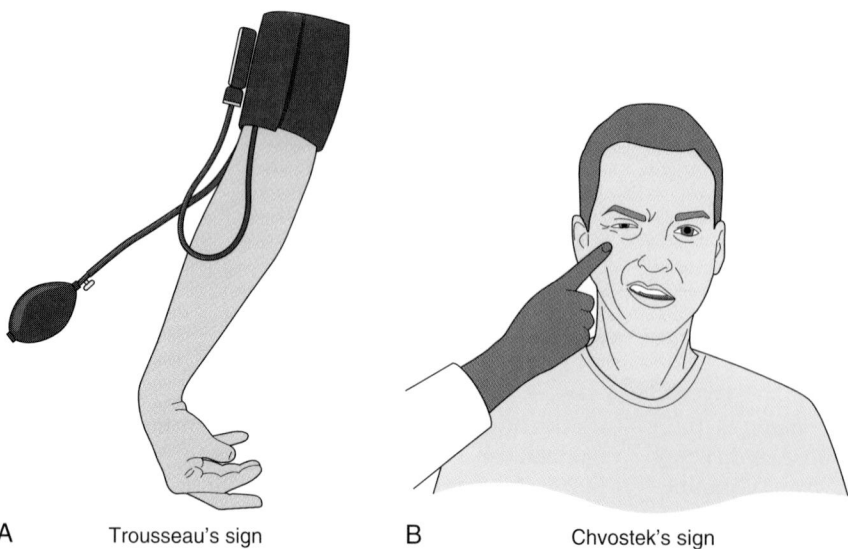

A   Trousseau's sign   B   Chvostek's sign

❧ **Figure 28–4**
Signs of hypocalcemia: Trousseau's sign *(panel A)* and Chvostek's sign *(panel B)*.

Hypercalcemia

Hypercalcemia, or an excess serum calcium, may result from overuse of calcium antacids, immobilization, malignancy, hyperparathyroidism, and thiazide diuretics. Acute hypercalcemia affects the hydration status by increasing renal loss of sodium and water, whereas chronic hypercalcemia impairs renal concentrating ability, decreasing ECF volume. Other symptoms include constipation, anorexia, lethargy, fatigue, depression, confusion, coma, cardiac arrhythmias, and renal lithiasis (Bove, 1996a; Graves, 1990).

Phosphorus Imbalances

Hypophosphatemia

Hypophosphatemia may result from increased renal losses during diuretic therapy or states of osmotic diuresis. It also occurs with hyperparathyroidism, malabsorption syndromes, or chronic administration of antacids. Phosphorus may also shift into the cell, particularly during refeeding following starvation or alkalosis, resulting in low serum levels. Symptoms associated with hypophosphatemia include weakness, mental confusion, irritability, anemia, bone brittleness, and respiratory arrest (Bove, 1996a; Graves, 1990).

Hyperphosphatemia

Hyperphosphatemia is usually associated with renal failure but may also occur from overuse of laxatives that contain phosphorus, a diet rich in phosphorus, and increased gastrointestinal absorption of phosphorus due to excess vitamin D intake. This imbalance is often associated with hypocalcemia, and symptoms of a decreased serum calcium level predominate (Bove, 1996a).

Magnesium Imbalances

Hypomagnesemia

Hypomagnesemia, or a decrease in magnesium, may occur without a decrease in the serum level of magnesium because less than 1% of magnesium is found in the serum. Clinical conditions associated with this imbalance include starvation, chronic diarrhea, malabsorption syndromes, diuretic therapy, chronic alcohol ingestion, hyperparathyroidism, acute myocardial infarction, congestive heart failure, and excessive sweating. Symptoms associated with hypomagnesemia include cardiac arrhythmias, coronary artery spasm, muscle weakness, muscle twitching and tremor, delirium, hyperreflexia, convulsions, coma, refractory hypokalemia, and hypocalcemia (Ferrin, 1996; Friday & Reinhart, 1991; Owens, 1993).

Hypermagnesemia

The primary risk factor for the development of hypermagnesemia is renal failure with low urine output. Other factors include adrenal insufficiency and the overuse of magnesium-containing medications or enemas. Symptoms associated with hypermagnesemia include weakness, hypotension, weak or absent deep tendon reflexes, slurred speech, drowsiness, lethargy, and cardiac arrhythmias. As the magnesium level continues to elevate, flaccid muscle paralysis, respiratory depression, apnea, coma, heart block, and cardiac arrest may develop (Felver & Pendarvis, 1989; Ferrin, 1996).

Acid-Base Balance

An **acid** is any substance that releases a hydrogen ion (H^+) into a solution, and a **base** is any substance that sequesters H^+. Within the human body, the physiologically correct balance for acids and bases is a relationship of 20 base bicarbonates to one carbonic acid (Russell, 1993).

Body acids are formed as end products of cellular metabolism and are either volatile (can be eliminated as CO_2) or nonvolatile. Carbonic acid is the only known volatile acid within the human body. Because the average person generates 50 to 100 mEq of acid per day, this same amount of acid must be neutralized or excreted to maintain pH balance (McCance & Huether, 1994).

Regulation of Hydrogen Ion Concentration

Regulation of acid-base balance is an important aspect of maintaining homeostasis. Acid-base balance refers to the regulation of H^+ concentration in the body fluids. The **pH** of a fluid reflects and is inversely proportional to H^+ concentration. In other words, as the pH increases, H^+ concentration decreases, and as the pH decreases, H^+ concentration increases. The normal pH of body fluids is 7.40, with a normal range of 7.35 to 7.45. Therefore, as H^+ concentration increases, the pH decreases below 7.40, and the fluid becomes acidotic. As H^+ concentration decreases, the pH increases above 7.40, and the fluid becomes alkalotic (Chenevey, 1987; McCance & Huether, 1994).

To maintain homeostasis, the pH must be maintained between 7.35 and 7.45. Even a slight variation in either direction could be fatal. Three mechanisms operate within the human body to maintain this delicate balance and include chemical buffers, the respiratory system, and the renal system (Fig. 28–5).

Chemical Buffers

The first compensatory mechanism is the blood buffer system, which is composed of pairs of weak acids and their bases. These buffer pairs can alternate from acid to base very quickly to stabilize the blood pH. The primary blood buffer is the sodium bicarbonate–carbonic acid buffer system, which buffers approximately 45% of all H^+ (York, 1987).

Regulation of acid-base balance in body fluids

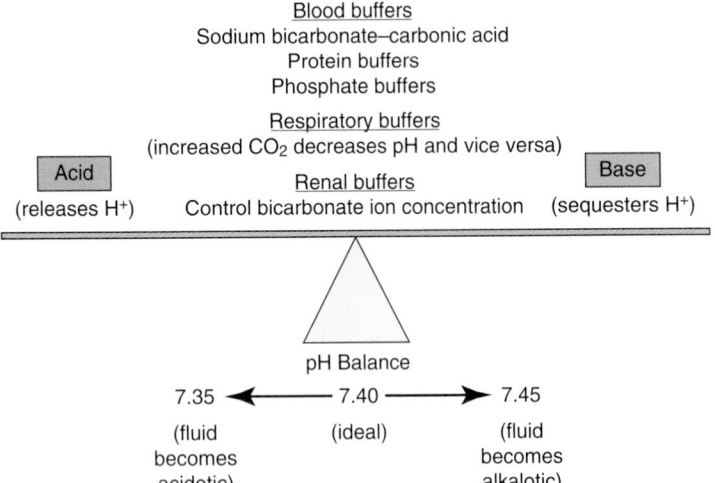

❧ **Figure 28–5**
Acid-base balance showing safe range supported by chemical buffers, respiratory system, and renal system.

When a strong acid such as hydrochloric acid (HCl) is increased, the bicarbonate–carbonic acid buffer system combines with this acid to produce sodium chloride and a weaker acid (carbonic acid). Carbonic acid further dissociates into carbon dioxide and water, and the lungs exhale excess carbon dioxide. Thus, the blood pH returns to normal. The following formula illustrates this process:

$$HCl + NaHCO_3 \rightleftharpoons H_2CO_3 + NaCl$$
$$H_2CO_3 \rightleftharpoons H_2O + CO_2$$

Two other chemical buffers include protein buffers and phosphate buffers. These buffers also work to absorb or produce H+ as needed to maintain blood pH. These buffers work within seconds whenever a change in pH occurs (Chenevey, 1987; York, 1987).

Respiratory Regulation

The respiratory system is a second compensatory mechanism that can regulate the pH through regulation of carbon dioxide levels. Carbon dioxide can combine with water to form carbonic acid. Therefore, an increase in CO_2 concentration in body fluids decreases the blood pH (acidemia), and a decrease in CO_2 concentration increases the blood pH (alkalemia). Respiratory compensation usually occurs within seconds of a change in blood pH (Chenevey, 1987).

As the pH decreases or becomes more acidotic, chemoreceptors in the medulla of the brain are stimulated, resulting in an increase in breathing and respiratory ventilation. This increase in ventilation results in loss of CO_2 from the lungs, and an increase in pH will occur. Conversely, as pH increases above normal, respiratory ventilation slows, CO_2 is retained, and the pH decreases (Chenevey, 1987; York, 1987).

Renal Regulation

The third compensatory mechanism is the renal system, which helps to control the bicarbonate ion concentration in body fluids. The kidneys, through a series of complex chemical reactions, regulate hydrogen ion concentration by increasing or decreasing bicarbonate. When the blood pH becomes acidotic, hydrogen ions, secreted into the renal tubule and excreted with urine, are exchanged for sodium ions, which then combine with bicarbonate to form the buffer sodium bicarbonate. As the blood pH becomes alkalotic, this process decreases, and hydrogen is retained while sodium bicarbonate and other buffer salts are excreted in the urine (Chenevey, 1987; York, 1987).

Thus, these three mechanisms help to maintain acid-base balance within body fluids. The chemical buffers and respiratory system work within seconds, whereas the kidneys take several hours to a day to regulate acid-base balance.

Disturbances in Acid-Base Balance

Changes in the concentration of hydrogen ions in the blood may lead to acid-base imbalances. When the pH of arterial blood is less than 7.35, acidemia occurs and is usually associated with a systemic increase in hydrogen ion concentration or acidosis. When the pH of arterial blood is greater than 7.45, alkalemia occurs and is usually associated with a systemic decrease in hydrogen ion concentration or alkalosis. Acid-base imbalances are usually categorized as respiratory acidosis, respiratory alkalosis, metabolic acidosis, and metabolic alkalosis (McCance & Huether, 1994). Table 28–3 summarizes acid-base imbalances.

Table 28-3

DISTURBANCES IN ACID-BASE BALANCE

IMBALANCE	CAUSATIVE FACTORS	MANIFESTATIONS
Respiratory acidosis	Hypoventilation—chronic obstructive pulmonary disease, pneumonia, overdose of barbiturates or sedatives	pH <7.35, $PaCO_2$ increased, restlessness, apprehension, lethargy, muscle twitching, tremors, convulsions, coma
Respiratory alkalosis	Hyperventilation—fever, mechanical overventilation	pH >7.35, $PaCO_2$ decreased, dizziness, confusion, tingling of extremities, convulsions, coma
Metabolic acidosis	Loss of HCO_3^- or increase in H^+—starvation, diarrhea, diabetic ketoacidosis, renal disease	pH <7.35, HCO_3^- decreased, headache, lethargy, coma, Kussmaul's respiration, anorexia, nausea, vomiting, diarrhea, cardiac dysrrhythmias
Metabolic alkalosis	Loss of metabolic acids—severe vomiting, nasogastric suction, diuretic therapy, excessive intake of sodium bicarbonate	pH >7.35, HCO_3^- increased, weakness, muscle cramps, hyperactive reflexes, slow respirations, confusion, convulsions

Respiratory Acidosis

Respiratory **acidosis** occurs as a result of retention of CO_2, resulting in an excess of carbonic acid. The $PaCO_2$ is increased, and the pH is decreased. Respiratory acidosis is associated with hypoventilation and may be the result of chronic obstructive lung disease, pneumonia, or overdose of barbiturates or sedatives. Manifestations of respiratory acidosis include restlessness and apprehension, followed by lethargy, muscle twitching, tremors, convulsions, and coma. The respiratory rate may be rapid initially and gradually becomes depressed (Brenner & Welliver, 1990; Hurray & Saver, 1992; McCance & Huether, 1994).

Respiratory Alkalosis

Respiratory **alkalosis** results in a deficit of CO_2 and therefore a deficit in carbonic acid. The CO_2 level is decreased, and the pH is increased. This imbalance is usually the result of hyperventilation and may be associated with fever or mechanical overventilation. Manifestations of respiratory alkalosis include dizziness, confusion, tingling of extremities, convulsions, and coma (Brenner & Welliver, 1990; Hurray & Saver, 1992; McCance & Huether, 1994).

Metabolic Acidosis

Metabolic acidosis results in a decrease in bicarbonate ions and a decrease in pH. This imbalance may be associated with either a loss of bicarbonate ions or an increase in noncarbonic acids. Causes of metabolic acidosis include starvation, severe diarrhea, diabetic ketoacidosis, or renal disease. Manifestations of this imbalance are headache; lethargy progressing to coma; deep, rapid respirations; anorexia; nausea; vomiting; diarrhea; abdominal discomfort; and cardiac

dysrhythmias (Brenner & Welliver, 1990; Hurray & Saver, 1992; McCance & Huether, 1994).

Metabolic Alkalosis

Metabolic alkalosis usually is associated with a loss of metabolic acids, resulting in an increase in bicarbonate and an increase in pH. This imbalance may be the result of severe vomiting, nasogastric intubation with suction, diuretic therapy, or excessive sodium bicarbonate intake. Manifestations of metabolic alkalosis may include weakness; muscle cramps; hyperactive reflexes; slow, shallow respirations; confusion; and convulsions (Brenner & Welliver, 1990; Hurray & Saver, 1992; McCance & Huether, 1994).

✦ Application of the Nursing Process

The nursing care of clients experiencing disturbances in hydration, electrolyte, or acid-base balance may be guided by the nursing process, which includes assessment, analysis, planning, implementation, and evaluation. During the assessment phase, data are gathered through the health history and physical examination, as well as analysis of pertinent laboratory data. Analysis of these data leads to the formulation of nursing diagnoses. Planning involves collaboration between client and nurse to identify client outcomes. Specific interventions are then implemented, and following implementation of these interventions, the client outcomes are evaluated and changes are made in the plan of care as indicated.

Assessment

The assessment phase includes both subjective and objective data gathering. Subjective data are obtained through the health history, whereas objective data are acquired through physical assessment and analysis of pertinent laboratory findings.

Nursing History

The nursing history is an important tool for obtaining subjective data related to hydration status, electrolyte balance, and acid-base balance. The history includes information related to the client's current and previous health status and family history, as well as psychological, spiritual, and sociocultural aspects of health.

Previous Health Experience

Begin with questions concerning the client's previous health and illness experience, including past experiences with health care providers and expectations of care, treatment, and staff. Also include any illnesses or surgeries the client may have had in the past, since many illnesses and surgeries predispose the client to disturbances in hydration and electrolyte and acid-base balance (Poyss, 1987).

In addition, determine if the individual is currently taking medications—prescription and nonprescription. Chronic use of laxatives and antacids, as well as long-term use of diuretics, may place the individual at risk for disturbances in fluid, electrolyte, and acid-base balance (Poyss, 1987).

Family History

Next determine the client's family history, which may provide information pertinent to the client's health status. A family history of illness, such as renal disease, heart disease, stroke, endocrine disorders, high blood pressure, or any chronic disease state, may indicate risk factors for the client to develop disorders affecting hydration, electrolyte balance, and acid-base homeostasis (Poyss, 1987).

Psychological History

Next determine any psychological factors that might place the individual at risk for hydration, electrolyte, and/or acid-base imbalances. Behavioral and emotional problems, such as chronic alcohol abuse, drug dependency, and denial of chronic illness like diabetes, are risk factors to be assessed (Horne *et al.,* 1991).

Spiritual and Sociocultural History

Assessment of spiritual beliefs and sociocultural practices may identify values or practices that may place the individual at risk for developing fluid, electrolyte, or acid-base imbalances. For example, a client who is a Jehovah's Witness is bleeding and refuses human blood products will need to be identified early so that care can be modified. Also, the client on a fixed income may be financially unable to obtain needed medication and may be at increased risk (Horne *et al.,* 1991).

Questions to Consider

Metheny (1992) designates specific questions to be considered in the nursing history (Box 28–1). Analysis of information from these questions, as well as from the history, may help identify individuals at risk for developing hydration, electrolyte, and acid-base imbalances.

Physical Examination

Assessment of vital signs and completion of a physical assessment yield objective data indicative of imbalances in hydration, electrolyte, and acid-base status.

Vital Signs

Changes in vital signs may signal changes in hydration and electrolyte balance. Body temperature, respiratory pattern, heart rate, and blood pressure should be determined every 4 hours or more frequently in the client at risk for imbalances (Metheny, 1992).

Temperature

Elevations in body temperature may lead to imbalances in hydration status through fluid and electrolyte loss due to increased sweating. Changes in body temperature may also be associated with fluid and electro-

---

Box 28–1

QUESTIONS TO INCLUDE IN THE NURSING HISTORY

Is any injury or disease process present that may disrupt fluid and electrolyte balance? If so, what type of imbalance is usually associated with this disease or injury?

Is the client receiving any treatment or medication that might disrupt fluid and electrolyte balance? If so, how does this therapy affect hydration and electrolyte balance?

Is an abnormal loss of body fluids occurring? What is the source of this fluid loss, and what types of imbalances are usually associated with this loss?

Is the client on any dietary restrictions? If so, how do these restrictions usually affect hydration status?

Does the client have an adequate intake of water and nutrients orally or by some other route? If not, how long has the intake been inadequate?

What is the total intake of fluids in comparison with the total output?

lyte imbalances. For instance, hyperosmolar fluid volume deficit may result in an increase in body temperature, whereas severe hypovolemia may result in a decrease in body temperature (Horne *et al.,* 1991).

Respiratory Pattern

Increases in respiratory depth, as well as increased production of respiratory secretions, may contribute to fluid volume depletion. Dyspnea, rales (crackles), or rhonchi may indicate increased fluid in the lungs due to fluid volume excess. Respiratory pattern may also change with acid-base imbalances. For instance, rapid, deep respirations (Kussmaul respirations) may occur with metabolic acidosis as the lungs attempt to normalize pH by blowing off CO_2 (Horne *et al.,* 1991).

Heart Rate

An increase in heart rate may occur with fluid volume deficit or excess. Also, changes in heart rate and rhythm may be associated with imbalances of potassium, calcium, or magnesium (Horne *et al.,* 1991).

Blood Pressure

Changes in blood pressure may also indicate imbalances in hydration and electrolytes. Fluid volume deficit may result in a decrease in blood pressure, whereas fluid volume excess may result in an elevation of blood pressure. Electrolyte imbalances may also result in a decrease in blood pressure (Horne *et al.,* 1991).

Orthostatic Vital Signs

Changes in heart rate and blood pressure as the client moves from lying to standing may also be assessed as an indication of fluid volume depletion. To perform the orthostatic test, take the client's blood pressure and heart rate while he or she is lying in bed. Then have the client stand, and retake the blood pressure and heart rate immediately and again at 1 minute. Most individuals will have a normal increase in heart rate on standing of less than 30 beats per minute and a decrease in systolic blood pressure of 10 to 12 mmHg. If the client's heart rate increases above 30 beats per minute or if the systolic blood pressure decreases by 15 mmHg or greater, volume depletion may be considered. In addition, the client may experience other orthostatic symptoms on standing, including syncope and pallor (Wandel, 1990).

The results of the orthostatic test should be interpreted with extreme caution in the elderly. Many factors other than fluid volume depletion may cause postural hypotension in this group. Conversely, the absence of abnormal orthostatic vital signs does not rule out a disturbance in hydration (Wandel, 1990).

Physical Assessment

The physical assessment is a detailed examination to look for changes that might indicate an imbalance in fluids, electrolytes, or acid-base function.

Weight

Acute changes in weight are usually indicative of acute fluid changes. Each kilogram of acute weight change suggests 1 L of fluid lost or gained, unless the individual is not eating or is not being maintained on enteral or parenteral nutrition. Weight gain does not necessarily indicate an increase in vascular volume but may indicate an increase in total body volume. The weight should be measured at the same time of day, preferably before breakfast, using the same scale with the individual wearing approximately the same clothing (Horne *et al.,* 1991).

Intake and Output

Intake and output should be measured and recorded for any client at risk for fluid and electrolyte imbalance (Box 28–2). Whereas the physician may order intake and output to be monitored, the nurse may also initiate this assessment if indicated. To ensure accuracy, liquid intake and output should be measured and recorded and all unmeasured volumes estimated and noted (Horne *et al.,* 1991).

Intake includes oral fluids, parenteral fluids, tube feedings, catheter irrigants, and medications. Output includes urine output, liquid feces, vomitus, nasogastric drainage, wound drainage, draining fistulas, excessive diaphoresis, and increased depth of respirations.

Integumentary Assessment

The skin is assessed for moisture, color, temperature, and turgor. The client's skin should appear well hydrated and full, without obvious perspiration. The presence of edema is also assessed. The oral cavity and eyes are also inspected for any changes (Horne *et al.,* 1991; Poyss, 1987).

The individual who has flushed, dry skin may have a fluid volume deficit. In addition, the client with profound fluid loss resulting in shock may have skin that is cool, clammy, and pale (Horne *et al.,* 1991).

To assess skin turgor, pinch the skin over the abdomen, forearm, sternum, dorsum of the hand, or the thigh (Fig. 28–6). With adequate hydration, the skin folds quickly return to normal. If poorly hydrated, the skin folds are slow to return to normal, and the skin appears "doughy." Skin turgor is not a reliable indicator of fluid loss in the elderly because of loss of elasticity with aging (Horne *et al.,* 1991; Poyss, 1987).

Assess infants for skin turgor, sunken eyeballs, and depressed anterior fontanel. Sunken eyes and dark skin around them, as well as depression of the anterior fontanel, can indicate a severe fluid volume deficit (Kee & Paulanka, 1994).

The individual should be free of localized or generalized edema. Edema, if present, is usually located in dependent areas of the body, such as the feet and legs if the client is standing. Assess for pitting edema over a bony surface, such as the tibia or sacrum, by applying pressure with a finger or thumb and noting the severity of the indentation after pressure is re-

---

Box 28–2

MEASURING AND RECORDING FLUID INTAKE AND OUTPUT

Sources of Fluid Intake

Oral fluids—include all fluids that are liquid at room temperature, as well as ice chips, which are recorded at approximately one half their volume

Parenteral fluids—record the exact amount of intravenous fluids given

Tube feedings—record the exact amount of tube feeding given, as well as any water used to flush the tube feeding or to flush following administration of medications

Catheter irrigants—record catheter irrigants that are not withdrawn when irrigating or lavaging a catheter

Medications—parenteral and liquid oral medications can be significant sources of fluids and should be recorded

Sources of Fluid Output

Urine output—urine output from a Foley catheter may be measured hourly or at least every 8 hours; all voidings should be measured and totaled at the end of each shift; to assess urine output from infants and toddlers, weigh diapers saturated with urine

Liquid feces—for individuals who are incontinent of urine or liquid feces, weigh the soiled pad or diaper to determine fluid loss: first, weigh a dry pad or diaper using a gram scale and document; then, weigh all soiled pads—each increase in weight by 1 g reflects approximately 1 ml of fluid loss

Vomitus—record the exact amount

Nasogastric drainage—record the exact amount

Wound drainage—document wound drainage by weighing the soiled dressings, by noting the type and number of dressings, or by directly measuring the drainage contained in a gravity or vacuum drainage device for wounds

Draining fistulas—document amount of dressings saturated or measure directly by collecting drainage in a stoma bag

Excessive diaphoresis—document excessive sweating on a scale of 1+ for noticeable sweating to 4+ for profuse sweating, or document by the amount of linen saturated with sweat

Increased depth of respirations—increased depth of respirations increases insensible fluid loss; however, this loss is usually not clinically significant

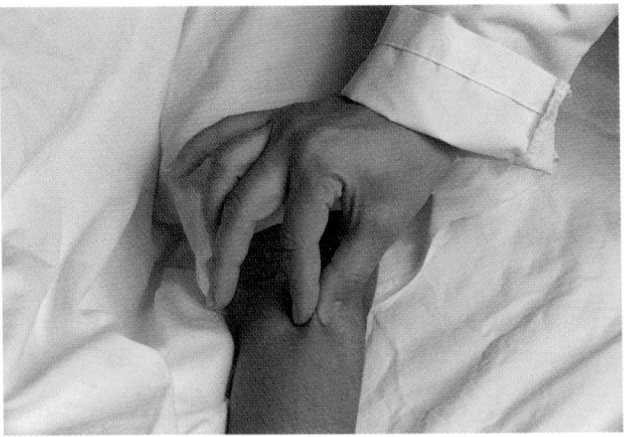

❧ **Figure 28–6**
Integumentary assessment for fluid volume deficit and fluid volume excess. Skin turgor is assessed by pinching the skin over the abdomen, forearm, sternum, dorsum of the hand, or the thigh. Poor hydration may be indicated if the skin folds are slow to return to normal, know as "tenting." Tenting is not a reliable indicator of fluid loss in the elderly, however, because of loss of skin elasticity with aging. Other indications of severe fluid volume deficit in infants are sunken eyes with dark skin around them, and depression of the anterior fontanel.

pink and moist. Pallor or dryness, as well as a red, rough, dry tongue, may indicate fluid volume deficit or hypernatremia (Poyss, 1987).

The eyes should appear alert, and the eyeballs should be moist. Changes, such as sunken eyeballs or periorbital edema, may indicate fluid imbalance (Poyss, 1987).

Cardiovascular Assessment

The cardiovascular assessment includes an assessment of capillary refill, pulse strength and volume, hand veins, and jugular veins.

Capillary refill may be used to evaluate arterial perfusion. Apply pressure over a toenail or fingernail. Normally, the nail blanches with pressure and then the color returns within 2 to 4 seconds after pressure is released. Refill taking longer than 4 to 6 seconds suggests poor arterial perfusion and may indicate decreased effective circulating fluid volume. Capillary refill may be delayed in the older adult secondary to local peripheral vascular disease (Horne *et al.*, 1991).

Pulse strength and volume are dependent on the volume of blood ejected by the left ventricle, as well as the strength of the left ventricular contraction. Therefore, a weak, thready pulse may indicate a reduction in intravascular volume, and a bounding pulse may signal a fluid volume excess. Pulse irregularity may also occur with abnormalities in potassium, magnesium, and calcium levels (Horne *et al.*, 1991).

Elevate the client's hand and forearm above the level of the heart to assess for fluid volume status. Usually, the hand veins empty in 3 to 5 seconds, and, when lowered, the veins refill in approximately the same time. With fluid volume depletion, the hand veins take longer than 5 seconds to fill, and with fluid

leased (Fig. 28–7). Pitting edema is rated according to severity on a scale of 1 to 4, with 1+ indicating barely detectable edema and 4+, deep, persistent pitting (Horne *et al.*, 1991; Poyss, 1987).

Thorough inspection of the oral cavity may reveal changes associated with hydration and electrolyte status. Usually the oral mucous membranes appear

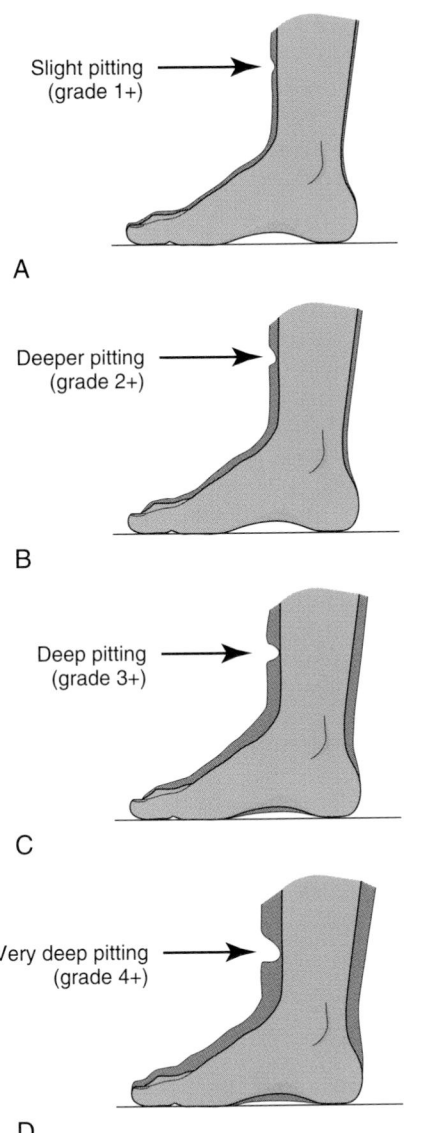

Slight pitting
(grade 1+)

A

Deeper pitting
(grade 2+)

B

Deep pitting
(grade 3+)

C

Very deep pitting
(grade 4+)

D

✦ **Figure 28–7**
To assess for edema, press with a finger or thumb over a bony surface and note whether an indentation remains (pitting edema) after the pressure is released. The severity of pitting edema is rated on a scale of 1 to 4, with 1+ indicating barely detectable edema and 4+ indicating deep, persistent pitting.

volume excess, the hand veins take longer than 5 seconds to empty (Poyss, 1987).

The degree of jugular venous distention provides an estimate of central venous pressure and fluid volume status. Elevate the head of the bed to 30 or 45 degrees and measure the distance between the level of the sternal angle and the point as which the internal and external jugular veins collapse. Optimally, this distance should be 3 cm or less. Intravascular volume excess may be indicated with distension above 3 cm, whereas decreased jugular venous distention or absence of distension with the client fully reclined may indicate fluid volume deficit (Horne *et al.*, 1991).

Neurological Assessment

The neurological assessment includes noting any changes in sensorium, as well as any abnormalities in neuromuscular excitability. Early symptoms of fluid volume deficit in infants are irritability, purposeless movement, and an unusual high-pitched or whining cry. As the deficit worsens, lethargy and loss of consciousness may also occur.

Changes in serum osmolality or severe acid-base imbalances may result in changes in awareness, orientation, and level of consciousness. The severity of the symptoms depends on the acuteness and the degree of the change. For instance, a sudden drop in serum sodium may be more likely to result in coma than a gradual change, which allows the cells to adjust to the change in osmolality. Restlessness and confusion may occur with fluid volume deficit or with acid-base imbalance, and markedly increased calcium levels can affect sensorium. With serum calcium and magnesium imbalances, individuals may experience agitation, confusion, psychosis, situational depression, and emotional changes (Horne *et al.*, 1991; Kee & Paulanka, 1994; Poyss, 1987).

Changes in neuromuscular excitability may occur with calcium and magnesium imbalances. As the serum calcium and magnesium levels decrease, neuromuscular excitability increases, with hyperactive reflexes and possible tetany-type spasms. Conversely, as the serum calcium and magnesium levels increase, neuromuscular function decreases, with diminished reflexes, decreased muscle tone, and muscle flaccidity. With metabolic alkalosis, symptoms similar to those associated with hypocalcemia may develop. Abnormalities in potassium levels also result in neuromuscular symptoms. With hyperkalemia, tingling, paresthesias, weakness, and flaccid paralysis may occur. With hypokalemia, weakness, muscle cramps, tetany, and paralysis may occur (Horne *et al.*, 1991; Poyss, 1987).

Tetany, a severe muscle spasm, which can interfere with breathing and cause death, may occur with greatly diminished calcium levels. To determine if increased neuromuscular excitability is present, Trousseau's and Chvostek's signs should be assessed. To assess Trousseau's sign, apply a blood pressure cuff to the upper arm and inflate it past the systolic blood pressure (BP) for 2 minutes. Trousseau's sign is positive if contraction of the hand and fingers occurs, indicating carpal spasm (see Fig. 28–4). To assess Chvostek's sign, tap on the facial nerve just in front of the ear. Chvostek's sign is positive if unilateral contraction of the facial and eyelid muscles occurs. Positive Trousseau's and Chvostek's signs may occur with hypocalcemia and hypomagnesemia (Horne *et al.*, 1991; McCance & Huether, 1994; Poyss, 1987).

Gastrointestinal Assessment

The gastrointestinal assessment includes assessment of any gastrointestinal disturbances, the presence of thirst, and abdominal girth. Although gastrointestinal symptoms may occur with hydration and electrolyte disturbances, these same symptoms may be a cause of fluid and electrolyte imbalances.

Common gastrointestinal disturbances associated with changes in hydration, including deficits and excesses, are anorexia, nausea, and vomiting. Bowel motility may also be altered with potassium or calcium imbalances, resulting in either diarrhea or constipation. Remember that vomiting and diarrhea may further enhance hydration and electrolyte imbalances (Horne *et al.*, 1991).

Symptomatic thirst develops when a loss of body water occurs and resolves once that loss has been corrected. Thirst indicates an increased serum osmolality and cellular dehydration, as well as decreased vascular volume. Thirst and polyuria (increased urinary output) are also associated with hypercalcemia and hypokalemia. Thirst may be diminished in the elderly and may be affected by social and emotional factors (Porth & Erickson, 1992).

Changes in abdominal girth may indicate retention of fluid in the gastrointestinal tract or in the peritoneal cavity (ascites). Measure abdominal girth daily in any individual with abdominal distention. To ensure consistency and accuracy, measure the abdominal girth at the same time each day using a nonstretchable tape measure. Be sure to mark the measurement site on the abdomen with indelible ink (Horne *et al.*, 1991).

Renal Assessment

Changes in urinary output should be monitored closely. A decrease in urine output may indicate a fluid volume deficit or the onset of renal failure, which could result in a fluid volume excess. An increase in urine output (polyuria) may be a contributing factor in the development of fluid volume deficit. For example, polyuria associated with diabetes mellitus or diabetes insipidus may result in a fluid deficit. Fluid deficits can also result from the overuse of diuretics (Horne *et al.*, 1991).

Changes in urinary output may also contribute to electrolyte imbalances. For instance, individuals who produce large volumes of urine are at risk of developing hypokalemia due to the loss of potassium in the urine. Conversely, individuals who produce very small volumes of urine are at risk of developing hyperkalemia due to the decreased excretion of potassium in the urine (Horne *et al.*, 1991).

When monitoring urine output, several factors need to be considered, including the following (Metheny, 1992):

1. The usual urine output in adults is 1 to 2 L/day

2. During periods of stress, the usual urine output is 750 to 1200 ml/day

3. If measured hourly, the usual urine output in adults is 40 to 80 ml/hour

4. During periods of stress, the usual urine output is 30 to 50 ml/hour

5. The elderly have a diminished renal concentrating ability and may need more fluid intake

6. A low urine volume with a high urine specific gravity indicates fluid volume deficit

7. A low urine volume with a low urine specific gravity indicates renal disease

Developmental Assessment

Developmental stage or client age may be a risk factor for the development of disturbances in hydration status. Infants and the elderly are at greater risk of developing hydration disturbances than are children and younger adults.

The infant has a proportionately high ratio of ECF to ICF; thus, the very young are predisposed to rapid losses of body fluid. Infants also have a limited fluid reserve capacity, which inhibits their adaptation to fluid losses. Immature renal structures and a high rate of metabolism further place the infant at risk for developing dehydration. Symptoms of this imbalance can occur quite rapidly in infants and can be very dramatic in their presentation (Kee & Paulanka, 1994).

The elderly are also at increased risk for developing fluid and electrolyte imbalances. Structural and functional changes that occur as a result of the aging process, as well as chronic diseases, decrease the aging adult's ability to maintain fluid and electrolyte balance (see box). Research also indicates that advancing age may be a risk factor for inadequate water intake (Horne *et al.*, 1991; Kee, 1995; Kee & Paulanka, 1994).

FLUID AND ELECTROLYTE BALANCE IN THE ELDERLY

Older adults have a reduced muscle mass, with an increase in total body fat. Because muscle tissue contains more water, a net reduction in total body water occurs.

With normal aging, a reduction in ICF occurs.

Compensatory mechanisms for water loss alter with aging. The ability of the nephron to concentrate urine is compromised; response to ADH secretion may not be as efficient; and thirst sensation may be diminished or absent.

Aging affects the ability of the kidney to regulate sodium. The aging kidney has a tendency to lose sodium, and with sodium loss, potassium is retained, making the older adult susceptible to hyponatremia and hyperkalemia.

Vitamin D synthesis into its active form is reduced with decreased absorption of calcium in the gastrointestinal tract. In response to decreased absorption of calcium, the parathyroid glands secrete PTH, mobilizing calcium from bones. These changes may be associated with the development of osteoporosis in the older adult.

Laboratory Assessment

Laboratory tests help to identify and to monitor fluid, electrolyte, and acid-base imbalances. Laboratory tests to determine hydration status include serum osmolality, hematocrit, blood urea nitrogen, serum albumin, urine osmolality, urine specific gravity, and urine sodium. Laboratory tests to determine electrolyte balance include serum sodium, potassium, calcium, phosphorus, and magnesium (Table 28–4). Laboratory tests to determine acid-base status include arterial blood gases (Table 28–5) and calculation of the anion gap using sodium, chloride, and bicarbonate levels.

Serum Osmolality

The serum osmolality measures the solute concentration of the blood and primarily reflects the concentration of sodium and its accompanying anions. The normal range for serum osmolality is 280 to 300 mOsm/kg (Chernecky et al., 1993; Horne et al., 1991; McFarland & Grant, 1994).

Hematocrit

The hematocrit measures the volume of red blood cells in relation to plasma and is the percentage of whole blood that is composed of red blood cells. Changes in plasma volume are reflected by changes in the hematocrit. Thus, the hematocrit decreases with fluid volume excess and increases with fluid volume deficit. Normal ranges for hematocrit are 37 to 47% for women and 40 to 50% for men (Chernecky et al., 1993; Horne et al., 1991).

Table 28–5

ARTERIAL BLOOD GAS VALUES

MEASUREMENT	NORMAL VALUE	RANGE
pH	7.40	7.35–7.45
$PaCO_2$	40	35–45
PaO_2	—	80–100
SaO_2	—	96–98%
HCO_3^-	24	22–26 mEq/L

Blood Urea Nitrogen

Urea is produced by the body as a byproduct of protein metabolism and is excreted by the kidneys. Because urea production occurs at a fairly steady rate, an increase in blood urea nitrogen (BUN) might indicate decreased renal function. However, urea excretion varies with water excretion, and in fluid volume deficit, decreased water excretion results in decreased urea excretion and a concomitant rise in BUN. The normal range for BUN is 6 to 20 mg/dL (Horne et al., 1991; McFarland & Grant, 1994).

Serum Albumin

Albumin, a small plasma protein produced by the liver, acts osmotically to help hold the intravascular volume in the vascular space. Decreased albumin may result in the development of edema as a result of a decrease in the plasma oncotic pressure. As this pressure decreases, fluid moves out of the vascular compartment into the interstitial space, resulting in a generalized edema. The normal range for serum albumin is 3.5 to 5.5 g/dL (Horne et al., 1991; McFarland & Grant, 1994).

Urine Osmolality

The urine osmolality is a measure of the solute concentration of the urine and is determined by the nitrogenous wastes (urea, creatinine, uric acid) in the urine. Urine osmolality may vary with hydration status. For instance, with fluid volume deficit, the urine osmolality increases, and with fluid volume excess, the urine osmolality may decrease. The usual range of urine osmolality is approximately 50 to 1400 mOsm/kg (Chernecky et al., 1993; Horne et al., 1991).

Urine Specific Gravity

The weight of a solution in relation to water is the specific gravity. The urine specific gravity evaluates the kidneys' ability to excrete or conserve water. Specific gravity may increase with fluid volume deficit and may decrease with fluid volume excess. However, several factors may give a falsely high urine specific grav-

Table 28–4

LABORATORY TESTS FOR HYDRATION AND ELECTROLYTE STATUS

LABORATORY TEST	NORMAL VALUE
Serum sodium	135–145 mEq/L
Serum potassium	3.5–5.3 mEq/L
Serum calcium	4.5–5.5 mEq/L or 9–11 mg/dl
Serum phosphorus	2.5–4.5 mEq/L
Serum magnesium	1.5–2.5 mEq/L
Serum osmolality	280–300 mOsm/kg
Hematocrit	Women: 37–47% Men: 40–50%
BUN	6–20 mg/dl
Urine osmolality	50–1400 mOsm/kg
Urine specific gravity	1.001–1.040
Urine sodium	50–130 mEq/L

ity and include glucose, protein, dextran, radiographic contrast material, and certain medications. The usual range for urine specific gravity is 1.001 to 1.040 (Chernecky *et al.*, 1993; Horne *et al.*, 1991, although a range of 1.012 to 1.025 is considered to reflect normal hydration (Methany, 1992).

Urine Sodium

Urine sodium levels may be measured to evaluate fluid volume status, hyponatremia, and acute renal failure. Urine sodium levels usually increase with increased sodium intake and decrease with a decrease in effective circulating blood volume. Urine sodium levels may also be increased with diuretic use and advanced renal failure. Urine sodium can be measured from a 24-hour specimen or from a random spot specimen. The usual range for urine sodium from a random specimen is 50 to 130 mEq/L (Horne *et al.*, 1991; McFarland & Grant, 1994).

Serum Electrolytes

Table 28–4 contains the normal values for sodium, potassium, calcium, phosphorus, and magnesium. Assessment of serum electrolytes is essential for any client with alterations in hydration or acid-base status.

Arterial Blood Gases

Arterial blood gases (ABGs) are utilized to determine the acid-base and oxygenation status of the client, as well as to identify any abnormalities in acid-base balance. Normal values for ABGs are shown in Table 28–5.

The pH designates the H^+ concentration and is inversely proportional to H^+. As the H^+ increases, the pH decreases or becomes more acidotic, and as the H^+ decreases, the pH increases or becomes more alkalotic.

The $PaCO_2$ measures the amount of CO_2 in arterial blood and, thus, the potential carbonic acid content. Changes in the rate of alveolar ventilation produce changes in the $PaCO_2$. When less CO_2 is removed, the $PaCO_2$ increases and the pH decreases. When more CO_2 is removed, the $PaCO_2$ decreases and the pH increases.

Changes in the HCO_3^- level denote the amount of bicarbonate or base in arterial blood. Thus, an increase in HCO_3^- results in an increase in pH, and a decrease in HCO_3^- results in a decrease in pH.

The PaO_2 is the percentage of oxygen in arterial blood, and the SaO_2 is the saturation of hemoglobin with oxygen (Lowenstein, 1993; McCance & Huether, 1994).

Interpretation of ABG using a five-step analysis technique may yield useful information concerning the client's acid-base status (Stringfield, 1993). Box 28–3 outlines the steps in ABG interpretation.

Acid-base abnormalities usually are categorized as respiratory acidosis, respiratory alkalosis, metabolic ac-

---

Box 28–3

FIVE-STEP ANALYSIS TECHNIQUE FOR ARTERIAL BLOOD GAS INTERPRETATION

1. Identify any abnormality in pH. If the pH is above 7.45, alkalosis is present, and if the pH is below 7.35, acidosis is present
2. Identify any abnormality in $PaCO_2$. Compare abnormal level to the pH. If the $PaCO_2$ is moving in the opposite direction of the pH level, a respiratory cause for the acid-base imbalance should be considered
3. Identify any abnormality in HCO_3^-. Compare any abnormal level with the pH. If the HCO_3^- is moving in the same direction as the pH level, a metabolic cause for the acid-base imbalance should be considered
4. Determine whether compensation has occurred. Compensation occurs when the pH has returned within the normal range. However, the $PaCO_2$ or the HCO_3^- abnormality will still be present
5. Make an interpretation

---

idosis, or metabolic alkalosis. Table 28–6 indicates the ABG changes associated with these acid-base abnormalities, as well as ABG changes with compensation (Hurray & Saver, 1992; York, 1987).

With respiratory alkalosis, the pH increases, the $PaCO_2$ decreases, and the HCO_3^- remains within normal limits. To compensate for this abnormality, the

---

Table 28–6

ARTERIAL BLOOD GAS CHANGES WITH ACID-BASE IMBALANCE AND COMPENSATION

IMBALANCE	pH	$PaCO_2$	HCO_3^-
Respiratory acidosis	<7.35	>45	Normal
Compensated	Low normal	>45 (A)	>26 (C)
Respiratory alkalosis	>7.45	<35	Normal
Compensated	High normal	<35 (A)	<22 (C)
Metabolic acidosis	<7.35	Normal	<22
Compensated	Low normal	<35 (C)	<22 (A)
Metabolic alkalosis	>7.45	Normal	>26
Compensated	High normal	>45 (C)	>26 (A)

A = abnormality; C = compensation.

kidneys begin to excrete bicarbonate. With compensation, the pH returns to the high normal range, the $PaCO_2$ remains decreased, and the HCO_3^- decreases (Hurray & Saver 1992; York, 1987).

With metabolic acidosis, the pH decreases, the $PaCO_2$ remains within normal limits, and the HCO_3^- decreases. To compensate for this abnormality, the rate and depth of respiration increases, and the lungs blow off CO_2. With compensation, the pH returns to the low normal range, the $PaCO_2$ decreases, and the HCO_3^- remains decreased (Hurray & Saver, 1992; York, 1987).

With metabolic alkalosis, the pH increases, the $PaCO_2$ remains within normal limits, and the HCO_3^- increases. To compensate for this abnormality, the respirations slow, and the lungs begin to retain CO_2. With compensation, the pH returns to the high normal range, the $PaCO_2$ increases, and the HCO_3^- remains elevated (Hurray & Saver, 1992; York, 1987).

Anion Gap

The anion gap may be used to determine different types of metabolic acidosis. The anion gap is the difference between the sum of sodium and potassium and the sum of chloride and bicarbonate. The normal anion gap is 10 to 12 mEq and is determined as follows:

$$\text{Anion Gap} = (Na^+ + K^+) - (Cl^- + HCO_3^-)$$

In metabolic acidosis, a normal anion gap is noted with bicarbonate loss, and an elevated anion gap is noted with increased levels of noncarbonic acids (McCance & Huether, 1994).

Nursing Diagnosis

Although many nursing diagnoses are applicable for the client with disorders of hydration, electrolyte, or acid-base homeostasis, this chapter concentrates on the diagnoses for problems with hydration.

Fluid Volume Deficit Related to Decreased Intake or Increased Output

The defining characteristics for this nursing diagnosis include dry skin and mucous membranes, weakness, decreased skin turgor, thirst, altered body temperature, decreased urine output, concentrated urine, and hypotension (Rios *et al.*, 1991).

Fluid Volume Excess Related to Fluid Retention, Increased Intake, or Decreased Output

The defining characteristics for this nursing diagnosis include dependent edema, dyspnea, fatigue, rales, change in mental status, restlessness, and weight gain (Rios *et al.*, 1991).

Planning

The planning phase of the nursing process includes determining client outcomes for each nursing diagnosis and formulating the nursing care plan (see Sample Care Plan). The client outcomes are written for each nursing diagnosis and should be mutually agreed on by the client, family, and health care team.

The primary outcome for fluid volume deficit is that the client will maintain adequate fluid intake and fluid balance as evidenced by

1. Pink, moist oral mucous membranes, with skin warm and well hydrated
2. Skin turgor intact, with skin folds returning to normal within 2 to 5 seconds
3. No complaints of weakness
4. Body temperature within normal limits of 98.6°F (37°C)
5. No complaints of thirst
6. Blood pressure within normal limits for that client
7. Urine output adequate and at least 30 to 50 ml/hour
8. Urine specific gravity within normal limits of 1.001 to 1.040

The primary outcome for fluid volume excess is that the client will maintain adequate fluid output and fluid balance as evidenced by

1. Absence of or reduction in dependent edema
2. No complaints of dyspnea, with respirations at 12 to 18 breaths per minute
3. No complaints of fatigue, with increased ability to carry out activities of daily living independently
4. Bilateral breath sounds equal and clear to auscultation
5. Awake, alert, and oriented to person, place, and time
6. Absence of restlessness
7. Body weight stable, with no acute gain

Implementation

Following planning, specific nursing interventions are implemented to assist with attainment of client outcomes. These interventions may be general in nature or more specific, such as intravenous therapy and administration of blood products.

General Interventions

General interventions may be independent or interdependent nursing activities and include measures to assess for hydration imbalances as well as measures to enhance adequate hydration.

Fluid Volume Deficit

Interventions appropriate for the client experiencing problems with fluid volume deficit include assessment of fluid status and replacement of fluids, either through oral or intravenous sources (Cullen, 1992). The nursing care plan includes general nursing interventions with appropriate rationales for the client experiencing fluid volume deficit.

SAMPLE NURSING CARE PLAN

CLIENT WITH A FLUID VOLUME DEFICIT

An 80-year-old client is admitted to the medical unit following 3 days of vomiting and diarrhea. Nursing assessment reveals poor skin turgor, dry mucous membranes, complaints of thirst, recent weight loss of 2 lb over the past 3 days, hematocrit of 56%, and BUN of 30 mg/dl.

Nursing Diagnosis: Fluid Volume Deficit related to fluid loss

Expected Outcome: Client will have adequate fluid intake and fluid balance following treatment.

Action	Rationale
1. Assess the client for indications of dehydration, such as poor skin turgor, delayed capillary refill, weak or thready pulse, thirst, dry mucous membranes.	1. Obtain a baseline assessment for purposes of comparison. Also assists in evaluating success of therapy.
2. Measure intake and output every 8 hours.	2. Intake and output records provide information on sources of fluid loss and inadequate intake.
3. Obtain daily weight at the same time using the same scale.	3. Change in body weight is the most sensitive indicator of fluid volume status.
4. Assess vital signs every 4 hours.	4. Changes in blood pressure, temperature, and heart rate may occur with changes in fluid volume status.
5. Instruct client on fluid intake measures, either oral or IV, if unable to retain oral fluids.	5. Fluid intake is needed to correct fluid deficit. Usually, IV fluids are ordered until oral fluids can be retained. Client needs instructions about the purpose of fluid therapy, as well as the type and amount of oral fluids needed to correct fluid volume deficit.
6. Document care and instructions on client record.	

Fluid Volume Excess

Nursing interventions for the client with fluid volume excess include assessment of fluid volume status, administration of diuretics as indicated, and careful monitoring of sources of fluid intake. These measures include the following (Cullen, 1992):

1. Assess intake and output every shift to determine excess intake, decreased fluid output, or both
2. Weigh daily and assess trends in weight change; an increase in daily weight may be indicative of fluid volume excess
3. Assess respiratory pattern for dyspnea, tachypnea, or shortness of breath; these symptoms may be associated with fluid volume excess, with fluid accumulating in the lungs
4. Assess breath sounds for crackles
5. Assess for peripheral or dependent edema
6. Administer diuretics as indicated to decrease ECF volume
7. Monitor laboratory values, including serum electrolytes, BUN, urine and serum osmolality, urine specific gravity, albumin, and total protein
8. Assess vital signs every 4 hours
9. Turn the client with dependent edema frequently to promote skin integrity

Intravenous Fluid Administration

The administration of intravenous (IV) fluids may be necessary for the client experiencing imbalances in hydration, as well as electrolyte and acid-base imbalances. The purposes of IV therapy include the following (Kee & Paulanka, 1994):

1. Provision of maintenance requirements for fluids and electrolytes
2. Replacement of previous losses of fluids and electrolytes
3. Management of concurrent losses of fluids and electrolytes
4. Provision of nutrition in cases in which nutritional needs cannot be met orally
5. Provision of a means for administration of medications and the transfusion of blood and blood components

Types of Intravenous Solutions

Intravenous fluids may be classified according to their tonicity, as well as their composition and use.

Tonicity

All IV solutions contain solute particles, including electrolytes or nonionizable particles, such as urea or glucose. In the healthy body, the number of cations and anions are equal, and when added together, cations and anions equal 310 mEq/L in ECF. IV solutions may be isotonic, hypotonic, or hypertonic, depending on their concentration of anions and cations in comparison with ECF.

Isotonic solutions are equal to ECF anion and cation concentrations, and the osmolality of isotonic solutions is approximately 310 mOsm/L. Because these solutions are almost equal in osmolality to ECF, they remain in the vascular compartment when administered, and fluid does not move into or out of the cells. Thus, these isotonic solutions increase the ECF volume (Vonfrolio, 1995).

Hypotonic solutions have an osmolality less than 280 mOsm/L and have less osmolality than ECF. Because these solutions have a greater concentration of free water molecules than inside the cell, water moves from the vascular compartment into the cells. These solutions should be administered slowly to prevent cellular edema (Jones, 1991; Vonfrolio, 1995).

Hypertonic solutions have an osmolality greater than 310 mOsm/L, which is greater than that of ECF. These solutions have a lower concentration of free water than ICF and pull water from the cell into the circulatory system (Vonfrolio, 1995). Examples of isotonic, hypotonic, and hypertonic solutions are given in Table 28–7.

Hydrating Solutions

Hydrating solutions provide free water and calories, as well as varying amounts of sodium chloride (NaCl). These IV fluids are useful for daily maintenance of body fluids, rehydration, and establishing effective renal output. These solutions include such IV fluids as 5% dextrose (D) in 0.45% NaCl (half-normal saline) and 5% D in 0.33% NaCl (one-third normal saline). When the D is metabolized, free water is then

available to the body (Kee & Paulanka, 1994; Mathewson, 1989).

Crystalloid Solutions

Crystalloids are IV solutions that contain electrolytes. These solutions have the potential to form crystals capable of diffusing through capillary endothelium and becoming distributed throughout the ECF compartment instead of just the vascular compartment. These solutions may be used for fluid volume replacement. Two examples of this type of IV solution are 0.9% NaCl and lactated Ringer's solution. Lactated Ringer's solution resembles the electrolyte composition of normal blood serum and plasma (Kuhn, 1991; Mathewson, 1989; Metheny, 1992).

Colloid Solutions

Colloids, also called plasma expanders, have the ability to expand a depleted blood volume by exerting a colloidal pressure similar to that of plasma proteins. When these fluids are infused, the colloidal pressure increases in the vascular bed, and fluid is pulled from the interstitial compartment into the vascular compartment, thereby increasing the total blood volume. Dextran and albumin are examples of colloid solutions in use today. Dextran is a colloidal solution used to increase plasma volume. There are two types of dextran: dextran 40, which is a short-lived plasma volume expander, and dextran 70, which is a long-lived plasma volume expander. Albumin is a plasma protein that maintains oncotic pressure in the vascular compartment (Kee & Paulanka, 1994; Kuhn, 1991).

Nutritional Solutions

Total parenteral nutrition (TPN) is a hyperosmolar-hypertonic solution designed to meet the complete

Table 28–7

TONICITY AND INTRAVENOUS SOLUTIONS

TONICITY	OSMOLALITY	INTRAVENOUS FLUIDS	INDICATIONS	NURSING
Isotonic	310 mOsm/L	Dextrose 5% in water, lactated Ringer's, normal saline (0.9%)	To expand ECF volume	Monitor fluid volume status
Hypotonic	<280 mOsm/L	½ normal saline (0.45%)	To provide free water, sodium, and chloride to aid the kidneys in excretion of solutes	May lead to ECF depletion, decreased BP, increase in ICF, and cell damage; monitor fluid status closely
Hypertonic	>310 mOsm/L	Dextrose 5% in saline, dextrose 5% in lactated Ringer's, 3% saline	Expand blood volume by shifting ECF into blood plasma, replace sodium, maintain fluid intake	Rapid infusion may cause circulatory overload and dehydration, monitor fluid status

nutritional needs of selected clients who cannot maintain their nutrition via the enteral route. TPN solutions contain dextrose, proteins in the form of amino acids, selected electrolytes, vitamins, and trace elements (Kee & Paulanka, 1994).

Administration of Intravenous Fluids

Administration of IV fluids is a nursing responsibility. Knowledge of infusion systems assists the nurse in safe administration of IV fluids and in identification and correction of problems should they arise.

Administration Sets

The administration set delivers IV fluid from the plastic or glass IV solution container to the client. Numerous types of administration sets are available that deliver various rates of IV solution per minute (Fig. 28–8).

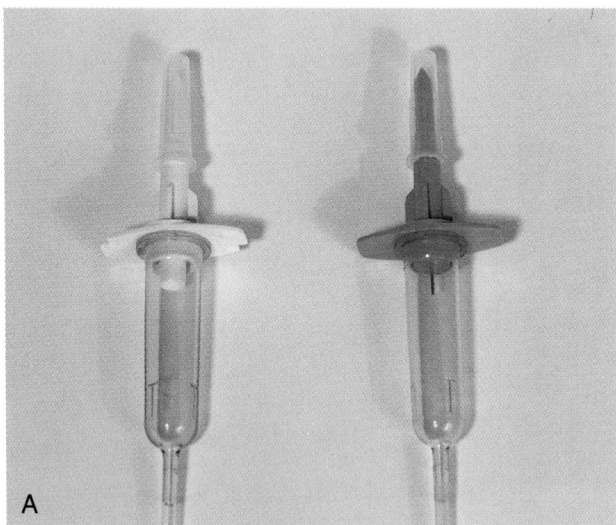

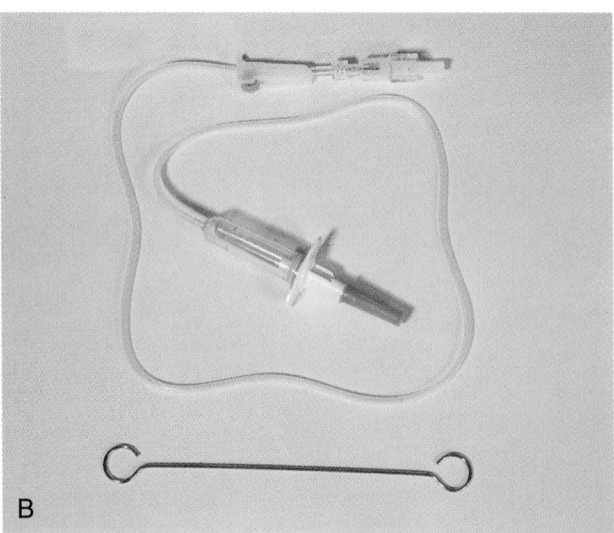

Figure 28–8
Intravenous sets. **A,** Macrodrip (white) and microdrip (blue) IV sets. **B,** Tubing for IV piggyback indicator.

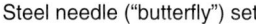

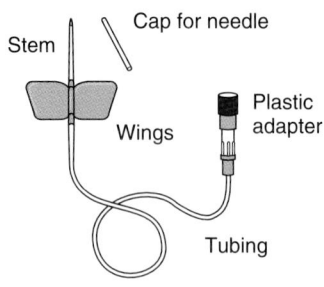

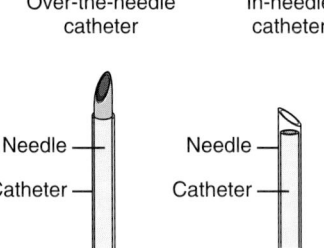

Figure 28–9
Intravenous cannulas: steel needle ("butterfly"), over-the-needle catheter, and in-the-needle catheter.

The regular or macrodrip administration sets are the basic administration sets for infusion of primary parenteral fluids. The drop factor for these sets varies from 8 to 20 drops per milliliter, depending on the manufacturer.

The microdrip administration sets maintain the parenteral infusion at a minimal flow rate. These sets have a much smaller diameter than the regular administration sets and deliver 50 to 60 drops per milliliter (Metheny, 1992).

Intravenous Cannulas

Intravenous solutions or medications are introduced into the venous system by means of either a steel needle or a plastic catheter (Fig. 28–9). The plastic catheter may be either an over-the-needle device or an in-needle catheter.

The steel needle or butterfly set consists of a wing-tip needle with a metal cannula, plastic or rubber wings, and a plastic catheter or hub. The infusion needle is 0.5 to 1.5 in long, with needle gauges of 16 to 26.

The over-the-needle catheter consists of a plastic catheter mounted over a needle. After the venipuncture is made, the catheter is guided off the needle and into the vein. The needle is available in gauges of 8 to 22 and in lengths of 1.5 to 8.0 in.

The in-needle catheter or through-needle catheter consists of a needle of 1.5 to 3.0 in in length and a plastic catheter of 8 to 36 in in length and a gauge of 8 to 22. After venipuncture is made, the catheter is guided through the needle into the vein, and the needle is then removed from the catheter.

These infusion devices are primarily utilized for short-term IV therapy and are inserted into the peripheral venous system by the nurse (Kee & Paulanka, 1994; Metheny, 1992).

Intermittent Infusion Sets

An intermittent infusion set may be used when intravascular accessibility is desired for the intermittent administration of medications by either IV push or IV piggyback. Any of the IV cannulas may be converted into an intermittent infusion set by the aseptic attachment of a Luer-locking, resealable injection cap. Following attachment of this injection cap, patency of the IV cannula is maintained through periodic flushing with normal saline solution.

When administering medication through the intermittent infusion set, first inject 1 to 2 ml of isotonic saline into the cannula to confirm placement of the cannula, and then administer the prescribed medication or infusion. Following administration of the medication, flush the cannula again with 1 to 2 ml of isotonic saline to maintain patency (Metheny, 1990; Peterson & Kirchhoff, 1991).

Needleless or Needle-Free Systems

Needleless or needle-free systems decrease the nurse's exposure to contaminated needles. A number of these devices are available for use with IV administration and include recessed needles and blunt plastic cannulas, as well as one-way valves that eliminate needles altogether (Booker & Ignatavicius, 1996).

Central Venous Catheters

Central venous catheters are placed in the large central veins, such as the superior vena cava, to deliver hyperosmolar solutions, to measure central venous pressure, and to infuse TPN or multiple IV infusions or medications. These catheters are radiopaque, and their position is determined by x-ray following insertion. These catheters may have a single, double, or triple lumen. Central venous catheters may be inserted peripherally and threaded through the basilic or cephalic vein into the superior vena cava, centrally through the internal jugular or subclavian veins, or surgically by tunneling through subcutaneous tissue into the cephalic vein (Greene & Gerlach, 1994; Kee & Paulanka, 1994).

Intravenous Flow Rate

The physician orders IV therapy, including the type of fluid for infusion and the amount to be administered in a specified period. Maintenance therapy for adults is usually 1500 to 2000 ml of fluid per 24 hours or 62 to 83 ml/hour. Replacement fluids with maintenance therapy for adults are usually 2000 to 3000 ml of fluid per 24 hours or 83 to 125 ml/hour. Hydration

therapy for adults is usually 1000 to 3000 ml of fluid per 24 hours or 60 to 120 ml/hour.

Fluid requirements for infants and children are calculated according to the body weight in kilograms. Typically, the infant weighing 1 to 10 kg needs 100 ml of fluid per kilogram per 24 hours. The infant or child weighing 11 to 20 kg needs 100 ml of fluid plus 50 ml per kilogram for each kilogram above 10 per 24 hours. The child weighing 21 kg or above needs 100 ml of fluid plus 20 ml per kilogram for each kilogram above 20 per 24 hours (Kee & Paulanka, 1994).

The fluids may be delivered via an infusion pump or by gravity. If gravity flow is utilized, the nurse calculates the IV infusion rate using either a one- or a two-step method. First, check the manufacturer's specifications for how many drops (gtt) per cubic centimeter (cc) or milliliter (ml) that the infusion set delivers. The number of drops per milliliter varies with manufacturer and ranges from 8 to 20 gtt/ml for macrodrip chambers and from 50 to 60 gtt/ml for microdrip chambers.

In the two-step method, the nurse first calculates the volume of IV fluid to be delivered per hour using the following formula:

$$\frac{\text{total volume}}{\text{time in hours}} = \text{volume per hour}$$

The nurse then calculates the drops per minute using the second part of the formula:

$$\frac{\text{volume to be infused (ml/h)} \times \text{gtt/ml (IV set)}}{\text{time in minutes (60 min/1 h)}} = \text{gtt/min}$$

For example, the physician's order reads 1000 cc normal saline (NS) to run over 8 hours, and the infusion set delivers 20 gtt/ml. Using the two-step method, the nurse would calculate as follows:

$$\text{Step one:} \quad \frac{1000 \text{ ml}}{8 \text{ h}} = 125 \text{ ml/h}$$

$$\text{Step two:} \quad \frac{125 \text{ ml/h} \times 20 \text{ gtt/ml}}{60 \text{ min (1 h)}} = 42 \text{ gtt/min}$$

Using the one-step method, the nurse may calculate the IV flow rate as follows:

$$\frac{\text{volume to be infused} \times \text{gtt/ml}}{\text{hours to administer} \times \text{min/h}} = \text{gtt/min}$$

In the example given here, the drops per minute using the one-step formula would be calculated as follows:

$$\frac{1000 \text{ ml} \times 20 \text{ gtt/ml}}{8 \text{ h} \times 60 \text{ min}} = 42 \text{ gtt/min}$$

If the IV fluids are to be delivered using an infusion pump, the nurse calculates the volume to be infused in an hour and enters that number on the pump (Kee & Paulanka, 1994).

For delivery of IV fluids to infants and children, either an infusion pump or a microdrip chamber set

(60 gtt/ml) should be used. The IV flow rate should be checked every 15 minutes for an infant or a child younger than 6 years and every 30 minutes for a child 6 years or older. To ensure safety, only 2 hours of the calculated solution should be in the solution container or set (Kee & Paulanka, 1994).

Initiation of Peripheral IV Therapy

Prior to initiation of IV therapy, the nurse informs the client and family of the need for therapy. Appropriate teaching is then initiated, and any questions regarding the initiation and infusion of IV fluids or medications are answered.

The first step in initiation of peripheral IV therapy is to select the proper site for the infusion. Veins in the hand, forearm, and the antecubital fossa are suitable sites for IV therapy (Fig. 28–10). Additionally, veins in the scalp and feet may be suitable for IV therapy in infants. Veins in the lower extremities in adults are not suitable sites for IV therapy due to the risk of thrombus formation and possible pooling of medications in areas of decreased venous return (Metheny, 1992). Box 28–4 indicates guidelines for selecting a site for IV infusion.

After the site has been selected, the cannula should be selected. Factors to consider when selecting the appropriate IV cannula include the purpose of the IV infusion; the expected duration of therapy; the client's age and clinical condition; and the condition, size, and availability of veins (Metheny, 1992).

Usually the over-the-needle catheter is preferable for rapid IV infusion and is more comfortable for the client. The butterfly infusion set may commonly be used in children and the elderly, whose veins are likely to be small or fragile. For prolonged infusions, the in-needle catheter, with its longer, narrower catheter is preferred (Kee & Paulanka, 1994).

Following teaching and selection of site and IV cannula, the nurse inserts the cannula according to facility protocol (Procedure 28–1).

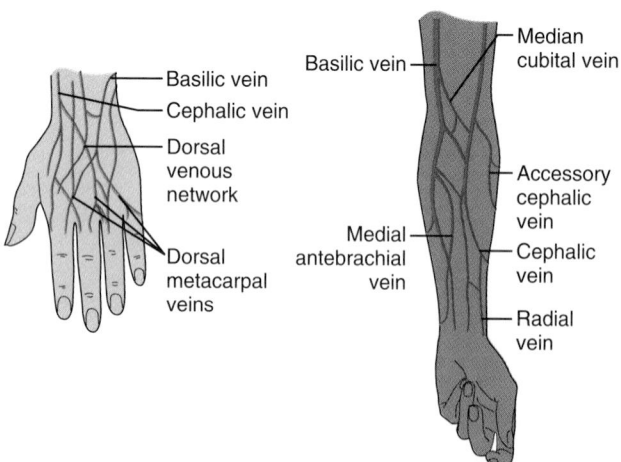

❧ **Figure 28–10**
Possible sites for IV cannula insertion. In infants, veins in the scalp and feet may be used.

Maintenance of the Venipuncture Site

Each health care facility has written guidelines for maintenance of the IV site. These guidelines help to prevent complications, such as infiltration, phlebitis, thrombophlebitis, infection, air embolus, catheter embolus, and allergic reactions, and also help to maintain adequate IV therapy (Irvine *et al.*, 1993). Box 28–5 illustrates general guidelines for maintenance of the venipuncture site.

The nurse is responsible for maintenance of the venipuncture site and for maintenance of adequate IV therapy. Refer to Procedures 28–2 and 28–3 for details.

Text continued on page 821

PROCEDURE

28–1

INSERTION OF A PERIPHERAL ACCESS LINE

Equipment Needed:

Intravenous solution
IV tubing
Over-the-needle catheter
IV start kit (if no kit available,
    gather alcohol preps, beta-
    dine preps, tourniquet, 2 ×
    2 gauze, and tape)
Intermittent device
IV pole
Clean gloves

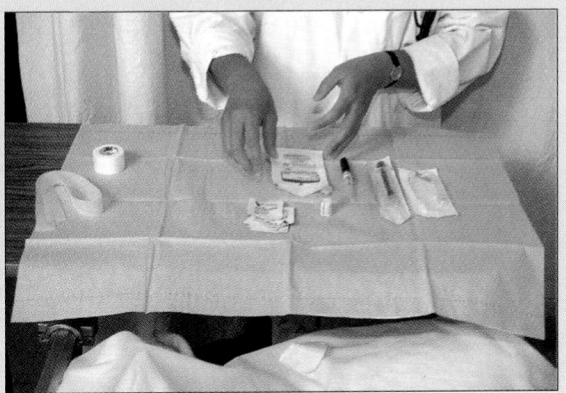

Intervention	Rationale
1. Check the physician order for type of IV fluid(s) and rate.	1. To obtain appropriate IV fluids and equipment.
2. Instruct the client and family about the need for IV fluids, IV start procedure, and possible complications.	2. To inform client and family about benefits and risks of IV infusion.
3. Gather the equipment. Draw up saline to flush the intermittent device.	3. To have all necessary equipment assembled prior to starting the IV.

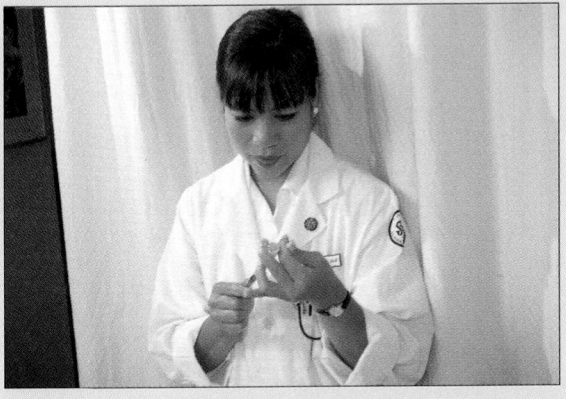

Step 3. *Draw up saline.*

4. Wash your hands with soap.	4. To prevent infection.
5. Inspect the IV container for any leaks and the IV solution for any particles. If there are leaks or the solution is cloudy, then discard.	5. To help ensure that the solution is sterile and to prevent infection.
6. Connect the IV tubing to the solution, and prime the tubing.	6. To remove air from the system and prevent air embolism.
7. Place clean gloves on both hands.	7. To prevent transmission of bloodborne diseases.

Continued

PROCEDURE

28–1

INSERTION OF A PERIPHERAL ACCESS LINE
(Continued)

Intervention	**Rationale**
8. Remove the tourniquet from the IV start kit and place at least 2 in above the IV start site, making sure that it impedes venous flow but not arterial flow.	**8.** To help distend the vein. If unable to visualize vein, may place the arm in a dependent position or gently rub the site to further distend the vein.

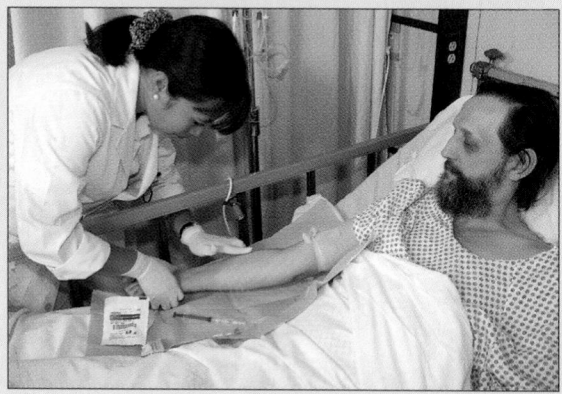

Step 8. *Tapping for vein.*

9. Select the site and clean for one full minute using a circular motion from inside to outside. Clean with 70% alcohol, Betadine solution, or both. If Betadine is used, ask about iodine allergy prior to use.	**9.** To clean the site prior to IV insertion and to prevent infection.

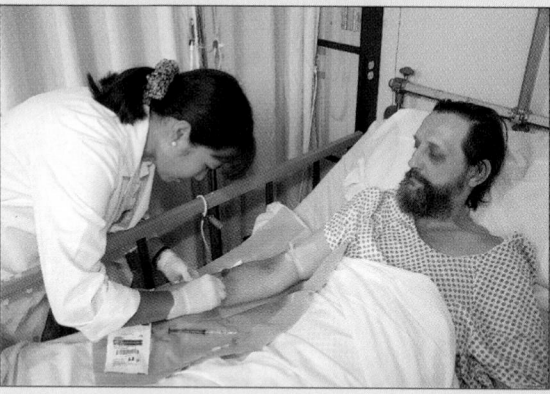

Step 9. *Cleaning site.*

PROCEDURE

28–1

INSERTION OF A PERIPHERAL ACCESS LINE
(Continued)

Intervention	Rationale
10. Insert the needle and cannula into either the top or side of the vein.	**10.** To access the venous system.

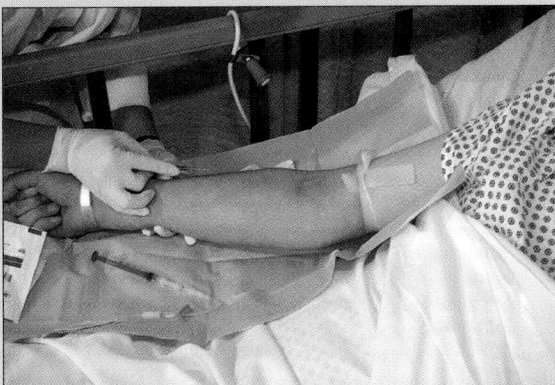

Step 10. *Inserting needle.*

Intervention	Rationale
11. When a flashback of blood enters the hub of the cannula, thread the cannula over the needle into the vein and remove the needle. *Never partially withdraw the needle from the cannula and then reinsert it.*	**11.** A flashback of blood indicates entry into the vein. *Withdrawing the needle partially and then reinserting may cause the catheter to break.*

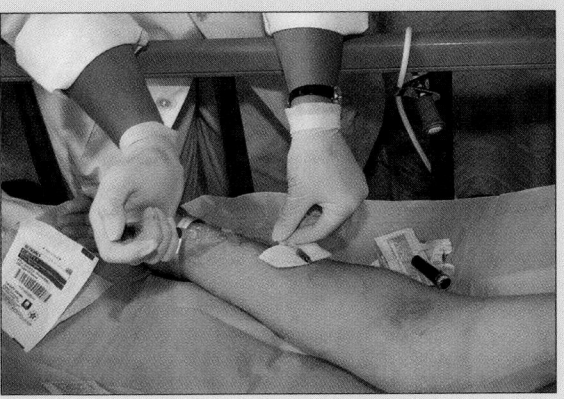

Step 11. *Secure needle.*

Continued

PROCEDURE

28–1

INSERTION OF A PERIPHERAL ACCESS LINE
(Continued)

Intervention	**Rationale**
12. Remove the tourniquet, connect the intermittent device to the cannula, and flush the device with 2 ml saline.	**12.** To ensure that the IV catheter is patent.

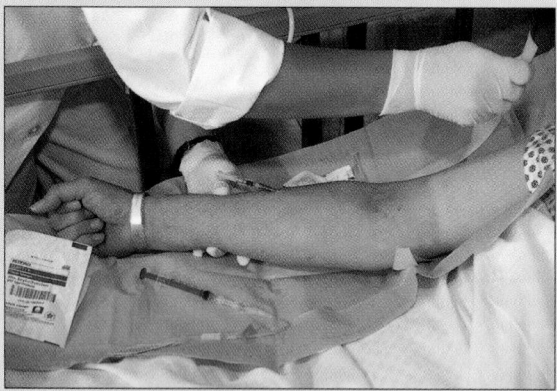

Step 12. *Release tourniquet.*

13. Secure the cannula with tape and apply a dry sterile dressing to the insertion site.	**13.** Taping the cannula prevents movement and possible dislodgement from the vein. A sterile dressing helps prevent infection.

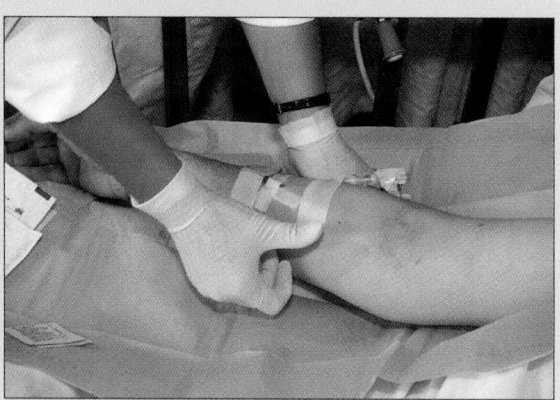

Step 13. *Secure the cannula.*

14. Clean the port of the intermittent device with alcohol, connect the IV tubing to the port, and start the infusion.	**14.** To deliver the intravenous solution as ordered.
15. Label the dressing with the type, gauge, and length of cannula; date and time of insertion; and initials of the nurse starting the IV.	**15.** To ensure communication regarding the IV among personnel caring for the client.
16. Document the site; type, gauge, and length of cannula; and date and time of insertion in the nurses' notes.	**16.** To provide adequate documentation of nursing interventions.

PROCEDURE

28–2

MONITORING THE INTRAVENOUS INFUSION

Equipment Needed:

Watch with second hand
Clean gloves

Intervention	**Rationale**
1. Check the IV flow rate every hour.	**1.** To ensure that the IV fluids are infusing at the prescribed rate.

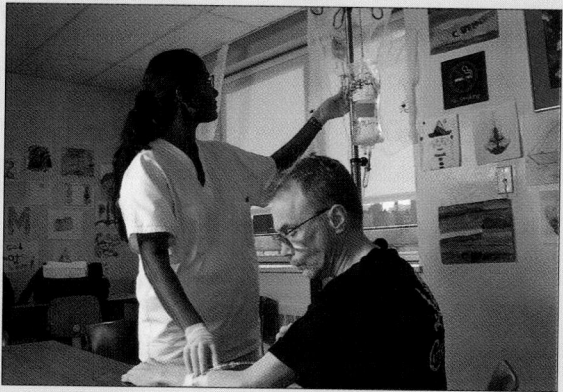

Step 1. *Checking IV flow rate.*

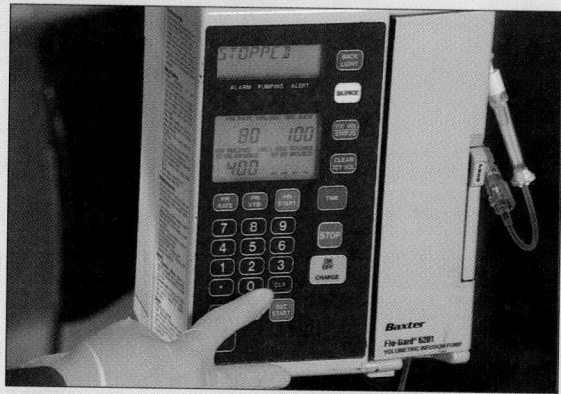

Step 2. *Checking drip on infusion.*

2. Check the IV solution that is currently infusing.

3. Check the IV administration set for any loose connections. Check to make sure the IV catheter is taped securely.

4. Check the IV insertion site for redness, swelling, and patency. If red or swollen, remove the IV catheter and restart in the opposite arm.

2. To ensure that the correct IV solution is infusing.

3. To ensure a closed system and to prevent complications such as infection, air embolism, or dislodgement of the catheter.

4. To detect any complications and to ensure the correct delivery of IV solution.

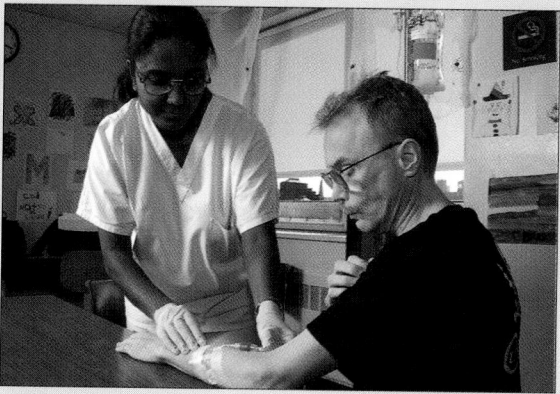

Step 4. *Check IV site for redness or complications.*

5. Assess the client's vital signs, appearance, and response to therapy every 4 hours or more often if indicated.

6. Document in the client's medical record the type of IV solution, flow rate, IV site appearance, and client response every 4 hours or more often if indicated.

5. To determine the client's response to IV therapy and to detect any complications.

6. To provide appropriate documentation of IV therapy and to provide a means of communication among members of the health care team.

PROCEDURE

28–3

USING AN INTERMITTENT DEVICE

Equipment Needed:

Two 3-cc syringes with 1-in
   needle or needleless sys-
   tem
Clean gloves
IV medication
Saline vial
Alcohol preps
Tape

Intervention	Rationale
1. Gather the equipment.	**1.** To have all the necessary equipment available prior to starting the procedure.
2. Explain the procedure to the client and wash your hands.	**2.** Teaching provides the client with information and reduces anxiety. Washing hands prevents infection.
3. Put on clean gloves, draw up 1 to 3 cc saline in the syringe, clean the injection cap with alcohol, and inject the saline into the port. *If the client complains of pain, if you are unable to flush the port, or if you note any swelling while flushing, stop and remove the IV cannula.*	**3.** To prevent infection and to flush the injection cap to ensure patency of the IV cannula prior to administering medications. *Complaints of pain, inability to flush, or swelling indicate that the IV cannula is no longer patent and must be removed. Never force flush the intermittent device (INT).*

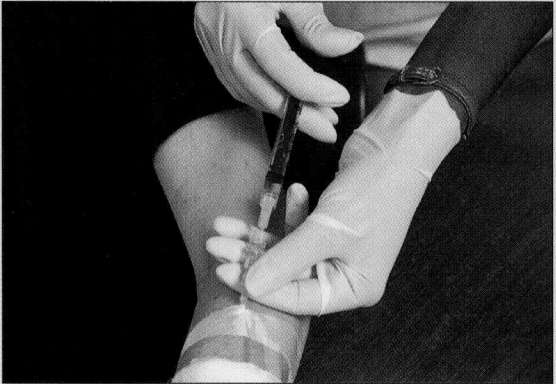

Step 3. *Inject saline into cannula.*

4. Administer the IV medication.	**4.** To deliver the medication.

USING AN INTERMITTENT DEVICE
(Continued)

Intervention	Rationale
5. Draw up 1 to 3 cc saline in the syringe, clean the port of the injection cap with alcohol, and flush with the saline.	**5.** To maintain patency of the IV cannula when not in use.

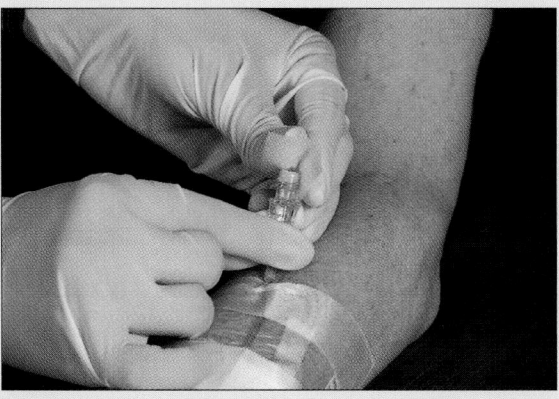

Step 5. *Cleaning INT cap with alcohol.*

6. Document the procedure.	**6.** To provide adequate documentation of the procedure in the client's record.

Prevention and Management of Complications of Intravenous Therapy

Although many clients receive IV therapy, this common form of treatment is not risk free. Several complications may occur with IV infusions, including infiltration, phlebitis, thrombophlebitis, infection, too rapid infusion of fluids, air embolus, catheter embolus, and allergic reactions (Bohony, 1993).

The most common complication associated with IV therapy is infiltration. Complete infiltration occurs when the cannula slips out of the vein, and the IV fluid infuses into the interstitial tissue. The arm is swollen, tender, and cool to touch, and there is no blood return with this type of infiltration. Incomplete or partial infiltration occurs when the tip of the cannula remains in the vein or the vessel wall does not seal around the cannula, allowing some of the IV fluid to infiltrate. The arm is swollen, tender, and cool to touch, but there is blood return with this type of infiltration. If infiltration occurs, remove the IV cannula immediately and restart the IV, preferably in the other extremity (Bohony, 1993; Bostrom-Ezrati *et al.,* 1990).

Phlebitis, or irritation of the vein, is a second complication that can occur with IV therapy. With this complication, the vein is hard, and the skin is red, swollen, tender, and warm. A blood return occurs, and the IV infusion may or may not be sluggish. If you suspect phlebitis, remove the IV immediately, notify the physician, and apply warm soaks to the affected area.

Thrombophlebitis is clot formation, along with inflammation of the vein. The site appears red and may be tender and warm. The IV infusion is sluggish. Never irrigate the IV cannula if you suspect that thrombophlebitis has occurred. Instead, remove the cannula immediately, notify the physician, and restart the IV in the opposite extremity (Bohony, 1993).

An IV site infection may lead to a systemic infection and is a serious complication of IV therapy. Periodic dressing changes, as well as solution and tubing changes, may prevent IV site infection. Suspect IV site infection if the infusion is sluggish and the IV site is hot, red, and painful but not hard or swollen. If you suspect IV site infection, change the site and the entire administration system using aseptic technique (Bohony, 1993; Booker & Ignatavicius, 1996).

If the IV infusion is administered too rapidly, speed shock or fluid volume overload may occur. Speed shock occurs when large volumes of fluid are given in a short time or when IV medications are given too rapidly. Symptoms include flushed face, severe headache, chest pain, irregular pulse, decreased

BP, loss of consciousness, and cardiac arrest. Stop the infusion immediately, notify the physician, and monitor the client's vital signs frequently. Symptoms of fluid overload occur gradually and include increased BP, distended jugular veins, rapid breathing, dyspnea, moist cough, and crackles. Keep the client warm, elevate the head of the bed, and assess for edema. To prevent these complications, monitor IV fluid rates, administer medications slowly, and never try to catch up an IV infusion if it gets behind schedule (Bohony, 1993).

An air embolism may occur whenever the IV system is disconnected (with administration set changes) or if there is a faulty connection that allows air to enter the system. Symptoms of air embolism include a sudden drop in BP and increase in pulse after a tubing change. If you suspect air embolism, place the client on his or her left side and lower the head of the

bed. Inspect the IV administration set for a disconnection or leak.

The tip of the IV cannula may break off during IV insertion or removal, resulting in the possibility of an embolus. Inspect all cannulas on removal, and if they are not intact, place a tourniquet on the extremity, notify the physician, and request an x-ray to confirm catheter embolism.

Allergic reactions may also occur as complications of IV administration. The client may be allergic to the IV cannula or to specific medications administered intravenously. If the client is allergic to the cannula, the vein develops a red streak, and the site is painful. If the client is allergic to the medication, the IV site will suddenly turn red, and the client will complain of itching and develop a rash. If an allergic reaction occurs, use a different type of IV cannula and discontinue the medication (Bohony, 1993). Table 28–8

Table 28–8

COMPLICATIONS OF INTRAVENOUS THERAPY AND NURSING INTERVENTIONS

COMPLICATION	MANIFESTATIONS	NURSING CARE
Local		
Infiltration	Arm swollen, tender, cool to touch; may or may not have blood return	Remove IV catheter and restart IV in the other extremity
Phlebitis	Vein hard with skin red, swollen, tender, warm; blood return present; IV infusion may or may not be sluggish	Remove IV catheter, notify the physician, apply warm soaks to the IV site
Thrombophlebitis	Site red, tender, warm; IV infusion sluggish	Never irrigate the IV catheter, remove the IV catheter, notify the physician, restart IV in opposite extremity
IV site infection	Site hot, red, painful but not hard or swollen; IV infusion sluggish	Remove IV catheter, restart in opposite extremity, change entire administration system
Catheter embolus	Decrease in BP; pain along vein; weak, rapid pulse; cyanosis of nail beds; loss of consciousness	Remove the IV catheter and inspect, place a tourniquet high on limb of IV site, notify physician, obtain x-ray, prepare for surgery to remove pieces
Systemic		
Infection	Fever, chills, general malaise	Change the infusion system, notify the physician, obtain cultures as ordered
Speed shock	Flushed face, severe headache, chest pain, irregular pulse, decreased BP, loss of consciousness, cardiac arrest	Stop the infusion, notify the physician, monitor vital signs frequently
Circulatory overload	Increased BP, distended neck veins, rapid breathing, dyspnea, moist cough, crackles	Elevate the head of the bed, keep warm, assess for edema, slow the infusion rate, notify the physician
Air embolus	Sudden drop in BP, increase in pulse	Place on left side and lower head of the bed, inspect IV infusion system for disconnection or leak, notify the physician
Allergic reaction	Catheter—red streak along vein, pain at IV site Medication—site red, itching, rash	Remove IV catheter, restart IV using different type of IV catheter, notify the physician, discontinue the medication

summarizes complications of IV administration, including indications of and nursing interventions for these complications.

Administration of Blood and Blood Products

Transfusion therapy is indicated for the restoration of blood volume, correction of insufficient oxygen-carrying capacity, or maintenance of blood coagulation. Transfusion therapy is the administration of whole blood or any blood component (Booker & Ignatavicius, 1996).

Blood Components

Blood consists of cells and plasma. The cellular components include erythrocytes (red blood cells

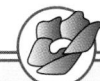

COMMUNITY BASED CARE

INTRAVENOUS THERAPY

When clients receive intravenous fluids and medications at home, they can be involved in their care, have reduced risk of infection, and remain in familiar surroundings. Intravenous medications include antibiotics for infections, chemotherapy drugs, analgesics for pain management, and diuretics or more complex drugs to support cardiac function. Certain blood transfusions may also be administered. Hydration fluids or parenteral nutrition can replace fluid and electrolytes lost from nausea and vomiting for clients experiencing chemotherapy side effects or hyperemesis during pregnancy.

Usually the home care nurse's goals are to provide teaching and support so the client or caregiver can self-administer the therapy. Exceptions to self-care include most chemotherapy drugs and blood transfusions, which are administered by the nurse. The nurse's ability to effectively assess barriers to learning and implement effective teaching methods is critical. For example, anxiety is a common response to learning "invasive" procedures. Decrease anxiety with a calm, unhurried approach. Demonstrate procedures while explaining the rationale for key steps. Involve the client initially in small, easy-to-perform steps, such as opening or closing catheter clamps.

Essential teaching topics include

1. Intravenous fluid/medication actions, dosage, schedule, side effects, and adverse reactions

2. Care of the intravenous catheter, including site care and flushing with heparin or normal saline to maintain patency

3. Administration method, whether it be gravity drip or specialized infusion pump

4. Home safety, including safe storage and disposal of supplies, infusion pump alarms and actions to take, and signs and symptoms requiring immediate reporting

[RBCs]), leukocytes (white blood cells [WBCs]), and thrombocytes (platelets). The plasma consists of 90% water and 10% solutes. Whole blood can now be separated into a variety of products for transfusion therapy (Booker & Ignatavicius, 1996).

Whole Blood

Advances in component therapy have made the use of whole blood rare today. It is primarily indicated for acute, massive blood loss that requires replacement of RBCs and plasma for volume expansion. However, if anemia is treatable with medications such as iron, vitamin B_{12}, recombinant erythropoietin, and folic acid, the client should probably not receive whole blood. Whole blood is composed of RBCs, plasma with plasma proteins, clotting factors, and 63 ml of anticoagulant preservative. The volume in one unit of whole blood is 450 ml blood and 63 ml anticoagulant, approximately 500 ml per unit. Whole blood may be stored up to 21 days (Booker & Ignatavicius, 1996; National Institutes of Health [NIH], 1990).

Packed Red Blood Cells

Packed RBCs are indicated for clients with severe anemia to increase oxygen-carrying capacity. This blood component should not be used for volume expansion. There are two types of PRBCs: RBCs with citrate phosphate-dextrose-adenine (CPDA-1) solution as an anticoagulant and preservative (final hematocrit, 80%) and RBCs with 100 ml additive solution (final hematocrit, 55–60%). The volume in one unit of PRBCs varies with the type of anticoagulant additive used and may be from 250 to 500 ml per unit. PRBCs with CPDA-1 may be stored up to 35 days, whereas PRBCs with additive solution may be stored up to 42 days (NIH, 1990).

Leukocyte-Poor Red Blood Cells

Leukocyte-poor RBCs have had the leukocytes (WBCs) removed through centrifugation, filtration, addition of sedimenting agents, or washing. These RBCs are indicated for clients who have had nonhemolytic febrile reactions. Removal of the WBCs makes the transfusion more comfortable for the client, with decreased risk of a febrile reaction (Booker & Ignatavicius, 1996).

Fresh Frozen Plasma

Fresh frozen plasma (FFP) is indicated to increase the level of clotting factors in clients with a demonstrated deficiency. FFP should not be used for volume expansion. FFP is composed of water, carbohydrate, and proteins (albumin, globulins, antibodies, and all clotting factors). If frozen within 6 hours of collection, all clotting factors are preserved. The volume in one unit of FFP is 200 to 250 ml per unit. FFP may be stored for 12 months. After thawing, it must be transfused within 24 hours or factors V and VIII will be lost (NIH, 1990).

Platelets

Platelets are indicated for control or prevention of bleeding associated with platelet deficiencies. Platelets are transfused for platelet counts under 20,000/mm³ and for bleeding with a platelet count under 50,000. Platelets should not be given to clients with immune thrombocytopenia purpura unless life-threatening hemorrhage occurs. A unit of platelets contains platelets and 50 to 70 ml plasma. The volume in one unit of platelets is 50 to 70 ml per unit. Platelets are stored at room temperature with gentle agitation for 5 days. They must be transfused within 4 hours once initiated (NIH, 1990).

Cryoprecipitate

This blood component is given to correct deficiencies of factor VIII (hemophilia A, von Willebrand's disease), factor XIII, and fibrinogen. Each bag is prepared from one unit of whole blood and contains 80 to 100 units of factor VIII, 250 mg of fibrinogen, and 20 to 30% of factor XIII present in the original unit. These clotting factors are suspended in plasma and then frozen. Each unit contains 10 to 20 ml or 5 to 10 ml, depending on the method of preparation. Cryoprecipitate may be stored for 12 months. Single units must be transfused within 6 hours after thawing, and pooled units, within 4 hours of pooling (NIH, 1990).

Granulocytes

A transfusion of granulocytes (WBCs) may be indicated to treat clients with neutropenia who have serious infections unresponsive to antibiotics. The long-term benefit of WBC therapy is still being evaluated. One unit contains granulocytes, variable amounts of lymphocytes, RBCs, plasma, and platelets. Granulocytes with platelets have a volume of 200 to 400 ml per unit, and granulocytes without platelets have a volume of 100 to 200 ml per unit. Granulocytes should be infused as soon as they are available because their survival time is less than 24 hours (NIH, 1990).

Transfusion Reactions

Blood transfusion is a type of transplantation—transfer of living tissue from one person to another. All blood products carry the risk of transfusion reactions and disease transmission. Clients may have reactions to both the cellular and noncellular components of blood. Table 28–9 summarizes transfusion reactions, symptoms, and preventive measures.

Erythrocyte Reactions

Erythrocyte reactions include acute hemolytic reactions and delayed hemolytic reactions. An acute hemolytic reaction results in the destruction of RBCs as a result of an antigen-antibody reaction. Antibodies in the recipient's plasma agglutinate and hemolyze donor red cells. These reactions are most frequently caused by ABO mismatch. The most common initial sign is fever with chills. A vague uneasiness and back pain also occur early. Other symptoms include red or dark-colored urine, dyspnea, hypotension, and shock. The primary cause of this type reaction is improper identification, in which the client receives the wrong blood (Gloe, 1991; Huston, 1996).

Delayed hemolytic reactions may occur 2 to 14 days after transfusion. The transfused RBCs possess an antigen to which the recipient has already been immunized in the past. Fever is the most common presenting symptom, which develops several days after transfusion. Other signs are chills, back pain, chest pain, dyspnea, hypotension, and shock. The client's hemoglobin level also decreases. To prevent this type of reaction, obtain new samples for compatibility testing within 48 hours of transfusion to detect new serum antibodies that may have developed after transfusion (Gloe, 1991).

Leukocyte Reactions

Leukocyte reactions include transfusion-induced graft-versus-host disease (GVHD), fever without hemolysis, and noncardiogenic pulmonary edema. GVHD disease is very rare and usually occurs in clients with cell-mediated immunodeficiency. GVHD occurs when donor immunocompetent lymphocytes become engrafted and replicate within immunocompromised recipients. These transfused cells may then react against the foreign tissue of the recipient. This reaction may occur in clients who have had bone marrow transplants, who have received chemotherapy with bone marrow suppression, or who have acute leukemia or lymphoma. Symptoms of GVHD begin 4 to 30 days after transfusion, with a high fever followed by a diffuse, erythematous, maculopapular skin rash. The rash progresses to a generalized erythroderma. Other signs include anorexia, nausea, vomiting, profuse diarrhea, liver enlargement, jaundice, and pancytopenia. To prevent GVHD in susceptible clients, administer irradiated blood, which inactivates lymphocytes without damaging other blood components (Gloe, 1991).

Fever without hemolysis is one of the most common types of transfusion reactions and is most frequently noted in clients who have had multiple transfusions or are multiparous. It may be caused by recipient antibodies reacting against antigens present on the cell membranes of transfused lymphocytes, granulocytes, or platelets. Fever is the primary symptom. To decrease the incidence of this type of reaction, transfuse leukocyte-poor RBCs (Gloe, 1991).

Noncardiogenic pulmonary edema occurs from alterations in permeability of the pulmonary capillary bed. Fluid accumulates in the air spaces and intersti-

Table 28–9

BLOOD TRANSFUSION REACTIONS

TYPE	BLOOD PRODUCT	MANIFESTATIONS	PREVENTION
Acute hemolytic	RBCs due to ABO mismatch	Fever, chills, uneasiness, back pain, dark-colored urine, dyspnea, hypotension, shock	Proper identification of the client to receive the blood
Delayed hemolytic	RBCs	Fever 2 to 14 days after transfusion, chills, back pain, chest pain, dyspnea, hypotension, shock, decreased hemoglobin	Obtain new samples for compatibility testing within 48 hours of transfusion to detect new serum antibodies
GVHD	WBCs	Begin 4 to 30 days after transfusion, fever, rash, anorexia, nausea, vomiting, profuse diarrhea, enlarged liver, jaundice, pancytopenia	Administer irradiated blood to inactivate lymphocytes
Fever without hemolysis	Lymphocytes, granulocytes, or platelets	Fever	Transfuse leukocyte-poor RBCs
Posttransfusion purpura	Platelets	Decreased platelet count, bleeding	No preventive measures, but usually self-limiting
Circulatory overload	Whole blood, PRBCs	Dyspnea, headache, coughing, cyanosis, peripheral edema	Administer blood component as slowly as possible
Urticaria	Usually plasma	Rash with pruritus	Pretreatment with an antihistamine
Citrate toxicity	Citrate in stored blood	Tingling in fingers and around mouth, nervousness, muscle cramps, hyperactive reflexes, convulsions, hypotension, cardiac arrest	Slow the rate of transfusion
Hyperkalemia	Stored blood	Nausea, muscle weakness, diarrhea, paresthesias, apprehension, slow pulse, electrocardiogram changes, cardiac arrest	No preventive measures, but monitor client's serum K^+ if receiving several units of blood
Allergic reaction	Immunoglobulin E antibodies fixed to mast cells	Flushing, nausea, vomiting, diarrhea, hypotension, loss of consciousness, respiratory stridor	Cannot be detected by pretransfusion testing; stop transfusion, give epinephrine and steroids
Disease transmission	Any blood component	Symptoms associated with particular infectious agent	Donor screening prior to blood collection, testing blood for hepatitis B and C, HIV

tium of the lungs, resulting in inadequate ventilation. Blood volume and cardiac return also decrease, but there is no evidence of heart failure. Symptoms of this type of reaction include respiratory distress, chills, fever, cyanosis, and hypotension. No specific measures prevent this reaction (Gloe, 1991).

Platelet Reactions

Transfusion reactions may also occur when platelets are transfused. The most common reaction is a febrile reaction, and a rare reaction is posttransfusion purpura. A febrile reaction is usually associated with reactions between recipient antibodies and leukocyte elements in the transfused platelets. Symptoms include fever, which may occur during or within an hour after transfusion, chills, and malaise. To prevent this type of reaction, premedicate the client with antipyretics (Gloe, 1991).

Posttransfusion purpura is a rare reaction that occurs approximately 1 week after transfusion; the client develops acute hemorrhagic thrombocytopenia. Symptoms include a decreased platelet count, with evidence of bleeding. Although no preventive measures exist, this type of reaction is usually self-limiting (Gloe, 1991).

Other Adverse Effects

Other adverse effects of blood transfusion include circulatory overload, urticaria, citrate toxicity, hyperkalemia, anaphylactic reactions, and disease transmission. Circulatory overload may occur in the very young, the elderly, clients with cardiac disease, or clients with expanded blood volume. Symptoms occur during or soon after the transfusion and include dyspnea, severe headache, coughing, cyanosis, and peripheral edema. To prevent circulatory overload, administer the blood component as slowly as possible (Gloe, 1991).

Urticaria is a reaction to the blood or blood components and is related to the amount of plasma transfused. If hives are unaccompanied by any other sign, the blood product does not have to be discarded or discontinued. The primary symptom is a rash with pruritus. If the client is prone to this type of reaction, pretreatment with an antihistamine is warranted (Gloe, 1991).

Stored plasma contains citrate, and as blood is transfused, the plasma level of citrate rises. At higher levels, citrate toxicity may occur with a decrease in the client's serum calcium level. Symptoms include tingling in the fingers and around the mouth, nervousness, muscle cramps, hyperactive reflexes, convulsions, hypotension, and cardiac arrest. To prevent this adverse effect, slow the rate of transfusion (Gloe, 1991).

When blood is stored for more than 48 hours, potassium begins to leak from RBCs, and potassium levels greatly increase after 4 days of storage. Symptoms of hyperkalemia include nausea, muscle weakness, diarrhea, paresthesias, apprehension, slow pulse, electrocardiographic changes, and cardiac arrest (Gloe, 1991).

Anaphylactic reactions are mediated by immunoglobulin E antibodies fixed to mast cells. When incompatible antigens come in contact with these antibodies, an allergic reaction ensues. These reactions are characterized by flushing, nausea, vomiting, diarrhea, hypotension, loss of consciousness, and respiratory stridor. These reactions are not caused by transfusing red cell–incompatible blood and cannot be detected by pretransfusion testing. Treatment of an allergic reaction includes stopping the transfusion and administering epinephrine and steroids (Gloe, 1991).

Transmission of infectious diseases may occur as a delayed transfusion complication. Viral hepatitis, human retroviruses (including human immunodeficiency virus [HIV]), and cytomegalovirus may be transmitted via blood transfusion. To prevent transmission of these diseases, the blood bank has designed donor selection criteria to eliminate potential carriers of these diseases. In addition, the blood bank now tests donated blood for hepatitis B and C and for antibodies to HIV. Due to the variable incubation period of viruses such as HIV, these tests do not identify blood contaminated with infectious agents with 100% accuracy, and transfusion therapy carries a risk of transmission of infectious diseases (Booker & Ignatavicius, 1996).

Management of a Transfusion Reaction

When a transfusion reaction occurs, the transfusion should be stopped immediately and the physician notified. If complications from the transfusion of blood or blood components result in death, the blood bank is required by law to notify the Food and Drug Administration (FDA) by telephone within 24 hours. In addition, the blood bank must file a written report of the investigation of the reaction with the FDA within 7 days (Booker & Ignatavicius, 1996; Harovas & Anthony, 1993a). Box 28–6 includes recommendations for managing a transfusion reaction.

Options for Transfusion Therapy

Several options are available today for the transfusion of blood and blood components. Blood donations may be either homologous or autologous.

Box 28–6

RECOMMENDATIONS FOR MANAGING A TRANSFUSION REACTION

1. Stop the transfusion and notify the responsible physician

2. Keep the IV line open with normal saline; if the normal saline is connected to the blood transfusion system by a Y connector, do not infuse the normal saline through the blood tubing; instead, hang the normal saline with new IV tubing

3. Check all labels, forms, and client identification to determine if the client received the correct blood component

4. Report the suspected reaction to the blood bank personnel immediately

5. Send the required blood samples, the discontinued bag of blood, the administration set, attached IV solutions, and forms and labels to the blood bank

6. Send other laboratory samples, such as urine to detect an acute hemolytic reaction, as directed by the physician or the blood bank

Text continued on page 830

PROCEDURE

28–4

TRANSFUSION OF BLOOD COMPONENTS

Equipment Needed:

Clean gloves
IV pole
250-ml bag of 0.9% saline
Y site blood tubing with filter

If no IV access is available, obtain IV start equipment and an 18- or 19-gauge IV catheter.

Intervention	Rationale
1. Explain the procedure to the client and obtain a transfusion history. If positive for any reaction, notify the physician and blood bank.	**1.** To inform the client of any risks and benefits of the transfusion and to determine any previous adverse effects with transfusion therapy.
2. Gather clean gloves, IV pole, 250-ml bag of 0.9% saline, and Y site blood tubing with filter. If no IV access is available, obtain IV start equipment and insert an 18- or 19-gauge IV catheter.	**2.** To have all necessary supplies prior to starting the blood transfusion.
3. Obtain the blood from the blood bank, following agency policy. Check the laboratory requisition slip with the information on the unit of blood. With the laboratory technician, check the client's name, the identification number, ABO and Rh types, blood bank identification number, and expiration date.	**3.** To obtain the correct blood product for transfusion and to prevent blood transfusion reaction caused by improper identification of the blood product.

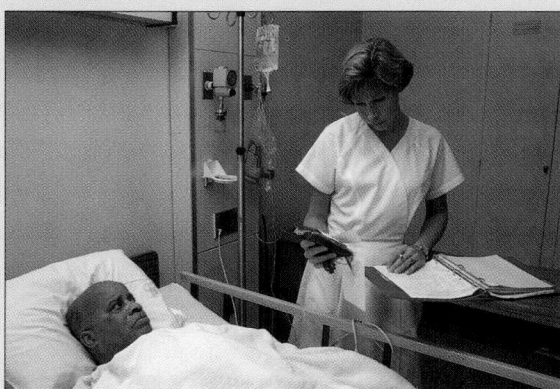

Step 3. *Nurse checks chart, blood.*

Continued

PROCEDURE

28–4

TRANSFUSION OF BLOOD COMPONENTS
(Continued)

Intervention	**Rationale**
4. Take the client's vital signs and assess skin for moisture, rashes, or flushing.	**4.** To obtain baseline data to detect any changes that might indicate a transfusion reaction.

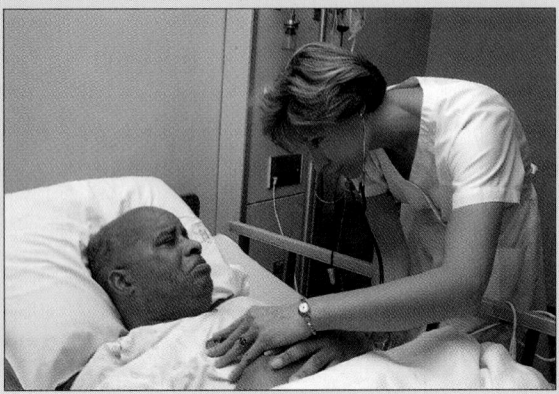

Step 4. *Nurse monitors client.*

Intervention	**Rationale**
5. With a second nurse or physician, compare the client's ABO group and Rh type with the blood bag's tag and label. Compare the client's name and ID number on the bag with the client's identification bracelet. Ask the client to state his or her full name. If there is any discrepancy, do not transfuse the blood product.	**5.** To ensure proper identification of the client receiving the blood product and to prevent transfusion reactions.
6. Wash your hands and put on clean gloves.	**6.** To prevent transmission of infectious diseases.
7. Close all three roller clamps of the Y site tubing, spike the 0.9% normal saline, gently squeeze the drip chamber, open the roller clamp on the Y tubing below the 0.9% normal saline and the one below the filter, and prime the tubing.	**7.** To remove air from the blood administration set and to cover the filter with fluid to prevent blood from falling onto a dry filter, which could damage the cells.

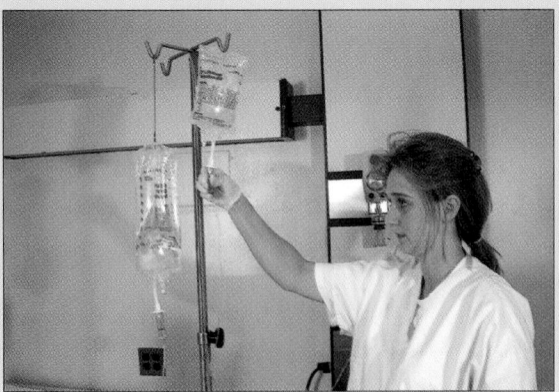

Step 7. *Squeeze drip chamber.*

PROCEDURE

28–4

TRANSFUSION OF BLOOD COMPONENTS
(Continued)

Intervention	Rationale
8. Carefully spike the blood bag with the other arm of the Y site tubing and keep the roller clamp to this arm of the tubing closed.	**8.** To have the blood product ready to transfuse.

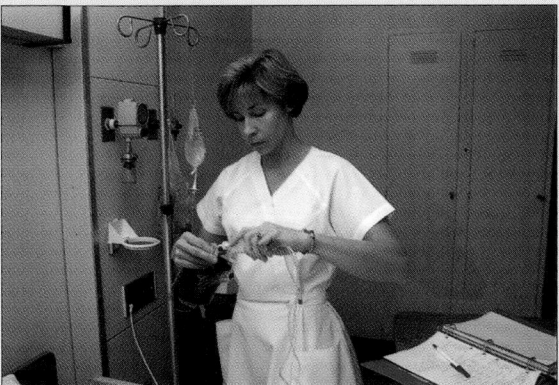

Step 8. *Nurse spikes blood bag.*

Intervention	Rationale
9. Connect the Y site tubing to the IV catheter and open the roller clamp below the filter and the one to the 0.9% normal saline and begin to infuse the 0.9% normal saline slowly.	**9.** To ensure that the IV catheter is patent and to flush any fluid or medication out of the IV catheter.
10. Close the roller clamp to the arm of the Y site tubing to the 0.9% normal saline, open the roller clamp on the arm connected to the blood product, and start the transfusion slowly at no more than 20 gtt/minute. Stay with the client for the first 15 minutes.	**10.** To assess and detect any indications of transfusion reaction because potentially dangerous reactions usually occur within the first few minutes of transfusing a blood product.

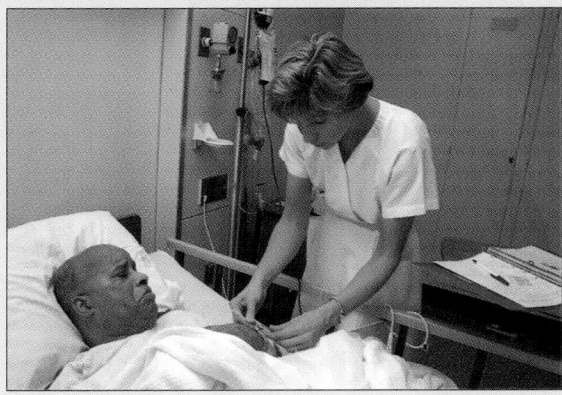

Step 10. *Nurse starts transfusion.*

Continued

PROCEDURE

28–4

TRANSFUSION OF BLOOD COMPONENTS
(Continued)

Intervention	Rationale
11. Take the client's vital signs, and if no change in client's condition is seen, adjust the infusion to the rate prescribed by the physician. All blood products should be completed within 4 hours of initiation.	**11.** To assess for indications of an adverse reaction and to prevent breakdown of blood product after removal from controlled refrigeration.
12. Monitor client's vital signs according to facility policy. When the blood product has infused, infuse another 10 to 20 ml of 0.9% normal saline, put on clean gloves, close the roller clamp below the filter, disconnect the Y site blood tubing from the IV catheter, and continue with prescribed IV therapy.	**12.** To assess for any adverse reactions, monitor client frequently. Flush with 0.9% normal saline to ensure that no blood is present in the IV catheter prior to continuing with prescribed IV therapy.

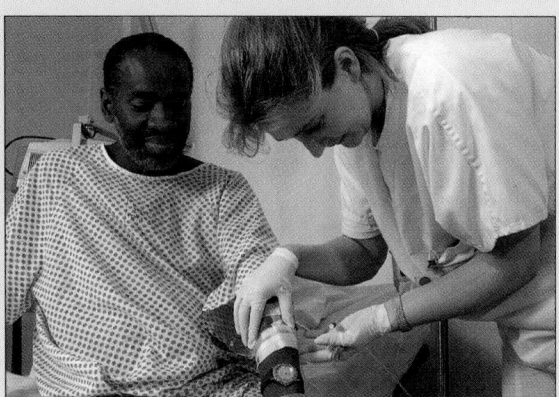

Step 12. *Monitor site/client during infusion.*

13. Document on the blood product requisition slip the date and time of transfusion, amount transfused, vital signs before and after transfusion, any reaction, and signature of two nurses checking the blood product and client identification. Document in the client record the date and time of transfusion, amount and type of blood product, blood bank unit number, amount of 0.9% normal saline infused, status of IV catheter, client's tolerance of the procedure, name and title of the person performing the procedure.	**13.** To accurately document the blood transfusion procedure and to ensure proper identification of the client and blood product.

Homologous Blood

Homologous blood is blood collected from volunteer donors for transfusion to another individual. These donors may be from the community or from the client's family. Assessment of blood donors prior to collection of blood includes a history to screen for HIV, including high-risk behavior and practices and circumstances that should make the donors refrain from donating. Certain illnesses, such as hepatitis or malaria (whether the disease is active or not), render the donor's blood unacceptable. Prior to making homologous blood available for transfusion, the blood

bank tests a sample for ABO and Rh type, as well as for infectious diseases (Booker & Ignatavicius, 1996).

Designated Blood

Designated blood is blood collected from a donor designated by the intended recipient. Compatibility testing is required, and the donor must meet all the requirements as those giving homologous blood. Evidence suggests that designated blood may be no safer than homologous blood collected from community blood donors because the donor may be reluctant to disclose information regarding disease or sexual practices (NIH, 1990).

Autologous Blood

Autologous blood is blood collected from the intended recipient. Self-donation may be done prior to planned surgery or procedures in which blood therapy may be needed. Autologous RBCs may also be salvaged during surgery and then transfused back to the client. Autologous therapy eliminates the risks of immune transfusion reactions, alloimmunization, and transmission of viral diseases (Johnson & Bowman, 1992; NIH, 1990).

Steps for Safe Transfusions

Each health care facility has policies and procedures for the safe administration of blood and blood products. Procedure 28–4 outlines steps for the safe administration of blood and blood products. Some general guidelines to keep in mind when blood is to be transfused include the following (Harovas & Anthony, 1993b; National Blood Resource Education Program's Nursing Education Working Group, 1991):

1. Obtain the client's transfusion history
2. Select a large-gauge needle or catheter, such as an 18- or 19-gauge needle for adults
3. Administer blood components through the appropriate-size filter to remove debris and blood clots
4. Follow health care facility protocol to obtain the blood product from the blood bank
5. Properly identify the blood and the client
6. Take vital signs according to health care facility protocol throughout the transfusion
7. Use only normal saline as the starter solution
8. Start the transfusion slowly and stay with the client during the first 15 minutes of the infusion
9. Maintain the prescribed transfusion rate; most blood products should be infused no longer than 4 hours
10. Monitor the client for any adverse reaction
11. Start the transfusion within 30 minutes after obtaining it from the blood bank refrigerator; never store any blood component on a nursing unit or in an unmonitored refrigerator
12. If blood is to be warmed prior to transfusion, use the coil tubing provided by the blood bank; never warm blood in a microwave oven, and never heat blood components to a temperature higher than 100.4°F (38°C)
13. Do not infuse drugs and blood through the same blood administration set and never add drugs to blood components

Evaluation

Evaluation of client outcomes should be an ongoing process. The nursing care plan may be revised depending on attainment, partial attainment, or no attainment of client outcomes.

For the client with fluid volume deficit, evaluation would indicate if the client maintains adequate fluid intake and fluid balance. Indicators of attainment of this outcome would include the following assessment findings:

1. Pink, moist oral mucous membranes with skin warm and well hydrated
2. Skin turgor intact, with skin folds returning to normal within 2 to 5 seconds
3. No complaints of weakness or thirst
4. Body temperature, BP, and pulse within normal limits
5. Urine output adequate and urine specific gravity within normal limits

For the client with fluid volume excess, evaluation would indicate if the client maintains adequate fluid output and fluid balance. Assessment findings that indicate attainment of this outcome include

1. Absence of or reduction in dependent edema
2. No complaints of dyspnea or fatigue
3. Bilateral breath sounds equal and clear to auscultation
4. Client is awake, alert, and oriented to person, place, and time
5. Body weight stable with no acute gain

Summary

This chapter introduces the concepts of hydration, electrolyte, and acid-base regulation. Body fluids are distributed between two compartments: the ECF compartment, including intravascular and interstitial fluids, and the ICF compartment. Body fluids contain water, nonelectrolytes, and electrolytes. Electrolytes are chemical substances that dissociate into electrically charged particles called ions when placed into a solution. Positively charged electrolytes are cations and include sodium, calcium, potassium, and magnesium. Negatively charged electrolytes are anions and include bicarbonate, chloride, phosphate, and sulfate. Water and particles move through the semipermeable cell membrane via diffusion, osmosis, active transport, and filtration.

Disturbances in fluid balance may result from fluid volume excess or fluid volume deficit. Electrolyte imbalances may be due to either an increase or a decrease in serum concentration of an electrolyte. These imbalances include hyponatremia or hypernatremia, hypokalemia or hyperkalemia, hypocalcemia or hypercalcemia, hypophosphatemia or hyperphosphatemia, and hypomagnesemia or hypermagnesemia.

Regulation of acid-base balance refers to the regulation of H^+ concentration in body fluids. Three mechanisms operate within the human body to maintain acid-base balance: chemical buffers, the respiratory system, and the renal system. Disturbances in acid-base balance result in acidosis (too much H^+) or alkalosis (too little H^+).

Assessment of the client with a disturbance in hydration, electrolyte, or acid-base balance includes the nursing history, physical examination, and analysis of laboratory findings. Nursing diagnoses for the client with disturbances in hydration include Fluid Volume Deficit related to decreased intake or increased output and Fluid Volume Excess related to fluid retention, increased intake, or decreased output.

Nursing interventions for the client experiencing disturbances in hydration include general interventions such as measuring intake and output, obtaining daily weight, assessing for symptoms of fluid volume deficit or overload, administering oral or IV fluids, and monitoring vital signs and pertinent laboratory values. IV fluid therapy may be initiated to provide maintenance requirements, to replace previous fluid losses, to manage concurrent losses of fluids or electrolytes, to provide nutrition, and to provide a means for administration of medications.

Blood transfusion is a type of transplantation—transfer of living tissue from one person to another—with the risk of transfusion reactions and disease transmission. Blood transfusion therapy is indicated for the restoration of blood volume, treatment of shock, treatment of chronic anemia, and maintenance of blood coagulation.

Evaluation of client outcomes is an ongoing process and indicates if the client maintains adequate fluid intake, adequate fluid output, and fluid balance.

CHAPTER HIGHLIGHTS

✦

- ✦ Body fluids are distributed between the ECF compartment and the ICF compartment and contain water, nonelectrolytes, and electrolytes.

- ✦ Electrolytes are essential for promotion of neuromuscular irritability, maintenance of body fluid osmolality, regulation of acid-base balance, and distribution of body fluids between the fluid compartments.

- ✦ Sodium is the primary cation in the ECF and is the major determinant of plasma osmolality and ECF fluid volume.

- ✦ Potassium is the primary cation in the ICF and plays a major role in nerve conduction, muscle contraction, and myocardial membrane responsiveness.

- ✦ Water and electrolytes are regulated by several mechanisms in the body, including thirst, hormonal secretion, and renal function.

- ✦ Edema is an accumulation of fluid in the interstitial spaces and is a problem of fluid distribution—not necessarily of fluid volume excess.

- ✦ An excess of ECF volume is usually associated with hypoosmolality and hyponatremia. Symptoms of fluid volume excess include confusion, convulsions, weakness, nausea, muscle twitching, headache, and weight gain.

- ✦ Fluid volume deficit may be isotonic, hypotonic, or hypertonic. Symptoms of fluid volume deficit include thirst, dry skin and mucous membranes, increased temperature, weight loss, and concentrated urine.

- ✦ Acid-base imbalances are usually categorized as respiratory acidosis, respiratory alkalosis, metabolic acidosis, and metabolic alkalosis.

- ✦ Acute changes in body weight are usually indicative of acute fluid changes. Intake and output should be measured and recorded every 8 hours for any client at risk for fluid and electrolyte imbalance.

- ✦ Intravenous fluids are classified according to their tonicity, as well as their composition and use.

- ✦ Intravenous fluids may be delivered via macrodrip or microdrip administration sets, may be introduced into the venous system by means of either a steel needle or a plastic catheter, and may be delivered into either the peripheral or central venous circulation.

- ✦ The physician orders IV therapy, including the type of fluid for infusion and the amount to be administered in a specified period.

- ✦ Each health care facility has written guidelines for maintenance of the IV site to help prevent complications and to maintain adequate IV therapy.

- ✦ Complications of IV therapy include infiltration, phlebitis, thrombophlebitis, infection, too-rapid infusion of fluids, air embolus, catheter embolus, and allergic reactions.

- ✦ Blood components that may be transfused include whole blood, PRBCs, FFP, platelets, cryoprecipitate, and granulocytes.

- ✦ Types of transfusion reactions include erythrocyte reactions, leukocyte reactions, and platelet reactions. Other adverse affects include circulatory overload, urticaria, citrate toxicity, hyperkalemia, anaphylactic reactions, and disease transmission.

- ✦ Several options are available today for the transfusion of blood and blood components, including homologous blood transfusion, autologous blood transfusion, and designated blood transfusion.

- ✦ Each health care facility has policies and procedures for the safe administration of blood and blood products, which include properly identifying the blood and the client, measuring vital signs, maintaining the prescribed transfusion rate, and monitoring for any adverse reactions.

Study Questions

1. The cation found in greatest concentration in the ECF and responsible for fluid balance is

   a. sodium
   b. potassium
   c. chloride
   d. calcium

2. Water moves across a semipermeable membrane by the process of

   a. diffusion
   b. osmosis
   c. active transport
   d. facilitated transport

3. M. B., a 66-year-old, client, is at risk for fluid volume overload. In planning care for M. B., the nurse should

   a. measure intake and output every 24 hours
   b. force fluids up to 2000 ml/day
   c. weigh daily
   d. anticipate the need for a central venous catheter

4. Respiratory acidosis is associated with

   a. overproduction of lactic acid
   b. pH greater than 7.45
   c. hyperventilation
   d. hypoventilation

5. The client has an intravenous solution infusing into the right hand. On assessment, the nurse notes that the hand is swollen, cool to the touch, and pale. The nurse's first action would be to

   a. notify the physician about the client's arm
   b. discontinue the IV catheter and restart in the other arm
   c. discontinue the IV fluids
   d. instruct the client to report any pain in the hand

Critical Thinking Exercises

1. Mr. M., age 72 years, was cutting grass and became unconscious. He is admitted with dehydration. Discuss the factors in the elderly that contribute to dehydration and some probable assessment findings you would find on assessing Mr. M.

2. Ms. P. is admitted with fluid overload with shortness of breath and edema. Discuss some nursing interventions and the outcome criteria you would assign for Ms. P.

References

Bohony, J. (1993). 9 common IV complications and what to do about them. *American Journal of Nursing, 93*(10), 45–49.

Booker, M. F., & Ignatavicius, D. D. (1996). *Infusion therapy: Techniques and medications.* Philadelphia: W. B. Saunders.

Bostrom-Ezrati, J., Dibble, S., & Rizzuto, C. (1990). Intravenous therapy management: Who will develop insertion site symptoms? *Applied Nursing Research, 3*(4), 146–152.

Bove, L. A. (1996a). Restoring electrolyte balance: Calcium and phosphorus. *RN, 59*(3), 47–51.

Bove, L. A. (1996b). Restoring electrolyte balance: Sodium chloride. *RN, 59*(1), 25–28.

Brenner, M., & Welliver, J. (1990). Pulmonary and acid-base assessment. *Nursing Clinics of North America, 25,* 761–770.

Brown, R. G. (1993). Disorders of water and sodium balance. *Postgraduate Medicine, 93,* 227–228, 231–232, 234.

Calhoun, K. A. (1990). Serum potassium concentration abnormalities. *Critical Care Nursing Quarterly, 13*(3), 34–38.

Chenevey, B. (1987). Overview of fluids and electrolytes. *Nursing Clinics of North America, 22,* 749–759.

Chernecky, C. C., Krech, R. L., & Berger, B. J. (1993). *Laboratory tests and diagnostic procedures.* Philadelphia: W. B. Saunders.

Cullen, L. (1992). Interventions related to fluid and electrolyte balance. *Nursing Clinics of North America, 27,* 569–597.

DeAngelis, R., & Lessig, M. L. (1992). Hyperkalemia. *Critical Care Nurse, 12*(3), 55–59.

DeAngelis, R., & Lessig, M. L. (1991). Hypokalemia. *Critical Care Nurse, 11*(7), 71–72, 74–75.

Felver, L., & Pendarvis, J. H. (1989). Home study program: Electrolyte imbalances . . . intraoperative risk factors. *AORN Journal, 49,* 989, 992–998, 1000.

Ferrin, M. S. (1996). Restoring electrolyte balance: Magnesium. *RN, 59*(5), 31–43.

Friday, B. A., & Reinhart, R. A. (1991). Mg metabolism: A case report and literature review. *Critical Care Nurse, 11*(5), 63–72.

Gloe, D. (1991). Common reactions to transfusions. *Heart Lung, 20,* 506–514.

Graves, L., III (1990). Disorders of calcium, phosphorus, and magnesium. *Critical Care Nursing Quarterly, 13*(3), 3–13.

Greene, L. M., & Gerlach, C. J. (1994). Central lines have moved out. *RN, 57,* 26–30.

Harovas, J., & Anthony, H. H. (1993a). Managing transfusion reactions. *RN, 56*(12), 32–37.

Harovas, J., & Anthony, H. H. (1993b). Your guide to trouble free transfusions. *RN, 56*(11), 27–35.

Horne, M. M., Heitz, U. E., & Swearingen, P. L. (1991). *Fluid, electrolyte, and acid-base balance: A case study approach.* St. Louis: Mosby-Year Book.

Hurray, J. M., & Saver, C. L. (1992). ABG interpretation. *AORN Journal, 55,* 178, 180–185, 188–192.

Huston, C. J. (1996). Hemolytic transfusion reaction. *American Journal of Nursing, 96*(3), 47.

Innerarity, S. A. (1992). Hyperkalemic emergencies. *Critical Care Nursing Quarterly, 14*(4), 32–39.

Irvine, L. L., et al. (1993). We put IV therapy down on paper. *RN, 56*(1), 34–37.

Isley, W. L. (1990). Serum sodium concentration abnormalities. *Critical Care Nursing Quarterly, 13*(3), 82–88.

Johnson, G. M., & Bowman, R. J. (1992). Autologous blood transfusion. *AORN Journal, 56,* 282–292.

Jones, D. H. (1991). Fluid therapy in the PACU. *Critical Care Nursing Clinics of North America, 3*(1), 109–119.

Kee, C. C. (1995). The renal system and its problems in the elderly. In M. Stanley, & P.G. Beare (Eds.), *Gerontological nursing* (pp. 228–240). Philadelphia: F. A. Davis.

Kee, J. L., & Hayes, E. R. (1990). Assessment of patient laboratory data in the acutely ill. *Nursing Clinics of North America, 25,* 751–759.

Kee, J. L., & Paulanka, B. J. (1994). *Fluids and electrolytes with clinical applications* (5th ed.). Albany, NY: Delmar Publishers.

Kuhn, M. M. (1991). Colloids vs crystalloids. *Critical Care Nurse, 11*(5), 37–51.

Lowenstein, J. (1993). *Acid and basics: A guide to understanding acid-base disorders.* New York: Oxford University Press.

Mathewson, M. (1989). Intravenous therapy. *Critical Care Nurse, 9*(2), 21–23, 26–28, 30–36.

McCance, K. L., & Huether, S. E. (1994). *Pathophysiology: The biologic basis for disease in adults and children* (2nd ed.). St. Louis: Mosby.

McFarland, M. B., & Grant, M. M. (1994). *Nursing implications of laboratory tests* (3rd ed.). Albany, NY: Delmar Publishers.

Metheny, N. M. (1992). *Fluid and electrolyte balance: Nursing considerations* (2nd ed.). Philadelphia: J. B. Lippincott.

National Blood Resource Education Program's Nursing Education Working Group (1991). Transfusion nursing: Trends and practices for the '90's. *American Journal of Nursing, 91*(6), 42–56.

National Institutes of Health. (1990). *Transfusion therapy guidelines for nurses* (HIH Publication No. 90-2668 a). Washington, D.C.: Department of Transfusion Medicine.

Owens, M. W. (1993). Keeping an eye on magnesium. *American Journal of Nursing, 93*(2), 66–67.

Perez, A. (1995b). Hypokalemia. *RN, 58*(12), 33–35.

Peterson, F. Y., & Kirchhoff, K. T. (1991). Analysis of the research about heparinized versus nonheparinized intravenous lines. *Heart Lung, 20,* 631–642.

Porth, C. M., & Erickson, A. (1992). Physiology of thirst and drinking: Implication for nursing practice. *Heart Lung, 21,* 273–284.

Poyss, A. S. (1987). Assessment and nursing diagnosis in fluid and electrolyte disorders. *Nursing Clinics of North America, 22,* 773–783.

Rios, H., Delaney, C., Kruckeburg, T., Chung, Y., & Mehmert, P. A. (1991). Validation of defining characteristics of four nursing diagnoses using a computerized data base. *Journal of Professional Nursing, 7,* 293–299.

Russell, J. M. (1993). Successful methods for arterial blood gas interpretation. *Critical Care Nurse, 11*(4), 15–19.

Stringfield, Y. N. (1993). Back to basics: Acidosis, alkalosis and ABG's. *American Journal of Nursing, 93*(11), 43–44.

Vonfrolio, L. G. (1995). Would you hang these IV solutions? *American Journal of Nursing, 95*(6), 37–39.

Wandel, J. C. (1990). The use of postural vital signs in the assessment of fluid volume status. *Journal of Professional Nursing, 6,* 46–54.

Weldy, N. J. (1992). *Body fluids and electrolytes: A programmed presentation* (6th ed.). St. Louis: Mosby-Year Book.

York, K. (1987). The lung and fluid-electrolyte and acid-base balance. *Nursing Clinics of North America, 22,* 805–814.

Bibliography

Aaronson, L., & Seaman, L. P. (1989). Managing hypernatremia in fluid deficient elderly. *Journal of Gerontological Nursing, 15*(7), 29–36.

Barta, M. A. (1987). Correcting electrolyte imbalances, part 1. *RN, 50*(2), 30–34.

Butler, S. (1989). Current trends in autologous transfusion. *RN, 52*(11), 44–55.

Calloway, C. (1987). When the problem involves magnesium, calcium, or phosphate. *RN, 50*(5), 30–36.

Falco, S. A., & McCormach, A. S. (1992). Intravenous therapy: Attitudes of nurses and implications for managers and educators. *Geriatric Nursing, 13,* 207–209.

Folkes, M. E. (1990). Transfusion therapy in critical care nursing. *Critical Care Nursing Quarterly, 13*(2), 15–28.

Goodinson, S. M. (1990). The risks of IV therapy. *Professional Nurse, 5,* 235–236.

Holder, C., & Alexander, J. (1990). A new and improved guide to IV therapy . . . protocols for intravenous therapy. *American Journal of Nursing, 90*(2), 43–47.

Karb, V. B. (1989). Electrolyte abnormalities and drugs which commonly cause them. *Journal of Neuroscience Nursing, 21,* 125–129.

Ludlow, M. (1993). Renal handling of potassium. *AANA Journal, 20*(1), 52–58.

Matz, R. (1993). Mg: Deficiencies and therapeutic uses. *Hospital Practice, 28* (4A), 70–82, 85–87, 91–92.

Metheny, N. M. (1990). Why worry about IV fluids? *American Journal of Nursing, 90*(6), 50–57.

Perucca, R., & Micek, J. (1993). Treatment of infusion-related phlebitis: Review and nursing protocol. *Journal of Intravenous Nursing, 16,* 282–286.

Workman, M. L. (1992). Fluid and electrolytes. *AACN Clinical Issues in Critical Care Nursing, 3,* 653–723.

Chapter 29

FLUID-GAS TRANSPORT: OXYGENATION

DINA M. CULPEPPER,
RN, MSN, CCRN

MARIA MENDOZA,
RN, EdM, CS, CCRN

KEY TERMS

✦

adventitious
airway resistance
arterial blood gas (ABG)
asthma
atelectasis
crepitus
cyanosis
diffusion
dyspnea
expiration
hemoptysis
hypoxia
inspiration

intrapulmonary pressure
lung compliance
orthopnea
oxygenation
pleura
pulmonary function tests
regulation
thoracentesis
tidal volume
transport
ventilation
vital capacity

LEARNING OBJECTIVES

✦

After studying this chapter, you should be able to

✦ Trace the route of a given volume of air from the time it is inhaled through the nose until it enters the lungs

✦ Describe the anatomical structures involved in the respiratory process

✦ Distinguish between inspiration and expiration and describe the mechanics of each

✦ Explain the various lung volumes and capacities

✦ Discuss the common diseases of the respiratory system

✦ Discuss psychosocial factors that affect the respiratory system

✦ Describe developmental factors that affect the respiratory system

✦ Use the nursing process to assess the respiratory status of a client

✦ Identify nursing diagnoses related to the respiratory system

✦ Identify an appropriate plan of action, based on the nursing assessment of the respiratory system

✦ Describe altered breathing patterns

✦ Describe how to promote healthy breathing

✦ Describe various methods to administer oxygen

✦ Use the appropriate life-saving techniques for maintaining a patent airway when necessary

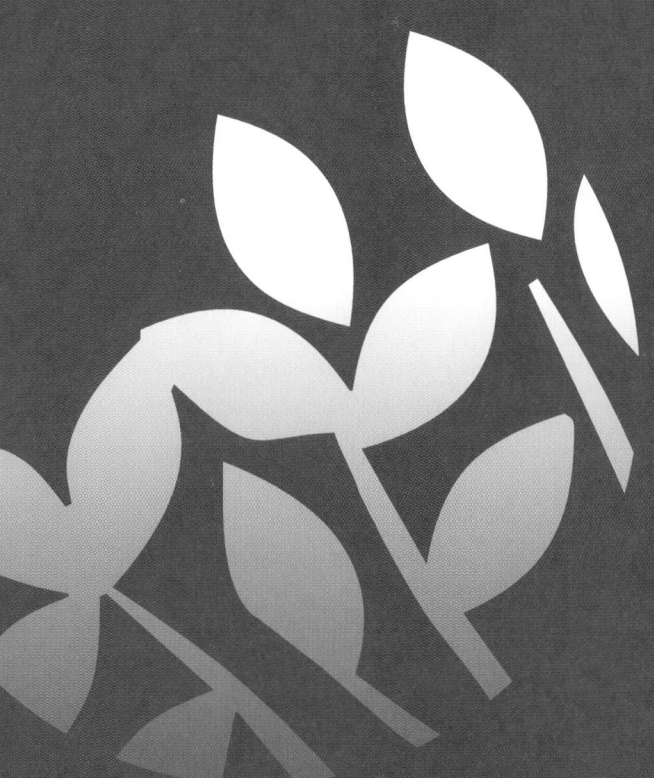

The cells of the body require a steady supply of oxygen to perform their basic metabolic activities. Along with this steady supply of oxygen, there must be a mechanism for removing carbon dioxide that is produced as a by-product of cellular activities. Oxygen is made available and carbon dioxide is eliminated through a process called **oxygenation.**

The respiratory system provides the mechanism by which tissues receive their oxygen supply. The respiratory system is influenced by multiple factors, including physiological, psychological, developmental, and environmental.

The role of the nurse in relation to oxygenation is to identify those factors that affect oxygenation and incorporate this information into a plan of action designed to maintain or improve the client's respiratory status.

With the focus of health care rapidly moving toward health promotion and disease prevention, nursing's role will increasingly become that of health educator and advocate of healthy behaviors that promote optimal oxygenation of tissues.

Anatomy and Physiology

The respiratory process is divided into two phases: external respiration (or the exchange of gases between the atmosphere and the lungs) and internal respiration (or the exchange of gases at the cellular level). There are four mechanisms involved in the respiratory process:

- Ventilation, or the movement of gases in and out of the lungs
- Diffusion of oxygen and carbon dioxide between the alveoli and the blood
- Transportation of oxygen and carbon dioxide to and from the cells
- Regulatory processes of breathing

Respiratory Structures

Oxygenation is made possible through the respiratory system. The respiratory system consists of the conducting airways, the gas exchange airspaces, and the pulmonary vasculature.

Conducting Airways

The conducting airways extend from the nose to the terminal bronchioles. These airways serve mainly as pathways for gases and do not participate in gas exchange. The pathways that do not participate in gas exchange are referred to as anatomical dead space. The upper conducting airways are the nose, the sinuses, the mouth, and the pharynx. The lower conducting airways consist of the larynx, the trachea, the bronchi, the bronchioles, and the terminal bronchioles (Figs. 29–1 and 29–2.)

Air enters the nose during normal breathing, where it is filtered, warmed, and humidified. The upper nasal passages are lined with coarse hairs that filter dust and large particles from the air. The inner nasal passages are lined with a vascular mucous membrane. The mucous membranes have an extensive blood supply that warms the air inhaled to within 2 to 3% of body temperature. These mucous membranes also humidify the air as it passes over them. The membranes of the nasal cavity and the delicate portions of the lung are protected from becoming frozen or dried out through this humidifying process.

The mouth serves as an alternative air passageway when the nose is obstructed or plugged or when a large amount of air exchange is needed, such as during running or aerobic exercise. The mouth and the nose are connected by an opening called the pharynx. The pharynx is divided into three parts: nasopharynx, oropharynx, and laryngopharynx (see Fig. 29–1). The pharynx communicates with the nasal cavity, mouth, middle ear, larynx, and epiglottis. The pharynx is a muscular structure lined with a mucous membrane. This mucous membrane is continuous with the structures with which it communicates. The nasopharynx is located immediately behind the nasal cavity and is continuous with it through the internal nares. The nasopharynx is also lined with a mucous membrane. The oropharynx is a continuation of the nasopharynx that extends to the laryngopharynx. Both the oropharynx and the laryngopharynx serve as a passageway for air to enter the larynx (see Fig. 29–1).

The larynx is the structure that divides the upper and the lower airway and is sometimes called the "watchdog" of the lungs. The opening into the larynx is the glottis. The epiglottis is attached to the thyroid cartilage. The primary function of the epiglottis is to cover the glottis during swallowing to prevent entry of food or foreign materials into the airway. The larynx connects the laryngopharynx with the trachea and comprises incomplete rings of cartilage. It is responsible for speech via the vocal cords and for transporting air to and from the lungs. The laryngeal muscles contract to close off the airway when a foreign object passes its way. This contraction leads to coughing, which helps expel the object. When the larynx is paralyzed, there is the danger of aspirating substances into the lungs.

The trachea is a tube that is about 10 to 12 cm (4–5 inches) long, extending from the larynx to the level of the seventh thoracic vertebra. It connects the larynx with the major bronchi of the lungs (see Fig. 29–2). Horseshoe-shaped cartilages keep the trachea from collapsing during negative pressure caused by inspiration. A mucous membrane that contains numerous goblet cells and cilia lines the trachea. The cilia beat upward and tend to carry foreign particles and excessive mucus secretions away from the lungs to the pharynx. The trachea divides into the right and left mainstem bronchi at the point called the **carina.** The carina is a special structure lined with nerve endings. Coughing and bronchospasm may result when the carina is stimulated (see Fig. 29–2).

The primary bronchi divide into secondary bronchi to supply the three lobes in the right and the two lobes in the left. The secondary bronchi further subdivide into the segmental bronchi, which supply the bronchopulmonary segments of the lungs (see Fig. 29–2). The bronchi continue to branch off until they become very small conducting airways, called the terminal bronchioles and the respiratory bronchioles (Fig. 29–3). Both lungs contain a total of about 35,000 terminal bronchioles. These terminal bronchioles further divide into terminal respiratory units, or acini, where gas exchange occurs. Acini are composed of respiratory bronchioles, alveolar sacs, and alveoli, and each one has a network of pulmonary arteries and veins.

The bronchi are made up of smooth muscles controlled by the autonomic nervous system via the vagus nerve, which innervates with the brain stem. Parasympathetic innervation of the respiratory smooth muscles results in bronchial constriction, and sympathetic stimulation leads to bronchial relaxation.

The lungs are cone-shaped organs with the pointed tip or apex extending into the top of the thoracic cavity behind the clavicle. The base of the lungs is broad and concave and rests atop the convex surface of the diaphragm. The hilus of the lung is on the medial surface. The bronchi and blood vessels enter and leave the lungs at the hilus. The costal surface, which lies against the ribs, is rounded to match the curvature of the ribs. The right side is divided into three lobes: upper or superior, middle, and lower or inferior. The left side is divided into two lobes: upper and lower (see Fig. 29–2).

The lungs are enclosed in a double-walled sac called the pleura. The surface of the pleura that adheres firmly to the lung's surface is called the visceral pleura. The surface that adheres to the walls of the thoracic cavity is the parietal pleura. Between the two layers of the pleura is a narrow, fluid-filled space called the pleural cavity. The lubricating fluid in the pleural cavity is the pleural fluid. Pleural fluid reduces the friction of respiration.

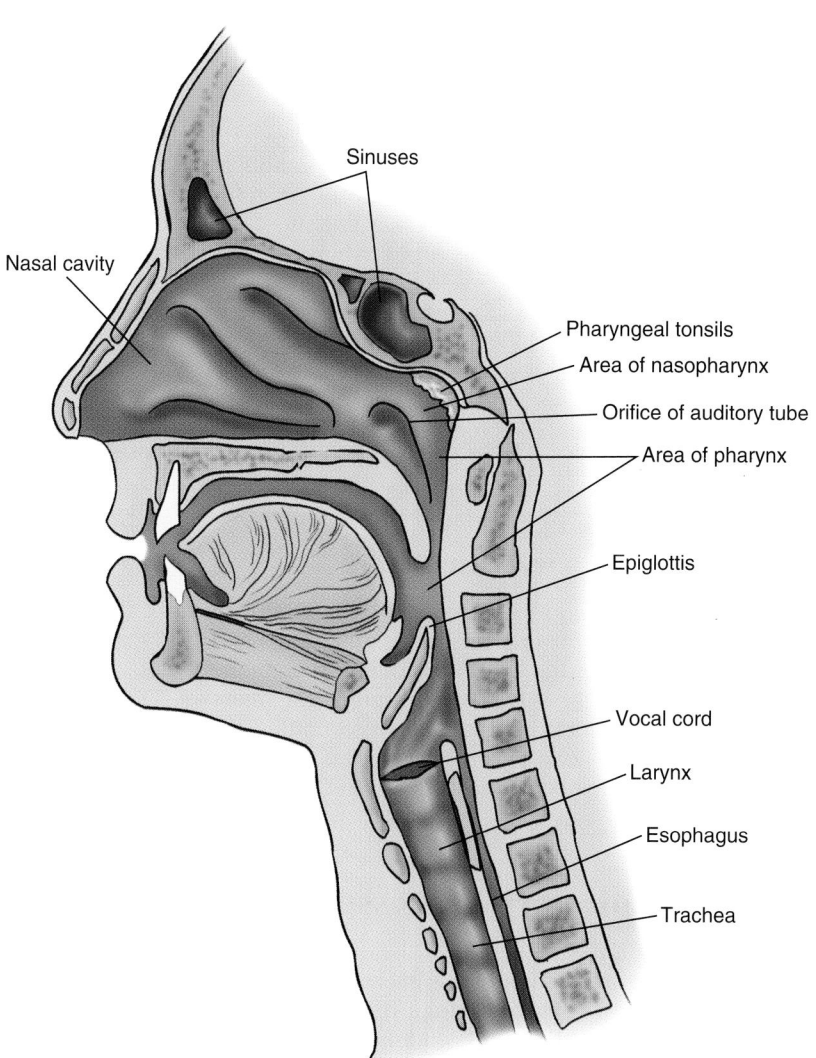

♦ **Figure 29–1**
The upper airway shown in cross-section. The larynx divides the upper and lower airway and connects the pharynx with the trachea.

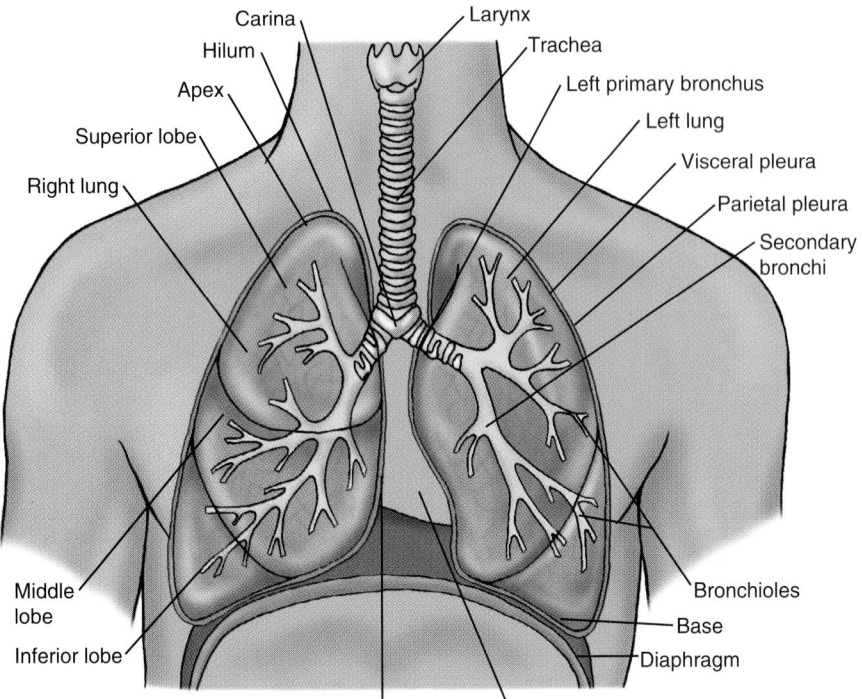

✦ **Figure 29–2**
The lower airway and thoracic cavity, showing the trachea and lungs.

Gas Exchange Airways

The bronchioles, alveolar ducts and sacs, and alveoli are the sites of gas exchange. The air that fills these structures is referred to as alveolar volume.

The functional units of the lungs where gas exchange occurs are called the acini. Each acinus contains structures that allow for gas exchange. These structures are the bronchiole and the alveolar ducts and sacs. Also contained in the acini is a network of capillaries. Thus, the surface of the acini is known as the alveolar-capillary membrane. The capillary bed is very permeable to oxygen, carbon dioxide, water, and electrolytes.

Pulmonary Vasculature

Deoxygenated blood is carried by a pulmonary artery that branches off into the tiny capillaries. These capillaries are part of the alveolar-capillary membrane. Blood is oxygenated as it passes through the membrane and is recollected by pulmonary venules that exit through a pulmonary vein. The pulmonary vein then returns oxygenated blood back to the left atrium of the heart.

Respiratory Processes

The respiratory process is divided into two phases: external respiration and internal respiration. External respiration is the exchange of gases between the atmosphere and the lungs. Internal respiration is the exchange of gases at the cellular level. There are four parts or steps in the process of respiration: ventilation, diffusion, transport, and regulation.

Ventilation

Ventilation is a mechanical event concerned with the movement of gases into and out of the lungs. This movement of air is dependent on several factors, including patent airways, an intact neuromuscular component, and intact skeletal structures of the thoracic cage.

The respiratory muscles include the diaphragm, intercostals, and accessory muscles (scalene and sternocleidomastoid muscles). Nervous innervation of the diaphragm comes from the phrenic nerve roots that arise from the third, fourth, and fifth cervical vertebrae (C3, C4, and C5). Injuries affecting C3 through C5 result in cessation of breathing. The intercostal muscles are innervated from the thoracic level of the spinal cord.

During the process of inspiration, the diaphragm contracts and pulls downward. The external intercostal muscles also contract and elevate the ribs. These movements increase the size of the thorax and stretch the lungs, causing decreased thoracic pressure. As the pressure in the lungs becomes less than the atmospheric pressure, air flows into the lungs, because the movement of gases is always from an area of greater pressure to one of lesser pressure (Boyle's law).

Expiration, unlike inspiration, is a passive event caused by the relaxation of the diaphragm and the respiratory muscles to their resting state. This relaxation causes a squeezing action on the lungs and a resulting increase in alveolar pressure above the atmo-

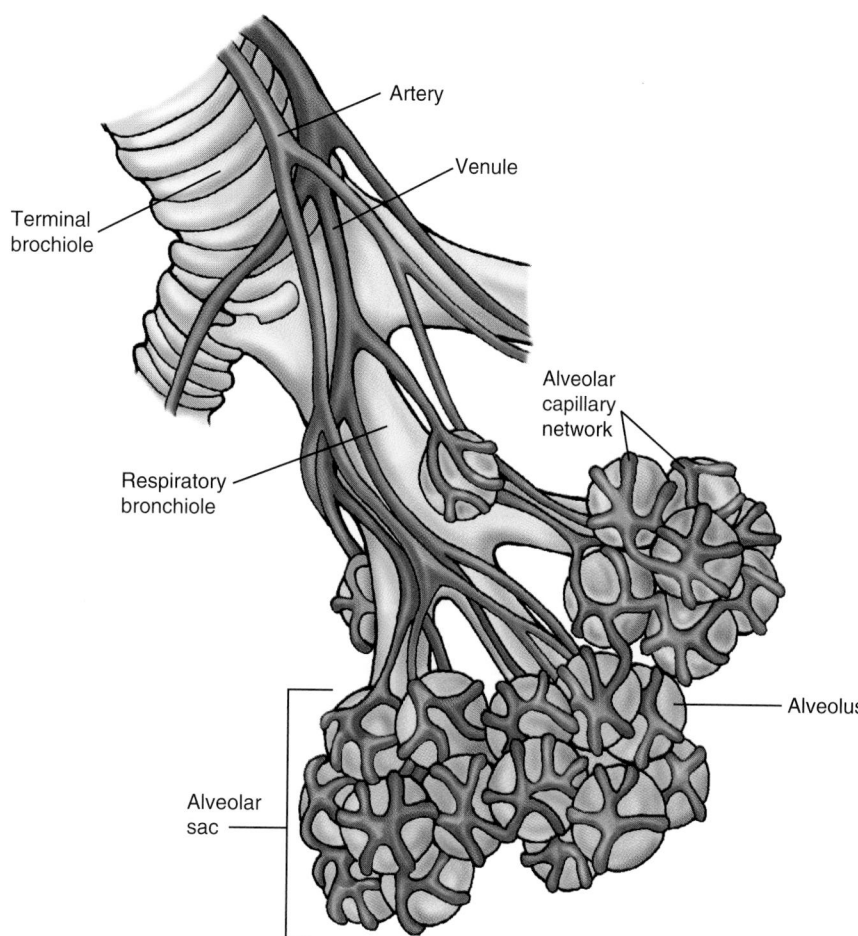

✦ **Figure 29–3**
The lungs contain approximately 35,000 terminal bronchioles. Each terminal bronchiole divides into terminal respiratory units called acini, where gas exchange takes place. Each acinus is composed of respiratory bronchioles, alveolar sacs, and alveoli, each with a network of pulmonary arteries and veins.

spheric pressure. To equalize pressure between the lungs and the atmosphere, air flows out of the lungs. When the diaphragm is not functioning, breathing is assisted by the contraction of the respiratory accessory and abdominal muscles, resulting in the pulling down on the ribs and the pushing up on the diaphragm, respectively.

✦ **Work of Breathing.** Because expiration is a passive process, the work of breathing occurs during inspiration and may be affected by any of the following.

• Lung compliance describes the elasticity of the lungs. It characterizes the ease with which the lung can be inflated against its elastic forces. Compliance is decreased in pulmonary fibrosis, pulmonary congestion, and edema. Compliance is increased in the elderly and in persons with emphysema, because of changes in the elastic tissue.

• Surface tension of the liquid film that lines the alveoli is an important factor in lung inflation. This liquid substance, known as surfactant, reduces the surface tension in the alveoli and keeps them from drying up. Premature infants may have immature alveolar cells that are not capable of producing adequate surfactant. Surfactant production may be impaired in adults with shock lung or adult respiratory distress syndrome.

• Airway resistance refers to the factors that impede airflow into the lungs. Airway obstruction, pulmonary edema, and bronchospasm can produce marked increase in airway resistance.

✦ **Pulmonary Volumes and Capacities.** There are four different pulmonary volumes: tidal volume, inspiratory reserve volume, expiratory reserve volume, and residual volume. The sum of these volumes equals the total lung capacity (TLC), or the maximum volume that the lungs can be expanded. The combination of two or more of these volumes is called lung capacity (Fig. 29–4).

• *Tidal volume* (TV) is the amount of air inhaled and exhaled during normal quiet breathing. This can be determined by direct spirographic measurement and is normally about 500 ml.

• *Inspiratory reserve volume* (IRV) is the extra volume of air that can be inspired in addition to the normal tidal volume. This volume is approximately 3,000 ml.

• Following a normal passive expiration of tidal volume, the additional air that can be forced out is the *expiratory reserve volume* (ERV).

• *Residual volume* (RV) is the volume of air always in the

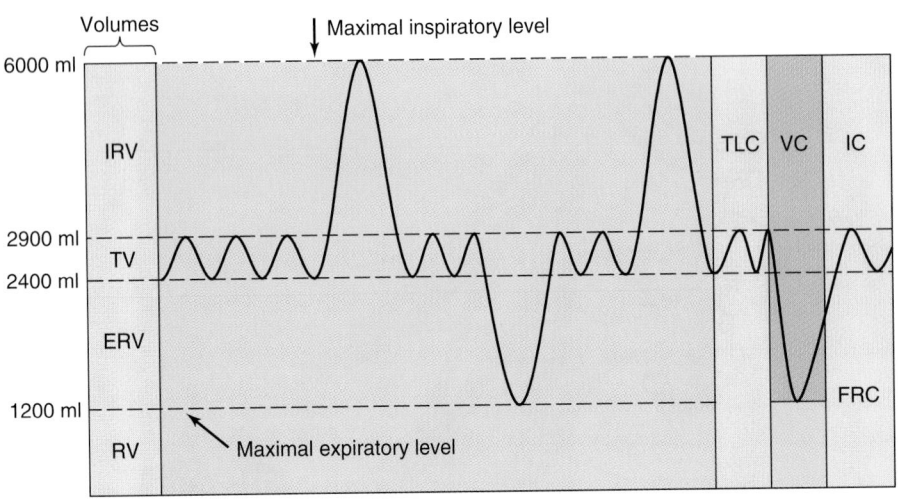

Figure 29–4
Components of lung volumes. (ERV = expiratory reserve volume; FRC = functional reserve capacity; IC = inspiratory capacity; IRV = inspiratory reserve volume; RV = residual volume; TLC = total lung capacity; TV = tidal volume; VC = vital capacity.)

lungs that cannot be exhaled. This volume is approximately 1200 ml.

- *Vital capacity* (VC) is the maximum volume of air that can be exhaled after maximum inspiration. The sum of the IRV and the ERV equals the VC.

- *Inspiratory capacity* (IC) is the maximum amount of air that can be inhaled. It equals the TV plus the IRV.

- *Functional residual capacity* (FRC) is the amount of air remaining in the lungs after a spontaneous expiration. The FRC is calculated by adding the ERV and the RV.

- *Total lung capacity* (TLC) is the maximum volume of gas the lungs can hold. The TLC is approximately 6000 ml and comprises the IRV, TV, ERV, and RV.

- *Forced vital capacity* (FVC) is the amount of air that can be forced out of the lungs on expiration.

Diffusion of Gases

Diffusion is the movement of gases from the alveolar-capillary membrane to the pulmonary capillary bed and vice versa, and it is the second step in the process of respiration. Gas diffuses from an area of higher concentration to an area of lower concentration. This is referred to as moving down the concentration gradient.

Diffusion is affected by several variables. It is directly affected by the surface area available for gas diffusion, the difference in the concentration of gases from one area to another, and the solubility of the diffusing gas. An increase in any of these factors directly increases the movement of gases across the membrane. Diffusion may be inversely affected by the thickness of the membrane, which determines the distance the gas has to travel, and by the molecular weight of the gas. The rate of diffusion is decreased if any of these factors is increased.

Under normal conditions, the diffusion of oxygen and carbon dioxide across the alveolar-capillary membrane is very fast. This is because the normal lung surface area is large (80 m²), and the alveolar-capillary membranes are normally one-cell thick (about 0.5 μm). Also, the difference in the pressure gradient of oxygen between the mixed venous blood and the alveoli is very wide, which allows the diffusion to occur rapidly from an area of high concentration to one of lower concentration.

Transport

The transportation of gases is the third step in the process of respiration and involves the movement of oxygen and carbon dioxide to and from the cells. About 97% of oxygen is transported to the tissues by hemoglobin in the form of oxyhemoglobin. A relatively small amount is dissolved in plasma.

Oxygen transport is largely dependent on the following:

- Amount of oxygen entering the lungs
- Blood flow to the alveoli and to the cellular level
- Adequacy of diffusion
- Capacity of the blood to carry oxygen

Carbon dioxide is a by-product that is produced as cells use oxygen. A small portion (5%) of this gas is transported in the dissolved state to the lungs. About 65% of carbon dioxide is carried to the lungs in the form of bicarbonate. The remaining 30% is combined with reduced hemoglobin to form carbaminohemoglobin.

Respiratory Regulation

Precise regulation of the respiratory process ensures an adequate supply of oxygen to meet the demands of the body. The two regulatory mechanisms are the neural and chemical regulators. Neural regulation includes the control of respiratory rate, depth, and rhythm by the central nervous system. Chemical regulation includes the control of the depth of respiration by carbon dioxide and hydrogen ion concentrations. These respiratory center regulators receive and respond to information from different sensory systems in the body.

Central and peripheral chemoreceptors provide information about the concentration of oxygen, carbon dioxide, and hydrogen ions in the blood. Mechanoreceptors in the lungs identify the degree of inflation (and probably deflation) of the lungs. Proprioceptors in the muscles of the thorax and abdomen provide information about the degree of contraction of these respiratory muscles.

✦ **Nervous Control of Respiration.** Located within the brain stem is the medulla, which contains the respiratory center. Inspiration is the result of impulses initiated by neurons. When the rate of impulses increases, the respiratory rate increases. Likewise, an increase in the strength or amplitude of impulses increases the tidal volume.

The dorsal aspect of the medulla oblongata contains the inspiratory center. Neurons in this area receive input directly from the chemoreceptors and mechanoreceptors.

The apneustic center, located in the pons portion of the brain stem, prevents the interruption of these inspiratory impulses. If the apneustic portion takes control over the otherwise balanced respiratory pattern, apneustic breathing patterns result. Conditions in which the apneustic center takes over include narcotic overdose or anesthesia. Apneustic breathing is characterized by short pauses following some expirations in an otherwise normal breathing pattern (Table 29–1).

Control of expiration is in the pneumotaxic center, also located within the pons. Neurons in this area send impulses that limit inspiration. If the pneumotaxic center takes over, the respiratory pattern that occurs is irregular, with deep and shallow breathing (see Table 29–1).

✦ **Chemical Control of Respiration.** Central chemoreceptors in the medulla are sensitive to changes in carbon dioxide and hydrogen ion concentrations. Increased carbon dioxide and hydrogen ion concentration (acidotic state) are potent stimuli of the inspiratory center, which results in increased ventilation.

Peripheral chemoreceptors are located in the carotid and aortic bodies. They respond to a decrease in oxygen content (oxygen bound to hemoglobin) and to carbon dioxide and hydrogen ion alterations. For example, in hypoxia, hypercapnia, or acidosis, the sensory nerve endings of the carotid bodies are stimulated. Impulses are conducted by the glossopharyngeal nerves to the inspiratory center in the medulla, leading to an increase in inspiratory rate.

The Hering-Breuer (stretch) reflex is a feedback mechanism in which stretch receptors in the smooth muscle of the airways send messages to the inspiratory center in the medulla. This response protects against overinflation of the lungs. For example, during strenuous exercise, lung expansion increases to take in as much air as needed by the body. This expansion causes an increased firing rate of the pulmonary stretch receptors and movement of nerve impulses along the afferent fibers of the vagus to inhibit the inspiratory center, thus permitting expiration and lung deflation.

Common Problems With Oxygenation

The chief respiratory complaints encountered by the nurse include dyspnea, asthma, chest pain, anorexia, cough, orthopnea, and hemoptysis. Each of these complaints must be thoroughly explored in relation to the client's statements, history, physical examination, and diagnostic tests.

Dyspnea, or shortness of breath, is a sensation that occurs when breathing becomes difficult and is out of proportion to the activity being performed. Nor-

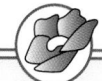

COMMUNITY-BASED CARE

OXYGEN THERAPY

Oxygen therapy may be part of the home care regimen for both adult and pediatric clients. Common indications for therapy include hypoxemia from chronic obstructive pulmonary or cardiac disease, sleep apnea, and cystic fibrosis. Oxygen may be administered using a nasal cannula or tracheostomy collar or with the newer transtracheal oxygen catheter. Sources of home oxygen include compressed gas in a tank, liquid oxygen, and, most often, the oxygen concentrator. The concentrator extracts oxygen from room air, runs on electricity, and serves as an "endless" oxygen supply unless an electrical shortage or malfunction occurs. An oxygen tank must always be available for back-up and as a mobile oxygen source when the client travels outside of the home.

The durable medical equipment company is responsible for delivery, initial safety teaching, and maintenance of the equipment. The home care nurse monitors client condition and continues teaching during home visits. Monitoring includes cardiopulmonary assessment, pulse oximeter checks (oxygen saturation), and coping. Support and education are essential in helping the client adjust to oxygen therapy. Some clients are fearful and anxious because of their oxygen dependence. Other clients' body image may be affected by the "external" evidence of their disease. Key teaching topics include

1. Benefits of oxygen—often, improved sleep, appetite, and energy levels

2. Oxygen flow rate, frequency of use, duration, and possible side effects

3. Safety issues—keeping oxygen source away from heat and flammable materials

4. Resources and telephone numbers for questions and troubleshooting

Table 29–1

VENTILATORY RATE AND PATTERN

VENTILATORY PATTERN	RATE	TIDAL VOLUME	COMMENTS
Normal (eupnea)	12–20/min	350–500 ml (adults)	Regular; occasional signs; inspiration to expiration (I:E) ratio, 1:2
Bradypnea	<12/min (slow)	Variable; depending on cause	Regular; I:E ratio, 1:2
Tachypnea	>20/min (rapid)	Shallow; small tidal volume with each breath	Regular; I:E ratio, 1:1; may be associated with CO_2 retention
Hyperventilation Central neurogenic hyperventilation if owing to lesions of lower midbrain or upper pons Kussmaul's breathing if owing to diabetic coma	>20/min (rapid)	Deep; large tidal volume	Usually regular; I:E ratio, 1:1; may be associated with CO_2 loss
Cheyne-Stokes	Variable	Variable; cyclical pattern: shallow before and after apnea, deep with hyperventilation	Regular-irregular pattern: crescendo-decrescendo pattern
Apnea	Absence of breathing	None	May be temporary or an emergency situation

mally, breathing becomes difficult with heavy exertion, but this should not occur during rest, when doing daily activities of living, or when walking.

Asthma is characterized by attacks of paroxysmal dyspnea with wheezing. The wheezing is caused by spasmodic contraction of the bronchi. Asthma may be induced by an allergen, vigorous exercise, irritant particles, or physiological stress.

Chest pain can have many implications. It is im-

portant to investigate the type of chest pain by using leading questions during the interview. Complaints of chest pain can be caused by many different factors.

Anorexia and weight loss are common complaints of clients with chronic respiratory problems such as chronic obstructive pulmonary disease, bronchogenic carcinoma, and tuberculosis.

Cough is an important normal defense mechanism of the respiratory system. It maintains clear airways.

However, coughing may also be a sign of a respiratory problem. Common pulmonary causes of cough are cigarette smoking, allergic reactions, respiratory infections, and bronchogenic carcinoma.

Orthopnea is shortness of breath that occurs when in a supine position. Orthopnea is an abnormal finding and may be caused by cardiac or respiratory problems.

When a client coughs up blood, the condition is called hemoptysis. Blood-tinged sputum may be present when coughing is violent in nature, causing superficial irritation of the upper respiratory tract mucous membranes.

Application of the Nursing Process

Assessment

Nursing History

The assessment of the client with an alteration in respiratory function begins with an interview to obtain a health history. When the client is unable to communicate, the history may be obtained from a parent or other relative, a friend or significant other, or a caregiver. If the data are not obtained directly from the client, the source of information should be noted on the chart (Bates, 1995). After the nurse collects the relevant data, a physical examination is conducted. To ensure a comprehensive picture of the client's respiratory function, the laboratory and diagnostic test results are analyzed in correlation with both subjective and objective findings.

➤ **History of Present Illness.** The history of present illness includes biographical data (age, sex, marital status, occupation, education, religion, and ethnic background) and an analysis of the presenting symptom. Ask about the client's chief complaint or the reason for the visit. Find out when and how the symptoms developed and how lifestyle is affected. Investigate each symptom thoroughly by asking leading questions (Box 29–1).

Document the chief complaint using the client's own words. This style of documentation provides an accurate description of the complaint as perceived by the client rather than by the interviewer (Bates, 1995).

The presenting complaint of clients with respiratory alteration may be varied. Common respiratory symptoms include dyspnea or shortness of breath, chest pain, cough, fever, anorexia, and weight loss (Wilson & Thompson, 1990).

The client may report an increasing shortness of breath associated with activities of daily living that previously did not cause shortness of breath—for example, walking up the same number of steps. Because dyspnea is a subjective sensation, the nurse can objectively quantify the degree of respiratory difficulty by

---

> **Box 29–1**
>
> ### ASSESSMENT QUESTIONS
>
> **General**
> - What brought you to the hospital/clinic/doctor's office?
> - How long have you had this symptom?
> - Where does it occur? What part of the body is affected? (Ask the client to localize symptoms by pointing to the body parts[s] affected.)
> - Does the symptom radiate or affect other parts?
> - How bad is the symptom? (severity)
> - Is the symptom diminishing, unchanging, or getting worse? Describe.
> - How does it develop? Is the onset gradual or sudden?
> - What provokes the symptom? (anxiety, body position, walking, eating)
> - How often does the symptom occur? What relieves it? (rest, medication, treatment, changing body position)
> - How long does the symptom last?
> - To what extent does the symptom affect normal daily living?
>
> **Specific to Oxygenation**
> - Have you noticed any change in your breathing pattern?
> - Do you have a history of heart or blood circulation problems? If so, describe.
> - Do you smoke? If so, how much?
> - Does a family member smoke?
> - Are you exposed to smoke or pollutants at work?
> - Are you exposed to any animal dander or feathers?
> - Have you had or do you have allergies, a cold, asthma, tuberculosis, bronchitis, pneumonia, or emphysema?
> - Have you been exposed to anyone with the above?
> - Do you have a cough? How much? How often?
> - Do you cough up sputum? Is the cough productive or dry?
> - If the cough is productive, how much sputum is produced?
> - Describe the color, amount, thickness, and odor of the sputum.
> - Is there blood in the sputum?
> - Are you awakened at night feeling short of breath?
> - Do you sleep with additional pillows? If so, how many?

---

using a grading system (Box 29–2). Orthopnea may indicate that the client has a respiratory or cardiac dysfunction, such as pulmonary hypertension or left ventricular failure. Other conditions that may lead to orthopnea include diaphragmatic paralysis, massive

---

Box 29–2

GRADING DYSPNEA

Grade 1 Dyspnea with mild exertion such as climbing a flight of stairs or running a short distance

Grade 2 Dyspnea while walking a short distance on level ground at a normal pace

Grade 3 Dyspnea while performing daily activities of living such as dressing, eating, combing hair, shaving, or bathing

Grade 4 Dyspnea at rest

Grade 5 Orthopnea

---

obesity, or chronic obstructive pulmonary disease. To quantify orthopnea, ask the client how many pillows are used to breathe easily during sleep.

Obtain a thorough history from clients presenting with a chief complaint of chest pain. Differentiating a complaint of chest pain is paramount in determining the cause. A sharp, stabbing substernal pain may indicate that the client has developed a spontaneous pneumothorax or collapsed lung. A burning sensation in the trachea that worsens with deep breathing or coughing may be associated with oxygen toxicity or aspiration. A stabbing, knifelike pain that increases with deep breathing or coughing may indicate pulmonary infarction owing to occlusion of the pulmonary artery, pneumothorax, or pleurisy from inflammation of the pleura. Localized chest pain and tenderness may occur with blunt chest trauma. When assessing the possible cause of chest pain, consider associated factors such as effects of breathing, posture, or body position on the pain.

A cough is a normal defense mechanism, but it may be associated with respiratory problems. Ask when the cough started, how long the client has had it, the type of cough (*e.g.*, hacking, dry, productive), if it comes intermittently or is constant, what time of day it occurs, and the precipitating factors. When cough is associated with sputum, find out the amount of sputum produced each day using common measurements, such as a teaspoon or tablespoon. Also determine the color and consistency of the sputum, the presence of blood, unusual odor, and the time of day when sputum is produced.

Hemoptysis, or blood-tinged sputum, may be upsetting for the client. There are serious disorders that can cause blood-tinged or frank bloody sputum, such as pneumonia, lung abscess, pulmonary edema, carcinoma of the lung, tuberculosis, pulmonary embolism, or bronchiectasis. A distinction between hemoptysis and hematemesis, vomiting blood from the stomach, should be made. Hemoptysis is characterized by bright red or pink frothy blood mixed with sputum. Hematemesis is characterized by dark red blood that may or may not be mixed with undigested food materials and often has a coffee-ground appearance. If necessary, a litmus paper test can be done to distinguish one from the other. Blood from the lungs produces a negative litmus paper test (blue color remains), and blood from the stomach produces a positive result (paper turns pink).

A client presenting with anorexia may also complain of weakness and fatigue. Anorexia is a common complaint of clients with chronic respiratory problems. Most of a client's energy is directed toward breathing, and intake of adequate nutrition may be poor. Assessment includes the history of recent weight loss, pattern of weight loss (*e.g.*, drastic or progressive), the client's usual weight, and the present weight and height. The ideal weight for the client should be determined for comparison using a reference table for normal weights.

An elevated temperature or fever often indicates respiratory infection or tissue necrosis from an embolus or carcinoma. Chills may or may not accompany the fever. At times, night sweats, which are common in pulmonary tuberculosis, may also occur in response to the elevated temperature. Obtain an accurate temperature reading as part of the assessment process. False low oral temperature readings may occur in mouth breathers and clients who are receiving humidified oxygen. Under these conditions, a rectal temperature reading is preferable.

✦ **Past Medical and Surgical History.** The past medical and surgical history helps explain existing symptoms and identifies a client's risk for developing respiratory problems. This history includes previous illnesses, injuries, and immunizations. Note the dates of significant treatments, diagnostic tests, and surgeries, and why and where they were done. Include the length of hospitalization or confinement, if any.

Focus on primary respiratory problems such as asthma, emphysema, or bronchitis. Investigate secondary problems that may precipitate or complicate respiratory functioning. For example, childhood illnesses such as infantile eczema, atopic dermatitis, or allergic rhinitis may precipitate asthmatic attacks. Inquire about chronic respiratory problems such as chronic sinus infection or postnasal discharge, because these may lead to bronchitis. Investigate other conditions that might lead to respiratory complications, such as cardiac problems, neurological alterations, and immune deficiency problems.

Record relevant immunizations such as BCG (immunization for tuberculosis used predominantly in Europe), DPT (diphtheria-pertussis-tetanus), flu vaccine, and pneumococcal vaccine. Include dates of immunization.

✦ **Family History.** The relevant family history determines the client's risk for hereditary or infectious respiratory diseases. The initial investigation centers on immediate blood relatives such as parents, siblings, and children. Positive findings from this group should instigate further data collection that includes maternal and paternal grandparents, aunts, and uncles. Investigate the occurrence of cancer, heart disease, chronic respiratory diseases (asthma, emphysema, bronchitis), and infectious diseases (tuberculosis, pneumonia, influenza). Hereditary respiratory disorders include cystic fibrosis. Ascertain if the client is living with anyone who has an infectious disease. Document the current state of health of each family member, and note their ages and cause of death, if deceased.

✦ **Social and Personal History.** The client's psychosocial profile must be included in the interview. These data provide knowledge about the client's lifestyle, occupation, ethnicity, home and community environmental factors, family support, and economic status, which may influence the client's current state of health and his or her ability to cope with health problems.

Investigate social habits that affect respiratory functions, such as use of tobacco, alcohol, and illegal substances. Collect both quantitative (how much and how long) and qualitative (type of substance and mode of administration) data. For example, ascertain how much tobacco the client uses daily for how many years and whether the tobacco is smoked or chewed. Cigarettes are usually quantified by the number of packs consumed a day and how long the habit has existed. Ask a client who uses illegal drugs about the type of drug used, how it is administered (*e.g.*, inhaled, taken orally, or taken intravenously), amount of daily consumption, and how long this habit has been in existence.

Physical Examination

The four techniques used in the physical assessment of a client with alteration in oxygenation are inspection, palpation, percussion, and auscultation (Jarvis, 1996). In order to assess subtleties of color and breathing patterns, natural lighting is necessary. Encourage the client to relax by providing privacy, and avoid interruptions. The nurse must be familiar with the chest landmarks for locating underlying structures during the examination and must be able to accurately describe any abnormal findings in relation to anatomical and topographical landmarks (Fig. 29–5). The major anterior landmark is the sternal angle or angle of Louis. The sternal angle is about 5 cm (2 inches) from the suprasternal notch. The second ribs articulate with the sternal notch. Underneath each rib are the interspaces, or intercostal spaces, which are numbered consecutively like the ribs. Therefore, finding the second rib makes it easier to locate the other ribs by palpating obliquely downward and posteriorly. In the posterior chest, the spinous processes may be counted and palpated starting with C7 or T1. These spinous processes, also known as vertebra prominens, visibly protrude when the neck is flexed forward. The scapula may also be used as a landmark posteriorly, because its inferior angle lies at approximately the same level as the seventh rib (see Fig. 29–5).

There are several imaginary lines on the anterior, lateral, and posterior chest walls. The anterior lines are

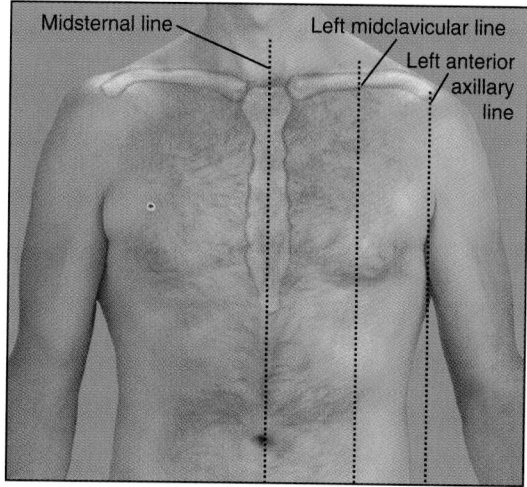

Anterior

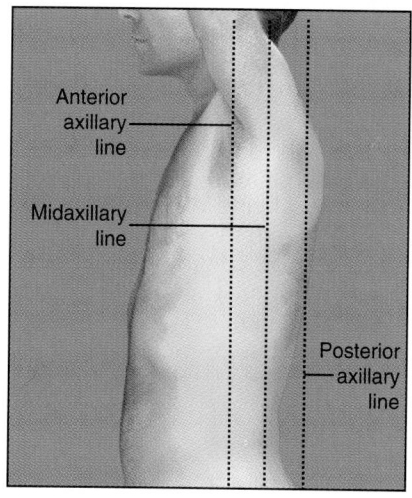

Lateral

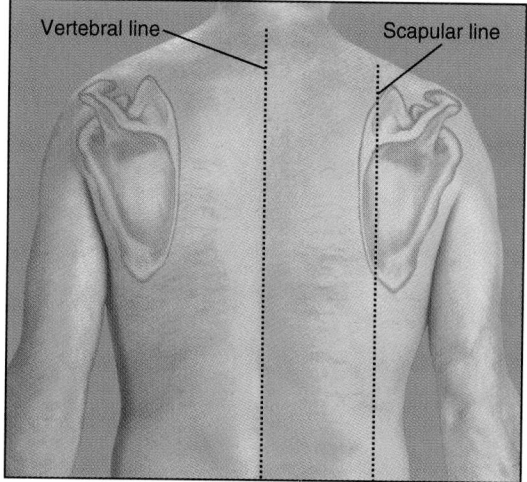

Posterior

✦ **Figure 29–5**
Anatomical and topographical landmarks of the thorax.

referred to as the midsternal line, the right and left midclavicular lines, and the right and left anterior axillary lines. Laterally, the imaginary lines are the midaxillary lines, the anterior axillary line, and posterior axillary line. Posterior lines are the vertebral line and the right and left scapular lines (see Fig. 29–5).

✦ **Inspection.** The inspection of the respiratory system starts from the time the nurse first sees the client. The color of skin, level of alertness and orientation, activity tolerance, posture, and pattern of breathing can easily be observed during the initial client contact. These features reveal a great deal about the client's oxygenation status. Refer to Table 29–1 for ventilatory rates and patterns.

The skin and mucous membranes are observed for cyanosis, which is considered a late sign of hypoxia. The lips (circumoral cyanosis), tip of the nose, earlobes, and mucous membrane inside the oral cavity are the best areas to check for bluish discoloration.

Carefully note the rate, rhythm, depth, and effort of breathing. Normal breathing should be quiet and regular, about 12 to 20 times a minute in adults. Obtain the respiratory rate with the client resting quietly. Clients may alter their respiratory patterns if they are aware that they are being observed. Anxiety may affect the rate and depth. Therefore, assess the client's respiratory rate after obtaining the pulse. Continue to palpate the radial artery while observing the rise and fall of the chest. Count the respiratory rate for 30 seconds to 1 minute. A respiratory rate that is quiet and regular is termed eupnea. An abnormally slow respiratory rate is called bradypnea, and an abnormally rapid respiratory rate is called tachypnea. In addition to counting the respiratory rate for a full minute, assess the depth and pattern of breathing. Occasionally, a sigh may be observed. A sigh is a deep inspiration followed by a slow audible expiration. Signs of breathing difficulty include flaring of the nostrils, supraclavicular retractions, contraction of the sternomastoid or other muscles during inspiration, and leaning forward to facilitate breathing. Note audible respiratory sounds such as wheezing, stridor, or noisy breathing associated with clogged nasal passages. Pursed-lip breathing indicates expiratory difficulty found in chronic obstructive pulmonary disease. The trachea should be midline. If it is displaced laterally, it may indicate pleural effusion, tension pneumothorax, or atelectasis. A deviated trachea, whatever the cause, is an emergency situation.

Chronic problems may be noted by inspecting the fingernails and alterations in the shape of the thorax. Clubbing of the nails indicates a chronic cardiorespiratory problem, such as fibrotic lung disease, cystic fibrosis, or congenital heart disease with cyanosis (Fig. 29–6). The anteroposterior diameter of the chest (barrel chest) may be increased in chronic obstructive pulmonary disease, although this may be a sign associated with aging (see Fig. 29–6).

✦ **Palpation.** Palpate the chest wall to identify areas of tenderness, masses, crepitus, tactile fremitus, and diaphragmatic excursion (Fig. 29–7A). Normally, the sternum, costal cartilages, ribs, intercostal spaces, and

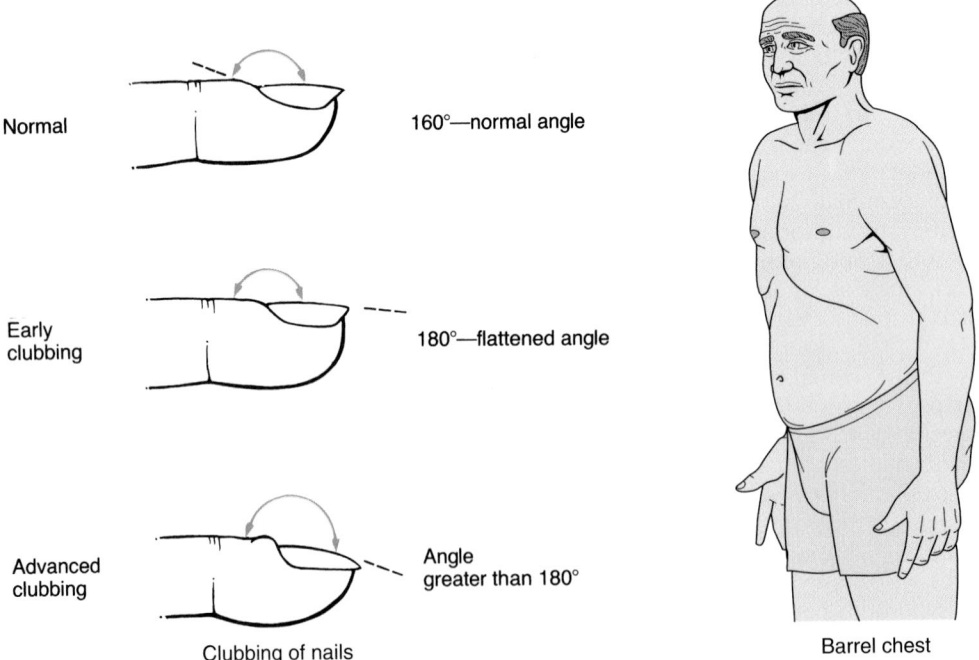

✦ **Figure 29–6**
Clubbing of the nails and barrel chest may indicate chronic respiratory problems. Nail clubbing is associated with fibrotic lung disease, cystic fibrosis, and congenital heart disease with cyanosis. Barrel chest—increased anteroposterior diameter of the chest—may be a sign of chronic obstructive pulmonary disease (although it may also be a sign of aging).

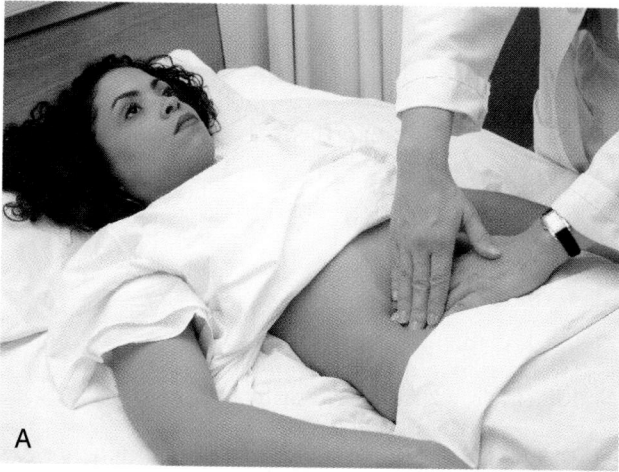

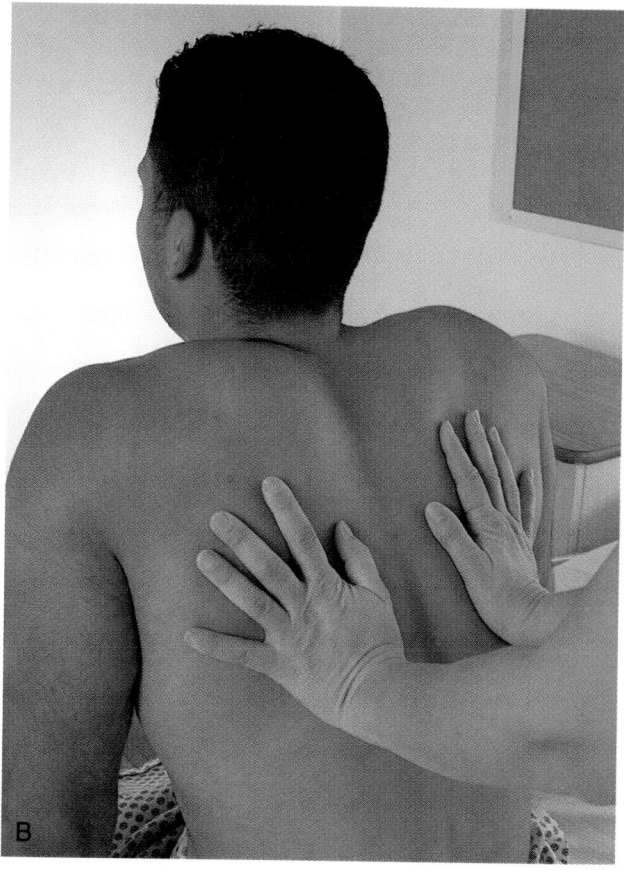

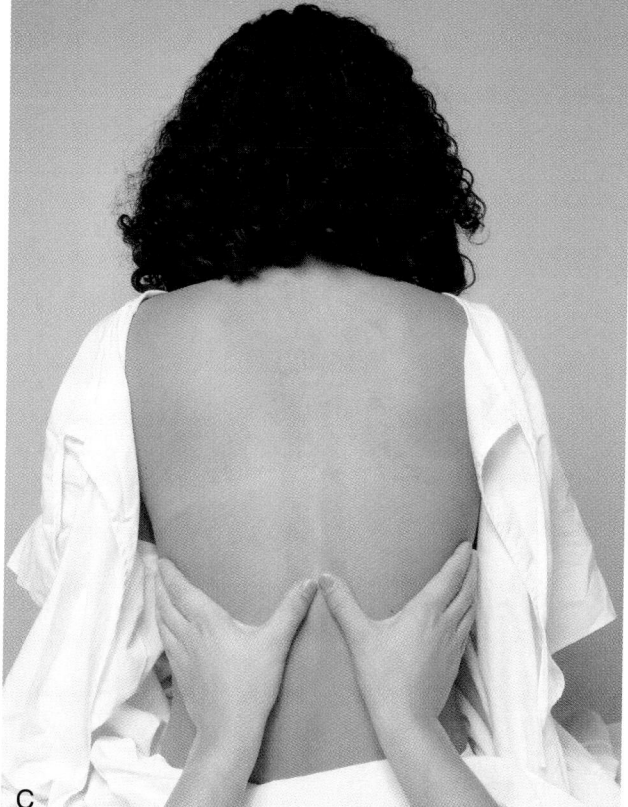

❧ Figure 29–7

A, Palpation of the chest wall to assess for areas of tenderness, masses, or crepitus. *B*, Palpating for fremitus, the vibration of the chest wall produced during vocalization. Ask the client to say "ninety-nine" or "one-two-three" while palpating with both hands, as shown. Abnormally increased or decreased fremitus may indicate a pathological condition. *C*, Assessing for chest expansion. Asymmetrical or decreased expansion may indicate a disease condition.

spine should not be tender on palpation. There should be no palpable masses or crepitus. Crepitus is a cracking sound produced when air is present in the subcutaneous tissue. It may occur if air from chest tubes or mechanical ventilation leaks out in the subcutaneous tissues. The fingertips are used to palpate for tenderness or crepitus.

Tactile fremitus, which is the vibration of the chest wall produced during vocalization, is assessed by pal-

pating the chest wall. Ask the client to say words such as "ninety-nine" or "one-two-three." Palpation is done using both hands (heel or palmar surface of the hand) to compare the vibration between left and right sides. Fremitus can be palpated in all areas of the lung fields. It is increased in the major airways, such as the trachea and mainstem bronchi. It is usually decreased or absent over the precordium. Abnormally increased fremitus may be present in conditions such as pneumonia with consolidation, atelectasis, lung tumor, pulmonary infarction, and fibrosis. Abnormally decreased or absent fremitus may be noted in conditions such as pleural effusions, pleural thickening, collapsed lung, bronchial obstruction, and emphysema (Fig. 29–7B).

Chest expansion can be roughly estimated by palpation. To do this, place the thumbs at about the level of and parallel to the 10th ribs, with the hands grasping the lateral rib cage. Slide the hand medially to raise loose skin folds between thumbs and spine. Instruct the client to inhale deeply. Divergence of the examiner's thumbs should be observed during inspiration. Also feel for the range and symmetry of respiratory movement. Asymmetrical and decreased chest expansion may indicate chronic fibrotic disease, pleural effusion, lobar pneumonia, or client splinting related to pleural pain (Fig. 29–7C).

❧ Percussion. Percussion of the lungs determines whether they are air filled, fluid filled, or solid. Normal adult lungs produce a resonant tone on percussion. Children's lungs are normally hyperresonant. Hyperresonance may also be produced in those with emphysema and pneumothorax. Dullness is the tone elicited from solid masses or when there is fluid in the lungs. Bilateral comparisons of the left and right sides of the thorax must be done during percussion. The anterior and the posterior thorax should also be percussed. Do not percuss over the sternum, ribs, or scapula.

Diaphragmatic excursion, which is the distance between the levels of dullness with deep inspiration and full expiration, can also be determined by percussion. Note the level of diaphragmatic dullness while the client is breathing normally. During quiet respiration, the lower border of the lungs is at the level of the 10th thoracic spinous process. An abnormally high level may suggest pleural effusion or atelectasis. Next ask the client to take a deep breath and hold it; continue to percuss until resonance is replaced by dullness. Note the difference between the two levels of dullness. Normally it ranges from 3 to 5 cm (1.5 to 2 inches). The right diaphragm is slightly higher owing to the presence of the liver.

Table 29–2

NORMAL VERSUS ADVENTITIOUS BREATH SOUNDS

TYPE	CHARACTERISTICS	COMMENTS
Normal Lung Sounds		
Normal	Low-pitched, soft, breezy sounds normally heard over the lung fields	Usually longer and louder during inspiration than during expiration
Vesicular	Medium intensity and pitch normally heard over lesser bronchi, bronchioles, and lobes	Equal inspiratory and expiratory phases
Bronchiovesicular	Loud, high-pitched, and hollow; normally heard over the main bronchi	Longer and louder expiratory phase than inspiratory phase
Bronchial	Loud, high-pitched, and hollow; normally heard over the manubrium	Longer and louder expiratory phase than inspiratory phase
Tracheal	Very loud, high-pitched sound heard over the trachea in the neck	Inspiratory and expiratory phases are about equal
Adventitious Breath Sounds		
Crackles (rales)—fine, medium, or coarse	Soft, high-pitched, discontinuous popping sounds heard during inspiration (early or late)	May be caused by fluid in airways or opening of collapsed alveoli; early obstructive pulmonary disease; late or restrictive pulmonary disease
Sonorous wheezes (rhonchi)	Deep, low-pitched, rumbling sound heard during expiration	May be caused by air moving through narrowed air passages; narrowing may be caused by secretions, tumors or spasms
Sibilant wheezes (wheezes)	Continuous, musical, high-pitched whistling sounds heard during inspiration and expiration	May be caused by narrowed bronchioles such as in asthma and bronchospasm
Pleural friction rub	Harsh, crackling sound similar to rubbing two pieces of leather together; heard during inspiration or expiration; loudest over anterior chest wall	May be caused by inflammation of pleural lining or loss of pleural fluid

✦ **Auscultation.** Auscultation of the lungs provides information about the airflow through the tracheobronchial tree. It helps detect obstruction of airflow in and out of the lungs as well as abnormalities such as adventitious or abnormal lung sounds. During auscultation, try to picture the underlying lung segment. The client should be in a sitting position or, if on bed rest, in a side lying position. Instruct the client to take slow, deeper-than-normal breaths with the mouth open. Observe for hyperventilation, which may lead to lightheadedness. Auscultation is done in a systematic manner, from the apices down to the bases, comparing side to side. Normal breath sounds should be clear (Table 29–2).

Diagnostic Studies

Diagnostic tests are used to assess the body's ability to exchange oxygen and carbon dioxide by measuring the adequacy of ventilation and oxygenation. Diagnostic studies are useful in identifying infectious or irritating processes that may interfere with adequate respiratory functioning. Certain diagnostic tests are also useful in identifying abnormal cell growth. The physician may order several different tests to enhance the findings from the physical examination and the history. Such tests may include venous or arterial blood samples, sputum specimens, pulmonary function tests, radiographic images, and throat cultures.

The complete blood count (CBC) includes the red blood cell (RBC) count, corpuscular indices, white blood cell (WBC) count, differential white cell count (diff), hemoglobin (Hgb), and hematocrit (Hct). The detection of anemia, evidenced by a decreased hemoglobin and hematocrit, is important in clients who have respiratory alterations. The presence of anemia decreases the oxygen-carrying capacity of the blood and therefore hinders oxygenation. Clients with chronic obstructive pulmonary disease may have an increased hemoglobin and hematocrit. This increase is called polycythemia and is a response to chronic hypoxia. An elevated WBC level can provide clues to possible infections in the lungs.

The arterial blood gas (ABG) reveals direct information about the status of arterial oxygenation and the acid-base balance. Arterial oxygen supply is determined by measuring the partial pressures of oxygen (PaO_2) and carbon dioxide ($PaCO_2$) in arterial blood. The arterial blood gas also measures saturation, or the percentage of hemoglobin carrying oxygen compared with the total amount of circulating hemoglobin (SaO_2), as well as the pH and bicarbonate level of the blood. Table 29–3 contains the normal arterial blood gas values.

Arterial blood is generally obtained from the radial artery with a needle and syringe. The syringe is usually preheparinized to prevent clotting of the blood specimen. After obtaining the blood, apply firm, direct pressure for approximately 5 minutes to stop the bleeding and prevent hematoma formation.

Blood cultures provide significant clues to pathogenic organisms that may invade the bloodstream and interfere with the oxygen-carrying capacity of red blood cells. Blood cultures also provide important information about appropriate antibiotic treatment. It is essential that all blood cultures be obtained before initiating any antibiotic regimen.

The pulse oximeter is a noninvasive monitor used intermittently or continuously to monitor the arterial oxygen saturation (SpO_2) (Sonnesso, 1991). A sensor is placed on an area where pulsating arteriolar blood is present, such as the finger, toe, earlobe, or nose. A normal SpO_2 is 95 to 100%. An SpO_2 less than 70% is life threatening and requires immediate attention (Szaflarski, 1989) (see Procedure 29–1).

In order to diagnose bacterial, fungal, or viral pulmonary diseases, skin tests are often performed. The most frequently performed skin test is the Mantoux test or tuberculin test, which detects present or previous infection with *Mycobacterium tuberculosis*. The test is performed by injecting 0.1 ml of purified protein derivative intradermally. If it is injected subcutaneously, a false-negative reaction may occur. The injection is performed on the inner forearm. The site is circled with a pen and documented clearly in the chart. The reaction is read 48 to 72 hours after the injection.

The amount of induration (hard swelling) is measured in millimeters and documented. An indurated area of 10 mm or greater is a positive reaction and indicates past or present infection. An induration of 5

Table 29–3

ARTERIAL BLOOD GASES

VALUE	NORMAL	ACIDOSIS	ALKALOSIS
pH	7.35–7.45	Below 7.35	Above 7.45
PaO_2	95–100 mm Hg	N/A	N/A
$PaCO_2$	35–45 mm Hg	Above 45	Below 35
HCO_3^-	22–24 mEq/L	N/A	N/A
N/A = not applicable.			

PROCEDURE

29–1

PULSE OXIMETRY

Pulse oximetry is a noninvasive monitoring technique that allows continuous measurement of arterial oxygen saturation of functional hemoglobin. This is important in situations in which early detection of SpO_2 changes is critical in the appropriate management of the client. It may also be used to evaluate the client's response to various activities that affect oxygenation, either positively or negatively (e.g., suctioning, turning and positioning, ventilator setting changes).

The pulse oximeter contains a sensor with two light-emitting diodes (red and infrared) and a photodetector. This sensor may be applied in areas where there is pulsating arteriolar blood, such as finger, toe, nose, or earlobe. The photodetector picks up fluctuating light signals registered by the pulsations. These signals are calculated into a digital display of percent saturation of hemoglobin (SpO_2) and pulse rate. Pulse amplitude is also shown.

Equipment:

Pulse oximeter
Monitor
Compatible sensor
Extension cable
Alcohol wipes
Nail polish remover

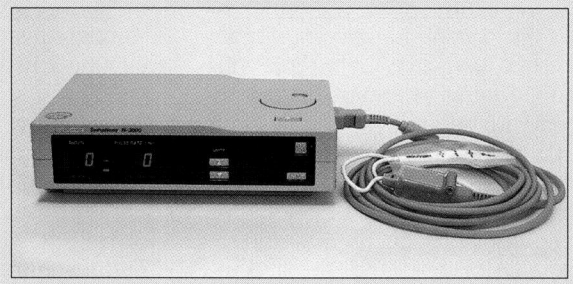

Action	Rationale
1. Wash hands. Take equipment to bedside.	**1.** Reduces spread of microorganisms.
2. Explain procedure to client and/or family.	**2.** Reduces anxiety and gains client's cooperation.
3. Plug oximeter into grounded wall outlet.	**3.** Minimizes electrical interference.
4. Assess digits for capillary refill and warmth. Check for arterial pulse. Avoid extremity with a blood pressure cuff, an arterial or intravenous line, an arteriovenous fistula or a pressure dressing. Note: If the client has poor peripheral perfusion, apply sensor to the nose or earlobe.	**4.** Accurate measurement of oxygen saturation (SpO_2) is dependent on adequate arterial pulsation.
5. Remove any nail polish if using the fingernails or remove any excess skin oil if applying the sensor to the nose.	**5.** Prevents blocking of the light transmission, which may lead to unreliable readings.

PULSE OXIMETRY
(Continued)

6. Apply the sensor according to the manufacturer's instructions. Check to make sure that the light-emitting diodes (LEDs) are alighted with the photodetector (PD).

6. Facilitates sensing of signals.

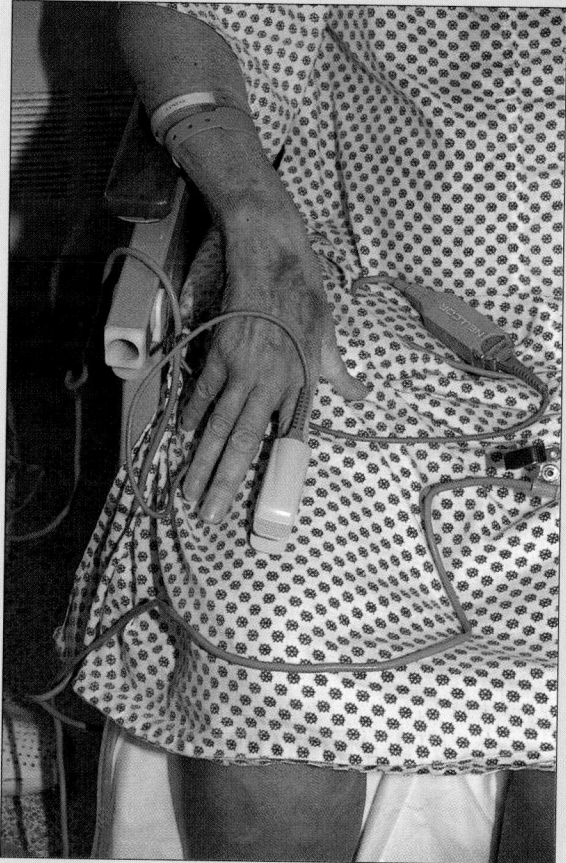

Step 6.

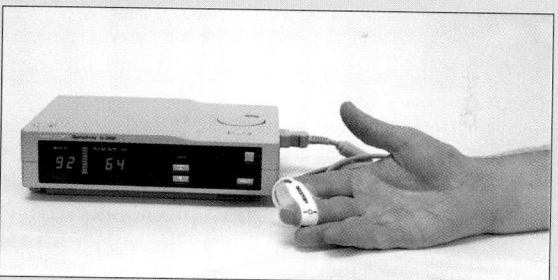

Step 9.

7. Cover the sensor with an opaque cloth, such as a blanket, to shield it from ambient light.

8. Connect the sensor to the extension cable.

9. Switch the power on. The monitor should show a self-test display. After a few seconds, an SpO$_2$ value and pulse rate will appear on the screen.

10. Set the low rate and high rate alarms according to institutional policy, the client's condition, or the physician's order.

11. Note and document the initial readings.

12. Wash hands.

7. Prevents optical interference from an external light source.

8. Completes the set-up of the system.

9. Verifies unit is operating correctly.

10. Alerts the staff of potential life-threatening readings.

11. Establishes a baseline.

12. Reduces spread of microorganisms.

to 9 mm is a doubtful reaction but may be positive if the client has had close contact with an infected person and radiographical evidence or signs and symptoms suggestive of tuberculosis are present. Indurations less than 4 mm are considered negative.

Sputum cultures are ideally obtained from the mucus located deep within the bronchus. Saliva (clear fluid excreted from salivary glands) is not an acceptable specimen for sputum cultures. A record of the amount, color, consistency, and odor of sputum should be documented with the specimen and submitted to the laboratory in a timely manner. Sputum cultures reveal valuable information about infectious organisms and sensitivity to appropriate antibiotics. Sputum specimens are also useful in detecting the presence of the tubercle bacillus germ that causes tuberculosis. For acid-fast bacillus (AFB) smears, a serial collection method of three consecutive early-morning specimens is necessary. Sputum specimens also yield information about malignancies (abnormal cell growth). As with AFB smears, sputum cytology studies require three consecutive early-morning specimens for optimal results.

Throat cultures are obtained from the oropharynx and tonsillar regions of the throat with a sterile swab to identify the presence of any invading organisms. If pathogenic organisms are identified, the appropriate antibiotic regimen is chosen, based on the culture and sensitivity results. Throat cultures are obtained with a special cotton-tipped swab applied directly to the oropharynx region.

Diagnostic tests to visualize structures of the respiratory system include chest radiographs (x-ray studies), fluoroscopy, and pulmonary angiography. Nuclear studies go beyond the capabilities of conventional radiographs to give more detailed information about the respiratory structures or masses.

Chest radiographs or x-rays are used to detect areas of density or hypersecretion, the presence of masses, and increased vascularity markings. Chest x-rays are also used to identify pneumothorax, cavitation, or lung abscess. Ideally, the evaluation consists of a posteroanterior (PA) view and at least one lateral view with the client standing or sitting up straight.

Computerized axial tomography is a noninvasive three-dimensional x-ray that further distinguishes minor differences in the radiodensities of soft tissues. Higher-density substances appear white, and lower-density substances appear dark.

Fluoroscopy uses the different x-ray absorption capacities of body structures to provide useful diagnostic images on a fluorescent screen (Fig. 29–8). Dense structures such as bones permit few x-rays to be absorbed, so bones appear as light areas on the screen. Soft tissues are less dense and allow greater absorption of x-rays, so soft tissues appear dark in contrast to nearby bony structures. In body structures that do not contrast naturally (*e.g.*, the abdomen), contrasting agents must be introduced into the body structure to achieve visualization.

Pulmonary angiography is a radiographical study in which a radiopaque material is injected into an artery or vein to allow visualization of the vascular system of the lungs. This test is most often used to identify the presence or absence of a pulmonary embolism or clot.

Nuclear studies such as the lung scan may be classified as perfusion scans or ventilation scans. With a perfusion scan, radioactive dye is administered intravenously. The dye allows for visualization of various fields of the lungs. Perfusion scans measure the integrity of blood vessels and assess the blood flow to the pulmonary tissues. The ventilation scan, often performed after the perfusion scan, uses a radioactive inert gas that is inhaled through a tight-fitting facial mask or nasal cannula. Ventilation scans detect abnormalities that occur during the ventilation process. Ventilation and perfusion scans are used to diagnose various pathologies of the lungs, including cancer, chronic obstructive pulmonary disease, pulmonary edema, and pulmonary infections.

Ultrasonography is a noninvasive diagnostic test that uses high-pitched sound waves to reveal information about the size, shape, and consistency of internal structures. Ultrasonography is also useful in identifying fluid, lesions, or masses in lung tissue.

Pulmonary function tests (PFTs) measure the functional ability of the lungs by identifying a restriction of or obstruction to airflow, or a combination of both. PFTs are extremely useful in identifying lung abnormalities, tracking the course of the disease process, and evaluating the effectiveness of various medications and/or treatment regimens over time. In routine PFTs, the client's lung size and breathing ability are compared with values for normal individuals who are similar to the client in age, sex, height, and race. The spirometer is the primary instrument used in this test. Spirometry provides an easy and inexpensive method to measure lung volume with relatively little risk to the client. In addition to simple spirometry, spirometry with gas dilution is also used as a diagnostic technique. The functional residual capacity can be calcu-

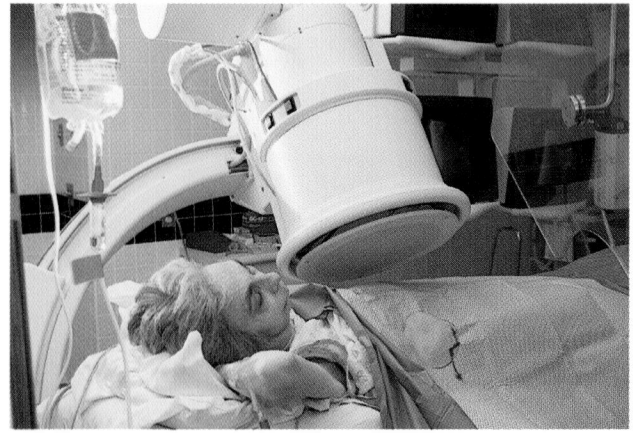

✦ **Figure 29–8**
Fluoroscopy and other types of radiographic imaging can provide useful information in diagnosing pulmonary problems.

lated with this method. In order to assess gas distribution throughout the lungs, helium or oxygen is inhaled in a known concentration. Helium does not cross the alveolar-capillary membrane, so the total amount of helium does not change.

Body plethysmography is also part of pulmonary function testing. The client sits in an airtight chamber or body box and breathes through a mouthpiece. Various lung volumes and capacities can be calculated using body plethysmography (Wilson & Thompson, 1990).

Nursing care prior to pulmonary function testing includes withholding bronchodilators and restricting meals for 4 to 6 hours before the test. If the client has dentures, they should be worn to facilitate a good seal around the mouthpiece. Inform the client that the test is painless.

Endoscopic and surgical procedures are also used to identify specific types of lesions. Diagnostic surgical procedures include biopsy and thoracentesis. Endoscopic procedures include direct laryngoscopy and bronchoscopy.

Endoscopic and surgical procedures require an informed consent. The client is asked not to eat or drink anything after midnight the night before the procedure. For endoscopic procedures, the throat is numbed with a spray and a fiberoptic endoscope is inserted into the trachea. Careful monitoring of the client's vital signs, including the SpO_2, is critical. After the procedure, the client is kept NPO (nothing by mouth) until the gag reflex returns.

Direct laryngoscopy is used to view the larynx directly under magnification to investigate abnormal signs associated with the larynx, such as hoarseness greater than 2 weeks' duration. Growths on the larynx such as polyps and nodules can be biopsied for pathological study. Foreign bodies that have lodged in the larynx can also be removed with direct laryngoscopy.

Bronchoscopy is the direct viewing of the trachea and tracheobronchial tree by means of a standard metal bronchoscope or a fiberoptic bronchoscope. Bronchoscopy is used in the diagnosis of such conditions as hemoptysis, lesions, masses, and abnormalities seen on the chest radiograph. Bronchoscopy may also be used to treat conditions that affect oxygenation, such as lung abscess, pneumonia, or aspiration, or to débride mucosal eschar and remove foreign bodies.

Biopsy is used to differentiate malignant and nonmalignant growth of a mass located in or around respiratory structures. Another indication for a biopsy is when a client's diagnosis remains undetermined despite a complete diagnostic analysis. The physician can visualize certain areas and obtain a biopsy if necessary. If a biopsy is obtained during a bronchoscopy, it is termed a closed chest biopsy. Open chest biopsies are performed in the operating room through a thoracotomy.

Thoracentesis is the surgical perforation of the chest wall and pleural space for diagnostic and/or therapeutic purposes. Excess fluid or air can accumulate in the pleural cavity as a result of injury or disease

and interfere with oxygenation and respiration. Through thoracentesis, the excess fluid or air can be removed from the pleural cavity. Chemotherapy agents can also be injected into the pleural cavity for the therapeutic relief of pain or dyspnea that can be symptomatic of pleural pressure.

An informed consent is required for a thoracentesis to be performed. Prior to the procedure, the client's vital signs are assessed. Auscultate all lung fields to establish a baseline. Observe the client's respiratory rate and depth, presence of cough, and characteristics and amount of sputum.

If possible, the client is positioned sitting up with the arms supported on a bedside table. If the client is unable to sit up, positioning is in a side-lying position dependent on the site of the thoracentesis.

After the physician has completed the procedure, the vital signs are reassessed. Frequent observation of the respiratory rate and depth, complaints of shortness of breath, tracheal position, and lung sounds is imperative.

Document the amount of drainage or air removed or any medications administered. Clearly label all specimen containers and send them to the laboratory promptly. Document the client's tolerance of the procedure.

See Procedure 29–2 for preparation of the client for thoracentesis and Procedure 29–3 for closed chest drainage.

Psychosocial Assessment

The psychosocial assessment captures relevant and important information about the client as a person. Some aspects of the client's lifestyle may affect the respiratory function. Stress may also exacerbate some respiratory conditions. Components of a client's psychosocial assessment that impact oxygenation include lifestyle, environmental concerns, smoking, substance abuse, nutrition and exercise, anxiety, and the family.

Lifestyle focuses on the personal habits of the client as they affect health. Specific to the assessment of oxygenation includes physical exercise or activity. Activity increases the rate and depth of respirations and consequently the oxygen supply to the body. Sedentary individuals are less able to respond to respiratory stressors because they lack the alveolar expansion and deep-breathing patterns seen in physically active individuals.

Environmental conditions such as heat, cold, altitude, and pollution all impact oxygenation. Persons at higher altitudes have increased respiratory rates and depths because of the lower atmospheric partial pressure of oxygen. Heat causes vasodilation, which increases oxygen demands. The increased oxygen demand results in an increased heart rate and respiratory rate to meet the demands of the body. Conversely, cold causes vasoconstriction, which decreases oxygen demand. This decrease in the demand for oxygen re-

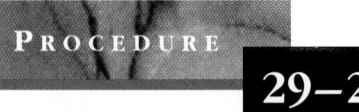

PROCEDURE

29–2

PREPARATION FOR THORACENTESIS

Thoracentesis is the removal of fluid through a needle or instilling chemotherapeutic medications into the pleural space.

Complications include hemothorax, pneumothorax, air embolism and subcutaneous emphysema.

Informed consent is required before the procedure begins.

Equipment:

Thoracentesis tray

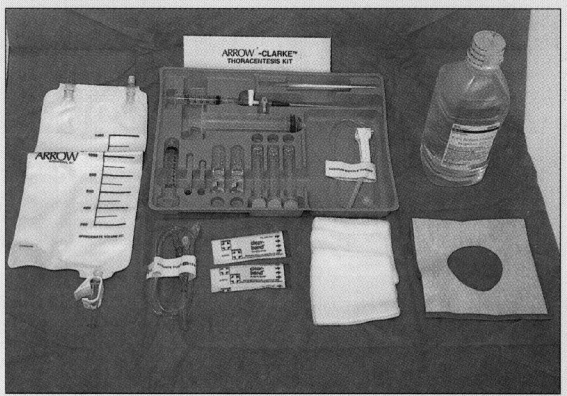

Action	Rationale
1. Wash hands before bringing equipment to bedside.	1. Reduces the transmission of microorganisms.
2. Position the client sitting on the side of the bed with arms resting on a table.	2. This is the optimal position for access to the area by the physician.
3. Obtain vital signs; auscultate lung fields.	3. Establishes a baseline before the procedure begins.
4. Assist physician as needed.	4. Provides client reassurance and continued monitoring of client's tolerance of procedure.
5. Label specimens and send to lab promptly.	5. Aids in obtaining accurate results.
6. Reassess vital signs; auscultate lung fields.	6. Identifies client's response to the procedure.
7. Continue to assess for sudden shortness of breath, tachycardia, tachypnea, deviated trachea.	7. Signs of pneumothorax, tension pneumothorax, air embolism.
8. Reposition client.	8. Provides comfort.

sults in a slower heart rate and respiratory rate. Pollution introduces contaminants and irritants into the respiratory system. Irritants can initiate an inflammatory process, which can interfere with oxygenation. The inflammatory process can result in bronchoconstriction. Individuals with a prior history of lung disease, such as asthma or bronchitis, could experience an exacerbation of the illness when exposed to pollutants. People living in crowded conditions such as inner-city housing have increased shared airspaces and are at increased risk for contracting communicable diseases that affect oxygenation. Communicable diseases include the common cold, influenza, and tuberculosis.

Smoking is a known irritant and carcinogen of the lung. Smoking initiates an inflammatory process that interferes with oxygen ventilation and perfusion. Risk of lung cancer increases with the amount and number of years smoked. Inhaled nicotine causes vasoconstriction of blood vessels and paralyzes the ciliary bodies, which assist with the movement of lung secretions. As a result, there are decreased surface areas and increased mucus accumulation. Additionally, the carbon monoxide in cigarette smoke combines with hemoglobin more readily than does oxygen and decreases the amount of circulating oxygen that is available to the body's tissues.

Cigarette smoking is a dangerous habit and remains the primary cause of preventable death and morbidity in the United States. Low-birth-weight infants and perinatal mortality have been linked to maternal smoking during pregnancy. Young children ex-

CLOSED CHEST DRAINAGE

Chest tubes are designed to drain fluid, blood, or air from the pleural cavity. They reestablish the negative pressure that facilitates reexpansion of the lungs. Chest tubes are inserted during surgery or emergently after chest trauma. After the chest tube is inserted, it is sutured to the skin and taped securely.

Informed consent should be obtained unless the tube is inserted in an emergency life-saving situation.

Equipment:

One-, two-, or three-bottle
system or commercial
three-chamber drainage
system
Sterile water
Chest tube insertion tray
Chest tube size as requested
(adult: 16 to 24 gauge to
drain air, 28 to 36 gauge to
drain liquid)
Tape

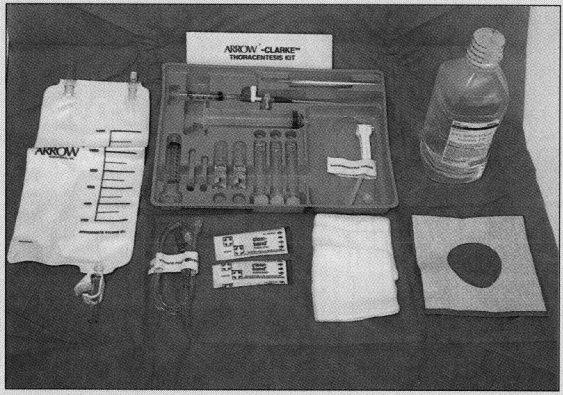

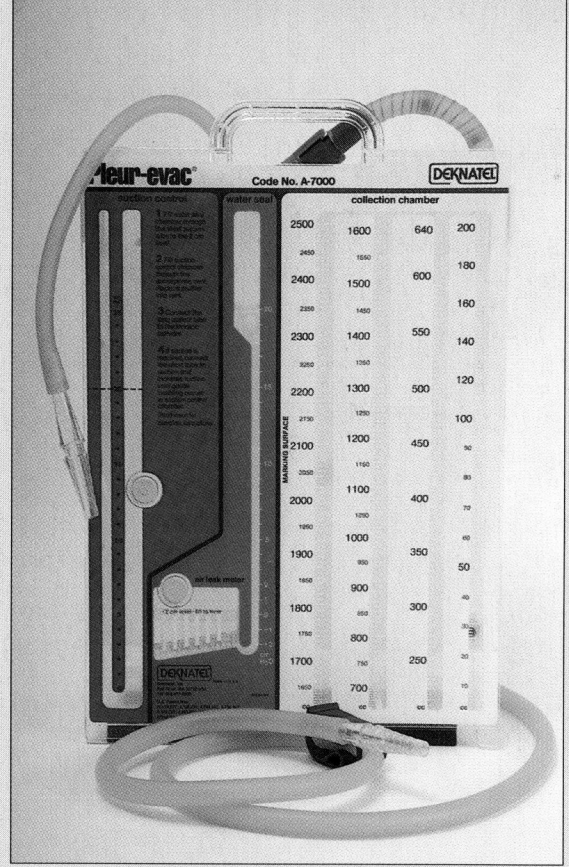

Step 6.

Continued

PROCEDURE

29–3

CLOSED CHEST DRAINAGE
(Continued)

Action	Rationale
1. Assess vital signs and respiratory rate, rhythm, and depth; auscultate lung fields.	**1.** Establishes a baseline.
2. Set up drainage system as ordered by physician.	

One Bottle (Water Seal/Drainage)

Action	Rationale
a. Maintain sterility and unwrap bottle and tubing.	**a.** All chest tube systems must be kept sterile.
b. With sterile water, fill bottle to 2 cm level. Rod should be submerged 2 cm. Never cover air vent with water.	**b.** Depth of rod determines degree of negative pressure.
c. Attach submerged tube to client's chest tube.	**c.** Provides drainage port.
d. Tape all connectors securely.	**d.** Avoids connectors becoming disconnected.
e. Observe for fluctuations in the water seal bottle.	**e.** Determines that drainage is occurring.

Two Bottle

Action	Rationale
a. Open both bottles with sterile technique. Prepare second bottle in the same manner as the first.	**a.** Prevents contamination.
b. The bottle closest to the client is for collection of drainage.	**b.** Identification prevents error.
c. The second bottle is the water seal and may be connected to suction if ordered.	**c.** Preparation allows suction to be instituted quickly.
d. Connect the two bottles by rubber tubing.	**d.** Creates closed connection.
e. Securely tape all connections.	**e.** Prevents leakage.
f. Observe for fluctuations and record amount/characteristics of drainage.	**f.** Determines that drainage is occurring and provides data for comparison.

Three Bottle

Action	Rationale
a. Open all three bottles with sterile technique. Prepare first two bottles as described in the two-bottle setup.	**a.** Prevents contamination.
b. The third bottle is used as a suction control bottle. The third bottle has a long tube with the end submerged in sterile water. The depth of water determines the amount of suction. For example, if 20 mm Hg suction is ordered, the water level will be 20 cm.	**b.** Allows changes as needed to control amount of suction.
c. Connect the third bottle to a suction control source.	**c.** System is ready for suctioning.

Care of Chest Tube Systems

Action	Rationale
3. Inspect all tubing for leaks and kinks.	**3.** Identifies problems quickly.
4. Keep chest tubes below level of chest.	**4.** Prevents drainage from flowing back into pleural space.
5. In the event of breakage or disconnection, two clamps should be kept at the bedside.	**5.** If tubing is clamped, it is only temporary until disconnection is corrected.

Continued

PROCEDURE

29–3

CLOSED CHEST DRAINAGE
(Continued)

6. Monitor amount, color, and consistency of drainage.

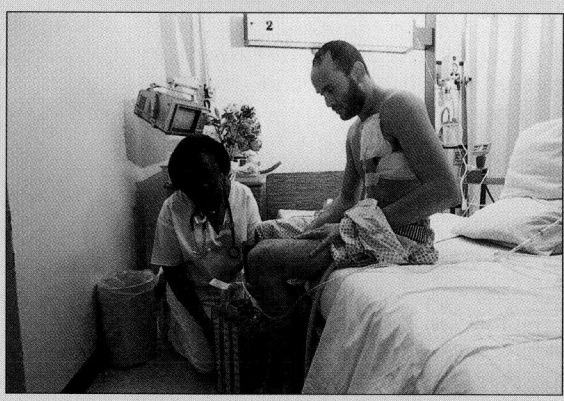

6. Notify physician if amount of drainage increases significantly.

7. Water seal level should rise with inhalation and fall with exhalation.

7. If the client is on mechanical ventilation, this will be opposite, owing to positive pressure from the ventilator.

8. If the chest tube is to suction, the water seal chamber will bubble continuously.

8. Visual confirmation of suction.

9. If there is no suction, detection of a pleural air leak is noted if the water seal chamber bubbles on exhalation.

9. Visual confirmation of problem.

Removal of Chest Tubes

10. Place the client in semi-Fowler position or on his or her side.

10. Reduces drainage.

11. Disconnect suction, if on.

11. Reduces drainage.

12. Chest tube sutures will be clipped by physician.

12. Removal of chest tubes is performed by physician.

13. Physician instructs the client to take a deep breath and hold it.

13. Stabilizes chest cavity.

14. Chest tubes are quickly removed.

14. Lessens discomfort.

15. Petroleum gauze dressing is applied over the wounds and taped securely.

15. Protects the wound and promotes healing.

16. Continue to assess for drainage from dressing, sudden chest pain, or shortness of breath.

16. Identifies complications at outset.

---

posed to environmental tobacco smoke are at risk for developing respiratory complications (American Thoracic Society, 1996).

Research indicates that individuals exposed to sidestream or secondhand smoke from cigarettes are also at risk for developing lung cancer and cardiovascular disease. Exposure to secondhand smoke reduces the blood's ability to deliver oxygen to the heart and compromises the myocardium's ability to use oxygen. Nonsmokers exposed to secondhand smoke in everyday life exhibit an increased risk of both fatal and nonfatal cardiac events (Glantz, & Parmley, 1995).

Substance abuse of narcotics such as morphine sulfate, heroin, cocaine, and meperidine hydrochloride depresses the respiratory center, which results in a decreased respiratory rate and depth. Smoking marijuana affects oxygenation in the same manner as cigarette smoking.

Allergens in food may also affect respiratory function. For example, dairy products tend to overstimulate mucus production. Poor nutritional status affects respiratory healing after an insult or injury. Obesity increases the incidence of dyspnea because of the additional weight and pressure on the diaphragm. As stated earlier, physically active individuals have a greater depth and rate of respiration than sedentary individuals.

Anxiety and decreased oxygenation tend to become a cyclical process. Lack of oxygenation increases the respiratory rate and depth and therefore increases the body's demand for oxygen. Clients who have an underlying respiratory problem associate difficulty breathing with the possibility of death, which increases anxiety further. Therefore, mechanisms to reduce the individual's anxiety, in addition to improving oxygenation, must be considered for the effective treatment of respiratory abnormalities.

Family and social factors also have an impact on oxygenation. An individual with a supportive family and friends tends to display more positive coping mechanisms when dealing with illness. Positive coping behaviors generally increase the individual's ability to recover and the willingness to change negative lifestyle factors that may be interfering with oxygenation.

Developmental Assessment

Age, developmental level, and the physiological changes of aging all have unique effects on oxygenation.

Premature infants are at increased risk for hyaline membrane disease, which results from a deficiency in surfactant production. Surfactant is normally produced in the latter stage of fetal development. Therefore, premature infants with immature lung development may have absent or insufficient amounts of surfactant. An inadequate amount of surfactant production causes unequal inflation of alveoli on inspiration and collapse of alveoli on end expiration. Therefore, the neonate is unable to maintain lung expansion, which results in atelectasis (Wong, 1993).

Infants and toddlers are at risk for increased upper respiratory infections because of their immature immune systems and exposure to other children who have immature immune systems. Common upper respiratory infections include tonsillitis, epiglottitis, influenza, pharyngitis, rhinorrhea, and the common cold. Infants are at risk for foreign body obstruction owing to their small tracheas and immature muscle control (Wong, 1993).

School-age children are commonly at risk for respiratory infections if they have a prior history of respiratory illness such as asthma or bronchitis. School-age children may begin risk-taking behaviors such as smoking and inhaling other substances, which can directly affect oxygenation (Wong, 1993).

Adolescents have increased risk of respiratory illnesses and diseases related to factors such as inadequate nutrition, poor dietary practices, cigarette smoking, and experimentation with other drugs or substances. Positive or negative peer pressure influences the adolescent's health promotion activities. The decision to smoke cigarettes or engage in other substance abuse is strongly influenced by peers.

Young and middle adults have risk factors related to lifestyle behaviors that are developed earlier in life. High-risk lifestyle behaviors include a sedentary lifestyle, smoking, increased stress levels, poor coping strategies, and poor dietary and exercise patterns.

Older adults have a natural decrease in immunity secondary to the aging process. The elderly are at increased risk for respiratory infections from such factors as decreased mobility or other coexisting diseases. Other changes that occur within the respiratory system of the older adult include increased anteroposterior diameter (barrel chest), progressive kyphoscoliosis, decreased cough ability, and decreased elasticity of the lung tissues.

Nursing Diagnosis

Nursing diagnoses are identified from the interpretation of data obtained through the nursing process. The nurse conducts the history, performs a physical examination, considers all related factors affecting oxygenation, and then formulates a diagnosis. The nursing diagnosis serves as the blueprint or plan of action that the nurse will implement to improve or maintain the oxygenation status of the client. Possible nursing diagnoses that may be related to oxygenation are listed in the accompanying box. The first three diagnoses listed are discussed in more detail.

Ineffective Airway Clearance

Ineffective airway clearance is a state in which an individual is unable to clear secretions or an obstruction from the respiratory tract in order to maintain airway patency. Focused assessment areas include a weak, ineffective cough with or without sputum; thick, tenacious sputum; rales; rhonchi; cyanosis; dyspnea; and a decreased lung expansion. Risk factors related to ineffective airway clearance include deceased energy and fatigue, tracheobronchial infection, percep-

NURSING DIAGNOSIS RELATED TO OXYGENATION

Ineffective airway clearance
Ineffective breathing pattern
Impaired gas exchange
Anxiety
Activity intolerance
Fatigue
Fear
Powerlessness
Sleep pattern disturbance
Social isolation
Risk for infection
Inability to sustain spontaneous ventilation

tual/cognitive impairment, trauma, edema of the upper airway structures, and bronchospasm.

Ineffective Breathing Pattern

An ineffective breathing pattern is a state in which an individual's respiratory pattern does not enable adequate lung inflation or deflation. Focused assessment areas include an abnormal respiratory rate, depth, and pattern; dyspnea; shortness of breath; tachypnea; fremitus; cyanosis; nasal flaring; pursed-lip breathing; prolonged expiratory phase; use of accessory muscles; decreased chest expansion; and abnormal arterial blood gases. Risk factors related to an ineffective breathing pattern are neurological impairment, pain associated with breathing, musculoskeletal impairment, and fatigue.

Impaired Gas Exchange

Impaired gas exchange is a state in which the individual experiences a decreased passage of oxygen and/or carbon dioxide between the alveoli of the lungs and the vascular system. Focused assessment areas include confusion, somnolence, restlessness, irritability, hypercapnia, hypoxia, cyanosis, diaphoresis, orthopnea, and decreased hemoglobin saturation. Risk factors related to an impaired gas exchange are a ventilation-perfusion imbalance; altered oxygen supply; altered blood flow; alveolar-capillary membrane changes, leading to a decrease in or loss of lung surface for gas diffusion; and secretions or fluid in alveoli, decreasing the gas diffusion.

Planning

Planning is the interim process between formulating a nursing diagnosis and implementing interventions. Based on the assessment and the collection of data, priorities of care are set. Planning involves deciding how to intervene and which processes need to be restored. Nurses employ various strategies to improve oxygenation at different levels. Each nursing care plan is individualized based on the client's age and physiological, psychological, and emotional needs. The client and his or her family and/or significant other should participate in the formulation of the plan of care.

The expected outcomes for a client with oxygenation problems are:

- To maintain a patent airway
- To maintain adequate ventilation

SAMPLE NURSING CARE PLAN 29-1

THE CLIENT WITH ASTHMA

A 17-year-old girl with a lifelong history of asthma comes to the emergency room for "an asthma attack." Her respiratory rate is 38, and she has musical inspiratory and expiratory wheezes throughout all lung fields. She is using her accessory muscles for respiration. Her mother states that she lost her inhaler the day before and they have not gotten a replacement.

Nursing Diagnosis: Ineffective breathing pattern related to decreased lung expansion and anxiety.

Expected Outcome: The breathing pattern will be effective and the airways will remain patent.

Action	Rationale
1. Observe for a change in the respiratory rate and depth.	1. Determines the adequacy of breathing.
2. Observe for nasal flaring, pursed-lip breathing, and use of accessory muscles.	2. Identifies increased work of breathing.
3. Observe for a change in level of consciousness.	3. May indicate hypoxia.
4. Monitor arterial blood gases.	4. Identifies oxygenation status as well as acid-base balance.
5. Measure the lung capacity, specifically tidal volume.	5. Demonstrates volume of air being moved in and out of the lungs.
6. Administer oxygen as ordered.	6. Provides additional oxygen for gas exchange and decreases the work of breathing.
7. Position the client in a high-Fowler position.	7. Optimizes diaphragmatic contraction.
8. Administer bronchodilators as ordered.	8. Dilates the bronchi, which increases the airway diameter.
9. Encourage the use of relaxation techniques.	9. Relieves anxiety and reduces the work of breathing.

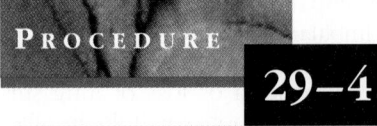

PROCEDURE

29–4

HEIMLICH MANEUVER

The Heimlich maneuver is recommended for removing foreign body airway obstruction. Air forced from the lungs creates an artificial cough intended to expel a foreign body from the trachea. It may be necessary to repeat the abdominal thrusts several times.

If the victim exhibits good air exchange and has a forceful cough, do not interfere. Poor air exchange is characterized by a weak, ineffective cough, high-pitched inhalations, and possibly cyanosis. The individual may be unable to speak, breathe, or cough. The individual may hold the neck with the hands—this is the universal distress signal when choking.

Action	Rationale
Victim Sitting or Standing: Conscious	
1. Verify that the victim cannot breathe; look for universal signal. Ask: "Are you choking?"	1. Verifies that the victim needs assistance.
2. Stand behind the victim.	2. Allows correct application of maneuver.
3. Make a fist with one hand.	3. Permits exertion of focused pressure.
4. Place thumb of fist against abdomen, slightly above navel and well below xiphoid process.	4. Avoids damage to internal organs.
5. Grasp fist with other hand and press fist into abdomen with a quick upward thrust.	5. The intention is to remove the object.
6. Repeat until the object is expelled or the victim becomes unconscious.	6. Each thrust should be separate and distinct.
7. If the victim becomes unconscious, lay him or her in the supine position on the floor.	7. Allows continuation of maneuver.
Victim Lying Down: Conscious	
1. Kneel astride the victim's thighs.	1. Places rescuer in natural midabdominal position.
2. Place heel of one hand against abdomen above navel and well below xiphoid process.	2. Avoids damage to internal organs.
3. Place second hand directly on top of first hand.	3. Increases thrust.
4. Press abdomen with quick upward thrusts.	4. Attempts to dislodge object.
Victim Becomes Unconscious	
1. Open mouth and perform finger sweep.	1. Do finger sweep only if the victim is unconscious; never in a seizure victim.
2. Perform Heimlich maneuver up to five times.	2. Repetitive motion may dislodge object.
3. Open mouth and perform finger sweep.	3. Object may have been forced up into oropharynx, where it can be removed.
4. Attempt to ventilate.	4. Use the head tilt–chin lift method.
5. If unable to ventilate, reposition and try again.	5. Ensures adequate positioning.
6. Repeat Heimlich, finger sweep, and ventilation attempts.	6. Continue until object is removed or ventilations are successful.
7. If victim resumes breathing, place in recovery position.	7. Airway is more likely to remain open.

- To maintain tissue perfusion and cellular oxygenation
- To reduce anxiety/fear
- To maintain an effective breathing pattern without fatigue or dyspnea

See the Nursing Care Plan 29–1 for a client with asthma.

Implementation

Patent Airway

Maintaining a patent airway is essential. Most clients do not have difficulty maintaining a patent airway and breathing spontaneously. However, upper airway

Text continued on page 863

PROCEDURE

29–5

ADULT CARDIOPULMONARY
RESUSCITATION

If the person is discovered pulseless and apneic, follow institutional policy for notifying personnel. If the victim is found pulseless and apneic in the community, activate the Emergency Medical System (EMS) via 911 if available. Remember: Airway, Breathing, Circulation.

Action	Rationale

One Rescuer

1. Determine unresponsiveness.
2. Place victim in a supine position.
3. Open the airway with the heal tilt–chin lift maneuver.
4. Place ear on mouth and nose and look, listen, and feel for respirations.
5. If the person is breathing but unconscious, place him or her in the rescue position.
6. If the victim is not breathing, obtain a barrier device. Note: Pocket masks are strongly encouraged.
7. Place mask or shield over mouth and nose and deliver two breaths.
8. If the victim has a pulse, deliver 10 to 12 breaths/minute. Rescue breathing should continue until the person spontaneously breathes or help arrives.
9. Check for pulse at carotid artery for 5 to 10 seconds.
10. If no pulse, begin chest compressions.
11. Place heel of one hand over lower half of sternum, and place other hand on top. Lace fingers together.

1. Ensures need for CPR.
2. Airway management and breathing are easier to achieve.
3. If there is possibility of neck injury, use the jaw-thrust maneuver.
4. This evaluation should take 3 to 5 seconds.
5. Rescue position maintains patent airway.
6. Observe universal precautions.
7. Masks prevent spread of microorganisms.
8. Maintain oxygenation of victim.
9. Pulse may be slow, irregular, very weak, or rapid.
10. Chest compressions facilitate circulation.
11. Rescuer should be kneeling next to the victim with his or her knee slightly below the victim's shoulder.

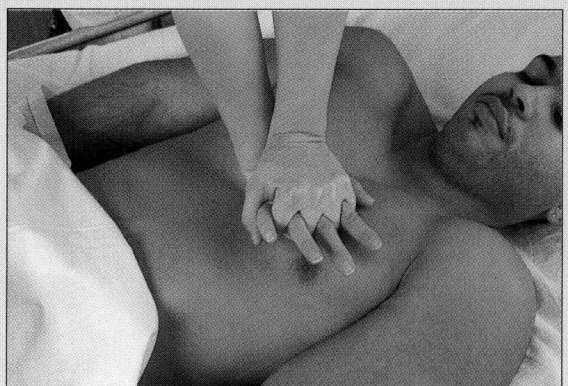

Step 11.

12. Straighten arms and lock elbows. Keep shoulders directly over hands.
13. Compress chest 1½ to 2 inches. Perform 15 chest compressions at a rate of 80 to 100/minute.

12. Maintains effective position, avoids damaging internal organs.
13. Delivers compressions at optimal depth and rate.

Continued

PROCEDURE

29–5

ADULT CARDIOPULMONARY RESUSCITATION
(Continued)

14. After the 15 compressions, deliver two slow rescue breaths. Perform four complete cycles of 15 compressions and two ventilations.

15. After four cycles, reassess. If the person is still pulseless and apneic, continue CPR. If pulse has returned but respirations have not, begin rescue breathing. If effective breathing and pulse have returned, place the victim in the recovery position.

Two Rescuers

1. Two-rescuer CPR is preferable. One rescuer performs chest compressions while the other performs rescue breathing.

2. The compression-ventilation cycle is 5:1. After five chest compressions, one breath is delivered.

3. When the rescuer performing chest compression becomes fatigued, the rescuers should change positions. Note: An Ambu bag may be used at any time.

14. Ensures adequate compression and ventilation.

15. Continued assessment of victim is essential.

1. It is more effective and less fatiguing.

2. Ensures optimal circulation and ventilation.

3. Allows rescue attempt to continue longer.

CHILD CARDIOPULMONARY RESUSCITATION

Hypoxemia and airway occlusion are the common causes of cardiopulmonary arrest in children. Establishment and maintenance of a patent airway are the most important components of resuscitation.

Action	Rationale
1. Establish unresponsiveness.	**1.** Determines need for CPR.
2. Open airway with head tilt–chin lift or jaw thrust technique.	**2.** Airway management and breathing are easier to achieve.
3. Look, listen, and feel for airflow. If spontaneously breathing, place in recovery position.	**3.** Maintains patent airway.
4. If the child is not breathing, form a mouth-to-mouth or mask seal and deliver two slow breaths.	**4.** Use of pocket mask or BVM is recommended.
5. Check for pulse at carotid artery if child is older than 1 year.	**5.** Peripheral pulse may be impossible to obtain.
6. If pulse is present, deliver rescue breathing at a rate of 20/minute.	**6.** Child's rate of respiration differs from adult's.
7. If no pulse is palpable, begin chest compression.	**7.** Chest compressions facilitate circulation.
8. Use one hand to maintain head position and the other hand for compressions.	**8.** Child requires less force of compression than adult.
9. Place heel of hand on lower half of sternum, avoiding the xiphoid process.	**9.** Avoids damage to internal organs.
10. Compression should be 1 to 1½ inches. Rate is 100/minute.	**10.** Adaptations for age are made.
11. Compression-ventilation cycle is 5:1.	**11.** Ensures optimal circulation and ventilation.
12. After 20 cycles, reassess the child. If pulse has returned, deliver rescue breathing. If child is still pulseless and apneic, continue CPR.	**12.** Continued assessment of victim is essential.

INFANT CARDIOPULMONARY RESUSCITATION
(Continued)

Action	Rationale
1. Establish unresponsiveness.	1. Determines need for CPR.
2. Open airway with head tilt–chin lift or jaw thrust technique.	2. Airway management and breathing are easier to achieve.
3. Look, listen, and feel for airflow.	3. If spontaneously breathing, place in recovery position.
4. If the infant is not breathing, form a mouth-to-mouth or mask seal and deliver two slow breaths.	4. Use of pocket mask or BVM is recommended. Deliver just enough air to make chest rise.
5. Check for pulse at brachial artery.	5. This point is easier to assess.
6. If pulse is present, deliver rescue breathing at a rate of 20/minute.	6. Adaptations made for age.
7. If no pulse is palpable, begin chest compression.	7. Chest compressions facilitate circulation.
8. Use one hand to maintain infant's head position.	8. Maintains airway so ventilations can be given without delay.

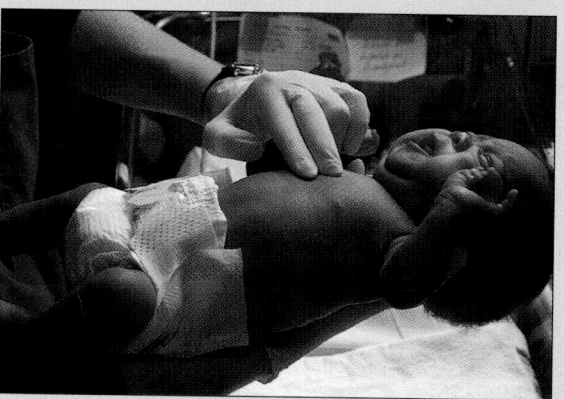

Step 8.

Action	Rationale
9. Place index finger just below level of the nipples. Place middle finger next to index finger. Avoid compression of xiphoid process.	9. Avoids damage to internal organs.
10. Compression should be 0.5 to 1.0 in. Rate is at least 100/minute.	10. Infant rates differ from those of adult or child.
11. Compression-ventilation cycle is 5:1.	11. Ensures optimal circulation and ventilation.
12. After 20 cycles, reassess the infant. If pulse has returned, deliver rescue breathing. If infant is still pulseless and apneic, continue CPR.	12. Continued assessment of victim is essential.

obstruction can result from foreign materials such as food, vomitus, or blood clots. An unconscious client in a supine position may have a blocked airway from the posterior displacement of the tongue.

Management of the client with a foreign body airway obstruction who is unable to cough effectively includes the use of subdiaphragmatic abdominal thrusts, or the Heimlich maneuver (see Procedure 29–4). Procedure 29–5 describes cardiopulmonary resuscitation for adults, children, and infants.

Positioning

Positioning of clients to facilitate optimal airway expansion is crucial. Clients experiencing dyspnea should be placed in a high-Fowler position. An un-

Text continued on page 867

PROCEDURE

29–6

INSERTION OF OROPHARYNGEAL AIRWAY

The oropharyngeal airway is a semicircular rigid device used to hold the tongue away from the posterior wall of the pharynx. It facilitates suctioning of the pharynx and prevents the client from biting and occluding an endotracheal tube. It is used only in unconscious clients because it may stimulate the gag reflex, leading to vomiting and laryngospasm in a conscious or semiconscious client.

Adult sizes are from 80 to 100 mm. Children's sizes are from 4 to 10 cm.

Equipment:

Appropriate size airway
Suction setup and equipment
Yankauer tip suction catheter

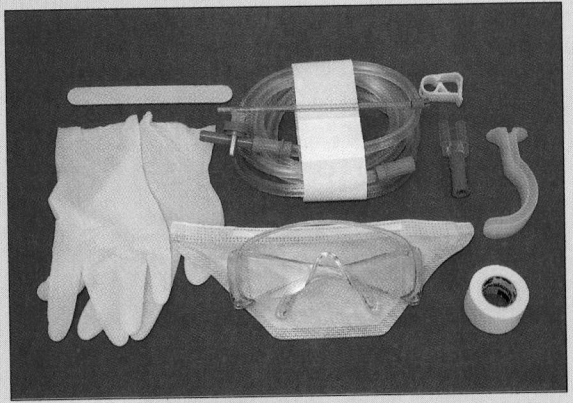

Action	**Rationale**
1. Wash hands.	1. Reduces the spread of microorganisms.
2. Select appropriate size airway.	2. An airway that is too long may press the epiglottis against the entrance of the larynx, producing complete airway obstruction.
3. Don gloves.	3. Follows safety guidelines.
4. Clear mouth and pharynx of secretions, blood, or vomitus using a Yankauer suction catheter.	4. Avoids aspiration.
5. Hold oropharyngeal airway curved upward and insert into mouth.	5. Avoids pushing the tongue posteriorly.

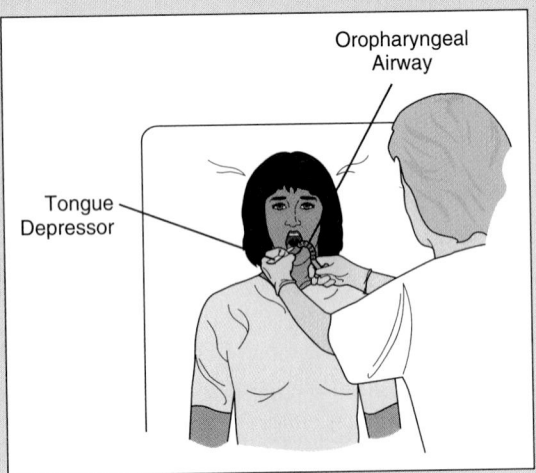

Oropharyngeal Airway

Tongue Depressor

INSERTION OF OROPHARYNGEAL AIRWAY
(Continued)

6. As airway approaches the posterior wall of the pharynx, rotate it 180° into proper position.

6. Avoids pushing tongue against posterior wall of oropharynx and occluding trachea.

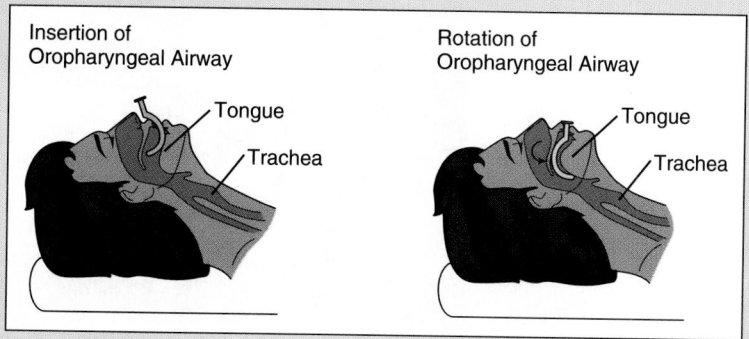

Insertion of Oropharyngeal Airway
— Tongue
— Trachea

Rotation of Oropharyngeal Airway
— Tongue
— Trachea

7. Maintain proper head position.

8. Secure oropharyngeal airway with tape.

7. Allows proper functioning of device.

8. Prevents airway from being dislodged.

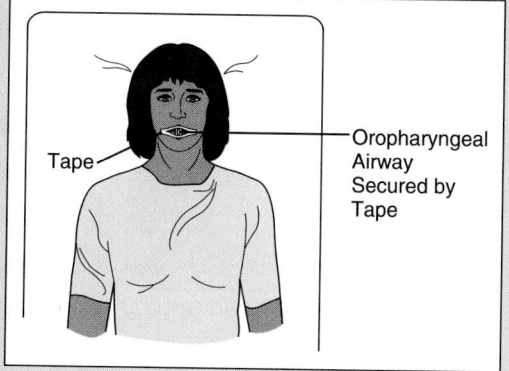

Tape —

— Oropharyngeal Airway Secured by Tape

9. Remove gloves and wash hands.

9. Reduces spread of microorganisms.

INSERTION OF NASOPHARYNGEAL AIRWAY

The nasopharyngeal airway is made of soft rubber or plastic. It is used when insertion of an oropharyngeal airway is technically difficult or impossible. It can be used in a semiconscious client who does not tolerate an oropharyngeal airway.

Adult sizes are from 6.0 internal diameter (i.d.) to 9.0 i.d.. Children's sizes are from 12 French to 36 French.

Continued

PROCEDURE

29–6

INSERTION OF NASOPHARYNGEAL AIRWAY
(Continued)

Equipment:

Appropriate size airway
Water-soluble lubricant
Suction setup and equipment
Yankauer suction catheter

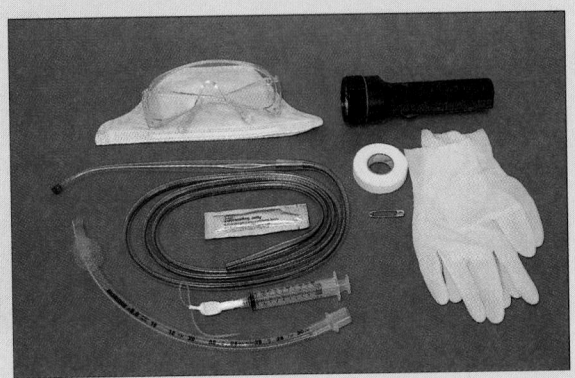

Action	Rationale
1. Wash hands.	1. Reduces the spread of microorganisms.
2. Select appropriate size nasopharyngeal airway.	2. If the tube is too long, it may enter the esophagus, causing gastric distention.
3. Don gloves.	3. Follows safety guidelines.
4. Clear mouth and pharynx of secretions, vomitus, or blood using a Yankauer suction catheter.	4. Prevents aspiration.
5. Lubricate end of airway with water-soluble lubricant.	5. Eases insertion and prevents injury to nasal mucosa.
6. Check nares for any deviation of septum and select nare that is patent. Gently insert the airway close to the septum along the floor of nostril into posterior pharynx behind the tongue.	6. Avoids trauma and eases insertion.

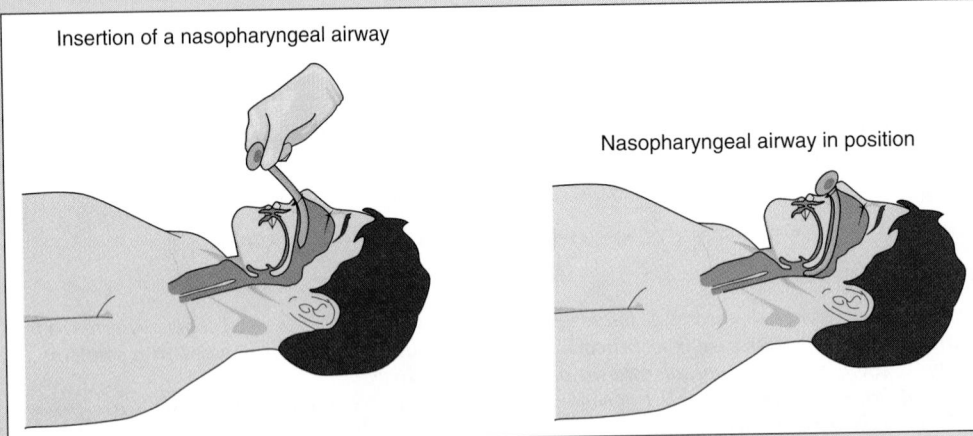

Insertion of a nasopharyngeal airway

Nasopharyngeal airway in position

7. Check for bleeding from insertion, and suction if needed.	7. Insertion may cause bleeding and possible aspiration of clots into the trachea.
8. Remove gloves and wash hands.	8. Reduces the spread of microorganisms.

conscious client who is spontaneously breathing and has a pulse should be placed in the recovery position (Chandra & Hazinski, 1994). The recovery position is a side-lying position that prevents the tongue from occluding the airway. If the client cannot be placed in a recovery position, an artificial airway, such as an oropharyngeal or nasopharyngeal airway, should be inserted (see Procedure 29–6).

Breathing Exercises

Effective breathing techniques improve ventilation and oxygenation by opening up the alveoli and preventing them from collapsing. Some clients who have had chest or abdominal surgery or have sustained chest trauma have a tendency to breathe in a shallow manner because of discomfort or pain induced by deep inhalation and exhalation. Other clients may have physiological problems that prevent them from breathing effectively, such as neuromuscular weakness of the respiratory muscles and diaphragm, a chronic debilitating disease, or chronic obstructive pulmonary disease. In these instances, clients have to be taught effective breathing techniques to ensure adequate ventilation and oxygenation and to prevent respiratory complications.

Pursed-lip breathing and diaphragmatic breathing are two techniques that are commonly taught. Clients who have chronic obstructive pulmonary disease should be taught how to use the abdominal muscles to overcome the resistance to airflow caused by narrowing of the airways. For abdominal breathing, instruct the client to lie on his or her back with the knees bent and abdominal muscles relaxed. If the client is unable to lie supine, the exercise can be performed in a sitting position. Instruct the client to use the abdominal muscles while inhaling through the nose. Breathing through the mouth causes the inhalation of gulps of air, which leads to more air trapping and difficult exhalation. Have client press his or her abdomen with both hands during this process to facilitate deep inhalation, then exhale slowly through pursed lips (whistle position), taking at least twice the time of inhalation. Pursed-lip exhalation helps create resistance to airflow, thus increasing bronchial pressure and minimizing collapse of the alveoli. With continued use of this exercise, it eventually becomes a normal breathing pattern for the client.

Deep breathing and coughing are indicated for postoperative clients who have undergone general anesthesia. Clients who have been immobilized or partially immobilized in bed benefit from this exercise. Deep breathing and coughing prevent atelectasis, which may lead to postoperative hypostatic pneumonia. Clients who have undergone abdominal or thoracic surgery should be taught how to splint. Splinting is a technique that stabilizes the incision when coughing, thereby decreasing pain. A pillow or folded blanket is placed on the abdomen or chest and is held tightly as the client deep-breathes and coughs. Often an incentive spirometer is used to help motivate the client to maximize lung inflation. The client assumes a comfortable sitting or lying position, follows the same technique as in abdominal and pursed-lip breathing, and is encouraged to cough two or more times during exhalation. This exercise has to be done at least hourly during waking hours and every 2 to 4 hours during the night.

Incentive Spirometer

An incentive spirometer is a device used to measure airflow during inhalation. There are two types available on the market: flow oriented and volume oriented. The flow-oriented spirometer is a clear plastic disposable device with a colored ball or disc that moves as the client inhales. The client is encouraged to maximally inhale and sustain it as long as possible. Motivation is provided by the height achieved by the ball or disc and the length of time it is kept elevated. The volume-oriented spirometer measures the specific volume of air inhaled as indicated by the rise of the cylinder.

The effectiveness of the incentive spirometer lies in the client's ability to use the device correctly. Provide adequate client teaching, supervised follow-up, and return demonstrations to ensure that the client knows the correct technique. In addition, remind the client to use the device on a routine basis, such as every 2 hours, to maximize its effectiveness. Incorporating the use of the spirometer into the scheduled daily nursing activities compels the client to adhere to its regular use. Encouraging the client to keep track of his or her progress motivates continued compliance. Provide positive reinforcements to increase success in the use of the spirometer. Procedure 29–7 details the use of the incentive spirometer.

Chest Physiotherapy

Chest physiotherapy consists of chest percussion and vibration. These techniques are used to dislodge and mobilize secretions from small, distal airways to larger, proximal airways, where the secretions can be expelled by coughing or suctioning. In conjunction with postural drainage, chest percussion is effective in removing secretions. It is recommended that chest percussion and vibration be done early in the morning before breakfast, because this is when there are large amounts of secretions. The procedure should never be done immediately after a meal. Chest percussion and postural drainage are indicated for conditions such as cystic fibrosis, bronchiectasis, lobar atelectasis, and retained secretions. These techniques are contraindicated in clients who are unable to tolerate the various position changes and in conditions in which the physiological status is adversely affected by position changes. Examples of contraindications for chest phys-

PROCEDURE

29–7

INCENTIVE SPIROMETRY

Incentive spirometry is used postoperatively to encourage deep breathing. It does not replace other coughing and deep-breathing exercises.

Equipment:

Commercial incentive
  spirometer

Action	**Rationale**
1. Wash hands.	1. Reduces the spread of microorganisms.
2. Assist the client to a seated or semi-Fowler position.	2. Encourages maximum lung expansion.
3. Instruct the client to seal his or her mouth around the mouthpiece and to inhale through the mouth similar to using a straw.	3. Ensures correct functioning.

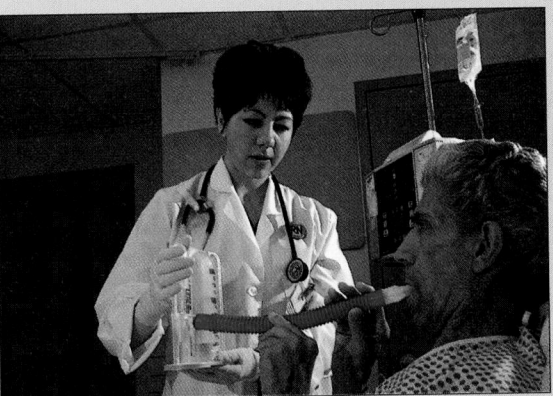

Step 3.

4. Encourage a deep ventilatory effort.	4. Allows a more successful use of the spirometer.
5. Ask the client to hold a deep breath for a few seconds before exhaling.	5. Helps prevent pulmonary complications.
6. Instruct the client to use the device every 3 to 4 hours or as ordered.	6. Continuous use helps prevent postoperative pulmonary complications.

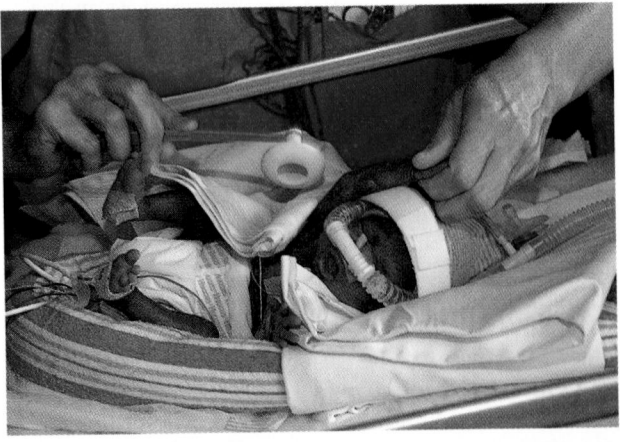

❥ **Figure 29–9**
A small cup is used instead of a cupped hand to percuss infants and small children in chest physiotherapy.

iotherapy include increased intracranial pressure, acute myocardial infarction, acute chest trauma, lung abscess, bronchopulmonary fistula, hemorrhage, eye surgery, and gastric reflux.

Chest percussion is the application of pressure over the affected area of the lung to aid in moving secretions. This is done by lightly striking the chest wall with a cupped hands. With infants and small children, a small cup such as a medication cup may be used to percuss the chest wall (Fig. 29–9).

Chest vibration is the application of vibratory movements over the affected area of the lung. This increases the velocity of air movement over the affected area and helps loosen secretions. Position both hands, one on top of the other, over the affected lung segment. Instruct the client to take a deep breath, and during expiration, create vibratory movements

Text continued on page 871

CHEST PHYSIOTHERAPY

Chest physiotherapy includes percussion, vibration, coughing, and deep breathing. It may be used in conjunction with postural drainage. It is an effective technique to loosen and move secretions into large airways to facilitate removal.

Do not perform chest physiotherapy immediately after the client has had a meal.

Action	Rationale
1. Wash hands.	1. Reduces the spread of microorganisms.
2. Explain the procedure to the client and/or family.	2. Reduces anxiety and gains the client's cooperation.
3. Place the client in a position so that the affected lobe is up. (See illustrations of positions.)	3. Promotes drainage.
4. Place the hands in a cupped position. Gently strike the chest wall with the cupped hands, alternating left and right.	4. Loosens secretions.
5. To perform vibration, place both hands over the affected lung segment and have the client take a deep breath. During expiration, gently vibrate the hands over the chest wall.	5. Increases velocity of air and helps loosen secretions.
6. Ask the client to cough at the end of expiration.	6. Helps expel loosened secretions.
7. If the client is unable to cough, suction out secretions.	7. Removes loosened secretions.

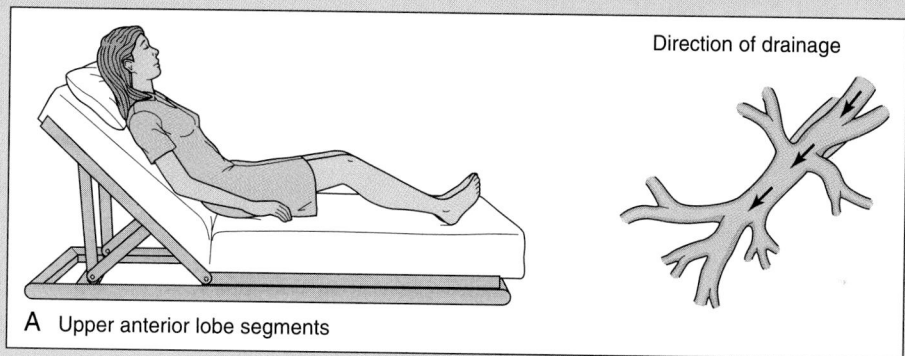

Direction of drainage

A Upper anterior lobe segments

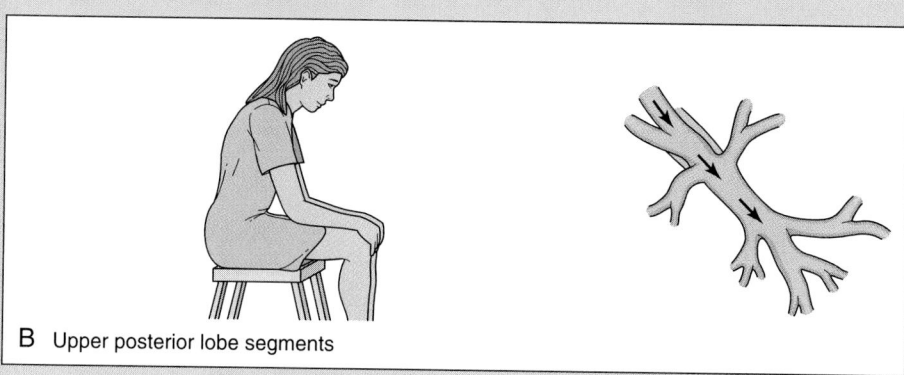

B Upper posterior lobe segments

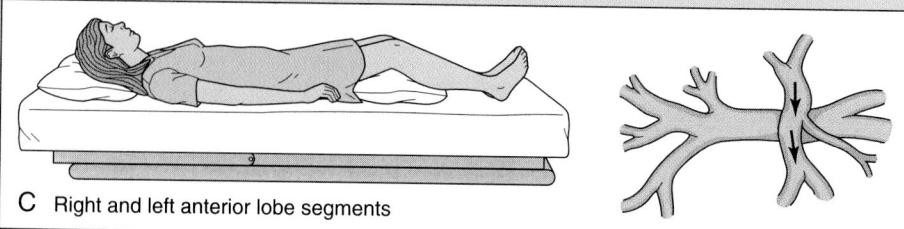

C Right and left anterior lobe segments

Continued

CHEST PHYSIOTHERAPY
(Continued)

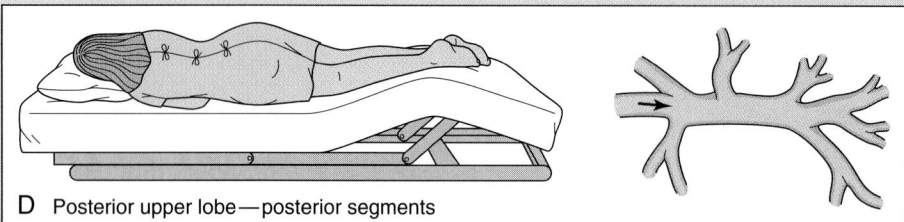

D Posterior upper lobe—posterior segments

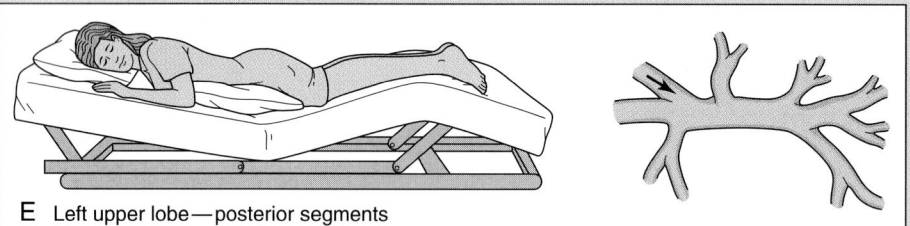

E Left upper lobe—posterior segments

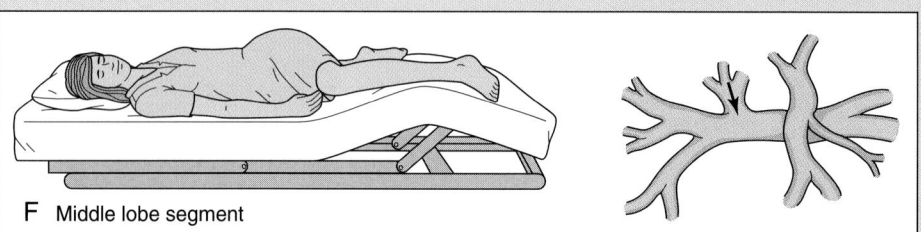

F Middle lobe segment

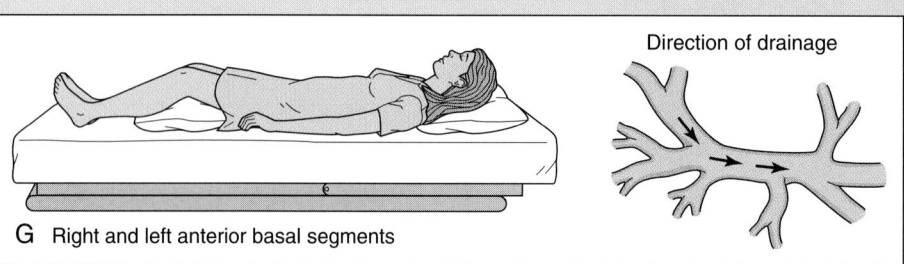

Direction of drainage

G Right and left anterior basal segments

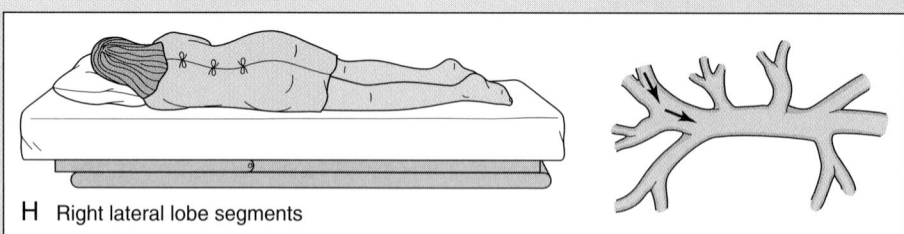

H Right lateral lobe segments

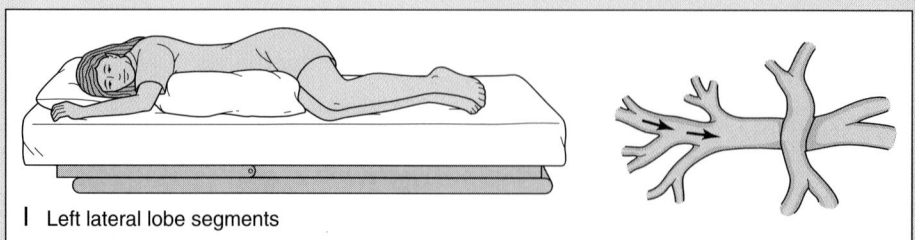

I Left lateral lobe segments

CHEST PHYSIOTHERAPY
(Continued)

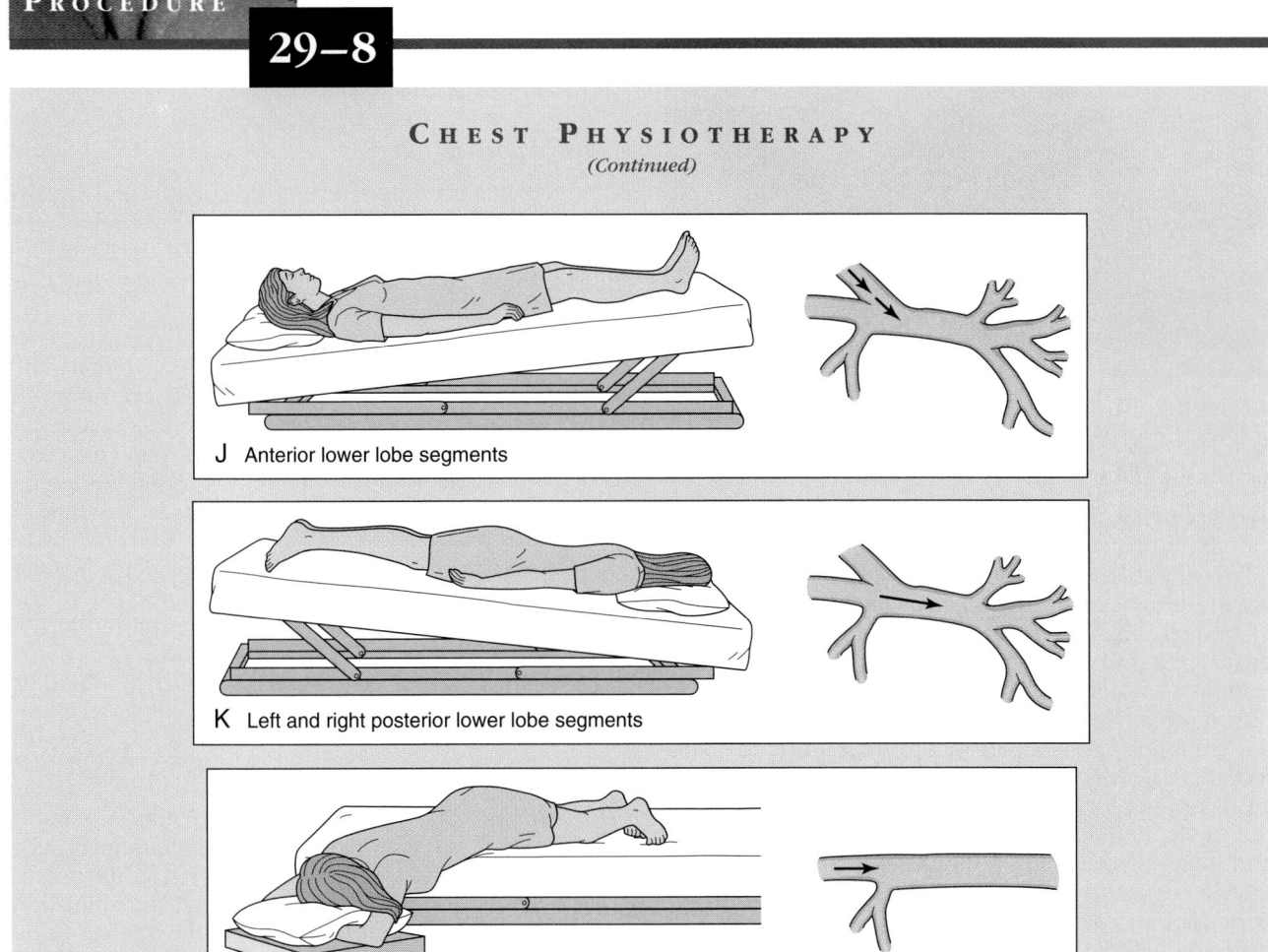

J   Anterior lower lobe segments

K   Left and right posterior lower lobe segments

L   Bronchi and trachea

with the hands over the chest wall. If the client is able, he or she should cough at the end of expiration. If the client is unable to cough or has a weak cough, the secretions are suctioned out mechanically.

Postural drainage is used in conjunction with percussion and vibration coughing and deep breathing. These interventions effectively loosen and move secretions into the large airways, where they can be coughed up or suctioned out. Postural drainage is indicated for clients with pneumonia, cystic fibrosis, or an ineffective cough owing to neuromuscular conditions such as quadriplegia, myasthenia gravis, and Guillain-Barré syndrome. Postural drainage is contraindicated in clients with cyanosis or dyspnea caused by chest physiotherapy, those with prolonged bleeding and clotting times, extremely obese clients, and those predisposed to pathological fractures.

In order to perform postural drainage, the client is placed in specific controlled positions that facilitate drainage of secretions from particular lung segments.

The client should remain in each position for at least 5 minutes. Procedure 29–8 identifies the 12 positions and which areas of the lungs are drained and details the method for performing chest physiotherapy with postural drainage.

Respiratory Medications

Respiratory medications are used in many different forms, including oral drugs, intravenous drugs, lozenges, and nebulized inhalers (Fig. 29–10). Some of these medications are available over the counter; others are available only by prescription.

Bronchodilators

Bronchodilators include sympathomimetics, xanthine derivatives, and muscarinic antagonists. Sympathomimetic drugs are further classified as nonselective adrenergic, nonselective β-adrenergic, and selective β_2-adrenergic drugs. Epinephrine, epinephrine bitartrate inhalation, racepinephrine inhalation solution,

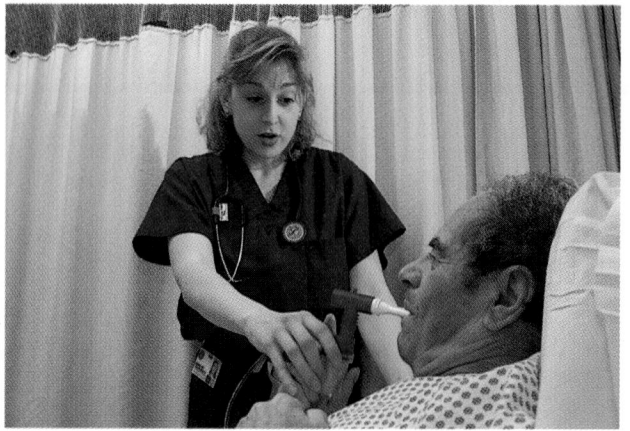

❧ **Figure 29–10**
Nurse teaching a client how to use a hand-held nebulizer.

and ephedrine are examples of nonselective adrenergic agents that exert their effect on the blood vessels, heart, and bronchial smooth muscles. These medications are indicated for the acute and temporary relief of bronchial asthma and reversible bronchospasm. Exercise extreme caution when administering these medications to clients with hypertension, diabetes, seizure history, advanced age, or prostatic hypertrophy.

Nonselective beta-adrenergic drugs exert their effect primarily on the heart and bronchial smooth muscle. Isoproterenol is an example and is indicated for the acute and temporary relief of bronchial asthma and reversible bronchospasm. When administering this inhalation medication, use caution in clients with hypertension, coronary artery disease, advanced age, and hyperthyroidism.

Selective beta-2-adrenergic drugs include albuterol, bitolterol, isoetharine inhalation, metaproterenol sulfate, and tributaline sulfate. These medications exert their effects primarily on bronchial smooth muscle, with minimal cardiac stimulation. These drugs are also used for acute and temporary relief of bronchial asthma, reversible bronchospasm, and prevention of bronchospasm. Precautions when using these medications are the same as for the nonselective beta-adrenergic medications.

The xanthine derivatives include theophylline, aminophylline, and oxtriphylline. These medications work in two ways. The primary action is relaxation of bronchial and smooth muscles (bronchodilation and vasodilation). In addition, these medications inhibit the release of bronchoconstricting substances such as histamine. The xanthine derivatives are prescribed for the relief or prevention of bronchial asthma and reversible bronchospasm. Caution should be exercised when administering these medications to clients with myocardial infarction, angina, severe hypoxia, hypertension, and congestive heart failure.

Muscarinic antagonists block the contraction of airway smooth muscles and the mucus secretion that results from parasympathetic stimulation. Ipratropium bromide is an example of a muscarinic antagonist.

This medication is used for bronchospasm associated with chronic obstructive pulmonary disease. Muscarinic antagonists should be used cautiously in clients with prostatic hypertrophy, bladder neck obstruction, or narrow-angle glaucoma.

Mucokinetic Drugs

Mucokinetic drugs include mucolytics and expectorants. These medications foster the removal of excessive respiratory tract secretions. To facilitate removal, the secretions are thinned and ciliary action is promoted.

Acetylcysteine is a mucolytic drug that reduces the thickness and stickiness of pulmonary secretions. By reducing the viscosity, secretions can be removed more effectively by coughing, postural drainage, or suctioning. The amount of secretions may increase, and if the client is unable to remove secretions with coughing, suctioning will be necessary to maintain a patent airway.

Expectorants liquefy and loosen mucus, soothe bronchial mucosa, and increase cough production. Examples of expectorants include guaifenesin, terpin hydrate, ipecac syrup, and potassium iodide. Use of expectorants is based on traditional practice; there is little evidence of their efficacy.

Corticosteroids

Corticosteroids have been used for many years to treat asthma and chronic obstructive pulmonary disease, even though the method of action is unknown. These medications decrease airway inflammation when administered parenterally or in the aerosol form. The dose of corticosteroids is slowly reduced over time and never abruptly discontinued.

Systemic corticosteroids include prednisone and methylprednisolone. These medications are indicated for bronchial asthma, status asthmaticus, and aspiration pneumonitis. Administer these medications cautiously in clients with peptic ulcer, heart disease, hypertension with congestive heart failure, diabetes, and glaucoma.

Beclomethasone, dexamethasone, flunisolide, and triamcinolone are aerosol corticosteroids. These aerosol inhalers are used for the control of bronchial asthma in conjunction with bronchodilator therapy. These medications are used only to prevent bronchial asthma attacks and are not useful for controlling an acute attack.

Antitussives

Antitussives are indicated for symptomatic relief of coughing and are available in narcotic and nonnarcotic forms. The narcotic form contains codeine. Coughing is a normal physiological mechanism designed to clear the airway of secretions. Therefore, cough suppressants should not be used indiscriminately and are generally indicated for mechanical or chemical respiratory tract irritation. Codeine is a narcotic, and although the abuse potential is low, psychological and/or physical dependence can occur with prolonged use.

Nonnarcotic antitussives include benzonatate, dextromethorphan, dextromethorphan-benzocaine, and diphenhydramine. Some of these preparations are available over the counter and are indicated for the control of a nonproductive cough. They are contraindicated when the cough is accompanied by excessive secretions.

Antihistamines

Antihistamines do not prevent the release of histamine but rather competitively bind with the receptor sites, which antagonizes the effects of histamine release. Diphenhydramine, tripelennamine, chlorpheniramine, and promethazine are examples of antihistamines. These medications do not treat the underlying cause of histamine release but provide symptomatic relief. Antihistamines are indicated for allergic rhinitis, rhinorrhea, sneezing, conjunctivitis, and oropharyngeal irritation. These medications should be used cautiously in clients with prostatic hypertrophy, narrow-angle glaucoma, and bladder neck obstruction.

Antibiotics

Penicillin, nafcillin, cephalosporin, tetracycline, streptomycin, and other antibiotics are used to treat respiratory infections. Selection of the antibiotic is based on the infecting agent, identified by culture when possible. After the specimen for culture is obtained, the antibiotic treatment begins.

Vaccines

Vaccines available to prevent respiratory infections include the pneumococcal and influenza vaccines. The pneumococcal vaccine protects against 23 of the most prevalent pneumococcal types. Antipneumococcal antibodies are produced, which prevent pneumococcal disease. Older individuals and those with chronic illnesses should receive the pneumococcal vaccine. Any individual with a febrile respiratory illness should not receive the vaccine until the illness has subsided. This vaccine is administered only once.

The United States Health Service formulates the influenza vaccine annually. This vaccine contains antigens to various strains of influenza that are expected to be prevalent in the upcoming year. The influenza vaccine is indicated yearly for individuals at risk for influenza-related complications. Health care workers are also encouraged to receive the vaccine to avoid transmitting the infection to high-risk individuals. The vaccine should be withheld from individuals with febrile respiratory infections until the illness has subsided.

Inhalers deliver a fine mist or spray of medication that is inhaled into the lungs. There are several different types of inhalers available. Metered-dose or hand-held inhalers contain a prescribed medication that is inhaled through a mouth- or nosepiece. Clients must be taught how to use the metered-dose inhaler in order to achieve the full effects of the drug. The inhaler is shaken five times before use. The mouthpiece cover is removed, and the lips are placed tightly around the mouthpiece. The client should exhale fully before placing the inhaler in the mouth. While taking a deep breath in, the inhaler is depressed once. This is equal to one dose. Breath holding after inhalation may increase deposition in the lower airways. Wait at least 1 to 2 minutes between doses. Refer to Nursing Care Plan 29–1 for steps that might be taken with a client experiencing an ineffective breathing pattern.

Supplemental Oxygen

Additional oxygen may be required for some clients. Indications for supplemental oxygen include hypoxemia, heart failure, pulmonary tumors that occlude gas exchange spaces, and surgery. Oxygen should never be withheld from any client in an emergency situation, such as cardiopulmonary arrest.

Oxygen is a medication and is administered with a physician's order. Like other medications, oxygen can have side effects and toxic effects. In an emergency situation, the nurse can initiate oxygen therapy according to the institutional policy.

Supplemental oxygen is administered through an oxygen mask, cannula, or oxygen tent. See Table 29–4 for specific types of masks, concentrations of oxygen delivered, and indications. Procedure 29–9 describes methods of administering oxygen.

An endotracheal tube is inserted for many different reasons, including surgical procedures, cardiopulmonary arrest, respiratory distress, or inability to maintain a patent airway along with poor respiratory effort (*e.g.,* as a result of a drug overdose). Clients with an endotracheal tube are placed on a ventilator and cared for in a critical care unit. Procedure 29–10 details how to assist in the insertion of and care for a client with an endotracheal tube. Only physicians, respiratory therapists, paramedics, and specially trained nurses

HEALTH PROMOTION AND PREVENTION

MAINTAINING OPTIMAL OXYGENATION

* Breathe through the nose.
* Do not smoke.
* Exercise regularly.
* Avoid exposure to secondhand smoke.
* Make sure that ovens, fireplaces, and wood stoves are properly ventilated.
* Support a pollution-free environment.
* Wear appropriate masks when working around substances that are irritating to the respiratory mucosa.

(certified registered nurse anesthetist) may insert an endotracheal tube.

Clients who must be on a ventilator for an extended period may have a tracheostomy tube surgically inserted, which may enable the client to be weaned from the ventilator quickly. Clients can also be on a medical-surgical floor or go home with a tracheostomy tube. Care of a client with a tracheostomy tube is described in Procedure 29–11.

Clients who are semiconscious or unconscious and have an endotracheal or tracheostomy tube in place require suctioning to remove excess secretions and maintain a patent airway (Carroll, 1994). These clients may have a weak cough effort or no cough effort at all. Suctioning is described in Procedure 29–12.

Clients who are dependent on oxygen are sent home with oxygen (Herrick & Yeager, 1989). Medical supply companies provide the oxygen setup and dem-

Text continued on page 889

Table 29–4

TYPES OF OXYGEN DELIVERY SYSTEMS

MASK TYPE	O₂ CONCENTRATION DELIVERED	INDICATIONS	DESIGN/HOW IT WORKS
Nasal cannula	Low-flow oxygen device that delivers a fractional inspired oxygen of 24–44%	Correct or prevent hypoxemia	Mixes room air with oxygen delivered through two plastic prongs inserted into the nares; delivered oxygen is humidified to prevent drying out the nasal mucosa
Simple face mask	Low-flow oxygen system that delivers moderate concentrations of oxygen (40–60% at 5–8 L/min)	Used for clients who can't use a nasal cannula; for example, those who have a nasal obstruction	Designed with a series of small holes or exhalation ports on both sides; entrains room air through these ports, thus reducing the oxygen concentration delivered; keep flow of oxygen at a minimum of 5 L/min to flush carbon dioxide from the mask
Venturi mask	Delivers a precisely controlled low to moderate concentration of oxygen from 24–50% regardless of variations in respiratory rate	Especially useful in delivering oxygen to clients with chronic obstructive pulmonary disease because of its precise control	Designed with multiple exhalation ports on both sides of the mask and a removable interchangeable adapter (jet diluter); the amount of oxygen concentration is controlled by changing the size of the jet diluter
Partial rebreather mask	Delivers oxygen concentration from 35–60% at 6–10 L/min	Generally used in clients requiring moderate concentrations of oxygen	Does not have a one-way valve but conserves the first third of the client's exhaled air, which flows into the reservoir bag, and the remaining two thirds are exhaled through the exhalation ports; the first third of exhalation is high in oxygen concentration because it comes from the trachea and bronchi, which do not participate in gas exchange
Non-rebreather mask	Delivers high concentrations of oxygen (up to 100%)	Used for clients who need high concentrations of oxygen	Has a one-way valve between the mask and bag; the bag gets filled up with pure oxygen, and when the client inhales, the one-way valve lifts up to allow the client to inspire oxygen

ADMINISTERING OXYGEN VIA NASAL CANNULA

A nasal cannula is a low-flow system that mixes oxygen with room air. This system is acceptable for clients with minimal or no respiratory distress.

The following table identifies the oxygen flow rate with the percentage of oxygen that is being delivered:

O_2 Flow (L/min)	Percentage
1	24
2	28
3	32
4	36
5	40
6	44

Equipment:

Oxygen supply (cylinder or piped in from wall)
Valve handle to open cylinder or oxygen flowmeter
Nasal cannula tubing
Humidifier

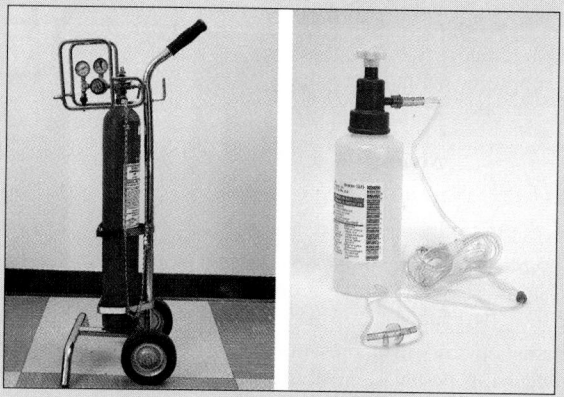

Oxygen tank

Nasal cannula attached to humidifier

Action	**Rationale**
1. Wash hands.	1. Reduces the spread of microorganisms.
2. Attach humidifier to oxygen source.	2. Humidified oxygen prevents drying of nasal mucosa.
3. Attach tubing to the humidifier.	3. Establishes connection.
4. Gently place prongs in each nare; loop around ears and slide clip to gently tighten.	4. Provides stability and greater comfort.

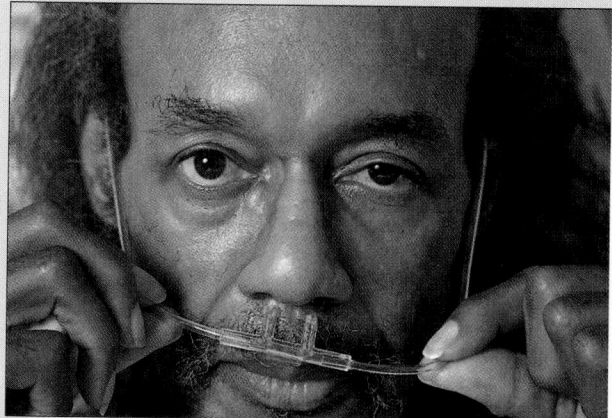

Step 4. *Placing prongs in nose*

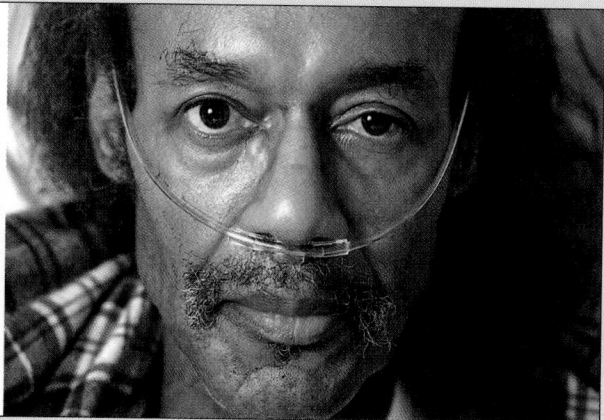

Step 4. *Nasal cannula in place*

Continued

PROCEDURE

29–9

ADMINISTERING OXYGEN VIA NASAL CANNULA
(Continued)

5. Adjust flowmeter to L/min as ordered or according to institutional policy.

6. Wash hands.

5. Ensures that proper amount of oxygen is delivered.

6. Reduces the spread of microorganisms.

ADMINISTERING OXYGEN VIA SIMPLE AND PARTIAL REBREATHING MASKS

Masks are used for clients who cannot use a nasal cannula and/or need moderate amounts of oxygen concentration.

Equipment:

Flowmeter connected to oxygen source
Humidifier
Simple or partial rebreathing mask

Action	**Rationale**
1. Wash hands.	**1.** Reduces the spread of microorganisms.
2. Explain procedure to the client and/or family.	**2.** Reduces anxiety and gains the client's cooperation.
3. Connect flowmeter and humidifier to oxygen source. Attach the simple mask or partial rebreathing mask as ordered by the physician.	**3.** Humidity prevents the drying effect of oxygen to the mucosal lining.
4. Turn flowmeter on to deliver prescribed concentration of oxygen. If using partial rebreathing mask, use the following guidelines:	**4.** Oxygen is a drug. A physician's order is needed to administer oxygen unless it is part of a standard approved protocol by the institution.

Percentage	O$_2$ flow (L/min)
35	6
40	7
45	8
50	9
60	10

Note: Allow oxygen to fill the bag, if using partial rebreathing mask.

Ensures that oxygen-enriched gas is delivered.

5. Place mask so that it covers the client's mouth and nose. Pull elastic to ensure a snug fit.

6. Wash hands.

7. Place a "No Smoking" sign in a visible area.

5. Ensures that prescribed concentration of oxygen is delivered.

6. Reduces the spread of microorganisms.

7. Promotes safety, because oxygen supports combustion.

ADMINISTERING OXYGEN VIA OXYGEN TENT

An oxygen tent is a convenient method for delivering oxygen to children. The tent covers the entire bed and delivers oxygen through an inlet port.

Equipment:

Oxygen tent setup
Flowmeter with oxygen source
Oxygen humidifier and heater

29–9

ADMINISTERING OXYGEN VIA OXYGEN TENT
(Continued)

Action	Rationale
1. Explain the procedure to the child in an age-appropriate manner and to the parents.	**1.** Reduces child and parental anxiety.
2. Set up the tent according to institutional policy.	**2.** Ensures correct and safe set up.
3. Set oxygen flow to correspond with oxygen percentage ordered:	**3.** Ensures ordered oxygen percentage is delivered.

Percentage	O_2 (L/min)
30–40	10
40–50	12
50	15

Action	Rationale
4. Tuck the tent in snugly around the mattress.	**4.** Reduces oxygen loss.
5. Plan nursing care so that the tent is opened as little as possible.	**5.** Reduces oxygen loss.
6. If tent has been opened for an extended period of time, turn up flow for a few minutes.	**6.** Flushes tent with oxygen to raise oxygen and mist concentration.
7. Monitor child's hair, clothing, and linens frequently for moisture.	**7.** Moisture condenses in tent and will chill the child.
8. Monitor temperature of humidifier frequently.	**8.** Keep oxygen humidifier/heater between 34.4°C (94°F) and 35.6°C (96°F).

ADMINISTERING OXYGEN VIA BAG-VALVE-MASK DEVICE

Bag-valve-mask (BVM) devices are also called Ambu bags. Use of the BVM may be cumbersome for beginners and is best used when two people are available. The mask must form a tight seal around the client's mouth in order to deliver adequate oxygen. The mask may be removed and an adapter used when bagging an individual who has a tracheostomy or is endotracheally intubated.

Equipment:

Oxygen source with flow-
  meter
Self-inflating BVM
Appropriate size mask

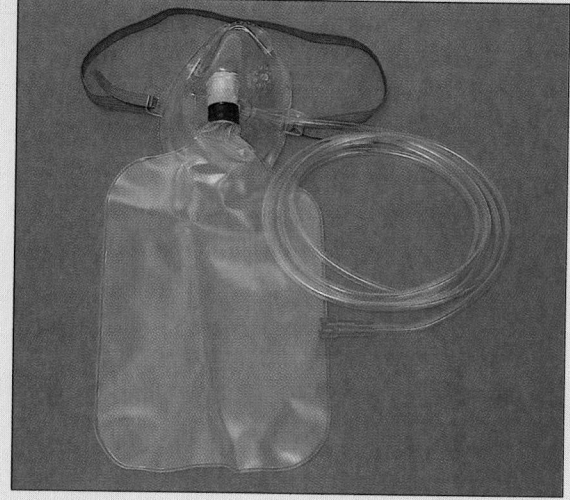

Action	Rationale
1. If the victim is unconscious, an oropharyngeal airway should be inserted.	**1.** Maintains patent airway.

Continued

PROCEDURE

29-9

ADMINISTERING OXYGEN VIA BAG-VALVE-MASK DEVICE
(Continued)

2. Position the head with the head tilt–chin lift method.

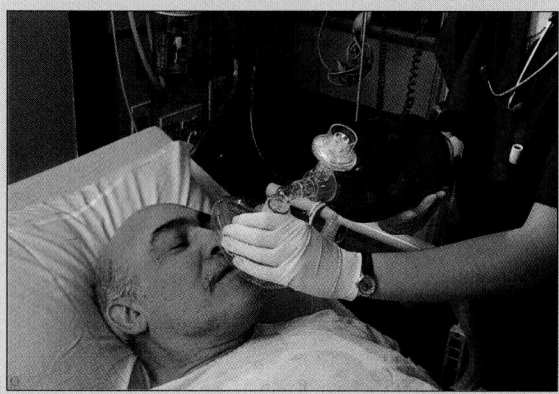

Step 2. *Using Ambu-bag*

3. Tightly seal the mask around the victim's nose and mouth.

4. Verify that the oxygen tubing is connected to the oxygen source and that the flowmeter is at 10 to 15 L/minute.

5. If two people are available, one holds the mask and one compresses the bag.

6. If only one person is available, the mask is held tightly with the nondominant hand while the dominant hand compresses the bag. Place the last and ring finger on the mandible and hold the mask tightly with the rest of the hand.

7. Head positioning must be maintained.

2. If there is a risk of neck injury, use the jaw thrust method.

3. A tight seal must be maintained to deliver an adequate tidal volume.

4. Avoids kinks in the tubing, which decrease the amount of oxygen being delivered.

5. Effective ventilations are more likely if two people are available.

6. Tight seal must be maintained to deliver oxygen.

7. Ensures delivery of adequate oxygen and tidal volume.

PROCEDURE

29–10

ENDOTRACHEAL TUBE INSERTION AND CARE

Equipment:
Endotracheal tube (ETT) with soft cuff and 15-mm adapter
Oropharyngeal airway
Stylet
Laryngoscope handle and blade with working light (either MacIntosh [curved blade] or Miller [straight blade])
Suction setup and equipment
Topical anesthesia (spray form)
10-cc syringe with Luer-Lok tip for checking cuff inflation
Self-inflating resuscitation bag with mask (bag-valve-mask)
Oxygen source
Tape, tincture of benzoin, scissors
Lubricant
Sterile gloves and other personal protective equipment such as mask, goggles, gowns, as needed

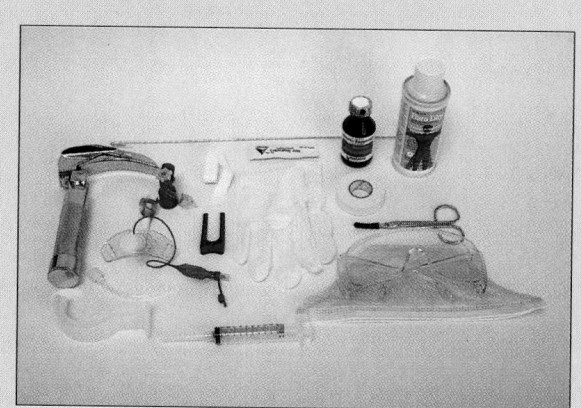

Action	Rationale
1. The physician or nurse explains the procedure to the client or family as appropriate.	1. Decreases anxiety and fosters client cooperation.
2. Bring equipment to bedside.	2. Ensures all equipment is readily available.
3. Wash hands. Don gloves and mask. Use protective goggles as needed.	3. Routine universal precautions.
4. Remove the client's dentures or removable plates/bridges. Place denture in cup with proper label.	4. Avoids confusion and loss of dentures.
5. Place the client in a supine position with the head extended and neck flexed, unless there is a neck injury. In this case, the jaw thrust maneuver is used or a nasotracheal intubation is preferred.	5. Aligns the axis of the mouth, pharynx, and trachea to facilitate intubation.
6. Check ETT cuff by inflating with air using 10-cc syringe. Deflate cuff after testing.	6. Verifies that cuff is not defective.
7. Prepare the laryngoscope by locking the blade in place, and make sure the light is on.	7. Establishes that equipment is working properly.
8. Insert stylet into ETT and make sure end is about 1 inch above the end of the tube.	8. Allows for flexibility of the tube during insertion. Proper insertion of stylet prevents trauma to trachea during insertion.
9. Lubricate tip of tube with water-soluble lubricating jelly.	9. Allows ease of insertion.
10. Hyperventilate and hyperoxygenate the client using a self-inflating BVM connected to 100% oxygen.	10. Minimizes hypoxia during insertion.

Continued

PROCEDURE

29–10

ENDOTRACHEAL TUBE INSERTION AND CARE
(Continued)

11. Suction oropharynx.

12. The physician chooses to do an orotracheal or nasotracheal approach. The insertion should take 30 seconds or less. If unable to intubate within 30 seconds, the procedure should be stopped, the client hyperventilated, and another attempt made.

13. Once the client is intubated, hyperventilate and hyperoxygenate. Observe for the rise and fall of the chest.

14. Auscultate breath sounds bilaterally and over the epigastric area.

15. Level of tube insertion is noted, and the tube is taped securely in place. Tincture of benzoin may be used to firmly adhere the tape.

16. Insert an oropharyngeal airway or bite block if necessary.

17. Obtain portable chest x-ray done.

18. Connect the client to mechanical ventilation as ordered by physician.

19. Assess the client's status and need for safety precautions such as restraints.

20. Assess respiratory status every 2 hours and the following as needed: respiratory rate, respiratory pattern, symmetrical chest expansion, breath sounds, arterial blood gases.

21. Suction endotracheal tube as needed.

22. Provide mouth care with mouthwash or peroxide solution. Suction out solution from the mouth.

23. ETT should be rotated to other side of mouth daily.

11. Maintains a patent, visible insertion pathway.

12. Ventilation should not be stopped for more than 30 seconds.

13. Minimizes hypoxia.

14. Audible breath sounds bilaterally confirm the passage of the ETT into the trachea. Absence of breath sounds indicates passage of the tube into the esophagus.

15. Checks that the tube has not moved from its previous position.

16. Prevents the client from biting tube.

17. Verifies placement of ETT.

18. Maintains adequate oxygenation.

19. Prevents accidental extubation.

20. Monitors client adequately and maintains professional quality.

21. Keeps airway patent.

22. Peroxide helps soften debris. Regular mouth care reduces oral microorganisms.

23. Prevents trauma and necrosis from tube pressure.

PROCEDURE

29–11

TRACHEOSTOMY TUBE CARE

The client is suctioned through the tube in preparation for tube care (Procedure 29–12).

Equipment:

Sterile water or saline solution
1:1 solution of H_2O_2 (hydrogen peroxide) and saline
Tracheostomy care kit
If tracheostomy has disposable inner cannula, obtain correct size
Gauze 4 × 4s
Gloves and other personal protective equipment, such as goggles, gowns, and mask
Precut tracheostomy gauze

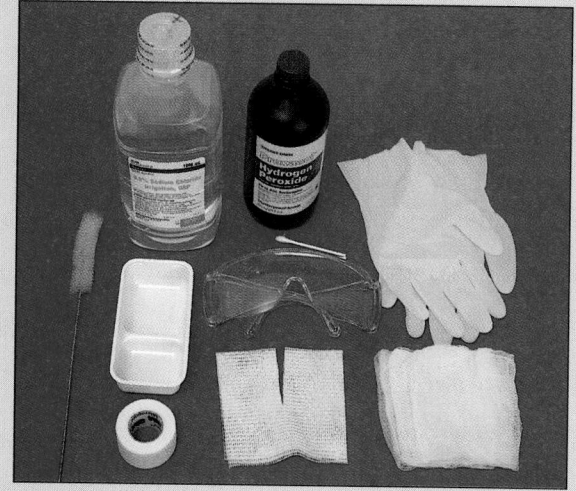

Action	Rationale
1. Wash hands.	1. Reduces the spread of microorganisms.
2. Explain the procedure to the client and/or family.	2. Decreases anxiety and fosters client cooperation.
3. Don personal protective equipment as needed.	3. Reduces the spread of microorganisms.
4. Disconnect the client from oxygen source or ventilator. Unlock and remove inner cannula. If inner cannula is disposable, throw away in appropriate waste container. If permanent, place in peroxide and saline solution.	4. Reduces the spread of microorganisms.

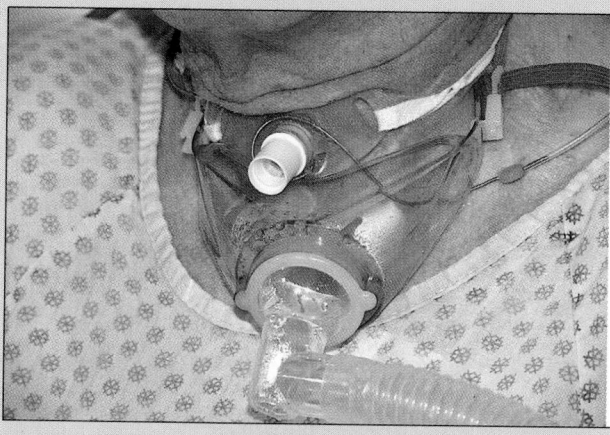

Step 4. *Removing O_2 from tracheostomy tube*

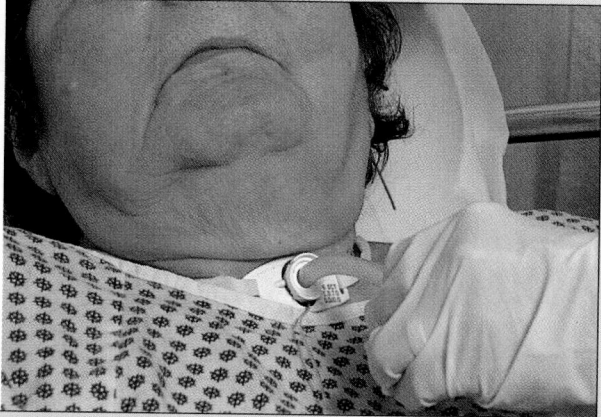

Removing inner cannula

5. Replace oxygen source or tracheostomy collar. If the client is on a ventilator, reattach the outer cannula to the ventilator.

5. Maintains oxygenation.

6. If the inner cannula is disposable, sterilely open new cannula, grasp at connector end, and gently reinsert into tracheostomy. Lock into place.

6. Provides clean appliance.

Continued

PROCEDURE

29–11

TRACHEOSTOMY TUBE CARE
(Continued)

7. If inner cannula is permanent, use pipe cleaner and brush to clean inner cannula. Rinse with plain sterile saline or water. Dry with sterile gauze.

7. Removes dried-up secretions and debris.

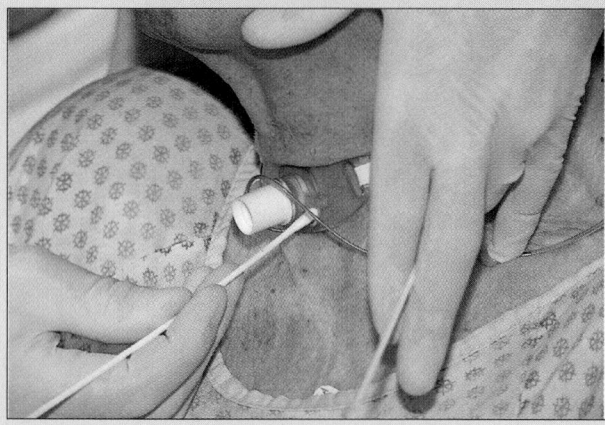
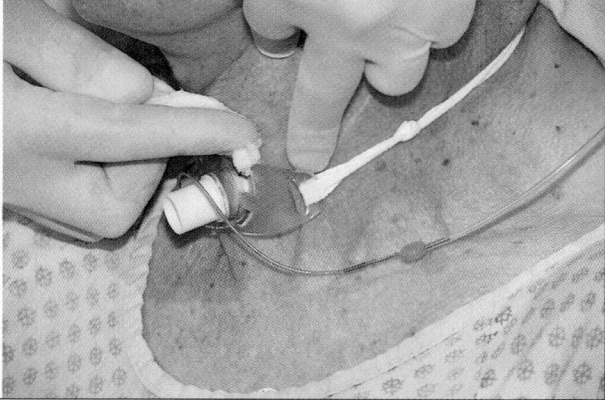

Step 7. *Cleaning under tracheostomy tube*

8. Disconnect from oxygen source or ventilator. Insert inner cannula and lock into place. Reconnect to oxygen or ventilator.

8. Provides clean appliance.

9. Suction the client through the tracheostomy tube if needed.

9. Clears the airway.

10. Clean stoma site and outer cannula with 4 × 4 gauze soaked in saline or hydrogen peroxide (check institutional policy). Dry with sterile gauze.

10. Removes dried-up secretions, old blood, and other debris from the stoma.

11. Check stoma for signs of irritation, tenderness, ulceration, and infection.

11. The stoma (especially a new stoma) is a potential site for infection.

12. Obtain assistance in changing trach ties. Cut and remove old ties while assistant holds the trach in place.

12. Prevents accidental extubation.

13. Apply new ties.

13. Secures tracheostomy in place.

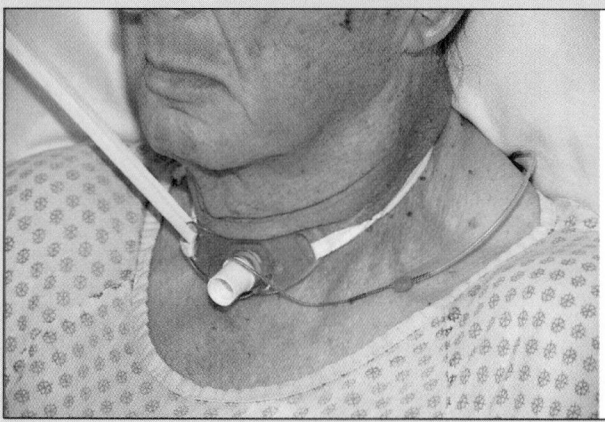
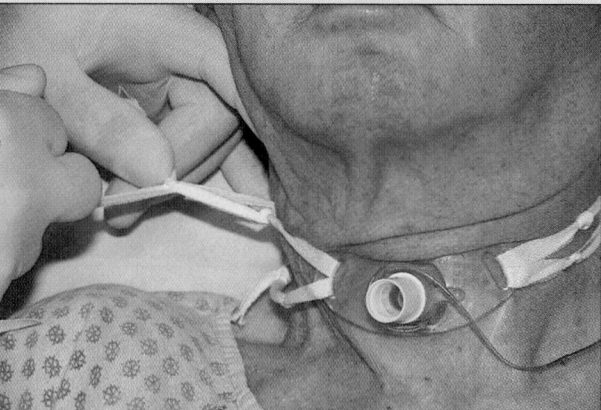

Step 12. *Attaching new tracheostomy tube ties*

PROCEDURE

29–11

TRACHEOSTOMY TUBE CARE
(Continued)

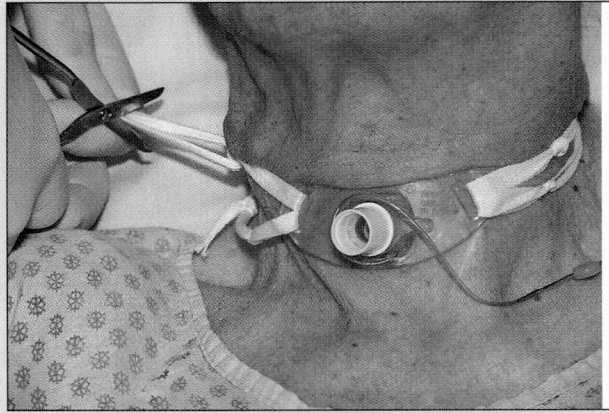

Cutting off excess on ties

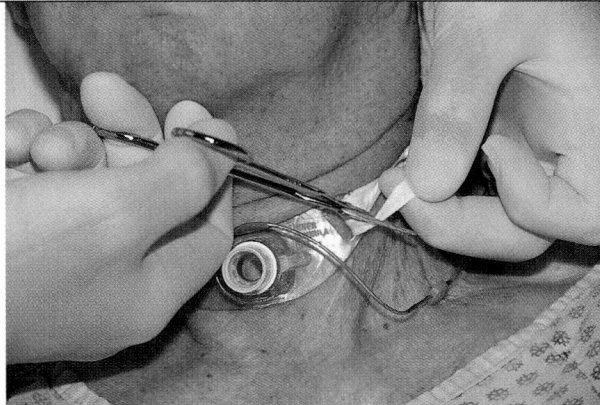

Removing old tracheostomy ties

14. Lift faceplate slightly to insert a clean precut tracheostomy gauze. Note: Use only precut gauze.

14. The gauze absorbs secretions that may irritate the stoma. Cutting gauze with scissors frays the edges and may emit lint, which may cause irritation to the stoma wound and get into the tracheal opening.

15. Remove and discard gloves and dispose of appropriately. Dispose of other supplies.

15. Reduces the spread of microorganisms.

16. Wash hands.

16. Reduces the spread of microorganisms.

PROCEDURE

29–12

SUCTIONING

Suctioning is done only as needed, because it can cause airway trauma and hypoxemia and increase the risk of atelectasis.

Hyperoxygenate the client before each suction pass. Apply suction (negative pressure) for less than 15 seconds at a time to decrease hypoxemia.

Use the appropriate amount of negative pressure for suctioning. The recommended amounts of negative pressure per suction manometer settings are as follows:

Age Group	Setting (mm Hg)
<1 year	60–80
1–8 years	80–120
Adult	120–150
>75 years	80–120

Use appropriate suction catheter size. Catheters that are too large can cause trauma during insertion, atelectasis, and hypoxemia. Catheters that are too small can cause increased airway resistance. The general recommendations are as follows:

Age Group	Catheter Size
Children <10 years	10 French
Adults	14 French
>75 years	10 French

Continued

PROCEDURE

29–12

SUCTIONING
(Continued)

The nasopharynx should be suctioned before the oropharynx, because the nasopharynx is cleaner.

Equipment:

Suction kit with or without suction catheter (if kit is not available: water-soluble lubricant, sterile gloves, sterile basin or container for sterile water or saline)

Sterile water or saline solution (100 ml)

Appropriate size suction catheter

Suction setup (suction source, vacuum regulator, connecting tubing, suction canister)

O_2 delivery system with bag-valve-mask and self-inflating resuscitation bag

Other personal protective equipment as needed (gown, mask, goggles)

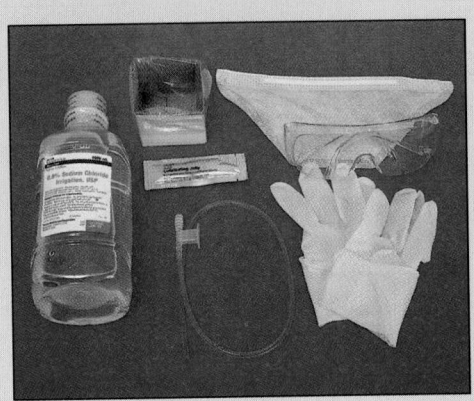

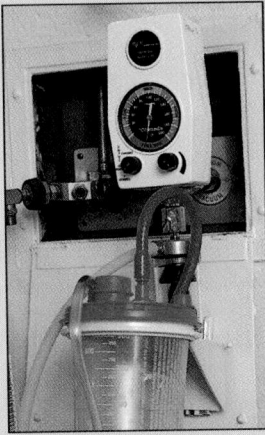

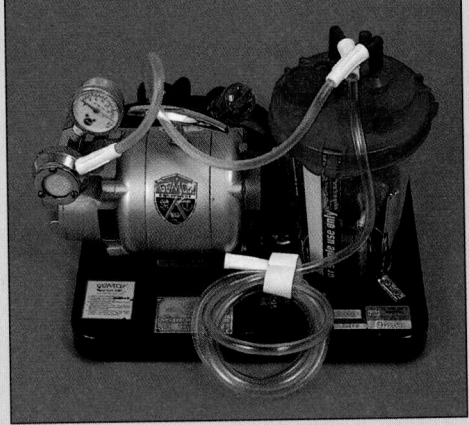

Action	Rationale
Oropharyngeal and Nasopharyngeal Suctioning	
1. Wash hands before bringing all the necessary equipment to the bedside.	1. Reduces the spread of microorganisms.
2. Explain the procedure to the client and/or family.	2. Reduces anxiety and gains the client's cooperation.
3. Set up suction apparatus. Set regulator to appropriate negative pressure.	3. Decreases hypoxia and airway trauma.
4. Secure the connecting tube to suction machine and place other end within easy reach.	4. Allows quick access.
5. Open sterile catheter package using sterile technique. Use the inside of the wrapping as a sterile field.	5. Reduces the spread of microorganisms.
6. Set up the sterile water or saline solution in a sterile basin if there is no unit dose provided.	6. Maintains sterile solution.
7. Open the water-soluble lubricant and squeeze onto sterile catheter package. Do not touch the sterile field.	7. Maintains asepsis.

SUCTIONING
(Continued)

8. Using the bag-valve-mask attached to a manual resuscitation bag connected to a 100% oxygen source, hyperoxygenate the client at least three times.

9. Don sterile gloves. If needed, other protective attire such as mask, goggles, and gown should be used.

10. Pick up the catheter with the dominant hand. Pick up the connecting tube with the nondominant hand.

11. Suction a small amount of saline.

12. Lubricate the distal end of the catheter with water-soluble lubricant.

Nasopharyngeal Suctioning

13. Verify patency of nasal airway by feeling for air movement over the flange.

14. Without applying any suction, gently insert the catheter through the patent nostril medially and downward along the passageway.

15. Rotate the catheter while slowly withdrawing it with the dominant hand. Apply intermittent suction during withdrawal.

8. Minimizes hypoxemia during suctioning.

9. Maintains sterile technique and protects the nurse against cross-contamination.

10. Allows dominant hand to remain sterile during the procedure.

11. Tests the suction equipment.

12. Lessens mucosal trauma during insertion.

13. Ensures smooth unobstructed airway insertion and prevents trauma during insertion.

14. Follows normal anatomical contour of nasal passageway.

15. Applying intermittent suction reduces the chance of hypoxemia.

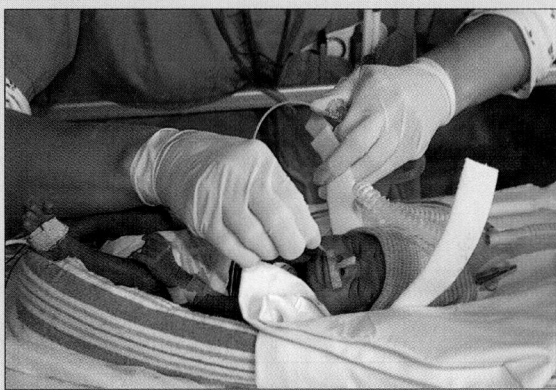

Step 15.

16. Repeat suctioning if needed to clear secretions. Note: Provide 1 to 2 minutes of rest between passes. Hyperoxygenate and hyperventilate between passes.

17. Rinse catheter and connecting tubing with sterile water or saline.

18. Coil catheter around fingers of dominant hand. Pull glove off the dominant hand and over the catheter coiled inside. Pull off other glove in the same manner.

19. Dispose of catheter and gloves and remainder of disposable supplies in appropriate receptacle.

20. Reposition the client and assess cardiopulmonary status. Replace oxygen therapy, as appropriate.

21. Wash hands.

16. Prevents hypoxemia.

17. Removes thick secretions in the tube.

18. Reduces the spread of microorganisms.

19. Reduces spread of microorganisms.

20. Possible complications of suctioning include hypoxia, and vasovagal stimulation, leading to dysrhythmias.

21. Reduces the spread of microorganisms.

Continued

SUCTIONING

(Continued)

22. Without applying suction, gently insert catheter into mouth and advance the tip to about 3 to 4 inches into the pharynx. Note: A Yankauer (tonsilar tip) catheter may be used to suction the mouth. If used, insert into mouth along gum line to pharynx. Avoid stimulating the gag reflex. Yankauer catheters may be reused. For infants and children, a bulb syringe may be used to suction the upper airway.

22. Follows normal anatomical contour of the oropharyngeal passageway.

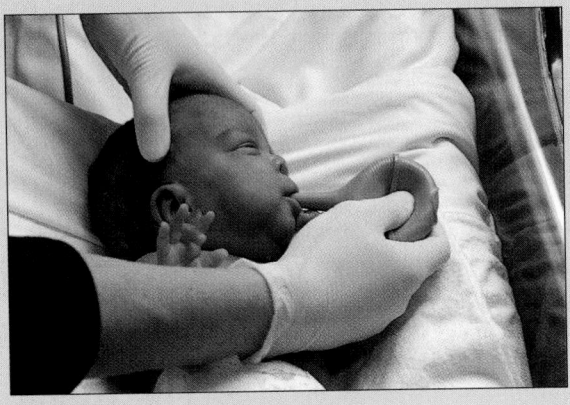

Step 22.

23. Follow steps 15 through 21. Note: Hyperoxygenation and hyperventilation may not be needed if suctioning is restricted to the oral cavity.

SUCTIONING VIA THE ENDOTRACHEAL AND TRACHEOSTOMY TUBE

Endotracheal and tracheostomy suctioning is done to maintain a patent airway in an intubated client. Suctioning is done only as needed, because repeated suctioning of the lower airway can predispose to atelectasis, hypoxemia, infection, and airway trauma.

Appropriate sized catheters should be used. The catheter should not be larger than half the diameter of the endotracheal or tracheostomy tube.

Refer to earlier in Procedure 29–12 for the recommended amount of negative pressure to use for suctioning.

Use additional personnel to assist with hyperoxygenation and hyperventilation of the client to reduce the incidence of accidental extubation.

Equipment:

Suction kit with or without suction catheter

If kit is not available: water-soluble lubricant, sterile gloves, sterile basin or container for sterile water or saline

Sterile water or saline solution (about 100 ml)

Appropriate size suction catheter

Suction setup (suction source, vacuum regulator, connecting tubing, suction canister)

O_2 delivery system (100% oxygen) with self-inflating resuscitation bag with adapter

Other personal protective equipment as needed

(See photos with above Equipment list.)

PROCEDURE

29–12

SUCTIONING
(Continued)

Action	Rationale
1. Wash hands.	**1.** Reduces the spread of microorganisms.
2. Bring all necessary equipment to the bedside.	**2.** Ensures that all equipment is readily available.
3. Explain the procedure to the client.	**3.** Reduces anxiety and gains the client's cooperation.
4. Set up suction apparatus. Set regulator to appropriate negative pressure.	**4.** Decreases hypoxia and airway trauma.
5. Secure the connecting tube to suction machine and place other end within easy reach.	**5.** Allows easy access.
6. Open sterile catheter package using sterile technique. Use the inside of the wrapping as a sterile field.	**6.** Reduces the spread of microorganisms.
7. Set up the sterile water or saline solution in sterile basin if there is no unit dose provided. Fill container up with 100 ml of the solution.	**7.** Maintains sterile solution.
8. Open the water-soluble lubricant and squeeze onto sterile catheter package. Do not touch the sterile field.	**8.** Prevents contamination.
9. Don sterile gloves. If needed, other protective attire such as a mask, goggles, and gown should be used.	**9.** Follows universal precautions.
10. Pick up the catheter with the dominant hand. Pick up the connecting tube with the nondominant hand. (The dominant hand should remain sterile during the procedure.)	**10.** Maintains sterile technique.
11. Suction a small amount of saline.	**11.** Tests the suction equipment.
12. Lubricate the distal end of the catheter with water-soluble lubricant.	**12.** Lessens mucosal trauma during insertion.
13. Disconnect the client from the ventilator or oxygen device with the nondominant hand. "Bag" (*i.e.,* hyperoxygenate) the client manually at least three times using the nondominant hand. Note: If available, a second person can do these steps.	**13.** Hyperoxygenates and hyperventilates the client and reduces hypoxemia.

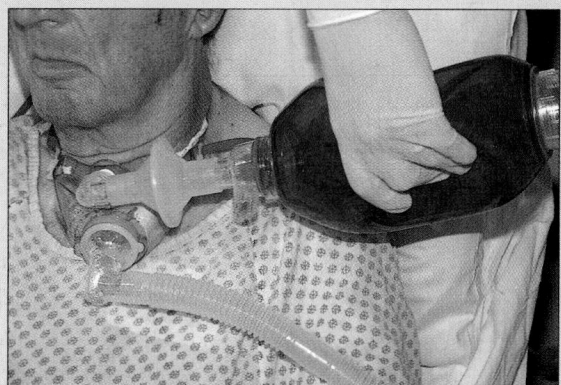

Step 13.

Continued

SUCTIONING
(Continued)

14. Without applying any suction, gently insert the catheter through the artificial airway with the dominant hand.

14. Prevents trauma.

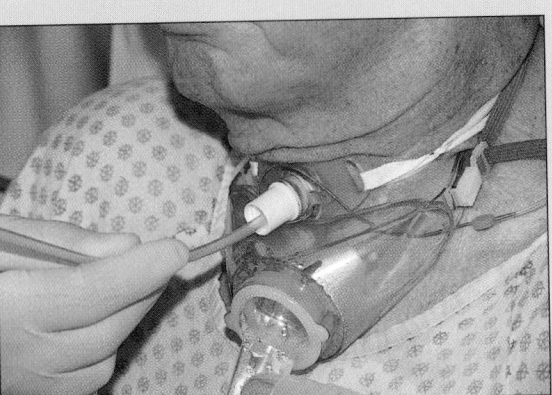

Step 14.

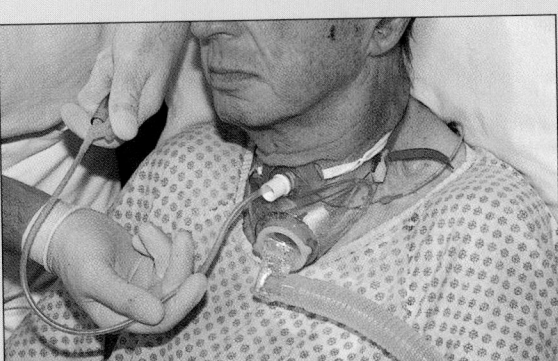

Step 15.

15. Rotate the catheter while slowly withdrawing it with the dominant hand. Apply intermittent suction during withdrawal of the catheter.

15. Prevents hypoxemia and mucosal trauma.

16. Hyperoxygenate and hyperventilate before suctioning again.

16. Prevents hypoxemia.

17. Rinse catheter and connecting tubing with sterile water.

17. Removes thick secretions in the tubing.

18. Repeat suctioning if needed.

18. Clears secretions.

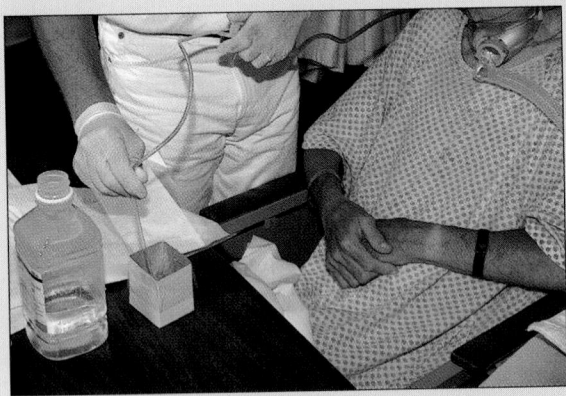

Step 17.

19. Reconnect to ventilator as appropriate and replace oxygen therapy. Reassess cardiopulmonary status.

19. Possible complications of suctioning include hypoxia and vasovagal stimulation, leading to dysrhythmias.

20. Coil catheter around fingers of dominant hand. Pull glove off the dominant hand and over the catheter coiled inside. Pull off other glove in the same manner.

20. Reduces the spread of microorganisms.

21. Dispose of catheter and gloves and remainder of disposable supplies in appropriate receptacle.

21. Reduces the spread of microorganisms.

onstrate to the client and family how to set the correct flow rate. Encourage the family to keep the medical supply company's phone number in an easily accessible location in the event that the equipment malfunctions. Clients and families should be taught about safety regarding oxygen. No one should smoke around the oxygen system, and the oxygen unit should be kept away from open flames, gas stoves, or kerosene heaters. The oxygen system should be kept in an upright position to avoid leaks. An all-purpose fire extinguisher should be kept nearby at all times. Encourage the family to contact the nearest fire station and inform it that oxygen is being used in the home. In most cases, the fire department will monitor the equipment and provide additional safety information (McCauley & Boller, 1987).

Clients should be taught health promotional behaviors that will help maintain optimal oxygenation (see the box on page 873).

Evaluation

The evaluation process is ongoing. Adjustments to or changes in the client's care are based on the client's response to the interventions. It is imperative to identify why a goal is or is not being met. For example, to evaluate if the goals are being met for a client with asthma, the tidal volume and lung capacities should be within normal limits, the lung fields should be clear, and the client should remain alert and oriented.

Summary

To provide effective nursing care for clients with respiratory problems, the nurse must understand the anatomy and physiology of the respiratory system and its structures, as well as psychosocial and developmental factors that affect oxygenation. Nurses must also be familiar with diagnostic studies that evaluate oxygenation. Using the nursing process, the student learns to assess the client's respiratory status; formulate a nursing diagnosis related to the oxygenation needs of the client; and plan, implement, and evaluate specific nursing interventions based on the diagnosis. Whether the nurse is at the bedside or delivering care in the home, identifying subtle clues to a client's oxygenation status is crucial.

CHAPTER HIGHLIGHTS

♦

♦ The four mechanisms involved in the respiratory process are ventilation, diffusion, transportation, and regulation.

♦ The functional units of the lung where gas exchange occurs are the acini.

♦ The pulmonary artery carries unoxygenated blood to the lungs, and the pulmonary vein carries oxygenated blood to the heart.

♦ Client complaints related to oxygenation include dyspnea, asthma, chest pain, anorexia, cough, orthopnea, and hemoptysis.

♦ Common respiratory symptoms include dyspnea, chest pain, cough, fever, anorexia, and weight loss.

♦ The physical examination technique for the respiratory system is inspection, palpation, percussion, and auscultation.

♦ Blood tests commonly ordered for clients with respiratory complaints include a complete blood count, arterial blood gas, and blood cultures.

♦ The most frequently performed skin test is the Mantoux test or tuberculin test.

♦ Frequently performed endoscopic and surgical procedures include direct laryngoscopy, bronchoscopy, biopsy, and thoracentesis.

♦ Commonly identified nursing diagnoses related to oxygenation are ineffective airway clearance, ineffective breathing pattern, and impaired gas exchange.

♦ The most important nursing intervention is to maintain a patent airway.

♦ Positioning the client to facilitate optimal airway expansion is crucial.

♦ Respiratory medications include bronchodilators, mucokinetic medications, corticosteroids, antitussives, antihistamines, antibiotics, and vaccines.

♦ Supplemental oxygen may be administered through nasal cannula, mask, or tent.

Study Questions

1. An arterial blood gas is ordered for a 25-year-old woman in the emergency room with status asthmaticus. After obtaining the blood, which of the following measures is essential for the nurse to implement?

   a. transport the blood to the lab
   b. hold pressure on the site for at least 5 minutes
   c. apply a sterile dressing
   d. monitor the client's blood pressure

2. A 59-year-old man is admitted to the floor with a chest tube in the right midaxillary line. Essential equipment to be kept at the bedside includes

   a. sterile water
   b. emesis basin
   c. incentive spirometer
   d. clamps and petroleum gauze pads

3. The nurse assesses a client's respiratory rate at 36. This rate is termed

a. tachypnea
b. tachycardia
c. eupnea
d. bradypnea

4. A 56-year-old man is admitted to the emergency room with a complaint of shortness of breath. To promote respiratory expansion and comfort, the client should be placed in which position?

a. supine
b. Trendelenburg
c. high-Fowler
d. side-lying

5. The amount of air inhaled and exhaled during normal quiet breathing is termed

a. residual volume
b. vital capacity
c. inspiratory capacity
d. tidal volume

Critical Thinking Exercises

1. Ms. D. is extremely short of breath and wheezing due to an acute exacerbation of asthma. She is sitting, leaning forward, and using accessory muscles. Respiratory treatments of metaproterenol sulfate are prescribed, and she is relieved in the emergency department. Discuss the teaching you would do with Ms. D. regarding inhaler use.

2. Mr. T. has developed a spontaneous pneumothorax. The nursing diagnoses of Breathing Pattern, Ineffective and Gas Exchange, Impaired are assigned. Develop a treatment plan for Mr. T. related to oxygen therapy and chest tube management.

References

American Thoracic Society. (1996). Cigarette smoking and health. *American Journal of Respiratory Critical Care Medicine, 153*(2), 861–865.

Bates, B. (1995). *A guide to physical examination and history taking* (6th ed.). Philadelphia: J. B. Lippincott.

Carroll, P. (1994). Safe suctioning PRN. *RN, 57*(5), 32–36.

Chandra, N. C., and Hazinski, M. F. (1994). *Textbook of basic life support for health care providers.* Dallas, TX: American Heart Association.

Glantz, S. L., & Parmley, W. W. (1995). Passive smoking and heart disease. Mechanisms and risk. *Journal of the American Medical Association, 273*(13), 1047–1053.

Herrick, T. W., & Yeager, H. (1989). Home oxygen therapy. *Annals of Family Practice, 32*(2), 157–159.

Jarvis, C. (1996). *Physical examination and health assessment* (2nd ed.). Philadelphia: W. B. Saunders.

McCauley, C. S., & Boller, L. R. (1987). The hazards of home oxygen therapy. *New England Journal of Medicine, 316*(2), 107–108.

Sonnesso, G. (1991). Are you ready to use pulse oximetry? *Nursing 91, 91*(8), 60.

Szaflarski, N. L. (1989). Use of pulse oximetry in critically ill adults. *Heart and Lung, 18*(3), 444–454.

Wilson, S. F., & Thompson, J. M. (1990). *Respiratory disorders.* St. Louis: Mosby-Year Book.

Wong, D. L. (1993). *Whaley and Wong's essentials of pediatric nursing* (4th ed.). St. Louis: Mosby.

Bibliography

Ahrens, T. S. (1993a). Changing perspectives in the assessment of oxygenation. *Critical Care Nurse, 13*(4), 78–83.

Ahrens, T. S. (1993b). The cutting edge in pulmonary critical care. *Critical Care Nurse (Supplement), 13*(3), 4–5.

Apps, M. C. (1992). A guide to lung function tests. *British Journal of Hospital Medicine, 48*(7), 399–401.

Arbour, R. (1993). Weaning a patient from a ventilator. *Nursing 93, 93*(2), 52–56.

Bach, J. R., & Beltrame, F. (1992). Alternative approaches to home mechanical ventilation. In M. Rothkopf & J. Askanazi (Eds.), *Intensive homecare* (pp. 173–198). Baltimore: Williams & Wilkins.

Bates, B. (1995). *A guide to physical examination and history taking* (6th ed.). Philadelphia: J. B. Lippincott.

Boggs, R. L., & Wooldridge-King, M. (1993). *AACN procedure manual for critical care* (3rd ed., pp. 1–220). Philadelphia: W. B. Saunders.

Boutotte, J. (1993). T. B. the second time around. *Nursing 93, 93*(5), 42–49.

Branson, R. D. (1993). The nuts and bolts of increasing arterial oxygenation: Devices and techniques. *Respiratory Care, 38*(6), 672–689.

Carpenter, K. D. (1993). A comprehensive review of cyanosis. *Critical Care Nurse, 13*(4), 66–71.

Chameides, L., & Hazinski, M. F. (Eds.). (1994). *Textbook of pediatric advanced life support.* Dallas, TX: American Heart Association.

Chulary, M. (1987). Hyperinflation/hyperoxygenation to prevent endotracheal suctioning complications. *Critical Care Nurse, 7*(2), 100–104.

Corley, M., et al. (1993). The myth of 100% oxygen delivery through manual resuscitation bags. *Journal of Emergency Nursing, 19*(1), 45–47.

Crimlisk, J. T., & Blansfield, J. S. (1993). Using $ETCO_2$ to confirm endotracheal tube placement. *Nursing 93, 93*(3), 77–81.

Cummins, R. O. (1994). *Textbook of advanced cardiac life support.* Dallas, TX: American Heart Association.

Czarnik, R. E., et al. (1991). Differential effects of continuous versus intermittent suction on tracheal tissue. *Heart and Lung, 20*(2), 144–147.

Erickson, R. (1989a). Mastering the ins and outs of chest drainage: Part 1. *Nursing 89, 19*(5), 36–44.

Erickson, R. (1989b). Mastering the ins and outs of chest drainage: Part 2. *Nursing 89, 19*(6), 46–50.

Eubanks, D. H., & Bone, R. C. (1990). *Comprehensive respiratory care: A learning system.* St. Louis: Mosby.

Fluck, R. R. (1985). Suctioning—intermittent or continuous. *Respiratory Care, 30*(10), 837–838.

Grossbach, I. (1993). Case studies in pulse oximetry monitoring. *Critical Care Nurse, 13*(4), 63–65.

Guyton, A. C. (1991). *Textbook of medical physiology.* (8th ed., pp. 402–451). Philadelphia: W. B. Saunders.

Henneman, E. (1991). The art and science of weaning from mechanical ventilation. *Focus on Critical Care, 18*(6), 490–501.

Hess, D. (1993). Techniques and devices for monitoring oxygenation. *Respiratory Care, 38*(6), 646–671.

Higgins, J. (1990). Pulmonary oxygen toxicity. *Physiotherapy, 76*(10), 588–592.

Kranzley, N. L. (1991). *Quick reference to respiratory critical care nursing.* Gaithersburg, MD: Aspen Publishers.

Krebel, A. (1991). Weaning from a mechanical ventilator: Current controversies. *Heart and Lung, 20*(4), 321–331.

Macey, B. A., & Landstrom, L. L. (1993). Replacing a chest

tube drainage collection device. *Nursing 93, 93*(3), 95–96.

Marino, W. D., & Kvetan, V. (1992). Home positive pressure ventilatory support. In M. Rothkopf and J. Askanazi (Eds.), *Intensive homecare* (pp. 159–172). Baltimore: Williams & Wilkins.

Martin, L., & Khalil, H. (1990). How much reduced hemoglobin is necessary to generate central cyanosis. *Chest, 97*(1), 182–185.

Mathews, R. J., et al. (1992). Airway monitoring and ventilation: What the future holds. *Nursing 92, 92*(2), 48–59.

Mergaert, S. (1994). S.T.O.P. and assess chest tubes the easy way. *Nursing 94, 94*(2), 52–53.

Noll, M., et al. (1990). Closed tracheal suction systems: Effectiveness and nursing implications. *AACN Clinical Issues, 1*(2), 318–320.

Pierson, D. J. (1992). What constitutes an order for mechanical ventilation, and who should give the order? *Respiratory Care, 37*(9), 1124–1130.

Poole, S. (1993). A requirement not to be overlooked: Nutritional aspects of respiratory disease. *Professional Nurse, 8*(4), 252, 254–256.

Redick, E. L. (1993). Closed system, in-line endotracheal suctioning. *Critical Care Nurse, 13*(4), 47–58.

Springfield, Y. N. (1993). Back to basics: Acidosis, alkalosis and ABGs. *American Journal of Nursing, 93*(11), 43–44.

Stiesmeyer, J. K. (1991). What triggers a ventilator alarm? *American Journal of Nursing, 91*(10), 60–64.

Stiesmeyer, J. K. (1993). A four-step approach to pulmonary assessment. *American Journal of Nursing, 93*(8), 22–28, 31–32.

Taber's Cyclopedic Medical Dictionary (17th ed.). (1993). Philadelphia: F. A. Davis.

Thompson, K. S., et al. (1991). Building a critical path for ventilator dependency. *American Journal of Nursing, 91*(7), 28–31.

Willens, J. S. (1993). Strengthen your life support skills. *Nursing 93, 93*(4), 54–58.

CIRCULATION

LINDA ULAK, EdD, RN, CCRN, CS

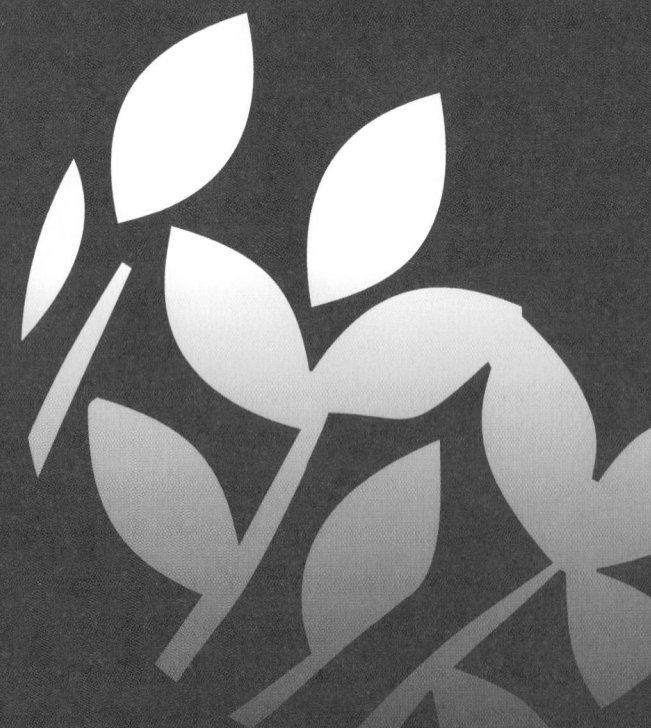

LEARNING OBJECTIVES

✦

After studying this chapter, you should be able to

✦ Explain the normal cardiac and systemic circulation

✦ Verbalize the significance of the differences between arteries and veins

✦ Describe systole and diastole in the cardiac cycle

✦ Discuss factors that contribute to normal cardiac output and tissue perfusion

✦ Demonstrate proper procedure for cardiovascular assessment

✦ Discuss rationales for variations from normal assessment findings

✦ Discuss cardiovascular changes that occur across the lifespan

✦ Utilize the nursing process in developing a plan of care for the client

✦ Explain basic tests that are performed in a cardiac examination

✦ Initiate a plan of care for the cardiac client

Circulation comprises an array of nursing concerns, from chronic difficulties like cold extremities to life-threatening ones like myocardial infarcts. The nurse is responsible for monitoring and documenting changes in circulation as a guidepost to the ongoing care of the client. The nurse must also act as an educator, teaching the client the important links between care of the circulatory system (*e.g.*, exercise, maintaining low cholesterol levels, weight control, no smoking) and overall health.

In this chapter, the circulatory system is reviewed. We examine its two major components: the cardiac and systemic circulation. Both systems are responsible for similar functions; *i.e.*, providing oxygen, nutrients, and other substances to cells while removing waste products.

Cardiac Circulation

The cardiac circulation takes blood to and from the heart. The heart is a four-chambered organ, weighing approximately 1 lb in an adult. It is positioned in the chest between the lungs in the mediastinal region. The heart chambers are right atrium, left atrium, right ventricle, and left ventricle (Fig. 30–1).

The atria are located at the top of the heart, which is called the base of the heart. The ventricles are lo-

cated at the bottom of the heart, called the apex. The ventricles are larger and have thicker walls than the atria. The reason for this is that the blood flows somewhat passively into the ventricles and therefore thick walls for contraction are necessary. The left ventricular wall has a thickness of 13 to 15 mm; the thickness of the right ventricle is 3 to 5 mm. The left ventricle requires this muscle mass to enable it to pump blood into the rest of the circulatory system. The left ventricle is the high-pressure chamber of the heart, as it must supply blood to the entire body; the right ventricle pumps blood only into the lungs.

Located between the atria and the ventricles are the tricuspid and mitral atrioventricular valves. These valves serve as one-way flow devices. The tricuspid valve, located on the right side of the heart, has three cusps. The mitral valve, on the left side of the heart, has two cusps. These leaflets, or cusps, prevent the backflow of blood from the ventricles into the atria. When functioning properly, these valves ensure forward flow of blood from the atria to the ventricles.

The semilunar valves prevent blood from flowing backward from the lungs or aorta into the ventricles. The pulmonic valve is located at the entrance to the pulmonary artery from the right ventricle. The aortic valve is at the entrance of the aorta from the left ventricle (see Fig. 30–1). When functioning properly, these valves ensure forward flow of blood from the ventricles into the aorta and pulmonary arteries.

The cardiac cycle is divided into two distinct cy-

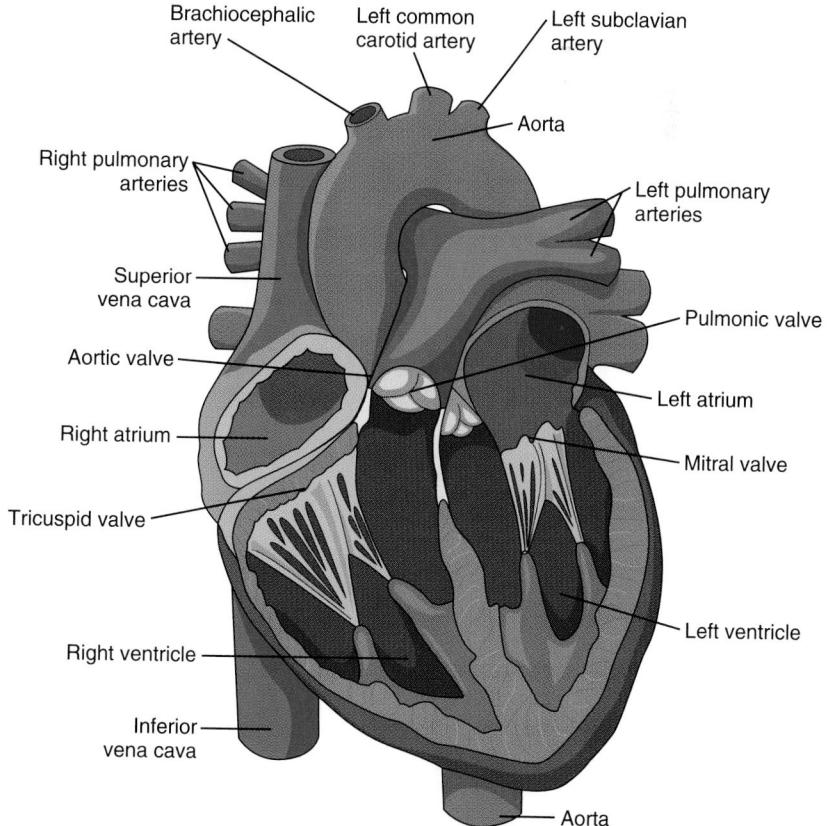

Figure 30–1
Anatomy of the heart.

cles: systole and diastole. **Systole** is the contraction of the ventricles, which forces blood through the pulmonic and aortic valves into the pulmonary arteries and aorta. The volume of blood that is ejected with each contraction is termed **stroke volume. Diastole** is often referred to as the resting phase of the heart. During this phase, blood moves from the atria through the atrioventricular valves into the ventricles. When the atria contract (atrial systole), the atria push remaining blood into the ventricles. This is important because the volume increases **cardiac output** significantly and reduces blood left in the atria, which could result in clot formation. Cardiac output is defined as heart rate times stroke volume. The entire process—the contraction and the relaxation that follows prior to another contraction—is a complete **cardiac cycle.** This one cardiac cycle sounds like "lub-dub" during auscultation of the heart.

Coronary Vessels

The heart has its own coronary circulatory system comprising coronary arteries and veins; these provide essential elements, such as nutrients and oxygen, to cardiac cells in the myocardium. The major coronary arteries are the right and left coronary arteries. Each branches several times, covering the entire surface area of the heart.

The left coronary artery divides into two major branches: the left anterior descending artery and the circumflex artery. The left anterior descending artery provides blood to the majority of the left ventricle and a portion of the right ventricle, as well as the wall (septum) separating the ventricles. The circumflex artery travels laterally along a groove that separates the left atrium and ventricle and also extends toward the back of the heart. The right coronary artery provides circulation to the posterior surface of the heart.

In addition to these major blood vessels are coronary collateral arteries, which are connections between branches of the coronary arteries. The value of the collateral circulation is questionable. It is not clear whether collateral circulation is more highly developed in certain individuals due to coronary ischemia (such as a person with longstanding angina) or whether it represents a protective feature to allow for better circulation.

Heart Rate

Neural, hormonal, and chemical factors affect the heart rate. The average adult heart rate is 70 beats per minute, although age, activity, and general condition may alter the rate. An adult heart rate between 60 and 100 beats per minute is considered acceptable. Infants and children have higher normal resting heart rates. Newborn infants, until the age of 3 months, have heart rates between 100 and 220, and children until age 2 have rates between 80 and 150. As the child matures, the heart rate approximates that of an adult.

Systemic Circulation

The systemic circulation, which supplies blood to the body, contains approximately 84% of the total blood volume; the rest is equally divided between the cardiac and respiratory circulation systems (Fig. 30–2). In the systemic circulation, blood moves from the arterial to the venous side of circulation along a pressure gradient, with hydrostatic and oncotic pressures causing fluid to move in and out of the vascular system. Hydrostatic pressure is the force within the vascular system that causes blood to move out of the vascular system. Oncotic pressure is related to the amount of proteins in the intravascular system, which hold the fluid within the vascular system. Oncotic pressure is normally greater than hydrostatic pressure, which ensures adequate vascular volume. An example of increased hydrostatic pressure is demonstrated when you examine the lower extremities of a person who has been standing or sitting with his or her feet down for many hours. The feet and legs are "puffy" or edematous, because the hydrostatic force was so great that it forced fluid from circulation into the interstitial spaces.

Arterial blood flow is pulsatile; higher pressures

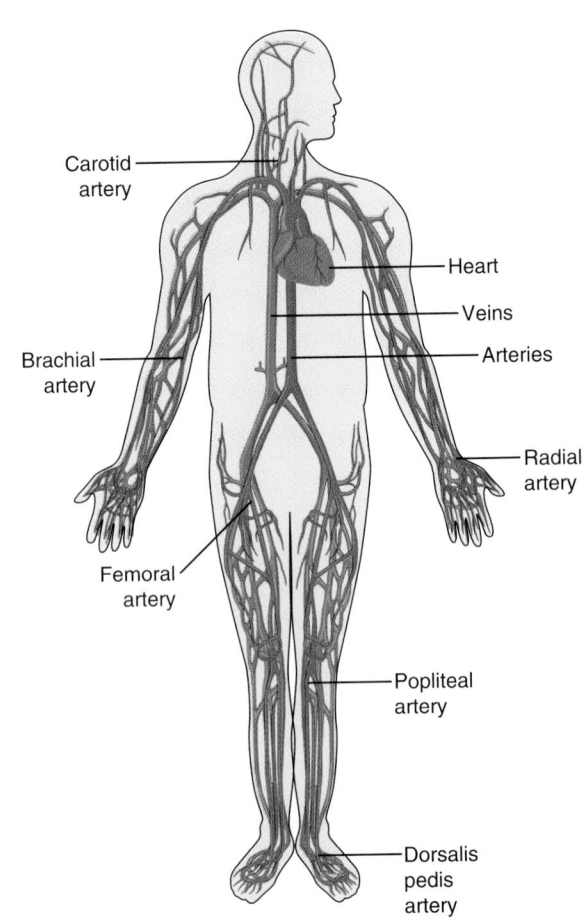

Carotid artery

Brachial artery

Femoral artery

Heart

Veins

Arteries

Radial artery

Popliteal artery

Dorsalis pedis artery

❧ **Figure 30–2**
The circulatory system.

are the systolic pressures, and the lower values are diastolic pressures. Capillaries and veins are nonpulsatile and have considerably lower pressures than the diastolic arterial pressure. The difference in pressure gradients is the force that provides for the forward blood flow in the systemic circulation.

Blood vessels, except for capillaries, have three layers: tunica externa (outermost), tunica media (middle layer) and tunica intima (inner layer). Arteries are thick-walled vessels with a large amount of elastic fiber, which allows them to stretch during systole (ventricular contraction) and to recoil during diastole (ventricular relaxation). The arteries depend on the sympathetic nervous system for vasoconstriction and dilation to maintain blood pressure. Therefore, an individual with a severed spinal cord and paralysis in the legs would have no sympathetic nervous system innervation to his or her legs; the result would be decreased vasoconstriction and pooling of blood in the legs. Arteries, unlike veins, do not have valves to prevent backflow. They are dependent on pulsation (blood pressure) to keep the blood moving forward.

Veins and venules are much thinner walled than arteries and can expand and collapse as required. In this way, they can serve as a reservoir for blood storage. This is an important compensatory mechanism because it can alter the amount of blood returned to the heart as necessary. If a person has too great a volume of blood returning to the heart, the veins can dilate and decrease the return, as in the case in a person with congestive heart failure. In heart failure, the heart is unable to pump blood adequately from the heart, and it backs up in the venous system. In the same manner, if the heart has too little blood returning to it, such as in a person who is hemorrhaging, the veins constrict and increase flow back to the heart in an attempt to maintain a normal blood pressure. Vasoconstriction causes the extremities and skin to be cool to touch and pale in color.

The venous system is low pressured and therefore depends on factors such as intraabdominal pressure and muscle activity to assist in moving blood back to the heart from elsewhere in the body. Exercise increases blood return to the heart. The peripheral veins, unlike the arteries, have valves that prevent back flow of blood and that also assist in returning the blood to the heart.

The capillary system is where the exchange of gases, nutrients, and cellular wastes occurs between tissue and the bloodstream. The walls of the capillaries are thin, with only a single layer of endothelial cells surrounded by a basement membrane. This minimal interface allows for adequate exchange of particles along the capillary system. Fluid movement in the veins, like that in the arteries, is controlled by pressure gradients. Fluids are pushed out of the capillaries on the arterial side while they are pulled back on the venous side. This allows for the transfer of nutrients and oxygen from the vascular system into the cells and waste product removal from the cells into the vascular system for disposal from the body.

Factors Affecting Circulation

Age

The aging process has a profound affect on both heart rate and blood pressure. As noted earlier, the normal heart rate for an infant may be as rapid as 220 beats per minute, whereas, for an adult the normal rate is between 60 and 100. There are many physiological changes that take place in the cardiovascular system as a person ages. Some of these changes result in improved cardiac function, while others result in decreased responsiveness to changes.

With advancing age, some specific changes that occur in the cardiovascular system include left ventricular hypertrophy, mitral and aortic valve thickening, increased myocardial stiffness, increased connective tissue in the heart, calcification of heart valves, arteriosclerosis, atherosclerosis, and elevated arterial systolic blood pressure. The arteries become stiff and less compliant as a person ages. This results in an increased workload for the left ventricle to overcome the resistance caused by the arteries. With advanced age, the baroreceptors, which normally respond to a low blood pressure by increasing blood pressure, are not as readily able to respond to pressure changes, which can result in postural hypotension (Baker, 1990). This significant change is the reason that the elderly should have their blood pressure checked when lying supine and in an upright position to detect orthostatic hypotension (Byra-Cook *et al.*, 1990).

Race

Hypertension is reported to be both more prevalent and more severe in the African-American population than in whites. Diastolic pressures are significantly greater for African-American than for white men and women in age groups 35 years and older. African-American women are 24% more likely to die of coronary artery disease than are white women, and the death rate from stroke in these women is 83% higher (Sandmaier, 1992). Actual cause for the elevated blood pressure is unknown at this time. It does not seem to be related to elevated renin levels; therefore, therapies other than renin interventions, such as diuretics, low-sodium diet, and calcium channel blockers, work well. Recent research has found that African-American clients demonstrate a significant impairment in the ability to vasodilate. These findings suggest that physiologic differences exist and that lack of access to health care providers, dietary issues, and compliance issues cannot entirely account for the higher rates of cardiovascular disease–related disorders in African-Americans (Drown, 1994).

Gender

Mortality rates in men have decreased from coronary heart disease since the 1950s but have increased in women (Flavell, 1994). More than 500,000 women die each year in the United States from coronary heart disease (Wenger *et al.*, 1993). Until menopause, estrogen gives women some protection against developing coronary artery disease. As a result, premenopausal women who have no other risk factors are less likely than men to develop a myocardial infarction or atherosclerosis (Kitler, 1991; Stampfer *et al.*, 1991). However, after menopause, the risk of women developing cardiac disease rises to the point of equal risk to men by the age of 75. Overall, approximately 10 million American women of all ages suffer from heart disease. According to Sandmaier (1992), 1 in 10 women 45 to 64 years of age has some form of heart disease, and this increases to 1 in 4 women 65 years of age or older.

Heredity

Although many cardiac conditions seem to have no hereditary basis, it is possible that heredity plays a role in the development of certain major disorders such as cerebral vascular accidents, myocardial infarctions, and hypertension. This family history is most important when developing the patient profile.

Lifestyles and Habits

Many factors that the individual experiences throughout the day affect blood pressure and heart rate. Some of these include smoking, over-the-counter and prescription medications, caffeine intake, and alcohol consumption. Cigarette smoking has been described as the most important health risk factor in the country. Approximately 26 million American women smoke. Women who smoke are two to six times as likely to develop a myocardial infarction as nonsmoking women (Haskell *et al.*, 1994). Smoking cigarettes increases heart rate, blood pressure, and peripheral vascular resistance. Together, this increases the workload of the heart and, over time, could result in heart failure. Many medications—not only those used for cardiac conditions—affect heart rate, rhythm, and blood pressure. Some common examples are cold, sinus, and thyroid medications. Caffeine intake in any form also increases heart rate and blood pressure and may lead to dysrhythmia. Caffeine intake can be lowered by drinking decaffeinated coffee, tea, and colas or by substituting other beverages for colas. Lastly, alcohol consumption has been demonstrated to have both beneficial and harmful effects. Some of the beneficial effects are lowered incidence of atherosclerosis and lower cholesterol levels, and harmful effects include elevated blood pressure and increased cardiac output at rest. Recent studies have reached opposing conclusions concerning mortality and morbidity among those who consume light to moderate amounts of alcohol (Haskell *et al.*, 1994).

Body Position

Because blood is a fluid and depends on many factors, including gravity, body position affects blood pressure. When an individual is lying supine, the force of gravity does not need to be overcome; therefore, stroke volume is increased because the heart and blood vessels are essentially at the same level. However, an individual who is sitting upright in a chair feels the effect of gravity. The legs are lower than the heart, and blood must overcome gravity to return to the heart. The result could be decreased venous return and a resulting increased blood pressure as the cardiovascular system compensates for this (Kennedy, 1990).

Temperature

A consistent body temperature is required for normal functioning of the body. Heat is a product of metabolic processes and absorption of heat from the environment when atmospheric temperatures are higher than body temperature. The autonomic nervous system attempts to maintain the normal body temperature by means of vasodilation or vasoconstriction. If body temperature is rising, the autonomic nervous system is activated, causing an increased diameter of a vessel due to relaxation of the vessel's smooth muscle. This allows blood to flow freely into capillaries near the body's surface, which allows heat to radiate into the surrounding air. The opposite occurs when the environmental temperatures are cold: Blood vessels constrict, causing the blood to flow more deeply within the body, resulting in prevention of environmental cooling.

Coping and Stress Tolerance

Factors such as stress, pain, and anxiety may all result in an increased blood pressure and heart rate. This is a result of vasoconstriction from the autonomic nervous system and direct stimulation of the adrenal gland, which releases epinephrine. If these emotions are extreme, the opposite physiological effects are possible.

Chronic Conditions Affecting Circulation

Angina pectoris is a chest pressure or pain sensation, frequently described as squeezing, burning, uncomfortable epigastric pain or gaslike pain. This pain may be or is often located in the precordial area and can radiate to the left shoulder, jaw, arm, or neck (Fig. 30–3). The duration of pain is usually less than 5 minutes and can be relieved by rest or nitroglycerin, a vasodilator. Angina occurs when myocardial **ischemia** (deficiency of blood) develops as the result of myocardial oxygen demand being greater than the supply. Some common causes of angina are physical exertion, exposure to cold, stress, coronary artery obstruction, and coronary vasospasm.

Myocardial **infarction** (commonly called a heart attack) is the death of cardiac tissue, caused by either a decrease in oxygen supply to the heart or excess myocardial demand for oxygen. In the year 1992, the

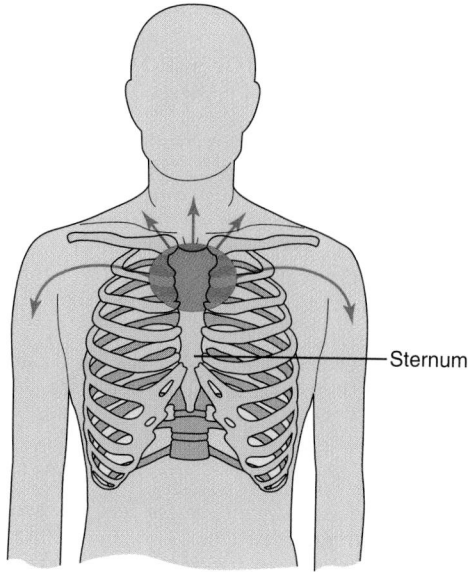

ANGINA PECTORIS

Location of pain usually
• Is substernal
• Is middle or lower sternum or retrosternal
• May radiate to the neck, jaw, shoulders,
  or arms

❧ **Figure 30–3**
Angina pectoris is the result of myocardial oxygen demand being
greater than the supply. Physical exertion, stress, exposure to cold,
coronary artery obstruction, and coronary vasospasm are common
causes of angina.

American Heart Association (1992) estimated that 1.5
million individuals suffered a myocardial infarction
and that 1 million individuals survived the event. Coronary artery disease remains the leading cause of a
myocardial infarction. Other causes are provided in
Box 30–1. Risk factors for a myocardial infarction include smoking, hypertension, diabetes mellitus, obesity, and high cholesterol levels. These risk factors are
the same in the general population as for those individuals with coronary artery disease (CAD). Typical
symptoms include chest pain, which may radiate as in
angina pectoris. Additional symptoms include tachycardia, anxiety, cool pale skin, fatigue, and weakness.
The pain of a myocardial infarction is not relieved by
rest or nitroglycerin.

The elderly are at risk for a myocardial infarction
secondary to the development of atherosclerosis. As
the cardiac vessels narrow from increasing atherosclerosis, it is easier for **thrombus** formation to occur,
resulting in occluded coronary circulation.

A *cerebral vascular accident* (CVA) is commonly
referred to as a "stroke." The term is used to connote
neurological changes that arise from compromised
blood flow to the brain. There are many causes for
CVA, including thrombotic causes (related to atherosclerosis) and infarction. Risk factors for CVA include
advanced age, diabetes mellitus, heart disease, hypertension, and atherosclerosis. Specific signs and symptoms of CVA are determined by the area of the brain
involved. They include loss of consciousness, sensory
deficits, aphasia, visual disturbances, motor impairment, and cognitive impairment.

Hypertension is diagnosed by two or more
blood pressure readings with a systolic pressure of 140
mmHg or greater or a diastolic pressure of 90 mmHg
or greater. In the elderly, hypertension is defined as a
systolic blood pressure of 160 mmHg or greater and a
diastolic of 90 mmHg or greater. The prevalence of
hypertension (systolic and diastolic) in the elderly
population of the United States ranges from 44 to 63%
for whites and 60 to 76% for African-Americans (Selig,
1991). Hypertension is viewed as the "silent killer"
because frequently there are no symptoms of the disease until a catastrophic event occurs, such as kidney
failure or CVA. Refer to Box 30–2 for hypertension
risk factors.

Box **30–1**

CAUSES OF MYOCARDIAL INFARCTION

Coronary thrombus

Coronary vessel spasm

Tachycardia, which decreases coronary artery blood
    flow

Anemia

Hypoxia

Atherosclerosis

High stress levels

Lack of exercise

Box **30–2**

RISK FACTORS FOR HYPERTENSION

Age: Increases in likelihood after age 50

Race: African-Americans have higher incidence than
general population

Family history: If one or more parents have hypertension, likelihood increases in their children

Heart disease, kidney disease: Heart and kidney disease increase risk

Obesity: Increases strain on the heart, frequently leading to hypertension

High-sodium diet: Sodium increases blood volume,
resulting in increased work for the heart

High cholesterol: Causes blockage of blood vessels

Smoking: Causes vasoconstriction

Application of the Nursing Process to Circulatory Disorders

Assessment

Nursing History

The health history for cardiovascular assessment must focus on current, as well as past, problems related to circulation. In addition, family history, health practices, and teaching needs may be identified through the health history.

Current Health History

In this area, it is important to ascertain the client's interpretation of the functioning of his or her cardiovascular system. Important areas to include in this section are the presence or absence of

1. Chest pain or discomfort
2. Palpitations or irregular pulse
3. Dizziness
4. Edema
5. Medications: prescribed or over the counter
6. Fatigue or weakness
7. Shortness of breath on exertion

Each of these areas should be carefully reviewed with the client to obtain a complete history, which will help guide the physical examination. Questions should be open ended to provide the client with an opportunity to fully explain and describe answers. Sample questions are provided in Box 30–3.

The first set of questions is concerned with eliciting the client's cardiac condition and determining if there is any reason to suspect any current conditions such as angina or myocardial infarction.

The second group of questions focuses on heart rate and rhythm from the client's perspective. This information provides the nurse with information that may provide insight into cardiac irregularities or the effect of exercise or stress on the heart.

The third group of questions seeks out information in relation to decreased cardiac output, decreased blood volume, and abnormalities about blood pressure. Medications such as antihypertensives or tricyclic antidepressants can frequently cause postural hypotension, especially in the elderly.

Questions in group four provide the nurse with information about both the heart and the peripheral vascular system. They can provide clues into adequacy of circulation and activity levels.

The last questions relate to medication use, both prescription and over the counter, as both could affect blood pressure, heart rate, and sodium intake. Many clients do not consider over-the-counter medication

---

Box 30–3

SAMPLE QUESTIONS FOR HEALTH HISTORY

1. Do you have any chest pain, pressure, or discomfort? If you do, does it radiate anywhere? How severe would you rate your pain on a scale of 0 to 10, with 10 being the worst pain that you ever had? How long have you been having pain/pressure like this? What do you do when you have this pain? What makes the pain worse? What makes the pain better?

2. Do you ever feel that your heart is beating too rapidly or skipping beats? Do you ever feel that your heart is beating too slowly?

3. Do you feel dizzy when you stand up? Do you get light-headed if you get out of bed too quickly?

4. Do you notice that your legs or feet are swollen at the end of the day? Are they swollen at other times? When you take your socks and shoes off, is there an imprint left behind? When you awaken, are your legs or feet swollen? Do your legs or feet ache? Are they a different color than normal? Are there any sores that do not heal on your feet or legs?

5. What medications do you take? Do you take any nonprescription medications? How often and what is the dose of each medication? Have any of your medications been changed recently?

---

use as an important part of their health history, although it can have significant cardiovascular affects.

Past Health History

The past health history determines any signs or symptoms of disease that the client may have had. Sample questions in this area include

* Do you have any history of, or have you ever been told that you have, high blood pressure, heart disease, stroke, angina, or heart attack?
* Were you ever told that you have a heart murmur or valve problem?
* Were you ever told that you have high cholesterol levels or diabetes?

This information provides guidance and direction for the nurse when he or she conducts the physical examination and the review of systems. These questions may also provoke anxiety for the clients so the nurse must provide follow-up information and guidance in these areas.

Review of Systems

In the review of systems, the nurse asks the client about each specific body system. Carefully directed questions regarding the cardiovascular system help the nurse to gather information about specific areas to be assessed and to assist in developing a plan of care.

Sample questions to include in this area are in Box 30–4.

Some of the questions in this area may be viewed as sensitive areas by the client and therefore require the nurse to be understanding. For example, frequently clients state that they are social drinkers when asked about their alcohol intake. This does not provide adequate information for the health care team to plan the client's care. Many clients do not consider beer and wine to be alcohol, so it is important to question the client specifically about these areas. This information is important because of the specific effects that alcohol may have on nutrition and the cardiovascular system. It is best to ask these questions toward the end of the review of systems, because by then a respectful nurse-client relationship has already been established.

Family History

The client needs to review with the nurse any pertinent family history that may affect cardiovascular health. Sample questions to ask the client in this area are

* Does anyone in your family have heart disease? If so, how are they being treated for it?
* When were they first told that they had this problem?
* Does anyone in your family have high blood pressure, angina, stroke, or myocardial infarction?

Physical Assessment

The physical examination of the chest for cardiovascular assessment involves inspection, auscultation, and palpation. Percussion is sometimes used, but not as a routine assessment tool in the cardiovascular assessment.

Inspection of the Chest

The purpose of inspection of the chest in a cardiovascular examination is to observe abnormal lifts or heaves, symmetry, and general appearance. Lifts or heaves are visible thrust seen during inspection of the chest wall. Normally none are seen, except in thin individuals. The precordium, the anterior of the chest wall overlying the heart and its related structures, should not have any visible pulsation to the right of the sternum. If present, it could represent an aortic aneurysm or rotation of the heart. A forceful pulsation on the left or displaced apical pulse below the fifth intercostal space or laterally from the midclavicular line may indicate ventricular hypertrophy.

The chest is viewed for symmetry in size and shape. The breasts are one exception to the rule of symmetry, because some variance does normally exist in breast size and symmetry. The nurse also notes the coloring of the chest, inspecting for pallor, cyanosis, or jaundice. Additionally, visibly distended veins on the chest should be noted, as these could indicate cardiac or liver abnormalities.

Abnormal findings during inspection of the chest may include barrel chest, scoliosis, kyphosis, use of accessory muscles of respirations, and venous distention.

Inspection of the Extremities

The extremities are inspected for color, hair growth, size, and symmetry. The nurse assesses the color of the extremities compared with the rest of the body and notes areas of increased pigmentation. Nail beds are inspected for color and for whether they are normal, pale, or cyanotic. Normal color of nail beds in all individuals is a pinkish color, similar to the color of the mucous membranes of that individual. Pallor of the nail beds may indicate anemia or shunting of blood away from the extremities to the vital organs, seen in conditions such as in shock. It could also indicate arterial insufficiency or occlusion and must be combined with an assessment of pulses. Cyanosis indicates inadequate oxygenation of blood or stagnant venous return.

Box 30–4

SAMPLE QUESTIONS FOR REVIEW OF SYSTEMS

Describe your diet.

What did you eat yesterday?

What types of foods do you like to eat?

Are there special foods that you like to eat?

Are there certain foods that you cannot eat?

If so, why can't you eat them?

Has your weight changed within the past 3 months?

Have your sleeping patterns changed within the past 2 months?

Do you get up during the night to go to the bathroom? How many times?

How many pillows do you sleep on?

Has this number changed recently?

Do you feel rested when you awaken?

What type of exercise do you do? How often?

Do you have any pain or pressure in your chest when you exercise?

Do you get short of breath during exercising?

Do your legs cramp or throb when you are exercising or walking?

How many cigarettes or cigars do you smoke a day?

When is the last time you smoked?

If you quit, how long has it been since you quit?

What did you do to quit?

How much alcohol do you drink each day?

What types of drinks do you enjoy?

How much beer or wine do you drink per week?

The nail beds are examined for shape and general condition. Clubbing of the nail, in which the angle between the nail and the nail bed is increased, indicates chronic respiratory problems. If nails are brittle or thickened, this may indicate inadequate cardiovascular functioning, resulting in decreased perfusion to the tissue.

Areas of increased pigmentation, especially of the lower extremities, is extremely significant. Increased pigment in the lower extremities may indicate venous insufficiency. It is significant because this is usually related to **varicosities**, which are abnormally dilated blood vessels usually seen in the lower extremities. Venous blood pools in the extremities, causing a buildup of waste products in the cells. This makes tissue breakdown a higher probability because of decreased tissue oxygenation.

Hair growth pattern should be symmetrical in the extremities. Proper tissue oxygenation and nutrition to tissue is necessary for the hair follicle to grow. A lack of hair on the extremities may indicate vascular insufficiency or inadequate **perfusion** from decreased blood flow to an area.

The shape of the extremities should be symmetrical. However, many factors, such as hypertrophy resulting from repetitive exercises to one extremity or neurological deficit resulting in atrophy of an extremity, may alter their size and shape.

Auscultation

Heart Sounds

During auscultation, the nurse assesses for heart rate, rhythm, heart sounds, and murmurs. There are four classical precordial landmarks: aortic area, pulmonic area, tricuspid area, and mitral or apical area (Fig. 30–4).

The aortic area is located to the right of the sternum at the second intercostal space; the pulmonic area is located to the left of the sternum at the second intercostal space; the tricuspid area is located to the left of sternum at the fifth intercostal space; and the mitral or apical area is located at the fifth intercostal space, at the midclavicular line. The areas of auscultation are located not where the actual valves are located, but in the direction of the blood flow through the specific valve.

The sounds auscultated at these areas provide information about the general cardiac condition in addition to the volume and blood flow as it passes through the valve. For example, auscultating the aortic valve provides information regarding adequacy of blood flow through the aortic valve in addition to the general condition of the valve. In addition, auscultating over the mitral area (apical) reflects the general condition of the left ventricle.

The nurse listens in a systematic method to all of the areas. Each area should be auscultated for several seconds so the nurse can distinguish first and second heart sounds, rate, rhythm, and the presence or absence of a murmur. Each area is auscultated with the diaphragm of the stethoscope so the nurse can hear high-pitched sounds (S_1, S_2), as well as with the bell so he or she can hear low-pitched sounds (S_3, S_4).

The nurse listens for the normal cardiac sounds, identified as S_1 and S_2, with the diaphragm of the stethoscope. The first heart sound, S_1, heard as a single heart sound, is heard over the mitral and tricuspid areas. It represents the closing of the mitral and tricuspid valves. S_2 is heard over the aortic and pulmonic areas and represents closing of the aortic and pulmonic valve.

Identifying which sound is S_1 and which is S_2 can be made easier by careful auscultation and practice. The auditory gap between S_1 and S_2 is shorter than between S_2 and S_1. S_1 is frequently thought of as lub and S_2, as dub; thus "lub-dub" is heard. Each of these sounds may also have a split due to closing of valves at slightly different rates. The left ventricle of the heart contracts more forcefully than the right, allowing for faster left ventricular emptying. This enables the valve on the left (mitral) to close quicker than that on the right (tricuspid). This type of splitting effect is normal.

The nurse must also auscultate for extra heart sounds, such as third and fourth heart sounds, and adventitious sounds, such as murmurs. The third heart sound is considered abnormal, except in young children or people with high cardiac outputs, such as athletes. Instead of "lub-dub," the sound is "Ken-Tuc-Ky" with S_3 as the extra sound after ventricular contraction. The third sound represents early, rapid filling of the ventricle. Causes include tricuspid or mitral valve insufficiency, which allows blood to leak backward into the ventricle, as well as congestive heart failure secondary to excessive vascular volume. The third heart sound is best heard at the mitral or tricuspid area with the bell of the stethoscope.

The fourth heart sound, S_4, is never considered normal. It is an atrial abnormality, with the S_4 occurring prior to S_1. Instead of "lub-dub," one hears "Tennes-see," S_4, S_1, S_2. The S_4 occurs after atrial contrac-

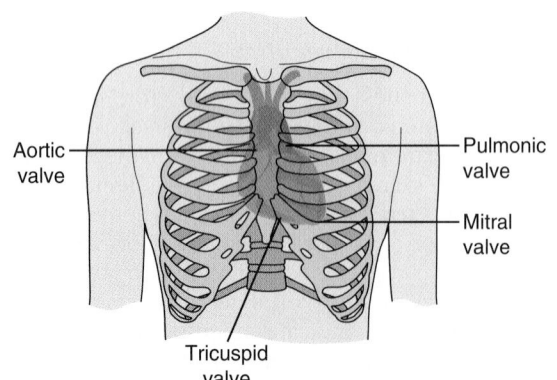

Figure 30–4
The four classic precordial landmarks. The sounds auscultated in these areas provide general information about the heart's condition, as well as information about the volume and flow of blood as it passes through each valve.

Aortic valve

Pulmonic valve

Mitral valve

Tricuspid valve

tion, and the sound is the result of blood rapidly flowing into the ventricle. Causes include hypertension, aortic stenosis, and pulmonic stenosis. **Stenosis** is the narrowing of an area within a vessel that makes it more difficult for blood to flow through the area. The fourth heart sound is best heard at the apical area using the bell of the stethoscope.

Murmurs

Murmurs are abnormal cardiac sounds that may occur at any point in the cardiac cycle. The three main causes of murmurs are (1) an increased blood flow through either normal or abnormal cardiac valves, (2) backward flow through an incompetent valve, and (3) forward flow through a constricted valve.

It is necessary to describe murmurs as completely as possible to aid in the diagnosis and the severity of the murmur. The seven items in Box 30–5 must be consistently evaluated and documented. Timing refers to when the murmur occurs in relation to systole and diastole. For example, a murmur may be referred to as systolic, diastolic, or pansystolic. *Intensity* refers to grading the loudness of the murmur. The acceptable scale is from I to VI, with I being barely audible, and grade VI being very loud (see Box 30–5). *Quality* describes the pattern and pitch of the murmur. Three common patterns are crescendo (increasingly loud), decrescendo (decreasing in loudness), and crescendo-decrescendo (increasing to a peak and then decreasing in loudness). Location refers to the site at which the murmur is audible. Examples are mitral or tricuspid murmurs. *Radiation* describes where the sound is transmitted. Murmurs radiate in the direction of blood flow. Therefore, for example, a pulmonic murmur radiates upward toward the subclavian area. *Ventilation* describes whether the murmur is affected by the respiratory cycle. *Position* describes whether the murmur is affected by position change, such as turning to the side or sitting forward. Other adventitious sounds include cardiac friction rubs, opening snaps, and ejection clicks.

Blood Pressure

A client with variations in blood pressure (it is either too high or too low) may need frequent blood pressure monitoring, such as at 15-minute intervals. Frequency of measurement depends on overall client condition and the regimen prescribed for the client.

It is important to use a blood pressure cuff of the size appropriate for the client. The blood pressure cuff may have indications on it from the manufacturer that will indicate whether the size is appropriate. See Procedure 30–1 for steps in obtaining blood pressure readings.

Occasionally a client will need careful monitoring of his or her blood pressure once discharged home (Fig. 30–5). Although a client can learn to take a blood pressure using a normal cuff and stethoscope, it is probably easier for the client to use a blood pressure home monitoring device. Instructions for use come with the device. A device with a memory and printout of the client's blood pressure is very useful because the client can bring a report of his or her blood pressures to the health care provider as needed.

At times, it may be necessary to obtain a blood pressure in the leg. Reasons for using the lower extremity may include the presence of intravenous lines in both arms, surgery on the arms, or bilateral mastectomy.

Box **30–5**

DESCRIPTORS FOR MURMUR IDENTIFICATION

Timing: Systolic, diastolic, pansystolic

Intensity: Rated from grade I through VI
  Grade I: Barely audible with a stethoscope on the chest
  Grade II: Still quiet, but audible with a stethoscope
  Grade III: Moderately loud; requires a stethoscope to hear
  Grade IV: Loud; can palpate a thrill
  Grade V: Very loud; can hear with stethoscope partially off of the chest; thrill is palpable
  Grade VI: Extremely loud; may be heard with stethoscope completely off of the chest; thrill always palpable

Quality: Crescendo, decrescendo, crescendo-decrescendo

Location: Valve involved

Radiation: Location of sound

Ventilation: Affect of respiration: increased or decreased

Position: Affected by change of position

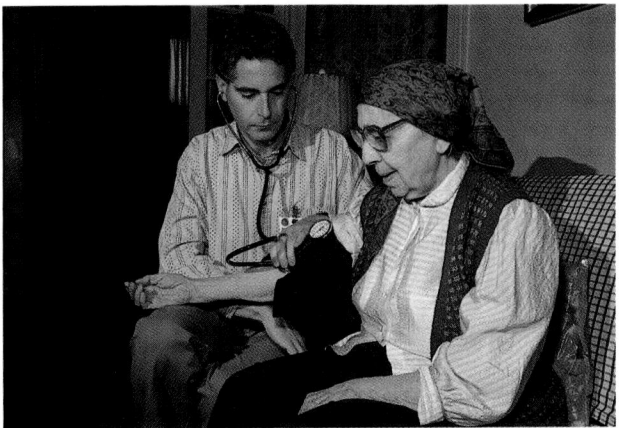

✦ **Figure 30–5**
At times, a client may need careful blood pressure monitoring after discharge. This can be done in the client's home by a community care nurse, as shown here, or the client can be instructed to use a home blood pressure monitoring device.

PROCEDURE

30–1

OBTAINING A BLOOD PRESSURE

Purpose:

Evaluate the client's blood pressure

Monitor effect of medication and treatments on the cardiovascular system

Assessment:

Identify factors that may alter blood pressure (*e.g.,* age, medication, activity, emotional response)

Assess appropriate site to obtain blood pressure; presence of fracture, cast, shunt, or mastectomy would preclude the use of a particular arm

Determine appropriate-size blood pressure cuff

Equipment:

Stethoscope
Sphygmomanometer
Paper and pen

Action	Rationale
Arm	
1. Wash hands and explain procedure to the client	**1.** To prevent the spread of infection and aid cooperation
2. Assist client to a comfortable position with the forearm supported at heart level	**2.** Blood pressure increases when the arm is below heart level and increases when above heart level
3. Expose the arm, ensuring that remaining clothing is not restricting blood flow to the arm; wrap the cuff snugly around the upper arm approximately 2 cm above the antecubital space, placing the center of the cuff bladder over the brachial artery	**3.** Restricting blood flow would result in false readings

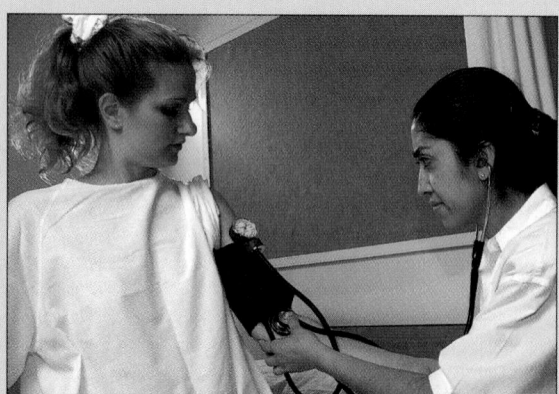

Step 3. *Cuff in place*

OBTAINING A BLOOD PRESSURE

(Continued)

Action	Rationale
4. If using a manometer, place it vertical at eye level.	**4.** To prevent distortion of the reading of the column
5. Palpate the brachial or radial artery with your fingertips; with the valve of the bulb closed, inflate the cuff until the pulse is no longer palpable	**5.** This localizes the pulse
6. Inflate the cuff 30 mmHg higher and slowly release the valve, noting the number when pulse reappears; deflate the cuff while leaving cuff in place if comfortable for the client	**6.** This identifies approximate systolic blood pressure
7. After 1 to 2 minutes, palpate the brachial pulse; place the earpieces of the stethoscope in your ears and place the diaphragm of the stethoscope over the site	**7.** Preparation for taking blood pressure reading

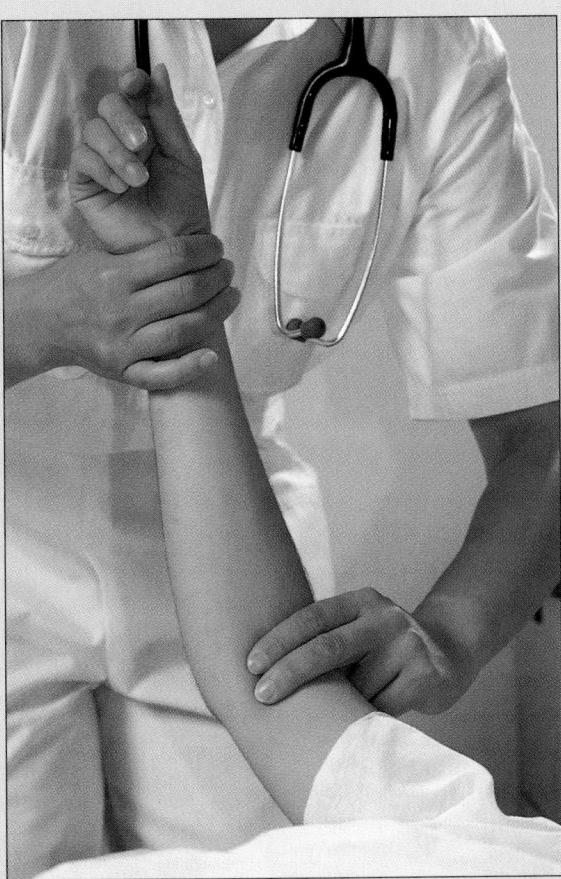

Step 7. *Palpating brachial pulse*

Action	Rationale
8. With the valve of the bulb closed, inflate the cuff to 30 mmHg higher than the reading when the blood pressure disappeared; slowly release the valve so that the pressure drops by 2 to 4 mmHg each second	**8.** Permits more precise identification of first Korotkoff sound
9. Listen and identify when the first clear Korotkoff sound is heard	**9.** This is the systolic blood pressure
10. Continue to slowly deflate the cuff pressure, noting when the sound muffles or dampens (fourth Korotkoff) and when it totally disappears (fifth Korotkoff); fully deflate the cuff and remove it if appropriate	**10.** The American Heart Association recommends the use of the fifth Korotkoff sound as the diastolic pressure for adults and the fourth Korotkoff sound in children

Continued

OBTAINING A BLOOD PRESSURE
(Continued)

Action	Rationale
11. Record the blood pressure as systolic/diastolic pressure (*e.g.*, 120/70); if third sound is recorded, it should be recorded as systolic/fourth Korotkoff sound/fifth Korotkoff sound (*e.g.*, 120/90/70); indicate which site was used for monitoring the blood pressure	11. Provides written data for analysis and comparison

Leg

1. Wrap the appropriate-size blood pressure cuff around the thigh; place the stethoscope in the popliteal space and proceed as in taking the blood pressure in the arm

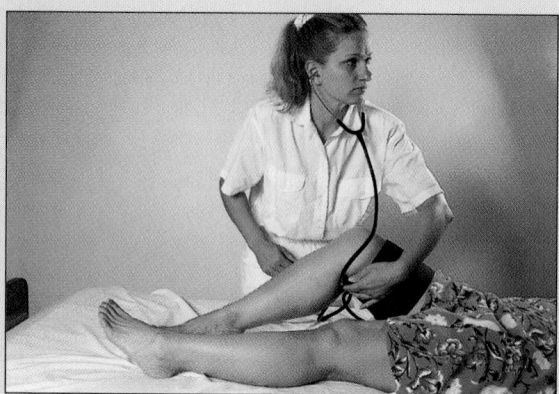

Step 1. *Cuff on thigh*

Palpation

The precordium is palpated for thrills over the valvular locations. Thrills are abnormal, turbulent blood flow through the cardiac valves. It is important to note their presence so that they may be auscultated during the appropriate part of the examination. The apical pulse is palpated at the left midclavicular line in the fifth intercostal space.

Peripheral pulses should be assessed in a systematic manner. Pulses must be assessed bilaterally to determine symmetry and equality. Essential characteristics to be assessed include rate, strength, and rhythm. Peripheral pulses commonly assessed are temporal, carotid, brachial, radial, femoral, popliteal, tibial, and pedal. The carotid pulse must be assessed only one side at a time to prevent stimulation of baroreceptors and decreased cardiac output. Besides pulses, the nurse must also check color and warmth of the extremities. Any absent pulse, with decreased warmth and abnormal color, is a serious condition indicating

arterial occlusion and warrants immediate intervention (Baker, 1991; Blank & Irwin, 1990; Hubner, 1988).

As the heart contracts during systole, it exerts a blood flow (pressure) through the arteries. Blood pressure is determined by the amount of blood, the tone (peripheral vascular resistance) of the arteries, and cardiac output. When taking a blood pressure, you may hear five phases of **Korotkoff sounds** (blood pressure). However, only phase 1 and phase 5, the systolic and diastolic, are usually recorded in practice. For an explanation of each sound, refer to Box 30–6.

Pulses

The nurse must be familiar with methods of obtaining a pulse. When first learning to obtain an apical pulse, count the number of beats for an entire minute. Once secure in identification of the apical rate, you can auscultate the heart for 30 seconds or 15 seconds and multiply by the appropriate number to obtain a rate per minute, as long as the rhythm is regular.

BOX 30–6

KOROTKOFF SOUNDS

Phase I: Initial, faint tapping sound that increases to a loud tap

Phase II: Sound changes to a softer swishing

Phase III: The sound again becomes crisp in nature

Phase IV: Muffled sounds with a blowing quality

Phase V: Sound totally disappears

(See Procedure 30–2 for methods of obtaining a pulse.)

The carotid pulse is felt with the tips of the forefingers, just lateral to the trachea and to the center of the angle of the jaw and the edge of the sternocleidomastoid muscle. Do not palpate both carotid pulses at the same time, as this could cause compromised blood flow to the brain.

The brachial pulse is palpated with the tips of the forefingers medial to the biceps tendon. This is easily identified at or just above the elbow. The brachial pulse is routinely used in newborn assessment. This pulse is located in the antecubital area, usually in the medial aspect of the arm. The radial pulse is located at the wrist on the radial side (lateral) just proximal to the thumb. The ulnar pulse is also located at the wrist on the ulnar side (medial) proximal to the little finger. This pulse is sometimes more difficult to palpate than the radial pulse but should be routinely assessed.

The femoral pulse can be palpated midway between the iliac crest and the symphysis pubis. It is necessary to press firmly and deeply to obtain this pulse. The popliteal pulse is more easily palpated with the knee flexed. Using both hands, palpate deeply behind the knee in the popliteal space. The posterior tibial pulse can be located behind the medial malleolus of the ankle. The dorsalis pedis pulse is located on the dorsum of the foot. Both the posterior tibial and dorsalis pedis pulse are sometimes difficult to obtain and may be absent, especially in the elderly, as a result of atherosclerosis.

The client should be taught how to take his or her own radial pulse if being discharged on cardiac medications or if the condition necessitates it. Sometimes the client may need to learn to take the carotid pulse. When teaching the client to take the carotid pulse, ensure that he or she takes the pulse on one side of the neck to avoid decreasing blood flow to the head and stimulating carotid receptors. Have the client demonstrate the procedure to the nurse prior to discharge.

At times, a pulse deficit may exist in which the apical pulse may be greater than the radial pulse. Therefore, you must assess for a pulse deficit in all individuals displaying signs of decreased cardiac output caused by cardiac disease, electrolyte imbalance, or a history of **dysrhythmia** (abnormal cardiac rhythm) (Procedure 30–3).

Capillary Refill

Capillary refill is tested by applying pressure over the fingernail or toenail and causing blanching of the nail. On release of the pressure, color **(capillary refill)** should take place within 3 seconds. If capillary refill takes longer than 3 seconds, there is decreased perfusion to the area, which could indicate decreased cardiac output or inadequate circulation such as is commonly seen in clients with arteriosclerosis.

Diagnostic Tests

The following are examples of diagnostic tests that provide important information about the client's cardiovascular status.

Cardiac Enzymes

This is a blood test that assists in the differentiation between angina and myocardial infarction. Enzymes are present in many cells throughout the body and are not cardiac specific. On death of cells, the enzymes are released from the cells and enter cardiac circulation. Enzymes such as creatinine phosphokinase (CPK), lactic dehydrogenase (LDH), and aspartate aminotransferase (AST) are located widely in the body. However, these enzymes have subtypes of themselves called isoenzymes. Some of these isoenzymes exist only in certain types of tissue. There are specific forms of these isoenzymes that are only located in the heart. As a result, cardiac isoenzymes are used to determine the degree of cardiac necrosis.

The CPK enzyme has three forms, one of which (CPK-MB) is specific for cardiac tissue. LDH isoenzymes may also be used to determine cardiac necrosis. There are five LDH isoenzymes, LDH_1 through LDH_5. Normally, LDH_1 is present in smaller amounts than LDH_2. When LDH_1 levels are greater than LDH_2 levels, this is known as a flipped pattern and is indicative of a myocardial infarction.

There is no special client preparation for this isoenzyme test. It can be performed at any time regardless of activity, meals, or medication. The nurse must ensure that the blood specimen is drawn at the specific time ordered. As with most tests, the specimen should be sent to the laboratory immediately or placed on ice for examination at a later time. Client teaching should focus on the reporting of chest pain or any discomfort associated with cardiac ischemia, because cardiac enzymes are tested in relation to cardiac events. Protocols for isoenzyme testing vary from every 8 hours for 24 hours to once a day for 3 days after cardiac symptoms.

Complete Blood Count

The complete blood count (CBC) is a blood specimen that evaluates the red and white blood cells for size, shape, and number. Specifically related to the cardiovascular examination, the nurse must assess the red blood cell count (RBC), hemoglobin, hematocrit, platelets, and white blood cell count (WBC). Refer to

Text continued on page 909

PROCEDURE

30–2

OBTAINING A PULSE

Purpose:

To obtain a baseline measurement of both heart rate and rhythm

To evaluate the response of the heart to various therapeutic modalities

To evaluate blood flow to an extremity

Assessment:

Obtain client history

Identify factors that may influence pulse (*e.g.*, age, gender, smoking, volume status, pain, anxiety)

Identify appropriate site for obtaining the pulse

Equipment:

Watch with a second hand
Paper and pen
Stethoscope
Doppler and gel (optional)

Action	Rationale
Apical Pulse	
1. Wash hands and explain procedure to the client	1. To protect client from infection and alleviate anxiety
2. Position client in a supine and sitting position; expose the client's left side of the chest	2. This allows easy access and a clear area for auscultation
3. If necessary, warm the diaphragm of the stethoscope in your hand for 10 to 15 seconds	3. This will be more comfortable for the client and decrease chilling
4. Insert the earpieces of the stethoscope into your ears and place the diaphragm over the apex of the client's heart; this is usually at the fifth intercostal space, left midclavicular line	4. This allows for hearing high-pitched sounds, such as S_1 and S_2; in women it may be necessary to lift the breast to find the appropriate area

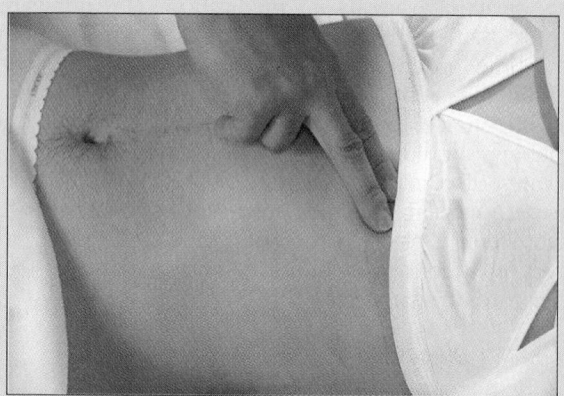

Step 4. *Apical pulse*

5. Assess the heartbeat for both rate and regularity	5. Heart rate is normally between 60 and 100 beats per minute and regular in rhythm

PROCEDURE

30-2

OBTAINING A PULSE
(Continued)

Action	Rationale
6. If rhythm is regular, count the heartbeat for 30 seconds and multiply by two; if the rhythm is irregular, count for a full minute	**6.** If the heart rate is irregular, the rate may vary greatly; for accuracy, take the pulse for a full minute
7. Replace the client's gown	**7.** This ensures privacy
8. Record the pulse on your paper and then in the appropriate client record	**8.** This will assist in the accurate transmission of assessment findings

Upper Extremity Pulse

Action	Rationale
1. Wash hands and explain the procedure to the client	**1.** This protects the client from infection and alleviates anxiety
2. Position client so that his or her arm is comfortably flexed across the chest or at the side	**2.** This position will allow you to locate the pulse more easily
3. Place fingertips of your first two or three fingers at the client's wrist along the groove at the base of the thumb	**3.** This is the location of the radial pulse

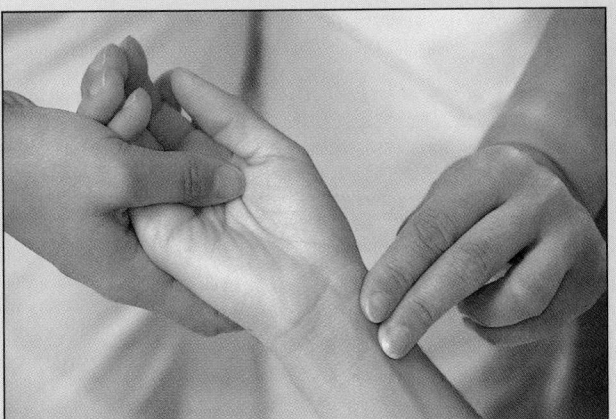

Step 3. *Radial pulse*

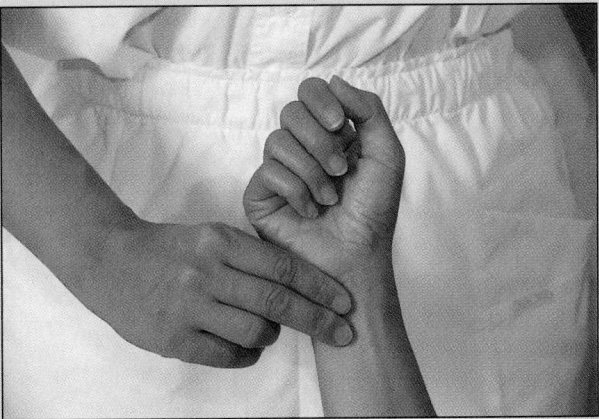

Step 3. *Ulnar pulse*

Action	Rationale
4. Apply moderate pressure against the radial artery to occlude the pulse, then gradually release pressure until the pulse is felt	**4.** Releasing the pressure allows you to feel the pulsation against your fingers
5. Assess the pulse for both rhythm and strength	**5.** Pulse should feel regular and strong

6. If pulse is not present or is weak, use a Doppler
    Apply gel to pulse site
    Turn on the Doppler by depressing the appropriate button or turning the switch "on"
    Place probe against the skin of the pulse site and reposition until sound is heard
    If pulse is regular, count for 15 to 30 seconds; if irregular, count for 60 seconds
	6. This allows you to "listen" to the blood flowing through the artery

7. To take an ulnar pulse, the procedure is the same as for taking the radial pulse, except palpate it on the ulner side of the wrist.	

Continued

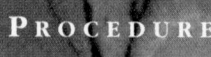

PROCEDURE

30–2

OBTAINING A PULSE
(Continued)

Action	Rationale

Lower Extremity Pulse

1. The same procedure as for the upper extremities is used except on any of the lower extremity pulses: femoral, popliteal, posterior tibial, or dorsalis pedis

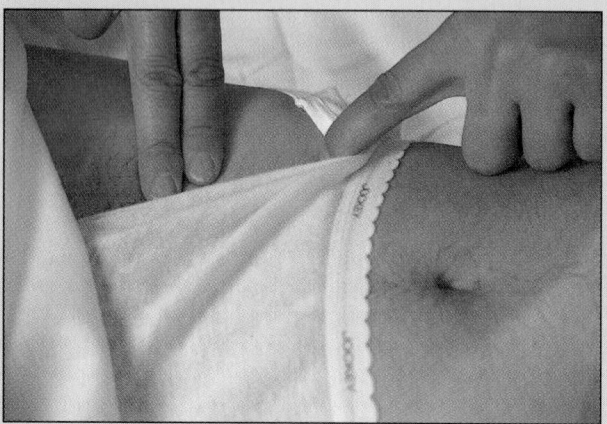

Step 1. *Femoral pulse*

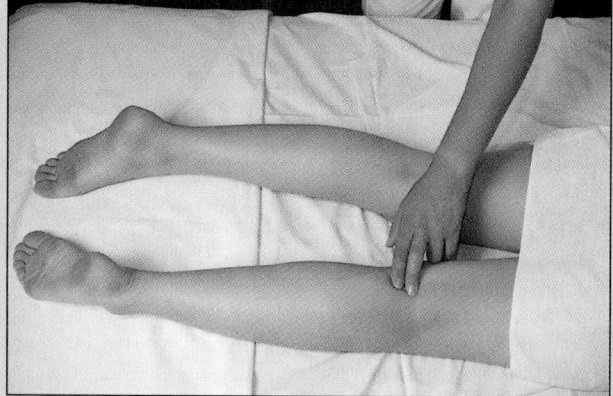

Step 1. *Popliteal pulse*

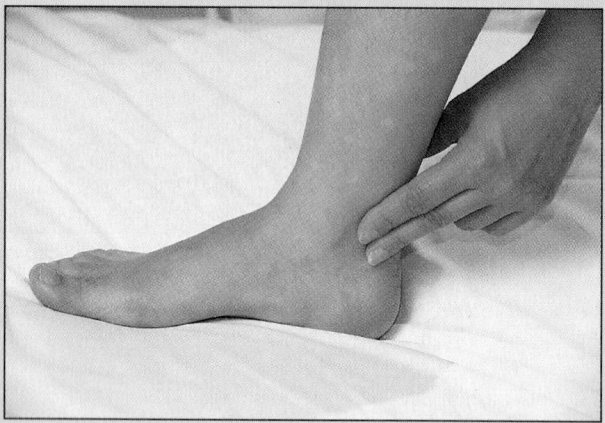

Step 1. *Posterior tibial pulse*

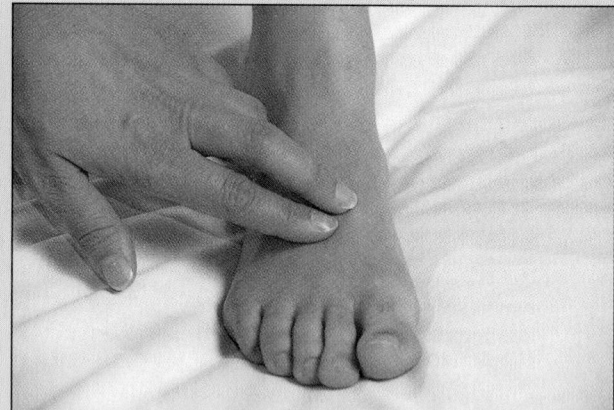

Step 1. *Dorsalis pedis pulse*

PROCEDURE

30–2

OBTAINING A PULSE
(Continued)

Action	Rationale

Carotid Pulse

1. The same procedure is used for the carotid pulse; however, only one carotid pulse may be palpated at a time

1. Cerebral blood flow may be compromised if both pulses are palpated at the same time

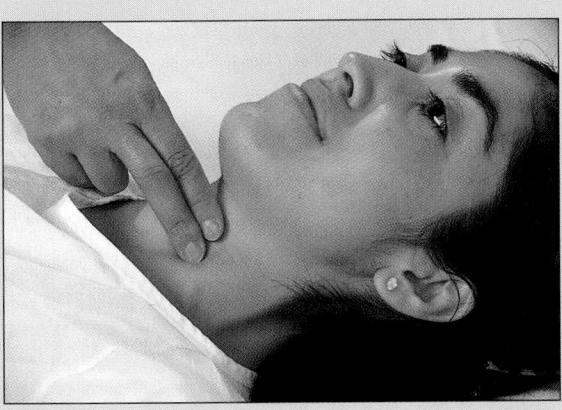

Step 1. *Carotid pulse*

Table 30–1 for normal values. The RBC, hemoglobin, and hematocrit are important for determining the oxygen-carrying capacity of the blood. With normal values, the tissues in the body are able to obtain adequate oxygen, provided the rest of the systems are normal. If values are low, oxygen-carrying capacity is diminished, which will decrease oxygen availability to tissues. This could increase the likelihood of angina in a person with atherosclerosis. If values are high, the viscosity of the blood may be too high, leading to increased blood clot formation, which could lead to myocardial infarction or CVA.

Platelets are assessed for adequacy in number. A low platelet count may result in spontaneous bleeding or hemorrhaging. The nurse would need to carefully assess the client for any signs of bleeding, both overt and covert. A high platelet count may lead to increased clotting ability, which could result in myocardial infarction or CVA.

The WBC is assessed for elevation to detect any infection or inflammatory process within the body. In terms of a cardiac assessment, after a myocardial infarction or in pericarditis, the WBCs are elevated due to an inflammatory process.

There is no special preparation for these laboratory tests other than explanation of the test to the client.

Lipid Profile

The lipid profile involves the collection of a blood specimen that is examined for total cholesterol and its three components: high-density lipoprotein cholesterol (HDL-C), low-density lipoprotein cholesterol (LDL-C), and triglyceride. Total cholesterol provides information about the overall cholesterol level in the blood, made up of HDL-C, LDL-C, and very low–density lipoprotein. When a total cholesterol level is reported, specific values for each type of cholesterol are not provided. This test is used as a screening procedure for individuals at risk for heart disease. Adults should have cholesterol levels checked at least every 5 years (National Cholesterol Education Program, 1993). Refer to Box 30–7 for cholesterol values.

High-density lipoprotein cholesterol provides a value for the "good" cholesterol, which is believed to have a beneficial effect within the body. This cholesterol removes cholesterol from cells and transports it to the liver, where it is secreted in bile (Hulley *et al.*, 1992). The higher the HDL-C, the more benefit for the client. A HDL level below 35 mg/dl is considered too low.

Low-density lipoprotein cholesterol provides a value for the "bad" cholesterol. LDLs carry blood cholesterol from the blood to the cells of the body, and a high LDL level is directly related to coronary heart

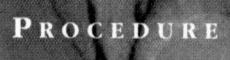

PROCEDURE

30–3

ASSESSING FOR PULSE DEFICITS

Purpose:

To determine if there is a difference between apical and radial pulses

Assessment:

Identify clients at risk for a pulse deficit (*e.g.*, elderly clients, those with history of dysrhythmia)
Assess for altered cardiac output

Equipment:

Watch with second hand
Stethoscope
Paper and pen

Action	Rationale
1. Wash hands and explain procedure to the client	**1.** This prevents the spread of infection and alleviates anxiety
2. Position the client for comfort while allowing easy access to the client's chest and radial pulse	**2.** Increases cooperation
3. After warming stethoscope, apply to apex of the heart	**3.** This allows the apical pulse to be taken
4. Second examiner places fingers on the client's radial pulse	**4.** This allows the radial pulse to be taken at the same time
5. Place watch where both examiners can view it; agree on when to start counting the pulse and do so for a full minute	**5.** This allows for the simultaneous counting of both pulses
6. Reposition the client	**6.** Ensures client comfort
7. Record the findings in the appropriate client records	**7.** Documents data for use and comparison

disease. For this test, the lower the value, the better for the client. An LDL level below 130 mg/dl is desirable. LDL levels of 130 to 159 mg/dl are borderline high. Levels of 160 mg/dl or above are high levels and are indicative of a high risk for coronary heart disease.

Triglycerides provide a means of storing fat in the body. They may also play a role in the development of CAD. Triglycerides in food are made up of saturated, polyunsaturated, and monounsaturated fats. The liver also produces triglycerides. When alcohol is consumed or when excess calories are taken in, the liver produces more triglycerides. It has not been determined whether high triglycerides cause narrowing of the arteries (Fig. 30–6) or are just associated with other risk factors like low levels of HDL-C and being overweight. It is desirable to have low triglyceride levels.

These lipid profile laboratory tests are sensitive to dietary intake. Therefore, it is recommended that the client not eat anything for at least 8 hours prior to the test. Based on the results of the lipid profile, dietary teaching may be necessary. Changing eating habits may be all that is necessary to lower LDL values. Sample dietary changes include cutting back on foods rich in fat, especially saturated fat, and in cholesterol. Weight loss for overweight persons also will lower cholesterol levels. Losing extra weight, quitting smoking, and increasing activity may boost HDL-C levels. To reduce triglyceride levels, a low-fat, low-calorie, weight-controlled diet and increased exercise is recommended.

Electrocardiography

The **electrocardiogram** (ECG) is a noninvasive method of viewing electrical activity of the heart. However, it does not provide information regarding the mechanical, contractile ability of the heart.

An ECG is typically performed with 12 leads,

	NEWBORN	CHILD	MALE ADULT	FEMALE ADULT
RBC*	4.8–7.1	4.5–4.8	4.6–6.2	4.2–5.4
Hemoglobin, g/dl	14–24	11–16	13.5–18	12–16
Hematocrit, %	44–64	35–41	40–54	38–47
Platelets†	140–300	150–450	150–450	150–450
WBC‡	9–30	5–13	5–10	5–10

Table 30–1

NORMAL COMPLETE BLOOD COUNT VALUES

*Million/mm³.

†One billion/mm³.

‡1000/mm³.

which provide 12 distinct views of the electrical activity of the heart. More advanced cardiac testing may involve an 18-lead ECG. Electrodes for the standard 12-lead ECG that measure the electrical activity of the heart are placed on the four extremities, in addition to six chest leads. The ECG provides the clinician with useful information about the client, such as heart rate and rhythm, areas of ischemia, and electrical blocks within the cardiac conduction system (Fig. 30–7). Serial ECGs, performed at least daily for 3 days after the patient has angina are useful in determining progression to a myocardial infarction.

Client preparation includes an explanation of the test to enhance cooperation during the procedure. The leads may be attached to the client temporarily with adhesive, gel, or straps. As a result, the client may have feelings of coolness or tightness on the extremities or chest. The client will have his or her chest exposed, so it is necessary to provide for privacy by closing doors or shutting curtains. During the ECG, the client must be still and quiet because the ECG records all muscle activity—not only cardiac muscle activity. The nurse must gain the cooperation of the client during the procedure.

Exercise Stress Testing

Exercise **stress testing** provides a means of determining cardiac function under a prescribed amount of induced physical stress. The most frequently used method of performing a stress test is by means of a treadmill; however, the clinician may instead use a step test or bicycle ergometer.

During testing, the client performs the specific exercise, usually walking on a treadmill, while the ECG and blood pressure are monitored. The amount of exercise is increased gradually until a predetermined level of exercise is attained, a predetermined heart rate is obtained, or the client develops chest pain. The development of chest pain, severe shortness of breath, ECG changes, or a decrease of blood pressure is highly suggestive of coronary heart disease. Stress tests may also utilize the infusion of medications such as thallium or persantine, which assist in detecting abnormal blood flow or activity within the heart.

Box 30–7

CHOLESTEROL VALUES

Total Cholesterol

Desirable: <200 mg/ml

Borderline high: 200 to 239 mg/ml

High risk: >239 mg/ml

High-Density Lipoprotein Cholesterol

Desirable: >34 mg/ml

Low-Density Lipoprotein Cholesterol

Desirable: <130 mg/ml

Borderline high: 130 to 159 mg/ml

High risk: >159 mg/ml

Triglyceride

Desirable: <250 mg/ml

Normal artery

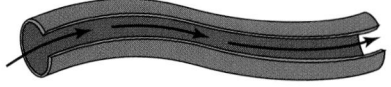

Artery with fatty buildup

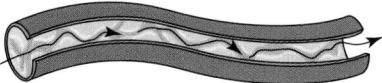

✦ **Figure 30–6**
Triglycerides (saturated, polyunsaturated, and monounsaturated fats) may play a role in the development of coronary artery disease. It has not yet been determined whether high triglyceride levels cause narrowing of the arteries or are associated only with other risk factors such as low levels of HDL-C.

Normal Sinus Rhythm

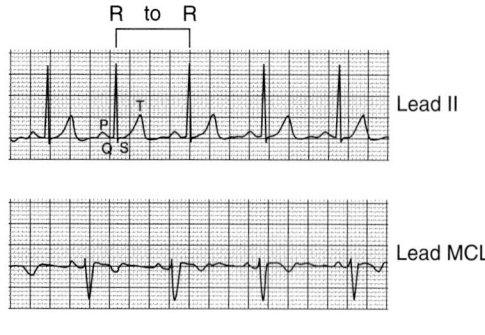

Lead II

Lead MCL₁

Normal Conditions With Normal
Sinus Rhythm

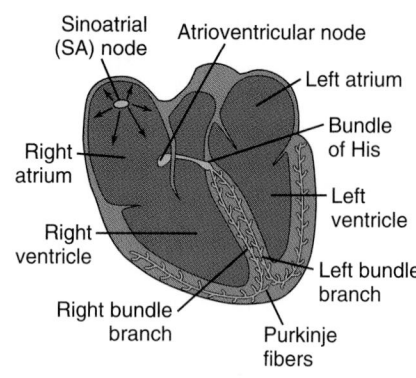

Normal Sinus Rhythm

P waves: Similar, 1:1 with QRS
Rate: Atrial: 60–100 beats per min
    Ventricular: 60–100 beats per min
Rhythm: Atrial–regular
    Ventricular–regular
P–R Interval: 0.12–0.20 sec
QRS Interval: 0.04–0.10 sec
Q–T Interval: 0.32–0.44 sec

A

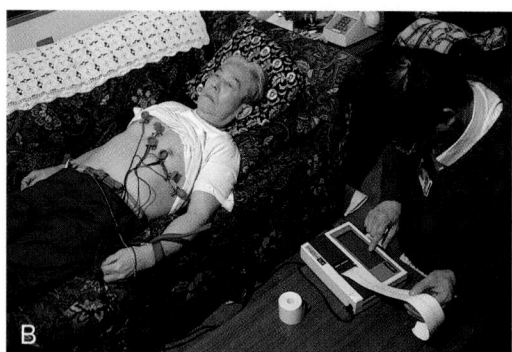

❯ **Figure 30–7**
The ECG provides information about heart rate and rhythm and reveals areas of ischemia and electrical blocks. *A*, The ECG reading on the left shows normal electrical activity; the diagram of the heart on the right shows the sources of the electrical impulses produced on the electrocardiogram. *B*, ECG being performed in a patient's home by a community nurse. The nurse explains to the patient that he may experience a sensation of coolness or tightness where the leads are attached, depending on whether gel, adhesive, or straps are used. The nurse also needs to ensure that the client remains still and quiet during the procedure so that the ECG will record only cardiac muscle activity and not other muscle activity.

Client preparation prior to the procedure includes imparting adequate knowledge of the test, physical preparation, and knowledge of what to report during the test. The client needs to be prepared with the proper clothing, such as well-fitting shoes or sneakers, to perform on the testing machinery.

Doppler Studies

Doppler studies utilize ultrasound waves, which are sent from a probe to body areas and are reflected back to the skin surface. Doppler studies can be useful in determining appearance and function of cardiac structures, as well as blood flow in the peripheral circulation. An echocardiogram is an example of a

Doppler study that looks at the valves of the heart and the functioning of the myocardium.

Special preparation for the client include teaching him or her about what to expect during the test. Because gel is applied to the examination area to transmit the ultrasound waves, clients frequently feel chilled. No pain is felt during this procedure, but the client will feel the pressure of the Doppler probe.

Arteriograms

Cardiac catheterization is a type of **arteriogram.** It is an invasive procedure involving the placing of special flexible catheters within the chambers of the heart and the three coronary vessels. Contrast ma-

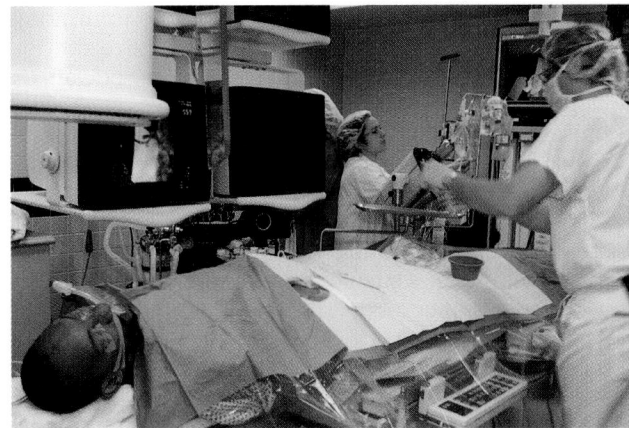

Setting up for angiogram

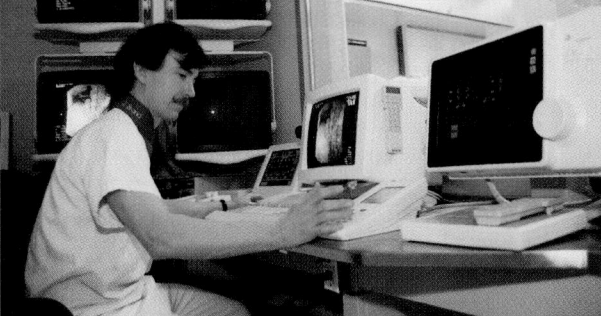

Angiogram control room

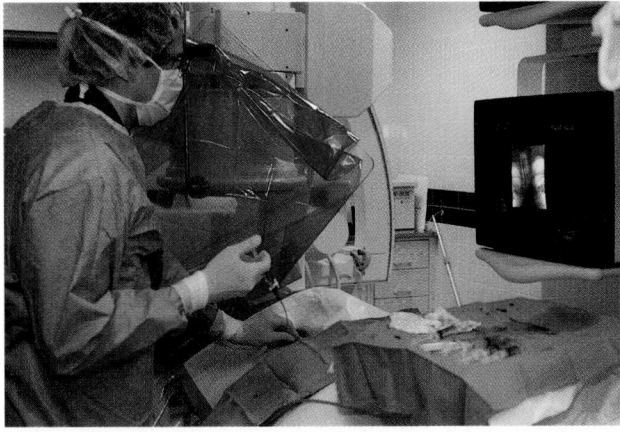

Catheterization

Reading angiogram result (CT scan above)

❧ Figure 30–8
Arteriography yields information about the patency of coronary and other blood vessels. Flexible catheters are placed into blood vessels; in cardiac catheterization, catheters are placed within the chambers of the heart and the three coronary vessels. Contrast material (dye) is injected and its flow observed. Because the dye can precipitate an allergic reaction or kidney failure as well as dehydration, the patient must be carefully assessed before and during the procedure, and adequate fluid resuscitation must be initiated after the procedure.

terial (dye) is injected into the coronary vessels. As the contrast material is injected, its flow is observed and the patency of the coronary vessels can be determined (Fig. 30–8). Sample precardiac catheterization teaching instructions can be found in Box 30–8. Preprocedure teaching of the client should include an explanation of the procedure and the information that although the client may receive a medication to relieve anxiety, he or she will remain awake during the procedure.

Cardiac catheterization may be performed using access from a cutdown site in the arm or percutaneously, usually from the femoral site. With either method, the client must not bend the extremity used after the procedure for several hours. Protocols vary in each institution regarding when the client is allowed to bend the extremity or get out of bed after the cardiac catheterization. In the past, a cardiac catheterization was only performed within the hospital setting; however, presently many of these procedures are being performed on an outpatient basis or even out of hospital setting. Sample postcardiac catheterization instructions are found in Box 30–9.

Arteriograms can also be used to determine the patency of other blood vessels in the peripheral vascular system. These are invasive procedures involving placing catheters into blood vessels and instilling contrast material. Because contrast materials can cause allergic reactions and kidney damage, the client must be carefully questioned for allergy history—especially reaction to iodine and shellfish. Use of newer contrast materials has lessened the likelihood of an allergic reaction. Kidney failure can also result from the high concentration of these materials. The contrast materials have a high osmotic value and can therefore pull fluids from interstitial and cellular spaces, resulting in dehydration. Nursing implications postprocedure include adequate fluid resuscitation via oral or intravenous fluids, which will cause a dilutional effect and replace lost volume.

Holter Monitor

A **Holter monitor** is a device that records each cardiac electrical impulse over an extended period,

---

Box 30–8

PATIENT INSTRUCTIONS: PRECARDIAC CATHETERIZATION

Although you may receive a medication prior to the procedure, the medication will not make you sleep.

You will be brought to the cardiac catheterization laboratory on a stretcher or in a wheelchair, as you would be brought to an operating room.

The cardiac catheterization laboratory will have several monitors, cameras, and other high-technology equipment.

Individuals in the room may include the cardiologist, medical physician, catheterization laboratory nurse, and technician.

The extremity to be used for the cardiac catheterization will be cleansed and draped with sterile towels.

The site will be numbed with a local anesthetic, and the appropriate vessels identified.

The physician will thread the catheter into the heart and obtain pressure readings. Afterwards, the catheter will be advanced into the various coronary arteries to look for patency and possible constriction of the vessels.

Contrast material will be injected to assist in the viewing of the vessels. A feeling of heat may be felt at this phase of the test and will pass quickly.

Pictures of the contrast flowing into the coronary arteries will be taken for review by the staff after the procedure so that the best course of treatment may be determined.

After the procedure, the catheter is removed, a dressing is applied, and pressure is applied to the site for several minutes.

Box 30–9

PATIENT INSTRUCTIONS: DOS AND DON'TS AFTER CARDIAC CATHETERIZATION

DO NOT bend the site where the catheterization was performed until instructed to do so.

If you feel any wetness or see any bleeding, DO notify your nurse immediately.

DO NOT elevate the head of the bed until your nurse tells you that you can. Usually, patients may have the bed elevated slightly (15 degrees).

DO NOT get out of bed until you are told to do so.

Do report any chest pain or pressure immediately.

DO report any redness or swelling at the catheterization site immediately.

---

usually 24 hours. The client is able to perform normal activities wearing a recording device the size of a portable radio around his or her neck or in a pocket. The client is connected to the device with leads similar to those for a 12-lead ECG. The major difference is that the leads are only on the chest, not on the arms or legs. Nursing care emphasizing client teaching about this test is important. Clients should record all of their activities and symptoms and the time they occur in a log to allow coordination of the events with the electrical events recorded. The client must be instructed not to remove any of the leads. Activity is not curtailed during the Holter monitoring (Fig. 30–9).

Chest X-Ray

The chest x-ray may be performed on a single-view or a multiple-view film. A single view is an anterioposterior x-ray in which the client is positioned in front of an unexposed film plate (Fig. 30–10). The

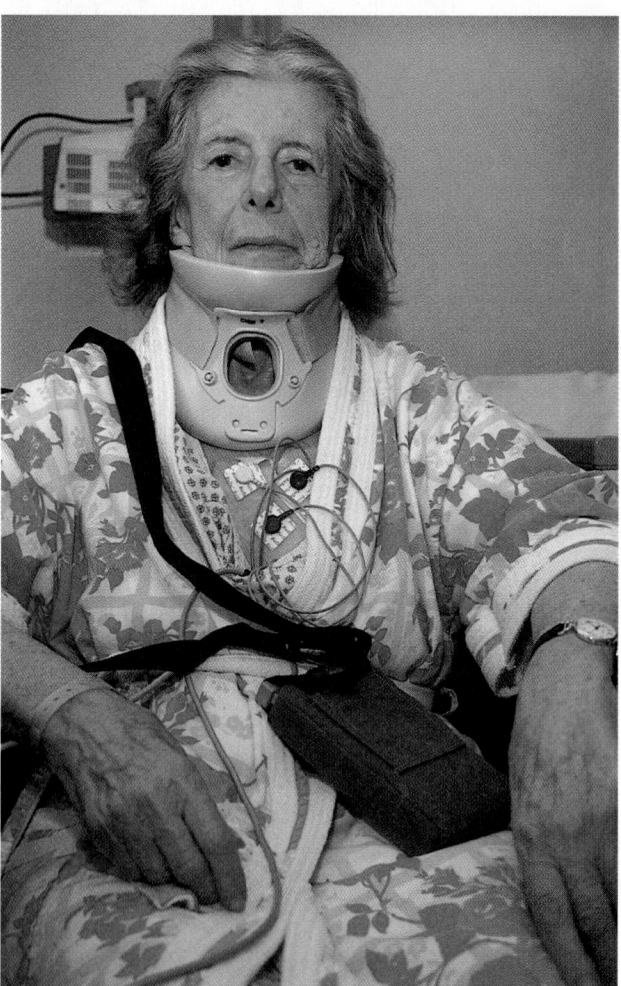

❥ **Figure 30–9**
Client wearing a Holter monitor, which records cardiac electrical activity over an extended period of time, such as 24 hours. The client performs normal activities wearing the device and records all of her activities and symptoms and the time they occurred in a log. When the text is complete, the client's log is compared with the electrical event recorded. Nursing care emphasizes client teaching.

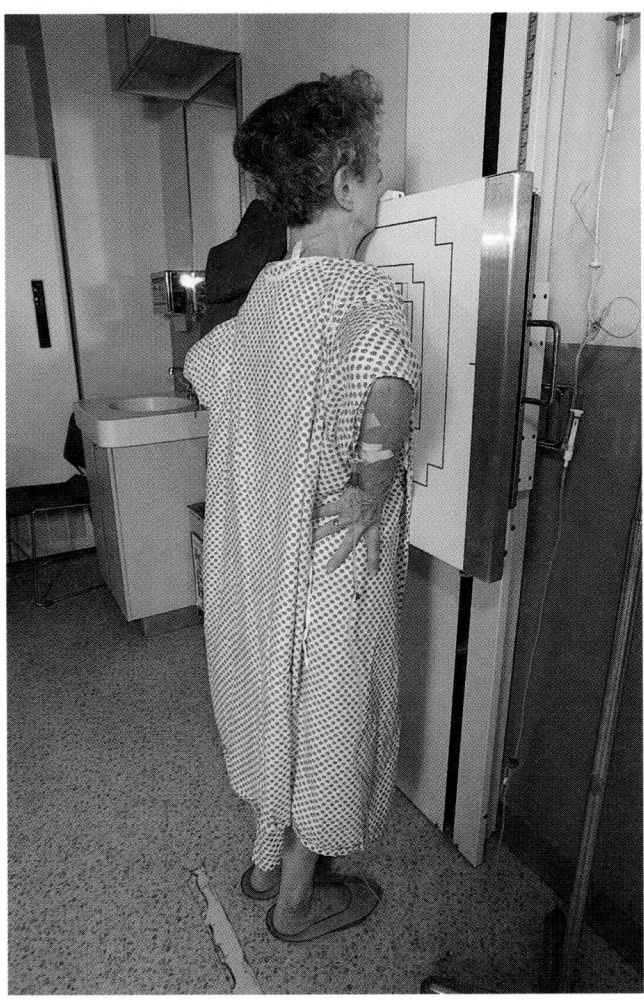

Client positioned for AP view

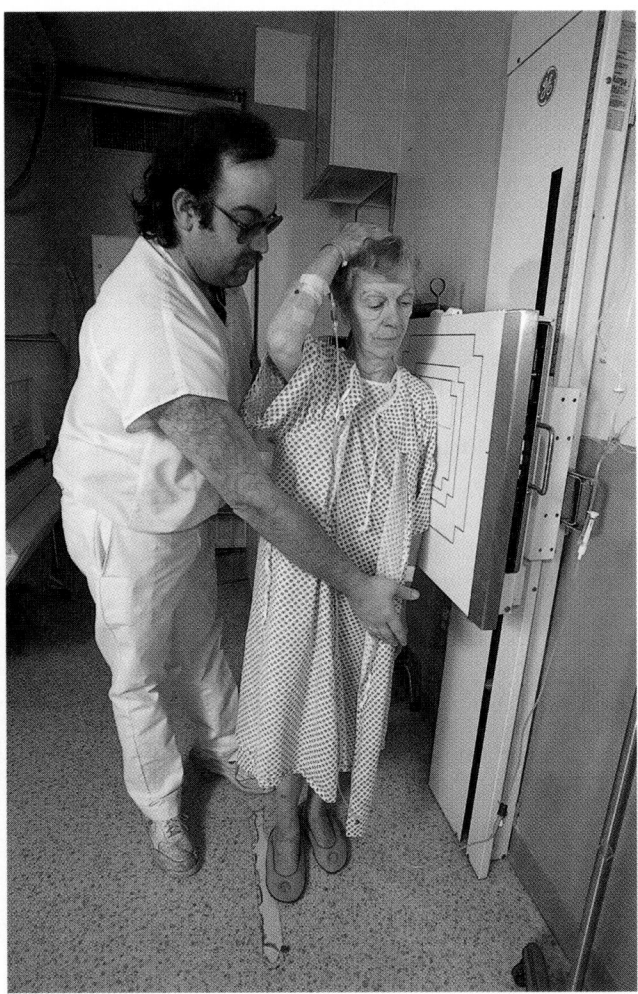

Technician positions client for lateral view

♦ **Figure 30–10**
Chest x-rays provide information about cardiac size and movement of the diaphragm. The physician may request both anteroposterior (AP) and lateral views. The client may need to be reassured that the amount of radiation is not harmful, even if the x-rays are performed daily while the client is critically ill.

chest x-ray may also be taken from the lateral view, in which the client would stand perpendicular to the film plate. This test may provide information about the lungs, as well as about cardiac size and location and calcification of valves and vessels.

The x-ray is taken during full inspiration, and the client must hold his or her breath to do this. This causes the structures of the lungs to be more clearly visible and provides information about movement of the diaphragm and cardiac size. One fear that clients sometimes express in regard to x-rays is radiation exposure. However, the amount of radiation that a client is exposed to during single x-rays, even if performed daily while he or she is critically ill, is not harmful.

Psychosocial Assessment

Preparation

The nurse must prepare the client for all of the necessary tests. This means that the nurse must teach the client about the purpose of the tests, what is involved in conducting the tests, what the client can do to assist in the testing, and what the results mean for that client. Often, the client will receive pieces of information from other health care members, but it is the nurse who must ensure that the client has a correct understanding, which leads to informed choices.

Impact of Diagnosis

A diagnosis of a cardiovascular problem is often viewed as life threatening by clients. Initially, any diagnosis is difficult to accept. Restrictions, such as to the diet or activity, and a medication regimen may be necessary and may alter previous lifestyles. Some clients react to a diagnosis with denial. They cannot believe that there is anything really wrong with them or that they need to change their lifestyle.

Impact of Chronic Condition

A chronic condition for which there is no cure—only abatement of symptoms—forces the client to make choices in his or her life. Some of these choices are following a specific diet, having frequent health care evaluations, and taking medications long term. Often, the client feels powerless or hopeless because of lack of control. The family of the client often attempts to coerce him or her to follow a restricted diet or ensure that he or she takes medications as prescribed. All of these factors could lead to role strain, hopelessness, and powerlessness.

Developmental Assessment

Age affects normal values for both the client's pulse and blood pressure. The elderly tend to develop high blood pressure due to a variety of reasons. The renin-angiotensin-aldosterone system is more readily activated in an older adult than in a younger person because the body is unable to recognize changes in fluid balance. Arteries become less compliant, causing higher resistance for the heart to overcome. When assessing the pulse, it is necessary to relate it to the overall condition of the client rather than in isolation. For example, if the pulse is 40 beats per minute, assess whether the client has any signs or symptoms of decreased cardiac output: dizziness, lightheadedness, confusion, decreased urine output, or low blood pressure.

Nursing Diagnosis

Many factors, including age, stress, exercise, physical and psychological condition, and activity level can affect pulse and blood pressure.

The normal adult pulse rate ranges from 60 to 100, whereas normal blood pressure is a systolic measurement of 100 to 140 mmHg and a diastolic of 60 to 90 mmHg. Initial blood pressures should be taken in both arms to determine if there are differences in the arms, which could indicate a major medical condition. Differences of pressures of greater than 10 mmHg could indicate coarctation of the aorta.

Blood pressure can be position sensitive. This means that the client's position—sitting, standing, or lying down—changes the blood pressure dramatically. To evaluate for orthostatic or postural hypotension, take the client's blood pressure while he or she is supine and in a sitting and a standing position. Wait 3 minutes before rechecking the blood pressure in each position. If there is more than a 20-mmHg pressure difference in systolic or diastolic pressure, then orthostatic hypotension is suspected. Orthostatic hypotension may be the result of several factors, such as hypovolemia from dehydration or bleeding, or medication. The pressure differences indicate that the cardiovascular system is unable to compensate by vaso-constriction to maintain normal blood volume in relation to the size of the vasculature.

There are many potential nursing diagnoses for a client with a cardiovascular problem. See the Nursing Diagnoses box for a selective list of nursing diagnoses related to the cardiovascular system.

Decreased Cardiac Output

This may be related to the physiological effect of a myocardial infarction, hemorrhage, or heart failure as a result of hypertension. The heart is reaching the point at which it is no longer able to meet the oxygen demands of the body. Focused assessments should include heart rate and rhythm, any abnormal cardiac sounds (e.g., murmurs), extra heart sounds, general skin color and temperature, color of extremities, presence of edema, venous distention, level of consciousness, and urine output.

Risk for Impaired Skin Integrity

As perfusion decreases, especially to extremities, so does cellular nutrition and oxygenation. The tissue environment is altered, resulting in cellular damage as evidenced by cyanosis, edematous extremities, and the development of pressure areas. Focused assessments to include are altered color of the skin (pallor or redness), presence of edema, and altered pigmentation. A neurovascular assessment must be completed to determine risk of decreased circulation to an area. This assessment examines the presence of pain, pallor, paresthesia, pulse, and position.

Risk for Altered Tissue Perfusion

As in the previous diagnosis, blood flow may become inadequate to maintain normal functioning of tissue. In addition, there may be inadequate tissue perfusion to essential organs. Focused assessments

---

POSSIBLE NURSING DIAGNOSES RELATED TO THE CARDIOVASCULAR SYSTEM

Decreased Cardiac Output

Risk for Impaired Skin Integrity

Impaired Tissue Perfusion

Powerlessness/Hopelessness

Activity Intolerance

Altered Health Maintenance

Body Image Disturbance

Individual Coping: Ineffective

Family Coping: Compromised, Ineffective

should include capillary refill, pulse rate and rhythm, level of consciousness, urine output, presence of chest pain or pressure, and color of extremities. Blood work, including serum electrolytes, enzymes, and iso-enzymes, as well as system-specific tests, should be examined.

Activity Intolerance

Limitation of activities may occur when the client can no longer perform activities of daily living in the usual manner. Normal activities such as shopping or walking up one flight of steps may become impossible to accomplish. This may be so progressively limiting that a client with activity intolerance is unable to get out of bed or to bathe without assistance. Focused assessments should include heart rate and rhythm, respiratory rate, use of accessory muscles, and blood pressure.

Powerlessness or Hopelessness

Whether the medical diagnosis is acute or chronic, the client may develop a feeling of lack of control over his or her condition and the future. The client can become dependent on health care providers or significant others rather then assuming an active role in his or her care. Focused assessments should include exploration of feelings, goals for the future, and plans for daily activities.

Caregiver Role Strain

The cardiac-compromised client may assume a dependent role, despite previous independence. As significant others attempt to demonstrate their care and concern to the client, the client may feel overwhelmed by them. Roles change due to illness. The "provider of the family" may no longer be able to function in this role. Focused assessment should include clients' and

---

SAMPLE NURSING CARE PLAN

A CLIENT WITH HYPERTENSION

A 38-year-old man comes to the clinic with a "history of high blood pressure" and is complaining of an occipital headache. His blood pressure is 190/100 mmHg. The nurse questions the client regarding his medications, to which he replies "I take the pills when I get a headache." He has no other significant health care problems. His father died at age 45 of a myocardial infarction, and his mother has had multiple episodes of heart failure.

Nursing Diagnosis: Altered Tissue Perfusion Related to Uncontrolled Blood Pressure.

Expected Outcomes: Client will attain a blood pressure of 130 to 140/70 to 85.

Action	Rationale
1. Assess physical status of the client	1. Obtain baseline information regarding the client's health care status
2. Reduce stressors in the environment	2. Creating a calming environment will decrease stimulation of the reticular activating system
3. Assess what he knows about medication	3. Obtain a baseline of client's understanding and what further teaching is necessary
4. Assess what he knows about hypertension, including myths and realities	4. Obtain information on what client already knows so that knowledge base can be expanded; it is a myth that blood pressure is only high if the person has a headache.
5. Provide verbal and written instructions about the specific medication	5. Client may not understand verbal or written language; assess what client is able to understand
6. Advise routine blood pressure checkups in the clinic	6. Blood pressure must be closely monitored when not under control
7. Refer to dietitian for follow-up on low-sodium diet	7. Referral can provide a more thorough information base and follow-through
8. Teach client and family about the importance of frequent, close monitoring of blood pressure and the advantages of monitoring units	8. Incorporating a significant other into the plan of care can assist the client in follow-through of the home medical regimen
9. Document blood pressure and all findings, including teaching and counseling provided	9. Provides for follow-up of client's needs
10. Have client record frequency of headaches and record blood pressure	10. To establish if client does develop headaches with too high blood pressure

family members' description of stress and strain in their lives and exploration of their feelings and concerns.

Altered Health Maintenance

In the best of circumstances, the client may try to adhere to the prescription of care. However, other factors may influence the client's ability to follow through with the prescription. It may be difficult for an elderly client to keep scheduled, physician appointments if he or she cannot drive or does not have a significant other to drive him or her. Others may have a difficult time following a low-sodium diet because of the expense of purchasing special foods that the rest of their family will not eat. Focused assessments should include exploring with the client reasons for not being able to comply with the necessary changes in his or her life.

Planning

The nurse, based on the assessment of the client, must set priorities of care. It is essential that life-threatening conditions (safety) be recognized and dealt with immediately. It serves no purpose if the nurse plans all of the care without considering the specialized needs of the individual. Each individual needs his or her own plan of care based on his or her age, religion, culture, socioeconomic status, and emotional and psychological needs.

The nurse plans care of clients based on client needs. Certain types of cardiovascular problems can be avoided or minimized by altering lifestyles as required. Those areas to be addressed with the clients include weight loss, control of blood pressure, dietary changes (such as lowering cholesterol and sodium), exercise, and cessation of smoking (see Sample Nursing Care Plan for a Client with Hypertension and Sample Nursing Care Plan for a Client After a Myocardial Infarction).

Implementation

The nurse plays a crucial role in all phases of cardiovascular care. Ongoing assessment and monitoring of the client's physiological status by checking the client's pulses and taking the client's blood pressure should be continued after initial assessments. The nurse functions in a variety of roles when caring for the client. The nurse is constantly teaching the client and significant others about the therapeutic regimen.

SAMPLE NURSING CARE PLAN

A CLIENT AFTER A MYOCARDIAL INFARCTION

A 76-year-old unmarried woman had a myocardial infarction 2 days ago. She has no other significant medical history. Her medical plan includes cardiac rehabilitation with progressive activity. She will need nutritional and exercise education to assist in losing 30 lb to reach her ideal body weight. She has no shortness of breath, is on room air, has a respiratory rate of 18 breaths per minute, and has a blood pressure of 140/86.

Nursing Diagnosis: Risk for Activity Intolerance Related to Recent Myocardial Infarction, Overweight Status and Age.

Expected Outcome: Client will be able to perform at least 80% of activities of daily living without demonstrating evidence of shortness of breath by discharge.

Action	Rationale
1. Determine baseline vital signs before all increases in activity	1. To establish what increases may occur with activity
2. Increase activity each day	2. To determine ability to tolerate increased activity
3. Assess knowledge of nutrition by having client keep 3-day diet diary	3. Diary assists in understanding patterns and eating habits
4. Analyze diet with client for proper nutrition	4. Review recommended fat, protein, and carbohydrate values
5. Encourage client to increase activity and to lose weight slowly (1–2 lb/wk)	5. Gradual weight loss will allow body to adjust to change and not fatigue the client
6. Teach client to weigh herself once a week	6. Expect weight loss of 1 to 2 lb/week
7. Teach client to perform activities but to stop if any fatigue or shortness of breath occurs	7. Monitoring is important to prevent client from overexertion

Health promotion focuses on nutrition, drug therapies, and exercise as approaches to better healthy lifestyles.

Nutrition

Maintenance of normal cardiovascular functioning has been found to be highly dependent on limiting the amounts of sodium and fats in the diet. Clients should be instructed to read labels and note the amount of sodium and fat that is in foods. Because sodium has a role as an etiological factor in the development of hypertension, the recommended daily intake of sodium for healthy adults should be under 6 g, although the daily minimum requirement is 500 mg. Overall fat content should be less than 30% of the total daily calories (Mahan & Escott-Stump, 1996). Table 30–2 provides a listing of relative sodium and cholesterol levels and content of some common foods. See Chapter 27 for a more detailed discussion of nutrition.

Cardiovascular Medications

A variety of cardiovascular medications are prescribed to control, alleviate, or prevent common circulatory problems. These drugs are used for emergency situations and for maintenance therapy. Table 30–3 provides a listing of common classifications for cardiovascular drugs. The nurse needs to be knowledgeable about the purpose of these drugs, their actions, recommended administration protocols, and expected side effects.

Cardiotonics

Cardiotonics, or cardiac glycosides, are drugs that are naturally occurring compounds from the leaves of the *Digitalis purpurea* plant. These drugs are prescribed to treat chronic heart failure and such cardiac

Table 30–2
FOODS WITH HIGH/LOW SODIUM AND CHOLESTEROL

HIGH	LOW
Sodium	
Canned vegetables	Homemade soups
Canned soups	Fresh vegetables
Processed meats	Nonprocessed
Cheeses	meats
	Yogurt
Cholesterol	
Shrimp	Fruits
Lobster	Vegetables
Organ meats	Grains
Egg yolk	Cereals
Ice cream	Skim milk
	Sherbert

arrhythmias as atrial flutter and fibrillation and paroxysmal atrial tachycardia.

In heart failure, the myocardium becomes weakened, and the heart is unable to eject adequate amounts of blood to meet the energy needs of the body. Eventually the client develops congestion of the lungs, edema of the peripheral tissues, and a decrease in urinary output. Cardiotonics function to increase the contractility of the cardiac muscle **(myocardium),** which subsequently increases cardiac output. This lessens fluid accumulation and increases urine output. Cardiac glycosides also have an effect on the electrical impulse generation and conduction within the heart through their indirect parasympathomimetic action on the vagus. Increased vagal tone results in slowing of the heart rate and decrease in conduction through the atrioventricular node.

The prototype cardiotonic is digoxin (Lanoxin), which can be administered both orally and parenterally. Larger doses of digoxin are administered as part of a loading or digitalizing dose to achieve a rapid onset and therapeutic blood level. Once the therapeutic blood level is achieved, the client takes a maintenance dose. The client's serum blood levels of digoxin and potassium and electrocardiogram should be monitored, as toxicity of digoxin can easily occur. Common side effects include anorexia, vomiting, weakness, fatigue, malaise, visual changes, cardiac changes, and confusion.

Antiarrhythmics

Cardiac **arrhythmias** are abnormal rhythms resulting from disorders involving impulse generation or impulse conduction and are related to a variety of pathophysiological conditions. Arrhythmias can be classified by the site involved, such as sinus (for sinoatrial node), atrial, or ventricular arrhythmias; by the change in heart rate, such as bradycardia (rate lower than 60 beats per minute in adults) or tachycardia (rates higher than 100 beats per minute); or by the conduction disturbance, such as heart block. The type of antiarrhythmic that is prescribed depends on the site involved and the type of disturbance.

Common antiarrhythmic drugs include quinidine, which is used to control supraventricular arrhythmias such as atrial flutter and fibrillation; procainamide (Pronestyl), which is used to treat ventricular arrhythmias; lidocaine, which is an anesthetic and is used as a parenteral medication to treat ventricular arrhythmias; flecainide (Tambocor), which is used to treat supraventricular and ventricular arrhythmias; propranolol (Inderal), which is used to slow ventricular response in atrial fibrillation; and calcium channel blockers (such as verapamil), which are used to treat paroxysmal supraventricular tachycardia.

Antihypertensives

Antihypertensives are a large class of drugs that includes central-acting sympatholytics, β-adrenergic

Table 30-3

COMMON CARDIAC MEDICATIONS

CLASSIFICATION	EXAMPLE	EFFECT
Cardiotonic	Digoxin	Increases contractility Decreases heart rate
Calcium channel blockers	Verapamil	Decreases heart rate and blood pressure
Beta-adrenergic blockers	Inderal	Decreases heart rate and blood pressure
Central vasodilators	Aldomet	Decreases blood pressure
Peripheral vasodilators	Apresoline	Decreases blood pressure
Diuretics	Furosemide	Increases urine output Decreases blood volume Decreases blood pressure
Electrolyte supplements	K-Lor	Maintains normal conduction of the heart

blockers, vasodilators, calcium channel blockers, and angiotensin-converting enzyme (ACE) inhibitors. Any one or a combination of these drugs is used to treat high blood pressure, generally agreed to be a situation in which the systolic blood pressure is above 140 mmHg and diastolic blood pressure is above 90 mmHg.

Central sympatholytic drugs (or central vasodilators) decrease sympathetic stimulation of the peripheral vasculature, which promotes vasodilation and decreases norepinephrine production, which reduces renin production by the kidney. The prototype drug in this category is methyldopa (Aldomet), and the drug is available in both oral and parenteral forms. The most common side effect of Aldomet is drowsiness, and clients may complain of lightheadedness when they first start taking the drug.

β-Adrenergic receptor–blocking agents (or β-blockers) work by blocking sympathetic stimulation of the heart, which decreases heart rate and cardiac output, and by blocking the release of renin, which decreases peripheral vascular resistance. β-Blockers are used cautiously with clients who have asthma, insulin-dependent diabetes mellitus, and congestive heart failure. Side effects of β-blockers include postural hypotension, drowsiness, headache, dyspnea, and nausea. Common β-blockers include propranolol (Inderal) and labetalol (Normodyne).

Direct vasodilators reduce blood pressure through their direct effect on the smooth muscle of the vasculature. This results in a decrease in arterial vascular resistance, which lowers blood pressure. Hydralazine (Apresoline), minoxidil (Minodyl), and sodium nitroprusside (Nipride) are common direct vasodilators. Nipride is used parenterally and in emergency situations only. Common side effects include headache, nausea, vomiting, tachycardia, hypotension, edema, and angina.

Calcium channel blockers work to block the effect of calcium ions on the vascular muscle, thus decreasing peripheral vascular resistance and blood pressure. Common calcium channel blockers include diltiazem (Cardiazem), verapamil (Calan), and nifedipine (Pro-

cardia). As discussed previously, calcium channel blockers also work as antiarrhythmics.

Angiotensin-converting enzyme inhibitors act primarily by preventing the conversion of angiotensin I to angiotensin II. This reduces vasoconstriction and decreases total peripheral vascular resistance. Common types of ACE inhibitors include enalapril (Vasotec) and captopril (Captoprin). Side effects that can occur include severe hypotension, chest pain, palpitations, nonproductive cough, nausea, vomiting, and dizziness.

Antilipidemics

Hyperlipidemia is widely known to be a major contributing factor in the development of coronary artery and peripheral vascular diseases. Antilipidemic drugs are used to lower the amount of lipids and cholesterol in the circulating blood. Common antilipidemics include cholestyramine (Questran), lovastatin (Mevacor), gemfibrozil (Lopid), and clofibrate (Atromid-S). These drugs should be used cautiously with clients who have biliary obstruction, liver disease, or hypoprothrombinemia.

Diuretics

Diuretics act to increase excretion of fluid from the body. Different categories of diuretics exist, classified according to where they have their primary effect. The most common diuretics are the thiazide diuretics and the loop diuretics. Thiazide diuretics act on the distal convoluted tubule to prevent water reabsorption. Hydrochlorothiazide (HydroDIURIL) is a commonly used thiazide diuretic. Loop diuretics are the most potent diuretics and work on the loop of Henle to prevent sodium reabsorption. Furosemide (Lasix) is the prototype loop diuretic.

Because diuretics deplete blood volume, hypotension is a common side effect. Other serious side effects of thiazide and loop diuretics result from hypokalemia. Careful monitoring of the client's serum potassium level is required, especially if the client is also taking digoxin (Lanoxin). Serious life-threatening arrhythmias can occur if the client develops hypokalemia.

Electrolyte Supplements

Potassium chloride is often administered to clients who are taking cardiovascular and diuretic drugs in combination. Hypokalemia is a common side effect of these drugs. Potassium chloride is available in both oral and parenteral forms. Oral forms are available as liquids, powders, capsules, or tablets. Parenteral potassium chloride should always be diluted in a larger volume solution and never be administered as a bolus. Serious life-threatening arrhythmias could occur if potassium is administered as a bolus.

Exercise

Daily exercise, such as walking or stair climbing, has been found to be a component of a healthy lifestyle in preventing coronary artery disease. Clients who lead a predominantly sedentary lifestyle should be encouraged to start exercising on a daily basis. Climbing two flights of stairs instead of taking the elevator and walking a mile a day instead of driving the car are two examples of activities that could easily be included in one's daily schedule without much difficulty. Ideally, an individual should exercise at least 20 minutes a day 3 days per week as part of a healthy lifestyle in preventing coronary artery disease.

Miscellaneous Activities

Other factors have been shown to be integral in preventing coronary artery and peripheral vascular diseases. Individuals who smoke cigarettes should be encouraged to stop, as nicotine has a negative impact on the caliber of blood vessels, leading to hypertension. Engaging in stress management and relaxation techniques can have a positive effect on reducing stress and therefore on reducing vascular changes. Women who are menopausal and are given exogenous estrogen have lower incidences of coronary artery disease than women who do not.

Evaluation

The nurse, in implementing the plan of care for the cardiac client, must incorporate the knowledge gained in the history and physical assessment. From the time of the client admission into the health care system to the time of discharge, the nurse uses the nursing process in assessing, planning, diagnosing, implementing, and evaluating the progress of the client. The entire nursing process is ongoing and in constant need of review.

Teaching clients and significant others the importance of frequent monitoring and the importance of follow-up with the health care team is essential. Hypertension, for example, can be controlled to prevent catastrophic results. However, this is aided by follow-

COMMUNITY BASED CARE

OPEN HEART SURGERY

Cardiac surgery clients are being sent home as early as 4 days after open heart surgery. Although the home environment promotes recovery and decreases the risk of nosocomial infections, clients may recall little postoperative or discharge instruction and may not be prepared for their return home. The risk of congestive heart failure, pulmonary complications, cardiac dysrhythmias, and wound complications also remains a threat. Home care by nurses with extensive knowledge and cardiac assessment skills is an important component of any early discharge program.

Goals of care include early detection and reporting of potential complications, client education, and emotional support. The home care nurse usually sees the client for two to five visits and coordinates referral to outpatient cardiac rehabilitation after home care. With each nursing visit, a head-to-toe assessment is performed, including

1. Cardiovascular status: vital signs, daily weight, peripheral perfusion, and heart tones to identify any murmurs, pericardial rubs, or dysrhythmias

2. Respiratory status: decreased breath sounds, pleural effusion, pulmonary emboli

3. Gastrointestinal and nutritional status: appetite, intake, elimination

4. Incisions: sternal, legs, chest tube and pacer wire sites

5. Pain management

6. Activity level tolerance

Teaching topics include

1. Medications

2. Pulse counting

3. Pain control

4. Incisional care and signs and symptoms of infection

5. Coughing and deep breathing exercises and use of incentive spirometry

6. Diet—low fat, low cholesterol

7. Home activity and exercise program guidelines, restrictions, and signs and symptoms of activity intolerance

ing a prescribed regimen. Therefore, the nurse takes on the role of counselor to support, encourage, and monitor the client's progress. The evaluation process must be ongoing, and the nurse needs to evaluate and make changes in the plan of care as the client's condition changes. The nurse must be able to assess any changes in the client's condition that might require an alteration in the plan of care, document the changes, and communicate these changes to other health care staff.

Summary

Assessment of the circulatory system is an ongoing process. Although vital signs are an important portion of this process, the assessment includes much more. As in all other systems, the initial assessment is based on the client's history and presenting symptoms. This information helps to guide the practitioner into areas that require more substantive assessment.

The circulatory system consists of both central and peripheral circulation. Although separate assessments are performed on each, the systems are interrelated and dependent on each other. Information from one system affects the other. As the nurse refines his or her assessment skills, assessments become more complete and yield better information. Many of the assessment findings gathered by the nurse become areas of client teaching, such as cholesterol screening or medication administration.

CHAPTER HIGHLIGHTS

✦

✦ The cardiac circulation (supplying the heart) and the systemic circulation (supplying the body) are responsible for providing oxygen and nutrients to cells and for removing waste.

✦ Arteries are thicker walled than veins and carry blood enriched with oxygen away from the heart. Veins are thin-walled and low-pressured vessels. Valves within the veins help ensure a unidirectional blood flow.

✦ Systole is the time when blood is forced out of the heart into the systemic circulation. Diastole is the resting phase of the heart, the time of ventricular filling.

✦ Cardiac output is dependent on heart rate and stroke volume. However, many factors, such as exercise, age, and blood volume, influence the cardiac output.

✦ Many changes occur throughout the body as a result of increased age. Blood vessels become less elastic and therefore increase the patient risk for high blood pressure and stroke. In addition, the vessels become narrowed as a result of atherosclerosis, which could further compromise blood flow to the heart, other organs, and peripheral circulation.

Study Questions

1. The nurse assesses Mr. Wilson's apical rate to be 90 beats per minute, but the radial pulse is 74 beats per minute. You know that this is indicative of

a. high blood pressure
b. pulse deficit
c. low blood pressure
d. high venous pressure

2. Susan Hart, 35 years old, is on beta-blocker medication to lower her blood pressure. Because beta-blockers lower both blood pressure and heart rate, she needs to learn how to take her pulse. Methods of teaching her this procedure include

a. feeling her apical pulse with her hand for 1 minute
b. palpating her popliteal pulse for 15 seconds
c. palpating her radial pulse for 30 seconds
d. percussing her apical pulse for 1 minute

3. Your client is nervous about the "cardiac catheterization" that she will be undergoing tomorrow. She tells you that she heard from her friend that it is a very dangerous procedure and that she will be incapacitated for 1 week afterwards. You would want to teach her that following a cardiac catheterization

a. she may need to lay flat in bed for several hours but then will be allowed out of bed
b. she may sit in a chair or walk to the bathroom within a half hour
c. she can be discharged from the facility within one half hour
d. she may sit upright in bed to eat

4. When taking a blood pressure, the nurse should first

a. palpate a systolic blood pressure
b. palpate an apical pulse
c. palpate a diastolic pulse
d. palpate a radial pulse

5. When auscultating heart sounds, the nurse should

a. use the bell of the stethoscope only
b. use both the bell and the diaphragm
c. listen to ERB's point
d. listen to the aortic and pulmonic valves

Critical Thinking Exercises

1. Mr. W. is admitted with a diagnosis of chest pain. Myocardial infarction (heart attack) has been ruled out. He is 50 years old, has a history of hypertension, has smoked two packs of cigarettes per day for 15 years, is obese, and has a stressful job as a bus driver. Assess Mr. W's needs for teaching regarding lifestyle alterations.

2. S_1 and S_2 are normal heart sounds. Ms. T. has developed an S_3. Discuss the pathophysiology of S_3 in relation to S_1 and S_2.

References

American Heart Association. (1992). *Heart and stroke facts.* Dallas: AHA.

Arnstein, P. M., Buselli, E. F., & Rankin, S. H. (1996). Women and heart attacks: Prevention, diagnosis, and care. *Nurse Practitioner: American Journal of Primary Health Care, 21*(5), 57–58, 61–62, 64.

Baker, E. (1990). Low blood pressure. *Nursing, 20*(11), 34–39.

Baker, J. (1991). Assessment of peripheral arterial occlusive disease. *Critical Care Nursing Clinics of North America, 3*(3), 493–498.

Blank, C., & Irwin, G. (1990). Peripheral vascular disorders: Assessment and intervention. *Nursing Clinics of North America, 25*(4), 777–794.

Byra-Cook, C., Dracup, K. A., & Lazik, A. J. (1990). Direct and indirect blood pressure in critical care patients. *Nursing Research, 39*(5), 285–289.

Drown, D. (1994). Physiological differences in vascular reactivity in the African-American population. *Progress in Cardiovascular Nursing, 9*(4), 41.

Flavell, C. (1994). Women and coronary disease. *Progress in Cardiovascular Nursing, 9*(4), 18–27.

Haskell, W., Alderman, E., Fair, J., Maron, D., Mackey, S., Superko, H., Williams, P., Johnstone, I., Champagne, M., Krause, R., et al. (1994). Effects of intensive multiple risk factor reduction on coronary atherosclerosis and clinical cardiac events in men and women with coronary artery disease: The Stanford Coronary Risk Intervention Project (SCRIP). *Circulation, 89*, 975–990.

Hubner, C. (1988). Nursing management of the patient with an ischemic limb. *Progress in Cardiovascular Nursing, 3*(4), 115–121.

Hulley, S. B., Walsh, J. M., Newman, T. B., (1992). Health policy on blood cholesterol. *Circulation, 86*(3), 1026–1029.

Kennedy, W. C., Jr. (1990). Vital signs: Reading the essentials. *Journal of Emergency Medical Services, 15*, 26–30, 34, 36–39.

Kitler, M. E. (1991). Differences in men and women in coronary artery disease, systemic hypertension and their treatment. *American Journal of Cardiology, 266*(4), 566–568.

Mahan, L. K., Escott-Stump, S. (1996). *Krouse's food, nutrition and diet therapy* (9th ed.). Philadelphia: W. B. Saunders.

National Cholesterol Education Program. (1993). *The second report of the Expert Panel on Detection, Evaluation, and Treatment of High Blood Cholesterol in Adults. Adult Treatment panel 11.* NIH Publication No. 93-3095. Bethesda, MD: National Institutes of Health, National Health, Lung, and Blood Institute.

Sandmaier, M. (1992). *The healthy heart handbook for women.* United States Department of Health and Human Services Publication No. 92-2720. Washington, DC: National Institutes of Health.

Selig, P. (1991). The prevention and screening of cardiovascular disease: An update. *Nurse Practitioner Forum, 2*(1), 14–18.

Stampfer, M. J., Colditz, G. A., Willett, W. C., et al. (1991). Postmenopausal estrogen therapy and cardiovascular disease. *New England Journal of Medicine, 325*(11), 756–762.

Wenger, N. K., Speroff, L., Packard, B. (1993). Cardiovascular health and disease in women. *New England Journal of Medicine, 324*(4), 247–256.

Bibliography

American Heart Association. (1994). *Heart attack: Still America's no. 1 killer. Stroke: Still America's no. 3 killer.* Washington, DC: AHA.

Amsterdam, E., Hayson, D., & Kappagoda, C. (1994). Non-pharmacologic therapy for coronary atherosclerosis: Result of primary and secondary prevention trials. *American Heart Journal, 128*, 1344–1352.

Bilodeau, M., & Capasso, V. (1990). Peripheral arterial thrombolytic therapy. *Critical Care Nursing Clinics of North America, 2*(4), 673–680.

Chan, V. (1990). Content areas for cardiac teaching: Patients' perceptions of the importance of teaching content after myocardial infarction. *Journal of Advanced Nursing, 15*, 1139–1145.

Expert Panel on Detection, Evaluation, and Treatment of High Blood Cholesterol in Adults. (1993). Summary of the second report of the National Cholesterol Education Program. *Journal of the American Medical Association, 269*(23), 3015–3023.

Friedman, M. (1993). Stressor and perceived stress in older females with heart disease. *Cardiovascular Nursing, 29*(4), 25–29.

Gehring, P. (1992). Vascular assessment. *RN, 55*(1), 40–48.

Harley, J. (1993). Preventing diabetic foot disease. *Nurse Practitioner: American Journal of Primary Health Care, 18*(10), 37–44.

Herr, K. (1992). Night leg pain in the elderly. *Geriatric Nursing: American Journal of Care for the Aging, 13*(1), 13–16.

Hulley, S. B., Walsh, J. M., Newman, T. B. (1992). Health policy on blood cholesterol. *Circulation, 86*(3), 1026–1029.

Kuhn, J., & McGovern, M. (1992). Peripheral vascular assessment of the elderly client. *Journal of Gerontological Nursing, 18*(12), 35–38.

Malasanos, L., Barkauskas, V., & Stoltenberg-Allen, K. (1990). *Health assessment.* St. Louis: Mosby-Year Book.

Neill, K. (1993). Ethnic pain styles in acute myocardial infarction. *Western Journal of Nursing Research, 15*(5), 531–547.

Owens, J. F., Matthews, K. A., Wing, R., et al. (1992). Can physical activity mitigate the effects of aging in middle-aged women? *Circulation, 85*(4), 1265–1269.

Shoemaker, W. (1992). Monitoring and management of acute circulatory problems: The expanded role of the physiologically oriented critical care nurse. *American Journal of Critical Care, 1*(1), 38–53.

Wallace, D., Lockhart, J., & Boyle, D. (1995). Service use by elders with heart disease. *Research in Nursing and Health, 18*(4), 293–301.

Wingate, S. (1991). Women and coronary heart disease: Implications for the critical care setting. *Focus on Critical Care, 18*(3), 212–220.

Wingate, S. (1990). Post-MI patients' perception of their learning needs. *Dimensions of Critical Care Nursing, 9*(2), 112–118.

Chapter 31

BOWEL ELIMINATION

NANCY BERGER, RN,C, MSN

MICHELLE L. FOLEY, RN,C, MA

KEY TERMS

✦

cathartic
colonoscopy
deglutition
dyschezia
enteral
feces
flatulence

flatus
hemorrhoids
impaction
incontinence
ostomy
tympanites

LEARNING OBJECTIVES

✦

After studying this chapter, you should be able to

✦ Discuss the anatomy and physiology of the gastrointestinal system

✦ List and explain the factors that affect defecation

✦ Explain altered nutritional intake patterns

✦ Identify common bowel elimination problems

✦ Assess client elimination patterns

✦ Identify primary and secondary nursing diagnoses

✦ List nursing strategies that promote regular bowel elimination

✦ Discuss medications used for the client who has altered bowel elimination

✦ Describe the procedure for administering an enema

✦ Discuss the types of bowel diversions and the nursing care of clients with ostomies

✦ Evaluate the effectiveness of nursing care

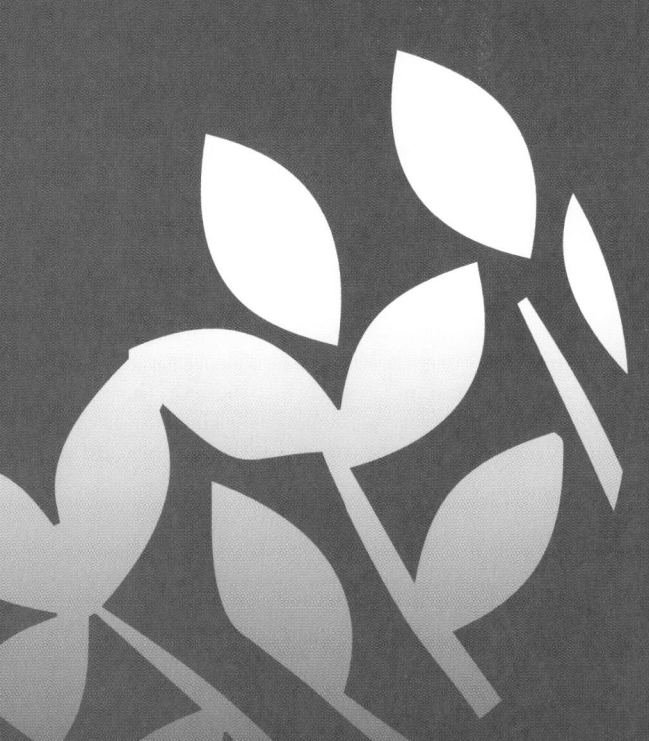

Bowel elimination is a natural process essential to human functioning. The regular elimination of bowel waste products is individualized and is generally based on a pattern established over many years. For some clients, having a daily bowel movement in the morning is the expected norm; for other clients, a bowel movement every 2 to 3 days at any time of the day is the expected norm. The elderly are especially prone to "bowel consciousness," and a deviation from their normal pattern can be viewed as being detrimental to their health and well-being.

Some alterations in bowel elimination can result from disease or can be the cause of disease. The nurse must be prepared to assist clients in returning to regular bowel elimination. Alterations in elimination are uncomfortable and often embarrassing for clients. An understanding, competent, and supportive nurse can be invaluable to the client experiencing these problems.

Anatomy and Physiology of the Gastrointestinal System

The gastrointestinal (GI) system is responsible for providing food and fluid to the body. This system is critical to energy production and sustenance (see Fig. 27–1).

Mouth

The mouth, also known as the oral or buccal cavity, contains the tongue, teeth, hard and soft palates, cheeks, the salivary gland ducts, and other structures. Taste buds are located at the sides, rear, and tip of the tongue. Food is chewed, shaped, and pushed to the back of the mouth as a bolus. **Deglutition,** also known as swallowing, moves the bolus from the mouth to the stomach.

Esophagus

The esophagus is a collapsible, muscular tube that is approximately 9 to 10 in (22–25 cm) long. The food mixes with mucus and is propelled through the esophagus by peristaltic waves. The bolus passes through the lower esophageal sphincter into the stomach.

Stomach

The stomach is divided into four sections: the cardia, the fundus, the body, and the pylorus. The body is the large, central portion of the stomach. The bolus of food mixes with gastric secretions, maceration occurs, and the result is a semiliquid called chyme. Peristaltic waves intensify as digestion proceeds. As the chyme moves toward the pyloric area, the pyloric

sphincter opens, and a small amount of chyme is ejected into the duodenum. A small amount of absorption occurs within the stomach (some water, alcohol, certain drugs [such as aspirin], and some electrolytes). The major function of the stomach is that of food reservoir.

Small Intestine

The small intestine starts at the pyloric valve and ends at the ileocecal valve. It consists of three parts: the duodenum, the jejunum, and the ileum. The small intestine is approximately 21 ft (6–7 m) long and is coiled throughout the abdominal cavity. The chyme is mixed with pancreatic enzymes, bile, and intestinal enzymes by segmentation. Segmentation is a contracting motion that enables chyme to come into contact with the mucosa for absorption. Peristalsis is the movement that propels food through the intestinal tract (Fig. 31–1). Absorption of nutrients and water is the major function of the small intestine.

Large Intestine

The large intestine is approximately 5 ft (1.5 m) long; it starts at the ileocecal valve and ends at the anus. The major parts of the large intestine are the cecum, ascending colon, hepatic flexure, transverse colon, splenic flexure, descending colon, sigmoid (or S-shaped) colon, rectum, anal canal, and anus. Chyme is propelled through the colon by haustral churning and peristalsis (see Fig. 31–1). Water, all except 3 to 4 oz (90–120 ml), is absorbed in the large intestine. The remaining solid material is called **feces.** Food that is consumed is generally passed through the intestinal

Digestive processes

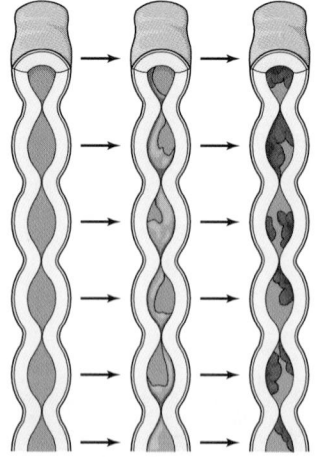

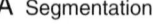

A Segmentation **B** Haustral churning

❧ **Figure 31–1**
Water and nutrients are absorbed in the digestive process in the small and large intestines. Material passes through the small and large intestines by the processes of segmentation, peristalsis, and haustral churning.

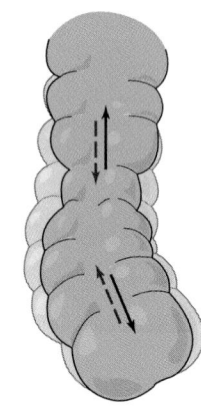

tract within 24 to 48 hours (although some food can remain in the system for up to 4 days). Because feces includes elements other than what is received from food, it is possible to have a bowel movement even if one has had nothing by mouth (NPO).

Fecal material is pushed into the rectum by a strong movement called mass peristalsis. As feces fills the rectum, the rectal wall becomes distended, and nerve impulses are sent to the brain and spinal cord. These impulses return back to the descending and sigmoid colon and rectum, which intensify peristaltic waves. The internal anal sphincter is relaxed, allowing feces to enter the anal canal. When one sits on a toilet or bedpan, the external sphincter relaxes voluntarily, emptying the rectum (Fig. 31–2). This emptying of the rectum is known as defecation.

Accessory Organs

The accessory organs of digestion include the liver, the gallbladder, and the pancreas.

Liver

The functions of the liver include bile production; detoxification; storage of vitamins, minerals, and glycogen; and coagulation. Bile is secreted into small ducts that join to form the right and left hepatic ducts. These larger ducts merge to form the common hepatic duct, which leaves the liver and joins the cystic duct from the gallbladder. These two ducts form the common bile duct. The common bile duct, along with the pancreatic duct, enters the duodenum at the ampulla of Vater. Bile aids in fat digestion, and urobilinogen, an end product of bilirubin breakdown, gives feces their color.

Gallbladder

The major function of the gallbladder is to store and concentrate bile. The gallbladder holds approximately 40 to 70 ml of bile. Bile is released into the small intestine when chyme, containing high levels of fat, enters the duodenum. When the small intestine is empty, the sphincter of Oddi closes, and bile remains in the gallbladder for storage.

Pancreas

The pancreas has both exocrine and endocrine functions. The exocrine functions include enzyme production for the metabolism of fats, carbohydrates, and protein; an alkaline pancreatic juice is produced that buffers the duodenal wall and enhances digestion. Endocrine functions include the production of glucagon and insulin. The pancreas lies behind the stomach and is attached to the duodenum by the pancreatic duct. As chyme enters the small intestine, pancreatic secretions are released and the digestive process continues.

Factors That Affect Defecation

Age and Development

Bowel characteristics change as an individual grows and develops. Infants have no voluntary control of elimination due to a lack of neuromuscular development, which does not usually occur until the age of 2 or 3 years. Infants tend to have more frequent and loose stools than older children because food passes quickly through the infant's GI tract due to quick peristalsis.

How the infant is fed also determines the stool characteristics. Breast-fed infants tend to have frequent, yellow or golden, soft, mushy bowel movements. This is because human milk is more easily digested than cow's milk, making it easier for the stool to be digested and passed through the intestinal tract. Infants who drink cow's milk have more formed and yellowish brown stools. Cow's milk has more casein than human breast milk. This higher percentage of casein results in larger, harder stools (Wong, 1995). Formula-fed infants also have formed stools that are pale yellow to light brown.

Young children develop voluntary bowel control (usually by the age of 3 years), and their stools become less frequent, more regular, and more formed. When the child becomes an adolescent, the intestines undergo rapid growth. Because of rapid growth spurts of puberty, adolescents often are hungrier than younger children and increase their diet. Although adolescents may eat more, what they are eating may not necessarily be nutritious; *e.g.,* they may buy food from vending machines or fast food restaurants. Because of the active pace of adolescents, eating patterns may not be consistent, which could contribute to altered bowel elimination patterns.

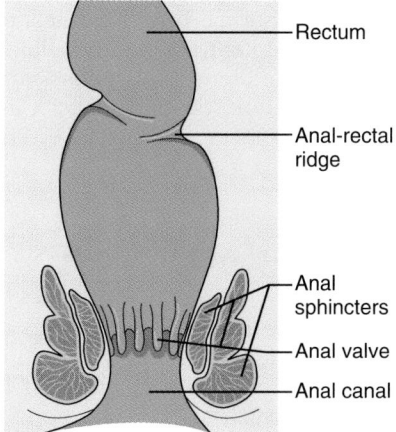

Rectum and the anal canal

- Rectum
- Anal-rectal ridge
- Anal sphincters
- Anal valve
- Anal canal

❧ **Figure 31–2**
Anatomical structures involved in defecation: anus, rectum, and internal and external sphincters.

Young and middle-aged adults may also experience alterations in bowel elimination. These age groups tend to have busy and rapidly paced lifestyles. Because of this, they may not always eat nutritious foods. Fast foods, which may be high in fat but low in fiber, and insufficient food intake due to "lack of time" could contribute to altered bowel patterns. Bowel activity may also be affected by not spending enough time on elimination needs.

As one ages, many changes that affect bowel elimination occur (see box). The following mechanisms contribute to impaired digestion and elimination in the older adult:

* As teeth are lost, chewing ability is decreased.
* The amount of digestive enzymes in the saliva and the volume of gastric acid decrease with aging, making food harder to digest.
* A decrease in the enzyme lipase causes an inability to digest fat-containing foods.
* Decreased peristalsis occurs due to decreased activity and exercise.
* Because the esophagus empties slower, discomfort may occur at the epigastric area.

Many older adults also suffer from incontinence. This occurs because muscle tone is lost in the perineal floor and anal sphincter.

Many older people are prone to constipation. A decrease in physical activity is a contributing factor, as is slowed nerve impulses. Many elderly individuals are less aware of the need to have a bowel movement. Many others suffer from perceived constipation. For example, a person who has routinely had one bowel movement a day for most of his or her adult life might notice that he or she is moving the bowels only every other or every third day. Educating these clients about the changes that occur with age can help them realize that what they are experiencing is normal. However, many clients have difficulty with these changes and feel they should have a bowel movement every day. As a result, a higher incidence of laxative and enema abuse is seen in the elderly than in any other age group.

GASTROINTESTINAL PROBLEMS AFFECTING OLDER ADULTS

* Atony of the smooth muscle of the colon
* Decreased abdominal muscle tone
* Decreased anal sphincter control
* Decreased fiber and fluid intake
* Decreased chewing ability
* Decreased exercise and physical activity
* Laxative and enema abuse

Diet

What clients eat tends to have an influence on bowel activity. Fiber (the indigestible residue in our diet) provides bulk in fecal material. Bulk-forming foods absorb fluid, which increases stool mass. This causes the bowel walls to stretch, stimulating peristalsis and initiating the defecation reflex. Foods high in fiber, therefore, encourage bowel activity. Some foods that are high in fiber include grains (*i.e.,* breads and cereals), raw and cooked fruit, and green and raw vegetables.

Foods that are gas producing also stimulate peristalsis by distending the intestinal walls, which increases motility. Some foods that tend to be gas producing include beans, onions, cabbage, and cauliflower. Spicy foods also increase peristalsis. Other foods, such as chocolate, bran, alcohol, and coffee, have a laxative effect. This is why a person who has a cup of coffee and a bowl of bran flakes for breakfast can expect to have a bowel movement soon after the meal has been completed.

Some people suffer from a condition called lactose intolerance, which is the inability to digest milk products. This can result in abdominal distention, cramps, flatulence, and diarrhea. Lactose (which is a simple sugar found in milk) is usually broken down by the enzyme lactase. Individuals who do not produce lactase are unable to digest lactose. Avoiding foods that contain lactose is the primary method of treating this condition. Supplements such as Ensure or Sustacal can also be added to the diet. Lactase supplements, which are commercially available, can also assist with digestion. Available in liquid or tablet form, these supplements should be taken with the first bite of food at meals.

Fluid Intake

Fluid liquefies intestinal contents so that they can pass more easily through the colon. A decreased fluid intake, therefore, slows food passage, and an increased fluid intake usually speeds up the passage of food. To maintain a normal bowel elimination pattern, adults need to drink 1400 to 2000 ml of fluid per day.

In addition to the amount of fluids, elimination is also affected by the type of fluid that a client drinks. Hot fluids and fruit juices, for instance, soften stool and increase peristalsis.

Diagnostic Procedures

Some procedures require that a person not have any food or fluids for many hours prior to the examination or test. In addition, many procedures require bowel cleaning (via enemas or cathartics) before the procedure is begun, such as a colonoscopy or barium enema. Diagnostic procedures can alter a client's bowel elimination, at least temporarily. For instance, a person who undergoes a lower GI series would need an enema after the procedure to evacuate any residual barium. Elimination patterns may also change related to the stress of an examination (and the awaiting of test results).

Anesthesia and Surgery

Patients who undergo surgery, even if the surgery is not to the GI system, can have an alteration in bowel elimination (see box). A client who has had local or regional anesthesia suffers no direct effect to his or her GI system. However, general anesthesia causes a temporary cessation of peristalsis. Inhaled anesthetics block the parasympathetic impulses to the intestinal musculature, slowing down peristalsis.

When someone has surgery to the GI system, direct manipulation of the bowel might occur. This manipulation temporarily stops peristalsis, which could result in a paralytic ileus. If this condition occurs, it generally lasts for 24 to 48 hours and can cause detrimental effects. Ambulating the postoperative client is important to decrease the possibility of this potential complication.

Activity

Physical activity promotes peristalsis. Immobility, on the other hand, depresses motility. This is why it is so important to encourage the hospitalized or ill client to be out of bed as much as possible. In addition, weak abdominal and/or pelvic floor muscle tone can cause an impaired ability to increase intraabdominal pressure and a decreased control of the external anal sphincter. Both of these factors, in turn, impair bowel elimination.

Psychological Factors

When a client is stressed, impulses from the parasympathetic division of the autonomic nervous system cause an increase in the digestive process and peristalsis within the GI tract to provide the body with the nutrients needed for defense. This causes distention of the intestinal mucosa, leading to diarrhea. For example, this is why many students develop diarrhea when they are nervous about an upcoming examination.

When one feels depressed, on the other hand, the autonomic nervous system decreases impulses from its parasympathetic portion, which decreases peristalsis, leading to constipation.

Lifestyle

Because bowel training is a normal part of growth and development, parents who are assisting their children in this task should treat it as a normal and healthy process rather than as being "dirty." Bowel elimination is an integral part of everyone's life and should be thought of as a natural process.

Most people normally have a bowel movement

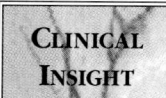

CLINICAL INSIGHT

Preventing Constipation in Postoperative Vascular Surgery Clients

A quality assurance and improvement study was done at a large midwestern tertiary care hospital with the purpose of preventing constipation in postoperative vascular surgery clients. This area was selected because the vascular unit had many older clients who were either bedbound or minimally mobile; both situations increase their chance of developing constipation or fecal impaction.

In a prestudy analysis, it was realized that 59% of the clients had an alteration in bowel elimination. Thirty four percent of the clients had a fecal impaction, and 59% requested laxatives or enemas to assist them in bowel elimination.

After compiling information from numerous other research studies, four interventions were developed for the clients on this unit who were assessed as being at high risk for constipation to assist with bowel elimination. The interventions included (1) the use of a dietary fiber supplement, (2) encouraging intake of 1500 to 2000 ml fluid per day (except if contraindicated by other underlying medical conditions), (3) giving maximum privacy and putting clients in an upright position when having a bowel movement, and (4) encouraging clients to do abdominal strengthening exercises while in bed. A multidisciplinary approach would be used, including nurses, dieticians, and physicians.

The study was followed over several years. All clients admitted were assessed to determine who was considered to be at high risk for developing constipation. The determination was based on such factors as history of bowel elimination, preadmission versus present activity levels, intake and output, use of medications, and dietary intake, to name a few. Those who were determined to be at high risk were included in the protocol described here (with the exception of doing abdominal strengthening exercises).

Using a combination of hygiene measures, increased fluid, and increased dietary intake of fiber, the incidence of constipation on this client unit decreased from 59% to approximately 9%. The incidence of impaction was eliminated, and requests for laxatives and enemas decreased from 59% to approximately 8%.

Research brief based on article by Hall, G. R., Karstens, M., Rakel, B., Swanson, E., & Davidson, A. (1995). Managing constipation using a research-based protocol. *MedSurg Nursing, 4*(1), 11–14.

after breakfast, when the gastrocolic and duodenocolic reflexes cause mass peristaltic waves to occur. However, one's daily schedule, including occupation, activity, and leisure time, plays a part in establishing and maintaining normal elimination patterns. One should never ignore the urge to defecate; however, if a client is not near a bathroom or if something else interferes with bowel timing, defecation may need to be delayed.

Medications

Nurses must be aware of the medications that their clients receive or take at home. This is absolutely imperative when dealing with the GI system because so many medications affect the GI system and therefore bowel elimination.

Some medications, such as narcotics, opiates, antacids containing aluminum, and anticholinergics, can decrease peristalsis in the GI tract, thereby causing constipation. Antibiotics can cause diarrhea because they disrupt the normal bacterial flora in the GI tract. They can also make the stool appear more green or gray than normal. A person who takes iron pills might have black stool. Any medication that causes GI bleeding (such as aspirin or anticoagulants) could cause the stool to look pink, red, or black. This is why it is so important to be aware of medication side effects and to teach clients about them as well.

Laxatives and cathartics soften stool and promote peristalsis. Chronic use of cathartics, however, causes the large intestine to lose tone, which decreases one's responsiveness to bowel stimulation. Laxative overuse, on the other hand, can cause severe diarrhea, which can lead to dehydration and electrolyte depletion.

Preexisting Medical Conditions

A person who suffers from a long-term illness or neurological disease that impairs nerve transmission could end up with decreased muscle tone. In this case, the person might suffer from constipation or incontinence. Diseases of the colon or rectum or a damaged spinal cord can contribute to constipation. Conversely, a person with a GI infection, malabsorption syndrome, cancer, diverticulitis, or hyperthyroidism can experience diarrhea.

Clients should also be aware of any changes in the pattern or consistency of their stool. For instance, a "ribbon-shaped" stool could indicate an intestinal blockage.

Pregnancy

Pregnant women may experience alterations in bowel elimination. A growing fetus in the uterus causes pressure on the large intestine, which can decrease GI motility, causing flatulence. Pressure is exerted on the veins of the rectum and anus as well, leading to hemorrhoids. Constipation during late pregnancy may also occur from an increase in progesterone and steroid metabolism, from displacement of the intestines due to an enlarged uterus, and as a side effect of oral iron supplements taken during pregnancy.

Pain

Conditions such as hemorrhoids, abdominal or rectal surgery, or a vaginal delivery can cause pain during defecation. To avoid pain, an individual often suppresses the urge to have a bowel movement. This leads to constipation, which creates even more discomfort.

Culture

Cultural values are an aspect affecting bowel elimination. It is important to perform a cultural assessment that includes questions about nutritional habits and bowel habits. If clients have alterations in bowel elimination, such as constipation or diarrhea, ask how they alleviate the alteration. It is important to provide clients with privacy and sufficient time for toileting.

Altered Nutritional Intake Patterns

The preferred method of nutritional intake is oral ingestion. If clients are unable to eat, then **enteral** tube feedings may be instituted. Enteral nutrition is the delivery of nutrients directly into the stomach, duodenum, or jejunum. Enteral feedings may be used as total nutritional support or as supplemental support.

If digestive and absorption abilities are functional, then enteral feedings are preferred over parenteral feedings. Enteral feedings cost less, cause fewer complications, and require less client monitoring. The most common complication of enteral tube feedings is diarrhea, which can result from several factors, including lactose intolerance, rapid infusion rate, concomitant drug therapy, bolus feedings, malabsorption, and use of hypertonic formulas. Strategies to prevent diarrhea include reducing the infusion rate, starting the feedings at half strength and slowly increasing the strength, adding antidiarrheal agents to the formula, changing to continuous feedings, adding fiber to the formula, and administering the feeding at room temperature.

Document the feeding type, amount, and rate and the client's response. Monitor the client's intake and output, weight, skin turgor, stools, and laboratory values.

Common Bowel Elimination Problems

Constipation

When the passage of feces through the large intestine is slowed from a decrease in gastric motility, more fluid is absorbed from the fecal mass, leaving a dry, hard stool. The passing of this type of stool is called constipation.

It is important to realize that constipation is not a disease but a symptom. Many individuals who claim to be constipated actually have a decrease in the frequency of the stools, while the consistency of the stools remains unchanged. The bowel elimination problem of constipation is therefore very individualized and often misinterpreted. Because of this, constipation can be considered a subjective matter, based on changes from one's regular habits (McLane & McShane, 1991). For example, if a person normally moves his or her bowels twice a week, this would not be considered to be constipation, whereas a person who has a bowel movement every day would consider himself or herself to be constipated if the pattern changed to every few days.

Several other symptoms may occur in the person complaining of constipation. Besides assessing the stool itself, the nurse should be alert to these corresponding signs and symptoms. The client may have complaints of anorexia, lower back pain, or a headache and may experience irritability, straining or difficult defecation **(dyschezia),** flatus or rectal fullness, and/or nausea and vomiting. These occur because of the enlarged mass of stool within the lower intestine. The client may also experience general fatigue due to the straining on defecation. Because of the stool sitting within the lower intestine, the client may have abdominal distention, decreased bowel sounds, or a palpable mass in the lower left colon.

There are many potential causes of constipation, including (but not limited to) decreased fluid or fiber intake, decreased exercise or activity, taking medications with constipating side effects, delayed defecation when the urge is present, mental stress or depression, pregnancy, abuse of laxatives or enemas, and a decrease in neurological status. The nurse must be alert to all of these potential conditions (see Box 31–1).

If a client's history indicates the presence of any of these potential causes of constipation, teaching must be initiated by the nurse.

The ultimate goal for a client with constipation is to have a soft, formed bowel movement without strain or discomfort according to the previous pattern.

Diarrhea

The passage of liquid and unformed stools, usually at frequent intervals, is called diarrhea. Diarrhea is a symptom of multiple disorders that affect digestion, absorption, and secretion in the GI tract. The intestinal contents pass through the intestines too fast to allow water to reabsorb from them. If the colon is irritated, increased mucus is produced, contributing to this watery feces. Diarrhea can be a protective mechanism. If irritants such as toxins are in the intestinal tract, having diarrhea gets rid of the irritants by increasing intestinal secretions. Diarrhea can occur for a number of reasons (see Box 31–1).

BOX 31–1

COMMON CAUSES OF CONSTIPATION AND DIARRHEA

Constipation

- Irregular bowel habits
- Ignoring the urge to defecate
- Lower-fiber diet but with high intake of animal fat and rich desserts
- Low fluid intake
- Laxative or enema abuse
- Lack of regular exercise
- Lengthy bed rest or inactivity
- Aging process
- Certain medications, such as opiates, iron, anticholinergics, tranquilizers
- Neurological conditions (such as a spinal cord tumor) that block nerve impulses to the colon
- Environmental changes
- Mental stress or depression
- Pregnancy

Diarrhea

- Anxiety and stress
- Food allergies or food intolerances
- Intestinal infection
- Certain medications such as antibiotics, laxatives, iron
- Colon disease (such as Crohn's disease)
- Surgical alterations (such as colon resection or gastrectomy)
- Laxative use
- A bacterial, fungal, viral, or protozoal infection in the intestines or alteration in the normal bacterial intestinal flora

---

Clients who have diarrhea tend to have complaints of nausea, vomiting, and abdominal cramps because of bowel irritability. The nurse should also assess for the presence of hyperactive bowel sounds, fever, and anal excoriation. The client should be asked if the diarrhea is acute, chronic, or recurrent and if any incontinence is experienced.

When diarrhea occurs, the body loses water, potassium, sodium chloride, and bicarbonate, all of which are necessary body components. A loss of fluid and electrolytes that results from diarrhea can therefore be dangerous. Elderly people and infants are especially at risk for fluid and electrolyte imbalance. If a person has persistent diarrhea, intravenous or oral replacement of fluids and electrolytes must occur.

The first step in assessing for diarrhea is to identify those clients at risk. Questions such as the following should be included in the assessment:

COMMUNITY BASED CARE

Constipation

Constipation is a common problem in the community. Many clients are at risk for constipation from

1. Decreased tone and muscle weakness associated with aging, immobility, inactivity

2. Clinical conditions—neurogenic diseases including stroke and spinal cord injury and metabolic diseases such as hypothyroidism

3. Medications, including analgesics and certain antacids

4. Mechanical factors such as inadequate dietary fiber

Prevention of constipation is always the goal. Establish a goal for bowel movement frequency with the client, usually four to seven times per week. Have the client establish a routine time to use the toilet or commode. Instruct on the importance of adequate dietary roughage, fluids, and exercise. Often, eating an extra piece of fruit daily can resolve the problem. Stool softeners and fiber products may also be helpful. They are best taken with a full glass of fluids, followed by something warm to drink. "Cocktails," such as Power Pudding, are a natural and effective way to decrease constipation:

Puree in blender: 1.5 cups pitted prunes, 1 cup applesauce, 0.5 cup unprocessed bran, and 0.75 cup prune juice. Refrigerate. Makes 15 0.25-cup servings.

Numerous clients who overuse laxatives will be encountered. Wean clients from laxatives on which they have become dependent slowly for greater success and compliance.

Teach the client regarding signs and symptoms to report to the home care nurse or physician:

1. Blood in the stools

2. Pain with evacuation

3. No stool in 4 days

4. Excessive cramping

5. Excessive straining

6. Uncontrolled voiding of stool

• Have you recently traveled outside of the country? (The water supply in some countries may not be as purified as ours, and the foods may be different, both of which could irritate the GI system.)

• Have you had any new foods or medication recently? (The client may be sensitive to a new food or medication.)

• What dietary changes have occurred recently? (For instance, is the client eating more greasy or fast foods?)

• Do you take laxatives? If so, what kind and how often? (Laxatives increase peristalsis.)

• Is there a personal or family history of GI disease? (Some GI diseases may be familial.)

• What stresses have occurred in your life lately? (Stress tends to increase parasympathetic impulses, which leads to increased GI motility.)

To decrease the risk for or incidence of diarrhea, the nurse and client together can try to decrease causative factors with the ultimate goal of "a regular formed bowel movement." Many actions can easily be incorporated into the client's daily routine (see box).

Although diarrhea is a side effect of many medications, clients need to be aware that they should not stop taking the medication because of the unpleasant side effects. They should be taught that once the medication is discontinued, the diarrhea generally dissipates within a few days.

If diarrhea becomes severe, an antidiarrheal medication might be ordered. Opiates (e.g., codeine, paregoric, Lomotil bismuth liquid) decrease intestinal muscle tone, which helps to slow the passage of feces.

Fecal Incontinence

Fecal **incontinence** is the inability of the anal sphincter to control the discharge of feces and gas. The most common causes are weakness of the external or internal anal sphincters and impairment of anal and rectal sensation. These can occur, for instance, from a spinal cord injury, a cerebrovascular accident (stroke), multiple sclerosis, tumors at the anal sphincters, or muscle flaccidity.

There are many ramifications for an individual who has incontinence. Fecal incontinence is emotionally distressing and can cause embarrassment, which

HEALTH PROMOTION AND PREVENTION

MANAGING DIARRHEA

• Drink at least eight glasses of water a day to prevent dehydration

• Limit fatty foods, such as processed meats and dairy products

• Increase intake of foods high in soluble fiber, such as skinless fruits or potatoes

• Avoid alcohol

• Limit caffeine

• Limit amounts of cold beverages

• Limit foods high in insoluble fiber, such as raw fruits and vegetables and whole grain breads and cereals

• Be aware of and limit foods that cause diarrhea

• If taking medications that cause diarrhea, confer with doctor or nurse practitioner

• Use soft toilet paper or cotton balls to wipe perianal area if it is irritated

could lead to social isolation. This is especially upsetting to the elderly, who might already be isolated from their peers because of other factors. Fecal incontinence can also lead to skin breakdown because of the acidic nature of stool. Therefore, it is equally important to deal with the emotional and physical outcomes of incontinence.

It is important to obtain a bowel history and explore the history of the incontinence. When did the incontinence begin? What changes in the client's life can be correlated with the incontinence? What other medical or psychological history might the client have that could affect bowel elimination? Potential causes should be identified. The nurse should assess the effects of the incontinence on the client's self-concept. Along with nursing interventions (see "Implementation") emotional support should always be offered.

Impaction

Fecal **impaction** is the prolonged retention or accumulation of fecal material, which forms a hardened mass in the rectum. Because of this, normal stool cannot be expelled. Fluid may seep around the hardened mass, and the client may complain of a constant oozing of diarrhea or a ribbonlike stool. Impaction is generally caused by unrelieved constipation. People who are at risk for impaction are those who are debilitated, unconscious, or confused or who have had a barium swallow or enema but have not passed the barium. (Barium is a chalky emulsion that solidifies in time if not evacuated.)

Besides passing liquid or ribbon-shaped stool, the client may complain of anorexia, cramping, rectal pain, or abdominal distention related to the stool that cannot be removed from the colon. The stool also may be palpated through the abdomen. The impaction can generally be palpated on digital rectal examination. The nurse should be aware of the possible need for a doctor's order to do a rectal examination on a client, depending on institutional policy.

It is always best to prevent an impaction from occurring. Once an impaction is diagnosed, it needs to be removed to prevent further discomfort and complications. Oil and cleansing enemas often are helpful in relieving an impaction. If these do not offer relief, the mass must be manually disimpacted.

Flatulence

Air or gas in the GI tract is known as **flatus.** The three causes of flatus are swallowed air, gas that leaves the bloodstream and enters the intestine, and bacteria acting on chyme in the large intestine.

Most gases that are swallowed are expelled through the mouth by belching. **Flatulence,** which is excessive gas in the intestines, causes the intestines to stretch and distend, a condition called **tympanites.** Air and gases that build up within the stomach cause gastric distention. Most gases that are formed in the large intestine are absorbed through the intestinal capillaries into the bloodstream. Bacterial action on nonabsorbable carbohydrates, such as lactulose and sorbitol, also causes the bowel wall to stretch and distend. Any gas that is passed through the gastrointestinal system and is expelled through the anus is called flatus.

One of the easiest ways to decrease flatulence is to avoid consuming irritating and gas-forming foods and beverages, such as lentils, dried beans, broccoli, onions, brussel sprouts, cauliflower, and beer. Activities such as drinking through a straw, drinking carbonated fluids, sucking on hard candy, and chewing gum increase the swallowing of air. Decreasing these practices results in less air being swallowed and, subsequently, less flatulence.

When intestinal motility is decreased enough, flatulence could become severe. This occurs commonly in clients who have abdominal surgery, are immobile, and use opiates. The air that remains in the GI tract causes abdominal cramps to often accompany flatulence. Interventions should be aimed at encouraging the escape of flatus. The client should be encouraged to move around in bed (if bed rest is necessary) or to ambulate if able because these interventions help to promote peristalsis and the passing of flatus.

Hemorrhoids

Hemorrhoids, also known as piles, are abnormally distended veins that generally result from an increase in venous pressure during defecation. Internal hemorrhoids are inside the rectum and are moist and red. External hemorrhoids are protrusions of skin outside the anus. Hemorrhoids may occur in clients who have chronic liver disease, are pregnant, have congestive heart failure, or strain on defecation.

Hemorrhoids can be completely asymptomatic. When hemorrhoids become inflamed and tender, a client may complain of itching, burning, and pain. Bleeding may occur from venous stretching.

Often, hemorrhoids do not require treatment and spontaneously shrink. External hemorrhoids may be treated with astringents, which shrink the tissues. If they cause discomfort, hemorrhoids may be treated with local anesthetics. Local heat, such as provided by sitz baths, is also soothing for external hemorrhoids. Internal and external hemorrhoids may also be removed surgically.

If the hemorrhoids are enlarged, care must be taken when inserting a thermometer or suppository into the rectum. The goal for a client with hemorrhoids is to have soft-formed stools. Stool softeners are useful to decrease the irritation that would come from passing hard stools. If the person has pain while having a bowel movement, the urge may be ignored, causing constipation, which would further irritate the hemorrhoids.

Application of the Nursing Process Related to Bowel Elimination

Assessment

Nursing History

To determine whether a person is at risk for a bowel elimination problem, a nursing history is essential. A major component of the nursing history is to obtain information about the individual's normal or usual patterns of bowel elimination.

The nursing history should include information on dietary intake, appetite, digestion, bowel elimination patterns, medications taken, and both a personal and family history of any GI problems (Box 31–2). In relation to diet and appetite, it is helpful to know what the client's usual dietary pattern is, including what he or she eats and what changes (if any) he or she has noticed. For example, does the client find that he or she is eating more or less than usual lately? Has a weight gain or loss occurred? Was this weight change intentional or not? Does he or she ever have vague or mild complaints of heartburn, an upset stomach, indigestion, nausea, or vomiting? Because most people have experienced these symptoms at one time or another, they are easily dismissed as being "harmless or meaningless" symptoms. However, these symptoms could indicate serious problems, especially if associated with other complaints.

In this country, elimination is considered to be a private matter, and most people have difficulty discussing this topic. The nurse must obtain this information, as well as the rest of the history and physical, in a private area. The nurse needs to ask about the client's routine bowel habits. How often does the client have a bowel movement? What time of day? What color and consistency are the bowel movements? Has the client noticed any changes in the pattern? Does the client use any artificial aids in maintaining elimination, such as laxatives or enemas? If so, how often? Is the client taking any kind of medication? Many medications (such as antibiotics) have GI side effects, and the nurse must know this information to better assess the client.

If the client is a child, the parents should be included in obtaining the nursing history. If the child is able to speak and understand, the child should be able to contribute to the history as well. For an older child, questions such as those listed in the previous paragraph should be asked. For younger children, the nurse should obtain information about the color, consistency, and number of stools. If the stools are bulky, have a bad odor, or float in the toilet, this could indicate a malabsorption problem. What age was the child toilet trained? This gives clues as to developmental problems. Does the child have any accidental bowel movement when ill? Some children regress when they do not feel well, but this may not necessarily indicate a GI problem. Is the underwear ever soiled? This could be an indication of incontinence. Has the child been vomiting or having difficulty gaining weight? These could be a sign of an obstruction, such as pyloric stenosis.

The nurse also needs to ask general questions regarding the client's health care habits:

* Does the client smoke? (Using tobacco affects taste perception and could affect the appetite. It also predisposes one to oral cancer.)
* Does the client drink alcohol? (Alcohol can irritate the lining of the stomach.)
* Does the client ingest caffeine? (Caffeine can also irritate the lining of the stomach and increases intestinal motility.)
* What is a typical day like? (For example, a sedentary lifestyle has been associated with constipation.)
* Is the client's job stressful? (Stress is associated with diarrhea.)
* Has he or she traveled to a foreign country lately? (Because foods differ in various parts of the world, a change in foods ingested could create a change in bowel activity.)

The nurse should also ascertain if the client ever had surgery of the GI tract.

Physical Assessment

After obtaining the pertinent health history, the nurse proceeds with the physical assessment, which involves the examination of the mouth, abdomen, and rectum. The client should be told that the examination should not be painful, although some discomfort might be experienced. The examination area should be private, warm, well lit, and quiet.

The assessment begins with the mouth, using the techniques of inspection and palpation. Mucous membranes should be moist, smooth, without lesions, and pink. The mucous membranes of dark-skinned pa-

---

Box 31–2

BOWEL HISTORY

Pattern: How often? What time of day?

Description: How does stool look (*e.g.*, color, consistency)?

Type of diet: What is normal daily intake? What type of fluids? How much? How is your appetite? Have you changed your diet recently?

Exercise: Usual pattern?

Medications taken: Routine? How long? Are medications taken to assist with bowel elimination?

Stress: Is there a stress at home or outside the home?

Family history: Is there any family history of GI problems?

Have there been any recent changes in any of the above?

tients normally have a bluish tint. Assess for missing, broken, loose, and repaired teeth. The tongue and lips should be examined for any inflamed or irritated areas. While examining the mouth, the nurse should note any breath odors because certain breath odors could indicate a problem with the GI system. For instance, a fecal odor emanating from the mouth could be an indication of an intestinal obstruction or ketoacidosis.

The abdomen should be assessed next. The client should be encouraged to urinate first and should be lying supine with the head on a small pillow to prevent abdominal muscle tensing. The chest and genitals should be covered, with the abdomen exposed. If a client complains of orthopnea (difficulty breathing when lying down) or has difficulty lying flat, the head and trunk may be elevated and the knees slightly flexed to promote relaxation of the abdominal muscles. Abdominal assessment of a child up to the age of 2 or 3 years can be done on the parent's lap. This will help the child feel more secure and relaxed. Relaxation can be enhanced by giving the child a bottle or pacifier to suck on during the examination.

Inspection

Assessment of the abdomen proceeds from inspection to auscultation to percussion to palpation. Inspection of the abdomen should occur while looking at the client from the foot of the bed as well as from the client's side. The abdomen should be inspected for contour, shape, skin integrity, appearance of the umbilicus, and visible pulsations. When supine, the abdomen generally appears slightly rounded. Slender clients have a flat or slightly concave abdomen, and obese clients tend to have a protruding abdomen. An infant's abdomen appears rounded and dome shaped because abdominal musculature is not fully developed. A young child's abdomen appears potbellied and becomes more convex by the time the child is 5 or 6 years old. The skin should appear smooth and intact, with varying amounts of hair. Assess for any discoloration surrounding the umbilicus. A bluish tinge could indicate an intraabdominal bleed. Observe for peristalsis, which is generally not seen on observation. If it is present, it could be an indication of an intestinal obstruction. In assessing for an umbilical hernia, the nurse should have the client raise the head and shoulders while remaining supine. A protrusion is noted if a hernia is present.

Auscultation

The nurse should warm his or her hands and stethoscope before proceeding with the next step of auscultation. This is done before percussion and palpation because these assessment techniques can alter intestinal activity and bowel sounds. The techniques of auscultation and percussion are the same for all age groups. Auscultation gives information about bowel motility and the underlying vessels and organs. The diaphragm of the stethoscope should be used in listening to the four abdominal quadrants.

Bowel sounds are produced from the movement of fluid and air in the GI tract and are soft, bubbling sounds that are usually heard every 5 to 15 seconds. Hypoactive bowel sounds (those heard less frequently than every 15 seconds) or absent bowel sounds could occur postoperatively and might be a sign of paralytic ileus. They also could occur when the bowel is full of feces, and motility slows down. Borborygmus, or "growling," occurs when bowel sounds are abnormally intense and frequent (hyperperistalsis) and is usually assessed when one is hungry. High-pitched and hyperactive bowel sounds could indicate a small intestine obstruction or an inflammatory disorder.

Percussion

Percussion is used to determine the size and location of abdominal organs and detects excessive accumulation of fluid and air in the abdomen. An air-filled stomach or abdomen is tympanic. An infant's abdomen may be more tympanic on percussion than an adult's because infants swallow air when crying or feeding. Dullness is assessed over the liver and spleen. This dullness also is found if an intestinal obstruction or a mass is present.

The abdomen might also be distended, which causes it to feel tight. This could be a sign of a tumor, excess fluid or gas, or severe malnutrition. Distention is sometimes difficult to assess. For instance, a heavy client may have an abdomen that appears and feels tight. In this case, it is best to ask the person if this is how the abdomen routinely is, or if this is a change for the client. If distention is suspected, abdominal girth needs to be monitored. This is done using a tape measure, usually at the level of the umbilicus, while the client is supine. The area used should be marked with a felt-tipped pen so that all staff members measure in the same place for accuracy.

Palpation

Palpation, the last assessment technique for the abdomen, involves checking for the presence, degree of, and location of pain and masses. The abdomen should be mentally divided into either four quadrants or nine sections (Fig. 31–3). Dividing the abdomen into four quadrants is the more common and easier method. Using the nine-section method allows for more precise identification of organ location. When palpating a young child's abdomen, the feet should be slightly elevated and the knees flexed; this helps to promote more relaxation of the abdominal musculature. A firm, rather than a soft, touch should be used, as some children may feel "ticklish" in the abdominal area. It is important for the nurse to know if any areas are painful because these should be assessed last. Touching painful areas first tenses the abdominal muscles, making other assessments either inaccurate or difficult.

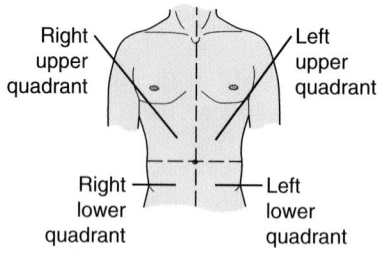

Quadrants of the abdomen

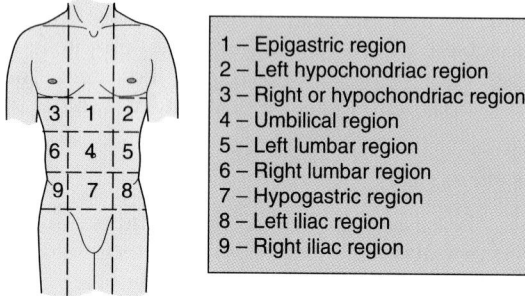

1 – Epigastric region
2 – Left hypochondriac region
3 – Right or hypochondriac region
4 – Umbilical region
5 – Left lumbar region
6 – Right lumbar region
7 – Hypogastric region
8 – Left iliac region
9 – Right iliac region

Regions of the Abdomen

❧ **Figure 31–3**
For systematic assessment of the abdominal organs, the abdomen is mentally divided into four sections (quadrants) or nine sections. The quadrant method is simpler and more commonly used. The nine-section method allows for more precise identification of organ location.

The rectal examination is the last part of the physical related to the GI system. This can be uncomfortable both physically and psychologically. It is usually done only for clients who are older than 40 years but should be included in the physical assessment of anyone with a history of bowel elimination changes or anal area discomfort or of an adult man with urinary problems. Inspection and palpation are done during examination of the rectal area.

If the client is ambulatory, the best positioning for a rectal examination is with the client standing with toes pointed inward and bending forward over an examination table. If the client is unable to get out of bed, the knee-chest position can be used. Because this is a difficult position for either a pregnant or an elderly client, the left lateral Sims position, in which the knees are drawn up and the buttocks are near the edge of the bed, is acceptable. Infants and young children should be placed on the back. The feet should be held together, with the knees and hips flexed onto the child's abdomen. Positions for rectal examination are shown in Figure 31–4.

During inspection, the anus and surrounding area should be exposed. The skin around the anal opening should appear intact and darker than the surrounding skin. The nurse should observe for any breaks in skin integrity, discharge, fissures, inflammation, lesions, scars, prolapse, hemorrhoids, or polyps. The client should then be asked to strain, as if having a bowel movement. This helps in assessing for internal hemorrhoids, polyps, or a rectal prolapse.

The nurse should then palpate the external and then the internal area. However, an internal rectal examination should not be done on a client who re-

Positions for rectal examination

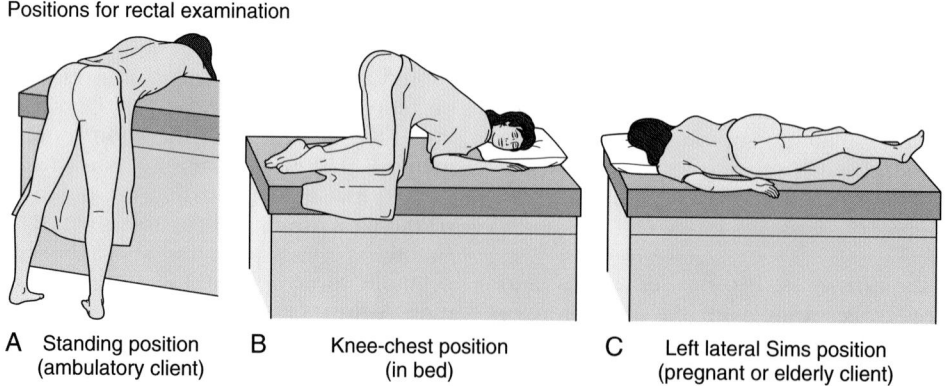

A Standing position
(ambulatory client)

B Knee-chest position
(in bed)

C Left lateral Sims position
(pregnant or elderly client)

❧ **Figure 31–4**
Positioning for rectal examination. An ambulatory client should stand with toes pointed inward and should be bent forward over a chair or examination table (A). The knee-chest position (B) can be used for a bedridden client. For an elderly or a pregnant client, the best position is the left lateral Sims (C), with knees drawn up and buttocks near the edge of the bed.

cently suffered from a myocardial infarction. A gloved finger covered with a water-soluble lubricant should be inserted 2.5 to 3 in (6–7.5 cm) into the rectum. The client should be encouraged to breathe through the mouth to decrease discomfort. If a constriction occurs, the nurse should not try to force his or her finger into the client's rectum. The nurse should rotate the finger, checking for sphincter tone and assessing for nodules, tenderness, irregularities, or impaction. The mucous membrane should feel smooth and soft. If mucus, blood, or stool is found on the gloved finger, this (as well as all findings) should be documented.

If possible, the nurse should assess the client's stool. Normal characteristics in the adult are that the stool is brown, formed, soft, semisolid, moist, and cylindrical, approximately 1 inch in diameter. Stool is composed of small amounts of undigested roughage, sloughed dead bacteria, and epithelial cells, as well as fat, protein, digestive juices, and inorganic material. The normal odor of stool is from the products of bacterial breakdown of protein in the colon, which are called indole and skatole.

The nurse should be aware of any abnormal stool characteristics (Table 31–1). For instance, a black or tarry stool could indicate an upper GI bleed or may be from ingestion of foods high in iron. Reddish stools could be an indication of lower GI bleed or could simply be found after the client ingested beets. Pale stool may be from the inability to adequately absorb fats. If pus is found or the stool has a pungent odor, this could be an indication of an intestinal infection. A narrow or pencil-shaped stool could indicate an intestinal obstruction.

It is important for the nurse to include the history and physical assessment findings when formulating a plan of care.

Diagnostic Studies

Many clients who present with GI symptomatology must undergo diagnostic examinations to ensure accurate diagnosis of their problem. The nurse plays an integral role in these testing measures.

Direct Visualization

Direct visualization of the GI system can occur by passing an instrument through the mouth or the rectum. These instruments can inspect the mucosa, blood vessels, and internal body organs. A fiberoptic endoscope is an optical instrument with a lens viewer and a light source. It is a long and flexible tube that allows the physician to observe the GI system and to obtain biopsy specimens. Because the tube is flexible, less trauma and discomfort occurs than if a rigid instrument were used. A rigid instrument is sometimes necessary when exploring the sigmoid colon and rectum. Unfortunately, the use of a rigid tube produces some discomfort.

As with any other procedure, clients need to be educated about any GI diagnostic procedures that they may have. The nurse is usually the one who initiates

---

Table 31–1

STOOL CHARACTERISTICS

	NORMAL	ABNORMAL	POSSIBLE RATIONALE FOR ABNORMALITY
Color	Adult—brown Infant—yellow	Black or tarry (melena) Red White or clay-colored Fatty and pale Green	Upper GI bleed; diet high in red meat or dark green vegetables; iron intake Hemorrhoids; lower GI bleed; ingestion of beets Absence of bile; after barium studies Malabsorption of fat Intestinal infection
Odor	Aromatic (depends on what one eats)	Very strong, noxious	Blood in feces or intestinal infection
Consistency	Soft but formed	Liquid Hard	Reduced absorption; increased motility Decreased motility; dehydration; laxative abuse
Frequency	Adult—daily to several times a week	More than normal	Hypermotility
	Infant—several times a day	Less than normal	Hypomotility
Shape	Cylindrical	Ribbonlike, narrow	Obstruction
Constituents	Undigested food, water, dead bacteria, bile pigment, fat, cells from intestinal mucosa	Mucus Pus Blood Foreign bodies Fat	Inflammation Infection GI bleed Swallowed foreign objects Malabsorption

this teaching. If the client is having a procedure done on an outpatient basis, the physician may initiate the teaching. The nurse, however, needs to reinforce any teaching when the client presents in the outpatient setting to make sure that preprocedure requirements have been met and to ensure that the client fully understands what to expect.

An esophagogastroduodenoscopy (EGD) is done to visualize the lining of the esophagus, stomach, and upper duodenum. A fiberoptic endoscope is inserted through the mouth. This procedure is used to check for hernias, obstructions, tumors, vascular changes, inflammation, or ulcers. It can also be used to remove foreign bodies or polyps. A review of the nursing care of a client undergoing an esophagogastroduodenoscopy can be found in Box 31–3.

Direct visualization of the lower intestine occurs with the use of a scope inserted through the anus. A proctoscopy is done to explore the anus and rectum, and a sigmoidoscopy allows the physician to look at the anus, rectum, and sigmoid colon. Together, these procedures are called a proctosigmoidoscopy. A **colonoscopy** allows visualization of the lining of the large intestine using a fiberoptic endoscope.

A proctosigmoidoscopy or colonoscopy might be done if the client has complained of changes in bowel habits; lower abdominal or perineal pain; or mucus, blood, or pus in the bowel movement. These procedures can check for inflammation, infections, ulcerative bowel disease, hemorrhoids, fistulas, or abscesses. A review of the nursing care of a client undergoing direct visualization of the lower GI tract can be found in Box 31–4.

All of the procedures described here are generally done in the radiology department or in a day surgery setting. However, if the client's condition is unstable it is possible to do these procedures at the bedside. The client is awake during all of these procedures because the risk of problems if general anesthesia is used is increased. An intravenous line is started, and intravenous sedation in the form of diazepam (Valium), midazolam HCl (Versed), or meperidine HCl (Demerol) is generally given (Renkes, 1993) so that the client generally does not remember the procedure on its completion. The client's blood pressure, electrocardiogram, and oxygen saturation (measured with a pulse oximeter) are monitored throughout the procedure. The client may hear alarms sounding during the procedure, even if all goes well, so he or she needs to be made aware of this prior to the start of the procedure. Emergency equipment must always be accessible.

Indirect Visualization

Sometimes direct visualization of deeper GI structures is not possible. In these cases, indirect x-ray examinations would be used. A contrast medium would either be ingested orally or instilled rectally, depending on whether the upper or lower GI tract needs to be examined. The most common contrast medium used is barium, a white and chalky radi-

---

Box 31–3

NURSING INTERVENTIONS FOR CLIENT UNDERGOING ESOPHAGOGASTRODUODENOSCOPY

Preprocedure

- Validate that signed consent is present
- Preprocedure teaching regarding nothing by mouth after midnight (or 6 to 12 hours before procedure, depending on institutional policy)
- Teaching
  Procedure lasts anywhere from 10 to 30 minutes
  Dentures and jewelry should be removed
  A mouth guard (oral airway) may be placed to protect the teeth
  Explanation of procedure:
    An anesthetic spray will be given to help pass and keep tube in throat
    Spray tastes bitter and numbs the back of the throat and mouth
    May feel gagging sensation and will be unable to talk
    Breathing is not affected by the spray
- Reassure
  Because client will be given sedative before the procedure, he or she may not remember it

During Procedure

- Provide emotional support
- Obtain baseline and monitor vital signs
- Administer intravenous sedation
- Observe for respiratory or other complications or problems
- If cautery is needed, apply ground pad to client
- Maintain towel or basin near mouth to catch secretions; suction mouth as needed
- Maintain client on left side
- Label and send specimens to lab

Postprocedure

- Give nothing by mouth until gag reflex returns
- Explain that hoarseness and sore throat may persist for a few days but may be treated with fluids, warm normal saline gargles, or throat lozenges
- Assess for and teach about adverse effects, such as respiratory distress, infection, or perforation (pain, vomiting blood, or persistent dysphagia)
- Document client response

---

opaque substance that "coats" the area being assessed. Oral barium is usually flavored for improved taste. Indirect visualization is helpful in detecting inflammatory disease, obstructions, ulcers, tumors, a hiatal hernia, or other structural changes.

An upper GI series (or barium swallow) visualizes the lower esophagus, stomach, and duodenum. It is

Box 31–4

NURSING INTERVENTIONS FOR CLIENT UNDERGOING DIRECT VISUALIZATION OF LOWER GASTROINTESTINAL TRACT

Colonoscopy

Preprocedure

- Validate that signed consent is present
- Teaching
  Need for oral osmotic solution to evacuate bowel without losing excessive electrolytes (e.g., polyethylene glycol electrolyte solution [goLYTELY])
  Solution tastes salty, so it is better if taken chilled; it should not be diluted (do not add ice)
  Drink 8 oz every 15 minutes until a full gallon is taken
  Should not drink small quantities constantly because this will not clean out the system as well
  Diarrhea usually begins 30 to 60 minutes after the first glass
  Bowels usually empty within 4 hours
  Clear fluids should be given the evening before procedure, and nothing is given by mouth the day of the procedure
  May need oral laxatives (pills) the evening before
  Explanation about procedure
    Include that the client will be given a sedative but still might feel the urge to pass flatus and have a bowel movement during procedure
    Many feel that the preparation for colonoscopy is more tiring than the procedure itself

During Procedure

- Provide emotional support
- Obtain baseline and monitor vital signs
- Administer intravenous sedation
- Maintain client draped and on left side with knees flexed
- Observe for respiratory distress (from intravenous sedation)
- Label and send specimens to laboratory

Postprocedure

- Assess vital signs
- Resume usual diet
- Encourage client to pass flatus if necessary
- Assess for and teach about adverse effects, such as rectal bleeding, abdominal pain (may indicate bowel perforation), fever, pain, malaise, distention (may indicate infection)
- Teach client that if polyp was removed, there may be blood in the stool
- Document client response

Proctosigmoidoscopy

Preprocedure

- Validate that signed consent is present
- Depending on hospital policy, enema or laxative night before procedure
- Depending on hospital policy, clear liquids or light meal evening before procedure
- Teach about procedure
  May feel discomfort and need to have bowel movement
  May feel gassy because air is instilled for better visualization

During Procedure

- Provide emotional support
- Maintain client draped; place in knee-chest or left lateral position
- Encourage client to bear down as scope is passed through anal sphincter
- Label and send specimens to laboratory

Postprocedure

- Same as for colonoscopy

---

commonly performed on clients who present with difficulty swallowing, epigastric burning or pain, weight loss, or a history of GI bleeding.

A lower GI series (or barium enema) visualizes the lower colon and is commonly performed on clients with altered bowel habits; lower abdominal pain; or mucus, pus, or blood in the stool. At times it is necessary to do both an upper and a lower GI series. If this is the case, the lower is done first because the barium takes longer to pass through the intestinal tract when an upper GI series is done than when the lower GI is done. It is extremely important for the client to pass the barium, as it becomes hardened within the GI tract if not passed. It is also necessary to realize that if the client has active GI bleeding or ulcerative colitis, a standard bowel preparation may not be tolerable. Bowel preparations may be irritating to the GI system and may exacerbate an episode of bleeding or colitis.

Nursing implications for the client undergoing an upper and lower GI series may be found in Box 31–5.

Stool Specimens

Medical aseptic technique must be utilized when obtaining a stool specimen. Because 25% of the solid portion of stool is bacteria from the colon, the nurse should wear gloves when in contact with another person's stool. The nurse is responsible for accurately obtaining, labeling, sealing, and sending the fecal specimen. It is important that urine, vaginal drainage,

---

Box **31–5**

NURSING INTERVENTIONS FOR CLIENT UNDERGOING UPPER AND LOWER GASTROINTESTINAL SERIES

Upper Gastrointestinal Series

Preprocedure

- Validate that informed consent is present

- Validate that client has maintained a low-residue diet (if possible) for 2 to 3 days and that client has received nothing by mouth since midnight

- Explain procedure to client
  Will drink 16 to 20 oz of barium contrast
  Procedure takes several hours to complete
  Will be on x-ray table, which rotates, changing client's position at times
  Discomfort minimal, except for the "hard" examination table on which client is placed

- Place client in hospital gown

Postprocedure

- Procedure is very tiring, so encourage rest afterward

- Encourage fluids to help expel barium

- Cathartics often are given to help expel barium (if barium is not passed within 2 to 3 days, doctor must be notified)

- Check stools for barium (appears chalky white)

- Client may resume previous diet immediately following procedure

- Document client response

Lower Gastrointestinal Series

Preprocedure

- Validate that informed consent is present

- Validate that client has maintained a low-residue diet (if possible) for 2 to 3 days and that client has had only clear fluids for 12 to 24 hours (depending on institutional policy); ensure that enema or cathartic has been given (as per hospital policy)

- Explain procedure to client
  Barium instilled via rectum (500–1500 ml)
  May feel fullness and cramping during this, but deep breathing helps to decrease discomfort
  Procedure takes 30 to 45 minutes; client will need to change position during examination

- Place client in hospital gown

Postprocedure

- Encourage fluids to expel barium and counteract dehydrating effects of cathartics

- Observe stools for barium

- Client may resume previous diet immediately following procedure

- Document client response

---

and toilet paper not be mixed with the stool specimen.

When obtaining a sample, 1 in of formed stool or 15 to 30 ml of liquid stool is generally sufficient. If any visible areas of blood, mucus, or pus are noted, these are the areas that should be tested. It is generally better to sample a fresh specimen and send it to the laboratory immediately. If this is not possible, the sample should be refrigerated (unless contraindicated by a specific test). Some specimens must be sent to the laboratory warm, such as those required for ova and parasites testing because bacteriological changes that occur at room temperature might affect results.

If it is suspected that a client has pinworms, clear cellophane tape should be placed on the anal area for a few seconds, removed, and then placed on a slide. This type of specimen should be taken first thing in the morning, before the client has a bowel movement or bath, because pinworms go to the anal area at night and enter the rectum during the day.

A common specimen that is obtained is a stool for guaiac, which monitors for hidden or occult blood. The guaiac test is useful for assessment of bleeding within the GI tract (see Procedure 31–1).

Nursing Diagnosis

Assessment of the client's GI tract may indicate an actual or a potential elimination problem. Alterations in bowel elimination may also affect other aspects of human functioning; therefore, clients can have primary and secondary diagnoses. Possible nursing diagnoses related to bowel elimination are listed in the box.

Planning

Once a diagnosis is established, the client and nurse mutually set goals and identify expected outcomes for restoring regular bowel elimination patterns (see Sample Nursing Care Plan). The plan of care should include the client's routines and habits. If these habits contributed to the problem, the nurse utilizes the opportunity to teach the client. Include the family and other health team members, such as the enterostomal therapist, in the plan of care when indicated. Examples of expected outcomes include

> The client's elimination pattern will be regular within 1 week
> The client's skin around the ostomy will remain intact
> The client will identify high-fiber foods within 3 days

Implementation

When implementing nursing interventions that will help to promote normal defecation and bowel habits, the nurse needs to be able to deal with his or her own feelings regarding bowel elimination. For example, does the nurse accept bowel elimination as a normal part of life, or is the nurse unable to openly

PROCEDURE

31–1

TESTING STOOL FOR OCCULT BLOOD

Equipment:

Hemoccult sample collection
card
Hemoccult developing solu-
tion
Disposable gloves
Wooden applicator

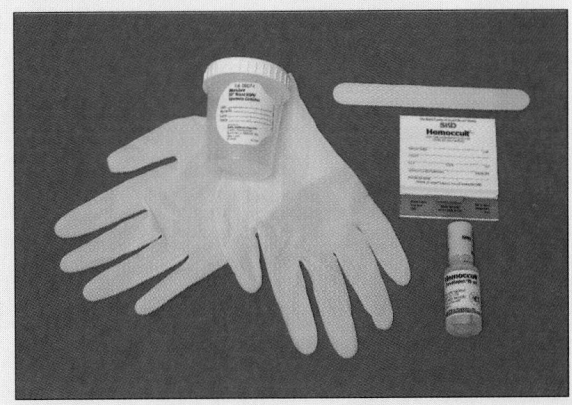

Nursing Action	**Rationale**
1. Assess diet and medications that the client has taken for the past 2 to 3 days.	1. Some medications, such as steroids, may give false readings. Red meats give a false positive.
2. Explain the procedure to client.	2. To ensure compliance and to educate client.
3. Wash hands and don clean gloves.	3. To prevent contamination with feces.
4. Using the wooden applicator, collect stool specimen, making sure it has not been contaminated by urine, menses, water, or toilet paper.	4. These contaminants might alter test results.
5. Open flap of test kit, and using thin wooden stick provided in Hemoccult test kit, make a thin smear in first box.	5. A thick smear may not allow guaiac developer to work accurately.

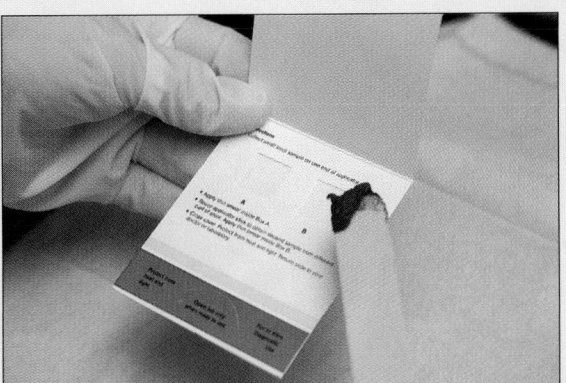

Step 5.

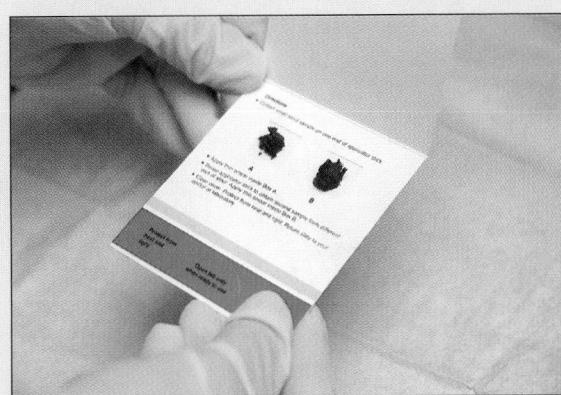

Step 6.

6. Take another sample (from a different area of stool) and make a thin smear in second box (using other side of wooden applicator).	6. By using another area, the chance of detecting blood is increased.

Continued

PROCEDURE

31–1

TESTING STOOL FOR OCCULT BLOOD
(Continued)

Nursing Action	**Rationale**
7. Close the flap on the test kit, turn it over, and open flap on other side.	7. This is where the guaiac developer will be placed.

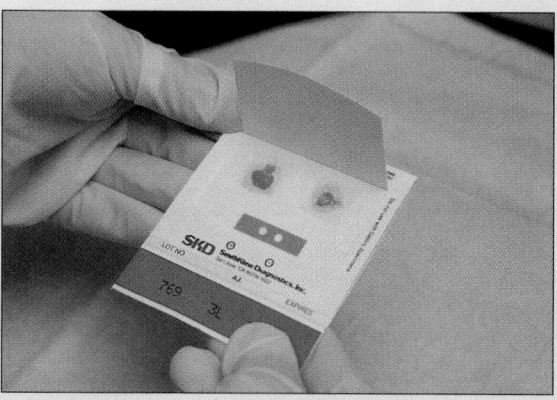

Step 7.

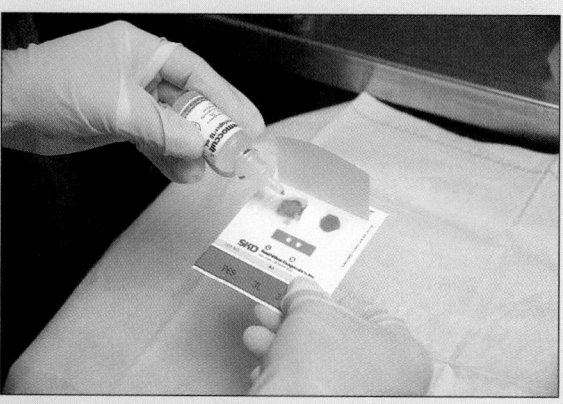

Step 8.

8. Place two drops of Hemoccult developing solution in each box and one drop between positive and negative control areas.	8. If blood is present, the developer will react with the stool.
9. After 30 to 60 seconds, compare test results with the control area.	9. A positive test result, which means that blood is present, will show a blue color.

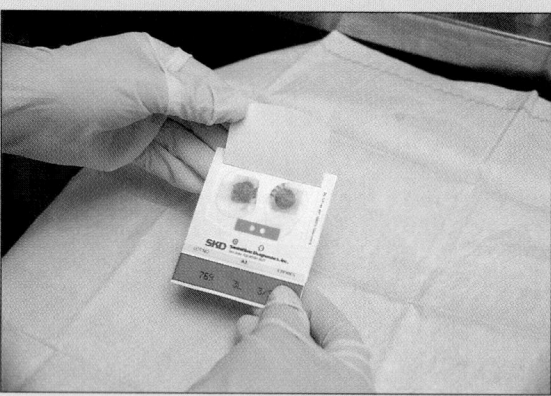

Step 9.

10. Discard test kit and wooden stick in appropriate container.	10. To decrease chance of contamination.
11. Remove gloves and wash hands.	11. To decrease chance of contamination.
12. Explain results to client.	12. To keep client informed.
13. Document results in the chart.	13. To communicate test results.

discuss the matter, considering it a "dirty" topic? It is important for the nurse to recognize his or her own feelings before being able to assist the client.

The nurse can do many things to assist the client with promotion of regular bowel habits (see box). For instance, for the hospitalized client, the call bell should be answered promptly. For a client in a home setting, bathroom facilities should be accessible and

NURSING DIAGNOSES RELATED TO BOWEL ELIMINATION

North American Nursing Diagnosis Association–approved diagnoses that are primary include

* Constipation
* Colonic Constipation
* Perceived Constipation
* Diarrhea
* Bowel Incontinence

Secondary diagnoses include

* Anxiety related to ostomy, diarrhea, or constipation
* Body Image Disturbance related to ostomy
* Growth and Development, altered, related to bowel training
* Individual Coping, Ineffective, related to ostomy or bowel incontinence
* Knowledge Deficit related to ostomy, diarrhea, or constipation
* Pain related to ostomy, diarrhea, or constipation
* Self Care Deficit: toileting related to bowel incontinence
* Sexual Dysfunction related to ostomy or bowel incontinence
* Skin Integrity, Risk for Impaired, related to ostomy or bowel incontinence
* Fluid Volume Deficit, Risk for, related to ostomy or bowel incontinence

HEALTH PROMOTION AND PREVENTION

PROMOTING ELIMINATION

* Do not ignore the urge to defecate
* The nurse should allow sufficient time and privacy
* Establish and maintain a regular exercise regimen
* Drink 2 to 3 L of fluid a day
* Include high-fiber foods in your daily diet, such as vegetables, fruit, and whole grains
* Avoid routine use of laxatives or enemas
* Maintain either a squatting or sitting down and leaning forward position when defecating

convenient to use. For example, a person who has had a hip fracture repaired needs to use an elevated toilet seat at home. Often, special devices or services can be arranged for before the client is discharged from the hospital. For example, the elderly client may have difficulty getting up or down from a low toilet seat, and railings may need to be installed in the bathroom at home.

The promotion of privacy, timing, diet, and exercise is essential in assisting the client to maintain or regain regular elimination habits. As with all other health maintenance, the family should be included in the plan of care, and explanations should be given when necessary.

Privacy

In our society, bowel elimination tends to be a private matter. At home, a person can close and lock the bathroom door without being disturbed. This "luxury" may not be afforded to the ill client, whether at home or in the hospital. If a client is able to get out of bed and use the bathroom, then this should be allowed. The bathroom door should be kept shut (or just slightly ajar if there is a potential safety issue). The nurse or caretaker can stay close by. For the bedridden client who is able to get on and off of a bedpan independently, the bedpan should be left within easy reach. If the client is bedridden, the curtains and door should be closed to enhance privacy. However, this situation is far from ideal because many hospital rooms are semiprivate, and the client could experience embarrassment from the odors and sounds associated with defecation.

Timing

Most people have a certain time of day when they have a bowel movement. Mass colonic peristalsis generally occurs about 1 hour after meals. Most people tend to have a bowel movement after breakfast, when the gastrocolic and duodenocolic reflexes cause mass propulsive movements in the large intestine. It is important for the nurse to know the client's habits and not to schedule procedures or treatments during this time. For example, the nurse should not plan to give the client a bath 30 to 60 minutes after breakfast if this is when the client usually has a bowel movement. Many clients feel uncomfortable about requesting time to have a bowel movement and may not broach the topic with the nurse.

The client needs to pay attention to the "urge of defecation" and try not to ignore it. If the client ignores the defecation urge then feces stays in the rectum. Although the urge disappears, the defecation reflex brings this feeling back later. Because the longer the stool stays in the intestine, the more water gets absorbed from it, ignoring the urge could lead to constipation. The client should not be rushed when this urge occurs.

Diet

There are several dietary measures that can help promote regular bowel elimination. For instance, un-

SAMPLE NURSING CARE PLAN

THE CLIENT WITH A BOWEL ELIMINATION PROBLEM

Mr. J., 72 years old, is admitted to the hospital complaining of severe back pain. His admitting diagnosis is "severe lumbosacral strain, etiology unknown." The physician has written the following orders:

Complete bed rest

Regular diet

Buck's traction with 8 lb of weight—may remove at bedtime and for morning care

Bedside commode

Robaxin, 1.5 g orally four times a day

Peri-Colace, one capsule orally at bedtime

Percocet, one tablet orally every 4 hours as needed

Mr. J. has a fair appetite but does not like hospital food. Mrs. J. will bring food from home, but she states that her husband likes to eat "mostly pasta and sauce." He also likes garlic bread, grilled cheese, meatloaf, oatmeal, baked beans, tuna, ice cream, and tea. He does not like the way most vegetables taste, and fruit "gives people the runs." Mr. J. is retired; he enjoys bingo, watching television, and reading. He likes to play with his six grandchildren. Today is Mr. J.'s third hospital day, and he is complaining of a stomach ache and cramps. He states, "I'm very regular. I go every morning after my cup of tea." Abdominal assessment reveals hypoactive bowel sounds, and the abdomen is slightly distended. Mr. J. has remained in bed since admission.

Nursing Diagnosis: Constipation related to immobility, as evidenced by complete bed rest, dietary intake, hypoactive bowel sounds, a slightly distended abdomen and the statement "I haven't gone to the bathroom in 2 days."

Expected Outcome: Mr. J. will resume regular bowel habits by time of discharge.

Objective: Mr. J. will increase his fluid and fiber intake starting today.

Action	Rationale
1. Teach client about the need for fiber in the diet.	1. Increased fiber improves muscle tone and helps to promote elimination.
2. Encourage client to drink at least 2000 ml of fluid daily.	2. Increased fluid softens stool and aids in stool passage.
3. Encourage client to increase his consumption of vegetables, fruit, bran, and other high-fiber foods.	3. Increases muscle tone and promotes elimination.
4. Allow sufficient time and privacy for client when urge to defecate occurs.	4. Maintains privacy and promotes relaxation, which may aid in defecation.
5. Encourage client to use bedside commode every morning after breakfast.	5. Because client's usual pattern is to have a bowel movement every morning, he should be encouraged to sit on the commode instead of lying in bed for a more "natural" position.
6. Document stool characteristics whenever client has a bowel movement.	6. To determine and monitor effects of interventions.

less contraindicated, 2 to 3 L of fluid should be taken each day. Fluids that contain alcohol or caffeine should not be counted as fluid because they do not contribute to the body's fluid need and have little nutritional value. Someone who is constipated should increase the amount of fluid taken each day, unless contraindicated. He or she should concentrate on drinking hot fluids and fruit juices, especially prune juice, because these types of fluids help to stimulate peristalsis. Liquids also help to lubricate the stool, making it easier to pass. A person with diarrhea also needs fluids to replace what has been lost. People may not want to drink more fluid because they may think that the fluid will result in more diarrhea. They need to be taught about the consequences of fluid and electrolyte loss that can occur with diarrhea.

Those with diarrhea should avoid excessively hot and cold fluids because these tend to increase peristalsis. Weak tea, bouillon, water, gelatins, and clear soup are helpful for those with diarrhea. If the client is unable to tolerate oral fluids and excessive diarrhea is present, intravenous fluids probably need to be initiated.

Adequate amounts of fiber, such as vegetables, fruits, and grains, must also be ingested. For those who are constipated, foods such as bran products, whole grains, breads, cereals, and raw fruit (such as raisins, apples with peels, and prunes) are excellent, as they are high in fiber. Vegetables are also helpful, as they have a high water content. For those who are elderly or have difficulty chewing, foods can be chopped and pureed. Eating hot meals also helps to stimulate peristalsis, allowing stools to pass easier.

For those who are experiencing diarrhea, bland foods should be encouraged, as they are easily absorbed. Foods and fluids that are high in potassium should also be encouraged (*e.g.,* orange and apple juice, bananas) to replace potassium loss from diarrhea. Highly spiced and high-fiber foods should be avoided because they aggravate the diarrhea. Foods such as pasta, lean beef, chicken, fish, and milk products are low-fiber foods and should be encouraged if possible.

Low-fat, high-fiber, and bulk-forming foods should be encouraged for everyone, depending on their health and dietary allowances, because these have been found to decrease the risk of colorectal cancer (American Cancer Society, 1993; Van Horn *et al.,* 1991). High-fiber foods decrease cancer risk because insoluble fiber or roughage helps to move foods faster through the GI tract, which decreases the amount of time that carcinogens are in contact with the GI mucosa. Saturated fat is more unhealthy than unsaturated fat. Decreasing one's fat intake to less than 30% of the total kilocalories eaten helps to decrease the incidence of cancer (Peckenpaugh & Poleman, 1995) (Box 31–6).

Box **31–6**

WARNING SIGNS AND RISK FACTORS OF COLON CANCER

The incidence of colon cancer has increased in both sexes.

Change in character, consistency, frequency, color of stool

Positive test for occult blood

At higher risk with high-fat, low-fiber diet

Be alert to family history of colon cancer

Age 40 years or older

History of polyps, colitis, Crohn's disease

Rectal bleeding

Exercise

An exercise regimen is imperative in maintaining regular bowel habits. Regular exercise, done several times a week, promotes GI motility. Activities such as walking, bicycling, and swimming are excellent for stimulating bowel motility. For someone who is bedridden, range of motion exercises should be done to stimulate intestinal motility.

A person who has weak abdominal and pelvic muscles—the muscles needed for defecation—can strengthen these muscles by doing isometric exercises. The following are examples of helpful exercises:

* When in a supine position, tighten the abdominal muscles by pulling the abdomen in. Hold for 10 seconds, then relax. If able, this should be repeated 5 to 10 times, four times a day.
* The thigh muscles should be tightened up 5 to 10 times, four times a day. This helps those who are bedridden and must use a bedpan.

If activity and exercise are insufficient, one develops a poor appetite, poor muscle tone, and sluggish intestinal motility. Even a person who is confined to bed rest should have exercise. For instance, turning a client frequently can help to stimulate peristalsis and expel flatus. A person who has difficulty walking long distances but is able to walk around the room should do so. Just walking around the room (as opposed to lying in bed) is a method of increasing intestinal motility and decreasing the risk of constipation.

Promotion of "Normal" Defecation

Positioning

The position that is most helpful in defecating is either squatting or sitting down and leaning forward. For clients who have joint or muscle-wasting diseases, a regular toilet seat may be too low; instead, a raised toilet seat, which fits over a regular toilet seat, should be used. An elderly person who has difficulty sitting on a low toilet would also benefit from a raised seat. These devices can be easily obtained for the home. Using a footstool helps to increase hip flexion.

Sometimes a client is unable to walk to the bathroom but is able to get out of bed. For such clients, a bedside or portable commode can be used (Fig. 31–5). A commode is a portable toilet with armrests. It may have a receptacle underneath it for bowel movements and urine, or it may have an area beneath for a bedpan.

A person who is unable to get out of bed requires the use of a bedpan. There are two types of bedpans: a standard, or regular, bedpan, which is shaped like a regular toilet, and a fracture bedpan, which is smaller and shallower (see Fig. 31–6). A fracture bedpan is used for clients who are unable to raise their buttocks because of a physical problem or whose condition does not allow them to raise their buttocks as high as a regular bedpan requires. A client with a fractured hip, for instance, would need to use a fracture bed-

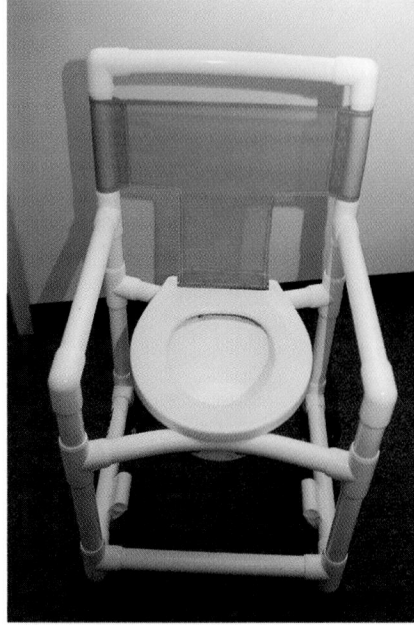

Portable commode.

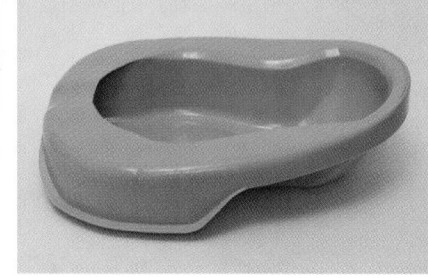

Standard bedpan.

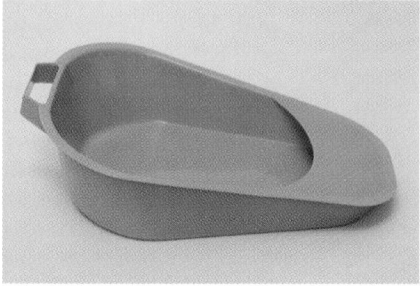

Fracture bedpan.

✦ **Figure 31–5**

For the client who is unable to walk to the bathroom, a bedside commode or a bedpan may be used.

pan. When a client sits on a regular bedpan, the buttocks rest within the rim (as on a regular toilet). If a fracture bedpan is used, the larger (deeper area) is positioned toward the foot of the bed.

It can be very tiring to use a bedpan, so the client may require some assistance. An overbed trapeze helps the client to get on and off of a bedpan. Having to use a bedpan can be very embarrassing because of the lack of privacy during bowel movement. If a client in the home setting has difficulty using a bedpan and cannot get up to go to the bathroom, the family or another caregiver needs to know how to assist with bowel elimination. A family member or assigned caregiver may need to be taught the proper technique for placing and removing a bedpan. Procedure 31–2 explains how to assist a client on and off a bedpan.

Bowel Training

A bowel training program may be used to help establish normal defecation. It can be helpful for those who are incontinent, suffer from constipation, or tend to have frequent impactions. To be considered for a bowel training program, a person needs to have some neuromuscular control. The client cannot have an impaction at the time of initiation of the program—the impaction should be relieved before a bowel training program begins. A potential candidate for bowel training also must have the desire to reestablish a regular bowel program and must want to be actively involved in the process. Consideration must be given to food, fluid, "normal" defecation habits, and exercise. Time, patience, and consistency are integral components of a bowel training program, on the part of both the

client and the caretaker. The nurse must remember that the plan of care must be individualized to the client's needs.

The first step is to determine the client's usual bowel habits and factors that help or hinder defecation. This requires good assessment skills on the part of both the client and the nurse. Times of incontinence should be recorded, as this gives an indication as to when normal defecation times occur. A plan of care can then be discussed with the client. This plan should include adequate fluid and fiber intake, a workable and realistic exercise routine, and a planned time for defecation. A daily routine should be set up, and this needs to be adhered to for at least 2 to 3 weeks before any type of regular pattern can be expected to return. Box 31–7 offers an example of what a bowel training program might entail.

The ultimate goal of care is to eliminate incontinent episodes and decrease or eliminate excoriated skin. Some nursing interventions to assist in the care of the incontinent person include

- Providing skin care. The anal area should be assessed for skin breakdown, and the area should be kept dry and clean. The perianal and rectal area need to be cleaned after each incidence of incontinence. Warm water and soap may be used (avoiding contaminating the urethral and vaginal area). Dry the area thoroughly. Ointments or creams (such as zinc oxide) may be applied to the anal and perianal area.

- Performing frequent linen changes when soiling occurs. Absorbent pads or incontinence pads may be utilized.

- Questioning clients frequently regarding the need to have a bowel movement. By asking and perhaps placing a cli-

PROCEDURE

31–2

ASSISTING A CLIENT ONTO AND OFF A BEDPAN

Equipment:

Toilet paper
Disposable gloves
Wash basin
Clean bedpan
Soap
Towels
Covering for bedpan
Waterproof, absorbent pads
Wet wash cloths or wipes

Onto Bedpan

Nursing Action	Rationale
1. Close curtains.	1. To ensure privacy.
2. Assess the client's mobility and strength.	2. To see how much help the nurse will need to offer.
3. If a metal bedpan is to be used, warm it by running warm water over it, and dry it.	3. The metal may be too cold for the client to sit on.
4. Wash hands and don clean gloves.	4. To maintain universal precautions when coming into contact with body fluids and excretions.
5. Raise the bed to a comfortable position for the nurse and position the bed flat if client is able to tolerate this.	5. Maintains correct body mechanics.
6. If client is able to assist, fold down top linen to thighs. Make sure that gown covers private area but does not fall into bedpan.	6. To maintain privacy and dignity.
7. Assist client to side-lying position. Place bedpan appropriately and roll client onto back.	7. To position client onto bedpan.

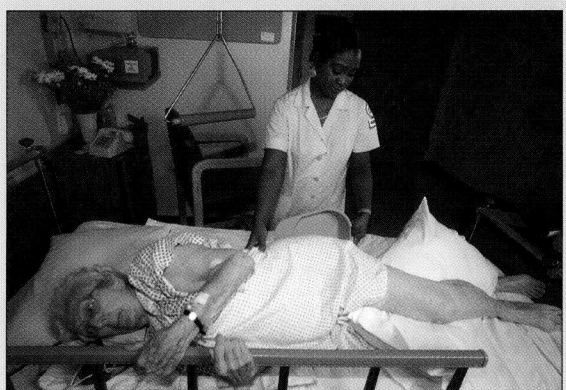

Step 6.

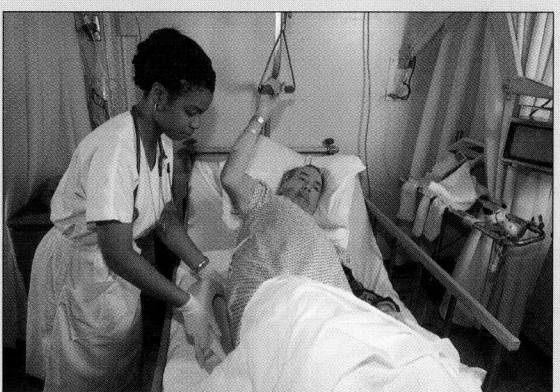

Step 7.

8. Powder can be applied to lower back and buttocks.	8. To prevent bedpan from sticking to skin.
9. Cover client.	9. To maintain privacy and dignity.
10. Unless contraindicated, raise head of bed to semi-Fowler's position.	10. To relieve strain on the back and maintain a more natural position.

Continued

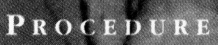

PROCEDURE

31–2

ASSISTING A CLIENT ONTO AND OFF A BEDPAN

(Continued)

Nursing Action	Rationale
11. Raise side rails if client is at risk for falling; lower bed.	11. To maintain safety.
12. Remove gloves and discard.	
13. Leave call bell and toilet paper within client's reach.	13. To maintain safety and personal hygiene.

Off Bedpan

Nursing Action	Rationale
1. Wash hands and don gloves.	1. To maintain universal precautions when coming into contact with fecal material.
2. If client is able, have him or her raise buttocks so bedpan can be removed. Hold bedpan steady.	2. So as not to spill contents.
3. Cover bedpan and place it on nearby chair.	3. To decrease embarrassment.
4. If client is unable to assist, raise bed to comfortable height for nurse.	4. To maintain correct body mechanics.
5. Put bed in flat position and fold down linens to thighs. Turn client off of bedpan while holding bedpan securely. If client turns away from you, put side rail up.	5. To prevent spilling of contents and to maintain safety.
6. Cover bedpan and place it on nearby chair.	6. To decrease embarrassment.
7. If client has wiped self, offer handwashing (wipes or wet wash cloths may be used).	7. To maintain proper hygiene.
8. If client is unable to wipe self, wrap toilet paper around your hand and wipe from front to back. Only use toilet paper once. Continue until area is clean. If no specimen is needed, toilet paper may be placed into bedpan. If sample is needed, put toilet paper into another receptacle for disposal.	8. To prevent spread of microorganisms from GI to genitourinary or reproductive tract. To prevent contamination of specimen.
9. Ensure that rectal area is clean and dry.	9. To prevent skin breakdown.
10. Wash client's hands.	10. To maintain hygiene.
11. Spray area with room freshener. Use caution if client has respiratory problem or is sensitive to odors.	11. Room freshener may be irritating to some clients.
12. Empty and clean bedpan (obtain sample first if needed).	
13. Replace bedpan to bedside stand. Do not leave on overbed tray.	13. For easy accessibility and to prevent food from being contaminated.
14. Discard gloves and wash hands.	14. To prevent spread of microorganisms.
15. Document bowel movement and describe findings.	15. Accountability.

ent on a bedpan more frequently, client complications may be avoided, and the nurse may save time.

• Instituting a bowel training regimen.

• Using a suppository or daily cleansing enema, which may decrease the incidence of incontinence because the lower colon is regularly emptied.

Negative feedback should never occur if the client is unable to successfully have a bowel movement at this time. Remember that patience is extremely important (from both the client and the caregiver) and that positive feedback does help when success has been attained.

Administration of Prescribed Medications

Whenever possible, a person should try to treat alterations in bowel elimination by methods other than

Box 31–7

BOWEL TRAINING REGIMEN

- Offer a stool softener or cathartic suppository every day approximately 30 minutes before the regular defecation time
- Offer client a hot drink or some fruit juice
- Place client on commode or toilet when he or she feels the urge to defecate
- Allow adequate time and privacy
- Encourage client to lean forward while sitting, bear down (but without straining), flex the thighs and apply manual pressure over the abdomen
- Document client response and progress

the use of medication. If all else fails or the problem is severe and requires immediate attention, prescribed medications can be administered.

Antidiarrheals

Some of the most effective antidiarrheal agents are opiates and opiate derivatives. These decrease the incidence of diarrhea by inhibiting peristaltic waves. This decreases intestinal muscle tone and, in turn, slows the passage of feces. The dosage given would be less than what is given to control or alleviate pain. Medications such as codeine, paregoric, and diphenoxylate hydrochloride with atropine sulfate (Lomotil) fall into this drug classification. These types of medications may be used to treat acute, nonspecific diarrhea or for diarrhea from toxic chemicals or pathogens.

Opiates and their derivatives, such as diphenoxylate hydrochloride with atropine sulfate (Lomotil) can be habit forming and many can cause drowsiness. Medications such as loperamide (Immodium), which can be purchased without a doctor's prescription, can also cause dizziness and fatigue. It is imperative for the nurse to educate a client properly about the actions as well as the side effects of medications taken to control diarrhea.

Adsorbents are a type of antidiarrheal that act by absorbing gas or toxic substances from the bowel. They also coat the walls of the GI tract. Kaolin and pectin are two common medications that are in this drug class. Adsorbents are generally taken after each loose bowel movement until the diarrhea is controlled. Clients must be cautioned when taking this type of medication because adsorbents interfere with the absorption of several other drugs, including digoxin, quinidine, and clindamycin.

Bismuth subsalicylate (Pepto-Bismol), another over-the-counter medication, is also used as an antidiarrheal. Despite the fact that this does not need a prescription, the client must be educated as to its use and side effects. Pepto-Bismol inhibits GI secretions. It

is also a salicylate and, if taken in large amounts, it can enhance the effects of oral anticoagulants, causing bleeding. Clients must be cautioned about using Pepto-Bismol if they are taking any type of aspirin products, antiinflammatories, or anticoagulants.

In addition to drug therapy, chronic diarrhea that lasts more than 3 or 4 weeks usually requires fluid and electrolyte replacement.

Cathartics and Laxatives

Before someone suffering from constipation initiates the use of a cathartic or laxative, increasing the amount of fiber and fluids ingested, as well as doing regular exercise, should be attempted. Habitual use of laxatives can actually cause constipation and is a very hard "habit" to break. Laxative abuse in our country is very common, especially in the elderly population. Many elderly people are unaware of the physiological changes that occur as they age and think that something is "wrong" if they do not move their bowels every day. Therefore, to assist their bowel elimination, many elderly clients rely on laxatives. However, laxatives should be used only occasionally or as a last resort in the treatment of constipation. For instance, they are generally safe to take when food intake is temporarily poor or activity is limited.

Because many laxatives may be obtained over the counter and because advertising promotes their usage, many people take them when they should not. A cathartic is absolutely contraindicated if someone has nausea, cramps, vomiting, or undiagnosed abdominal pain.

A **cathartic** or laxative may be used for the treatment of constipation or as a preparatory measure in cleaning out the bowels before GI testing or surgery. The same drug may have either a laxative or a purgative effect, depending on the dosage. A purgative effect produces frequent bowel movements, soft liquid stools, and, at times, abdominal cramping. A laxative effect is similar but milder than a purgative effect.

Several types of laxatives and cathartics are available (Table 31–2):

Bulk-forming agents increase fluid, gas, or solid bulk in the intestines, which distends them, initiating reflex bowel activity

Chemical irritants or stimulants irritate intestinal mucosa, causing rapid movement of contents

Lubricants soften and delay drying of feces

Saline or osmotic agents bind with water in the intestines to increase fluid bulk and lubricate feces

Wetting agents (stool softeners) decrease the surface tension of feces so that water can penetrate the feces

Hyperosmotic agents increase osmotic pressure in the bowel, which increases peristalsis via local irritation (a glycerin suppository is an example)

Cathartics may be administered either orally or via rectal suppository. If given rectally, the action of cathartics occurs by one of three mechanisms:

Table 31-2

CATHARTICS

TYPE	EXAMPLE	ONSET OF ACTION	NURSING IMPLICATIONS
Bulk forming	Metamucil	12–24 h	Give with at least 8 oz of fluid (can cause impaction and obstruction) Need to swallow quickly when mixed with fluids; otherwise, it solidifies Least irritating of all cathartics May interfere with the absorption of calcium and iron
Chemical irritant/ stimulant	Bisacodyl Cascara Castor oil ExLax	6–8 h (Dulcolax supposi- tory works within 30 min)	Prolonged use can cause fluid and electrolyte imbal- ances May cause cramps Bisacodyl is enteric coated so must be swallowed whole Can lead to loss of intestinal tone with overuse ExLax may turn urine and feces pink
Lubricant	Haley's MO Mineral oil	6–8 h	If aspirated, could get pneumonia Regular use interferes with the absorption of fat-solu- ble vitamins such as A, D, E, and K, so is better to give on empty stomach Mixing with juice decreases unpleasant taste
Saline (osmotic)	Epsom salts Magnesium citrate Milk of magnesia	1–3 h	Not recommended for someone with renal disease or congestive heart disease Can cause fluid and electrolyte imbalance and dehy- dration
Wetting agents (Stool softeners)	Colace	Several days	Used when the goal is to prevent straining

* As a stimulant to the nerve endings in the rectal mucosa
* By softening feces
* By releasing gases that distend the rectum

Suppositories

A suppository melts at body temperature and is generally effective within 30 minutes. For bowel elimi- nation, it is best to administer a suppository either after breakfast or 30 minutes before the patient's regu- lar defecation time. A suppository that acts by affect- ing the nerve endings is good for those with weak muscle tone or poor nerve innervation. If it acts by releasing CO_2, approximately 200 ml of gas is liber- ated, causing distention, which stimulates the intes- tines and initiates elimination impulses. The proper method for inserting a rectal suppository can be found in Procedure 31–3.

Antiflatulents

An antiflatulent such as simethicone (Mylicon) is used to treat conditions of excessive gas. It acts by dispersing gas pockets within the GI tract and is usu- ally given after meals and at bedtime.

Administration of Enemas

An enema is the instillation of fluid (and, at times, medication) into the large intestine. The purpose is to assist in the elimination of feces and flatus. Enemas require a physician's order, and indications include

cleansing the bowel prior to surgery, childbirth, or diagnostic tests; removal of impacted feces; and as a part of bowel retraining. Before using enemas at home, clients should talk to their health care provider. Enemas should not be used to maintain bowel regu- larity because this action promotes dependence.

There are several types of enemas, including cleansing, carminative, retention, and return flow. En- ema volume depends on the age of the client. For example,

Infant, toddler: 50 to 150 ml (normal saline only)

Preschool child: 200 to 300 ml

School-age child: 300 to 500 ml

Adult: 500 to 1000 ml

Cleansing enema solutions include tap water, soap suds, saline, and hypertonic saline. These enemas stimulate peristalsis and evacuation by irritating the colon or distending the colon with fluid:

Tap water (hypotonic): Stimulates defecation; not to be repeated

Saline (isotonic): Stimulates defecation; mix 1 teaspoon of table salt in 500 ml tap water

Fleet's (hypertonic): Pulls fluid from interstitial spaces; distention produces defecation; only 4 to 6 oz; do not use for infants or dehydrated clients

Soap suds (irritant): Use with tap water or saline; use only pure castile soap—1 teaspoon soap to 1000 ml fluid

If the physician orders enemas until clear, the

PROCEDURE

31–3

INSERTION OF A RECTAL SUPPOSITORY

Equipment:

Disposable gloves
Suppository
Water-soluble lubricating jelly

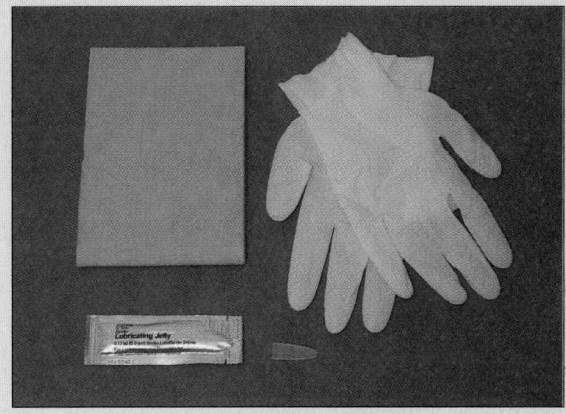

Nursing Action	Rationale
1. Explain procedure to client.	**1.** For client understanding and compliance.
2. Wash hands and don clean gloves.	**2.** To maintain universal precautions.
3. Position client on side and drape appropriately.	**3.** For ease of insertion and to maintain privacy.
4. Lubricate glove and suppository.	**4.** For easier insertion.
5. Separate buttocks while asking client to breathe through the mouth while the suppository is inserted.	**5.** To assist the client in relaxing rectal muscles.
6. Insert suppository approximately 4 in. Do not insert into fecal mass.	**6.** To place it past the internal anal sphincter. Inserting into fecal mass will not break it up.

Rectal internal
sphincter

4 in

Step 6.

7. Encourage client to retain suppository for 30 to 45 minutes or as long as possible.	**7.** For better results.
8. Document client response.	**8.** Accountability.

nurse may administer up to three large-volume enemas in succession. Use caution with tap water enemas, which can lead to fluid and electrolyte imbalances as a result of excessive absorption of the
hypotonic solution. These enemas may be ordered as
high or low. High enemas clean the entire large intestine. The client lies on the left side, then turns supine,
then turns to the right side. The height of the enema
bag is 18 in (45 cm) above the client's hips. Low
enemas cleanse the sigmoid colon and rectum. The
client remains on the left side, and the bag is held at
the regular height of 12 to 18 in (30–45 cm) above
the client's hips.

Carminative enemas are used to relieve distention
and to help expel flatus. The most common types are
the milk and molasses (equal amounts) enema and the
1,2,3, or MGW, enema (1 oz of magnesium sulfate, 2
oz of glycerin, and 3 oz of water).

Retention enemas are administered for several different reasons. It is very important for the client to be
able to retain the fluid for up to several hours. Oil
retention enemas are given to lubricate the rectum and
to soften feces for easier passage. Medicated enemas
are given to administer medications, such as sodium
polystyrene sulfonate (Kayexelate) or neomycin sulfate, that are absorbed by the rectal mucosa.

Return flow, high colonic, or Harris flush enemas
are used to help relieve flatus. After the solution is
instilled, the bag is lowered, and the fluid is siphoned
back into the bag. Repeating this process dispels flatus
and stimulates peristalsis.

Most enemas are administered using disposable
equipment or clean reusable equipment. This is a
clean, rather than sterile, procedure because the colon
contains bacteria. The nurse uses gloves to prevent
transmission of fecal bacteria. Enemas are given with
the solution warmed to 105 to 110°F (40–43°C); for
children, keep the temperature at 100°F (37.7°C). The
size of the rectal tube used in enema administration
varies with age:

Infant: #10 to #12 French

Toddler: #12 to #14 French

School-age child: #16 to #18 French

Adult: #22 French or larger

The length of administration time depends on the
volume of fluid. For example, 1000 ml of fluid should
be given over 15 to 20 minutes. If the client experiences cramping, slow the infusion down, lower the
bag, and instruct the client to breathe deeply through
the mouth. Instruct the client to retain the enema for
as long as possible, and then assist the client onto the
bedpan or commode or into the bathroom. Document
how the client tolerated the procedure and the results
of the enema. See Procedure 31–4, which outlines
administration of an enema.

Digital Disimpaction

The purpose of disimpaction is to manually break
up and remove an impacted mass. It is generally nec-

essary to obtain a doctor's order before doing a digital
disimpaction. This is not a pleasant procedure for the
client. It is very uncomfortable, may irritate the rectal
mucosa, and can cause rectal bleeding. It can decrease
the heart rate from the effects of vagal stimulation.
Therefore, it should be done cautiously with cardiac
clients and elderly individuals.

The client needs an explanation before and during
the procedure as to the process. The client should be
placed in a side-lying position and appropriately
draped. A bedpan should be handy in which to place
the obtained stool masses. The nurse should wash his
or her hands, raise the bed up to a comfortable position (while maintaining one side rail up), and don
clean gloves. A clean pad should be placed under the
client. The nurse's forefinger should be lubricated generously and gently inserted into the rectum. The client
should take deep breaths during this procedure to
encourage relaxation. The nurse then works the forefinger into and around the mass to break it up (Fig.
31–6). Because this is an uncomfortable and sometimes long procedure, it needs to be done slowly and
at the client's pace.

Rectal Tubes

A method that helps gas to escape from the GI
tract is by the insertion of a rectal tube. This helps to
stimulate peristalsis and provides a passageway for the
escape of flatus. The nurse should place a waterproof
pad under the client's buttocks. The rectal tube should
be lubricated before insertion and is inserted approximately 4 to 6 in (10–15 cm) in an adult and 2 to 4 in
(5–10 cm) in a child. If any pain is felt on insertion or
resistance is met, the nurse should stop the procedure
and inform the doctor. After the rectal tube is inserted,
it is taped to the buttocks (Fig. 31–7). It should not
be left in longer than 20 minutes because it will not
act as a stimulant for peristalsis after this time, but it
may be reinserted several hours later if insufficient
relief was obtained. When a rectal tube is inserted to
relieve flatus, the client should be encouraged to assume various positions (*e.g.,* lying on the belly, knee-
chest position) to help move the flatus.

In some institutions, a Foley catheter with the balloon inflated may be used in lieu of a rectal tube.
However, this can be dangerous because the inflated
balloon could damage the rectal sphincter and mucosa.

Fecal Incontinence Pouches

Fecal incontinence pouches (rectal pouches) are
being used more frequently for incontinent clients.
These collect and contain the stool and are especially
useful for a person whose skin is prone to breakdown. Some of the advantages of a pouch compared
with a diaper, disposable underpad, or indwelling
catheter are as follows (Bosley, 1995):

• Soiled diapers involve changing and cleaning the skin.
This can be degrading to the incontinent person. With a
pouch, these tasks are avoided.

Text continued on page 956

PROCEDURE

31–4

ADMINISTERING AN ENEMA

Equipment:

Disposable enema set
Water-soluble lubricant
Bath thermometer
Bath blanket
Disposable gloves
Intravenous pole
Waterproof pad
Necessary additives (soap, salt)
Washcloth, soap, towel
Bedpan (or commode) and toilet tissue

Solution as ordered by physician:
Temperature:
    For adult: 105 to 110°F (40–43°C)
    For children: 100°F (37.7°C)
Amount: Varies depending on type of solution, age of the person, and the client's ability to retain the solution; average cleansing enema for an adult may range from 750 to 1000 ml

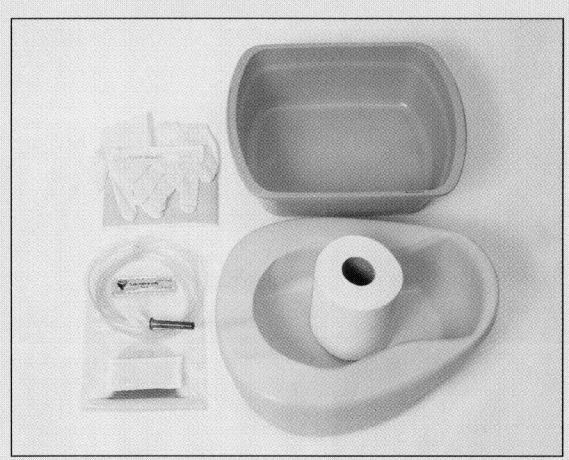

Nursing Action	Rationale
1. Explain the procedure to the client.	**1.** Reduces anxiety and promotes cooperation.
2. Assemble the equipment and the appropriate solution and additive if ordered.	**2.** Organization facilitates task performance.
3. Wash hands.	**3.** Minimizes risk of infection.
4. Provide privacy by closing curtains around bed or closing door to room.	**4.** Reduces embarrassment.
5. Raise bed to appropriate working height and raise side rail on opposite side.	**5.** Promotes use of good body mechanics and client safety.
6. Assist client into left side-lying (Sims) position with right knee flexed. Position clients with poor sphincter control on bedpan in comfortable dorsal recumbent position.	**6.** Allows enema solution to flow downward by gravity along natural curve of sigmoid colon and rectum, thus improving retention of solution. Clients with poor sphincter control cannot retain all enema solution.

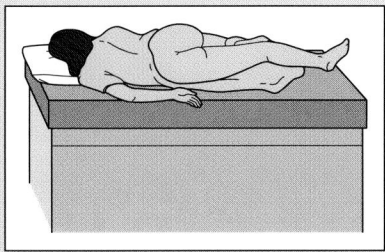

Step 6.

7. Place waterproof pad under hips and buttocks.	**7.** Prevents soiling linen.

Continued

PROCEDURE

31–4

ADMINISTERING AN ENEMA
(Continued)

Nursing Action	Rationale
8. Cover client with bath blanket, exposing only rectal area.	**8.** Provides warmth, reduces exposure of body parts, and allows client to feel more relaxed and comfortable.
9. Don gloves.	**9.** For infection control.
10. Place bedpan or commode in easily accessible position. If client will be expelling contents in toilet, ensure that it is free.	**10.** Used in case client cannot retain enema solution.
11. Administer enema using disposable enema bag (for administering a prepackaged enema, go to "Prepackaged Hypertonic Enema"):	
a. Raise container, release clamp, and allow solution to flow long enough to fill tubing.	a. Removes air from tubing.

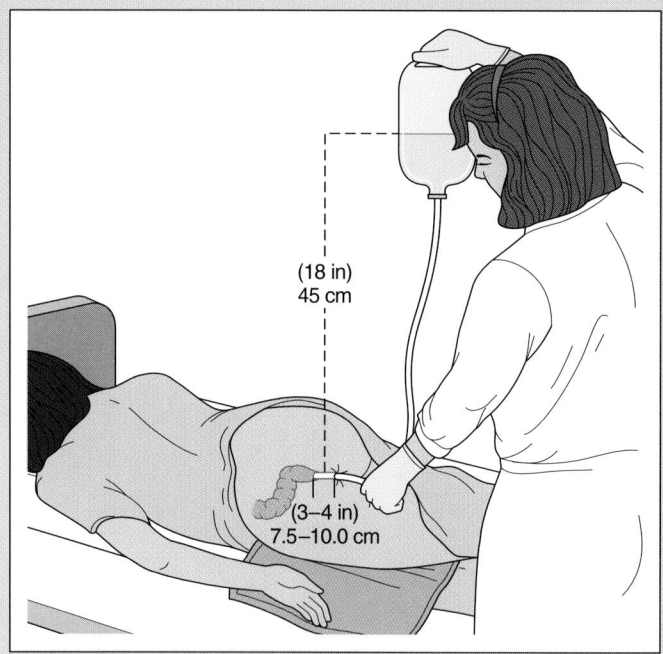

(18 in)
45 cm

(3–4 in)
7.5–10.0 cm

Step 11.

b. Reclamp tubing.	b. Prevents further loss of solution.
c. Lubricate 7.5 to 10 cm (3–4 in) of tip of rectal tube with lubricating jelly.	c. Allows smooth insertion of rectal tube without risk of irritation or trauma to the mucosa.
d. Gently separate buttocks and locate anus. Instruct client to relax by breathing out slowly through mouth.	d. Breathing out promotes relaxation of external sphincter.
e. Insert tip of rectal tube slowly by pointing tip in direction of umbilicus. Length of insertion for adults is 7.5 to 10 cm (3–4 in)	e. Prevents trauma to rectal mucosa from accidental lodging of tube against rectal wall. Insertion beyond proper limit can cause bowel perforation.

PROCEDURE

31–4

ADMINISTERING AN ENEMA
(Continued)

Nursing Action	**Rationale**
f. Hold tubing in rectum constantly until end of fluid instillation.	f. Bowel contraction can cause expulsion of rectal tube.
g. Open regulating clamp and allow solution to enter slowly, with container at client's hip level.	g. Rapid infusion can stimulate evacuation of rectal tube.
h. Raise height of enema container slowly to appropriate level above anus (high enema: 45 cm [18 in]; low enema: 30 cm [12 in]). Infusion time varies with volume of solution administered (*e.g.,* 1 L in 15–20 minutes).	h. Allows for continuous, slow infusion of solution. Raising container too high causes rapid infusion and possible painful distention of colon.
i. Lower container or clamp tubing if client complains of cramping or if liquid escapes around rectal tube.	i. Temporary cessation of infusion prevents cramping, which may prevent client from retaining all fluid, altering effectiveness of enema.
j. Clamp tubing after all solution is infused.	j. Prevents entrance of air into rectum.
12. Place toilet tissue around tube at anus and gently withdraw the tube.	12. Provides for comfort and cleanliness.
13. Explain to client that feeling of distention is normal. Ask client to retain solution for 5 to 10 minutes or as long as possible while lying in bed.	13. Solution distends the bowel. Length of retention varies with type of enema and client's ability to contract anal sphincter. Longer retention promotes more effective stimulation of peristalsis and defecation.
14. Discard enema container and tubing in proper receptacle.	14. Controls transmission and growth of microorganisms.
15. Assist client to bathroom or help to position client on bedpan.	15. Normal squatting position promotes defecation.
16. Observe character of feces and solution (caution client against flushing toilet before inspection).	16. When enemas are ordered "until clear," it is essential to observe contents of solution passed.
17. Assist client, as needed, to wash anal area with warm soap and water.	17. Fecal content can irritate skin. Hygiene promotes comfort.
18. Inspect character of stool and fluid passed.	18. Determines whether stool is evacuated or fluid is retained.
19. Remove gloves by pulling them inside out and discarding in proper receptacle.	19. Prevents transmission of microorganisms.
20. Wash hands.	20. Reduces transmission of infection.

21. Record pertinent information:
  a. Type and volume of enema given
  b. Color, amount, and consistency of fecal return
	21. Communicates pertinent information to all members of health care team. Prompt recording improves documentation of treatment.

Prepackaged Hypertonic Enema

1. Remove plastic cap from rectal tip. Tip is already lubricated, but apply more jelly as needed.	1. Lubrication provides for smooth insertion of rectal tube without causing rectal irritation or trauma.
2. Gently separate buttocks and locate anus. Instruct client to relax by breathing out slowly through mouth.	2. Breathing out promotes relaxation of external sphincter.
3. Insert tip of bottle gently into rectum. Advance tip 7.5 to 10 cm (3–4 in) in the adult.	3. Prevents trauma to rectal mucosa.
4. Gently squeeze the bottle to empty contents into the rectum and colon. Maintain pressure on the container and withdraw from the rectum.	4. Releasing pressure will cause the liquid to be drawn back into the colon.
5. Go back to step 13 and continue.	

Breaking up impaction

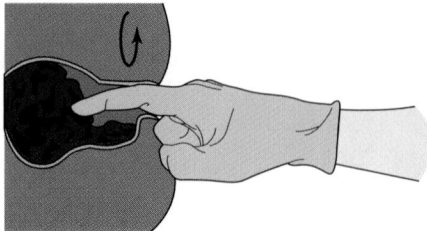

Removing feces

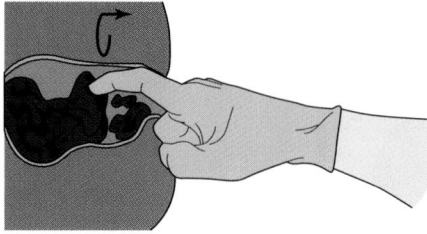

❧ **Figure 31–6**
When oil and cleansing enemas are not successful in relieving a fecal impaction, manual disimpaction is required.

- If the pouch is correctly applied, stool will not leak so skin will not become irritated. With other devices, soiled underpads can increase the risk of skin breakdown.
- An indwelling catheter (which some institutions use) is invasive and questionably safe. It can also obstruct feces simply by its presence.

The nursing care involved for a person with an incontinence pouch includes

- Assessing and documenting the skin integrity
- Maintaining fecal drainage by keeping the drainage bag below the level of the anus or by emptying the drainage bag when necessary
- Changing the bag every 72 hours (or sooner if leakage occurs)
- Explaining the purpose and care of the pouch to the client and significant others

The following are the steps involved in applying a fecal incontinence pouch:

1. Explain the procedure to the client
2. Assist the client to the side-lying position with knees drawn up to expose the anus (if possible, get assistance in spreading the buttocks)
3. Clean and dry the skin (it is best to apply the pouch to skin that has not broken down yet)
4. Shave (or clip) any excess hair from the area
5. Apply a protective skin sealant and allow it to dry
6. Cut the opening of the pouch larger than the anus (because the anus expands during defecation)
7. Apply the pouch after removing the paper backing
8. Hold the pouch against the skin for approximately 30 seconds (to enhance sticking)
9. Attach drainage bag, if necessary

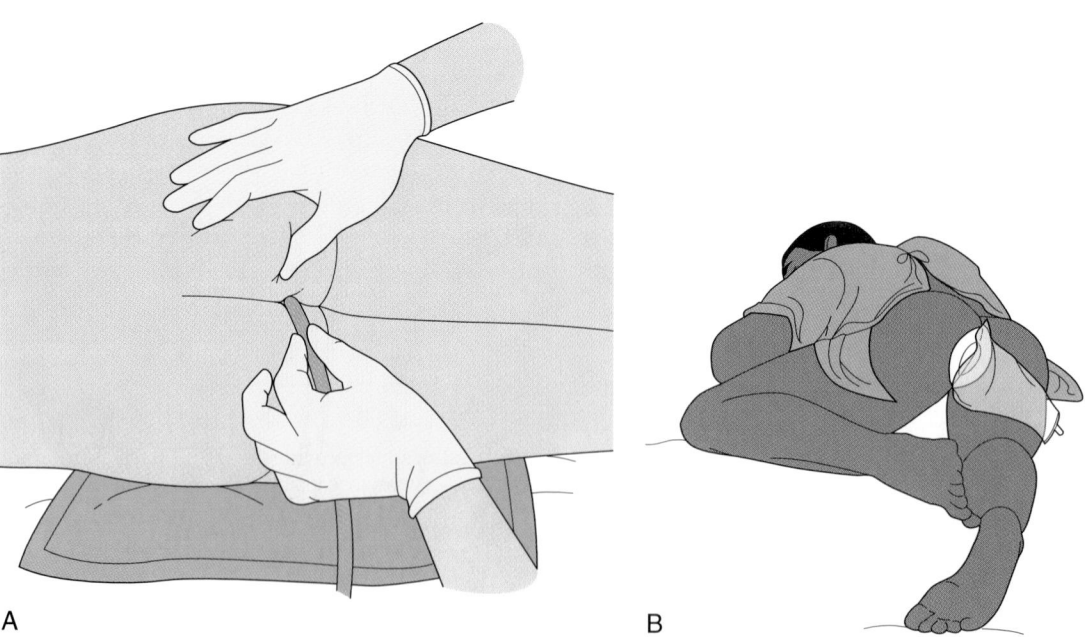

A   B

❧ **Figure 31–7**
A, Rectal tubes allow intestinal gas to escape and help stimulate peristalsis. The tube is lubricated before insertion and is inserted approximately 4 to 6 inches in an adult, and 2 to 4 inches in a child. The tube is taped to the buttocks and should be left in place no longer than 20 minutes.
　　B, A fecal incontinence pouch (rectal pouch) may be used for an incontinent client instead of a diaper, disposable underpad, or indwelling catheter. The rectal pouch is especially useful for a person whose skin is prone to breakdown. The bag must be changed every 72 hours or sooner if leakage occurs.

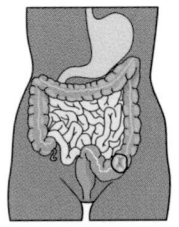 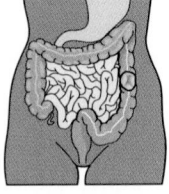 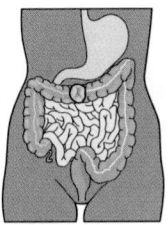 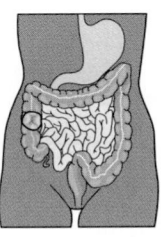 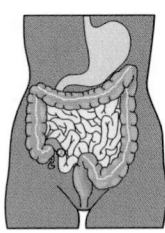

| Sigmoid colostomy | Descending colostomy | Transverse colostomy | Ascending colostomy | Ileostomy |

❥ **Figure 31–8**
Anatomical locations of bowel diversion ostomies and ileostomies.

Bowel Diversions—Ostomies

There are many types of ostomies. The word ***ostomy*** means artificial opening. This opening is created by a surgical procedure and is named by anatomical location. A colostomy is an opening into the colon. Clients may have an ascending colostomy, a transverse colostomy (single or double barrel), a descending colostomy, or a sigmoid colostomy. An ileostomy is an opening into the ileal portion of the small intestine (Fig. 31–8).

Ostomies can be either temporary or permanent. Temporary ostomies are performed to allow healing of the intestinal tract after traumatic injury or inflammatory diseases. Permanent ostomies are performed when the rectum or anus is nonfunctional, such as with an imperforate anus or a disease such as cancer.

The location of the ostomy determines the consistency of the stool. Ileostomy drainage is more liquid due to water resorption occurring in the large intestine. Clients with ileostomies wear appliances at all times. Sigmoid colostomy stools are formed and much easier to regulate. Clients with this type of ostomy may not have to wear an appliance continually.

Odor is a minimal problem with ileostomies and can be controlled with sigmoid colostomies. Odor is a major problem with ascending and transverse colostomies. Instruct the client on techniques for odor control, such as the use of baking soda or charcoal in the ostomy bag. Clients should be encouraged to consume dark green vegetables for their chlorophyll content, and they should avoid gaseous, odorous foods.

Stoma and Skin Care

Assess the stoma frequently (Box 31–8). The color should be pink to dark red. Initially, the stoma may be edematous, but as healing progresses, the size of the stoma should decrease. Carefully inspect the skin around the stoma; the peristomal area must remain intact. The fecal material from a colostomy or ileostomy is very irritating, and if not treated immediately, the area will break down. The peristomal skin should be washed and dried thoroughly. Before applying the appliance, pouch, or bag, measure the size of the stoma. An accurate fit will decrease or eliminate leakage problems. Apply a skin barrier around the stoma. This can be a powder, such as karaya, or a wafer or

ring. The bag should be emptied as needed. The entire appliance should be changed once every 4 to 7 days. If skin irritation or breakdown is a problem, the appliance should be changed more frequently and the peristomal area should be assessed and treated. See Procedure 31–5 for details about changing an ostomy appliance.

Colostomy Irrigation

Some clients who have a sigmoid or descending colostomy choose to irrigate the stoma to regulate the function of the colostomy. Ileostomies are not irrigated because the fecal material is liquid. Irrigations are similar to enemas in technique of administration. Irrigation equipment includes an irrigation bag, an irrigating catheter with stomal cone, lubricant, and a long irrigating sheath or drainage bag. The purpose of the cone is to prevent trauma to the stoma. Irrigations, unlike enemas, may be used to promote regular evacuation patterns. A client with a sigmoid colostomy may not require an appliance if evacuations are regular. An irrigation takes about 1 hour per day, and the client should choose the time of day. Some clients with a sigmoid colostomy prefer to control elimination via dietary regulation.

Promotion of Self-Concept

Clients need assistance when bowel elimination patterns are changed. For clients with ostomies, body
Text continued on page 961

Box **31–8**

STOMA ASSESSMENT

Color: pink to dark red

Location: ileal, ascending colon, transverse, descending colon, sigmoid

Size: initially edematous; should reduce in size within 4 to 6 weeks after surgery

Type: loop or end; single or double barrel

Skin: peristomal skin should be dry, clean, and intact

Report abnormal color, excessive edema, pain, or bleeding immediately.

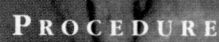

PROCEDURE

31–5

CHANGING AN OSTOMY APPLIANCE (DISPOSABLE)

Equipment:

Disposable gloves
Bedpan (or client may go into bathroom)
Pen or pencil
Tail closure or clamp
Stomal measuring guide
Tissue or gauze pad
Cleaning materials, including tissues, warm water, mild soap, washcloth or cotton balls, towel
Clean ostomy appliance with optional belt
Peristomal skin paste or powder
Skin barrier (liquid protective covering or peristomal pectin wafer skin barrier)
Moistureproof bag (for disposable pouches)
Scissors
Tape

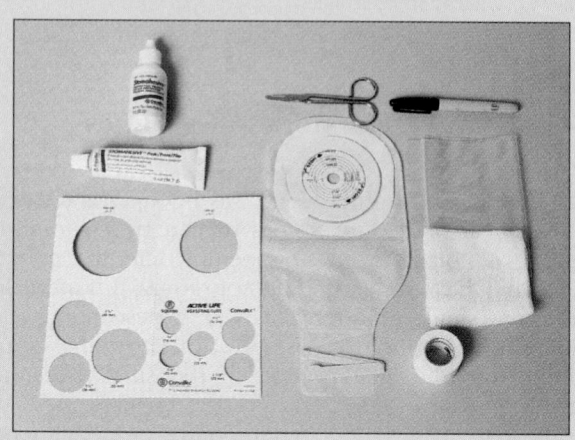

Nursing Action	**Rationale**
1. Select the appropriate time.	**1.** Avoid meal time and visiting times and after medications that stimulate bowel function.
2. Explain the procedure to the client and significant other.	**2.** Helps the client and significant other to understand ostomy care; projects a positive attitude, and encourages the client to assist with care.
3. Prepare equipment, provide privacy, wash hands, and don disposable gloves.	**3.** Organization facilitates task performance. Decreases risk of infection. Client will feel more comfortable.
4. If pouch is full, remove clamp and empty contents into bedpan.	**4.** Prevents spillage on skin.

PROCEDURE

31–5

CHANGING AN OSTOMY APPLIANCE
(DISPOSABLE)
(Continued)

Nursing Action	**Rationale**
5. Remove old appliance as one piece.	**5.** Reduces trauma.

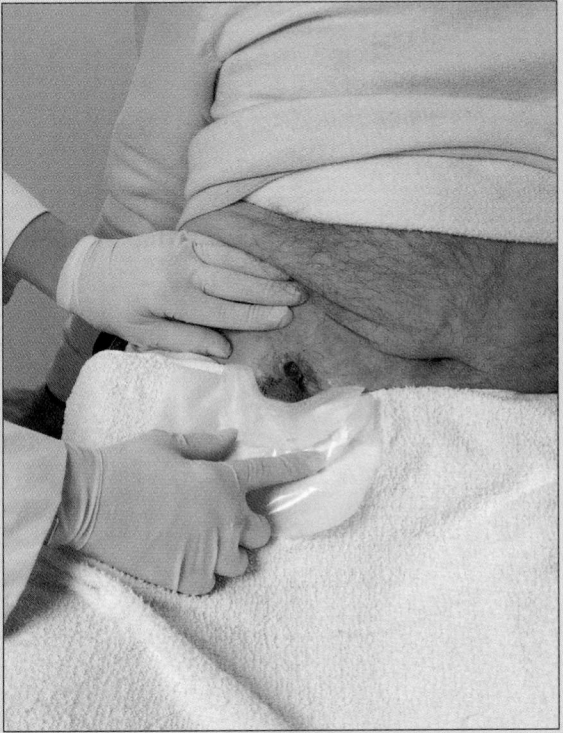

Step 5.

6. Wash skin gently with skin cleanser or with regular soap and water. Remove secretions from skin.

6. Secretions act as irritant to skin. Bacteria in fecal secretions can enter incisional area (new colostomy) and cause infection.

7. Rinse soap off thoroughly. Blot dry.

7. The presence of any soap residue could result in film or residue being left behind. These residues can result in chemical reactions or burns and can cause premature leakage because of interference with pouch adhesion. After rinsing well, blot dry gently to avoid trauma to stoma, which normally bleeds easily.

8. If blood appears after washing, reassure client that small amount is normal. Clarify what is abnormal.

8. Minimizes anxiety. Bowel has rich vascular supply. Client must be able to recognize complications.

9. Observe condition of skin and stoma. Encourage client to make these observations daily.

9. Allows for early monitoring of complications. Client observation aids in acceptance and adjustment; client also develops habit of observing for skin-stomal problems, which are more easily correctable if detected and reported early.

Continued

CHANGING AN OSTOMY APPLIANCE
(DISPOSABLE)
(Continued)

Nursing Action	Rationale
10. Measure the stoma with the stomal measuring guide. Trace the exact measurement of the stoma on the back and in the center of the skin barrier. Cut out the circle from the skin barrier.	**10.** You will need to measure the stoma frequently during the postoperative period because the stoma will continue to shrink in size, with the majority of the shrinkage occurring during the first 2 to 3 months.

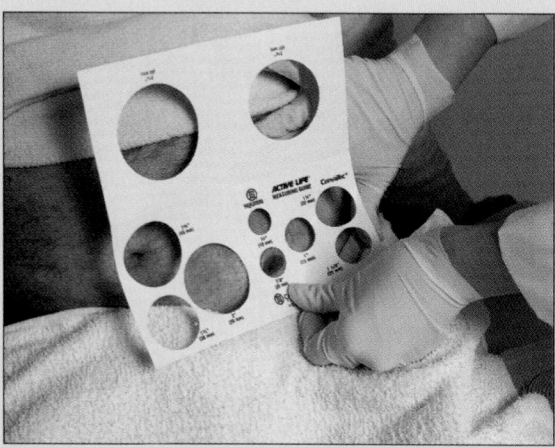

Step 10.

11. If abdominal crease is present or if contour is irregular, fill in with paste-type barrier. Allow paste to dry thoroughly.	**11.** Provides smooth surface for application of skin barrier and pouch's faceplate.

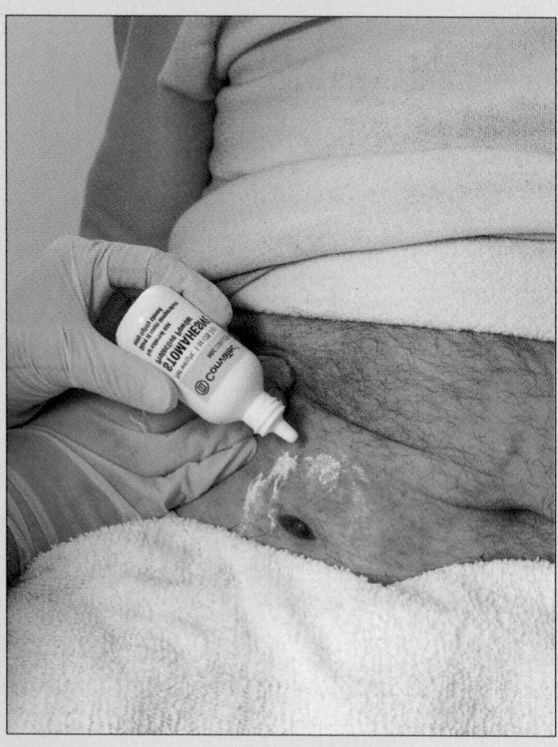

Step 11.

PROCEDURE

31–5

CHANGING AN OSTOMY APPLIANCE (DISPOSABLE)
(Continued)

Nursing Action	Rationale
12. Remove the paper backing to expose the sticky adhesive side. Center the skin barrier over the stoma and gently press it onto the client's skin, smoothing the barrier well.	**12.** Provides an improved leakproof barrier. Provides an accurate fit. Creates a wrinkle-free, secure seal onto the skin.

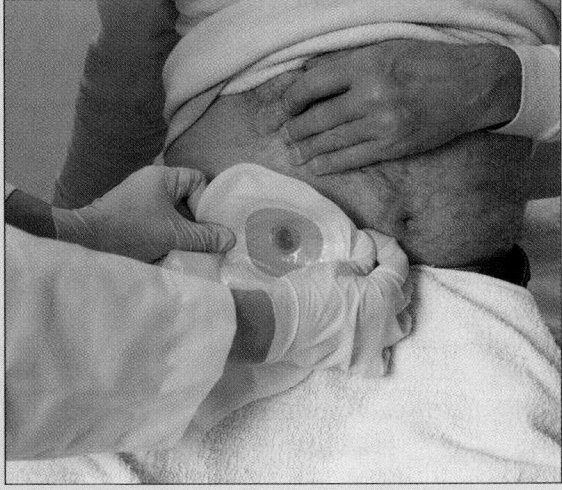

Step 12.

13. Apply hypoallergenic tape as needed to edges of faceplate over skin barrier. If client prefers, use the optional belt.	**13.** Adds extra reinforcement.
14. Fold bottom edges of pouch over to fit clamp. Secure clamp.	**14.** Prevents leakage of pouch contents.
15. Dispose of old appliance in moistureproof bag and dispose in trash chute. (Be sure this is not reusable appliance, because they should be washed and re-used several times.)	**15.** Avoids odor lingering in room, which is unpleasant to client and staff.
16. Remove soiled gloves and dispose in proper receptacle.	**16.** Reduces transmission of infection.
17. Wash hands.	**17.** Reduces transmission of infection.
18. Assist client to comfortable position if necessary.	**18.** Ensures client comfort.
19. Record pertinent information: type of pouch and skin barrier, amount and appearance of feces, and condition of stoma and surrounding skin.	**19.** Documents care and provides data for later determining changes in client's condition.

image has been altered, and clients should be encouraged to verbalize their feelings, fears, needs, and concerns. The nurse should have the client participate with care, and the client should proceed with assuming self-care.

The nurse can further assist the client and family or significant other through the following nursing strategies:

1. Provide information about diet, exercise, appliances, sexual activity, and odor control

2. Suggest that the client talk to a member of an ostomy club

3. Provide positive reinforcement for the progress that the client achieves, no matter how small

4. Provide privacy and allow for grieving

5. Demonstrate understanding, caring, and acceptance

Some ileostomy clients may be candidates for use of an internal intestinal reservoir or pouch. The client should discuss this option with his or her physician.

Evaluation

During this phase of the nursing process, the nurse assesses the effectiveness of the care plan. The expected outcomes are the basis for evaluation. The nurse compares the client's response to the outcomes, and if needed, the care plan is revised or modified. Some expected outcomes for clients with alterations in bowel elimination include

- The client establishes and maintains a regular bowel pattern
- The client's skin remains clean, dry, and intact
- The client expresses a positive self-image
- The client explains the relationship between food and fluid intake and bowel regulation
- The client does not experience diarrhea or constipation
- The client maintains weight and fluid and electrolyte balance
- The client demonstrates correct use of ostomy appliances and equipment
- The client states three ways to prevent constipation

Summary

This chapter has identified a variety of altered bowel elimination problems. These problems affect all age groups and both sexes. Regular bowel elimination requires maintenance of GI function. The overall goal is to return to the client's expected norm of bowel function.

Clients depend on the nurse to assist them in maintaining bowel elimination. The nurse can utilize the strategies of assessment, planning, implementation, teaching, and evaluating to help clients in reaching their goals.

CHAPTER HIGHLIGHTS

✦

- ✦ The GI system is composed of the mouth, esophagus, stomach, small intestine, large intestine, and anus. Accessory organs include the liver, gallbladder, and pancreas.
- ✦ Patterns of fecal elimination vary, but a regular pattern of fecal elimination (with formed, soft stools) is essential.

- ✦ Many factors, such as age and development, diet and fluid intake, diagnostic procedures, anesthesia and surgery, activity, psychological factors, lifestyle, medications, pain, and culture, affect defecation.
- ✦ Common bowel elimination problems include constipation, diarrhea, flatulence, incontinence, impaction, and hemorrhoids. Each problem has specific characteristics, contributing causes, and treatment modalities.
- ✦ Bowel elimination problems can affect skin integrity, nutritional status, fluid and electrolyte balance, and self-concept.
- ✦ Nursing assessments related to bowel elimination should include a thorough nursing history and physical examination of the mouth, abdomen, and rectum.
- ✦ North American Nursing Diagnosis Association–approved nursing diagnoses that are specific to bowel elimination include Constipation; Constipation, Colonic; Constipation, Perceived; Diarrhea; and Bowel Incontinence. Related diagnoses include Anxiety; Body Image Disturbance; Growth and Development, Altered; Individual Coping, Ineffective; Knowledge Deficit; Pain; Self Care Deficit; Sexual Dysfunction; Skin Integrity, Risk for Impaired; and Fluid Volume Deficit, Risk for.
- ✦ Regular bowel elimination should be promoted in both ill and well clients by encouraging proper positioning, timing, privacy, nutrition, and exercise.
- ✦ A bowel training program may be utilized to help manipulate factors within the client's control to achieve a soft, formed stool at regular intervals.
- ✦ Clients need to understand the importance of heeding the urge to defecate.
- ✦ Medication may be needed to assist a client in maintaining or regaining regular bowel elimination. These medications may include laxatives, cathartics, antiflatulents, or antidiarrheals.
- ✦ Although they have valid uses, laxatives are frequently abused.
- ✦ Clients with ostomies require special care. The location of an ostomy influences the consistency of stool.

Study Questions

1. When administering enteral feedings, the head of the bed should be

   a. flat
   b. elevated 10 degrees
   c. elevated 20 degrees
   d. elevated 30 degrees

2. Which one of the following reasons is NOT a purpose for enemas?

a. to maintain bowel regularity
b. to assist in elimination of feces
c. to assist in elimination of flatus
d. to instill medications

3. A client has a transverse colostomy, and she is very upset about "the awful odor." The nurse should suggest that the client consume which of the following vegetables to help decrease odor?

a. cabbage
b. spinach
c. carrots
d. potatoes

4. Which of these conditions contributes to bowel elimination changes in the elderly?

a. increased peristalsis
b. decreased chewing ability
c. easier accessibility to high-fiber foods
d. quicker emptying of stomach and esophagus

5. The correct order in which to assess the abdomen would be

a. inspection, auscultation, percussion, palpation
b. inspection, palpation, percussion, auscultation
c. auscultation, palpation, percussion, inspection
d. palpation, percussion, auscultation, inspection

Critical Thinking Exercises

1. Mary is immobile following a cerebrovascular accident. She is incontinent of stool. Discuss ways to manage Mary's incontinence.

2. Dan has an ostomy following emergency surgery for Crohn's disease. Discuss your assessment and documentation of the ostomy.

References

American Cancer Society. (1993). *Cancer facts and figures—1993*. Atlanta: American Cancer Society.
Bosley, C. L. (1995). Applying perianal pouches with confidence. *Nursing '95, June,* 58–61.
Hall, G. R., Karstens, M., Rakel, B., Swanson, E., & Davidson, A. (1995). Managing constipation using a research-based protocol. *MedSurg Nursing, 4* (1), 11–14.
McLane, A., & McShane, R. (1991). Constipation. In M. Maas, K. Buckwalter, & M. Hardy (Eds.), *Nursing diagnosis and interventions for the elderly* (pp. 147–158). Redwood City, CA: Addison-Wesley.
Peckenpaugh, N. J., & Poleman, C. M. (1995). *Nutrition: Essentials and diet therapy* (7th ed.). Philadelphia: W. B. Saunders.
Renkes, J. (1993). GI endoscopy: Managing the full scope of care. *Nursing '93, June,* 50–55.
Van Horn, L., Moag-Stahlberg, A., *et al.* (1991). Effects on serum lipids of adding instant oats to usual American diets. *American Journal of Public Health, 81* (2), 183–188.
Wong, D. L. (1995). *Whaley and Wong's nursing care of infants and children* (5th ed.). St. Louis: Mosby.

Bibliography

Baer, C. L., & Williams, B. R. (1992). *Clinical pharmacology and nursing* (2nd ed.). Springhouse, PA: Springhouse.
Betz, C. L., Hunsberger, M., & Wright, S. (1994). *Family-centered nursing care of children* (2nd ed.). Philadelphia: W. B. Saunders.
Burns, P. E., & Jaireth, N. (1994). Diarrhea and the patient receiving enteral feedings: A multifactorial problem. *JWOCN, 21* (6), 257–262.
Carpenito, L. J. (1995). *Nursing care plans and documentation: Nursing diagnoses and collaborative problems* (2nd ed.). Philadelphia: J. B. Lippincott.
Celik, A. F., & Katsinelos, P. (1995). Constipation and incontinence in the elderly. *Journal of Clinical Gastroenterology, 20* (1), 61–70.
Davis, J., & Sherer, L. (1994). *Applied nutrition and diet therapy for nurses* (2nd ed.). Philadelphia: W. B. Saunders.
Donald, J. J., & Burhenne, H. J. (1993). Colorectal cancer: Can we lower the death rate in the 1990's? *Canadian Family Physician, 39,* 108–114.
Donowitz, M., Kokke, F., & Saidi, R. (1995). Evaluation of patients with chronic diarrhea. *The New England Journal of Medicine, 332* (11), 725–729.
Floch, M. H., & Wald, A. (1994). Clinical evaluation and treatment of constipation. *The Gastroenterologist, 2* (1), 50–60.
Fruto, L. V. (1994). Current concepts: Management of diarrhea in acute care. *JWOCN, 21* (5), 199–205.
Hogstel, M. O., & Nelson, M. (1992). Anticipation and early detection can reduce bowel elimination complications. *Geriatric Nursing, January/February,* 28–33.
Iyer, P., Taptich, B. J., & Bernocchi-Losey, D. (1995). *Nursing process and nursing diagnosis* (3rd ed.). Philadelphia: W. B. Saunders.
Lennard-Jones, J. E. (1993). Clinical management of constipation. *Pharmacology, 47* (1), 216–223.
McConnell, E. A. (1995). Clinical do's and don'ts: Testing stool for occult blood. *Nursing '95, June,* 26.
McKenry, L. M., & Salerno, E. (1995). *Mosby's pharmacology in nursing.* St. Louis: Mosby.
Nair, P., & Mayberry, J. F. (1994). Vegetarianism, dietary fibre and gastrointestinal disease. *Digestive Diseases, 12,* 177–185.
Ross, D. G. (1993). Subjective data related to altered bowel elimination patterns among hospitalized elder and middle-aged persons. *Orthopaedic Nursing, 12* (5), 25–32.
Seidel, H. M., Ball, J. W., Dains, J. E., & Benedict, G. W. (1995). *Mosby's guide to physical assessment* (3rd ed.). St. Louis: Mosby.
Shollenberger, D. (1994). Giving enemas safely. *Nursing '94, September,* 32X–32Z.
Sparks, S. M., & Taylor, C. M. (1995). *Nursing diagnosis reference manual* (3rd ed.). Springhouse, PA: Springhouse.
Wald, A. (1993). Constipation in elderly patients: Pathogenesis and management. *Drugs and Aging, 3* (3), 221–231.
Wald, A. (1994). Constipation and fecal incontinence in the elderly. *Seminars in Gastrointestinal Disease, 5* (4), 179–188.
Watson, J., & Jaffe, M. S. (1995). *Nurse's manual of laboratory and diagnostic tests* (2nd ed.). Philadelphia: F. A. Davis.

Chapter ✦ 32

URINARY
ELIMINATION

BARBARA J. COHEN EdD, RN

KATHLEEN T. FLAHERTY MA,
RN, CRRN

KEY TERMS
✦

bacteriuria
benign prostatic
  hyperplasia
calculi
catheterization
closed-system
  catheterization
Credé maneuver
cystitis
detrusor muscle
diuresis
dysuria
enuresis
frequency
functional incontinence
hematuria
hesitancy

hydronephrosis
hydroureter
Kegel exercises
micturition
mixed incontinence
neurogenic bladder
nocturia
overflow incontinence
reflux
residual urine
retention of urine
stress incontinence
total incontinence
urge incontinence
urinary incontinence
urinary urgency

LEARNING OBJECTIVES
✦

After studying this chapter, you should be able to

✦ Recall the structures and functions of the urinary system

✦ Describe the process of urination

✦ Explain the key factors influencing the ability to urinate

✦ Assess for alterations in patterns of urinary elimination

✦ Explain the purposes of laboratory procedures used to assess urinary elimination

✦ Formulate appropriate nursing diagnoses based on assessment data

✦ Identify client goals and expected outcome criteria when planning nursing care for individuals at risk for or experiencing alterations in urination

✦ Provide appropriate nursing interventions for individuals experiencing alterations in urination

✦ Evaluate effectiveness of nursing interventions to achieve client goals based on expected outcome criteria

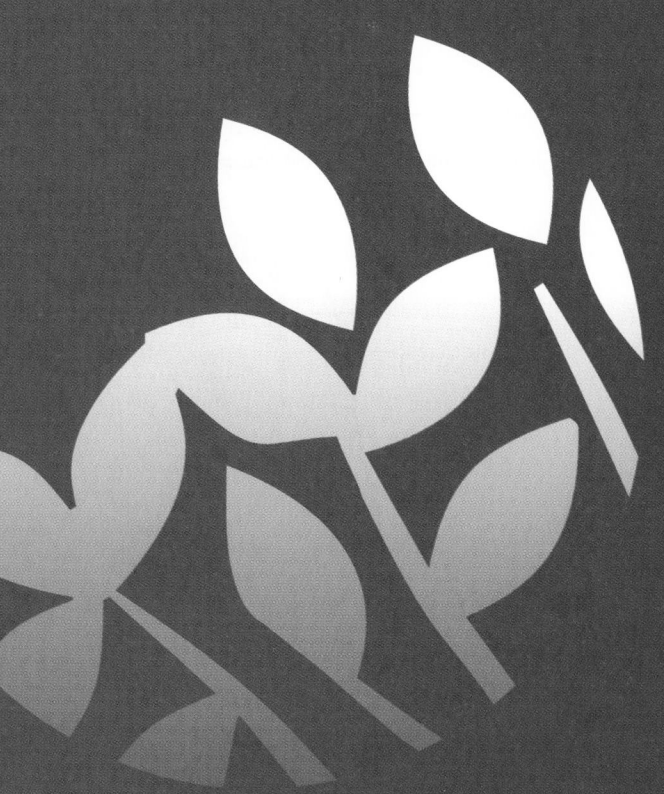

A basic human need is to have the ability to maintain physiological homeostasis. The urinary system helps to achieve this balance through the production and excretion of urine. Urine contains water-soluble waste products of metabolism, toxins produced by or taken into the body, and excessive fluids and electrolytes. *Voiding,* **micturition,** and *urination* are interchangeable terms used to indicate the elimination of urine from the body.

Nurses have an important role in helping clients maintain the ability to eliminate urine. Through the use of the nursing process, nurses provide therapeutic and psychosocial interventions that involve health education, early detection, and treatment of alterations in urinary elimination. These interventions also involve helping individuals to cope with changes in their patterns of voiding. Before using the nursing process, the nurse must understand the process of urination and the multiple factors that influence the production and elimination of urine.

Structures and Process of Urination

The urinary system consists of the kidneys, ureters, the urinary bladder, and the urethra. In males, it includes the organs of reproduction, because semen and urine are both passed through the urethra (Figs. 32–1 through 32–3).

Kidneys

The kidneys are paired, bean-shaped organs approximately 11 cm long, 5.0 to 7.5 cm wide, and 2.5 cm thick. They are located behind the peritoneal cavity, one on each side of the vertebral column (12th thoracic to third lumbar vertebrae). The right kidney is positioned slightly lower than the left kidney because of the position of the liver. A person can live with only one kidney as long as the remaining kidney is able to carry on the vital functions needed to sustain life (*i.e.,* production of renin, erythropoietin, and an active form of vitamin D; maintenance of fluid, electrolyte, and acid-base balance; excretion of the waste products of protein metabolism; and excretion of toxic substances in the blood).

When protein foods (such as milk, meats, eggs, and cheese) are metabolized, nitrogen substances are formed as waste products. Blood urea nitrogen (BUN) is the waste product of protein metabolism. Other waste products excreted in urine include uric acid, ammonia, and creatinine.

Each kidney contains more than a million functional units, called nephrons, which permit filtration of fluid and particles from the blood (Fig. 32–4). In the

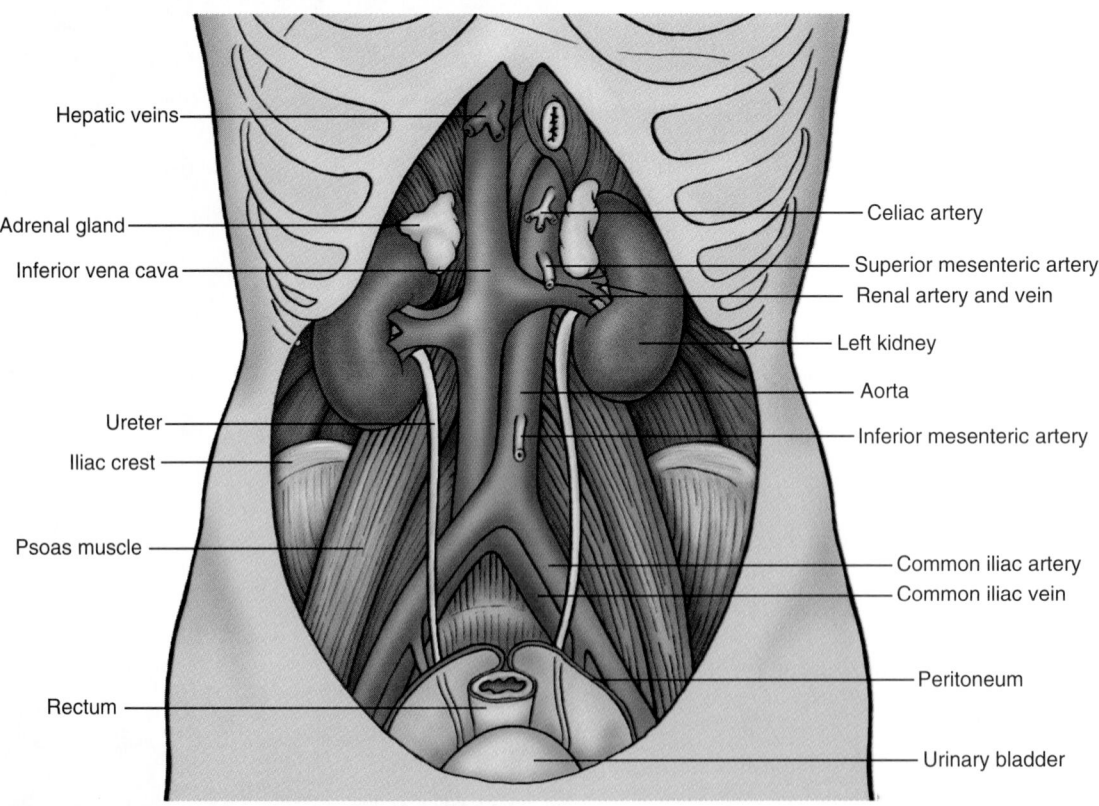

Figure 32–1
Anatomical structures of the urinary tract. (From Monahan, F. D., Drake, T., & Neighbors, M. [1994]. *Nursing care of adults.* Philadelphia: W. B. Saunders.)

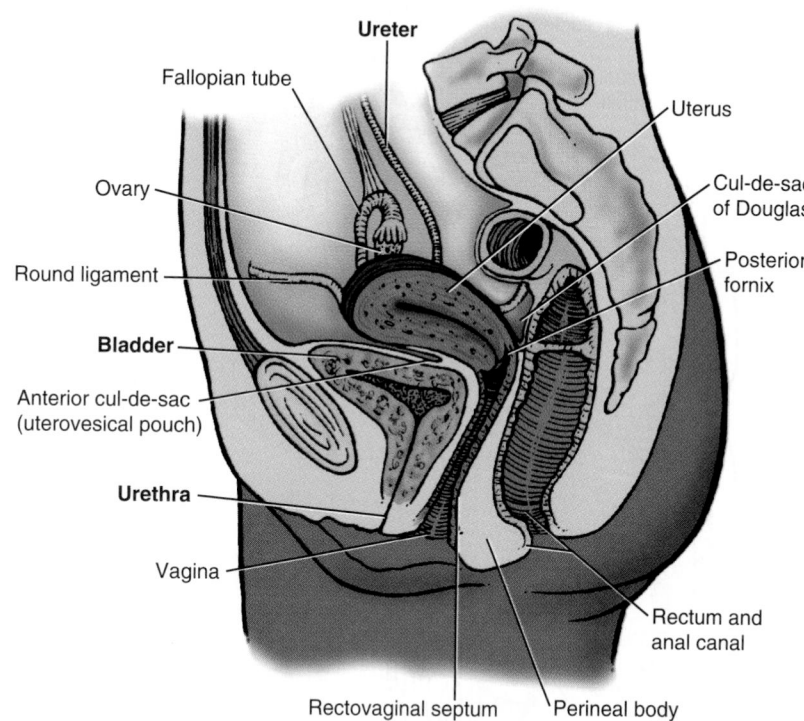

✦ **Figure 32–2**
The female urogenital system. (From Monahan, F. D., Drake, T., & Neighbors, M. [1994]. *Nursing care of adults*. Philadelphia: W. B. Saunders.)

tubular structures of the nephron, urine is formed from the waste products in the blood. This begins with the filtration of protein-free plasma through the glomerular capillaries into Bowman's capsule. In adult individuals who have an adequate blood flow and renal function, about 125 ml of fluid are filtered each minute; this is referred to as the glomerular filtration rate. The glomerular filtrate moves into the tubular segments of the nephron. Nutritionally important sub-

stances are reabsorbed (placed back into the systemic circulation). Substances that are not needed by the body (*e.g.,* excessive fluid and electrolytes) are secreted as urine. The kidneys are able to produce either a concentrated or dilute urine, depending on the composition and volume of the extracellular fluids.

One indicator of kidney function is the amount of urine excreted per hour. The minimum amount of urine needed to maintain kidney function in children

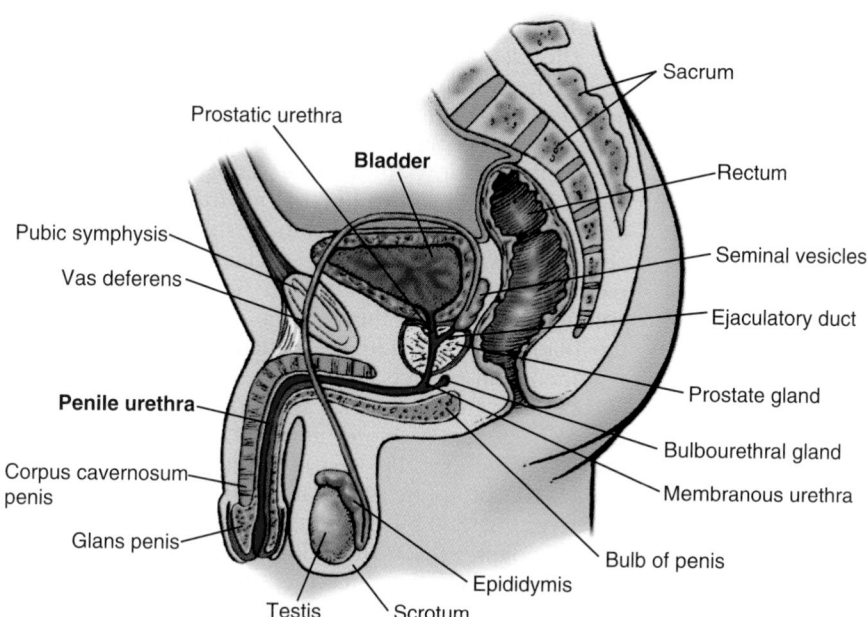

✦ **Figure 32–3**
The male urogenital system. (From Monahan, F. D., Drake, T., & Neighbors, M. [1994]. *Nursing care of adults*. Philadelphia: W. B. Saunders.)

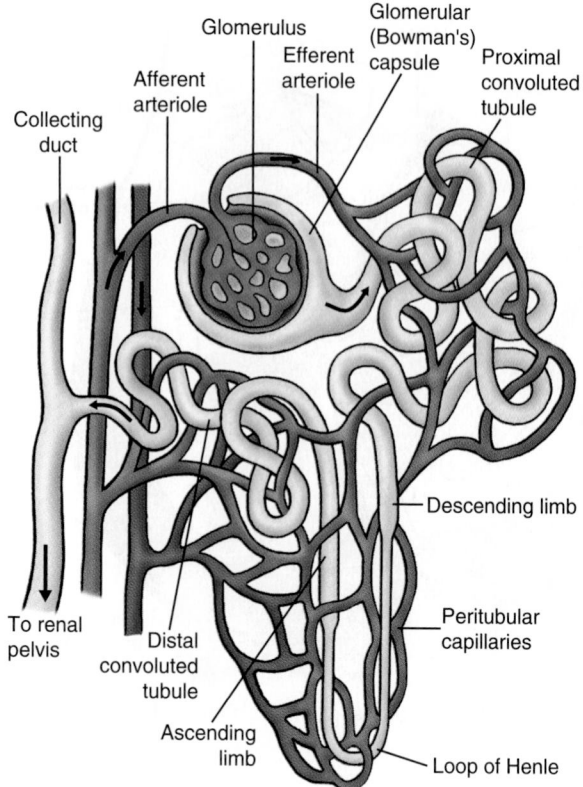

◆ Figure 32–4
The nephron. (From Monahan, F. D., Drake, T., & Neighbors, M. [1994]. *Nursing care of adults.* Philadelphia: W. B. Saunders.)

is 1 ml per kg of body weight per hour (Betz *et al.,* 1994). In adults, the minimum amount of urine output is 30 ml per hour. Usually the average output of urine in the adult is 60 ml per hour and 1500 ml per day (Porth, 1994).

Adequate kidney function is essential to urine production. Kidney diseases may originate in the kidneys or develop as the result of other conditions in the body, such as diabetes. The inability of the kidney to function is known as renal failure, which may be acute or chronic. Acute renal failure is abrupt in onset. If recognized early and treated appropriately, it is often reversible. Acute renal failure can be caused by prerenal, intrarenal, or postrenal factors (Table 32–1.) Chronic renal failure develops slowly and is the end result of irreparable damage to the kidneys.

Urine collects in the pelvis of the kidney. As the urine distends the pelvis, the muscle wall contracts and pushes the urine into the ureters. Kidney damage can occur if urine is not permitted to flow out of the renal pelvis into the ureters. This may happen if a urinary tract obstruction is below the level of the pelvis of the kidney. The obstruction may be in the ureters, bladder, bladder neck, or urethra. A bladder obstruction may be due to hyperplasia (overgrowth) of prostatic tissue, tumors, or calculi (stones). Calculi located in the ureters or kidneys can also result in an obstruction to the flow of urine.

Ureters

The ureters, which are two muscular tubes approximately 25 to 30 cm long and 1.25 cm wide, carry the urine from the renal pelvis (ureteropelvic junction) to the urinary bladder. Urine flow in the ureters is accomplished by peristaltic action of the ureters plus the force of gravity. The ureters enter the posterior wall of the urinary bladder, the ureterovesical junction, at an oblique angle. A fold of membrane serves as a valve where the ureters enter the bladder. The oblique angle, the mucous fold, and peristalsis normally prevent a **reflux** (backflow) of urine into the ureters when the bladder contracts.

Problems of the ureters are usually associated with obstructions, increased pressure in the bladder, and congenital anomalies. Distention of one or both ureters due to the backflow of urine is known as **hydroureter.**

Urinary Bladder

The urinary bladder is a hollow muscular sac that acts as a reservoir for urine before it is excreted from the body via the urethra. The position of the bladder varies with the state of fullness, age, and gender. In infants, the bladder is found within the abdomen. Just before puberty, it assumes its position in the pelvis behind the symphysis pubis. The bladder does not migrate; instead, changes in growth and development of the bony pelvis occur (Gray, 1995).

The bladder is composed of several layers: mucosa, submucosa, detrusor muscle, and serous layer. The mucosal layer has multiple folds (rugae); this allows the bladder to stretch as it fills with urine. The submucosa layer contains connective tissue that connects the mucous and muscular layers, and the serous layer coats the superior portion of the bladder and is formed by the peritoneum (Bullock & Rosendahl, 1992).

The bladder contains a network of smooth muscle fibers, the **detrusor muscle,** which is the muscle of micturition. The trigone of the bladder is an area at the base of the bladder formed by the two ureters and the urethra. Below the bladder and the urethra is an internal urethral sphincter; below that is an external urethral sphincter. These sphincters are formed by circular muscles, which, when stimulated, allow urine to pass from the bladder into the urethra. The external sphincter surrounds the urethra distal to the base of the bladder. The external sphincter helps to maintain continence in periods of high bladder pressure.

Bladder capacity varies with individuals. The bladder can generally store about 1000 to 1800 ml of urine. As the bladder becomes distended with urine, stretch receptors are stimulated. In adults, this occurs when 150 to 300 ml of urine fill the bladder (Bullock & Rosendahl, 1992). In children, a quantity of 50 to 200 ml of urine stimulates the stretch receptors. Once this volume stimulates the stretch receptors, reflex

Table 32–1

CAUSES OF ACUTE RENAL FAILURE

PRERENAL ACUTE RENAL FAILURE	

Conditions that are systemic and affect the amount of blood reaching the kidneys	Hypovolemia
	    Dehydration
	    Water and electrolyte losses (vomiting, diarrhea, nasogastric suctioning, intestinal obstruction, uncontrolled diabetes mellitus)
	    Hemorrhage
	    Fluid shifts (*e.g.,* burns)
	Septic shock
	Heart failure
	Interruption of renal blood flow caused by surgery

INTRARENAL ACUTE RENAL FAILURE	

Disorders that occur within the kidneys	Acute tubular necrosis
	    Prolonged renal ischemia
	    Exposure to nephrotoxic agents
	        Aminoglycosides (e.g., gentamicin, kanamycin, colistin)
	        Heavy metals (*e.g.,* lead, mercury)
	        Organic solvents (*e.g.,* carbon tetrachloride, ethylene glycol)
	        Radiopaque contrast media
	Intratubular obstruction
	    Uric acid crystals
	    Hemolytic reactions (*e.g.,* blood transfusion reactions)
	    Precipitated proteins resulting from multiple myelomas
	    Acute glomerulonephritis

POSTRENAL ACUTE RENAL FAILURE	
Problems that occur once the urine leaves the kidney	Ureteral obstruction (*e.g.,* calculi, tumor, clots) Bladder outlet obstruction (*e.g.,* prostatic hyperplasia, urethral strictures)

Data from Huether, S. E., & McCance, K. L. (1996). *Understanding pathophysiology.* St. Louis: Mosby-Year Book; Porth, C. M. (1994). *Pathophysiology concepts of altered health states,* (4th ed.). Philadelphia: J. B. Lippincott.

contraction of the bladder and relaxation of the internal sphincter occur, resulting in emptying of the bladder. Contraction of the external sphincter, a learned behavior, prevents micturition. Proper neurological functioning is also essential to control micturition. The bladder is protected from infection by the phagocytic abilities of its mucous membrane lining, the unidirectional flow of urine, its high concentration of urea, its high osmolarity, and the acidity of the urine. The constituents of the urine inhibit or kill bacteria.

Urethra

The function of the urethra is to serve as a passageway for urine from the bladder to the meatus, the external opening of the urinary system. The length of the urethra in men is 17 to 23 cm; in women, it is approximately 2.5 to 3.5 cm. The short urethra in women and its anatomical location (anterior to the vaginal opening and posterior to the clitoris), as well as its proximity to the rectum, place women at risk for infections of the urethra and bladder. The turbulent flow of urine as it passes through the urethra provides some defense against infections.

Prostate Gland

In males, the prostate gland lies just below the bladder and surrounds about an inch of the urethra. The primary function of this walnut-sized gland is to secrete a thin, milky, alkaline fluid needed to nourish and transfer sperm as they are ejaculated. This fluid helps to neutralize the acidic fluid of the male urethra (Schlosser, 1992). The prostate gland's location and the passing of prostatic secretions through the urethra permit the prostate gland to affect the body's ability to excrete urine. With aging, a normal hypertrophy (enlargement) of the prostate occurs, which can obstruct the flow of urine from the bladder. The length of the urethra and the prostatic secretions (which possess antibacterial properties) decrease the risk of urethral infections in men.

Process of Urination

The process of urination involves structural and innervation competence. *Innervation competence* refers to the functioning of the voiding reflex centers and the voiding control center. The voiding reflex centers involve the spinal nerves and the spinal and motor tract dealing with involuntary control. The voiding control center (cerebral cortex) controls voluntary voiding and makes an individual cognitively aware of the need to urinate and the action to be taken. The process of urination is illustrated in Figure 32–5.

Factors Affecting Urination

Many factors affect urination. All of these factors need to be considered when assessing a client's patterns of urination:

* The physiological integrity of the urinary system
* Developmental level
* Intake of fluids, foods, medications, and toxic substances
* Fluid lost by other routes
* Sensory-motor innervation defects
* Mobility level and muscle tone
* Mental and emotional status

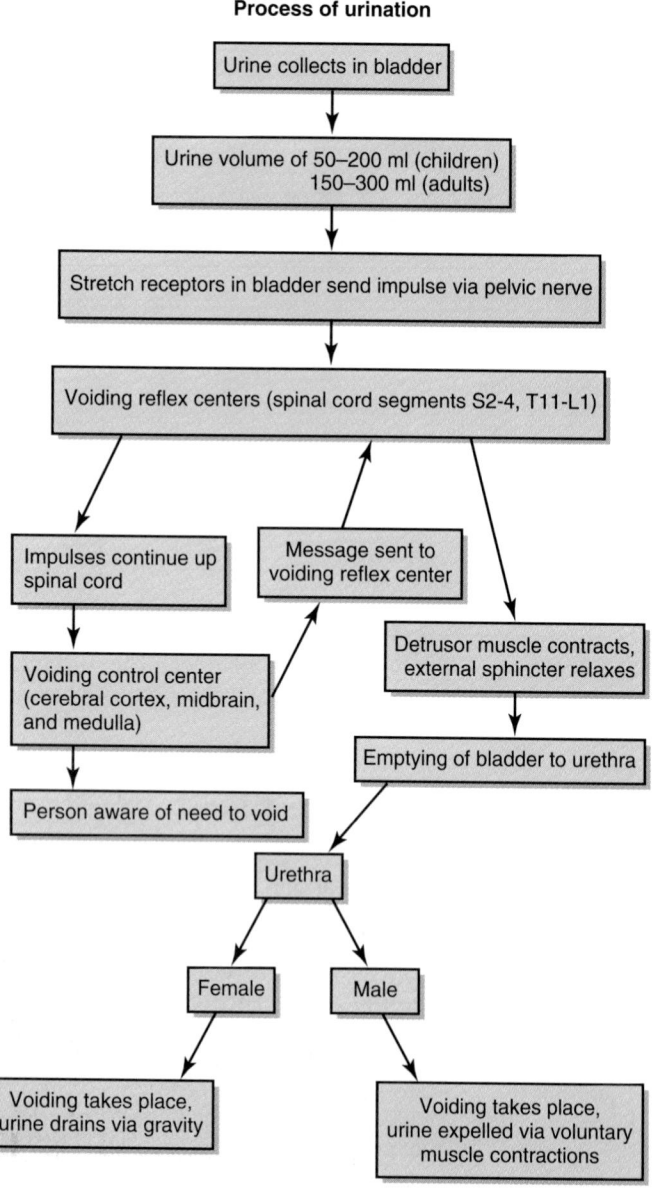

Process of urination

Urine collects in bladder

↓

Urine volume of 50–200 ml (children) 150–300 ml (adults)

↓

Stretch receptors in bladder send impulse via pelvic nerve

↓

Voiding reflex centers (spinal cord segments S2-4, T11-L1)

Impulses continue up spinal cord

Message sent to voiding reflex center

Voiding control center (cerebral cortex, midbrain, and medulla)

Detrusor muscle contracts, external sphincter relaxes

Person aware of need to void

Emptying of bladder to urethra

Urethra

Female   Male

Voiding takes place, urine drains via gravity

Voiding takes place, urine expelled via voluntary muscle contractions

❧ **Figure 32–5**
The process of urination.

- Sociocultural influences
- Gender

Physiological Integrity of the Urinary System

The urinary system can be viewed as a single system, with urine forming in the kidneys and flowing as a continuous stream to the urinary meatus, where it is excreted. Therefore, a disorder in one component of the system affects the other components. A problem in one structure usually affects the structure above it, so problems of the genitourinary tract usually result in complications in ascending structures. The physiological integrity of the urinary system is disrupted by infections, obstructions, congenital anomalies, and inherited disorders.

Developmental Level

The urinary system undergoes changes with aging. Prior to the first 2 years of life, the urinary tract has not matured sufficiently to concentrate urine effectively (Bullock & Rosendahl, 1992). As a result, when an infant is dehydrated, the kidneys are not able to compensate and conserve fluids, and severe dehydration can occur quickly.

As the adult ages, the kidneys become smaller, and the number of reserve nephrons decreases. Accompanying changes in the circulatory system (vascular changes and a decrease in cardiac output) result in decreased renal functioning. Although the kidneys can maintain homeostasis of fluids and electrolytes, they are slower to respond to changes in fluid composition or periods of stress. Also occurring with aging is diminished bladder muscle tone, which results in increased frequency of urination. This occurs because of physical changes in the structure of the bladder, decreased bladder capacity, and weakening of muscles of the pelvic floor. A result of this is **urinary incontinence** (involuntary loss of urine) and **retention of urine** (inability to void or empty the bladder completely). Incontinence can occur at any age, but its prevalence increases with age.

Developmental level affects toilet training. The timing when toilet training is initiated can vary from 10 months to 5 years of age. A realistic expectation for physical control of urination is 18 months to 3 years of age. Physiological control of the urethral sphincters is achieved at 18 to 24 months. However, the child must be psychologically ready to master voluntary control. The child must recognize the urge to urinate, be motivated to please the parent, and communicate the urge to urinate to the parent (Wong, 1995). Bladder control in children varies, but it is usually seen between the ages of 2 and 5 years. Daytime control is achieved earlier than nighttime control. Bladder control at night may not be achieved until the child is 5 years of age (Wong, 1995).

Intake of Fluid, Food, Medications, and Toxic Substances

Fluid intake refers to all liquids taken into the body, including liquids ingested by mouth, administered by tube feeding, and given intravenously. The amount of fluid intake influences urine output. For example, the client who is dehydrated has decreased urine output.

Foods vary in the amount of fluid they contain. Examples of foods high in fluid content are raw fruits and vegetables (*e.g.,* lettuce, carrots, celery), milk, and cooked cereal.

Individuals who ingest large amounts of fluids containing caffeine have an increased urine output, because a physiological effect of caffeine is **diuresis** (increased excretion of urine by the kidneys). Examples of liquids containing caffeine are coffee, tea, and some soft drinks (such as cola).

Foods that are high in sodium result in fluid retention. Examples of foods high in sodium are salt-preserved foods (such as salted or smoked meat), buttermilk, sour cream, broth, bouillon, and canned soups.

Medications also influence the amount of urine output, the color of urine, and the presence of abnormal constituents in urine. Diuretic drugs result in increased urine volume and urine excretion by acting on certain sites along the nephron tubules to interfere with sodium reabsorption. Examples of diuretics are furosemide (Lasix), hydrochlorothiazide (Hydrodiuril), bumetanide (Bumex), and torsemide (Demadex).

Analgesic drugs such as opiates and opiate derivatives (which include morphine) and meperidine (Demerol) may cause urinary retention or difficulty in urination. Both types of drugs cause an increase in the tone of the detrusor muscle, urinary bladder, and vesical sphincter (Smith & Reynard, 1995). Also, opiates depress the central nervous system and may make a client inattentive to the stimuli arising in the bladder.

Several drugs alter the color of urine. Examples include phenazopyridine (Pyridium), which is used for urinary tract analgesia and turns the urine orange-red; and nitrofurantoin (Furadantin, Macrodantin), an antiinfective agent effective in urinary tract infections (UTIs), which turns the urine brown or rust-yellow (Shlafer, 1993). Levodopa also turns the urine brown (Chernecky *et al.,* 1993). Anticoagulant drugs, such as heparin or coumadin, can cause blood in the urine (hematuria), which is observed as urine that becomes pink, red, or dark brown in color (McKenry & Salerno, 1989).

A variety of substances have the potential to have a nephrotoxic effect on kidney cells (do damage to the nephron of the kidney and decrease renal functioning). The most common nephrotoxic substances are medications, especially antibiotics. Examples of antibiotics that may damage the kidneys include gentamicin, tobramycin, kantamycin, and the sulfonamides.

The dosages of specific medicines may be considered nephrotoxic. Therefore, nurses need to understand the effects drugs may have on the kidney and be aware of any existing kidney problem that the client is experiencing, perhaps due to aging or existing pathology.

The client's age must be considered because renal blood flow and glomerular filtration rate decrease with age. In addition, many drugs are taken chronically by the elderly, and " . . . for any given dose and dosing interval, the steady-state blood level is likely to be higher in older people. In addition, the differences among individuals are frequently greater than any average "age-related' differences" (Smith & Reynard, 1995, p. 610).

Toxic substances in the environment are also responsible for causing kidney damage. These substances may be ingested or inhaled or may enter the body through the skin surface. For example, heavy metals, such as lead and mercury; solvents such as carbon tetrachloride; and pesticides have been associated with kidney damage (Porth, 1994). Ingestion of toxic materials is more likely to occur in children.

Fluid Lost by Routes Other Than Urine

It is important for nurses to encourage and monitor fluid intake to ensure that fluid intake is equal to fluid output. In addition to being lost in urine, fluid is also lost through respiration, perspiration, and feces. When individuals report that their urine production has decreased, it is important to assess if their fluid intake has changed or if excess fluid is being lost by other routes, such as through the gastrointestinal tract (*e.g.,* diarrhea, vomiting) or through the skin (*e.g.,* diaphoresis). Refer to Table 32–2 for average urine output in children and adults.

Fluid deficits in the body may occur as a result of third space losses or trauma. Third space losses occur from changes in the distribution of body fluids (*e.g.,* extracellular fluid that collects in an area that is physi-

ologically unavailable to the body, such as in injured tissues) (Porth, 1994; Price & Wilson, 1992). Examples of third space losses from trauma include the collection of fluid as the result of a burn or muscle trauma. Hemorrhage can also result in fluid loss, with a subsequent decrease in the amount of urine produced. Refer to Chapter 28 for further discussion of fluid shifts.

Sensory-Motor Innervation Defects

Sensory-motor innervation of the bladder and urethral structures regulates bladder emptying and urinary continence (see Fig. 32–5). The type of urological deficits that may occur depends on what aspect of innervation has been disrupted. Innervation of the bladder can be interrupted at any point along the sensory neural pathway, motor neural pathway, or both neural pathways of the brain and spinal cord. Nerves supplying the bladder and urethra and the motor area of the cerebrum must be intact for maintenance of urinary control. The two main categories for classifying neurogenic bladder disorders (any urinary disorder caused by a disruption of innervation to the bladder) are detrusor muscle hyperreflexia and detrusor muscle areflexia.

Detrusor Muscle Hyperreflexia

Detrusor muscle hyperreflexia (autonomic, spastic, neurogenic bladder) occurs when a spinal cord lesion is above the voiding reflex centers. (The voiding reflex centers are located in the sacral [S2 through S4] and thoracolumbar [T11 through L1] segments of the spinal cord [Porth, 1994].) Voluntary control of urination is lost, but reflex contraction of the bladder is maintained. Bladder reflexes are uncoordinated with bladder filling and sphincter opening and closure. This leads to frequent spontaneous bladder spasms, incomplete emptying of the bladder, urinary stasis within the bladder, potential urinary tract infections, hypertrophy of the trigone (the triangular area of the bladder bounded by the ureters and urethra), vesicoureteral reflux, and renal damage.

Detrusor Muscle Areflexia

Detrusor muscle areflexia (atonic, flaccid, autonomous neurogenic bladder) occurs when a spinal cord lesion is at the sacral level, S2 to S4, or from peripheral trauma. Voluntary control and reflex urination are absent, which results in distention of the bladder and urinary retention.

Many diseases (*e.g.,* Parkinson's disease, cerebrovascular accidents, spinal cord trauma, multiple sclerosis, and diabetes mellitus) result in sensory-motor innervations defects.

Mobility Level and Muscle Tone

Without exercise, abdominal and pelvic muscles weaken. This can lead to impairment of detrusor con-

---

Table 32–2

AVERAGE 24-HOUR URINE OUTPUT— CHILDREN AND ADULTS

AGE	URINE OUTPUT, ml
2 mo–2 y	500–600
1–3 y	500–600
5–8 y	650–1000
14 y to adulthood	1500

Data from Porth, C. M. (1994). *Pathophysiology concepts of altered health states* (4th ed.). Philadelphia: J. B. Lippincott; Hoyler-Grant, C. (1995); Hoyler, G. C. (1995). Health assessment of the pediatric urology patient. In Kaslowicz, K. A. (Ed.), *Urologic nursing: Principles and practice.* Philadelphia: W. B. Saunders.

tractions and inadequate control of the external sphincter of the bladder. Contraction of the abdominal muscles increases intraabdominal pressure, which increases pressure within the bladder. The muscles of the pelvic floor help support the bladder and maintain urinary continence.

Lack of mobility is a major predisposing factor for development of renal calculi. **Calculi,** or stones, can be formed as a result of calcium leaving the bones during long periods of immobility. Individuals who are paralyzed or who are on prolonged bed rest are at risk for calculi formation.

Prolonged use of an indwelling catheter decreases bladder tone. An indwelling catheter continuously drains the bladder of urine, and the bladder does not fill. Therefore, the detrusor muscle is not stimulated to contract. When a muscle is not used, it loses its tone and becomes flaccid. Once the indwelling catheter is removed, the client may have difficulty regaining control of urination.

Ability to use the toilet requires some degree of mobility. Deficits in the ability to walk to a toilet, to lower oneself to a sitting position, to stand from a sitting position, or to remove clothing to urinate present obstacles to voiding. Individuals who require assistance in using a toilet may not want to ask for help, or help may not be available. This may result in functional incontinence.

Decreased mobility also places individuals at risk for alterations in eliminating feces. Fecal impaction (hardened, dry stool in the rectum) may press on the urethra and impede the flow of urine. This may lead to urinary retention with overflow incontinence (dribbling of the overflow of urine).

Mental Status

Individuals who are mentally confused or disoriented may be incontinent of urine. Confusion may be caused by a physiological disorder, a change in physical environment, or drugs.

Physiological disorders may contribute to mental confusion. For example, insufficient oxygen to the brain (which may occur in chronic pulmonary disease) can result in decreased mental alertness. Long-term use of sedative hypnotics, such as flurazepam (Dalmane) and diazepam (Valium), contributes to confusion in the elderly.

Individuals, particularly children and the elderly, who are in an unfamiliar environment may become incontinent. The reason may be as simple as not knowing where the toilet is located. Finding oneself in an unfamiliar environment may also cause anxiety. Anxiety may stimulate or inhibit urination. Increased **frequency** (an increase in the number of times per day that one voids, more than usual voiding pattern) and **urinary urgency** (intense and immediate need to void) are associated with the parasympathetic responses to stressful situations (fight or flight). Anxiety may also result in urinary retention as a result of tightening of the perineal muscles. Depression also contributes to changes in urinary patterns and is associated with incontinence. Depression may decrease the person's motivation to get to a toilet when the sensation to void occurs (Case-Gamble, 1990).

Sociocultural Influences

What is accepted as the norm in voiding practices varies among cultures and between genders. These variations include privacy, socialized behaviors, and use of intrusive procedures.

In North America, one expects private toilet facilities designated for either male or female users. Women expect privacy for toileting. Men are not provided with, nor do they expect, privacy when urinating. In many countries, communal facilities are the norm and are used by both men and women.

Nurses need to explore how their clients feel about privacy and then respect their preferences whenever possible. However, client safety should never be compromised. Providing a call bell or closing a bathroom door without locking it provides privacy while ensuring the nurse quick access to the client. When possible, curtains should be closed around a client who is toileting, and visitors and nursing personnel should leave the room.

Patterns of urinary elimination are highly individualized. In general, the expectation is that an adult individual voids four to six times per day. The times of voiding can be influenced by an individual's expectations and lifestyle. Time for urination is frequently allocated during school or work breaks (*e.g.,* school recess, coffee breaks, meal times). Most individuals urinate shortly after awakening from sleep and prior to bedtime. These times need to be considered when providing bladder training.

In some cultures, any procedure that is intrusive to the body may be viewed negatively (*i.e.,* not be seen as being therapeutic). For example, the Chinese yin and yang beliefs state that health is promoted through spiritual and physical harmony. Any procedure that is intrusive detracts from body harmony. Procedures such as urinary catheterization or diagnostic testing may be considered a threat to this harmony (Ebersol & Hess, 1990).

Gender

Female gender is considered a risk factor for urinary tract infection and some types of urinary incontinence, and male gender is a risk factor for some types of urinary incontinence and obstructions of the bladder and kidney.

Women have a higher incidence of UTIs because of the urethra's length and its close anatomical position to the vagina and rectum. The incidence of incontinence in women is twice that of men (Wyman, 1992). Women have a shorter urethra that exerts less resistance to bladder pressure. The enlarged uterus during pregnancy adds pressure to the bladder, and incontinence is frequently experienced. During and after menopause, a deficiency of estrogen causes a thinning of the urethral mucosa. In addition, with aging a loss of the posterior ureterovesical angle occurs in women, which prompts involuntary urine loss. Women who have multiple vaginal births or surgery that involves the perineum and pelvic structures are at risk for incontinence of urine.

Young boys have a higher incidence of enuresis than do girls. Suggested causes include a maturational delay in the development of the bladder musculature's ability to withstand the pressure of a large urine volume and toilet training that occurred too early. Obstructions of the bladder and kidney are seen more frequently in men. Benign prostatic hyperplasia (BPH) and formation of calculi (stones) contribute to this.

Common Alterations of the Urinary Tract

The four common alterations of the urinary tract are infections, obstructions, retention, and incontinence.

Urinary Tract Infections

An infection can occur anywhere in the urinary tract. Most lower tract infections are attributed to an ascending infection of gram-negative bacteria. Once part of the urinary tract is infected, the entire system is compromised. The most dangerous outcome is pyelonephritis (infection of the kidney).

Within the hospital, inserting instruments into the urethra and bladder for diagnostic purposes or for dilating the urethra or inserting a urinary catheter into the bladder places the client at risk for a nosocomial infection (an infection acquired during hospitalization). In catheterized clients, the incidence of infection is more than 50%, and some hospitals report rates as high as 100% (Matassarin-Jacobs, 1993). Furthermore, the length of time a urinary catheter remains in the client increases the risk of infection. In one study, it was reported that 50% of the clients who had a catheter left in their bladder for 10 days had urinary tract infections (Ader *et al.*, 1990). Donegan (1996) stated that ". . . virtually all patients will acquire **bacteriuria** (presence of organisms without accompanying white cells) after 10 days of catheter use" (p. 1965). In women, the two most common UTIs are **cystitis** and urethritis. Prostatitis is the most frequently seen UTI in men. Many risk factors are associated with UTI (Table 32–3).

A UTI may be present whether the client manifests symptoms or not. Common symptoms of bladder and urethral inflammations are **dysuria** (burning or pain on urination), frequency of urination, urgency, voiding small amounts, inability to void, incomplete

emptying of the bladder, and suprapubic tenderness. Hematuria, low back pain, malaise, nausea, vomiting, abdominal pain, fever, chills, and flank pain also may occur. The urine may appear dark yellow to amber in color, be cloudy or bloody, and smell foul. Pathogenic microorganisms may be in the urinary tract without any signs and symptoms of infection being present for months or years (Moore *et al.*, 1993; Smeltzer & Bare, 1996; Stamm & Turck, 1983).

Obstructions

When an obstruction in the urinary tract occurs, the flow of urine is impeded. Blockage to urine flow may be partial or complete. The effects of the obstruction are related to the degree of blockage. An obstruction may cause a "backflow" of urine from the bladder to the ureters and kidneys, which may result in a hydroureter (dilation of the ureter to accommodate increased urine volume in the ureter) or hydronephrosis (distention of the renal pelvis and calices with urine). Obstructions contribute to the cause of urinary tract infection and the formation of calculi, but damage to the renal tissue is the most serious result of an obstruction.

Obstructions have multiple and varied causes, such as congenital defects in structure or position, tumors, formation of calculi (stones), and strictures resulting from an inflammatory process (Fig. 32–6). The

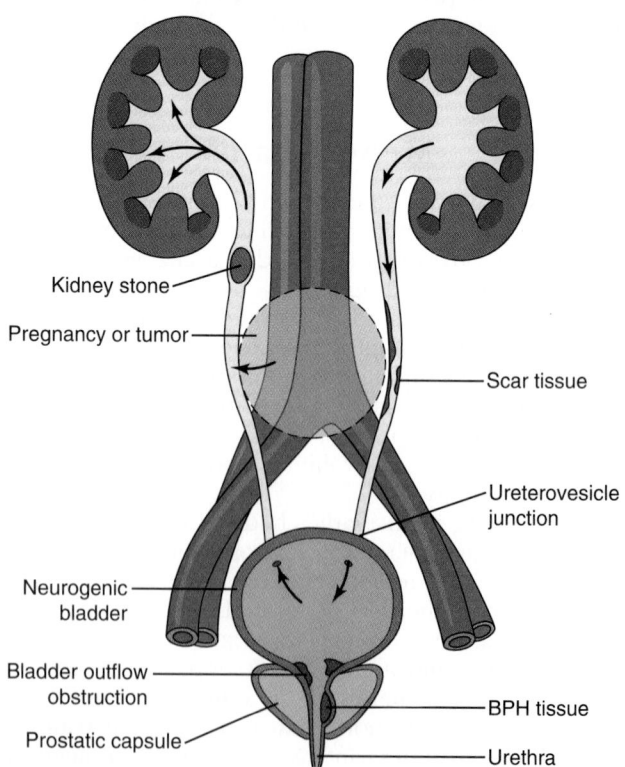

Kidney stone

Pregnancy or tumor

Scar tissue

Ureterovesicle junction

Neurogenic bladder

Bladder outflow obstruction

BPH tissue

Prostatic capsule

Urethra

꙳ Figure 32–6

Obstructions in the urinary tract. *A,* Tumor. *B,* Stone. *C,* Stricture. *D,* Benign prostatic hyperplasia. *E,* Fecal impaction.

Table 32-3

RISK FACTORS FOR URINARY TRACT INFECTION

RISK FACTOR	RATIONALE
Gender (female clients have a higher incidence of UTIs than male clients)	Location and short length of urethra; poor hygiene and trauma during intercourse introduce bacteria into the urethra; pregnancy also places women at greater risk; the antibacterial properties of prostatic fluid and the length of the urethra in male clients may account for the lower incidence of UTIs in men under 50 years of age; after that time, benign prostatic hypertrophy increases the risk of UTIs
Inadequate hydration	Concentrated urine fosters bacterial growth
Immobility	Promotes bone demineralization with ensuing stone formation and obstructive disorders, increasing the risk of UTIs
Age (risk increases with age)	Decreased mobility, poor personal hygiene, and relaxation of pelvic musculature contribute to UTIs
Poor hygiene after toileting	Bacteria from feces can enter urethra
Presence of indwelling urinary catheter or poor asepsis in insertion, irrigation, or care of catheter	Route for ascending urinary infection; insertion of catheter can cause trauma to mucous membrane; break in aseptic technique during insertion can result in introduction of bacteria to urethra
Urinary retention (*e.g.,* neurogenic bladder)	Stasis of urine results in a favorable medium for bacterial growth
Bubble baths	Introduction of bacteria into urethra
Contaminated hands of health personnel and contaminated hospital equipment	Introduce bacteria into urethra

most common causes of obstructions are urinary calculi and BPH.

Benign prostatic hyperplasia is almost a universal phenomenon in older men and is considered part of the aging process. Approximately 51% of the male population have BPH when they are 60 to 69 years old (Huether & McCance, 1996). The incidence continues to increase with age. Ninety-five percent of men older than 70 years are affected (Cotran, *et al.,* 1994). The etiology of BPH is unknown, but it is associated with changes in hormone levels.

Urinary Retention

Urinary retention is the inability to empty the bladder completely. Factors contributing to urinary retention include weakened detrusor muscles, which leads to high urethral pressure; hypertonic sphincters, which may be related to anxiety; inhibition of the micturition reflex arc, which may be caused by the use of drugs (antidepressants/antipsychotics, anticholinergics/antispasmodics, opiate analgesics, antihistamines, anti-Parkinsonism drugs, and antihypertensives); neurological disorders, which result in weak or absent sensory or motor impulses; and urethral blockage caused by fecal impaction, surgical site swelling,

postpartum edema, rectal or vaginal packing, presence of calculi, tumors, or an enlarged prostate gland (Voith, 1988).

Retention of urine in the bladder leads to urinary stasis, which places an individual at risk for a UTI. Stasis of urine alters the pH, and normally acidic urine becomes alkaline. Alkaline urine favors bacterial growth. In addition, a distended bladder decreases the blood flow to the bladder, making it less resistant to gram-negative bacilli from the urethra.

Urinary Incontinence

Urinary incontinence is the loss of voluntary control of voiding. Incontinence is a symptom, not a disease. It is considered one of the most costly, underreported and underdiagnosed health problems in the United States (McCormick *et al.,* 1992). Incidence rates vary from 8 to 51% in individuals who reside independently in the community and from 38 to 55% in those residing in long-term care facilities (Appleby, 1995; Herzog & Falty, 1990; Mohide, 1986). Frequently, individuals do not report that they are incontinent or seek the help of health care professionals in assisting them with this problem. The reasons include

1. Embarrassment over urinary loss and fear of odor
2. Feelings of isolation and depression
3. An attitude that incontinence is an unavoidable result of the aging process
4. Fear of surgery
5. Insufficient teaching of health care professionals that incontinence can be prevented, diagnosed, and treated effectively
6. Fear of institutionalization (Appleby, 1995; McCormick *et al.,* 1992; Turner & Plymat, 1988; Wyman, 1992)

Statistics regarding the prevalence of incontinence are not precise because of underreporting. Urinary incontinence is upsetting to the individual who experiences it and, when applicable, to the caretakers. It is considered the predominant reason for institutionalization of the elderly (Kaschak Newman *et al.,* 1991).

Urinary incontinence can be transitional or chronic. Treatment of the underlying cause usually resolves the problem of transitional incontinence. (Refer to Table 32–4 for common causes of transitional incontinence.) According to the Agency for Health Care Policy and Research ([AHCPR], 1992a, b), incontinence may be classified as stress, urge, functional, mixed, overflow, reflex, and total.

Functional incontinence occurs in clients with normal bladder and urethral functioning who have an involuntary loss of urine due to sensory, motor, cognitive, or environmental barriers. Examples include physical immobility, visual impairments, confusion, emotional disorders, restraints, bedside rails, and poor lighting (see Clinical Insight Box).

Stress incontinence is involuntary loss of urine in amounts of less than 50 ml, usually during periods of increased intraabdominal pressure such as during laughing, coughing, sneezing, and lifting heavy objects. Stress incontinence is associated with a weakening of the pelvic muscles, specifically the pubococcygeal and transverse perineal muscles. When intraabdominal pressure increases and exerts pressure on the bladder, the weakened pelvic muscles do not maintain closure of the urethral sphincter; thus, incontinence occurs. Weakened sphincter tone and a decreased urethrovesicular angle may contribute to stress incontinence. Stress incontinence occurs predominantly in young to middle-aged women who have experienced multiple pregnancies, traumatic childbirth, or gynecological procedures, or who are obese. In older women with postmenopausal estrogen deficiencies, thinned out urethral mucosa contributes to decreased urethral sphincter tone. Occasionally, men may have stress incontinence related to damage to the proximal urethra after undergoing prostate surgery (AHCPR, 1992; Appleby, 1995; Doenges & Moorehouse, 1993; Kaschak Newman *et al.,* 1991; McCormick *et al.,* 1992; Turner & Plymat, 1988; Voith, 1988).

Urge incontinence is involuntary loss of urine occurring after a sudden and strong urgency to void. The client may lose urine in small amounts of less than 100 ml or in sudden massive amounts of greater than 500 ml. Usually urge incontinence is associated with urinary frequency (voiding more often than every 2 hours). The client may complain of the urge to void followed by the inability to reach a toilet in time. Urge incontinence may be due to detrusor hyperreflexia with impaired bladder contractility; decreased bladder capacity (associated with abdominal surgeries or prolonged use of Foley catheters); irritation of bladder stretch receptors, causing spasm (associated with UTI or neuropathy); increased urine production (associated with use of diuretics, alcohol, caffeine, and increased fluids); and overdistension of the bladder or prolapsed bladder, uterus or rectum (AHCPR, 1992a, b; Appleby, 1995; Kaschak Newman *et al.,* 1991; McCormick *et al.,* 1992).

Table 32–4

CAUSES OF TRANSITIONAL INCONTINENCE

COMMON CAUSES	RATIONALE
Delirium (confusional state)	Decreases an individual's awareness of the urge to void Correction of the confusional state will diminish the incidence of incontinence
Dehydration	Concentrated urine irritates the bladder wall, which can lead to episodes of incontinence
UTI	Irritation of the mucous membrane of the bladder and urethra may occur; with symptoms of frequency and dysuria, elderly individuals may not be able to reach the toilet in time
Urinary retention	The adverse effect of some medications and prostate enlargement interfere with emptying of the bladder; this can result in overflow incontinence
Fecal impaction	Stool impaction causes pressure on the bladder, which can lead to either urge or overflow incontinence; removal of the impaction resolves the urinary incontinence
Atrophic vaginitis	Results from postmenopausal estrogen depletion (*i.e.,* inflammation, and thinning of mucosal wall of bladder and urethra); symptoms of dysuria, burning on urination, urgency, agitation (in confused patients) and sometimes leaking of urine occur; treated with conjugated estrogen

Data from Agency for Health Care Policy and Research. (1992a, b). Kaschak Newman, D., Lynch, K., Smith, D. A., & Cell, P. (1991). Restoring urinary continence. *American Journal of Nursing, 91* (1), 28–36.

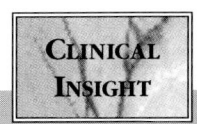

Incontinence

CLINICAL INSIGHT

The relationships of functional, urological, and environmental characteristics of 131 older women to their frequency of incontinence were investigated. The women all lived in the community and ranged in age from 55 to 90 years. The mean duration of incontinence was 10.3 years.

Functional status included speed of walking and responses to a subscale of the Activities of Daily Living Scale. Urological characteristics consisted of bladder capacity, subjects' perceived ability to delay voiding, and urodynamic abnormalities. The severity of incontinence referred to the number of times involuntary loss of urine occurred during 1 week. Environmental factors included the distance to the toilet from other rooms in the home and existing physical obstacles to reaching the toilet, such as furniture, loose rugs, and poor lighting.

All subjects underwent a comprehensive physical evaluation, functional assessment, urinalysis, and blood chemistry determination. Following urodynamic assessment, subjects were grouped into diagnostic groups. One group, consisting of 90 women, was diagnosed as having genuine stress incontinence. The second group, 41 women, was assessed as having detrusor instability with or without accompanying genuine stress incontinence.

In this study, the subjects with detrusor instability had significantly more impaired physical function, slower gait speeds, small bladder capacities, and less ability to delay voiding than subjects with genuine stress incontinence alone. Physical functional status and urological characteristics, including urodynamic diagnosis, did not predict incontinence severity. The authors reported that their findings confirm, in part, that mobility and the environment influence urinary incontinence.

From Wyman, J. F., Elswick, R. K., Jr., Ory, M. G., Wilson, M. S., & Fantl, J. A. (1993). Influence of functional, urological and environment characteristics on urinary incontinence in community-dwelling older women. *Nursing Research, 42* (5), 270–275.

Mixed incontinence is a combination of stress and urge urinary incontinence (AHCPR, 1992). It occurs when both the sensation and exertion to void occur simultaneously, resulting in leakage of urine.

Overflow incontinence involves loss of urine associated with an overdistended bladder. The client may complain of constant dribbling of urine; sensation of bladder fullness; small, frequent voiding; dysuria; and a weak urinary stream. The client does not completely empty his or her bladder, with postvoid residual being greater than 150 ml. Overflow incontinence is most commonly caused by urinary retention secondary to some type of obstruction of the urinary system,

e.g., an enlarged prostate. This type of incontinence may also be associated with atonic bladder caused by neurological problems or medications (AHCPR, 1992a, b; Appleby, 1995; Kaschak Newman *et al.,* 1991; McCormick *et al.,* 1992).

Total incontinence is an unpredictable and continuous loss of urine. This may be caused by neurological impairments such as spinal cord injury, cerebral lesions, and diabetic neuropathy, which prevents the transmission of the voiding reflex or triggers voiding at unpredictable times. Total incontinence has also been associated with bladder fistulas (abnormal tube-like passages within the bladder; *e.g.,* an opening between the vagina and bladder). Uninhibited bladder spasms, nocturia, lack of bladder filling sensation, and unawareness of incontinence may occur with total incontinence (Appleby, 1995; Doenges & Moorehouse, 1993).

Enuresis

Enuresis is ". . . involuntary or inappropriate voiding in a child at an age when bladder control is expected" (Lawrence, 1995, p. 599). Although enuresis may occur during the day or at night, it occurs more frequently during the night (nocturnal enuresis). It may occur in children who have never achieved consistent urinary control (primary enuresis) or in children who have had a period of bladder control before enuresis started (secondary enuresis) (Lawrence, 1995).

No one specific cause for enuresis has been identified. Contributing factors are psychogenic and physical. Examples of psychogenic factors are temporary regression related to a stressful situation (*e.g.,* the birth or death of a family member, starting school, and separation from parents during hospitalization). Several examples of physical factors are a maturational lag in the central nervous system, a small bladder capacity, structural defects of the urinary system, UTI, and diabetes (Wong, 1995).

Application of the Nursing Process

Assessment

Nursing History

A client's health history is important in identifying existing or potential urinary tract disorders. The symptoms reported with urinary tract problems include changes in the characteristics of urine (amount, color, odor), changes or disturbances in voiding patterns (frequency, amount, inability to control voiding), pain (during voiding, back pain, pain in testicles or labia), and gastrointestinal problems (nausea, vomiting, anorexia). However, many clients with disorders of the urinary tract may not report any symptoms.

Table **32–5**

HEALTH HISTORY

QUESTIONS	IMPLICATIONS
Characteristics of Urine	
About how much urine do you pass each time you void?	Small amount of urine excreted but need to urinate frequently is associated with obstructions and retention of urine.
Please describe what your urine looks like (*e.g.,* Color? Is it cloudy?)	Diuretics, foods high in fluid, and beverages high in caffeine increase fluid output.
Does your urine have an unusual odor?	Cloudy and/or foul-smelling urine suggests presence of a UTI, kidney disease, or other existing pathology (see Table 32–7).
Difficulty in Urinating and Voiding Patterns	
How often do you urinate?	Increased urge to urinate occurs in UTIs and obstructions (*e.g.,* BPH).
Do you need to get up at night to urinate?	Nocturia seen in BPH and in clients taking diuretics.
Is it difficult to initiate a stream of urine?	Difficulty in initiating a stream of urine seen in BPH.
Do you need to strain (like you are having a bowel movement) to start urinating?	The need to increase intraabdominal pressure to void is a symptom of obstruction.
Do you feel as though there is urine in the bladder after you urinate?	Symptom of obstruction and retention of urine.
Is it painful to urinate? (Please describe the pain; *e.g.,* burning).	Indication of UTI.
Urinary Incontinence (Involuntary Loss of Urine)	
Do you lose urine involuntarily?	Helps determine presence and type of urinary incontinence.
What precipitates the loss of urine (*e.g.,* sneezing, coughing, laughing)?	
If you are losing urine, what measures have you taken to treat the incontinence (*e.g.,* absorbent pads, fluid restrictions, dietary changes, exercises, medications)?	Baseline data about what has been tried and what works.
How successful are these measures in controlling urine loss?	
How many children did you give birth to? (Need to differentiate between vaginal and caesarean deliveries.)	Supporting structure of pelvic floor may be compromised. This may result in stress incontinence of urine.
Did you ever have any gynecological surgery?	
Do you need help with toileting (*e.g.,* walking to the bathroom, removing clothing, sitting or standing)?	Self-care abilities related to toileting may contribute to incontinence.
Pain Not Associated With Urinating	
Do you have abdominal pain? back pain? pain in upper thigh? pain in testicles? labia pain? Please describe type of pain (*e.g.,* severe, dull aching, stabbing, radiating).	Type and location of pain provide information about disorders. Bladder disorders may cause suprapubic pain. A severe colicky pain that radiates from the upper back to the testicles or labia may indicate an obstruction of the ureter by a calculus.
Diet History	
What is your typical intake of food and fluid for a 24-hour period?	Certain foods and beverages promote urination (*e.g.,* caffeine, food with high fluid content).
Drug History	
What medications are you currently taking? (This includes prescribed drugs and over-the-counter medication.)	Medication can alter the amount of urine voided and characteristics of urine voided.
Previous Family and Client History of Disorders of Urinary Tract	
Did you ever pass a kidney stone?	Lifestyle and diet may predispose an individual to calculi.
Do you have a family history of kidney disease or problems? (Have client elaborate naming the disease or problem and relationship of the individual involved to the client.)	Some diseases are hereditary (*e.g.,* polycystic kidneys). Some disorders are not hereditary but related to a family disposition (*e.g.,* calculi).

	Table 32–5

HEALTH HISTORY
(Continued)

QUESTIONS	IMPLICATIONS
Systems Other Than Urinary Tract	
Are you aware of the need to urinate? (Nurse may have to further assess mental status.)	Confusion may alter perception of need to urinate.
Did you ever have a stroke or head injury or were told you had a neurological disorder (*e.g.,* multiple sclerosis)?	May be damaged innervation to the bladder. A cerebral lesion may eliminate control of urination.
Do you experience nausea, vomiting, loss of appetite, abdominal cramps?	Gastrointestinal symptoms may be associated with kidney disorders such as pyelonephritis and obstructions. The urinary and gastrointestinal tracts have common autonomic and sensory innervation. The kidneys lie in close proximity to the organs of the gastrointestinal tract. The peritoneum covers the anterior surface of both kidneys (Smith, 1992).
Are you able to walk to the bathroom by yourself?	
Are you able to remove clothing yourself?	
Are you experiencing or do you experience constipation?	Feces in the rectum and sigmoid colon press on the bladder and may cause an obstruction of urine and subsequent overflow incontinence.
Sexual History	
Are you currently sexually active?	Risk factor associated with UTI and sexually transmitted disease.
How often do you have sex?	
What type of protection do you use during sex?	
Did you ever have a sexually transmitted disease?	Sexually transmitted disease may result in UTI and obstruction of urinary tract.
Environmental	

Accessibility of bathroom:
  Climb stairs?
  Distance?
  Presence of grab bars on toilet?
  Elevated toilet?
  Lighting?	

Data from Bates, B. (1995). *A guide to physical examination and history taking* (6th ed.) Philadelphia: J. B. Lippincott; Grinspun, D. (1993). Bladder management for adults following head injury. *Rehabilitation Nursing, 18* (5), 300–305; Kaschak Newman, D., Lynch, K., Smith, D. A., & Cell, P. (1991). Restoring urinary continence. *American Journal of Nursing, 91* (1), 28–36.

After eliciting data about the areas noted here, the nurse should also obtain information about the client's food and fluid intake (assessment of intake and output information to ascertain if fluid intake is greater than fluid output through voiding), past medical history, and family history. Samples of questions that are included in a health history and the rationale for asking these questions are provided in Table 32–5.

When collecting a history from a child with enuresis, Lawrence (1995) suggests assessing the following areas:

- Age when child attained urinary control
- Length of time the child maintained urinary control
- Average duration of dry intervals
- Events surrounding the loss of control (*e.g.,* unaware of loss of urine, participation in strenuous physical activity)
- Time of day or any particular place when the loss of urine occurs
- Frequency of nocturnal enuresis
- Methods employed to manage their child's enuresis
- Family history of enuresis
- Existing stress in the child's life (*e.g.,* marriage, divorce, death)

Physical Examination

In this chapter, assessment focuses on the kidneys, bladder, and urinary meatus.

Kidneys

Percussion and palpation are used in examining the kidneys. The right and left costovertebral angles are percussed to detect tenderness in the kidneys. Reports of pain or tenderness may indicate kidney infection. However, pain may also be related to musculoskeletal conditions. Percussion involves placing a palm of one hand over the right costovertebral angle and striking the other hand against the palm by using the ulnar surface of the wrist (Fig. 32–7A). This maneuver should be repeated at the left costovertebral angle (Bates, 1995).

Deep palpation is required to feel the outer aspect of the adult kidney (see Fig. 32–7B). A normal left kidney is rarely palpable because of the position of the spleen. A normal right kidney may be palpable, particularly in thin, relaxed female clients. The kidney should feel smooth and firm. Enlarged kidneys may be caused by polycystic disease, hydronephrosis, cysts, and tumors (Bates, 1995).

A two-hand maneuver is used to "capture" the kidney between the two hands. The examiner's left hand is placed below and parallel to the 12th rib, with the fingers reaching for the costovertebral angle. The right hand is placed over the left costal margin. The client should be instructed to take a deep breath. The examiner should lift as if trying to dislodge the kidney. This procedure is repeated on the opposite side of the client.

Bladder

The bladder of the adult may be visualized, particularly if the client is thin. The curvature caused by the

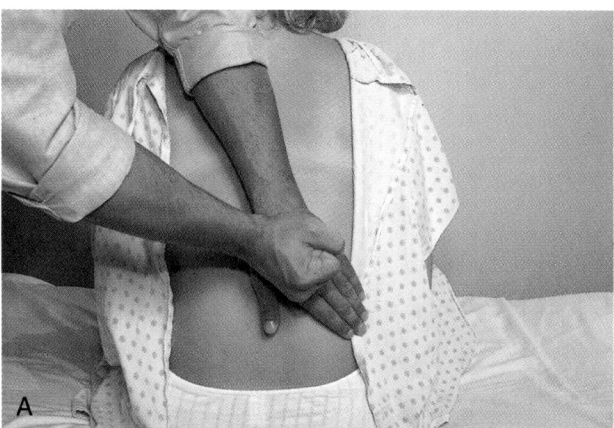
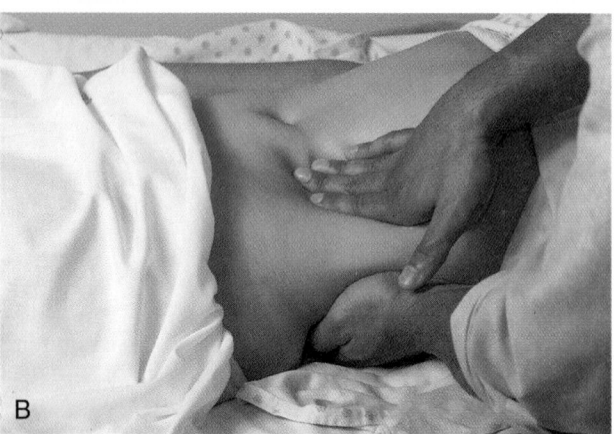

❧ Figure 32–7
A, Percussion of the kidney. B, Deep palpation.

bladder may be seen above the suprapubic bone. The bladder should be palpated and percussed. If it is distended, it can be percussed and palpated more than two finger breadths above the pubic symphysis. Percussion of the bladder involves tapping the area of the abdomen from the suprapubic bone to the umbilicus. The presence of a distended bladder yields a dull sound. An infant's bladder is often felt and normally percussed to the level of the umbilicus.

Prostate

On rectal examination, an enlarged prostate can be palpated. A benign enlargement of the prostate is smooth, hard, elastic, and nontender.

External Meatus

The meatus should be inspected for redness, swelling, and discharge. This may involve retracting the foreskin in an uncircumcised male client. When examining a female client, signs of redness and swelling in the labia and vulva should be noted.

Other Body Systems

In investigating problems of the urinary tract, other body systems must be examined. These include the gastrointestinal system (ability to ingest adequate food and fluids), the musculoskeletal system (muscle tone and activity level), the integumentary system (skin breakdown related to urinary incontinence, evidence of sexually transmitted disease, edema associated with fluid retention), and the neurological system (neurological disease affecting the sacral nerves or nerve routes). Examples of data to consider when collecting a health history and conducting a physical examination on a incontinent client are illustrated in Table 32–6 (types of incontinence and assessment data). Medications that can be associated with transitional incontinence are diuretics, sedative-hypnotics, calcium channel blockers, α-adrenergic agents, sympathomimetics, and anticholinergics.

Diagnostic Procedures

Diagnostic procedures include urine examinations, visualization of the urinary tract, and urodynamic studies. Whenever a diagnostic test is to be performed, information must be offered to the client. This information should include the name of the procedure, the purpose of the procedure, preparation that is necessary and the rationale, procedures employed during the diagnostic study, risk(s) involved, and postprocedure care.

Urine Examinations

There are several types of urine examinations to evaluate the status of the urinary tract.

Table 32–6

TYPES OF INCONTINENCE AND ASSESSMENT DATA

NURSING DIAGNOSIS AND DEFINITION	RELATED FACTORS	SUBJECTIVE DATA	OBJECTIVE DATA
Stress incontinence is a loss of less than 50 ml of urine, concurrent with the urge to void; usually associated with increased intraabdominal pressure	Obesity, multiparity, prolonged catheterization, chronic overdistension, degenerative changes in pelvic support structures associated with increased age and menopause	Complains of loss of urine with activities such as vomiting, coughing, sneezing, lifting, and aerobic exercises; may complain of urgency and frequency at least every 2 h	Weak sphincter tone, weak pelvic muscles, increased urethrovesicular angle, damaged external sphincter
Urge incontinence is an involuntary loss of urine occurring soon after a strong desire to void	Irritation of bladder stretch receptors, causing detrusor spasm (associated with infection, neuropathy); decreased bladder capacity (associated with pelvic inflammatory disease, multiple abdominal surgeries, and indwelling urinary catheter); increased urine production (associated with increased fluid intake, alcohol or caffeine intake, or use of diuretics); concentrated urine (can irritate the bladder); overdistension of the bladder	Client reports inability to reach toilet in time; may also report putting off voiding; complains of symptoms of urgency, frequency (at least every 2 h) and nocturia; use of diuretics, caffeine, and/or alcohol increases fluid output, which increases the risk of incontinence; complains of symptoms of UTI	Client is incontinent of urine after urge to void; voiding in small amounts of less than 100 ml or in large amounts of greater than 500 ml; may have a distended bladder; leakage of urine when rising from a chair is common
Reflex incontinence is an involuntary loss of urine that occurs in a predictive pattern in response to a specific bladder volume	Neurological impairment (*i.e.,* multiple sclerosis, spinal cord injury above the S2 to S4 segments); cerebral lesion that eliminates control of urination	No awareness of bladder fullness, urge to void, or incontinence	Voids in large amounts; uninhibited bladder spasms at regular intervals; presence of bladder distension and may have residual urines
Functional incontinence is an involuntary and unpredictable loss of urine in the absence of actual bladder dysfunction	Sensory or cognitive deficits (use of sedatives, unresponsive to urge to void; motor or self-care deficits (*e.g.,* difficulty with getting to toilet and removing clothing); environmental barriers (*e.g.,* poor lighting, bed side rails, inability to locate bathroom, reluctant to use call bell or bedpan)	Incontinent of urine before reaching toilet or commode; complains of difficulty with locating bathroom and has trouble with toileting skills	May be disoriented to place, lethargic; difficulty with dexterity and motor skills; voids in large amounts

Table continued on following page

Table **32–6**

TYPES OF INCONTINENCE AND ASSESSMENT DATA
(Continued)

NURSING DIAGNOSIS AND DEFINITION	RELATED FACTORS	SUBJECTIVE DATA	OBJECTIVE DATA

Total incontinence is an unpredictable and continuous loss of urine	Anatomical malformation
	  Fistula
	Congenital anomalies
	  Strictures
	  Hypospadias
	  Epispadias
	  Ureterocele
	  Megalocystis
	Disorders of urinary tract
	  Infection
	  Trauma
	  Urethritis
	Neurological disorders or trauma
	  Spinal cord injury, tumor, infection
	  Brain injury, tumor, infection
	  Cerebrovascular accident
	  Multiple sclerosis
	  Diabetic neuropathy
	  Alcoholic neuropathy
	Treatment related
	  After prostatectomy
	  Extensive pelvic dissection
	  After indwelling catheter
	  General or spinal anesthesia
	Situational (personal, environmental)
	  Unable to communicate needs; stress or fear; decreased attention to bladder cues (confusion, depression); dehydration
		Constant urinary flow at unpredictable times; nocturia—at least two or three times per night; lack of awareness of bladder filling or incontinence	Bladder distention is not present without uninhibited bladder spasms; incontinence persists despite treatments

Urinalysis

Urinalysis refers to the examination of urine to determine the presence of abnormal substances indicative of disease. The time of day a urine specimen is obtained must be considered when interpreting results. The first morning specimen is usually considered the optimal specimen because it is more concentrated and relatively free of dietary influences and changes due to physical activities. Although for most urine testing a freshly voided random (taken at any time during the day) specimen is utilized, a urinalysis should be performed on a midstream urine, also called a clean voided or clean catch urine, that has been collected in a *clean* container.

Urine specimens should be analyzed shortly after they are obtained or should be stored in a refrigerator until they are sent to the laboratory. If urine is not stored properly, then changes, such as alterations in the glucose level, pH, and color, may occur (Watson & Jaffe, 1995).

Urine is inspected for general characteristics (color, clearness, odor), measurements (*e.g.,* pH, specific gravity, red blood cells, white blood cells), chemical determinations (*e.g.,* glucose, ketones, blood, protein, bilirubin), and microscopic examination of sediment (*e.g.,* red blood cells, white blood cells, casts, crystals). (Refer to Table 32–7 for routine urinalysis, significance of findings, and nursing implications; also refer to Procedure 20–2).

Text continued on page 986

Table 32–7

ROUTINE URINALYSIS

	SIGNIFICANCE	NORMAL VALUE	NURSING IMPLICATIONS
General Characteristics			
Color	Color usually related to concentration and the client's level of hydration; the color may change in many disease states; *e.g.,* dark cola color in hepatitis; color may also be affected by drugs	Pale yellow to amber	Color should be assessed using a fresh sample in a good light against a white background; the color of urine will deepen if allowed to stand at room temperature for any length of time
Turbidity (cloudiness)	Caused by colloidal particles or by suspended precipitate or sediments; cloudy urine may indicate abnormalities (*e.g.,* presence of white blood cells, red blood cells, bacteria, and epithelial cells); excessive alkaline or acidic pH of urine may alter the clarity	Fresh urine is normally clear or slightly cloudy	Instruction of clients required to ensure that specimen collected does not include substances such as prostatic fluid, menstrual blood, vaginal discharges, and fecal material (see Procedure 32–2)
pH	Indicates the ability of the renal tubules to maintain the hydrogen ion (H^+) concentration in the plasma and extracellular fluid	4.5–7.8; pH can vary widely	Dietary and drug history should be assessed; certain foods (*e.g.,* meat, cranberries) will produce an acidic urine; a diet high in vegetables and citrus fruits will produce alkaline urine; example of a drug producing acidic urine is methamine mandelate (Mandelamine); sodium bicarbonate and potassium citrate will result in alkaline urine
Specific gravity	Indicates hydration status (dehydration or overhydration); also reflects presence of constituents as protein or glucose (elevated values) or kidney infections, severe renal damage, and diabetes insipidus (decreased values)	1.016–1.022	15 ml of urine needed for test
Odor	Ingestion of certain foods and drugs will affect the odor; fruity odor may indicate ketonuria (seen in diabetes mellitus or starvation); fishy odor is usually associated with bacterial infection	Faint (not fruity, musty, fishy, or fetid)	A fresh urine specimen should be used; as urine is allowed to stand, the urea breaks down, causing a strong ammonia odor

Table continued on following page

Table 32-7

ROUTINE URINALYSIS
(Continued)

	SIGNIFICANCE	NORMAL VALUE	NURSING IMPLICATIONS
Chemical Determination			
Protein (albumin)	Presence of persistent protein in the urine (proteinuria, also called albuminuria) is seen in renal disease or systemic disorders; *e.g.*, multiple-myeloma or extensive destruction of muscle fiber; proteinuria may also be seen in individuals who are dehydrated or right after strenuous exercise	Negative	Ensure urine specimen is not contaminated with vaginal or prostatic secretions; provide instruction regarding collection of urine
Bilirubin (results from breakdown of hemoglobin)	Presence of bilirubin in the urine indicates liver disease or extrahepatic biliary obstruction	Negative; 0.02 mg/dl	Only fresh specimens should be used since light and room air will give false negative results; urine that has a high bilirubin tends to be tea or cola colored
Urobilinogen (results from breakdown of hemoglobin)	Increase in urine urobilinogen may be seen in liver disease or hemolytic disorders.	01.0–1.0 Ehrlich U/dl	
Glucose	Glycosuria (glucose in the urine) is usually abnormal and caused by diabetes mellitus; however, sugar may appear in the urine after a heavy meal, with emotional stress, or with ingestion of certain drugs	Negative	The first voided specimen of the morning should not be used; urine that was in the bladder overnight may contain excessive glucose because of food ingested the prior evening and increased concentration of urine; allowing the urine to stand at room temperature may produce false positive results; certain drugs may also cause false positive results; *e.g.*, ascorbic acid, penicillin, levodopa
Ketone bodies (acetone)	Excess production (ketonuria) of ketones is primarily associated with diabetes; ketones are formed as a result of fat primarily being used as body fuel instead of carbohydrates; this may occur when there is an impaired ability to metabolize carbohydrates, inadequate carbohydrate intake, and increased metabolic demand	Negative	Take a drug and diet history; false positive results may occur in individuals receiving drugs such as levodopa, paraldehyde, and pyridium

Table 32-7

ROUTINE URINALYSIS
(Continued)

	SIGNIFICANCE	NORMAL VALUE	NURSING IMPLICATIONS
Chemical Determination			
Blood	Blood in the urine (hematuria) visible to the eye indicates bleeding somewhere in the urinary tract; color may range from pink tinged to brownish-black; hematuria may occur after strenuous exercise; occult blood (not detected with the eye alone) (hemoglobinuria) is related to conditions outside the urinary tract where an extensive destruction of erythrocytes occurs	Negative	Ensure urine not contaminated with menstrual blood; when menstruation is occurring and a urine specimen must be obtained, have the client place a tampon in the vagina prior to obtaining a urine specimen; take a drug history; for example, salicylates, anticoagulants, and sulfonamides may cause hematuria
Microscopic Examination			
Cells			
Erythrocytes	Although red cells may occasionally be found in the urine, persistent occurrence may indicate renal disease; there are several nonrenal diseases that may result in red blood cells in the urine, such as acute appendicitis, diverticulitis, and infectious disease; strenuous exercise may also damage the mucosa of the bladder	0–1 in high-power field 1 or 2 in low-power field	Menstrual blood may lead to a false positive result (see Procedure 32–2); take a drug history, because salicylates, anticoagulants and sulfonamides may cause hematuria
Leukocytes	White blood cells may come from anywhere in the genitourinary tract; a large number of leukocytes indicates bacterial infection	0–5 in high-power field	Once leukocytes are detected, a urine specimen for culture and sensitivity should be collected (see Procedure 32–2)
Epithelial cells	Derived from lining of urinary tract, including the renal pelvis and the renal tubules	A few cells are normal; large number of cells may indicate kidney pathology	
Casts			
	Gel-like substances formed in renal tubules and collecting ducts; excessive numbers may indicate renal disease	0–4 Hyaline casts at low-power field; a few casts normal; excessive numbers may indicate renal disease	Prepare client if additional diagnostic tests are ordered

Table continued on following page

Table 32–7

ROUTINE URINALYSIS
(Continued)

	SIGNIFICANCE	NORMAL VALUE	NURSING IMPLICATIONS
Crystals			
	Formed by salts that precipitate; drug therapy or radiographic dyes may cause precipitation of crystals	Small amount	Affected by temperature; some crystals precipitate at room temperature, whereas others precipitate if urine is stored in the refrigerator; crystal formation tends to occur in urine that is concentrated

Data from Chernecky, C. C., Krech, R. L., & Berger, B. J. (1993). *Laboratory tests and diagnostic procedures.* Philadelphia: W. B. Saunders; Fischbach, F. T. (1988). *A manual of laboratory diagnostic tests* (3rd ed.). Philadelphia: J. B. Lippincott; Watson, J., & Jaffe, M. S. (1995). *Nurse's manual of laboratory and diagnostic tests* (2nd ed.). Philadelphia: F. A. Davis.

Urine Culture and Sensitivity

A urine specimen for culture and sensitivity is ordered if a UTI is suspected or to monitor the responses to treatment for UTIs. The urine is cultured to type and number of organisms present in the urine. The urine is then tested to determine which antibiotics to which the organisms are susceptible. *A sterile specimen container must be used when collecting urine for a culture and sensitivity test.*

The combination of pyuria and significant bacteria in the urine (more than 100,000 organisms per ml of urine) suggests an infection. If the client presents with a urethral discharge, a stained smear of the discharge or a blood test may be obtained to rule out venereal disease.

A urine specimen may also be collected when the client has a urinary catheter in place (Fig. 32–8; also see Procedure 20–2).

Residual Urine

A **residual urine** refers to the amount of urine remaining in the bladder immediately after voiding. To obtain an estimate of residual urine, a catheter is passed into the client's bladder immediately after the client has voided. The amount of urine collected via catheterization is measured and recorded. A normal finding is considered when 50 ml or less of urine is left in the bladder of an adult. In clients who require frequent assessment of residual urine, a portable ultrasound device may be used, which is used to scan the bladder and display the amount of urine left in the bladder. The client should void immediately prior to the scan. An abnormal presence of urine in the bladder may indicate sphincter impairment, strictures, or problems with bladder innervation.

Other Urine Examinations (see Table 32–7)

In some cases, a urine specimen analysis is performed by the nurse rather than a laboratory. Tests for glucose, ketones, protein, pH (hydrogen ion concentration), and **hematuria** (blood in the urine) are frequently conducted by nurses or by clients themselves with the use of a dipstick or tablet (Fig. 32–9). Testing with a dipstick means immersing a dipstick in urine for the length of time designated by the manufacturer of the dipstick. The dipstick is then examined at a time interval determined by the manufacturer. For example, in testing urine for protein, Albustix and Combistix is the most commonly used dipstick test (Price & Wilson, 1992). The end of the stick is dipped in urine and removed immediately. The urine is shaken off by tapping the stick on the side of the container. The result is then compared with the color chart on

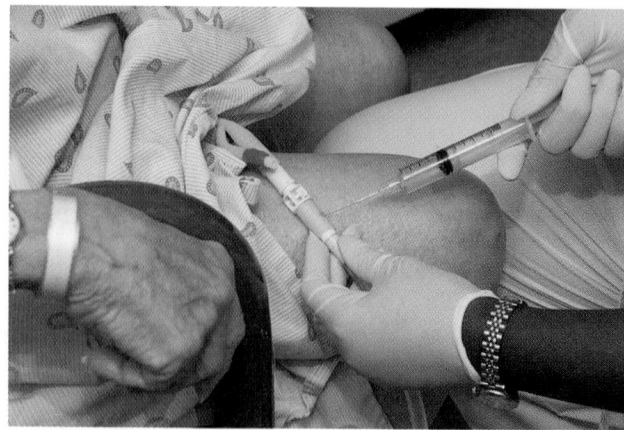

❯ **Figure 32–8**
Urine is obtained from a catheter port.

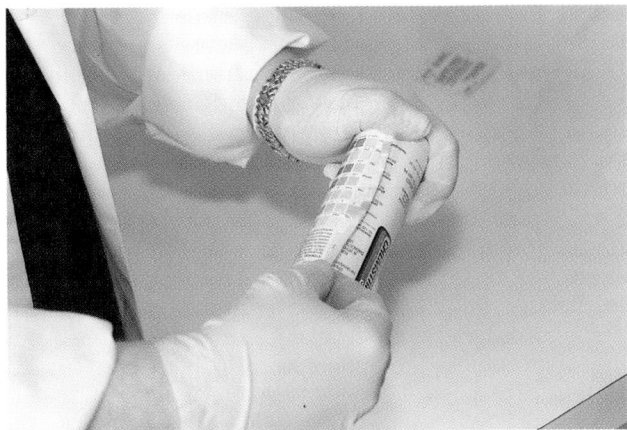

✦ **Figure 32–9**
Urine samples with reagent sticks.

the label. When using the tablet method, the designated number of drops of urine to be placed on the tablet and the time interval to assess the color of the tablet are assigned by the manufacturer of the tablet.

Usually, urine specimens being tested for glucose (glycosuria) are collected before meals and at bedtime. The presence of glycosuria (glucose in urine) depends on the amount of glucose in the blood. Glucose spills into the urine once the blood sugar is around 160 to 180 mg/dl. This is known as the renal threshold of glucose.

Testing for ketones (the metabolic end products of fat and protein metabolism) can also be done using a dipstick or tablet. Ketones in the urine (ketonuria) indicate that the body is using fat as the major source of energy. This happens when insufficient glucose is available for the energy. Abnormal values range from 20 to 80 mg/dl or higher.

Urine pH may be tested by using a commercial strip of paper designed to indicate the acidity or alkalinity of liquid (*e.g.,* Squibb Nitrazine paper) or a dipstick test. It is important to use fresh urine only because the urine becomes more alkaline if allowed to stand (due to breakdown of urea to ammonia). The test strip should be removed promptly and the color compared with the standard provided by the manufacturer (Price & Wilson, 1992).

Normally, only small amounts of protein are present in the urine. Proteinuria in amounts greater than 150 mg per day is considered pathological. False positive readings may result from urine that is highly alkaline, concentrated, or containing many white blood cells or vaginal secretions (Gibbs, 1995). The end of the dipstick is dipped in urine and removed immediately.

Normally, blood is not present in the urine. Both hematuria and hemoglobinuria (a product of red blood cell destruction) are detectable by the dipstick. False positive results can be caused by high levels of ascorbic acid in urine, presence of bacterial enzymes, and contamination of urine with povidone-iodine (Gibbs, 1995).

Specific Gravity

The specific gravity of urine is determined by measuring the density of urine compared with the density of distilled water, which has a specific gravity of 1.000. The range of urine specific gravity depends on the state of hydration and varies with urine volume and the load of solids to be excreted. Specific gravity helps evaluate the concentrating and filtration status of the kidneys and the hydration status of the body.

The range for normal values of specific gravity of urine in adults is between 1.016 and 1.022 (Chernecky *et al.,* 1993). A urine specific gravity above 1.025 indicates that the urine is concentrated, and below 1.010 indicates that the urine is dilute. An increased specific gravity (concentrated urine) is seen in conditions such as congestive heart failure, dehydration, proteinuria, and glomerulonephritis. A decreased specific gravity (dilute urine) is seen in diabetes insipidus (a condition that causes excessive diuresis), overhydration (*e.g.,* excessive intravenous fluid administration), hypothermia (low body temperature), and malignant hypertension. The specific gravity is determined by floating a hydrometer or urinometer in a cylinder of urine.

The urinometer should be dry and clean before use. The cylinder should be filled about three fourths full of urine (at least 15 ml of urine is needed). The urinometer is inserted into the cylinder and then is given a gentle spin to avoid errors of surface tension and to prevent it from adhering to the sides of the cylinder. When the spinning stops, the urinometer is read. The urinometer, which is calibrated in units of 0.001, is read by determining the bottom of the meniscus, which should be read at eye level (Chernecky *et al.,* 1993; Price & Wilson, 1992) (Fig. 32–10).

Visualization of the Urinary Tract

Through the use of radiology, ultrasonic studies, nuclear magnetic resonance, and cystoscopy, the urinary tract can be visualized.

Kidney, Ureter, Bladder

A KUB is an x-ray film of the kidneys, ureters, and bladder that gives images of the size and position of these organs and the presence of calculi (Fig. 32–11). A KUB is usually ordered before more extensive radiological studies are performed. The use of contrast medium (radiopaque substance) permits visualization of body structures. The contrast material used in a specific examination may be ingested orally, injected intravenously, or administered by enema.

Usually a KUB requires no physical preparation for clients; however, some physicians order a bowel preparation (enemas or laxatives/cathartics) to ensure better visualization of the organs of the urinary system, because fecal material and gas in the gastrointestinal tract can interfere with visualization. Restriction of food or fluids is not required prior to this x-ray.

Urinometry

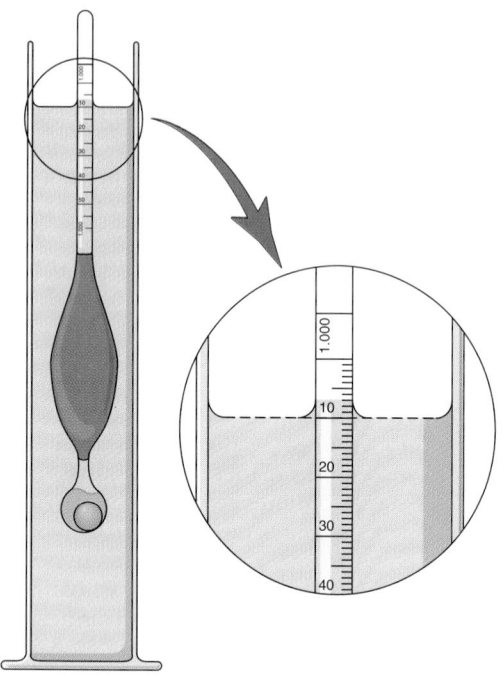

❧ **Figure 32–10**
A urinometer is displayed. The meniscus is shown.

Intravenous Pyelography (Excretory Urography)

An intravenous pyelogram (IVP) permits visualization of the kidneys, ureters, bladder, and urethra. This is an invasive procedure and uses contrast radiopaque dye injected intravenously. As the contrast material passes through the kidney and collecting system, x-rays are taken, allowing visualization of the urinary system. Prior to an IVP, a careful client history must be obtained. An existing pregnancy, a history of allergies (particularly to iodine and shellfish), and any health problems need to be identified prior to the administration of the contrast medium. Clients who have severe asthma or a history of sensitivity to the radiographic dye may be medicated with corticosteroids.

For several hours (usually 8) prior to an IVP, the client is not permitted any fluids or food orally. The client may be placed on intravenous therapy to maintain hydration and to provide an intravenous access for the test. The contrast media that is used decreases systemic blood flow and increases blood viscosity. Therefore, if conditions exist in which blood flow is already compromised (*e.g.,* vascular disease, diabetes mellitus, multiple myeloma, and renal insufficiency), the client is at risk for renal failure (McConnell & Zimmerman, 1983). Preparation of the bowel is usually given for the reasons noted for x-ray of the kidneys ureter and bladder. An IVP should be scheduled so that it precedes any contrast studies of the gastrointestinal tract, such as a gastrointestinal series or barium enema. Existing contrast medium present in the gas-

trointestinal tract interferes with visualization of the organs of the urinary system. Clients should be informed that they may experience transient side effects, such as flushing, metallic taste, and headache following injection of the contrast material. Clients need to be monitored for any anaphylactic or severe response to the dye (*e.g.,* respiratory difficulty and urticaria). Appropriate drugs, oxygen, and resuscitation equipment should be readily available.

Postprocedure care includes assessing for reaction to the dye for 24 hours and ensuring that the client drinks at least three 8-oz glasses of water to flush out the dye, unless contraindicated (Chernecky *et al.,* 1993).

Cystoscopy

A cystoscopy permits direct visualization of the bladder. An instrument with an optical lens is inserted through the urethra into the bladder (Fig. 32–12). This procedure can be performed under either local or general anesthesia. The preparation depends on the type of anesthesia and whether x-rays are needed. If general anesthesia is to be administered, then it is

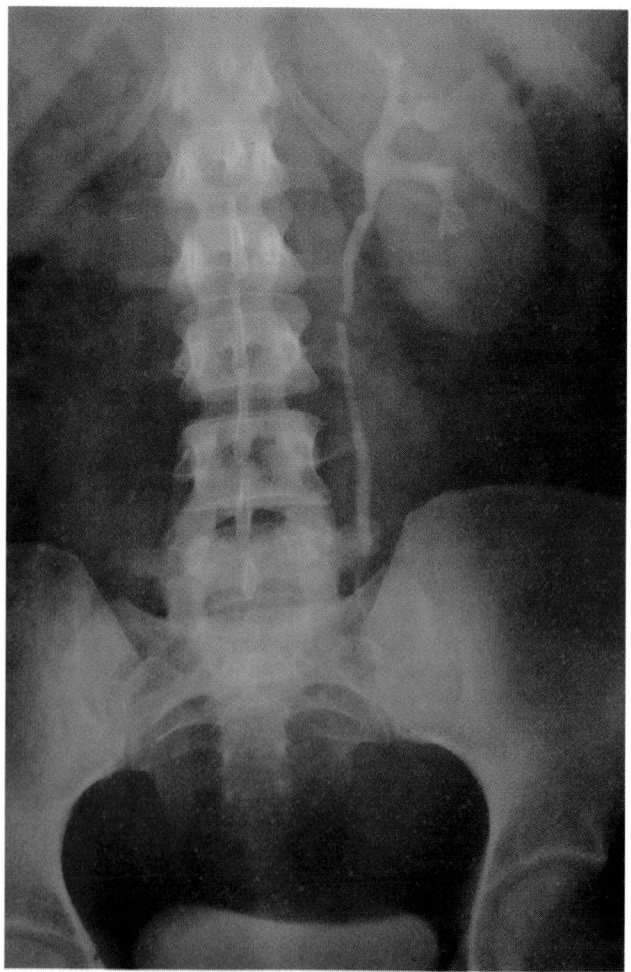

❧ **Figure 32–11**
X-ray film of a client with one kidney.

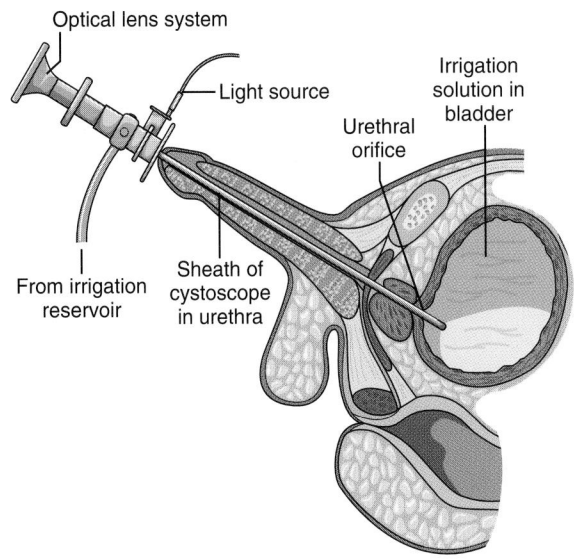

Optical lens system

Light source

Irrigation solution in bladder

Urethral orifice

From irrigation reservoir

Sheath of cystoscope in urethra

♦ Figure 32–12
Cystoscopy.

necessary that nothing be taken orally 8 hours prior to administration of anesthesia. This is done to prevent the client from aspirating gastric contents into the lungs if vomiting occurs while the client is anesthetized. If an x-ray is obtained, preparation of the bowel is needed, as discussed previously. During a cystoscopy, a retrograde pyelogram, retrograde cystogram, or biopsy may be performed.

Following a cystoscopy, the nurse should monitor

* Vital signs (the frequency to do this is based on whether the client received general anesthesia): If general anesthesia was administered, vital signs should be taken every 15 minutes four times, then every 30 minutes twice, then every 2 hours twice; if the client received a local anesthetic, vital signs are taken until they return to baseline or for 30 minutes (Chernecky *et al.,* 1993)
* Fluid intake and output for 24 hours
* Presence of hematuria: Pink urine is normal initially, but it should clear; hematuria should not last more than 4 to 6 hours, and bright red bleeding and clots are abnormal
* Presence of painful urination (dysuria); dysuria lasting more than 4 to 6 hours is abnormal

Routine postoperative care, including promoting such activities as deep breathing and coughing, should be given if general anesthesia was administered. Common sensations reported by clients are bladder spasms, a feeling of bladder fullness, low back pain, burning, and frequency of urination. These sensations occur as a result of irritation of the bladder during cystoscopy. Analgesics may be ordered for bladder spasms. Tub or sitz baths may help decrease genital area discomfort (Chernecky *et al.,* 1993).

Retrograde Pyelogram

This diagnostic test necessitates a cystoscopy, in which a catheter is passed from the urethra to the

bladder and then to the ureters and renal pelvis. Contrast media is injected into the renal pelvis or ureters. This procedure is useful in the diagnosis of ureter obstruction. Risk factors are the same as those associated with instrumentation of the urinary tract (*i.e.,* trauma and infections). If a ureteral catheter is left in the client following the procedure, drainage from the ureteral catheter must be monitored separately, in addition to the drainage from a catheter left in the bladder. This procedure is being used less frequently because of improved techniques in excretory tomography.

Cystography and Ureterography

A retrograde cystogram permits x-rays of the bladder after instillation of a radiopaque fluid into the bladder. The presence of diverticula of the bladder (outpouching of the wall of the bladder), vesicoureteral reflux, and fistulas (abnormal tubelike openings), between the bladder and vagina can be visualized.

Voiding Cystourethrogram

This diagnostic test is used to visualize bladder and urethral obstructions. A Foley catheter is inserted into the bladder, and a radiopaque dye is injected into the bladder via the catheter. X-rays are taken during and after voiding. Urethral stenosis and bladder neck obstruction may be seen. A voiding cystogram may reveal ureteral reflux when other procedures do not because of increased bladder pressure at the time of voiding.

Renal Computed Tomography or Computerized Axial Tomography Scan

Tomography provides a three-dimensional image by multiple x-ray beams, a scanner system, and a computer. The purpose is to detect and evaluate renal pathology, such as tumors, obstructions, calculi, polycystic kidney disease, congenital anomalies, and abnormal fluid accumulation around the kidneys (Loeb, 1993). Intravenous contrast medium may or may not be used. If contrast material is used, the client needs to fast for 4 hours before the test so that the contrast medium is not diluted. Preparation of the bowel may also be ordered.

Radioisotopic Studies

Kidney scanning assists in providing information about the kidneys. Radioisotopes used for this purpose are usually administered intravenously. Images produced by a scintillation camera show the distribution of the isotope in the kidneys, which can assist in the diagnosis of tumors.

The use of radioisotopes also provides information about the valve at the ureterovesicular junction. A radioisotope is instilled into the bladder with saline via a catheter until the bladder is filled. The client then voids. Through the use of a scintillation camera, images provide information about vesicoureteral reflux and gross anomalies (Watson & Jaffe, 1995).

Ultrasonic Studies

Ultrasonic studies allow for deep structures of the body to be visualized when high-frequency sound waves are reflected into internal tissues of the body and reflected back to a transducer. A transducer is a device that translates pressure or temperature to an electrical signal. Ultrasonic studies are noninvasive procedures and are valuable when excretory urography is ruled out, such as occurs when a client has an allergy to contrast material.

Ultrasonography may be performed to assess the kidneys, ureters, bladder, and urethra. Ultrasonography may identify changes in size, structure, or position of the kidneys. Bladder ultrasonography allows the visualization of the size and contour of the bladder by providing an outline of the organ when it is full of urine (Watson & Jaffe, 1995). To test for a residual urine with a bladder scan, the client should void prior to the scan.

Urodynamic Studies

These diagnostic procedures consist of several tests to evaluate urinary bladder function, including neuromuscular function (cystometry), urinary flow rate (uroflowmetry), and urethral pressure and closing ability (urethral pressure profile) (Watson & Jaffe, 1995).

A cystometrogram measures bladder filling and emptying and is used to help diagnose motor and sensory abnormalities, obstructive abnormalities, and infectious disorders (Watson & Jaffe, 1995) (Fig. 32–13). During the procedure, the client is requested to void in a supine position and to lie still. A catheter is inserted into the bladder, and sterile normal saline, distilled water, or carbon dioxide is instilled into the bladder. Pressure and volume readings are recorded. The client is requested to void, and again pressures are taken in the bladder. After voiding, the bladder is emptied of any fluid, and the catheter is removed. Characteristics of voiding, such as volume voided and presence of dribbling, straining, or **hesitancy** (difficulty with initiating urinary flow and a decrease in the force of the stream of urine), are noted.

The procedure should be performed using sterile technique to avoid infections. After the procedure, the client is advised to increase fluid intake and report any changes in his or her voiding pattern. It is important to monitor the client for any signs of UTI, such as burning, frequency, or urgency.

A uroflowmetry is used to evaluate urinary flow rate while the client is voiding. This procedure does not require the insertion of a urinary catheter or instillation of gas or solutions. The female client sits and the male client stands and voids into a commode. The volume of urine excreted and the frequency of urination are recorded on a graph. Aftercare and assessment are the same as for any urodynamic study (Watson & Jaffe, 1995).

A urethral pressure profile measures pressure changes along the urethra when the bladder is at rest. This test is indicated to determine external urethral sphincter competency, cause of stress incontinence in women, and obstruction of urinary flow associated with hypertrophic prostatic gland and to evaluate the effect of drug therapy on urethral sphincter control. A double-lumen catheter connected to a transducer is inserted into the bladder. Fluid or gas is constantly infused into the bladder. Urethral pressures are measured when the catheter is withdrawn (Watson & Jaffe, 1995).

Provocative stress testing provides direct visualization of leakage of urine from the meatus. A full bladder is required. The client is instructed to relax and cough when placed in the lithotomy position. The test is repeated with the client standing. Urine loss with coughing indicates stress incontinence. Delayed leakage of urine or persistent leakage after the coughing indicates possible detrusor overactivity (McCormick et al., 1992).

The urine stream interruption test assesses the effectiveness of the pelvic floor muscles in impeding urine flow. This test quantifies the length of time it takes for a women to interrupt the flow of urine. A full bladder is needed prior to the test. Therefore, clients are instructed to drink three 8-oz glasses of liquid prior to the test.

Nursing Diagnosis

Based on assessment data, a nursing diagnosis is formulated. Nursing diagnoses may indicate actual or potential alterations in urinary elimination. Problems outside of the urinary tract that are precipitated by an alteration in urinary elimination may exist (e.g., skin

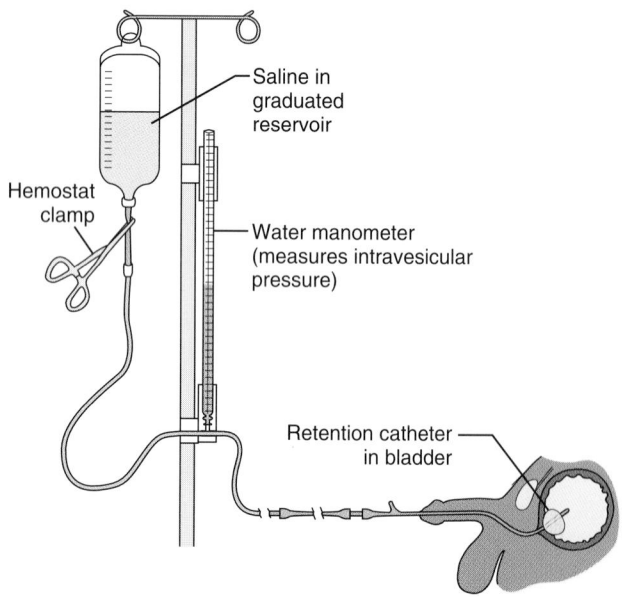

Saline in
graduated
reservoir

Hemostat
clamp

Water manometer
(measures intravesicular
pressure)

Retention catheter
in bladder

❧ **Figure 32–13**
A cystometrogram.

SAMPLE NURSING CARE PLAN

THE CLIENT WITH URINARY RETENTION

D. L., a 56-year-old woman, is 2 days postoperative following abdominal surgery. Her Foley catheter was removed 6 hours ago. She states that she feels some pressure and has the urge to urinate. She has attempted to void but only "dribbles very small amounts" about every half hour. On palpation, the nurse notes bladder fullness above the symphisis pubis.

Nursing Diagnosis: Urinary retention related to decreased bladder tone secondary to effect of indwelling catheter.

Client Goal: D. L. will regain her usual voiding pattern.

Expected Outcome Criteria:
1. D. L. will demonstrate techniques to promote voiding.
2. D. L. will void and have a postvoid residual of less than 50 ml.
3. D. L. will void adequate amounts of urine every 3 to 4 hours.
4. D. L. will be continent of urine.
5. D. L. will not have sensations of bladder pressure.

Nursing Interventions	Rationale
1. Assess for signs and symptoms of bladder fullness: 　a. Client complaints of dysuria, pressure, and feelings of fullness. 　b. Palpate for bladder distention above the symphis pubis. 　c. Monitor intake and output.	Provides baseline data needed for evaluating effectiveness of interventions and subsequent planning of further interventions. Fullness above the symphisis pubis indicates that a volume of at least 250 ml of urine is in the bladder.
2. Encourage client to void using micturition techniques, including: 　a. Providing privacy. 　b. Letting the client hear the sound of running water in the bathroom. 　c. Having the client attempt to void in the bathroom instead of using a bedpan. 　d. Pouring warm water over the perineal area. 　e. Stroking the lower abdomen or inner thigh.	Providing privacy facilitates relaxation of the perineal muscles. Voiding techniques stimulate the afferent (sensory) loop of the micturition reflex and the sphincter relaxes.
3. Insert a straight catheter (on physician's order).	Used to empty the bladder if the client has not voided within 6 to 8 hours after the Foley was removed.
4. Continue to monitor for achievement of expected outcomes, including: 　a. Bladder distention. 　b. Urine output—postvoid residuals, time and amount of voiding, color, odor and continence. 　c. Client's complaints of dysuria and pressure. 　d. Client demonstrating micturition techniques. 　e. Fluid intake adequate to meet client's hydration needs.	Evaluation of the client's expected outcomes assists the nurse and the client to plan further interventions to successfully meet the client's urinary elimination needs.

breakdown, body image disturbance, poor self-esteem). Refer to the Nursing Diagnosis Box for examples of North American Nursing Diagnosis Association–approved nursing diagnoses related to urinary elimination.

Planning

The process of identifying expected outcomes (measurable goals expected to be achieved) should be client centered and is an integral component of developing a plan of care. This means that the client should

be encouraged to participate in planning realistic outcomes. By incorporating the client's lifestyle and health beliefs into the plan of care, the potential for meeting the outcomes is greater. Overall outcomes for clients with potential or actual alterations in urinary elimination include

1. Promotion or restoration of the client's normal urinary elimination patterns (Sample Nursing Care Plan for the Client With Urinary Retention)

2. Prevention of complications associated with therapies used to treat urinary disorders (Sample Nursing Care Plan for the Client With a Urinary Tract Infection)

SAMPLE NURSING CARE PLAN

THE CLIENT WITH A URINARY TRACT INFECTION

J. A., a 24-year-old woman, reports that she is experiencing suprapubic pain and burning on urination. She has been voiding very small amounts and has the urge to void every half hour. Further history taking reveals that she has recently started using a diaphragm and spermicidal cream for birth control. She has sexual intercourse on a regular basis and has a previous history of recurrent UTIs associated with coitus. Physical assessment findings show no signs of fever and a nondistended bladder, and the urine is cloudy and foul smelling.

Nursing Diagnosis:	Altered urinary elimination related to irritation of bladder mucosa.
Client Goal:	J. A. will resume her normal voiding pattern without irritation to the bladder mucosa.
Expected Outcome Criteria:	1. J. A. will verbalize the signs and symptoms of UTI and the interventions to treat her infection.
	2. J. A. will void without pain or burning on urination within 24 hours.
	3. J. A. will be free of symptoms of urgency, frequency, dysuria within 3 days after treatment has begun.
	4. J. A. will verbalize an understanding of the risk factors that make her susceptible to infection.
	5. J. A. will verbalize measures to prevent recurrent infection.
	6. J. A. will state the early signs and symptoms of UTI and interventions she should implement.

Nursing Interventions	Rationale
1. Obtain a urine specimen for culture and sensitivity (see Collecting Urine Specimens).	Identifies the pathogen causing the infection. The specific antibiotics to be used for treatment of the infection will also be identified.

2. Teach client to monitor urine for
  a. Output.
  b. Color.
  c. Odor.
  d. Presence of cloudiness, blood, mucus, casts, and crystals.
  e. pH.
	Used to measure client responses to interventions.

3. Instruct client on medication regimen: a. Start taking a broad-spectrum antibiotic as ordered by physician until the urine culture and sensitivity results are obtained.	Antibiotic therapy should be initiated as soon as possible after the urine specimen is obtained.
b. Change to an antibiotic that treats the specific pathogen identified in urine culture.	Broad-spectrum antibiotics should be discontinued when the urine culture and sensitivity results are read. Administration of broad-spectrum antibiotics can increase the risk of resistance to antibiotics (Langford, 1994).
c. Take urinary tract analgesics as prescribed by physician (*i.e.,* Pyridium, Azo Gantrisin).	Used to treat the pain and burning on urination.
d. Complete the full course of antibiotics (usually 7–10 days, depending on the specific antibiotic).	Prevents recurrence of UTI.
e. Acidify or alkalinize urine if needed for specific antibiotics (refer to acid/ash diet table).	Required for certain antibiotics to be effective (*i.e.,* acidify urine for Hiprex [methenamine] and Mandelamine [methenamine]; alkalinize urine for Bactrim [trimethodine] and Septra [trimethodine]).
4. Encourage client to increase fluids to at least 2 to 3 L every 24 hours.	Aids in flushing the bladder and dilutes the urine (extremely important if the client is taking sulfa drugs, since they can cause crystal formation in the concentrated urine).
5. Instruct client on importance of follow-up urine culture 1 week after completion of antibiotics.	Evaluation of effectiveness of antibiotic regimen.

Continued

SAMPLE NURSING CARE PLAN

THE CLIENT WITH A URINARY TRACT INFECTION
(Continued)

Nursing Interventions	Rationale
6. Teach client risk factors that increase susceptibility to UTI for her:	
a. Sexual activity.	The motion of coitus aids in moving organisms from the urethra to the bladder.
b. Poorly fitted diaphragm.	Exerts pressure on bladder, which causes urinary retention and stasis.
c. Improper use of spermicidal creams.	Can cause an alkaline urine, which is a medium for bacterial growth, especially *Escherichia coli;* also alters the normal vaginal flora.
7. Teach client preventive measures:	
a. Ingest foods that acidify urine (*e.g.,* meat, whole grains, eggs, cheese, cranberries, prunes, and plums).	Acidic urine is a poor medium for bacterial growth.
b. Monitor urine pH.	Should be 5.5 or less to be acidic.
c. Increase fluids to at least 2 to 3 L every 24 hours.	Dilutes urine, ensures adequate output, and prevents urinary stasis.
d. Cleanse perineum prior to sexual intercourse and void immediately after coitus.	Decreases risk of pathogen entry into the urinary tract.
e. Proper usage of diaphragm and spermicidal cream.	Prevents urinary retention and alkaline urine.
f. Drink one to three glasses of cranberry juice daily.	Cranberries synthesize and excrete hippuric acid into the urine, which provides a bacteriostatic effect. Cranberries make urine clearer, decrease white blood cell count, and decrease the smell of urine (DeGroot-Kosolcharoen, 1995).

Implementation

Promotion of Normal Urination

Interventions to maintain normal urinary elimination patterns include maintaining adequate fluid intake and promoting voiding habits.

Fluid Intake

An adequate fluid intake is needed to maintain the normal body functioning. An adequately dilute urine helps to prevent bladder irritation, UTIs, and formation of calculi. In instances of excessive fluid loss (*i.e.,* vomiting, diarrhea, diaphoresis [excessive perspiration]), additional fluid must be provided to balance this loss. Fluid intake can be fostered by providing foods high in fluid content and fluids that the client prefers. Parenteral fluids may be required. Increasing fluid intake is contraindicated for individuals who are on fluid restrictions, such as those with renal failure or congestive heart failure.

To prevent the need to urinate at night **(nocturia),** fluids should be restricted 2 hours prior to bedtime.

Promoting Normal Voiding Habits

Nursing interventions should be directed toward stimulation of the micturition reflex and muscle relaxation. Helping clients assume a "normal" position to void helps stimulate urination. The normal position for female clients to void is sitting or squatting. These positions stimulate pelvic and intraabdominal muscle contraction and facilitate the flow of urine by gravity drainage. When a female client cannot use the toilet, a bedside commode or bedpan may be required. Bedpans are either standard in shape or are not as deep as standard, with one side being narrower (a fracture bedpan). A commode is a portable toilet (*i.e.,* a bedpan or pail is inserted under a movable chair). Bedpans are placed by having the client turn onto his or her side. The bedpan is placed at the buttocks. The client rolls onto to the bedpan and is then placed in a sitting position. Fracture bedpans are used if the client has limited mobility. The fracture pan is slid into place with the client in a supine position.

Male clients prefer to stand when voiding. This position enables urine to flow through the urethra by gravity. If the male client cannot use the bathroom, a urinal is provided. If the male client is unable to get out of bed and stand alone, he may need to be as-

EXAMPLES OF NORTH AMERICAN NURSING DIAGNOSIS ASSOCIATION–APPROVED NURSING DIAGNOSES: URINARY ELIMINATION

Urinary Elimination, Altered, Related to

* Dehydration
* Bladder infection
* Sensory motor impairment
* Mechanical trauma

Urinary Retention Related to

* Fecal impaction
* Medication
* Inhibition of reflex arc
* Urethral blockage

Incontinence, Functional, Related to

* Mobility deficit (*e.g.,* difficulty removing clothes)
* Altered environment (*e.g.,* poor lighting, side rails, reluctance to use call bell, inability to locate toilet)
* Cognitive deficit (inattentive to voiding signals)

Incontinence, Stress, Related to

* High intrauterine pressure (*e.g.,* from obesity, pregnancy)
* Weak pelvic muscles and structural supports

Incontinence, Urge, Related to

* Decreased bladder capacity
* History of pelvic inflammatory disease, indwelling urinary catheter

Incontinence, Reflex, Related to

* Neurological impairment (e.g., spinal cord injury)

Incontinence, Total, Related to

* Neurological impairment
* Anatomical malformations (*e.g.,* fistula)

Infection, Risk for, Related To

* Indwelling urinary catheter
* Urinary stasis

Skin Integrity, Risk for Impaired, Related to

* Incontinence
* Urinary diversion
* Use of condom catheter

Body Image Disturbance

* Incontinence
* Urinary diversion

masks sound of urination for clients who may be embarrassed); (2) applying slight hand pressure over the pubic area (increases pressure on bladder); (3) leaning forward while sitting on the toilet or bedpan (increases intraabdominal pressure); (4) stroking the inner thigh of the female client, which stimulates the sacral reflex; (5) assisting a client to the bathroom when he or she has the urge to void, because delay may result in loss of the desire to void or incontinence of urine; (6) encouraging the client to urinate during the times when he or she ordinarily urinates; and (7) forcing fluids (increases production of urine).

Promoting relaxation and providing privacy help decrease stress and anxiety. Anxiety characterized by generalized muscle tension can interfere with perineal relaxation, which may lead to retention of urine in the bladder.

Sensory stimulation can assist the client to relax. Some ways to do this are pouring warm water over the female client's perineum, placing the client's hands in a pan of warm water, and providing music. Warming a bedpan is another method for promoting muscle relaxation and provides physical comfort.

Comfort measures should be provided prior to voiding. Relieving physical discomforts, (*e.g.,* giving pain medication), and providing appropriate emotional support promote relaxation. This should enable the client to concentrate on voiding.

Adequate time should be allowed for clients to void without feeling pressured to do so. With mental pressure to void, muscle relaxation cannot occur. Some clients cannot void when other people are present in the room. After ensuring that the client is safe and the call bell is within reach, the client should be left alone.

Interventions for Clients With Urinary Tract Infections

Once a UTI has been diagnosed, therapies employed include drugs, increasing fluid intake, relieving discomfort, and client education about preventing subsequent UTIs.

Drug Therapy

Medications commonly used to treat UTIs include the cephalosporins (*e.g.,* Cipro [ciprofloxacin]) and the sulfonamide or sulfonamide combination products (*e.g.,* Gantrisin [sulfisoxazole] and Septra DS). Sulfonomides may crystallize in the renal tubules if their concentration is too high. The risk of this happening can be reduced if the urine volume or urine pH increases. It is important to maintain an output of at least 1.5 ml per day for an adult (Shlafer, 1993).

A drug history of allergy to medications must be obtained prior to commencing therapy.

Fluid Intake

Increasing fluids (eight glasses of liquid a day) flushes out the bacteria and prevents concentration of drugs in the kidneys. Sometimes increased fluid is

sisted to a standing position, which facilitates using a urinal.

A number of measures can be used to stimulate the micturition reflex. These include (1) running water in the sink (auditory stimulation for voiding, also

contraindicated. For example, excessive fluid intake interferes with adequate urinary concentration of some drugs.

Relief of Pain

A variety of measures are used to alleviate discomfort. Urinary analgesics, such as Pyridium (phenazopyridine hydrochloride), may be prescribed. Clients should be cautioned that Pyridium changes the urine to an orange-red color and may stain fabrics.

Client Education

Information regarding prevention or recurrence of UTI needs to be provided by nurses. Refer to the Health Promotion and Prevention Box and Sample Nursing Care Plan for the Client With Urinary Retention.

Interventions for Obstructions of the Urinary Tract and Retention of Urine

A primary goal to alleviate urinary retention is to facilitate the flow of urine. Interventions are designed to alleviate the problem causing urinary retention (see Sample Nursing Care Plan for the Client With a Urinary Tract Infection). For example, if the retention of urine is caused by an obstruction, an attempt is made to remove the obstruction. Acute urinary retention caused by benign prostatic hyperplasia may be temporarily relieved by drainage of the urine via urethral or suprapubic catheterization. In urethral catheterization, an indwelling catheter is placed through the urethra in the bladder. Suprapubic catheterization means that the catheter is placed directly into the bladder through the abdomen. The urethra is therefore bypassed. It may be necessary to remove the prostate gland by surgery.

When the reason for the obstruction is calculi, interventions include diet therapy, relieving pain, and removing the stone. The specific diet prescribed depends on the composition of the stone. Usually the diet consists of moderate calcium, restricted or moderate phosphorus, and high fluid intake. Clients need to be given instructions about the need to increase fluid intake and adhere to their drug and diet regimen to avoid reoccurrence of calculi.

Pain control is usually accomplished with narcotic analgesics such as morphine or meperidine hydrochloride. A calculus may be removed by an open surgical technique or a procedure performed with endoscopic instruments or destroyed by extracorpal shock wave lithotripsy (a noninvasive procedure whereby the stone is crushed by shock waves produced outside of the body). The reader is referred to a textbook on medical-surgical nursing for a discussion of these procedures.

When retention of urine occurs, medications may be used to promote bladder emptying. Other drugs may be prescribed to promote bladder storage of urine; for example, when the client is incontinent of urine. Please refer to Table 32–8 for medications used to promote emptying of the bladder and medications prescribed to promote bladder storage.

Bladder Decompression

Emptying the bladder of urine may call for the **Credé maneuver** or catheterization. The Credé maneuver is used in clients who have a flaccid bladder. This technique consists of a manual compression of

Table 32–8

MEDICATIONS USED TO TREAT URINARY DYSFUNCTIONS

MEDICATION	TYPE	ACTION
Outcome: To Promote Bladder Emptying		
Urecholine (bethanechol) Duvoid (bethanechol)	Cholinergic	Enhances bladder contraction and tone
Dibenzyline (phenoxybenzamine hydro-chloride) Minipress (prazosin hydrochloride)	Adrenergic blocker	Decreases urethral sphincter tone, which decreases outflow resistance
Dantrium (dantrolene sodium) Lioresal (baclofen) Valium (diazepam)	Antispasmodic Skeletal muscle relaxant	Increases relaxation of external sphincter
Outcome: To Promote Bladder Storage		
Pro-Banthīne (propantheline bromide) Ditropan (oxybutynin)	Anticholinergic Antispasmodic	Inhibits detrusor contractions and increases bladder capacity
Imipramine Ephedrine Sudafed (pseudoephedrine)	Alpha-adrenergic	Increases urethral resistance; contracts bladder neck
Urispas (flavoxate hydrochloride) Bentyl (d. cyclomine)	Smooth muscle relaxant and mild anticholinergic	Relaxation of detrusor muscle
Conjugated estrogen	Estrogens	Restores urethral mucosa's tone, vascularity, and responsiveness; increases bladder outlet resistance
Procardia (nifedipine)	Calcium channel blocker	Increases bladder capacity used for detrusor instability

Agency for Health Care Policy and Research. (1992a, b).; Kaschak Newman, D., Lynch, K., Smith, D. A., & Cell, P. (1991). Restoring urinary continence. *American Journal of Nursing, 91* (1), 28–36; McCormick, K. A., Kaschak Newman, D., Colling, J., & Pearson, B. D. (1992). Urinary incontinence in adults. *American Journal of Nursing, 92* (10), 75–88.

the bladder with the hands, which forces expulsion of urine from the bladder. The Credé maneuver is contraindicated in clients who have normal bladder tone or bladder spasm because of the possibility of causing urethral damage and urinary reflux to the kidneys.

Catheterization of the bladder may be indicated if other measures prove ineffective. Urinary catheterization is used to treat acute or chronic urinary retention, for incontinence for which other treatment measures were ineffective; and for accurate measurement of urine in clients who are comatose or critically ill.

Catheterization consists of introducing a latex or silicone catheter through the urethra into the bladder. Two types of catheterization can be employed: straight catheterization (intermittent) or retention catheterization (indwelling). When intermittent catheterization is desired, the catheter is inserted into the bladder to obtain urine and then immediately removed. A single-lumen (opening) catheter is used.

Intermittent catheterization is indicated when assessment of residual urine is needed, for collection of sterile urine specimens, and for alleviation of acute postoperative urinary retention (*i.e.,* when a client

does not void 6 to 8 hours after surgery). Intermittent catheterization is also used in clients with neurogenic bladders, with spinal cord injury, or with multiple sclerosis. Intermittent catheterization is frequently performed by clients in their own home (see box).

Many research studies have compared the use of clean versus sterile technique with self-intermittent catheter insertion. The literature indicates that the incidence of UTIs is less when clean technique is used, compared with sterile technique; therefore, clean technique is advocated over sterile technique (Moore, 1991; Perkash & Giroux, 1993; Wyndale & Maes, 1990).

Retention catheterization is also referred to as continuous, Foley, or indwelling catheterization. The catheter is inserted into the bladder and is held in place by an inflatable balloon. Continuous drainage of urine is permitted. For this purpose, a two-lumen catheter is used. One lumen is used for urine drainage, and the other permits inflation of the balloon once the catheter is in place. A three-way Foley catheter is also used as a retention catheter. The third lumen is used to instill a sterile irrigating solution into the bladder (Fig.

32–14). The irrigating solution may be run continuously as a bladder irrigation (Fig. 32–15). The continuous bladder irrigation is usually run after prostatectomy to prevent the tubing from being clogged with blood clots and mucous.

CLEAN INTERMITTENT CATHETERIZATIONS

Purpose of Clean Intermittent Catheterizations
* Mimics normal bladder emptying
* Prevents stasis of residual urine in bladder
* Prevents ischemia of bladder wall

Procedure for Self-Intermittent Catheterizations
* Clean procedure is most commonly recommended
* Wash hands; use clean disposable gloves
* Cleanse perineal/meatal area with mild soap and water prior to and after catheterization
* Use straight catheters (single lumen) or coudé catheter for insertion
* Use mirror to visualize urethral area in female clients
* May reuse clean catheter until it becomes rigid
* Remove catheter after urine has completely drained
* Frequency depends on client's needs (usually 4–6 hours)
* Apply external condom catheter if needed between catheterizations

Care of Catheters
* Wash catheter with soap and water; rinse well; dry thoroughly with paper towels
* Store in dry container (*e.g.*, plastic bag, small jar)
* Reuse catheter for up to 4 weeks (catheter should be soft, clean, and intact for use)

Drainage Bag Care With Use of Condom Catheters
* Prepare a bleach solution (15 ml bleach to 150 ml water)
* Clean drainage bag with cool tap water, agitate for 10 seconds, and empty
* Instill 30 ml bleach solution and immediately empty
* Instill remaining bleach solution, agitate for 30 seconds, and empty
* Air dry drainage bag for next use

Data from McCash, D. C., & Kirchhoff, K. T. (1993). Decontamination of vinyl urinary drainage bags with bleach. *Rehabilitation Nursing, 18* (5), 292–295; McCormick, K. A., Kaschak Newman, D., Colling, J., & Pearson, B. D. (1992). Urinary incontinence in adults. *American Journal of Nursing, 92* (10), 75–88; Rainville, N. C. (1994). The current nursing procedure for intermittent urinary catheterization in rehabilitation facilities. *Rehabilitation Nursing, 19* (6), 330–333.

The size of the catheter is designated according to the size of the diameter of the lumen. Measures are given using a French scale of numbers. The larger the number, the larger the lumen is. Therefore, a catheter marked 14 Fr has a larger diameter than a catheter marked 12 Fr. The size of the balloon for Foley catheters is also indicated on the catheter itself. Sizes range from 5 cc to 30 cc; *i.e.,* the balloon is fully inflated with 5 cc or more of sterile water. The most frequently used sizes are 5-cc and 10-cc balloons. The shape of the catheter facilitates passage through the urethra into the bladder. Although most catheters are straight, the coudé is a round-tip catheter. It is used when a retention catheter must be passed through urethral, prostatic, or bladder neck blockage. Please refer to catheterization procedure (Procedure 32–1).

Numerous hazards are associated with the long-term use of an indwelling catheter. Among the most common hazards are UTIs, obstructions secondary to encrustation of the catheter, urethral erosion, hematuria, pain, and bladder spasms. The incidence of UTIs increases with prolonged catheter use; *i.e.,* more than 7 to 10 days. It is recommended that catheters be changed within this time frame and that a closed urinary drainage system be maintained to prevent UTIs. Whenever possible, avoidance of the use of indwelling catheters is advocated (Ader, *et al.,* 1990; AHCPR, 1992b).

Care of the meatus is needed to reduce the risk of infections. Conti and Eutropius (1987) reported no significant difference in the development of bacteria in the urine with the use of antiseptic soaps or ointments compared with mild soap and water. Perineal care should be provided using soap and water during bathing and after each bowel movement to prevent fecal

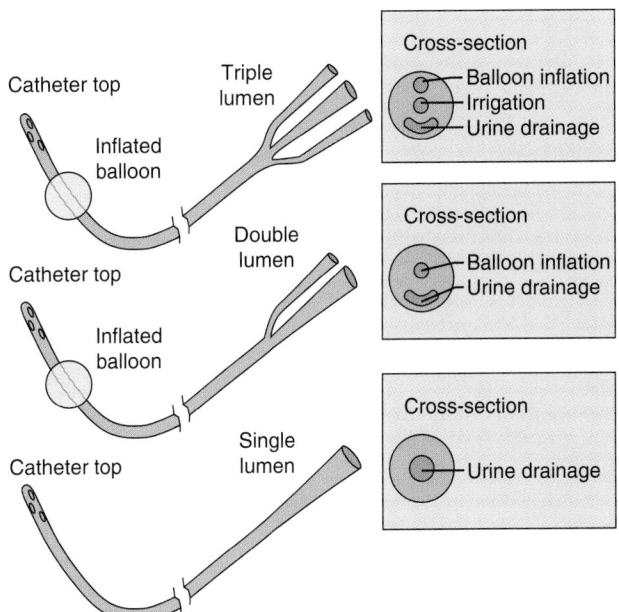

✦ **Figure 32–14**
Single-lumen, double-lumen, and triple-lumen catheters.

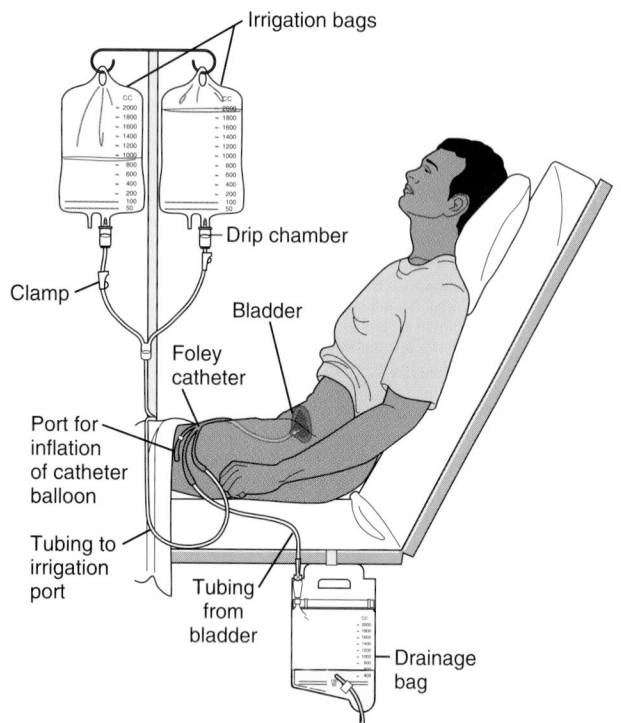

❧ **Figure 32–15**
Continuous bladder irrigation.

contamination. Nurses should check with agency policies regarding accepted practice for the institution.

Retention catheters should be removed as soon as possible. To remove a retention catheter, the client is positioned in a supine position. Fluid from the balloon is aspirated using a syringe. The catheter should not be removed until the balloon is emptied of all of the fluid used to inflate it. If the balloon is still inflated when the catheter is removed, it can cause trauma to the urethra. The catheter is gently withdrawn and placed in a red bag receptacle (universal precautions). A sample of urine may be collected prior to removing the catheter for determining the sensitivity of the organisms to specific antibacterial drugs. Perineal care should be provided once the catheter is removed.

Periodic clamping of the catheter prior to its removal has not been effective in bladder retraining and is not advised. Removing catheters during the daytime is helpful because it gives the client an opportunity to void when more staff members are available to assist with toileting. Measures to promote voiding were discussed previously. If voiding has not occurred within 8 hours after the catheter is removed, the physician should be notified and intermittent catheterization performed. This is repeated every 6 hours. Postvoided residual urines may be obtained, and fluid intake and output should be recorded. As the client progresses in his or her ability to void, the length of time between intermittent catheterization is increased until the client is urinating adequate amounts with minimal residuals (*i.e.,* less than 50 ml) (Resnick, 1993).

Urinary Diversions

A urinary diversion is a surgical routing of the flow of urine from the kidneys to a site other than the bladder. This means that urine will exit the body directly from the kidney pelvis, from the ureters, or from an artificially created pouch. The reasons for diverting urine include cancer of the bladder, prostate, urethra, and vagina; neurogenic or nonfunctioning bladders; radiation injury to the urinary structures; and severe trauma to the bladder or other structures of the urinary system. Urinary diversion may be temporary or permanent. Permanent diversions are essential in those instances in which total loss of the bladder has occurred.

Temporary diversions are used to promote rest and healing of the affected urinary structures. The main types of urinary diversions include cutaneous ureterostomy, ileal conduit, a pouch or reservoir, and nephrostomy tubes. Refer to Table 32–9 for a brief description of each type of procedure, advantages, and appropriate nursing interventions. Refer to Chapter 31 for care of ostomies.

Interventions for Clients with Incontinence

Nursing interventions for urinary incontinence should be planned with the client and caregivers when appropriate. Collaborative efforts should be directed at promoting continence with the client's needs and lifestyle and preventing complications of incontinence. One of the major nursing foci with bladder training is client and family teaching or teaching and supervision of ancillary personnel. In helping incontinent clients, nurses need to provide information regarding behavioral approaches, prescribed medications, amounts and types of fluids to ingest, and dietary intake. It is essential that the nurse also provide emotional support to the client and family as they learn self-management techniques to achieve continence (see the following Sample Nursing Care Plan).

There are several behavioral approaches to promote continence that nurses can teach clients. These are summarized in Table 32–10.

External Collection Devices

External condom catheter devises are used for male clients with complete spontaneous loss of urine. These devices should be used as a temporary measure until a bladder training regimen for the client is started (AHCPR, 1992b). Common problems with female external collection devices are inadequate fitting, leakage, discomfort, and skin irritation.

Before applying an external collection device it is important to assess the condition of the skin and the presence of bladder distention. Pubic hair surrounding the genital area is removed to prevent skin friction and urinary leakage. It is also necessary to ensure that the skin of the perineal and genital area is clean and dry.

Condom catheters, also called Texas catheters, are

Text continued on page 1007

32–1

INSERTING AN INDWELLING CATHETER

Equipment:

Sterile catheterization kit containing
Sterile gloves
Sterile drapes (one fenestrated)
Cotton balls or gauze squares
Antiseptic solution
Forceps
Prefilled syringe (usually filled with sterile water)
Water-soluble lubricant
Catheter of appropriate size (*e.g.*, #8 or #10 for children; #14, #16, or #18 for adults)
Sterile specimen container if necessary
Sterile drainage tubing and collection bag (may be preconnected to catheter)
Gooseneck lamp or flashlight
Bag or receptacle for disposing of used cotton balls or gauze squares
Bath blanket
Waterproof absorbent pad
Basin with warm water, soap, wash cloth, and towel
Disposable gloves

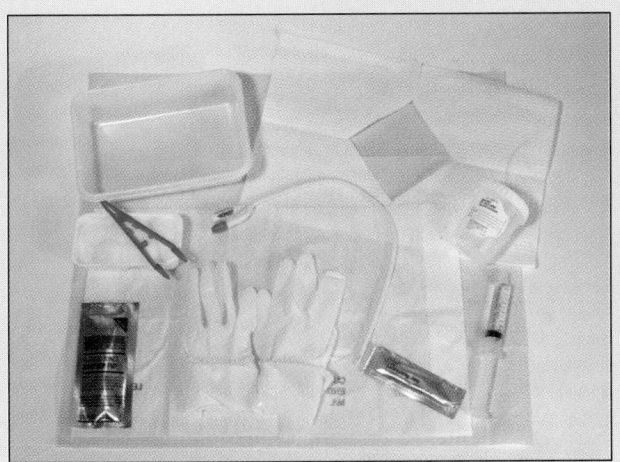

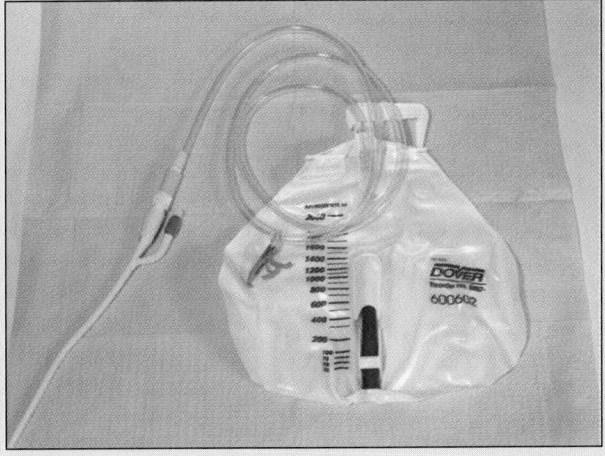

Continued

PROCEDURE

32–1

INSERTING AN INDWELLING CATHETER

(Continued)

Nursing Interventions	Rationale
1. Prepare the client: a. Explain the reason for catheterization. b. Assess for allergies to antiseptic solution. c. Inform client that there may be a sensation of pressure during catheter insertion, but that the procedure is painless. d. Inform client that he or she may feel an urge to void during catheter insertion and for a short time afterward. e. Teach the client how he or she can participate during the procedure and in catheter care.	**1.** Client teaching helps to decrease anxiety and promotes active participation in care. Relieving anxiety facilitates catheter insertion by relaxing urinary sphincters. Avoid reaction to antiseptic solution.
2. Wash hands before procedure.	**2.** Decreases transmission of microorganisms.
3. Facing client, stand on left side of bed if you are right handed and on right side if left handed.	**3.** Provides position of comfort for nurse to successfully catheterize client (easier dexterity or visualization in this position).
4. Position client as follows: a. Female client: dorsal recumbent position, with legs abducted, knees flexed, and hips externally rotated. Place pillow under buttocks to elevate pelvis. (For clients with severe leg spasms or arthritis, position in side-lying position with upper leg flexed at knee and hip.) Visualize urethral meatus from the back. b. Male client: supine position with thighs slightly abducted, legs in extension.	**4.** Provides good visualization of perineal structures.
5. Place waterproof pad under client's buttocks.	**5.** Prevents soiling of bed linens.
6. Cover client's legs with bath blanket, exposing only the perineal area.	**6.** Promotes comfort and privacy.
7. Apply disposable gloves and wash and dry perineal area.	**7.** Reduces microorganisms at perineal area. Protects client and nurse.
8. Position gooseneck lamp or get assistance with flashlight.	**8.** Provides visualization of perineal structures.
9. Open sterile catheterization kit and catheter if packaged separately.	**9.** Maintain sterile technique throughout procedure.
10. Put on sterile gloves.	**10.** This is a sterile procedure.
11. Drape the client with the sterile drapes: a. Place the first drape (female client) as an underpad (under the client's buttocks), with plastic side down or (male client) apply drape over thighs just below penis. To keep your gloves sterile, keep the drape edges cuffed under your gloves. b. Place fenestrated drape over perineal area, exposing only the labia or penis.	**11.** Maintains sterile environment.
12. Place sterile kit and its contents on sterile drape: a. Female clients: between legs. b. Male clients: on thighs.	**12.** Maintains sterile field.

PROCEDURE

32–1

INSERTING AN INDWELLING CATHETER
(Continued)

Nursing Interventions

13. Organize equipment in sterile kit:
   a. Open package of antiseptic solution and pour over cotton balls.
   b. Open lubricant package and apply lubricant to catheter (3 in for female clients, 6 in for male clients).
   c. Open top of specimen cap and leave it on loosely.

14. Test catheter balloon by injecting solution from pre-filled syringe into balloon valve on catheter. Aspirate fluid from balloon and leave syringe on catheter port.

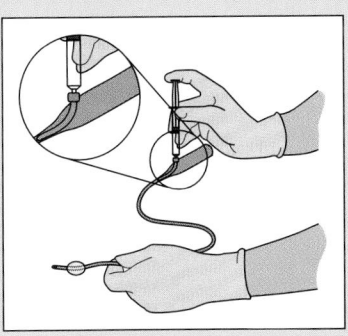

Step 14.

15. Cleanse urethral meatus.
   a. Female clients:
      1. Position nondominant hand on labia and separate labia to fully expose urethra meatus.
      2. Keep this hand in place during the rest of the procedure.
      3. With dominant "sterile" hand, pick up cotton balls with sterile forceps. Using one stroke, wipe from meatus to anus and dispose of cotton ball in receptacle. Use a new cotton ball for each wipe; cleanse each side of labia minora and then straight down the meatus.
   b. Male clients:
      1. If client is not circumsized, gently retract foreskin with nondominant hand.
      2. Grasp penile shaft, just below glans.
      3. Retract urethral meatus between thumb and forefinger.
      4. Keep this hand in place during the rest of the procedure.
      5. With dominant "sterile" hand, pick up cotton balls with forceps.
      6. Wipe the meatus first and then the surrounding areas. Use a new cotton ball for each wipe.

Rationale

13. Prepare all equipment using sterile gloves before touching client.

14. Assesses integrity of balloon for proper inflation and leaks.

15.

Reduces the number of microoragnisms in perineal area. During catheter insertion, fewer organisms will enter the urethra.

Reduces the number of microorganisms in perineal area. During catheter insertion, fewer organists will enter the urethra.

Continued

INSERTING AN INDWELLING CATHETER
(Continued)

Nursing Interventions	Rationale
16. Insert catheter.	**16.**
a. Female clients:	
1. Gently insert catheter into meatus until urine flows. Advance catheter another 5 cm (2 in). This ensures that the catheter is advanced into the bladder. If resistance is met, ask client to take a deep breath, and slowly insert catheter. *DO NOT* insert catheter if resistance exists.	Forceful pressure can cause trauma to urethral meatus. This ensures that the catheter is advanced into the bladder, for proper balloon inflation. Deep breathing can help to relax the external sphincter.
2. If no urine appears, the catheter may be in the vagina. Leave this catheter in place. Obtain another catheter, recleanse client's perineal area, and advance catheter until urine flows: child, 2.5 cm (1 in); adult: 5.0 to 7.5 cm (2 in). Remove catheter from vagina.	The misplaced catheter in vagina serves as a landmark. This will help in identifying the meatus.
3. Release labia and hold catheter securely with your dominant hand.	Prevents catheter from slipping out of bladder from sphincter or bladder contraction.
b. Male clients:	
1. Lift penis to a position perpendicular to body (90-degree angle) and exert slight traction upward.	Straightens urethral canal.

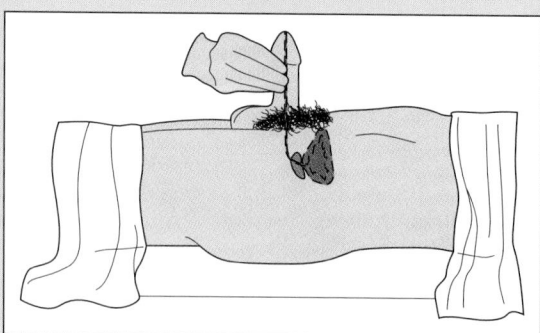

Step 16b1.

Nursing Interventions	Rationale
2. Ask client to take a deep breath.	Relaxes external urethral sphincter.
3. Insert catheter to the bifurcation (where balloon lumen separates from catheter).	Male urethra length ranges from 6 to 9 in. In some cases, however, the urethra may be longer. To prevent urethral trauma and hematuria from balloon inflation into the urethra, catheters are inserted to the bifurcation. After balloon inflation, the catheter is gently pulled back into place with the balloon resting on the bladder neck wall.
17. Collect a urine specimen if needed:	**17.**
a. Pinch the catheter and place drainage end over sterile container.	Maintains sterility for specimen collection for testing.
b. Release pinch and collect adequate amount of urine for test (*e.g.*, urine culture and sensitivity [3 ml], urinalysis [15–30 ml]).	
c. Securely place top on specimen container and label later.	
d. If catheter is preattached to drainage bag, collect specimen from drainage bag after catheterization.	Drainage bag is sterile, and specimen can be obtained from it at this time. Urine is a fresh sterile sample.

PROCEDURE

32–1

INSERTING AN INDWELLING CATHETER
(Continued)

Nursing Interventions	**Rationale**
18. Empty or partially drain urine from bladder (refer to institutional policy for amount to drain).	**18.** Whether to drain urine in amounts of greater than 1000 ml has been a controversial issue. Past practice advocated clamping the Foley after 750 to 1000 ml of urine drained. It was thought that rapid emptying of large amounts of urine would induce engorgement of the pelvic blood vessels and hypovolemic shock. Current research advocates for *complete emptying* of the distended bladder. Clients did not clinically display vital sign changes, diaphoresis, mental status changes, or hematuria and were more comfortable after catheterization. Complete bladder emptying was found to be as safe as threshold clamping.
19. Inflate the balloon (if indwelling catheter). Inject the required amount of fluid into the balloon as indicated for the specific balloon size (5–30 ml).	**19.**
20. Attach the catheter to the collecting tube of the drainage bag (if catheter was not preconnected to a urinary drainage bag).	**20.** Provides a closed sterile urinary drainage system.
21. Attach drainage bag to bed frame with hook or strap provided. Keep bag off the floor and below the level of the bladder.	**21.** Urine flows by gravity to drainage bag. By keeping the bag off the floor, you are preventing microorganism contamination.

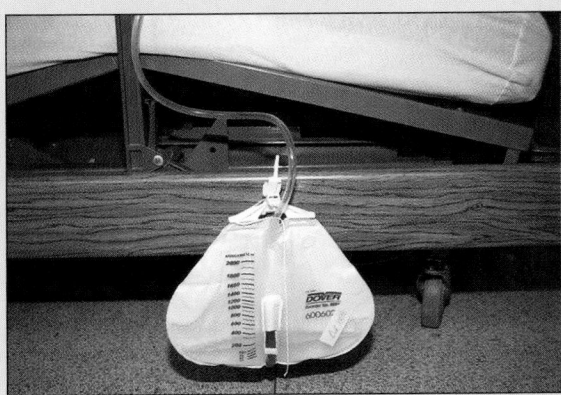

Step 21.

Continued

INSERTING AN INDWELLING CATHETER
(Continued)

Nursing Interventions	Rationale

22. Anchor the catheter using nonallergenic tape.
  a. Female clients, tape to the inside thigh.
  b. Male clients: tape to the abdomen with penis positioned upward toward abdomen.
	22. Taping prevents trauma to the urethra with catheter movement.
	By taping the catheter to the lower abdomen in male clients, pressure is decreased at the junction of the penis and scrotum and reduces tissue necrosis. The catheter balloon may be placed in the urethra instead of the bladder. Pain and potential trauma will occur if the balloon is inflated in the urethra. (*Safety precaution for male clients: Inflation of balloon is done with catheter inserted to bifurcation [see step 16b].)
	Indicates that the balloon is inflated properly and is anchored in bladder.
	Decreases resistance of catheter on the bladder neck wall.

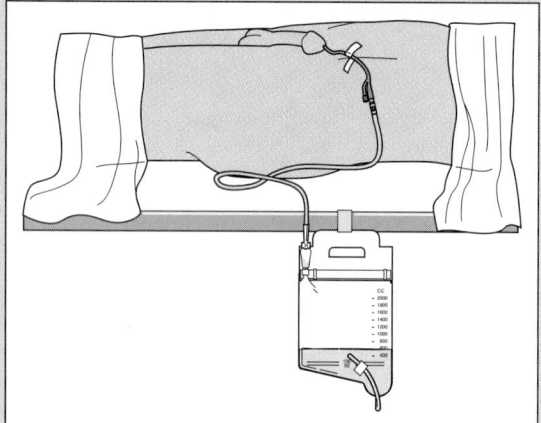

Step 22b.

c. Allow some slack in catheter length so movement does not cause tension on catheter.

d. If the client complains of discomfort during inflation, deflate the balloon by aspirating the fluid and advance the catheter further. Reinflate the balloon.

e. Apply gentle traction on catheter until you feel resistance.

f. Release the traction on the catheter and move the catheter slightly back into bladder and remove the syringe.

23. Coil excessive drainage tubing and place beside the client. The remaining tubing should run in a vertical line down to the drainage bag. Fasten the straight tubing to the bottom sheet with tape or clip provided with drainage set.	**23.** Prevents kinking of tube and provides free flow of urine by gravity.
24. Remove equipment that was used from bedside.	**24.** Prevents transmission of bacteria.
25. Assist client to a comfortable position and wash and dry perineal area (remove excess lubricant and antiseptic solution from perineal area).	**25.** Provides client comfort and good skin care.
26. Wash hands after procedure.	**26.** Use of universal precautions prevents cross-contamination.

27. Chart pertinent data:
  a. Insertion date and time.
  b. Characteristics of urine (amount, color, odor, presence of sediment, blood).
  c. Catheter and balloon size used.
  d. Whether a specimen ws obtained.
  e. Client's response to intervention.
	27. Documentation needed to provide information to other health care providers.

Table 32–9

METHODS OF URINARY DIVERSION

TYPES	NURSING ACTIONS	ADVANTAGES	DISADVANTAGES

Cutaneous ureterostomy necessitates wearing an external appliance
Unilateral ureterostomy: a single ureter is brought through the abdominal wall to the skin surface
 	
Unilateral ureterostomy
 	
Bilateral ureterostomy: both ureters are brought through the abdominal wall to the skin surface; two drainage appliances are required
 	
Bilateral ureterostomy
 	
Double-barreled ureterostomy: both ureters are brought through the abdominal wall to the skin surface, and the two stomas are placed close together; this requires only one drainage appliance
 	
Double barreled ureterostomy
	Assess
	  Urine output (patency of ureter)
	  Skin breakdown around stoma
	Patient teaching: skin care
	  Inspect for infection
	  Application and changing appliance
	  Odor control
	  Measures to prevent UTIs
	Promote coping skills: address sexuality issues
	  Changes in body image
	  Changes in self-esteem
		Relatively easy, rapid surgery; considered appropriate for patients with limited prognosis; avoids potential intestinal and peritoneal complications	Wearing an external appliance(s); potential complications, urinary obstruction, infection, and skin breakdown

Table continued on following page

Table 32–9

METHODS OF URINARY DIVERSION
(Continued)

TYPES	NURSING ACTIONS	ADVANTAGES	DISADVANTAGES
Transureterostomy: one ureter is connected to the other ureter, and a single stoma is created		Able to wear a single appliance	
Loop ureterostomy: the midsection of each ureter is brought to the skin surface of the flank area; two drainage appliances are needed		Allows for conversion to normal urinary functioning after healing has occurred	
Ileal conduit (also referred to as ileal loop, ureteroileostomy; Bricker procedure); usually a segment of the ileum is used; ureters joined to ileum or colon or jejunum; distal end of conduit brought through abdominal wall as stoma	Same as for cutaneous ureterostomy	Stoma is larger and more easily fitted with an appliance	Presence of stoma, altered body image, wearing an external appliance, prolapse of stoma and adjacent hernia, skin problems (*e.g.,* infection, ulceration, odor, calculi), obstruction at the ileal ureter surgical connection

Table 32–9

METHODS OF URINARY DIVERSION
(Continued)

TYPES	NURSING ACTIONS	ADVANTAGES	DISADVANTAGES
Reservoir or pouch: a reservoir or pouch does not require an external appliance; the client needs to learn how to catheterize himself or herself through the abdominal opening; this requires emptying every 4–6 h; the client is fully continent of urine; the stoma is flush with the skin; structure prevents ureteral reflux ascending infection	Patient teaching: self-catheterization every 4–6 h and at bedtime; drain urine from pouch; check for pouch distention		
Kock pouch (also referred to as continent vesicotomy; is a surgically created urinary bladder): approximately 60 cm of the ileum is resected; this is folded and sutured so that a pouch is formed; the ureters are implanted into the pouch; a nipple is created so that urine will not drain out of the opening on the abdomen nor back into the ureters		Fully continent of urine, stoma flush with skin, external appliance not necessary, prevents ureteral reflux and ascending infection	Self-catheterization required every 4–6 h and at bedtime; due to extensive length of surgery, is not advised for poor surgical risks (*e.g.,* very ill clients or those over 55 years of age); slippage of continence-providing valves; complications may include urinary obstruction, incontinence, urinary reflex, and possible pyelonephritis, bacteria, absorptive difficulties, and electrolyte imbalances
Indiana pouch: a segment of the sigmoid colon is used instead of ileal segment to form a reservoir		The colon has thicker musculature; fewer of the complications	Larger stoma
Nephrotomy tube: tubes are inserted into the pelvis of the kidneys; this may be used as a temporary procedure if the ureters are being repaired; it may be permanent if the ureters are removed; a high risk of infection and calculi	Assess for infection at nephrotomy site (systemic and site infection) and output of urine; prevent injury and infection: never irrigate; be careful not to dislodge tubes; keep drainage system closed; maintain fluid intake of at least 2000 ml/d		

From Matassarin-Jacobs, E. (1993). Nursing care of clients with disorders of the ureters, bladder and urethra. In *Luckman and Sorensen's medical-surgical nursing: A psychophysiologic approach* (4th ed., p. 1473). Philadelphia: W. B. Saunders.

available in a wide range of types and sizes. Some condom catheters are nonconstricting and are made of a double-sided adhesive nonlatex material. They are secured on the shaft of the penis and connected to a collecting bag by a urinary drainage tube (Procedure 32–2). The condom catheter must be secure enough to remain on the penis while not constricting blood flow. Nursing care should focus on promotion of skin

SAMPLE NURSING CARE PLAN

THE CLIENT WITH STRESS INCONTINENCE

M. K., a 37-year-old mother of four children, reports involuntary loss of urine whenever she sneezes, coughs, laughs, or exercises. Incontinence of urine began after the birth of her first child as an occasional "dribbling" of urine. Loss of urine has progressively increased after each pregnancy. M. K. currently wears absorbent protective pads on a continuous basis. She stated her fears of smelling like urine and changes protective pads four times a day.

Nursing Diagnosis: Stress Incontinence related to weak pelvic muscles and structural supports secondary to multiple pregnancies.

Client Goal: M. K. will be continent of urine during periods of increased intraabdominal pressure.

Expected Outcome Criteria:
1. M. K. will verbalize an understanding of her condition and interventions to manage bladder incontinence during follow-up home visit.
2. M. K. will correctly identify and contract the pelvic muscles during follow-up home visit.
3. M. K. will perform 10 Kegal exercise cycles (10-second contraction/relaxation cycles) three times a day for first 2 weeks.
4. M. K. will perform 20 Kegal exercise cycles three times a day within 3 weeks.

Nursing Interventions	Rationale
1. Assess client's voiding pattern. Request M. K. to keep a 24-hour diary of her voiding patterns, including:	
a. Amount of urine voided.	With stress incontinence, client can lose amounts of urine as high as 50 ml with any activity that increases intraabdominal pressure.
b. Frequency of incontinence.	
c. Events stimulating incontinence.	Activities that stimulate incontinence include sneezing, coughing, laughing, and exercise (*e.g.*, jogging, tennis, and aerobics).
d. Number of absorbent pads saturated with urine in 24 hours.	
2. Assess client's fluid intake (amount and type) by requesting that M. K. keep a 24-hour diary of her fluid intake.	Fluid intake of caffeine or alcohol promote diuresis and stress incontinence.
3. Palpate and percuss the bladder.	With stress incontinence, bladder will not be distended.
4. Perform a pelvic examination:	Assess for weakened structural support of pelvic organs.
a. Are abdominal and gluteal muscles used to contract the pelvic muscle?	
b. Assess period of time M. K. can contract the pelvic muscle.	
5. Prepare M. K. for provocative stress test.	Decreases anxiety and foster active participation in examination.
6. Assess M. K.'s self-management techniques for stress incontinence.	Self management techniques may include
	a. Emptying bladder frequently.
	b. Limiting fluid intake.
	c. Use of absorbent pads.
	d. Restricting activities.

THE CLIENT WITH STRESS INCONTINENCE
(Continued)

Nursing Interventions	Rationale
7. Teach M. K. about the need to	
a. Void every 3 hours.	Decreases pressure on bladder.
b. Avoid caffeine and alcohol intake.	Diuretic effect of these fluids can stimulate diuresis and subsequent incontinene.
c. Restrict fluid intake 2 to 3 hours prior to bedtime.	Avoids nocturia.
d. Avoid aerobic activities such as jogging, and substitute with low-impact exercise (*e.g.,* swimming).	Aerobic exercises increase intraabdominal pressure.
e. Perform Kegal exercises (see Table 32–10).	Strengthens pelvic muscles.
f. Start and then stop urinating two or three times each time she voids.	Assists in localizing the pubococcygeal muscle and strengthens pelvic muscles.
g. Perform sit-ups with knees bent.	Increases abdominal muscle tone. Abdominal muscles are used in voiding.
h. Change absorbent pads frequently and wash the perineal area with each pad change.	Warm saturated pads are a medium for bacterial growth and possible UTI; urine in contact with the skin can promote skin breakdown.
8. Listen to M. K.'s concerns regarding her incontinence and provide emotional support.	Incontinence may place restrictions on a person's lifestyle and can cause embarrassment and changes in body image.

Table 32–10

BEHAVIORAL APPROACHES TO PROMOTE CONTINENCE

DESCRIPTION OF APPROACH	PURPOSE	CLIENT TEACHING
Bladder training consists of client education, scheduled voiding, and positive reinforcement	Promotes Gradual distention of the bladder with adjustment of fluid intake Increased bladder capacity through delayed voiding and increased intervals between voiding Used to treat urge and stress incontinence	Resist sensation of urgency by using a relaxation breathing technique Initially postpone voiding for 5 min and gradually increase the postponement time Void according to a timed schedule rather than when there is an urge to void Start with a 2-h interval schedule while awake and gradually increase to 3–4 h
Timed voiding: fixed timed schedule for voiding is established	Used primarily in hospitals and nursing homes to promote continence in clients	Clients are assisted with bathroom or bedpan on a fixed time schedule; *e.g.,* every 2 h
Habit training: scheduled voiding at regular intervals; attempt to match person's natural voiding schedule	To promote continence by use of a schedule based on client's habits	Clients are assisted with bathroom or bedpan; schedule is based on client's voiding pattern; *e.g.,* after meals and at bedtime
Prompted voiding consists of Monitoring of client's continence at regular intervals Prompting—person is asked to use the toilet at regular intervals Praising—initially the person is praised for attempts at toileting; gradually, the person is praised for continence and not just for voiding attempts	Used as a supplement to habit training. Effective approach with cognitively impaired, developmentally disabled or dependent persons in a nursing home.	Clients are taught to: Differentiate their incontinence/continence state Request toileting assistance from caregivers

Table continued on following page

Table **32–10**

BEHAVIORAL APPROACHES TO PROMOTE CONTINENCE
(Continued)

DESCRIPTION OF APPROACH	PURPOSE	CLIENT TEACHING
Kegel exercises (pelvic muscle exercises) used to improve the tone and function of perineal muscles through exercise	Used in treatment of stress incontinence in female clients; improved urethral closure Reduce incontinence in men following prostatic surgery Improved continence in women who have had multiple surgeries Urge incontinence	Client is taught to "draw in" the perivaginal muscles as if to control urination or defecation without using abdominal, thigh, or buttock muscles; emphasis on maintaining the muscle contraction for an equal amount of time as relaxation; counting and breathing techniques have helped with this exercise; initially the length of contraction time may be 3s; gradually, the person attempts to reach a goal of 10-s contraction and relaxation cycles; frequency and duration of exercises have not been agreed on in the research; in general, 30–80 times per day for up to 6 w is recommended
Bent knee sit ups may be used as an adjunct treatment to Kegel exercises	Increased abdominal muscle tone	
Vaginal cones used as an adjunct to pelvic muscle exercises; set of cones of identical shape and volume but increasing in weight	Increased pelvic muscle strength; provide feedback to client on effectiveness of her pelvic muscle contraction	Woman places cone intravaginally and attempts to retain the cone by pelvic muscle contraction; as she is successful with one cone, she progresses to the heavier cones
Biofeedback techniques used as a learning technique to help with improving continence; biofeedback methods include visual and auditory stimulation, which gives feedback on physical responses; for example, vaginal, anal, and abdominal electromyography readings can be done as feedback for the client as she learns Kegel exercises	Improved continence as a result of client's ability to use biofeedback methods	
Electric stimulation is an external device used to control intermittent electrical currents to the pelvic floor via anal or vaginal electrode probes; electrical currents can be adjusted to client's tolerance level	Used primarily to treat stress and urge incontinence; improves sphincter control, detrusor contractibility, and detrusor stability	May be used an adjunct to teaching pelvic floor exercises or be surgically implanted; prepare client for surgery if implantation is performed

Data from Agency for Health Care Policy and Research. (1992a, b).; Appleby, S. L. (1995). A home health perspective on the management of urinary incontinence. *Journal of Wound, Ostomy and Continence Nurses, 22* (3), 145–152; McCormick, K. A., Kaschak Newman, D., Colling, J., & Pearson, B. D. (1992). Urinary incontinence in adults. *American Journal of Nursing, 92* (10), 75–88; Wyman, J. F. (1992). Managing incontinence: The current bases for practice. In S. G. Funk, E. M. Tornquist, M. T. Champagne, & R. A. Wiese (eds.), *Key aspects of elder care* (pp. 135–154). New York: Springer.

integrity, maintenance of urinary drainage, and promoting client self-esteem. The catheter should be changed daily and the skin of the penis cleansed and dried. Recent research findings have reported no difference in changing condom catheters every other day as compared with daily (Stelling & Hale, 1996). Further research regarding the frequency for changing condom catheters is needed.

Text continued on page 1013

PROCEDURE

32–2

APPLYING A CONDOM CATHETER

Equipment:

Bath blanket
External condom catheter
Velcro strap or elastic tape
Bedside and leg drainage bags
    with extension tubes
Disposable gloves
Wash cloth, towel, mild soap
    and basin of warm water

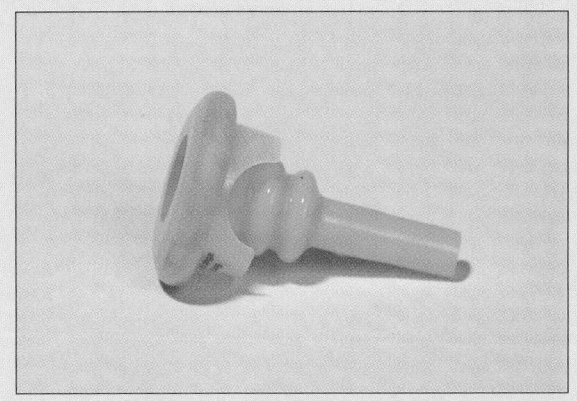

Nursing Interventions	Rationale
1. Prepare the client:	**1.**
a. Explain the reason for using a condom catheter.	Client teaching helps to decrease anxiety and promotes active participation in care.
b. Describe how the condom catheter provides a free flow of urine to a drainage bag.	
c. Inform the client that if he feels the urge to void, he should tell the nurse.	If the client feels the urge to void, bladder training should be attempted.
d. Teach the client how he can participate during the procedure and in skin care.	
2. Procedure preparation:	**2.**
a. Wash hands and don gloves before procedure.	Decreases transmission of microorganisms; universal precautions.
b. Facing client, stand on left side of bed if you are right handed and on right side if you are left handed. Assist client to prone position.	Position facilitates easier dexterity for applying condom.
c. Place a bath blanket on client.	Provides client privacy.
3. Provide skin care to genital area:	**3.**
a. Assess the penis for skin irritation, contact dermatitis, swelling, excoriation, or discoloration.	Application of the condom catheter is contraindicated if any skin alterations are seen.
b. Gently retract foreskin (if present) and wash the genital area with mild soap and warm water.	Decreases the risk of skin irritation and excoriation after the condom is applied.
c. Dry skin thoroughly and place foreskin (if present) back in position.	
d. Measure the circumference of the penis, using the measuring device provided by the condom catheter manufacturer.	Ensures proper condom catheter size.

Continued

PROCEDURE

32–2

APPLYING A CONDOM CATHETER
(Continued)

Nursing Interventions	**Rationale**
4. Apply the condom catheter:	4. Use of nonlatex condoms (*i.e.*, silicone, styrene) is recommended for clients who have latex allergies.
a. Before applying, roll the condom outward onto itself.	Prevents the adhesive inside the condom from self-adhering.

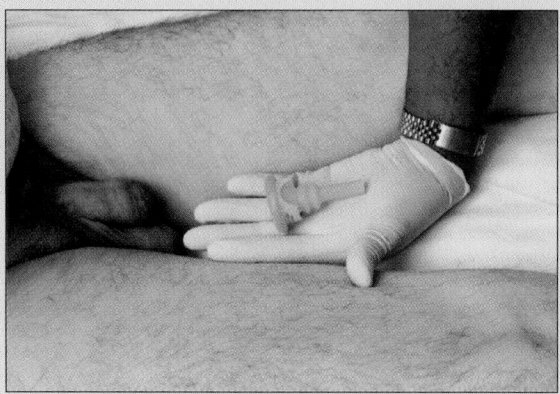

Step 4a.

b. Gently push back the pubic hair away from the penile area; shave pubic hair if necessary.	Pubic hair can provide space for urine to leak out of the condom; also prevents hair loss and skin irritation during condom catheter removal.
c. Roll the condom smoothly over the penis and leave 2.5 cm (1 in) space between the tip of the penis and the rubber or plastic connecting tube.	Prevents skin friction and resulting irritation of the tip of the penis and facilitates urinary drainage.

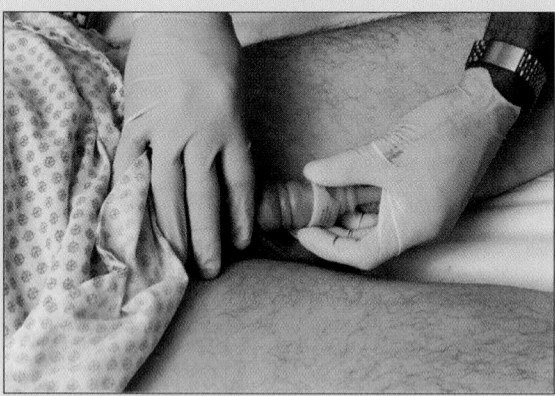

Step 4c.

32–2

APPLYING A CONDOM CATHETER
(Continued)

Nursing Interventions	Rationale
d. Secure the condom catheter to the penis with a Velcro strap or elastic tape using spiral technique.	Condom should be on firmly but not too tightly to prevent restricted circulation to the penis. *CAUTION:* DO NOT use adhesive tape to secure the condom catheter. It does not stretch and can restrict circulation to the penis.

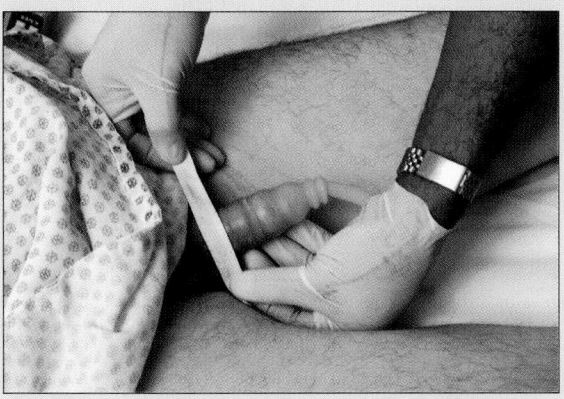

Step 4d.

Nursing Interventions	Rationale
5. Attach the urinary drainage bag: a. Attach the drainage bag to the condom.	5. Select the appropriate type of drainage bag that will facilitate urinary flow by gravity.
b. Make sure that the condom is not twisted. c. Attach the urinary drainage bag to the bed frame if the client is to remain in bed.	Prevents obstruction of urinary drainage. Promotes urinary flow via gravity.
d. Attach the urinary drainage bag to the client's leg if he is getting out of bed to sit in a chair or to ambulate.	Prevents twisting of condom and maintains the extension tube's position.
e. Remove gloves and wash hands.	Universal precautions.
6. Examine the penis 30 minutes after applying the condom catheter. Assess area at least every 2 hours thereafter.	6. Assess for urinary flow and check the penis for signs of impeded circulation (swelling and discoloration).

7. Change the condom daily and provide skin care:
  a. Remove the Velcro strip or elastic tape and roll off the condom.
  b. Cleanse the genital area with mild soap and water.
  c. Assess the genital area for irritation, excoriation swelling, and discoloration.
	7. Prevents skin irritation and excoriation; allows for early detection of skin breakdown and circulatory impairment.

Absorbent Products

Absorbent products may be used to manage urinary incontinence when other treatment measures are ineffective or as a supportive measure to manage urinary odor and wetting of clothes during treatment trials. Products that are frequently used include small perineal pads (similar to sanitary napkins but with a coating to prevent urine leakage), larger or full-length pads, diaperlike garments, and bed pads. Although products may help the individual with stress incontinence to engage in their normal activities without feeling embarrassed about soiling or odor, there are negative factors to consider. Early dependency on absorbent products can encourage the individual to have a feeling of security. This in turn may decrease the individual's motivation to seek any treatment for the incontinence. Use of absorbent products should be considered as a last resort after other measures are tried.

Absorbent products can contribute to the development of a UTI and to the irritation and breakdown of skin due to the acidity of urine. A saturated pad provides a warm environment, thereby fostering bacterial growth and subsequent infection. The risk for decubitus formation is especially high in the elderly due to their thinner layer of adipose tissue and decreased mobility. Plastic liners are often used in bed pads and absorbent pads. The plastic fosters skin breakdown because the urine is maintained in close contact with the skin instead of being drawn away. Absorbent products need to be changed frequently. Frequent skin care is also required, including cleansing the skin with soap and water and drying it thoroughly after each episode of incontinence. The use of skin ointment (*e.g.,* hydrocortisone 1%) in a petrolatum base applied to clean, dry skin is beneficial. The petrolatum base creates a water vapor barrier.

Some of the factors to consider in using absorbent products are the functional abilities of the client; type and severity of incontinence; gender of incontinent individual; availability of caregivers; effectiveness of treatments to control incontinence; and client preference (AHCPR, 1992a, b).

Children With Incontinence

Interventions designed to eliminate primary enuresis may be focused on the children themselves or on their parents. Techniques that are child centered include medications (*e.g.,* Minaprine, imipramine, and other tricyclic antidepressants). These drugs have antimuscarinic actions on the bladder, causing urinary retention (Shlafer, 1993). Rewards are also employed to change the child's behavior. In a research study by Ronen and Abraham (1996), retention control training (RCT) was found to be effective in treating young children close to the final stage of bladder development. RCT provides training in motor and cognitive skills. Through exercises, RCT aims to increase the child's awareness of internal stimuli, strengthen the bladder, and facilitate retention (*e.g.,* stopping the flow of urine immediately after starting to empty the bladder). An example of a parent-centered technique is to change parents' responses to the child's bed wetting.

The following measures (Lawrence, 1995) are suggested when a child is incontinent:

1. Implementing a voiding schedule, urinating before bedtime
2. Placing a night light in the bathroom
3. Reducing the child's fluid intake 1 to 3 hours before bedtime
4. Educating parents that others have the same problems and that embarrassment, shame, and guilt are not unusual feelings experienced by children
5. Providing skin care and controlling odors
6. Knowing how prescribed drugs work and when to administer them. Examples of drugs prescribed include imipramine (Tofranil), which causes a local constriction on the bladder neck and relaxes the detrusor muscle; oxybutynin chloride (Ditropan) to relieve bladder irritability;

Table **32–11**

TYPES OF SURGICAL INTERVENTIONS FOR ALTERATIONS IN URINATION

TYPE OF PROCEDURE	COMMENTS
Bladder neck suspension (*i.e.,* transvaginal or transabdominal suspension of bladder neck)	Performed when an urethrocele exists; effectively treats stress incontinence
Sling procedures (*i.e.,* urethral sling—a piece of tissue, muscle, vaginal wall, or synthetic material is used to create a sling to elevate and compress the urethra)	Helps place the urethra in a more natural position and facilitates closure during bladder filling; effective in restoring continence; in some instances, self-catheterization may also be indicated due to urinary retention

Periurethral bulking
  Injections
    Polytetrafluoroethylene (Teflon) or collagen materials are injected in the periurethral area
	Used to increase urethral compression. Particles of polytetrafluoroethylene have migrated to lymph nodes and lungs; this may result in the development of a tumor; the most common side effects are urinary retention, infection, and urethral erosion

Placement of artificial sphincter: sphincter consists of a reservoir of fluid, a pump, and a cuff to compress the urethra during bladder filling; for urination to occur, the pump is compressed and the fluid enters the reservoir; this causes the sphincter to relax and the urine drains	Used most commonly for ureteral insufficiency after prostatectomy with severe incontinence; side effects include infection, mechanical failure, and urethral injury

Data from Chalker, R., & Whitmore, K. E. (1990). *Overcoming bladder disorders.* New York: Harper & Row; Kaschak Newman, D., Lynch, K., Smith, D. A., & Cell, P. (1991). Restoring urinary continence. *American Journal of Nursing, 91* (1), 28–36; McCormick, K. A., Kaschak Newman, D., Colling, J., & Pearson, B. D. (1992). Urinary incontinence in adults. *American Journal of Nursing, 92* (10), 75–88.

and desmopressin acetate (deamino-D-arginine-vasopressin [DDAVP]), an antidiuretic. Drugs may also be given if the cause of enuresis is a urinary tract infection.

Surgical Procedures for Alterations in Urination

A number of procedures have been designed to relieve incontinence. As in any surgical procedure, the risk factors, success rate for correcting the specific urinary alteration, the client's condition, and potential changes in lifestyle after surgery need to be considered. Surgery is usually performed after other less-invasive treatments have been ineffective. When an anatomical anomaly is present, surgery may be the most effective treatment (Table 32–11)

COMMUNITY BASED CARE

URINARY CATHETERS

Long- and short-term urinary catheterization may be indicated for certain clients. Clean, intermittent self-catheterization may be used to manage persistent urinary retention. The client is taught to regularly insert the catheter into the bladder and empty it, usually three or four times per day. Although the procedure may initially produce anxiety, most clients are able to learn the procedure. If the client lacks the necessary manual dexterity, the procedure is taught to a willing caregiver. Catheters are cleaned after each use, usually with soap and water, and allowed to thoroughly dry. Catheters may be reused until they begin to crack or develop an odor.

Although intermittent catheterization is preferred, some clients may not be able to manage the procedure, and some may be too debilitated. In these cases, indwelling urethral or suprapubic catheters may be placed. Usually, the home care nurse inserts the catheter, utilizing sterile technique. The catheter is usually changed every 4 to 8 weeks. Complications from indwelling catheters include infection, trauma, discomfort, and blockage. Client and caregiver instruction is essential. Teaching includes

1. Good handwashing when handling the urinary drainage system

2. Daily care of drainage bag and tubing, including how to empty, how and when to cleanse, maintaining a closed system

3. Daily care and cleansing of the urinary meatus

4. Signs and symptoms of a malfunctioning drainage system, such as leaking, pain, or bladder distention

5. Emergency removal of catheter

6. Safety precautions, including measures to prevent accidental dislodgement and reducing risk of infection

7. Dietary implications, including increased fluid intake

Evaluation

Evaluation involves an appraisal of client goal achievement. The client-specific expected outcome criteria are used to measure the client's individualized goal attainment. It is important to also evaluate the effectiveness of the interventions to reach the goals, whether the goals could be realistically achieved, and plan revisions to the plan of care with the client if necessary. Examples of goals and expected outcome criteria are provided in the three care plans presented earlier. These outcome criteria should be used to evaluate goal achievement.

In the client with Urinary Retention related to decreased bladder tone secondary to effect of indwelling catheter, the nurse would monitor for attainment of the expected outcomes by assessing for bladder distention, monitoring urine output, and assessing post-void residuals as per the physician's orders. The client would also be involved in the evaluation process. The client could keep a voiding diary to record the urinary elimination pattern and periods of continence and incontinence. Evaluating the client's ability to perform micturition techniques and whether they effectively stimulate voiding for this client are also important data areas to assess.

In a client with Altered Urinary Elimination related to irritation of bladder mucosa, the nurse would evaluate achievement of these outcomes by assessing for signs and symptoms of UTI. The effectiveness of client teaching of risk factors, signs and symptoms, preventive measures, and interventions for UTIs should be evaluated by having the client verbalize what was learned. Written instructions would help the client remember pertinent information at home. After completion of antibiotics, the client should have a follow-up urine examination for culture and sensitivity.

During follow-up home visits to the client with Stress Incontinence related to weak pelvic muscles and structural supports secondary to multiple pregnancies, the nurse would evaluate whether the client can correctly contract the pelvic muscles without use of thigh, buttocks, or abdominal muscle contraction by pelvic examination. The client is encouraged to participate in the evaluation process through the use of a voiding diary, monitoring the amount and types of fluid ingested and evaluating the effectiveness of using **Kegel exercises** are (pelvic muscle exercises in which the person contracts and relaxes the perivaginal muscles without contracting abdominal or inner thigh muscles and buttocks) during periods of increased intraabdominal pressure.

Summary

The effects seen when an individual experiences impairment of the urinary system may include changes in self-esteem, body image, and ability to function independently. Nurses are in a unique position to help clients maintain their ability to eliminate urine and to prevent the complications associated with urinary retention and incontinence. An understanding of the process of urination (from production in the kidneys to excretion via the urethra) is prerequisite to the assessment, planning, and provision of interventions and evaluation of client outcomes.

The scope of the nurse's role ranges from educating clients (and family members) about prevention of urinary problems to providing care postoperatively when surgery is performed to divert urine, to promoting self-care. Educating clients about factors that can lead to or worsen incontinence is important (such as the effects of obesity, medications, lack of exercise, or overuse of caffeine). Providing information and support during diagnostic tests, teaching clients how to perform self-catheterization, and discussing the types of urinary drainage devices and absorbent products on the market are also important components of the nursing role.

◼   ◼

C H A P T E R   H I G H L I G H T S

✦

✦ A disruption in one part of the urinary system (kidneys, ureters, bladder, urethra) can affect the structure and function of other parts of the urinary system.

✦ The amount of urine excreted per hour is one indicator of kidney function. In adults, a urine output of less than 30 ml per hour may indicate that kidney function is compromised.

✦ Factors affecting urination include the physiological integrity of the urinary system; intake of fluids, foods, medications, and toxic substances; fluids lost by other routes; sensory motor innervation defects; mobility level and muscle tone; mental and emotional status; gender; and sociocultural influences.

✦ Urine that is dilute (not concentrated) helps reduce the risk of bladder irritation, UTIs, and formation of calculi.

✦ Infections, obstructions, retention, and incontinence are common alterations of the urinary tract.

✦ Women have a higher incidence of UTIs and incontinence than men. A higher incidence of enuresis is seen in young boys.

✦ Urinary tract infections may be present without symptoms.

✦ A sterile specimen container must be used when collecting urine for a culture and sensitivity test.

✦ A urine specimen is *never* taken from a urinary drainage bag.

✦ Urinary catheterization is used to treat acute or chronic urinary retention, for incontinence in which other treatment measures were ineffective, and for accurate measurement of urine in clients who are comatose or critically ill.

✦ To prevent the flow of urine from a urinary drainage bag into the bladder, the drainage bag should always be placed below the level of the bladder.

✦ Incontinence is considered the predominant reason for institutionalization of the elderly.

✦ Behavioral approaches to promote continence include bladder training, timed voiding, habit training, prompted voiding, Kegel exercises, and biofeedback techniques.

Study Questions

1. What is the functional unit of the kidney?

   a. Bowman's capsule
   b. bladder
   c. ureter
   d. nephron

2. What is the minimum amount of urine required in an adult to maintain kidney function?

   a. 50 ml per hour
   b. 30 ml per hour
   c. 100 ml per hour
   d. 10 ml per hour

3. How do the kidneys change as the adult ages?

   a. the kidneys respond more slowly to changes in fluid and electrolyte composition
   b. the kidneys have an increased number of reserve nephrons
   c. the kidneys increase in size and can become edematous
   d. kidney perfusion improves

4. Which of the following drug classifications has a side effect of urinary retention?

   a. diuretics
   b. laxatives
   c. anticholinergics
   d. sedatives

5. A client had his Foley catheter removed 4 hours ago and has not voided. Which of the following nursing actions would the nurse perform FIRST?

   a. call the physician for an order for an intermittent catheterization
   b. perform the Credé maneuver every 15 minutes
   c. force fluids to 2 L every 24 hours
   d. palpate at the symphis pubis

Critical Thinking Exercises

1. Ms. K. is experiencing stress incontinence. Discuss methods to control this problem and outcome criteria for Ms. K.

2. Ms. L. is discharged with a catheter. Discuss teaching you would give Ms. L. regarding care of her catheter.

References

Ader, K., Brown Pierce, L. L., & Salter, J. P. (1990). Urinary tract infections: A quality assurance rehabilitation nursing perspective. *Rehabilitation Nursing, 15* (4), 193–196.

Agency for Health Care Policy and Research, Urinary Incontinence Guideline Panel. (1992a). *Quick reference guide for clinicians. Urinary incontinence in adults.* AHCPR Pub. No. 92-0041. Rockville MD: Agency for Health Care Policy and Research, Public Health Service, U.S. Department of Health and Human Services.

Agency for Health Policy and Research, Urinary Incontinence Guideline Panel. (1992b). *Urinary incontinence in adults: Clinical practice guideline.* AHCPR Pub. No. 92-0038. Rockville MD: Agency for Health Care Policy and Research, Public Health Service, U.S. Department of Health and Human Services.

Appleby, S. L. (1995). A home health perspective on the management of urinary incontinence. *Journal of Wound, Ostomy and Continence Nurses, 22* (3), 145–152.

Bates, B. (1995). *A guide to physical examination and history taking* (6th ed.). Philadelphia: J. B. Lippincott.

Betz, C. L., Hunsberger, M. M., & Wright, S. (Eds.). (1994). *Family-centered nursing care of children* (2nd ed.). Philadelphia: W. B. Saunders.

Bullock, B. L., & Rosendahl, P. P. (1992). *Pathophysiology adaptations and alterations in function* (3rd ed.) Philadelphia: J. B. Lippincott.

Case-Gamble, M. K. (1990). Urinary incontinence in the elderly. In P. Ebersol & P. Hess. (1990), *Toward healthy aging: Human needs and nursing responses* (3rd ed., pp. 311–322). St. Louis: C. V. Mosby Inc.

Chalker, R. & Whitmore, K. E. (1990). *Overcoming bladder disorders.* New York: Harper & Row.

Chernecky, C. C., Krech, R. L., & Berger, B. J. (1993). *Laboratory tests and diagnostic procedures,* Philadelphia: W. B. Saunders.

Conti, M. T., & Eutropius, L. (1987). Preventing UTIs: What works? *American Journal of Nursing, 87* (3), 307–309.

Cotran, R. S., Robbins, S. L., & Kumar, V. (1994). *Pathologic basis of disease* (5th ed.). Philadelphia: W. B. Saunders.

DeGroot-Kosolcharoen, R. (1995). Thirteen ways to protect your patient from bacteriuria. *Nursing 95, 25* (4), 30.

Doenges, M. E., & Moorehouse, M. F. (1993). *Nurse's pocket guide: Nursing diagnoses with interventions* (4th ed., pp. 45–59). Philadelphia: F. A. Davis.

Donegan, N. (1996). Management of patients with infectious disease. In S. C, Smelzer & B. G. Bare (Eds.), *Medical-surgical nursing* (8th ed., pp. 1954–1998). Philadelphia: Lippincott-Raven.

Ebersol, P., & Hess, P. (1990). *Toward healthy aging: Human needs and nursing responses* (3rd ed.). St. Louis, C. V. Mosby.

Fischbach, F. T. (1988). *A manual of laboratory diagnostic tests* (3rd ed.). Philadelphia: J. B. Lippincott.

Gibbs, T. D. (1995). Health assessment of the adult urology patient. In K. A. Karlowicz (Ed.), *Urologic nursing principles and practice* (pp. 41–85). Philadelphia: W. B. Saunders.

Gray, M. L. (1995). Genitourinary embryology, anatomy and physiology. In K. Karlowicz (Ed.), *Urologic nursing principles and practice* (pp. 3–32). Philadelphia: W. B. Saunders.

Grinspun, D. (1993). Bladder management for adults following head injury. *Rehabilitation Nursing, 18* (5), 300–305.

Herzog, A. R., & Falty, N. H. (1990). Prevalence and incidence of urinary incontinence in the community-dwelling population. *Journal of the American Geriatric Society, 38,* 273–281.

Huether, S. E., & McCance, K. L. (1996). *Understanding pathophysiology.* St. Louis: Mosby-Year Book Inc.

Kaschak Newman, D., Lynch, K., Smith, D. A., & Cell, P. (1991). Restoring urinary continence. *American Journal of Nursing, 91* (1), 28–36.

Langford, R. (1994). Keeping control. *Nursing Times, 90* (27), 58–59.

Lapides, J., Diokno, A. C., Silber, S. J. & Lowe, B. S. (1972). Clean intermittent catheterization in the treatment of urinary tract disease. *Journal of Urology, 107,* 458–461.

Lawrence, C. A. (1995). Pediatric voiding disorders. In K. A. Karlowicz (Ed.), *Urologic nursing, principles and practice* (pp. 593–619). Philadelphia: W. B. Saunders.

Loeb, S. (Ed.). (1993). *Illustrated guide to diagnostic tests student version.* Springhouse, PA: Springhouse.

Matassarin-Jacobs, E. (1993). Nursing care of clients with disorders of the ureters, bladder and urethra. In J. M. Black and E. Matassarin-Jacobs, *Luckman and Sorensen's medical-surgical nursing: A psychophysiologic approach* (4th ed., pp. 1442–1486). Philadelphia: W. B. Saunders.

McCash, D. C., & Kirchhoff, K. T. (1993). Decontamination of vinyl urinary drainage bags with bleach. *Rehabilitation Nursing, 18* (5), 292–295.

McConnell, E. A., & Zimmerman, M. F. (1983). Care of patients with urological problems. Philadelphia: J. B. Lippincott.

McCormick, K. A., Kaschak Newman, D., Colling, J., & Pearson, B. D. (1992). Urinary incontinence in adults. *American Journal of Nursing, 92* (10), 75–88.

McKenry, L. M., & Salerno, E. (1989). *Mosby's pharmacology in nursing* (17th ed.). St Louis: C. V. Mosby.

Mohide, A. (1986). The prevalence and scope of urinary incontinence. *Clinics in Geriatric Nursing,* (2), 639–656.

Moore, K. N. (1991). Intermittent catheterization: Sterile or clean? *Rehabilitation Nursing, 16* (1), 15–18, 33.

Moore, K. N., Kelm, M., Sinclair, O., & Cadrain, B. (1993). Bacteriuria in intermittent catheterization users: The effect of sterile versus clean reused catheters. *Rehabilitation Nursing, 18* (5), 306–309.

Perkash, I., & Giroux, J. (1993). Clean intermittent catheterization in spinal cord injury patients: A follow-up study. *Journal of Urology, 149,* 1068–1071.

Porth, C. M. (1994). *Pathophysiology concepts of altered health states* (4th ed.). Philadelphia: J. B. Lippincott.

Price, S. A., & Wilson, L. M. (1992). *Pathophysiology clinical concepts of disease processes* (4th ed.). St. Louis: Mosby-Year Book.

Rainville, N. C. (1994). The current nursing procedure for intermittent urinary catheterization in rehabilitation facilities. *Rehabilitation Nursing, 19* (6), 330–333.

Resnick, B. (1993). Retraining the bladder after catheterization. *American Journal of Nursing, 93* (11), 46–49.

Ronen, T., & Abraham, Y. (1996). Retention control training in the treatment of younger versus older enuretic children. *Nursing Research, 45* (2), 78–82.

Schlosser, S. P. (1992). Normal and altered male reproductive function. In B. L. Bullock & P. P. Rosendahl (Eds.), *Pathophysiology adaptations and alterations in function* (3rd ed.). Philadelphia: J. B. Lippincott.

Shlafer, M. (1993). *The nurse, pharmacology, and drug ther-*

apy, Redwood City, CA: Addison-Wesley Nursing (a division of Benjamin/Cummings Publishing.)

Smeltzer, S. C., & Bare, B. G. (1996). *Brunner and Suddarth's textbook of medical-surgical nursing* (8th ed.). Philadelphia: Lippincott-Raven.

Smith, C. M., & Reynard, A. M. (1995). *Essentials of pharmacology,* Philadelphia: W. B. Saunders.

Smith, D. R. (1992). *General urology* (13th ed.). Los Altos, CA: Lange Medical.

Stamm W. E., & Turck, M. (1983). Urinary tract infection, pyelonephritis, and related conditions. In R. G. Petersdorf, *et al.* (Eds.) *Harrison's principles of internal medicine* (10th ed., p. 1652). New York: McGraw-Hill.

Stelling, J. D., & Hale, A. M. (1996). Protocol for changing condom catheters in males. *SCI Nursing, 13* (2), 28–34.

Turner, S. L., & Plymat, K. R. (1988). As women age: Perspectives on urinary incontinence. *Rehabilitation Nursing, 13* (3), 132–135.

Voith, A. M. (1988). Alteration in urinary elimination. Concepts, research and practice. *Rehabilitation Nursing, 13* (3), 122–131.

Voith, A. M. (1986). A conceptual framework for nursing diagnosis: Alterations in urinary elimination. *Rehabilitation Nursing, 11* (1), 18–21.

Watson, J., & Jaffe, M. S. (1995). *Nurse's manual of laboratory and diagnostic tests* (2nd ed.). Philadelphia: F. A. Davis.

Wong, D. L. (Ed.). (1995). *Nursing care of infants and children* (5th ed.) St. Louis; Mosby-Year Book.

Wyman, J. F. (1992). Managing incontinence: The current bases for practice. In S. G. Funk, E. M. Tornquist, M. T. Champagne, & R. A. Wiese (Eds.), *Key aspects of elder care* (pp. 135–154). New York: Springer.

Wyman, J. F., Elswick, R. K., Ory, M. G., Wilson, M. S., & Fantl, J. A. (1993). Influence of functional urological and environmental characteristics on urinary incontinence in community-dwelling older women. *Nursing Research, 42* (5), 270–275.

Wyndale, J., & Maes, D. (1990). Clean intermittent self catheterization: A 12-year follow-up. *Journal of Urology, 143,* 906–908.

Bibliography

Baker, J., & Norton, P. (1996). Evaluation of absorbent products for women with mild to moderate urinary incontinence. *Applied Nursing Research, 9* (1), 29–33.

Boyle, J. S., & Andrews, M. A. (1989). *Transcultural concepts in nursing care,* Glenview, IL: Scott, Foresman and Company.

Brink, C. A. (1996). The value of absorbent products and containment devices in the management of urinary incontinence. *Journal of Wound, Ostomy and Continence Nurses, 23* (1), 2–4.

Brooks, M. J. (1995). Assessment and nursing management of homebound clients with urinary incontinence. *Home Healthcare Nurse, 13* (5), 11–16.

Carpenito, L. J. (Ed.). (1992). *Nursing diagnosis application to clinical practice* (4th ed.). Philadelphia: J. B. Lippincott.

Charbonneau-Smith, R. (1993). No touch catheterization and infection rates in select spinal cord injured population. *Rehabilitation Nursing, 18* (5), 296–299, 305.

Cook, E. A., & Thigpen, R. (1993). Identification and management of cognitive and perceptual deficits in the rehabilitation patient. *Rehabilitation Nursing, 18* (5), 310–313.

Crandall, B. I. (1989). Acute renal failure. In B. T. Ulrich (Ed.), *Nephrology nursing concepts and strategies* (pp. 45–59), Norwalk, CT: Appleton & Lange.

Fiers, S. (1995). Management of the long-term indwelling catheter in the home setting. *Journal of Wound, Ostomy and Continence Nurses, 22* (3), 140–144.

Guyton, A. C. (1992). *Human physiology and mechanisms of disease,* Philadelphia: W. B. Saunders.

Harris, M. D. (1995). Incorporating the agency for healthcare policy and research. *Home Healthcare Nurse, 13* (4), 17–18.

Johnson, V. Y., & Gary, M. A. (1995). Urinary incontinence: A review. *Journal of Wound, Ostomy and Continence Nurses, 22* (1), 8–16.

Kunin, C. M., Chinn Q. F., & Chambers, S. (1987). Morbidity and mortality associated with indwelling urinary catheters in elderly patients in a nursing home: Confounding due to presence of associated diseases. *Journal of the American Geriatric Society, 35* (11), 1001–1006.

Kurtz, M. J., Van Zandt, K., & Burns, J. L. (1995). Comparison study of home catheter cleaning methods. *Rehabilitation Nursing, 20* (4), 212–214, 217.

Lewis, N. A. (1995). Implementing a bladder ultrasound program. *Rehabilitation Nursing, 20* (4), 215–217.

McConnell, E. A. (1994). How to apply a self-adhesive condom catheter. *Nursing 94, 24* (11), 26.

McConnell, E. A. (1995). Inflating an indwelling urinary catheter balloon. *Nursing 95, 25* (12), 13.

McIntosh, L. J., & Richardson, D. A. (1994). 30 minute evaluation of incontinence in the older women. *Geriatrics, 49* (2), 35–44.

Qualey, T. L. (1995). An approach to elderly incontinence. *Nursing Management, 26* (4), 48Q–48T.

Quigley, P. A., & Riggin, O. Z. (1993). A comparison of open and closed catheterization techniques in rehabilitation patients. *Rehabilitation Nursing, 18* (1), 26–33.

Resnick, B. (1995). A bladder scan trial in geriatric rehabilitation. *Rehabilitation Nursing, 20* (4), 194–196.

Resnick, B., Slocum, D., Ra, L., & Moffett, P. (1996). Geriatric rehabilitation: Nursing interventions and outcomes focusing on urinary function and knowledge of medications. *Rehabilitation Nursing, 21* (3), 142–147.

Skoner, M. M. (1994). Self management of urinary incontinence among women 31 to 50 years of age. *Rehabilitation Nursing, 19* (6), 339–347.

Stanley, M., & Gauntlett Beare, P. (1995). Gerontological nursing. Philadelphia: F. A. Davis.

Trout, S., Dattolo, J., & Hansbrough, J. F. (1993). Catheterization: How far should you go? *RN, 56* (8), 52–54.

Wells, T. J. (1990). Pelvic (floor) muscle exercise. *Journal of the American Geriatrics Society, 38,* 333–337.

Williams, S. R. (1989). *Nutrition and diet therapy* (6th ed.). St. Louis: Times Mirror/Mosby College Publishing.

Wyman, J. F., (1988). Nursing assessment of the incontinent geriatric outpatient population. *Nursing Clinics of North America, 23* (1), 169–179.

Unit ✦ VII

APPLICATION OF THE NURSING PROCESS TO PSYCHOSOCIO-CULTURAL NEEDS

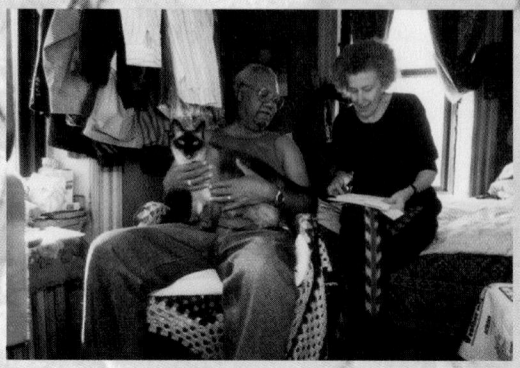

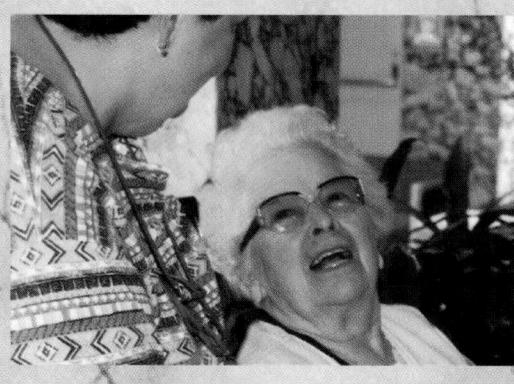

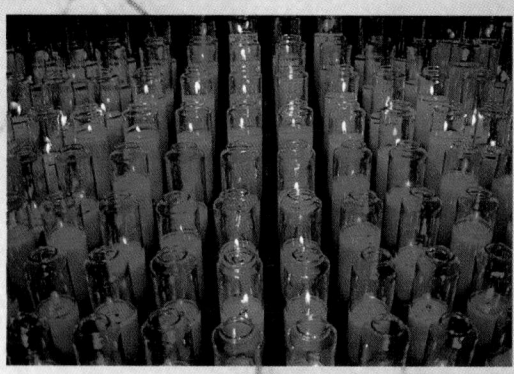

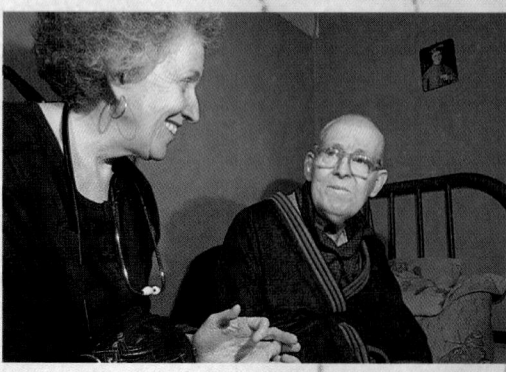

Parish nursing is both ambiguous and obvious in its "holistic" approach to nursing. Students of various nursing schools and colleges rotate through our program as part of their public health education. When orienting these future nurses, parish nursing is presented as a non–hands-on approach to nursing; almost immediately, the student nurse's demeanor becomes awkward. This is because nurses are accustomed to doing versus being.

Acute loneliness is not a medical diagnosis; however, many suffer from this human condition. When asked what primary skills best serve the parish nurse and his or her clients, I respond "good listening skills." In listening, we can become a healing presence to each person. We become the health counselor, advocate and link to community resources and services, and a minister of health to the churches within the parish community.

The most challenging services of the parish nurse are to teach preventative medicine and supervise volunteers. With well-trained and committed volunteers, the parish nurse can serve as a resource and refuge for volunteer services. By being available to volunteers and their pastors, the parish nurse can combine and ally both in the needs of the parish community.

We have established a 9-week certificate program (Faith and Action Training Program), with a full-time program coordinator and a qualified professional faculty. Pastors of faith communities are invited to send their volunteers to learn skills in commitment, confidentiality, listening, and when to refer.

Serving the people in a holy and holistic manner is to me the essence of the parish nurse.

Anna M. "Pat" Dougherty, RN
Pat Dougherty is trained in clinical pastoral education and is a certified chaplain in the National Association of Catholic Chaplains. For the past 5 years, she has been the parish nurse coordinator at Saint Agnes Medical Center, Philadelphia, Pennsylvania, serving the churches of South Philadelphia.

Chapter 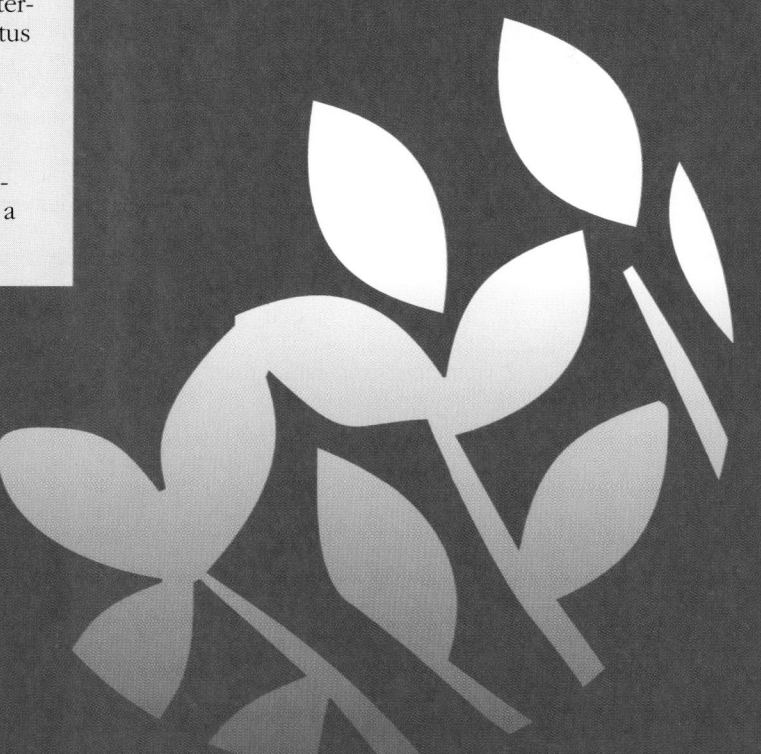 33

KEY TERMS

♦

anxiety
crisis
locus of control

self
self-concept
self-esteem

LEARNING OBJECTIVES

♦

After reading this chapter, you should be able to

♦ Define self

♦ Discuss the development of stress in an individual

♦ Identify and discuss the elements that constitute one's self-concept

♦ Discuss high and low self-esteem and factors that contribute to each

♦ Discuss the effects of anxiety on clients' thoughts, feelings, and behavior

♦ Discuss crisis and describe how nursing intervention can prevent a change in health status from developing into a crisis

♦ Define self-sustaining and self-enhancing goals

♦ Use the nursing process effectively with clients to support self-esteem and encourage a positive self-concept

SELF-ESTEEM AND SELF-CONCEPT

♦

LINDA WILLIAMSON PEREZ,
RNC, MS, CS, NP

I have said that the soul is not more than the body,
And I have said that the body is not more than the soul.
And nothing, not God, is greater to one than one's
self is.

—Walt Whitman

Who am I? This excellent and ageless question is asked by individuals throughout their lives. What is my purpose? What should I be doing? Does my living, my suffering, my dying mean something? What does it mean? Each individual struggles to find his or her own answers.

Why should nurses concern themselves with understanding their clients' self-concept? What difference does it make to the nurse if the client's level of self-esteem is high or low? How does the nurse's self-concept influence the way the nurse practices his or her profession? A careful reading of this chapter will provide answers to these questions.

Self

Before discussing self-concept and self-esteem, it is important to have an understanding of what the term *self* means.

When someone says "I am in charge" or "I will be there" or "I like the color green," that person is talking about someone who is distinct from others. "I" am not you or them or even us. Each person is, in a fundamental way, a separate entity. The self is a conception of one's own person, distinguished from other objects in the external world, as a separate whole being (Haber et al., 1987). Although people are to greater and lesser degrees interdependent and connected with others, each person can distinguish himself or herself from others.

Developmental research has revealed that infants do not have the ability to distinguish themselves from their primary caregivers. The infant exists as a tiny universe unto itself. Everything the baby sees, feels, and hears is the baby. Around 11 months of age, the infant begins to realize that it is separate and sometimes alone. The fear that this realization engenders is relieved when the primary caregiver comes back (see Chapter 16).

By the age of 2 years, children relish their individuality and pepper their speech liberally with "I do it" and "Mine!" As children grow, learn, and develop, they realize how they are connected to others (*e.g.,* membership in a family, cultural heritage, citizenship, neighborhood) yet how distinct they remain. As is discussed in Chapter 36, individuality and uniqueness are valued quite highly in some cultures, whereas connection and loyalty to one's family and society are prized in others. Nurses need to know and respect the cultural values of their clients, even if they don't readily understand or agree with them.

Another useful way to define self is to say that one's self is who one is. By early adulthood, most people have developed a characteristic response pattern that is fairly stable. Even with mere acquaintances, one can usually tell if they are acting "out of character." A person knows if an article of clothing or piece of furniture is "not me," because it is not in that person's typical pattern of responses to buy something in that style or price range. **Self,** then, can be defined as the total of one's characteristic response patterns, which includes what one does and how one does it, along with physical attributes—in short, everything that makes a person unique.

Self-Concept

If self is who one is, then what is self-concept? **Self-concept** is who one thinks he or she is. The self-concept has four aspects: body image, personal identity, role performance, and interpersonal competence.

Body Image

Body image is the mental idea a person has of his or her body. A person's body image is based on past as well as present experience. Body image consists of one's assessment of how one appears, functions, and feels.

✦ **Appearance.** How do I look? What do I look like? I look big, small, scarred, attractive, plain. A person's body image can be an accurate or an inaccurate assessment of his or her actual appearance. Most people have a fairly accurate sense of what they look like. A minor discrepancy between how a person really looks and how that person thinks he or she looks is usually not a problem. Severe distortions in body image, however, can have life-threatening consequences, as in the disorder anorexia nervosa. People with this condition perceive themselves to be grossly overweight when in fact they are emaciated. This inaccurate perception leads them to further starve themselves.

✦ **Functioning.** Does my body do what I need it to do? Does it move when I want it to? Does it excrete waste effectively and discreetly? Is my body separate from and subordinate to my mind? Does my body need and deserve care, including food, rest, and exercise, or do I take for granted that my body will do what I want it to do when I want to do it? The way a person answers these questions is a strong indication of what his or her body image is.

✦ **Feeling.** Does my body hurt? Do I feel weak and tired, or strong and energetic? Am I angry at my sick or disabled body for betraying me, or am I angry at myself for perhaps neglecting or abusing my body? These components of body image can and do assume different priorities at different ages and under changing circumstances. For example, an 8-year-old may be most concerned with how fast he or she can run (functioning). At age 16, the young woman or man may be most interested in how attractive she or he is to others (appearance). At any age, a person with a health problem may be preoccupied with the presence of signs and symptoms (function, appearance, and feeling).

Personal Identity

Personal identity is how we know ourselves. In most situations, people know what they like, whom and what they dislike, what they are good at, and what they need and want. Personal identity may fluctuate, but most adults have a solid sense of what they can expect from themselves. "I'm not myself" is a phrase we use when we have behaved uncharacteristically.

An individual's locus of control is part of his or her personal identity. **Locus of control** refers to who or what a person believes is in control of his or her life, circumstances, and environment (Haber et al., 1987). A person who has an *internal locus of control* believes that what happens in his or her life is determined primarily by his or her own actions. "I make things happen. I can usually prevent bad things from happening to me, but if something should go wrong, I can probably fix it." Someone who has an *external locus of control* believes that fate, chance, authority figures, or something else, outside of himself or herself, is responsible for what happens. "Things happen to me. It doesn't matter what I do. What will be will be, and I can't do a thing about it."

This aspect of self-concept is particularly important with regard to a person's health care–seeking and health-promoting behaviors. People who view the world as a challenge, who view themselves as in control, and who have a commitment to themselves seem to stay healthier under stress than people with the reverse traits (Ornstein & Swencionis, 1990) (Fig. 33–1). Consider the person who has had a heart attack. An individual with an internal locus of control is more likely to adjust his or her diet, level of activity, and methods of handling stress than is a person with an external locus of control, who may attribute his or her health problems to bad luck, a lousy job, or a demanding family.

Role Performance

An individual's role and the way he or she fulfills them are important parts of self-concept. People learn which roles are open to them and which ones they are expected to accept from their families and cultural groups and the society they live in. Each individual occupies several roles (consecutively and simultaneously) throughout his or her lifetime. Some of these roles are dependent on age and stage of life (*e.g.,* baby of the family, eldest child, grandfather, widow). Other roles depend on ability, inclination, and preparation (*e.g.,* professional nurse, family caregiver, wage earner). The priority assigned to the various roles an

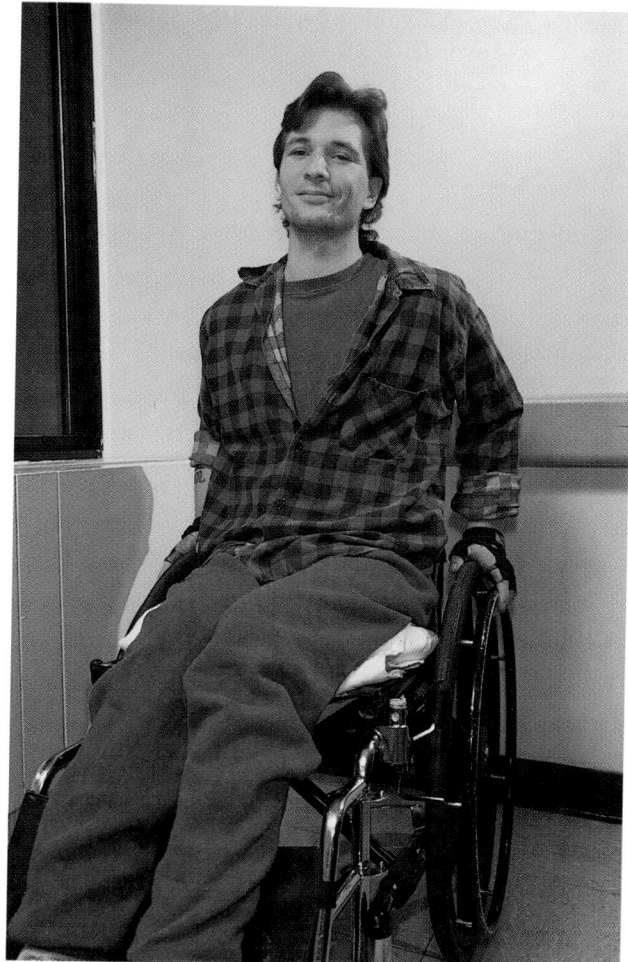

✦ **Figure 33–1**
People with an internal locus of control view the world as a challenge and see themselves as in control, despite crises and setbacks.

individual fulfills varies with time and circumstances. For example, the father of an infant may consider his role as sole financial support of his family to be more crucial than his role as a caregiver for the infant while the child's mother is on maternity leave. When the mother returns to work, the father may have to assume more responsibility for the child's care and therefore view his caregiver role as having gained importance.

Interpersonal Competence

The interpersonal competence aspect of self-concept is a person's assessment of how successful he or she is in relationships with other people. People define "success" in relationships differently. An individual who believes that success means being in control in a relationship will judge himself or herself to be successful if he or she is in control of most relationships. An individual who views being cared for as the best part of a relationship will feel successful in relationships in which he or she is cared for. A person who prefers to be the caretaker in relationships with others is likely to have difficulty accepting care and therefore poses a special challenge for nurses.

Self-Esteem

Self-esteem can be defined as what one thinks of oneself, how a person evaluates his or her worth. A person who has a positive opinion of himself or herself is said to have high self-esteem. This individual's self-concept may include less than perfect assessments, however, such as, "I look skinny" or "I'm not a good athlete" or "I'm disorganized." A person can still have high self-regard if he or she recognizes other strengths and talents and can accept being imperfect. Positive feelings about oneself facilitate involvement in relationships with others, motivate one toward achievement, and provide one with a sense of worth and power (Corkille-Briggs, 1975).

Those who do not hold themselves in high regard are said to have low self-esteem. Low self-esteem results when there is a large discrepancy between a person's ideal self (who a person thinks he or she should be) and self-concept (who a person thinks he or she is). When the ideal self is a glorified vision that is unrealistic and unattainable, the individual will have negative feelings and incorporate these into the self-concept: "I am an ineffective and unsuccessful person."

Self-esteem is how a person feels about himself or herself, an overall self-judgment, a reflection of how much he or she likes his or her particular person (Corkille-Briggs, 1975). An individual's self-judgment influences creativity, integrity, stability, and the use made of aptitudes and abilities. An individual's self-esteem is an evaluation of the self-concept (Fig. 33–2). Keep in mind that although most people have days when they don't like themselves very much, self-esteem is usually consistent for an individual and is based on positive reflections received as a child from significant adults. Self-esteem is actually a filter through which the person views himself or herself. A person with low self-esteem can even view an achievement as a failure. For such an individual, winning second prize is the same as losing. Self-esteem is not forged for all time, although once established, it is not easily disturbed (Corkille-Briggs, 1975).

Development of Self-Concept

In Chapters 15–19, theories of development and family interaction are discussed in detail. Harry Stack Sullivan, a theorist who paid particular attention to the development of the self, postulated that the self develops in relation to social norms and behavior patterns. Significant others serve as intermediaries between the

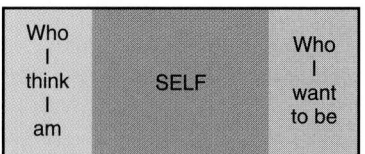

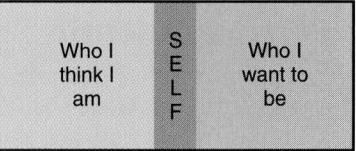

✦ **Figure 33–2**
A person's self-esteem is affected by who he or she wants to be and who he or she thinks he or she is.

person and the culture (Sullivan, 1953). The primary influences in the development of the self are parents and siblings. Extended family members also affect the child's developing sense of self. Later on, teachers and other community members contribute to the child's development. The developing person's perception of the verbal and nonverbal responses of others, the actual responses of others, and the person's internalization of these perceived responses contribute to the nascent self (Fig. 33–3). The mechanism by which a child's self-concept and self-esteem are developed through interactions with the people around him or her is captured in this well-known poem.

Children Learn What They Live

If a child lives with criticism he learns to condemn.
If a child lives with hostility he learns to fight.
If a child lives with ridicule he learns to be shy.
If a child lives with shame he learns to feel guilty.
If a child lives with tolerance he learns to be patient.
If a child lives with encouragement he learns confidence.
If a child lives with praise he learns to appreciate.
If a child lives with security he learns to have faith.
If a child lives with approval he learns to like himself.
If a child lives with acceptance and friendship he learns to find love in the world.
                        —Copyright ©1972 Dorothy Law Nolte

A person's self-concept remains fairly stable but is subject to modification as the environment and personal situation change. Changes in health, particularly illness with or without hospitalization, can affect a person's self-concept dramatically.

Why should nurses be concerned with the self-concept and self-esteem of their clients? The client's self-concept and level of self-esteem strongly influence his or her response to health problems. The mental self-image that the client has determines his or her ability and willingness to participate in his or her own care and make the best use of the resources available. Although an accurate self-concept and high level of self-esteem are valuable assets any time, they are especially so when a person is coping with the demands of illness, hospitalization, and medical treatment.

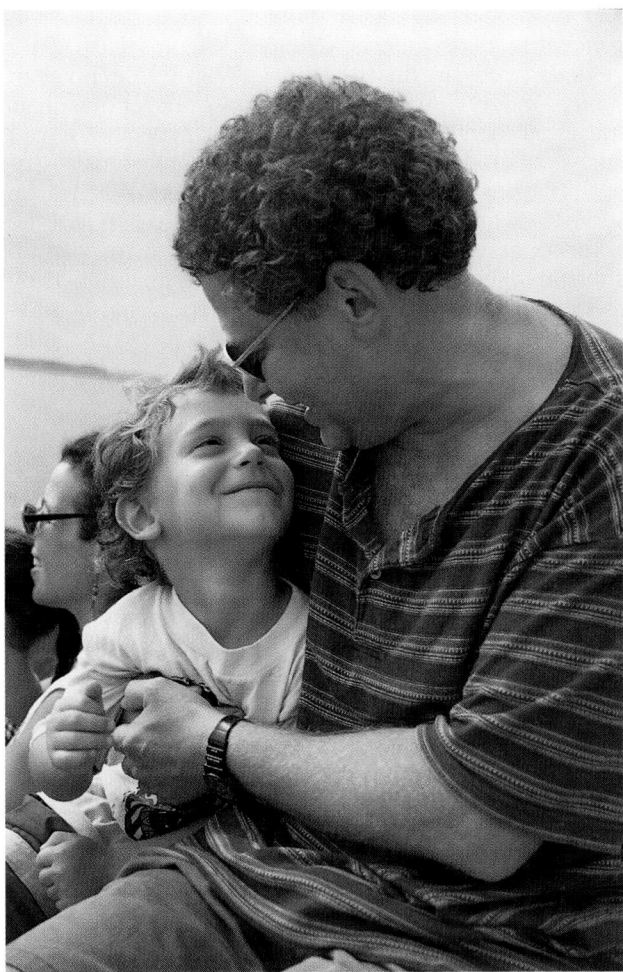

🌿 **Figure 33–3**
Parents are a primary influence on the development of a child's self-concept. Security, praise, and affection contribute to a positive self-concept.

Self-Concept and Self-Esteem in Elders

Supporting the self-concept and self-esteem of elderly clients is especially challenging and rewarding for nurses. Although illness and hospitalization can be harrowing for anyone, these experiences pose a tremendous threat to the self-esteem and self-concept of elders.

Loss is a predominant theme in characterizing the emotional experiences of older people (Butler & Lewis, 1986). This is easily understood when one looks at the changes that elders are compelled to deal with: loss of spouse, loss of friends, decline in health, less financial security, and so forth. Most elders adjust to these losses with grace and wisdom. Acute or chronic illness, however, can mean additional losses, such as loss of stamina, mobility, sexual potency, and memory. A lifetime of achievements, relationships, joys, and sorrows can be masked by sudden or progressive health problems. To make matters worse for

elderly clients, many health care professionals are "ageist," or prejudiced against old people. These health care providers assume that older adults are confused, unintelligent, or perhaps worst of all, cute, and treat them as if they were dull, wrinkled children. Nurses can assess their own ageist attitudes and correct them by doing the following exercise:

> Memorize the following brief directions and close the book. Don't open the book until you have completed the exercise.
>
> Write the word ELDERLY in large letters on a piece of paper. Then write down the first ten words that come to mind when you hear and see that word. When you've finished, turn the paper over. Now take a fresh piece of paper and write the word ELDER in large letters. Now write down the first ten words that come to

COMMUNITY-BASED CARE

ROLE REVERSAL

Role reversal is often a concern for older couples. When his or her spouse becomes ill or disabled, a husband or wife may face new responsibilities. For example, if the husband can no longer manage the family's finances or drive, the wife may have to deal with the checking account, taxes, and decisions about investments, lawn work, household repairs, and transportation. On the other hand, if a wife cannot manage her responsibilities, her husband may be faced with cooking, washing, ironing, planning meals, and shopping for groceries. Assuming responsibility for unfamiliar tasks can cause tremendous stress for older people who are already coping with added caretaking burdens and may have physical and memory problems of their own.

The nurse may suggest community services to assist older people who are dealing with unfamiliar responsibilities:

1. Resource directory: Refer to the community service guide and United Way listing in the telephone book.

2. Finances: Bank employees can teach clients about managing their accounts. Local volunteers (*e.g.,* Area Agency on Aging [AAA]) may assist with tax and other financial questions. A financial advisor can help with investment accounts.

3. Senior services: AAA, other local organizations, and churches may offer chore services, lawn care, and housekeeping at a reasonable cost. They may provide free or reduced-cost transportation.

4. Health care and respite: Home care agencies provide homemakers, home care aides, and companions to assist with housekeeping, personal care, and meals.

5. Meals: Most communities offer mobile meals; call United Way.

6. Support groups: Many groups are available. Consider "friendly visitor programs" that offer phone support.

mind when you see and hear the word ELDER. Now compare the lists.

Most people associate the word elderly with words like frail, irritable, sick, confused, and stubborn; in contrast, associations with the word elder include words such as wise, adviser, counselor, and respected. Perhaps some older clients are cranky, irritable, and helpless. What changes in their self-concept and self-esteem might result if they were treated like elders? What can nurses do to enhance the "elder status" of their clients? The accompanying box provides a summary of interventions designed to do just that.

Anxiety

Anxiety is the feeling of pervasive dread associated with a threat to the self-concept. By its very nature, a

---

ASSISTING ELDERS TOWARD IMPROVED SELF-ESTEEM

* Address your clients as Mr., Mrs., Miss, or Ms. and their surnames, unless they request that you call them by another name. These titles convey respect, whereas endearments such as grandma, grandpa, and sweetie do not.

* Find out as much as you can about your clients. Talk with them about what they do or did for a living. If your client is retired, talk about his or her hobbies and favorite pastimes. Your client will feel valued and supported, and you can learn a great deal from those who have "been there and done that."

* Listen actively to your clients' stories. Elders are generous with their lives when they know that a nurse is really interested. Illness and medical treatment can be so stressful and overwhelming that it's hard to remember life BMD (before my diagnosis). When your clients talk about their lives with you—their joys and sorrows, their achievements and regrets—you have the opportunity to remind them of what they've accomplished. You can and should express your admiration for what your clients have done and endured and your confidence that they will get the help they need to cope with their present problems.

* Encourage elders to make their own choices about the times and types of nursing care they receive. Allow plenty of time to provide care to your older clients. This may mean giving them care after you have completed caring for your younger clients. Trying to rush an elder is frustrating for the nurse and anxiety provoking for the client, so don't do it.

---

real or perceived health problem threatens the self-concept in all its aspects. Clients ask themselves: Will I be disfigured by this treatment? Will I lose my hair (body image)? Must I undress in front of strangers (personal identity)? Will I be able to enjoy the things I enjoyed before becoming ill (function, personal identity, role performance)? Will I still be me? Will I even survive? What about my customary roles? Will I be able to parent my child and make love to my partner after this illness or treatment? Will I be abandoned by or be a burden to those I love (interpersonal competence)? Will the nurses and doctors recognize how important I am? Do I still deserve respect and consideration? Will they listen to me and take what I say seriously, or must I just do what I'm told to do?

Usually, the client does not have the answers to these questions; perhaps no one does. In this case, the person can experience serious threats to his or her self-concept. The level of anxiety experienced depends on how serious the perceived threat is, how important the threatened aspects of the self-concept are to the individual, and how much of his or her self-esteem depends on those aspects.

CASE STUDY   **Mrs. Lewis Feels Worthless**

Mary Lewis, a 65-year-old widowed grandmother, had a stroke that left her with right hemiparesis. Mrs. Lewis has become increasingly anxious during her hospitalization having difficulty sleeping, crying spells, and complaints of nervousness. She confides to the nurse that because she cannot babysit for her daughter's children anymore, she is of no use to anyone. Mrs. Lewis's primary concerns are her perceived change in role, interpersonal competence, and personal identity rather than her appearance and loss of function related to hemiparesis.

Anxiety, which is always a result of a real or perceived threat to the self-concept, affects the way a person thinks, feels, and functions. *Trait anxiety* refers to the level of anxiety that an individual experiences even when not acutely stressed. A person's level of trait anxiety is the usual degree to which his or her self-concept is threatened. A person who often feels nervous or whom others might describe as "high-strung" has a high level of trait anxiety. *State anxiety* is the anxiety that a person experiences in a situation that poses a specific threat, such as a physical examination or a nursing final examination. Clearly, a person who has a high level of trait anxiety will be more uncomfortable when confronted with a situation that provokes state anxiety, such as illness or medical treatment, than someone who has a low level of trait anxiety.

Mild anxiety leads to a sense of vigilance and alertness, during which the individual is open to the environment and takes in information and processes it fairly accurately. In fact, mild anxiety may be beneficial. Mild anxiety about cervical cancer causes many women to have gynecological examinations and Pap smears, as recommended by their primary care providers. A woman who experiences moderate anxiety when she experiences unusual vaginal bleeding will probably call her physician and request an appointment as soon as possible. In its most severe form, however, anxiety can lead to crippling panic.

CASE STUDY | **Mrs. Green Ignores Irregular Vaginal Bleeding**

Janet Green, a 43-year-old married mother of two, first noticed irregular vaginal bleeding 6 months ago. She has been experiencing pain when having intercourse and bleeding afterward. Mrs. Green's mother died at age 35 of what was described to her as "female problems." Mrs. Green hasn't told anyone about her symptoms. Her last gynecological examination and Pap smear were 15 years ago as part of her postpartum checkup. Lately, Janet has been telling her husband and sister that she thinks she is going through menopause but denies any need for medical intervention. She confides this to a nurse at a blood pressure screening at her church.

Depending on the level of trait anxiety and the degree of threat to self-concept that a health problem poses, a client may experience mild to panic levels of anxiety. A moderately anxious person experiences alterations in thinking, feeling, and functioning and probably experiences one or more of the physiological manifestations of anxiety listed in Box 33–1. These symptoms are the result of activation of the autonomic nervous system, which accompanies anxiety. As a person's anxiety level increases, the alterations in thinking, feeling, and functioning and the physiological manifestations usually become more profound.

Nurses must remember that the more anxious a person is, the more difficulty he or she will have in concentrating and attending to the environment. This difficulty in concentration is the foundation of the alterations in thinking (including memory, perception, and judgment), feeling, and functioning that so many clients have.

CASE STUDY | **Mr. Rowan Forgets to Collect His Urine**

The nurse asks Gerald Rowan to save his urine so that it can be collected for 24 hours. She explains the rationale for this and shows him the container, reminding him once more before leaving the room. When she returns, she finds that Mr. Rowan has saved none of his urine; furthermore, he categorically denies that she ever mentioned anything to

---

> **Box 33–1**
>
> ## COGNITIVE, AFFECTIVE, BEHAVIORAL, AND PHYSIOLOGICAL MANIFESTATIONS OF ANXIETY
>
> **Cognitive**
> Difficulty concentrating
> Impaired memory
> Perceptual alterations—time and situation
> Impaired judgment
> Lack of insight
> Hypervigilance/suspicion
>
> **Affective**
> Anger
> Irritability
> Tearfulness
> Fear
>
> **Behavioral**
> Restlessness
> Agitation
> Easily startled
> Hyperventilation
> Flight
> Rapid speech
> Physical tension
>
> **Physiological**
> Rapid pulse
> Diaphoresis
> Shortness of breath
> Faintness
> Diarrhea, nausea
> Chest pain
> Lump in throat
> Gasping/sighing
> Urinary frequency
> Abdominal pain

him about saving it, "although you're always ordering me around."

The nurse recognizes that Mr. Rowan does not remember her instructions because his high level of anxiety prevented him from concentrating on what she was telling him. In this situation, the nurse could review the rationale for saving the urine and write down any special instructions to leave with him. A question about his work or family may give him a way to relax and think about something other than his illness. Then before leaving, the nurse could post discreet signs in the bathroom and on the urinal to help Mr. Rowan remember.

An anxious person's perception of time can be inaccurate. Someone who is in pain may tell a caregiver that she called for pain medication an hour ago when it has only been 10 minutes. This inaccurate perception of the passage of time is likely related to the level of anxiety combined with physical discomfort.

Anxiety also affects the *client's mood.* He or she may be angry, irritable, and demanding or withdrawn and depressed. The nurse may bear the brunt of the person's angry feelings, simply because he or she is there most of the time with the client. The nurse should remember that anger that is out of proportion to the circumstances is often an indication of the client's level of anxiety and is nothing personal. This awareness makes it easier for the nurse to intervene professionally and effectively with an angry client.

| CASE STUDY | **Mr. Baker Lashes Out After Genital Surgery** |

Lucy Modesto, RN, enters Jared Baker's room and brightly says, "Good morning." Mr. Baker, a 22-year-old man who had an orchiectomy the day before, replies, "It would be a good day if I were still a man." Mr. Baker refuses to look at his dressing or assist in washing his genital area. When Ms. Modesto suggests that Mr. Baker should stop being so pessimistic, he screams at her to leave the room and uses profane language to describe Ms. Modesto and all the nursing staff. Ms. Modesto calmly states that she can see that he is upset and will return shortly to see if he wants to talk about what is bothering him.

In this situation, the nurse's first response to the client was dismissive of his concerns. She quickly realized that her client was very angry, and her subsequent response showed respect for his feelings as well as her own. Ms. Modesto realized that she was too upset to interact effectively with her client. Her comment showed her concern for him and her willingness to help him at a later time.

| CASE STUDY | **Mr. Rodriguez Is Diagnosed With Diabetes** |

Miguel Rodriguez, a 55-year-old obese, newly diagnosed diabetic, curses and throws his lunch tray on the floor. Jane King, his primary nurse, asks, "What made you upset, Mr. Rodriguez?" Mr. Rodriguez replies that he can't believe that he will have to live on such small portions of food for the rest of his life.

By listening to Mr. Rodriguez's feelings, the nurse shows understanding for the frustration he feels. The nurse may inquire about how Mr. Rodriguez usually copes with problems he faces and try to draw parallels to this current problem. Expressions of praise and respect for the client's efforts can reinforce and motivate the client.

After assessing the impact of his illness on his self-concept, the nurse might refer Mr. Rodriguez to a registered dietitian who can help him identify foods he likes and new ways to prepare them. It is also useful to draw the family into a discussion of favorite foods or basic ethnic food items, to give him support in moving toward a healthier diet. Arranging follow-up with a home care agency is important to reinforce teaching done in the stressful hospital environment.

Because anxiety has such a profound impact on how a person feels and thinks, it always affects his or her behavior. In many cases, people who act out of anxiety may be embarrassed by their behavior. In such cases, anxiety leads to behavior that further threatens the self-concept and can lead to even more anxiety. The nurse needs to focus on the client's feelings and express understanding and a willingness to help. Expressing irritation and anger at a client's behavior may heighten the person's anxiety, leading to even more inappropriate behavior.

Crisis

Crisis is a state of disequilibrium that results when a person is confronted with a hazardous circumstance that, for the time being, he or she can neither escape nor solve with customary problem-solving resources (Caplan, 1964). Crises are usually precipitated by situations related to real or perceived loss, such as illness or a change in status or responsibilities. The term *maturational crisis* refers to an event that is related to normal growth and development. Maturational crises are usually predictable: the first day of kindergarten, adolescence, new parenthood, retirement. *Situational crises* are events that are precipitated by unanticipated stressors such as illness (with or without treatment), death of a loved one, or any physical or psychological trauma. A person who is undergoing a maturational crisis may also experience a situational crisis. For example, a boy who was first diagnosed with diabetes mellitus when he was 8 years old may be compliant with treatment until his teenage years. Then he may rebel, because being among peers and being able to act like others is important at this stage of life.

Not all health problems precipitate crises. Although a crisis is never pleasant, if successfully negotiated, it can actually lead to a higher level of functioning, an enhanced self-concept, a higher level of self-esteem, and decreased levels of anxiety.

Aguilera and Messick's (1982) model of crisis assessment proposes that a person who has adequate situational support, an accurate perception of the precipitating event, and effective coping mechanisms will be able to deal with and perhaps grow through the experience (Fig. 33–4). The lack of these balancing

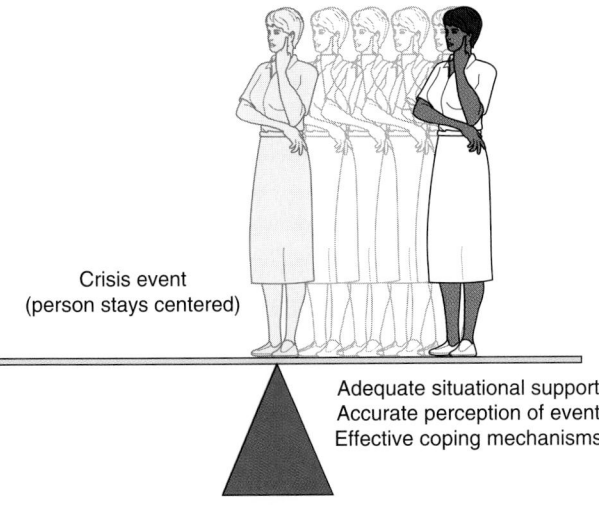

Crisis event
(person stays centered)

Adequate situational support
Accurate perception of event
Effective coping mechanisms

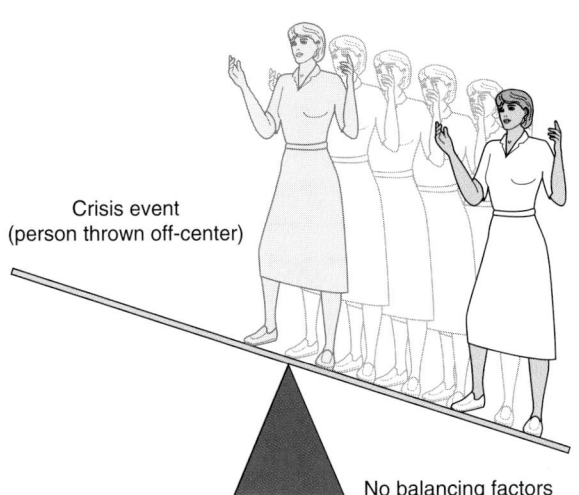

Crisis event
(person thrown off-center)

No balancing factors

✦ **Figure 33–4**
Balancing factors can help a person stay centered in a crisis situation. A realistic perception of the crisis and support from others will help the person cope.

factors predicts a crisis for which more intensive interventions may be necessary.

Application of the Nursing Process in Relation to a Client's Self-Concept

Assessment

The assessment of a client's self-concept, level of self-esteem, and level of anxiety is done at the same time as the basic nursing assessment. It is important to note that if the nurse wants the client to reveal himself or herself, the nurse's "self" must really be present. If the nurse appears rushed or distracted, the client will not reveal the personal information needed to make a thorough and accurate assessment. Whether the assessment is being performed in the client's home, a clinic, a same-day surgery suite, or a hospital room, the nurse identifies himself or herself by name and shakes the client's hand. It is important to make eye contact, to relate in a calm manner, and to practice active listening. Speech must be clear and slow enough to be understood.

❧ **Assess Who the Client Is—Self.** Note the client's reactions during the interview. How does the client relate to family and significant others? Who is the client most concerned about? Does the client defer to relatives for answers to questions? Does the client appear relaxed or nervous? Is he or she talkative or reticent? Does the client ask for clarification when necessary or seem overly compliant? What does he or she do for a living? Where does he or she live, and with whom? Observe the client's appearance. Is his or her grooming meticulous, adequate, or careless? Attention to these details gives the nurse a sense of the characteristic response patterns of this individual. As in every assessment, the process is continuous, and the nurse's understanding of the client becomes richer after each interaction.

❧ **Assess Who the Client Thinks He or She Is— Self-Concept, Body Image.** What is the client's mental picture of himself or herself, and how accurate is that perception? Ask for the client's weight and height before weighing and measuring him or her. Ask if there are parts of the body that the client would like to change.

❧ **Personal Identity.** Notice what surrounds the client at home or what he or she has brought to the hospital. Books, religious articles, photographs, handcrafts, trophies, and so forth reveal what this person values about himself or herself. The toys, games, and clothing that children and adolescents have can reveal who they are. Ask the person what he or she likes to do, what he or she does well. Find out what the client usually does when he or she doesn't feel well. Ask if there is anything the nursing staff should know to help take care of the client. Listen to the client describe his or her health problems to determine whether the client has an internal or external locus of control. Did this illness just happen? Can the client aid in his or her recovery or take complete responsibility for it? Does the client think that nothing that he or she does will have an impact on his or her recovery and that the only option is to wait and see what happens?

❧ **Role Performance.** Ask what the person would be doing if he or she weren't in the hospital or incapacitated at home. Are there any duties or obligations that he or she has not been able to fulfill since becoming ill? Is someone else fulfilling those roles, and if so, how well are they doing? Is the client worried that those substituting will do a poor job, or is the client more concerned that they will do a good job and that he or she will not be missed?

♦ **Interpersonal Competence.** Does it seem important to the client to make a good impression on the nurse, or does the client try to show the nurse that he or she is the boss and that the nurse works for him or her (or at least for the client's doctor)? Ask whether the client anticipates visitors or wants any restrictions on visitors or phone calls. This information provides a sense of how "attached" the client is to others.

Self-Esteem

It is not easy to assess an individual's self-esteem. A seemingly successful person may have a negative self-image because of unrealistic expectations. In contrast, a person who seems to be unsuccessful may be able to appreciate his or her talents and abilities and have a high level of self-esteem. The nurse should listen carefully to the client's spontaneous verbalizations regarding how he or she will cope with the current health problem. Statements such as "I'm not surprised, I must deserve this illness," or "What does it matter if I get well or not?" indicate low self-esteem.

Anxiety

During the interview and examination, the nurse is looking for the signs and symptoms of anxiety listed in Box 33–1. What parts of the nurse-client interaction seem to have provoked anxiety? Observe the client's physical responses and be aware of what is said and how it is said. Are the client's hands sweating? Does the client complain of frequent urination, stomach cramps, headache, or palpitations (exclusive of current health problems)?

Listen to the client's speech. Is it halting, rapid, slow, or disjointed? Does the client lose his or her train of thought easily or forget things the nurse just said? Does the client ask a lot of questions, or does the client expect the nurse and family members to take care of things? What does the client choose to talk about: job, children, concerns about pain, privacy, or prognosis? These spontaneous verbalizations give the nurse a good idea of which aspects of the self-concept are being threatened and how serious that threat seems to the client.

The nurse also needs to determine what the person's previous experience with health care providers has been. If the client is satisfied with the care received in the past, he or she will probably be less anxious than if there were unsatisfactory experiences with nurses and physicians.

It is important to assess for congruence of affect and thinking. Affect can easily be defined as the expression on a person's face. Usually an individual's facial expression is a fairly accurate reflection of what he or she is feeling and thinking. When someone tells a sad story, we expect that person to look sad. When

we hear a joke, we expect the person telling it to laugh along with us at the punch line. Incongruence of affect and thinking may indicate high levels of anxiety. In such a situation, the anxiety experienced by the person is so intense that it is unbearable, and the person cuts off the emotional response to the threat. Remember that a client who relates with indifference that he or she has a serious illness is probably acutely anxious.

Culture

In all assessments, be aware of cultural differences, and do not draw conclusions about the behav-

CULTURAL DIVERSITY AND SELF-ESTEEM/ SELF-CONCEPT

A basic working definition of culture is that it encompasses beliefs and behaviors that are learned and shared by members of a group (Galanti, 1991). The culture that a person is born into will have a strong influence on what he or she values. Your clients' self-esteem depends on how well they think they live up to the expectations and obligations that their cultural groups hold up as standards. Health problems can limit an individual's or a family's ability to fulfill a "cultural imperative" and cause a self-esteem disturbance. Consider the impact of the following situation on the client's self-esteem:

Large families are the rule and are considered both a blessing and an obligation in Orthodox Jewish communities. Susan Gold is a 20-year-old woman who developed complications during the delivery of her first child and required a hysterectomy. When the community health nurse visits the Gold home, she finds Susan tearful and anxious. She tells the nurse that she feels like a failure and that her whole life is ruined. Susan's mother tells the nurse that the whole family would like to be more supportive of Susan, but they don't know what to do to help her in this family tragedy. Susan's 20-year-old husband is so disappointed that he will not be able to father a large traditional family that he cannot even talk about it with his father and brothers.

Nursing Implications

The nurse should encourage Mrs. Gold's expression of her feelings without attempting to minimize her grief or suggesting that she be grateful for the healthy son she has. Her mother can be assisted in identifying coping mechanisms that the family has utilized when dealing with previous disappointments and pain and encouraged to try them in this situation. The family can be encouraged to seek out the support of their Rabbi and religious congregation. All highly developed cultures include mechanisms such as rituals, traditional teachings, and group support for dealing with personal suffering and loss. Experiencing the support of their cultural group can help the Golds reestablish their equilibrium and incorporate their "small family status" into their self-concepts in a healthy way.

ior of a person who comes from an ethnic or cultural group whose traditions are unfamiliar (see accompanying box and Chapter 36).

Nursing Diagnosis

There are several nursing diagnoses that relate to self-concept and self-esteem (see box). The following are common diagnoses that have already been illustrated in this chapter:

- Ineffective individual coping related to a high anxiety level, as evidenced by avoiding appropriate health care: Mrs. Green, the 43-year-old woman who has had irregular vaginal bleeding for 6 months and refuses to see her primary care provider, for fear that she will be diagnosed with terminal cancer.
- Decisional conflict related to maturational conflict, as evidenced by recent noncompliance with treatment: A teenage boy with insulin-dependent diabetes mellitus who becomes noncompliant with diet, exercise, and medication.
- Self-esteem disturbance related to effect of health problem on role performance: Mrs. Lewis, the 65-year-old woman who is no longer able to babysit for her grandchildren and says, "I'm of no use to anyone anymore."
- Anxiety related to serious illness, as evidenced by the client's difficulty in following simple directions: Mr. Rowan, the man who does not remember instructions to collect urine for 24 hours.
- Altered thought processes related to cumulative stress of injury, unfamiliar environment of hospital, and surgery, as evidenced by inaccurate perception of time: A client who reports that she had to wait an hour for pain medicine when in fact the nurse provided medication within 10 minutes of her call.
- Grieving related to real or perceived loss of function, beauty, and/or interpersonal competence: Mr. Baker, the 22-year-old man who says after an orchiectomy, "I'm not a man anymore."
- Knowledge deficit related to lack of accurate information: Mr. Rodriguez, the 55-year-old newly diagnosed morbidly

obese diabetic, who states, "I can't believe I'll have to eat such small portions for the rest of my life."
- Hopelessness related to lack of situational support: Mrs. Gold, the 20-year-old Orthodox Jewish woman 1 week after a hysterectomy, whose husband and other family members are unable to console and reassure her because of their own grief.

Planning

Nurses always involve clients in goal setting (see Nursing Care Plan 33–1). Nowhere is this more important than when working with clients who have self-concept and self-esteem disturbances and associated nursing diagnoses. Two categories of goals can be formulated: self-sustaining and self-enhancing goals.

❧ **Self-Sustaining Goals.** Self-sustaining goals are usually short term and refer to the safety and comfort of the client.

CASE STUDY	Mr. Lyons Has AIDS

Harry Lyons, a 34-year-old man who has been HIV-positive for 5 years, has just been told that his CD4 count is 100 and he now has AIDs. He is in the hospital for treatment of *Pneumocystis carinii* pneumonia and has told the nurse that he wants to kill himself and get it over with. His nursing diagnosis is Risk for self-injury related to serious illness, as evidenced by statement of suicidal intent. An appropriate self-sustaining goal for Mr. Lyons would be: Mr. Lyons will not harm himself while in the hospital.

CASE STUDY	Ms. DeMarco Needs to Lower Her Cholesterol

Carol DeMarco, a morbidly obese 47-year-old woman, learned last week that her cholesterol level is 400. Ms. DeMarco told the nurse that her mother died of a myocardial infarction at age 45 and that she was destined to "go the same way." The visiting nurse observes that Ms. DeMarco continues to consume a fatty diet and formulates the nursing diagnosis of Ineffective individual coping related to inaccurate perception of her condition. An appropriate self-sustaining goal is: Ms. DeMarco will express understanding of the need for a low-fat diet and decrease her fat intake.

❧ **Self-Enhancing Goals.** Self-enhancing goals relate to improved coping and improved self-esteem secondary to discovering previously unknown strengths and developing new coping mechanisms.

> ## NURSING DIAGNOSES RELATED TO SELF-ESTEEM AND SELF-CONCEPT
>
> Altered thought processes
>
> Anxiety
>
> Chronic low self-esteem
>
> Decisional conflict
>
> Grieving
>
> Hopelessness
>
> Ineffective individual coping
>
> Knowledge deficit
>
> Posttrauma response
>
> Powerlessness
>
> Self-esteem disturbance
>
> Situational low self-esteem

SAMPLE NURSING CARE PLAN

AN ADOLESCENT DIAGNOSED WITH INSULIN-DEPENDENT DIABETES

John Moss, a 15-year-old boy, was first diagnosed with insulin-dependent diabetes mellitus at the age of 8. Recently he has become noncompliant with his diet and blood glucose monitoring. He told the nurse that he didn't want to be different from the other kids anymore.

Nursing Diagnosis: Anxiety related to threat to personal identity and interpersonal competence, secondary to maturational crisis evidenced by the statement, "I'm tired of being different from everyone else."

Self-Sustaining Goal: John will comply with prescribed diet, exercise, blood glucose monitoring, and insulin administration.

Self-Enhancing Goal: John will acknowledge that his well-controlled diabetes does not interfere with his enjoyment of age-appropriate activities and relationships with others.

Action	Rationale
1. Encourage expression of feelings. Listen nonjudgmentally.	1. Establishes trust. Lecture-type education will further distance an adolescent client from the nurse.
2. Explore age-appropriate adjustment to client treatment plan with primary care provider and client (*e.g.*, additional exercise, decreased frequency of monitoring).	2. Flexibility and client input provide a sense of control and competence and enhance compliance.
3. Refer client to support group for diabetic teenagers.	3. Enhances personal identity and provides situational support. Client can learn new coping strategies from people in a similar situation.
4. Explore normal adolescent development with family members.	4. Clarifies family's misperceptions of client's behavior, thereby decreasing stress and anxiety for the entire family.

CASE STUDY | **Ms. Cruz Needs to Cope With Asthma**

Gloria Cruz, a 28-year-old single woman, was seen in the emergency department for treatment of an asthma attack. While there, she asks if the nurse knows anything about stress management for people with asthma. An appropriate self-enhancing goal for Ms. Cruz is: Ms. Cruz will attend stress management training and use techniques effectively.

Implementation

The client's plan of care depends on the nursing diagnoses and the client's individual goals. All interventions that support the positive aspects of the self-concept and decrease anxiety are appropriate.

Each interaction with the client is an opportunity to support his or her self-concept.

- Ask the client what he or she wants to be called, and address the client that way.
- Provide the level of nursing care that the person requires to be comfortable. For example, a client with chronic obstructive pulmonary disease who is out of bed may still need help bathing. Without that help, the client may feel unclean, uncomfortable, and helpless. The nurse's calm and patient manner lets the client know that he or she deserves care.
- Create a climate in which the client can tell that the nurse's concern is genuine. This can be accomplished by talking with the client about some of the personal facts he or she has shared about job, family, and so forth. Encourage the client to discuss thoughts and feelings.
- Make every effort to adjust the health care routine to the client's preferred routine. For example, if a business executive reads the newspaper each morning after breakfast and before bathing, plan to assist the client in bathing after he or she reads the paper. Accommodating the client's routine supports his or her personal identity.
- Ensuring a person's privacy, offering choices whenever possible, and encouraging the use of personal clothing, toiletries, and cosmetics are all helpful in supporting the individual's self-concept.
- The nurse's honest expression of admiration and respect for each client and family as they go through the process of illness, recovery, adjustment, or dying bolsters the client's and family's sense of competence and self-esteem.

A client who is overwhelmed by health problems and experiencing high levels of anxiety is in danger of experiencing a crisis. The nurse can help the client tap into or develop the balancing factors associated with crisis prevention or effective resolution by doing the following:

- Provide situational support. Encouraging the client to express feelings and being accessible and open to the client's requests and need for attention are not easy for the busy nurse. A caring attitude and a willingness to support the client can be conveyed during caregiving activities. Be honest with the client and don't make promises that may be impossible to keep, such as "I'll be right back" or "I'll be here as soon as you call me." A broken promise may destroy the trust the client has for the nurse and make it more difficult for the nurse to support the client.

- Promote an accurate perception of the event. The client needs to express his or her feelings and fears. The nurse who knows what the client's fears are can help the client distinguish these fears from the facts associated with the health problem. Clients and their families need accurate and adequate information if they are to avoid the anxiety that is associated with uncertainty and misinformation. The nurse who remembers that anxious people have trouble remembering will encourage the client to write down questions (and the answers to them) in a notebook to which the client and the family can refer.

- Encourage effective coping mechanisms. People come to the health care setting or system with a variety of experiences and coping mechanisms. The hospital or clinic environment is so different from what they are familiar with that they may assume that they have no repertoire of skills to call on to help them get through this experience. The nurse should ask the client what he or she usually does to cope with stress. If the client usually listens to music, encourage visitors to bring in a radio or tape player. Or if a client's sister is his closest support but he doesn't want to upset her by letting her know about his illness, the nurse may encourage the client to think about what his sister would want to know and how she would feel about being able to support him. The surgical client who prides himself on having a high tolerance for pain needs education about pain management in order to cope with the postoperative experience.

Additional client teaching tips are listed in Box 33–2.

Evaluation

The client must be continually reassessed during his or her relationship with the nurse. As the illness and treatment progress or the client's health status changes, self-concept and self-esteem may be threatened.

✦ **Self-Sustaining Goals.** The client should be safe and participating in his or her own care as much as possible. If the client's anxiety remains so high that it interferes with his or her ability to do so, the plan must be reevaluated and probably changed.

✦ **Self-Enhancing Goals.** If the self-enhancing goals have been achieved, the client will have an improved sense of his or her own competence and ability to

---

Box 33–2

CLIENT TEACHING TIPS

Client education is a lot trickier than you might think. Many nurses are frustrated because the time spent teaching seems like time wasted when so many clients just don't seem to "get it." To maximize the effectiveness of your client teaching, you should remember that client education is an ongoing process that may begin in the hospital but continues at home. Don't forget that anxiety affects a person's ability to concentrate and to absorb and remember information. The more anxious your client is, the less he or she will learn from you—unless you

- Schedule your teaching when your client is well rested and comfortable.

- Take your time. Present your information in a calm, unhurried manner. Expect that your client may have trouble understanding the material and go slowly. Give him or her time to ask questions, but don't be surprised if the client can't think of any, until you leave the room.

- Make the information easily accessible and understandable. If you know that your client can read and write, you can write the information down. Whether you have preprinted teaching sheets or just some clearly written notes you have made, go over the material with the client (in person) and then give it to the client so that he or she and family members can read it again and again. If your client is not fluent in English, make sure that your verbal and written instructions are well translated into the client's language. Use common sense in this area; avoid using well-meaning roommates, family members, or nonprofessional staff members as translators. Your client and your teaching are important and deserve accurate interpretation.

---

handle life's challenges. A person who has a diminished sense of self-esteem and confidence may require crisis intervention on an outpatient basis in a mental health clinic or private practitioner's office.

Summary

Nursing would be a much easier profession if all clients cooperated with their nurses' efforts to care for them. Instead, many of them are noncompliant, inattentive, withdrawn, disruptive, or rude. This chapter has provided a better understanding of why clients do the things they do.

A nurse who does not assess the effect that the client's condition has on his or her self-concept is bound to provoke the anger and frustration, or neglect the anxiety and fear, that the client is experiencing. A nurse who assesses the client's self-concept and self-esteem can plan care that is designed to keep anxiety to a minimum and promote a sense of competence and control.

■   ■

CHAPTER HIGHLIGHTS

✦

✦ The term self-concept refers to who a person thinks he or she is. The self-concept has four aspects: body image, personal identity, role performance, and interpersonal competence.

✦ An individual's self-concept and self-esteem influence his or her response to health problems.

✦ Any change in health status, such as acute illness, trauma, hospitalization, or disability, can be a threat to a person's self-concept.

✦ Anxiety is the result of one or more threats to the self-concept and may be associated with dysfunctional coping with health problems and the development of a crisis.

✦ Nurses can intervene in several ways to support the self-concept of their clients, decrease their anxiety, and decrease the likelihood of crisis development.

✦ Nurses formulate self-sustaining and self-enhancing goals with their clients who are experiencing disturbances in self-concept and self-esteem. Self-sustaining goals are usually short term and refer to the safety and comfort of the client. Self-enhancing goals relate to improved coping and self-esteem as a result of having discovered or developed previously unknown strengths and coping mechanisms.

Study Questions

1. A person experiencing a severe degree of anxiety related to a health problem can be expected to

   a. seek appropriate health care in a timely manner
   b. comply with prescribed treatment
   c. deny the problem and rationalize the presence of signs and symptoms
   d. complain about care provided

2. The client least likely to experience a crisis as a result of illness or injury is someone who

   a. is preoccupied with a maturational crisis
   b. has an external locus of control and little situational support
   c. has high levels of trait anxiety and low self-esteem
   d. has an internal locus of control and low levels of trait anxiety

3. George Donohue, a 79-year-old retired police detective, resides in a nursing home. He has mild dementia and loves to talk with people. He tells the nurse that he

doesn't feel important anymore. The intervention that is most likely to enhance Mr. Donohue's self-esteem is

   a. escorting him to the activity area, where he can join the residents playing the tambourine
   b. telling him how handsome he is for a man of his age
   c. encouraging him to talk about his days on the police force
   d. calling his out-of-state relatives and telling them to visit more often

4. Mary Lee is a registered nurse working in an area where the population is culturally diverse. It is important that she

   a. take anthropology courses to understand the cultures of all her clients
   b. provide the same care in the same way to all clients to promote fairness
   c. respect the values and health care practices of her clients and their families
   d. care for clients of her own or similar ethnic/racial background

5. Mr. Stern, a 55-year-old married, overweight businessman who smokes cigarettes, is brought by ambulance to the emergency department with crushing chest pain. Education about "heart smart" living is likely to be most effective if provided

   a. in the emergency department shortly after his arrival
   b. in the coronary care unit after his pain has subsided
   c. at home with his wife present
   d. at his first follow-up appointment with his cardiologist

Critical Thinking Exercises

1. Ms. S. is 4.5 months pregnant and married, with a history of one miscarriage. She is discharged to home with a diagnosis of "incompetent cervix." She is placed on bedrest and gains 60 lb during the pregnancy. Discuss the implications on her self-esteem.

2. Mr. G. is a 29-year-old Hispanic man admitted with a new spinal cord injury. He is refusing to eat. Discuss the impact of the injury on his self-concept and a plan to help him cope with the crisis.

References

Aguilera, D. C., & Messick, J. H. (1982). *Crisis intervention: Theory and methodology* (4th ed.). St. Louis: C. V. Mosby.

Butler, R., & Lewis, M., (1986). *Aging and mental health* (3rd ed.). Columbus, OH: Charles E. Merrill.

Caplan, G. (1964). *Principles of preventive psychiatry*. New York: Basic Books.

Corkille-Briggs, D. (1975). *Your child's self esteem*. Garden City, NY: Doubleday.

Galanti, G. A. (1991). *Caring for patients from different cultures*. Philadelphia: University of Pennsylvania Press.

Haber, J., et al. (1987). *Comprehensive psychiatric nursing* (3rd ed.). New York: McGraw-Hill.

May, R. (1950). *The meaning of anxiety*. New York: Ronald Press.

Miller, J. (Ed.). (1959). *Complete poetry and selected prose by Walt Whitman*. Boston: Houghton Miffin.

Ornstein, R., & Swencionis, C. (1990). *The healing brain, a scientific reader.* New York: Guilford Press.

Sullivan, H. S. (1953). *The interpersonal theory of psychiatry.* New York: W. W. Norton.

Bibliography

Bensink, G. W., et al. (1992). Institutionalized elderly; relaxation, locus of control, self esteem. *Journal of Gerontological Nursing, 18*(4), 30–36.

Duffy, M. E. (1993). Determinants of health promoting lifestyles in older persons. *Image, Journal of Nursing Scholarship, 25*(1), 23–28.

Erdos, D. (1992). Redefining identity when appearance is altered. *Dermatology Nursing, 4*(1), 41–46.

Field, L. K., et al. (1992). The relationship of internally directed behavior to self reinforcement, self esteem and expectancy values for exercise. *American Journal of Health Promotion, 7*(1), 21–27.

Fraiberg, S. H. (1959). *The magic years: Understanding and handling the problems of early childhood.* New York: Charles Scribner's Sons.

Greenblatt, F. (1992). Maintaining self esteem in long term care residents. *Journal of Long Term Care Administration, 20*(4), 78.

Heidrich, S. M., et. al. (1992). The role of self in adjustment to cancer in elderly women. *Oncology Nursing Forum, 19*(10), 1491–1496.

Hogstel, M. (Ed.). (1991). *Geropsychiatric nursing.* St. Louis: C. V. Mosby.

Hosking, P. (1993). Utilizing Roger's theory of self concept in mental health nursing. *Journal of Advanced Nursing, 18*(6), 980–984.

Killeen., M. R. (1993). Parent influences on children's self esteem in economically disadvantaged families. *Issues in Mental Health Nursing, 14*(4), 323–326.

King, G. A., et al. (1993). Self evaluation and self concept of adolescents with physical disabilities. *American Journal of Occupational Therapy, 47*(2), 13–40.

Le Mone, P. (1992). Analysis of a human phenomenon: Self concept. *Nursing Diagnosis, 3*(2), 48–53.

Medora, N. P., et al. (1993). Variables related to romanticism and self esteem in pregnant teenagers. *Adolescence, 28*(109), 155–170.

Misk, V. (1993). Body image in women treated for breast cancer. *Nursing Research, 42*(3), 153–157.

Muller, R. L., et al. (1992). The effect of leukemia and its treatment on self esteem in school age children. *Maternal Child Nursing Journal, 20*(304), 155–165.

O'Brien, M. T. (1993). Multiple sclerosis: The relationship among self esteem, social support and coping behavior. *Applied Nursing Research, 6*(2), 54–63.

Pletsch, P. K., et al. (1991). Self image among early adolescents: Revisited. *Journal of Community Health Nursing, 8*(4), 215–231.

Popkess-Varolter, S., et al. (1992). Compounded problem: Chronic low back pain and overweight in adult females. *Orthopaedic Nursing, 11*(6), 31–35.

Ramer, L. (1992). Self image changes with time in the cancer patient with a colostomy after operation. *Journal of Enterostomal Nursing, 19*(6), 195–203.

Satir, V. (1967). *Conjoint family therapy.* Palo Alto, CA: Science and Behavior Books.

Siegel, B. S. (1986). *Love, medicine and miracles.* New York: Harper & Row.

Smits, M. W., et al. (1992). Correlates of self care among the independent elderly: Self-concept affects well being. *Journal of Gerontological Nursing, 18*(9), 8–13.

Strauman, T. J., et al. (1993). Self discrepancy and natural killer cell activity; immunological consequences of negative self evaluation. *Journal of Personality and Social Psychology, 64*(6), 1042–1052.

SENSORY STIMULATION

LISA D. BRODERSEN, MA, CCRN

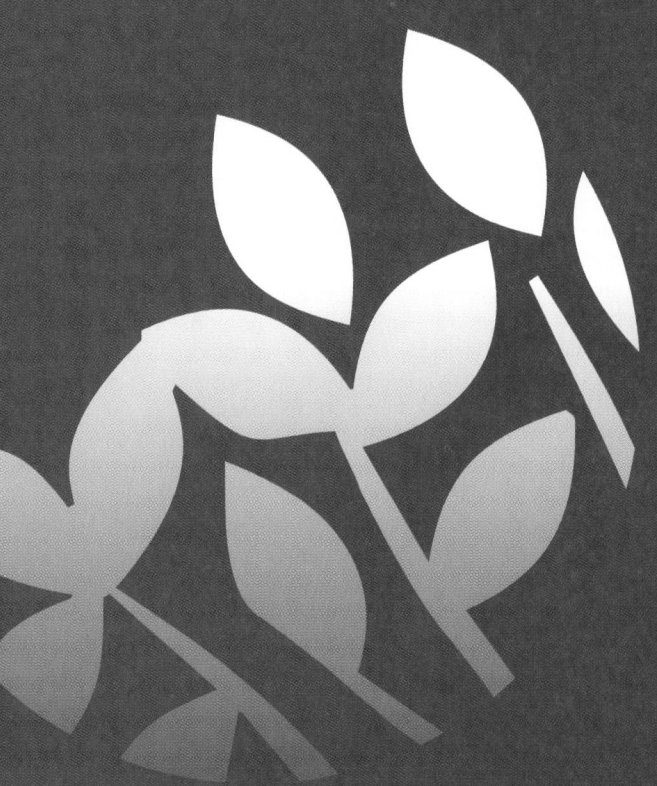

LEARNING OBJECTIVES

✦

After studying this chapter, you should be able to

✦ Define terms and discuss concepts related to sensory stimulation

✦ Explain the stimulus-response process

✦ Describe structures of the nervous system involved in the stimulus-response process

✦ Discuss factors that influence the effectiveness of human responses to stimuli

✦ Describe nervous system components involved in higher-level thought processes

✦ List barriers to accurate sensory perception

✦ Discuss the influence of physical and psychological maturity on human responses to stimuli

✦ Describe manifestations of altered sensory perception

✦ Develop nursing diagnoses, plan outcomes, and describe interventions for persons experiencing actual or potential alterations in sensory perception in the following situations: inadequate sensory stimulation, excessive stimuli, barriers to accurate sensory perception

The human body is subjected to multiple and varied stimuli at all hours of the day. Stimuli are events or changes that provoke or excite a nerve (Guyton, 1991). Stimuli are received by the central nervous system through sensory receptors. When a stimulus reaches a sensory receptor, it becomes an impulse and is routed to a specific area of the central nervous system, where it is interpreted and assigned meaning. This process is called perception. Perception influences a person's *response* to the stimulus (Guyton, 1991; Roy, 1984).

Responses are behaviors elicited by stimuli. Human responses are the result of physical and mental adjustments that promote adaptation to the internal and external environment. Adaptation to environmental stimuli is necessary for survival, growth, and development. The internal environment refers to all the structures, organ systems, and tissues inside the body and their functions. The external environment consists of the social and cultural systems we live in and interact with, including all people, living things, and objects in our world (Roy, 1984). The systems that constitute the internal and external environments are interdependent, with each system perpetually receiving and responding to stimuli from other systems and stimulating other systems as well.

Humans constantly interact with their internal and external environments, receiving and responding to a relentless barrage of stimuli. The stimulus-response interaction between human body systems enables humans to meet basic survival needs and maintain a stable internal environment. It also determines the extent to which humans use their physical and intellectual capabilities to modify and adapt to their external environment. Essentially, how people behave at each moment in time is the product of a continuous stimulus-response process.

It might seem that humans have little time to do anything but attend to each stimulus that their bodies are subjected to. Fortunately, the human nervous system takes care of many responses without requiring constant attention and awareness. Responses are either voluntary or involuntary. Voluntary responses require conscious awareness and decision-making. Putting on a jacket in response to feeling cold is a voluntary behavior. In contrast, involuntary responses occur automatically and do not require conscious awareness (Guyton, 1991; Roy, 1984). For example, no conscious decision is involved when blood vessels in the skin constrict and goose bumps form in response to cold. Breathing and eye blinking are other involuntary responses.

Human responses to stimuli depend on two basic conditions: the ability to receive the stimuli through body structures that enable seeing, hearing, smelling, tasting, feeling, and awareness of body position, and the ability to send information about the stimuli to parts of the nervous system that can process and interpret it before initiating behavior in response to those stimuli.

Going through the motions of living from day to day can become a problem if there is a sudden change in the character of the stimuli a person is normally subjected to, or if the person's ability to receive and respond to stimuli is altered. Each person has a unique range of tolerance for variations in the amount, intensity, and frequency of stimuli. When that range of tolerance is exceeded, the person must alter his or her usual response patterns in order to adapt to the change (Roy, 1984). For example, putting on a jacket in response to a cool breeze may be an effective adaptive response until the breeze becomes a strong wind or the environmental temperature drops. Eventually, vasoconstriction, goose bumps, and the jacket will not be enough to maintain a desired level of comfort and a stable body temperature. The person's body temperature will decrease, and shivering may occur. If further adaptive measures are not pursued (*e.g.*, putting on a hat and a warmer coat or seeking shelter), shivering may lead to metabolic abnormalities, and the person may become seriously ill.

◆ Response to Stimuli

Ineffective Response to Stimuli

Human responses are not always effective; in other words, the response does not necessarily promote survival or facilitate growth and development (Roy, 1984). Ineffective responses may result in injury, illness, loss of independence, increased health care expenses, or even death (Lipowski, 1990; Weddington, 1982; Williams *et al.*, 1985).

Ineffective or maladaptive responses are the result of sudden changes in the character of stimuli or alterations in the ability to perceive stimuli accurately (Gordon, 1990). These alterations produce barriers to accurate sensory perception. Barriers are similar to risk factors (*i.e.*, conditions or events that interfere with perception and response to stimuli). It is essential that nurses understand barriers to accurate sensory perception in order to provide interventions that promote the most effective responses (Carpenito, 1992).

Alterations in the Character of Stimuli

When the amount, intensity, and quality of stimuli exceed a person's range of tolerance, perception becomes impaired and adversely influences behavioral responses. In such situations, a person's senses are often deprived of certain stimuli and overloaded by other stimuli (Fig. 34–1). Too much or too little exposure to all types of stimuli may cause anxiety, fatigue, boredom, and confusion (Spies Pope, 1995).

Sensory deprivation and sensory overload refer to conditions in which the amount, intensity, and quality of sensory stimuli exceed a person's range of adapt-

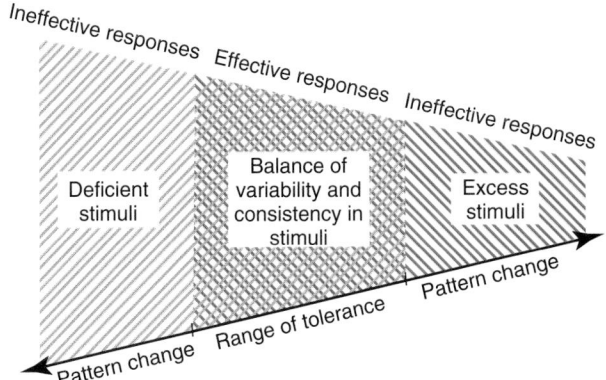

✦ Figure 34–1
If the amount, intensity, or quality of stimuli exceeds a person's tolerance, the person's perception becomes impaired. Overloaded by some stimuli and deprived of other stimuli, the person may become anxious, fatigued, bored, or confused.

ability, impair perception, and adversely influence responses (Roy, 1984). Sensory deprivation is the condition in which stimuli are deficient or meaningless and exceed a person's minimal level of tolerance. Sensory overload is the state of excessive stimulation that exceeds an individual's maximal level of tolerance (Gordon, 1991).

The quality and frequency of auditory, visual, tactile, olfactory, and proprioceptive stimuli influence the development of sensory deprivation and overload. Excessive auditory stimulation is often a factor in sensory overload. People depend on auditory stimuli for entertainment, information, and safety. Sounds in the environment warn of potential danger, provide reassurance, and bring enjoyment. However, sounds can be irritating and obnoxious as well. In an environment such as a hospital, noise frequently surpasses the Environmental Protection Agency's hospital noise-level recommendations (Halm & Alpen, 1993). Rest may be impossible for a hospitalized person who is subjected to the simultaneous sounds of device alarms, the hospital paging system, and staff conversations and routines.

As a person's senses are besieged by one type of excessive or obnoxious stimuli, other senses may simultaneously be deprived of stimuli. Immobility may restrict a person to limited and unvaried scenery. Illness separates the client from the social interaction and touch supplied by significant others. Other illness-related conditions may deprive the client of olfactory and gustatory stimuli provided by food and vegetation. A person who has had surgery for a gastrointestinal problem may have a nasogastic tube and restricted oral intake, which eliminates food as a source of stimuli. If the client requires critical care following surgery, even fresh flowers cannot provide olfactory stimuli, because most surgical intensive care units do not allow flowers owing to infection control restrictions. Refer to Box 34–1 for conditions and events that may precipitate sensory deprivation or sensory overload. ✦

Alterations in the Ability to Perceive Stimuli

For human responses to occur, stimuli must be received and processed by the nervous system. Stimuli reach the nervous system through sensory organs such as the ears, eyes, nose, tongue, and skin.

When sensory organs fail to deliver stimuli to the nervous system, auditory (sound), gustatory (taste), olfactory (odor), tactile (touch), and proprioceptive (body position) information may be missed. Sensory organ impairment occurs as a consequence of injury, illness, or aging. Loss of sensory information alters the context or scenario in which the sensory stimuli are received. That context is the basis for behavior, judgments, and decision-making (Warren, 1996). For example, when a person places his or her foot in water that is too hot, a reflex response occurs—the foot is quickly removed, even before the judgment is made that the water is too hot and cooler water must be added. If the same person has lost his or her sense of feeling in the extremities, the heat from the water is not perceived. Hence, the context of the situation is altered; no reflex withdrawal of the extremity from the water occurs, and a burn injury to the extremity results. When the ability to perceive stimuli is altered, appropriate adaptive responses are replaced by maladaptive responses. Box 34–2 contains examples of maladaptive and adaptive responses caused by alterations in sensory perception.

Neural Structure and Function

The process of receiving and interpreting stimuli is called perception (Christenson, 1990; Guyton, 1991). Stimuli are received by the neural structures in the nervous system and perceived through the process of neural function. Neural structure refers to the anatomical properties of the nervous system, including neurons, sensory receptors, nerve fibers, the spinal cord, and brain structures. Neural function refers to the basic nervous system functions of reception, transmission, interpretation, perception, and response to stimuli (Ackerman, 1993; Guyton, 1991). Perception is not based on information received from only one source but is the sum or integration of visual, auditory, tactile,

olfactory, and proprioceptive sensations from multiple sources (Warren, 1996). The basic nervous system functions are as follows:

* Reception is the process of receiving stimuli through sensory receptors in the eyes, ears, tongue, nose, skin, and tissues and organs inside the body. When stimuli are sensed by a sensory receptor, a sensory signal is created.
* Transmission is the process of conducting the sensory signal to specific structures in the nervous system that process the signal.
* Interpretation is the process of translating the sensory signal in a specific area of the nervous system and comparing it with any memories gained from previous experience.
* Perception is the culmination of the other steps in the process. It is the point at which meaning is assigned to the sensory signal and responses are initiated.
* Response is the behavior elicited by the stimulus. It is an attempt to continue or stop the stimulus.

The structures of the nervous system are categorized as the central nervous system (CNS) or the peripheral nervous system (PNS). The CNS includes the brain and spinal cord. The brain is divided into higher and lower structures. The PNS includes the cranial and spinal nerves, the autonomic nervous system (ANS), and the somatic nervous system (SNS). Basic structures common to both the CNS and PNS include neurons and sensory receptors. They are located in every organ and nearly all the tissues in the body. They function to enable the stimulus-response process to occur. Table 34–1 reviews the structure and function of the nervous system.

Stimuli are received by sensory receptors, transmitted across synapses from neuron to neuron, and routed to structures in the CNS. Some interpretation of stimuli takes place at the level of the spinal cord, resulting in a reflex motor response. More sophisticated or higher-level interpretation of stimuli occurs in higher brain structures such as the cerebral cortex.

Higher-level processes involve the use of cognitive ability, which is the capacity to think, reason, and make decisions. A person must be conscious in order to use the cognitive abilities characteristic of higher-level thought processes (Ackerman, 1993; Geary, 1994). Cognitive abilities include orientation, attention, concentration, memory, judgment, and reasoning.

Orientation refers to a person's ability to know where he or she is at any given time and the purpose for being there. Orientation also includes general knowledge about the external environment, including the identity of other people, locations, and objects. Attention is the ability to focus or concentrate on specific stimuli. Concentration is the ability to sustain attention on a particular task or problem without being distracted by less salient or nonrelevant stimuli (Glick, 1993). Attention and concentration enable humans to learn and store information in higher brain structures so that it can be retrieved and used later. Memory is the process of storing information. It enables us to use past experience and learning to reason and make

---

Box 34–2

ADAPTIVE AND MALADAPTIVE RESPONSES TO ALTERED SENSORY PERCEPTION

Maladaptive Responses

* An elderly Japanese woman functions adequately within her ethnic community but relies on her extended family to translate when she must communicate with English-speaking citizens. When she is hospitalized for a broken hip, she becomes agitated and confused.
* A diabetic client with diminished sensory nerve function in his extremities burns his foot while taking a bath.
* A premature infant becomes apneic, hypotensive, and hemodynamically unstable at the mere touch of her nurse.

Adaptive Responses

* A man who lost his sight in an accident 2 years ago is able to live in his own apartment and walk to the grocery store three blocks away by using his senses of hearing, touch, and proprioception and by using assistive devices for the sight impaired.
* A diabetic person with neuropathy of the lower extremities learns to use a thermometer to check the temperature of the bath water before getting in.
* A premature infant cries, becomes red, and extends its extremities for a few seconds following a heel stick but is able to regain a flexed posture and quiet state.

Table 34–1

STRUCTURES AND FUNCTIONS OF THE CENTRAL NERVOUS SYSTEM (CNS)

STRUCTURE	COMPONENTS	FUNCTION
Basic structures		
Neurons (basic functional units)	Dendrites, axons, synapses	Conduct nerve impulses by secreting neurotransmitters. Dendrites bring electrical impulses to the neuron, and axons conduct impulses to other neurons toward the CNS. A synapse is a coupling between two neurons where neurotransmitters are secreted, enabling impulse transmission.
Sensory receptors	Exteroceptors, interoceptors, proprioceptors	Receive various types of stimuli. Exteroceptors receive stimuli from outside the body (*e.g.,* temperature, odors, light, sound); interoceptors receive internal or visceral stimuli (*e.g.,* cramps, fullness, muscle aches); proprioceptors detect body position, posture, and movement.
CNS		
Spinal cord	Ascending and descending nerve tracts	Conducts impulses from sensory receptors to the brain; initiates reflex motor responses, conducts voluntary motor impulses from the brain.
Brain	Cerebrum	Contains the cerebral cortex, which determines the source and meaning of all stimuli, initiates voluntary motor responses, and conducts higher-level thought processes.
	Diencephalon (thalamus, hypothalamus)	Thalamus: Transmission of pain, temperature, and generalized touch and pressure impulses to cerebral cortex; general location and meaning of stimuli. Hypothalamus: Coordinates autonomic nervous system (ANS) activities, including heart rate and smooth muscle regulation, and releases regulating factors that stimulate secretion of hormones; location of centers for mind over body, emotion, coordination, rage, aggression, thermoregulation, appetite, and thirst.
	Cerebellum	Coordinates subconscious movement of skeletal muscle, posture, balance, and proprioception. Transmits motor impulses to correct movement to maintain balance and coordination.
	Brain stem (medulla, pons, mesencephalon)	Medulla: Pathway for conduction of motor and sensory impulses between the brain and spinal cord; regulates involuntary changes in heart rate, respiratory rate, and blood vessel shape, as well as swallowing, vomiting, coughing, sneezing, and hiccuping. Pons: Participates in taste perception, salivation, facial expressions, eyeball movement, chewing, equilibrium, respiratory rhythm, and sensations of the structures of the head and face. Mesencephalon: Contains ascending sensory fibers and descending motor fibers; regulates reflex eye movement and head and trunk adjustments in response to auditory stimuli.
Peripheral Nervous System		
Cranial and spinal nerves	Afferent and efferent nerve fibers	Afferent fibers carry stimuli information from receptors in the muscles, tissues, and organs to the CNS. Efferent fibers carry response signals from the CNS to muscles and glands.
	Somatic nervous system	Consists of efferent neurons that conduct impulses from the CNS to skeletal muscle tissue and produce voluntary movement.
	Autonomic nervous system	Consists of efferent neurons that convey information from the CNS to smooth muscle tissue and glands to produce involuntary responses. Controls arterial blood pressure, gastrointestinal motility, urine production, sweating, and body temperature

judgments. The ability to reason and form judgments enables sophisticated responses to stimuli in the form of decisions, mathematical calculations, problem solving, and abstract thinking (Baggerly, 1991; Glick, 1993).

Normal thought processes are necessary for accurate perception and effective response to many types of stimuli. Thought processes permit memories, emotions, personality, and intelligence to influence voluntary motor responses and ANS activity (Guyton, 1991; Tortora & Anagnostakos, 1987). The first condition that must be met in order for higher-level thought processes to occur is consciousness, a state of arousal or wakefulness controlled by lower brain structures (Ackerman, 1993; Geary, 1994). A person's state of consciousness is controlled by a network of neurons called the reticular activating system (RAS). The RAS allows a person to sleep, wake up, and pay attention to stimuli. Almost any sensory stimulus, internal or external, can activate the RAS, but some stimuli are more potent than others. Based on the strength and type of stimulation, different areas of the RAS are activated, which in turn activates specific areas of the cerebral cortex. A person may not be awakened by the sound of raindrops against a window, for exam-

ple, but thunder and lightning are likely to produce arousal from sleep. This selective activation of specific cortical areas probably plays an important role in our ability to attend to certain stimuli while ignoring other stimuli (Ackerman, 1993; Geary, 1994; Guyton, 1991).

In summary, barriers to accurate sensory perception are caused by the character (*i.e.,* amount, frequency, and intensity) of stimuli or problems in perceiving stimuli. Barriers can be classified into one of three domains: environmental, physiological, and psychological (Inaba-Roland & Maricle, 1992; Lipowski, 1990; Roberts & Lincoln, 1988). Refer to Box 34–3 for a summary of environmental, physiological, and psychological barriers to accurate sensory perception. In addition to barriers, other factors influence a person's perception and response to stimuli. These factors include stage of maturity or growth and personal preferences, values, and beliefs.

The Influence of Maturity and Aging

The manner in which people receive, perceive, and respond to stimuli is affected by physiological and

---

Box 34–3

BARRIERS TO ACCURATE SENSORY PERCEPTION

Physiological Barriers

Neural Structure Alteration

Trauma to the CNS: head or spinal cord injury

Infection of the CNS: meningitis, encephalitis, AIDS, neurosyphilis

Cerebral vascular accident

Tumor of the brain, spinal cord, or peripheral nervous system

Chronic disease: diabetes mellitus, Alzheimer's

Pain from trauma, surgery, inflammation, infection

Sensory Deficits

Vision deficits: refractive errors, cataracts, retinopathy

Tactile deficits: neuropathy

Auditory deficits: sensorineural or conductive hearing loss

Olfactory and gustatory deficits

States That Impair Tissue Perfusion

Hypotension: shock, heart failure, cardiac dysrhythmias

Altered thermoregulation: hyper- and hypothermia

Acute or chronic respiratory failure

States Producing Metabolic or Chemical Disruptions

Malnutrition: vitamin deficiencies, hypoalbuminemia

Fluid and electrolyte imbalance: hyper- and hypovolemia; abnormal sodium, potassium, phosphorus, magnesium

Hepatic failure

Renal failure

Endocrine dysfunction: pituitary disorder; thyroid, pancreatic dysfunction (diabetes)

Chemical substances: withdrawal, overdose, or change in usual pattern of ingestion (*e.g.,* salicylate toxicity)

Environmental Barriers

Sensory deprivation

Sensory overload

Interrupted or deficient sleep

Culture care deprivation

Psychological Barriers

Altered affect states: anxiety, depression, fear

Mental illness

History of dementia

History of acute confusion during hospitalization

Underdeveloped or ineffective coping skills

Preoccupation with physiological problems: constipation, chronic or acute pain

---

Adapted from Wilson, 1993.

psychological maturity. Most infant responses are related to physiological needs. A normal infant relies completely on its caregivers in the external environment to meet its basic needs. Hunger is a stimulus that elicits crying. By crying, the infant is able to inform caregivers that it is hungry or uncomfortable. The baby responds to holding, feeding, and rocking by becoming content and sleeping (Fig. 34–2). In contrast, a premature infant is less efficient at responding and adapting to stimuli. Responding to hunger by crying could result in dangerous blood pressure changes and physiological instability. Responding to nutritional needs is especially difficult for a premature infant who has no ability to suck (D'Apolito, 1991).

As children mature, they become more sophisticated in their ability to respond to stimuli and progressively less dependent on caregivers. As the CNS matures, attention span lengthens and experiences are memorized. Children begin to attend selectively to certain stimuli while disregarding other less relevant stimuli.

A child's perception of the environment influences physiological responses. Hospitalization presents many perceived threats and taxes the child's limited ability to respond effectively. The psychological stress experienced by an ill or injured child in an unfamiliar environment can impair the ability to recover (Kidder, 1989).

As a person matures, the ability to integrate physical and cognitive skills permits greater control over the environment, as responses become the product of past experience rather than trial and error (Baggerly, 1991; Kidder, 1989). However, as a person nears the end of life, the effects of maturity can actually become barriers to sensory perception.

Over the life span, many factors affect a person's ability to receive and respond to stimuli. Lifestyle, environmental, and genetic factors influence sensory organ function and the ability to respond as people age. Accidents and injury to sensory organs can impair or eliminate the ability to see, speak, move, or hear. Sensory and motor function can also be lost through the process of aging and illness. Such changes may be gradual, allowing for adjustments to sensory deficits (see Fig. 34–2). Other changes are sudden, resulting in loss of independence and a period of disorganization or maladaptation (Christenson, 1990). For example, gradual vision loss as a person ages permits physical and psychological adjustment over time. In contrast, an 85-year-old person who suffers a cerebral vascular accident resulting in sudden blindness or vision impairment may have difficulty returning to independent living and may be forced into institutional or assisted living. Box 34–4 discusses causes of visual and auditory sensory deficits.

The effects of the aging process reduce the efficiency of adaptation to noxious internal and external environmental stimuli and increase the risk for maladaptive responses. Elderly persons often have chronic illnesses that impair their health and capacity for adaptation. Although heart disease is the most common

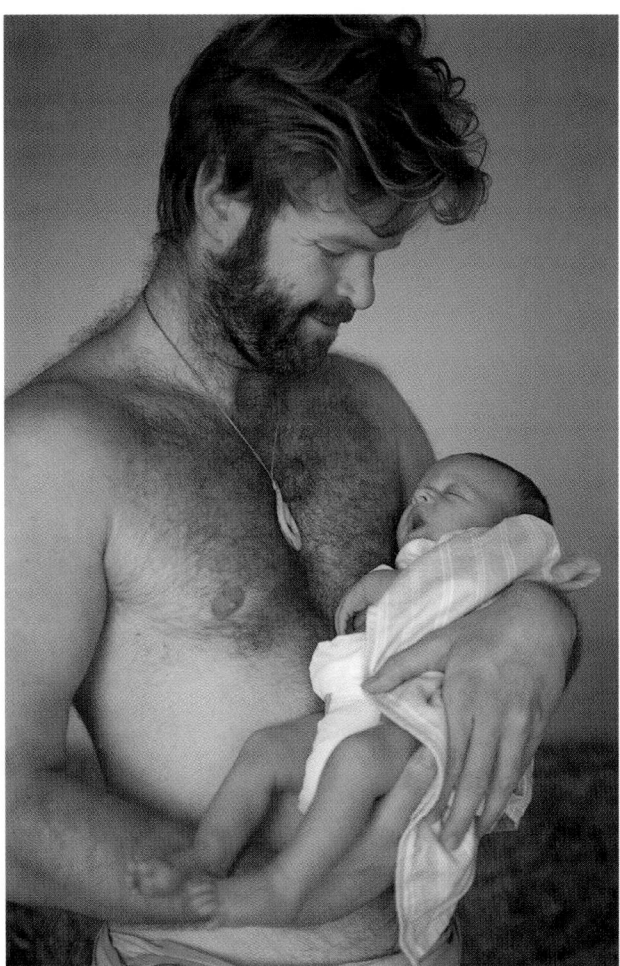

Father holding infant

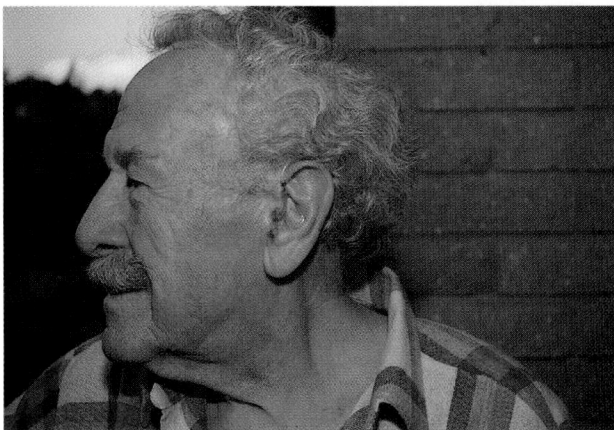

Older man with hearing aid

✦ **Figure 34–2**
Human response to stimuli varies across the life span. Infants depend on holding and touching for comfort and security. Older adults may depend on special devices to restore loss of sensory organ function that occurs with aging.

cause of morbidity in the elderly, 55% of the elderly have one or more medical conditions in addition to heart disease. Multiple chronic diseases such as hypertension, diabetes, atherosclerosis, and obstructive pul-

Box 34–4

CAUSES OF AUDITORY AND VISUAL SENSORY LOSS

Hearing Loss

Sensorineural Hearing Loss

• Deterioration in the neural structure and function of the inner ear and nerve pathways to the brain

• Damage to inner ear structures; *e.g.,* damage to the cochlea causes hearing impairment for high-frequency sounds (common in older persons), and damage to the organ of Corti results in hearing impairment for low-frequency sounds

• Damage to the organ of Corti from excessive exposure to loud sounds

• Damage to the eighth cranial nerve from antibiotics or other chemical exposure, causing nerve deafness for all sound frequencies (Guyton, 1991)

Sensorineural hearing loss can be detected by performing a Weber test (see Table 34–2).

Conductive Hearing Loss

• Conditions that physically obstruct sound transmission from the external and middle ear to the inner ear; *e.g.,* structural damage in the middle ear owing to chronic infection or diseases or cerumen (ear wax) impaction (see Procedure 34–1 for a description of how to remove excess cerumen).

• Conductive hearing loss can be detected by performing a Rinne test (see Table 34–2).

Visual Deficits

Optical Defects

Myopia (Nearsightedness). Images are focused in front of the retina and blurred when they reach the retina.

Hyperopia (Farsightedness). Images are focused behind the retina and remain out of focus on the retina.

Presbyopia. Lens change that becomes noticeable in one's early 40s, caused by reduced elasticity of the lens; results in loss of near vision focus.

Astigmatism. Because of irregular curvatures of the lenses, images do not focus on the retina.

Oculomotor Control Defects

Specific cranial nerve problems (III, IV, VI) occur, causing impaired movement of one or more of the extra-ocular muscles, resulting in decreased speed, control, and coordination of eye movements.

Visual Field Deficits

There is loss of vision in one or more of the peripheral areas within which objects may be seen when the eye is staring straight ahead, owing to cerebral vascular accident, brain lesion, or tumor.

Structural Changes Associated With Deteriorating Vision

Cornea

• Becomes opaque and transmits light less efficiently

• Requires more intense light in order to see an image

• Distinguishing colors and contrasts is more difficult

• Focusing on images is more difficult

Lens

• Becomes thicker, less pliable, more dense

• Less able to produce a sharp image of near objects on the retina

Ciliary Body

• Becomes thicker

• Becomes blocked, preventing the watery fluid that maintains retinal pressure from draining and resulting in glaucoma (increased pressure in the eye)

Retina

• Changes in blood supply with age cause retinal deterioration

• Diminished resolution of fine details and contrast

• Spatial discrimination ability is lost

• Impaired color perception

• Hampered contrast discrimination

Optic Nerve

• Thickens and degenerates and reduces the number and speed of messages to the brain

• Decreased discrimination of light, *i.e.,* space and frequency

---

monary disease have a deleterious effect on the capacity to adapt to the stress of additional physiological, environmental, and psychological barriers (Frantz & Ferrell-Torry, 1993; Kern, 1991).

Poor cardiac function predisposes the elderly to poor tissue perfusion. Decreased cardiovascular reserve, coupled with the stress and increased metabolic demands of acute illness and hospitalization, results in decreased cerebral blood flow, resulting in impaired brain function.

During an acute illness, the adrenal glands secrete more cortisol in response to the physiological and psychological stress. The elderly degrade cortisol less efficiently, resulting in elevated blood levels. Elevated cortisol levels have been associated with impaired higher-level processes (Lipowski, 1990).

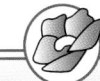

Aging is accompanied by diminished neurological control. Peripheral nerve function is decreased, and there are fewer neurotransmitters. Sensory deficits impair perception and the ability to assign meaning to environmental cues (Williams *et al.,* 1979).

Personal Preferences, Values, and Beliefs

As people grow and mature, they develop the beliefs, preferences, values, customs, traditions, and language that define their culture. There may be transcultural differences in how people respond to stimuli, because stimuli have different meanings across generations and cultures (Kloosterman, 1991). For example: A sound that one person experiences as unpleasant will be perceived louder for that person than for a person who likes the sound (Fucci *et al.*, 1993). What a teenager defines as music may be perceived as obnoxious noise to an elderly person (Spies Pope, 1995). Pain has different meaning and a less debilitating effect in people from Eastern cultures than in those from Western cultures (Kodiath & Kodiath, 1995).

Transcultural variations in responses to stimuli have not been adequately studied, but theoretically, the cultural influence could actually be a barrier to accurate sensory perception. For example, when a 75-year-old Asian man who speaks no English becomes ill and requires hospitalization in the midwestern United States, there will probably be few people in the hospital environment who speak his language or understand his values and beliefs. His ability to interpret and assign meaning to the immediate environment is influenced by his culture. Failure to address the health care needs defined by his culture that will help him get well leads to cultural care deprivation. Cultural care deprivation is a deficiency in the supportive and assistive measures that a person believes will lead to improved health and wellness (Kloosterman, 1991). (See also Chapter 36.)

♦ Manifestations of Altered Sensory Perception

Manifestations of altered sensory perception range from a simple misinterpretation of sensory stimuli to severe cognitive and psychomotor behavior impairment. Each response carries a certain degree of seriousness, based on the potential consequences. The consequences of maladaptive responses range from mild inconvenience to risk of death. In contrast, if a person is able to cope with changes in stimuli or sensory alterations, adaptive behaviors will result. The goal of nursing is to promote adaptive responses. This can be achieved by recognizing and intervening when maladaptive responses occur.

Sensory deprivation and sensory overload represent stressful situations to which people of all ages respond both physiologically and psychologically. Physiological responses include pupil dilation, elevated heart rate and blood pressure, sodium and water retention, and elevated serum cortisol. Fear, anxiety,

The Phenomenon of Acute Confusional State (ACS)

The phenomenon of ACS became the focus of medical and nursing research in the 1960s with the advent of cardiac surgery (Blachy & Starr, 1964). Easton and MacKenzie described ACS (delirium and ICU psychosis) as "components or manifestations of sensory perceptual alteration related to sensory overload" (1988, p. 230).

In ACS, consciousness varies from lethargy to hyperalertness and agitation. Cognitive impairment is demonstrated. The client is unable to understand or remember instructions. For example, an acutely confused person with intravenous infusions and a urinary bladder catheter may repeatedly get out of bed unassisted, despite instructions to request assistance with activity. The person may be disoriented to person, place, or time, failing to recognize significant others or remember the reason for hospitalization (APA, 1994; Inaba-Roland & Maricle, 1992; Lipowski, 1990).

Disturbances in affect are apparent. The confused person may demonstrate anxiety, euphoria, depression, or apathy (APA, 1987; Easton & MacKenzie, 1988; Geary, 1994). Symptoms of psychoses, including illusions, delusions, hallucinations, or paranoia, may be experienced.

Nurses and physicians may contribute to the development of these symptoms by depersonalizing the client. Health care providers may assume that the victim of ACS cannot comprehend appropriately, so they focus their attention on the monitoring equipment and the person's surroundings rather than on the person. They may fail to address the client directly and may talk *about* the client instead of *to* the client (Halm & Alpen, 1993). The depersonalized client may feel left out, unrecognized, and detached. Because of this, equipment used for physiological support and monitoring may be misperceived, resulting in illusions and delusions. Persons experiencing ACS have reported feeling like they were being held prisoner and that care providers were in a conspiracy against them. Restraints, wires, and tubing attached to the client have produced the illusion of being bound and gagged (Easton & MacKenzie, 1988; Sullivan-Marx, 1995). Paranoid feelings lead to lack of cooperation with nursing care such as refusals to take medications or eat. One of the dangers of this aspect of ACS is the potential for a person to misinterpret internal stimuli such as pain or the need for elimination. The person's inability to perceive or articulate symptoms or needs correctly may result in inadequate analgesic administration or inappropriate sedation if the client should become restless or incontinent (Inaba-Roland & Maricle, 1992; Williams et al., 1985). Another dangerous aspect of ACS that could result in client injury is altered psychomotor behavior. Examples of altered psychomotor behavior include repeated attempts to get out of bed, resistance to repositioning in bed, and pulling at and removing tubing and throwing off the bed linens (Sullivan-Marx, 1994; Wilson, 1993). Episodes of severe psychomotor hyperactivity tempt health care providers to use physical or chemical restraints.

A person's sleep-wake cycle is often disrupted during ACS. Deviations from the person's normal pattern include nocturnal insomnia and sporadic, brief periods of sleep during the day (Foreman & Zane, 1996; Lipowski, 1990).

Researchers have attempted to identify specific barriers associated with the development of ACS, but a consistent pattern or grouping of barriers has not been demonstrated. Generally, the nursing profession accepts theories that describe the influence of environmental, psychological, and physiological barriers on neural function (see Box 34-3). The presence of one or more of these barriers contributes to a change in brain metabolism, which is the use of nutrients, oxygen, and other chemicals necessary for normal brain function (Mentes, 1995; Wilson, 1993). With the change in brain metabolism, an imbalance in neurotransmitters (*i.e.,* acetylcholine and dopamine) occurs. Neurotransmitters are chemicals necessary for transmitting sensory information and for proper functioning of the brain and nervous system (Lipowski, 1990).

The onset of ACS is sudden, and the duration is brief. Usually, ACS resolves after a few days or weeks (Easton & MacKenzie, 1988; Lipowski, 1990). The severity and presentation of symptoms may fluctuate throughout the day. For example, the client may appear to have normal cognitive functioning during the day but develop symptoms of disorientation and paranoia as evening approaches (APA, 1994; Mentes, 1995).

The incidence of ACS is widely variable and dependent on the population studied. The reported incidence of ACS is 10 to 18% for all hospitalized clients (Trzepacz, Sclabassi, & Van Thiel, 1989; Williams et al., 1979) and 13 to 50% for conscious clients in critical care units (Easton & MacKenzie, 1988; Geary, 1994). The reported incidence of ACS is 10 to 44% in the general surgical population (Lipowski, 1990; Williams et al., 1979) and from 10 to 83% in the cardiac surgical population (Blachy & Starr, 1964; Budd & Brown, 1974; Kornfeld, Zimberg, & Malm, 1965; Sadler, 1981). ACS is not absent in the pediatric population. It generally occurs with conditions such as high fever, head trauma, chemical ingestion, epilepsy, migraines, and central nervous system infections (Amit, 1988; Schwartz & Rodriguez, 1991).

The behaviors manifested during an episode of ACS are distressing for the person experiencing it as well as for the significant others and health care providers involved in the person's care. ACS interferes with the person's ability to follow instructions, communicate needs, and cooperate with interventions. Clients with ACS require increased nursing surveillance and may need chemical or physical restraints (Fish, 1991; Williams et al., 1985). Persons with ACS are predisposed to longer hospitalizations and increased morbidity and mortality (Francis et al., 1990; Levkoff et al., 1992; Lipowski, 1990).

disrupted sleep patterns, and psychotic behavior are some of the psychological responses to sensory deprivation and sensory overload (Halm & Alpen, 1993). An acute confusional state (ACS) is a severe manifestation of altered sensory perception. ACS is a transient condition with an abrupt onset. It is characterized by confusion, disorientation, agitation, and impaired higher-level thought processes (Foreman & Zane, 1996). Refer to the accompanying box for a detailed discussion of ACS.

An infant or child's growth and development may be adversely affected by sensory deprivation or overload. For example, overstimulation, unnecessary handling, and improper positioning in the intensive care environment cause physiological instability (*e.g.*, inadequate blood pressure, poor oxygenation, and abnormal neurological development) in premature infants. The amount and type of stimulation needed change as the infant progresses through each developmental stage. Infants require a certain amount of sensory stimulation from a consistent source, such as a parent, for normal psychosocial growth and development (Gardner-Cole *et al.*, 1990; Long, Lucey, & Philip, 1980).

Physical growth and development are also dependent on adequate sensory stimulation. For example, a toddler who suffers from chronic otitis media may have conductive hearing loss, which may cause delays in verbal development. Amblyopia, or lazy eye, results from inadequate transmission of visual stimuli to the brain and usually involves only one eye. It must be detected and treated before the age of 7 years to restore normal sensory development in the affected eye. The treatment is to cover the unaffected eye and force the affected eye to receive and transmit visual stimuli to the brain (Moore, 1994).

Application of the Nursing Process

Assessment

Baseline Assessment

A thorough and accurate assessment of a person's baseline sensory status is essential so that barriers can be detected before the person suffers any consequences of impaired sensory perception. The assessment process includes collecting demographic information, a health history, an inventory of personal habits, and current symptoms and performing mental status and neurological examinations. Refer to Box 34–5 for a summary of information collected during the initial assessment.

The assessment process also includes obtaining subjective information from the client's family members or significant others. If the client is a child, the parents or primary caregivers should be present to provide a history. Old records of previous encounters with the person are reviewed. Information regarding the person's sensory status (*e.g.*, hearing or vision deficits and any sensory aids used) is obtained. An account of the current problem, current medications, recent and remote CNS trauma or infection, comorbid conditions, and the contributory health status of family members are recorded. Subjective data on recent changes in cognitive function, environment, and emotional state are also relevant.

Mental Status Assessment

The physical examination begins while collecting the client profile by observing the client's level of consciousness, facial expression, affect, speech, and language. Some clues to cognitive function may surface during the nursing history, but further testing may be needed to identify occult deficits that may interfere with accurate sensory perception. Box 34–6 describes the components of a mental status examination.

The criteria for determining mental status must be tailored to age-appropriate behaviors and cultural variations. Mental status in an infant or nonverbal child can be assessed by observing how the child interacts with parents and caregivers. A toddler can tell the nurse his or her name and parents' names. How toddlers and older children engage in play and sleep patterns may provide important clues to mental status. For persons with language, speech, or hearing barriers, the services of someone qualified to interpret and translate are necessary.

Sensory-Motor Function

Sensory-motor assessment provides information about the function of cranial nerves, spinal nerves, and integrated brain functions (Fig. 34–3). Sensory-motor assessment includes an evaluation of motor function, reflexes, and the functions of the special senses. Assessment of reflexes and peripheral sensation indicates the status of spinal nerve function and their ability to transmit sensory impulses to the brain and motor impulses to the muscles. Each spinal nerve transmits sensation and motor impulses to specific areas of the body, called dermatomes (Fig. 34–4).

Cranial Nerve Function

Assessment of the cranial nerves provides information regarding the sensory and motor function of the structures that receive stimuli through the special senses—the ears, eyes, nose, tongue, and skin—and through movements of the neck, face, throat, tongue, and eyes (Ackerman, 1993). Refer to Table 34–2 for a guide to cranial nerve assessment. Tactile (touch), gustatory (taste), olfactory (smell), and proprioceptive (body position) senses should all be assessed with the client's eyes closed.

Box **34–5**

CLIENT PROFILE: BASELINE ASSESSMENT

Demographic Data

Age

Education level

Occupation

Language spoken

Past Health History

Illness

Injury

Stressful events

Current Health Status

Chief complaint

Chronic illness

Routine medications (over the counter and prescription)

Sensory deficits in hearing, vision, taste, smell, touch, and proprioception

Personal Habits

Diet

Exercise

Sleep pattern

Leisure activities

Chemical ingestion (alcohol and drug abuse, caffeine, nicotine)

Methods of dealing with problems (coping)

Social

Family structure

Support systems (spiritual, cultural, organizational)

Relationships: monogamous or marital relationships, friendships

General Appearance

Hygiene

Affect or mood

Posture

Verbal and motor behavior

Mental Status (see Box 34–6)

Consciousness

Attention

Orientation

Memory

Reasoning

Judgment

Cranial Nerve Evaluation (see Table 34–2)

Motor Function

Cerebellar function: balance and coordination (Romberg, stair stepping, heel-to-toe walk)

Gait: symmetry, grace, precision

Muscles: tone, size, strength

Sensory Function

Superficial and deep touch, pressure, thermal, pain, vibration, and position (proprioception) senses

Discriminative sensations, *e.g.,* point discrimination

Reflexes (*e.g.,* Table 34–3 and Fig. 34–5)

Superficial

Deep tendon

Sensory Function

The sensory functions of most of the special senses are covered by the cranial nerve assessment. Superficial touch, temperature, and pain sensations are tested by stimulating the dermatomes. Superficial touch and pain can be tested with sharp and blunt stimulation using a toothpick and a cotton swab. If necessary, deep pain and pressure may be tested by pinching the trapezius or quadriceps muscles. Test tubes filled with cool and warm water can be placed against the client's skin to test thermal sensation. Vibration is tested by applying a vibrating tuning fork to a bony prominence (*e.g.*, elbow, knee, ankle, tibia, tips of toes). After the client no longer senses the vibration, the tuning fork is placed on the identical area of the examiner's body. If the examiner, who is assumed to have normal sensory function, still feels the vibration, it may be an indication that the person has diminished vibratory sense (Levin, 1991). Proprioception, or position sense, is tested by having the client, whose eyes are closed, identify the position of body parts while the examiner puts them through their ranges of motion (Pedretti, 1996).

The integration of the sense of touch and cerebral cortex function enables people to identify objects by touch and discriminate where they are being touched even when they cannot see the stimulus. This ability, referred to as point discrimination, is tested by touching the client simultaneously in two different areas of the body (two-point remote) and in two places on one body part (two-point near) while the client's eyes are closed. The client must identify the locations being touched and that two different stimuli are occurring in one area. Next, a common object, such as a button or coin, is placed in the client's hand, and the client is asked to identify the object without looking at it.

Box 34–6

ASSESSMENT OF HIGHER-LEVEL THOUGHT PROCESSES

Orientation

Observe:

Response to familiar people and strangers

Cooperation with instructions

Response to pain

Knowledge of general information

Ask the Person:

What is the day, month, year, and season?

Where are you, and why you are here?

What city are we in?

Who is the president?

Where is the capital?

What is the weather like in Hawaii?

Who is Ronald McDonald?

Attention

Observe:

Response to stimuli in the immediate environment

Ability to converse without being distracted

Ability to follow instructions

Ask the Person to:

Describe a favorite toy or pet

Discuss current news events

Follow a series of simple instructions, *e.g.,* get out of bed, put on your robe and slippers, wash your hands, and sit in the chair

Concentration

Observe:

Ability to sustain attention to complete a task

Ask the Person to:

Count forward and backward by nines, ending and beginning with 54 (older child or adult)

Play a game of tic-tac-toe (child)

Count backward from 10

Spell "word" backward

Memory

Observe:

Response to visitors

Whether the client recognizes nurses who have provided care for more than one shift

Ask the Person to:

Repeat and memorize three words at the beginning of the exam and recall them later in the exam

Recall his or her wedding anniversary and the birthdates of children, names of pets, schoolteacher's name last year

Judgment

Observe:

Accuracy of answers

Difficulty in answering questions

Ask the Person:

If the baby is in the bathtub and you need to answer the front door, what would you do?

Why shouldn't you play with matches?

Reasoning

Observe:

Logic of answers

Difficulty in answering questions

Ask the Person:

What does this mean: the grass is always greener on the other side of the fence?

Which item does not belong in this group: refrigerator, stove, dishwasher, toilet?

Note: Such an assessment of higher-level thought processes requires a fully alert and conscious client. Questions should be modified according to age, developmental level, and cultural background. The criteria for acceptable responses should also be modified, depending on the availability of orienting devices such as clocks and calendars. A relative should be consulted to verify answers to personal questions.

Reflexes

Assessment of superficial (cutaneous) and deep tendon reflexes provides information about the sensory-motor function of the spinal cord and some cranial nerves. Refer to Table 34–3 for a guide to reflex assessment. Figure 34–5 illustrates how some deep tendon reflexes are tested.

Nursing Diagnosis

The way people respond to stimuli is a primary concern to nurses. A state in which "diminished, exaggerated, distorted, or impaired responses" accompany a "change in the amount or patterning of oncoming stimuli" is called a sensory/perceptual alteration. Sensory/perceptual alteration is a nursing diagnosis cate-

Text continued on page 1055

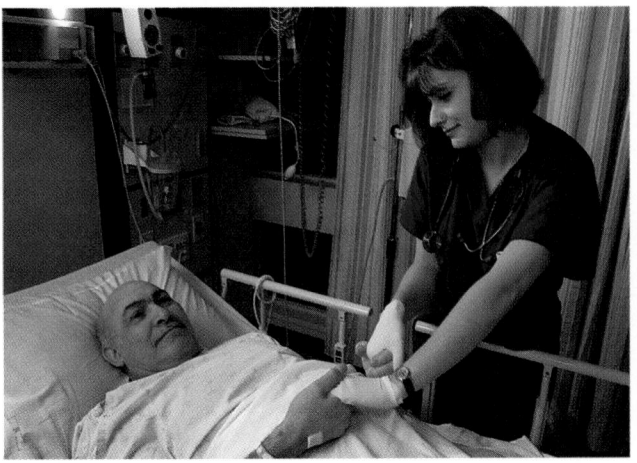

Assessing motor function

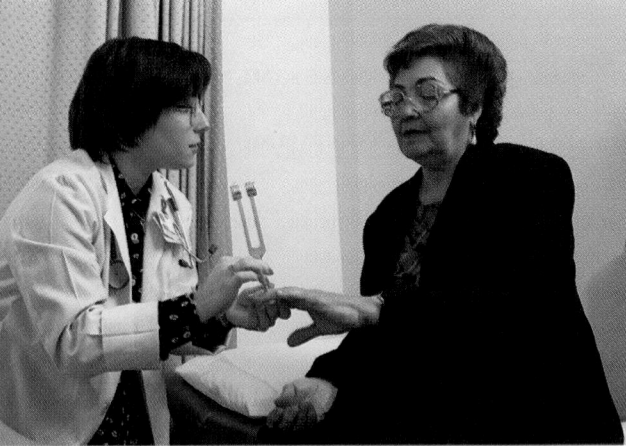

Assessing sensory function

❥ **Figure 34–3**
Sensory-motor assessment provides information about the function of cranial nerves, spinal nerves, and integrated brain functions.

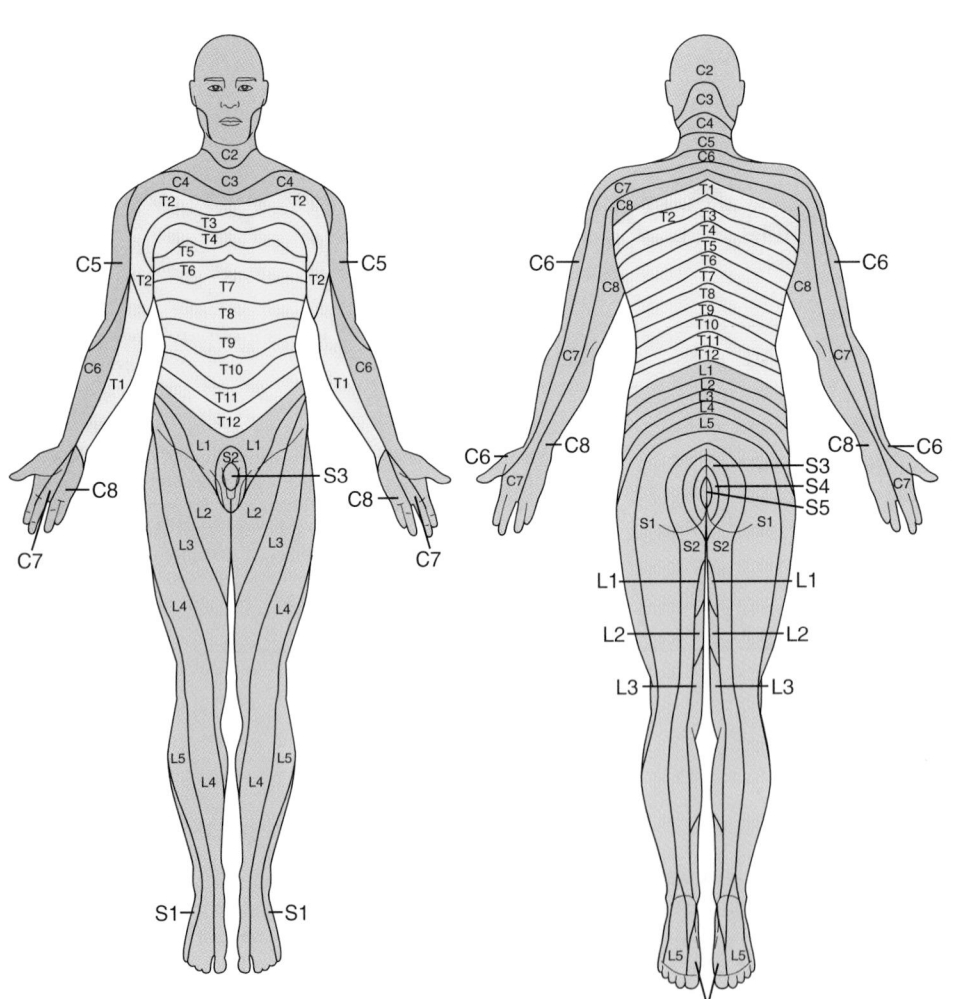

❥ **Figure 34–4**
Dermatomes, areas of the body innervated by the various spinal nerves.

Table 34–2

CRANIAL NERVE ASSESSMENT

CRANIAL NERVE	FUNCTION	ASSESSMENT
I: Olfactory	Sensory: reception and interpretation of odors	Test one nostril at a time. Ask the person to distinguish between common odors (*e.g.,* cinnamon, garlic, an orange).
II: Optic	Sensory: vision reception, acuity, and visual fields (peripheral vision)	Test visual acuity with a Snellen chart. To assess visual fields, ask the client to train both eyes on your (the examiner's) eyes, then hold your hands out as shown about 30 cm above eye level with your index fingers extended. Ask the client to state which index finger you move. This process is repeated with the examiner's hands approximately 30 cm below eye level.

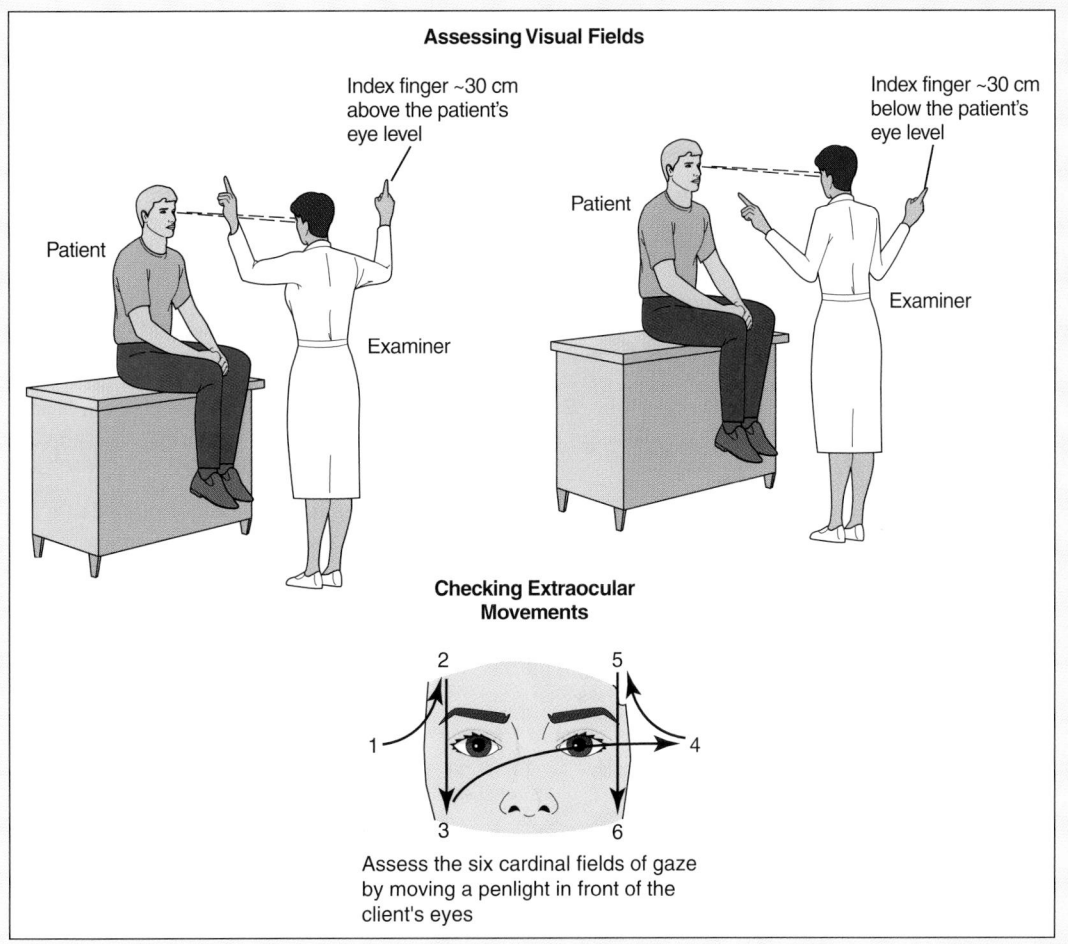

Assessing Visual Fields

Index finger ~30 cm above the patient's eye level

Index finger ~30 cm below the patient's eye level

Patient

Patient

Examiner

Examiner

Checking Extraocular Movements

Assess the six cardinal fields of gaze by moving a penlight in front of the client's eyes

| III. Oculomotor | Motor: raises eyelids, extraocular movements; pupil constriction via parasympathetic stimulation | Symmetry or droopiness (ptosis) of eyelids, pupillary light response, pupil accommodation |

Table continued on following page

Table **34–2**

CRANIAL NERVE ASSESSMENT
(Continued)

CRANIAL NERVE	FUNCTION	ASSESSMENT

Inferior oblique (CN III)

Superior rectus (CN III)

Medial rectus (CN III)

Lateral rectus (CN IV)

Superior oblique (CN IV)

Inferior rectus (CN III)

The six muscles used in eye movement and the cranial nerves that innervate these muscles

CRANIAL NERVE	FUNCTION	ASSESSMENT
IV: Trochlear	Motor: extraocular eye movement, downward and inward eye movement	Extraocular movements: Instruct the client to follow your hand with only the eyes as you move it through the six cardinal fields of gaze. Observe for nystagmus.
V: Trigeminal	Sensory: sensation of eyes, eyelids, forehead, nose, jaw, nasal and oral mucosa, teeth, tongue, ears, facial skin Motor: chewing, clenching, teeth grinding	Observe for facial atrophy and tremor. Palpate the strength of jaw opening and closing (which involves the temporal and masseter muscles). Sensation of forehead, cheeks, and jaws: Touch the forehead, cheek, and jaw. Have the client indicate when touch is felt. Differentiate between sharp and dull sensations with the pointed and blunt ends of a toothpick. Corneal (blink) reflex—see Table 34–3. The sensory function involving facial sensation is indicated by divisions 1 (ophthalmic), 2 (maxillary), and 3 (mandibular).

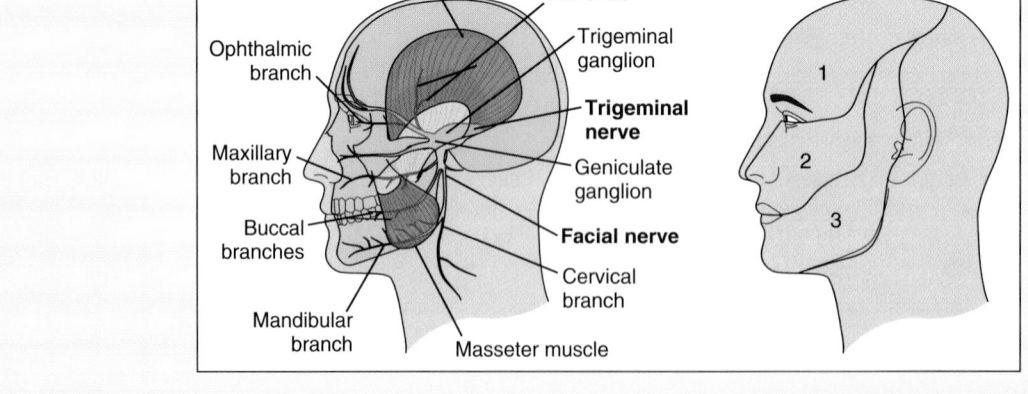

Cranial Nerves V and VII and Branches

Temporal muscle
Temporal branches
Trigeminal ganglion
Ophthalmic branch
Trigeminal nerve
Maxillary branch
Geniculate ganglion
Buccal branches
Facial nerve
Cervical branch
Mandibular branch
Masseter muscle

Sensory Function

1—Ophthalmic
2—Maxillary
3—Mandibular

CRANIAL NERVE	FUNCTION	ASSESSMENT
VI: Abducens	Motor: lateral eye movement	See oculomotor assessment. Note whether the client can sustain a lateral gaze for a few seconds without extreme nystagmus.

Table 34–2

CRANIAL NERVE ASSESSMENT
(Continued)

CRANIAL NERVE	FUNCTION	ASSESSMENT
VII: Facial	Sensory: taste on proximal ⅔ of tongue and sensation to pharynx Motor: facial expressions (not jaw), eyelid movement, mouth shapes for speech Salivation and tearing	Taste: See CN IX assessment. Check for facial symmetry when the client smiles, whistles, clenches teeth, raises eyebrows (noting symmetry of wrinkles on forehead), blinks, closes eyes tightly (watch eye movement), and looks up at the ceiling.

Checking for Facial Symmetry

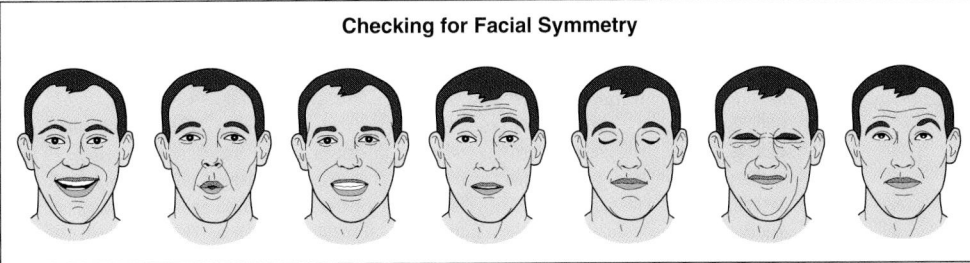

VIII: Acoustic or vestibulocochlear	Sensory: hearing, equilibrium	Note the client's ability to hear a whisper, a watch ticking within 2 feet, and normal conversation. Perform the Rinne and Weber tests. *Rinne test:* Place the stem of a vibrating tuning fork on the client's mastoid process until he or she can no longer hear the sound; then quickly move the tuning fork next to the client's ear and note if the sound is still heard. A positive (normal) Rinne test is when the sound is heard twice as long via conduction through air as through bone. (Note: test each ear individually.) *Weber test:* Place the stem of a vibrating tuning fork on top of the client's forehead and note if he or she is able to hear the sound in both ears. Equilibrium: Perform the Romberg test: Note the client's ability to stand up steadily with heels together, arms extended to the front, and eyes open. Repeat the test with eyes closed.

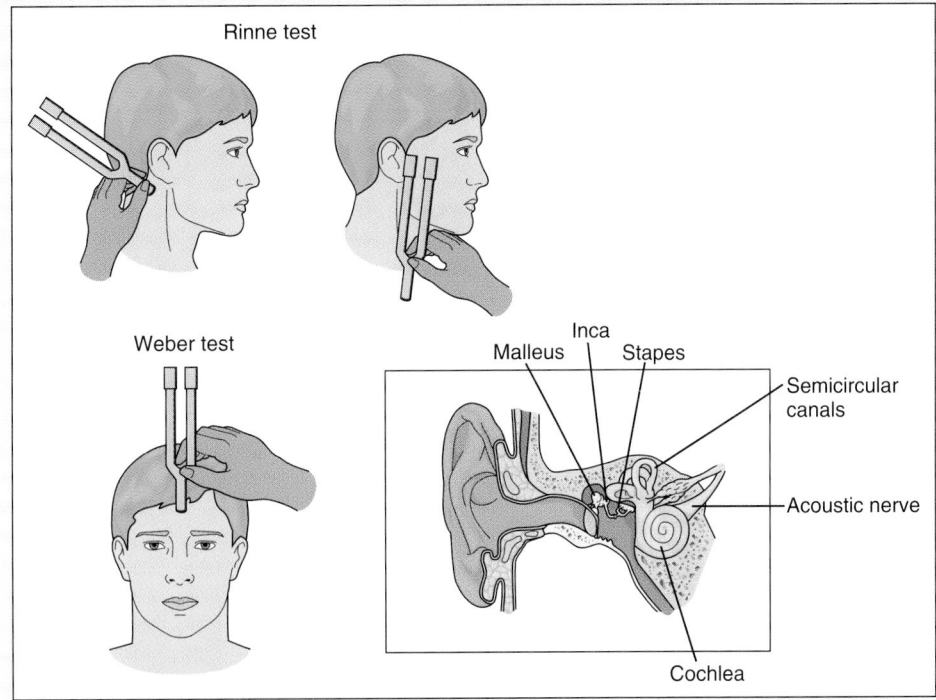

Table continued on following page

Table **34—2**

CRANIAL NERVE ASSESSMENT
(Continued)

CRANIAL NERVE	FUNCTION	ASSESSMENT
IX: Glossopharyngeal	Sensory: touch to nasopharynx, soft palate, tonsils; taste on distal ⅓ of tongue Motor: swallowing and phonation Carotid reflex and salivation	Palatal reflex and gag reflex—see Table 34–3. Note ability to swallow sips of water without choking.
X: Vagus	Sensory: touch to exterior ear, behind ear, and sensation to thoracic and abdominal viscera Motor: swallowing and phonation; secretion of digestive enzymes; peristalsis; carotid reflex; involuntary action of heart, lungs, and digestive tract; uvula and soft palate movement	Gag and swallow (pharyngeal reflex) Note the symmetry of the soft palate and uvula movement as the client says "ahh." (The uvula normally moves centrally.) Then touch the pharyngeal wall behind the pillars. The uvula should lift. Ask the client to compare the sensation on both sides of the uvula. Note voice quality (clear vs. hoarse)

XI: Spinal accessory	Motor: movement of sternocleidomastoid, upper trapezius muscles for shoulder movement and neck rotation	Note client's ability to shrug shoulders against resistance from examiner's hands and then by having client turn his or her head from side to side against opposing pressure from examiner's hand

Table continued on following page

Table 34-2

CRANIAL NERVE ASSESSMENT
(Continued)

CRANIAL NERVE	FUNCTION	ASSESSMENT

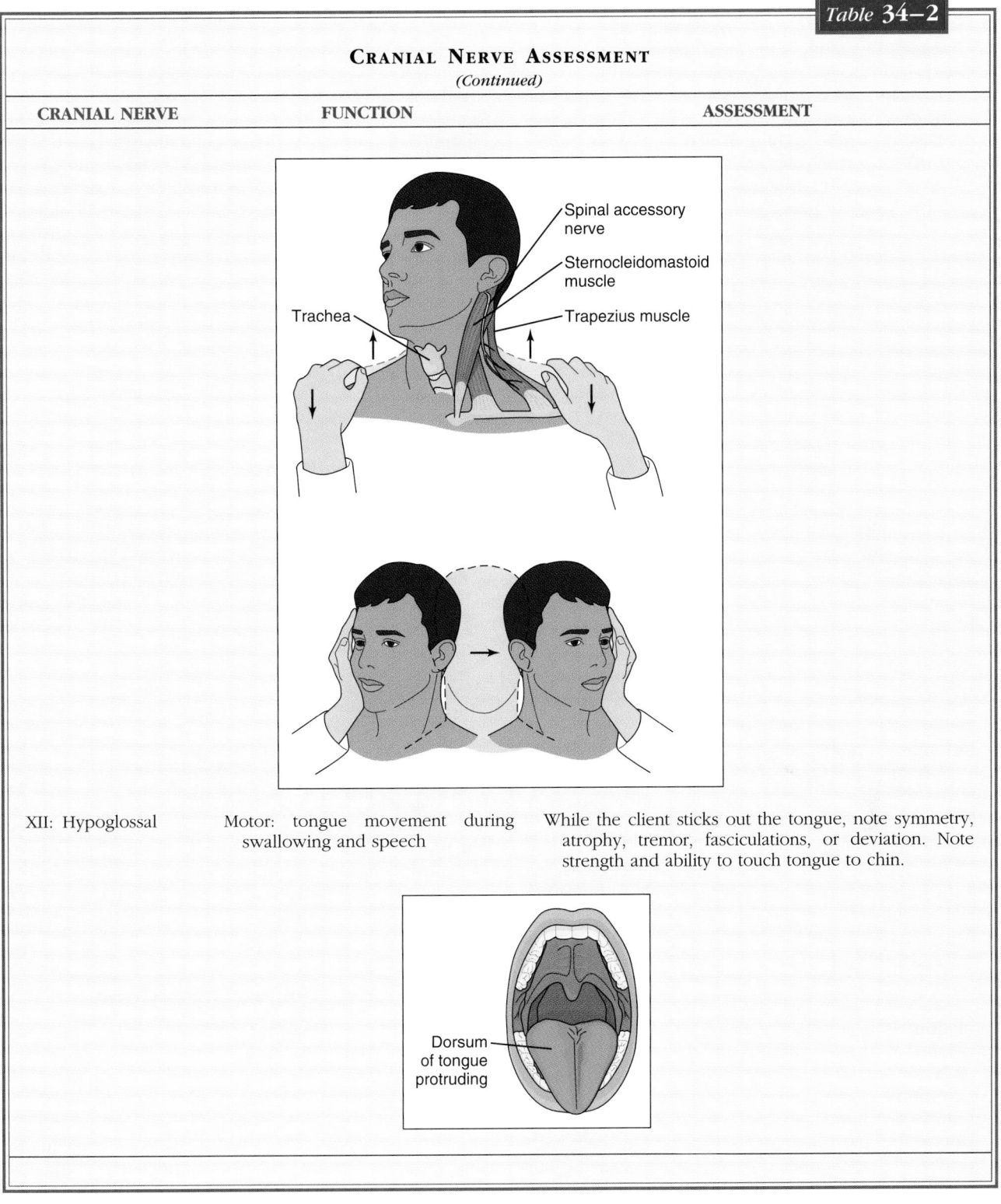

XII: Hypoglossal	Motor: tongue movement during swallowing and speech	While the client sticks out the tongue, note symmetry, atrophy, tremor, fasciculations, or deviation. Note strength and ability to touch tongue to chin.

gory that describes a sudden temporary adverse behavioral response to a change in the pattern of normally encountered stimuli (NANDA, 1990, p. 92).

The ineffective responses to stimuli listed in Box 34–2 are diagnostic cues to nursing diagnoses (Gordon, 1991). Risk factors for, or barriers to, accurate sensory perception are identified in Box 34–3. The number and severity of behavioral manifestations and the presence of secondary sequelae need to be considered when selecting appropriate nursing diagnoses for ineffective responses to sensory stimuli. For example, the appropriate diagnosis for a 56-year-old man in an acute confusional state in the intensive care unit after heart surgery is sensory/perceptual alteration, input excess. The unfamiliar technology, personnel, routines, and atmosphere in the intensive care environment provide the right conditions for concurrent sensory overload and deprivation. His ability to cope with these stressors is influenced by existing physiological risk factors or barriers (*e.g.*, anemia, electrolyte imbalance, interrupted sleep, and fluid balance) imposed by heart surgery. Secondary diagnoses might include altered thought processes, self-care deficit, and risk for injury, all warranted by the disability imposed by the acute confusional state.

The primary diagnosis for a woman who has neuropathy and retinopathy as a result of long-term or poorly managed diabetes mellitus would be sensory/perceptual alteration: impaired function of the special senses. Because her sensory deficits prevent her from accurately perceiving thermal, tactile, and visual stimuli and place her at risk for accidents and injury, she also has a risk for injury directly related to her sensory deficits.

Once the appropriate nursing diagnoses have been determined, interventions to achieve desired outcomes are identified. Examples of nursing diagnoses appropriate for clients who are at risk or actually experiencing sensory/perceptual alterations are provided in the accompanying box.

Planning

Nurses need to identify and try to prevent manifestations of altered sensory perception. Persons who are actually experiencing or are at risk for alterations in sensory perception are identified in the assessment phase of the nursing process.

Community vision and hearing screenings are helpful in identifying people with visual and auditory deficits. Well-child health checks and routine vision and hearing screenings in public schools can identify deficits at an early age, before growth and learning are affected.

Data compiled during the assessment provide information about a person's cognitive function, sensory function, social interaction, communication ability, activity level, independence, and chemical agent history. An inventory of the person's physiological, psychological, and environmental barriers should be taken. What sensory disabilities does the person have to deal with? The quality and number of orienting cues in the current environment (*e.g.*, windows, clocks, calendars, and sources of outdoor light) should be noted (Fig. 34–6). Recent social disruptions should be identified, and abnormal laboratory values and active disease processes should be considered (Inouye *et al.*, 1993; Williams *et al.*, 1985). The more barriers the person has, the greater his or her risk for altered sensory perception (Wilson, 1993). See Nursing Care Plan 34–1 for a client with a hip fracture.

Implementation

Persons at risk may benefit from the timely implementation of preventive interventions and avoid the morbidity and loss of independence associated with sensory/perceptual alterations. Nursing interventions should be directed at (1) identifying persons at risk, (2) optimizing sensory function, (3) modifying or correcting the etiology, and (4) promoting adaptation by preventing injury and restoring optimal functioning. As discussed, the range of tolerance to extremes in sensory stimuli and alterations in normal patterns of stimuli is individual. An attempt should be made to tailor interventions to each client based on his or her unique responses to stimuli. The client's age, developmental stage, values, and beliefs must be considered when interpreting assessment data and planning interventions (Albers Evans & Cunningham, 1996; McSweeney & Zhan, 1994).

Research-Based Intervention

Research is needed to identify strategies that are effective in preventing or reducing the negative impact of excessive or deficient environmental stimuli in persons who are at risk for sensory/perceptual alterations. There is little recent research on interventions, and existing research covers only a few client populations. Consequently, interventions are often implemented on a trial-and-error basis, based on nursing experience and common sense (Agostinelli *et al.*, 1994). Nursing studies in the last decade have tested interventions such as providing eyeglasses, hearing aids, calendars, television and radio access, lighting and room temperature adjustments, privacy, and personal belongings and pajamas to hospitalized medical and surgical clients. These strategies sometimes have a positive effect on the prevention or elimination of manifestations of sensory/perceptual alteration (Nagley, 1986; Scherubel & Tess, 1994; Wanich *et al.*, 1992; Williams *et al.*, 1985). A thorough discussion of the interventions follows.

Environmental Structuring

♦ **Optimizing Sensory Organ Function.** The goal of environmental structuring is to prevent or correct sensory deprivation and overload and to minimize the effects of sensory deficits (Manion, 1990). The first step is to identify sensory impairments and investigate the cause. Cerumen (ear wax) impaction is a common and easily corrected cause of conductive hearing loss in the elderly (Hasel & Erickson, 1995; Zivic & King, 1993). Impacted cerumen should be removed by a skilled practitioner before further evaluation of hearing deficits takes place (see Procedure 34–1).

Once correctable causes of sensory dysfunction are identified, the next step is to make sure that sensory aids such as hearing aids and eyeglasses are available and functioning properly. Performing the physical assessment (*e.g.*, sensory organ assessment or

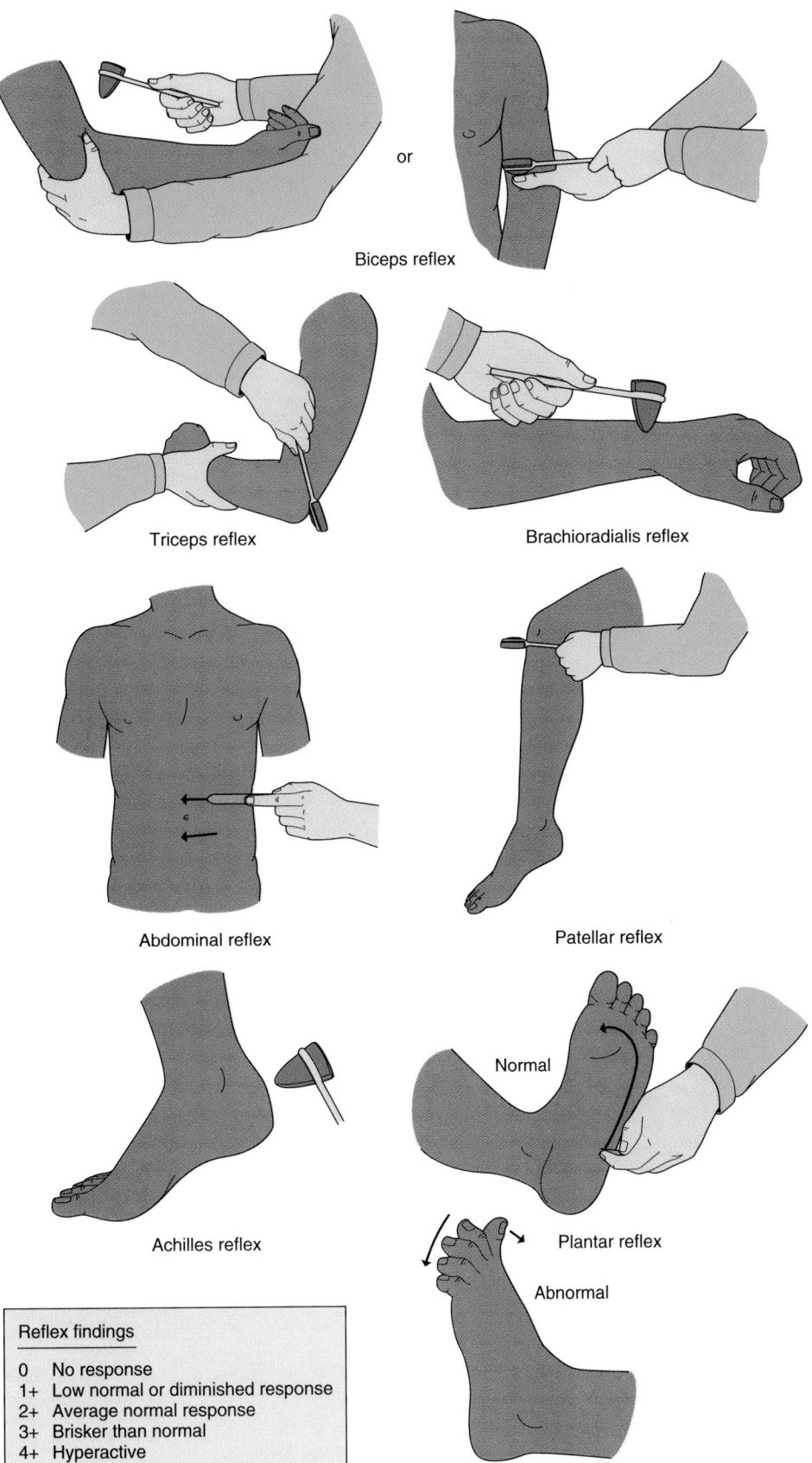

Biceps reflex

Triceps reflex

Brachioradialis reflex

Abdominal reflex

Patellar reflex

Achilles reflex

Normal

Plantar reflex

Abnormal

Reflex findings

0	No response
1+	Low normal or diminished response
2+	Average normal response
3+	Brisker than normal
4+	Hyperactive

❥ **Figure 34–5**
Testing deep tendon reflexes. (See also Table 34–3.)

Table 34–3

TESTING REFLEXES

REFLEX	LEVEL OF SPINAL CORD OR NERVE	ASSESSMENT	NORMAL RESPONSE
Deep tendon reflexes			
Biceps	C5-6	Examiner supports client's forearm on own forearm while placing thumb on client's biceps tendon just above elbow fossa. Strike directly through examiner's thumb. (See Fig. 34–5.)	Flexion of forearm into upper arm
Triceps	C7-8	Flex client's arm at elbow with palm toward body and pull it slightly across chest. Strike triceps tendon above elbow with a direct, nonglancing blow. (See Fig. 34–5.)	Triceps muscle should contract and extend at the elbow
Brachioradialis	C5-6	With client's forearm resting in lap, strike the radius 1–2 in. above the wrist. (See Fig. 34–5.)	Flexion and supination of forearm
Patellar	L2-4	Client sits on exam table dangling legs over edge. Examiner places hand over quadriceps muscle and strikes tendon just below the patella. (See Fig. 34–5.)	Extension of lower leg and contraction of quadriceps
Achilles	S1-2	Dorsiflex foot and strike Achilles tendon. (See Fig. 34–5.)	Plantarflexion of foot
Superficial (cutaneous) reflexes			
Corneal	CN V	Create a light breeze directly in front of the person's eyes by fanning the air. Observe for spontaneous blinking throughout the exam.	Spontaneous blinking or blinking in response to fanned air
Palatal	CN IX	Stimulate (touch) the soft palate (roof of mouth) with a tongue blade	Swallowing
Pharyngeal	CN X	Stimulate (touch) the pharynx (back of throat near uvula) with a tongue blade	Swallowing or gagging
Abdominal	T8-12	Lightly and briskly stroke the abdomen diagonally toward the umbilicus in all four quadrants. (See Fig. 34–5.)	Contraction of abdominal muscles and deviation of umbilicus toward stimulus; obesity may hide this reflex
Cremasteric (male)	L1-2	Lightly stroke the inner aspect of each thigh.	Ascension of testicle on side of stimulus
Plantar	L2-4	Using a dull, pointed object, such as the handle end of a reflex hammer, stroke the sole of the foot from the heel, up the lateral side, and across the ball of the foot. (See Fig. 34–5.)	Normal: plantarflexion of all toes Abnormal: +Babinski sign—dorsiflexion of the great toe and fanning of the other toes

cranial nerve assessment) with the client's sensory aids in place will detect device deficiencies and/or malfunctions. Eyeglasses and hearing aids are expensive, and proper care ensures optimal function and prolonged use. Box 34–7 provides suggestions for hearing aid care and support of a person with a hearing aid.

✦ **Sensory Assistive Devices.** After sensory organ function has been optimized (*e.g.*, proper eyeglass

Potential for Injury Related to Sensory Organ Deficits

Outcomes: Avoids injury, uses sensory aids, demonstrates caution and use of methods to prevent errors. Able to use emergency communication equipment.

Interventions: Optimize sensory function with eyeglasses, hearing aids; use auxiliary devices (see Box 34–8). Maintain safety: hand rails, ambulation assist devices, large lettering on signs. Remove unnecessary equipment from hallways and ambulation areas. Persons with neuropathy should check footware for proper fit and presence of foreign objects. Adjust water heater to maximum temperature of 110–115°F. Assess environment for presence of smoke detectors and/or smoke or heat alert devices.

Self-Care Deficit Related to Altered Cognitive Function, Inaccurate Perceptions

Outcomes: Regains or maintains level of independence enjoyed prior to the change in normal pattern of stimuli.

Interventions: Assess ability to bathe, dress, and feed self. Encourage attempts at self-care. Provide assist devices such as walkers, hand rails, toilet seat elevators, and hand rails.

Sensory/Perceptual Alteration Sensory Excess, Infant and Child

Outcomes: Consolable or able to self-quiet, able to use gaze aversion and hand to mouth to maintain quiet state. Cooperative, less fearful, oriented, shows interest in normal play activities.

Interventions: Eliminate negative stimulation, assist infant to maintain flexed position and achieve hand to mouth, swaddle and rock, provide nonnutritive sucking, support and educate parents.

Sensory/Perceptual Alteration Sensory Deficit, Infant and Child

Outcomes: Interacts with environment, achieves age-appropriate developmental tasks.

Interventions: Vestibular stimulation, preparatory sensory information, support system enhancement; provide personal belongings, play age-appropriate games.

Sensory/Perceptual Alteration Sensory Excess, Adult

Outcomes: Oriented, relaxed, intact cognitive function, adequate sleep.

Interventions: Delirium management: relieve pain, restore and maintain sense of control, assist person to pay attention and concentrate.

Sensory/Perceptual Alteration Sensory Organ Deficit, Adult

Outcomes: Maintains level of self-care and independence. Avoids injury and inaccurate judgment. Uses sensory aids.

Interventions: Facilitate visiting by family and normal social contacts. Expose to normal changes in light, newspapers, music, tape recordings of family voices. Provide orienting tools: newspaper, calendar, clock. Provide sensory aids.

Altered Thought Processes

Outcome: Intact mental status.

Interventions: Identify and eliminate etiology. Provide reality orientation and orienting cues. Maintain safety.

Altered Growth and Development, Infant

Outcomes: No sensory deficits, performs age- or ability-appropriate activities.

Interventions: Environmental modification to eliminate detrimental sensory stimuli. Enhance support systems. Use individualized developmental assessment and planning. Teach parents appropriate stimuli for developmental stage. Provide age-appropriate toys (*e.g.,* mobile).

---

prescription and adequate hearing aid function), sensory augmentation should be considered. People with sensory impairments can use services, devices, and methods that enhance their ability to give and receive information (see Box 34–8). Services include sign and foreign language interpretation, video- and audiotaped information, and printed material. There are telecommunications devices that enable television, radio, and telephone use and enhance the ability to hear conversation. Note writing, pictorial communication, lipreading, and hand gestures are examples of communication methods that can be used with sensory-impaired people (Beveridge, 1994).

In the community, social services, visiting nursing services, state and/or local commissions for the blind and deaf, and local telecommunications service carri-

ers are resources. In the inpatient health care setting, these services are available through social services, rehabilitation services, and communications services (switchboard).

✦ **Manipulating the Quality of Stimuli.** After sensory organ function has been optimized by treating correctable causes and using augmentation devices, external stimuli should be modified. For example, three environmental factors that affect vision are illumination, contrast, and pattern. Box 34–9 lists interventions to optimize the perception of visual stimuli.

✦ **Modifying the Variety of Stimuli.** Environmental structuring in the home or institutional health care setting includes replacing detrimental sensory input

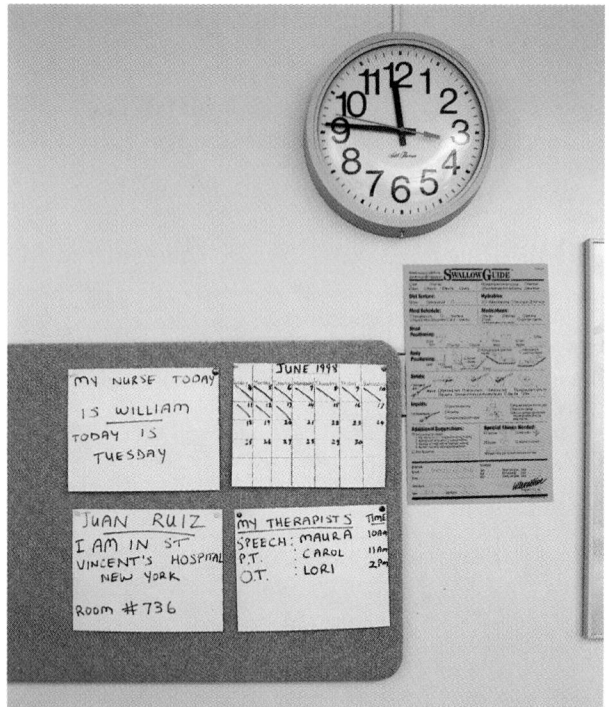

✦ **Figure 34–6**
Orienting cues, such as a clock, a calendar, and notes identifying
hospital personnel, can help prevent altered sensory perception.

with tolerable variations in visual, auditory, olfactory, tactile, and proprioceptive stimuli (Thomas, 1990). The environment of a sensory-impaired person should be designed to decrease exposure to extremes in sensory stimuli. Persons who have been relocated to unfamiliar environments should not be deprived of personal belongings and contact with significant others (Nagley, 1986; Wanich *et al.*, 1992). Strategies for providing therapeutic visual stimulation should be designed. Such strategies include using art, patterns, textures, shapes, and lighting that research has shown to be nonirritating (Christenson, 1990; Thomas, 1990).

Attempts should be made to vary the environment by taking the person to planned activities in different rooms, if the client's physical condition permits. Going for walks and going outdoors should be incorporated into daily routines. Planning several activities, with each one occurring in a designated room, can help provide a balance of variation and routine and avoid sensory overload. Moving from room to room or going outdoors can provide variations in visual, thermal, olfactory, and proprioceptive sensations as well. Appropriate auditory stimuli incorporate the client's choice of music, television, radio, or tape recordings of familiar, meaningful voices. Sources of tactile stimulation include back rubs, hand-holding, hugs, and petting animals (Fig. 34–7). When possible, the opportunity to experience different aromas should be provided. The smell of freshly cut grass or baking is a source of pleasant olfactory stimuli. Special sweet snacks and hard candy are sources of gustatory stimu-

lation, which can be modified to fit dietary restrictions (Christenson, 1990; Thomas, 1990). Box 34–10 summarizes interventions that promote optimal tactile, olfactory, and gustatory senses.

Rhythmic motion may provide a beneficial source of stimulation and relaxation. Vestibular stimulation is an intervention designed to stimulate the eighth cranial nerve using rhythmic motions such as rocking, swinging, being pushed in a stroller or wheelchair or pulled in a wagon, or lying on a water mattress. These activities provide rhythmic motions that diminish the perception of excessive environmental stimuli while providing a source of tolerable and soothing stimulation. In children, the benefits of vestibular stimulation include a calming effect and enhanced cognitive, physical, and social development (Leners, 1990). It is theorized that active rocking in older adults may produce relaxation and decrease sympathetic nervous system activity, but research has not supported this idea (Houston, 1993).

Alternative strategies are needed for persons who are confined to their rooms because of critical illness or isolation for protection or quarantine. Research on such interventions is needed. Old research has shown that the mere presence of windows may decrease manifestations of sensory/perceptual alteration in general surgical clients (Wilson, 1972), and clocks, calendars, and television help maintain orientation after heart surgery (Budd & Brown, 1974).

Alternative methods of communicating with health care personnel are needed for persons who are unable to vocalize because of language barriers (non-English-speaking), disease processes (aphasia, dysarthria), or medical treatment (endotracheal intubation, jaw immobilization). These clients should be provided with a means of communicating through interpreters, hand signals, nods, writing, or the selection of symbols or common phrases from a communication chart (Halm & Alpen, 1993). Refer to Box 34–11 for a discussion of barriers to verbal communication and services available to overcome them.

Loss of contact with significant others is a barrier to accurate sensory perception. Family and friends can be prepared to assist in the prevention and treatment of sensory/perceptual alteration. Research has shown that teaching the wives of male cardiac surgical patients about postoperative care, equipment, and the need for touch and orientation produces a desirable effect on orientation, behavioral appropriateness, confusion, delusions, and sleep (Chatham, 1978). Premature infants benefit from enhancement of parental support. Parents should be taught to understand the meaning of infant physiological and behavioral responses and how environmental stimulation affects physical and cognitive development (Als *et al.*, 1988; Lawhon, 1986).

✦ **Reducing Excess Stimuli.** Strategies for avoiding sensory overload include removing or buffering excess sensory stimuli. Sources of excess stimuli include noise, lighting, odors, people, and pain.

SAMPLE NURSING CARE PLAN

DIABETIC CLIENT WITH A HIP FRACTURE

Situation: An 84-year-old diabetic woman with a hip fracture is admitted to the general medical surgical floor after total hip replacement. On the first postoperative day, you enter her room to find her sitting at the side of her bed, her IV stretched tight and urinary bladder catheter coiled up on the floor. She is grimacing and diaphoretic. She asks, "Why did you tie my arm to the fence?" and begs, "Shoot that snake before it bites me." When you try to help her lie down, she resists, tries to hit you, and swears loudly.

Nursing Diagnosis: Sensory/perceptual alteration: input excess and sensory organ dysfunction.

Expected Outcomes: Normal thought process, calm affect, cooperates with caregiver, avoids further injury, satisfied with pain control.

Action	Rationale
1. Provide any sensory aids normally used (eyeglasses, hearing aid).	1. Use of corrective lenses and hearing aids optimizes visual and auditory perception.
2. Provide orientation cues (clock, calendar, newspaper, signs, and exposure to outdoor light changes).	2. Orienting items helps restore normal environmental cues.
3. Assess the client's awareness and perception of pain and provide adequate relief measures.	3. Adequate pain management reduces psychological and physiological stress and preoccupation with pain; reduces strain on tolerance.
4. Simulate routines in sleep (e.g., promote nocturnal sleep by adjusting lighting, decreasing noise, and modifying care routines to allow 60- to 90-minute sleep periods).	4. Promotes normal sleep patterns and reduces strain on tolerance to alterations in stimuli exposure.
5. Maintain safety: physical or chemical restraints.	5. Safety measures reduce the risk of injury secondary to impaired judgment.
6. Treat the client politely and with respect and do not speak about the client as if he or she were absent.	6. Avoids depersonalization and risk of delusions.
7. Acknowledge fears; do not minimize or deny perceptions.	7. Provides unconditional positive regard and trust.
8. Identify and modify etiological factors causing acute confusional state (ACS).	8. Barriers may be modified or eliminated, reducing strain on tolerance.
9. Reduce exposure to monotonous and irritating stimuli (e.g., noise and odors). Attempt to provide exposure to pleasant stimuli (e.g., flowers, music, art, human touch).	9. Reduces risk of sensory input excess or deficit.
10. Encourage the presence and assistance of significant others, and maintain consistent pattern of caregivers.	10. Maintains contact with familiar people.
11. Provide personal belongings (e.g., pictures of family, rosary, pajamas).	11. Maintains contact with personal items and identity. Maintains some sense of control.
12. Prepare for environmental change by explaining smells, touches, pressures, discomfort, positions, tastes, and sights that accompany a procedure or event.	12. Allows the client time to mentally prepare for the event and reduces risk for misperceptions, anxiety, and sensory overload.
13. Provide objective information on the purpose and duration of treatments and activities.	13. Increases knowledge, cooperation, and sense of control.
14. Promote mobility as frequently as appropriate. Provide regular turning and out-of-bed activity.	14. Reduced mobility is associated with ACS.
15. Prepare for discharge by assessing the need for home care personnel and any mobility or sensory assist devices that may be needed.	15. Discharge planning makes the transition to home less chaotic.

Data from Albers Evans, Jones Kenny, & Rizzuto, 1993; Christenson, 1990.

PROCEDURE

34–1

CERUMEN REMOVAL BY CURETTE OR IRRIGATION

Equipment: otoscope
curette
otological syringes or 20 to 50-cc syringes with flexible angiocatheter attached
water jet dental irrigating device (Water Pik)
body temperature water
emesis basin
towel

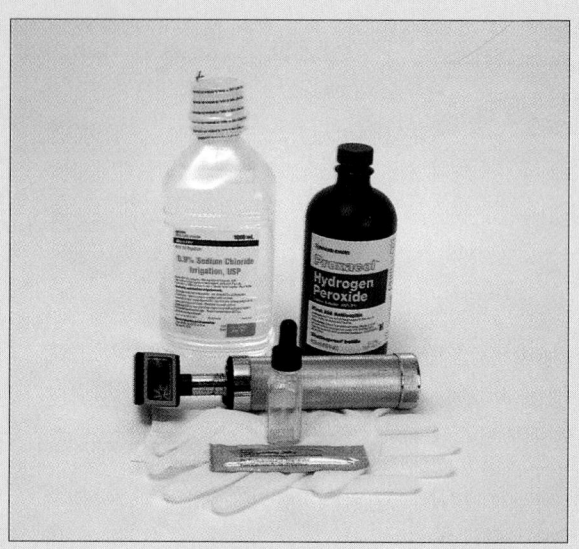

Removal of Cerumen by Curette

Action

1. Use otoscope to visualize. Insert curette distal to impaction and gently pull wax outward.

Removal of Cerumen by Irrigation

Action

1. Examine the ear with an otoscope.

2. Explain the procedure to the client and caution against sudden movements.

3. If client is a child or not responsible for his or her actions, obtain assistance with head immobilization.

4. Check the temperature of the irrigating solution; it should be body temperature or 37°C.

5. Cover the client's shoulders with a towel and position an emesis basin or suitable drainage receptacle against the neck under the ear lobe. Have the client assist with holding the basin if able.

6. Tip the client's head toward the shoulder on the side being irrigated.

7. Fill the syringe with irrigating solution and purge the air. Place the tip of the irrigating device barely inside the external meatus. The tip should still be visible.

8. Pull up and back on the pinna to straighten the ear canal.

9. Direct the stream of the fluid toward the posterior wall of the ear canal.

Rationale

1. Blind removal is never attempted, owing to the risk of perforating the eardrum or lacerating the ear canal.

Rationale

1. Confirms presence of cerumen and identifies infection or abnormalities in the tympanic membrane that may contraindicate lavage.

2. Teaching provides reassurance and decreases anxiety, reduces risk of injury.

3. Decreases risk of sudden head movement and injury to ear canal and tympanic membrane.

4. Temperature extremes can cause injury, nausea, vomiting, dizziness.

5. Prevents the client from becoming unnecessarily wet and catches irrigation debris.

6. Allows irrigation solution to run out into basin.

7. Prevents excessive insertion of the irrigation device tip and decreases risk of injury.

8. Allows the irrigation solution to be directed to the posterior wall of the ear canal.

9. Avoids direct pressure and injury to the tympanic membrane.

PROCEDURE

34–1

CERUMEN REMOVAL BY CURETTE OR IRRIGATION

(Continued)

Action	Rationale
10. Inject the fluid slowly, maintaining a steady stream, or in short pulsatile squirts.	**10.** Both injection methods loosen and flush out cerumen.
11. Stop the irrigation if the client complains of pain, dizziness, or nausea.	**11.** These are signs of intolerance and/or injury.
12. Intermittently examine the ear canal during the procedure, checking for residual cerumen. Continue irrigating as long as the client is comfortable and cerumen remains in the ear.	**12.** Confirms success or failure of procedure.
13. Dry the canal gently with a cotton-tipped swab.	**13.** Residual moisture is a source for infection.
14. Add a chemical to the ear canal such as acetic acid and benzethonium chloride or 70% isopropyl alcohol.	**14.** Chemically dries and restores proper ear pH.
15. Instruct the client that cerumen production is normal. Advise to avoid inserting objects such as bobby pins or paper clips into the ear. Instruct to use a damp washcloth wrapped around a fingertip to clean the ear canal instead of inserting cotton swabs into the ear.	**15.** Objects can injure the ear canal or eardrum.

Document the following:

Irrigation device used and the type, temperature, and amount of irrigation solution

Ceruminolytic agents used, amount, and frequency

Appearance of the ear canal and tympanic membrane before and after the procedure

Improvement or deterioration in hearing

Tolerance of the procedure (*e.g.,* pain, nausea, vomiting, vertigo)

Amount and appearance of cerumen or debris removed from ear canal

Noise. Noise levels in caregiving environments may reach detrimental levels (Baker, 1993; Halm & Alpen, 1993). Noise should be monitored and maintained at tolerable levels. Sources of avoidable noise include personal conversations and laughter among staff, dropping of metal objects, and toilet flushing (Baker, 1993; Thomas, 1990).

Lighting. Unvaried harsh lighting can also contribute to sensory overload. Lighting should be bright and indirect, and attempts to simulate routines of normal light exposure should be made (Geary, 1994; Kolanowski, 1992).

Odors. Odors in the client's environment may also have a negative sensory impact. Smells that permeate carpet and curtains should be eliminated (Christenson, 1990). The quality of the odors that the client is exposed to should be monitored and controlled.

Box 34–7

SUPPORTING A CLIENT WITH A HEARING AID

Hearing Aid Care

Cleaning

Clean it daily with a dry soft toothbrush and soft tissue. Don't use water, alcohol, or any liquid to clean the hearing aid. Don't insert toothpicks, pins, or sharp objects into the hearing aid openings to clean it. Avoid exposing the hearing aid to cosmetics, hair sprays, oils, and lotions. Remove the hearing aid when bathing. After bathing or showering, make sure the ear is completely dry before inserting the hearing aid, because moisture is detrimental to the electronic circuitry.

Batteries

Keep batteries in a cool, dry place. Keep extra batteries in supply. When not in use, turn the hearing aid off and remove the battery. Check and replace the battery frequently.

Storage

The hearing aid should be worn at all times when awake, except when bathing or swimming. When not in use, keep the hearing aid in a cool, dry place, and avoid temperature extremes.

Volume

Adjust the hearing aid volume to the minimal adequate level to avoid feedback, squeaking, or whistling.

Nursing Support

- Assist with proper insertion. Practice insertion and removal until the client feels confident and comfortable handling the hearing aid.

- Help the client learn to insert the battery correctly. If the battery is inserted incorrectly or has reached the end of its life, the hearing aid will not function. Identify locations where batteries can be purchased and keep extras in supply.

- Teach the person how to adjust the hearing aid volume after it is properly inserted. If the client has hearing aids for both ears, differentiate the right from the left.

- If whistling occurs, check the position and make adjustments to improve fit.

- Sometimes hearing aids whistle during telephone use. If this occurs, instruct the client to angle the receiver away from the ear until the whistling stops.

- Encourage the client to use the hearing aid at all times.

- Frequently check ears for cerumen buildup and remove regularly.

- Point out the benefits of hearing aid use, *e.g.,* improved ability to receive auditory stimuli and participate in conversations. Even people with sensorineural hearing loss may benefit from sound amplification provided by a hearing aid.

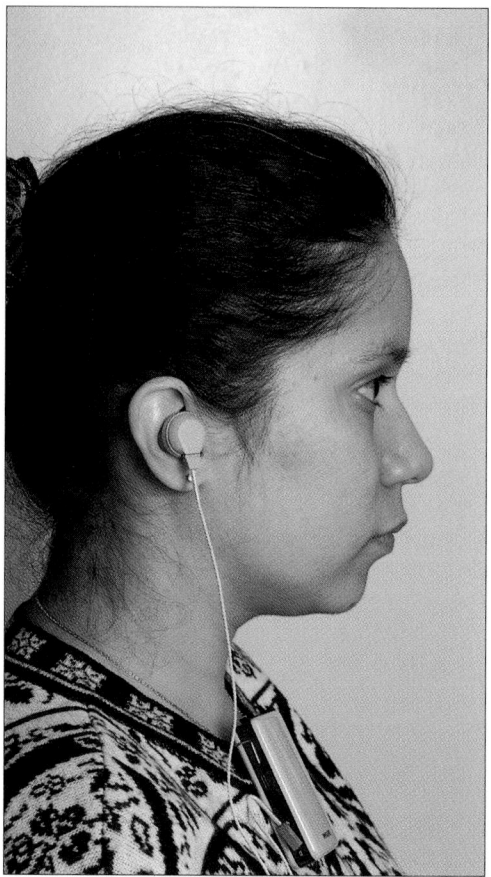

Client wearing a hearing aid

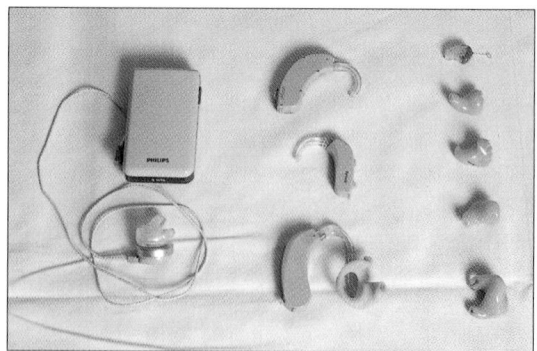

Types of hearing aids

Box 34–8

SENSORY ASSIST DEVICES, TECHNIQUES, AND SERVICES FOR PEOPLE WITH SENSORY IMPAIRMENTS

Deaf or Hearing-Impaired Persons

Sign Language Interpreters

Diagnostic, Treatment, and/or Decision-Making Situations

When decisions about health care treatment options or diagnostic information must be exchanged, the use of a qualified interpreter is advised. A qualified interpreter is a person who is specially trained and possibly certified in interpreting American Sign Language and English. These people are listed in the Registry of Interpreters for the Deaf and adhere to a code of ethics that includes maintaining confidentiality, impartiality, and discretion in sign language interpretation situations.

Nonmedical Situations

Interpretation assistance from family members, friends, or inpatient facility volunteers is appropriate in nonmedical situations. For example, nonregistered interpreters could help a deaf person select diet menu items or translate preferences about the furniture arrangement.

Volunteer Interpreters

Inpatient and outpatient health care facilities should keep lists of employees and local volunteers who are willing to translate for clients with language barriers. Volunteers should be briefed on the principles of confidentiality. Use of volunteer interpreters instead of qualified interpreters should be reserved for nonmedical situations or when general information will be exchanged, *e.g.,* menu selection, environmental comfort preferences, daily routine preferences, weather information, and current events.

Auxiliary Aids

TDD

A telecommunications device for the deaf (TDD) is a typewriter-like device used with a standard telephone that allows deaf persons to use the telephone.

Volume Control Telephone

A volume control telephone is a telephone handset that has been modified to provide receiver amplification.

Telecaption Closed-Caption Decoder

The telecaption closed-caption decoder is a device that is either attached to or located within a television set. It generates printing on the bottom of the television screen (like subtitles), so that hearing-impaired persons can follow the dialogue.

Amplified Listening Devices

An amplified listening device (ALD) can enhance a hearing-impaired person's ability to hear words spoken during one-on-one conversations. The device can also be used to amplify TV or radio sound and to augment hearing aid performance.

Visual Aids and Methods

Presenting information visually when an interpreter is not available can be an effective communication means. Visual methods are also useful tools that speech-impaired persons can use to convey information when sign language is not an option.

Note Writing and Picture Communicating

Note writing requires the ability to read and simple equipment such as a tablet and pen or a dry-erase board. For persons who are debilitated, holding a pen or pencil may be a challenge. These people may find it easier to control a medium- or broad-point felt-tip marker. Nurses should keep in mind that for many deaf persons, American Sign Language is their primary language and English is their second language, which may hinder their ability to communicate effectively by writing notes. For these people, picture communicators may be more appropriate. A picture communicator features simple pictures of common questions and basic human needs. For example, if the client points to a picture of a clock, the nurse knows that the client wants information about the time. A picture of a bedpan or commode indicates that the client needs to use the toilet. Picture communicators may also display the alphabet, so that partial or full spelling can be used to convey a thought or a question.

Lipreading

Some hearing-impaired persons are able to lip-read. Lipreading can be an adequate means of communicating on a routine, uncompromised basis. However, illness or injury may expose a person to environmental change and unfamiliar terminology that can't be recognized by lipreading. It is important to note that illness may impair the ability to lip-read. Nurses should confirm that clients understand what they are told by asking them to reflect or summarize the information they are given.

Gesturing

Gesturing refers to nonverbal communication with facial expressions and body movements that may serve as an adjunct to note writing and speaking with hearing-impaired persons. People with language or speech barriers may also find gestures helpful, particularly when trying to convey symptoms that have universal expressions or gestures. For example, hands clutching the throat indicate choking, whereas a furrowed brow, open eyes, and sad mouth indicate discomfort or pain.

Printed Material

Printed material can be used to convey health-related information or to provide diversional activity. Examples include written instructions for diagnostic test preparation or poetry or fiction material. Printed material requires the ability to read, and it may be necessary to arrange an interpreter to ascertain a deaf person's understanding of printed material.

Continued on following page

Box 34–8

SENSORY ASSIST DEVICES, TECHNIQUES, AND SERVICES FOR PEOPLE WITH SENSORY IMPAIRMENTS
(Continued)

Telecommunication Relay Services

This service is available through local telephone service carriers. It allows deaf, hearing-impaired, and speech-impaired people to communicate with one another by telephone with the assistance of an agent, who relays the conversation.

Vision-Impaired Persons

A simple magnifying glass may be helpful to a person with poor vision. Special magnifying devices are also available for computer screens. Audiotaped information is an excellent communication method for vision-impaired people. Audiovisual material may also be helpful, as long as gestures are not heavily relied on to convey the content. Telephone dials and clocks with large numbers, books on tape, and braille or large-print reading material help vision-impaired people maintain their independence. Some telephone service carriers waive directory assistance and operator dialing assistance charges for vision-impaired people, because large-print telephone directories are usually not available. There are also devices that enable visually impaired people to use computers. Software programs provide magnification. Magnifiers and filters can be attached to the screen to provide enlargement of text and graphics. Even blind people can use computer output in auditory or tactile form. Devices such as screen readers can verbalize information on the computer screen. Special printers can actually print in braille.

Data from Beveridge, 1994; Erber, 1994.

Box 34–9

INTERVENTIONS TO OPTIMIZE THE PERCEPTION OF VISUAL STIMULI

Visual Aids

* Ensure that appropriate corrective lenses are worn.
* Provide a magnifying glass to read labels.

Communication

* Identify yourself and anyone accompanying you to the client.
* Explain your purpose for being there.
* Speak to the client face-to-face in close proximity so that he or she can see you and receive clues from your body language.
* When conversing in a social situation, refer to people in the group by name, not pronouns (*i.e.,* he or she).
* Describe the size, shape, and colors of items used in personal care activities.
* Design signs and posters with large lettering on contrasting background and nonglossy paper.

Environment

* See that auxiliary lighting and furniture are properly placed so that light is distributed evenly throughout the room and chairs are positioned near windows to take advantage of natural lighting.
* Minimize glare from windows by using blinds or shades.
* Use night-lights in bedrooms and bathrooms.
* Install dimmer light switches to allow gradual increases or decreases in illumination and avoid sudden changes in light intensity that may be difficult to adjust to.
* Provide color and contrast in the environment. At certain distances, older people need three times as much color contrast as younger people to see patterns clearly.
* Paint doorways, doorknobs, and floor borders a contrasting color from the walls. Furniture and walls should contrast in color. Brightly colored accessories (*e.g.,* vases and lamps) make furniture easier to locate.
* Use the clock technique for describing the position of food on the plate (*e.g.,* your mashed potatoes are at 12 o'clock).
* Position medication in the client's visual field. Determine the client's ability to set up his or her own medications. Arrange assistance from friends, relatives, or visiting nurses.
* Obtain a telephone with large, raised, color-contrasted numbers and a programmable automatic dialing feature.
* Use a clock with oversized numbers and contrasting background.
* Provide large-print books, books on tape, and card games modified for vision-impaired persons.

Data from Kavanaugh & Tate, 1996; Christenson, 1990.

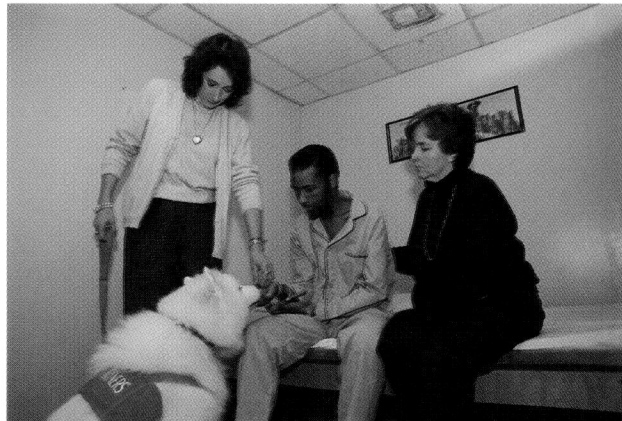

Figure 34–7
"Pet therapy" can provide much-needed tactile stimulation for sensory-deprived clients.

Personnel. Interventions should attempt to eliminate unnecessary exposure to unfamiliar hospital personnel and should strive for continuity in primary caregivers. Environmental services, laboratory, and other ancillary personnel should always identify themselves to the client, and the purpose of all equipment should be explained. Machines such as ventilators, balloon pumps, and pneumatic stockings should be removed when they are no longer needed (Easton & MacKenzie, 1988). Clients should be provided with explanations of environmental stimuli that they are subjected to (Halm & Alpen, 1993).

Nurses caring for infants in the intensive care environment should be educated about the importance of ongoing individual developmental assessment and the planning of care to avoid stressing the infant's physiological system and contributing to developmental and sensory deficits. Behavioral and physiological cues should be used to guide infant care and enable the infant to use self-regulating strategies. Protection from light and noise and positioning to maintain a flexed, stable posture are appropriate environmental modifications for premature or ill infants (D'Apolito, 1991; Gardner-Cole *et al.*, 1990).

Pain. Pain has been identified as a barrier to accurate sensory perception. In fact, pain was a major predictor of acute confusion in a study of elderly postsurgical clients (Duggleby & Lander, 1994). It is not clear whether pain precipitates acute confusional states or whether the state prevents the accurate perception of pain. Persons experiencing acute confusional states may deny that pain or discomfort is occurring, even though other physiological signs may be apparent (Inaba-Roland & Maricle, 1992). It is imperative that nurses assess for the presence of pain, especially in surgical clients. Assessment of pain should use age- and developmentally appropriate tools. In addition to regularly administered analgesia, interventions that promote muscle relaxation and anxiety relief should be implemented (Jacox, 1992).

Box 34–10

STRATEGIES TO OPTIMIZE TACTILE, GUSTATORY, AND OLFACTORY, STIMULATION

Tactile Impairment

Cause: Peripheral neuropathy, or delayed transmission of nerve signals owing to damage to the nerve fiber from disease or trauma. The person may not be able to perceive pain or feel temperature differences. People with diabetes mellitus can develop peripheral neuropathy.

Prevent injury
* Check bathwater and dishwater temperature with a thermometer
* Inspect extremities for injury
* Wear properly fitted shoes

Prevent sensory deprivation
* Therapeutic touch and massage therapy
* Regular turning and repositioning

Optimize skin integrity
* Prevent skin dryness
* Avoid excess moisture

Gustatory Impairment

Causes: Cranial nerve IX damage, tongue injury or disease

Enhance taste of food
* Serve adequately seasoned fresh foods
* Serve food at appropriate temperature
* Encourage sips of water between bites of food

Olfactory Impairment

Causes: Cranial nerve I damage, nasal allergies, viruses, or other diseases that occlude the nasal passages

Optimize the ability to sense odors and aromas
* Serve adequately seasoned fresh foods
* Provide sources of olfactory stimulation (*e.g.,* exposure to vegetation such as fresh flowers or cut grass)
* Treat viruses and illnesses that affect the patency of nasal passages

---

Efforts should be made to prepare persons for planned procedures involving various sensory experiences. Objective descriptions of sensory stimuli associated with health-related events and procedures should include the purpose and duration of the event or procedure and sights, sounds, tastes, touches, and body position encountered during the event (Christman *et al.*, 1992; Holt, 1993). Providing age-appropriate information to children before planned hospitalizations and procedures may reduce fear, anxiety, and ineffective physiological and behavioral responses (Thomas,

Box 34—11

SUPPORT FOR PERSONS WITH VERBALIZATION BARRIERS

Types of Verbalization Barriers

Although the inability to speak is not a sensory disorder, it does impair a person's ability to communicate. *Communication* is the process of sending and receiving verbal and nonverbal messages. *Language* is a system of symbols and signs that represent our thoughts. *Articulation* is the expression of thought through speech. *Speech* is the auditory expression of language and is one vehicle by which responses to stimuli are expressed.

Speech impairment may be classified into three categories: aphasia, dysarthria, and language barrier. There are two types of aphasia. *Expressive aphasia* is the inability to articulate speech because the words cannot be transferred from the cerebral cortex into a motor response. The person understands what is said to him or her and knows how he or she wants to respond, but can't. Damage to Broca's speech center in the brain results in expressive aphasia. *Receptive aphasia* is the inability to understand the spoken word when articulation is still possible. People with receptive aphasia can't understand what is said to them but can speak clearly, although their conversation is usually illogical. Damage to Wernicke's speech center in the brain can result in receptive aphasia. A cerebral vascular accident, tumor, or head trauma could cause damage to Broca's and Wernicke's speech centers. *Dysarthria* is the inability to articulate owing to altered structure or function of the speech organs (*e.g.*, larynx, cranial nerves V, VII, or IX). A *language barrier* exists when a person does not speak the same language as other people whom he or she must attempt to communicate with.

Interventions for People With Verbalization Barriers

Aphasia

In addition to audiovisual materials, picture communicators, gesturing, and note writing are useful communication methods for people with speech impairments. Nurses should consider the etiology of the speech impair-ment before selecting a communication device. For example, note writing may be ineffective for a person who can receive and understand information but can't articulate a response owing to expressive aphasia secondary to a cerebral vascular accident (damage to Broca's area). For expressive aphasia, use pantomime, ask closed-ended questions, encourage open-ended answers, and use note writing. For receptive aphasia, decrease environmental distractions when attempting to communicate; speak slowly and divide tasks into small steps.

Dysarthria

Exercise patience as the person attempts to verbalize. Encourage note writing, gesturing, and exercises to optimize the function of muscles used for forming speech.

Language Barriers

The AT&T Foreign Language Translation Service is available 24 hours a day to assist people who do not speak English or who have only a limited command of the language. The service is capable of either oral or written translation of over 140 languages and/or dialects. The service should be used when health care decision-making situations arise (*e.g.*, to describe medical procedures, present treatment options, obtain informed consent for treatment, and deliver special care instructions). Almost any type of organization that conducts business with non–English-speaking clients can benefit by having a Language Line account. In the inpatient setting, the institution's switchboard makes the proper connection with Language Line. The nurse, doctor, or health team member describes to the interpreter what the client needs to know about the treatment or procedure. The interpreter then repeats the information that he or she will tell the client so that inaccuracies can be detected before the information is conveyed. Personal interpretation through Language Line without a customer account is available. The toll-free number may be obtained by calling AT&T or a local telephone service carrier.

1990). Studies support the effectiveness of sensory preparation in decreasing the distress, restlessness, tension, confusion, and need for sedation associated with health-related procedures (Christman *et al.*, 1992).

Managing Acute Confusional States

When a client exhibits severe manifestations of sensory/perceptual alteration, or acute confusional state, additional interventions are needed to manage the constellation of alterations characteristic of ACS.

Reality orientation is the "promotion of a patient's awareness of personal identity, time and environment" (McCloskey & Bulechek, 1992, p. 404). Reality orientation is an essential supplement to helping acutely con-fused clients and can be implemented during normal conversation. For example, the nurse might enter a hospitalized client's room saying, "Good morning, Mr. Doe. I noticed your breakfast tray being prepared. Would you like me to open your curtains so you can see the sunshine? It's only going to be 75° today. That is really cool for the Fourth of July in central Iowa. Would you like to watch the space shuttle launch on CNN?" (Holt, 1993). It is important to avoid ignoring the other components of an acutely confused person's thought processes. Recent research emphasizes the need to enhance the concentration, attention, and memory aspects of thought process rather than trying to reorient clients (Foreman, 1991). This is accomplished by making tactile and eye-to-eye contact with the client while delivering step-by-step instructions.

Orienting cues in the form of calendars, clocks, and written instructions are also recommended (Agostinelli *et al.*, 1994).

Impaired orientation, reasoning, and judgment increase the acutely confused client's risk of injury. A safe environment should be provided by removing potentially harmful objects, such as scissors or sharps, from the client's range of reach. Side rails and physical and chemical restraints should be used if the client attempts to ambulate unassisted or remove intravenous access devices or other necessary equipment. The need for safety must be carefully weighed against the client's right to freedom and self-determination (Quinn, 1993). Careful documentation of behaviors indicating that the client is a danger to self or others should accompany the use of restraints. The use of a bed alarm and sitter should be considered as adjuncts or alternatives to physical restraints (Schott-Baer *et al.*, 1995).

Neuroleptics (haloperidol) and benzodiazepines (lorazepam, midazolam hydrochloride) are recommended as appropriate and effective chemical agents in the treatment of severe manifestations of sensory/perceptual alteration (Crippen, 1994; Fish, 1991). Haloperidol is the neuroleptic of choice in critically ill clients, because it does not have respiratory depressant side effects and is not addictive (Sanders & Stern, 1993). Although it may cause extrapyramidal symptoms (*e.g.*, abnormal movements of the arms, face, and neck and laryngospasm), it is generally well tolerated. The sedative and antipsychotic properties of lorazepam make it a good choice (Crippen, 1994; Fish, 1991). Haloperidol and lorazepam may actually complement each other when given simultaneously, requiring lower doses of each medication (Geary, 1994).

Facilitating accurate communication is essential. Simple, direct instructions regarding treatments and nursing care should be given. Clients who are unable to speak, such as mechanically ventilated clients or those who are simply too weak to verbalize, need to be provided with alternative means of communication. Enabling the client to write or use symbols and providing interpreters for non–English-speaking clients are examples. In addition, clients should be given unconditional positive regard, and their fears should not be ignored or invalidated. Caring and reassurance should be provided for illusions and hallucinations.

Above all, the nurse must act as an advocate for the acutely confused client, even when frustrated. It is essential to resist the urge to reprimand or scold acutely confused and agitated clients. Nurses must realize that these clients are victims of their altered perceptions and deserve to be treated courteously, even when they become a danger to others as well as themselves.

Evaluation

When the nurse evaluates a client with a diagnosis related to altered sensory stimulation, the specific outcomes must be addressed and, if necessary, adapted to the client's long-term needs. Many clients suffer long-term conditions that require attention to emotional as well as physical well-being. Networking, informing the client of community resources, and teaching the client about the value of support groups are all important aspects of nursing care.

In acute situations, such as with ACS or in the intensive care neonatal unit, evaluation involves close monitoring of mental status and vital signs. The astute nurse observes for often subtle, nonverbal as well as verbal signs that indicate whether the client is adapting to and coping with the environment.

Summary

Perception and response to stimuli may be voluntary or involuntary. Response to stimuli depends on (1) the ability to receive the stimuli through body structures that enable seeing, hearing, smelling, tasting, feeling, and awareness of body position and (2) the ability to send information about the stimuli to parts of the nervous system that can process and interpret it before initiating behavior in response to that stimuli.

Human responses are not always effective. Ineffective or maladaptive responses are the result of sudden changes in the character of stimuli or alterations in the ability to accurately perceive stimuli. Changes in the character of stimuli and/or the ability to perceive it present barriers to accurate sensory perception. Barriers are risk factors (*i.e.*, conditions or events) that interfere with perception and response to stimuli.

Age and culture can also affect the ability to perceive stimuli accurately. Adverse physiological responses and ineffective emotional or behavioral responses are manifestations of altered sensory perception.

The nursing process is used to identify persons at risk for or those actually experiencing sensory/perceptual alteration, plan preventive or therapeutic nursing interventions, and evaluate outcomes. Interventions for sensory/perceptual alteration include strategies to modify or correct the etiology, restore or maintain an optimal level of independence, and promote adaptation.

CHAPTER HIGHLIGHTS

✦ Stimuli are events or changes that provoke or excite a nerve. Stimuli are transmitted on nerves to the central nervous system, where they are interpreted. This process is called perception.

✦ Responses are behaviors elicited by stimuli. Human responses are the result of physical and mental adjustments that promote adaptation to the internal and external environment.

✦ The internal environment refers to the structures, organ systems, and tissues inside the body and their functions. The external environment refers to the people, living things, and objects in the world.

✦ Sensory deprivation and sensory overload represent changes in the character of stimuli.

✦ Neural structure refers to the anatomical properties of the nervous system, including neurons, sensory receptors, nerve fibers, the spinal cord, and brain structures. Neural function refers to the basic nervous system functions of reception and transmission.

Study Questions

1. Stimuli are

    a. structures in the nervous system
    b. false beliefs
    c. events or changes that provoke or excite a nerve

2. The stimulus-response process consists of

    a. reception, transmission, interpretation, perception, and response
    b. reception, diffusion, recognition, perception, and response
    c. reception, transmission, awareness, cognition, and response

3. Manifestations of altered sensory perception include

    a. confusion, disorientation, agitation
    b. second-degree burn on the foot of a diabetic client who did not realize that the bathwater was too hot
    c. disrupted sleep
    d. all of the above

4. Barriers to accurate sensory perception do not include

    a. sensory overload
    b. separation from family members
    c. inadequate oxygen
    d. being able to see a clock

5. The following are services, methods, and assistive devices for people with sensory organ impairments

    a. sign language interpreters, telecommunication device for the deaf (TDD), note writing
    b. eyeglasses, hearing aids, loud talking
    c. fluorescent-colored lettering, bright lighting, squinting

Critical Thinking Exercises

1. Ms. N. is an 83-year-old woman admitted to the coronary care unit following an acute myocardial infarction (heart attack). She has never been hospitalized before except for during childbirth. The coronary care unit is very busy; alarms are constant, lights are never dimmed, and open visitation is allowed. Ms. N. is on vital signs every 2 hours. The staff of the unit are in upheaval, and many temporary personnel are being utilized. Discuss the impli-

cations of this situation on the sensory perception of Ms. N.

2. Ms. Z. is sent home following a new diagnosis of retinitis pigmentosa. Her doctor estimates that Ms. Z. has about 6 months of poor eyesight left before she is totally blind. She has few visitors and no close family who live nearby. Discuss the sensory needs of Ms. Z. at her home.

References

Ackerman, L. L. (1993). Alteration in level of responsiveness: A proposed nursing diagnosis. *Nursing Clinics of North America, 28*(4), 729–746.

Agostinelli, B., Dimers, K., Garrigan, D., & Waszyski, C. (1994). Targeted interventions: Use of the Mini-Mental State Exam. *Journal of Gerontological Nursing, 20*(8), 15–23.

Albers Evans, C., & Cunningham, B. A. (1996). Caring for the ethnic elder. *Geriatric Nursing, 17*(3), 105–110.

Albers Evans, C., Jones Kenny, P., & Rizzuto, C. (1993). Caring for the confused geriatric surgical patient. *Geriatric Nursing, 14*(5), 237–241.

Als, H., Lawhon, A., Gibes, R., Duffy, F., McAnulty, G., & Blickman, H. (1988). Individualized behavioral and environmental care for the VLBW preterm infant at high risk for bronchopulmonary dysplasia and intraventricular hemorrhage. Study II: NICU outcome [abstract]. Presented at the meeting of the New England Perinatal Society, Woodstock, VT.

American Psychological Association (APA). (1994). *Diagnostic and statistical manual of mental disorders* (4th ed.). Washington, DC: Author.

Amit, R. (1988). Acute confusional state in childhood. *Child's Nervous System, 4,* 255–258.

Baggerly, J. (1991). Sensory perceptual problems following stroke: The invisible deficits. *Nursing Clinics of North America, 26*(4), 997–1005.

Baker, C. (1993). Annoyance to ICU noise: A model of patient discomfort. *Critical Care Nursing Quarterly, 16*(2), 83–90.

Beveridge, T. (1994). Patients with vision, hearing, speech, communication, and language barriers. *Mercy Hospital Medical Center Standard Practice Bulletins,* April.

Blachy, P., & Starr, A. (1964). Post-cardiotomy delirium. *American Journal of Psychiatry, 121,* 371–375.

Budd, S., & Brown, W. (1974). Effect of a reorientation technique on postcardiotomy delirium. *Nursing Research, 23*(4), 341–348.

Carpenito, L. (1992). *Nursing diagnosis: Application to clinical practice* (4th ed.). Philadelphia: J. B. Lippincott.

Chatham, M. (1978). The effect of family involvement on patients' manifestations of postcardiotomy psychosis. *Heart and Lung, 7*(6), 995–999.

Christenson, M. (1990). Adaptations of the physical environment to compensate for sensory changes. In E. D. Taira (Ed.), *Aging in the designed environment* (pp. 3–30). New York: Howorth Press.

Christman, N., Kirckhoff, K., & Oakley, M. (1992). Concrete objective information. In G. M. Bulechek & J. C. McCloskey (Eds.), *Nursing interventions: Essential nursing treatments* (pp. 140–150). Philadelphia: W. B. Saunders.

Crippen, D. (1994). Pharmacologic treatment of brain failure and delirium. *Critical Care Clinics, 10*(4), 733–766.

D'Apolito, K. (1991). What is an organized infant? *Neonatal Network, 10*(1), 23–29.

Duggleby, W., & Lander, J. (1994). Cognitive status and post-operative pain: Older adults. *Journal of Pain Symptom Management, 9*(1), 19–27.

Easton, C., & MacKenzie, F. (1988). Sensory-perceptual alterations: Delirium in the intensive care unit. *Heart and Lung, 17,* 229.

Erber, N. (1994). Communicating with elders: Effects of amplification. *Journal of Gerontological Nursing, 20*(10), 6–10.

Fish, D. (1991). Treatment of delirium in the critically ill patient. *Clinical Pharmacy, 10,* 456–466.

Foreman, M. (1991). The cognitive and behavioral nature of acute confusional states. *Scholarly Inquiry in Nursing Practice, 5*(1), 3–16.

Foreman, M., & Zane, D. (1996). Nursing strategies for acute confusion in elders. *American Journal of Nursing, 96*(4), 44–51.

Francis, J., Martin, D., Kapoor, W. (1990). A prospective study of delirium in hospitalized elderly. *JAMA, 26*(8), 1097–1101.

Frantz, R., & Ferrell-Torry, A. (1993). Physical impairments in the elderly population. *Nursing Clinics of North America, 28*(2), 363–371.

Fucci, D., Petrosino, L., Hains, D., & Banks, M. (1993). The effect of preference for rock music on magnitude-estimation scaling behavior in young adults. *Perceptual and Motor Skills, 76,* 1171–1176.

Gardner-Cole, J., Begish-Duddy, A., Judas, M. L., & Jorgensen, K. M. (1990). Changing the NICU environment: The Boston City Hospital model. *Neonatal Network, 9*(2), 15–23.

Geary, S. M. (1994). Intensive care unit psychosis revisited: Understanding and managing delirium in the critical care setting. *Critical Care Nursing Quarterly, 17*(1), 51–63.

Glick, O. J. (1993). Normal thought processes: An overview. *Nursing Clinics of North America, 28*(4), 715–728.

Gordon, M. (1990). Toward theory-based diagnostic categories. *Nursing Diagnosis, 1*(1), 511.

Gordon, M. (1991). *Manual of nursing diagnosis.* St. Louis: C. V. Mosby.

Guyton, A. C. (1991). *Textbook of medical physiology* (8th ed.). Philadelphia: W. B. Saunders.

Halm, M., & Alpen, M. (1993). The impact of technology on patients and families. *Nursing Clinics of North America, 28*(2), 443–457.

Hasel, K., & Erickson, R. (1995). Effect of cerumen on infrared ear temperature measurement. *Journal of Gerontological Nursing, 21*(12), 6–14.

Holt, J. (1993). How to help confused patients. *American Journal of Nursing, 93,* 32–36.

Houston, K. (1993). An investigation of rocking as relaxation for the elderly. *Geriatric Nursing, 14*(4), 186–189.

Inaba-Roland, K., & Maricle, R. (1992). Assessing delirium in the acute care setting. *Heart and Lung, 21*(1), 48–55.

Inouye, S., Viscoli, C., Horwitz, R., Hurst L., & Tinetti, M. (1993). A predictive model for delirium in hospitalized elderly medical patients on admission characteristics. *Annals of Internal Medicine, 119*(6), 474–481.

Jacox, A. (1992). Pain control. In G. M. Bulechek & J. C. McCloskey (Eds.), *Nursing interventions: Treatments for nursing diagnoses* (pp. 221–231). Philadelphia: W. B. Saunders.

Kavanaugh, K., & Tate, B. (1996). Recognizing and helping older persons with vision impairments. *Geriatric Nursing, 17*(2), 68–71.

Kern, L. (1991). The elderly heart surgery patient. *Critical Care Nursing Clinics of North America, 3*(4), 749–756.

Kidder, C. (1989). Reestablishing health: Factors influencing the child's recovery in pediatric intensive care. *Journal of Pediatric Nursing, 4*(2), 96–103.

Kloosterman, N. (1991). Cultural care: The missing link in severe sensory alteration. *Nursing Science Quarterly, 4*(3), 119–122.

Kodiath, M., & Kodiath, A. (1995). A comparative study of patients who experience chronic malignant pain in India and the United States. *Cancer Nursing, 18*(3), 189–196.

Kolanowski, A. (1992). The clinical importance of environmental lighting to the elderly. *Journal of Gerontological Nursing, 18*(1), 10–14.

Kornfeld, D. S., Zimberg, S., & Malm, J. (1965). Psychiatric complications of open-heart surgery. *New England Journal of Medicine, 273,* 287–292.

Lawhon, G. & Melzar, A. (1988). Developmental care of the very low birth weight infant (case study). *Journal of Perinatal Nursing, 2*(1), 56–65.

Leners, D. (1990). Vestibular stimulation. In M. Craft & J. Denehy (Eds.), *Nursing interventions for infants and children* (pp. 274–284). Philadelphia: W. B. Saunders.

Levin, M. (1991). Diabetic foot lesions. In J. Young, R. Graor, J. Olin, & J. Bartholomew (Eds.), *Peripheral vascular diseases* (pp. 669–712). St. Louis: Mosby-Year Book.

Levkoff, S., Evans, D., Liptzin, B., Cleary, P., Lipsitz, L., Wetle, T., Reilly, C., Pilgrim, D., Schor, J., & Rowe, J. (1992). Delirium: The occurrence and persistence of symptoms among elderly hospitalized patients. *Archives of Internal Medicine, 152,* 334–340.

Lipowski, Z. (1990). *Delirium: Acute confusional states.* New York: Oxford University Press.

Long, J., Lucey, J., & Philip, A. (1980). Noise and hypoxemia in the intensive care nursery. *Pediatrics, 65*(1), 143–145.

Manion, J. (1990). Preparing children for hospitalization, procedures, or surgery. In M. Craft & J. Denehy (Eds.), *Nursing interventions for infants and children* (pp. 74–92). Philadelphia: W. B. Saunders.

McCloskey, J., & Bulechek, G. (1992). *Nursing interventions classification (NIC).* St. Louis; Mosby-Year Book.

McSweeney, E., & Zhan, L. (1994). Cultural and pharmacologic considerations when caring for Chinese elders: Knowledge of traditional Chinese medicine is necessary. *Journal of Geronontological Nursing, 20*(10), 11–16.

Meador, J. (1995). Cerumen impaction in the elderly. *Journal of Gerontological Nursing, 21*(12), 43–45.

Mentes, J. C. (1995). A nursing protocol to assess causes of delirium: Identifying delirium in nursing home residents. *Journal of Gerontological Nursing, 21,* 26–30.

Moore, B. (1994). Pediatric cataracts: Diagnosis and treatment. *Optometry and Vision Science, 71*(3), 168–173.

Nagley, S. (1986). Predicting and preventing confusion in your patients. *Journal of Gerontological Nursing, 12*(3), 27–31.

North American Nursing Diagnosis Association (NANDA). (1990). *Taxonomy 1 revised—1990.* St. Louis, North American Nursing Diagnosis Association.

Pedretti, L. (1996). Evaluation of sensation and treatment of sensory dysfunction. In L. Pedretti (Ed.), *Occupational therapy: Practice skills for physical dysfunction* (pp. 213–226). St. Louis: Mosby-Year Book.

Quinn, C. (1993). Nurses' perceptions about physical restraints. *Western Journal of Nursing Research, 15*(2), 148–162.

Roberts, B., & Lincoln, R. (1988). Cognitive disturbance in

hospitalized and institutionalized elders. *Research in Nursing and Health, 11,* 309–319.

Roy, C. (1984). *Introduction to nursing: An adaptation model* (2nd ed.). Englewood Cliffs, NJ: Prentice-Hall.

Sadler, P. (1981). Incidence, degree, and duration of post-cardiotomy delirium. *Heart and Lung, 10*(6), 1084–1092.

Sanders, K., & Stern, T. (1993). Management of delirium associated with use of the intra-aortic balloon pump. *American Journal of Critical Care, 2*(5), 371–377.

Scherubel, J., & Tess, M. (1994). Measuring clinical confusion in critically ill patients. *Journal of Neuroscience Nursing, 26*(3), 146–150.

Schott-Baer, D., Lusis, S., & Beauregard, K. (1995). Use of restraints: Changes in nurses' attitudes. *Journal of Gerontological Nursing, 21*(2), 39–44.

Schwartz, R., & Rodriguez, W. (1991). Toxic delirium possibly caused by loperamide. *Journal of Pediatrics, 118,* 656–657.

Spies Pope, D. (1995). Music, noise, and the human voice in the nurse-patient environment. *Image: The Journal of Nursing Scholarship, 27*(4), 291–296.

Sullivan-Marx, E. M. (1995). Psychological response to physical restraint use in older adults. *Journal of Psychosocial Nursing, 33*(6), 20–25.

Sullivan-Marx, E. M. (1994). Delerium and physical restraint in the hospitalized elderly. *Image: Journal of Nursing Scholarship, 26*(4), 295–300.

Thomas, K. (1990). Environmental Manipulation. In M. Craft & J. Denehy (Eds.), *Nursing interventions for infants and children* (pp. 259–273). Philadelphia: W. B. Saunders.

Tortora, G., & Anagnostakos, N. (1987). *Principles of anatomy and physiology* (5th ed.). New York: Harper & Row.

Trzepacz, P., Sclabassi, R., & Van Thiel, D. (1989). Delirium: A subcortical phenomenon? *Journal of Neuropsychiatry, 1*(3), 283–290.

Wanich, C., Sullivan-Marx, E. M., Gottlieb, G., & Johnson, J. (1992). Functional status outcomes of nursing intervention in hospitalized elderly. *Image, 24,* 201–207.

Warren, M. (1996). Evaluation and treatment of visual deficits. In L. W. Pedretti (Ed.), *Occupational therapy: Practice skills for physical dysfunction* (4th ed., pp. 193–212). St. Louis: C. V. Mosby.

Weddington, W. (1982). The mortality of delirium: An under-appreciated problem? *Psychosomatics, 23,* 1232–1235.

Williams, M., Campbell, E., Raynor, W., Musholt, M., Mlynarczyk, S., & Crane, L. (1985). Predictors of acute confusional states in hospitalized elderly patients. *Research in Nursing and Health, 8,* 31–40.

Williams, M., Holloway, J., Winn, M., Wolanin, M., Lawler, M., Westwick, C., & Chin, M. (1979). Nursing activities and acute confusional states in elderly hip-fractured patients. *Nursing Research, 28,* 25–35.

Wilson, L. (1993). Sensory perceptual alteration: Diagnosis, prediction and intervention in the hospitalized adult. *Nursing Clinics of North America, 28*(4), 747–766.

Wilson, M. (1972). Intensive care delirium. *Archives of Internal Medicine, 130,* 225–226.

Zivic, R., & King, S. (1993). Cerumen-impaction management for clients of all ages. *Nurse Practitioner, 18*(3), 29–37.

Bibliography

American Association of Critical-Care Nurses. (1990). *Outcome standards for nursing care of the critically ill.* Laguna Niguel, CA: Author.

Andersson, E., Knutsson, I., Hallberg, I., & Norberg, A. (1993). The experience of being confused: A case study. *Geriatric Nursing, 14*(5), 242–247.

Beck, K., Heacock, P., Rapp, C., & Shue, V. (1993). Cognitive impairment in the elderly. *Nursing Clinics of North American, 28*(2), 335–347.

Beumont, P., & Large, M. (1991). Hypophosphataemia, delirium and cardiac arrhythmia in anorexia nervosa. *Medical Journal of Australia, 155,* 519–522.

Bowman, A. (1992). Relationship of anxiety to development of postoperative delirium. *Journal of Gerontological Nursing, 18*(1), 24–30.

Campbell, E. B., Williams, M. A., & Mlynarczyk, S. M. (1986). After the fall—confusion. *American Journal of Nursing, 86*(2), 151–154.

Clarke, S. P. (1994). Increasing the quality of family visits to the ICU. *Dimensions in Critical Care Nursing, 14*(4), 200–212.

Courts, N. F. (1996). Salicylism in the elderly: A little aspirin never hurt anybody! *Geriatric Nursing, 17*(2), 55–59.

Dickson, L. (1991). Hypoalbuminemia in delirium. *Psychosomatics, 32*(3), 317–323.

Eiser, C., & Patterson D. (1984). Children's perceptions of hospital: A preliminary study. *International Journal of Nursing Studies, 21*(1), 45–50.

Fleming-Owens, J., & Hutelmyer, C. (1981). The effect of preoperative intervention on delirium in cardiac surgical patients. *Nursing Research, 31*(1), 60–62.

Foreman, M. (1986). Acute confusional states in hospitalized elderly: A research dilemma. *Nursing Research, 35*(1), 34–37.

Foreman, M. (1989). Confusion in the hospitalized elderly: Incidence, onset, and associated factors. *Research in Nursing and Health, 12,* 21–29.

Foreman, M. (1990). Complexities of acute confusion. *Geriatric Nursing, 11,* 136–139.

Foreman, M. (1991). The cognitive and behavioral nature of acute confusional states. *Scholarly Inquiry in Nursing Practice, 5*(1), 3–16.

Foreman, M., Gillies, D., & Wagner, D. (1989). Impaired cognition in the critically ill elderly patient: Clinical implications. *Critical Care Nursing Quarterly, 12*(1), 61–73.

Foreman, M., & Grabowski, R. (1992). Diagnostic dilemma: Cognitive impairment in the elderly. *Journal of Gerontological Nursing, 18*(9), 5–12.

Francis, J., Martin, D., & Kapoor, W. (1990). A prospective study of delirium in hospitalized elderly. *JAMA, 263*(8), 1097–1101.

Fulmer, T., & Walker, M. (1990). Lessons from the elder boom in ICUs. *Geriatric Nursing, 11*(3), 120–121.

Gillick, M. R., Serrell, N. A., & Gillick, L. S. (1982). Adverse consequences of hospitalization in the elderly. *Social Science and Medicine, 16,* 1033–1038.

Glass, P., Avery, G., Kolinjavadi, N., Subramanian, S., Keys, M., Sostek, A., & Friendly, D. (1985). Effect of bright light in the hospital nursery on the incidence of retinopathy of prematurity. *New England Journal of Medicine, 313*(7), 401–404.

Glick, O. J. (1993). Normal thought processes: An overview. *Nursing Clinics of North America, 28*(4), 715–728.

Golinger, R., Peet, T., & Tune, L. (1987). Association of elevated plasma anticholinergic activity with delirium in surgical patients. *American Journal of Psychiatry, 144*(9), 1218–1220.

Hart, D., & Bossert, E. (1994). Self-reported fears of hospitalized school-age children. *Journal of Pediatric Nursing,* *9*(2), 83–90.

Jitapunkul, S., Pillay, I., & Ebrahim, S. (1992). Delirium in newly admitted elderly patients: A prospective study. *Quarterly Journal of Medicine, 83*(300), 307–314.

Kroeger, L. (1991). Critical care nurses' perceptions of the confused elderly patient. *Focus on Critical Care, 18*(5), 395–401.

Lipowski, Z. (1983). Transient cognitive disorders: Delirium, acute confusional states in the elderly. *American Journal of Psychiatry, 140,* 1426–1436.

Luis, S., Hydo, B., & Clark, L. (1993). Nursing assessment of mental status in the elderly. *Geriatric Nursing, 14*(5), 255–259.

McCartney, J., & Boland, R. (1994). Anxiety and delirium in the intensive care unit. *Critical Care Clinics, 10*(4), 673–680.

Miller, C. (1993). Interventions for sleep pattern disturbances. *Geriatric Nursing, 14*(5), 235–236.

Moran, S. (1987). Innovative geriatric care. *Nursing Management, 18*(6), 26–28.

Morency, C., Levkoff, S., & Dick, K. (1994). Research considerations: Delirium in hospitalized elders. *Journal of Gerontological Nursing, 20*(8), 24–30.

Nagley, S., & Deaver, A. (1988). What we know about treating confusion. *Applied Nursing Research, 1,* 80.

News Watch. (1993). Duke University test predicts delirium in ICU patients. *Geriatric Nursing, 14*(5), 233–234.

North American Nursing Diagnosis Association. (1988). NANDA approved nursing diagnostic categories. *Nursing Diagnosis Newsletter, 15*(1), 43–45.

Orem, D. (1991). *Nursing: Concepts of practice* (4th ed.). St. Louis: C. V. Mosby.

Padula, C., & Willey, C. (1993). Tobacco withdrawal in CCU patients. *Dimensions in Critical Care Nursing, 12*(6), 305–312.

Quinless, F., Cassese, M., & Atherton, N. (1985). The effect of selected preoperative, intraoperative, and postoperative variables on the development of postcardiotomy psychosis in patients undergoing open heart surgery. *Heart and Lung, 14,* 334–337.

Schibler, K., & Fay, S. (1990). Sleep promotion. In M. Craft & J. Denehy (Eds.), *Nursing interventions for infants and children* (pp. 285–302). Philadelphia: W. B. Saunders.

Schor, J., Levkoff, S., Lewis, A., Lipsitz, A., Reilly, C., Cleary, P., Rowe, J., & Evans, D. (1992). Risk factors for delirium in hospitalized elderly. *JAMA, 267,* 827–831.

Tess, M. (1991). Acute confusional states in critically ill patients: A review. *Journal of Neuroscience Nursing, 23*(6), 398–402.

Trzepacz, P., Brenner, R., Coffman, G., & vanThiel, D. (1988). Delirium in liver transplantation candidates: Discriminant analysis of multiple test variables. *Biological Psychiatry, 24,* 3–14.

Tueth, M., & Cheong, J. (1993). Delirium: Diagnosis and treatment in the older patient. *Geriatrics, 48*(3), 75–80.

Westwater Foot, A., & Holcombe, J. (1994). Acoustic neuroma: Suggestions for helping the patient adapt after translabyrinthine surgery. *Journal of Neuroscience Nursing, 26*(3), 162–165.

Williams, M., Campbell, E., Raynor, W., Mlynarczyk, S. & Ward, S. (1985). Reducing acute confusional states in elderly patients with hip fractures. *Research in Nursing and Health, 8,* 329–337.

Williams, M., Ward, S., & Campbell, E. (1988). Confusion: Testing versus observation. *Journal of Gerontological Nursing, 14*(1), 25–29.

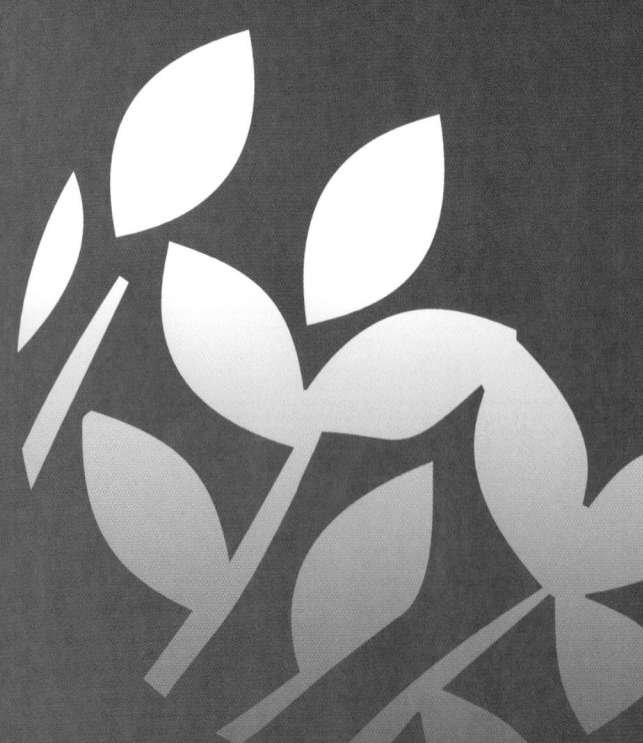

SPIRITUALITY

VERNA BENNER CARSON,
PhD, RN, CSP

Spirituality . . . the term is increasingly seen in health-related literature, and there is a growing sense that Western medicine is deficient in addressing the spiritual aspects of health. Yet despite this growing awareness regarding the role of spirituality in health, the term remains a difficult one to define. People attempt to pin it down with definitions that focus on who we are as people and how we relate to the Transcendant Spirit, or God (however we may define God). Spirituality reflects what is occurring in our spirit. We cannot see or point to our spirit, nor can we see or point to God's spirit. Yet, according to a 1993 Gallup poll (The Way We Live, 1994), most Americans accept the existence of both. Many of us are certain that we can evaluate whether someone is either low or high spirited; many individuals have the same certainty regarding their ability to recognize the presence and work of God's spirit. Many of us claim to know of the spirit and what it does, just as we know of the wind but we are not able to catch it, hold it, or examine it in our hands. It seems somehow paradoxical that a term so elusive could also be viewed as so essential to all human concerns and especially to health concerns, but, indeed, it is essential.

It is also essential to be clear about what **spirituality** is not. It is not the same as religion. Spirituality is like an umbrella that encompasses many different religions. For some individuals, their religious beliefs provide the expression for their spirituality; for others, their spirituality has nothing at all to do with religion. Such individuals may not belong to an organized faith tradition, or they may see their faith tradition serving purposes other than spiritual ones. It is important for nurses to know that it is not necessary for a person to belong to a religious group to be spiritual or to believe in God. Some people describe themselves as spiritual, and yet they do not include a relationship with God as part of that spirituality. Such individuals might define their spirituality in humanistic terms and believe that if there is divinity, it resides only within the human heart. It is important for nurses to acknowledge this broad view of spirituality to appreciate the many varieties of spiritual expressions they will encounter in clients. A nurse's thinking must not limit spirituality to a client's response to the questions "Are you a member of an organized religion?" "If so, which one?" Such an approach not only is narrow but also does not even provide information about the client's commitment to a particular faith (Burkhardt & Nagai-Jacobson, 1994; Carson, 1994a, 1994c).

The purpose of this chapter is to examine spirituality and religion and their impact on nursing care. To do so, we look at the concept of spirituality as a world view and examine the relationship of religion to world view. We examine the universal components of spirituality, the importance of spirituality to health and healing, spiritual development across the life span, the major religions and their health-related beliefs, nursing approaches to meeting spiritual and religious needs, and, finally, the application of the nursing process to clients in spiritual distress.

♦ Definitions

A helpful way of looking at spirituality is to consider it as a world view. This approach allows a more exact description of spirituality. A world view is simply a way of looking at and thinking about all that happens in life—an attempt to look at the "big picture" and to make sense out of what we see. A world view usually includes our beliefs about the nature of the universe, our place in it, our responsibility to others and the environment, and a sense of how we fit into history. All of these descriptions are also true of spirituality (Sire, 1994).

According to Dr. Barbara Hoshiko (*World view as a model of spirituality.* Key Note Presentation at University of Maryland Conference, May 7, 1993), looking at spirituality as a world view provides a way of examining all belief systems—those that are organized into a religion and those that are not—and clearly analyze where the client is feeling spiritual distress. For instance, if a nurse is working with a client who belongs to a religious faith unfamiliar to the nurse, the model suggests the areas that the nurse needs to assess to diagnose spiritual distress. The model consists of six mutually interactive relationships of the client to

The Ultimate Other

Himself or herself

Neighbors

The environment in terms of producing and consuming natural resources and other goods

Time past

Time future

A disturbance in one relationship affects other relationships in the individual's world view. Hoshiko suggests that nurses map the relationships in a diagram similar to Figure 35–1.

Let us look at a client example using the world view model. An individual is in the terminal stages of an illness and is expressing guilt about times in his past when he was unfaithful to his wife. He believes that he has not only harmed his wife but offended his God. He believes that he is unworthy of forgiveness and is damned to hell for eternity. In this individual's spiritual world view, there are disturbances in several relationships, including the relationships with the Ultimate Other, self (feelings of guilt and unworthiness), other (his wife), and time (his belief that he will spend eternity in hell). In this example, the nurse is able to make some statements of a spiritual nature about this individual, including the statement that he is experiencing significant spiritual pain. It is not possible, however, to draw any conclusions about his religion.

All religions are undergirded by a spiritual world view, but a spiritual world view can and does exist outside of religion. **Religion** is humanity's attempt to structure spiritual issues; to codify beliefs; and to es-

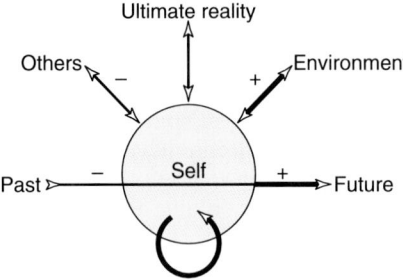

✦ **Figure 35–1**
The nurse can map a client's world view in terms of six spiritual relationships: with self, with others, with past, with future, with environment, and with ultimate reality. The meaning of each of the six basic relationships is dynamic, constantly changing, and varies on two continua: (1) intensity (strong to weak) and (2) valence (friendly to hostile). A *broad line* indicates strong intensity; a *narrow line* indicates low intensity; and an *absent line* (not shown in this example) indicates no relationship. A *plus sign* indicates a positive valence for a relationship, and a *minus sign* indicates a negative relationship. (Courtesy of Barbara R. Hoshiko, PhD, RN.)

tablish rules, rituals, and practices (Carson, 1993b). There are a variety of spiritual world views. However, all spiritual world views include

* A sense of connectedness to others
* A sense of connectedness to a transcendant force
* A search for meaning and purpose in life

Spiritual world views differ in the ways that people define the nature and character of the transcendant force and how they determine what is most important in their own lives. Let us look at specific world views to explain this. A theistic spiritual world view holds that the universe was created by a benevolent, creator God who made all people in His image to love and serve Him and each other. **Theism** is associated with the Judeo-Christian God of the Scriptures and with the Jewish, Christian, and Islamic religions. An individual professing a theistic spirituality might say that the most important relationship is with God and that purpose in life comes from loving and serving God and each other (Karns, 1991; Sire, 1994).

A monistic spiritual world view **(monism)** espouses that there is one energy source; this energy source is the same in everything and everyone. This belief that "all is one and one is all" leads to a pantheistic spiritual world view. **Pantheism** states that god is in everyone and everything. Therefore, "I am god and you are god." Monism and pantheism undergird the Eastern religions, including some sects of Hinduism and Buddhism. An individual professing a monistic and pantheistic spirituality might describe meaning and purpose in life as striving to achieve oneness with the energy force by diminishing the self (Pacwa, 1992; Sire, 1994).

A polytheistic spiritual world view includes belief in many gods. **Polytheism** is practiced in many nativistic religions and in some sects of Hinduism. An individual who believes in many gods may define the

meaning and purpose of life in terms of the efforts made to appease the gods. These efforts, usually in the form of sacrifices, are to ensure good fortune and to ward off evil (Sire, 1994). A humanistic spiritual world view states that human beings are ultimate. In **humanism,** issues of purpose and meaning in life are concerned with human achievements.

The Nurse's Spirituality

Every nurse brings to the caring situation his or her own spiritual world view. The nurse's personal beliefs may be challenged by what the client says, what the client practices, and how the client lives. To cope effectively with spiritual challenges and to be a spiritual caregiver, it is important for nurses to examine what they believe and what undergirds their own values and to recognize what, if any, are their spiritual "hot buttons" that call forth a judgmental response. Once the nurse has identified potentially sensitive spiritual issues, it is important to plan how those issues will be handled. Without this self-examination and anticipatory planning, it is difficult for nurses to offer clients nonreactive listening and empathy.

Some nurses are very uncomfortable with spirituality; it may not be an area that they have personally developed, or they may be experiencing spiritual distress themselves. Other nurses may be struggling with issues related to their own religion and feel ill at ease exploring either spiritual or religious issues with clients. Still other nurses may have strong religious beliefs and experience difficulty accepting beliefs that are different. Yet, some nurses are able to easily weave spiritual interventions throughout their nursing care.

Spiritual care is so important that it is essential for nurses to be clear where they stand in relationship to this issue so that they do not block the client's expression of spiritual need or impose their own interpretation or belief system on the client. Spiritual caregiving does not require that nurses agree with clients' beliefs. Spiritual caregiving does not depend on the religiosity of nurses, nor does it depend on a nurse's theological knowledge. What is required of the nurse is genuine concern for the client, a willingness to put aside personal feelings and really listen to what the client is saying, the ability to respond and ask questions that encourage the client's exploration of spiritual concerns, a sense of personal humility with regard to the nurse's ability to have all the answers, and a willingness to involve the skills of others in the health care team to meet the client's spiritual needs.

A common question voiced by nurses is whether it is ever appropriate to share their own beliefs. There are times when this is appropriate. However, there are certain caveats regarding personal disclosure. First, a statement of personal beliefs must never be coercive or intimidating to the client. Second, the client must

SPIRITUAL CAREGIVING CHALLENGE

Jane Walker was assigned to admit Mr. Jack Dorsey to her unit for treatment of AIDS. Ms. Walker knew from reading Mr. Dorsey's chart that he had been convicted of raping several children. Before going into his room to complete the admission assessment, she expressed her reservations about working with him to her head nurse. "How am I going to give him care? The thought of what he has done just makes me sick!" The head nurse was empathetic but encouraged Ms. Walker to do her best and offered to meet with her at the end of the day to discuss her feelings. When Ms. Walker entered the room, she found an emaciated middle-aged man reading the Bible. Ordinarily, she would have picked up on the Bible as a cue for assessing spiritual needs. Not this time. Her reaction was one of disdain: "How can he be reading the Bible after the things that he has done?" She hurried through the assessment and gathered enough information to do a basic plan of care. She was careful not to make eye contact with Mr. Dorsey, and she did not inquire about spiritual needs. Later, in her discussion with the head nurse, she talked about her feelings of abhorrence for what he had done but also her sense that she had not provided him with good nursing care—especially in not asking about spiritual issues. The head nurse offered to assign Mr. Dorsey to someone else, but Ms. Walker chose to keep him as a patient. The next time she went into the room, she sat by his bed, looked him in the eyes, smiled, and said "I really didn't get to know you yesterday when I admitted you. I realize that I didn't even inquire about your reading the Bible. That usually cues me to explore spiritual needs with my patients. Well, perhaps we can do that today." Mr. Dorsey's eyes brimmed with tears as he spoke: "Thank you, I have felt absolutely worthless since I was admitted—the Bible was my only consolation—but I can sure use someone to talk to."

never feel that care is dependent on agreement with the nurse. Third, the nurse must state his or her beliefs in "I" terms; that is, "I believe . . .," rather than "You should believe. . . ." Box 35–1 presents a spiritual caregiving challenge faced by a nurse and the options considered.

Spirituality/World View: Impact on Health and Healing

People are whole and indivisible. This means that it is impossible to pinpoint the spirit, the personality, the will, or the values that an individual holds dear. When people hurt, they hurt all over. Something as simple as a corn on a toe can cause enough discomfort that

irritability, distractability, and even spiritual distress result. The problem is clearly located on the toe, but the impact is felt holistically. A hungry infant cries in distress, and his or her whole being is involved in the effort. The hunger pains are in the infant's stomach, yet the infant is red in the face, crying loudly, and moving his or her arms and legs. Why? Because hurting calls forth a holistic response. This implies that healing requires a holistic effort from those in the healing professions.

A model of human beings that describes the interaction of body, mind, and spirit was developed by Jean Stallwood and Dr. Ruth Stoll (1975) and is shown in Figure 35–2. It is a **holistic model of humanity.**

The model shows three concentric circles. The largest circle refers to the physical dimension of a person with five senses of seeing, hearing, touching, feeling, and smelling. The physical, or body, self is "world conscious." The next circle is the psychosocial

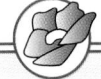

COMMUNITY BASED CARE

SPIRITUAL NEEDS

Assessment of spiritual needs is an important component of a holistic approach to care. A spiritual assessment includes

1. Religious affiliation
2. Meaningful religious/spiritual practices
3. Sources of strength in life
4. Coping strategies
5. Meaningful and important relationships

Although some health caregivers, nurses, and therapists may feel comfortable with the spiritual aspects of care, many others do not. Client needs may meet with a chaplain or other spiritual staff member. Chaplains who are available for counseling and prayer have always been a part of home care agency hospice programs. Often these chaplains served on a volunteer basis. Now chaplains may be employed as members of the agency interdisciplinary team. Spiritual services staff minister to the emotional, relational, and spiritual needs of an individual, recognizing the importance of healing people, not diseases. Although any client may benefit from the ministry of spiritual staff, certain types of clients do so more frequently. Terminal clients may be searching for meaning in their life. They yearn for someone to reflect on their life accomplishments with them. Lonely and depressed clients seek a comforting smile, a listening ear, or a hug of reassurance. Chronically ill clients may request sacraments at home, someone to pray with, and someone to offer encouragement as they deal with the powerlessness of their illness. When the agency or organization does not offer this service, it is important to identify other community resources for the client, such as pastors, parish nurses, and other community volunteers.

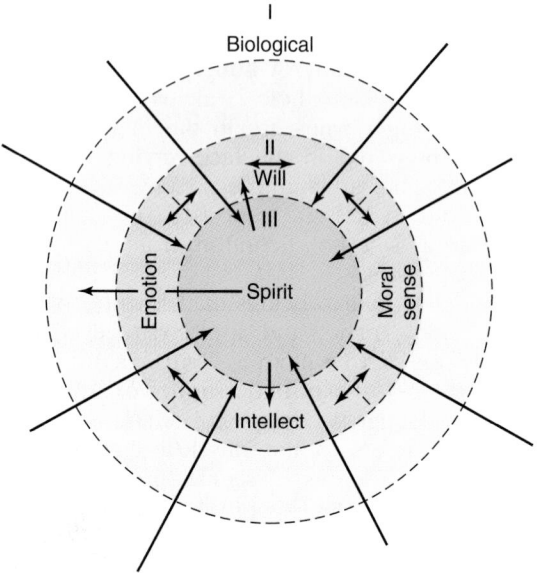

Figure 35–2
Conceptual model of the nature of humans. I = Biological: Five
senses, world consciousness. II = Psychosocial: self-consciousness,
self-identity. III = Spirit: God-consciousness, relatedness to deity.
(Reprinted with the permission of Simon & Schuster from CLINICAL
NURSING 3/e by Irene L. Beland and J. Y. Passos. Copyright © 1975
Macmillan Publishing Company.)

dimension, or that part of a person that gives one
"self-consciousness" and personality through the emotions, the intellect, the moral sense, and the will. The
innermost circle, the spirit, is the most difficult to comprehend because of its mystery and indefinable nature. The spirit is the core of the person; within this
spiritual core lies the potential for awareness of and
relatedness to the Transcendant.

Because the human person is and functions as a
dynamic whole and not three separate dimensions,
each dimension influences and is influenced by the
other two. This is shown on the model by the broken
lines that make up the boundaries of the circles and
illustrates the flow between and among the three dimensions of a person. The model also depicts arrows
flowing into and out of the three circles. This demonstrates that the person is interacting with and is
strengthened by resources that exist outside of the
self. Therefore, when an individual is feeling depressed, the experience includes not only sadness but
also crying, sleeplessness, loss of appetite, slowed
thinking, lack of energy, conflict in personal relationships, and a spiritual void expressed as hopelessness
and despair about God's place in his or her life
(Carson, 1994c). With this in mind, any nursing approach that deals only with the mind or only with the
body is inadequate. A holistic approach includes the
use of an antidepressant medication, counseling regarding unresolved issues, teaching the causes and
effects of depression, encouragement that there is
hope because depression is treatable, attention to
physical problems, involvement of the family and/or

significant others in care, and discussion about ways
to alleviate the spiritual distress secondary to the sense
of being a burden and the sense that God has turned
away.

Spirituality Across the Life Span

We are spiritual just as much as we are physical and
emotional in our makeup. However, this does not
mean that we are always aware of the spiritual dimension within ourselves, nor does it mean that each dimension grows and develops at the same rate. Figure
35–3 depicts the inverse relationship between spiritual
development and physical and emotional development
from birth to death.

The cone on the left depicts the natural life of
physical and emotional development. The widest portion of the cone reflects the earliest years of life,
which are characterized by phenomenal changes that
occur in children as they grow and mature into adults.
The cone in the middle depicts the spiritual life. The
widest portion of the cone is closest to death, and the
point of the cone is at birth. This demonstrates that
spiritual development occurs slowly in the early years
of life and fully develops in the later years, approaching the end of life. The drawing on the right shows
the spiritual life cone superimposed on the natural life
cone, indicating that everything that is lost in the natural life through aging is gained in the spiritual life.

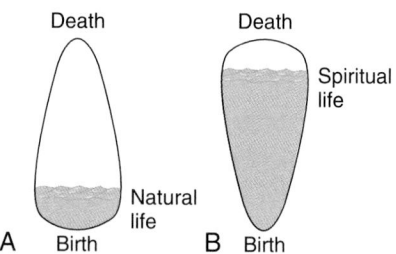
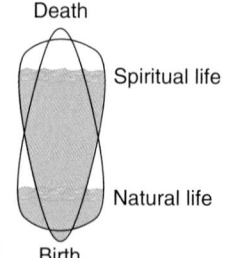

Figure 35–3
At birth, natural life predominates over spiritual life (panel A), and at
death this is reversed (panel B). The overlapping cones (panel C)
show that everything lost in the natural life through aging is gained
in the spiritual life.

Childhood

In some ways, spiritual development parallels cognitive and emotional development. That is, a child's spirituality is limited by his or her abilities to engage in abstract thinking, to recognize and express feelings, and to trust and to feel confident in his or her own skills. However, sometimes children display spiritual maturity beyond their years. Nurses who work with dying children frequently comment on the level of spiritual development present in the very young. How do we explain this? One explanation deals with the nature of God and God's ability to become known to a child who, according to developmental theory, is not ready for such knowledge. Many people would like to box spiritual development into a neat and tidy stage theory. Sometimes we are able to do so. But sometimes spiritual development does not follow a "regular" pattern; children can know God even when their parents and caregivers do not, and spiritual awareness can break through a life spontaneously without warning (Carson, 1989; Coles, 1990).

Adults are frequently amazed and surprised that children develop their own simplistic spiritual world views. Frequently the child's spiritual understandings are quite different from the world views held by their parents. Children are not able to comprehend the world in the same way that adults do; they have difficulty with abstract concepts such as spirit. Therefore, they frequently convert an adult spiritual world view into a reality that they can grasp. Preschool children may construct a world view that includes notions of God as either a benevolent, kind old man who answers all prayers or a mean, vengeful monster ready to exact punishment for transgressions. Because young children are self-centered, their spiritual world view places them front and center, with little room for others. They tend to be present oriented and lack understanding of time-related concepts such as "forever." Robert Coles (1990) believes that children are spiritual whether or not their parents encourage spirituality or provide religious experiences. The experiences provided by parents do not create the spirituality in the child but rather give the child's innate spirituality stimulus for growth and development.

Adolescence

With increasing maturity, children generally assume the spiritual world view of their parents. This world view may provide security or terror to the child, depending on the ideas that parents impart regarding the nature of the Ultimate Other. As children enter adolescence, they begin a process of separating from their parents and defining themselves as individuals. During this process, their spiritual world views are reviewed, critiqued, and modified, along with other values and beliefs that they had previously accepted without question from their parents. By the end of adolescence, many young people have returned to a spiritual world view that resembles what they had been taught as children (Carson, 1989).

Young Adulthood

It is difficult to draw generalities about spirituality during the late teen years and early 20s. Some young adults are very spiritual; they may be very involved in and committed to a particular faith tradition, or they may have committed to something less traditional but with personal meaning for them, such as sports, music, or the arts. During this stage of life, it is not uncommon for some individuals to have a genuine and transformative spiritual experience. People refer to such experiences as "conversions" or "awakenings." Some interpret these experiences as calls from the Transcendant; others interpret them in terms of the potential for self-fulfillment and self-actualization. Many young adults commit to a significant other during this time, and this relationship that calls forth mutual love and sacrifice may serve as the impetus for spiritual development. For other young adults, spirituality is a foreign concept, without meaning and relevance to their lives. They are caught up in living for the moment, struggling to launch a career, and beginning intimate relationships. The grand signficance of these events to their lives seems to hold little import. This lack of concern for spiritual issues may continue indefinitely.

The Family

Beginning a family is a spiritual turning point for many individuals, especially those who have not attended to their own spirituality. The responsibility for providing children with a foundation in values and beliefs can serve as the stimulus for adults to reexamine what they believe and how they wish to transmit these beliefs to their offspring. However, this reexamination does not always have the effect of making the adult more spiritual; sometimes it makes him or her more cognizant of teaching spiritual and religious values to children. The demands of a growing family, maintaining a home, and attending to a career leave many adults with little time to devote to their own spiritual needs. They may long for a bit of quiet time to spend in reflective contemplation about their own place in the universe. That time comes as children mature, leave home, and begin their own families. Childless couples or single individuals frequently make other commitments to the next generation (*i.e.*, volunteer work with children, church and community service) and may experience spirituality through these commitments.

Middle and Late Adulthood

In the middle to late adult years, faced with an empty nest and sometimes retirement, individuals begin to turn inward. Some consider this turning inward a middle-aged depression and avoid it. Others see it as a welcome change from the driven and frenzied lifestyle that they may have maintained while raising children or building their careers. For some, it represents their first spiritual awakening; for others, it may be a renaissance. They experience the pleasures of quiet reflection; their faith may be very much alive; and the outward expressions of their spirituality are sacrifice and service to others (Carson, 1989).

The older years bring with them growing awareness of the ravages of time on the body and the impact of cumulative losses over the years. The individual is faced with the spiritual task posed by the question, "Can I accept my life as I lived it?" The successful resolution of this task leaves the older person with a sense of unconditional acceptance. Religion, which takes on new meaning in the later years, and spirituality can facilitate a quiet acceptance that "I have lived a good life; I won some and I lost some, but all in all I did my best." For some people, there

can be appreciation that God has delighted in this one unique life (Lashley, 1992; Reed, 1991a, 1991b).

Health-Related Beliefs of Theistic and Pantheistic Religions

It is important to remember with regard to health-related beliefs and religion that not everyone who is raised in a certain faith tradition incorporates all the teachings of that particular tradition. Some individuals will totally ignore the teachings, others will accept them without question, and still others will pick and choose what to believe. Although it is possible to make generalizations about common health-related beliefs within a particular faith tradition, it is not possible

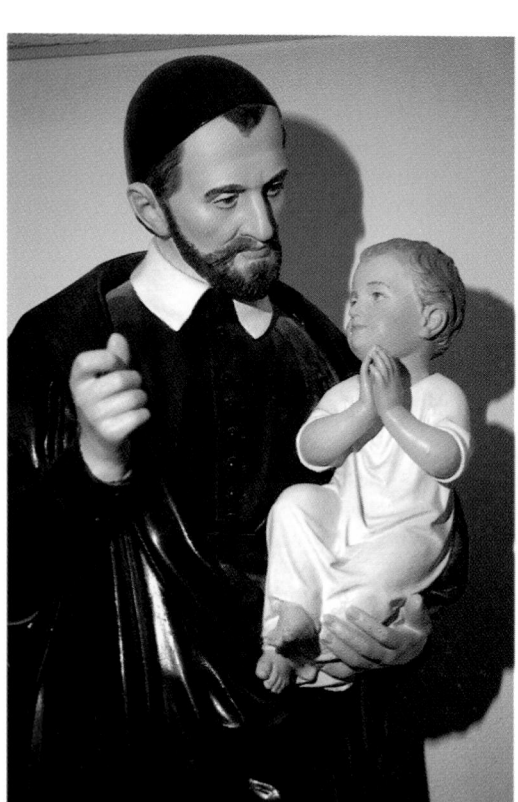

Christian icon

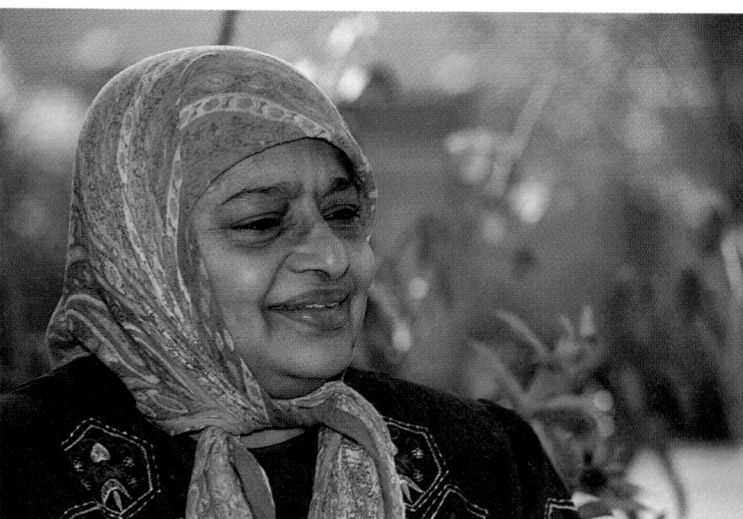

Muslim woman

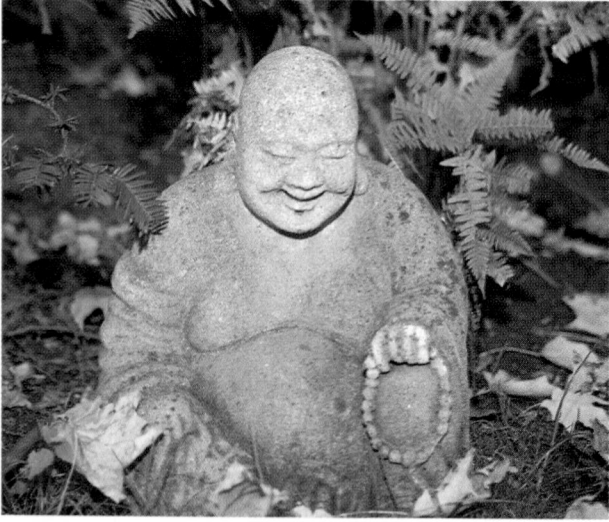

Buddhist icon

❧ **Figure 35–4**
An important aspect of nursing care is awareness of and respect for the religious beliefs and practices of patients and their families. Religious faith can assist patients in coping with life crises such as birth, illness, suffering, and death. In addition, religious beliefs often affect health practices. Patients who do not profess affiliation with a particular religion may have their own personal spiritual beliefs and needs.

to make generalizations about the degree to which individuals within a certain faith tradition adhere to these beliefs. Also, it is not essential that nurses become experts on the beliefs and practices of all religions. What is essential is that they have an awareness that these beliefs and practices can be important to the client's well-being and healing; a willingness to ask the client about these beliefs and practices, and a commitment to respect these beliefs and practices as part of nursing care (Fig. 35–4).

Religions With a Theistic World View

Theistic religions include Judaism, Christianity, and Islam. These religions are undergirded by a spiritual world view that is based on the God of the scriptures. Important to these religions are their moral codes, which stress honor of parents, honesty, kindness, generosity, and social concern and reject stealing, lying, slander, covetousness, and adultery. Although there are similarities among the theistic religions, they are not identical. Each religious group must be seen from the perspective of persons within that faith for a nurse to fully grasp the meaning of life for that individual.

The belief in a personal God offers a source of hope and confidence to individuals that assists them in coping with the crises of life, including birth, illness, suffering, and death. Sometimes these life crises serve to strengthen, shatter, or reawaken an individual's belief in God. The theistic religions offer solace and support through the belief in a personal God who is concerned with the suffering of His people. In addition, these religions include practices and rituals that surround each of these life crises, and it is these practices to which the nurse needs sensitivity. Interventions that are consistent with a theistic world view include the use of self to comfort and support another in a "God-like" manner; prayer to God for comfort, healing and forgiveness; meditation; religious reading; religious practices; and "doing good works." Let us briefly examine each of the theistic religions and their health practices.

Judaism

Judaism is the oldest continuous religion that is still practiced in Western civilization; it is the foundation for both Christianity and Islam. Jewish history is recorded in the Hebrew scriptures, which include the Pentateuch, or the five books of Moses; the Prophets; and other holy writings. The major tenets of Judaism include

1. God created the world according to His will and placed humans at the center of the universe to fulfill His supreme will

2. Humans are the focal point of God's creation and they are endowed with the capacity to do God's will

3. God created humans with a holy soul; therefore, they are inherently good and, as such, must worship God and strive to be as God is—merciful, compassionate, just, and kind

Every Jew does not practice his or her faith in the same manner. There are three major groups within Judaism, including Orthodox, Conservative, and Reform. The major difference among these groups lies in their interpretation of the laws of the Torah (Scripture), adherence to dietary laws, celebration of holy days, and Sabbath worship. Orthodox Jews have strict rules surrounding births, care of women, diet, observance of the Sabbath, deaths, birth control and abortion, organ transplants, shaving, head covering, and prayer. Conservative Jews may or may not subscribe to some of the same rules as the Orthodox Jew. The Reform Jew adheres to very few of the rules that govern the lives of the Orthodox Jew. It is important for nurses to ask questions such as "Do you follow any dietary rules that I should be aware of while you are in the hospital?" or "Do you have any religious practices that I should know about as we plan your care together?"

Christianity

Christianity is the largest religion in the world, based on numbers of people who adhere to Roman Catholicism, Eastern Orthodox, and the Protestant faiths. Christianity is also the most diverse of all religions in terms of stated beliefs. However, there are eight core beliefs that are held by all Christian faiths:

1. There is only one God and Creator, from whom all things take their origin.

2. This God is a self-revealing God, and He himself is active in the knowledge that Christians have of Him as Father, Son, and Holy Spirit.

3. In Jesus, the full meaning of the lives of Christians and of God's purpose for the universe is revealed. Christians are created to be in loving relationship with their God. Through the death of Jesus Christ, God is reconciled with His children. Through the resurrection of Jesus, He has brought into being a new order or new creation.

4. In Jesus, Christians see the way in which they ought to live; His life is the example to which every Christian is unconditionally bound and to which by His grace they are increasingly conformed.

5. The Cross of Jesus shows that to follow Him will certainly result in suffering; this is neither to be evaded nor resented.

6. The Christian faith may learn much from other faiths, but it is universal in its claims; in the end Christ must be acknowledged as Lord of all.

7. Death of the human body is not the end; Christ has revealed the eternal dimension as the true home of the spirit.

8. The Bible is the inspired word of God.

The Roman Catholic church places great importance on receiving the sacraments, especially baptism, the Eucharist, reconciliation, and the anointing of the sick. In the case of a newborn with a grave diagnosis, stillborns, and all aborted fetuses, emergency baptism is required. The nurse should call a priest to perform the baptism. However, if the infant's death might occur before the priest arrives, then the nurse or someone else can baptize the infant. The baptizing person pours warm water on the infant's head while saying, "I baptize you in the name of the Father, of the Son, and of the Holy Spirit." All information about the baptism is recorded on the chart, and the priest and family are notified.

Offering to call a priest so that a Roman Catholic client can receive the sacraments is an important intervention. Roman Catholic clients may engage in private devotions, such as saying the rosary; these devotions may play an important role in recovery. Roman Catholicism advocates natural family planning and prohibits artificial birth control. Organ donation and transplantation are allowed as long as the donor is not harmed or deprived of life.

The Eastern Orthodox Church was part of the Roman Catholic Church until 1054 A.D. The Eastern Orthodox believes that infants must be baptized within 40 days of birth. If immersion or sprinkling with water is not possible, the baby is moved through the air in the sign of the cross. This must be performed by an ordained priest or a deacon. Eastern Orthodox clients might desire to receive the Eucharist or annointing of the sick, which is provided by a priest. They observe certain days of fasting from meat and dairy products. Last rites are obligatory, and the priest should be notified while the client is conscious. The Eastern Orthodox Church does not support abortion, birth control, or euthanasia and discourages autopsies and organ donation.

The Protestant churches believe in the death and resurrection of Jesus Christ, and they view the Bible as the basic source of authority. They split away from the Roman Catholic Church in 1517. Because there are so many different denominations within Protestantism, the nurse needs to make sure that the assessment includes questions regarding specific religious practices that might have an impact on health. In general, the nurse needs to focus on the client's beliefs and practices regarding baptism, Holy Communion, annointing of the sick, dietary restrictions, and death rituals.

Islam

Islam is one of the largest and fastest-growing religions in the world. It is a religion that emphasizes brotherhood and sisterhood for all and the equality of races and social classes (Carson, 1989). Started by the prophet Mohammad, who received visions from the angel Gabriel while meditating in a cave near Mecca, Islam holds forth belief in one god, Allah. Muhammad received many other visions in his life, which were transcribed in what is now called the Qur' an (or Koran in English). These transcriptions include instructions for living a good life and attaining salvation. The major tenets of Islam include the following:

1. The belief in Allah, one God, who is all seeing, all hearing, all speaking, all willing, and all powerful is central to Islam

2. That Allah created the universe

3. That Salvation depends on total commitment to Allah

4. The existence of a group of creatures called jinn, which are half human and half angel; some jinn are good, and others are evil and harm people

5. That Allah has communicated through the ages to prophets, but that Allah's communication with Muhammed represents the completion of this process

6. That Allah will judge all; believers will reside eternally in Paradise, and nonbelievers will be sent to hell

7. That each individual is given free will by Allah; so each individual is free to choose or reject Allah; Allah respects the individual's right to choose but holds the person accountable for those choices

8. That religious duty is essential for all Muslims and that there are Five Pillars, which Muslims are expected to perform:

   a. Repetition of the creed "There is no God but Allah, and Muhammad is the messenger of Allah."

   b. Prayer five times each day—at dawn, midday, mid-afternoon, sunset, and bedtime; a believer rolls out a prayer rug and prays toward Mecca. Prior to prayer, hands, feet, and face must be washed with water; clean soil may be used for symbolic cleansing. Friday is the Muslim day of congregation, and it is observed through prayer, readings from the Koran, and a sermon.

   c. Muslims are expected to give alms of at least 2.5% of their wealth to help the poor, to maintain mosques, to support Imans (prayer leaders), and to support a government tax.

   d. Muslims are expected to fast from food and drink from dawn to dusk during the sacred 9th month of Ramadan. In addition, on the first day of the 10th month, 3 days of additional fasting are expected. This is called Eid-al-Fitr. Exemptions to the fasting rules are allowed for the sick, nursing mothers, young children, and travelers.

   e. A pilgrimage (haji) to Mecca once during a lifetime is strongly encouraged.

The Islamic religion has rituals and requirements in the areas of birth, diet, prayer time, care of women, and death. Caring for an Islamic client requires knowledge of these rituals and respect for the importance that these may hold for the individual. For instance, babies are bathed immediately after birth, before the mother holds the infant. The father or mother whispers the call to prayer in the baby's ears so that the first sounds it hears are about the Islamic faith. Pork and alcoholic beverages are forbidden, and other meats must be blessed and killed in a special way. A Muslim family will surround a dying loved one and read from the Koran while praying. The dying client is positioned to face Mecca and makes a confession of sinful behavior. After death, the Muslim family usually prefers to wash, prepare, and place the body in a position facing Mecca. Health care providers who assist in this final preparation must wear gloves. Burial is performed as soon as possible; cremation is forbidden. Autopsy is permitted only for legal reasons. Organ donation is also not permitted. Contraception is permitted by some Muslims and forbidden by others.

Abortion is forbidden. Prior to praying, Muslims must wash; clients may need assistance with this. Provision of privacy is important during prayer. Muslims consider the Koran to be sacred. Because of this, the Koran should not be touched by anyone who is ritually unclean. Muslim women are very modest and frequently wear clothes that cover all of the body; they prefer to be examined by female physicians. If there is any discussion regarding family planning, the husband must be present. Women are not allowed to sign a consent form or to make decisions regarding family planning. For 40 days after giving birth and during menstruation Muslim women are exempt from prayer because these times are seen as cleansing.

Religions With a Pantheistic World View

Pantheistic religions include Buddhism, some sects of Hinduism, and Taoism. The spiritual world view of these religions is based on a belief in the oneness of the universe. The material world is considered to be illusion; reality consists of only one impersonal element called Atman. Atman, which is energy, is the essence or the soul of every person. Atman is also Brahman, which is the essence or the soul of the cosmos. Because Atman equals Brahman, each person is, in essence, divine and is god. The goal of these religions is to become one with Brahman—to pass beyond one's personality, knowledge, and the concepts of good and evil. Accomplishment of this goal is not through belief, doctrine, or good works, but through techniques that emphasize quiet, solitude, and centeredness, such as chanting a mantra (a Sanskrit word given to the individual by a spiritual master) and meditation. In Eastern pantheism, death marks the end of personal existence—the Atman becomes reabsorbed into the Brahman. Time is not real in this world view—history is cyclical; thus, many who hold this world view believe in reincarnation (Carson & Arnold, 1996; Eshleman, 1992; Sire, 1994).

The interventions that are consistent with this world view involve very directed and focused modalities to create energy changes (to manipulate the divine Brahman) in the promotion of healing. These therapies include traditional Chinese medicine, acupuncture, imagery, therapeutic touch, therapeutic massage, relaxation, bioenergetics, and biofeedback. It is essential for the nurse to consider the world view of a client when considering a particular intervention. The world views of theism and pantheism are not only different but they are mutually exclusive; therefore, the interventions derived from one world view may not be acceptable to an individual who holds a different world view. Nurses must consider informed consent when offering a client a specific spiritual intervention. For instance, a Hindu client may not be comfortable with a nurse praying to Jesus for healing, and a Catholic client may not be comfortable with the practice of therapeutic touch. Spiritual interventions must be sensitive to the client's belief system, and the nurse should never impose his or her beliefs onto the client.

The beliefs and practices of the pantheistic faiths are not easily categorized. There are no specific rituals that accompany major life events. However, there are attitudes regarding health and health-related practices that beg for explanation. For instance, the Eastern or pantheistic world view discourages aggression and advocates moderation and balance. The concepts of the yin and yang are relevant to balance. *Yin* and *yang* represent polarities or opposites. The yin represents darkness, receptivity, stillness, intuition, and femininity; the yang represents brightness, action, creativity, and masculinity. However, these concepts must be considered as complementary rather than as antagonistic to one another; they are in constant dynamic interplay with one another and do not carry connotations of good and bad. Neither exists apart from the other or has meaning except in relation to the other.

Another concept espoused by a pantheistic world view is that of nonattachment or dispassion. According to this world view, much human misery stems from strong desires and attachments. Therefore, the move toward health is expedited by "letting go" of the need to grasp or possess. The concept of *karma,* which holds that for every action there is a corresponding reaction and for every effect, a preceding cause, has an obvious relationship to health. For instance, if people choose to consume unwholesome food, the impact is felt physically. If individuals give in to their emotions and say and do things that are wrong, such behavior results in a weakening of their strength of will. If humanity is an integral part of nature, then humanity is subject to the laws of nature. Choosing to obey these laws results in harmony with nature; disregarding the laws of nature leads to alienation. Therefore, health, which is an outcome of harmony, is within an individual's control.

Health-related practices growing out of a pantheistic world view include

1. The practice of Yoga—a system designed to achieve integration of mind, body, and spirit, which involves following a lifestyle of nonviolence, truthfulness, and not stealing; practicing physical postures; engaging in meditation; and controlling the breath

2. Use of herbs and spices as part of therapeutic nutrition

3. Evaluation of the pulse, which to the Eastern practitioner is more than a measure of cardiovascular function but also offers a glimpse into past health history as well as future health outlook

4. Use of acupuncture—a procedure that uses needles along the meridians (12 pathways of energy flow within the body) to manipulate, disperse, or reactivate the universal energy flow within the individual

5. Use of acupressure—a procedure using pressure application along the meridians to release blocked energy

6. Use of therapeutic massage—a procedure using massage to release blocked energy

Therapeutic Touch

Therapeutic touch, a nursing intervention developed by Dolores Krieger (1981), is *not* part of traditional Eastern practices; however, it derives from a pantheistic world view. According to Krieger, therapeutic touch is a conscious intentional spiritual intervention without a religious basis (Fig. 35–4). Macrea (1991, p. 18) states that "The practice of therapeutic touch involves the use of oneself (that is, one's own localized energy field) as an instrument to help whatever areas within the patient's field that have become obstructed and disordered by disease."

Essential concepts in therapeutic touch are the beliefs that everyone is a healer, that there is a life force present in every person that can be manipulated; and that this universal energy or life force seeks balance on all levels of body, mind, and spirit. By intentionally intervening in the energy field through placing hands around the client, a practitioner moves the life force to areas of depletion and clears blockages in the same field to allow a free and ordered flow of vital life energy and thus healing (Fish, 1996; Hamilton, 1991; Heidt, 1991).

The practice of therapeutic touch involves five phases (Krieger, 1979):

1. The nurse or practitioner centers the self
2. The practitioner assesses the client's energy field
3. The practitioner unruffles the energy field
4. The practitioner directs and modulates the energy
5. The practitioner recognizes when it is time to stop, based on the fact that there are no longer perceivable differences bilaterally in the client's energy fields

The assessment of the client's energy field is conducted through a manual sweep over his or her body. A number of sensations are felt by the practitioner in assessment; *i.e.,* uneven temperatures or feelings of vibrational stuckness in certain areas of the field. The sensations are subjective and qualitative to the observer. Macrea (1991, pp. 31–34) describes these cures in terms of

1. Healthy energy flow—evenly distributed and unbroken
2. Loose congestion—a cloud or wave of heat or heaviness
3. Light congestion—cold or no response to the vibrations
4. Deficit—a hollowness, or depletion of vibration
5. Imbalance—an area's vibrations not flowing in harmony with the whole

Assessment involves total interaction with the client's energy field in terms of listening, observing, and feeling to integrate one's understanding of the client's balance. The practitioner intuits the client's vibrations, so to speak. The healing practice involves a second sweep across the client's energy fields. This time the practitioner focuses on manipulating imbal-ances and transferring energy from the practitioner to the client in an effort to create balance (Hanley, 1991; Hover-Kramer, 1991).

There is a growing body of research focused on therapeutic touch; so far the results are inconclusive. Dolores Krieger cites Grad's studies (1963, 1965) as foundational to her own work on therapeutic touch. Grad's work, as well as the work of nurse researchers, was reviewed by Clark and Clark (1984), who concluded that the results of therapeutic touch research showed transient results, no significant results, or a need for replication of the studies. Janet Quinn (1989), a National Institutes of Health–funded nurse researcher, set out to test the theory of intentionality and energy exchange. Quinn hypothesized that clients who were treated with therapeutic touch would experience a decrease in anxiety, as measured by blood pressure, heart rate, and state-anxiety scores, compared with clients who were treated with a mimic therapeutic touch. The results were nonsignificant. Despite the equivocal research findings, many nurses who use therapeutic touch cite anecdotal evidence of its effectiveness in calming clients and providing a sense of peace.

The New Age Movement

Although the New Age Movement is not considered among the world's great religions, the effects of new age thinking are affecting health care and must be examined. **New Age spirituality** represents a pantheistic world view and an amalgam of Westernized Buddhism and Hinduism, Zen, Sufism, and Native American religion, mixed with humanistic psychology, Western occultism, and modern physics. There is great diversity among New Age thinkers regarding beliefs and practices. However, there are certain areas of commonality (Fish, 1996; Pacwa, 1992; Sire, 1994). These include the following:

1. Each person is divine.
2. Right and wrong are relative and are determined by the individual.
3. History is cyclical; individuals will reincarnate repeatedly, each time evolving into a more developed and perfect human being. Individuals are encouraged to engage in life regressions to examine past lives. This view of reincarnation differs from the Eastern teachings, in which the concept of reincarnation is intimately tied to karma; for instance, if a person has committed wrongful deeds, he or she might reincarnate as a lower life form or a human with greater suffering so that he or she can "work off" his or her karma.
4. We can control and change our own reality.
5. The use of occult practices—seances, for instance—is common.
6. Crystals are believed to contain healing powers and are used to promote health.

Nursing Approaches to Spirituality

A review of current and past literature testifies to nursing's leadership role among the health professions in recognizing the importance of and responding to spiritual needs in clients. Nursing has adopted a number of models, some of which are clearly theistic, some of which are pantheistic, and some of which are nonspecific. Let us briefly review these models.

Theistic Approaches to Spirituality

There are four theistic approaches to spirituality used by nursing. These approaches include spiritual needs, spiritual well-being, spiritual distress, and Dr. Betty Neuman's Systems Model. Each is discussed.

Spiritual Needs

Many nursing authors have defined **spiritual needs** of patients (Bensley, 1991). Although the definitions vary somewhat, there is a consistency in recognizing that spiritual needs stem from a relationship with a loving personal God who is forgiving and trusting. Furthermore, these needs influence how individuals meaningfully live out their lives and how they relate to themselves and to others. Spiritual needs include

1. Forgiveness—from God, self, and others
2. Unconditional love—from God, self, and others
3. Hope
4. Faith
5. Meaning and purpose in life

Box 35–2 gives an example of a spiritual needs approach that was integrated into psychiatric home care.

Spiritual Well-Being

The concept of **spiritual well-being** is defined as "the affirmation of life in a relationship with God, self, community, and environment that nurtures and celebrates wholeness" (Cook, 1980, p. XIII). Ellison and Paloutzian (1983), psychologists interested in spirituality, said that spiritual well-being consists of existential and religious well-being. They developed a 20-item Likert-type scale of Spiritual Well-Being (SWB). The scale consists of two subscales: Existential Well-Being (EWB) and Religious Well-Being (RWB). The EWB subscale measures the sense of well-being related to the person's sense of purpose in and satisfaction with life. The RWB subscale measures the sense of well-being experienced by a person in relationship with God.

The SWB scale has been used in several studies by nurse researchers to examine the role of SWB in college students; in clients with arthritis, breast cancer, or acquired immunodeficiency syndrome (AIDS); in hospice patients, and in relationship to hope (Carson, 1993a; Carson & Green, 1992; Carson et al., 1990; Fehring et al., 1987; Mickley et al., 1992; Miller, 1985). Although these studies demonstrated a positive, health-promoting role for SWB, none of the studies prove that SWB produces greater hope, less anxiety, or less loneliness. They only prove that these concepts are related.

The SWB scale is an easily administered and scored measure. The maximal score for each subscale is 60, and for the total SWB, the maximal score is 120. There are no precise norms; however, the measure allows a practitioner to discern an overall level of SWB, as well as to identify whether the client is experiencing either religious or existential distress (see Clinical Insight Box: Spirituality Research).

Box 35–2

SPIRITUAL NEEDS MET IN PSYCHIATRIC HOME CARE

The patient's name was Evelyn. She was dying of amyotrophic lateral sclerosis. The psychiatric home care nurse had received a referral because Evelyn was severely depressed. After completing an assessment, the nurse decided that the depression was appropriate given the prognosis that Evelyn faced. However, the nurse noted that Evelyn was experiencing distress because of unmet spiritual needs. She expressed concern that she had become a burden to her husband and two daughters. She did not understand why God continued to allow her to suffer. She asked "Has He forgotten me?" She was feeling that her life was meaningless and that she was no longer loved by God or her family. The nurse used a variety of spiritual interventions, including prayer, expressions of compassion, listening and communication strategies, accompanying Evelyn through her suffering, and cognitive reframing. The nurse was able to suggest that Evelyn's interpretation that she was a burden was open to other interpretations. For instance, the nurse noted that her husband and daughters, many neighbors, the oxygen therapist, church members, and even people whom Evelyn did not know well seemed to be drawn to her—not out of duty but out of desire. Could it be that caring for Evelyn offered others an opportunity to be kind and unselfish? Could it be that her suffering provided others a chance to minister? Over the course of 6 weeks, Evelyn became less depressed and more at peace. Finally, on the last visit Evelyn told the nurse "You know, I don't need you anymore. I am feeling better. You helped me in a way that no one else was able to do." The nurse received a call from Evelyn's husband a month later to tell her that Evelyn had passed away peacefully.

Reproduced by permission of the National Association for Home Care, from *CARING* magazine, volume XIII, no. 12 (November 1994). Not for further reproduction.

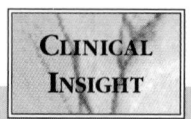

CLINICAL INSIGHT

Spirituality Research

A survey was conducted on various aspects of quality of life for 191 women who were long-term cancer survivors. The results indicated that women who had a positive philosophical or spiritual outlook were more likely to have good health habits and be supportive of others.

Nursing implication: Interventions by the nurse to promote spiritual well-being can have a positive impact on clients' long-term outlook.

Kurtz, M. E., Wyatt, G., & Kurtz, J. C., (1995). Psychological and sexual well-being, philosophical/spiritual views, and health habits of long-term cancer survivors. *Health Care for Women International, 16*(3), 253–262.

Spiritual Distress

Spiritual distress is an accepted nursing diagnosis (North American Nursing Diagnosis Association [NANDA] 1995) and falls under the human response pattern of valuing. This diagnosis is appropriately used when an individual experiences conflict regarding spiritual and/or religious values, practices, and/or beliefs. The diagnosis is broad enough to capture all world views, but in practice it is generally used to identify conflicts or disruptions in usual religious patterns. The diagnosis has been criticized as being bound to religiosity and a theistic world view.

Dr. Betty Neuman's Systems Model

Dr. Betty Neuman developed a systems model of nursing that includes a spiritual variable as one of the main variables operating in individuals (Neuman, 1989, 1994). Dr. Neuman, herself a devout Christian, states that a personal relationship with God is essential not only to spiritual health but also to overall health.

Pantheistic Approaches to Spirituality

There are many nursing articles based on pantheistic views of spirituality; generally the authors do not identify their spiritual world view. For instance, Heliker (1992) challenges the nursing diagnosis of Spiritual Distress as being traditional and bound by religiosity. Heliker further suggests the need for expansion of the nursing diagnosis of Spiritual Distress to include the Eastern world view, which suggests that people are energy fields in constant, open exchange with the environment. Rather than dismiss the theistic nature of the present nursing diagnosis, it seems more productive to recognize that spiritual distress can be concep-

tualized in different ways, according to an individual's world view.

Burkhardt and Nagai-Jacobson (1994) attempt to view spirituality from a theistic as well as a pantheistic world view. They suggest that spirituality is a force, manifested in the self and reflected in one's being, knowing, and doing. Caring relationships with oneself, others, nature, and God or the life force form the context within which spirituality is experienced. By articulating that one of the main relationships is with God or a life force, Burkhardt and Nagai-Jacobson have allowed a broad world view interpretation. However, in their view of spirituality, the "self" and "connections" are the key elements; placing the "self" as central is inconsistent with theism but consistent with a pantheistic world view.

Martha Rogers (1970) and Margaret Newman (1987), both nursing theorists, espoused models of nursing based on the assumption that individuals are energy fields constantly and freely exchanging energy across boundaries with the universal energy source. Rogers' model describing human beings as evolving four-dimensional energy fields has encouraged a generation of nursing students to explore topics such as precognition, out-of-body experiences, Eastern mysticism, and clairvoyance. Jean Watson's (1994) work on caring and spirituality is based on a pantheistic view of the world. Dolores Krieger (1979), who developed therapeutic touch, and Janet Quinn (1989), who has researched therapeutic touch and conducts workshops across the United States teaching nurses the technique of therapeutic touch, operate from a pantheistic world view. Finally, in the 1995 NANDA diagnoses, one of the new diagnoses is Energy Field Disturbance, a diagnosis that reflects a pantheistic world view.

Application of Nursing Process to Spirituality

Before applying the nursing process to the issue of spirituality, let us first take a look at a patient situation. Mrs. Jacobs is a 70-year-old woman admitted to the hospital last week for treatment of pneumonia. You notice that no one has visited her the whole week. She makes a lot of demands but is always pleasant. She frequently calls for a nurse. Everytime you go into her room, she appears sad, unsettled, and distracted. She complains that she is not sleeping well and has no appetite. You share your observations with Mrs. Jacobs: "You know I have noticed some things that concern me. You appear sad and distracted, Mrs. Jacobs. You ask me to come in a lot, but when I do you don't seem to feel any better when I am ready to leave your room than when I came in . . . That makes me think I am not really focusing on what the problem is. Could you tell me what is going on so that I can help you better?" Mrs. Jacobs starts to cry

OBSERVATIONS TO BE MADE IN A SPIRITUALITY ASSESSMENT

Nonverbal Behavior

1. Observe affect. Does the client's affect or attitude convey loneliness, depression, anger, agitation, or anxiety?

2. Observe behavior. Does the client pray during the day? Does the client rely on religious reading material or other literature for solace?

Verbal Behavior

1. Does the client seem to complain out of proportion to his or her illness?

2. Does the client complain of sleeping difficulties?

3. Does the client ask for unusually high doses of sedation or pain medication?

4. Does the client refer to God in any way?

5. Does the client talk about prayer, faith, hope, or anything of a religious nature?

6. Does the client talk about church functions that are a part of his or her life?

7. Does the client express concern over the meaning and direction of life? Does the client express concern over the impact of the illness on the meaning of life?

Interpersonal Relationships

1. Does the client have visitors or does he or she spend visiting hours alone?

2. Are the visitors supportive or do they seem to leave the client feeling upset?

3. Does the client have visitors from his or her church?

4. Does the client interact with the staff and other clients?

Environment

1. Does the client have a Bible or other religious reading material with him or her?

2. Does the client wear religious medals or pins?

3. Does the client use religious articles such as statues in observing religious practices?

4. Has the client received religious get-well cards?

5. Does the client use personal pictures, artwork, or music to keep his or her spirits up?

Data from Carson, V. B. (1989). *Spiritual dimensions of nursing practice*. Philadelphia: W. B. Saunders, p. 158.

here, but I'm afraid that she won't care even if she knows." You further inquire, "Can you tell me more about this, Mrs. Jacobs?" Mrs. Jacobs begins "I was furious with my daughter when she married a Catholic boy; I couldn't accept the fact that she was marrying outside of our Jewish faith. I cut her off from me. But really I cut myself off from her, her husband, and their children. And the funny thing is that I cut myself off from God as well. I don't think He is happy with me about this. He feels pretty distant."

Assessment of Spiritual Needs

There are a number of approaches to the assessment of spiritual needs. First, note all the observations of verbal and nonverbal behaviors and environmental and interpersonal cues that might be indicative of spiritual concerns. Refer back to Figure 35–1; note that the spiritual dimension is represented as the innermost circle. Because spirit is not able to be seen or directly touched, its presence is inferred from emotional and physical behaviors of the person. Box 35–3 includes observations that are made in a spirituality assessment.

In addition, the use of interview questions to focus specifically on spiritual needs and specific spiritual assessment tools such as the SWB scale (Ellison & Paloutzian, 1983) are very useful. Box 35–4 includes sample interview questions for assessing spirituality. Box 35–5 shows the SWB scale.

SAMPLE INTERVIEW QUESTIONS FOR ASSESSING SPIRITUALITY

Concept of God

Is religion or God important to you? If so, can you describe how?

Do you use prayer in your life? If so, does prayer benefit you in any way?

Do you believe God or a deity is involved in your personal life? If so, how?

What is your God or deity like?

Sources of Strength and Hope

Who are your support people?

Who is the most important person in your life?

Are people available to you when you are in need?

Who or what provides you with strength and hope?

Religious Practices

Is your religious faith helpful to you?

Are there any religious practices that are meaningful to you?

Has your illness affected your religious practices?

Are there any religious books or symbols that are helpful to you?

very softly and appears embarrassed to be seen crying. She states "I know I am being a baby; I feel alone here; I haven't seen my daughter in years and it is all my fault. I want to call her and let her know I am

Box 35–5

SPIRITUAL WELL-BEING SCALE

For each of the following statements, circle the choice that best indicates the extent of your agreement or disagreement as it describes your personal experience:

SA = strongly agree

MA = moderately agree

A = agree

D = disagree

MD = moderately disagree

SD = strongly disagree

1. I don't find much satisfaction in private prayer with God.	SA	MA	A	D	MD	SD
2. I don't know who I am, where I came from, or where I am going.	SA	MA	A	D	MD	SD
3. I believe that God loves me and cares about me.	SA	MA	A	D	MD	SD
4. I feel that life is a positive experience.	SA	MA	A	D	MD	SD
5. I believe that God is impersonal and not interested in my daily situations.	SA	MA	A	D	MD	SD
6. I feel unsettled about my future.	SA	MA	A	D	MD	SD
7. I have a personally meaningful relationship with God.	SA	MA	A	D	MD	SD
8. I feel very fulfilled and satisfied with life.	SA	MA	A	D	MD	SD
9. I don't get much personal strength and support from my God.	SA	MA	A	D	MD	SD
10. I feel a sense of well-being about the direction my life is headed in.	SA	MA	A	D	MD	SD
11. I believe that God is concerned about my problems.	SA	MA	A	D	MD	SD
12. I don't enjoy much about life.	SA	MA	A	D	MD	SD
13. I don't have a personally satisfying relationship with God.	SA	MA	A	D	MD	SD
14. I feel good about my future.	SA	MA	A	D	MD	SD
15. My relationship with God helps me not to feel lonely.	SA	MA	A	D	MD	SD
16. I feel that life is full of conflict and unhappiness.	SA	MA	A	D	MD	SD
17. I feel most fulfilled when I'm in close communion with God.	SA	MA	A	D	MD	SD
18. Life doesn't have much meaning.	SA	MA	A	D	MD	SD
19. My relation with God contributes to my sense of well-being.	SA	MA	A	D	MD	SD
20. I believe there is some real purpose for my life.	SA	MA	A	D	MD	SD

One other assessment strategy involves mapping the six relationships inherent in a world view (refer to Figure 35–1). Let us apply this strategy to Mrs. Jacobs. We can see that she has significant stress in the following relationships: (1) with her daughter and family; (2) with her God; (3) with herself (she feels lonely and guilty); (4) with the past (Mrs. Jacobs feels guilty and sad regarding lost with her daughter); and (5) with the future (Mrs. Jacobs fears that the future holds the promise of loneliness and estrangement from her daughter as well as from her God). We know that Mrs. Jacobs is Jewish and that her religious faith was important enough to her at one time to cut herself off from her own daughter when the daughter married a non-Jewish man. Now Mrs. Jacobs is experiencing significant spiritual distress because the consequences of her decision to sever ties with her daughter are more difficult than she had imagined. She is concerned that she made the wrong decision.

Nursing Diagnosis

After collecting and analyzing the data, your next step is to determine the appropriate nursing diagnosis or diagnoses for a particular client. In the case of Mrs. Jacobs, she is clearly suffering from spiritual distress. Five of the six possible world view relationships are disturbed; her spiritual distress is reflected in emotional behaviors of sadness and frequent demands, as well as in physical behaviors of inadequate rest and no appetite. The complete nursing diagnosis for Mrs. Jacobs is: Spiritual Distress related to disruption in relationships with her God and her daughter, as evi-

SAMPLE NURSING CARE PLAN

THE CLIENT IN SPIRITUAL DISTRESS

Mrs. Jacobs complains of feeling alone, "cut-off" from her daughter and her God, and guilty about a past decision to sever ties with her daughter when the daughter married a non-Jewish man.

Nursing Diagnosis:	Spiritual distress related to disruption in relationships with her God and her daughter as evidenced by Mrs. Jacobs statements of feeling lonely, guilty, and estranged from her God and her daughter.
Expected Outcome:	Mrs. Jacobs will state that she is feeling at peace regarding her relationship with her daughter and her God.

Nursing Action	**Rationale**
1. Assess level of spiritual well-being using SWB scale (Ellison & Paloutzian, 1983).	1. Provides baseline data regarding Mrs. Jacob's level of spiritual well-being; these data can be used to evaluate effectiveness of interventions.
2. Engage Mrs. Jacobs in discussion of her feelings about situation with daughter and her reasons for making decision to sever ties with her daughter over religious issue.	2. Allows Mrs. Jacobs to examine her own problem-solving process.
3. Ask Mrs. Jacobs to evaluate the earlier decision; would she make the same decision again? If no, why not?	3. Helps Mrs. Jacobs examine the significance of earlier decision and to consider alternative options.
4. Offer to bring in a rabbi for Mrs. Jacob's with whom to discuss her situation.	4. A referral to the client's spiritual advisor or leader may sometimes provide comfort, reassurance, and necessary guidance in decision making.
5. Ask Mrs. Jacobs to identify what she would like to change and ways that the change can occur. Ask her if there are spiritual or religious practices that might assist her in examining her situation.	5. This approach is empowering and supportive. Mrs. Jacobs is in control of decreasing her spiritual distress while the nurse guides the process and directs Mrs. Jacobs to consider all resources.
6. Encourage Mrs. Jacobs to act on her choices—whether to remain firm in her earlier decision with regard to her daughter or possibly to reach out to her daughter to reestablish the relationship. Encourage her to reach out to her God in prayer so that she does not feel so distant and removed from Him.	6. This approach encourages the client to actively evaluate her decision making and to make necessary changes; by making a clear choice, the client may feel peace that she has made the right choice for her.

Evaluation:	On the spiritual well-being scale, Mrs. Jacobs scored 82. The process of responding to the items on the SWB provided the opportunity for the nurse to discuss the situation between Mrs. Jacobs and her daughter. The nurse asked Mrs. Jacobs if the pain that she felt regarding her daughter influenced her responses to the SWB scale. Mrs. Jacobs agreed that this was true. She shared with the nurse the strong feelings she had experienced when her daughter married outside of the Jewish faith; she felt as if her daughter had turned her back on everything that had been taught to her. Now, after living with this decision, she has strong regrets. She says to the nurse, "I paid a steep price for sticking to principles . . . I have lost my daughter. If I had to do it over again, I would do it differently." In discussing options to this situation, Mrs. Jacobs asked the nurse if she would be willing to call her daughter and ask her to visit Mrs. Jacobs. The nurse agreed to do this and also offered to call the hospital rabbi. Mrs. Jacobs met with the rabbi, who talked and prayed with her. Her daughter came to visit and spent 2 hours with her mother. When the daughter left the room, Mrs. Jacobs thanked the nurse for helping her to reconnect with her daughter and said, "How can I ever repay you? You helped me get my daughter back, and I feel right with God again!"

denced by Mrs. Jacobs' statements of feeling lonely, guilty, and estranged from her daughter and her God. The expected outcome for Mrs. Jacobs is: Mrs. Jacobs will state that she is at peace regarding her relationships with her God and with her daughter.

Planning

The plan of care involves establishing short-term goals that logically lead to the expected outcome and deciding who will deliver the care to Mrs. Jacobs. Short-term goals might include

> Mrs. Jacobs will discuss the reasons for making her earlier decision regarding her daughter
>
> Mrs. Jacobs will evaluate her earlier decision regarding her daughter in light of her religious beliefs and the consequences of the decision
>
> Mrs. Jacobs will decide if there were other options she could have considered
>
> Mrs. Jacobs will consider what options presently exist for her to change her situation
>
> Mrs. Jacobs will act on her choices
>
> Mrs. Jacobs will express peace about her decisions

See the Nursing Care Plan.

Interventions

There are a number of appropriate interventions that can be used to meet spiritual needs, regardless of the client's world view. These include

1. The nurse's presence—being present to someone else as he or she communicates deep concerns is a powerful spiritual tool. This intervention communicates that the client is valued, cared about, and respected.
2. The nurse's communication and listening skills—being able to "tune in" to the client's authentic concerns requires that the nurse listen with his or her ears as well as his or her heart and respond based on the true meaning of the client's message. In the example of Mrs. Jacobs, excellent communication and listening skills were essential to discover the meaning of the behaviors of sadness, frequent use of the call light, inadequate sleep, and no appetite.
3. Compassion—the nurse's ability to accurately identify the client's feelings and communicate his or her understanding of the suffering conveyed by those feelings provides the client with reassurance that Mrs. Jacobs is not alone.
4. Cognitive reframing—being able to look at situations from a variety of perspectives allows clients to do the same. This is an important strategy when a client's spiritual distress stems from a feeling of meaninglessness. Nurses cannot make meaning for another person, but nurses can share different views of a particular situation that may provide flexibility as the client attempts to interpret events.
5. Accompaniment—the nurse's ability to accompany the client through suffering is important (Fig. 35–5).

There are some interventions that are appropriate from a theistic world view. These include

1. Prayer—offering to either pray for or with a client can be a tremendous comfort. Prayer is communication with God, and sometimes illness interferes with the client's ability to engage in conversation. The nurse's offer to pray facilitates the communication process between that individual and God, offers support, and strengthens the individual's faith and hope.
2. Reading religious material—offering to read religious material to a client may be very comforting. For instance, a client who believes that Holy Scripture is the inspired word of God may be very comforted by hearing the words of a favorite Psalm or other passage.
3. Respect for religious practices and rituals—inquiring about, respecting, and providing the opportunity and privacy to practice significant religious practices and rituals decreases anxiety in many clients and allows them to draw on religious sources of support in their healing.
4. Referral to a religious leader—inquiring whether the client would like to speak to a religious leader and facilitating this referral are important strategies in linking the client with sources of support that are outside of the health care team but are just as essential for healing.
5. Use of religious music—many clients find that listening to hymns and other music is both soothing and uplifting and are appreciative when someone recognizes and respects this as important.

Appropriate interventions from a pantheistic world view include the following:

1. Therapeutic touch
2. Acupuncture
3. Therapeutic massage
4. Acupressure

Evaluation

The last step of the nursing process involves the evaluation, which looks not only at the effectiveness of nursing interventions, but also at the accuracy and adequacy of the assessment. In the case of a spiritual need, the nurse might ask the following questions in evaluating the nursing process:

1. Did I specifically ask about spiritual matters?
2. Did I validate the observations that I made regarding spirituality?
3. Was I comfortable in meeting the client's spiritual needs? If not, did I delegate this aspect of care to someone comfortable with spiritual issues?
4. Was I attuned to the world view of the client? Was I respectful of this world view, even though it differed from my own?
5. Did I consider the world view of the client when choosing nursing interventions?
6. Were the short-term goals adequate?
7. Did the client achieve the expected outcome?
8. If the client did not achieve the expected outcome, how did I modify the plan?

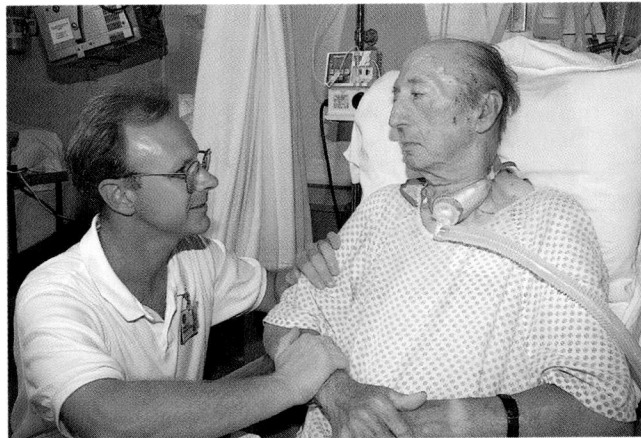

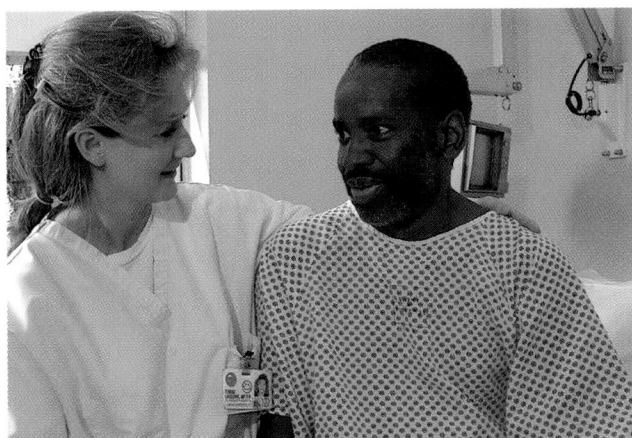

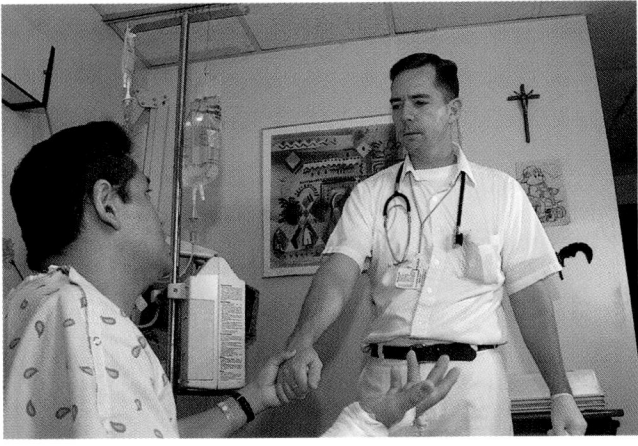

✦ **Figure 35–5**
Touch is an important aspect of reaching out to meet the spiritual needs of patients. Touch communicates to the patient that he or she is valued, cared about, and respected. Compassion can relieve stress and encourage the patient to express spiritual needs.

Summary

Examining spirituality as a world view provides a concrete method of discussing a concept that is difficult to define. This approach allows the nurse to identify and respond to spiritual distress without having to be an expert on all health-related religious practices. *Spirituality* is a broad term that encompasses religious belief but is not the same as religious belief. All people are spiritual by nature; however, not all are religious, nor do all share the same spiritual world view. Nurses need awareness of their own spiritual world views, as well as those of clients.

Spirituality is important to health and health care. When people are in spiritual distress, they are experiencing difficulty in one or more of six relationships, including the relationship to the Ultimate Other, to others and self, to the environment, and to time past, present, and future. The impact of this distress is holistic; spiritual pain is felt in the body as well as the mind and spirit of an individual. Conversely, an individual who is suffering from either a physical or a psychiatric illness experiences that suffering in his or her body and mind, as well as spirit. Therefore, nurses, as holistic caregivers, need to provide care for the body, mind, and spirit. This may mean making religious practices available to the client and/or family.

It may also mean listening, empathizing, and accompanying the client through suffering as he or she attempts to make sense out of the illness. It may involve a referral to a representative of the client's faith tradition. It may involve praying with the client or providing him or her with privacy so that he or she can pray as he or she sees fit. Whatever the specific intervention, the goal is to relieve spiritual distress so that the client's sense of well-being and, ultimately, the client's healing, can proceed.

■   ■

CHAPTER HIGHLIGHTS
✦

✦ Spirituality can be viewed as a world view—a way of understanding God, ourselves, others, the environment, and time.

✦ All religions are undergirded by a world view. The great religions of the world are either theistic, pantheistic, or polytheistic in their world views.

✦ Religions represent attempts by humankind to structure spiritual experiences.

✦ The universal aspects of spirituality include a desire to be connected with the Ultimate Other and search for meaning; the unique aspects of spirituality include how the Ultimate Other is defined and how we go about finding meaning in life.

✦ The Stallwood-Stoll model of spirituality is a mutually interactive model that includes spirituality and psychosocial and biological dimensions. Distress in any of the dimensions is felt in all of the dimensions. Therefore, any physical or psychosocial health issues have an impact on the spirit. Likewise, spiritual distress is felt by the body as well as the mind.

✦ The New Age Movement is not a religion but it is an eclectic spiritual world view borrowing from Hinduism, Zen, Sufism, and Native American religion and mixed with humanistic psychology, Western occultism, and modern physics. New Age thinking has begun to influence some areas of nursing regarding spiritual issues and interventions. The use of crystals is an example of a New Age Movement intervention.

✦ The theistic religions identify specific health-related practices that have an impact on care.

✦ The pantheistic religions support a philosophy of living that affects health.

✦ Therapeutic touch is an intervention developed by Dolores Krieger. The intervention is not religious but is based on a pantheistic world view. Acupressure, acupuncture, and therapeutic massage are also derived from a pantheistic world view.

✦ Prayer, Scripture or other religious reading, referral to a member of the clergy, and practice of specific religious rituals are all interventions derived from a theistic world view.

✦ Nursing approaches spirituality in one of three ways: spiritual needs, spiritual distress, or spiritual well-being.

Study Questions

1. An example of a theistic nursing intervention is

    a. therapeutic massage
    b. regression therapy
    c. prayer
    d. crystal therapy

2. *Pantheism* refers to

    a. a belief in many gods
    b. a belief that we are all god
    c. a belief in a personal creator god
    d. a belief that science is our god

3. Assessment of spiritual needs includes all of the following except

    a. finding out everything about the client's religion
    b. finding out the client's level of commitment to his or her religion

    c. finding out about the quality of the client's relationships
    d. finding out if the client has issues requiring forgiveness

4. The universal aspects of a spiritual world view include all of the following except

    a. the belief that there is one god
    b. a sense of connectedness with something greater than ourselves
    c. a search for meaning and purpose in life
    d. the belief that we are connected to others

5. Which of the following statements about spiritual development are incorrect?

    a. spiritual development somewhat parallels cognitive development
    b. children do not possess spiritual world views
    c. religious beliefs of parents have a strong influence on children
    d. the older years are characterized by renewed spirituality

Critical Thinking Exercises

1. You are caring for a 10-year-old girl whose parents refuse a blood transfusion that could save the girl's life. Discuss your spiritual feelings regarding this matter and how you would handle this situation.

2. You are asked to discontinue tube feedings and intravenous fluids for a 92-year-old woman with terminal cancer who is being cared for at her home. Her son has power of attorney and has arranged to do this with her physician. You are aware of the fact that the woman wished for everything to be done for her. You feel the son is trying to get his inheritance. What are the spiritual implications in this case? How would you intervene in this situation?

References

Bensley, R. J. (1991). Defining spiritual health: A review of the literature. *Journal of Health Education, 22*(5), 287–290.

Burkhardt, M. A., & Nagai-Jacobson, M. G. (1994). Reawakening spirit in clinical practice. *Journal of Holistic Nursing, 12*(1), 9–21.

Carson, V. (1994a). Caring: Rediscovering our nursing roots. *Perspectives in Psychiatric Care, 30*(2), 4–6.

Carson, V. (1994b). The importance of spirituality in psychiatric disorders. *Smooth Sailing, Winter,* 3–4.

Carson, V. (1993a). Prayer, meditation, exercise, and vitamin use: Behaviors of the hardy individual who is HIV+, diagnosed with ARC or AIDS. *Journal of the Association of Nurses in AIDS Care, 4*(3), 18–22.

Carson, V. (1994c). Spiritual care of Evelyn. *Caring Magazine, 13*(12), 25–28.

Carson, V. (Ed.). (1989). *Spiritual dimensions of nursing practice.* Philadelphia: W. B. Saunders.

Carson, V. (1993b). "Spirituality: Generic or Christian?" *Journal of Christian Nursing, 10*(1), 24–27.

Carson, V. B., & Arnold, E. C. (1996). *Mental health nursing: The nurse-patient journey.* Philadelphia: W. B. Saunders.

Carson, V., & Green, H. (1992). Spiritual well-being: A predictor of hardiness in the AIDS patient. *Journal of Professional Nursing, 8*(4), 209–220.

Carson, V., Soeken, K., Shanty, J., & Toms, L. (1990). Spiritual well-being and hope in the person with AIDS. *Perspectives in Psychiatric Care, 26*(9), 28–34.

Clark, P., & Clark, M. J., (1984). Therapeutic touch: Is there a scientific basis for practice? *Nursing Research, 33*(1), 37–40.

Coles, R. (1990). *The spiritual life of children.* Boston: Houghton-Mifflin.

Cook, T. C. (1980). Preface. In J. A. Thorson, & T. C. Cook. (Eds.), *Spiritual well-being of the elderly.* Springfield, IL; Charles C. Thomas.

Ellison, C. W., & Paloutzian, R. F. (1983). Spiritual well-being: Conceptualization and measurement. *Journal of Psychology and Theology, 11*(4), 330–340.

Eshleman, M. J. (1992). Death with dignity: Significance of religious beliefs and practices in Hinduism, Buddhism and Islam. *Today's OR Nurse, November,* 19–22.

Fehring, R. J., Brennan, P. F., & Keller, M. L. (1987). Psychological and spiritual well-being in college students. *Research in Nursing Health, 10,* 391–398.

Fish, S. (1996). Therapeutic touch: Healing science or metaphysical fraud? *Journal of Christian Nursing, 13*(3), 4–10.

Grad, B. (1969). Some biological effects of the laying-on-of-hands: A review of experiments with animals and plants. *Journal of the American Society for Psychical Research, 59,* 95–127.

Grad, B. (1963). A telekinetic effect on plant growth. *International Journal of Parapsychology, 5,* 117–133.

Hamilton, D. (1991). Vital energy: The antebellum health movement. *Journal of Holistic Nursing, Winter, 9*(3), 10–18.

Hanley, M. A. (1991). Therapeutic touch—The art of improvisation. *Journal of Holistic Nursing, Winter, 9*(3), 26–31.

Heidt, P. R. (1991). Therapeutic touch—The caring environment. *Journal of Holistic Nursing, Winter, 9*(3), 19–25.

Heliker, D. (1992). Reevaluation of a nursing diagnosis: Spiritual distress. *Nursing Forum, 27*(4), 15–20.

Hover-Kramer, D. (1991). Energy fields: Implications for the science of human caring. *Journal of Holistic Nursing, Winter, 9*(3), 5–9.

Karns, P. S. (1991). Building a foundation for spiritual care. *Journal of Christian Nursing, 8*(3), 10–13.

Krieger, D. (1979). *The therapeutic touch* (pp. 62–63). Englewood Cliffs, NJ: Prentice-Hall.

Krieger, D. (1981). *Foundations for holistic health nursing practices—The renaissance nurse.* Philadelphia: J. B. Lippincott.

Kurtz, M. E., Wyatt, G., & Kurtz, J. C., (1995). Psychological and sexual well-being, philosophical/spiritual views, and health habits of long-term cancer survivors. *Health Care for Women International, 16*(3), 253–262.

Lashley, M. (1992). Reminiscence. *Journal of Christian Nursing, 9*(3), 4–8.

Macrae, J. (1991). *Therapeutic touch.* New York: Alfred A. Knopf.

Mickley, J. R., Soeken, K., & Belcher, A. (1992). Spiritual well-being, religiousness and hope among women with breast cancer. *Image Journal of Nursing Scholarship, 28*(4), 267–272.

Miller, J. F. (1985). Assessment of loneliness and spiritual well-being in chronically ill and healthy adults. *Journal of Professional Nursing, 1,* 79–85.

NANDA nursing diagnoses: Definitions and classification 1995–1996. (1995). Philadelphia: North American Nursing Diagnosis Association.

Neuman, B. (1989). *The Neuman systems model.* New York: Appleton-Lange.

Neuman, B. (1994). *The Neuman systems model* (2nd ed.). New York: Appleton-Lange.

Newman, M. A. (1987). *Health as expanding consciousness.* St. Louis: Mosby-Year Book.

Pacwa, M. (1992). *Catholics and the New Age Movement.* Ann Arbor, MI: Servant Publications.

Poloma, M. M. (1993). The effects of prayer on mental well-being. *Second Opinion, 18*(3), 37–51.

Quinn, J. (1989). Therapeutic touch as energy exchange: Replication and extension. *Nursing Science Quarterly, 2*(2), 79–87.

Reed, P. G. (1991a). Spirituality and mental health in older adults: Extant knowledge for nurses. *Family Community Health, 14*(2), 14–25.

Reed, P. G. (1991b). Self-transcendence and mental health in oldest-old adults. *Nursing Research, 40,* 5–11.

Rogers, M. (1970). *An introduction to the theoretical basis of nursing.* Philadelphia: F. A. Davis.

Sire, J. (1994). *Why should anyone believe anything at all?* Downers Grove, IL: Intervarsity Press.

Stallwood, J., & Stoll, R. (1975). Spiritual dimensions of nursing practice. In I. L., Beland, J. Y. Passos (Eds.): *Clinical nursing* (3rd ed.). New York: Macmillan.

Watson, J. (1994). Myth, mystery, and metaphors for ecocaring. In E. A., Schuster, & C. L. Brown, *Exploring our environmental connections.* New York: National League for Nursing.

The way we live. *LIFE Magazine,* (1994). *March,* 54–63.

Bibliography

Bergin, A. E. (1991). Values and religious issues in psycho therapy and mental health. *American Psychologist, 46*(4), 94–403.

Carson, V. (1990). Spirituality and spiritual directions: Important issues to the persons with AIDS. *Journal of Christian Healing, 12*(3), 3–7.

Carson V. (1994). Value-Belief Pattern. In R. Ferri (Ed.). *Care planning for the older adult* (pp. 345–354). Philadelphia: W. B. Saunders.

Carson V., Soeken, K., & Belcher, A. (1991). The relationship among spiritual well-being, hardiness and ego strength in persons with AIDS. *Journal of Christian Healing, 13*(2), 21.

Carson, V., Soeken, K., & Grimm, P. (1988). Hope and its relationship to spiritual well-being. *Journal of Psychology and Theology, 16*(2), 159–167.

Carson, V., Winkelstein, M., Soeken, K., & Brunins, M. (1987). The effect of didactic teaching on spiritual attitudes. *Image, 18*(4), 161–164.

Ellis, A. (1992). Do I really hold that religiousness is irrational and equivalent to emotional disturbance? *American Psychologist, 47*(3), 428–429.

Ferraro, K. F., & Albrecht-Jenson, C. M. (1991). Does religion influence health? *Journal for the Scientific Study of Religion, 30*(2), 193–202.

Gartner, J., Larson, D. B., & Allen, G. D. (1991). Religious commitment and mental health: A review of the empirical literature. *Journal of Psychology and Theology, 19*(1), 6–25.

Larson, D. B., & Larson, S. S. (1991). Religious commitment and health: Valuing the relationship. *Second Opinion, 17*(1), 27–40.

Chapter 36

CULTURAL COMPETENCY IN NURSING

MARY BARB HAQ, PhD, RN, CS

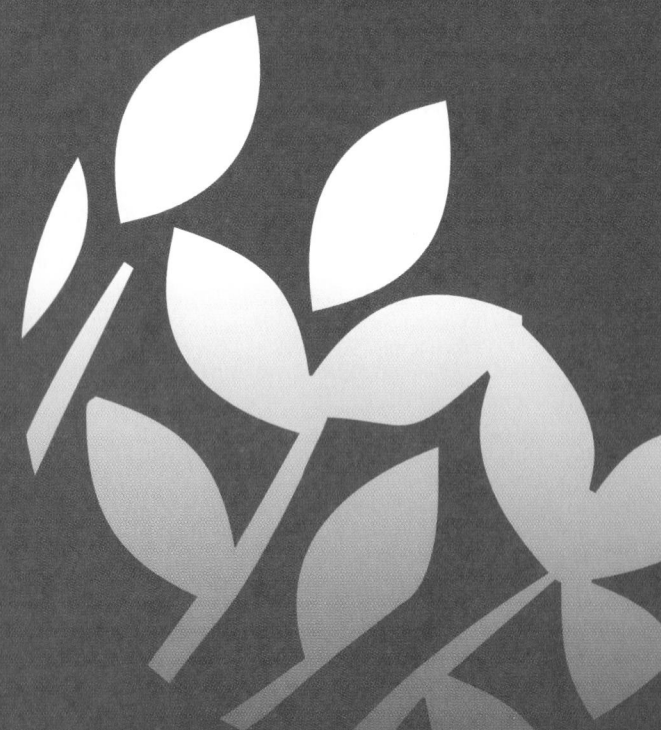

KEY TERMS
✦

acculturation
advocate
anthropology
assimilation
beliefs
cultural sensitivity
culture
culture brokering
culture shock
emigrant
ethnicity
ethnocentrism

folk illness
folk medicine
homeopathy
immigrant
migrant
prejudice
race
refugee
stereotyping
transcultural nursing
values
worldview

LEARNING OBJECTIVES
✦

After studying this chapter, you should be able to

✦ Define the key terms related to cultural competence

✦ Discuss the historical development of transcultural nursing

✦ Identify the factors that contribute to a pluralistic society

✦ Identify the demographics of the immigrant population in the United States

✦ Analyze the effects of immigration on the health care system

✦ Identify the demographics and risk factors of migrant workers in the United States

✦ Describe the differences in health status for different ethnocultural groups

✦ Analyze the relationship between cultural practices and increased risk of disease

✦ Conduct a competent cultural assessment

✦ Relate the culture of poverty to health status and access to health care systems

✦ Use the nursing process for culturally diverse clients

With recent increases in transportation, migration, and political strife around the world, many countries are finding that their populations are more diverse than ever. The United States has continued its history of immigration, with many people continuing to immigrate from the Third World and Latin America.

Nursing practice differs from other health professions in the delivery of care that is holistic and client centered. This client-centered focus is based on a complete and thorough understanding of cultural diversity. Nurses will continue to be challenged by an ever-growing ethnically and culturally diverse client population. The best preparation for this challenge is culturally competent nursing care practiced within a transcultural nursing context.

The interaction among the client, the nurse, and the environment is multifaceted. Nursing education prepares the beginning nurse in the necessary skills and knowledge to provide health care for all clients across the life span. Environmental aspects of care are closely interwoven in all aspects of nursing care. The concepts of culture and cultural diversity are aspects of a person's environment that need to be carefully assessed and understood when planning and providing holistic care.

An individual's **culture** encompasses the political, economic, social, religious, philosophical, technical, and environmental context of our lives (Leininger, 1990). An individual is born, lives, and dies within a cultural framework. One's culture guides all everyday decisions—who has the authority in the family, how meals are prepared, how we communicate, care of the sick and dying, care and feeding of the newborn, and so forth. A thorough and accurate understanding of culture contributes immensely to the ability to effectively complete the nursing process.

Ethnicity and culture are closely related. An individual's ethnicity is linked to his or her association with a group's customs and language. Sometimes it is easier to identify one's ethnicity than a specific culture because of the strong identification with one's ethnic group. Ethnicity is different from **race.** Our identification with a particular race is based on physical characteristics such as skin color and hair texture. These physical characteristics have evolved over time as humans adapted to the environment.

As we develop, we learn how to respond and adjust to other ethnocultural groups. Positive responses include cultural sensitivity, tolerance, acceptance, and **acculturation.** Minority cultures respond to the majority through a process of **assimilation.** Often it is difficult to identify one's culture clearly because of the assimilation process. Negative responses to people from different ethnocultural groups include **prejudice,** insensitivity, and avoidance. A person who believes that his or her culture is the only acceptable one or the best one is participating in **ethnocentrism.** This attitude is unacceptable in a multicultural society because of the negativity and derisiveness that can occur.

Cultural competence is based on a **worldview** and understanding of ethnocultural concepts. A nurse who is culturally competent fosters positive attitudes toward people from other cultures and facilitates health care within the individual's ethnocultural framework. The steady evolution of transcultural nursing to the more widely accepted phrase *cultural competency* has increased awareness and acceptance of this important role for nursing. As nurses have developed their **cultural sensitivity,** it has become apparent that cultural competency is necessary at the current level of nursing practice. Sensitivity is a lifelong process. It is not enough to teach and practice sensitivity. Professional nurses must plan, organize, and promote health within an individual's ethnocultural framework.

History of Cultural Diversity in Nursing Practice

The earliest documentation of the need for cultural awareness in the nursing profession is found in public health nursing literature of the early 1900s (Tripp-Reimer & Fox, 1990). Then, the United States was experiencing a tremendous influx of immigrants. Along with the increase in population, the diversity in cultures brought its own special health problems. Public health nurses became aware that an ethnocentric approach to the health care and education of various ethnocultural groups was insufficient. The emphasis was on assimilation, or adoption of American ways. In the 1950s, nursing education evolved to include the study of culture and social concepts. The profession progressed into its current holistic, individualized approach to client care.

In 1970, Madeleine Leininger developed the subspecialty of transcultural nursing. A series of national transcultural nursing conferences brought nurses together, along with anthropologists and social scientists, to develop and define the new field (Leininger, 1979). Knowing, understanding, and caring for clients according to their cultural values was a major new challenge for the profession. "Transcultural nursing refers to a learned subfield or branch of nursing which focuses on the comparative study and analysis of cultures with respect to nursing and health-illness caring practices, beliefs, and values with the goal to provide meaningful and efficacious nursing care services to people according to their cultural values and health-illness context" (Leininger, 1979, p. 15). Early goals to study and develop culturally derived nursing care as it related to the specific cultural needs of groups strengthened the organization.

National nursing organizations worked to incorporate the concepts of cultural sensitivity and diversity into the professional standards. In 1977, the National League for Nursing (NLN) mandated that cultural content be included in nursing curricula for accreditation.

The Transcultural Nursing Society (TNS), organized in 1974, is a worldwide organization for nurses interested in the advancement of transcultural nursing. The purposes of TNS are to (1) advance the body of knowledge; (2) share experiences in caring for clients from different cultures; (3) stimulate theory development and research; (4) discuss methods of applying transcultural concepts to care of families and world cultures; (5) exchange information; and (6) support quality-based consultation at the local, national, and international levels. The TNS offers a formal certification program in transcultural nursing.

In 1981, Leininger evaluated the progress of transcultural nursing. Areas for revision and exploration were identified. The subspecialty has been slowly recognized, and specific educational programs are few. In the 1990s and beyond, nurses will continue to develop their education and practice with cultural competency.

This chapter presents a broad discussion of the number and extent of the diverse cultures found within US society. Immigration, as it relates to diversity and health care needs, is also discussed. Nurses need information concerning the diverse nature of US society, especially as it relates to immigration. This broad view provides a solid foundation for application of the nursing process.

Demographic and Socioeconomic Characteristics of the United States' Population

To meet the demands of a pluralistic society, the nursing profession should be aware of the extent and location of the many ethnocultural groups found within US borders. Socioeconomic indicators, such as income, employment, and housing, along with demographic information, reveal information that has a direct impact on access to health care systems. These indicators are often the key to understanding the current health status of individuals and families. The best source for current indicator data is obtained from the US Bureau of the Census. The Census Bureau is mandated by law to conduct regular assessment of the US population every 10 years. Census reports, published by the government printing office (GPO), are located in larger public and university-affiliated libraries. Four of the largest demographic groups in the United States classified by the Census Bureau by race—white, black, Native American, and Asian–Pacific Islander—are discussed. The Hispanic classification, considered an ethnic group, is discussed separately.

In the 1990 census, 81% of the US population was white, 12% black, 1% Native American, and 3% Asian (US Bureau of the Census, 1992). Nearly 9% (21 mil-

lion) of the total population was Hispanic. Nearly 82% of all whites were married, compared with 69% of Hispanics and 47% of blacks. The black population had the largest percentage of female-headed households (46%), as compared with whites (13%) and Hispanics (24%). The highest percentage of college graduates was reported in the white population.

Family income estimates are also important health indicators. Seven percent of all whites reported a family income of less than $10,000; 25% of blacks and 18% of Hispanic families reported this income level. The largest groups living below the poverty level are blacks (29%), Hispanics (25%), and whites (8%). Families who identify themselves as black Hispanics are the largest group with income below the poverty level (35.4%).

The Hispanic population is the largest ethnocultural group in the United States (US Bureau of the Census, 1993). By the year 2050, it is projected to grow to 81 million. It is the fastest growing group, increasing 53% between 1980 and 1990. The Hispanic population encompasses all citizens from Mexico, Puerto Rico, Cuba, Central and South America, and Spain (Fig. 36–1). Use of the label can be misleading, because Hispanic persons speak many different languages and have various cultural practices. This steady population growth is boosted by higher birth rates and substantial immigration. Nearly 90% of all Hispanic persons live in 10 US states (Fig. 36–2). For example, 4 out of 10 people in New Mexico and 1 person in 5 in Arizona are Hispanic.

Effects of Immigration

Many people will continue to migrate beyond their borders as the need continues for economic opportunities, improved education, advanced health care, employment, and safety from political oppression. The United States has a long tradition of immigration that continues today (Fig. 36–3). The Immigration and Naturalization Service reported that a total of 23.5 million legal immigrants entered the country between 1881 and 1920 (US Bureau of the Census, 1993). Between 1950 and 1990, another 17.7 million immigrants legally entered the United States, primarily from Mexico and Latin America. Immigrant numbers from Canada and Europe steadily decreased to 919,000 in the 1980s.

In its early development, the United States opened its shores to all immigrants. There were many employment opportunities. Quotas were developed in the early 1900s as a means of limiting immigrants classified as undesirable. The groups with the smallest quotas were usually from non-European countries. The United States continues to set quotas for immigrant applications, as do other countries, especially in Europe. The effects of immigration are wide ranging. In the early decades, immigrants were expected to adopt American language, style of dress, cultural norms, values, and become educated in American traditions. Immigrants, adjusting to the pressure to conform, needed

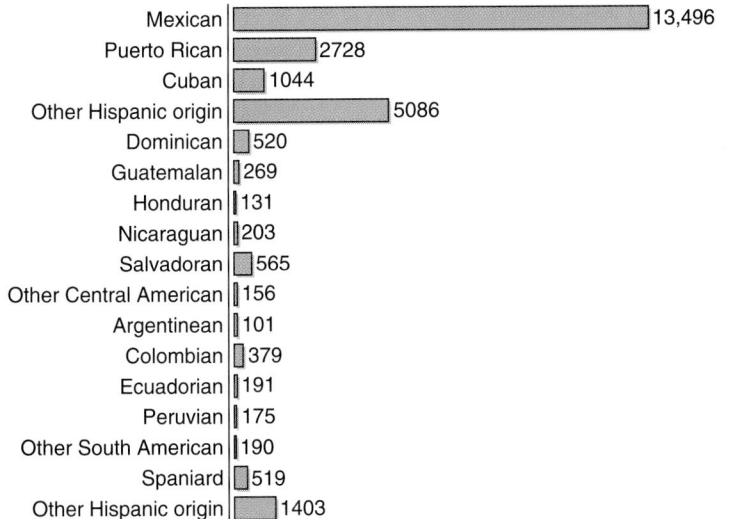

> **Figure 36–1**
> Hispanic population, by type of origin, 1990 (in thousands). (From US Department of Commerce, Bureau of the Census. [1993]. *Hispanic Americans today [current population reports].* Washington, DC: Government Printing Office.)

great amounts of patience, diligence, and hard work. Immigrants experienced culture shock, demonstrating signs of frustration, loneliness, feelings of isolation, and uneasiness. Environmental and health problems, such as overcrowded living conditions, overworking, and lack of knowledge and access to the health care system, have continued across generations.

Acculturation was generally easier for the second generation because of their English-speaking abilities and acquisition of American habits and traditions. The pressure to conform is slowly eroding as new groups of immigrants find US communities that resemble their own. Generations of immigrants have set up a network of heritage support systems, such as their own houses of worship, community centers, food stores, and health care providers.

Migrant Worker Populations in the United States

A migrant worker is a farmworker who travels across the country following the harvest season. The view of farm work as life in clean, outdoor air with

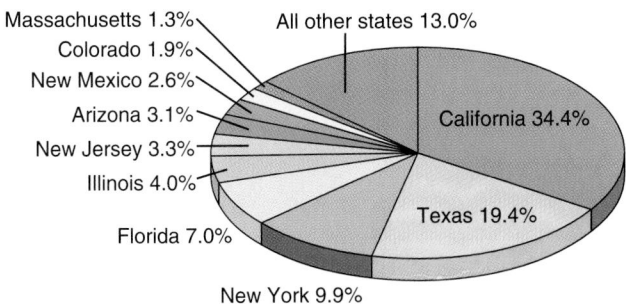

> **Figure 36–2**
> Hispanic population for selected states, 1990 (percent distribution). (From US Department of Commerce, Bureau of the Census. [1993]. *Hispanic Americans today [current population reports].* Washington, DC: Government Printing Office.)

plenty of fresh food was a popular misconception held by the public and nurses (Smith, 1986). In reality, migrants suffer a mixture of hardship, loneliness, poverty, illiteracy, and multiple health risks.

Because of the large numbers of illegal immigrant workers, it is difficult to collect accurate demographic information on this population. However, it has been determined that the average migrant worker is a young Mexican-American male who earns about $1800 for approximately 82 days (a season). Workdays last from sunup to sundown, with only Sunday off for rest and relaxation. Abuse and mistreatment of migrant workers continue, even with federal laws and protection from the Occupational Safety and Health Administration. Major health problems for this group include malnutrition (most significant), an alarmingly high rate of accidents, higher-than-normal incidences of respiratory and skin diseases, and a prevalence of parasitic disorders. Migrant workers experience long, hard days in hot temperatures with limited access to clean water and food, high exposures to toxic levels of chemicals and pesticides, heat-induced illnesses, no compensation for injuries, and substandard housing that often lacks bathing facilities and safe food storage. A survey of 936 migrant farmworkers documented a prevalence rate of diarrhea that is 20 times higher than that in the general population (Arab & Weiner, 1986). Extremely high levels of gastroenteritis and fevers of unknown origin were reported. Over 66% of the farm owners failed to provide toilets in the field or fresh water.

A change in the ethnocultural makeup of migrant workers has occurred as the homeless and unemployed travel rural areas in search of work. Whole families have been living in tent cities in park vacation areas. Nurses should have an understanding of the culture of migrancy as these families and individuals migrate between rural and urban areas. Assessment forms should include the possibility of migrant field work and its associated health risks, even in urban clients.

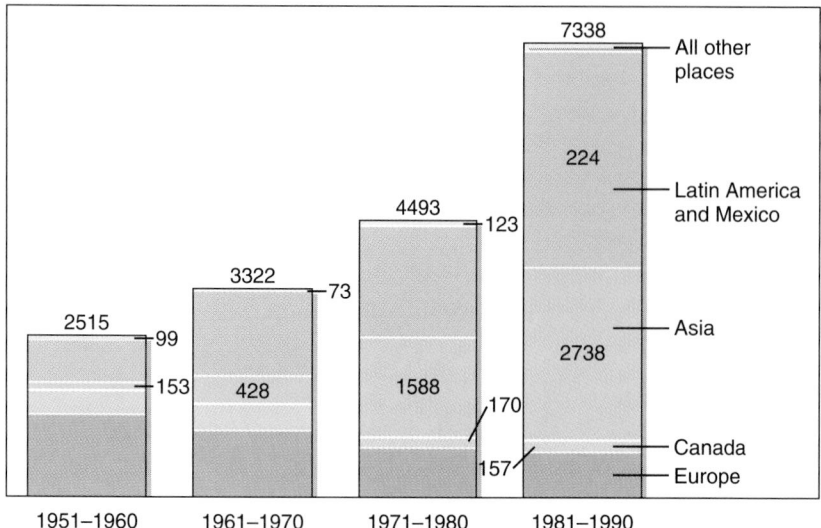

❧ **Figure 36–3**
Legal immigration in the United States by area of origin, 1951–1990 (in thousands). (From US Department of Commerce, Bureau of the Census. [1993]. *Hispanic Americans today [current population reports].* Washington, DC: Government Printing Office.)

Poverty in the United States

The terms "poverty population," "poor," and "below the poverty level" are used interchangeably. The definition of poverty was developed by the Social Security Administration in 1964. Two revisions of the definition occurred in 1969 and 1981. The threshold of poverty generally rises each year in relation to the annual consumer price index. A family of four is considered living in poverty with an annual income of $14,335 or less.

The Economics and Statistics Administration under the U.S. Department of Commerce analyzes and summarizes the income information received by the U.S. Bureau of the Census (1993). These Current Population Reports discuss the relationship between race and the culture of poverty (see Box 36–1).

The lifestyle, environment, and occupational factors associated with a life of poverty have been well established. Persons living in poverty generally share an environmental culture that includes tobacco addiction, alcohol/drug abuse, air/water pollution, and asbestos and lead exposure (Kerner, Dusenbury, & Mandelblatt, 1993). The poor are more likely to experience inadequate and poor variety in foodstuffs, inadequate sanitation, and lack of preventive medical services (Fig. 36–4). Medical services, such as prenatal care, childhood immunization, and chronic disease screening, would greatly improve their health status and reduce the characteristics of poverty.

Box **36–1**

UNITED STATES POVERTY STATISTICS

* 36.9 million persons lived in poverty in the USA in 1992

* The number of poor in 1992 was the highest since 1962

* The poverty rates for whites, blacks, Hispanics, and Asians have not significantly changed

* The region in America with the highest poverty rate is the South

* $5,751 is the amount of money it would take to raise the income of poor families above the poverty level

* About 28.5% of the poor reported the lack of medical insurance

* Hispanics were less likely to be insured than blacks or whites

---

U.S. Bureau of the Census (1993). *Poverty in the United States, 1992.* Current Population Reports, Series P60-185. Washington, DC: GPO.

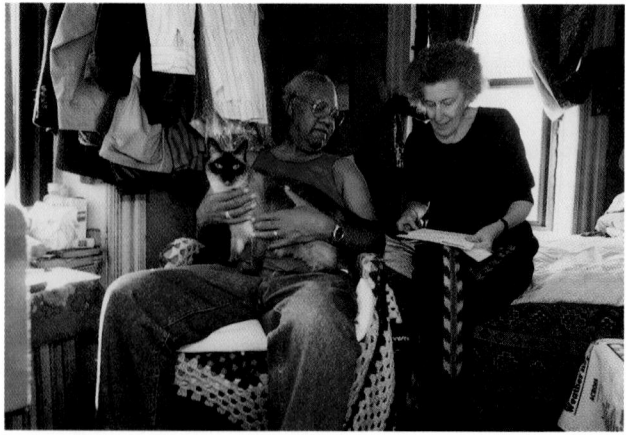

❧ **Figure 36–4**
The role of patient advocate is especially important with clients who live in impoverished conditions. Community hospital systems are trying to remove barriers to health care by developing neighborhood satellite and mobile clinics and emphasizing home health care.

Application of the Nursing Process

Cultural Assessment

As the first step that provides the foundation for professional nursing practice, assessments should be well planned, organized, professional, and display a high level of cultural sensitivity. The goals of a cultural assessment are to (1) understand the cultural context of the client and family, (2) develop and broker (*i.e.*, facilitate) culturally appropriate strategies for care, (3) encourage reciprocal learning between caregiver and client, and (4) clarify expectation of roles and outcomes. A competent cultural assessment identifies clients' strengths and weaknesses and subsystem resources. Assessment of known risk behaviors particular to ethnocultural groups should be included. An understanding of the worldview through proper analysis of demographics, vital statistics, and morbidity/mortality rates is essential.

Many assessment forms are published in the nursing literature that foster cultural sensitivity. Checklists that have closed-ended questions should be avoided. Basic interview skills can be modified to incorporate cultural competence and sensitivity (see Box 36–2). The Bloch Ethnic/Cultural Assessment Guide is a comprehensive approach to completing the assessment phase of the nursing process. Nurses should use the guide as a foundation for completing assessments with cultural sensitivity (see Box 36–3).

Working with the client, the nurse should always assess for the use of folk healers. Many cultures use folk or traditional healers to a varying degree. Clients continue to use folk healers even after admittance to health care systems. Folk healers are generally less expensive, more friendly, available to families, and seen as having ties to the spiritual world.

CASE STUDY — Hispanic Client Receiving Home Health Nursing

Mrs. Rojas is a 60-year-old Hispanic woman who has been living in the United States for the last 5 years. She has a history of colon cancer, hypertension, and cataracts. She has been admitted to the home health nursing agency with a primary diagnosis of anorexia and fecal impaction. Upon the initial assessment, the home health nurse finds that the client has been going to a *curandero* for the treatment of her *empacho*. Mrs. Rojas believes that the pain and cramps in her stomach are caused by balls of food clinging to the stomach wall. The treatment for the *empacho* consisted of massaging the stomach and pinching along the spine several times a day. The client has not taken the Dulcolax (laxative) and Colace (stool softener) that were prescribed by her primary physician. The nurse found a packet of herbs given to the client by her *curan-*

---

dero. The herbs are to be steeped in a tea for Mrs. Rojas to drink twice a day. During this home visit, Mrs. Rojas's abdomen is greatly distended with diminished bowel sounds; she is anorexic and still in great pain. The nurse is unable to determine what herbs are in the packet.

Possible Nursing Diagnoses

* Alteration in elimination related to client's folk beliefs and lack of compliance with prescribed medication
* Caregiver (nurse) knowledge deficit related to effects of herbal packet on normal gastrointestinal function

---

Families know that folk healers care and can be trusted. Folk healers also live and work in the communities of their culture, which gives them the same worldview as their clients. Folk healers use a form of folk medicine that is either natural or magicoreligious (occult). Natural folk medicine uses herbs, plants, minerals, and animal substances to treat and prevent illness (Table 36–1). Occult folk medicine uses charms, holy words, and actions to prevent and cure illness.

It would be impossible to list all the common home remedies according to ethnocultural group. The nurse should develop a broad understanding of the origin and use of common home remedies so that the right questions will be used during the assessment (Fig. 36–5).

Differences in Health Status

Minority groups have lagged behind in some health status indicators, such as infant and maternal mortality rates, death rates from chronic diseases, cancer 5-year survival rates, and presence of elevated high blood pressure (DHHS, 1990). The decision when, where, and how to seek health care is driven

Box 36–3

CULTURAL ASSESSMENT (BLOCH'S ETHNIC/CULTURAL ASSESSMENT GUIDE)

Cultural

Ethnic origin
* Does the client identify with a particular ethnic group (*e.g.,* Puerto Rican, African)?

Race
* What is the client's racial background (*e.g.,* black, Filipino, Native American)?

Place of birth
* Where was the client born?

Relocations
* Where has he or she lived (country, city)? During what years did the client live there and for how long? Has he or she moved recently?

Habits, customs, values, and beliefs
* Describe habits, customs, values, and beliefs the client holds or practices that affect his or her attitude toward birth, life, death, health and illness, time orientation, and health care system and health care providers. To what degree does the client believe in and adhere to his or her overall cultural system?

Behaviors valued by culture
* How does the client value privacy, courtesy, respect for elders, behaviors related to family roles and sex roles, and work ethics?

Cultural sanctions and restrictions
* *Sanctions*—What is accepted behavior by the client's cultural group regarding expression of emotions and feelings, religious expressions, and response to illness and death?
* *Restrictions*—Does the client have any restrictions related to sexual matters, exposure of body parts, certain types of surgery (*e.g.,* hysterectomy), discussion of dead relatives, and discussion of fears related to the unknown?

Language and communication processes
* What are some overall cultural characteristics of the client's language and communication process?

Language(s) and/or dialect(s) spoken
* Which language(s) and/or dialect(s) does the client speak most frequently. Where? At home or at work?

Language barriers
* Which language does the client predominantly use in thinking? Does he or she need a bilingual interpreter in nurse-client interactions? Is the client non–English-speaking or limited English-speaking? Is he or she able to read and/or write in English?

Communication process
* What are the rules (linguistics) and modes (style) of the communication process (*e.g.,* "honorific" concept of showing "respect or deference" to others using words common only to specific ethnic/cultural group)?

* Is there need for variation in technique of communicating and interviewing to accommodate the client's cultural background (*e.g.,* tempo of conversation, eye/body contact, topic restrictions, norms of confidentiality, and style of explanation)?
* Are there any conflicts in verbal and nonverbal interactions between client and nurse?
* How does the client's nonverbal communication process compare with other ethnic/cultural groups, and how does it affect the client's response to nursing and medical care?
* Are there any variations between the client's interethnic and interracial communication process or intracultural and intraracial communication process (*e.g.,* ethnic minority client and white middle-class nurse, ethnic minority client and ethnic minority nurse; beliefs, attitudes, values, role variations, stereotyping [perceptions and prejudice])?

Healing beliefs and practices
Cultural healing system
* What cultural healing system does the client predominantly adhere to (*e.g.,* Asian healing system, Raza/Latina Curanderismo)
* What religious healing system does the client predominantly adhere to (*e.g.,* Seventh Day Adventist, West African voodoo. Fundamentalist sect, Pentecostal)?

Cultural health beliefs
* Is illness explained by the germ theory or cause-effect relationship, presence of evil spirits, imbalance between "hot" and "cold" (yin and yang in Chinese culture), or disequilibrium between nature and human beings?
* Is good health related to success, ability to work or fulfill roles, reward from God, or balance with nature?

Cultural health practices
* What types of cultural healing practices does a person from the ethnic/cultural group adhere to? Does he or she use healing remedies to cure *natural* illnesses caused by the external environment (*e.g.,* massage to cure *empacho* (a ball of food clinging to stomach wall), wearing of talismans or charms for protection against illness)?

Cultural healers
* Does the client rely on cultural healers (*e.g.,* medicine men for Native American, Curandero for Raza/Latina, Chinese herbalist, hougan [voodoo priest], spiritualist, or minister for black)?

Nutritional variables or factors
* What nutritional variables or factors are influenced by the client's ethnic/cultural background?

Box 36–3

CULTURAL ASSESSMENT (BLOCH'S ETHNIC/CULTURAL ASSESSMENT GUIDE)
(Continued)

Characteristics of food preparation and consumption
* What types of food preferences and restrictions, meaning of foods, style of food preparation and consumption, frequency of eating, time of eating, and eating utensils are culturally determined for the client? Are there any religious influences on food preparation and consumption?

Influences from external environment
* What modifications, if any, did the ethnic group that the client identifies with have to make in its food practices in white-dominant US society? Are there any adaptations of food customs and beliefs from rural setting to urban setting?

Client education needs
* What are some implications of diet planning and teaching to a client who adheres to cultural practices concerning foods?

Sociological

Economic status
* Who is the principal wage earner in the client's family? What is the total annual income (approximately) of the family? What impact does economic status have on lifestyle, place of residence, living conditions, and ability to obtain health services?

Educational status
* What is the highest educational level obtained? Does the client's educational background influence his or her ability to understand how to seek health services, literature on health care, client teaching experiences, and any written material the client is exposed to in health care setting (*e.g.,* admission forms, client care forms, teaching literature, and lab test forms)?
* Does the client's educational background cause him or her to feel inferior or superior to health care personnel in the health care setting?

Social network
* What is the client's social network (kinship, peer, and cultural healing networks)? How do they influence health or illness status of the client?

Family as supportive group
* Does the client's family feel the need for continuous presence in the client's clinical setting (is this an ethnic/cultural characteristic)? How is family valued during illness or death?
* How does the family participate in the client's nursing care process (*e.g.,* giving baths, feeding, using touch as support [cultural meaning], supportive presence)?
* How does the ethnic/cultural family structure influence client response to health or illness (*e.g.,* roles, beliefs, strengths, weaknesses, and social class)?

* Are there any key family roles characteristic of a specific ethnic/cultural group (*e.g.,* grandmother in black and some Native American families), and can these key persons be a resource for health personnel?
* What role does family play in health promotion or cause of illness (*e.g.,* would the family be an intermediary group in client interactions with health personnel and making decisions regarding his or her care)?

Supportive institutions in ethnic/cultural community
* What influence do ethnic/cultural institutions have on the client's receiving health services (*e.g.,* institutions such as Organization of Migrant Workers, NAACP, Black Political Caucus, churches, schools, Urban League, community clinics)?

Institutional racism
* How does institutional racism in health facilities influence the client's response to receiving health care?

Psychological

Self-concept (identify)
* Does the client show strong racial/cultural identity? How does this compare with that of other racial/cultural groups or to members of dominant society?
* What factors in the client's development helped shape his or her self-concept (*e.g.,* family, peers, society labels, external environment, institutions, racism)?
* How does the client deal with stereotypical behavior from health professionals?
* What impact does racism have on a client from a distinct ethnic/cultural group (*e.g.,* social anxiety, noncompliance to health care process in clinical settings, avoidance of using or participating in health care institutions)?
* Does ethnic/cultural background have an impact on how the client relates to body image change resulting from illness or surgery (*e.g.,* importance of appearance and roles in cultural group)?
* Is there any adherence to or identification with ethnic/cultural "group" identity (*e.g.,* solidarity, "we" concept)?

Mental and behavioral processes and characteristics of ethnic/cultural group
* How does the client relate to his or her external environment in a clinical setting (*e.g.,* fears, stress, and adaptive mechanisms characteristic of a specific ethnic/cultural group)? Any variations based on the life span? What is the client's ability to relate to persons outside of his or her ethnic/cultural group (health personnel)? Is he or she withdrawn, verbally or nonverbally expressive, negative or positive, feeling mentally or physically inferior or superior?

Continued

Box 36–3

CULTURAL ASSESSMENT (BLOCH'S ETHNIC/CULTURAL ASSESSMENT GUIDE)
(Continued)

* How does the client deal with feelings of loss of dignity and respect in a clinical setting?

Religious influences on psychological effects of health/illness
* Does the client's religion have a strong impact on how he or she relates to health/illness influences or outcomes (*e.g., death/chronic illness, cause and effect of illness, or adherence to nursing/medical practices*)?
* Do religious beliefs, sacred practices, and talismans play a role in treatment of disease?
* What is the role of significant religious persons during health/illness (*e.g., ministers, Catholic priests, Buddhist monks, Islamic imams*)?

Psychological/cultural response to stress and discomfort of illness
* Based on ethnic/cultural background, does the client exhibit any variations in psychological response to pain or physical disability of disease processes?

Biological/Physiological

(Consideration of *norms* for different ethnic/cultural groups)
Racial-anatomical characteristics
* Does the client have any distinct racial characteristics (*e.g., skin color, hair texture and color, color of mucous membranes*)?
* Does the client have any variations in anatomical characteristics (*e.g., body structure [height and weight] more prevalent for ethnic/cultural group, skeletal formation [pelvic shape, especially for obstetrical evaluation], facial shape and structure [nose, eye shape, facial contour], upper and lower extremities*)?
* How do the client's racial and anatomical characteristics affect his or her self-concept and the way others relate to him or her?
* Does variation in racial-anatomical characteristics affect physical evaluations and physical care, skin assessment based on color, and variations in hair care and hygienic practices?

Growth and development patterns
* Are there any distinct growth and development characteristics that vary with the client's ethnic/cultural background (*e.g., bone, density, fat folds, motor ability*)?
* What factors are important for nutritional assessment, neurological and motor assessment, assessment of bone deterioration in disease process or injury, evaluation of newborns, evaluation of intellectual status, or capacity in relationship to motor/sensory development in children?
* How do these differ in ethnic/cultural groups?

Variations in body systems
* Are there any variations in body systems for a client from a distinct ethnic/cultural group (*e.g., gastrointestinal disturbance with lactose intolerance in blacks, nutritional intake of cultural foods causing adverse effects on gastrointestinal tract and fluid and electrolyte system, and variations in chemical and hematological systems [certain blood types prevalent in particular ethnic/cultural groups]*)?

Skin and hair physiology, mucous membranes
* How does skin color variation influence assessment of skin color changes (*e.g., jaundice, cyanosis, ecchymosis, erythema, and its relationship to disease processes*)?
* What are methods of assessing skin color changes (comparing variations and similarities between different ethnic groups)?
* Are there conditions of hypopigmentation and hyperpigmentation (*e.g., vitiligo, mongolian spots, albinism, discoloration caused by trauma*)? Why would these be more striking in some ethnic groups?
* Are there any skin conditions more prevalent in a distinct ethnic group (*e.g., keloids in blacks*)?
* Is there any correlation between oral and skin pigmentation and their variations among distinct racial groups when assessing the oral cavity (*e.g., leukoedema is normal occurrence in blacks*)?
* What are variations in hair texture and color among racially different groups? Ask the client about preferred hair care methods or any racial/cultural restrictions (*e.g., not washing "hot-combed" hair while in a clinical setting, not cutting very long hair of Raza/Latinas*).
* Are there any variations in skin care methods (*e.g., using Vaseline on black skin*)?

Diseases more prevalent among ethnic/cultural groups
* Are there any specific diseases or conditions that are more prevalent for a specific ethnic/cultural group (*e.g., hypertension, sickle cell anemia, G6-PD, lactose intolerance*)?
* Does the client have any socioenvironmental diseases common among ethnic/cultural groups (*e.g., lead paint poisoning, poor nutrition, overcrowding [prone to tuberculosis], alcoholism resulting from psychological despair and alienation from dominant society, rat bites, poor sanitation*)?

Diseases ethnic/cultural group has increased resistance to
* Are there any diseases that the client has increased resistance to because of racial/cultural background (*e.g., skin cancer in blacks*)?

© Bobbie Bloch. Used with permission.

Table 36-1

COMMON HOME REMEDIES AND HERBAL TREATMENTS

REMEDY/HERB	COMMON USAGE
Swamp root	Diuretic
Turpentine	To clean puncture wounds
Syrup of black draught	For constipation
Liniment	For arthritis, minor sprains, cough
Mustard plaster	For severe chest colds
Fennel seeds	To increase milk in nursing mothers
Licorice (powdered root)	For coughs
Garlic, onions	To prevent illness (eaten raw)
Ginseng root	To stimulate digestion, for sedation, to help frail babies

by one's cultural beliefs and practices. Also important is the level of assimilation into the larger society. Minority males have the shortest life expectancy in the United States. Death rates for minority babies during the first year of life are nearly double that for white babies. Heart disease is still responsible for a significant portion of the death rate in black males. (The classification of black is used according to the racial breakdown developed by the Bureau of the Census. This category includes African-Americans and others who identify their race as black, non-white, non-Asian, and so forth.)

Black Americans have higher incidences of oral, esophageal, pancreatic, and female breast cancers (Ries, Hanley, & Edwards, 1990) (Table 36–2). Liver cancer and hepatitis B are more common in people

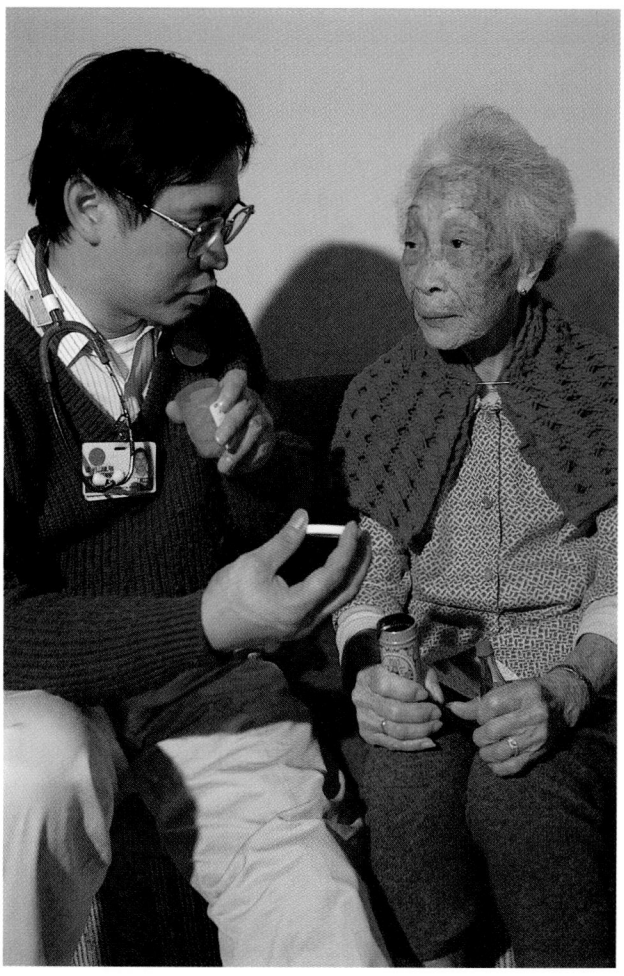

❧ **Figure 36–5**
Showing respect for a client's culturally based health beliefs will foster the client's trust and better enable the nurse to communicate and advise the client and family. Folk remedies and herbal cures can often be incorporated into a plan of care.

Table 36-2

SUSCEPTIBILITY TO DISEASES ACCORDING TO REGION OR GROUP AND RISK FACTORS

DISEASE	REGION OR GROUP	RISK FACTORS
Cancer		
Stomach	China, eastern Asia, South America	Use of nitrates
Colon/rectum	South America	Diet high in protein and animal fat
Liver	China	Infection with hepatitis B and C virus
Pancreas	China	Alcohol ingestion
Larynx	Northern Africa	Alcohol ingestion
	Latin America	Betel-quid chewing
Tuberculosis	Native American, black	Socioeconomic status
Hypertension	black	Socioeconomic status
Sickle cell anemia	black	Genetic disorder

from Southeast Asia. Nasopharyngeal cancers are found in approximately 40% of the southern Chinese population. Reports of high numbers of Epstein-Barr viral infections are found in Asia and Africa, owing to dietary habits such as the consumption of fermented, pickled, or preserved foods and a genetic predisposition. In developing countries, oral cancer rates continue to rise, owing to tobacco chewing practices (Boffetta & Parkin, 1994).

In Asia, the prevalence of risk factors such as tobacco and alcohol ingestion, micronutrient deficiencies, thermal injuries, and mycotoxin is important to understand. Many of these risk factors may be prevalent in new immigrants arriving in the United States. The tools for cancer prevention—early detection, screening, and prevention—must be used consistently in professional nursing. Scientific evidence defines the role of personal beliefs and negative health practices in cancer development. An analysis of the international incidence and epidemiology of diseases helps nurses understand the cultural implications. Specific information regarding cancer rates according to racial/ethnic grouping can be found in the American Cancer Society's subcommittee report titled the *National Advisory Committee on Cancer in the Socioeconomically Disadvantaged (SED)*. The variance between socioeconomic status, race/ethnicity, and cancer has clearly documented significant differences. Significant differences in the rates of bladder, prostate, and uterine cancer and multiple myeloma exist and are often closely related to occupational hazards. The association between occupational hazards such as toxic chemicals, fumes, and radiation and higher risk for certain cancers has been well documented. Occupations with these hazards are more likely to be manual labor, blue-collar jobs associated with lower socioeconomic groups.

The risk for exposure to HIV and the rate of AIDS cases are higher in minority groups. This is directly related to environmental and socioeconomic factors. Also, different beliefs about the origin and proper treatment of the disease have contributed to the increase in morbidity. Persons from disadvantaged groups are more likely to have higher cholesterol levels, have poorer perceptions of their individual health status, and miss more days from work because of illness or disability. Although blacks spent more days in the hospital, this group is less likely to visit a dentist or a physician's office regularly (DHHS, 1990). This lack of regular primary health care affects the system's ability to keep costs down.

The health status of the many ethnocultural groups in the United States varies. The Health Resources and Services Administration (HRSA) is mandated by law to identify health resources (Box 36–4) and service problems to ensure reasonable cost of and access to health care for all U.S. citizens. As part of the HRSA, the Division of Disadvantaged Assistance collects and analyzes specific data from groups who are disadvantaged by race, ethnicity, socioeconomic status, and gender.

Cultural Practices That Increase the Risk of Disease and Disability

As individuals, we learn how to prevent disease, reduce the risk of illness, and promote health within our cultural values, beliefs, and mores. Methods used to treat illnesses often have religious origins. The culturally competent nurse needs to be educated in all the possible alternative medicines, practices, beliefs, and health care providers (healers) within each ethnocultural group. Although it is impossible to identify all such information in this textbook, some examples are presented in the tables and boxes in this chapter. This broad discussion does not implying that a specific culture always shows a particular risk or practice. Stereotyping should always be avoided.

An efficient method that the nurse might use to identify specific behaviors that place a client's health at risk is risk assessment. Risk assessment is the process of identifying health behaviors or practices that place a person at a higher risk than normal for a specific disease or condition. The process of risk assessment also decides the level of health-promoting behavior. Certain ethnocultural groups, owing to their belief concerning the afterlife, fate, or the individual's power over health, are reluctant to practice health promotion. Accurate information used to guide a risk assessment comes from safety and nutrition experts, cancer specialists, and epidemiologists. Although it is impossible to identify one's risk for a specific disease or condition conclusively, the literature identifies behaviors or health practices associated with members of specific ethnocultural groups.

CASE STUDY — Health Promotion in an Indian Christian Family

Piara and Elizabeth, in their middle 30s, have lived in the United States for 5 years. They send monthly checks to their families in India. They use an ancient system of Ayurveda medicine for their health care. Referring to specific illnesses as spirits, they rarely use pain medicine. The wife, responsible for all household chores and child rearing, is stressed with caring for her two young children and the household. As a middle-class family in India, they would have servants to help her. Elizabeth uses little prepackaged or frozen food. Rice is eaten at almost every meal. The children are fed on a want basis; no time schedule is ever used. The family attends church two to three times a week beyond the normal Sunday services. Elizabeth complains of very long days and fatigue since moving to the United States. She becomes weepy when talking about her homeland and the family she left in India. She is unable to give any examples of specific time set aside for her rest and relaxation. The family attends many social events, and there is always the expectation that Elizabeth will assist and prepare many freshly cooked dishes. Elizabeth's sister-in-law speaks her dialect and lives several miles away. She does not drive a car at the present time.

Box **36–4**

RESOURCES RELATED TO CULTURE AND ETHNICITY

Transcultural Nursing Society
Madonna University
College of Nursing and Health
36600 Schoolcraft Road
Livonia, MI 48150-1173
(313) 591-8358

Council on Nursing & Anthropology
Nursing & Health Services
Salisbury State University
Salisbury, MD 21801

Office of Bilingual Education and Minority Language Affairs
Switzer Building, Room 5086
330 C Street, SW
Washington, DC 20202-6641

Office of Minority Health Resource Center
US Department of Health and Human Services
P.O. Box 37337
Washington, DC 20013-7337
1-800-444-6472

Multicultural Training Resource Center
1540 Market Street, Suite 320
San Francisco, CA 94102
(415) 861-2142

National Coalition of Hispanic Mental Health and Health
   Service Organizations (COSSMHO)
1501 16th Street, NW
Washington, DC 20036
(202) 387-5000

American Folklife Center
The Library of Congress
101 Independence Avenue, SE
Washington, DC 20540-4610
(202) 707-6590

Asian Health Service, Inc
310 9th Street, Suite 200
Oakland, CA 94607

Asian American Health Forum
116 New Montgomery, Suite 531
Sand Francisco, CA 94105
(415) 541-0866

Office of Minority Affairs
US Department of Health and Human Services
Public Health Service
Room 118-F, HHH Building
200 Independence Avenue, SW
Washington, DC 20201

American Indian Health Care Association
(612) 293-0233

Office of Migrant Education
US Department of Education
(202) 401-0740

Office of Migrant Health
US Department of Health and Human Services
(301) 443-1153

Migrant Legal Action Program
(202) 462-7744

Possible Nursing Diagnoses

- Altered health maintenance related to lack of physical activity and stress
- Fatigue related to social isolation and homesickness

It may be awkward for nurses to discuss some beliefs or behaviors. The nurse must make every effort to understand the cultural derivation of the practice or belief. Clients might not share this information during an initial assessment. Information such as that provided in Box 36–3 gives the nurse some idea of practices and beliefs to include in all assessments. For example, it is widely accepted in US culture that individuals may reduce their risk of developing certain cancers by improving their nutrition, taking advantage of early screening services, and reducing certain behaviors. This ready acceptance of health promotion behaviors may not occur in cultures that believe in fate and are oriented to the present.

❧ **Nutrition/Diet–Associated Risks.** Nutrition is a strong component of one's culture. Mealtimes, food preparation and storage methods, use of spices, and level of socialization at meals are all culturally derived. Who is the main meal provider? How is the meal served? Who gets to eat first and last? Are utensils used? Food is often used in social and religious rituals. Certain foodstuffs may be avoided or denied when one is ill, pregnant, recovering from childbirth, or menstruating. Large quantities of spices may be used, especially salt. Some nutritional practices cause an increased risk for nutrient or vitamin deficiencies, obesity, high cholesterol levels, and high rates of cardiac and hypertensive diseases and cancers. Different ethnocultural groups may use a method of classifying foods according to a hot/cold "humors" system. This system is meant to either protect the individual from sickness or treat individual symptoms such as fever, muscle spasm, and headaches. This method of food classification is similar to the belief that food has either a hot or a cold property. Having nothing to do with actual physical temperature, this property is related to the effects that food is believed to have on the body once it has been ingested.

Any group that ingests uncooked seafood is at great risk because of the common presence of *Clonorchis* and *Opisthorcis* parasites in the foodstuffs. Asians, such as Koreans, Japanese, Filipinos, and Chinese, depending on the generation, may eat uncooked seafood as a staple in their diet.

The Chinese are well known for their use of health foods and herb tonics to cure and prevent illness (Boyle & Andrews, 1989). This yin-yang theory signifies a balance of harmony with the universe. Yang represents male, hot, and light; yin signifies female, cold, and darkness. The nurse needs to identify clients who follow this method of classification. It is important to offer foods classified as yang when a client is suffering from a yin condition, and vice versa. Balance between yin and yang is necessary for good health.

Assessment of the method of food preparation also contributes to the early identification of health risks. The use of saturated fats, such as the ghee used by Indian and Pakistani cultures, has had a negative impact on the health and life expectancy of those populations (Haq, 1994). Ingestion of large amounts of smoked, pickled, uncooked meats is harmful yet widely practiced in other cultures. Recent reports from the Food and Drug Administration documented that the foods highest in fat content may be found in cultures that use large amounts of animal-based cooking oils. Frying is often the preferred method of meat cooking. Salted fat is sometimes added to cooking. Southern African-Americans use salted fat in the cooking of their vegetables such as beet greens, collards, kale, spinach, and turnip greens.

❥ Women's Right to Self-Determination. The nurse should never assume that there is equality among the sexes in all cultures. Some US social problems, such as spouse and child abuse, violations of personal rights, wage discrimination, and blocked job access, are also found in other cultures. Some Asians, Africans, and Native Americans arrange marriages for their children. Women from the Indo-Pakistani subcontinent experience tremendous pressure to produce male children. This pressure often leads to continuous pregnancies. Some Hispanic families encourage the educational development of male children but restrict female children to child rearing and household responsibilities. Violation of women's rights can be especially cruel when the woman has recently immigrated to a new country. Frequently, the woman lacks the language, driving, and social skills to obtain help for herself or her children if she has been a victim of abuse.

Assessment of the practice of female circumcision (infibulation) must be included in all health histories. It has been estimated that there are approximately 100 million women in the world who have undergone this form of genital mutilation. Although this practice is found in North America, middle Europe, Australia, and

26 African nations, it is rarely seen in Asia. Infibulation has been practiced for many centuries with social and religious undertones. Women who are circumcised suffer severe and lifelong physical, emotional, and psychological complications (Toubia, 1994) (Box 36–5). Nurses must understand the cultural importance of infibulation. Some societies rationalize the practice as an effective control of women's sexual desire, promoting fidelity. Using gentle and nonjudgmental communication styles, nurses must screen for this practice and its potential complications. Nurses should not assume that immigrant families stop this practice once they are in the United States. Although it is illegal and classified as child abuse, the practice continues. Nurses must never participate in reinfibulation practices once a woman has delivered a child in the United States.

Nursing Diagnosis and Analysis

Careful validation of assessment information contributes to the identification of a client's health or illness state. Several resources may be used at this stage. Family members, religious leaders, lay health care providers, and cultural consultants can often clarify information, leading to more accurate diagnoses and related factors.

Some nursing diagnoses used today are biased toward one culture—the culture of nursing (Eliason, 1993). As late as 1989, the North American Nursing Diagnosis Association's (NANDA) list of nursing diagnoses contained few defining characteristics or factors (Geissler, 1992). Analysis of the 1992 NANDA list still shows a lack of ethnoculturally derived nursing diagnoses. Examples of culturally derived nursing diagnoses developed in Geissler's (1992) study are *Impaired verbal communication related to cultural differences, Impaired social interaction related to sociocultural dis-*

> *Box* **36–5**
>
> ### HEALTH PROBLEMS OF CIRCUMCISED WOMEN
>
> Initial mutilation
> * Hemorrhage, severe pain, shock, death
> * Local infection, ulcers, delayed healing, tetanus, gangrene
>
> Chronic complications
> * Interference with urine and menstrual blood flow
> * Chronic pelvic conditions
> * Chronic back pain
> * Urinary tract infections and dermal cysts
> * Common syndrome of chronic anxiety and depression
>
> ---
> Data from Toubia, N. (1994). Female circumcision as a public health issue. *New England Journal of Medicine, 331*(11), 712–716.

sonance, and *Noncompliance related to patient value system.* These diagnoses require further testing and evaluation by NANDA. Geissler (1992) concluded that the use of formalized nursing diagnoses may lead to a lack of acknowledgment of other culturally relevant viewpoints, may be too generalized, and may mislabel culturally affected phenomena. The nurse should be careful to describe clearly the culturally relevant etiologies and related characteristics when using the NANDA list (see the accompanying box).

Planning

At this stage of the nursing process, the nurse must pay close attention to barriers of access of health care. Also critical is the need for an understanding of the unique culture that is found within health care institutions. Hospital routines may seem foreign and even bizarre to people of various cultures. Free, open visits by multiple family members may be normal in other countries. Nurses should be aware of sources of prejudice and discrimination in their work sites (Eliason, 1993). Guidelines for helping the nurse in planning care for culturally diverse clients are found in Box 36–6.

Along with traditional planning skills, the nurse needs to be aware of social and cultural barriers to reaching U.S. health care (see the accompanying case study). The nurse needs to negotiate a plan of care — bringing in all decision makers and persons with au-

thority in the culture. Attempts to reduce sociocultural barriers and to increase access and use must incorporate health beliefs and practices. Predominant barriers to health care found among all groups in the United States is the inability to pay, lack of transportation and child care, lack of understanding of treatment plans, inability to incorporate prescribed health plans into daily living practices, and cultural beliefs and practices (Russell & Jewell, 1992). Community hospital systems are trying to remove some of these barriers with the development of neighborhood satellite and mobile clinics. Health care availability, affective reactions, and sociodemographic factors have been established as significant barriers in the Hispanic population (Marks *et al.,* 1987). Individual, group, or community program planning must proactively remove potential and existing barriers. Use of cultural resources within the community is most effective. Nurses must never underestimate the need for free and open religious expression when illness is present. This need is more crucial when a client is dying or a death has occurred. An understanding of these beliefs and behaviors must be evident in the planning stage (see Box 36–7).

NURSING DIAGNOSES WITH POTENTIAL CULTURALLY RELATED FACTORS

Ineffective individual coping related to health care system's prevention of family visits and caregiving

Fear related to misunderstanding health care provider's use of touch and space

Risk for infection related to use of folk medicines in place of pharmaceuticals

Knowledge deficit related to beliefs regarding efficacy of health promotion behaviors

Noncompliance related to personal values or predominant culture's use of scientific methods

Altered nutrition related to beliefs concerning hot and cold properties of certain foods

Pain related to prevention of a person's demonstration of pain by health care providers

Relocation stress syndrome related to loss of family home and country of origin

Social isolation related to inability to communicate in common language

Spiritual distress related to prevention of practice of religious rituals in hospitals

---

CASE STUDY ### Advocacy for Culturally Diverse Client

Mumtaz Sharif, a 67-year-old Pakistani woman, comes to the emergency room (ER) with complaints of shortness of breath and chest pain. This is her first trip to the United States, where she has been visiting her son and his American-born wife. Mrs. Sharif speaks no English but appears to have a limited understanding of the language. A disruption occurs in the ER because she refuses to let the technician take an ECG and portable chest x-ray. Mrs. Sharif does not want to remove several layers of undergarments and two amulets that are around her neck. The son refuses to help, stating that his mother would never remove her clothing in front of one of her sons. The American-born wife is brought in to assist the client.

Nursing Diagnosis

Noncompliance with diagnostic treatment related to personnel's failure to meet modesty needs and lack of understanding

Expected Outcomes

• Client's modesty needs will be maintained.

• Client's use of religious amulets will be maintained.

• Client will understand the need for diagnostic tests.

Interventions

• Determine what layers of undergarments must stay on for client comfort.

• Establish the makeup of the religious amulets.

• Have the daughter-in-law help with removing clothes and applying electrodes.

• Have the client hold the amulets.

Box 36–6

GUIDELINES FOR RELATING TO CLIENTS FROM DIFFERENT CULTURES

1. Assess your personal beliefs surrounding persons from different cultures.
   * review your personal beliefs and past experiences
   * set aside any values, biases, ideas, and attitudes that are judgmental and may negatively affect care

2. Assess communication variables from a cultural perspective.
   * determine the ethnic identity of the patient, including generation in America
   * use the client as a source of information when possible
   * assess cultural factors that may affect your relationship with the client and respond appropriately

3. Plan care based on the communicated needs and cultural background.
   * learn as much as possible about the client's cultural customs and beliefs
   * encourage the client to reveal cultural interpretation of health, illness, and health care
   * be sensitive to the uniqueness of the client
   * identify sources of discrepancy between the client's and your own concepts of health and illness
   * communicate at the client's personal level of functioning
   * evaluate effectiveness of nursing actions and modify nursing care plan when necessary

4. Modify communication approaches to meet cultural needs.
   * be attentive to signs of fear, anxiety, and confusion in the client
   * respond in a reassuring manner in keeping with the client's cultural orientation
   * be aware that in some cultural groups, discussions with others concerning the client may be offensive and may impede the nursing process

5. Understand that respect for the client and communicated needs is central to the therapeutic relationship.
   * communicate respect by using a kind and attentive approach
   * learn how listening is communicated in the client's culture
   * use appropriate active listening techniques
   * adopt an attitude of flexibility, respect, and interest to help bridge barriers imposed by culture

6. Communicate in a nonthreatening manner.
   * conduct the interview in an unhurried manner
   * follow acceptable social and cultural amenities
   * ask general questions during the information-gathering stage
   * be patient with a respondent who gives information that may seem unrelated to the health problem
   * develop a trusting relationship by listening carefully, allowing time, and giving the client your full attention

7. Use validating techniques in communication.
   * be alert for feedback that the client is not understanding
   * do not assume that meaning is interpreted without distortion

8. Be considerate of reluctance to talk when the subject involves sexual matters.
   * be aware that in some cultures sexual matters are not discussed freely with members of the opposite sex

9. Adopt special approaches when the client speaks a different language.
   * use a caring tone of voice and facial expression to help alleviate the client's fears
   * speak slowly and distinctly, but not loudly
   * use gestures, pictures, and play acting to help the client understand
   * repeat the message in different ways if necessary
   * be alert to words that the client seems to understand and use them frequently
   * keep messages simple and repeat them frequently
   * avoid using medical terms and abbreviations that the client may not understand
   * use an appropriate language dictionary

10. Use interpreters to improve communication.
   * ask the interpreter to translate the message, not just the individual words
   * obtain feedback to confirm understanding
   * use an interpreter who is culturally sensitive

From Giger, J. N., & Davidhizar, R. E. (1995). *Transcultural nursing* (2nd ed.). St. Louis: Mosby. Used with permission.

Introduction of treatment plans when compromises are brokered take patience and diligence to overcome cultural conditioning (Kuhni, 1990). Other avenues for reducing barriers include involving the community, increasing the efficiency of service organizations, modifying services to allow for privacy and modesty needs, recruiting cultural representatives for health care training, developing coalitions with religious organizations, and using ethnocultural communication networks effectively. The nurse should strive to

Box **36–7**

SELECTED CULTURAL BELIEFS AND BEHAVIORS REGARDING DEATH AND DYING

General
- Death is a normal part of life (Native American, Asian)
- Death is passage from one realm of life to a better one (black)
- Death is passage into the next life (Asian)
- No belief in afterlife (Native American)

Violent death
- Violent death provokes stronger emotional outbursts than does a normal death (black)
- Violent death is punishment for misdeeds (Lao)
- Violent death creates a ghost to wander forever (Navajo, Cheyenne)

Suicide
- Suicide should be concealed because of shameful nature (Latino, Filipino)
- Suicide may be used to save family honor (other Asian)

Place of death
- Hospitalization means death is imminent (black, Asian, Native American)
- Death should occur at home (Hmong, Vietnamese)

Preparation and disposal of body
- Touching a dead body may bring misfortune (Navajo, Tlingit)
- Passing a child over a dead body may cure illness (black)
- Entire body must be disposed of together; autopsy may be resisted (Native American)
- Bodies should be cremated (Tlingit, Quechan)
- Bodies should be buried (Pueblo tribes)
- Bodies should be exposed to air on funeral platform (Sioux)
- The dying person should be dressed in funeral clothes before death (Tlingit)
- Family members should prepare the body for burial (Sioux)

- Bodies are prepared for burial by commercial mortuary (Latino)
- Bodies should be richly dressed and wrapped in new blankets (Navajo)
- Clothing of a dead person may contain evil spirits (Chinese)

Grief and mourning
- Emotional grieving lasts for 4 days, after which the name of the dead is never spoken (Cheyenne, Quechan, Navajo)
- White should be worn during the mourning period (Hmong)
- Black should be worn during the mourning period (Latino)
- Social activities should be restricted during the mourning period (Latino)
- The dead should be included in rituals commemorating ancestors (Vietnamese)
- The funeral and wake are a time to rejoice for the dead and comfort the living (black)
- Funeral mass is preceded by saying the rosary (Latino)
- The first Monday after death begins 9 days of evening prayer for the dead (Latino)

Participation and knowledge
- Dying clients should be protected from knowledge of impending death (Latino)
- Children should participate in the care of dying family members, funerals, and mourning (Native American, Latino)
- The eldest son should be present at the death of a parent (Chinese)
- Family members must be present for the spirit to leave the body (Native American)

From Clark, M. J. (1992). *Nursing in the community.* Norwalk, CT: Appleton & Lange. Used with permission.

---

include members of the cultural network (religious leaders, folk healers, and godparents) in planning for the treatment of illnesses. Specific goals of the planning phase are to remove barriers to health care, increase client knowledge; foster client satisfaction; show meaningful, culturally competent care; and reduce health risks.

Intervention

Many nursing interventions for culturally diverse populations are based on key principles of effective interpersonal communication, treating all clients with dignity and respect, and avoiding moral judgments. During all communication, it is crucial to establish who is the person responsible for decisions in the family. This person may be the client, spouse, family elder, or religious leader. The nurse must help the client distribute all pertinent health information to the family and persons helping with care decisions. It is important to stress and educate some cultures about the scope and importance of the nursing role. A professional demeanor must be maintained; avoid jokes and slang language. Keep all health education in simple terms, avoid jargon, and emphasize the effects of the condition and/or treatment.

Showing dignity and respect to all clients is a cornerstone of nursing practice. The nurse must avoid the tendency to overlook modesty needs. In some cultures, it may be unacceptable for a female nurse to bathe a man's genital areas. Male nursing students

COMMUNITY BASED CARE

CULTURAL DIVERSITY

Each of us has mental images about the world and the people who live in it. Our mental images influence how we think and what we do. Most of the time we are not aware of these images. We just assume that *our* world is the *real* world and that everyone holds similar views. These images limit our ability to see the many dimensions of the people who are from cultures different than ours. They also affect the development of our attitudes toward people of different cultures.

Long-standing values, attitudes, and/or lack of exposure to different cultures can have a negative impact on the quality of care we deliver. All ethnic groups or cultures may have specific needs that potentially require specific interventions. Increased awareness of cultural differences will improve the care that we provide. Consider food. Clients may be fed in the hospital and discharged on a specific dietary regimen. Once at home, dietary teaching becomes an important intervention. However, for teaching to be successful, the home care nurse or other professional must assess and incorporate the types of foods and spices normally used by the client in the teaching plan.

To be effective in the care you deliver, remember to

1. Examine your mental images
2. Seek feedback from others about your perceptions
3. Respect differences that are important to others
4. Integrate these actions into client care
5. Accept people as they are
6. Learn about the different cultures you encounter
7. Set aside cultural biases and avoid stereotypes

CASE STUDY   **Korean Client Receiving Home Health Nursing**

Mr. Lee is a 79-year-old Korean man diagnosed for many years with coronary artery disease, peripheral vascular disease, and insulin-dependent diabetes. He is admitted to home health care with a primary diagnosis of two stage III pressure sores on his toes; one toe is necrotic and has serosanguineous drainage. Mr. Lee and his 65-year-old wife live on the third floor above their small food market. Mrs. Lee is currently managing the food market. She has refused a referral for a home health aide. Mrs. Lee does all the daily household chores, along with bathing, feeding, and giving medication to her husband. Mr. Lee ambulates with a walker to the bathroom but otherwise stays in bed all day. Mrs. Lee answers all questions and serves as interpreter. Mr. Lee refuses to participate in his care. He reads a book while the nurse changes the dressings and teaches his wife how to care for him. Recently, the nurse found out that the family has been paying for all of Mr. Lee's 14 prescriptions from their savings account. One prescription is for Epogen, which costs $80 a vial. Mr. Lee uses one vial three times a week. Also, the nurse notes that Mrs. Lee clutches her chest as if in pain after walking down the stairs to open the front door. She is found to have signs of early congestive heart failure and exhaustion.

Possible Nursing Diagnoses

• Caregiver role strain related to expectations in Korean culture
• Knowledge deficit related to sources of state and federal health programs

---

may find that they are unable to care for pregnant clients because of their gender and lack of acceptance in their professional role. Folk medicines and traditional religious practices should be accepted as a natural part of the client's treatment, as long as they are not harmful or counterproductive. The family will see this as a sign of acceptance from the nurse. Clients and families should be familiarized with the hospital routine, rooms, and personnel. Nurses need to recognize spatial differences, as some clients will insist on keeping doors closed and curtains drawn. Individuals from other cultures may not readily accept the nursing assistant giving a bed bath to their loved one. Family members should be allowed to provide hygienic care if it is expected in their culture. The nurse may need to educate the family caregiver on skin care and signs and symptoms to observe for when completing hygienic care such as bathing and foot or mouth care.

The role of client advocate is important in professional nursing practice. The methods that the nurse uses in this role will shape the client-nurse relationship (Jezewski, 1993). The ideal client advocate is a nurse who is nonjudgmental and able to empower clients to exercise their individual rights to self-determination. For example, a Native American client may eat varying numbers of meals during the week. One day the person may have two meals, another day four meals, and none on one day of the week. This may be related to his or her understanding of harmony with the environment and to spiritual needs. The nurse needs to understand this practice, especially when educating a client who needs to take a certain medication at mealtimes. The nurse must try to explain the legal issues while helping the family partake in rituals that they require for religious or traditional reasons. Nurses are often challenged to help clients with religious rituals and prayers that may interfere with normal hospital routine. Clients have been known to lose prayer books and religious medals in linen hampers. Mealtimes can be disrupted if a Jewish client who keeps Kosher receives a meal tray containing both dairy and meat products. The dairy-meat combination is not acceptable, and a new meal tray will have to be obtained from the kitchen.

The need for advocacy is the strongest when one is faced with an individual, group, or community with limited economic, social, or political power. Transcultural conflicts should be removed at all levels of the health care system. An early intervention in every health care plan should be activity that fosters recognition and understanding of a client's cultural beliefs, values, and practices. The nurse initiates advocacy through the intervention of culture brokering (see the case study on page 1099). Defined by Jezewski (1993), culture brokering is the act of bridging, linking, or mediating between groups and individuals with different ethnocultural backgrounds. The purpose of the brokering is to remove conflicts, producing change and promoting acceptance. Bridging the cultural gap calls for mutual respect (West, 1993). The professional nurse needs excellent assessment, communication, political awareness, and activism skills, along with the ability to identify power sources. Courage and diligence are also needed if one is to be an effective cultural broker in health care.

Evaluations of Culturally Meaningful Outcomes

Nurses in acute care settings often have difficulty evaluating culturally meaningful outcomes (Box 36–8). Clients often find it difficult to modify or change behavior in stressful new environments such as acute care settings. One's culture and learned behavior provide a sense of normalcy and comfort in settings that are new, confusing, and stressful. Often, it is difficult to evaluate care outcomes within the present health care system. Clients are often admitted the day of surgery or procedures. Tremendous pressure is placed on all health care providers for early discharge and reduction of health care costs. The need for health care reform is driven by escalating costs and inefficiency within the system as a whole. The client population that suffers the most during this reform process may be the different ethnocultural groups. The effectiveness of cultural competency is built on the need for adequate time and resources to implement all stages of the nursing process. Exploration and definitive research of culture diversity concepts are ongoing. Jezewski (1993) suggested that research projects concerning culturally derived intervening conditions and refinement of the cultural brokering model are needed. Rooda (1993) stressed the need to continue the study of nursing attitudes toward and knowledge about clients of difference cultures. Removing barriers and improving access across cultural boundaries remain essential. In performing nursing studies, researchers must be more diligent about obtaining samples that mirror the larger society.

Box 36–8

EVALUATION OF CULTURAL COMPETENCE

During the evaluation phase of the nursing process, ask yourself the following questions:

1. Did I avoid any signs of cultural bias, ethnocentricity, and stereotyping in my behaviors and communication?

2. Did I demonstrate cultural sensitivity and competence in my assessment?

3. Was my communication style altered to coexist with the style used with this cultural group?

4. If I used an interpreter, did the interpreter help facilitate the communication and avoid interjecting his or her presumptions or biases?

5. Did I tailor my physical examination to screen for diseases and conditions that I know may be found in the group?

6. Did I spend enough time identifying cultural practices that may have increased the person's risk of disease and disability?

7. Did I take into account possible effects of recent immigration or migration?

8. In my diagnoses, did I clearly identify the related cultural factors?

9. Were the goals negotiated with the client and meaningful within the cultural context?

10. Was the planning done with the client using my culture brokering skills?

11. If the expected outcomes were not evident, was the nursing care plan modified?

12. If necessary, was the alternative health provider included in the care planning and implementation?

13. At the completion of the care, did the client experience safe, holistic nursing care that demonstrated cultural sensitivity and competence?

Summary

This chapter educates the professional nurse in the many concepts surrounding cultural competency. Cultural competency was born out of earlier concepts of cultural sensitivity and diversity. The nurse of the 21st century must have a broad worldview of the interrelatedness of the factors that affect individual, group, and community health. The nurse of the future will see each client in truly holistic terms, sharing in the development of health care programs under the umbrella of culture and ethnicity. The future of transcultural nursing remains strong. The 21st century will require nurses to have knowledge and skills in transcultural nursing that can serve as the basis for therapeutic nursing care (Leininger, 1991). Transcultural nursing concepts should guide the nursing profession in practice, education, and research endeavors. Advances are still needed in ethnographic research and design to increase our theoretical understanding of all culture-related concepts mentioned in this chapter.

CHAPTER HIGHLIGHTS

✦

✦ To be culturally competent, a nurse must foster a positive attitude toward persons from other cultures and facilitate health care within the individual's ethnocultural framework.

✦ Transcultural nursing has had its greatest development since 1970, when Madeleine Leininger spearheaded a movement to develop it as a subspecialty.

✦ Immigration status, ethnic background, and income level all have an impact on a person's access to and expectations of the health care system.

✦ Migrant workers are mostly concentrated in a few areas in this country. Their working and living conditions create tremendous health risks, but their access to the health care system is often minimal.

✦ Poverty affects access to health care both in terms of ability to pay for treatments and in terms of having the know-how to negotiate the health care system.

✦ When cultural practices and Western medical practices are in conflict, the nurse should identify the cultural practice or medicine being used and attempt to coordinate culturally meaningful practices with the regimen prescribed.

✦ Nurses will continue to evaluate their personal attitudes toward different ethnocultural groups and explore the impact of health care reform on care of diverse populations.

Study Questions

1. You are caring for an Asian woman at home who is currently taking digoxin, Lasix (furosemide), and Slow-K (potassium chloride) for a heart condition. You notice that she drinks an herbal tea each morning. Which of the following is your most appropriate intervention?

   a. assess the contents of the tea
   b. encourage her to continue drinking the tea to show your cultural sensitivity
   c. call her doctor right away
   d. encourage her to notify her doctor about the tea
   e. do nothing; we all drink different types of tea

2. A community health nurse states that all people living in the United States should learn to speak English. The nurse is displaying signs of:

   a. cultural blindness
   b. cultural sensitivity
   c. ethnocentrism
   d. cultural imposition

3. You have just given a talk on safe sex to a group of African-American teenagers. One of the young women yells from the back of the room, "It is against my religion to use birth control. How can I practice safe sex?" What is the proper response?

   a. "I'll tell you again, if you have sex with someone without using a condom, you increase your risk of contracting HIV."
   b. "We aren't talking about birth control issues today."
   c. "If you were practicing your religion properly, you wouldn't be having sex."
   d. "I understand that these are complicated issues. It is your choice to practice safe sex knowing what you learned in today's class about the transmission of HIV."

4. Which cultural group is likely to use the services of *curanderos* (folk healers) and *parteras* (lay midwives)?

   a. black Americans
   b. Arab Americans
   c. Mexican Americans
   d. Asian Americans

5. The "culture shock" that many immigrants experience after coming to the United States can be relieved by which of the following community health services?

   a. small group meetings of new immigrants and community leaders
   b. high school evening classes
   c. referral to a psychiatric nurse who specializes in relaxation techniques
   d. small group meetings at a cultural-specific community center with acclimated immigrants and new arrivals

Critical Thinking Exercises

1. You were told that your area contained 60% single-parent families, 40% of whom were below poverty socioeconomic status. The population consists of 30% Hispanics, 40% blacks, and 30% whites. How would these statistics influence your care of clients if you were a health department nurse?

2. Discuss the cultural assessment and nursing interventions of a client who is a 33-year-old Hispanic woman who is admitted for a diagnosis of new onset of seizures. The client speaks no English, and she has been refusing to eat for 3 days. She is not aware of diagnostic test results, which have revealed a brain tumor.

References

Arab, D. M., & Weiner, B. L. (1986). Infectious diseases and field water supply and sanitation among migrant field workers. *American Journal of Public Health, 76*(6), 694–695.

Boffetta, P., & Parkin, D. M. (1994). Cancer in developing countries. *CA: A Cancer Journal for Clinicians, 44*(2), 81–90.

Boyle, J. S., & Andrews, M. M. (1989). *Transcultural concepts in nursing care.* Glenview, IL: Scott, Foresman/ Little, Brown.

Clark, M. J. (1992). *Nursing in the community*. Norwalk, CT: Appleton & Lange.

Division of Disadvantaged Assistance, Bureau of Health Professionals. (1990). *Health status of the disadvantaged, chartbook, 1990*. U.S. Dept. HHS, Public Health Services. DHHS Pub. NO. (HRSA). HRS-P-DV 90-1. Washington, DC: GPO.

Eliason, M. J. (1993). Ethics and transcultural nursing care. *Nursing Outlook, 41*(5), 225–228.

Geissler, E. M. (1992). Nursing diagnosis: A study of cultural relevance. *Journal of Professional Nursing, 8*(5), 301–307.

Giger, J. N., & Davidhizar, R. E. (1995). *Transcultural nursing assessment and intervention*. St. Louis: Mosby.

Haq, M. B. (1994). Lady health visitors: Public health nursing education in Pakistan. *Journal of Cultural Diversity, 1*(2), 36–40.

Jezewski, M. A. (1993). Culture brokering as a model for advocacy. *Nursing & Health Care, 14*(2), 78–85.

Kerner, J. F., Dusenbury, L., & Mandelblatt, J. S. (1993). Poverty and cultural diversity: Challenges for health promotion among the medically underserved. *Annual Review of Public Health, 14*, 355–377.

Kuhni, C. Q. (1990). When cultures clash at the bedside. *RN, 53*(1)23–25.

Leininger, M. M. (1979). *Transcultural nursing*. New York: Masson International Nursing Publications.

Leininger, M. M. (1990). Transcultural nursing: A worldwide necessity to advance nursing knowledge and practice. In J. C. McClosky & H. K. Grace (Eds.), *Current issues in nursing* (3rd ed., pp. 534–541).

Leininger, M. M. (1991). Leininger's acculturation health care assessment tool for cultural patterns in traditional health and non-traditional life ways. *Journal of Transcultural Nursing, 2*(3), 40.

Marks, G. M., Solis, J., Richardson, J. L., Collins, L. M., Lourdes, B., & Hisserich, J. C. (1987). Health behavior of elderly Hispanic women: Does cultural assimilation make a difference? *American Journal of Public Health, 77*(10), 1315–1319.

Ries, L. A., Hankey, B. F., Edwards, B. K., eds. (1990). *Cancer Statistics Review, 1973–1987*. NIH Publication no. 90-2789. Bethesda, MD: National Cancer Institute.

Rooda, L. A. (1993). Knowledge and attitudes of nurses toward culturally different patients: Implications for nursing education. *Journal of Nursing Education, 32*(5), 209–213.

Russell, K. R., & Jewell, N. (1992). Cultural impact of health care access: Challenges for improving the health of African-Americans. *Journal of Community Health Nursing, 9*(3), 161–169.

Smith, K. G. (1986). The hazards of migrant field work: An overview for rural public health nurses. *Public Health Nursing, 3*(1), 48–56.

Toubia, N. (1994). Female circumcision as a public health issue. *New England Journal of Medicine, 331*(11), 712–716.

Tripp-Reimer, T., & Fox, S. S. (1990). Beyond the concept of culture: On how knowing the cultural formula does not predict clinical success. In J. C. McClosky & H. K. Grace (Eds.), *Current issues in nursing* (3rd ed., pp. 542–546). St. Louis: Mosby.

U.S. Bureau of the Census. (1992). *Statistical abstract of the United States, 1992* (112th ed.). Washington, DC: GPO.

U.S. Bureau of the Census. (1993). *Poverty in the United States, 1992*. Current Population Reports, Series P60-185. Washington, DC: GPO.

U.S. Department of Commerce, Bureau of the Census. (1992). *Exploring alternative race-ethnic comparison groups in current population surveys*. Current Population Reports, Series P23-182. Washington, DC: GPO.

U.S. Department of Commerce, Bureau of the Census. (1993). *Hispanic Americans today*. Current Population Reports, Series P23-183. Washington, DC: GPO.

U.S. Department of Health & Human Services, Bureau of Health Professions. (1990). *Health Status of the Disadvantaged Chartbook*. DHHS Publication no. (HRSA) HRS-P-DV 90-1, Washington, DC: GPO.

West, E. A. (1993). The cultural bridge model. *Nursing Outlook, 41*(5), 229–234.

Bibliography

Bell, R. (1994). Prominence of women in Navaho healing habits and values. *Nursing & Health Care, 15*(5), 232–240.

Bernal, H. (1993). A model for delivering culture-relevant care in the community, *Public Health Nursing, 10*(4), 228–232.

Bond, M. L., & Jones, M. E. (1994). Short-term cultural immersion in Mexico. *Nursing & Health Care, 15*(5), 248–253.

Brink, P. J. (1984). Value orientation as an assessment tool in cultural diversity. *Nursing Research, 33*(4), 198–203.

Brower, H. (1982). Advocacy: What is it? *Journal of Gerontological Nursing, 8*, 141–143.

Chin, J. L. (1991). Health care issues for Asian-Americans. *Journal of Multi-Cultural Community Health, 1*(2), 17–22.

Geissler, E. M. (1994). *Pocket guide to cultural assessment*. St. Louis: Mosby-Year Book.

Green, J. (1989). Death with dignity, Hinduism. *Nursing Times, 85*(6), 50–51.

Johnson, T. (1992). *Changing in minority demographics in the U.S.* Published in the proceedings of the Invitational Congress "Caring for the Emerging Majority: Creating a New Diversity in Nurse Leadership." Health Resources and Services Administration, Bureau of Health Professionals, Division of Nursing.

Leininger, M. M. (1994). Transcultural nursing education: A worldwide imperative. *Nursing & Health Care, 15*(5), 254–257.

National Center for Health Statistics. (1993). *Health, United States, 1993*. Hyattsville, MD: Public Health Service.

National League for Nursing. (1992). *An agenda for nursing education reform in support of nursing's agenda for health care reform*. New York: Author.

National League for Nursing. (1993). *Nursing data review 1993*. Pub. No. 19-2529. New York: Author.

Office of Migrant Education. (1992). *Directory of services for migrants and seasonal farmworkers and their families*. U.S. Department of Education. Washington, DC: Author.

Office of Minority Health. (1993). *Towards equality of well-being: Strategies for improving minority health*. U.S. Dept. of Health and Human Services, Public Health Service. Washington, DC: GPO.

Pope-Davis, D. B., Eliason, M. J., & Optive, T. M. (1994). Are nursing students multiculturally competent? An exploratory study. *Journal of Nursing Education, 33*(1), 31–33.

Porter, C. P., & Villarruel, A. M. (1993). Nursing research with African-Americans and Hispanic people: Guidelines for action. *Nursing Outlook, 41*(2), 59–67.

Princeton, J. C. (1993). Promoting culturally competent nursing education. *Journal of Nursing Education, 32*(5), 195–197.

Rosella, J. D., Regan-Kublinski, M. J., & Albrecht, S. A. (1994). The need for multicultural diversity among health professionals. *Nursing & Health Care, 15*(5), 242–246.

Schroeder, P. (1994). Female genital mutilation—A form of child abuse. *New England Journal of Medicine, 331*(11), 739–740.

Smith, B. E., Colling, K, Elander, E., & Latham, C. (1993). A model for multicultural curriculum development in baccalaureate nursing education. *Journal of Nursing Education, 32*(5), 205–208.

Solis, J. M., Marks, G., Garcia, M., & Shelton, D. (1980). Acculturation, access to health care, and use of preventive services by Hispanics: Findings from HANES 1982–84. *American Journal of Public Health, 80*(suppl), 11–18.

Spector, R. E. (1991). *Cultural diversity in health and illness* (3rd ed.). Norwalk, CT: Appleton & Lange.

Tripp-Reimer, T., Brink, P. J., & Saunders, J. M. (1984). Cultural assessment: Content and process. *Nursing Outlook, 32*(2), 78–82.

U.S. Bureau of the Census. *Statistical abstract of the United States, 1990.* (110th ed.). Washington, DC: GPO.

U.S. Department of Health and Human Services. (1991). *Healthy people 2000: National health promotion and disease prevention objectives.* 91-50212. Washington, DC: GPO.

Chapter 37

SEXUALITY

JUDY BRADBERRY,
RN, PhD, NCMT

KEY TERMS

✦

abortion
circumcision
contraception
gender
gestation
heterosexuality
homosexuality
infertility
menstrual cycle
nocturnal emission

premenstrual
    syndrome
puberty
sex
sexual abuse
sexual dysfunction
sexuality
sexually transmitted
    disease

LEARNING OBJECTIVES

✦

After studying this chapter, you should be able to

✦ Define human sexuality as a holistic concept

✦ Discuss the influence of culture on sexuality

✦ Discuss the influence of sexuality on health and health care

✦ Discuss the importance of nurses' sexual self-awareness

✦ Describe the major sexual development of each stage of the life cycle

✦ Identify components of both male and female genitals and their functions

✦ Discuss the role of nursing related to the issues of abortion, contraception, homosexuality, infertility, sexual abuse, sexually transmitted diseases, and sexual dysfunction

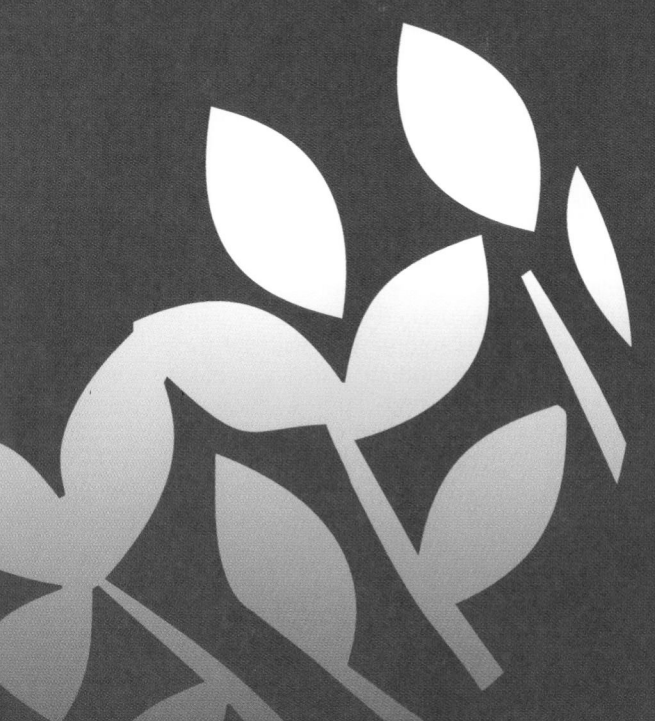

This chapter examines the concept of human sexuality as it relates to nursing care. Human sexuality is defined as a holistic component of the human experience, manifesting in physical and psychosocial ways. Emphasis is placed on the nurse's awareness of the role sexuality has on all human interactions.

"Sex," "sexuality," and "human sexuality" are all terms that carry multiple meanings, often charged with a variety of emotions. "Sex" can refer to something as clinical as whether a spider is male or female or to something as intimate, complex, and profoundly emotional as two people involved in passionate lovemaking. For many people, "sexuality" is a broader concept that incorporates behavioral expectations as well as a definition of biological functions. "Sexuality" is also used instead of simply "sex" to sound more formal or polite, to shroud the conversation, to be silly, or to be sensitive. For instance, if a young college student and her roommates had an interesting late-night conversation, she might say to a friend, "We talked all night about sex." If the same college student were discussing this textbook chapter with her grandmother, she might say, "We're learning about sexuality." The topic in these two hypothetical conversations is the same, but the tone of the communication is different because of the different situations. It is these subtle nuances that make it difficult to provide an exact definition of sexuality that fully describes all its multifaceted components. It is this subtle, sensitive nature that makes it difficult, yet imperative, for nurses to be able to communicate in a clear, professional manner regarding sexuality.

Here are a few definitions of sexuality: "the quality or state of being sexual; a. the condition of having sex; b. the condition of having reproductive functions dictated by the union of male and female . . . . c. the expression of the sex instinct: sexual activity . . . d. the condition, potential, or state of readiness of the organism with regard to sexual activity" (*Webster's,* 1986, p. 2082). Taber's (1989, p. 1668) defines sexuality as: "1. State of having sex; the collective characteristics that mark the differences between the male and the female. 2. Constitution and life of individual as related to sex; all the dispositions related to the love life whether associated with the sex organs or not."

Sexuality is interwoven with all the other aspects of our being, including our emotional, psychological, cultural, and spiritual natures. Masters, Johnson, and Kolodny (1993) clarify that "sexuality means a dimension of personality instead of referring to a person's capacity for erotic response alone" (p. 4). Sexuality is an integral aspect of each human being. I define human sexuality as the integral aspect of being that reflects the state of maleness or femaleness and is manifested in all components of being human.

Sexuality and a person's sex are different from gender. Sex is a relatively simple concept that refers strictly to the biological existence of maleness or femaleness. Gender, however, is the more complex, culturally influenced, subjective experience of being male or female. In US culture, one's gender and one's sex are usually seen as being the same, or at least it is thought that they should be the same.

Sexuality as a Holistic Concept

Sexuality and all other components of human life are inseparable, although our forms of communication force us to talk about sexuality as if it were something that could be taken apart from the rest of our humanness and divided into parts. Human sexuality as a concept is talked about as physiological, psychological, social, and cultural. In reality, all these parts are intertwined.

Because it is impossible to separate culture from the psychosocial components of our sexual natures, this chapter discusses human sexuality in the mainstream US culture. There are many subcultures, depending on ethnicity, socioeconomic status, race, religion, geography, age, and other variables. One way that the nurse can increase his or her ability to provide sexually appropriate care to a variety of clients is to become familiar with cultural differences among groups of people.

Our existence as male or female permeates every other component of life, from our most rudimentary biological functions to our most complex psychosociospiritual interactions. Even in a coma, an adult woman still experiences the hormonal fluctuations of the menstrual cycle. The balance of estrogens to androgens constantly influences such things as hair growth and fat deposits, whether we are aware of that influence or not. The subtle biological forces of the sex hormones are usually beyond our conscious control. Unless specific medical interventions are taken, nothing stops a man's beard from growing under the influence of androgens, and nothing stops the development of breast tissue in a pubescent girl under the influence of estrogens.

From the very beginning we are treated differently, depending on our femaleness or maleness. For example, because an infant's gender is usually not obvious without assessing the genitals, many boy babies in US culture are dressed in blue and girl babies in pink. Why is it important to know the gender of a newborn?

Nurses' Self-Awareness

Perhaps the most important thing for nurses to keep in mind about the complexity of human sexuality is that their own sexuality and the sexuality of everyone with whom they interact cannot be circumvented. It is possible to ignore how sexually attractive or unattractive someone is to another individual, but it is never possible to obliterate the sexuality of both parties in any interaction. Nurses must be aware of themselves and their clients as sexual beings. This does not mean that one is constantly aware of whether or not one is behaving in a sexually seductive manner. It may mean something as nonerotic having a different perspective on an ethical dilemma in health care because of one's gender. Gilligan and Antanucci (1988) found that women do hold a different ethical worldview than men. Because most nurses are female, this means that nurses are likely to have a different paradigm for ethical decision-making than other health care professionals, who are preponderantly male.

Role Relationships

Sexual self-awareness among nurses also may mean understanding that their role in the health care professions has been heavily influenced by male-female differences in society. The old traditional role of nurses as physicians' handmaidens rested largely on the fact that women were men's handmaidens at the time that nursing and medicine were in their infancy.

Feelings About Clients

Sexual self-awareness may be manifested in the way that nurses feel about certain clients. The actual physical nursing care administered to a homosexual man or to a woman having an abortion may not be affected by the nurse's negative feelings about those lifestyle choices, but the nurse's feelings are real and valid and may become clear through body language and choice of words.

Clarity in Communication

Clarity about one's own feelings helps the nurse make wise career choices. Obviously, if a nurse is uncertain how he or she feels about homosexuality, taking a position in a clinic in the midst of a predominantly gay community may not be the best career choice. No matter what job choices nurses make during their careers, it is almost inevitable that they will encounter individuals whose sexual behavior is different from their own. If the nurse can communicate clearly that he or she does not have the same sexual values as the client, appropriate nursing care can usually be delivered. If, however, the nurse is unaware of his or her feelings, both the nurse and the client may feel an uncomfortable sense of mistrust that would not be therapeutic.

Self-awareness, however, does not come easily or quickly. Nurses must incorporate self-examination for biases into their routine evaluation of professional growth. Sometimes our biases are obvious only by what we choose to ignore. Most nurses develop high levels of sexual self-awareness over time, through experience. To learn from experience, one must be willing to examine oneself honestly. Obviously, we need to know whether to use the male or female pronoun in reference to infants. However, it is also likely that we wish to know the gender of infants so that we can behave toward them in what we believe are gender-appropriate ways. We may not want to call a boy "pretty," as that is a word generally reserved for girls. Studies have shown that adults speak to, look at, and touch girl babies more frequently than boy babies (Fogel & Lauver, 1990, p. 61). It is common for newborn boys to be given stuffed footballs and newborn girls stuffed teddy bears, in anticipation of their expected gender roles. Expectations about our behaviors based on gender persist throughout our lives.

✦ Culture

The degree to which individual response to the environment is determined by biological sex or by early cultural conditioning is an unanswered question at this time. Our beliefs have changed drastically over the last century. In Victorian times, it was believed that humans' response to the world was almost totally biologically controlled. For example, it was believed that women were not capable of participating in business or scientific matters because their brains were too small (Caplan, 1987). During the height of the women's movement in the 1960s, it was believed that all differences were culturally induced. It was unpopular to suggest that differences in gender were biological at all. Recently, research has begun to reassess which of our ideas about who we are and how we ought to act, think, and feel as men or women are biological and which are cultural (Gorman, 1992).

Research is also being done to answer questions such as, "Are women better at assessing others' emotions?" and "Are men better at solving spatial problems?" (Gorman, 1992). The implications of these questions can lead to the assignment of roles to one sex or the other. The stereotype is that "men are smart and women are emotional," but common sense and observation of human behavior indicate that both men and women are both smart and emotional.

In most of US history, the "masculine" concepts of aggressiveness, intellectuality, practicality, and logicality have been valued. People have paid money and awarded honors to those who exhibited these characteristics. In contrast, to be called "emotional" or "intuitive" is generally considered negative and feminine. Parents caring for children, and nurses nurturing the sick, have been paid little or no money and seldom receive recognition for their acts. One contribution that nurses can make in meeting the challenge of valuing all humanness is to proudly claim all that we are and all that we do. Nurses as scientific decision-makers and technological manipulators demonstrate intellectuality and measurable activity while providing many immeasurable services such as nurturing and basic caregiving. Holding these services in high esteem ourselves will help the rest of the culture embrace these activities as honorable and worthy.

It is possible for a culture to acknowledge difference and still hold all characteristics in equal value. In most traditional Native American cultures, men were seen as more aggressive and women as more nurturing. However, both of these qualities were considered necessary for harmonious balance and were valued. Many tribes allowed women access to tribal councils and positions of authority and held the wisdom of female elders in extremely high esteem. Some tribes had both war councils and peace councils, with female elders making up the majority of the peace councils. Usually, the peace council had to give permission for the war council to take action, thereby making the "feminine" aspect of peacekeeping a superior cultural influence. Among Native American healers, women were often more highly respected, for their superior intuition gave them information about the patient that male healers might not observe with the five physical senses (Medicine Eagle, 1991).

Cultural Change

The last three decades in US culture have been a time of intense reexamination of our definitions of sexuality and all it means to us. Only a generation ago, the cultural norm was for adults (at least women) to abstain from sexual activity until married, to remain married to the same spouse throughout life, to have children, and to observe a rather strict division of labor. Men who cleaned house were snubbed as "sissy," and women who aspired to positions outside the domestic arena were treated disdainfully and regarded as "not real women." Contraceptive technology was at a point of development that made remaining childless throughout a sexually active adulthood very difficult. Because childbearing was the norm for married couples, even when oral contraceptives became available in the 1960s, social pressure for all married couples to reproduce was strong.

The feminist movement of the 1960s and 1970s caused Americans to question their assumptions about gender identity. Examination of the feminine role in the United States led to a drastic reconception of what it meant to be feminine. Literature is also reexamining our definitions of masculinity. Harris (1994) states that men moved from defining masculinity in terms of strength and aggressiveness to a more sensitive, nurturing model, in direct response to women's demand for change. Apparently, in the last two decades, men did what women have been doing for centuries, *i.e.*, defining themselves in reaction to others' demands. Harris states that men, like women, must create their own identities rather than simply react to others.

Other changes are reflected in the media. Issues such as abortion, homosexuality, out-of-wedlock pregnancy, and sexual abuse were not discussed in polite company until the 1970s, but they are aired on the news and TV shows routinely in the 1990s. Whether the change in our conversations reflects real change in behaviors and values is not clear. Some believe that

open discussion of all sexual matters frees us to solve problems, such as unwanted pregnancy and sexual abuse; others believe that such discussion encourages further problematical behavior.

Influence of Sexuality on Health Status and Health Care Seeking

The differing gender roles in the United States contribute to differences in health status, health care–seeking behaviors, and how one is perceived and treated by health care professionals. Obviously, many of the differences in health status are direct results of the biological status of being male or female. For example, males do not have premenstrual syndrome because they do not have menstrual cycles. Women do not have testicular cancer because they do not have testicles.

Lifestyle Factors

Many of the health differences observed between men and women go beyond pure biology. For instance, women have higher incidences of hypertension, diabetes, and arthritis than do men. Do these higher rates reflect genetic differences only, or are they influenced by lifestyle differences between men and women? Additionally, demographic and economic indicators demonstrate that women and children represent the fastest growing proportion of the very poor in the United States. The lack of financial resources, which is more likely to plague women than men, may result in the receipt of less health care (Swanson & Albrecht, 1993).

Life Expectancy

Although it is projected that life expectancy for women in the United States and most other developed countries is longer than men's life expectancy, the reverse is true in many undeveloped countries (Swanson & Albrecht, 1993). Perhaps this statistic represents better management of childbearing in technologically advanced countries, decreasing the possibility of young women dying as a consequence of childbearing.

Marital Status

The most interesting statistics about health in relation to gender are those involving marital status. Masters, Johnson, and Kolodny (1985) reviewed several studies that indicate that married men are healthier than single men, but that the reverse is true for women. It is hypothesized that married men are healthier than single men because they have more of their psychological needs met by having both families and careers, without the added stress of many of the familial obligations that women are expected to fulfill. Women, conversely, are less likely to enjoy overall good health if they are married, because they often have multiple role strain—working outside the home in addition to maintaining the traditional role of mother, wife, and homemaker. Alger (1991) reported that role overload for working married women can lead to increased family stress. With increasing evidence that high levels of stress can lead to a variety of health problems, this may partially explain married women's decreased health status compared with their single counterparts.

♦
Sexual Anatomy and Physiology

The biological state of being female or male influences all of an individual's anatomy and physiology to some degree. This section focuses on only a brief description of the genitals and their reproductive functioning. Genitals or genitalia are defined as reproductive or-

Table 37-1

	SEXUAL ANATOMICAL PARTS	
NAME	**DESCRIPTION**	**FUNCTION**
	Female	
Bartholin's gland	Two small glands just inside vagina	Secretes lubrication during arousal
Clitoris	Protrusion of innervated tissue inside labia minora	Most sensitive part
Fallopian tube	Tiny tubes extending laterally from uterus toward ovary	Transports ova from just outside ovary to uterus
Hymen	Membranous tissue over vaginal introitus	Covers vaginal opening
Introitus	Opening of the vagina	Allows penile penetration and childbirth
Labia majora	Hair-covered fatty tissue extending around the rest of external genitals	Provides cushioning during intercourse
Labia minora	Folds of hairless mucous membranes just inside labia majora	Provides protection to vagina and urethral meatus
Mons pubis	Fatty deposit over pubic bone	Provides cushioning during intercourse
Ova	Female gamete	Carries female genetic contribution to reproduction
Ovary	Firm, round, walnut-sized organs lateral to uterus	Produces hormones, releases ova
Skene glands	Small glands lateral to urethral meatus	Provides lubrication during intercourse
Uterus	Small, muscular organ just above vagina	Carries pregnancy
Vagina	Elastic, rugaed vault of mucous membranous tissue	Allows intercourse
	Male	
Corpus cavernosum	Columns of spongy tissue above the urethra	Allows penile erection
Corpus spongiosum	Column of spongy tissue on underside of penis	Allows penile erection
Cowper gland	Tiny gland below prostate gland	Secretes clear preejaculatory fluid
Ejaculatory duct	Tiny tubes between seminal vesicles and urethra	Part of passageway of seminal fluid to outside the body
Glans	Distal portion of penis	Highly sensitive
Foreskin	Fold of skin around glans that is removed in circumcision	Purpose undocumented
Penis	Highly vascular, highly innervated cylindrical organ	Allows intercourse
Prostate gland	Muscular and glandular organ at proximal end of urethra	Produces a minority of seminal fluid
Scrotum	Hair-covered, rugaed sac around testicles	Allows testicles to be carried away from direct body heat
Seminal vesicle	Small glands that join with ejaculatory duct	Produces majority of seminal fluid
Sperm	Male gamete	Carries male contribution to reproduction
Testicle	Round, firm, walnut-sized organs carried in scrotum	Produces sperm
Vas deferens	Tiny tube between the testicles and ejaculatory duct	Part of passageway of sperm to outside the body

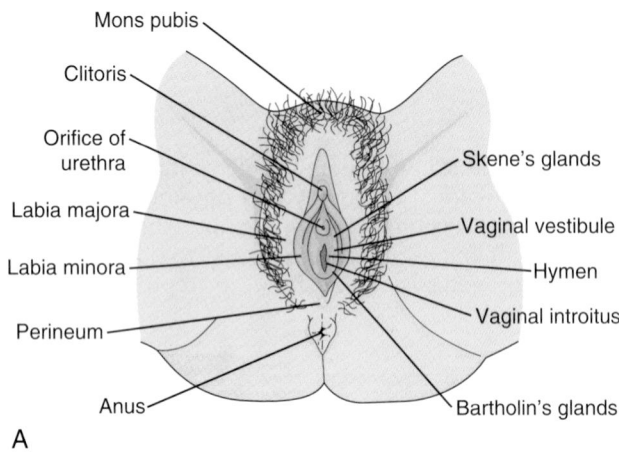

A

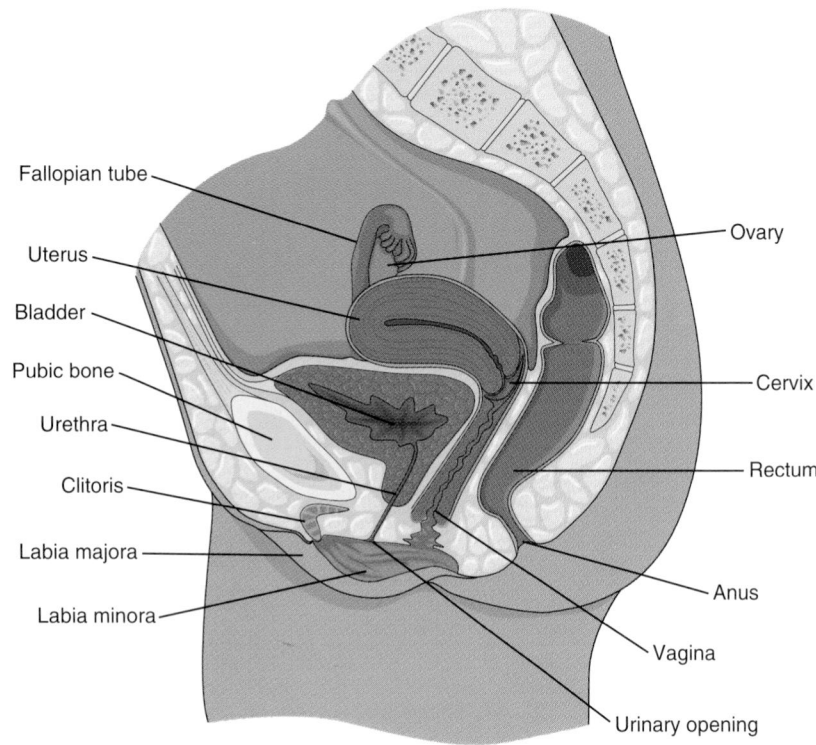

B

✦ **Figure 37–1**
Female reproductive anatomy. *A,* External.
B, Internal.

gans. I intentionally omit the breasts from this discussion, because they are used to feed the young of our species, not to create them.

Lay language has many names for the various parts of the sexual anatomy. Appropriate terminology should be used when talking with clients about sexual matters. Slang should be avoided in communicating with clients unless it becomes apparent that the client has no understanding of the terms being used by the nurse. In such a case, the nurse should explain, in a noncondescending manner, what is meant by the words he or she is using and then continue using appropriate terminology. Table 37–1 gives a brief description of the female and male reproductive anatomy. Figures 37–1 and 37–2 illustrate female and male reproductive anatomy.

♦
Sexuality Throughout the Life Cycle

Sexuality is an integral aspect of human life from before birth to death. The individual progresses through various developmental periods throughout the life cycle. Table 37–2 reviews the major milestones of each developmental stage according to Erikson, Freud, and Kohlberg. See also Chapters 15 through 17 for further discussion.

Infants

In the literature about sexuality during infancy, several significant ideas come to light. One is that the

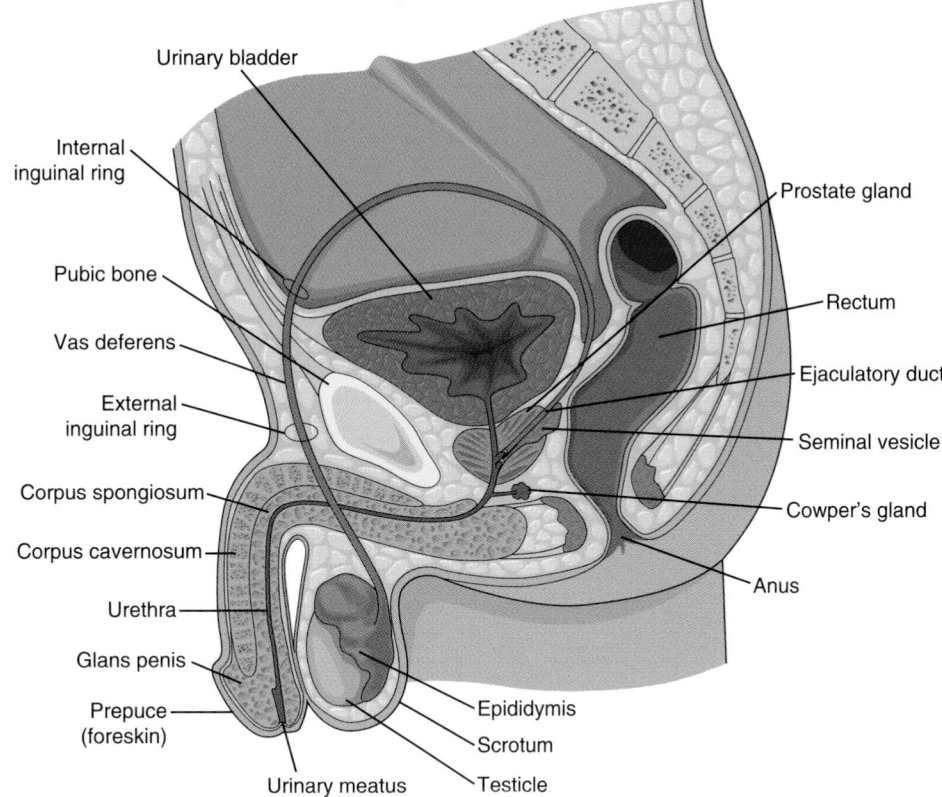

Urinary bladder

Internal inguinal ring

Pubic bone

Vas deferens

External inguinal ring

Corpus spongiosum

Corpus cavernosum

Urethra

Glans penis

Prepuce (foreskin)

Urinary meatus

Prostate gland

Rectum

Ejaculatory duct

Seminal vesicle

Cowper's gland

Anus

Epididymis

Scrotum

Testicle

❧ **Figure 37–2**
Male reproductive anatomy.

sensation of touch is critical during infancy; another is the discussion of love between the parent and child; and the last is the discussion of needs gratification.

The nursing implications for this stage are primarily in educating parents about normal growth and development of infants. After the nurse assesses what parents already know about child development, an appropriate educational plan can be implemented. Parents should be taught that touch is one of the infant's primary ways of learning. They need to understand that infant self-touching is not sexual in the same sense that adults interpret sexual touching.

Table **37–2**

DEVELOPMENTAL STAGES ACCORDING TO ERIKSON, FREUD, AND KOHLBERG

STAGE	ERIKSON	FREUD	KOHLBERG	NURSING CONSIDERATIONS
Infancy	Trust/mistrust	Oral	Prereligious	Parental education about the importance of touch and self-exploration for the infant
Toddler	Autonomy/shame and doubt	Anal	Punishment/ obedience	Parental education about toilet training in positive ways and development of gender identity
Preschool	Initiative/guilt	Oedipal	Self-interest	Parental education about curiosity at this age and appropriate responses to questions
School age	Industry/inferiority	Latent	Conventional	Assess for possible sexual abuse; educate parents about normalcy of same-sex play
Young adult	Intimacy/isolation	Genital	Postconventional	Education about STDs, family planning; support for establishment of adult lifestyle
Middle adult	Generativity/ stagnation	Genital	Postconventional	Support through lifestyle adjustments; facilitate support groups
Older adult	Generativity/ stagnation	Genital	Postconventional	Education about changing physical characteristics; support through lifestyle changes

Data from Pillitteri, A. (1995). *Maternal and child health nursing.* Philadelphia: J. B. Lippincott.

Nurses can also foster healthy sexual development in infants by providing secure, loving handling when caring for infants. This fosters a sense of trust in others, which is later reflected in all interactions, both of a directly sexual nature and of a nonsexual nature.

Toddlers

Toddlerhood is an extremely important period in the development of sexuality, especially because of the emphasis on toilet training. Owing to the anatomical proximity of the excretory organs and the sexual organs, attitudes about toilet training play a large role in how the child perceives his or her genitals. If toileting is treated as filthy, and infractions of toileting etiquette are punished harshly, the child may subsequently associate these attitudes with sexuality. Conversely, if toileting is treated as a natural function, and appropriate learning is reinforced in a timely fashion, the child will not be encumbered by negative associations between toileting and the genitals.

Many toddlers begin to masturbate during this time, which may be a source of anxiety for parents. With assistance from nurses, parents can be helped to see masturbation in toddlers as an opportunity for teaching anatomy and the concept of privacy, rather than as a behavior to be punished or ignored (Poorman, 1988).

Most toddlers can identify "boy" or "girl" between the ages of 2 and 3 years (Poorman, 1988, p. 32). Core gender identity, the idea that one is male or female, is thought to be solidified by age 3 (Masters *et al.*, 1985). During the toddler stage, individuals begin to imitate parental behavior. Most often, girls imitate their mothers, and boys imitate their fathers. This is significant in reinforcing gender roles considered appropriate by the person's culture.

Parental knowledge deficit related to sexual development in toddlers is a likely nursing diagnosis during this stage. The nurse should also assess for signs of appropriate self-esteem and body image in toddlers.

Preschoolers

Because children at this age have gained good mobility and language skills, they are increasingly independent. Their curiosity about sexuality also increases during this time, which is often manifested by examining one another's bodies and asking questions about parents' private behaviors, including bathroom behaviors, as well as some relational questions. The sex play that occurs between opposite-sex or same-sex peers is generally a learning experience rather than an erotic experience.

The primary nursing support that families need during this time is similar to that provided during the toddler stage. Parents need guidance about appropriate ways to answer preschoolers' questions about anatomy and physiology without going into detail that is incomprehensible to the child.

School-Age Children

Reinisch (1990) reports that the highest incidence of sex play occurs between children in the 6 to 10 age range. Because school age is also the time when children play mostly with same-sex peers, sex play with same-sex peers is not abnormal. This is also when children begin to develop their own sense of morality (Poorman, 1988). Thus, the rules they are being taught about sexual behavior become more important to them.

Poorman (1988) reports that children ages 6 and 7 may be at the greatest risk for sexual abuse by adults. It is critical for children of this age to be prepared to recognize a potential threat of sexual abuse and to report it to a trusted adult. Obviously, assessing for the possibility of sexual abuse among children in this age group is an important nursing function. Knowledge deficit about possible sexual abuse and ways to prevent it is another possible nursing diagnosis in this developmental stage.

Adolescents

Adolescence is perhaps the most significant time of life in regard to sexual development. Certainly, it is when sexual development is most obvious, because puberty occurs.

The most significant event in puberty for females is menarche, or the beginning of menstruation. The average age for menarche in the United States today is 12.8 years (Gorrie *et al.*, 1994). How a young woman feels about menarche depends on several factors, including any accompanying physical discomfort and how menstruation is perceived by her family and her culture. The accompanying box highlights research findings regarding some beliefs about women's cyclicity.

For young men, the most significant event of puberty is the first nocturnal emission, or "wet dream," in which seminal fluid is released during sleep, often accompanied by sexual dreams. If young men are prepared for these nocturnal emissions, which can occur frequently, and have been taught to view them as normal, they may not cause much anxiety. However, should they occur while spending the night with friends and the friends know of the emission, it can cause embarrassment.

In addition to hormonal changes, the adolescent undergoes major psychological changes during these years. It is usually during this time, after possible experimentation with both sexual preferences, that a commitment is made to a sexual preference. Pairing and dating also begin during this time. Swensen

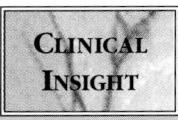

McFarlane and Williams' Study of Cyclicity

McFarlane and Williams (1994) indicate that the majority of American women report having premenstrual syndrome, although when examined they do not meet diagnostic criteria. They studied cyclicity among women and men in relation to menstruation (in the women subjects), day of the week, and lunar cycles. They found that although the majority of both male and female subjects experienced cyclicity in their lives, most of the women's cyclicity was not necessarily congruent with the menstrual cycle.

Nursing Implications

This study shows how powerful cultural beliefs can be in a woman's perception of her menstrual experience.

It is important for nurses to teach young women to view their sexually maturing selves as objectively as possible, in order to avoid entrapment in a belief that menstruation is the controlling factor in their lives.

Data from McFarlane, J. M., William, T. M. (1994). Placing premenstrual syndrome in perspective. *Psychology of Women Quarterly, 18,* 339–373.

(1992) found that among 183 adolescents in a large metropolitan area who were 15 years old or younger, 87% had experienced sexual activity.

Knowledge deficit related to sexuality during the adolescent period is a common nursing diagnosis. Assessment of what beliefs a client holds and what myths or misconceptions he or she has heard is essential when preparing an individual or community educational plan.

Perhaps the area of sexual education that needs the most emphasis during adolescence, as well as adulthood, is responsible decision-making in terms of disease prevention and family planning. Providing information on contraception and on the prevention of sexually transmitted diseases (STDs) is controversial in some communities and for some families. The nurse must always respect the client's right to make lifestyle decisions based on his or her personal moral and ethical values. Information can be made available to those who choose to receive it, but every individual has the ultimate responsibility for deciding how such information will be used.

Young Adults (Age 18–30)

It is during young adulthood that most people in the US culture marry and have at least one child, thus establishing intimacy with the spouse and the child.

Sexual intimacy is a significant aspect of life intimacy at this time.

Although people have generally committed to a sexual preference by the time they reach this age and may have committed to a significant relationship, they now have to enact what it means to them to be an adult man or woman. Decisions must be made and behaviors initiated about the degree to which one wishes to live within the cultural gender role. For example, in the United States, it is still the norm for men to work outside the home rather than to place their primary focus on child rearing and home management. Each man must decide for himself whether he chooses to live within this cultural norm. Because of these types of life issue questions and the challenges of balancing the multiple demands of adult roles, nurses are sometimes called on to act as empathic listeners for individuals or groups. Careful listening to what is said, how it is said, and what is not said is a valuable assessment tool for the nurse in this complex, sensitive area. Nurses with advanced preparation provide counseling to assist people with these kinds of questions.

Middle Adults (Age 31–65)

Adults during this time define themselves in terms of caring for the next generation, both in their own families and in the larger society through work. This tends to be a busy time of life for many adults, and sexual relationships may suffer from lack of time or energy. As a consequence, common nursing diagnoses include fatigue, risk for loneliness, and altered family processes. One way that the nurse can help such clients is by encouraging and supporting open communication between people about their needs and how they would like them to be met. In this role, the nurse is, in essence, a permission-giver for individuals to take care of themselves.

For women, one of the most significant sexual changes toward the end of this time is menopause, which is defined as the last menstruation. Like puberty, menopause is actually a process that takes several years to manifest and has many complex aspects. Menopause was historically seen as a negative experience by many people. Although many of the physical symptoms of insomnia, hot flashes, and irritability are still present for many women, men's and women's perception of how menopause affects a woman's sexuality is changing. Both women and men are beginning to see menopausal and postmenopausal women as maintaining their sexual attractiveness.

Consequently, nursing care is changing. The emphasis is on providing information about ways to minimize or cope with the symptoms of menopause, such as eating low-fat diets; exercising; and using alcohol, tobacco, and caffeine in small amounts, if at all.

Older Adults (Age 65 and Older)

Both men and women may have some changes in arousal patterns during the older years. Typically, these changes are more obvious in men and are addressed more often clinically and in the research literature because of the cultural injunction for men to "perform" sexually. Such challenges can be dealt with by education and by remaining open to exploring new and creative ways to enjoy sexual pleasure. The second important thing for aging individuals to know about their sexuality is that any sudden or major changes may be related to a health problem rather than to normal aging. They should report any such changes to their health care providers, so that any underlying pathology can be investigated (Reinisch, 1990).

Obstacles to older adults continuing to enjoy their sexuality include poor health, lack of appropriate partners as the male-female ratio changes owing to women's longer life spans, and the cultural perspective on sexuality among the aging. Perhaps the greatest of these obstacles has been the cultural rejection of the idea of older people being sexual. Our stereotype of both men and women during their older years is as sexless people. Nursing diagnoses for this age group are likely to include risk for loneliness, body image disturbance, and impaired adjustment to changing life roles. Nurses can assist older people to maintain the levels of sexual activity and sexual identity they desire by providing good general health information, facilitating group support meetings, and consistently presenting the information that sexuality and its expression are normal parts of all stages of life.

✦ Sexual Response Cycle

For sexual activity and reproduction to take place, something must occur to stimulate that activity. In this section, the terms "sexual interaction" and "sexual activity" refer to behaviors that are directly sexual, or that have sexual intercourse as a possible goal. Those things that cause sexual stimulation are called erotic and vary tremendously from culture to culture and from individual to individual. Thoughts and people can be considered erotic, as can material items such as lingerie or magazines and movies. Erotic stimulation can be physical or psychogenic. It can be self-induced or externally induced. It has been said that the brain is the most erotic part of the body, because it is with the brain that we respond to stimuli and evaluate whether something is erotic.

Those things considered erotic can stimulate a variety of behaviors, including heterosexual genital intercourse, heterosexual oral-genital intercourse, heterosexual anal-genital intercourse, homosexual oral-genital intercourse, or homosexual anal-genital in-

tercourse. Sexual activity is not limited to these behaviors, however. The nurse's role in discussing behavior with individuals is, as always, primarily educational and never judgmental about which behaviors are "normal."

Although there is vast variation in what stimuli are erotic, once an individual is initially aroused, a fairly predictable pattern of physiological events occurs during uninterrupted sexual activity. This sequence of events is called the sexual response cycle and is divided into four phases, which are similar, though not identical, in men and women.

Excitement

The excitement phase is primarily one of vasocongestion in the genitals. In men, this results in penile erection, as well as flattening and smoothing out of the scrotum. In women, the vasocongestion results in vaginal lubrication, flattening of the labia majora, ballooning of the outer portion of the vagina, and tumescence of the clitoris. Both sexes may experience nipple erection and a rashlike reddening of the chest area, called the sex flush. Both nipple erection and sex flush are much more common in women than in men (Fogel & Lauver, 1990).

Plateau

The plateau phase is in many ways a continuation and stabilization of the excitement phase. Vasocongestion of the genitals and nipple erection continue. The continued swelling of the outer portion of the vagina forms what is called the orgasm platform. The sex flush may spread to other areas of the body. Hyperventilation, tachycardia, and generalized increase in muscle tension are usually added to the physiological responses during this time.

Orgasm

The subjective experience of all four phases of the sexual response cycle varies from one individual to another but this variation is perhaps most pronounced during the orgasmic phase. One subjective experience that appears to be commonplace, however, is the loss of awareness of the environment as all focus is absorbed by the orgasmic experience. Physically, orgasm is the involuntary, rhythmic contraction of genital as well as other body muscles. It is important to note that orgasm is a total body–total mind experience, not a purely genital experience. Respiration, heart rate, and blood pressure all elevate during orgasm.

The genital contractions, which generally occur in both men and women at about 0.8-second intervals, are responsible for ejaculation of semen from the man. They are responsible for the sudden release of muscular tension and the beginning of the release of vasocongestion in the genitals. It is generally believed that it is this sudden release of tension that causes the intense sense of pleasure associated with orgasm (Fogel & Lauver, 1990; Masters *et al.*, 1985).

Resolution

Although individuals may feel that a sexual encounter comes to a physical termination with the end of orgasm, there is one more physical phase of the sexual response cycle. During the resolution phase, the body returns to its preexcitation state. Vasocongestion is relieved, along with the release of myotonia, resulting in detumescence of the penis and clitoris. The nipples return to the nonexcited state, the sex flush disappears, and all vital signs return to the preexcitement state. It is in the resolution phase that the greatest differences between women and men are seen. These differences are sometimes reflected in differences in the preceding phase. Men typically progress rather rapidly through the plateau and orgasm phases, followed by a period of complete resolution before any further excitation. Women, in contrast, sometimes experience multiple orgasms without appearing to experience resolution.

◆ Nursing Process

In the area of sexuality and sexual health, the nursing process is an effective tool for the professional. As always, the first step is to assess the overall situation related to the client's sexual health and related needs.

Assessment

Obviously, when doing a full health assessment, sexuality is an important aspect of health. However, in situations in which the nurse-client encounter is brief and focused on a specific health issue, discussion of sexuality may not be pertinent. Aspects of sexuality may vary in significance during an individual's life. For example, contraception may be one of the major health concerns of a young heterosexual individual but not a concern at all for a postmenopausal woman or a homosexual. Knowing what to assess, when, and how requires expertise acquired through study and experience. The depth of assessment and intervention in this sensitive area depends not only on the client's situation but also on the nurse's level of expertise. Nurses should always be willing to seek advice from colleagues or to refer clients to other professionals if they are unprepared to provide appropriate health care services. See Box 37–1 for examples of common sexual health assessment questions.

Nursing Diagnosis

Of course, nursing diagnoses are based on the individual assessment and may include a variety of diagnoses. Examples of nursing diagnoses that might

---

Box 37–1

COMMON SEXUAL HEALTH ASSESSMENT QUESTIONS

- People's ideas about themselves sexually change from time to time. How do you feel about yourself as a sexual person right now?
- What are your feelings about having children?
- Tell me about your relationship with your partner.
- Many people have questions about how their general health affects their sexuality. What questions do you have in this area?
- Sexuality is often an area that people have difficulty talking about, and miscommunication can be a problem. Have you experienced anything like this? Are there any questions you would like to ask?

---

be applicable in the area of sexuality are listed in the accompanying box.

Planning

Planning of care, including goal setting, methods of meeting goals, and methods of evaluating goal attainment, should include the client and take into consideration individual, familial, and cultural factors. The outcomes should be specific and measurable. It is important to involve the client in all stages of planning, implementing, and evaluating, because self-esteem and self-confidence can be determining factors in the success of interventions. See Nursing Care Plan 37–1.

POSSIBLE NURSING DIAGNOSES RELATED TO SEXUALITY

- Impaired adjustment related to divorce
- Body image disturbance related to testicular cancer
- Decisional conflict related to peer pressure to be sexually active
- Knowledge deficit related to sexually transmitted diseases
- Personal identity disturbance related to nonnormative erotic desires
- Rape-trauma syndrome; silent reaction related to date rape
- Altered role performance related to impotence
- Self-esteem disturbance related to sexual abuse
- Sensory/perceptual alteration (tactile) related to childhood sexual abuse
- Sexual dysfunction related to chronic disease
- Altered sexuality patterns related to death of partner

SAMPLE NURSING CARE PLAN

THE CLIENT WHO HAS SUFFERED A MYOCARDIAL INFARCTION

Anthony is a 45-year-old man who underwent coronary bypass surgery 6 months ago after a major myocardial infarction. During a checkup at his physician's office, in order to assess how Anthony is adapting to his cardiac condition, the nurse asks him to describe his life now compared with immediately before the surgery. Anthony says that he feels much better than he did, is enjoying his exercise program, and has even adapted to his low-fat diet. As the nurse explores further, she begins to sense that Anthony would like to discuss some aspect of his health that he does not know how to approach. The nurse investigates by stating, "Some of our clients tell us that it is difficult to adapt sexually after bypass surgery. What has this adjustment been like for you?" Anthony replies that he and his wife of 20 years enjoyed frequent sexual activity before his surgery but have had intercourse only a few times since his surgery. He seems saddened by this change in his sexual expression.

Nursing Diagnosis: Altered sexuality patterns related to coronary bypass surgery, as evidenced by client stating that frequency of sexual activity is much lower than it was preoperatively

Expected Outcome: Client will report greater sexual satisfaction at the next health assessment

Action	Rationale
1. Encourage client's verbalization regarding sexuality by maintaining professional demeanor, using scientific terms, and assuring him that your interest is based on your desire to provide professional assistance.	1. Many clients are not comfortable discussing sexuality unless they are assured that the health care provider is comfortable with the topic. (Example: Maintaining appropriate personal distance and eye contact with Anthony, the nurse might say something like, "You seem sad about this change in your sexual activity with your wife.")
2. Ensure privacy for the discussion by closing doors to a private room.	2. Clients should be provided with privacy to discuss all health matters, especially those of a sensitive nature such as sexuality. (Example: Although generalizations about the types of problems encountered may help the client feel less alone, each client should be reassured that his or her personal concerns will not be discussed with others by such statements as, "Everything we talk about in this professional relationship is completely confidential.")
3. Further assess the client's feelings about the identified problem.	3. Nursing intervention should always be based on thorough assessment, and the client's feelings regarding changed sexuality patterns are significant in directing the plan of nursing care. (Example: "Tell me more about your feelings about the decreased sexual activity you describe.")
4. Assess the client's perception of his partner's feelings about altered sexuality patterns, and involve the partner in further discussions if possible and if the client consents.	4. Sexuality patterns involve complex interactions between the client and his partner. Resolution of the problem is facilitated by involvement of both persons in discussions with health care professionals. (Example: "How is your wife feeling about these changes?)
5. Educate the client and his partner about the relationship of cardiac functioning and sexual activity.	5. Knowledge of the effects of sexual activity on cardiac functioning may alleviate fears of hurting the heart, which may be the cause of altered sexuality patterns. (Example: "If you would like, we can invite your wife to join us, and I can go over some information about how sexual activity affects your heart, the kinds of things some people are afraid of, and the kinds of activities that would be perfectly safe for you.")

SAMPLE NURSING CARE PLAN

THE CLIENT WHO HAS SUFFERED A MYOCARDIAL INFARCTION

(Continued)

Action	Rationale
6. Provide the client and his partner with written material describing cardiac function during sexual activity.	**6.** Clients often forget or misunderstand verbal instructions received in a fairly stressful situation. Written material allows the client to review the instructions as often as necessary in a comfortable environment. (Example: "I have some pamphlets that cover some common questions about sexual activity after bypass surgery. Please take these home so that you and your wife can go over them at your leisure. If you have other questions as you read, you can call me or we can discuss them at your next visit.")
7. Refer the client to coronary bypass support groups and/or further counseling.	**7.** Discussion with others who have had similar experiences is often helpful, because of a sense of connection and trust. Counseling by a psychologist or sex therapist may be needed in some cases. (Example: "Sometimes bypass support groups can be helpful in this area, as well as many other areas of life that change after surgery. Here is the phone number for a support group in your area. If this concern continues, I have other resources I can refer you to as needed.")
8. Document client concern and intervention provided.	**8.** Documentation of care increases continuity of care and describes care to third party payors.

Implementation

In clients with diagnoses related to sexuality, successful interventions require that nurses be aware of sexuality as an integral part of the person. Nurses must also provide a nonjudgmental presence, remembering that the person has a right to resolve sexual concerns according to his or her own values.

Two major roles of the nurse in implementing nursing care are to provide information and to create a supportive environment by listening to the client. The nurse needs to observe the client for unexpressed anxieties or feelings and be prepared to open the topic of sexuality as it applies to the client's situation.

Chronic Health Challenges

Chronic health challenges obviously span a broad spectrum of alterations, from things that may not be obvious to others to alterations that are the main focus of initial social interactions. A person with early-childhood onset of diabetes may experience some challenges in sexual functioning in adulthood as a result of the disease's effect on circulatory, nervous, and hormonal systems. This same individual, however, may have little alteration in sexual self-concept, because diabetes is not a disease that others readily see and focus attention on. Conversely, a person who has been blind since birth may have all other systems fully functional in adulthood. Yet learning about the self as

a sexual being is often difficult because of the different kinds of interactions one has with others as a result of blindness. These are examples of sexual dysfunctions of primarily physiological origins that may manifest in either physiological or psychosocial ways.

Acute-Onset Health Challenges

Acute-onset alterations in physical health may have different types of influences on a person's sexuality. Commonly, nurses are called on to assist persons in adapting to health alterations such as heart disease, cancer, diabetes, spinal cord injury, and a host of other injuries and diseases. Of course, it is not only the disease itself that influences a person's response but also his or her age, understanding of the disease, body parts affected, and previous sexuality. Nurses may encounter clients who have complaints of sexual dysfunction that are not directly related to the illness. In such cases, it may be that the individual never sought assistance with the dysfunction until he or she was already in contact with health professionals about another issue.

Nurses can be important to a person's understanding of how a disease or injury influences his or her sexuality by simply ensuring that the client fully understands the physiology of what has happened to him or her. This often clarifies misconceptions and defuses powerful myths. Another significant role that nurses play in helping clients adapt sexually to an injury or disease is to be an emotionally supportive sounding board for the client's feelings. Clients are often reluctant to talk to friends or family about such personal concerns but are helped greatly by the opportunity to verbalize their fears and worries. It is just as important for the nurse to listen as it is to talk. Impaired adjustment to changes in sexuality resulting from injury is a common diagnosis nurses might reach after assessing a client. Following are several examples of health alterations and the types of sexual concerns clients face.

Myocardial Infarction

Fogel and Lauver (1990) reviewed the literature related to reported sexual activity following myocardial infarction (MI). In general, clients who experienced MIs reported decreased sexual activity for as long as 4 years after the event. Initially, decreased sexual activity can be explained by a focus on matters of life and death. Survival of the self is a critical issue, rather than sexual expression or many other aspects of the pre-MI lifestyle. As time progresses, factors that frequently account for the continuation of sexual restraint include fear of causing another infarct or even bringing on sudden death, alteration in self-concept, and alteration in the relationship with the sexual partner. Often, partners share the same fears of hurting the MI client during sexual activity and take on the role of protector, setting limits on food intake, exercise, stress, and sexual activity. This protector role is often more parental than spousal, thus potentially undermining sexual feelings between the partners.

Education about normal cardiac function during sexual activity can do much to alleviate a client's fears about the possibility of having another MI as a result of sexual activity. Although studies conclusively indicate rather large increases in heart rate, respiratory rate, and blood pressure during orgasm, these increases are normal and can generally be as well tolerated as moderate exercise. Changes in vital signs during orgasm do not appear to be any different in MI clients than in the general population, nor are they any greater than vital sign changes brought on by stair climbing. Sometimes physicians use exercise tolerance in advising clients when to resume sexual activity. Another significant factor in cardiac safety during sexual activity is comfortable, familiar surroundings. In Fogel and Lauver's (1990) review, the literature indicated that men who have sexual intercourse with a partner other than a spouse are at greater risk of a cardiac incident than those engaging in marital sexual activity. Although the reports reviewed by Fogel and Lauver (1990) present conflicting information about vital sign changes with the MI client on top or on the bottom during sexual intercourse, it appears that the client being on the bottom demands less energy expenditure, perhaps decreasing oxygen demand. Nurses need to provide such information as part of discharge teaching when the client leaves the hospital and should be available on an ongoing basis for follow-up

discussion of postevent lifestyle, including sexual concerns.

Encouraging couples to communicate honestly with each other and helping them do so in a safe environment is often part of follow-up discussions. Because expression of affection and expression of sexual desire are often the same behaviors, such as touching, hugging, and kissing, partners often miscommunicate in this area. Perhaps a partner does not touch an MI client as frequently as he or she did before the event for fear that the touch will be interpreted as seductive or sexually demanding behavior. The client, however, may interpret this well-meaning restraint as a decrease in affection as a result of being "less of a person" after a cardiac event. (See Nursing Care Plan 37–1.)

Cancer

Cancer is another disease that often causes major changes in an individual's sexuality. As with cardiac problems, people's initial reaction to a diagnosis of any kind of cancer often focuses on matters of life and death, totally subverting all attention and energy away from sexuality. Many times, this continues for extended periods, depending largely on the severity of the diagnosis and the type of treatment involved. Nurses are often the most consistent caregivers as clients progress through different health care facilities to receive various types of treatments. Thus, the nurse is the most likely professional to address a client's concerns about sexuality as they change over time, depending on the course of the disease and the effects of treatments.

Cancer presently affects approximately one-third of the US population at some time in their lives. Because treatment modalities have improved in recent years, about half of those diagnosed with cancer experience long-term survival. Thus, these people are faced with the pleasant challenge of creating lives for themselves after treatment is finished. Consequently, Auchincloss (1991) believes that the most significant time for sexuality counseling is at the conclusion of oncology treatment. She states that if professionals never address sexuality, oncology clients "may even presume that the staff's silence means that their sex life is over" (p. 27). Although discussion of sexual concerns may not be all that is needed to alleviate the high rate of sexual dysfunction among cancer survivors, it is the beginning of assessing for problems that may need further referral. Sexual dysfunction after cancer may result from physical dysfunction of the genitals or of the neurological or circulatory systems, which may come about because of the disease or the treatment. Such dysfunctions may need to be treated medically. Other dysfunctions may arise in response to changes in self-concept or in relationships during the course of the disease and treatment. Such dysfunctions are best referred to a psychologist or sex therapist.

Breast cancer is perhaps the classic example of how the loss of a body part as a result of cancer affects a person's self-concept and thus sexuality. Fortunately, detection of and treatment for breast cancer have advanced in recent years, allowing more women to keep breasts that have been affected by cancer. However, many women still undergo loss of a body part, chemotherapy, radiation, and hormonal treatment, all of which may change body appearance, self-concept, and sexuality. Dest and Fisher (1994) state that nurses can help breast cancer clients minimize sexual dysfunction by good management of symptoms, such as vaginal dryness or nausea and vomiting, that may be caused by various types of treatment.

| CASE STUDY | A Woman Receiving Chemotherapy |

Ms. Hauser is a 38-year-old African-American woman who has been receiving chemotherapy after a simple unilateral mastectomy 3 months ago. She and her home health nurse have established a strong rapport over the months. One day, the nurse notices that Mr. and Ms. Hauser both seem tense, and Ms. Hauser is not her usual bright self. After Mr. Hauser excuses himself, the nurse asks Ms. Hauser if there is anything she would like to talk about. Ms. Hauser begins to cry, stating that she is not sure what is happening to the loving, intimate relationship she and her husband always enjoyed. Although he seemed to have adjusted to her mastectomy, and they resumed sexual activity several weeks after the surgery, he has recently expressed feelings of rejection because Ms. Hauser does not experience vaginal lubrication and complains of pain during intercourse. She states, "I know I feel the same way about him that I always have. I don't know why my body doesn't work the way it did before my surgery. Has my surgery changed the way I perform sexually?"

The nursing diagnosis in this case would be altered sexuality patterns related to chemotherapy-induced vaginal dryness. In this situation, the nurse can assist in several ways:

- Provide information about the cause of vaginal dryness to the client.
- Offer to provide the same information to the partner if the client desires.
- Provide information about the use of water-based vaginal lubrication.
- Provide further opportunity for the client to express her feeling about changes in sexuality related to health alteration.
- Evaluate by seeking information from the client regarding the problem at the next visit.

Spinal Cord Injury

Bertosa, Cellura, Pierce, and Rothacker (1993) state that approximately 12,000 Americans are permanently disabled by spinal cord injury (SCI) each year. Such individuals obviously require unique nursing care for extended periods. Many persons affected by SCI learn to deal with their disabilities quite independently and live relatively normal lives, except for the need to use certain equipment and techniques for mobility. Others are affected, either physically or emotionally, in a way that almost totally curtails their participation in an active life. The sexual needs of persons with SCI thus vary tremendously, depending on the degree of injury and the person's adaptation to the injury. Some things that need to be considered are the following.

Although most men with SCI are no longer able to maintain erections or impregnate a woman, some men may be able to have erections and participate in intercourse by having penile implants inserted. Many women with SCI continue to have normal fertility. Consequently, making choices about contraception continues to be a concern. Oral contraceptives are generally contraindicated because of the inability to feel signs of thrombophlebitis, which may be a risk factor secondary to immobility. Nurses working in obstetrics may have the opportunity to assist a woman with SCI during pregnancy and childbirth. Generally, such clients need more intensive bladder care, assistance with bowel care, meticulous attention to skin care, and assistance with positioning.

Although most clients with SCI are asensory in the genital area, they are not asexual. The psychosocial aspects of sexuality remain intact. They still need to be accepted as sexual beings by themselves and others. Although the stress of adapting to such a major injury and lifestyle change may cause relationship difficulties, the SCI itself is no barrier to maintaining or initiating sexually intimate relationships. In fact, some clients with SCI have reported sexual responsiveness in unaffected body parts, providing them with physical sensations of sexual arousal and satisfaction, as well as the ability to feel close to their partners during sexual activity (Masters *et al.*, 1985).

One way that nurses can help clients with SCI is by educating the population in general about the facts of SCI so that others have a more factually based perception of people with SCI. Common myths about disabled persons that foster lowered self-esteem include that those with SCI are asexual, that disabled persons should have relationships only with other disabled persons, and that disabled persons are childlike (Masters *et al.*, 1985). Nurses involved in any kind of community education regarding disability may dispel such myths by explaining the anatomy and physiology involved in SCI.

Issues Related to Sexuality

Pregnancy

Full discussion of human conception, gestation, and parturition is beyond the scope of this text. However, a brief overview of pregnancy is provided.

For conception to occur, a mature ovum must be fertilized by a mature sperm during the approximately 8 to 24 hours the ovum is viable after being released

1130 UNIT VII ✦ APPLICATION OF THE NURSING PROCESS TO PSYCHOSOCIOCULTURAL NEEDS

from the ovary. Fertilization is usually accomplished by the male ejaculating into the vagina and the sperm swimming through the uterus and into the fallopian tube in which the ovum is traveling. The fertilized egg, called a zygote, is the beginning of embryonic life. The genetic sex of the individual is determined at this time by whether the sperm that fertilized the ovum was carrying an X chromosome (female) or a Y chromosome (male). Thus, the sex of an infant is determined by the father.

Once fertilization has occurred, the zygote begins dividing into multiple cells that are at first undifferentiated from one another. (Differentiation of cell type begins early during gestation, however.) The mass of cells travels through the fallopian tube to the uterus in about 4 days and soon after attaches itself to the uterine lining, from which it obtains nourishment. Together, the ball of cells and the uterine lining create the placenta, the organ that sustains fetal life for the duration of pregnancy, which is an average of 266 days (Masters *et al.*, 1985).

Pregnancy is divided into three trimesters of approximately 13 weeks each. The experiences of the pregnant woman, as well as the development of the fetus, vary greatly during each trimester. For the fetus, the first trimester is considered critical, because it is during this time that organogenesis occurs. The second trimester is when fetal movement usually becomes strong enough to be perceived by the mother. The third trimester is one of rapid weight gain for the fetus.

For the expectant mother, the first trimester is often a time of numerous physical complaints, such as nausea, and a time of ambivalent emotions. The second trimester is often when pregnant women feel the best physically and experience fetal movement, giving the pregnancy a greater sense of reality. During the third trimester, like the first, the woman is often plagued by a variety of physical discomforts and is impatient for the pregnancy to end.

Although the pregnant woman and the fetus may be the individuals most directly affected in creation of new life, other family members are involved in and respond to pregnancy as it progresses. A wide range of individual and cultural variations among expectant fathers, grandparents, and siblings is observed among humans.

Abortion

Abortion is defined as the termination of pregnancy before the fetus reaches the age of viability, which is typically considered to be about 20 weeks (Gorrie *et al.*, 1994).

✦ **Spontaneous.** Spontaneous abortion is typically called miscarriage in lay terminology. Although this type of abortion has received little attention compared with therapeutic abortion, it is quite significant as a matter of sexual self-esteem. The incidence of spontaneous abortion is estimated to be as high as 20% of all

pregnancies (Bennett, 1992). The cause of many spontaneous abortions is unknown, leading to much fear among parents that they may have done something, or not done something, that led to the abortion. They may also fear the occurrence of spontaneous abortions in the future. The role of the nurse is to provide emotional support in the form of an empathic presence. There are no right or wrong statements to make in all cases. The nurse must sensitively assess the family's state and respond accordingly. Avoiding or denying the situation is not therapeutic.

✦ **Elective.** Elective abortion is intentional termination of pregnancy by medical or self-induced means. Elective abortion became legal in the United States in 1973 after the *Roe versus Wade* Supreme Court decision. Most individuals have rather strong feelings about elective (or therapeutic) abortion. One of the most important things that a nurse can do regarding this issue is to strive constantly for clarity about his or her own feelings about abortion. This is one area in which nurses may give nonverbal messages that conflict with verbal ones. The nurse may verbally state that he or she is able to provide unbiased care to a woman seeking an abortion or who has had an abortion, but lack of eye contact or appropriate touch may indicate that the nurse does not feel completely accepting of the client.

A nurse who chooses to work in family planning centers or abortion clinics must keep in mind that the decision to terminate a pregnancy is not an easy one for a woman to make. Sensitive listening and counseling are imperative to assist the woman to make a decision that is congruent with her beliefs, values, and lifestyle.

In addition to psychosocial aspects of nursing care, the woman needs expert physical care. Many women take for granted the safety of therapeutic abortion, yet there is risk of hemorrhage, infection, and ill effects from anesthesia. The nurse must assess for signs of the development of complications. Because most abortions are performed on an outpatient basis and the woman or her family is the primary care provider soon after the procedure, education about signs of complications that require attention is essential.

Abortion is both a women's and men's issue, because it is men who impregnate women. Perhaps one of the nurse's most powerful roles in this area is to provide education and other forms of empowerment that free men and women to behave in sexually responsible ways. Taking responsibility for one's sexual behavior can lead to fewer unwanted pregnancies, thus decreasing the demand for elective abortions. Family planning information and services are readily available to most Americans.

Contraception

Contraception, or family planning, is the act of doing something to decrease or obliterate the possibility of pregnancy occurring. Table 37–3 shows various types of contraception, their effectiveness rates, major advantages, and major disadvantages. Figure 37–3 shows a variety of contraceptive devices.

Many of the contraceptive methods can be categorized as barrier methods or hormonal methods. Generally, the barrier methods are more closely associated with sexual activity than are hormonal methods. Hormonal methods are not directly associated with inter-

course; the hormones are in the body whether or not the woman is sexually active.

The primary advantage of some barrier methods is that they may provide protection against the transmission of sexually transmitted diseases (STDs). Hormonal methods provide no protection from STDs. This may be an important consideration in a person's choice of contraceptive method. When counseling clients about family planning, it is important to reinforce the differ-

Table 37–3

EFFECTIVENESS, ADVANTAGES, AND DISADVANTAGES OF CONTRACEPTIVE TYPES

TYPE	EFFECTIVENESS	ADVANTAGES	DISADVANTAGES
Cervical cap	82%	Smaller than diaphragm Requires less spermicide No pressure on bladder Remains in place longer	Sizes limited May dislodge during intercourse Initial cost More difficult to insert than diaphragm Requires MD or NP to fit Must be refitted annually
Condom	88%	Protects against STDs Inexpensive Available Discreet	Cultural beliefs about use Must be checked for intactness
Depo-Provera (medroxyprogesterone acetate)	99%	Disassociated with sexual activity Requires thought only every 3 months	Physical side effects Must receive injection every 3 months
Diaphragm	82%	Can be inserted several hours before intercourse Few side effects	Initial cost Requires MD or NP to fit May cause pressure on bladder Requires repeated application of spermicide May be difficult to insert or remove
Intrauterine device	97%	Disassociated with sexual activity Requires thought only once a month	Initial cost Potential side effects May be spontaneously expelled
Natural family planning	80%	No side effects	Requires high levels of education and commitment
Norplant (levonorgestrel)	99.9%	Disassociated with sexual activity Requires no thought for 5 years	May cause side effects Insertion costly, requires MD or NP, and may cause discomfort Removal may be difficult
Oral contraceptive (pill)	97%	Disassociated with sexual activity	Must be taken regularly May cause side effects that are uncomfortable or dangerous
Spermicide	79%	Low cost Availability May provide some protection against some STDs	Must be used at time of intercourse
Sponge	72%	Few side effects Availability May provide some protection against some STDs	Must be used at time of intercourse
Sterilization	99.7%	Requires no further thought	Permanent in many cases Requires surgery with some pain and potential complications
Abstinence	100%	No cost Assured result	Lack of sexual intimacy in a relationship

*Effectiveness rates are based on actual user rates of effectiveness rather than theoretical rates, which are generally higher.
Data from Fogel, C., & Lauver, D. (1990); Gorrie, T., McKinney, E., & Murray, S. (1994).

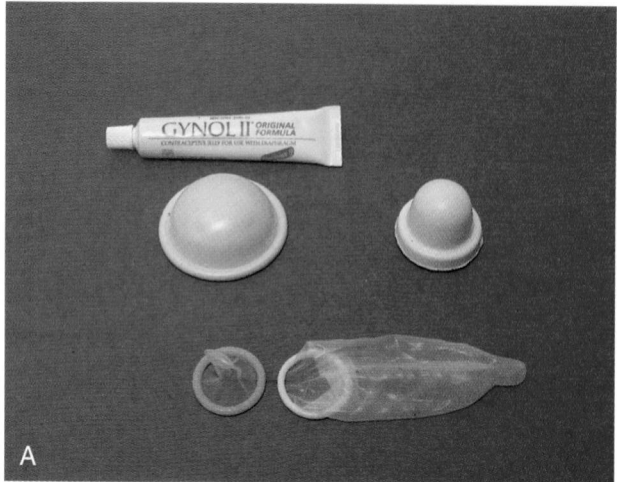

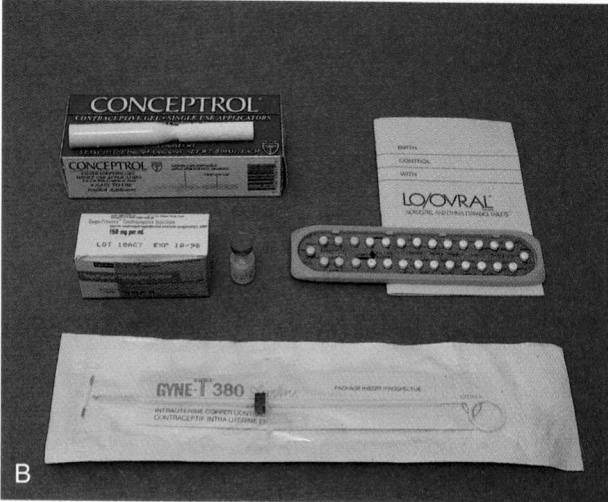

✦ **Figure 37–3**
Contraceptive devices. *A,* A diaphragm with gel *(top left),* a cervical cap *(top right),* and two condoms, one rolled and one unrolled. *B,* Contraceptive gel with applicator *(top left);* one variety of oral contraceptives, "the pill" *(top right);* Depo-Provera (Upjohn, Kalamazoo, Michigan) (box and vial; medroxyprogesterone acetate); and an IUD.

ence between the prevention of pregnancy and the prevention of STDs.

There are several considerations that a woman, or a couple, must keep in mind when choosing the best contraceptive method at a given time in life. Effectiveness is often the first factor people think of when considering different methods of contraception. However, there are other factors that may influence the choice. Some women may be unwilling to subject their bodies to the potential side effects of hormonal contraceptives, even though the effectiveness rate is generally very high. Other women may be interested in nonpharmacological methods but may have difficulty with the idea of touching their genitals. These women may find barrier methods such as cervical caps, diaphragms, or female condoms unacceptable. Complete assessment of the client's needs and feelings is essential in providing contraceptive counseling.

✦ **Cervical Cap.** Cervical caps are small latex cups that fit over the cervix to prevent sperm from reaching the fallopian tube, where fertilization usually takes place. Cervical caps must be used in conjunction with spermicides but do not require reapplication with each intercourse. One of the advantages of a cervical cap is that the small size allows a woman to leave it in place for longer than a diaphragm, without the risk of bladder irritation or toxic shock syndrome. The primary disadvantage is that a woman must plan ahead. First, she must be fitted for the cervical cap by a physician or nurse practitioner (NP). Many sexually active teenagers have difficulty with this aspect of contraception. Some women find planning ahead a deterrent to the enjoyment of spontaneous sexual expression. Others find manipulating their own genitals distasteful. Learning how to insert and remove the cervical cap requires thorough education and some practice.

✦ **Condom.** Condoms are the only form of contraceptive presently available for male use. In recent years, female condoms have also been developed. Although one might expect condom use to increase as the population becomes more educated about STDs, especially human immunodeficiency virus (HIV), some studies show that many people are continuing to engage in sexual intercourse without protection. DeBuono and colleagues (1990) report that the majority of sexually active college women are still not insisting on condom use on a regular basis. The incidence of condom use actually decreased among those having more than 10 sexual partners. Smith and Lathrop (1993) attribute the high incidence of unprotected sexual activity to a sense of denial among the population.

There continues to be a strong cultural conviction that intercourse with condoms is so unpleasurable as to be almost not worth having. Nurses are in a crucial position to help fight this misconception, which could prove fatal for some people. Education about how to properly place a condom on the penis and appropriate lubricants to use can increase the use of condoms.

✦ **Diaphragm.** Diaphragms, like cervical caps, are a barrier method that the woman inserts into the vagina so that it covers the cervix, thus blocking the entry of sperm into the fallopian tube. Some women experience an allergic reaction to the material from which the diaphragm is made and may experience bladder irritation and subsequent urinary tract infections as a result of diaphragm use. It is recommended that diaphragms not be left in place for longer than approximately 6 to 8 hours at a time. Because the woman should insert the diaphragm shortly before intercourse, it may interfere with spontaneous sexual activity.

✦ **Depo-Provera (Upjohn, Kalamazoo, Michigan).** Depo-Provera (medroxyprogesterone acetate) is an injection of progesterone hormones that a woman can receive every 3 months to provide highly effective contraception during the entire 3-month period. Because there are no estrogens, which can be associated with serious cardiovascular side effects, Depo-Provera is considered safe for most healthy women in their childbearing years. Many women experience some side effects, such as bleeding at irregular intervals during the cycle. Some women are hesitant to place a long-acting hormone in their bodies, but others enthusiastically embrace the high rate of effectiveness of this method, which requires little thought or action.

◆ **Intrauterine Device (IUD).** IUDs have come and gone out of favor with health care professionals and with consumers over the last generation. Although they are highly effective and require little effort on the part of the user, they sometimes cause side effects such as cramping or irregular bleeding. IUDs available in the United States in the 1990s include copper and progestin types, which have been shown to be much safer than earlier types of IUDs. The primary teaching that nurses need to provide for IUD users is that they must ensure that the device has not been expelled. Because this is most likely to occur during menses, the woman should make it a habit to feel for the IUD strings in her vagina after each period.

◆ **Natural Family Planning (NFP).** NFP consists of several different systems of fertility control without mechanical or chemical intervention. Some women use all aspects of NFP. NFP requires a high degree of commitment from the woman or the couple, because the woman must pay close attention to changes in her body, and sexual intercourse cannot occur during fertile times. Changes that the woman notes include changes in her basal body temperature (BBT), vaginal secretions, and moods and other feelings; she also keeps a menstrual diary, noting the dates of each period.

BBT, which must be taken immediately upon awakening in the morning, rises approximately 0.5 to 1° at the time of ovulation, after perhaps a slight decrease in BBT just before ovulation. The BBT remains at the elevated state until just before the next period, or longer if pregnancy occurs. Cervical mucus changes from thick to thin and elastic during the time of ovulation. (The ability to stretch the mucus between the fingers like egg white is called spinnbarkeit.) Other changes that a woman may notice around the time of ovulation include one-sided pain called mittelschmerz, increased appetite, or increased libido. Additionally, if a woman has regular cycles, she may estimate that ovulation will occur 14 to 16 days before the anticipated date of the next period. Intercourse is not considered safe for several days before and after ovulation. Although the ovum generally remains viable for less than 24 hours, sperm may still be alive in the female reproductive tract for 72 hours after the last ejaculate.

Lack of sleep, infection, certain medications, or sexual intercourse may alter temperature patterns, the cervical mucus, and other bodily experiences. Many people find it difficult to practice abstinence during fertile periods. It has many advantages, but NFP is not

one of the more effective methods of contraception for persons without high commitment.

◆ **Norplant.** Norplant (levonorgestrel) is a relatively new method of hormonal contraception in the United States. Six small rods with time-released progesterone are implanted in the woman's body, usually on the underside of the upper arm. This surgical procedure is done under local anesthestic in an outpatient setting. Most women report minor bruising and soreness for several days after insertion. This type of contraception provides highly effective protection against pregnancy for 5 years. The obvious advantage for women who are fairly certain that they do not want to have children in that time frame is that Norplant requires no further thought or action for 5 years after it is implanted. Although it is not associated with serious side effects, it does cause irregular bleeding in many women during the first months of use.

◆ **Oral Contraceptives Pill (OCP).** Oral contraceptives are generally a combination of estrogens and progestins. They come in a variety of combinations and strengths, so that even if a woman is unable to tolerate one prescription, she may be able to safely and comfortably use a different preparation. Some preparations require that a pill be taken every day of the month; others require that the user take one pill a day for 21 days and have 7 unmedicated days in each cycle. The pill is a popular contraceptive choice for many women because of its high effectiveness rate and short duration of action. Should a woman decide to become pregnant, she can generally do so as soon as she discontinues use of the pill. Pills do, however, have a number of side effects for many women. The most serious side effect, which makes pill use contraindicated in some women, is cardiovascular risk. Women with histories of stroke, hypertension, or thrombophlebitis are generally not considered candidates for OCPs. Because the risk of various types of cancers in women over age 35 who smoke and who use OCPs is higher than in the general population, many health care practitioners recommend other types of contraceptives for smokers in this age group.

Because use of OCPs requires daily action on the part of the client, thorough education is a high-priority nursing intervention. A nurse working with family planning clients must be an expert in medication interactions, so that accurate information can be given to clients. Many antibiotics decrease the effectiveness of OCPs, and women should be encouraged to use a back-up method, such as condoms, during any cycle in which they take antibiotics.

◆ **Sterilization.** Sterilization for women is called tubal ligation, and it is a surgical procedure in which the fallopian tubes are cut and the ends sealed so that future ova cannot reach the uterus (Fig. 37–4A). It is a relatively simple procedure, often done laparoscopically on an outpatient basis.

Vasectomy is the surgical procedure that sterilizes a man. This procedure cuts the vas deferens so that sperm cannot be ejaculated in seminal fluid (Fig. 37–4B). This procedure, like tubal ligation, is done on an outpatient basis, and the client can generally return to normal activities within several days, as can a woman after tubal ligation. One significant difference between vasectomy and tubal ligation is when they become effective. Tubal ligation is effective immediately. Vasectomy may not be effective for a month or more,

because sperm that are already in the reproductive tract at the time of the procedure will remain alive.

At the time of a sterilization procedure, a nurse must provide the client with thorough teaching about the procedure and about self-care after the surgery. Just as important is the nurse's role in providing counseling to individuals or couples considering sterilization as a method of contraception. Although modern techniques have made it possible to reverse both tubal ligations and vasectomies, it is much more complex than the original sterilization procedure and does not guarantee fertility. Consequently, clients considering sterilization must be fully informed about the probable permanence of the decision. People also frequently have questions about how sterilization may influence their sexual functioning, as well as their general health. Sterilization affects only the ability to reproduce. It does not alter a person's sexual feelings or performance. It also has not been demonstrated to have any significant effect on general health.

Although many people make an intellectual decision not to have children in the future, the loss of the capacity to reproduce may cause mild depression in some people, particularly if that individual has defined his or her personal self-worth in terms of reproductive capability. The nurse should help individuals anticipate how sterilization may influence their self-concept.

✦ **Other Methods of Contraception.** There are a few other techniques for decreasing the possibility of pregnancy that should be mentioned. None of these techniques is discussed in depth because of the low effectiveness rates. The first is coitus interruptus, or withdrawal. In this method, the man withdraws the penis from the vagina before ejaculation. This method obviously requires a great deal of awareness and control on the part of the man. Even when used expertly, however, it is not considered a reliable form of contraception, because some men express small amounts of seminal fluid before actual ejaculation.

Another unreliable form of child spacing is breast-feeding. Although breast-feeding does elevate prolactin levels, which interferes with the normal hormonal cycle to some degree, most American women do not nurse their infants often enough to keep prolactin levels high enough to prevent ovulation. Because there is a common belief that nursing a baby is a reliable form of family planning, it is imperative that maternity nurses educate their lactating clients that it is not an effective method.

Another form of contraception, usually reserved for victims of sexual assault, is the oral postcoital contraceptive pill. It must be used within 24 hours of intercourse and is associated with a high incidence of congenital anomalies if conception is not prevented.

The last form of contraception mentioned is abstinence from sexual intercourse. This, of course, has a 100% effectiveness rate. However, it is not a choice that many adults make for long periods in their lives.

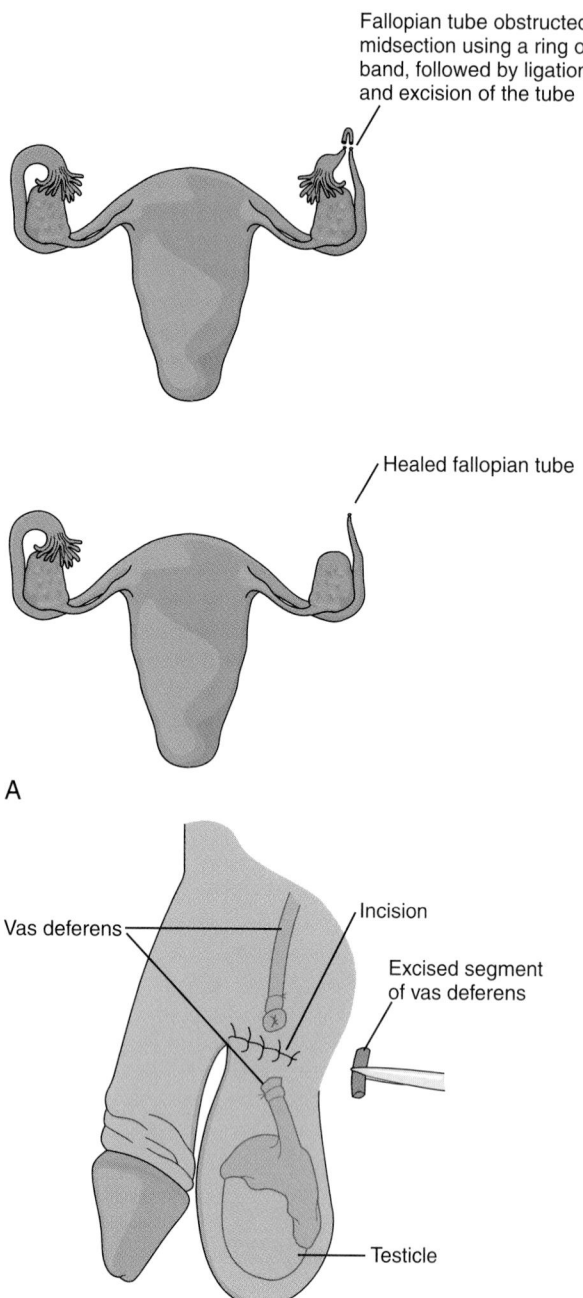

Fallopian tube obstructed in midsection using a ring or band, followed by ligation and excision of the tube

Healed fallopian tube

A

Vas deferens

Incision

Excised segment of vas deferens

Testicle

B

✦ **Figure 37–4**
Sterilization techniques. *A,* Female—tubal ligation. *B,* Male—vasectomy.

For this reason, it is considered to have a low user effectiveness rate.

Infertility

Infertility is defined as the inability to conceive after having regular sexual intercourse for 1 year without the use of contraceptives. Infertility can be primary, meaning that conception has never occurred, or secondary, meaning that conception has occurred in the past but does not easily recur (Gorrie *et al.,* 1994). Although this is the formal definition used by most authorities on infertility, many infertility specialists include in their practices those who conceive but are unable to carry a pregnancy to term. Another leniency in the definition is that, depending on the woman's age, infertility may be diagnosed, evaluated, and treated after only 6 months of unsuccessful attempts to conceive.

The incidence of people seeking infertility treatment appears to be rising. Presently, approximately 15% of all couples desiring to have a child meet the criteria for infertility. Suggested causes for the apparent rise in infertility include the incidence of STDs, which may cause pelvic inflammatory disease or other reproductive problems; lifestyle behaviors such as smoking and other drug use; environmental factors; or postponement of childbearing until the middle adult years.

Perhaps the greatest contributor to the rise in people seeking infertility treatment is the rise in awareness of new technology. A generation ago, childless couples had few options. Couples in the 1990s have numerous methods of assistance available to them (Gorrie *et al.,* 1994). The group of clients receiving infertility treatment is relatively homogeneous. Most infertility clients are middle- or upper-class couples, because infertility treatment is expensive and is viewed as elective health care.

✦ **Causes.** Causes of infertility are myriad and complex. It is estimated that biological factors in the man account for 35% of infertility, biological factors in the woman account for 35% of infertility, and a combination of factors in the man and the woman accounts for 30% of infertility. Twenty percent of infertility cases are never attributed to a specific cause (Gorrie *et al.,* 1994). Although problems that require dramatic, highly technological intervention have received the greatest media attention for about 20 years, many couples are infertile as a result of minor problems that can be corrected with minor changes in lifestyle. For example, men who wear constrictive garments around the genitals may be forcing the testes close to the body, thereby killing sperm with the high body temperature. Change in style of underclothing may be all that is needed to enhance fertility. One simple cause of infertility in women is that body fat is lower than optimal to achieve and maintain pregnancy. If a woman increases calorie consumption and/or decreases excessive exercise to achieve a higher percentage of body fat, pregnancy may soon follow. Nurses play a major role in the health care of couples experiencing infertility.

✦ **Health Needs.** Because childbearing is still the norm for married couples in the United States, there is often a great deal of subtle but powerful social pressure to have a baby. This, combined with what may be a natural instinct to reproduce the species, can lead to self-esteem disturbance, impaired verbal communication, social isolation, and ineffective individual coping for those who are not easily able to accomplish reproduction. As was mentioned in the discussion of sterilization, for some individuals, the matter of choice may be significant. Even if having a baby is not the ultimate life goal, most individuals want to know that they have a choice about this important aspect of life. Furthermore, being fully healthy and functional is highly valued in U.S. society. If one is not able to function like other members of the society in this sensitive area, that alone may cause self-esteem problems in an individual. Depending on the degree to which a person defines himself or herself as male or female by the ability to reproduce, infertility may be a minor problem or a major life crisis. Those for whom infertility treatment is quickly effective may be left with little or no effect from the experience of being infertile. Those who require more extensive treatment or who perceive their infertility as chronic are more likely to view infertility as a major factor in life (Sandelowski, 1994).

Because causes of infertility are often difficult to diagnose, one of the big psychological factors in infertility treatment is the avoidance of blame. Biological factors are generally things over which individuals do not have a great deal of control. Blame also deteriorates self-esteem and healthy relationships, thus further increasing health care demands. Nurses are often in prime positions to educate people about infertility, thus alleviating the blame and guilt that may arise from myths and misconceptions.

✦ **Nursing Role.** Nurses can play a significant role in facilitating and clarifying communication between partners. Many communities that have treatment facilities for infertility also offer support groups for people experiencing infertility. Nurses are frequently the facilitators of such groups. Nurses who embrace this role must be highly knowledgeable about the causes of infertility, treatments available, and therapeutic ways to support couples during treatment, which can last for years. With adequate education, nurses can provide couples with realistic hope without deluding them. Nurses may need to provide bereavement support to couples who lose a pregnancy or who eventually lose their dream of ever having their own child. In cases in which it is medically unlikely that a couple will successfully reproduce, nurses need to be prepared to provide adoption counseling to those who are willing to consider that option. Last, nurses who facilitate infertility support groups must be keenly aware of their own personal feelings and experiences about fertility and infertility.

Homosexuality

Up to this point in the chapter, sexual behavior has been described primarily in heterosexual terms — that is, sexual interaction between people of the opposite sex. This bias has been taken because it represents the predominant type of sexual expression and because heterosexuality accomplishes reproduction. However, in recent years, our culture has become more open to the reality that some people's sexual preference is for the same sex.

Homosexuality is the preference for sexual affiliation with members of one's own sex — males prefer males, and females prefer females. Homosexuality, or lesbianism among females, continues to be one of the most emotionally charged aspects of human sexuality. This is perhaps best typified by the public debates that raged when President Clinton suggested that homosexuals be allowed in the military in the early 1990s. Popular attention to acquired immune deficiency syndrome (AIDS) since the mid-1980s has brought increased public focus on the matter of homosexuality. AIDS was first identified exclusively as a "gay disease," because it was first reported only among homosexual men. The prevalence of AIDS among homosexual men, especially early in the epidemic, fueled the fire of prejudice against this group. However, the cohesive response of the homosexual community to this fatal disease has increased self-acceptance and self-esteem among many homosexuals and has put homosexuals in a more favorable light with many other groups.

Homosexuality has existed in all cultures throughout recorded history. In many cultures prior to the Middle Ages in Europe, homosexuality was not seen as a societal issue at all. Based on paintings and writings, it appears that homosexuality was not viewed as an aberration or a moral problem in many ancient cultures (Masters *et al.,* 1985).

Because being homosexual is considered unacceptable by many Americans, some homosexuals go to great extremes to deny and hide their sexual preference. Therefore, it is impossible to estimate accurately the number of homosexuals in the population. However, estimates indicate that there are more homosexual men than homosexual women. Although some homosexuals dress in clothing designed for the opposite sex, most do not. Dressing in clothing designed for the opposite sex is transvestism and is not the same as homosexuality.

There is also a group of individuals who are attracted to and engage in sexual activity with both sexes. These people are called bisexual.

✦ **Causes.** The cause or causes of homosexuality are unknown. Theories include biological or chemical imbalances, childhood experiences or traumas, or choice. Because the cause of homosexuality is not known, it is not known whether an individual has a choice about sexual preference. In general, studies have not demonstrated that familial patterns have much influence on the development of homosexuality. Some research has supported the idea that sexual preference can be predicted by the play preferences of preschool children; that is, boys who like to play with dolls and tea sets may be likely to be homosexual adults, and girls who choose trucks and toy soldiers may have a higher rate of lesbianism in adulthood. Other research, however, has shown that some individuals give no outward sign of sexual preference until well into adult life. Some people begin life as heterosexuals and "switch" sometime during adulthood, thus negating the theory that early childhood behaviors shape or even predict adult sexual preference (Masters *et al.,* 1985).

✦ **Health Needs.** The particular health needs of a homosexual depend on many other lifestyle choices. Just as in the heterosexual population, if an individual chooses to have unprotected sex with multiple partners, the risk of STDs, including AIDS, is a high-priority nursing problem. If, however, a homosexual individual practices safe sex, especially with only one partner, the risk of STDs for that person is not significantly different from that of a heterosexual practicing the same sexual protections.

One thing that does differ for homosexuals, however, is their sense of acceptance and trust in the health care system. Having been victimized by prejudice in the US culture for generations, it may be difficult for a homosexual to feel comfortable sharing his or her true identity and lifestyle with health care professionals. Working with homosexuals is one of the situations in which nurses must be aware of their own feelings.

Other ways in which nursing care of homosexuals may differ from nursing care of heterosexuals is that the constellation of significant others may differ. If, for instance, a homosexual's family of origin does not accept the individual, they may not be present during a health crisis. Such an individual, however, may have built a family of close friends who take on the supportive roles usually played by blood kin in health crises. It is imperative that nurses, who are often the monitors of visitors in health care settings, be open-minded in their definitions of "family." The nurse may also be called on to assist individuals with issues of self-concept and self-esteem, especially if the person is in the process of discovering and accepting his or her own homosexuality.

Sexual Abuse

Sexual abuse is a broad topic, defined in different ways because of the variety of behaviors it may cover. For purposes of this text, sexual abuse is defined as any sexual activity perpetrated by one person on another person who is either unwilling to participate in that sexual activity or who is incapable of making an informed decision about that sexual activity. Sexual abuse can occur between two adults, between an adult and a child, or between two children.

In the US culture, where sexuality is more openly discussed now than a generation ago, it seems that the incidence of sexual abuse, especially of children, is increasing. Sexual abuse is a form of violence, and violence is increasing in our culture, perhaps at least partly owing to the increase in the abuse of drugs that alter our perceptions of reality and free our inhibitions about expressing violent feelings.

Another reason that we may be experiencing a rise in the reporting of sexual abuse is that individuals are seeking psychological care more often for unrelated factors. In the process of therapy, many women regain memories of childhood sexual abuse that they had previously been unaware of. Loftus, Polonsky, and Fullilove (1994) report that of the 105 women studied during their treatment for substance abuse, 54% reported having been victims of childhood sexual abuse. Nineteen percent of these women indicated that they had experienced long periods of time when they did not remember the abuse.

✦ **Child Sexual Abuse.** Sexual abuse of children is most often perpetrated on girls by adult men, although sexual abuse of girls and boys by both men and women does occur (Masters *et al.,* 1985). Those who engage in sex with children are predominantly male. The majority are family or friends of the children they molest. When sexual encounters occur between family members who are either biologically or legally related, it is called incest. The psychological impact of a female child being sexually assaulted by a stepfather whom she trusts and views as a father may be as traumatic as sexual activity with a biological father.

Although physical force is often used, psychological coercion is most common. One of the worst ramifications reported by victims of childhood sexual abuse is the sense that they were totally alone in the world, as their molesters insisted that they divulge the secret to no one. De Chesnay and others (1988) identified "maternal distance" in 96% of the abusive families studied, indicating that children did not perceive that they had access to their mothers to protect them from abuse. Interestingly, the investigators also found that among incestuous families, those who were most geographically stable manifested the longest duration of abuse. They referred to these families as "pillars of the community," who serve as evidence that sexual abuse occurs in all socioeconomic groups.

Sexual abuse may occur at any age and take any form. Often the adult perpetrator exposes himself or herself to the child and may describe sexual fantasies to the child. Although such behavior does not do the physical harm that actual forced intercourse does, the

COMMUNITY BASED CARE

RAPE

Caring for women who have experienced sexual assaults is a challenge for nurses. It is essential that rape survivors be seen in the emergency department or rape crisis center as soon as possible following the assault, both to assist the victim and to obtain evidence. It is also important to provide privacy during physical examinations and to ask rape survivors to repeat details of the incident only one time. Describing the assault is usually very traumatic.

Typically, nurses who participate in both physical and emotional assessment and provide related interventions receive specialized training. Such training involves crisis intervention for the client and handling evidence for future prosecution. Care includes

1. Physical concerns: Identify the location and extent of any bruises, abrasions, or lacerations, especially on the face and neck. The client's clothing may be torn, dirty, and stained; it should be saved as evidence.

2. Laboratory tests: Include a blood test for human immunodeficiency virus and cultures and smears to assess for infection and sperm. The "human immunodeficiency virus" blood test should be repeated in 6 months.

3. Emotional concerns: Assess the rape survivor's feelings and emotions carefully. Rape survivors experience emotional stress related to an intrusion into a very personal, sensitive part of their sexual identity. They are psychologically fragile and will probably experience feelings of fear, guilt, and humiliation. Rape is an act of violence that can have lasting effects, especially on the woman's sense of security. Rape survivors should be referred for counseling as soon as possible.

It is important that the rape survivor reports the assault to the police immediately.

psychological trauma of being forced to participate in an activity that the child instinctively feels is wrong may be lifelong. One nursing implication related to childhood abuse is that clients may need ongoing support, counseling, and therapy, even if they begin to receive treatment fairly soon after the sexual abuse occurs. Unfortunately, because many families in which sexual abuse occurs are dysfunctional in other ways, it is not common for the child to receive immediate assistance. Warren and associates (1994) report that being sexually abused is often a major precursor to youths running away from home.

Patterns of incest may vary from a one-time incident to frequently repeated episodes over most of the child's life. The extent to which each individual is affected by the pattern of abuse depends on many factors, including the severity of the abuse, the timeliness of intervention, and other factors of support or devaluation that the child experiences during childhood.

✦ **Adult Sexual Abuse.** Adult sexual abuse involves two adults, but the element of force or coercion is the same as with child sexual abuse. One adult physically, psychologically, or economically forces another adult to engage in unwanted sexual activity. This may take the form of a male employer insisting that a female employee tolerate sexually explicit language (sexual harassment), or it may be a brutal physical sexual attack.

Sexual Harassment

Sexual harassment in the workplace or educational setting is strictly forbidden by law. However, the economic realities that many women face often make reporting sexual harassment extremely difficult. Economic opportunity and security are still considerably less for women than for men. Therefore, many women are financially unable to be without a job for any period of time while litigation is in progress. Further, a woman who prosecutes a sexually harassing employer may fear that she will be labeled as a "squealer" and will have great difficulty gaining future employment.

Rape

The most common type of sexual abuse talked about in our culture is rape, which is commonly defined as the forced insertion of the penis into the vagina without consent (Masters et al., 1985). Although this is still the legal definition in many states, rape is often more broadly defined to include forced anal or oral penetration. It is estimated that one in four women will be the victim of rape sometime in her life (Lonsway & Fitzgerald, 1994). The exact legal definition of rape varies from state to state, and the definition may be critical in determining the legal outcome if a victim presses charges against the perpetrator. The legal management of rape has gotten significantly better over the last generation but still requires improvement. Nurses are playing a critical role in changes that make women more willing and more able to take effective legal action against rapists. Many hospital emergency rooms have specially trained nurses who provide primary care to all rape victims who come to the facility. These nurses are able to provide expert physical care and highly sensitive emotional care, as well as to obtain physical evidence to be used later in court.

Rape-Trauma Syndrome

Much has been written about rape-trauma syndrome, which is a type of posttraumatic stress disorder. Although there is much individual variation in the pattern of feelings women experience after rape, typical responses include extreme fear, generalized anxiety, depression, and somatic complaints. This syndrome, if treated by trained professionals, resolves for many women between 6 months and 2 years following the event. Again, as with child abuse, reporting of the incident and seeking treatment are often not done. Consequently, many women who experience rape suffer at length.

The most critical thing for nurses to remember when dealing with rape victims is to be nonjudgmental. The implication that rape is at least partially the woman's fault is most acute in cases of "date rape." Kahn, Mathie, and Torgler (1994) found that almost half of a group of college women who had experienced nonconsensual sexual intercourse with a known man did not even define the experience as rape. This was attributed to the fact that women believe rape to be a brutal attack by a stranger rather than forced sex with an acquaintance. Date rape or acquaintance rape involves situations in which the man and woman are having a mutually agreed on relationship, up to a point. When the woman states that she is not willing to engage in further intimacy and the man rapes her, accusations are almost always made that she was "asking for it," was a "tease," or should not have been alone with him. Knowing that such accusations are likely to be leveled, many women never divulge the occurrence of date rape to anyone. It should be pointed out that our culture does not apply the same logic to other crimes.

Sexually Transmitted Diseases

Sexually transmitted diseases are a serious health concern. The number, type, and severity of STDs appear to have increased rather dramatically in recent history (1993 Sexually Transmitted Diseases Treatment Guidelines, 1993). As is the case with sexual abuse, some of the apparent increase may result from better reporting and better scientific knowledge than existed a generation ago. Some of the apparent increase may be a result of sexual activity among broader groups of people as travel is made easy and as cultural mores regarding sexual behavior change. Yet another contributor to the increase may be that many microorganisms are mutating and becoming resistant to the antibiotics that have been used for two human generations. It is critical that nurses assume the role of public educators about the risks of contracting a serious infection through sexual contact.

The Centers for Disease Control and Prevention defines STDs as "infections spread by the transfer of organisms from person to person during sexual contact" (1993 Sexually Transmitted Diseases Treatment Guidelines, 1993, p. 23). In-depth discussion of each of the diseases that fall into this category is beyond the scope of this chapter. Table 37–4 provides a brief overview of the major diseases prevalent in the United States today, their primary symptoms, and their primary treatments.

Sexual Dysfunction

Sexual dysfunction is a broad term used to describe a plethora of seemingly unrelated problems. Sometimes sexual dysfunction is minor and temporary, and sometimes it is major and lifelong. Sometimes it results from psychological issues, sometimes from physical causes, and sometimes from an interaction of both. For purposes of this text, sexual dysfunction is defined as a person's inability to feel sexually fulfilled without offending self or others. This definition ultimately allows each client to determine whether he or she is sexually dysfunctional. For example, if a person is a homosexual and has a sense of acceptance about this within himself, from significant others, and from the community, he would not define himself as sexually dysfunctional, because his sexual fulfillment is achieved in a way that is acceptable to himself and to those around him. However, if a person is a homosexual and does not have acceptance from himself or from significant others who may do physical or psychological harm, the client may define the state of homosexuality as sexually dysfunctional.

There are, of course, some types of behavior that the US culture defines as sexually dysfunctional because of a cultural agreement that others are harmed by it. Such things as rape and sexual abuse of children fall into this category. This text discusses sexual dysfunction that arises primarily out of psychological factors separately from that which results primarily from biological factors. Although this is the only convenient way to discuss such a phenomenon, the reader is reminded that psychological and biological realms are not truly divisible, and one is always in interaction with the other.

❧ Psychological Origins of Sexual Dysfunction.
As with all matters of health that have a primarily psychological function, it is impossible to make generalizations that cover each individual case. In some cases described in this text, the origin may have been childhood trauma. Other cases may have arisen from early adult issues related to incidents of a directly sexual nature or of a more general nature. For instance, some men who experience the dysfunction of being aroused only by rape may have been sexually abused as children. Others may not have experienced sexual abuse as children but may have been humiliated or physically abused by a dysfunctional female figure. Thus, the concepts discussed in this text represent only the most common scenarios in which sexual dysfunction exists. Nurses must always take care to individualize data collection and treatment planning when dealing with clients.

Impotence and Premature Ejaculation. In cultures in which sexual performance is valued, it is not uncommon for individuals to have anxieties about their performance. Sometimes, the very problem an individual has anxiety about manifests as a result of performance anxiety. Impotence and premature ejaculation are common examples of this in men. Impotence is the inability to maintain erection of the penis (Masters *et al.*, 1985). Sometimes men experience impotence only in certain situations, some of which may be related to physical factors such as fatigue or consumption of alcohol or other drugs. However, it is possible for a man to believe that one or several occasions of impotence are signs of dysfunction, aging, disease, lack of interest in the partner, or any number of frightening possibilities. This may increase his anxiety, which may interfere with adequate erections in the future, thus spiraling the problem from one incident of erectile dysfunction to anxiety about impotence to actual chronic impotence. It is critical that nurses who deal with this complaint take a thorough health history and

| | | *Table* **37-4** |

SEXUALLY TRANSMITTED DISEASES, SYMPTOMS, AND TREATMENTS

DISEASE	SYMPTOMS	TREATMENTS
Chlamydia	May be none or may cause genital discharge; blindness in neonate	Tetracycline
Gonorrhea	May be none or may cause genital discharge; blindness in neonate	Norfloxacin
HIV	Variety of symptoms that indicate immune system failure (eventually fatal)	Supportive treatment only
HPV	Genital warts	Cryotherapy, cautery, laser, or acid removal
Hepatitis B	Malaise and jaundice (can be fatal)	Generally supportive
Herpes simplex type II	Genital blisters	Acyclovir is helpful
Syphilis	Symptoms vary with stage, beginning with genital chancre (sore), followed by rash, followed by involvement of major body systems	Penicillin
Trichomoniasis	May be none or may cause genital discharge	Metronidazole

refer such clients to appropriate help. Treatment may include treatment for any coexisting disease such as diabetes or alcoholism, as well as psychological counseling and sex therapy.

Sex therapists (who *never* have sex with their clients) may offer suggestions about relaxation techniques, anxiety management techniques, and "sensate focusing" techniques. Sensate focusing techniques encourage individuals to focus their attention on the pleasure of various nonintercourse types of touch. In many cases, this is a useful technique for impotence, premature ejaculation, anorgasmia, and decreased libido (Masters *et al.,* 1985).

❧ Physiological Origins of Sexual Dysfunction.
Physiological origins of sexual dysfunction may at first appear easier to understand, predict, and treat than psychological causes. However, the complexity of the human body itself, coupled with the reality that the body is inseparable from the rest of human experience, makes such dysfunctions just as challenging as those of psychological origin. As indicated earlier, some dysfunctions, such as impotence and anorgasmy, may result from physiological causes.

Evaluation

Evaluation of the client with a diagnosis related to sexuality must address the specific outcomes outlined in the planning stage and determine whether and to what extent they were successful. The long-term needs of the client should always be assessed, and referrals to community or other resources (*e.g.,* a church support group for widowed elderly) may be appropriate.

As mentioned earlier, the nurse should also include a self-evaluation in this process. By reviewing one's own feelings about working with a client and one's ability or inability to provide care without judgment, the nurse is in a position to improve future nursing care.

Summary

Nursing care for individuals with any type of health alteration should include at least some acknowledgment of the person as a sexual being whose sexuality may be affected by the health alterations. Such acknowledgment, teaching, counseling, and referral at appropriate times may be significant factors in decreasing the incidence of sexual dysfunction as a direct result of the health alteration.

Self-evaluation is an important part of a nurse's preparation for assisting clients with sexuality issues. The nurse need not agree with the client's choices or preferences in order to provide effective nursing care. However, the nurse must recognize each person's

right to personal decisions in this area and must refrain from judgment in the nursing setting.

CHAPTER HIGHLIGHTS
✦

✦ Sexuality is a state of being male or female that encompasses the whole person—body, mind, and soul.

✦ Sexuality is influenced by the culture in which one lives.

✦ Sexuality exists throughout the life cycle, from embryonic life until death.

✦ Sexuality influences the health care needs of individuals, as well as the way they go about taking care of their health.

✦ The sexual response cycle includes the four stages of excitement, plateau, orgasm, and resolution.

✦ Sexually transmitted diseases, including HIV, are serious concerns related to sexuality.

✦ Pregnancy, contraception, infertility, and abortion are sexual issues that nurses may encounter in their careers.

✦ Nurses need to be aware of their feelings about such lifestyle choices as homosexuality so that their feelings will not undermine a therapeutic relationship.

✦ Sexual dysfunction may result primarily from psychological alterations or primarily from physiological alterations.

Study Questions

1. Sexuality is defined as
   a. the biological fact of being male or female
   b. having XX or XY chromosomes
   c. the holistic state of being male or female
   d. the ability to reproduce

2. Which of the following is true regarding the role of the nurse in sexual health care?
   a. the nurse must never let his or her feelings about sexuality show
   b. the nurse must be aware of his or her own sexual feelings in all client interactions
   c. sexuality should not be an issue in a professional relationship
   d. the nurse must always be direct in telling clients about his or her sexual feelings and beliefs

3. Which of the following is true of sexuality in adulthood?
   a. issues of sexual preference are always resolved by age 25

b. sexuality continues until death
c. sexual interest declines after age 45
d. reproduction is the most important aspect of sexuality during one's 30s

4. Which of the following is true of homosexuality?

a. it is a genetic disease
b. it is primarily a moral issue
c. it has existed in most recorded cultures
d. it can be treated

5. The role of the nurse in treating persons with a sexual dysfunction is to

a. provide education and support
b. provide medication only
c. avoid the issue
d. defer to physicians

Critical Thinking Exercises

1. Ms. T. is 19 years old and is not involved in a serious relationship presently. She is diagnosed with breast cancer, and a radical mastectomy is performed. She is undergoing chemotherapy as an outpatient and experiences anorexia and alopecia. Discuss the impact on her sexual development.

2. Nurse P. overhears a conversation during a home visit and begins to suspect sexual abuse of a 12-year-old child. Discuss the impact of sexual abuse on the sexual development of the child.

References

Alger, I. (1991). Marital therapy with dual-career couples. *Psychiatric Annals, 21,* 455–458.

Auchincloss, S. (1991). Sexual dysfunction after cancer treatment. *Journal of Psychosocial Oncology, 9*(1), 23–42.

Bennett, M. (1992). Abortion. In N. F. Hacker & J. G. Moore (Eds.), *Essentials of obstetrics and gynecology* (pp. 415–424). Philadelphia: W. B. Saunders.

Bertosa, H., Cellura, M., Pierce, L., & Rothacker, C. (1993). Women with spinal cord injuries require sensitive reproductive care. *Maternal–Child Nursing Journal, 18,* 254–257.

Caplan, P. (Ed.). (1987). *The cultural construction of sexuality.* New York: Tavistock Publications.

DeBuono, B., Zinner, S., Daamen, M., & McCormack, W. (1990). Sexual behavior of college women in 1975, 1986, and 1989. *New England Journal of Medicine, 322,* 821–825.

de Chesnay, M., Marshall, E., & Clements, C. (1988). Family structure, marital power, maternal distance, and paternal alcohol consumption in father-daughter incest. *Family Systems Medicine, 6,* 453–461.

Dest, V., & Fisher, S. (1994). Breast cancer, dreaded diagnosis, complicated care. *RN, 57*(6), 49–54.

Fogel, C., & Lauver, D. (1990). *Sexual health promotion.* Philadelphia: W. B. Saunders.

Gilligan, C., & Antanucci, J. (1988). Two moral orientations: Gender differences and similarities. *Merreill-Palmer Quarterly, 34*(3), 223–237.

Gorman, C. (1992). Sizing up the sexes. *Time, 139,* 42–49.

Gorrie, T., McKinney, E., & Murray, S. (1994). *Foundations of maternal newborn nursing.* Philadelphia: W. B. Saunders.

Harris, C. (1994). *Emasculation of the unicorn: The loss and rebuilding of masculinity in America.* York Beach, ME: Nicolas Hayes.

Kahn, A., Mathie, V., & Torgler, C. (1994). Rape scripts and rape acknowledgment. *Psychology of Women Quarterly, 18,* 53–66.

Loftus, E., Polonsky, S., & Fullilove, M. (1994). Memories of childhood sexual abuse. *Psychology of Women Quarterly, 18,* 76–84.

Lonsway, K., & Fitzgerald, L. (1994). Rape myths. *Psychology of Women Quarterly, 18,* 133–164.

Masters, W., Johnson, V., & Kolodny, R. (1985). *Human sexuality.* Boston: Little, Brown.

Masters, W., Johnson, V., & Kolodny, R. (1993). *Biological foundations of human sexuality.* New York: Harper-Collins College Publishers.

McFarlane, J. M., & Williams, T. M. (1994). Placing premenstrual syndrome in perspective. *Psychology of Women Quarterly, 18,* 339–373.

Medicine Eagle, B. (1991). *Buffalo Woman comes singing.* New York: Ballantine Books.

Pilliterri, A. (1995). *Maternal and child health nursing.* Philadelphia: J. B. Lippincott.

Poorman, S. (1988). *Human sexuality and the nursing process.* Norwalk, CT: Appleton & Lange.

Reinisch, J. (1990). *The Kinsey Institute new report on sex.* New York: St. Martin's Press.

Sandelowski, M. (1994). On infertility. *Journal of Obstetric, Gynecologic, and Neonatal Nursing, 23,* 749–752.

Smith, L., & Lathrop, L. (1993). AIDS and human sexuality. *Canadian Journal of Public Health, 84*(supplement 1), S14–S18.

Swanson, J., & Albrecht, M. (1993). *Community health nursing: Promoting the health of aggregates.* Philadelphia: W. B. Saunders.

Swensen, I. E. (1992). A profile of young adolescents attending a teen family planning clinic. *Adolescence, 27,* 647.

Taber's cyclopedic medical dictionary. (1989). Philadelphia: F. A. Davis.

US Department of Health and Human Services. (1993). *1993 Sexually transmitted diseases treatment guidelines.* Atlanta, GA: Centers for Disease Control.

Warren, J., Gary, F., & Moorehead, J. (1994). Self-reported experiences of physical and sexual abuse among runaway youths. *Perspectives in Psychiatric Care, 30*(1), 23–28.

Webster's third new international dictionary. (1986). Springfield, MA: Merriam-Webster.

Bibliography

Boutcher, F., & Gallop, R. (1996). Psychiatric nurses' attitudes toward sexuality, sexual assault/rape, and incest. *Archives of Psychiatric Nursing, 10*(3), 184–191.

Chrisler, J., Johnston, I., Champagne, N., & Preston, K. (1994). Menstrual joy: The construct and its consequences. *Psychology of Women Quarterly, 18,* 375–387.

Cooper, M. (1989). Gilligan's different voice: A perspective for nursing. *Journal of Professional Nursing, 5*(1), 10–16.

Eliason, M. J. (1996). Lesbian and gay family issues. *Journal of Family Nursing, 2*(1), 10–29.

Erikson, E. (1968). *Identity, youth and crisis.* New York: Norton.

Jones, S. (1994a). Assisted reproductive technologies: Genetic and nursing implications. *Journal of Obstetric, Gynecologic, and Neonatal Nursing, 23,* 492–497.

Jones, S. (1994b). Genetic-based and assisted reproductive technology of the 21st century. *Journal of Obstetric, Gynecologic, and Neonatal Nursing, 23,* 160–165.

Lederer, L. (Ed.). (1995). *Price we pay—The case against racist speech, hate propaganda, and pornography.* New York: Hill and Wang.

MacDonald, N., Wells, G., Fisher, W., Warren, W., King, M., Doherty, J., & Bower, W. (1990). High-risk STD/HIV behavior among college students. *Journal of the American Medical Association, 263,* 3155–3159.

Nobel Conference. (1988). *Evolution of sex.* San Francisco: Harper & Row.

Reynolds, V. (1991). *Mating and marriage.* Oxford: Oxford University Press.

LOSS, DEATH, AND GRIEF

MARGOT SCHOEPS, RN, MS, CS

LEARNING OBJECTIVES
✦

After studying this chapter, you should be able to

✦ Describe typical losses that humans navigate in the life span

✦ Identify specific losses associated with illness

✦ Discuss the process of grief and behaviors typical during mourning

✦ Identify the tasks of mourning

✦ Describe interventions that assist the client and family in coping with anticipated and actual death

✦ Apply the nursing process to the care of a dying person

✦ Discuss nurse responses to the death of clients

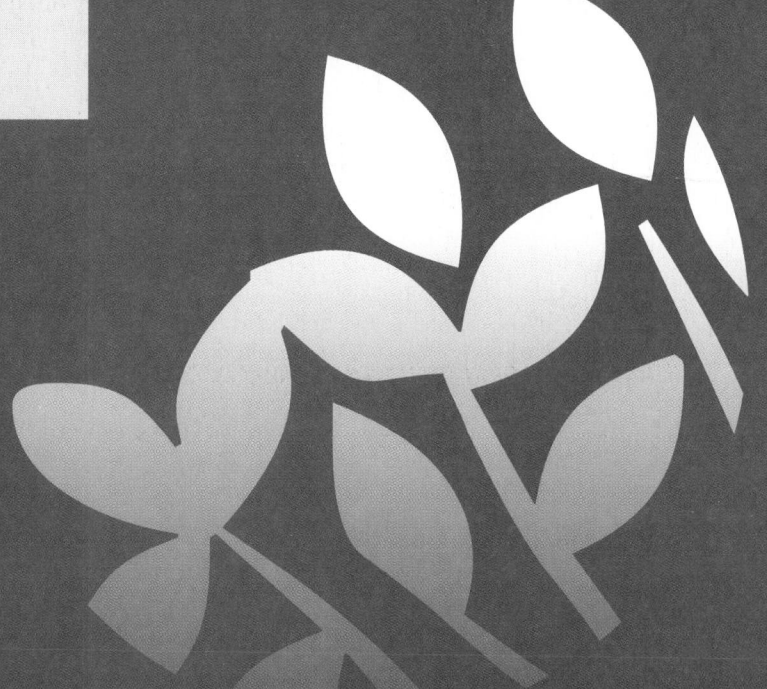

Although death has always been a part of life, societies vary in how they deal with the reality of death. In the United States, death was once an event that took place at home. Now the overwhelming majority of deaths take place in institutions. Frequently a client is isolated in unfamiliar surroundings and connected to machinery designed to sustain life but that, in fact, prolongs the dying process. It is often a nurse who is with the client during the final moments of life and who assists the family with acute grief.

The writings of Elisabeth Kübler-Ross in the 1950s articulated issues of death and dying to both health professionals and the public. Her articles and books kicked off a renewed examination of personal values and beliefs about death and an understanding of components of the experience of grief. Since that time, countless volumes have been written, and death and dying education has become widespread. Research has been conducted on the steps of recovery from loss, and theories on the response to grief abound. Hospice programs have re-created the concept of a family death. A strong "right to die" force has put the power of decision-making back into the hands of the client and family. Advocacy groups for the dying have formed, and issues of euthanasia and assisted suicide are being publicly debated.

This chapter examines loss within the context of a life span. It outlines nursing care of the dying client as well as interventions designed to ease suffering and promote healing even in the face of death. The emotions and behaviors associated with the process of grief are discussed. In addition, suggestions designed to help nurses cope with and grow from experiences of loss are offered.

Loss Throughout the Human Life Span

As a person emerges from the uterus of the mother, the first experience of loss is encountered. From that time on, each individual must face a series of losses, both desired and unwanted, until the final loss, which is death. Although the idea of loss tends to have a negative connotation, even the most desirable changes in life require that one give up the old way of being to arrive at another. Think of the infant who acquires the ability to walk. The child is now expected to demonstrate that skill even when he or she wants to be carried. The parents are thrilled with their child's new independence yet mourn with a mixture of emotions the loss of their child's infancy.

Throughout life there are developmental gains that can be made only by letting go of previous stages. The security of home is left for school and a larger world of relating. High school friends are left behind to be replaced by college or career relationships. The

nurse in training must leave the security of school to find the reward of "real" practice. Marriage requires letting go of one family in order to form a new family. And one cannot be coupled without exchanging some independence for new intimacy. Human relationships are a process of forming attachments and letting go of them. Life requires that persons move from one stage to another in a progression, always experiencing a loss so that it is possible to enter the next stage of development. It is a process of letting go in order to find new meaning.

> One who is well lives well.
> One who lives well loves well.
> One who loves well cries well.
> One who cries well becomes well.
> One who becomes well loves again and dies well.
>
> Sandra Bess (Kutscher & Kutscher, 1972, p. 216)

This quote aptly describes one of the many paradoxes of life and points to the role that loss, grief, and death play in the health of an individual. The emotions associated with human loss need to run their course. Each experience prepares one for the next loss, and each successive loss ultimately prepares one for the final loss of death.

Theories of loss and grief and of death and dying describe sequences and stages to help explain the suffering manifest in loss. Although the various theories can help explain what the professional observes, the theories should never become a recipe for the right way to grieve. Each person's experience is unique, even though grief is a universal human experience.

Judith Viorst, in her book *Necessary Losses* (1986), writes about the losses of childhood (separation of self from other), the impossible expectations we bring to relationships (with ensuing loss of self, loss of dreams, or loss of relationship), the loss of our own younger selves as we age, and the loss of people we love. She discusses the enhancement of living that comes with full awareness of death as an inevitable part of the glory of life. Death can be viewed as a curse laid on our lives or as a reality that enhances the meaning of our lived moments.

In *The Road Less Traveled*, M. Scott Peck begins with the following words:

> Life is difficult.
>   This is a great truth, one of the greatest truths. It is a great truth because once we truly see this truth, we transcend it. Once we truly know that life is difficult—once we truly understand and accept it—then life is no longer difficult. Because once it is accepted, the fact that life is difficult no longer matters.

This truism may serve the nurse well as a framework for viewing the losses of life. Few of us were raised with this philosophy, yet each of us has come to know the reality that life is difficult. Accepting loss with its accompanying emotions and transcending the experience to find a new sense of the mysteries and wonders of life become an important part of wellness.

Nurses must do that for themselves as well as help others in this task.

Loss as an Element of Illness

When a person encounters the first symptom of illness, he or she loses the security that is part of wellness. When an accident happens, victims experience a momentary or permanent interruption in their sense of safety in the world. There is no ultimate safety or security, yet until something happens, most of us go along as if shielded from the harsh possibilities in life. When someone we know is injured or ill, we likewise have our illusions of safety disrupted to a greater or lesser extent, depending on our vulnerability at the time, our relationship with that individual, and our identification with what has happened to him or her.

Nurses go a long way toward understanding the behavior of an ill or injured person when they keep in mind, at each stage of the nursing process, the concept of loss. Initially, what do persons give up when they engage with a health care provider? Independence, control, and privacy are three immediate threatened losses. One must also give up the image of oneself as healthy and may have to face the loss of role identification, income, or function or even the threatening prospect of loss of life. Think of the impact of the simple words, "Mrs. Jones, you have a tumor in your stomach," or "Mr. Smith, your son needs an operation." Every alteration in health status has its accompanying loss, both imagined and real, temporary or permanent.

In acute illness that is treated and cured, a person's sense of wellness may be quickly restored. However, he or she will never be restored to exactly the same self. A person who knows what it is to be ill may gain a greater appreciation of health. For the chronically ill, there are exacerbations and remissions and usually a general decline of health over months or often years. An accommodation process takes place as a person adapts to these losses, which can be referred to as "little deaths." There may be a prolonged period of anticipation of the end. In terminal illness, there is the shock of original diagnosis and then various accommodations as a person tries to find some sort of equilibrium. Responses to this process are as varied as the individuals, yet patterns can be observed.

Anticipated and Actual Loss

Anticipated loss can have as much impact as actual loss, in that it activates the response to loss, which is grief. As individuals struggle to face what is real versus what is imagined, they need help in sorting out the difference between the two. Their response to a threatened or actual loss depends on an array of factors, including age, perceived impact of the loss, prior experience with loss, other stressors present, supports available, cultural and religious patterns of behavior, and their repertoire of personal coping mechanisms. Guilt and blame may also play a role in the individual response to loss, as do such factors as how a person coped with prior losses and the cumulative effect of multiple losses.

Death as the Final Loss

Death has been described as the final stage of growth and development (Kübler-Ross, 1975) and as an inevitable aspect of the human experience. Yet it is often feared, shrouded with mystery, and talked about in whispers. The rate of death is one to one—one death for one life. We are all terminal. Like birth, death is a natural process. It can be eased by professionals who possess the capacity to care, the skill and knowledge to intervene to relieve suffering, and enough comfort with their own mortality to openly address the issues of dying. Whether equipped to handle the situation or not, the nurse is a key person in the care of both the client and the family in a variety of settings, including home, hospital, and long-term care institution. The nurse has a unique opportunity to make a profound difference in the experience of dying, as well as to influence the experience of those who must deal with the loss. In the process of helping, the nurse's life will be altered.

Talking About End-of-Life Decisions: Advance Directives

In 1990, the Patient Self-Determination Act was passed, requiring all institutions that receive Medicare or Medicaid funding to provide every adult client with written information on his or her right to be involved in treatment decisions, including the right to formulate an advance directive. The law further stipulates that such directives must be documented in the chart and that institutions have a responsibility to educate staff and the community on advance directives. How this actually happens in individual institutions varies, but it is clear that nurses are involved in the process. It is always the responsibility of the nurse to be aware of any advance directive documented in the chart and to read that documentation instead of relying on the interpretation of another staff member (Fig. 38–1).

Perhaps the most valuable contribution nurses can make in the area of advance directives is to get the client talking about what makes life worth living. Ideally, parents, children, and spouses will discuss end-of-life treatment and decisions before they are actually faced with an illness or injury. However, that frequently does not happen, and the burden of discussing end-of-life treatment options may fall to the physician, who often has a vested interest in preserving life at all costs and who may view death as a failure. Nurses who attend to the client on a 24-hour basis are most in touch with the client who begs, "Don't let them do this to me," or "Why do I have to go through all this when I can't ever get better anyway?" One client may say that life without full brain capacity is

Nursing SOAP Note

10/22/93   12 noon   Problem A: "Edema"

S: "I won't live much longer…I want all the usual emergency treatments…I wouldn't want a machine continued if there was no hope that I'd get better…I'm not sure if my Mom could actually carry out this request. I'll talk to her today."

O: Increased facial and neck edema. Discussed wishes for emergency treatment for sudden events (arrests). Does not want maintained by machines if no hope for recovery to current level of functioning. Dr. Jones notified.

A: Full code. Potential respiratory distress due to increasing edema

P: Continue to assess respirations. Facilitate autonomy in decision making.   *Marcia Bosek, RN*

Nursing Narrative Note

8 am	C/O neck swelling. Left cheek and entire neck obviously swollen. No C/O dysphagia. R=20 and easy. Lungs clear bilaterally. *Marcia Bosek, RN*
8:30 am	Dr. Jones notified of cheek and neck swelling. *Marcia Bosek, RN*
10 am	Informed of O$_2$ saturation tests q shift, instructed to notify nurse of respiratory distress. Discussion initiated by RN regarding wishes about emergency treatment for respiratory arrest. Stated: "I won't live much longer. I want all the usual emergency treatments. I wouldn't want a machine continued if there was no hope that I'd get better. I'm not sure if my Mom could actually carry out this request. I'll talk to her this afternoon." Provided with copy of DPOA and instructed on use. Verbalized understanding of process. *Marcia Bosek, RN*

❧ **Figure 38–1**
Sample documentation of verbal advance directives. (From Ignatavicius, D. D., Workman, M. L., & Mishler, M. A. [1995]. *Medical-surgical nursing: A nursing process approach* [2nd ed.]. Philadelphia: W. B. Saunders.)

not worth living, and another may indicate that life in any form is sacred and should be preserved. A client may talk about the mistake he or she made by having a feeding tube placed in his or her mother, thus prolonging her dying for many weeks. These discussions should be encouraged and documented, as they can give clear and convincing evidence of a client's feelings about matters related to the end of life.

Some nurses struggle with how to discuss Do Not Resuscitate (DNR) orders with a client or family. The topic can be introduced with questions such as, "Have you ever thought about what you would want done if your heart stopped beating?" or "How do you feel about some of the life-support technology we have today?" It may be particularly useful to point out to clients that just because a physician suggests a particular treatment does not mean that they have to accept it. They can take time to talk it over with family or to think about it. Some clients need to be left alone, away from family members trying to persuade them one way or another, in order to articulate their true feelings. Other clients can be enormously helped by full family involvement. Clients need to know that they are allowed to change their minds even after forms have been signed.

When the client lacks the capacity to make his or her own decisions, the family or health care proxy is approached. This should be done in such a way that those deciding for the client do not feel that they are in charge of deciding whether their loved one lives or dies. The real question is to what extent aggressive treatment should be continued. What are the possible benefits versus the cost in human suffering of the treatments available? To what extent might treatment only prolong an inevitable dying process? Families need to be given time and need to be aware that they can change their minds. Treatments can be started and discontinued if they do not produce a measurable benefit.

When clients or families make the decision that it is time to stop futile treatments, some staff members may struggle to accept that decision. It is not always easy to see food and hydration withdrawn or clients weaned from respirators when the inevitable outcome is death. Nonetheless, there can be comfort in respecting the wishes of the client and family, and there can be acknowledgment that a peaceful death is a desired goal. (See also Chapter 3, Values and Ethics in Nursing Practice.)

Most institutions have a mechanism in place for resolving ethical dilemmas concerning life and death decisions. Nurses should be aware of that mechanism. Nurses can also be proactive in avoiding ethical dilemmas by setting the stage for regular and frequent dialogue with clients and families, as well as with multidisciplinary colleagues concerning end-of-life decisions. A conference with the treating doctor, representative nurses, the family, and a social worker, clergy person, liaison nurse, or client representative can be invaluable.

One final form of advance directive that should be mentioned is that of organ donation (Fig. 38–2). Although most states provide for organ donation directives on driver's licenses, the question is actually left up to the survivors. Donation of eyes, skin, bones, live organs, or whole bodies (to scientific research) can be meaningful to those who live on and can salvage something hopeful out of a seemingly senseless sudden death. The nurse must be familiar with the procedures at his or her own facility. For live organs, there needs to be early involvement of transplant teams. These teams provide specially trained organ requesters to explain procedures and help the family sort through the issues involved in reaching a decision about this delicate matter. There are strict guidelines to be followed for determining the eligibility of donors and for maintaining viable organs until transplantation can be arranged.

Grief as a Response to Real or Threatened Loss

Remember that grief is an intense yet normal response to real or threatened loss. Whether isolated or in a community, the grieving person must navigate the waters of grief as an individual. What that process looks like depends on factors such as socioeconomic level, cultural influences, religion, family background, and an individual's personality and family dynamics. Although many generalizations about the cultural and religious differences of various groups can be made, there are individual variations even within homogeneous groups. The fewer assumptions made by the nurse, the better.

✦ **Figure 38–2**
A typical organ donor card. (Courtesy of Delaware Valley Transplant Program, Philadelphia, PA.)

Denial, bargaining, anger, depression, and acceptance are recognized stages that a person facing a life-threatening illness experiences. These stages are also seen in the grief response to loss. Not all stages are experienced by each individual, and the stages do not progress in any ordered fashion. Because grief can be so painful and overwhelming, it frightens most people. Many people wonder if they are grieving in the "right" way and if what they are experiencing is normal. As clients and families face the losses associated with injury or illness or the final loss of death, nurses can be particularly helpful by educating people about grief.

Lindemann (1944) describes a normal grief reaction as being characterized by five stages:

1. Somatic distress
2. Preoccupation with the image of the deceased
3. Feelings of guilt
4. Hostile reactions
5. Loss of patterns of conduct

Although Lindemann was describing grief caused by the death of a loved one, grief responses are regularly seen in the health care setting, because actual and threatened losses are part of the experience of all injured or ill persons. If "preoccupation with the image of the deceased" were replaced by "preoccupation with illness or injury," one could be describing a stage of the response to illness or to death. Therefore, it is important for nurses to be familiar with the physical, emotional, and behavioral characteristics of grief (see Box 38–1).

Stages of Grief

Nursing literature outlines the stages of coming to grips with death and dying. They are defined by Elisabeth Kübler-Ross as denial, anger, bargaining, depression, and acceptance. These stages can also be seen in persons coping with other health crises.

The first response to bad news is one of shock and disbelief. "Surely there is a mistake." "Wake me up, I must be having a nightmare." Denial serves as a buffer against the unexpected and difficult to comprehend news. It is a protective, unconscious defense mechanism that relieves the anxiety that arises when an individual is threatened with the possibility of death, disfigurement, disability, or pain. Denial can serve a person well until there is time to gather resources and replace the denial with partial acceptance. Some people never move beyond denial.

Allowing a client to maintain denial in the early phases of threatened loss does not mean giving him or her false hope or misinformation. Clients who use denial do not usually ask many questions and can immediately discount any information they do not feel ready to handle. Denial becomes dangerous for the client only when it prevents him or her from making an important reality assessment that is necessary for safety or realistic future planning. For instance, if a

---

Box **38–1**

CHARACTERISTICS OF NORMAL GRIEVING

Physical Characteristics

- Tightness in the throat or heaviness in the chest
- Frequent sighing and difficulty swallowing
- A loss of appetite and/or nausea with stomach pain
- A chronic feeling of fatigue, muscle weakness, numbness
- Feeling dizzy, short of breath, or headachy

Cognitive Characteristics

- Inability to concentrate
- Wandering thoughts with daydreaming
- Forgetfulness

Emotional Characteristics

- A sense of sadness that persists
- Feeling isolated and separated from others
- Feeling anger toward others whose lives seem happy
- Experiencing sudden changes of mood with frequent tears
- Yearning for life as it used to be
- Spending much time reviewing the past
- Feeling apathetic, with loss of interest in usual activities
- Guilt over real or imagined wrongdoing or over being happy sometimes
- Inability to concentrate or make decisions
- Anger at the deceased or at God
- Wishing to be dead

Behavioral Characteristics

- Difficulty either going to sleep or staying asleep
- Lowered interest in sexual activity
- Restlessness
- Sensing the presence of the one who died, sometimes hearing or seeing him or her
- An urge to fill the days with constant activity or busyness
- Decreased ability to socialize
- Hearing footsteps of the deceased or imagining seeing him or her on the street
- Tendency to use alcohol or drugs such as tranquilizers to a greater degree

---

client wants to sign out of the hospital against medical advice because he does not accept that he has had a heart attack, the denial must be confronted. But if a client with metastatic disease is denying the likelihood of death, that denial need not be addressed. Research has even suggested that those who are less preoccupied with their illnesses and have higher indexes of denial have longer survival rates (Andrykowski *et al.,* 1994).

Anger may be a first response to upsetting news, or it may take over when denial can no longer be maintained as the primary coping mechanism. The predominant theme of "why me?" or the blaming of doctors, nurses, and family members can be difficult to endure. The nurse may be criticized for responding too slowly to needs, for folding bed linens incorrectly, for inflicting pain, or for other perceived discrepancies or injustices. Anger at anyone who is healthy may prevail, and families can become angry merely because people around them are laughing and happy.

On a psychological level, anger is aimed at the correction of a perceived wrong (Averill, 1982). Anger is a signal that something is not right. The source of anger may be specific, as when a client is in pain and feels ignored, or it may be generalized, as when a client doesn't know what is wrong but is just in a bad mood. Staff also can experience angry feelings that need to be recognized. Nurses may harbor unspoken anger at clients when they do not do well with a prescribed treatment or when they fail to be kind to family members who are attempting to be supportive.

The nurse may redirect anger and set limits but must remember what lies behind the angry response. To become defensive when the family indulges in verbal attacks generally only increases the anger.

| CASE STUDY | **Nurse Responds Defensively to Anger of Family** |

Nurse Smith has been caring for a client with metastatic disease for several days. The client's condition has been steadily deteriorating, and the client's mother attacks Ms. Smith, saying, "You nurses have no concept of what a mother goes through. And why are you, an inexperienced young thing, taking care of my daughter?" The nurse responds, "I am 30 years old and have taken care of hundreds of clients without a complaint." The mother begins another round of more insistent attacks, now criticizing the nurse for treating her daughter "like just another number."

The fuel for this mother's attack is not the nurse involved but the anger that has been aroused by the increasing likelihood of the death of her daughter. "I know this must be an incredibly difficult time for you" is a response that is likely to reveal the thinly disguised sadness behind the anger. Although it is never easy to remain detached from the sting of a personal attack, the nurse must remember that even though it feels personal, the anger in this situation is not about the nurse.

Although not universally seen, a phase of bargaining is common. "Just let me live until my children are raised" or "If God will just let me recover from this injury I will never drink again" are typical "deals." The bargains are often a way for the client or family to deal with a sense of guilt for things done or undone in a lifetime. Sometimes a family bargaining for its loved one showers gifts on the staff. It is almost as if they believe that they can bargain for special care that will somehow preserve life. Although a gift of food is often accepted as a thank you from a family, excessive gift giving should be examined for what might lie behind such gestures.

Withdrawal and sadness are expected responses to illness, loss, or approaching death. Depression manifests itself in a variety of ways. Clients may verbalize hopelessness, weep openly, or remain quiet and withdrawn. The clinical signs of depression, such as loss of appetite, inability to sleep, and diminished psychomotor activity, may be apparent but dismissed owing to the client's physical condition. Making a distinction between grief with a depressed mood and a major depressive syndrome may be difficult and important. In the usual presentation of grief associated with loss, there is sadness without a significant decrease in self-esteem. In a major depression, in contrast, the person is more likely to feel worthless and undeserving of attention and affection. There is a big difference between "I wish I were dead so this would be over" and the desire to take action to harm oneself. If the nurse is unsure of how to interpret what may be suicidal ideation, he or she should in all cases seek further evaluation from a mental health professional.

Not all people experiencing loss reach a point of acceptance. They may stay stuck for prolonged periods in one of the other phases or only hint rarely at acceptance. Acceptance is not an all-or-nothing proposition but rather a stage that one moves toward gradually, as issues and struggles are resolved. Death does not wait for acceptance.

In her thematic analysis of individuals in bereavement, nurse Susan Carter (1989) reports five core themes in loss: being stopped, hurting, missing, holding, and seeking. She further describes three meta-themes about grief: change, expectation, and the inexpressibility of feelings. Change speaks to the inevitable alterations that take place after loss. Expectation refers to the pressure on the grieving individual to behave in prescribed ways. This sense of "oughtness" tends to be a burden that leads to a pretense of either grief or recovery, a reluctance to speak openly, and a heightened sense of aloneness. Inexpressibility speaks to how difficult it is to put into words the experience of grief.

Responding to Grief Reactions

As described in the section on stages of grief, there are certain behaviors that are typical of people experiencing actual or threatened loss. The nurse needs to know what to do with denial, anger, guilt, depression, and acceptance and how to help loved ones who may be struggling with similar responses to loss or to the responses they see in their loved one. Other specific responses to loss and the accompanying grief include anxiety and regression.

Denial

As mentioned previously, denial may be protective and frequently requires no intervention beyond making sure that accurate information has been given. It is often the case that client and family do not share the denial. For instance, a child may be perfectly aware of his or her approaching death, but the parents may be unable to give up the denial. The nurse can then be a nonjudgmental ear for both parties while attempting to get the client and family to talk directly to each other. A spouse may talk openly to the nurse about what to do about funeral arrangements yet need to deny the reality when talking to her husband about plans to bring him home.

Some clients and families view it as a betrayal of hope to acknowledge their acceptance of approaching death, because they interpret giving up as a lack of faith. At the same time, it is not uncommon for a family that is seemingly in denial to react with relative calm at the news of the death of a loved one. "I knew this was coming, but I just couldn't say it," or "I refused to accept it until I had no other choice," is a common response.

Anger

Anger never needs a justification, and there is little value in nurses trying to talk a client out of his or her anger. Instead, pulling up a chair and saying, "Tell me about your anger and frustration" may be particularly supportive. The anger is frequently a smoke screen for the sadness that lies just beyond the anger. A client may unconsciously be using anger to gain control of an out-of-control situation or to avoid the tears that would feel like an intensified loss of control.

Particularly difficult for families can be the anger directed at them or at the staff. "My father is never like this," says a tearful daughter who needs to be reminded that anger is a natural response to threatened or actual loss. In the case of children, anger is frequently directed at a parent. When a mother or father is the most vulnerable, she or he may have to endure the angry outburst of a child screaming, "If you won't take me home I'll hate you forever." Parents can be reminded that a child fending off the fear of abandonment may unconsciously reject the parent who could inflict the pain of abandonment. People threatened with loss often take out their frustrations on those who are most trustworthy in providing support. It does not mean that a parent needs to stand silently and be abused. Calling for a "time out" can be useful while parent and child collect themselves. A neutral person such as a nurse, social worker, play therapist, or another child may be able to provide distraction. Parents need a safe place to vent their own angers and frustrations so that they do not un-

consciously punish their angry children by rejecting them.

When clients become preoccupied with anger directed at themselves or others, they may benefit from a mental health evaluation and intervention. There may be unresolved issues from the past or deep-seated regrets triggering the anger.

Angry clients and families are frequently avoided, because the interactions are unpleasant. This avoidance, of course, only intensifies the anger, and the problem escalates. Having a client care conference concerning the angry client can be useful. Nurses and physicians need to verbalize their own negative feelings about the angry client or family before a unified approach can be developed. Otherwise, alienation will result and problems will intensify.

Guilt

Guilt is an internal process used by the mind to ensure that a person behaves in a certain way. When activated, guilt may be like a voice within the conscience that signals to a person that behavior needs correcting. Individuals experiencing guilt are usually preoccupied with the guilt-provoking situation and cannot forgive themselves. The guilt may be based on irrational assumptions or flawed thinking. The nurse's attempt to dismiss the guilt feelings with statements such as "Stop beating on yourself," or "You shouldn't feel guilty over something you couldn't control," usually do little to ease the client's guilt. The nurse needs to listen to the client nonjudgmentally, promote the notion that the client can change his or her behavior or way of thinking, limit self-punishing statements, correct myths and misconceptions, and promote rational thinking and problem solving. When asked what he or she could envision doing to relieve the guilt, the client may have a clear notion of how to reach closure. Writing to someone, talking on the phone, or arranging a visit may be possible and may ease the client's mind.

Complicating a grief response can be a sense of survival guilt. Survivors of a car crash or natural disaster may suffer from this form of guilt. Likewise, a spouse may report, "I should have died instead of him—he's the good one." Nurses sometimes report, "She shouldn't have had to go through this; it's not fair." Illness and death are not doled out with any sense of fairness that we can understand. Nonetheless, it can be useful for the nurse to explore the client's perception of why he or she acquired a certain illness or sustained a particular injury.

Sadness

The sadness that is part of grief has no easy remedy and needs to be expressed. It often comes over a person in waves, overwhelming him or her for a moment and then receding like the ocean. The words "be strong" give the message that tears are inappropriate. In fact, it takes courage and strength to allow the sadness to be expressed in tears. Men, women, and children need permission to cry. At the same time, the absence of tears does not mean that a person is not experiencing the sadness of loss. Some cultures encourage the expression of emotion, and others censure such expressions. Although there is a tendency to want to come up with the right words or actions to relieve the emotional suffering, it is best for the nurse to remain silent while allowing the client or family member to express the emotion. A nonverbal touch can communicate "I am with you. I see your pain. I care."

Nurses should never assume that they know what the person is sad or depressed about. A nurse coming upon a terminally ill client in tears may incorrectly assume that the client is thinking about his or her medical situation. In fact, when asked, the client may respond, "Oh, these are happy tears. I just got the nicest note from my grandson. He is going to grow up to be such a joy to my daughter." It is appropriate to ask about tears or other apparent sadness.

Anxiety

Anxiety is a diffuse feeling of apprehension or dread that occurs as a response to a perceived threat. It may range from a mild state to panic levels and often accompanies many of the stages of grief. An individual's ability to tolerate anxiety varies. Manifestations of anxiety may appear in the physical dimension as sweaty palms, palpitations, jitteriness, restlessness, upset stomach, and insomnia or in the psychosocial dimension as irritability, uncertainty, rumination, preoccupation, attention-seeking behavior, and aggression. Because unrelieved anxiety tends to escalate, the goal is to intercede early in the spiral and keep levels of anxiety manageable.

Anxiety deserves a careful examination from a developmental and psychodynamic perspective. Strain and Grossman (1975) report that anxiety emerges in an ill person because he or she experiences the situation as dangerous, and some basic fears and threats encountered during early childhood development are awakened. These include the fear of loss of sense of self as whole and competent, fear of strangers, fear of separation, fear of loss of love and approval, fear of bodily injury, fear of loss of developmentally achieved function, and fear of retaliation. The illness may be experienced as a punishment for previous transgressions for which the person carries a sense of shame.

In the repertoire of interventions for anxiety are all the interactive skills of the nurse, along with warm baths, back rubs, meditation, guided imagery, and thought-stopping techniques. In addition, antianxiety medications may be indicated. When the client or family is seeking attention as a way of relieving anxiety, the nurse needs to develop a consistent approach. It may be necessary to set up a mechanism for checking on the client at set intervals or to provide regular time for speaking with family members. Dependable structure goes a long way toward alleviating anxiety that is provoked by uncertainty.

Because nurses and doctors struggle when there is an anticipated death on a unit, they may be adding their own anxiety to an already charged situation. Deciding on a plan—what resuscitative efforts will be made, who will speak to the family, what notifications should be made—may provide needed structure to relieve staff anxiety about an approaching death.

Regression

Overwhelmed by physical and psychological stresses, a client or family member may face a loss with regression, returning to a previous level of development that feels more comfortable. The person may be tearful and clinging, seem incapable of doing ordinary things for himself or herself, or throw temper tantrums. Although the behaviors can be particularly annoying and often seem manipulative, it must be remembered that regression is a coping mechanism. The person is not aware of making a choice about the behavior, and the nurse must work to resist rejection or punishment for the regression. With consistent encouragement and praise for age-appropriate or higher-level functioning, the person can usually give up the regression.

The process of grief is summarized in Box 38–2.

BOX 38–2

PROCESS OF GRIEF AND BEHAVIORS TYPICAL DURING MOURNING

Process of Grief

- Shock and disbelief, manifest in denial, which is a coping mechanism
- Anger and resentment, which may be directed at the nurse
- Bargaining, which may not be universal
- Sadness and depression, manifest in waves of tears that need to be expressed
- Acceptance, which is gradual and may never be complete
- All loss as productive of change
- Expectations of others prescribe a way of grieving as well as a picture of recovery
- Emotions of grief are indescribable in words, though the feelings are recognized

Tasks of Mourning

- Hurting
- Finding meaning
- Letting go and reinvesting energy in life

Tasks of Mourning

The course of mourning, although not predictable, involves some characteristic tasks as well as the typical stages and behaviors discussed previously. Whatever the emotions or actions of the person experiencing the loss, the tasks at hand are to feel the hurt, accept the loss, and move on to a new understanding of the role of the lost object, person, or experience in the shaping of one's own life. This process may take months, years, or a lifetime. Resolution of mourning requires a letting go of what was and a renewed investment in life as it is at the present.

In the case of a death, the intensity of mourning depends on the relationship with the deceased, circumstances of the death, support networks, and inner resources of the bereaved. Violent death, sudden death, deaths in which there is no body recovered, and the death of a child can be particularly difficult, because these do not follow the "natural order" of what people expect. Prolonged dying, as is experienced in many chronic conditions, provides an opportunity for anticipatory grief but may intensify the mourning instead of making it easier. When loved ones have assumed the caregiver role over prolonged periods, they may be particularly lost when death finally occurs.

Even though the task of mourning may seem complete, certain landmarks in time may produce an intense reawakening of grief. A parent who experienced the death of a child at birth may feel intense pain when that child would have started school. Birthdays of the deceased, anniversaries of the death, and holidays may be celebrated with a mixture of sadness and joy. When individuals are hospitalized there is often an acute longing for someone who has died—someone who would have been there for the person in this time of need. "My mother has been gone 40 years already but I miss her so much today. She would have been here for me for this surgery." In some sense, the work of grief does not end, even though the intensity of feelings changes over time.

Nurse researcher Susan Carter (1989) writes about a contextual theme of bereavement—the theme of personal history. Each loss in life fits into a story that is one's life. A client's stories about the past—who has died, what losses he or she has endured, who the client has loved and lost—are essential to understanding the client. We are given precious few opportunities to tell our stories, yet that is a vital task in the process of mourning. It is one of the gifts the nurse can give—to listen to the stories of the client. There is healing in the telling and in the listening.

Role of the Nurse in Facilitating Grief Work at the Time of Death

When a client dies and family members are told, there is much the nurse can do to facilitate the grief process (see Box 38–3). Survivors will relive the final hours or days of their loved one again and again, replaying the words and actions of the nurse and other caregivers. Following are suggestions for the nurse:

1. *Acknowledge the loss.* Because they worry that they might say the wrong thing, nurses sometimes don't say anything. Once the family has been told of the death (usually by the physician), the nurse caring for that client needs to approach the family. Using the word "death" or "died" can help break through the shock and disbelief experienced. A simple "He died at one o'clock" or "I'm sorry we had to tell you that your mother died" makes the fact of death a reality. Physical touch or holding can say volumes at this time.

2. *Refrain from telling the family how they should feel.* There is no right or wrong way to respond to the news of the death of a loved one, and no assumptions about how the person is feeling should be made. Seemingly soothing words, such as "It's a blessing because she suffered so," may spark rage from family members. This rationalization of the pain of loss may be used by the family but should not be offered by caregivers. Likewise, "Now don't cry, and be strong" is less helpful than "You will get through this and there will be people to help."

3. *Allow for questions.* Although the doctor may have answered all questions at the time of the death notification, much of that conversation may need to be repeated by the nurse. Family members often want to know if their loved ones said anything, if they were in pain, if they were conscious. No questions are inappropriate. Answers should be simple and honest. This is not the time for complicated medical explanations or hypotheses about what happened. Questions that the nurse cannot answer should be referred to the appropriate person.

4. *Offer to take the family to the bedside.* Most experts agree that viewing the body exerts a beneficial influence on the acutely grieving family, creating a reality of death. However, the viewing is left to the discretion of the individuals involved. The nurse should prepare family members for what they will see by describing any changes in the appearance of the deceased since last seen by loved ones. The client and room should be prepared. Remove all tubes according to the institution's policy and clean up

---

Box **38–3**

NURSING INTERVENTIONS THAT ASSIST THE FAMILY IN COPING WITH DEATH

* Acknowledge the loss
* Refrain from telling others how to feel or judging responses
* Explore past coping and resources used
* Refrain from clichés that try to take away the pain
* Reinforce prior positive experiences of resolution of loss
* Give permission for grief
* Give assurance of healing over time

any bodily fluid or discharge. If there was a resuscitative effort made, emergency equipment can be removed, but sometimes it is better left in place if the family needs to see that every effort was made to revive the person. The client should be appropriately dressed in a clean gown with hands and face exposed. Glaring lights can be turned down and chairs made available if family members feel faint or want to sit at the bedside.

Some families may want a clergy person to be with them; others need to call family members to be with them for the viewing. There is no need to hurry this process. The family may want to be left alone at the bedside for a period of silence, prayer, or good-byes. If appropriate, show the family how to connect with their loved one by touching. In the case of an infant or small child, the nurse can offer the opportunity to hold the child.

5. *Allow the grieving family to be with their pain.* Although there is a desire to stop the hurting that is visible at this time, the skilled nurse offers a silent and reassuring presence. The person experiencing loss needs to feel that the listener can bear to hear the full power of their emotions and some reminiscing without judgment. Family members can be encouraged to talk about their loved one and thus begin their healing. The nurse should not say something just to make himself or herself feel better or more comfortable around the bereaved. Avoid clichés such as "I know exactly how you feel," "Her death was for the best," or "It was God's will."

6. *Instruct the family on how to proceed.* Death does not offer a rehearsal, and families usually do not know how to proceed. They may need to discuss how they will get home, who should be called, how to make funeral arrangements, and how they will get through the next few hours. The nurse, a social worker, or other support staff may help with phone calls.

7. *Offer resources.* Families need to know that the intense emotions of grief are normal but that professional help may be needed. The phone number of a crisis team or mental health bereavement resource might be useful. They should also be assured that they can call the unit later with any questions or to ask about bereavement resources.

8. *Arrange for any bereavement follow-up for the family.* If there is a bereavement follow-up program at the facility, the family should be told about that contact. In other cases, the nurse may want to call the family later or write a note. Hospice programs have a regular bereavement follow-up, and family members can be prepared for what to expect. For families, support is usually available during funeral preparations and burial, but after the rituals of mourning are over, they may particularly appreciate a note or call.

Perhaps the greatest gift a nurse can give at the time of death is a disciplined presence rather than doing something for the bereaved (Solari-Twadell *et al.,* 1995). Just remaining with the bereaved supports the notion of recognizing and honoring the role of suffering in recovery. There are no words to make it all okay again, yet the nurse must know that, as intense as the emotions of grief are, most people get through this period. Humans have much training in surviving loss, and they have an astonishing ability to heal and move forward.

Children and Grief

Children and teenagers need to participate in loved ones' dying in ways that are appropriate for their age, comfortable for the client and the rest of the family, and suited to their relationship to the dying person (see Box 38–4). Parents often ask if their children should visit the hospital and to what extent they should be included in the rituals of mourning. Regardless of age, if the child insists on visiting and being included, he or she should be allowed to do so if the parents are willing. Likewise, if the child does not want to participate, it is a mistake for the parents to

---

Box 38–4

HOW CHILDREN CONCEPTUALIZE DEATH AT VARIOUS AGES

Preschool

Children often think that death is a reversible process, like falling asleep and waking up or going away for a time and returning. Their images of death from television are of death without emotion. Because of their use of magical thinking, they may have myths about how they contributed to the death. Rather than showing emotions, they may act out their feelings, with an increase in clinging behavior or night fears. They need reassurance that others in their life are not going to "disappear." Although using the words "she is dead," they may with the next breath say, "I want to go see her."

Ages 6 to 9

This is a time of fascination with the concrete aspects of death, such as what happens to the body, how it is prepared for burial, whether the person can see, and how long decomposition takes. There is a better understanding of the finality of death. Sometimes there is a thought that death is contagious, and there is an accompanying desire to avoid someone they think or hear is very sick or dying. Death may be personified as Darth Vader or other figure.

Ages 9 to 12

At this age, children have similar concerns as adults. There is often an increased outward display of emotions of grief. They are beginning to understand some of the biological aspects of death and the fact that they too will die, sometime, somewhere.

Adolescence

Because their own emotional balance may be precarious, teens often suffer intensely in grief, as they do with other emotions. Some regress in behavior, and others act overly adult and repress emotion. There is often no sense that the intensity of feeling will subside, so teens are at a greater risk of suicidal preoccupation. Teens need to talk endlessly about their feelings and like to receive support from their peers.

force a child to visit, view the body, or attend the funeral.

In talking with children, especially young ones, it is important to use the words "death," "dying," and "dead" to explain that the body ceases to function. If one talks about death as "sleep," the child may become afraid to go to bed. Children may feel unrealistically responsible for a loved one's death. They need reassurance that death cannot be the result of their negative thoughts, feelings, wishes, or actions.

When helping families with children face the death of a loved one, the nurse can encourage parents to give clear, understandable information to their children. Kids need to feel involved and important, rather than abandoned. They may need help in identifying and understanding the grief of adults around them, and they need permission to still be interested in their usual activities—school, birthday parties, sports, and so forth. Although children may not talk directly about their feelings of loss, their behaviors may act out their anxieties. At the same time, because children are less inhibited, they can offer real words of wisdom and comfort to adults. "Don't be so sad, Mommy, because Grandma will always be with us because we loved her and she loved us," were the words of a 6-year-old.

The Elderly and Grief

All those who live long enough have the opportunity to grieve for family and friends. It is common for the elderly to wait to die or to be preoccupied with reading obituaries, attending funerals, and talking about "the end." In addition to preparing for their own deaths, they may be grieving for ambiguous losses, such as the loss of mental capacity, memory, or physical function, or for unfulfilled hopes. They may feel the pressure of being a burden or feel that they have outlived their time and that their families are waiting for them to die.

Particularly difficult for families is the grief associated with progressive dementia in loved ones or the "slow death" and progressive losses of chronic illness. The person as known may be gone long before the body dies. Helping families accept their own ambiguous feelings and stay invested in meaningful pursuits can be a particular challenge for the nurse.

The Nursing Process As It Relates to Care of the Dying Person

Assessment

The nurse working with a dying client and his or her family needs keen assessment skills to determine their physical, emotional, and spiritual needs. Physi-cally, key issues for the client are pain control, sleep and rest, and general discomforts.

Pain, which is discussed elsewhere, deserves special consideration in the dying. Nurses and families often say, "If only he weren't so alert. I can't stand to see him aware of what is happening." If, in fact, death is the final stage of growth, there is no reason for the client to be medicated into oblivion if there is no experience of physical pain. Actual physical pain should be adequately treated with all available medications and modes of delivery. Relief of pain may be the least and most we can do for the dying. Although clients frequently fear great pain, their pain often decreases as they approach death. Psychic and spiritual pain must be addressed separately, as must anxiety, which may intensify pain perception.

Sleep often eludes dying persons, as fears intensify through the dark and often lonely night. Questions to raise include the following:

* Does the client view sleeplessness as a problem?
* Are fears, intensified at night, preventing sleep?
* Is the person sleeping all day and lying awake at night?
* Are fears of abandonment in the absence of loved ones a concern?
* Is confusion more prevalent at night, and is it intensifying fears?
* Is fear of death creating hypervigilance in the client?

Discomforts of the dying person may include dry mouth owing to the inability to take in food or liquids, pressure sores owing to immobility, dry and itching skin owing to dehydration, and stiffness related to lying in one position. Physical assessment, as outlined in other chapters, is applicable for a dying client experiencing discomfort.

Emotionally, a key assessment is to distinguish between anxieties and fears. Anxiety is a diffuse, vague apprehension associated with feelings of uncertainty and helplessness. That is different from specific fears of loneliness, of suffering and pain, of loss of identity, or of regression. Distinguishing between specific fears and anxiety may be difficult, especially if the client is nonverbal.

Assessment of the dying person's psychological dimension may include some of the following:

* What is the client's knowledge regarding his or her disease and dying? Research and clinical experience tell us that people know when they are dying, although they may be selective in choosing with whom they share that knowledge (Kübler-Ross, 1974). Even if families and physicians keep their prognoses from them, clients frequently deduce the actual situation. They pick up cues from overheard comments, from changes in behavior, from changes in medical routines, or from changes in physical location. The tragedy in keeping the truth from the client is that the client too must keep up the charade.
* Does the client or family have the necessary information to make informed decisions? The family may be trying to protect the client, or the doctor may be withholding information in an attempt to spare them. Avoidance of hard

issues may be causing poor communication between the client and family or between health care professionals and the client or family.

- Are the client and family knowledgeable about the physical process of dying and what actually happens to the human body? Once the inevitability of death is accepted or at least openly talked about, information about the physiological changes that occur as death approaches may be useful. Although specific changes are dependent on the type of disease, Box 38–5 lists some of the most typical clinical signs of approaching death.

It is not only the professional clergy who are responsible for the spiritual assessment of the dying client. Nurses, because of their long hours with the client and family, their intimate knowledge of family dynamics, and their around-the-clock availability, should be able to answer the following questions:

- Are issues of religious conflict causing pain and suffering?
- Do the client and family find spiritual supports helpful?

Box 38–5

SIGNS AND SYMPTOMS OF APPROACHING DEATH

The decline in body systems causes physiological changes. Although specific changes are dependent on the type of disease, all terminal illness is accompanied by a progressive weakness and a lessened ability to cope with environmental demands. This internal disintegration probably precedes the emotional withdrawal of terminal clients. Some clinical signs of approaching death include the following:

1. Decreased level of consciousness, including coma.
2. Decreased desire for food and liquids.
3. Decrease in urine output and concentration of the urine.
4. Incontinence of bladder and bowel. As fluid intake decreases, the skin may become drier, and urine is likely to be more concentrated and less in volume.
5. Respirations slower and more shallow. They may have a starting and stopping quality, with periods of loud sucking breaths or short, shallow breaths at varying intervals.
6. Pulse rate changes, becoming either faster or slower.
7. Temperature changes, sometimes producing fever—often seen in dehydration.
8. Decrease in circulation. Hands and feet may be cool to the touch.
9. Increased restlessness. The person may become squirmy, as if trying to get away from something, or may pull at bedclothes and any constricting items.
10. Mental confusion. The person may begin talking to persons not in the room (often those who are already dead) or talking of going home.

- How do the client and family view death—as a relief from pain and suffering, as a failure, as an unnecessary evil, as a cruel fate, as the will of God?
- Are there cultural influences affecting how the client and family are responding?
- Is there unfinished business that requires the client's attention?
- Is the client questioning the significance of his or her life and the meaning of death?
- What important persons need to be seen by the client?
- Is place of death (*i.e.,* hospital vs. home) of significance to the client?

The specifics of spiritual assessment, planning, intervention, and evaluation are discussed in Chapter 35.

How are family members coping with potential death of a loved one? The nurse must assess their needs as well as the client's. Family members may be far behind or ahead of the client in accepting approaching death. Certain maladaptive coping patterns, such as increased use of alcohol and/or drugs (noted by alcohol on the breath or slurred speech and boisterous behavior), exhaustion, neglect of personal needs for food and rest, verbalization of thoughts about self-destruction, or recurrence of mental illness, must receive special attention (Davidson, 1984). Although it should not be assumed that a person with even a serious mental disorder will have difficulty with normal grieving, the added stress can be too much for someone who is already in precarious mental health.

The nurse may need additional help in assessing the coping ability of family members, especially when there is a known history of mental illness or evidence of maladaptive coping. When family members talk about wanting to die with their loved ones, the nurse needs to ascertain whether this is normal grief or the expression of suicidal ideation and/or intent. A more formal psychiatric assessment by a social worker or other mental health professional may be needed.

An additional aspect of assessment when working with dying clients and their families is for the nurse to determine how his or her own anxieties and/or feelings of inadequacy may interfere with appropriate nursing care. Medical staff often view death as a failure and may project some of their feelings of disappointment and frustration onto the nurse. The nurse too may have identification issues or recent losses that prevent skillful attention to the needs of a particular client or family. Awareness of personal limitations is vital, or avoidance of the needs of the client and family may result.

Dying is an individual process, even though it is a universal experience. There is no right or wrong way to experience or face death. It is not the nurse's place to impose his or her religious beliefs on the client or family or to burden them with the nurse's emotions regarding the impending loss. Although it is common for less experienced nurses to have difficulty separating their own emotions from those of the client and family, that is what is required and will become easier with experience.

When a client is dying on a unit, it is common to hear nurses make statements such as, "The husband should be here more often," or "They must not love her because they don't even cry." These judgments are unfair to the family. Staff can never know the full picture of family functioning or the makeup of relationships observed. Furthermore, the impending death of a family member is a crisis in family life and often dramatically alters usual behavior. The goal is to assess what is going on, not to pass judgment on it.

Nursing Diagnosis

Once the nurse has assessed the client and family, information is analyzed and unmet needs are determined. See the accompanying box for examples of nursing diagnoses related to the needs of a dying client and his or her family. This is by no means an exhaustive list of possible diagnoses or suggested related etiology.

Just because a person is dying does not imply that there is a problem. When persons involved are expressing emotions; making informed, reasoned decisions; and using coping mechanisms and resources to their advantage, the final stage of life is proceeding as intended.

NURSING DIAGNOSES RELATED TO NEEDS OF THE DYING CLIENT AND FAMILY

Ineffective airway clearance

Impaired physical mobility

Altered oral mucous membrane related to dehydration

Fear related to the dying process

Constipation

Diarrhea

Bowel incontinence

Altered urinary elimination

Ineffective coping related to awareness of impending death

Powerlessness

Body image disturbance related to disfigurement of disease processes or procedures

Risk for loneliness related to isolation from significant others

Knowledge deficit related to illness

Ineffective family coping related to role changes

Spiritual distress related to disrupted spiritual rituals

Spiritual distress related to questioning of meaning of suffering

Anticipatory grieving

Hopelessness

Planning

Deciding on realistic goals, both long and short term, for the dying client and his or her family requires that the nurse be continually aware that the goal is to move toward acceptance of the impending death and toward adaptation to the loss. These factors were discussed in the section on grief. Examples of general goals for nursing care of the dying client are as follows:

1. To minimize evidence of physical discomfort
2. To gain an understanding of the physiological changes occurring
3. To maintain a level of social interaction desired
4. To maintain trust in caregivers
5. To participate in decision-making regarding treatments and therapies
6. To develop a repertoire of coping skills to minimize anxiety
7. To express feelings related to impending death
8. To plan for future needs of the family
9. To move toward a sense of calmness and acceptance
10. To verbalize an increased ability to let go of unfinished business
11. To verbalize an increased comfort that survivors will find resources to continue life

See Nursing Care Plan 38–1.

Implementation

The physical needs of the dying person are addressed through pain relief, proper hygiene, provision of sleep and rest, and avoidance of unnecessary invasive procedures. The client's physical status may change rapidly, requiring the nurse to change the care provided.

Pain control for the dying client should be provided in the same way that it is provided for clients who are not terminal. The issues of addiction are meaningless in the face of approaching death. Some nurses and doctors worry that pain medication may hasten death by decreasing respiratory drive. Nonetheless, the actual goal of treatment—to keep the person comfortable—must be kept in mind. To withhold available relief would be as unethical as to administer drugs intended to hasten death. The goal is comfort and a peaceful death.

Drugs may be indicated for anxious clients. Sedatives, antianxiety medications, and narcotics may aid in clouding mental alertness and can help the frightened client. As peripheral circulation fails, the absorption of drugs given subcutaneously is impaired. Thus intravenous drugs or suppositories may prove more beneficial near the end of life. Frequently, an intravenous morphine drip is used because of the ease of titrating the desired dose to maintain comfort. Clients who are at home may be maintained on around-the-

SAMPLE NURSING CARE PLAN

A CLIENT WITH RECURRENT BREAST CANCER

A 32-year-old single woman has been diagnosed with recurrent breast cancer. A modified radical mastectomy and chemotherapy have been recommended. The client is found tearful and sitting in a dark room.

Nursing Diagnosis: Grief related to actual or anticipated loss

Expected Outcome: Client will grieve adaptively, as evidenced by expression of feelings, verbalization of concerns, and identification of support resources

Action	Rationale
1. Approach the client and acknowledge the tears with an offer to be with her.	1. Balancing the client's private and alone time with an opportunity to talk is respectful.
2. Unless the client asks to be left alone, ask her to talk about the emotions she is experiencing.	2. Talking about feelings is a way of discharging the emotions and sorting out thoughts.
3. Assess the significance of the loss to the client—the worst fear, the greatest concern, the view of the future.	3. Assuming what is of greatest concern to the client may lead to erroneous notions. Ask. This is a way to identify any myths.
4. Assess for somatic distress associated with emotions (headache, stomach pains, choking sensations, altered eating and sleep patterns).	4. Loss of sleep and inability to take in food or fluids are common with grief. Self-care needs to be encouraged.
5. Explore past coping with difficult events.	5. The greatest predictor of present and future coping is past coping.
6. Assess client support systems and encourage use of those resources, as well as offer any additional resources available to the client either now or in the future.	6. Perceived support is a modifier of the grief response.
7. Describe briefly the normal human responses to real or threatened loss, including psychological reactions over time and variety of responses. Include family or significant others in this teaching if possible.	7. Education about loss helps normalize the client's response. Inclusion of others fosters a wider circle of support for the client and attends to the needs of important family and friends.
8. Document client concerns, support given, response to support, and teaching.	8. Documentation is the only evidence of care given and is a communication tool for the treatment team.

clock long-acting morphine in oral or suppository form.

Despite the fact that medical and nursing staff spend much time and energy regulating pain medication, clients frequently indicate that they are in pain. Underlying psychological factors may lead to an exaggerated pain response and need to be addressed. The help of consultation/liaison psychiatrists, social workers, or psychiatric clinical nurse specialists may be indicated to sort out the interplay between psychological and physical pain.

Hygiene needs of the dying client may be partially met by family members who want to do something for their loved one. The nurse should carefully assess the client's and the family's comfort level with this, but including loved ones in the care of the dying may be therapeutic for both. Inappropriate use of the family can obviously produce resentment and mistrust of the nursing staff. For the family or nurse to "baby" the client by performing tasks that he or she is capable

and desirous of performing unnecessarily diminishes the client's self-esteem and contributes to regression.

Oral hygiene and mouth care become important as the client faces the inevitable dehydration of dying. Nutritional needs of the hospitalized client may be kept up with the use of intravenous access and/or tube feedings, but the dying person has increasing difficulty assimilating nutrition by any means. At home, the client may stop any efforts to drink or eat. This can be unbearable to families, who fixate on the need for food and water. They need to be helped to distinguish between the suffering of a healthy person deprived of food and water and the decreasing need for food and hydration in the dying. Although it is difficult to watch the wasting that is common as death approaches, the dying often beg their families to stop pushing them to eat or drink. The nurse may need to redirect the family to provide other forms of comfort that symbolize their caring and alleviate their sense of helplessness.

It is sometimes assumed that the dying person needs a quiet, darkened room away from the noise of everyday life. This may be the person's choice, but a hospitalized client may feel more secure if he or she is near the nursing station or with a roommate who can provide some escape from isolation. If placed in a room at the end of the hall, the dying client is all too easily avoided, as nursing and medical personnel yield to their natural tendency to sidestep an uncomfortable situation. Lights left on even at night may be a comfort to the client. Music may be therapeutic, and the background noise of a television may be desired. The home setting may allow a person to be at the very center of life in a busy household until his or her last breath.

The role of touch in caring for the dying should be emphasized. Nurses touch automatically in the multitude of cares they give. Clients talk about wanting to be held. Family members may be afraid to touch for fear of disturbing equipment or causing pain. One client reported, "They used to hug me, then they patted my shoulder or my head, and now they just wiggle my toe."

Invasive procedures such as blood drawing, certain tests, hemodynamic monitoring by A-lines, and even mechanical respirators may be considered burdensome to the dying client and not justifiable when considered from the standpoint of pain and suffering versus possible benefit. These kinds of difficult questions require attentiveness to the client's wishes as expressed directly or through the use of advance directives and health care proxies. The nurse can facilitate the necessary conversations among client, family, and treatment team. It is the right of a client to be involved in all aspects of care and to refuse all standard forms of treatment (see Box 38–6). Any form of monitoring or treatment can be stopped, and hospitals have protocols and guidelines for carrying out such decisions.

With a dying client, the nurse must strive for a balance between performing cares of comfort and protecting the client from unnecessary and potentially painful procedures. Being attentive to and recording client response to comfort measures are vital for shift-to-shift continuity and individualization of the client's care.

Sleep medications, antianxiety medications, gentle massage, guided imagery, alterations of the environment (lights, noise, proximity to the nurses' station), and the presence of loved ones are all ways to improve sleep. Taking time to pull up a chair and have a brief conversation with a dying client or to just sit for 5 minutes may be therapeutic for both the client and the nurse. The act of sitting down can make worlds of difference in client perception of being cared about and heard.

Psychosocial interventions for the dying client and his or her family all involve first establishing a therapeutic relationship of trust—not an easy matter in view of the gamut of emotions that go along with loss and anticipated death. Nonetheless, the nurse needs to

---

Box 38–6

THE DYING PERSON'S BILL OF RIGHTS

I have the right to be treated as a living human being until I die.

I have the right to maintain a sense of hopefulness, however changing its focus may be.

I have the right to be cared for by those who can maintain a sense of hopefulness, however changing this might be.

I have the right to express my feelings and emotions about my approaching death in my own way.

I have the right to participate in decisions concerning my care.

I have the right to expect continuing medical and nursing attention even though "cure" goals must be changed to "comfort" goals.

I have the right not to die alone.

I have the right to be free from pain.

I have the right to have my questions answered honestly.

I have the right not to be deceived.

I have the right to have help from and for my family in accepting my death.

I have the right to die in peace and dignity.

I have a right to retain my individuality and not be judged for my decisions, which may be contrary to beliefs of others.

I have the right to discuss and enlarge my religious and/or spiritual experiences, whatever these may mean to others.

I have the right to expect that the sanctity of the human body will be respected after death.

I have the right to be cared for by caring, sensitive, knowledgeable people who will attempt to understand my needs and will be able to gain some satisfaction in helping me face my death.

---

spend time with the client and family and pay particular attention to listening skills. Knowing what to say is not nearly as important as knowing when to listen and keep quiet. Given adequate time and a relationship of trust, the client and family will let the nurse witness their efforts to reconcile loss and impending death. They do not need advice, but rather the confidence that they can cope with the processes of letting go and grieving.

One of the common fears of the dying is that of being alone. "Don't leave me alone" could mean that the client wants family or medical personnel at the bedside or that he or she simply does not want to be isolated and abandoned. Elisabeth Kübler-Ross, who has written extensively about the experiences of dying persons, confidently tells clients that they will not die alone (Kübler-Ross, 1974). Based on her numerous conversations with people who have survived near-death experiences or been revived after cardiac arrest, she says that people never report a feeling of aloneness but either an experience of being with others whom they have known and who have preceded them in death or a vague sort of joining with a supreme being or "presence." Both clients and families may take comfort in this kind of information. Often there is a bedside vigil that goes on for hours or days, and then when a client is alone for a brief time, he or she dies. The timing involved with death often has meaning for the person dying as well as for the family that goes on living. For a family feeling guilty for not being there at the precise moment of death, it may be comforting to say, "The timing of moments of birth and death is out of our hands."

Nonverbal communication can be particularly useful in working with the dying. A touch or a hug can convey caring and confidence when words fail. Similarly, openers such as "Tell me about your mother" or "What kinds of things are coming to mind as you lie there?" can facilitate the kind of life review or storytelling that is indicated.

Clients and families often want to discuss their religious or cultural beliefs about dying, and this verbalization should be encouraged. Clergy may be a valuable resource for the client and family or for the nurse. A client's spiritual needs are most effectively met through interventions that are meaningful within his or her own spiritual frame of reference and not based on the nurse's spiritual beliefs. At times, a family or client may ask a nurse to participate in some religious ritual or to join them in prayer. The nurse is free to participate if doing so is acceptable to the nurse's personal values. If the nurse is uncomfortable with the request and declines to participate, he or she may find someone else on the staff who will participate.

Evaluation

The client is not part of the final evaluation of the effectiveness of interventions designed to promote the welfare of the dying. However, the nurse must ask whether the interventions promoted a death that was in keeping with the desires of the client and family. In evaluating the results of interventions, it is essential to keep in mind that the goal is not to eliminate the pain of loss, letting go, and facing death. These are human experiences that can be supported and eased, but the struggle can never be eliminated. Just as there is nothing that can erase the pain of the end of a runner's long race, the emotional pain of the final lap of life comes with a certain cost. To remain with a client and family and accept their process without judgment is the gift of the nurse. Were they kept informed along the way? Are loved ones knowledgeable about the grief process? Was respect given to the wishes of the client and family? Was physical pain relieved? These are important questions to ask in evaluating the role played by nursing.

One step of evaluation that should not be overlooked is for the nurse to question the effect of the death on the nursing staff as individuals and as a unit (see "The Nurse's Response to Death"). Some hospitals require a review process of all hospital deaths. A special review committee looks over the chart, evaluating with key persons on the health care team the interventions that were rendered. Such a forum can be especially useful when ethical decisions are involved. Quality control is as important at the end of life as in the rest of care.

Where to Die?

When it becomes apparent that a client is dying, the place of death becomes a consideration. In an intensive care unit (ICU), there are usually restrictive visiting hours, and the efforts of staff are geared toward saving lives and providing heroic measures. But if the client has been in the ICU for some time, the client and family have likely formed alliances with and a sense of trust in the staff. To move the client hours or days before death might be disruptive. However, when the intensive care bed is needed for an acutely ill person for whom heroic measures may be life saving, it is impossible to justify the use of that bed for a dying client.

When a DNR order is written, a client is frequently transferred out of the ICU—a move that can be interpreted by the client and family as giving up or abandonment. It is imperative to communicate that care of the client will be maintained regardless of setting. A DNR order says nothing about the withdrawal of care. It means only that cardiopulmonary resuscitation will not be initiated should the heart stop beating. Death will be accepted.

Typical staffing patterns of a general hospital are not always conducive to giving optimal attention to the needs of the dying client and his or her family. Another alternative to the general hospital is a hospice (Fig. 38–3). A hospice is a special institution, a unit in a facility, or a home care program that is devoted

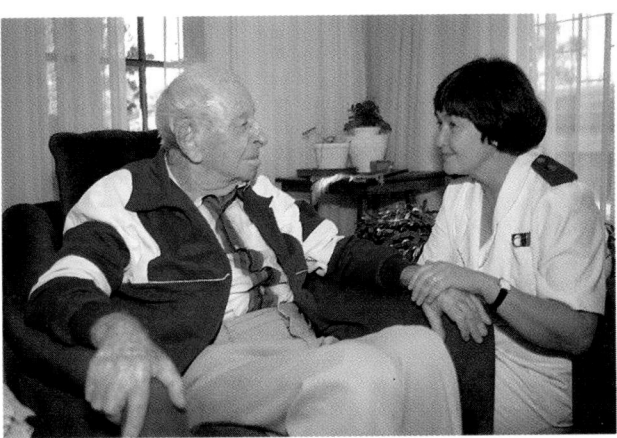

❧ Figure 38–3
Hospice nurse providing care for a dying person at home.

exclusively to the support of people actively involved in the dying process and their families. The hospice concept was begun in England and is being practiced in the United States and other countries. Sometimes a hospice home care program run by visiting nurses, allied health professionals, and volunteers can provide for the death of a client at home. The important thing to remember is that there are alternatives to be considered. Maintaining control over place of death can be the last wish of a client.

CASE STUDY | **Mrs. Manfried Directs Her Care**

Mrs. Manfried is a 52-year-old woman with end-stage heart disease. She has been in the intensive care unit many times over the last 2 years, and she and her family have always wanted everything possible done to promote life. With each hospitalization, she cannot wait to go home to her loving family. Aware that treatments are not helping her during this hospitalization, she insists on being dis-

charged home to die. The physicians insist that the medical care she is receiving (including intravenous Lasix [furosemide], oxygen, and the daily adjustment of a host of cardiac medications) cannot be maintained at home. She pleads, "I don't fear dying at home. I only fear I will die here hooked up to all of this stuff and away from the home I have loved all these years."

With the help of a psychiatric clinical nurse specialist, a social worker, a home care hospice team, and the family, this client was weaned off many of her technical cares and sent home, where she died after 2 days. Part of the role of the clinical nurse specialist and the social worker was to help the treating team—the doctors and nurses who had devoted so much time and effort to keeping their beloved Mrs. Manfried alive—accept the right of the client to say "Enough is enough" and to shift gears from maximal treatment to comfort measures only. The team was helped to let go and to recognize a situation in which doing less meant more.

Nurses in hospitals need to be familiar with home care programs and alternatives for the dying client. Often a hospice coordinator or other member of a hospice team is willing to visit a client and family in the hospital to discuss options.

COMMUNITY BASED CARE

HOSPICE NURSE

Hospice care allows a person to remain in his or her home with family and friends until he or she dies. Symptoms are managed by the client and family, with support and instruction from the hospice team. The team consists of the client, family/caregivers, physician, nurse, social worker, chaplain, volunteers, and professionals from any other disciplines needed to help the client and family. Equipment, medications, and supplies are brought into the home as needed for care.

All people come to the dying process with different experiences and expectations. Often, the client and the family members have different fears and expectations. The hospice nurse's ability to effectively assess the client and family's physical, emotional, and spiritual needs, plan with the team, and teach in a supportive way is critical to discovering and meeting the client and family's unspoken needs. Teach by listening carefully to the client and family. Allow silence in the conversation. Often, people are unable to learn simple procedures because of unspoken fear related to the procedure being taught. For example, if a client or caregiver is thinking about his or her mother who "died screaming in pain" 30 years ago, the nurse needs to allow the client and caregiver to talk about dying, teach modern pain management, and address any other fears or questions before attempting to teach the procedure. Involve other team members in making joint visits to allow private conversations with the client and family. As a hospice nurse, you become very important to the family during one of the most intimate moments of a family's life.

The Nurse's Response to Death

When there has been a death on a unit, nurses have a ritual that can give meaning to the loss—that of preparing the body for the morgue. This is a time to treat the body with full respect given to the living. Each hospital or care facility has a protocol for how bodies are to be prepared and wrapped, what tubes are to be left in place or removed, what identifying tags need to be in place, and any other details of the care of the deceased. The nurse should consider asking for the help of a coworker in preparing the body. During that time together, there is the opportunity to discuss the passing of this life—what it has meant to the caregivers.

Nurses sometimes wonder why some deaths are easy to accept and others cause considerable stress. Each nurse is affected differently, depending on his or her past experiences, the amount of time spent with the client or family, whether the deceased reminded him or her of anyone, what else is happening in the nurse's life, how many other deaths have occurred in a short time, and other factors. Expected deaths aren't necessarily any easier than unexpected deaths, because with long-term clients, bonds of intimacy have been formed.

There is no easy advice for nurses to cope with client loss. The process is the same as for all grief. To grieve is to hurt, to search for meaning, and to reinvest in the living. That takes time. The stories of clients become part of the story of the nurse's life, as he or she takes stock of what has been meaningful. A busy hospital unit does not necessarily allow time to process a loss, yet all nurses must make the time to do just that. Whether with a colleague, a friend, a counselor, or family, in a journal, or simply with thoughts, nurses need to reflect on how working with persons at the end of life shapes the caregiver's perspective. Mourning for the clients cared for involves the weaving of their stories into the nurse's own.

While having a reverence for life, nurses often become frustrated by caring for clients who are irreversibly comatose or vegetative or being maintained on a ventilator with tube feedings. Some clients with grim prognoses are revived again and again with poor outcomes and a slow death. One nurse says, "Why prolong the inevitable? It only makes it harder on everyone." Another nurse reports, "Life is precious, and miracles do happen." Personal and collective convictions on the complex issues of death and dying are formed through the firsthand experiences of the nurse. Nurses are in a unique position to be involved in the shaping of health care policy about advance directives, ethical decisions at the end of life, DNR policies, and allocation of scarce resources. By using a wealth of firsthand knowledge, the nurse can help shape the death experience for future clients and families.

An issue often ignored is whether it is all right for nurses to show emotion when working with grieving or dying people and their families. Many judge themselves or others harshly if there are caregiver tears over a sad situation or at the time of death. If the nurse is moved to tears with a client, there is no need to apologize to anyone. Although there is a difference between having one's eyes fill with tears and crying uncontrollably, tears communicate caring. Therapeutic involvement cannot occur unless the caregiver cares and gives. When attachments form—and they will—the emotions will be felt. To detach from either the emotion or its expression can result in a shutting down of all feelings—both sadness and joy. Tears do not necessarily mean a greater level of caring, and dry eyes can also express empathy and care.

Nurses sometimes want to attend services for a client they have cared for over a long period or a client whose death has caused personal stress out of the realm of normal. Although it is not wrong to attend, several questions need to be asked:

- Am I attending for my own need or because I think the family needs me there?
- Are there significant others who might better take over the role of support?
- Will my presence bring attention to me and away from the family that must live on?
- Is there another appropriate way for me to reach closure on the death?

Over time, most nurses develop a personal policy about whether they attend clients' funerals or wakes, and care facilities sometimes offer quarterly or annual interfaith memorial services for staff to remember those who have died. Although it is necessary to find a way to separate one's personal life from one's work, a nurse's life is influenced by the performance of caring service. Nonetheless, a balance must be found and maintained, or the nurse runs a high risk of becoming emotionally and physically drained.

Dealing with clients and families during the crisis of illness or injury or at the end of life can be rewarding work, enriching one's appreciation for wellness and life. It can fill one with an awareness of the fragility of human life as well as the amazing ability of humans to go through difficult times and still find new meaning and hope. It can hold the reward of the knowledge that one person can make a difference. Although not able to change the ultimate outcome— the fact of death—the nurse can dramatically alter human experience along the road of life.

✦ Summary

This chapter contains the elements of nursing that may be most challenging over time. Helping individuals deal with the multitude of losses associated with acute, chronic, or terminal illness requires the nurse to use a skill that is acquired only through experience. Knowledge of the elements of normal loss, grief, and mourning is an essential beginning to this skill. Also essential for the care of dying clients and their families is an acceptance on the part of the nurse that dying is a part of living. There is no prescribed way to face death and no recipe for coping with the multitude of emotions involved with letting go of life. Each individual's pain of loss is uniquely his or hers—a suffering to be honored.

■ ■

CHAPTER HIGHLIGHTS
✦

- ✦ All humans experience loss and its accompanying response, which is grief.
- ✦ There are patterns of grief, but individual expressions and timing are unique.
- ✦ The pain of grief is one of the prices of living.
- ✦ At times, the most therapeutic intervention of the nurse is to remain present and silent.
- ✦ Knowing when to be silent can be a more useful skill than knowing what to say.
- ✦ Sometimes in the care of the dying, doing less means more.
- ✦ Individuals have a right and a responsibility to communicate their end-of-life decisions.

✦ The nurse is affected by the experiences of caring for grieving clients and their families. The effect can be life affirming and uplifting.

Study Questions

1. When a client is in denial about his or her terminal illness and is refusing chemotherapy, it is important for the nurse to

   a. clarify what the client has been told
   b. remind the client of the possible benefits of chemotherapy
   c. arrange for the client to speak to someone else who has been through chemotherapy
   d. arrange for a clergy person to visit the client
   e. contact a hospice representative to speak to the client

2. When coming upon a tearful client who is dying, the nurse should

   a. respect the person's need for privacy and leave him or her alone
   b. call for a psychiatric clinical nurse specialist, social worker, or clergy person
   c. inquire what the tears are about
   d. put his or her hand gently on the client's shoulder and say calmly, "Don't give up hope, miracles do happen"
   e. offer tissues to the client and try to cheer him or her with some distracting conversation

3. Which of the following behaviors might be considered a normal response to just learning of the death of a loved one?

   a. staring blankly into space without saying a word
   b. screaming, dropping to the floor, and pounding one's fists
   c. shouting angrily at the person giving the news
   d. saying, "Oh, my God, I can't go on, I'll kill myself without them"
   e. all of the above

4. You are caring for a dying client who whispers to you, "Am I going to die?" How might you best respond?

   a. "Only God knows for sure who will die and when."
   b. "We are all going to die."
   c. "You will need to speak to your doctor about that issue."
   d. "Tell me more about your thoughts and concerns."
   e. Ignore the question, because no one would be able to handle that news.

5. Nurses dealing with dying clients need to

   a. change jobs periodically to get a more upbeat perspective
   b. attend the wakes or funerals for clients they liked
   c. toughen up so that the work doesn't get to them
   d. have a strong religious faith in order to survive the demands of the work
   e. know how to allow a person to be with his or her own emotional pain

Critical Thinking Exercises

1. Ms. T. lost a baby to sudden infant death syndrome. Ms. S. just experienced the loss of a 6-year-old son after he battled leukemia for a year. Discuss the differences in the grieving process of these two mothers.

2. The nursing supervisor of 9 years just went into cardiac arrest while making rounds while on duty. The attempts to revive her were unsuccessful. Discuss the grief work of the staff and the code team.

References

Andrykowski, M., Brady, M. J., & Henslee-Downey, P. J. (1994). Psychosocial factors predictive of survival after allogenic bone marrow transplantation for leukemia. *Psychosomatic Medicine, 56,* 432–439.
Averill, J. R. (1982). *Anger and aggression: An essay on emotion.* New York: Springer.
Carter, S. L. (1989). Themes of grief. *Nursing Research, 38*(6), 354–358.
Davidson, G. W. (1984). *Understanding mourning—A guide to those who grieve.* Minneapolis: Augsberb Publishing House.
Jackson, E. N. (1965). *Telling a child about death.* New York: Hawthorne-Dutton.
Kübler-Ross, E. (1974). *Questions on death and dying.* New York: Macmillan.
Kübler-Ross, E. (1975). *Death: The final stage of growth.* New York: Macmillan.
Kutscher, A., & Kutscher, L. (Eds.). (1972). *Religion and bereavement: Counsel for the physician—Advice for the bereaved—Thoughts for the clergyman.* New York: Health Sciences.
Lindemann, E. (1944). Symptomatology and management of acute grief. *American Journal of Psychiatry, 101,* 141–148.
Peck, M. S. (1978). *The road less traveled: A new psychology of love, traditional values, and spiritual growth.* New York: Simon & Schuster.
Solari-Twadell, P. A., Bunkers, S. S., Wangs, C. E., & Snyder, D. (1995). The pinwheel model of bereavement. *Image: Journal of Nursing Scholarship, 27*(4), 323–326.
Strain, J. J., & Grossman, S. (1975). Psychological reaction to medical illness and hospitalization. In *Psychological care of the medically ill: A primer in liaison psychiatry.* New York: Appleton-Century-Croft.
Viorst, J. (1986). *Necessary losses—The loves, illusions, dependencies and impossible expectations that all of us have to give up in order to grow.* New York: Simon & Schuster.

Bibliography

Blankenship, J. (1984). *In the center of the night—Journey through bereavement.* New York: B. P. Putnam's Sons.
Bluebond-Langnew, M. (1978). *The private words of dying children.* Princeton, NJ: Princeton University Press.
Colgrove, M. (1984). *How to survive the loss of a love.* New York: Bantam Books.
Council on Scientific Affairs, American Medical Association. (1996). Good care of the dying patient. *Journal of American Medical Association, 275*(6), 474–477.
Cowles, K. V. (1996). Cultural perspectives of grief: An expanded concept analysis. *Journal of Advanced Nursing, 23,* 287–294.

Cutillo-Schmitter, T. (1996). Managing ambiguous loss in dementia and terminal illness. *Journal of Gerontological Nursing, 22*(5), 32–39.

Davis, B. D., Cowley, S. A., & Ryland, R. K. (1996). The effect of terminal illness on patients and their carers. *Journal of Advanced Nursing, 23,* 512–520.

deGroot-Bollujt, W., et al. (1993). Bereavement: Role of the nurse in the care of terminally ill and dying children in the pediatric intensive care unit. *Critical Care Medicine, 21*(9 Suppl), S391–S392.

Dufault, K. J., & Martocchio, B. C. (1982). *Bereavement: The price of loving. Advances in geriatric and long-term care.* Villanova, PA: Pro Scientia.

Jevne, R. (1991). *It all begins with hope—Patients, caregivers, and the bereaved speak out.* San Diego, CA: LuraMedia.

Kramer, K., & Kramer, H. (1993). *Conversations at midnight—Coming to terms with dying and death.* New York: Avon Books.

Levine, S. (1982). *Who dies? An investigation of conscious living and conscious dying.* Garden City, NY: Anchor Books.

Miles, A. (1993). Caring for the family left behind. *American Journal of Nursing, 93,* 34–36.

Moffat, M. J. (Ed.). (1992). *In the midst of winter—Selections from the literature of mourning.* New York: Vintage Books.

Nouwen, H. (1980). *In memorium.* Notre Dame, IN: Ave Maria Press.

Nuland, S. (1993). *How we die—Reflections on life's final chapter.* New York: Alfred A. Knopf.

Oerlemans-Bunn, M. (1988). On being gay, single, and bereaved. *American Journal of Nursing, 79,* 472–476.

Schoenbeck, S. B. (1993). Exploring the mystery of near-death experiences. *American Journal of Nursing, 93,* 43–46.

Wheeler, S. R. (1996). Helping families cope with death and dying. *Nursing, 96,* 25–30.

Zack, M. V. (1985). Loneliness: A concept relevant to the care of dying persons. *Nursing Clinics of North America, 20*(2), 403–412.

Unit ✦ VIII

APPLICATION OF THE NURSING PROCESS TO SPECIAL SITUATIONS

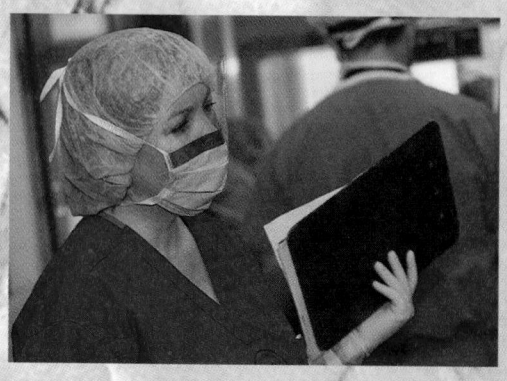

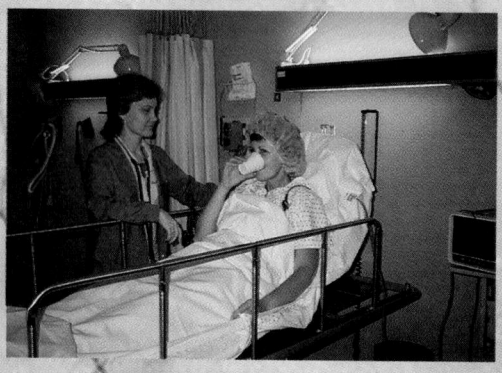

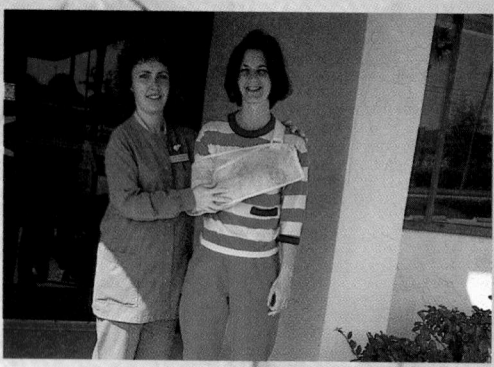

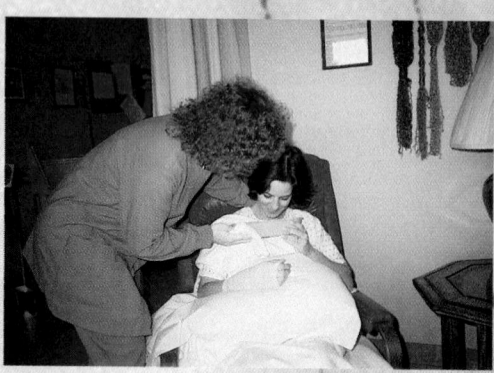

Ambulatory surgical nursing is a blend of many specialties, from medical/surgical to perianesthesia, intraoperative, and even home health. For the past 14 years, the close interactions with clients and their families have brought me great professional joy. My work involves preparing clients for procedures; helping them through procedures with dignity and comfort; and keeping them safe during the recovery period, when a nurse must be especially vigilant to potential changes in the airway, vital functions, surgical complications, anesthetic effects, client comfort, social needs, and more.

To describe this specialty succinctly is difficult because the clients and experiences are diverse, but the adjectives I would use are interactive, customer focused, friendly, comprehensive, fast paced, *and* responsible. *Positive, smiling, team-spirited nurses are the ones who will enjoy this specialty.*

An ambulatory surgical nurse must always consider clients in the context of their home settings. Is someone able to provide home care? Will my clients clearly understand— and follow— the preoperative instructions? Will safe transportation be available? Throughout the client's experience, providing understandable information is imperative, because the client and family are responsible for so much of the preparation and recuperation at home.

Education, careful assessment, and responsibility for follow-up are essential nursing keys. From the extra effort it takes to discover potential risk factors in the client's life and health history beforehand to the telephone call after the client's discharge, the nurse gains as much as he or she gives. The real "pay" is the human connection— the connection of true caring and making a difference. There is no better feeling than having a client who had been frightened preoperatively tell you how much your care meant to him or her as he or she is safely discharged after surgery.

Nancy Burden, BS, RN, CPAN, CAPA
Nancy Burden is Director of the Outpatient Center at Morton Plant Mease, Trinity Outpatient Center in New Port Richey, Florida and is certified in both postanesthesia and ambulatory perianesthesia nursing. Her early career in intensive care and "recovery room" nursing prepared her for the past 14 years in the ambulatory surgery field, where she has been a staff nurse, team leader, and director with responsibility for surgical, endoscopic, and pain management clients. No matter what her role, Burden describes the bedside as the most satisfying place to be.

Chapter 39

THE PERIOPERATIVE EXPERIENCE

BETTYANN HUTCHISSON,
RN, BSN, CNOR, CRCST

CHERI ACKERT BURR,
RN, MSN, CNOR, CRCST

KEY TERMS

◆

advance directives
anesthesia
aseptic technique
circulating nurse
durable power of
  attorney
endoscopic procedure
intraoperative phase

operating room (OR)
perioperative nursing
postanesthesia care
  unit (PACU)
postoperative phase
preoperative phase
scrub nurse

LEARNING OBJECTIVES

◆

After studying this chapter, you should be able to

◆ Define the scope of perioperative nursing
  practice

◆ List the types of surgery

◆ Discuss the roles of the surgical team

◆ Discuss the special needs of the surgical client

◆ Identify the "at-risk" client

◆ Describe nursing interventions for each phase
  of the perioperative experience

◆ Discuss the nursing process in the preoperative, intraoperative, and postoperative phases
  of the perioperative experience

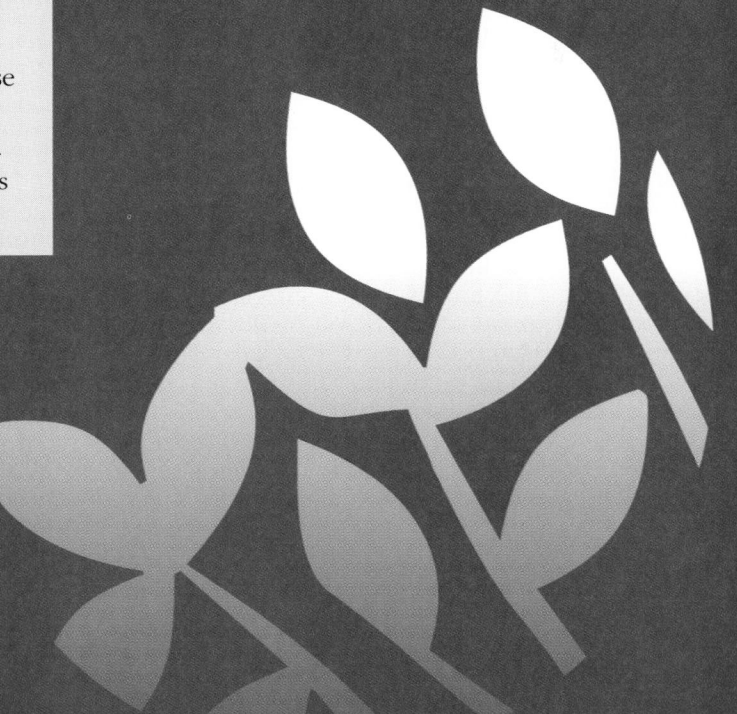

One of the most challenging areas of nursing practice is perioperative nursing. This field offers the nurse an opportunity to practice in many types of settings; *i.e.,* hospitals, day surgery centers, endoscopy centers, physicians' offices, and free-standing clinics. The perioperative role utilizes the nursing process, which includes multiple levels of assessment. The plans of care, interventions, and evaluations are constantly changing with the emergence of new knowledge and technology.

Perioperative nursing is a team effort that begins when a client decides to have a surgical procedure and ends when the client returns to an acceptable level of function or to some form of resolution of the initial problem. This chapter discusses the roles of the surgical team when caring for clients and their significant others during the surgical experience.

Today's perioperative nurse must be able to not only perform advanced technical skills necessary for intricate procedures but also provide physical and emotional support for the client and the client's significant others. The perioperative nurse must be able to develop rapid client rapport and trust, have highly effective assessment skills, and coordinate the plan of care and evaluation for the client.

The medical world did not believe it was necessary to train nurses in the prevention of infection until around 1880, when Lord John Lister discovered the importance of antisepsis in surgery. Shortly after this discovery, around 1889, Johns Hopkins University in Baltimore set up the first training program for **operating room (OR)** nursing, making OR nursing the first nursing specialty.

The advances of anesthesia allowed for extended operating times but also created a shortage of nursing personnel to work in the OR. This made it necessary to bring student nurses into the OR to assist with surgery. Student nurses continued to assist in the OR until about 1941. At this time, America entered World War II and the nurses left the hospitals to join the Armed Forces, leaving a void in the OR.

In 1949, several OR nurse managers met in New York City to discuss issues of concern. Training for OR nurses and what to do about the shortage of OR nurses were two of the topics discussed. This meeting became the first meeting of the Association of Operating Room Nurses (AORN). In 1960, AORN published its first official journal, entitled *OR Nursing* (now, *AORN Journal*). The primary focus of AORN is the education of OR nurses. In 1973, the organization adopted its first resolution, declaring a need to have a registered nurse in the OR. This OR nurse took on the role of consumer and client advocate.

The 1990s have been filled with challenges for the health care industry. The role of the OR nurse is changing and expanding, sometimes beyond our imaginations. Although OR nurses are now called perioperative nurses, the primary focus is still to act as client advocates who seek excellence in practice and to continue to act as vital individuals in the changing health care environment.

The Perioperative Experience

The perioperative experience is divided into three very distinct phases of care. The first or initial phase is the **preoperative phase.** This phase of care begins when the client decides to have surgery. It can occur in the physician's office, emergency department, or free-standing clinic and continues until the client arrives in the OR. The second, or **intraoperative, phase** begins when the client arrives at the door of the OR and ends when the client is delivered to the **postanesthesia care unit (PACU).** The third and final phase is the **postoperative phase** of care. This phase begins with the surgical client's admission to the PACU and ends when a return to an acceptable level of function or some form of resolution of the initial problem occurs. Recovery may take weeks, months, or sometimes years after discharge from the hospital and is dependent on a variety of factors, including the health status of the client and the type of surgery performed.

The perioperative nurse has a unique opportunity to utilize the nursing process to the fullest when caring for the surgical client through a variety of settings. The nursing care in the OR is a dynamic process. An ongoing, ever-changing process of data collection, planning, implementation, and reevaluation occurs. The process is never stagnant. Each phase of the perioperative experience utilizes the nursing process. The perioperative nurse has the opportunity to establish client rapport, determine client needs through preoperative assessment, and develop an individualized plan of care.

Surgical Classifications

Surgery can be a frightening and a potentially life-threatening experience for any person. There are several classifications or types of surgery.

Emergency surgery is a procedure that needs to be done immediately to save a life, a limb, or an organ. This may occur when a client sustains a traumatic injury following a motor vehicle accident. Imperative or urgent procedures are those that must be performed within 12 to 48 hours after determining the need for surgery. An elective procedure is performed for a condition that is not life threatening but will give the client a better prognosis or quality of life. It may or may not need to be done or may be offered as an alternative to noninvasive treatment.

Diagnostic surgery enables the surgeon and pathologist to establish or confirm the diagnosis of an illness or disease process. Diagnostic surgery usually involves some type of tissue biopsy from an organ, such as breast or prostate, or a biopsy from a suspicious-looking tissue mass. It may also involve a procedure to visualize the suspected unhealthy tissue, such as an endoscopic procedure. Palliative surgery relieves the symptoms of an illness but does not cure the disease. It can improve the quality of life and possibly ease chronic pain. Constructive surgery is performed to create a new or different body part or provide better function of an existing body part for the client. Reconstructive procedures improve appearance or function through partial or complete restoration or replacement of damaged tissue, such as cosmetic surgery, total joint replacements, repair of cleft palate, or when women have breast implants following removal of the breast (mastectomy). Curative procedures seek to cure illness or restore malfunctioning tissue by removing or altering diseased or damaged tissue, such as excising a tumor or removing a diseased gallbladder. Table 39–1 lists examples of surgical procedures for each classification.

Recent medical advances have changed the way surgical procedures are performed in the OR. Two of the advances in the OR that are discussed here are lasers and endoscopic surgery.

Laser Surgery

Laser is an acronym that stands for light amplification by stimulated emission of radiation. Albert Einstein first discussed stimulated emission of radiation in the early 1930s, but it was Dr. Theodore Maimon who designed the first Ruby Red laser in the 1960s (Ball, 1995).

The laser was first used in the OR for the treatment of vocal cord polyps and is still the treatment of choice today. The benefits of laser use in the OR include

1. Precision at the surgical site
2. Minimal blood loss
3. Minimal invasiveness of the procedures
4. A significant reduction in postoperative pain

5. A decrease in recovery time
6. The fact that general, regional, local, or topical anesthesia can be used

Several important safety issues must be addressed regarding the use of lasers in the OR. The first and most important is the potential for fire. The laser is a heat-related instrument that must be monitored. The perioperative team must be alert to signs of fire, location of fire alarms, and specific hospital protocols of what to do in the event of a fire. A fire during laser surgery can be prevented. Water should always be available on the surgical back table, and wet towels or sponges should be available to place around the laser site. A halogen fire extinguisher should be readily available.

One of the most important elements of a laser safety program is eye protection. Each type of laser light has a specific wavelength; therefore, each laser type has a different type of protective eyewear. The carbon dioxide laser has a wavelength of 10,600 nm and requires clear plastic or glass eyewear. Argon lasers have a wavelength of 488 nm and 518 nm and require eyewear with an orange tint. The neodymium:yttrium-aluminum-garnet laser has a wavelength of 1060 nm and requires eyewear protection with a green tint. The eyewear should have side shields, and a statement on the frame should describe the wavelength for which it can be used. Goggles can be purchased to fit over prescription glasses, or special goggles can be purchased that come with prescription lenses tinted to the different wavelengths. Microscopes and endoscopes can be fitted with special filters to prevent back-scattering of the laser beam. The client's eyes also must be protected. If the client is awake, then goggles should be worn by the client. Moistened eye pads should be taped over the client's eyes when he or she is anesthetized. The windows of the OR should be covered to prevent the transmission of the beam through the windows. A pair of goggles should be placed on the door to be used by anyone entering the room. Laser warning signs must be posted on all the outside doors to warn people of the hazard and to

Table **39–1**

CLASSIFICATION OF SURGICAL PROCEDURES

TYPE OF SURGERY	DEFINITION	EXAMPLES
Emergency	Done immediately to preserve life	Control of hemorrhage; tracheostomy
Urgent	Done within 24–48 hours; may prevent additional health problems	Vascular repair for obstruction; removal of malignant tumor
Elective	Based on client preference; not essential	Tonsillectomy; cataract surgery; facelift
Diagnostic	Makes or confirms diagnosis	Breast biopsy; exploratory laparotomy
Palliative	Relieves or reduces intensity of an illness	Colostomy; débridement of necrotic tissue
Constructive	Restores function in congenital anomalies	Cleft palate repair
Reconstructive	Restores function to traumatized or malfunctioning tissue; improves self-concept	Scar revision; internal fixation of a fracture
Curative	Cures illness by removal of damaged tissue	Removal of gallbladder

help reduce the traffic in the laser room. Lasers are very effective surgical instruments when used safely.

Endoscopic Procedures

An **endoscopic procedure** is defined as examination of a body cavity with the use of high-resolution video cameras (Fig. 39–1). Smaller incisions, less trauma to the tissue, and a faster recovery are a few of the benefits to the client having endoscopic surgery (Kneedler & Dodge, 1994). This procedure can be useful in surgical removal of the gallbladder, bowel resection, vaginal-assisted hysterectomy, thoracoscopy, and nasal sinus surgery, to name a few, and has created a new age in the performance of surgery. Table 39–2 lists surgical specialties using endoscopes and the procedures involving endoscopy.

Although abdominal endoscopic procedures are not the only type of endoscopic procedure, for the purposes of this text we only discuss abdominal endoscopy. General anesthesia is usually used because it allows the abdominal wall muscles to relax. The client is placed in the supine position, and the arms may be tucked at the sides. The abdomen is prepared with povidone-iodine (Betadine) solution, from nipple line to the symphysis pubis. This is done in preparation for the unlikely event of complications that would necessitate an open procedure. If the client has a lot of abdominal hair, a razor or clippers may be used to remove the hair before the skin preparation. The nurse needs to ensure that extra equipment, such as cameras, light cords, a carbon dioxide (CO_2) tank and tubing, and laparoscopic instruments, is available. An insufflation needle is inserted through the abdominal wall, and CO_2 gas is introduced into the peritoneum to allow visualization and to provide more room to separate the internal organs during the procedure.

Although there are many benefits from endoscopic procedures, the perioperative nurse must be aware that the client still is at risk for stress related to the surgical procedure. The same fear of the unknown is

Table 39–2	
AREAS OF SPECIALTY IN WHICH ENDOSCOPIC SURGERY IS USED	
Obstetrics and gynecology	Viewing of anatomy Diagnosis (minimally invasive) Lysis of adhesions Treatment of endometriosis Treatment of blocked fallopian tubes Assisting with vaginal hysterectomy
Sinus surgery	Viewing of anatomy Diagnosis (minimally invasive) Treatment for clearing sphenoid, front blockage
Gastroenterology	Viewing of anatomy Diagnosis (minimally invasive) Biopsy of polyps Cauterization of varices
Orthopedics	View of anatomy Diagnosis (minimally invasive) Repair of ligaments and tendons Repair of meniscus injuries Repair of patella pathology

present. The same complications of anesthesia are a possibility. Other complications can include puncture of the intestine or major vessels and the potential to become an open procedure. Clients who are at risk for complications in other types of surgery may be at similar risk for complications with endoscopic surgery.

✦ Anesthesia

Many factors are considered when choosing **anesthesia,** which involves the loss of sensation that may or may not involve the loss of consciousness. The anesthesiologist usually makes the decision to use local, regional, or general anesthesia but does consider the surgeon's needs and wishes, the procedure to be performed, the client position during surgery, the client's wishes, and the client's medical condition. Each administration of anesthesia has two objectives: to have the best possible outcome and to provide the best quality of anesthesia effect with the least amount of medication.

When the anesthesiologist interviews and assesses the client, he or she is assessing the client's medical condition, past surgical and anesthesia history, allergies, any physical limitations, prosthetic devices, and current medications. After reviewing the medical history, laboratory results, and diagnostic studies, the anesthesiologist assigns the client an anesthesia classifi-

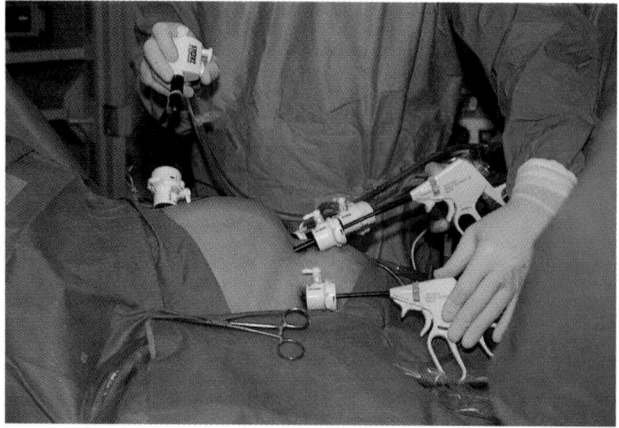

✦ **Figure 39–1**
Endoscopic equipment.

cation. This decision is discussed with the client and family members. The anesthesiologist also notifies the surgical team.

Anesthesia Classifications

Anesthesia classification is an evaluation of anesthetic morbidity and mortality related to the extent of systemic diseases and physiological medical abnormalities. The classification system includes

I. Healthy client: no physiological, psychological, biochemical, or organic disturbances

II. Mild systemic disease without functional limitation: cardiovascular disease with minimal restriction or activity, hypertension, asthma, chronic bronchitis, obesity, or diabetes mellitus

III. Severe systemic disease without functional limitation: cardiovascular or pulmonary disease that limits activity; severe diabetes with systemic complications; history of myocardial infarction, angina pectoris, or poorly controlled hypertension

IV. Severe, life-threatening systemic disease: severe cardiac, pulmonary, renal, hepatic or endocrine dysfunction

V. Moribund client: surgery is done as a last recourse or resuscitative effort; major multisystem or cerebral trauma, ruptured aneurysm, or large pulmonary embolus

E. Emergency surgery: for any client requiring emergency surgery, an E is added to the physical status

Type of Anesthesia

Several types of anesthesia can be used: general, spinal or epidural, and regional or local. Each type of anesthesia has advantages and disadvantages, risks, and special considerations. Box 39–1 lists common complications associated with each type of anesthesia.

General Anesthesia

The OR nurse and the postanesthesia care nurse need to be familiar with complications, length of effect, side effects, the potential for emergency situations, and knowledge of what the client may experience and expect on discharge.

General anesthesia was the first type of anesthetic used in surgery. In the beginning, its administration involved a great deal of guess work. The client was continuously assessed for changes in skin temperature, diaphoresis, and rigidity of muscles. As research and the specialty became more familiar, advances in equipment used for induction, monitoring, and the actual agents used for anesthesia were made. Today, general anesthesia is considered to be a safe procedure, although risks exist with any procedure. Table 39–3 outlines types of general anesthesia.

An anesthesiologist determines the route of administration (inhalation or intravenous injection) for each client. Regardless of which technique is used, the client passes through each of the four stages of anesthesia. These stages include

---

Box 39–1
COMPLICATIONS OF ANESTHESIA
General Anesthesia

Sore throat

Cut lip

Hypotension

Bronchospasm

Laryngospasm

Cardiac arrest

Respiratory failure

Possibly lost or cracked teeth

Numbness

Spinal and Epidural

Hypotension

Spinal headache

Urinary retention

Local and Regional

Anaphylactic reaction to drugs

Cardiac arrhythmias

Swelling or hemorrhage at injection site

Stage I: This stage begins with the administration of the anesthetic agent and ends with the client's loss of consciousness. This stage is known as the state of analgesia.

Stage II: This stage is known as the "excitement phase," when muscles become tense but the swallowing and vomiting reflexes are still intact. The client may have irregular breathing patterns. Breath holding is common during stage II.

Stage III: This stage is known as the "state of surgical anesthesia" and begins with the onset of regular breathing. Vital functions are depressed, eyes are fixed, and reflexes are depressed or temporarily lost. The surgeon begins the procedure during this phase.

Stage IV: This is the stage of complete respiratory depression.

During general anesthesia, the perioperative nurse's role is to assist the anesthesiologist with intubation and suctioning. The nurse also stands by the client's head and helps calm him or her.

Regional Anesthesia

Regional anesthesia involves blocking a specific set of nerve fibers or an individual nerve. The more familiar regional anesthetics include spinal, epidural, caudal, and peripheral nerve blocks (Fig. 39–2). Epidurals are frequently used in obstetrics during late labor and delivery. Spinal or epidurals are often used in high-risk clients undergoing pelvic and lower ex-

Table 39–3

ANESTHETIC AGENTS: ADVANTAGES AND DISADVANTAGES

TYPE	ADVANTAGES	DISADVANTAGES
Intravenous Induction Agents		
Thiopental sodium (Pentothal)	Quickly crosses blood-brain barrier; rapid and smooth induction	pH of 10.5, causing irritation when injected; histamine release causes flushing; possible skin rashes
Methohexital sodium (Brevital Sodium)	Is 2.5 times more potent than thiopental; can be used to produce short-term unconsciousness (retrobulbar, peribulbar, or other local injection); has amnesic effects; faster recovery of psychomotor function	Can cause hiccoughing, laryngospasm, cough, tremors, and involuntary muscle movement
Etomidate (Amidate)	Very short acting; can be used as an alternative to barbiturates; has few cardiovascular effects; has no histamine release	Myoclonia and dyskinesia may be observed; high incidence of pain on injection; nausea and vomiting postoperatively; cough and hiccoughs may occur during induction
Propofol (Deprivan)	Rapid recovery of consciousness and psychomotor abilities postoperatively; low incidence of nausea and vomiting; metabolized in the liver and excreted in the urine; twice as potent as thiopental	Pain on injection; hiccoughs and coughing on induction; involuntary small muscle movement
Dissociative Agents		
Ketamine (Ketalar)	Can be administered intramuscularly; can be used for combative clients who do not have an intravenous access; provides analgesia; normal protective airway is maintained	Produces cardiovascular stimulation, increasing heart rate, blood pressure, and cardiac output; emergence delirium, confusion, disorientation, bad dreams, hallucinations, and restlessness; must have a very quiet environment immediately postoperatively; use of benzodiazepine can prolong recovery
Inhalation Agents		
Oxygen	Sustains life; used on all general anesthetic clients; may be used on monitored anesthesia and local clients	
Nitrous oxide	When used with other inhalation agents, it decreases the amount of the other agent needed	Must be given in combination with oxygen; mild respiratory depression; mild myocarial depression; increases pressure inside air-containing spaces (*e.g.,* ear, bowel)
Halothane (Fluothane)	Good agent for bronchial asthma clients; rapid induction; used widely in pediatrics	Hypotension; decrease in myocardial contractile force; ventricular arrhythmias; local anesthesia with epinephrine needs to be monitored; return to consciousness is slower; shivering immediately postoperatively
Enflurane (Ethrane)	Cardiac output well maintained; cardiac rhythm remains stable; stable, nonflammable anesthetic gas	Possible hypocarbia in clients with history of seizures; respiratory depression
Isoflurane (Forane)	Stable, nonflammable gas; food muscle relaxant; no evidence of central nervous system activation of electroencephalogram or irritability is seen; very few hemodynamic changes	Excitement coughing; breath holding may occur when induction is too rapid
Desflurane (Suprane)	Rapid induction; rapid recovery	Similar to isoflurane

Table **39–3**

ANESTHETIC AGENTS: ADVANTAGES AND DISADVANTAGES
(Continued)

TYPE	ADVANTAGES	DISADVANTAGES
Depolarizing Muscle Relaxants		

Succinylcholine chloride (Anectine; Quelicin)	Rapid onset; short duration; rapidly metabolized in plasma	May be prolonged in clients whose pseudocholinesterase is atypical or deficient; may cause
		    Hypertension
		    Tachycardia
		    Bradycardia
		    Arrhythmias
		    Potassium release
		    Postoperative myalgia

Nondepolarizing Muscle Relaxants		
Atracurium besylate (Tracrium)	Intermediate acting; broken down in the plasma; good for clients with liver or kidney disease; no cumulative effect	Possible histamine release; bronchospasm; bradycardia; hypotension
Vecuronium bromide (Norcuron)	Intermediate onset, duration, and recovery; stable cardiovascular status	Some cumulative effect increases the duration of neuromuscular blockage
Tubocurarine chloride (Curare)	Paralysis of respiratory muscles	Arterial hypotension, especially in the elderly; use cautiously in clients with asthma and bronchitis
Mivacurium chloride (Mivacron)	Short acting; metabolized in the plasma; no cumulative effect	
Pancuronium bromide (Pavulon)	Most popular muscle relaxant; five times more potent than curare; little histamine release; paralysis of respiratory muscles	Sinus tachycardia; hypertension; excreted through the kidneys
Benzodiazepines		
Diazepam (Valium)	Gradual onset; few cardiovascular side effects; anticonvulsant; long acting; amnesia effects	Prolonged action due to storage in fatty tissue; pain at injection site; amnesic effects; long half-life (21–37 h)
Midazolam hydrochloride (Versed)	Short acting; water soluble; rapid hepatic clearance; half-life of 1–4 h; little venous irritation	Prolonged effects may occur in elderly clients
Reversal Agents		
Edrophonium chloride (Tensilon)	Reverses muscle weakness	Severe bradycardia
Naloxone hydrochloride (Narcan)	Narcotic antagonist; must be given in very small incremental doses	Cessation of analgesia; agitation; hypertension; noncardiogenic pulmonary edema; atrial and ventricular arrhythmias; cardiac arrest; possible nausea and vomiting
Neostigmine methylsulfate (Prostigmin)	Increases the response of muscles to nerve impulses	
Pyridostigmine bromide (Mestinon)	Increases the response of muscles to nerve impulses	

tremity surgery. Peripheral nerve blocks, such as an axillary block or bier block, are used for hand or arm surgical procedures. Ankle blocks are used for foot and toe surgeries. Table 39–4 lists common drugs used for local and regional anesthesia. It also describes onset and duration of the drugs, which is important in determining the agent to be used and the care to be given postoperatively.

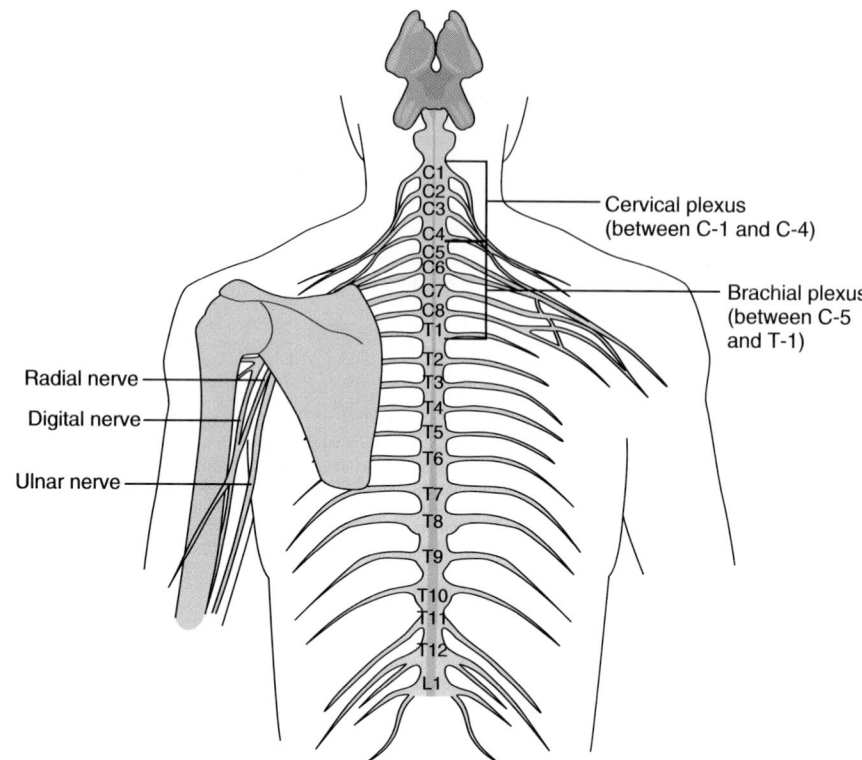

A

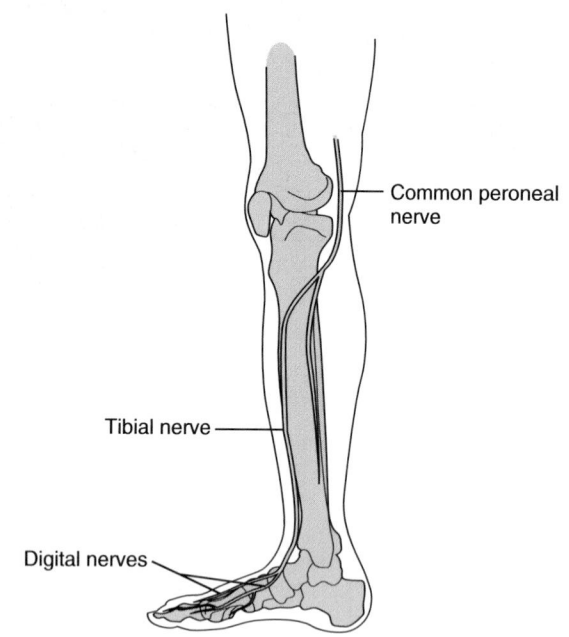

B

> ❧ **Figure 39–2**
> Sites of regional nerve blocks.
> *A,* Common upper extremity sites—
> radial nerve, digital nerve, ulnar nerve,
> and cervical plexus.
> *B,* Common lower extremity sites—
> common peroneal nerve, tibial nerve,
> and digital nerves.

Monitored Anesthesia

Monitored anesthesia is used in conjunction with a local anesthetic agent to provide a twilight sleep while the local anesthetic is injected into the surgical site or to decrease awareness during the procedure. The client has a medication injected intravenously to provide systemic analgesia and sedation and to depress the response of the client's autonomic nervous system. This technique is used for clients who may be critically ill or for any procedure that can be performed under local anesthesia. This method provides comfort for clients who may be extremely anxious. The client is monitored with blood pressure and oxygen satura-

Table 39-4

LOCAL AND REGIONAL ANESTHETIC AGENTS: ONSET AND DURATION OF ACTION

NAME OF DRUG	DURATION OF ACTION (NO EPINEPHRINE), MIN	DURATION OF ACTION WITH EPINEPHRINE, MIN	ONSET OF ACTION	DURATION OF ACTION
Bupivacaine hydrochloride (Sensorcaine; Marcaine)	120–240	240–480	Intermediate	Long
Chloroprocaine hydrochloride (Nesacaine)	15–30	30–90	Rapid	Short
Cocaine	10–55	None	Rapid	Short
Lidocaine hydrochloride (Xylocaine)	30–60	60–120	Rapid	Intermediate
Mepivacaine (Carbocaine; Polocaine; Cavacaine; Isocaine)	45–90	120–360	Intermediate	Intermediate
Procaine (Novocaine; Unicaine)	15–30	30–90	Rapid	Short
Tetracaine (Pontocaine)	120–240	240–280	Slow	Long

tion monitoring equipment, intravenous access, and electrocardiogram.

Local Anesthesia

Local anesthesia is usually used during minor procedures, such as superficial tissue biopsies, superficial cyst excision, insertion of pacemakers or arteriovenous grafts, and insertion of vascular access devices. With this type of anesthesia, the client can be immediately discharged to the nursing unit or to the same-day surgery unit, as care in the PACU is not usually required. However, if the client needs to be monitored after the procedure, the surgeon may request that the client go to the PACU for a short period.

Client Rights

The advent of modern medicine has been wonderful. Miracles happen every day. Lives are saved every day. However, modern medicine can frighten the average person. Life can be maintained by artificial support systems, and complicated surgeries can be performed that are not understood or wanted. Laws have been passed to protect the average person.

Informed Consent

Surgery cannot be performed until informed consent from the client has been obtained. It is the physi-

cian's responsibility to obtain an informed consent. Informed consent must cover the need for the procedure, describe the procedure to be performed, and document the risks involved and alternative treatments available. This explanation should be witnessed by another qualified health care worker.

If the client is a minor, is confused, has been medicated, or is mentally incompetent, another responsible party, such as a parent or significant other, must be present for the explanation and may need to be the person to sign the consent form. If it is an emergency situation and the client cannot sign and the next of kin is not available, then surgery may be performed with the concurring second opinion from another surgeon. Every effort must be made to obtain permission from a responsible family member. Telephone permission may be obtained and witnessed by two hospital employees on extension telephones.

All consent forms must be signed by the client and witnessed by a responsible person (usually a staff member) before preoperative medications have been given. If the client is illiterate, he or she can make a mark, witnessed by a staff member. The consent form must be timed, dated, and signed in ink.

Advance Directives

Written documentation that expresses the client's desires regarding medical interventions should the client become incapacitated are known as **advance directives** (Rosen, 1996). Two types of advance directives are living wills and durable power of attorney.

Living Wills

Most states now have laws stating that a competent adult can specify instructions, in writing or verbally, to his or her physician identifying specific situations in which artificial life-prolonging methods are not to be used (see Fig. 4–6). The client may also state when he or she would want to limit nutrients or fluids. Living wills only go into effect if the client develops an incurable or irreversible condition. This condition must be certified by two physicians. The nurse should become familiar with government regulations in the state in which he or she practices nursing.

Durable Power of Attorney

Many states allow competent adults the right to designate another person to make health care decisions if he or she becomes unable to communicate his or her wishes. This is called **durable power of attorney** and is different from a living will because the client does not have to be in a terminal condition to have the appointed person act on his or her behalf. For example, the client could be in a coma.

Nursing Process in Care in the Preoperative Phase

Assessment

During the preoperative phase, the nurse is in a critical position to assess the client and identify potential factors that might place the client at risk during the surgical procedure. The nurse's assessment is an essential component of the preparation required for the client.

Nursing History

The nursing history can provide valuable information. The nurse should begin with a simple visual inspection of the client. This is sometimes referred to as purposeful looking.

It is imperative that a nursing history be completed to provide the best and safest nursing care possible. Because time is limited, the nurse needs to have excellent interviewing skills and a strong knowledge base of the surgical procedure to obtain the information needed in a timely fashion. The nurse should begin by introducing himself or herself to the client. The nurse should find a quiet place for the interview. A separate room is ideal, but sometimes the nurse simply has to close the curtains in a semiprivate room to shut out the outside environment. The goal is to provide as much privacy as possible.

The nurse must actively listen to the client and look for nonverbal signals of anxiety, which could include lack of eye contact, poor posture, or inappropriate responses. If the client is very ill, then a family member or significant other should join the interview process to lessen the demand on the client while assisting the nurse to obtain necessary information.

The client provides good information if he or she senses a positive response from the nurse. For instance, the client may be anxious and can easily pick up on the fact that the nurse is preoccupied and in a hurry. The nurse should ensure that the client believes that he or she is the main focus. The nurse should use appropriate open-ended questions to enhance the interview and obtain needed information. Judgmental responses or questions are not appropriate. After collecting the data, the nurse should summarize the information for the client to offer a way to verify that both the nurse and the client have the same understanding of the procedure, activities, and outcomes. This also offers an opportunity for questions. The more pertinent information that can be gained, the better. Once the client has been administered anesthetic agents, it is impossible to get information.

A major focus of the nursing history is collecting information about the client to determine surgical risk factors. Factors that are to be included in the nursing history are

General Health

The general health of the client can affect the outcome of a surgical procedure. The perioperative nurse should look at and evaluate the appearance of the client. When people do not feel well, they ignore their outward appearance. A man who has not shaved or a woman who has not fixed her hair or nails may be too ill or tired to do so. Height and weight can be indicators of well-nourished or malnourished individuals. The client may say that he or she has not gained or lost weight, but the nurse may assess that the client's clothing does not fit properly; for example, it may be too tight.

Smoking Habits

The client who has a history of smoking can be at risk for pulmonary complications. The individual who smokes tends to have an increase in thickened mucous secretions in the lungs, thus decreasing the capability of air exchanges. These clients have more difficulty clearing and maintaining a patent airway during the postoperative period.

Alcohol Use

The client who has a history of excessive alcohol ingestion is at risk for anesthesia reactions. It is necessary to use more of the anesthesia and analgesic medications to keep the client comfortable. Alcohol can potentiate the effect of the autonomic nervous system response, such as causing a decrease in respirations. The client who abuses alcohol also can be at risk for malnutrition, liver damage, and overall decreased general health.

Age

Infants and elderly clients are at greater risk during surgical procedures than adolescent or middle-aged clients. Each group has special risks that must be evaluated and addressed for the most positive outcome to a surgical procedure.

Infants do not have a well-developed shiver reflex, so they have difficulty maintaining body temperature. This can lead to hypothermia or hyperthermia. Infants are also at greater risk for dehydration related to small volumes: Infants have less total blood volume than older children and adults, so they have less to lose before they are in crisis. The infant cannot respond to the need for increased oxygenation during the surgical procedure so must be monitored carefully throughout the procedure.

Elderly clients have gone through several physiological changes of aging that put them at risk for surgical complications. They have decreased circulation, possibly due to atherosclerosis, and this leads to longer healing processes and a potential for thrombophlebitis. Elderly clients also have a decreased cough reflex, which reduces their ability to clear their airway effectively. The elderly have sensory deficits that decrease their reaction time to external stimuli. The nurse must allow more time for them to understand what is expected of them. Questions should be short and simply stated; nurses should speak low and directly. The elderly have dry, inelastic skin, which can lead to easier skin breakdown and can slow the healing process. Initial and ongoing skin assessment is critical to the positive outcome of the elderly client.

Nutrition

Good nutrition is a necessary requirement of a good surgical recovery. Clients who are either overweight or malnourished are at risk for surgical complications.

Obese clients can have several risk factors that need to be addressed. Obese clients have poor circulation. This results in inadequate nutrients for tissue building, and perfusion of major organs, such as heart, lungs, and kidneys, is decreased. These clients can have an elevated blood pressure or respiratory difficulties, which can affect the position in which they must be placed during surgery and the recovery period.

The malnourished client is at risk for skin breakdown and poor wound healing. Vitamins and proteins are needed for wound healing—especially vitamin K, which is needed for blood clotting.

Attitude

The client's attitude is very important in contributing to a positive outcome for a surgical procedure. If a client is overly anxious, this can increase the surgical risk. For example, if a client is afraid that death will be the outcome of surgery, the nurse should notify the surgeon and anesthesiologist at once. The surgery may

need to be postponed until counseling can be obtained.

If the client had surgery in the past and experienced a bad outcome, then this client may have a negative attitude about this procedure. The previous negative experience could have included poor pain control, the degree of disability after the surgical procedure, poor family support, or a poor hospital experience.

Medication History

The client's use of drugs, whether prescribed or over the counter, can affect his or her reaction to surgery and anesthesia. Clients who have a chronic illness, such as diabetes or hypertension, require the continued use of some medications. Other medications can potentiate a negative reaction. For instance, steroids can alter the inflammatory response and affect the blood pressure, anticoagulants can place the client at high risk for hemorrhage, and diuretics can alter the fluid and electrolyte balance within the body (Box 39–2).

Physical Examination

A physical examination is performed for all clients having a surgical procedure. If the procedure is not an emergency, this examination will probably be performed in the physician's or health care provider's office. Some common health problems may place a client at risk for surgical complications and may even lead to cancellation of the procedure. These include

1. Cardiac conditions like angina pectoris, recent myocardial infarction, severe hypertension or hypotension, and severe congestive heart failure

---

Box **39–2**

THE AT-RISK CLIENT

The pediatric client is at risk for dehydration and airway complications

The geriatric client is at risk for decreased circulation and difficulty clearing the airway, and is at increased risk for skin breakdown

The obese client is at risk for poor wound healing, elevated blood pressure, and respiratory difficulties

The malnourished client is at risk for poor wound healing and increased skin breakdown

The client with multisystem diseases is at risk for poor wound healing, increased pain, and decreased circulation

The mentally or physically challenged client is at risk for increased anxiety, poor pain management, and decreased participation in self-care

Cultural barriers place the client at risk for increased anxiety, decreased cooperation, and decreased self-care (see Chapter 36)

2. Problems with blood clotting, which can lead to hemorrhage or shock

3. Upper respiratory infections or chronic lung diseases such as emphysema, which could place the client at risk for postoperative complications of severe lung infections

4. Diabetes mellitus, which can place the client at risk for poor wound healing, wound infection, or delayed healing

Vital signs should be taken and evaluated. Anxiety and fear can cause the blood pressure and heart rate to accelerate. While assessing the client, the nurse can gather more data specifically related to the client's normal pulse and blood pressure. The preadmission vital signs are used as a baseline in the intraoperative and postoperative assessment process.

Sociocultural Assessment

The cultural barriers that can affect surgery are countless. Does the client speak the same language as the surgical team? If not, is it possible to get an interpreter to assist the client? If the client comes from a culture that has strict rules for female dress, can she get enough privacy before anesthesia to feel safe or comfortable? Does the client's culture have taboos that the nurse needs to know about? The nurse must be aware of and understand that a client may not be cooperating because what is being asked of him or her is forbidden in his or her home culture or because he or she simply does not understand what is being asked. (Chapter 36 addresses culture and its implications for nursing care.)

Screening Tests

Several clinical screening tests may be ordered before any surgical procedure. These tests provide baseline information about the client or objective information about the client's risk for postoperative complications. Common screening tests that are done include complete blood count to evaluate the client's hematological status, chest x-ray to determine pulmonary function, electrocardiogram (a common test usually done on all clients over 40 years of age to evaluate cardiac function), and urinalysis to screen renal function.

Nursing Diagnosis

The nursing diagnoses for the client who is in the preoperative phase include actual and potential problems, based on the information gathered in the initial assessment. Examples of nursing diagnoses, appropriate for the preoperative client taken from the North American Nursing Diagnosis Association, may include, but are not limited to,

* Anticipatory Grieving related to loss of normal body image

* Anxiety related to the perioperative experience

* Fear related to effects of impending surgery, risk of death, loss of control during anesthesia, waking up during the operation, or the outcome of the procedure

* Knowledge Deficit related to preoperative routines or postoperative expectations

* Sleep Pattern Disturbance related to hospital environment or the stress of the surgical procedure

* Ineffective Individual Coping related to past experiences or a lack of problem-solving skills

Planning

The expected outcomes for all preoperative clients are basically the same. The approach to reaching these outcomes is individualized, depending on the assessment of the client (see Sample Nursing Care Plan). The client should be

Physically and emotionally prepared for surgery

Able to demonstrate deep breathing and coughing exercises

Able to verbalize understanding of the procedure and expectations for him or her in the postoperative phase

Able to maintain an adequate fluid and electrolyte balance in the intraoperative and postoperative phases

Implementation

Nursing interventions during the preoperative phase of the surgical procedure are provided to assist the client to achieve a positive outcome from the procedure by reducing anxiety and fear of the unknown and opening communication among the client, family, and health care team.

Preoperative Teaching

Preoperative teaching has a positive outcome for the surgical client. Shorter hospital stays, less pain medication needed, and increased compliance with planned interventions, activities, and therapies have all been documented with preoperative teaching (Hathaway, 1986; Healy, 1968). The literature also shows the importance of including the family in preoperative teaching. A decrease in the family's anxiety allows them to give support to the client and speed recovery and discharge (Moss, 1986). Preoperative teaching should include the following.

The Surgical Experience

The surgical procedure should be explained in detail to the client and family members. This should include risk factors, preadmission routine, the OR environment and routines, any skin preparations, positions, and expected outcomes.

Preoperative instruction should include medications that the client should take before coming to the hospital and any medication that might be given at the hospital. The client may be asked to bring medications that he or she takes at home with him or her.

Text continued on page 1183

SAMPLE NURSING CARE PLAN

THE CLIENT WITH AN ABDOMINAL HYSTERECTOMY

Sue Vitaz, age 58 years, is admitted to the hospital on the 7th of January for an abdominal hysterectomy on the 8th of January. She states that she has been having bloody discharge from her vagina for about 1 month, and the physician thinks that she has fibroid tumors. These tumors are not malignant. Mrs. Vitaz has no history of previous surgeries and has always been healthy. Her husband and two daughters accompanied her to the hospital. A physical assessment finds her height 5 feet, 3 in; weight, 128 lb; temperature, 98.8°F (37.1°C); respirations, 20; blood pressure, 126/82. Laboratory findings (done last week at the physician's office) include normal potassium, complete blood count, electrocardiogram, chest x-ray, and urinalysis. Mrs. Vitaz has many questions and states: "I'm very nervous about tomorrow."

Preoperative Phase

Nursing Diagnosis: Anxiety related to the surgical experience

Expected Outcome: The client will demonstrate a decrease in anxiety as evidenced by

Regular breathing

Ability to respond to simple questions

Ability to describe upcoming events of surgical procedures

Action	Rationale
1. Explain the surgical procedure to the client.	1. Correct information clarifies any errors and lets the client know what to expect.
2. Explain the sequence of events that will take place in the OR and holding area (*e.g.,* intravenous lines, OR protocols).	2. Lets the client know what to expect. Follows hospital policy and procedure.
3. Explain early postoperative client expectations (*e.g.,* turning, coughing, moving).	3. Cooperation is forthcoming when the client knows what to expect.

Nursing Diagnosis: Knowledge Deficit related to the surgical experience

Expected Outcome: Client Knowledge of the physiological and psychological responses to the surgical intervention, as evidenced by

Verbalization of procedure

Verbalization of client teaching

Demonstration of decrease in anxiety

Action	Rationale
1. Assess the client's knowledge of the surgical procedure, OR environment, and past surgical and medical experiences.	1. Lets the nurse know what needs to be explained and at what level this information needs to be shared.
2. Provide verbal information about the procedure and the environment.	2. Clarifies information and increases client knowledge base.
3. Instruct the client about OR routines and activities. a. Monitoring equipment (*e.g.,* electrocardiogram, pulse oximeter, blood pressure cuff, temperature). b. Personnel in the room.	3. Reduces fear when the client knows what to expect.

Continued

SAMPLE NURSING CARE PLAN

THE CLIENT WITH AN ABDOMINAL HYSTERECTOMY

(Continued)

Intraoperative Phase

Nursing Diagnosis: Risk for Injury related to positioning, retained extraneous objects, and chemical, physical, or electrical hazards

Expected Outcome: The client will demonstrate absence of adverse effects through

No retained extraneous objects

No chemical burns

No electrical burns

No physical changes in skin integrity

Action	Rationale
1. Assess for risk factors: age, weight, nutritional status, mobility, allergies, medical history, circulatory status, type of procedure, length of procedure, activity level.	1. Proper assessment provides safe actions for the client. Provides baseline values.
2. Monitor counts for correctness: sponges, needle, instruments.	2. Client will be free from extraneous objects.
3. Place electrocautery grounding pad correctly.	3. Prevents burns from electrical current.
4. Assess for allergies.	4. Prevents injury from incorrect medication.
5. Check electrical equipment for safety.	5. Client will be free from injury related to equipment.
6. Prevent pooling of preparation solutions.	6. Client will be free from chemical burns.
7. Position the client in correct anatomical alignment utilizing positioning.	7. Client will be free from injury related to positioning.

Nursing Diagnosis: Risk for Impaired Skin Integrity related to the surgical environment

Expected Outcome: The client will demonstrate maintenance of skin integrity by having no visible changes in skin integrity.

Action	Rationale
1. Pad bony prominences.	1. Protects those areas with greater potential for skin breakdown.
2. Place grounding pad correctly.	2. Prevents chance of electrical burns.
3. Assess for allergies.	3. Decreases risk of anaphylactic reaction.
4. Assess current skin integrity.	4. Baseline assessment.
5. Keep skin dry (except at preparation site).	5. Decreases risk of skin breakdown due to moisture.

Nursing Diagnosis: Risk for Wound Infection related to the surgical procedure

Expected Outcomes: The client will demonstrate absence of infection, as evidenced by

No redness

No swelling

No purulent drainage

Action	Rationale
1. Monitor aseptic technique of all surgical team members.	1. The practice of aseptic technique will keep the client infection free.
2. Practice aseptic technique.	2. Follow policy and procedure in hospital.

SAMPLE NURSING CARE PLAN

THE CLIENT WITH AN ABDOMINAL HYSTERECTOMY

(Continued)

Nursing Diagnosis: Risk for Fluid and Electrolyte Imbalance related to the surgical procedure

Expected Outcome: The client will demonstrate balance of electrolytes and fluids, as evidenced by

Hematocrit and hemoglobin within normal limits or presurgery acceptable limits

Intake and output balance

Blood pressure and pulse within normal limits for the client

Electrolytes within normal limits

No restlessness or confusion postoperatively

Action	Rationale
1. Monitor blood loss.	1. Replacement of lost fluid can be done if correct monitoring is maintained.
2. Monitor for fluid overload.	2. Decreases risk for hypovolemic shock.
3. Monitor intake and output.	3. Decreases risk for congestive heart failure and pulmonary edema.

Postoperative Phase

Nursing Diagnosis: Risk for Pain related to psychological and physical response to the surgical event, positioning, and immobility

Expected Outcome: Client will be free of pain, as evidenced by

Blood pressure within 20 mmHg of baseline

Heart rate 60 to 100 beats per minute

Respirations regular, nonlabored (12–28 per minute)

Absence of nausea and vomiting

Absence of nonverbal communication suggesting discomfort

Absence of chilling

Action	Rationale
1. Assess type, amount, and administration of anesthetic agents.	1. Prevents overmedication.
2. Assess physical response to discomfort.	2. All clients perceive pain differently and respond differently.
3. Assess verbal and nonverbal communication.	3. Determine client's ability to communicate pain because some clients wait until pain is unbearable to request medication, and then the medication does not work as well.
4. Palpate for bladder distention.	4. Bladder distention will cause more abdominal pain.
5. Administer pain medication and evaluate responses.	5. Presence of pain prolongs convalescence.
6. Position for comfort using warm blankets.	6. Cold produces more pain sensation, shivering, and discomfort.

Continued

SAMPLE NURSING CARE PLAN

THE CLIENT WITH AN ABDOMINAL HYSTERECTOMY
(Continued)

Nursing Diagnosis: Risk for Airway Obstruction related to preoperative sedation, anesthesia, or laryngospasm

Expected Outcome: Client will not show signs of airway obstruction, as evidenced by

Respiration spontaneous, regular, and quiet

Breath sounds clear

Symmetrical chest expansion

Absence of restlessness

No changes on the electrocardiogram

Client oriented to person, place, time, and situation

Action	Rationale
1. Assess for airway patency.	1. The number one priority in the perioperative experience is airway patency.
2. Assess rate, depth, rhythm or respirations.	2. Useful in early recognition of atelectasis, rates, and airway obstruction.
3. Determine types and times of anesthetic agents.	3. May affect respiratory status postoperatively.
4. Monitor for oxygen saturation greater than 95.	4. Oxygen levels less than 95 decrease oxygen tissue perfusion.
5. Assess for skin color.	5. Cyanosis is an early sign of poor circulation.
6. Assess for respiratory distress (confusion, restlessness, gasping).	6. Physiological emergencies.

Nursing Diagnosis: Risk for Fluid and Electrolyte Imbalance related to surgical procedure

Expected Outcome: The client will not show signs of fluid or electrolyte imbalance, as evidenced by

Intake and output balanced

Hematocrit and hemoglobin within normal limits or presurgery acceptable limits

Blood pressure and pulse within normal limits for the client

Electrolytes within normal limits

No evidence of restlessness or confusion

Action	Rationale
1. Monitor blood loss.	1. Large amounts of blood loss can lead to hypovolemic shock.
2. Monitor for fluid overload.	2. Fluid overload can lead to pulmonary edema and congestive heart failure.
3. Monitor intake and output.	3. This will assist in evaluating dehydration.

Nursing Diagnosis: Risk for Wound Infection related to the surgical procedure

Expected Outcome: The client will be free of infection, as evidenced by

No redness

No swelling

No purulent drainage

Action	Rationale
1. Practice aseptic technique.	1. Standard of care.
2. Monitor aseptic technique of all team members.	2. It is the responsibility of all nursing personnel to prevent nosocomial infections.

Nothing by Mouth Status

As a general rule, the client is told to withhold food and water after midnight the night before surgery. Nothing by mouth (NPO) status assists in preventing aspiration of stomach contents during the surgical procedure. If the stomach is empty then no gastric contents are present to vomit. During the preoperative assessment by either the perioperative nurse or the anesthesia personnel, the client may be instructed to take morning medications for hypertension or cardiac conditions with a few sips of water.

Infants are usually not kept without food and water for as long a time as adults. The age and weight of the child determines how long the child will be kept at an NPO status before the procedure.

Pain Management

The surgical client and family usually are concerned about pain management during the perioperative experience. It is normal to have pain after a surgical intervention. The client should be informed that pain medication will be ordered by the physician. Pain medications are usually ordered as needed and by the route appropriate for the client's condition. Medication is ordered by intramuscular injection or intravenous injection when the client is unable to take it orally,

but as the client becomes stronger and is able to take medication orally, the route is changed. The client should be instructed to ask for pain medication as needed and not to fear becoming addicted to it.

Intravenous Line

An intravenous infusion line is inserted into the client on the morning of the procedure. The intravenous line is used to maintain fluid and electrolyte balances during the surgical procedure. During major surgical procedures, an increase in fluid and blood loss usually occur. The intravenous line is used to help replace those losses and to administer medication. Procedure 28–1 explains the procedure and purpose of an intravenous line.

Skin Preparation

The client will be asked to take a shower the night before and the morning of surgery using an antimicrobial soap. The client will be asked to remove all nail polish and to report for surgery without makeup. No hairpins, barrettes, or clips with metal should be worn to the OR. Any hair accessories left in place could contribute to the loss of hair at the site due to pressure. Hair accessories or jewelry may also act as conduits when electrical cautery is used. Figure

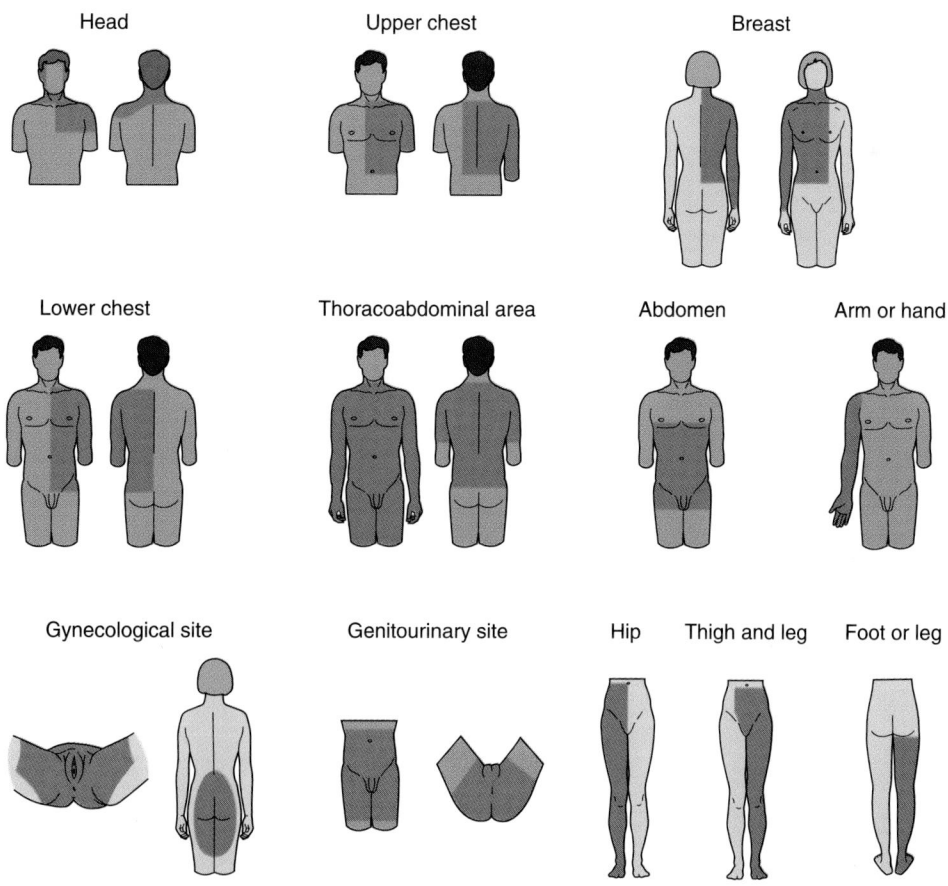

Figure 39–3
Common skin preparation sites for surgery.

PROCEDURE

39–1

HAIR REMOVAL

Explain the procedure and purpose of the procedure to the client and family.

Clinical Situation: The client will be shaved prior to the surgical procedure to remove hair and decrease bacteria present at the operative site.

Anticipated Response: No postoperative infection related to hair around the incision site will occur.

Equipment: *Gather before beginning*

Shave kit
Unsterile gloves
Disposable razor
Antimicrobial agent
Towels
Basins
Water
Impervious drapes

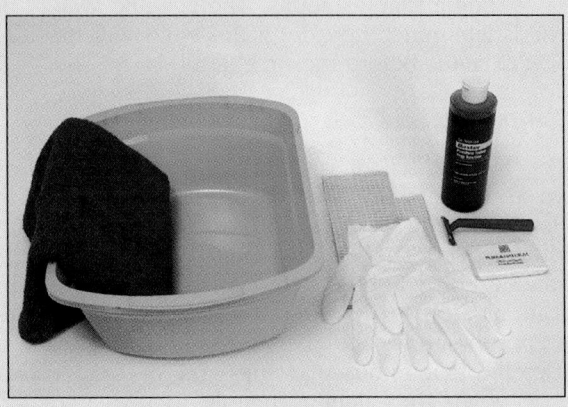

Action	**Rationale**
1. Allow for privacy of the client; make sure you have adequate lighting; and check for allergies, scars, or moles that may hinder hair removal. Gather correct equipment.	**1.** Prepares client for procedure.
2. Expose area to be shaved. Put on gloves. Place impervious drapes under client. Lather skin. Hold skin taut. Direct razor in the direction of hair growth. After shave is complete, rinse and dry the skin.	**2.** Gloves are used whenever there is a chance of coming into contact with blood or body fluids. Always shave in the direction of hair growth for a cleaner shave with less chance of nicks.

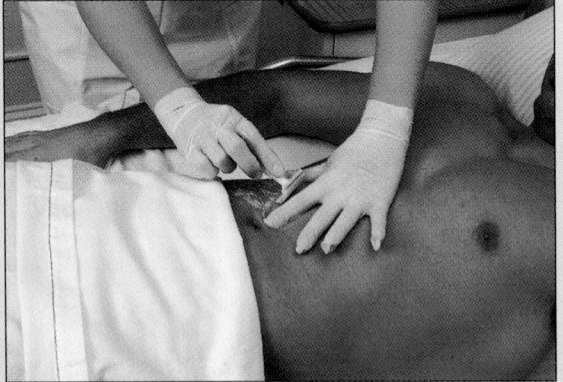

Step 2.

3. Depilatory creams: Perform skin test. If test is negative, apply cream according to manufacturer instructions; after specified time, remove cream and hair. Clean, rinse, and dry the skin.	**3.** A skin test is done to be sure client does not have an allergy to the cream that would cause the need to cancel the surgical procedure because of rash.

PROCEDURE

39–1

HAIR REMOVAL
(Continued)

Action	Rationale
4. Electric clippers: Long hair around the surgical incision may need to be cut with scissors before using electric clippers.	**4.** Long hair can jam the clippers.
5. Common agents for skin cleaning: Povidone-iodine (Betadine)	**5.** Action: Fast acting Nonstaining Slow release Can be used on mucous membranes Should not be allowed to pool (can cause skin burns) on skin or in body cavities
Hexachlorophene (pHisoHex)	Cumulative suppressive action Bacteriostatic effect Minimally active against gram-negative bacteria
Chlorhexidine (Hibiclens)	Effective against wide range of microorganisms Fast acting Nonstaining Few reported cases of allergic reactions Eye injuries associated with use Can cause ototoxicity if instilled into the middle ear

39–3 shows skin preparation sites for common surgical procedures. Procedure 39–1 on hair removal and Procedure 39–2 on surgical skin preparation explain the purpose and procedure for each of these activities.

In today's health care environment, few differences exist between inpatient and outpatient or same-day surgery preoperative or postoperative teaching techniques. Each client should go home with written instruction detailing limitations, procedures to be performed, and the correct dispensation of medications.

Positioning

It is essential for the nurse to make a good preoperative assessment before placing a client in any position. The nurse should place the client in the operative position during the preoperative assessment to be sure that no physical limitations would prevent the client from being placed in the desired position. This also helps the client to understand some of the muscle stiffness in the postoperative phase.

General Expectations

Minor symptoms like headache, sore throat, and general muscle aches are reasonable expectations of any surgical procedure. Warm gargles, lozenges, and warm baths can help alleviate these symptoms. Analgesia such as acetaminophen (Tylenol) or aspirin can

be used. Gentle stretching exercises can also relieve sore muscles. Before the client is discharged from the hospital or same-day clinic, the perioperative nurse assists the client in making follow-up appointments with the physician.

Diet

Because many clients are admitted on the morning of the surgical procedure, any dietary restrictions should be outlined in writing. Increased oral fluids are encouraged, especially after urological procedures and spinal anesthesia. However, alcohol is restricted for 24 hours because of its ability to potentiate the effects of sedation.

A common postoperative problem is nausea. If the client experiences nausea, he or she is instructed to lie flat with the head elevated, limit the amount of oral intake, and eat bland food such as crackers before taking oral medication.

Activity

The client is often instructed to limit activities. Returning to normal activity levels too soon can result in exhaustion, bleeding, or increased pain and swelling. The client needs to rest and follow the recommended schedule.

PROCEDURE

39–2

SURGICAL SKIN PREPARATION

Explain the procedure and purpose of the procedure to the client.

Clinical Situation: The surgical skin preparation is performed to reduce the risk of surgical wound infection by reducing the bacteria count of the skin.

Anticipated Response: The client will not develop a surgical wound infection.

Equipment: *Gather before beginning*

    Sterile preparation set
    Sterile gloves
    Sterile absorbent towels
    Antimicrobial agents

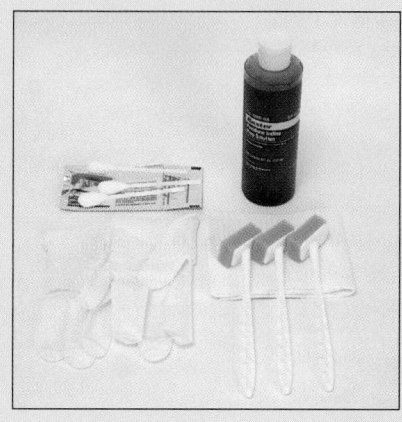

Action	Rationale
1. Check the physician order.	**1.** Helps to gather the correct equipment.
2. Select a broad-spectrum antimicrobial agent that will reduce and inhibit both transient and residual microorganisms. Ineffective against soaps and organic matter.	**2.** Decreases the potential for infection. The agent should be fast acting, easily applied, and long acting. It should be nonirritating.
3. After client is positioned, expose only area to be prepared.	**3.** Maintains client privacy and keeps client warm.
4. Put on sterile gloves and tuck sterile absorbent towels around the client.	**4.** Prevents pooling of solutions that could cause skin burns.
5. Begin cleaning at incision site and move out peripherally, never bringing a soiled sponge back toward the center.	**5.** Prevents contamination of incision site.

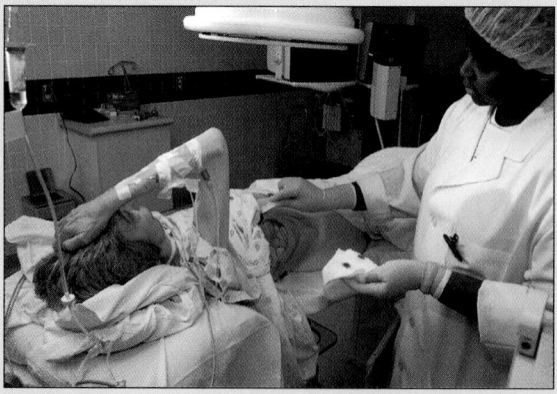

Step 5.

6. If a stoma will be in the preparation site, cover with a sterile dressing and prepare last.	**6.** Prevents contamination.

PROCEDURE

39–2

SURGICAL SKIN PREPARATION
(Continued)

Action	Rationale
7. If there is a second (graft) site, a second kit should be used, or the graft site should be prepared first.	7. Prevents contamination of the graft site, or if there is chance of malignancy, prevents the chance of seeding tumor in second site.
8. If preparing a malignancy, do not scrub vigorously; paint the area with solution paint or gel.	8. Prevents the spread of the tumor.
9. After the preparation is finished, blot the lather with absorbent towel, pick towel up at outer edge, being careful not to pull over prepared site.	9. Prevents contamination of the incision site.
10. Pull towels that were originally tucked around the client.	10. Prevents pooling of the solution, which can cause skin burns.
11. Apply antimicrobial solution, starting at the incision site and working out to the periphery.	11. Prevents contamination of the incision site.
12. If using a flammable agent (alcohol), allow the solution to dry and the fumes to evaporate before using the laser or electrosurgical unit.	12. Prevents fires.
13. Document the condition of the client's skin before and after the preparation, the agent used, and the area prepared.	13. Keeps team members informed to assist with ongoing care.

Infection Control

The client will be instructed to use good handwashing techniques before touching the dressing or wound to limit the potential for infection. The symptoms of infection should be written clearly for the client. These symptoms include fever over 101°F (38.3°C), chills, redness around the wound, swelling, foul odor, purulent drainage, or pain. Symptoms of an infection are not usually apparent for 36 to 48 hours postoperatively.

Urinary Status

The client should be instructed to notify the physician if he or she is unable to urinate. This can happen from the effects of anesthesia. Helpful hints to the client to stimulate urination include sitting in a tub of warm water, running water from the faucet, and having a quiet environment.

Transportation at Discharge

The driving restrictions following sedation and anesthesia must be discussed with and understood by the client. The client should refrain from driving for 24 hours following anesthesia and sedation and possibly for longer, depending on the type of surgery and the surgical procedure. This restriction makes it imperative that a responsible person be available to drive the client home. Any deviation from this procedure can prolong the discharge process. The client having surgery in the hospital setting can be admitted to the facility, but the ambulatory surgery setting does not provide this opportunity. Clients can experience serious postsurgical complications if they do not adhere to this instruction.

Leg Exercises

Venous return often is hampered during the surgical procedure because of altered circulation and possibly the position that the client is in during surgery. Stasis of blood in the lower extremities places the client at risk for thrombophlebitis. To prevent this complication, the client is instructed on the correct leg exercises to perform following surgery. These exercises are useful in improving circulation after the surgical intervention. A return demonstration is expected. Figure 39–4 discusses the purpose and explains in detail the correct leg exercises that should be practiced:

- Place the bed in the Fowler position
- Have the client bend the knee and raise the foot, hold the position for a few seconds, extend the leg, and lower it to the bed
- Instruct the client to repeat with opposite leg
- Instruct the client to trace circles with feet, one foot at a time
- Instruct the client to repeat five times

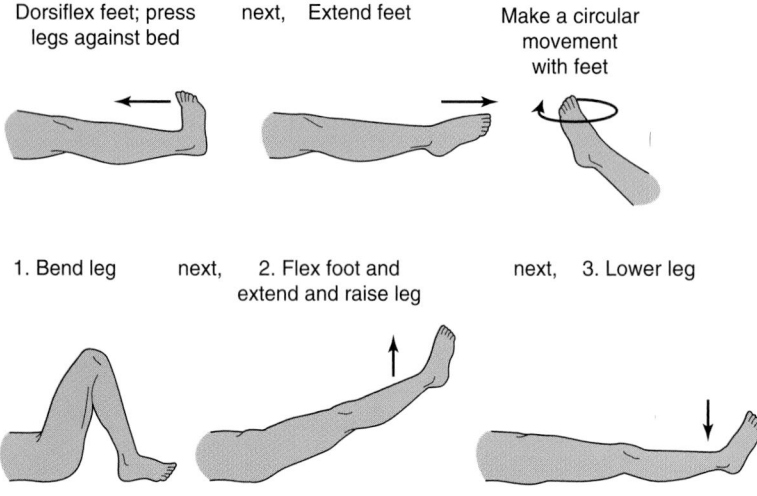

Dorsiflex feet; press legs against bed | next, | Extend feet | Make a circular movement with feet

1. Bend leg | next, | 2. Flex foot and extend and raise leg | next, | 3. Lower leg

Foot exercises
Alternately flex and extend feet four to five times
Make circular movement with feet four to five times
  to the left; then repeat to the right

Leg exercises
Repeat positions 1, 2, and 3 four to five times for each leg

Purpose
To stimulate circulation and prevent blood clots

Figure 39–4
Leg exercises.

Antiembolism stockings may be ordered for the client with identified venous circulation problems to the lower extremities. The stockings apply graduated compression to promote increased blood flow velocity in the recumbent client. This decreases the chance of thrombosis. Procedure 39–3 explains the application of antiembolism stockings.

Deep Breathing, Coughing, and Splinting

During surgery, the client's breathing pattern is limited, if not controlled, through artificial respirators. Mucus easily accumulates in the alveoli, further limiting lung expansion. When the alveoli are not fully or adequately expanded, they may collapse. This severely compromises the client's oxygenation.

Deep breathing, coughing, and splinting of the incision are important procedures to be taught to the client. By inhaling deeply, the client expands the air passages and prevents atelectasis and pneumonia. A frequent reason why clients do not deep breathe sufficiently is pain. Coughing loosens mucus from the respiratory tract. Splinting of the surgical wound provides support to the surgical incision and reduces the degree of pain. Clients can then breathe more deeply (Fig. 39–5). Use the following procedures:

* Place the client in a high Fowler position
* Place a small pillow or folded blanket over the surgical incision

* Instruct the client to take three slow breaths (inhaling through the nose and exhaling through the mouth) to stimulate a cough reflex
* Instruct the client to cough on the third deep breath to clear the secretions from the lungs

Nasogastric Tube

A nasogastric tube is usually inserted once the client is anesthetized if the client is to have a major surgical procedure. When connected to low suction, this tube empties the gastric contents and decreases the chances that the client will aspirate vomitus during

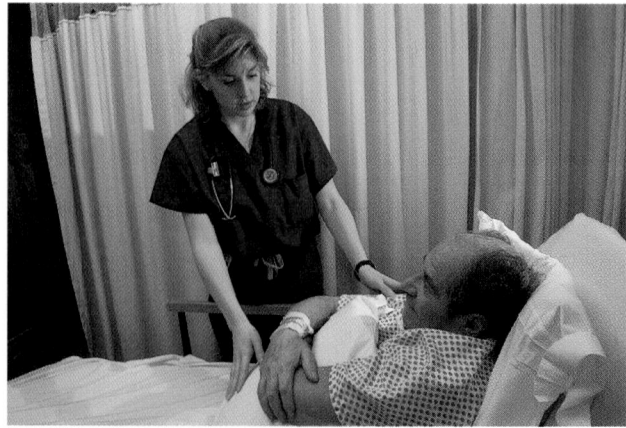

Figure 39–5
Deep breathing and splinting.

PROCEDURE

39-3

APPLICATION OF ANTIEMBOLISM STOCKINGS

Explain the procedure and the purpose of the procedure to the client.

Clinical Situation: The antiembolism stockings are applied to the legs to increase venous return and reduce swelling.

Anticipated Response: The client will not have venous pooling or swelling of the lower extremities and will have a decreased potential for thrombosis.

Equipment: *Gather before beginning*
> Measuring tape
> Size chart
> Correct size of antiembolism
>   stockings

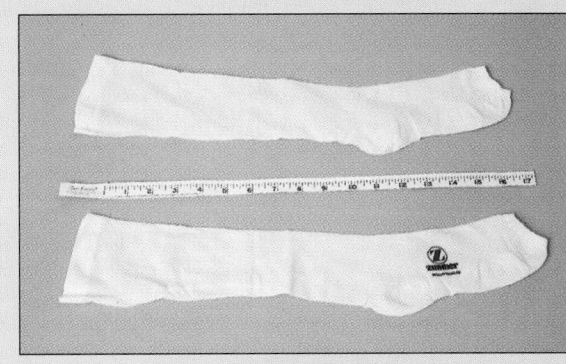

Action	Rationale
1. Check physician order.	1. Must have a physician order or standing order.
2. Provide privacy for measuring the client's legs.	2. Allows for dignity to be maintained.
3. Measure and apply in early morning.	3. Distention of the veins occurs after the client has been ambulatory for a period of time.
4. Elevate the lower extremities for 20 to 30 minutes if the client has been ambulating.	4. Reduces swelling and increases venous return.
5. Take measurements: For *knee-high stockings,* measure the circumference at the widest point of the calf (approximately 6 in. below the patella). Measure length from the heel to the popliteal space.	5. Correct measurements will allow the correct selection of stocking that will best benefit the client.

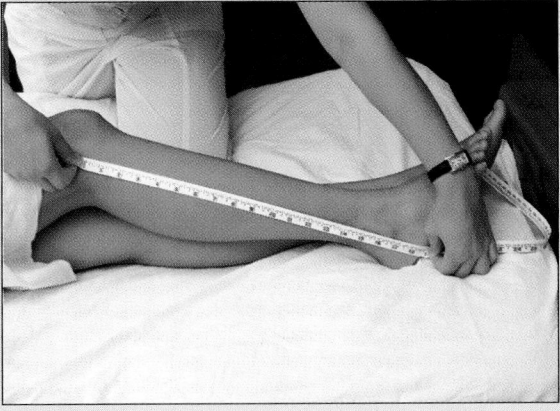

Step 5.

Continued

APPLICATION OF ANTIEMBOLISM STOCKINGS
(Continued)

Action	Rationale
For *thigh-high stockings,* measure the thigh approximately 6 in. above the superior aspect of the patella. Measure the length of the leg from the heel to the gluteal fold.	
For *waist-high stockings,* measure the calf and thigh as for other types of stockings. Measure the leg length from the bottom of the heel to the waist along the side of the body.	
6. Compare measurements with the chart provided on the package to select correct size.	**6.** Correct sizes provide the greatest degree of client benefit.
7. Have the client lie in a reclining position. Make sure skin is dry (may apply powder to the skin).	**7.** The easiest position to apply stockings. This makes application easier by decreasing friction.

Knee High

Action	Rationale
8. Turn the stocking inside out by inserting your hand into the stocking from the top and grabbing the heel pocket from the inside.	**8.** The stocking must be gathered to provide easier application.
9. Hook index and middle fingers of both hands into the foot section (similar to putting on a child's sock or shoe).	**9.** Makes application of stocking easier.
10. Face the client and have him or her point the toes as you pull the stocking up past the heel. Have the client bend the knee. Stretch the stocking as you continue upward. Make sure the heel is centered in the pocket.	**10.** Allows for stability while applying the stocking.

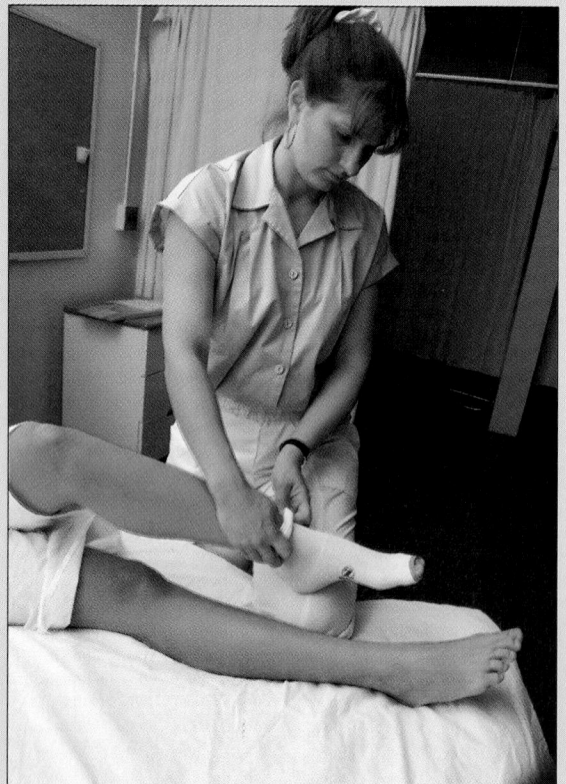

Step 10

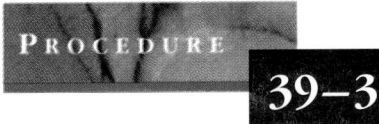

APPLICATION OF ANTIEMBOLISM STOCKINGS
(Continued)

Action	Rationale
Thigh High	
11. Straighten the knee to apply the stocking above the knee. Flex the knee to complete the rest of the thigh length. Make sure material is evenly distributed. The top should be 1 to 3 in. below the gluteal fold.	11. This application allows for maximum efficiency of the stocking. This decreases the potential for a tourniquet effect at the gluteal fold.
Waist High	
12. Have the client stand to finish applying the stocking. Extend the stocking up to the top of the gluteal fold. Carefully adjust the waist belt so that it does not interfere with wounds or external devices.	12. Allows for maximum benefit without interfering with drains or the incision site.
13. Check for equal smoothness over the whole leg.	13. Creases can cause painful lines and constrictions.
14. Stockings should be removed for 1 hour every 8 to 12 hours.	14. Allows the skin to breathe and decreases any irritation.

extubation. Depending on the type of procedure, this tube can remain in place postoperatively for days or weeks. Procedure 27–2 shows insertion of a nasogastric tube. (See Chapter 27.)

Evaluation

As with all nursing interventions, the nurse must evaluate all aspects of the preoperative assessment. There are numerous ways to accomplish this. Each area of the assessment is as important as any other. Prioritizing the interventions allows the nurse to accomplish as much as possible in the shortest amount of time. The nurse needs to remember that each client responds differently to the surgical experience. Some want to have a great deal of information and may ask many questions, while others only want it to be "over with" and may not want to know anything. It is very important for the nurse to be aware of the client's wishes and function accordingly.

The nurse must document the outcomes of the nursing interventions for the preoperative phase. When evaluating the client's understanding of the procedure, the nurse needs to remember that the client may explain the procedure in layperson's terms. He or she may not know what a "cholecystectomy" is but may be familiar with the term *gallbladder*. The client may only have a vague idea of the general area where the surgical site is but can point to the area. Some clients may be very specific and have a great deal of knowledge of the procedure.

Another opportunity for the nurse to evaluate the client's preoperative experience is to allow the client to verbalize thoughts and feelings about the information he or she has received. This is an excellent opportunity to hear the client's concerns and what he or she considers priorities, as well as learn just how successful the preoperative instruction was for the client.

A third way to evaluate the preoperative phase is to have the client do return demonstrations of the preoperative teaching. This allows the nurse to continue to establish rapport with the client as well as make corrections in the client's skills demonstration. This is also an excellent opportunity to "chit chat" with the client, helping to put him or her at ease.

Documentation

The last component of the preoperative evaluation is the documentation. This includes completing the preoperative checklist, sending the chart with the client, and notifying the operating room of any special concerns or omissions in the chart (Fig. 39–6).

Some special considerations may need to be communicated to the OR staff nurse. If the client is hard of hearing, hearing aids may need to be left in place. Dentures should be taken out before the client enters the OR. If this causes the client a great deal of stress, the dentures may be left in place, and the circulating nurse will be informed. Other special considerations are glasses; preoperative antibiotics, which need to be taken to the OR with the client; antiembolism stockings, which may need to be put on just prior to surgery or immediately after surgery; and if the client is a child, how far the parents can come with the child.

The last important documentation check is to verify that consent forms are correctly filled out, dated,

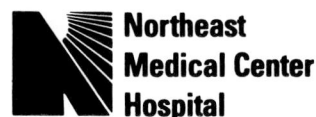

Northeast Medical Center Hospital

18951 Memorial North • Humble, Texas 77338

SURGICAL CHECK LIST

Floor Nurse's Check List

1. A. Surgical Procedure: _____
    _____
    B. Name of Surgeon: _____
2. Consent signed and witnessed: Yes _____ No _____
3. Sterilization signed and witnessed:
    (when required)   Yes _____ No _____
4. Surgical prep done by: _____
    Area: _____
5. History/Physical: Dictated _____ On Chart _____
6. Identification band checked   Yes _____ No _____
7. Allergies: _____
    Band checked: Yes _____ No _____
8. IV: Yes _____ No _____ IV count: _____
9. A: Test Done   B: Report on Chart

		A	B			A	B
1.	CBC	____	____	7.	PT-PTT	____	____
2.	H/H	____	____	8.	BUN	____	____
3.	UA	____	____	9.	K	____	____
4.	Preg.	____	____	10.	SGOT	____	____
5.	EKG	____	____	11.	Glucose	____	____
6.	Chest		____	12.	Blood Type/Screened/		
	X-Ray	____			Crossmatch	____	____

10. Voided: _____ Foley inserted: _____
11. Dentures removed: _____ Contacts removed: _____
12. Make-up, nail polish removed: _____
13. Jewelry & underwear removed: _____ TED Hose on: _____
14. Pre-Op Medication & Time given: _____
    _____ Time: _____
15. Medication record in chart: Yes _____ No _____
16. Condition after Pre-Op: Awake   Asleep   Drowsy
                                   Circle
17. Addressograph sent with patient: _____
18. Transported by stretcher/bed
    with side rails   Yes _____ No _____
Completed by: _____ , R.N.

OR 112 5/92

Operating Room Check List

1. Pt. understands: _____
    _____
    B. _____
2. _____
3. _____
4. _____
5. _____
6. _____
7. _____
    Band checked: Yes _____ No _____
8. IV: Yes _____ No. _____ IV count _____
9. A: Test Done   B: Report on Chart

	A	B		A	B
1.	____	____	7.	____	____
2.	____	____	8.	____	____
3.	____	____	9.	____	____
4.	____	____	10.	____	____
5.	____	____	11.	____	____
6.	____	____	12.	____	____

10. _____
11. _____ Contacts removed _____
12. _____
13. (a) _____ (b) _____
14. _____
    _____
15. Medication record in chart: Yes _____ No _____
16. _____
17. _____
18. _____
Completed by: _____ , R.N.

❥ **Figure 39–6**
Surgical checklist. (Courtesy of Northeast Medical Center Hospital, Humble, TX.)

HOLDING AREA PLAN OF CARE

Pre-Op Vital Signs	T	P	R	B/P	SaO2

Nursing Prompts	Time	Medication	Route	Initial
Unstable vital signs				
Hyperthermia				
Confusion				
Delay				
Intake/output				
Communication				
Anxiety, requiring intervention				
Education				

Pre-Operative Assessment

Activity:		Normal		Other	Color		Normal		Other

Describe: Describe:

Consciousness:		Awake		Drowsy	Skin:		Warm	Dry		Intact
		Responds appropriately				Other				
		Confused			Describe:					
		Unresponsive								
Respiration:		Normal, unlabored			Emotional Status:		Calm, informed		Other	
		Other			Describe:					

Describe:

DATE	TIME	FOCUS	D-DATA A-ACTION R-RESPONSE
			Signature: R.N.

❧ **Figure 39–6** *Continued*

and signed, *i.e.,* procedure, blood administration, sterilization, and photography if applicable. The transferring nurse will check that the physician's orders have been completed and signed off and the medication and vital sign graphics sheets are in the chart. All of this documentation is vitally important for the operating room nurse. Once the client is anesthetized any other information must come from the chart.

Nursing Process in Care in the Intraoperative Phase

The intraoperative phase of perioperative nursing begins when the client arrives at the door of the OR and ends when the client is delivered to the PACU or the same-day surgery unit or is returned to his or her room.

Many people with varying degrees of knowledge and expertise are involved in the care of the client during the intraoperative phase to achieve a positive outcome. The client and family members or significant other are probably the most important members of the team. Once the decision for surgery is made, the client becomes the central focus. The client is in the best condition to achieve expected outcomes when he or she has a positive attitude and a willingness to participate in the recovery. Family members or significant others are asked to give support and encouragement. They may also be asked to act as caretakers once the client returns home and still needs to reach complete recovery to a healthy state.

At least two nurses usually are present in the OR. The first is the **scrub nurse;** this can be a certified surgical scrub technician or a registered nurse. It is the scrub person's responsibility to maintain as clean an environment as possible. The scrub person does this by maintaining and monitoring **aseptic technique** while garbed in sterile gown, gloves, and mask. The scrub nurse also assists the physician during the procedure, passing instruments and monitoring the rest of the scrub personnel for breaks in aseptic technique. The second nurse is a registered nurse, also known as the **circulating nurse.** The main focus of this nurse is to be the client advocate. He or she does an initial assessment of the client, has all the needed supplies and equipment for the procedure, and provides client comfort measures before the start of the procedure. The circulator is responsible for the client's safety and privacy and is the link with the family or significant other during the intraoperative phase.

An anesthesiologist or certified registered nurse anesthetist is present in the OR if the client is to have general or monitored anesthesia. His or her primary responsibility is to administer anesthesia, manage the airway, and administer other medications. He or she also is responsible for monitoring and maintaining the physiological status of the client (Fig. 39–7).

The surgeon, who is the head of the surgical team, is responsible for explaining the procedure in detail to the client and family or significant other preoperatively, obtaining informed consent, communicating any special needs to the rest of the team, and performing the surgical procedure.

Medical students, student nurses, admitting personnel, laboratory technicians, x-ray technicians, orderlies, and nursing assistants are a few of the many people who are also involved in the positive outcome of any surgical procedure. A positive outcome for the surgical client can only be accomplished if the surgical group works as a team.

Assessment

During the intraoperative phase, the perioperative nurse is continually assessing the client (Fig. 39–8). Listening and observation skills are instrumental in collecting data during this phase. Listening to verbal exchanges between the surgeon and scrub nurse and between the surgeon and the anesthesiologist can give important information related to the progress of the procedure and difficulties encountered or any unplanned changes requiring immediate intervention.

Observation is another important tool for the nurse to use during the surgical procedure. Being familiar with the equipment and able to interpret the numerous monitors utilized during surgery allows the perioperative nurse to determine physiological status of the client. For example, the pulse oximeter is placed on the client to determine his or her oxygen levels. During surgery, the client's oxygen saturation should be maintained at 98% to 100%.

During the surgical procedure, the client will be monitored for safety with specific monitoring equipment. This equipment may include an electrocardiograph, which displays cardiac rhythm and activity, and an automatic blood pressure monitor, which helps the anesthesiologist monitor the physiological status of the client. Each of the monitoring devices has upper and lower alarm thresholds that inform the surgical team when the client's status has changed. For example, if the pulse goes over the upper limit of 100 beats a minute, the alarm rings.

During surgery, the perioperative nurse works with the anesthesiologist and surgeon by monitoring blood loss, possibly weighing sponges, monitoring urine output when appropriate, and keeping track of irrigation fluid used. Safety of the client and surgical team is also monitored. The use of electrical grounding devices and cautery pencil allows the surgeon to reduce bleeding and to dissect tissue while providing a safe, continuous electrical circuit. If the position of the client is changed during surgery, all monitoring attachments must be checked to identify changes and maintain safety monitoring.

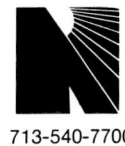

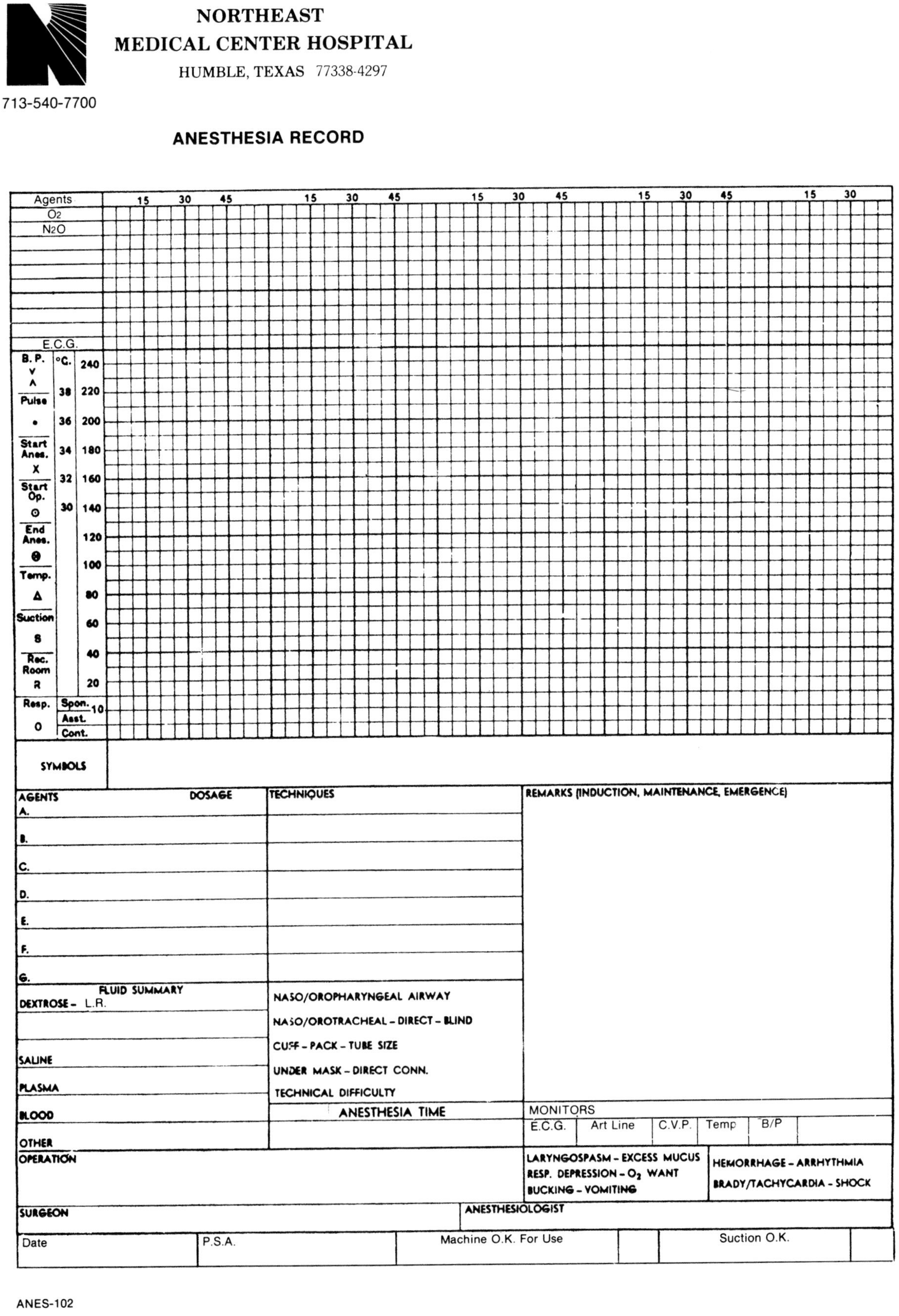

NORTHEAST
MEDICAL CENTER HOSPITAL
HUMBLE, TEXAS 77338-4297

713-540-7700

ANESTHESIA RECORD

Agents		15	30	45		15	30	45		15	30	45		15	30	45		15	30
O₂																			
N₂O																			

E.C.G.

B.P.	°C.					
v		240				
∧	38	220				
Pulse	36	200				
•						
Start Anes.	34	180				
X	32	160				
Start Op.	30	140				
⊙						
End Anes.		120				
⊕		100				
Temp.						
△		80				
Suction		60				
8						
Rec. Room		40				
R		20				
Resp.	Spon.	10				
	Asst.					
O	Cont.					

SYMBOLS

AGENTS	DOSAGE	TECHNIQUES	REMARKS (INDUCTION, MAINTENANCE, EMERGENCE)
A.			
B.			
C.			
D.			
E.			
F.			
G.			

FLUID SUMMARY

DEXTROSE – L.R.	NASO/OROPHARYNGEAL AIRWAY
	NASO/OROTRACHEAL – DIRECT – BLIND
	CUFF – PACK – TUBE SIZE
SALINE	UNDER MASK – DIRECT CONN.
PLASMA	TECHNICAL DIFFICULTY
BLOOD	ANESTHESIA TIME
OTHER	

MONITORS				
E.C.G.	Art Line	C.V.P.	Temp	B/P

OPERATION	LARYNGOSPASM – EXCESS MUCUS RESP. DEPRESSION – O₂ WANT BUCKING – VOMITING	HEMORRHAGE – ARRHYTHMIA BRADY/TACHYCARDIA – SHOCK

SURGEON	ANESTHESIOLOGIST	
Date	P.S.A.	Machine O.K. For Use	Suction O.K.

ANES-102

❧ **Figure 39–7**
Anesthesia record. (Courtesy of Northeast Medical Center Hospital, Humble, TX.)

Northeast Medical Center Hospital

PERIOPERATIVE RECORD

DATE: O.R.#   SCHEDULED ☐   ADDED ☐   EMERGENCY ☐
INPATIENT ☐   OUTPATIENT ☐   OBS ☐   MAJOR ☐   MINOR ☐

TIMES — HOLDING AREA: To O.R.:   ANES.:   INCISION: CLOSURE: To PACU:

ASSESSMENTS
AWAKE/ALERT ☐ DROWSY/PREMEDICATED ☐ OTHER _____
ALLERGIES: _____ NKA ☐
MOTOR/PHYSICAL IMPAIRMENTS _____ NONE ☐
LANGUAGE BARRIER ☐ NO ☐ YES _____
SKIN CONDITION: WARM ☐ DRY ☐ INTACT ☐
OTHER ☐ _____
Physician identified patient ☐   NPO ☐ YES ☐ NO

TEAM MEMBERS

SURGEON	CIRCULATOR
FIRST ASSIST.	CIRCULATOR
SECOND ASSIST.	SCRUB NURSE
OTHER	SCRUB NURSE
ANESTHESIOLOGIST	RELIEF
CRNA	RELIEF

LINES AND DRAINS

DESCRIPTION	ON ARRIVAL	HOLDING	INTRA-OP
PERIPHERAL IV's	☐	☐	☐
CENTRAL IV's	☐	☐	☐
ARTERIAL LINES	☐	☐	☐
FOLEY	☐	☐	☐
N.G. TUBE	☐	☐	☐
URETERAL CATH.	☐	☐	☐
WOUND DRAIN	☐	☐	☐
OTHER	☐	☐	☐
OTHER	☐	☐	☐
OTHER	☐	☐	☐

DIAGNOSIS
PRE-OP: _____
POST-OP: _____

ANES.
M.A.C. ☐   LOCAL ☐   GENERAL ☐   I.V. SEDATION ☐
SPINAL ☐   OTHER ☐   INTUBATED ☐   O₂ ☐

PROCEDURE

COUNTS

	OPEN	FIRST	FINAL
		CORRECT ☐ INCORRECT ☐	CORRECT ☐ INCORRECT ☐
RN		RN	RN
ST		ST	ST

M.D. NOTIFIED OF INCORRECT COUNT ☐ YES ☐ NO ☐ N/A

IMPLANTS

WOUND CLASS   W.C.I. ☐   W.C.II. ☐   W.C.III. ☐

CHART REVIEWED BY: _____ R.N.

POSITION
SUPINE ☐
PRONE ☐
LT ☐ RT ☐ LATERAL ☐   LITHOTOMY ☐
ARMS _____ EXTENDED ☐ _____ TUCKED ☐ _____
LEGS _____
SUPPORTS _____
SAFETY STRAP ☐ YES ☐ NO _____
WILSON FRAME ☐ CHEST ROLL ☐ BEAN BAG ☐ FX TABLE ☐
AXILLARY ROLL ☐ SHOULDER ROLL ☐ HORSESHOE HEADREST ☐

PREPS
BETADINE ☐ SCRUB ☐ SOLUTION ☐ ALCOHOL ☐ PHISOHEX ☐
AREA OF PREP _____
SHAVE: HOLDING AREA ☐ O.R. ☐ CLIPPERS/RAZOR USED ☐
AREA OF SHAVE _____

SUPPORTIVE DEVICES
ELECTROSURGICAL GENERATOR # _____ BI-POLAR # _____
GROUND PAD SITE _____ N/A ☐
SETTINGS _____ COAG. _____ CUT
K-THERMIA UNIT
UNIT # _____ TEMPERATURE SETTING _____ PAD TEMP. _____
LASER: CO₂ ☐ KTP ☐ OTHER ☐
USED: YES ☐ (See Attached Sheet) N/A ☐

MEDS/FLUIDS
NACL 1000CCX
H₂O 1000CCX
OTHER
OTHER
OTHER
OTHER

TOURNIQUET
PRESSURE SETTING _____ mmHG   SITE _____
TIME ↑ _____ TIME ↓ _____
TIME ↑ _____ TIME ↓ _____ TESTED: YES ☐ NO ☐

DRESSINGS
ADAPTIC ☐ TELFA ☐ 4X4s ☐ KERLIXFLUFFS ☐ KLING ☐
KERLIXROLL ☐ ACE WRAPS ☐ XEROFORM ☐ ELASTOPLAST ☐
PAPER TAPE ☐ DERMACEL TAPE ☐ OTHER ☐ _____
PLASTER CAST ☐ _____
FIBERGLASS CAST ☐ _____
PLASTER SPLINT ☐ _____
OTHER ☐

SPECIMENS

POST OP ASSESSMENTS

DESCRIPTION

I.V. SITE	OBSERVED ☐	NOT OBSERVED ☐
DRESSING SITE	DRY ☐	WET ☐
FOLEY PATENT	YES ☐	NO ☐
AIRWAY PATENT	YES ☐	NO ☐
O₂ + AmBu	YES ☐	NO ☐
ACCOMPANIED BY ANES. & R.N.	YES ☐	NO ☐

TRANSFERRED BY STRETCHER ☐   BED ☐
SIDERAILS ↑↑ ☐   N/A ☐
INTUBATED: YES ☐ NO ☐   EXTUBATED: YES ☐ NO ☐
PT. ADMITTED TO PACU ☐   SICU ☐   FLOOR ☐   OTHER ☐
SKIN: WARM ☐   DRY ☐   WET ☐   OTHER ☐
ABLE TO MOVE EXTREMITIES X: ONE ☐ TWO ☐ THREE ☐ FOUR ☐
REPORT GIVEN TO LICENSED NURSE: YES ☐ NO ☐

NURSES NOTES
(ALL NSG. ENTRIES TO BE SIGNED) _____

CHART COMPLETED BY: _____ R.N.

OR 113

✦ **Figure 39–8**
Perioperative record. (Courtesy of Northeast Medical Center Hospital, Humble, TX.)

Nursing Diagnosis

The nursing diagnoses associated with the client during the intraoperative phase of the perioperative experience include, but once again are not limited to,

* Risk for Injury related to positioning, anesthesia, environmental hazards, use of mechanical methods of achieving hemostasis, or the use of lasers
* Impaired Skin Integrity related to improper positioning, a nonhealing wound, or handling tissue with instruments during the procedure
* Risk for Fluid Volume Deficit related to intraoperative bleeding or the use of hyperosmotic agents
* Risk for Fluid Volume Excess related to administration of intravenous fluids during the procedure
* Risk for Wound Infection related to exposure to the surgical environment or use of microfibrillar collagen, hemostat, gelatin sponge, or oxidized cellulose

Planning

The expected outcomes for the intraoperative client are as follows:

The client will be free of injury related to burns, incorrect counts, and wound contamination

The client will maintain intact skin surfaces (except the incision)

The client will maintain appropriate fluid and electrolyte balances

Implementation

The nurse is involved in maintaining and caring for the client throughout the entire surgical procedure. Table 39–5 explains the responsibilities of the perioperative nurse during the intraoperative phase of the perioperative experience.

Grounding Pad

Placement of the grounding pad on the client is a very important safety consideration. The grounding pad allows electrical current, used throughout the procedure to control bleeding and tissue dissection, to pass harmlessly from the client. The pad is placed across the largest area of a muscle body, which is usually the thigh or buttocks. When placing the pad on the client, the nurse needs to consider surgical site,

Table 39–5

NURSING RESPONSIBILITIES DURING THE INTRAOPERATIVE PHASE

RESPONSIBILITY	INTERVENTION	RATIONALE
Supplies and equipment	Obtaining surgical instrument set; verifying sterilization integrity of sterile supplies; verifying availability of specialty equipment; verifying working status of the equipment	Decreases the potential for delays
Positioning aids	Obtaining Arm boards Stirrups Donuts Pillows Beanbags Safety belt Chest braces Shoulder braces Sandbags	Decreases potential for injury; provides correct anatomical alignment
Safety	Maintaining and monitoring aseptic technique of all team members; obtaining safety devices; performing counts; obtaining instruments: Sponges Sharps Miscellaneous, as required Applying grounding pad; monitoring electrical safety; monitoring for physiological changes: Cardiac arrhythmias Intake and output Blood loss	Decreases the potential for injury; maintains fluid and electrolyte balance; decreases the potential for infection

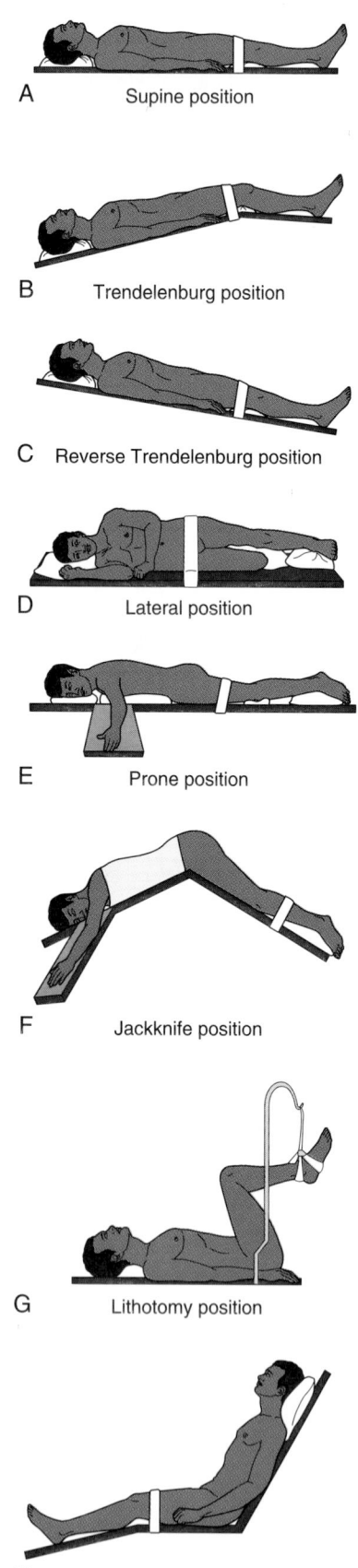

A   Supine position

B   Trendelenburg position

C   Reverse Trendelenburg position

D   Lateral position

E   Prone position

F   Jackknife position

G   Lithotomy position

H   Modified Fowler position

✦ **Figure 39–9**
Surgical positions.

implanted prosthetics, presence of a pacemaker, and positioning requirements. The grounding pad site is evaluated before and after placement for injury. Placement site and unusual circumstances, such as those mentioned here, are documented on the intraoperative record in the section for grounding pad placement.

Positioning

After induction of anesthesia, the client is positioned for surgery. The goal for positioning the client is to have the greatest accessibility to the surgical site without sacrificing the client's respiratory or circulatory function (McEwen, 1996).

It is the joint responsibility of the nurse, physician, and anesthesiologist to position the client correctly. This responsibility should not be taken lightly because all team members are held legally responsible for injuries that may be incurred due to incorrect positioning. The nurse needs to have knowledge of anatomy and physiology and of how positioning devices can affect the client. All clients should be placed in anatomical alignment for each position.

There are seven general types of positions in which a client may be placed during surgery: supine, Trendelenburg, reverse Trendelenburg, lithotomy, sitting, lateral, and prone (Fig. 39–9).

Supine is the most common position (see Fig. 39–9A). The client is placed on the OR bed flat on his or her back with the face upward and the head level with the heart. It is the position used for abdominal, ophthalmological, foot and hand, cardiac, and craniotomy procedures. Arm boards (padded), a donut, a pillow, safety straps, and a foot extender are the positioning devices needed to prevent injury. The complication of supine position is that pressure sores can develop on any area that bears weight, such as the heels and sacrum. The arms should be secured at the client's side or placed on padded arm boards. The client's skin should not come in contact with any metal from the table or positioning devices. A pillow should be placed under the client's knees to take pressure off the lower back.

The Trendelenburg position is a variation of the supine position (see Fig. 39–9B). The bed is flat, but the client's head is lower than the heart. This position is very useful in surgical procedures of the lower abdomen. The positioning devices are the same as for supine position, except that shoulder braces also may be used to prevent the client from sliding on the OR table. Complications could occur if the shoulder braces are not in the right position. The potential for brachial plexus nerve damage exists. Shearing can happen if the client's position changes without lifting help from the perioperative team members. Shearing is caused when the client is pushed or pulled while the skin is still in contact with the surface of the OR bed.

The reverse Trendelenburg position is also a variation of the supine position (see Fig. 39–9C). The bed is flat, but the head is higher than the heart. This position is used almost exclusively for head and neck procedures and for laparoscopic procedures. The positioning devices needed include arm boards, a donut, a pillow, safety straps, a shoulder roll or sandbag, and foot boards. The main complication to look for is peripheral pooling of blood in the lower extremities.

The lithotomy position is often used for gynecological or genitourinary surgery (see Fig. 39–9G). The client is flat on the back facing upward, and the feet are carefully positioned in stirrups. Special positioning devices include stirrups, holders to attach to the OR bed, arm boards, and a safety strap. In this position, the client is at risk for strained lumbosacral muscles, saphenous vessel and nerve damage, and perineal nerve damage. The potential for severe hypotension also exists. Both legs need to be raised and lowered together. Potential for crushing damage to fingers can occur if the nurse does not pay special attention to the break in the table when the client's arms are positioned at his or her side.

The sitting position (see Fig. 39–9H) is the position of choice for shoulder procedures and craniotomies. The OR bed is placed in a high Fowler position, with the feet dependent. The positioning devices include a headrest, safety straps, pillows, and arm boards. Complications can include corneal abrasions and neck injuries. There is a risk for an air embolism when the client is positioned in the sitting position. The anesthesia personnel will use special equipment to assist in safe monitoring of the client.

The lateral position is used for orthopedic, kidney, and some thoracic surgeries (see Fig. 39–9D). The client is positioned on the right or left side, with the operative site up. Positioning devices include arm boards, donuts, a pillow, sandbags, shoulder pads, an axillary roll, safety straps, and bean bags. Potential complications include decreases in chest expansion and circulation. Blood can pool in dependent limbs. Pressure sores at the hip and ankle of the dependent limb and damage to the brachial plexus also may occur if the client is not positioned correctly.

The prone position is used for the dorsal approach required in spinal cord procedures, such as a laminectomy (see Fig. 39–9E). The client lies face down on the OR bed. Positioning devices include chest rolls, a donut, pillows, and safety straps.

The jackknife position is a variation of the prone position, with the client flexed at the waist.

Complications include airway inaccessibility; potential for facial skin breakdown; and tissue damage to knees, ankles, and chest. Potential exists for corneal abrasions, decreased blood pressure, decreased chest movement, and femoral artery occlusion. The client is anesthetized in a regular bed and then turned to the prone position. The anesthesiologist coordinates the move to the OR bed because he or she is responsible for maintaining a patent airway. The regular bed will be kept in the room in case a need arises to turn the client to the supine position.

Skin Preparation

Hair should not be removed unless it directly interferes with the surgical incision. If it is decided to remove the hair around the incision, then the hair should be removed immediately before surgery. The time between the hair removal and incision impacts the potential for wound infection. Shaving the hair should not be performed in the OR because the airborne hair and skin debris can contaminate the sterile field. Therefore, shaving is usually performed in the preoperative holding area or in the client's room.

Hair removal may be accomplished by a depilatory cream, a wet razor shave, a dry razor shave, or the use of electric clippers. The choice is usually made by the surgeon according to his or her preference. An antimicrobial skin scrub is performed by the circulating nurse after the client is positioned and before sterile drapes are applied. Each surgical procedure involves specific body surfaces that must be prepared to remove transient microorganisms from the skin and to decrease the risk of infection. Procedure 39–2 explains the purpose and the procedure for surgical skin preparation.

Female clients having facial procedures and pediatric clients usually do not need to be shaved due to lack of facial and body hair. Always avoid shaving the eyebrows on any client, as eyebrows do not usually grow back.

Evaluation and Documentation

All evaluations and documentation for the client during the intraoperative phase are completed on the intraoperative record (see Fig. 39–8). It is very important that every block and space on the intraoperative record be completed. If the information requested does not apply, then a diagonal line through the block or space or the designation N/A (not applicable) is used. The client may be unable to respond to questions because of the medication given intraoperatively, so it is important that the client does not leave the OR unless an identification band is in place.

Nursing Process in Care in the Postoperative Phase

The postoperative phase of perioperative nursing care can be subdivided into two phases: immediate postoperative nursing care and nursing care after discharge from the PACU.

Immediate Postoperative Nursing Care

The postoperative phase begins with the surgical client's admission to the PACU or the postoperative

Table 39–6

NURSING RESPONSIBILITIES IN THE IMMEDIATE POSTOPERATIVE PHASE

RESPONSIBILITY	INTERVENTION	RATIONALE
Vital signs	Blood pressure; heart rate; respirations; temperature; pulse oximeter	Provides admission baseline evaluation; determines changes since leaving the OR
Intake and output	Intravenous fluids; urine; nasogastric; vomitus; drains	Measuring intake and output helps to determine if the client is hemodynamically stable; kidney function is not impaired
Oxygen	Venturi mask; nasal cannula; T piece for endotracheal tube	Life requirement
Level of consciousness	Call the client by name; orient the client to place; give simple verbal commands: Open your eye Lift your head Cough Swallow	Determines awareness; determines muscle control after anesthesia; determines swallowing control; determines cough reflex
Mobility	Ask the client to move all extremities	Assesses level of mobility; assesses residual anesthetic; determines differences in preoperative and postoperative mobility status
Comfort level	Administer pain medication; provide warm blankets; keep the client in correct anatomical alignment; provide muted environment; orient client	Relieves pain, allowing the client to relax and to begin the healing process; provides emotional support; decreases muscle soreness; increases respiratory and circulatory function
Dressing status	Assess for drainage; assess for placement	Provides information about potential hemorrhage
Drains	Assess amount and quality of drainage	Maintains correct intake and output; provides information about potential infection or hemorrhage

surgical floor. Ideally, the client is accompanied by anesthesia personnel or the surgeon. Pertinent information should be communicated to the PACU nurse, including procedures performed, allergies, drains, medications given during the procedures, where the family members are located, and any other information that could affect the client's recovery.

Assessment

Because all anesthetics are depressants, it is assumed that the initial care for all clients in the PACU is the same. An initial assessment of the cardiorespiratory system should be the PACU nurse's first concern. The nurse should first determine if the client's airway is patent. Associated with this is checking if the respirations are unlabored. The nurse should perform a quick check of all dressings and drains for gross bleeding and check and record the client's blood pressure, pulse, and rate of respirations.

After the initial observations are made, as shown in Table 39–6, a systematic assessment should be performed for each postoperative client (Fig. 39–10).

Respiratory Status

Respiratory function should be assessed by observing the rate and character of the respirations. Also, the client's skin color should be noted. The normal adult has a resting rate of respiration in the range of 16 to 20 breaths per minute. The normal respiration rate in infants and children can be 20 to 35 breaths per minute. The respirations should be quiet and unlabored. The most frequent respiratory complications postoperatively are hypoventilation, obstruction of the airway, aspiration of mucus, and atelectasis (collapse of the lung).

Inspection

Observe the client's chest for equal bilateral expansion. Pain is usually the cause for deviations in chest expansion. Signs of respiratory distress would include nasal flaring and the use of accessory muscles. The depth of respirations is equally as important as the rate of respirations. Shallow respirations are a sign of continuing depression from anesthesia or preoperative medications.

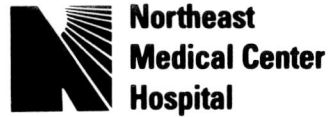

Northeast Medical Center Hospital

POST ANESTHESIA PLAN OF CARE

Name _____ Rm # _____ Hospital # _____ Date _____

Surgeon _____ Anes. Person _____ Anes. _____ Anes. Time_____

Time Of
Arrival _____ Allergies _____ Time Of
Consciousness _____

Operation _____

IV Fluids, cc on arrival _____ Stretcher Locked ☐ Side Rails Up ☐

POST ANESTHESIA RECOVERY SCORE	IN	MINUTES 30	60	90	OUT
ACTIVITY					
Able to move 4 extremities vol. or on com'd =2					
Able to move 2 extremities vol. or on com'd =1					
Able to move 0 extremities vol. or on com'd =0					
RESPIRATION					
Able to deep breath and cough freely =2					
Dyspena or limited breathing =1					
Apneic =0					
CIRCULATION					
BP+20 of Preanesthetic level =2					
BP+20-50 of Preanesthetic level =1					
BP+50 of Preanesthetic level =0					
CONSCIOUSNESS					
Full Awake =2					
Arousable on calling =1					
Not responding =0					
COLOR					
Pink =2					
Pale, dusky, blotchy, jaundiced, other =1					
Cyanotic =0					
TOTAL					

HOB _____ FOOT _____

NIBP Cuff Site _____
  Pulse present on dismissal ☐

Bilateral Breath Sounds, Clear & Equal _____

CODE: Blood Pressure • Pulse X Respiration O

TIME 0 15 30 45 1HR 15 30 45 2HR 15 30 45 3HR
(graph grid 20–200)

SaO2

Airways - none, oral, nasal, Ett, _____	
02, yes no FT N/C T-tube _____ L _____ %	
Ventilator V$_T$ _____ Sa02 _____ Rate _____	
Resp, Deep & Reg. _____	
Skin, Warm & Dry, Core Temp. _____	
EKG Monitor yes no Rhythm _____	
IV, A/L patent, no redness/swelling	
site _____ site _____	
TED, Ice Bag, Post Op Shoe, Sling, 5 Lb. Sand Bag	
Drsg, dry/intact site _____ site _____	
Drains secured - JP, Hemovac, Foley, N/G,	
Chest, Penrose _____	
Pulses pedal dorsalis R_____ L_____	
tibialis R_____ L_____	
Other	
Card Cath site dry, no hematoma _____	
Level of sensation adm _____ d/c _____	

All fluids, OR & PACU	Begun	End	Amt. Infused	X	INTAKE	OUTPUT
				X		
				X		
				X		
				X		
				X		
				X	TOTAL_____	TOTAL_____

RELIEF SIGNATURE_____ ( ) R.N.   SIGNATURE_____ ( ) R.N.

PACU 169 10/91

❧ **Figure 39–10**
Postanesthesia plan of care. (Courtesy of Northeast Medical Center Hospital, Humble, TX.)

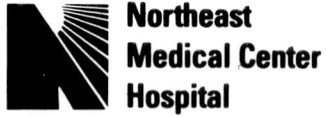

**Northeast
Medical Center
Hospital**

NURSING DIAGNOSIS PROMPTS

Temperature	Safety
Comfort/Pain	Education
Breathing	Neurovascular Status
Drainage/Output	Airway
Anxiety	Other

TIME	MEDICATION	ROUTE	INIT.

NEUROVASCULAR STATUS		IN	MINUTES			OUT
			30	60	90	
COLOR						
Pink	2					
Pale/Dusky	1					
Cyanotic	0					
SKIN TEMP						
Warm	2					
Cool	1					
Cold	0					
CAPILLARY REFILL						
Less than 3 seconds	2					
3 — 5 seconds	1					
Over 5 seconds	0					
MOTION						
Full motion	2					
Partial motion	1					
Unable to move	0					
SENSATION						
Full sensation	2					
Partial sensation	1					
No sensation	0					
TOTAL						

DATE	TIME	FOCUS	D-DATA A-ACTION R-RESPONSE

TRANSFER	VIA
Bed	Ambulance
Stretcher	Ambulatory
Wheel Chair	Davis Roller

Patient transferred to _____ in _____ condition.

Report to licensed nurse._____

VITAL SIGNS _____ SIGNATURE _____ R.N.

PostAnesth2

❥ **Figure 39–10** *Continued*

The nurse should place his or her hand in front of the client's airway (this could be an artificial airway or the mouth and nose) and feel the amount of exhaled air. The nurse should also check the client's skin color. Cyanosis is a late sign of severe tissue hypoxia. Restlessness, confusion, and anxiety are early signs of carbon dioxide retention and hypoxia.

Palpation

Examination by touch gives information about the temperature, moisture, and turgor of the skin, as well as edema. Crepitation (a crackling sensation) may result from air escaping from the respiratory system and entering the subcutaneous space. This may be seen in clients with pneumothorax. The normal spoken voice can produce a sound known as fremitus (a vibration of the chest wall felt by placing a hand over the chest that vibrates during speech). Fremitus may indicate collapse of lung tissue, presence of a lung lesion, or accumulation of mucus.

Percussion

The normal sound heard when the lungs are percussed is resonance, which is a sound of moderate to loud intensity that is low pitched and hollow, heard over the peripheral lungs. A hyperresonant sound is heard over hyperinflated lungs and could signify emphysema. Dullness, or a soft, high-pitched, thudlike sound, is percussed over solid organs (*e.g.,* heart, liver) or indicates consolidation or filling of the alveolar or pleural spaces by fluid, a common problem associated with pneumonia.

Auscultation

Normal respirations are quiet to the ear. The most common cause of changes in breath sounds is an accumulation of fluids in the lungs. Rales, or crackling sounds, are always considered abnormal. They can indicate congestive heart failure or bronchitis. Wheezes (musical rales), which are more prominent during expiration, can indicate bronchitis, cystic fibrosis, asthma, or foreign body aspiration. Wheezing can also indicate bronchospasm. *Stridor,* a term used to characterize a high-pitched crowing sound that occurs with difficult inspiration, may indicate laryngospasm, which may lead to complete or partial closure of the trachea. This sometimes occurs in clients who have had an endotracheal tube, which can cause irritation to the larynx, inserted. It is also seen in children with croup and aspiration of a foreign object. A gurgling sound indicates mucus accumulation. The most effective way to clear secretions is to encourage the client to cough in a purposeful manner.

Cardiovascular Status and Perfusion

Three components of the circulatory system should be evaluated: the heart as a pump, the blood, and the arteriovenous system.

Inspection

The overall condition of the client must be observed. Inspect for skin color, skin turgor, peripheral cyanosis, edema, dilation of the neck veins, and shortness of breath. Also, check the incision site for blood loss, and record the amount lost during the surgical procedure.

Arterial Blood Pressure and Heart Rate

Blood pressure, or the force exerted by the blood against the vessel wall, reflects the balance among cardiac output, blood volume, peripheral vascular resistance, and blood viscosity. Hypertension, or high blood pressure, is caused by a lack of elasticity and thickening of the arterial wall, resulting in a decrease in blood flow to vital organs. Hypotension, or low blood pressure, occurs when dilation of the arteries in the vascular bed, loss of blood, or failure of the heart to pump correctly occurs.

Stress and medication are just two factors associated with surgical procedures that can influence blood pressure. Fear, pain, and anxiety initiate sympathetic stimulation and a rise in blood pressure. Medications, such as diuretics (which reduce reabsorption of sodium and water by the kidney), calcium channel blockers (which reduce peripheral vascular resistance), and narcotics lower blood pressure.

Several factors affect the heart rate. Pain and anxiety cause sympathetic stimulation and increase the heart rate. Increasing tachycardia is also an early sign of shock and should be investigated. A decrease in heart rate is due to a parasympathetic stimulation and is seen in clients in severe or chronic pain. Medications can be responsible for both increases and decreases in heart rate. Therefore, it is the responsibility of the perioperative nurse to be aware of the actions and side effects of all medications that the client is taking and will be given as a surgical client.

Central Nervous System Status

All anesthetics are depressants that affect the central nervous system. The postoperative assessment includes gross evaluation of behavior, consciousness, intellectual performance, reflexes, and emotional status. As a client emerges from anesthesia, the nurse is responsible for reorienting the client and encouraging his or her wakefulness.

The use of fluorinated anesthetics has made emergence from anesthesia generally quiet and uneventful. The nurse tells the client where he or she is, that the surgery is over, and what time it is. With continuous information, the client should become oriented rather quickly. If the client becomes less oriented, it can be an early sign of impaired oxygen delivery, and action should be taken quickly to reverse the process.

Temperature

The assessment of body temperature is often ignored in the PACU. However, both hypothermia and hyperthermia are associated with physiological changes that can interfere with recovery. Clients at either end of the age continuum are at greater risk for developing temperature abnormalities. Normal body temperature may vary from 35.9°C to 38.0°C (96.6°F–100.4°F).

Fluid and Electrolyte Balance

Imbalance in fluids and electrolytes can occur in the postoperative client because of NPO status, fluid loss during the procedure, and stress. The normal body response to stress during the surgical procedure is renal retention of water and sodium.

Fluid Intake

The normal adult oral fluid intake is 2000 to 2200 ml a day. The client who is not able to take fluids orally must be given replacement intravenous fluids.

Intravenous Fluids

Most postoperative clients enter the PACU with an intravenous line in place. The anesthesia personnel keep an open line to administer medications and replace fluid lost during the procedure. The intravenous site should be checked to be sure that the needle is still in the vein. Also, watch for kinking or disconnection of the tubing. Pediatric clients may require a protective device over the intravenous site or soft restraints to prevent them from dislodging the needle.

Oral Fluids

Oral fluids are restricted postoperatively until laryngeal and pharyngeal reflexes are fully returned. Always start with small amounts of ice chips, as they are less likely to cause nausea.

Fluid Output

Normal urine output for an adult is about 1500 ml of urine a day. If the postoperative client has an indwelling urethral (Foley) catheter in place, the minimum expected output for an adult is about 30 ml per hour. Urine output that is less than this indicates an inadequate circulatory blood volume. A careful check of the urine output alerts the nurse to overhydration or dehydration. A lower urinary output can be expected immediately postoperatively as the body's reaction to stress from the surgical procedure. The color of the urine should be noted. Urine that is dark amber can be indicative of dehydration. Blood-tinged urine may indicate bladder or renal system trauma.

Recording of fluid output includes drainage from the incision site and drainage from any tubes inserted during the procedure. The amount, color, and odor of all fluid output should be noted and charted.

Wound Status

The nurse should check for drainage at the wound site. If drainage is occurring, the nurse should mark the dressing with ink to determine the amount of drainage or to determine changes in drainage between assessment periods. The nurse should follow the physician's orders or the policy and procedures of the nursing unit for the first dressing change. During all dressing changes, aseptic technique should be followed to prevent a wound infection. An open or healing wound is susceptible to bacterial growth.

Level of Comfort and Pain

The nurse should assess the client's level of pain, including where the pain is, how the client would describe it, and how intense the pain is. It is helpful to ask the client to rate the pain on a scale of 0 (no pain) to 10 (severe pain). The client's ability to rate

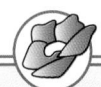

COMMUNITY-BASED CARE

MASTECTOMY AND LUMPECTOMY

When clients undergo procedures such as mastectomy or lumpectomy and are hospitalized for only 24 to 48 hours, the majority of their preoperative and postoperative care may be delivered in their homes. Preoperative preparation and teaching may be completed during a home visit prior to the surgery or, alternatively, may occur in the outpatient department. After surgery, the need for assessment and continued teaching is critical. Postoperatively, one or two home visits are made by the home care nurse, usually beginning the day after hospital discharge. The nurse assesses the client's vital signs, incision, pain control, and drain output. Surgical drains usually stay in place for a week to 10 days. Instruction includes how to empty and measure output until the drains are removed. Drain removal may be performed by the home care nurse or by the physician during a follow-up appointment. Additional teaching includes

1. Signs and symptoms of infection; when to notify the physician

2. Arm care to reduce risk of infection and lymphedema, including avoidance of blood pressure measurements and venipuncture of the affected arm

3. Activity and exercises to facilitate recovery; referral for occupational therapy to start 2 to 3 weeks after surgery is common

Psychosocial issues, including body image disturbance, a sense of loss, and fear related to the diagnosis of cancer, must also be addressed. The nurse assesses client coping and provides emotional support to both the client and family. Resources are identified, such as where to obtain a prosthesis and where to attend support groups or other programs in the area.

pain is considered stable from rating to rating and enables the nurse to evaluate the client's comfort level.

Tubes

The nurse should regularly assess the status of any tubes that the client may have, including

Intravenous line: Check the location of the needle, rate of flow, patency, and amount of fluid left in the bag, and note the type of fluid infusing

Nasogastric tube: Connect to low-Gomco suction and note the type and color of drainage

Chest tube: Connect to suction (pleurovac or other) and record the amount and color of drainage

Bladder catheter: Check that the catheter is not clamped or kinked and that urine is freely draining and note the color and amount of the drainage

Psychological Assessment

Almost all surgical clients experience anxiety about the procedure, anesthesia, and recovery. The physical signs and symptoms of anxiety are the same as those of any stressor the body is experiencing. The PACU nurse must be able to differentiate the symptoms of anxiety from those of other causes. A calm, confident nurse in a quiet environment can do much to relieve the stress of the surgical client. It is important to remember that hearing is the first sense to return after anesthesia; therefore, care should be taken to avoid yelling at the client, as this will create more stress for him or her.

If the client becomes anxious, the nurse will observe restlessness and increased blood pressure. Anxiety also increases pain sensation and the demand for oxygen. This is frequently manifested by tachycardia and tachypnea.

A flow sheet is maintained. The client is assessed on admission and then every 15 minutes thereafter unless more frequent evaluations are indicated.

Nursing Diagnosis

Nursing diagnoses for the client in the postoperative phase of the perioperative experience include, but are not limited to,

* Pain related to the surgical procedure
* Risk for Ineffective Breathing Pattern related to transfer to and from the surgical unit, intravenous sedation, anxiety, pain, smoking history, or improper position of the client during transfer
* Risk for Injury related to impaired physical mobility or devices used to assist recovery (tape for dressings)
* Risk for Ineffective Airway Clearance related to effects of anesthesia, history of smoking, or pain
* Risk for Infection related to impaired skin integrity (*e.g.*, from an incision), knowledge deficit (*e.g.*, how to care for drains and dressings), or urinary tract (*e.g.*, from dehydration, catheter)

* Self Care Deficit related to activity restrictions, restrictive devices (*e.g.*, chest tubes, urinary catheters), or pain management
* Other potential complications include hemorrhage, hypovolemic shock, paralytic ileus, and urinary tract infection.

Planning

The expected outcomes for the postoperative client are

An absence of infection, with no signs of redness, swelling, and pain on movement, no signs of nosocomial infection, and no signs of urinary tract infection

A verbal description of decrease in pain

A balanced intake and output of fluid

Effective deep breathing and coughing

Implementation

Respiratory Function

The primary goal of the postoperative nursing team is to maintain respiratory function. The nurse encourages the client to breathe deeply and cough about every 2 hours. The client with an abdominal incision tends to limit the depth of inspiration because of operative pain. When inspiratory effort is weak and tidal volume is decreased, alveoli are not aerated well. Secretions pool and can lead to hypostatic pneumonia. A decrease in gas exchange at the alveoli causes hypoxemia. An abdominal splint, made from a small pillow or blanket, is useful in reducing the pain involved in deep breathing and coughing.

Many hospitals are using incentive spirometry for postoperative ventilation therapy (see Procedure 29–7). An incentive spirometer is an apparatus that allows the client to use a mouthpiece and breathe as deeply as possible. The client is instructed to hold that breath for 3 seconds and then exhale. The goal is to work toward increasing inspiratory effort and tidal volume. The client should be instructed to refrain from using incentive spirometry at mealtimes to decrease the chance of nausea.

Positioning

The nurse should position the client for comfort utilizing correct body alignment. Positioning should allow for maximum respiratory status and comfort to decrease pain. This can be accomplished with pillows to support extremities, providing support while the client is turned on his or her side, and keeping the head elevated.

Pain Management

For in-house clients, during the first 24 hours after surgery the nurse should administer narcotics for pain relief in conjunction with positioning and other therapeutic measures. Nursing interventions include changes in position and back rubs. Medicate the client

Table 39–7

NURSING RESPONSIBILITIES IN POSTOPERATIVE PLANNING AND IMPLEMENTATION

RESPONSIBILITY	INTERVENTION	RATIONALE
Maintain respiratory function	Encourage coughing and deep breathing every 2 h; encourage use of incentive spirometer; monitor vital signs every 4 h; encourage leg exercises; encourage early ambulation	Anesthesia can decrease respiratory function
Maintain adequate intake and output	Measure intake and output; encourage fluids	Anesthesia can depress bladder tone
Maintain nutrition	Encourage fluids; listen for bowel sounds	Anesthesia depresses peristalsis
Maintain wound healing	Use aseptic technique when changing dressings	Altered nutrition and circulation can cause infection
Provide comfort	Encourage rest; administer pain medication; assist in changing positions	Shortens hospital stay

for nausea and vomiting. Nursing interventions include wiping the client's face with a cool towel, encouraging the use of mouthwash, and repositioning the client for comfort. Encourage the client to request pain medication before the pain intensifies to the point where the medication is ineffective. Table 39–7 outlines the nursing responsibilities and goals for the postoperative client.

Fluid Balance

The postoperative nurse is also concerned with prevention of fluid and electrolyte imbalances. Maintaining adequate intake and output records is essential. A decrease in fluid volume can lead to decreased blood pressure, increased temperature, cardiac arrhythmias, and pale, cool extremities.

An increase in fluid volume can lead to pitting edema, dyspnea, orthopnea, moist breath sounds, increased blood pressure, and distended neck veins.

Nutrition

The third goal of the postoperative nurse is to maintain nutrition. Encourage fluids, especially after urological procedures or procedures that involve the use of contrast media. It is important to listen for bowel sounds before giving food by mouth. Anesthesia can depress peristalsis.

Wound Healing

The postoperative nurse must also concentrate on promotion of wound healing. The surgical client is at risk for infection because of altered nutrition and circulation. To prevent infection, the primary technique is hand washing. Hand washing is the most important activity in preventing primary infections or cross-contamination.

Evaluation

Many institutions use a form of the Post Anesthesia Recovery Room Score for criteria for discharge (Box 39–3). These criteria include

1. The client has regained consciousness and is oriented to time and place
2. The airway is clear, and danger of aspiration is past
3. Circulatory and respiratory vital signs are stabilized

Box 39–3

POSTANESTHESIA ASSESSMENT CHART

Activity
0 = Unable to lift head
1 = Moves two extremities
2 = Able to move four extremities

Respirations
0 = Apneic
1 = Labored or limited respirations
2 = Can take deep breath and cough well

Circulation
0 = Has abnormally high or low blood pressure
1 = Blood pressure within 20–50 mmHg of preanesthesia level
2 = Stable blood pressure and pulse

Neurological status
0 = Not responsive
1 = Responds to pain
2 = Stupor
3 = Responds to verbal stimuli
4 = Drowsy
5 = Awake and alert

Color
0 = Cyanotic
1 = Pale, blotchy
2 = Pink

Documentation

All aspects of the immediate postoperative phase are recorded on the postanesthesia plan of care. An example of this form is given in Figure 39–10.

Nursing Care After Discharge From the Postanesthesia Care Unit

Postoperative care for the surgical client involves many areas of preparation. Before the client returns to the clinical unit from surgery, the nurse prepares the room to receive the client. Many factors must be considered when preparing the room. The nurse must have some familiarity with the surgical procedure that has been performed to allow him or her to have a basic plan for selecting needed supplies and equipment. The nurse should also utilize the client report from the PACU to include any additional requested supplies or equipment.

The first step in preparing the room is to have the client's bed clean and made up. This step allows minimal movement for the client immediately postoperatively and allows for a more efficient transfer of the client from the transport gurney. Chux pads or other positioning equipment should be available or already in place if possible.

Equipment and supplies that the nurse should consider for the postsurgery client include intravenous poles, an emesis basin, suction, oxygen (nasal prongs or a mask), tissues, and any other specialty equipment. When deciding what equipment and supplies might be needed, the nurse should consider the type of surgery. Will any drains be used? Will the drains be connected to intermittent wall suction, or will a closed reservoir system be used? Another consideration should include postoperative medications to be administered, including intravenous fluids, pain medication, antibiotics, or other prescribed medications. The nurse should be prepared for any treatments that may be needed, such as respiratory therapy, range of motion, exercises, use of antiembolism stockings, use of continuous range of motion machines, or use of overhead traction with trapezius bar. As nurses gain experience, they will begin to anticipate individual needs for the postoperative client.

Assessment

A nursing assessment is performed immediately on the client's arrival in the room (Box 39–4). This assessment includes the following.

> ## Box 39–4
>
> ### AMERICAN SOCIETY OF POST ANESTHESIA NURSES (ASPAN) RECOMMENDATIONS FOR ASSESSMENT
>
> 1. Vital signs
>   A. Respiratory rate and competency, airway patency, breath sounds, type of artificial airway, mechanical ventilator and settings
>   B. Blood pressure—cuff or arterial
>   C. Pulse—apical, peripheral, cardiac monitor pattern
>   D. Temperature—oral, tympanic, rectal, axillary, or digital through dermal or internal sensors
>   E. Oxygen saturation level—pulse oximeter
> 2. Pressure readings—central venous, arterial blood, pulmonary artery wedge, and intracranial pressure if indicated
> 3. Position of the client during surgery
> 4. Condition and color of the skin
> 5. Circulation—peripheral pulses and sensation of the extremity(ies) as applicable
> 6. Condition and location of dressings
> 7. Condition of the suture line (if no dressing)
> 8. Type and patency of drainage tubes, catheters, and reservoirs
> 9. Amount and type of drainage
> 10. Muscular response and strength
> 11. Pupillary response as indicated
> 12. Fluid therapy, location of lines, type and amount of solution infusing (including blood or expanders)
> 13. Level of consciousness
> 14. Level of physical and emotional comfort
> 15. Numerical score if used (see Postanesthesia Assessment Chart in Box 39–3)
>
> ---
>
> From the American Society of Post Anesthesia Nurses (1995). Resource 7. *Standards of Perianesthesia Nursing Practice* (pp. 42, 43). Thorofare, NJ: American Society of PostAnesthesia Nurses.

Respiratory Status

The rate and depth of respirations and color and temperature of the skin are assessed. The respiratory status is maintained by encouraging the client to breathe deeply and cough and to use incentive spirometry. Actions and results of treatment should be documented to provide a progressive plan of care. Documentation should include what treatment is being used, who helped the client with the treatment, whether it was a health care member or the family of the client, what levels were reached, and specifically how the client responded to the treatment.

Neurological Status

The nurse must determine the neurological status of the client. To do this, questions should be asked to determine orientation to name, time, place, date, or any other questions that should be asked to determine orientation. Movement should be assessed. This can be done easily when the client is transferred to the bed from the gurney. Make sure that directions are given so that the client can understand them. Documentation should include all aspects of your neurological assessment.

Cardiovascular Status

Vital signs, color, and temperature of the skin are assessed. The cardiovascular status is maintained by checking the pulse. Immediately postoperatively, the pulse is slightly tachycardic. A rate of 110 beats per minute or higher is called tachycardia and is symptomatic of fever, blood loss, and anxiety. A rate of 60 beats per minute or less is called bradycardia, and unless other symptoms are noted, bradycardia is usually considered normal. Remember that it may be appropriate to ask the client his or her normal heart rate, as this gives a baseline for the assessment. Usually, this is done if a heart rate is outside the "normal" limits; the normal limits are 60 to 100 beats per minute.

Wound Status

The nurse should check for drainage at the wound site. If drainage is occurring, the nurse should mark the dressing with ink to determine the amount of drainage or to determine changes in drainage between assessment periods. The nurse should follow the physician's orders for the first dressing change or the policy and procedure of the nursing unit for dressing changes. During all dressing changes, aseptic technique should be followed to prevent a wound infection. An open or healing wound is a ready source for bacterial growth.

Level of Comfort and Pain

The nurse should assess the client's level of pain. This includes where the pain is, how the client would describe it, and how intense the pain is. It is helpful to ask the client to rate the pain on a scale of 0 (no pain) to 10 (severe pain). The client's rating is considered stable from rating to rating and enables the nurse to evaluate the client's comfort level.

Tubes

The nurse should regularly assess the status of any tubes the client may have, including

Intravenous: Check the location of the needle, rate of flow, patency, and amount of fluid left in the bag, and note the type of fluid infusing

Nasogastric: Connect to low-Gomco suction, and note the type and color of drainage

Chest: Connect to suction—Pleurovac or other—and record amount and color of drainage

Bladder catheter: Check that it is not clamped or kinked and urine is freely draining, and note the color and amount of the drainage

Nursing Diagnosis

Nursing diagnoses for the client in the postoperative phase of the perioperative experience include, but are not limited to,

Pain related to surgical procedure

Risk for Ineffective Breathing Pattern related to transfer to and from the surgical unit, intravenous sedation, anxiety, pain, smoking history, or improper position of the client during transfer

Risk for Ineffective Airway Clearance related to effects of anesthesia, history of smoking, or pain

Risk for Injury related to impaired physical mobility or devices used to assist recovery (*e.g.,* tape for dressing)

Risk for Infection related to impaired skin integrity (*e.g.,* incision), knowledge deficit (*e.g.,* of drains and dressings), or urinary tract (*e.g.,* dehydration, catheter)

Self Care Deficit related to activity restrictions, restrictive devices (*e.g.,* chest tubes, urinary catheters), or pain management

Potential complications include hemorrhage, hypovolemic shock, paralytic ileus, and urinary tract infection.

Planning

The expected outcomes for the postoperative client are

An absence of infection, with no signs of redness, swelling, or pain on movement; no signs of nosocomial infection; and no signs of urinary tract infection

A verbal description of decrease in pain

A balanced intake and output

Effective deep breathing and coughing

Implementation
Respiratory Function

During the ongoing postoperative period, maintaining respiratory function continues to be a primary goal. The client needs to be encouraged to continue with deep breathing and coughing exercises, especially if he or she had major abdominal or thoracic surgery. These clients are at risk for developing hypostatic pneumonia over the days following the surgery if adequate aeration does not occur.

The client should continue to use the incentive spirometer as discussed previously. In addition, getting out of bed and ambulating early improves the client's respiratory function. In most instances, clients who have major surgery are transferred out of bed on the first postoperative day. The distance that the client ambulates should increase with each episode. The nurse should ensure that clients who need assistance in ambulating are provided with that assistance.

Positioning

The client's comfort should be a primary basis for how he or she is positioned postoperatively, unless specifically contraindicated. For instance, clients who have cranial surgery are limited both to how high the head of the bed can be raised and to which side they may be repositioned. The nurse should carefully check the physician's orders for any restrictions about the client's position.

Maintaining Comfort

Clients will continue to experience pain or discomfort for a period of time following their discharge from the PACU. Clients who have had major surgery may have a patient-controlled analgesic pump for a period of time. For other clients, less-potent analgesics may be prescribed. The nurse should administer prescribed analgesics and provide alternative comfort measures, such as positioning, back rubs, or hygiene measures, that will promote comfort for the client. It is important for the nurse to remember that pain perception is subjective, and the client's need for comfort is essential during this time. The nurse should not be concerned about overmedicating clients. Clients who receive adequate comfort measures do well postoperatively.

Clients who are being discharged home should receive instructions about analgesia and other, nonpharmacological comfort measures. If the client has a prescription for a medication, the nurse should review with the client the importance of getting the prescription filled and the necessity of taking the medication to relieve pain. Included in the instructions should be a list of side effects for which the client should carefully monitor.

Fluids and Nutrition

Clients who have ambulatory surgery and are discharged home should be instructed about taking adequate fluids during the early postoperative period. Even if they do not start to eat solid food shortly after discharge, it is essential that they understand the importance of drinking sufficient amounts of fluids and urinating adequately. Clients should be given a detailed list of what is permissible for them to have and what to observe for during this period.

Clients who remain in the hospital for a longer period should be carefully monitored by the nurse for their fluid balance. Many clients have intravenous infusions for a period of time if they are unable to drink sufficient amounts of oral fluids. A major concern for these clients during this period is the possibility of developing a fluid and electrolyte imbalance. The nurse should closely monitor vital signs and intake and output. Clients with an insufficient fluid intake develop a decreased blood pressure; pale, cool extremities; concentrated urine; and increased body temperature. Manifestations of fluid overload include dyspnea, rales (crackles), increased blood pressure, and distended neck veins.

Clients who have had major abdominal surgery often have a nasogastric tube connected to suction for a period postoperatively until peristalsis returns. The nurse should closely monitor the client's bowel sounds and whether the client is passing flatus. Once the client has bowel sounds and the nasogastric tube is removed, the client is then usually started on clear oral fluids and progressed to a regular diet. The nurse should ensure that the client is able to tolerate the fluids and food and does not develop abdominal distention. Carefully note whether the client becomes nauseated and begins to vomit. If vomiting persists, the client may need to have the nasogastric tube reinserted and have intravenous fluid initiated so that dehydration does not occur.

Wound Healing

The client remains at risk for a wound infection until the wound has adequately healed. For the client who is discharged home, the nurse should provide detailed instructions about care of the wound. Generally, clean technique will usually suffice for a client who is performing self-care of the wound.

For the client in the hospital, the nurse should be vigilant about the prospect of preventing wound infections. Hand washing is the most important measure in preventing and controlling wound infections. Infections of the wound are a major factor in delaying the client's progress and account for many delayed discharges. (See Chapter 23 for a more detailed discussion on the care of wounds and complications associated with wound healing.)

Discharge Teaching

Discharge planning should begin during the postoperative period before the client enters the hospital to have the surgical procedure. Especially important is planning for the client who is going to be discharged home following the surgery. For instance, driving instructions need to be reviewed with the client, and the importance of having a person with him or her needs to be emphasized.

Discharge instructions about home care and emergency medical attention should be given verbally and in writing so that the client can take them with him or her. For ambulatory surgical clients, this is usually provided during the preoperative period and then reviewed again postoperatively. Because these clients have minimal time with the nurse, it is essential that they receive good perioperative teaching and instructions. These instructions must include, but are not limited to,

• The physician's office telephone number
• The hospital's telephone number
• Future physician appointments (the date and time)
• Review of medications and treatments

- Guidelines related to the specific surgery
- Activity
- Dressing and wound care
- Signs of complications

Evaluation

The client should state that he or she has no pain postoperatively. The surgical incision should heal without infection. The client should not develop pneumonia or atelectasis.

Summary

The perioperative experience begins when the decision is made to have surgery and ends with the client's return to the highest level of wellness possible. During the three phases of the experience, the perioperative nurse works in conjunction with the client and family to orchestrate the care and recovery of the client. Preoperatively, the nurse is responsible for assessing the preparation of the client and family for the surgical procedure. Intraoperatively, the nurse assists the surgeon and the surgical team to produce a safe and positive outcome. Postoperatively, the nurse assists and encourages the client to achieve a positive outcome and return to the highest level of health and activity possible.

CHAPTER HIGHLIGHTS

✦

- ✦ Perioperative nursing consists of three distinct phases: the preoperative, intraoperative, and postoperative phases.
- ✦ During the preoperative phase, the nurse prepares the client and family for the intraoperative and postoperative phases. An assessment of the client is also performed to include actual and potential problems.
- ✦ During the intraoperative phase, the nurse works with the surgeons and other team members to provide a safe environment for the client.
- ✦ During the postoperative phase, the nurse assists the client to return to the highest level of function possible.
- ✦ Surgical procedures are classified according to urgency and purpose.
- ✦ The benefits of laser surgery include minimal blood loss, reduction in pain, and decrease in recovery time.

- ✦ The number of minimally invasive surgical procedures are increasing as health care management looks for alternatives to hospitalization after surgery.
- ✦ Endoscopic procedures allow the surgeon to examine a body cavity with a video camera. Smaller incisions, less trauma to tissue, and faster recovery are a few of the benefits.
- ✦ General, regional, or local anesthesia is used in most surgical procedures.
- ✦ Surgery is not performed unless informed consent is obtained from the client.
- ✦ Advance directives are integral components of the perioperative experience, allowing the client's wishes to be honored.
- ✦ Preoperative teaching has a positive outcome for the surgical client.
- ✦ After induction of anesthesia, the client is positioned for greatest accessibility to the surgical site without sacrificing respiratory or circulatory function.
- ✦ Hair should not be removed unless it interferes with the surgical incision.
- ✦ Each type of surgical procedure has its individual risk factors. Many clients have multiple risk factors, which vary depending on their general health condition.
- ✦ The nursing process is an important component of the perioperative experience.

Study Questions

1. Surgery performed to relieve symptoms of an illness but that does not cure the disease is known as

   a. elective
   b. constructive
   c. palliative
   d. diagnostic

2. The anesthesia classification that describes a client as one with severe systemic disease without functional limitations: cardiovascular disease that limits activity, severe diabetes with systemic complications, or poorly controlled hypertension would be a class

   a. I
   b. II
   c. III
   d. IV

3. The anesthesia involving blocking a specific set of nerve fibers or an individual nerve is known as

   a. general anesthesia
   b. regional anesthesia
   c. monitored anesthesia
   d. local anesthesia

4. A complication of spinal anesthesia is

    a. laryngospasm
    b. spinal headache
    c. cracked tooth
    d. bronchospasm

5. The scope of nursing practice throughout the surgical experience is

    a. perioperative nursing
    b. postoperative nursing
    c. preoperative nursing
    d. intraoperative nursing

Critical Thinking Exercises

1. Kari is scheduled for a radical mastectomy at age 39 years. Discuss preoperative and postoperative teaching for Kari.

2. Following ostomy surgery, Mr. T. returns to the room with an intravenous line, patient-controlled analgesia pump, a nasogastric tube, and a Foley catheter. Document critical aspects you would include in your postoperative notes.

References

Ball, K. A. (1995). *LASERS: The perioperative challenge* (2nd ed.). St. Louis, MO: C. V. Mosby

Hathaway, D. (1986). Effect of preoperative instruction on postoperative outcomes: A meta-analysis. *Nursing Research, Sept/Oct*, 269–275.

Healy, K. (1968). Does preoperative instruction make a difference? *American Journal of Nursing, 68*(1), 62–67.

Kneedler, J. A., & Dodge, G. H. (1994). *Perioperative client care: The nursing perspective* (4th ed.). Boston: Blackwell Scientific Publications.

McEwen, D. (1996). Intraoperative positioning of surgical patients. *AORN, 63*(6), 1059–1086.

Moss, R. (1986). Overcoming fear. *AORN, 43*(5), 1107–1114.

Rosen, L. Self-determination (Part I). *Today's Surgical Nurse*, July/August, 1996, 46–47.

Bibliography

Association of Operating Room Nurses. (1990). *Core curriculum for the RN first assistant*. Denver: Association of Operating Room Nurses.

Association of Operating Room Nurses. (1990). *Perioperative nursing documentation*. Denver: The Association of Operating Room Nurses.

Association of Operating Room Nurses. (1991). *Monitoring the client receiving local anesthesia*. (2nd ed.). Denver: Association of Operating Room Nurses.

Association of Operating Room Nurses. (1994). *1994 Standards and recommended practices*. Denver: Association of Operating Room Nurses.

Atkinson, L. J., & Kohn, M. L. (1986). *Berry and Kohn's introduction to operating room technique* (6th ed.). New York: McGraw-Hill.

Benz, J. D. (1992). Pharmacist's corner, injectable local anesthetics. *AORN Journal, 55*(1), 274–284.

Burden, N. (1993). *Ambulatory surgical nursing*. Philadelphia: W. B. Saunders.

Carpenito, L. J. (1992). *Nursing diagnosis, application to clinical practice* (4th ed.). Philadelphia: J. B. Lippincott.

Craft, M. J., & Denehy, J. A. (1990). *Nursing interventions for infants and children*. Philadelphia: W. B. Saunders.

Drain, C. B., & Christoph, S. S. (1987). *The recovery room: A critical care approach to post anesthesia nursing* (2nd ed.). Philadelphia: W. B. Saunders.

Gauthier, D. K., O'Fallon, P. T., & Coppaage, D. (1993). Clean vs sterile surgical skin. *AORN Journal, 58*(3), 486–495.

Genitron, J. D. (1992). A comparison of three anesthetic agents. *AORN Journal, 55*(6), 1562–1570.

Gregory, B., Lewis, J., & Ward, S. (1992). *Quality improvement in perioperative nursing*. Denver: Association of Operating Room Nurses.

Groah, L. K. (1990). *Operating room nursing*. San Mateo, CA: Appleton & Lange.

Guendermann, B. J. (1990). Surgical asepsis revisited. *Today's OR Nurse, October*, 10–13.

Haines, N. (1992). Same day surgery: Coordinating the education process. *AORN Journal, 55*(2), 573–580.

Hallstrom, R., & Beck, S. L. (1993). Implementation of the AORN skin shaving standard: Evaluation of a planned change. *AORN Journal, 55*(3), 498–506.

Hill, J. M. (1991). Time saving formats for client care planning in outclient surgery units. *Journal of Post Anesthesia Nursing, 6*(3), 181–184.

Jepsen, O. B., & Bruttomesso, K. A. (1993). The effectiveness of preoperative skin preparations: An integrative review of the literature. *AORN Journal, 58*(3), 477–484.

Kim, M. J., McFarland G. K., & McLane A. M. (1993). *Pocket guide to nursing diagnosis* (5th ed.). St. Louis: Mosby-Year Book.

Kjervik, D. K., & Weisensee, M. G. (1992). Empowering older people is a perioperative nursing challenge. *AORN Journal, 55*(4), 1086–1089.

Laufman, H. (1990). What's happened to aseptic discipline in the OR? *Today's OR Nurse, October*, 15–19.

Leclair, J. (1990). A review of antiseptics. *Today's OR Nurse, October*, 25–28.

Leske, J. S. (1992). Practice-based perioperative research: Meeting the challenges. *AORN Journal, 55*(3), 172–173.

Long, V. C., & Phipps, W. J. (1993). *Essentials of medical-surgical nursing: A nursing process approach* (3rd ed.). St. Louis: C. V. Mosby.

Longinow, L. T., & Rzeszewski, L. B. (1993). The holding room: A preoperative advantage. *AORN Journal, 57*(4), 914–924.

Marriner-Toomey, A. (1991). Standard care plans for the post anesthesia care unit. *Journal of Post Anesthesia Nursing, 6*(1), 26–32.

Milner, D. G. (1990). Anesthesia: The perioperative nurse's role. *Today's OR Nurse, August*, 24–29.

Murphy, E. K. (1992). OR nursing law, advance directives and the client self-determination act. *AORN Journal, 55*(1), 270–272.

Oetker-Black, S. L. (1993). Preoperative preparation. *AORN Journal, 57*(6), 1402–1415.

Perkins, J. J. (1969). *Principles and methods of sterilization in health sciences*. Springfield, IL: Charles C Thomas Publishers.

Phippen, M. L., & Wells, M. P. (1995). *Perioperative nursing handbook*. Philadelphia: W. B. Saunders.

Phippen, M. L., & Wells, M. P. (1994). *Perioperative nursing practice*. Philadelphia: W. B. Saunders.

Position statement on the role of the RN in the management of clients receiving IV conscious sedation for short-term therapeutic, diagnostic or surgical procedures. (1992). *AORN Journal, 55*(1), 207–210.

Reichart, M. (1993). Laparoscopic instruments, client care, cost issues. *AORN Journal, 57*(3), 637–655.

Ronk, L. L., & Girard, N. J. (1994). Risk perceptions, universal precautions compliance: A descriptive study of nurses who circulate. *AORN Journal, 59*(1), 253–266.

Rothrock, J. C. (1990). *Perioperative nursing care planning.* St. Louis: C. V. Mosby.

Schmaus, D. C., Nelson, S. L., & Davis, D. L. (1987). *Positioning the surgical client.* Denver: Association of Operating Room Nurses.

Scott, S. M., Mayhew, P. A., & Harris, E. A. (1992). Pressure ulcer development in the operating room: Nursing implications. *AORN Journal, 56*(2), 242–250.

Selman, S. W., & Mistretta, E. F. (1992). Perioperative concerns of the older adult undergoing total joint replacement. *AORN Journal, 55*(2), 618–622.

Chapter 40

COMMUNITY-BASED CARE

MICHELE C. CLARK, PhD, RN

POLDI TSCHIRCH, PhD, RN, CS

KEY TERMS

✦

community-based
nursing
primary prevention

public health nursing
secondary prevention
tertiary prevention

LEARNING OBJECTIVES

✦

After studying this chapter, you should be able to

✦ Identify the implications of trends in health care reform for community-based nursing

✦ Define community-based care and public health

✦ Differentiate nursing practice in community-based care and public health

✦ Discuss the nursing role in a variety of community-based settings

✦ Describe the application of case management principles in community-based nursing

✦ Identify complementary roles of multidisciplinary teams

✦ Describe how the nursing process is applied to practice in community-based settings

✦ Use the nursing process for specific community-based nursing problems

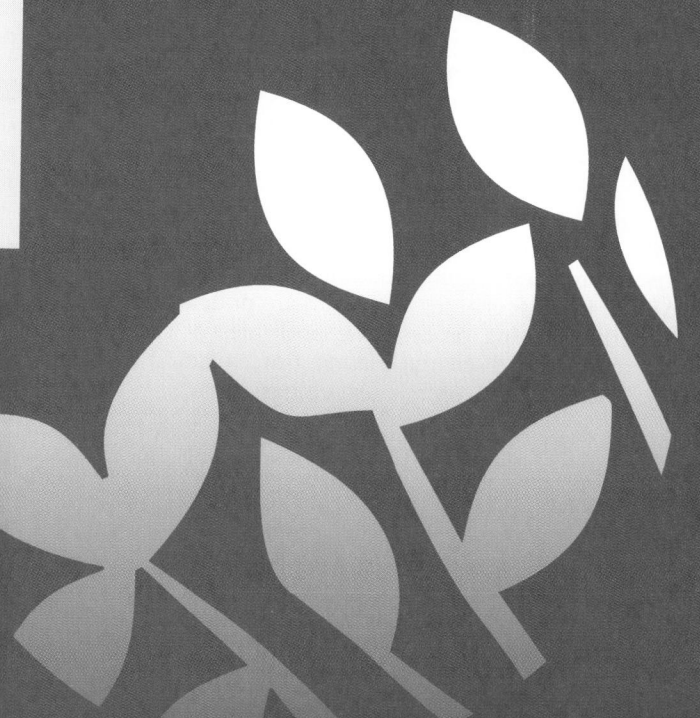

Nurses have a long tradition of bringing nursing care to clients and families in the settings where they live and work. Florence Nightingale's scheme for district nursing in the latter half of the 19th century, Lillian Wald's creation of the school nurse role in 1902, and Mary Breckinridge's Frontier Nursing Service founded in 1925 (which sent nurses on horseback into rural Appalachia), were all nursing innovations focused on promoting access to care for underserved populations by bringing nurses into the communities they served. Public health, occupational health, and school health have long been recognized as essential community-based services. Current trends in health care reform are contributing to an increased interest in the community as a site for care delivery, as spiraling health care costs have focused attention on issues of access, cost, and quality of care. The US health care system has been characterized by a focus on acute care, intensive use of technology, and a highly specialized workforce. A common theme in many reform proposals is an increased emphasis on community-based services.

A significant change observed by the nursing profession is the movement of many health care services from the hospital to the community. Community-based nurses include all levels of prevention as they work with clients and families to maintain the client's maximum level of functioning within the home and community. The nursing process serves as the organizing framework for nursing care delivery in all settings. It guides community-based nursing in adapting plans of care to client or family lifestyle, values, and home environments. Educating clients for self-care and adapting care to the home environments are major emphases.

Nursing case management is becoming a popular framework within which to manage clients' needs in and out of the hospital. Case management is used in community-based care to provide coordination for clients who need a variety of services to be maintained safely at home. An important role of the case manager is to facilitate movement across levels of care. Discharge planning is an integral part of this process. It ensures that the treatment plan prescribed at a hospital or ambulatory care setting can be safely and effectively provided within the home. The information provided in this chapter supports an understanding of how the nursing process, the principles of case management, and discharge planning are adapted to care for clients within community settings.

◆ Health Care Reform and Community-Based Care

Socioeconomic Trends Affecting Health Care Delivery

Changes in health care delivery and financing are currently and will continue to be influenced by social change. Demographic changes include an aging population, decline in population of younger age groups, increasing racial and ethnic diversity, and changes in the family unit. The proportion of the US population older than 64 years is expected to increase from 12.2% in 1987 to 21.8% by 2030, while the age group younger than 5 years will decline from the 1990 level of 18.4 million to 16.9 million in 2000, stabilizing at approximately 16 to 17 million until 2050 (Pew Health Professions Commission, 1993). School-age and college-age groups have decreased steadily since 1987, with numbers expected to increase but not exceed 1987 levels by 2000 to 2010. Cultural diversity will pose new challenges to health care delivery. By 2005, Hispanic and African-American populations will be nearly equal in size and will represent 26% of the total US population. Because of higher poverty rates, African-American and Hispanic populations in general receive fewer health services. On the basis of indicators such as life expectancy and infant mortality, these two groups have a lower health care status than does the larger population.

Changes in the family unit also have implications for health care service delivery. The cultural norm of the traditional intact family with two married adults with children no longer represents the reality of many within our society. Major changes in family structure have occurred in the past two decades: The rate of married women in the workforce with children younger than 5 years reached 63.8% in 1989. Approximately half of all marriages end in divorce, and one in three children will spend part of their lives in one-parent households headed by women (Pew Health Professions Commission, 1993).

Additionally, the US economy is under pressure from global competition and a large debt burden. Economic trends that have driven health care reform activity in recent years include the shift from a manufacturing to a service and information base, with resulting disruptions in employment, a widening gap between the richest and poorest Americans, budget deficits, and resultant pressure to reduce public spending. Federal

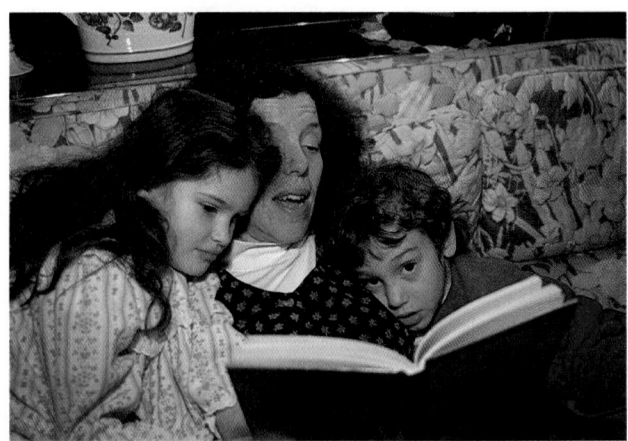

❧ **Figure 40–1**
A mother reads a bedtime story to her children.

spending on health and social welfare programs, which expanded tremendously over the past four decades, is increasingly at risk. Budget pressures have created an urgent need for spending reductions, threatening programs that provide health and social services and exacerbating problems of access to care for low-income citizens.

Patterns of Health and Illness

Healthy People 2000 (US Department of Health and Human Services [USDHHS], 1991) identifies a number of trends in the health status and disease patterns of Americans. Major areas of concern relate to infant mortality, lifestyle and behavior, diseases of aging, environmental hazards, and the reemergence of infectious disease. Groups identified as especially vulnerable include people with low incomes; members of African-American, Hispanic, Asian, and Native American racial and ethnic minority groups; and people with disabilities. Whereas this report documents overall health improvements achieved as a result of preventive efforts, it identifies a significant continuing burden of preventable illness, injury, and disability. The overarching goals for all Americans articulated in *Healthy People 2000* that provide a framework for the proposed initiatives include increasing the span of healthy life, reducing health disparities among population groups, and achieving access to preventive services.

The health trends and issues identified in *Healthy People 2000* (USDHHS, 1991) reflect the limitations of our current health care delivery system, as well as the impact of demographic change, lifestyles, and disease patterns on the health status of Americans. Since World War II, health care delivery, research, and health professions education have been oriented toward illness treatment, development of increasingly sophisticated diagnostic and treatment technologies, and creation of a highly skilled, highly specialized workforce. Although this system has produced signifi-

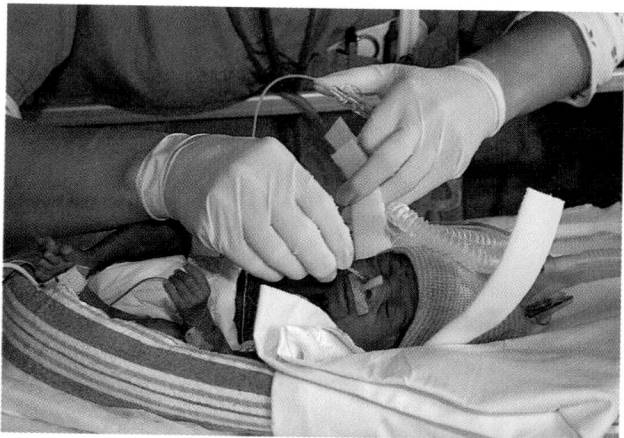

Figure 40-2
An infant in the neonatal intensive care unit.

Box 40-1

THE CHARACTERISTICS OF THE EMERGING HEALTH CARE SYSTEM

* Orientation toward health—emphasis on prevention, wellness, and individual responsibility for health behaviors

* Population perspective—focus on risk factors affecting the community, including physical and social environment

* Intensive use of information—reliance on information systems to provide complete, easily assimilated client information, as well as access to relevant information on current practice

* Focus on the consumer—encouragement of client partnerships in treatment decisions, facilitated by availability of information on outcomes

* Knowledge of treatment outcomes—emphasis on determination of the most effective treatment under different conditions and dissemination of this information to those involved in treatment decisions

* Constrained resources—pervasive concern over increasing costs, coupled with expanded use of mechanisms to control or limit expenditures

* Coordination of services—increased integration with providers with concomitant emphasis on teams to improve efficiency and effectiveness across all settings

* Reconsideration of human values—careful assessment of the balance between expanding capability of technology and the need for humane treatment

* Expectations of accountability—growing scrutiny by a larger variety of payers, consumers, and regulators coupled with more formally defined performance expectations

* Growing interdependence—further integration of domestic issues of health, education, and public safety, combined with a growing awareness of the importance of US health care in a global context

Pew Health Professions Commission Report. (1993). *Health professions education for the future: Schools in service to the nation.* San Francisco: The Pew Health Professions Commission.

cant advances in clinical knowledge, it has done so through a supply-driven system with limited mechanisms for controlling health care costs. Despite health care expenditures exceeding 15% of the Gross Domestic Product in 1995 (nearly one trillion dollars), it is estimated that approximately 40 to 45 million people are uninsured (Pew Health Professions Commission, 1993). This high level of expenditure has failed to yield proportional health benefits and is proving unsustainable in the current economic climate. Health care reform proponents have focused on the structural changes needed to address pressing issues of cost, access, and quality.

Nursing and Health Care Reform

Many of these themes are evident in *Nursing's Agenda for Health Care Reform* (American Nurses Association, 1991), which spells out the nursing profession's recommendations for a restructured health care system. A central assumption of this document is that reform of health care financing mechanisms must be accompanied by a shift in the orientation of health care toward consumer needs, a wellness and care focus, and delivery of care in community-based sites to increase access. It advocates for a federally defined package of essential services available to all, financed through an integration of public and private resources. Delivery of primary care services, increased consumer responsibility for health, and utilization of the full range of providers to deliver cost-effective care at the appropriate level are some of the other essential elements of nursing's platform. Cost reductions are expected to result from the use of research-based outcome measures that improve care effectiveness, ensure appropriate leveling of care, and improve disease prevention.

The vulnerable groups targeted by the nursing profession for increased levels of service represent those identified by *Healthy People 2000* (USDHHS, 1991): the poor, the minorities, and the uninsured. Managed care is seen as an essential element of reform, although restructuring to accommodate consumer choice and health promotion is deemed necessary. Case management is proposed as a tool to provide holistic, coordinated care for individuals with complex health needs. Not surprisingly, the *Agenda* (American Nurses Association, 1991) places nurses in a central role in the implementation of these reforms. A major criticism of the current system is its failure to address financial and regulatory barriers that prevent the full utilization of nurses' abilities.

The Pew Commission predicts that within another decade, 80 to 90% of the insured population will receive their care through the emerging systems of integrated care that combine levels of services and also intensively manage service delivery, focusing on cost reduction, consumer satisfaction, and improved health care outcomes. The Commission anticipates that as many as half of the nation's hospitals will close, with a loss of 50 to 60% of hospital beds. In addition, massive expansion will occur in the delivery of primary care services in ambulatory and community settings. A surplus of physicians and nurses will occur as demand for specialty care shrinks and hospitals close. Allied health professions will consolidate into multiskilled professions.

Clearly, the professional practice environment for nurses is undergoing rapid and far-reaching change. The Pew Commission (1995) has identified several "Competencies for 2005" for the health professional, which are listed in Box 40–2. This definition of competencies has major implications for community-based nursing. Major emphasis is placed on the health of communities, client and family involvement in health care decisions, and health promotion and disease prevention, all of which are important features of community-based nursing practice. Nursing is particularly well positioned for the reformed health care system because of its long-standing commitment to wellness, client-centered care, client education, and community-based care.

BOX 40–2

COMPETENCIES FOR 2005

- Care for the community's health
- Provide contemporary clinical care
- Participate in the emerging system
- Accommodate expanded accountability
- Ensure cost-effective care and use technology appropriately
- Practice prevention and promote healthy lifestyles
- Involve patients and families in the decision-making process
- Manage information and continue to learn

From Pew Health Commission. (1995). *Critical challenges: Revitalizing the health professions for the twenty-first century.* San Francisco: The Pew Health Professions Commission.

Community-Based Nursing Care

In essence, health care reform strives to provide universal access to high-quality care, keep health care costs reasonable, maintain consumer choice for services, and find fair ways to finance this new health care system (Primomo, 1995). In response to these needs, community-based care has emerged as a widely recognized strategy to achieve these goals. One significant change observed by the nursing profession is the movement of many health care services away from the hospital toward the community. For example, in the past, clients with large wounds demanded special hospital care. Presently, these same clients can receive the same care in their homes. Wound care, physical assessment, and well-child examinations are now frequently done in the home. Unfortunately, with more health services becoming community based, the roles of public health nursing and community-based nursing are becoming blurred. Funding sources of public and private agencies are asking nurses to differentiate community-based nursing from public health nursing.

Public Health Nursing

In public health nursing, the population of interest (e.g., children, pregnant mothers, the homeless) is de-

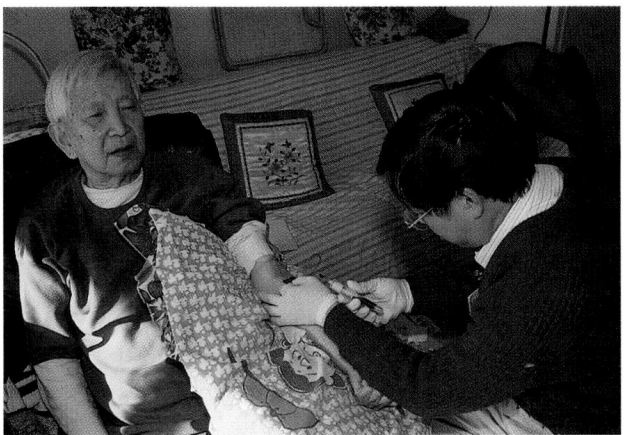

Figure 40–3
A home care nurse draws blood from a client.

fined as the community (Williams, 1997). Therefore, the focus of public health nurses becomes protecting this subgroup or population of interest from disease, injury, disability, and premature death, primarily through primary prevention measures. Primary prevention measures might include teaching mothers about infant feeding, immunization schedules, and accident prevention. Public health nurses center their nursing activities around health promotion and disease prevention.

Although many public health nurses' activities are concerned with primary prevention, they are also involved in secondary and tertiary prevention (Bechtel *et al.*, 1995; Williams, 1997) measures. In secondary prevention, case finding and screening for early detection of disease become the focus of many health care professions. As an example, a public health nurse might monitor the health of pregnant women for early signs of toxemia. The nurse might perform hearing and vision screenings in schools. These screening ac-

tivities are important in maintaining the health of the community.

Public health nurses are also involved in tertiary prevention by providing care to limit disabilities and to rehabilitate persons with chronic conditions. Many public health programs guarantee care for children with certain disabilities. For example, in certain geographical areas, the public health department may have a special program for children with asthma. These children would come to a clinic for care and then might be visited by a public health nurse working with the school nurse to ensure that these asthmatic children maintain their highest level of functioning.

Community-Based Nursing

Focus of Practice

In community-based nursing, the individual, not the larger population of interest, is the client and major focus of nursing practice. Health care in community-based sites is episodic, requiring nursing care to be family centered to ensure that the family is competent to provide the client's care safely in the home (Zotti *et al.*, 1996). Therefore, the nursing care plan formulated by a community-based nurse is directed not only by the medical and nursing needs of the client but also by the family's values, beliefs, and stresses. For example, one client who is a newly diagnosed diabetic, living with his wife and 10-year-old daughter, may identify family food preferences that are in opposition to his new diabetic diet. Attention to this family's food preferences highlights for the nurse how such considerations can influence compliance or noncompliance with a treatment plan. The nurse and family will work in partnership to incorporate a diet that is reasonable to this family's traditions and tastes. Such nurse and family collaborations, which are the

		Table **40–1**
PRIMARY CHARACTERISTICS OF PUBLIC HEALTH NURSING AND COMMUNITY-BASED NURSING		
	PUBLIC HEALTH NURSING	**COMMUNITY-BASED NURSING**
Focus of Practice	Population aggregates	Individual/family
Practice Goals	Primary prevention	Secondary/tertiary prevention
Practice Roles	Community education	Individual/family education
	Case management	Case management
	Wellness/prevention program development and implementation	Direct care
Practice Settings	Public health departments	Home
		Clinics
		Schools
		Workplace
Client Profile	All age groups	All age groups with focus on individual/ families
	Focus on aggregates (*i.e.,* newborns, pregnant women)	

heart of community-based nursing, ensure that medical and nursing treatment can successfully be continued in the home, workplace, or school.

Practice Goals

Unlike public health nursing, in which the main goal is primary prevention, community-based nursing practice aims to manage individuals' acute or chronic conditions, or to practice tertiary prevention. Community-based nursing practice differs significantly from public health nursing in goals, types of clients, roles, services, and even in many special activities (Primomo, 1995). Individuals receive their tertiary care in community-oriented primary care clinics, health maintenance organizations (HMOs) individual homes, workplaces, or schools (Zotti *et al.,* 1996). Although community-based nurses also practice primary and secondary prevention, as explained in the previous section, they become involved with the client during an acute or chronic episode related to health status. Thus, their initial and primary nursing activity is involved with tertiary care and prevention as it relates to the chronic condition.

Practice Roles

In community-based practice, nurses take on a number of different roles, depending on the community setting in which they practice, as well as the treatment plans that they are trying to implement. These roles may include educator, counselor, direct care provider, and case manager. As each client's various care needs emerge, different roles for the nurse become appropriate. For example, a nurse working in a community clinic specializing in rehabilitation may be required to exhibit a number of professional roles. Suppose a rehabilitation practitioner works with a client with right-sided weakness because of a recent stroke. This nurse, specializing in rehabilitation, may need to educate the family and the client about strengthening exercises for the affected extremities (Rice & Rappl, 1996). The nurse may also need to familiarize the family with new medications that the client is now required to take. Furthermore, once the nurse begins to educate the client and the family on these nursing concerns, the nurse may find it necessary to take on the role of counselor, focusing on the family and the client's grief related to physical losses suffered because of the stroke. These grief concerns may actually be important to address before other areas of the treatment plan can be initiated. Individual circumstances that arise in practice dictate the appropriate roles that the practicing community based nurse needs to assume.

Practice responsibilities also influence which roles the nurse will use in the practice setting. For example, the primary responsibilities of nurses working as case managers might include managing different community resources needed to facilitate the client's healing. They may not be involved with direct care but will rather refer the client to health care agencies to get the needed care. The case manager thus becomes an important leader, working directly with other members of the interdisciplinary team to ensure that the client receives the best care for his or her needs.

Practice Settings

Because practice sites for the community-based nurse can include the client's home, work, school, or place of recreation, an understanding of how the many systems of work, school, play, and home affect the client's rehabilitation and illness behavior is imperative (Jenkins & Sullivan-Marx, 1994). By understanding the many systems with which a client interacts daily, the nurse is able to develop and direct a more holistic and individualized plan of care. For example, a client discharged from a primary care–oriented community clinic with an injured hand caused by repairing and servicing telephone lines might have difficulty meeting his little league coaching duties or finishing repairs on his roof. The nurse could incorporate in her care plan strategies so that the man could meet at least some of these responsibilities safely despite this injury. Additionally, the nurse would work with this family to problem solve about how these obligations could be met in other ways.

Client Profile

Although they certainly have distinct differences, public health nursing and community-based nursing do intersect at many points. Like public health nursing, community-based nursing is concerned with the care of individuals across the life span. Community-based services address individuals, such as infants, children, adolescents, adults, or older adults. These clients can be seen in a variety of settings, including specialty ambulatory clinics, primary care community-oriented clinics, home health care agencies, and managed care organizations (Clark, 1992). Because community-based nurses primarily care for acute or chronic conditions, their nursing practice focuses on ensuring compliance with medical and nursing treatment plans through education and training. Public health nurses, however, *may* care for individual clients, but their interest in this care is how it reflects high-risk groups or aggregates in the community.

Cultural Influence on Clients' Behaviors

Both the community-based nurse and the public health nurse work with a variety of cultures. However, the community-based nurse works on an individual basis with each client and family. Community-based nursing care requires the nurse to be sensitive to the many cultural differences seen in practice so that care plans are tailored to clients' and families' individual preferences and needs (Jackson, 1996). If a community-based nurse were working with both an elderly African-American and an Italian-American recently diagnosed with congestive heart failure, the nurse would observe that the two clients probably have very different dietary concerns related to their cultural and ethnic backgrounds. When formulating and suggesting a required low-salt, low-fat diet, the nurse should consider these cultural factors.

Client Responsibilities

Both the public health nurse and the community-based nurse support individual and family autonomy. In community-based care, however, clients managing acute or chronic conditions do so under the direction of health care professionals, usually in their homes. Clients and their families are primarily responsible for performing the needed medical and nursing care. In the past, a client newly diagnosed with diabetes would be hospitalized to stabilize blood sugars and to be educated on diabetic treatment protocols. Now this care is more often administered in community clinics, HMOs, or at home. Community-based nurses understand that as family members become incorporated into the treatment plan, they are more able to support the clients' care once health care professionals are absent. By being involved in the treatment plan, the family unit becomes more independent and responsible for the care of the client.

Funding for Community-Based Care

Community-based care is financed through a variety of mechanisms, utilizing both public and private funds. Public funds play a large role in provision of community-based care. Medicare and Medicaid are government-sponsored programs established in 1965 to improve access to care for the elderly, poor, and disabled. A significant portion of community-based care is financed through these programs. Medicare, the federally financed health insurance for those over 65 years old, provides payment for home health care ser-

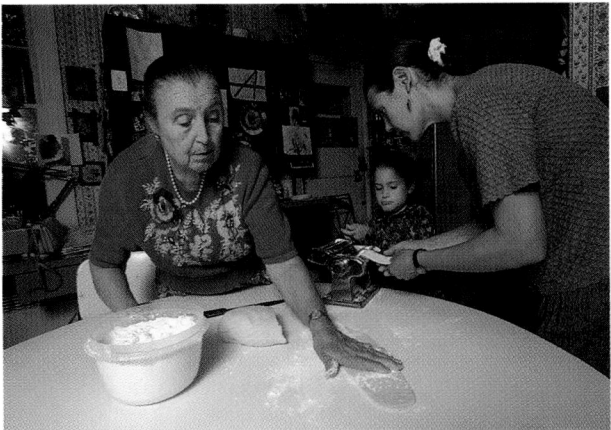

✦ **Figure 40–4**
Three generations of Italian-Americans make a pasta dinner together.

vices, hospice care, and some medical equipment and supplies. Medicaid, funded by both the federal government and state governments and administered by the states, provides funds for home health care and some primary and preventive services for citizens in certain low-income groups. Public funds, usually at the state and local level, are used to finance the services provided by public health departments, such as well-child clinics and immunization and screening programs. The community-based services provided by school nurses are funded by local tax revenues as part of school budgets. Private insurance plans also may provide coverage for home health care and clinic-based services.

Funding for community-based services comes from a mix of public and private funds, with public funds being the largest source. Often, public and private funding sources review documentation to analyze the care given and the client's response to treatment as well as to decide on reimbursement. For example, for reimbursement in the community-based service of home health care, the client record must demonstrate that the nurse provides skilled nursing services to the client. These would include teaching or training, observation, evaluation and assessment, direct care, and management of the client's care plan. If these skilled services are not evident in the client record, Medicare, the payer for home health care, cannot reimburse the nurse for his or her home visit. Box 40–3 provides an example of documentation with skilled nursing assessment and teaching.

Types of Community-Based Settings

Community-based care may be provided to individuals or groups using the principles of primary, secondary, or tertiary care, with a focus on tertiary care (Zotti, *et al.*, 1996). Because community-based care is often directed toward a specific group of people who have special or common needs, a variety of settings are used to meet the medical and nursing needs of the client.

Community-based nursing care's focus is twofold: (1) to meet the health care needs of individuals when they are in a particular health care facility and (2) to meet these same individuals' unique health care needs as they move among different health care settings. The community-based nurse often must "manage the case"—that is, know the different community resources that the client can use to meet his or her health and rehabilitation needs.

A nurse working in a community-based primary health clinic needs to be aware of the many health-related services that his or her client can access. Let us suppose that a client, Mr. Black, has been diagnosed with diabetes mellitus and had an amputation of the

Box 40–3

HOME HEALTH NURSING NOTES

Clinical Findings

Temp 99	BP 140/80	Pulse 88/regular	Resp 16	Height 5 ft 6 in	Usual weight 156 lb	Weight on admission 200 lb

GENERAL APPEARANCE: *65-year-old Hispanic male who is cooperative and alert*

PRIMARY DIAGNOSIS: *Myocardial infarction (heart attack)*

SECONDARY DIAGNOSIS (ASSESSMENTS PERTINENT TO CARE)
Because of diagnosis and associated condition, client complains of feeling very depressed. Presently on a new medication for the depression.

CLIENT/CAREGIVER ABILITY TO LEARN/DO CARE:
Wife very motivated and interested in giving her husband good care.

BARRIERS TO LEARNING: *None*

HANDS-ON CARE/TEACHING THIS VISIT: *Assessed nutritional status and caloric requirements and instructed the client in a 1200-calorie diet for weight loss. Instructed client on a low-cholesterol, low-fat, sodium-restricted diet, as ordered by the physician. Assisted client in identifying work stressors and instructed him on relaxation techniques to use not only at work but also at home.*

BP = blood pressure; Resp = respirations; Temp = temperature.

---

right foot 6 weeks ago. The nurse at the community-based clinic needs to know that in addition to coming to the clinic to have the healing of the surgical area monitored, Mr. Black is also being fitted for a prosthesis at a local specialty clinic and is seeing an endocrinologist for his diabetes. Although a community-based case manager may arrange this other care, complete information about the case is vital to the community-based nurse in the primary care facility caring for Mr. Black because it will influence his or her planning for client education, scheduling for direct care in the clinic, and monitoring how well Mr. Black is following up on the other needed community resources. This type of total care requires an autonomous and independent professional nurse who will be aware of the many health care needs of the client.

Community-based nurses are required to use many different skills to ensure that clients reach their maximum level of health. They often work autonomously, practicing their skills in a variety of diverse settings and programs. The setting of their care may vary (Table 40–2), but community-based nurses are focused on the complete health care picture of the client, including the other health care resources that are being used.

Parish Nursing

Nationally, it is estimated that there are over 2000 parish nurses representing the Catholic, Protestant, and Jewish congregations (Kiser, *et al.*, 1995). The parish nurse practice theory was developed by Granger Westberg, who combined medicine and theology within a holistic health care framework. Parish nurses are creating health ministries in communities, estab-

lishing partnerships with the residents so that physical, mental, and spiritual health care needs can be considered as the nurse and client work together to address these individual needs. The role of the parish nurse can include that of health counselor, educator, referral source, and interpreter of the relationship between faith and health. Some examples of ac-

Table 40–2

COMMUNITY-BASED PRACTICE SETTING

SETTING	DESCRIPTION
Parish nursing	Health ministries that focus on both physical and spiritual needs of community
Nursing centers	Clinics operated by nurses, often for individuals in underserved communities
School-based clinics	School-based sites for primary care, where care is usually provided by an advanced practice nurse
Block nursing	Neighborhood-based support services, primarily for elders with limited family support
Home health nursing	Nursing care provided in home that includes direct care (i.e., wound care, tube feedings), nursing assessment, and education
Hospice	Care for a terminally ill client focused on comfort care for clients and families, usually delivered in the home

tivities that parish nurses may pursue are providing blood sugar and blood pressure screenings (possibly after a church service), organizing food pantries, and presenting health education programs for members of the congregation.

Nursing Centers

Community-based nursing centers have a potential for delivering cost-effective health care to high-risk populations (Scott & Moneyham 1995). These clinics are organized and usually administered by nurses for individuals living in an underserved community, with the purpose of improving access to health care services. The primary care providers are usually advanced nurse practitioners. However, a variety of nurses with different skills are also employed in these centers. Community-based nursing centers are usually located in areas that are visible, safe, and close to public transportation, so that they are easily accessible to the populations they are serving. Examples of individuals served by these centers might be pregnant women, the frail elderly, and children with asthma.

School-Based Clinics

School-based clinics are relatively new sites for primary care, where the advanced nurse practitioner usually provides the care. Primary care includes physical assessments, laboratory tests, the prescription of medications, and medical treatment for general medical problems. When client problems are complex, they are usually referred to a specialist.

School-based clinics should not be confused with school health clinics where school nurses provide health services for children with minor illnesses. School-based clinics are centers where primary care is delivered to a group of people (beyond students) living in a specific geographical area. The school is often a preferred site because of its central location. Addi-

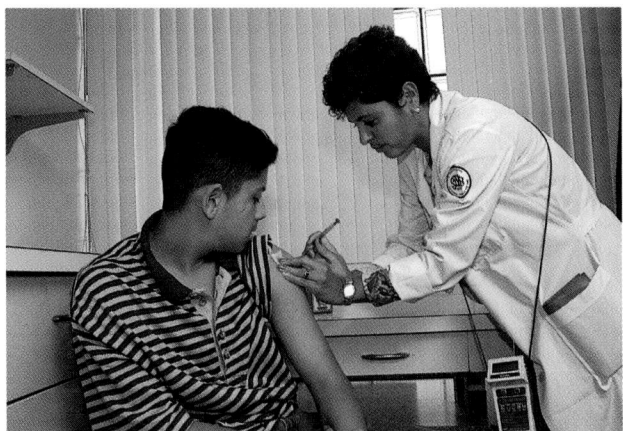

♣ Figure 40–5
A teenage boy receives a vaccination for hepatitis B in a school-based clinic.

tionally, a school is a structure that can be more efficiently used if many activities take place in it. School-based clinics may be organized by a health department, neighborhood center, or local community agency to provide needed services to a particular population.

Block Nursing

Twenty years ago in St. Paul, Minnesota, Marjorie Jamison created a program based on her belief that if a frail elder knew that a nurse lived close by, the frail elder would use him or her during a medical or family crisis (Knollmueller, 1994). Hence, nurses who are part of Jamison's useful program contact appropriate elders and become available to them until referral to formal agencies is appropriate. This program is particularly helpful to elders who are poor, ill, and alone, with little support. Block nursing began in St. Paul, Minnesota and has spread to other areas in the state.

Home Health Nursing

Home health nursing became a part of health care services in 1883 when Lillian Wald established the Henry Street Settlement in New York City (Rice, 1996). However, when Title XVIII and Title XIX of the Social Security Act were passed in 1965, home care services became a type of care that was offered through these legislative programs. Presently, Medicare beneficiaries represent the largest group of home health care services users.

Certain requirements need to be met by the Medicare recipient to become eligible for this particular community-based (home health care) service. Clients must be homebound and have an unstable condition or an acute episode that can be medically managed safely in the home intermittently. The nursing care that is provided in the home must include one of the following nursing activities: direct nursing care (e.g., wound care), nursing assessment to evaluate the client's unstable condition, and education as it relates to the client's diagnosis. If the client and nursing criteria are met, the physician can order home health care services to be provided for the client. Because of increasing technological advances, many treatments formally done in the hospital (e.g., intravenous antibiotic therapy, enteral feedings, administration of total parenteral nutrition, and wound care) are now done in the home. This movement toward family-focused care has allowed clients to remain in the familiar surroundings of their home while they complete their healing and rehabilitation.

Hospice

Since the founding of the St. Christopher's Hospice in southern London, modern day hospice has become a familiar philosophy that includes medical and emotional support to assist clients and families approach a loved one's death (Campbell, 1986). The community-based nurse is part of a multidisciplinary team whose purpose is to deal with the client's holistic needs in the final stages of his or her life. The nurse's role includes pain control, as well as assessing vital signs, skin, appetite, and elimination (Zerwekh, 1989).

A primary goal of hospice care for the nurse and the multidisciplinary team is to provide comfort care for the client and the family; that is, the focus of care is on pain control for a peaceful death and support for the caregiver during this very final and important process. Therefore, no heroic measures are appropriate for the hospice client. The community-based nurse supports the multidisciplinary team in providing the supportive care where a dignified and peaceful death can occur.

A variety of community-based settings exist in which nurses provide health care services to clients and their families. In a community-based setting the nurse usually administers to the client for a short time. Therefore, it is important that the nurse have some assurance through her assessment and provision of client education that the client or the family can provide the necessary care needed to maintain or maximize the client's highest level of rehabilitation. The community-based nurse considers the holistic needs of the client and may coordinate community resources to meet the client's many health care needs.

Community-Based Nursing Case Management

Nursing case management is becoming a popular framework within which to manage clients' needs in and out of the hospital. Community-based nursing management concerns nurses who are case managers for a group of clients outside the hospital setting (Rogers *et al.*, 1991). The community-based case manager can manage and coordinate a number of different client needs in a variety of settings. Institutions and insurance companies have created the nursing case management role to arrange, coordinate, and explicate how a variety of services are facilitating the rehabilitation and health of the client. This coordination prevents clients' care from becoming fragmented through services that might otherwise be duplicated or missed.

Case managers are often assigned to clients who need a variety of community services to be maintained safely at home. For example, a community-based case manager may coordinate services for a client diagnosed with chronic obstructive pulmonary disease (COPD). The case manager may want to suggest home health care for client education and medication administration. A special support group may be helpful for the client's spouse. The client may need community support in acquiring transportation to physician appointments. The community-based case man-

ager may arrange all of these services as well as be available to report to each service the needs of this client. Community-based case managers are receiving more responsibility for the community-based client, who is often living at home. These case managers are required to work autonomously, problem solving and deciding how to best meet the health care needs of clients residing alone or with families in the community.

Community-Based Care Team Members

Nurse

Nurses play a vital role in interdisciplinary community-based care. The focus of professional nursing is the "diagnosis and treatment of human responses to actual or potential health problems through such services as case finding, health teaching, health counseling, and provision of care supportive to or restorative of life and well-being" (ANA, 1995, p. 6). Nurses participate in community-based care in a number of ways. They function as home health nurses and work in public health departments, schools, and occupational health settings. In these settings, they perform services that assist clients and families to manage their own health needs. As clients are discharged earlier from hospitals, home health nurses provide interventions such as wound care and intravenous therapy in homes. They perform interventions, monitor client condition, educate family members as care providers, and coordinate resources. Nurses in public health departments perform a wide variety of services, including immunization programs, well-child care, and supervision of drug therapy for clients with tuberculosis. Nurses in school and occupational settings provide health screening and health promotion activities, as well as some primary care services. They often function as case managers in home health and public health arenas. Nurse practitioners play a vital role in delivery of primary care services in the community, working with client case loads that involve diagnosis and management of common acute conditions and chronic stable conditions that are managed in ambulatory care settings.

Dietitian

The registered dietitian supports the community-based care of clients by providing nutritional care, which includes evaluation of nutrition status, dietary patterns, and diet plans, as well as counseling on nutritional needs.

Occupational Therapist

The occupational therapist provides vital services for community-based care. The focus of occupational therapy practice is the education or reeducation of clients in everyday skills needed to function at home, school, work, and in the community. Occupational therapists assist clients to recover abilities impaired through illness or injury or to adapt to these limitations. They work with clients in hospital, clinic, and home settings. For example, the occupational therapist may assist a wheelchair-bound client to rearrange her kitchen and adapt cooking methods so that she can prepare meals.

Pharmacist

The pharmacist works with clients to meet their medication therapy needs in community-based care. In addition to supplying prescribed medications, pharmacists offer counseling on medication management (including over-the-counter preparations), monitor the client's drug therapies, and notify physicians of potential problems like drug interactions.

Physical Therapist

The physical therapist focuses on functional mobility, working with clients to restore mobility lost through disease or injury. Physical therapists, like occupational therapists, promote recovery of impaired abilities and help clients adapt to altered mobility. Working on prevention of further injury or loss of function and assisting clients to learn use of adaptive devices, physical therapists utilize their skills in institutional, clinic, and home settings. For example, the physical therapist may support a stroke victim with an exercise regimen at home or help a wheelchair-bound client learn to transfer from chair to bed.

Physician

The physician has highly developed skills in diagnosis and treatment of disease. Certain specialties within medicine are focused on community-based care, including occupational health and family medicine. Physicians establish treatment plans that clients and families implement at home. They also work collaboratively with nurses, providing care in a variety of community-based settings.

Social Worker

The social worker focuses on the important task of enabling individuals, families, and communities to obtain social services, such as access to programs like Medicaid, nursing home placement, and vocational rehabilitation, to name just a few. Social workers may serve as case managers, coordinating community resources for individuals and families. They are educated as counselors and client advocates.

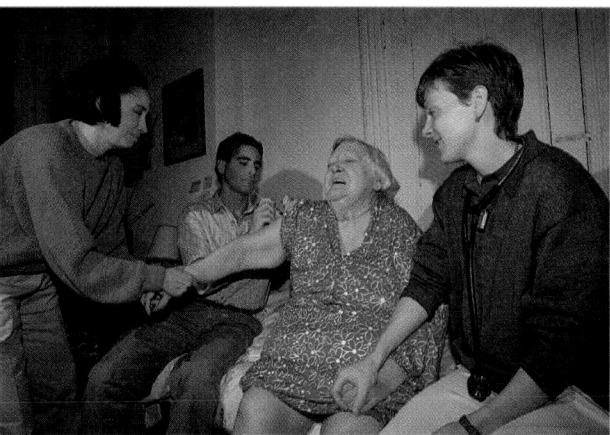

❥ **Figure 40-6**
A nurse gives an influenza shot during a team visit with an elderly client.

Speech Pathologist

The speech pathologist assists clients who have experienced impaired communication related to problems of dysphagia, phonation, and decreased ability to express and/or receive communication. Speech pathologists work with clients on restoring abilities lost through illness or injury, through rehabilitative efforts or use of assistive aids for communication.

Discharge Planning

One of the case manager's important roles is to facilitate client movement across levels of care; for example, from hospitalization to home to ambulatory care. Discharge planning is an integral part of this process. All community-based nurses must incorporate discharge planning skills into their practice. The purpose of discharge planning is to ensure that the treatment prescribed at a hospital or community-based clinic can safely and adequately be provided by either the client or the family in the home (Clark, 1992; Kelly & McClelland, 1989). Hospitalized clients are often discharged from the hospital to the community-based service of home health care. For clients being discharged from any hospital or community-based facility, discharge planning is appropriate. Although hospitals or community-based sites may have varying requirements about how to ensure safe continuity of care of community clients, discharge planning in varied settings still shares some common elements.

The primary goal of discharge planning is to support continuing, uninterrupted services until the client reaches full health and rehabilitation potential. The discharge planning process begins with the identification of health needs and coordination of related resources. An important health care goal is to ensure that when a client is discharged from an acute care center or a community-based site, any adaptations related to his or her health needs promote maximal health maintenance (Kersten & Hackenitz, 1991).

Initial planning involves assessing the client's and family's needs, determining the nursing care plan, and identifying community resources that promote the client's maximal functioning and independence. The community-based nurse needs to evaluate the family and client's understanding of the diagnosis, prognosis, and actual care required. With this initial information, community-based nurses can start to work with the client and family, training and evaluating their ability to continue the prescribed care at home. Because family members will eventually become the principal providers of care, it is important for them to be able to identify their own learning needs. Family members must also be aware of when it is appropriate to seek medical or health care resources in the community.

In the discharge planning process, planning and coordination of community-based services often become an interdisciplinary effort. Often, the primary physician, primary nurse, and social worker, as well as community resource providers, must work together to provide the necessary care in the community.

Assessment

For adequate discharge planning to be initiated, an accurate assessment of the client, family, and environment is imperative. The assessment should include a medical record review as well as a client interview. The medical record will apprise the nurse of the history and physical examination. Nurse and physician progress notes offer an overview of the client's progress and prognosis. The medical record will present the laboratory and radiology reports, physical therapy reports, and information from the dietitian and the pharmacist. All of these data become important to the nurse when planning how this client can receive the best care possible in the next care facility.

Client Interview

If the client is hospitalized, a client interview should be instituted early in his or her hospital stay. If the client is in a clinic or on home health care, the nurse should initiate an interview before the client's discharge to the next care facility or home. It is often helpful to ascertain how a client managed at home prior to being hospitalized or using the community-based clinic.

Evaluating the client's present functional abilities is also important for successful discharge. The nurse needs to establish how well the client can perform the necessary activities of daily living (ADL) (Table 40–3). Included in these basic and necessary functions are feeding, bathing, dressing, and toileting. During the discharge process, these, as well as the instrumental

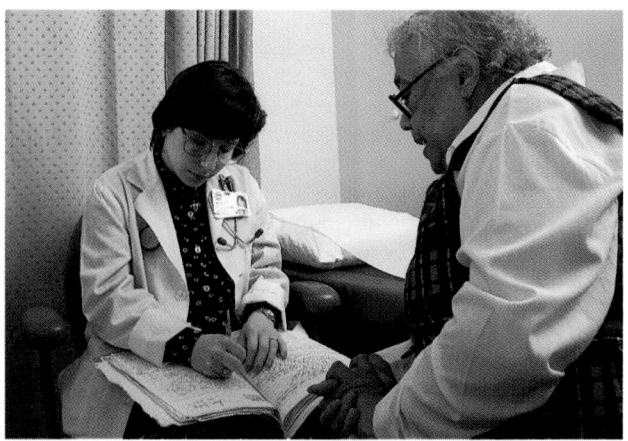

✦ **Figure 40–7**
A nurse interviews a client prior to discharge from the hospital.

activities of daily living (IADL) (Box 40–4), need to be considered when developing plans for the client to go home. When clients exhibit significant disabilities in ADL or IADL, the nurse can evaluate whether extra medical equipment or special arrangements need to be made to discharge the client home. During the initial discharge interview, the nurse should assess four areas to ensure the client's safety: the client's level of cognitive functioning, training needs, housing requirements, and equipment needs.

Mental Status

First, evaluate the *mental status* of this client. If the client is confused, assess his or her cognitive functioning. Use the short mini-mental examination. If the client is cognitively impaired, the family members will need to be included when instructing the client about his or her disease and treatment. Evaluating the client's mood, picking up on feelings such as anger or fear toward the medical staff or a family member, also helps in formulating educational approaches to prepare a client to continue treatment in his or her home.

Training

After the client's environmental needs have been established, client and/or caregiver *learning* must be considered. Will the client or caregiver need to learn about diet, transfer methods, medications, or treatments? What level of instruction would be most appropriate for this client? An important component to address with learning needs is the presence of feelings in the client that may adversely affect his or her readiness to learn. The client may be experiencing pain, anger, depression, or fear, all of which will affect his or her ability to learn. In a community-based clinic or doctor's office, clients may be experiencing pain as well as anger. However, unless the client or the primary caregiver can learn the necessary skills to maintain the client at home safely, the nurse may need to

Table 40—3

ACTIVITIES OF DAILY LIVING EVALUATION FORM

Name _____ Date of evaluation _____

For each area of functioning listed below, check description that applies. (The word *assistance* means supervision, direction, or personal assistance.)

1. Bathing—either sponge bath, tub bath, or shower

☐ Receives no assistance (gets in and out of tub by self if tub is usual means of bathing) · ☐ Receives assistance in bathing only one part of the body (such as back or leg) · ☐ Receives assistance in bathing more than one part of the body (or not bathed)

2. Dressing—getting clothes from closets and drawers, including underclothes and outer garments, and using fasteners (including braces if worn)

☐ Gets clothes and gets completely dressed without assistance · ☐ Gets clothes and gets dressed without assistance, except for assistance in tying shoes · ☐ Receives assistance in getting clothes or in getting dressed, or stays partly undressed

3. Toileting—going to the "toilet room" for bowel and urine elimination; cleaning self after elimination and arranging clothes

☐ Goes to "toilet room," cleans self, and arranges clothes without assistance (may use object for support, such as cane, walker, or wheelchair, and may manage night bedpan or commode, emptying same in morning) · ☐ Receives assistance in going to "toilet room" or in cleansing self or in arranging clothes after elimination or in use of night bedpan or commode · ☐ Does not go to room termed "toilet" for the elimination process

4. Transfer

☐ Moves in and out of bed, as well as in and out of chair without assistance (may be using object for support, such as cane or walker) · ☐ Moves in or out of bed or chair with assistance · ☐ Does not get out of bed

5. Continence

☐ Controls urination and bowel movement completely by self · ☐ Has occasional "accidents" · ☐ Supervision helps keep urine or bowel control, catheter is used, or is incontinent

6. Feeding

☐ Feeds self without assistance · ☐ Feeds self, except for getting assistance in cutting meat or buttering bread · ☐ Receives assistance in feeding or is fed partly or completely by using tubes or intravenous fluids

From Katz, S. *et al.* (1963). Studies of illness in the aged. *Journal of the American Medical Association, 185,* 914–919. Copyright 1963, American Medical Association.

work with the client and caregiver for a referral to another community-based or hospital facility to sustain the needed treatment.

Housing

Evaluate whether the client's *housing* and environment supports treatment and healing (Box 40–5). This assessment might include the furniture. Is it arranged to maximize safety? Is the home on the first floor or is it upstairs? Is a bathroom accessible? Who helps with meals and laundry? Is the client homeless? For a client who is being discharged with major disabilities, these important questions can dictate whether he or she can be discharged to the primary residence or if he or she needs other community support.

Equipment

Once a client's housing and educational needs have been established, it is important to identify if any *equipment* (*e.g.,* walker, wheelchair, bath bench) is necessary to help maximize independent functioning. Additionally, equipment (such as a glucometer) may be needed to help monitor the current physical problem. After identifying what equipment is needed, the nurse should determine if this equipment can be transferred safely to the client's home. If possible, ask the client how he or she might use the medical equipment. This would also be an opportune time to discuss with the client how he or she plans to incorporate the new plan of care and treatment into daily life.

It is important to verify, through the primary care-

Box 40–4

INSTRUMENTAL ACTIVITIES OF DAILY LIVING

Category

A. Ability to use telephone
  1. Operates telephone on own initiative—looks up and dials numbers, etc. _____
  2. Dials a few well-known numbers _____
  3. Answers telephone but does not call _____
  4. Does not use telephone at all _____

B. Shopping
  1. Takes care of all shopping needs independently _____
  2. Shops independently for small purchases _____
  3. Needs to be accompanied on any shopping trip _____
  4. Completely unable to shop _____

C. Food preparation
  1. Plans, prepares, and serves adequate meals independently _____
  2. Prepares adequate meals if supplied with ingredients _____
  3. Heats and serves prepared meals or prepares meals but does not maintain adequate diet _____
  4. Needs to have meals prepared and served _____

D. Housekeeping
  1. Maintains house along or with occasional assistance (*e.g.,* "heavy work—domestic help") _____
  2. Performs light daily tasks such as dishwashing, bedmaking _____
  3. Performs light daily tasks but cannot maintain acceptable level of cleanliness _____
  4. Needs help with all home maintenance tasks _____
  5. Does not participate in any housekeeping tasks _____

E. Laundry
  1. Does personal laundry completely _____
  2. Launders small items—rinses socks, stockings, etc. _____
  3. All laundry must be done by others _____

F. Mode of transportation
  1. Travels independently on public transportation or drives own car _____
  2. Arranges own travel via taxi, but does not otherwise use public transportation _____
  3. Travels on public transportation when assisted or accompanied by another _____
  4. Travel limited to taxi or automobile with assistance of another _____
  5. Does not travel at all _____

G. Responsibility for own medications
  1. Is responsible for taking medication in correct dosages at correct time _____
  2. Takes responsibility if medication is prepared in advance in separate dosages _____
  3. Is not capable of dispensing own medication _____

H. Ability to handle finances
  1. Manages financial matters, independently budgets, writes checks, pays rent and bills, goes to bank, collects and keeps track of income _____
  2. Manages day-to-day purchases, but needs help with banking, major purchases, etc. _____
  3. Incapable of handling money _____

Modified from Lawton, M., & Brody, E. (1969). Assessment of older people: Self-maintaining and instrumental activities of daily living. *The Gerontologist, 9,* 179–186.

---

giver or another family member, that the client understands how the equipment works. Sometimes clients exaggerate their understanding and abilities to use equipment because of their fear of not being allowed to return home.

Environmental Adaptations

For the discharging hospital or community-based nurse, the client's environment can present the most challenging problems. Within the client's immediate environment, it is essential to create a therapeutic space for the client to improve and strengthen his or her abilities to function safely and independently. In evaluating the environment, always ask about the client's immediate neighborhood. Is it safe? Is he or she close to needed services (*e.g.,* store, pharmacy, school)? Inquire about the immediate household. Is the lighting around the stairwells good? Are there handrails on both sides of the staircases? Is the front door accessible to this particular client? What modifications need to be put in place to make the home accessible to this particular client? Through the interviewing process, the discharge nurse evaluates the

Box 40–5

GUIDELINES FOR HOME ASSESSMENT CHECKLIST

General Household

1. Is good lighting available, especially around stairwells?

2. Are there handrails (which can be easily grasped) on both sides of the staircases, designed to indicate when top and bottom steps have been reached?

3. Are top and bottom steps painted in easily seen colors? Are nonskid treads used?

4. Are the edges of rugs tacked down?

5. Is a telephone present? Does the telephone have numbers that are easily readable? Are emergency numbers written in large print and kept near the telephone?

6. Are electrical cords, footstools, and other low-lying objects kept out of walkways?

7. Are electrical cords in good condition?

8. Is furniture arranged to allow for free movement in heavily traveled areas?

9. Is furniture sturdy enough to give support?

10. Is furniture designed to accommodate easy transfers on and off?

11. Is the temperature of the home within a comfortable range?

12. What are the heating and cooling devices in the home? Do they have protective screens?

13. Are smoke detectors present? Where? Do they have good batteries in them? When were the batteries changed? (especially in the kitchen and bedroom)

14. Are there rapidly closing doors?

15. Are there alternative exits from the house?

16. Are basements and attics easy to get to, well lighted, and well ventilated?

17. Are slippers and shoes in good repair? Do they fit properly and have nonskid soles?

Kitchen

18. Are loose extension cords, small sliding rugs, or slippery linoleum tiles present? (Suggest the use of rubber-backed, nonskid rugs and nonskid floor wax.)

19. Is the cooking stove gas or electric?

20. Are large, easily readable dials present on the stove or other appliances, with the "on" and "off" positions clearly marked?

21. Are refrigerators in good working order? Are refrigerators placed on 18-in platforms to avoid client having to bend over?

22. Are spaces for food storage adequate? Are shelves at eye level and easily reachable?

23. Is a sturdy stepladder present for reaching?

24. Are electrical circuits overloaded with too many appliances?

25. Are electrical appliances disconnected when not in use?

26. Are sharp objects (such as carving knives) kept in special holders?

27. Are kitchen chairs sturdy, with arm rests and high backs?

28. Is stove free from flammable objects?

29. Are pot holders available for removing pots and pans from the stove?

30. Is baking soda available in case of fire?

Bathroom

31. How wide is the bathroom door?

32. Are there grab bars in the bath, in the shower, and around the toilet?

33. Are toilet seats high enough to get on and off without difficulty?

34. Can the bathroom door be easily closed to ensure privacy? (Avoid locks.)

35. Are there nonskid rubber mats in the bath, in the shower, and on the floor?

36. Is there good lighting in the area of the medicine cabinet?

37. Are internal and external medications stored separately and safely? (especially important with young grandchildren present in the house)

38. Do medication containers have childproof tops? Are they labeled in large print? Is a magnifying glass present for reading medication instructions?

39. Have all outdated medications been discarded?

40. Do you notice any medications (both prescription and over the counter) that could cause adverse side effects or drug interactions that the client is unaware of?

41. Can the water temperature be easily regulated?

42. Are electrical cords, outlets, and appliances a safe distance from the tub?

43. Are razor blades kept in a safe place?

44. Is a first aid kit available?

Bedroom

45. Is there adequate lighting from the bedside to the bathroom?

46. Are lights easily accessible? (If not, suggest keeping a flashlight by the bedside or using a flashlight for entry into dark rooms if light switch is not within easy reach.)

47. Are beds in good repair?

48. Are beds at the proper height to allow for easy transfer on and off without difficulty?

49. Do bedroom rugs have nonskid rubber backings?

From Tideiksaar R. (1983). Ritter Department of Geriatrics and Adult Development, The Mount Sinai Medical Center.

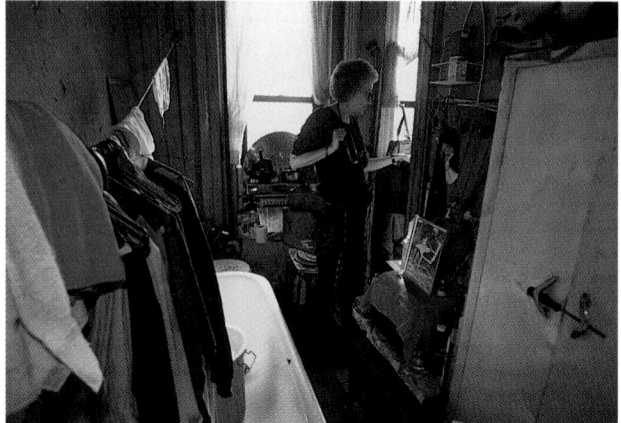

❯ **Figure 40–8**
A home care nurse evaluates the client's home environment for treatment support.

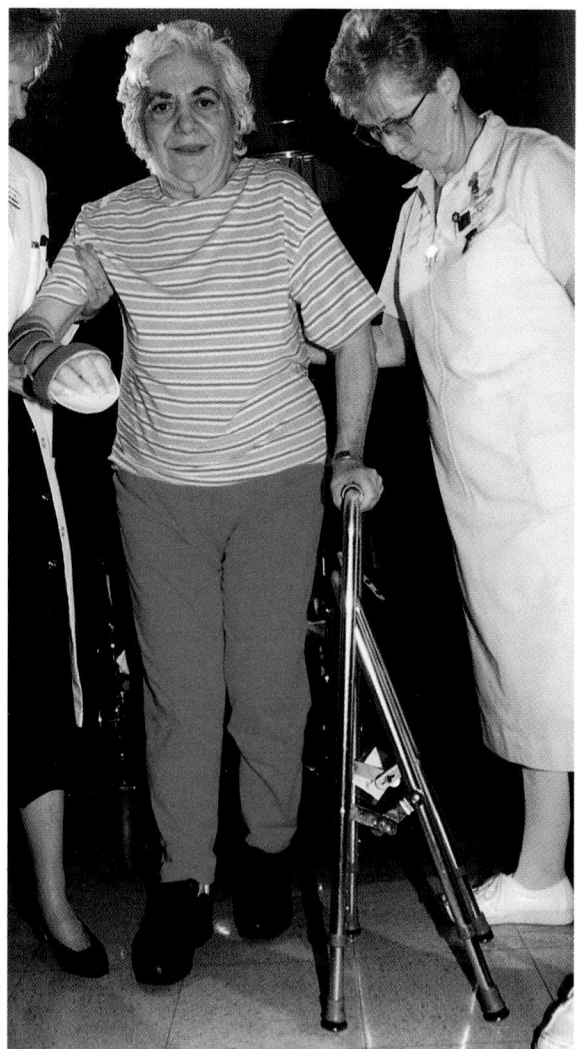

❯ **Figure 40–9**
A client practices using her new walker with the assistance of two nurses.

physical environment of the home to determine whether it accommodates the client's highest level of functioning.

In addition, it is the nurse's responsibility to evaluate whether the family *can* care adequately for the client returning home. The nurse needs to interview the client and family to establish how well the family and client can incorporate the plan of treatment in the home. Additionally, an assessment of the family's learning needs is necessary to ensure that the family has the necessary skills to support the needed therapy or treatment. Keep in mind the caregiver's abilities and limitations. How many people are living in this household, and what are their needs? What effect will the client's arrival home generate? The answers to these questions will give the nurse more information on how to plan for the client's discharge needs. With attention to a thorough discharge planning, the healing process can continue beyond the institutional or community-based setting, into the home environment.

Role In Community-Based Nursing

Community-based nurses include all levels of prevention in their practice as they work with individuals and families to maintain a client's maximum level of functioning in the home and community setting. For example, a community-based home health care nurse might be involved in administering direct care for a leg ulcer on an elderly client diagnosed with congestive heart failure, which would meet the requirements for tertiary care. The nurse might also be involved in screening for household hazards to prevent injury and falls (secondary prevention), as well as educating the client on the importance of hydration during the hot humid summer months (primary prevention) (Clark,

1991). The community-based nurse needs to plan his or her care to include all of the client's health needs.

Application of the Nursing Process

The nursing process provides a reasoning framework for nurses that guides practice in all settings with all populations. Nurses in institutional and community settings use the nursing process to guide the planning and delivery of care. The application of the nursing process to community-based care ensures that all nursing interventions are focused on the identified client goals. The nursing process may have variations in terminology related to the process but usually includes the following steps: assessment, nursing diagnosis, planning, interventions, and evaluation. In community-based nursing, information, plans, and nursing interventions are important because the environment where the care is being delivered and the family who will support the care are an integral part of the care plan.

Assessment

In assessing a client in a community-based area, the nurse needs information about the client's family, friends, and others who may be present in the environment where care will be provided once the client leaves the community-based clinic (Humphrey, 1994). Therefore, the client's support system always needs to be included. The nurse also needs information on the family's ability to support the prescribed treatment plan when the client is at home. For example, an elderly woman may not be able to assist her husband with necessary dressing changes on an arm because of her own disabling arthritis, and the wife of a client newly diagnosed with cardiac disease on a special diet may not want to create menus that consider her husband's dietary restrictions.

In addition to information on the present physical status of the client, the community-based nurse considers physical assessment data from the medical facility from which the client came. The nurse needs to be aware of all the medical information available to him or her as well as his or her own physical assessment findings before he or she is able to move to developing a nursing diagnosis that relates to the physical needs of the client.

The community-based nurse also needs to know if the home environment is adequately safe for the prescribed treatment given to the client in the community-based clinic. Generally, the home environment needs to provide shelter, water, and electricity. When doing an environmental assessment for safety and support of the prescribed treatment, the nurse should consider the age of the client and the presence of children or frail elderly spouses or parents—factors that dictate the areas of concern. For example, an elderly client with cardiac disease who needs a walker for support and has been sent home on a new diet and medications will have markedly different safety concerns than a new young mother being released to home and needing instruction on how to care for her cesarean abdominal scar. With the elderly client, the nurse might assess the home environment for adequate lighting so that the client can see his or her medications. She or he would also need to evaluate whether electrical cords, footstools, and other low-lying objects are kept out of walkways. Because the client has a walker, the nurse may be interested in whether the furniture is sturdy enough to accommodate the weight of the client when he or she is transferring on and off the walker. For the young mother with the abdominal scar, the nurse would assess whether the home provides safety and security for the baby, a place to store the dressing supplies for the mother's healing cesarean scar, and an arrangement

of furniture facilitating easier lifting and moving of the baby. Evaluation of homes demands a particular focus that depends on the client's disabilities and unique needs.

Nursing Diagnosis

From the assessment data, the nurse would then develop a nursing diagnosis. Nursing diagnoses evolve from client problems (Humphrey, 1994). Whereas an understanding of the client's identified problems is a standard and useful approach in developing care plans, the community-based nurse also needs to be aware of client strengths. It is often these strengths that guide the nursing interventions. For example, if a terminally ill client was being discharged home with a 70-year-old spouse, a nursing diagnosis might be "Caregiver Role Strain." Although the nurse would be aware of the signs and symptoms of caregiver strain, interventions, in trying to prevent caregiver role strain, would always consider this spouse's strengths. The 70-year-old spouse's strengths might include organizational skills, spirituality, and active work in a supportive church congregation. By considering these strengths, the nurse might be able to develop better ways in approaching the identified nursing diagnosis of caregiver strain. For example, helping this elderly caregiver use the church congregation so someone can sit with the client when the spouse is shopping may help alleviate some of the caregiver role strain. The nurse is also concerned with potential problems. This same man may have a nursing diagnosis of "Risk for Injury, due to balance and coordination problems." Being able to foresee potential problems is important for the professional nurse working in the home or any community-based setting.

Planning

Based on the nursing assessment and nursing diagnosis, the community-based nurse develops a plan of action specific to the needs of the client as well as to the abilities of the family or support system that will be assisting the client with the prescribed treatment and care (Jaffe & Skidmore-Roth, 1993). Because the client will need to continue his or her care in the home independent of health care presence, the nurse needs to involve the client and the family when developing nursing interventions specific to the client's needs. This allows both the nurse and client to collaboratively develop realistic goals based on the client's physiological status and support from his or her immediate family or community. For example, a nurse may want an elderly client with chronic obstructive pulmonary disease and who is often in bed to sit up in a chair three times a day. However, this may prove problematic because the client's spouse is elderly with arthritic pain in the shoulders. Working with the spouse, the nurse and spouse agree that the client can be put in a chair once a day when their son comes to check on them. The spouse will put the client back in bed 1 hour later because the spouse feels comfortable moving the client from the chair to the bed. The spouse also agrees to remind the client to turn every 3 hours while the client is awake.

Evaluation

Finally, the nurse must evaluate the plan for its effectiveness in reaching client goals. Because the family or support persons are often involved in the client's care, they need to be included in the evaluation. The nurse, family, and client need to decide if the objectives of the care were met and, if not, why not. With this information, the nurse and family can revise interventions and set up activities that will better meet the client and family needs (Jaffe & Skidmore-Roth, 1993).

As one example of how a care plan may change after evaluation, consider a young client requiring dressing changes twice a day owing to an industrial accident that injured the leg. The nurse discovers that healing has been delayed because the client's morning dressings are changed only intermittently. Further investigation reveals that the spouse is busy getting the children dressed and off to school and is unable to assist the client in placing the dressing on areas that the client cannot reach. When the nurse realizes the difficulties this couple is having, the plan is revised. The nurse, with permission from the client, decides to arrange for the occupational nurse at the client's employment site to do the morning dressing, allowing the spouse to be free to help the children get ready for school. The evaluation may be the most important step in ensuring the client has met with a workable plan, as it offers the nurse one more chance to revise his or her interventions to better meet the client's nursing goals.

◆ Community-Based Care Exemplar

To assist families and clients in safely continuing treatment in the home setting, community-based nurses apply critical thinking and problem-solving skills in addressing client and family needs. The nursing process provides nurses with a reasoning framework that guides practice in all settings with all populations. Nurses in institutional and community settings use the nursing process to guide the planning and delivery of care. The skills that are unique to nursing practice in community-based sites are discussed as they relate to the special health care needs of our case study, the Jones family. The nursing process is the structure used to organize the nursing care.

CASE STUDY

Mrs. Jones, a 36-year-old divorced working parent, lives with her 10-year-old son and widowed 72-year-old father (Mr. Evans) in a three-bedroom home in a small suburban community. Mr. Evans, who has had type II (non–insulin-dependent) diabetes for the past 10 years, has recently been admitted to the hospital because of difficulty controlling blood glucose levels. He now has a type I (insulin-dependent) diabetes and will be discharged in 2 days on Humulin 70/30 25 units subcutaneously each morning and 15 units each evening.

Mrs. Jones sees herself as basically healthy and the primary support for the family. Mrs. Jones' son Paul is a fifth grader who performs well in school and is active in sports. He was diagnosed with asthma in infancy and was hospitalized twice before age 3 for acute asthmatic episodes. He periodically experiences wheezing and shortness of breath, more frequently in spring.

Mr. Evans will be discharged from the hospital in 2 days. His primary nurse and the unit case manager share the discharge plan with the nurse from the home health agency who will provide care for Mr. Evans at home. They highlight the following assessment findings as significant in the formulation of nursing diagnoses.

Assessment

Box 40–6 summarizes Mr. Evans' physical findings. The primary hospital nurse shares with the community-based home health care nurse the interpretation of the physical assessment data, identifying a pattern of blood glucose levels ranging from normal to moderately increased and excessive weight for height and body size. He has been instructed on insulin self-administration and has correctly prepared and administered his required dosage for the past 3 days. He has also been educated on finger-stick blood glucose monitoring and has performed this procedure correctly without prompting from the nurse. He was able to describe the symptoms of hypoglycemia and the actions that he would take if he experienced them. Unfortunately, Mr. Evans' functional and lifestyle data reflect preferred eating patterns that conflict with prescribed diet. The hospital nurse informs the home health nurse that Mr. Evans often goes to the cafeteria for the food he enjoys, like hamburgers and onion rings. The nurse feels that his daily habits may require adjustments to his medication and meal schedule.

Functional and psychosocial data for Mr. Evans are as follows:

- Eating patterns
  Lots of fried foods
  Irregular meals
  Dislikes diet restrictions
- Leisure activities
  Concerned about medication schedule affecting his daily fishing outings
- Reaction to diagnosis
  Having difficulty verbalizing concerns

Box 40–6

PHYSICAL FINDINGS

Blood pressure: Stable at 150/85

Pulse: Regular 88

Temperature: 97.6

Open lesion on right heel: 2 cm, round, stage I

Heart: Regular rate, no murmurs

Lungs: Clear all areas

Abdomen: Soft bowel sounds in all four quadrants

Urine: Clear, normal

Lower extremities: Diminished sensation

Height: 5 ft, 8 in

Weight: 240 lb

Nursing Diagnoses

Based on this assessment data, the primary hospital nurse has identified as priority diagnoses for the discharge plan (1) Management of Therapeutic Regimen, Risk for Ineffective, and (2) Nutrition: More than Body Requirements, Altered. The home health nurse concurs. A principal reason that the nurse will be following up on Mr. Evans is to ensure that he is able to translate the sound instruction he received from the primary hospital nurse on diabetic self-management into action at home.

Planning

The primary nurse and case manager worked with Mr. Evans to identify outcomes of care for his hospital stay and longer-term outcomes to be achieved after his discharge. The in-hospital stage focused on stabilizing his condition and introducing him to diabetes self-management. The outcomes to be achieved after discharge include

- Complete healing of stage I ulcer
- Proper foot care
- Achievement of target weight—180–200 lb
- Correct self-administration of medications
- Appropriate monitoring, corrective action

The nursing staff feels confident that Mr. Evans has acquired the essential knowledge base for taking care of his foot lesion and managing insulin. They are somewhat concerned about how he will handle regulating his diet and medication schedule because he is accustomed to staying out fishing for hours, eating junk food, and drinking beer.

The nursing actions the home health nurse plans to perform to achieve desired outcomes include

- Assessment of foot ulcer
- Monitoring of blood sugar
- Completing a 24-hour diet history
- Assessing Mr. Evans' symptom management
- Observing insulin self-administration

Note that the nursing plan relates directly to Mr. Evans' presenting problems and medical diagnoses. The nurse has talked with both Mr. Evans and his daughter, Mrs. Jones, to arrange a visit for the morning after his return home.

Implementation

The home health nurse arrived at the Evans' home at 8:00 A.M. on the day after Mr. Evans was discharged. The nurse spoke with his daughter before she left for work. The house is neat, clean, and comfortable. Mrs. Jones shows the nurse the tackle box in which Mr. Evans' medications and syringes are kept. A medication schedule is taped into the lid, and there is a daily medication record that Mrs. Jones developed on her computer at work. Mrs. Jones looks very tired and is coughing a great deal during the conversation. In discussing how Mr. Evans is managing his diet, Mrs. Jones indicates that she prepares meals only at night and will rely on her father to prepare his own breakfast and lunch. She is preparing separate evening meals because she and her son don't like the food on Mr. Evans' diet. She was taught how to give him his injections but hasn't yet. "I'm really afraid of that needle."

Mr. Evans comes in from the garage to greet the nurse, who notes that he is in his stockinged feet. He performs his fingerstick blood glucose measurement without assistance, obtaining a reading of 172 mg/dl. While the home health nurse observes, he correctly draws up and administers his 25-unit daily dose of Humulin 70/30 by subcutaneous injection. He cannot find his glasses and had some difficulty seeing the syringe markings. The nurse's physical assessment focuses on skin integrity and circulation in Mr. Evans' lower extremities. The lesion on his foot is clean and dry but has not decreased in size. She also checks his blood pressure, which is 154/82, and weight, which is 240 lb. She spends some time talking with him about his knowledge of symptoms of hypoglycemia and hyperglycemia and symptom management. In reviewing his diet for the previous 24 hours, Mr. Evans indicates that he skipped dinner to get out to the fishing pier but brought some oranges, a bag of pretzels, and some beer.

Evaluation

Based on the data from this initial home visit, the home health nurse concludes that Mr. Evans is performing his glucose monitoring and insulin injections correctly and is able to describe symptoms and symptom management. The nurse is concerned that he does not wear his glasses while preparing his insulin. Two additional concerns are his inattention to proper foot care and his eating patterns.

Revisions

Based on the data collected during this visit, the home health nurse revises the problem list identified in the discharge plan, adding two new nursing diagnoses: Individual Coping, Ineffective, and Knowledge Deficit. The nurse spent time on this visit encouraging Mr. Evans to discuss his love of fishing and ways in which he can arrange his eating patterns to accommodate his activities. They made a list of nutritious items that are easily carried or packed in an ice chest. The nurse also reviewed principles of proper foot care and left teaching material for him to review.

The similarities between the hospital-based and community-based nursing concerns include the need for monitoring of Mr. Evans' condition and education for self-care. These differences are in emphasis rather than in area of concern. The nurse in the hospital setting makes continuous observations of client status. The setting provides the opportunity for more control over assessment data, monitoring procedures, and management of complications. This nurse initiates education and has some family contact but less opportunity for family intervention.

The community-based nurse places greater emphasis on client education, because the client and family have primary responsibility for monitoring and managing complications. The continuous monitoring available in the hospital setting is not an option in the home. Because the daughter is the secondary caregiver, the home health nurse will provide more counseling for her, particularly in the area of managing caregiver stress. Also emphasized is incorporation of client lifestyle into the treatment plan. The hospital-based nurse cannot observe the client's home environment and lifestyle. This dimension, which is essential to the client's ability to manage his disease, is best addressed by the community-based nurse.

✦ Summary

Health care reform trends have led to increased emphasis on delivery of community-based services. Nurses who practice in the growing field of community-based care will require highly developed skills in collaboration with clients, families, and multidisciplinary teams to support this practice. Nurses perform the roles of educator, counselor, direct care provider, and case manager in community settings. The nursing process provides the reasoning framework for practice, allowing the nurse to develop individualized plans of care appropriate to community-based settings. As health care delivery increasingly moves into the community, these skills will be essential for all nurses.

CHAPTER HIGHLIGHTS

✦

✦ Implications of health care reform for community-based nursing

✦ Differentiation of public health nursing and community-based nursing

✦ Practice roles in community-based settings

✦ Case management in community-based nursing

✦ Roles of the interdisciplinary team in community-based care

✦ Application of the nursing process in community settings

Study Questions

1. A home health care nurse has been asked by the physician to evaluate Mr. Black's home. Mr. Black suffered a stroke that left him paralyzed on the left side, and he is being discharged home from the hospital with a quadripod cane tomorrow. Which of the following would be appropriate for the nurse to consider FIRST?

   a. size of the bathroom
   b. availability of grocery stores in the neighborhood
   c. location of throw rugs and electrical cords
   d. availability of transportation to the physician's office

2. Mrs. B., an 80-year-old woman with a hip replacement, is being evaluated for discharge from the rehabilitation unit in 4 days. To assess Mrs. B.'s cognitive functioning, the nurse will administer a mini mental examination. The nurse explains to Mrs. B. that this will be a simple test. Mrs. B. starts to cry and says "I always do horrible on tests, please don't make me take this one." The MOST APPROPRIATE action for the nurse at this time would be to

   a. further discuss Mrs. B's fear of testing
   b. inform the client on the importance of the examination in preparing for discharge
   c. incorporate the questions of the mini mental examination in the general interview
   d. take three points off the final score of the mini mental examination because of the client's refusal to take it

3. A home health care nurse is scheduled for a first visit to a 68-year-old client who is a newly diagnosed with diabetes. Which of the following activities would need to be completed before the admission visit?

   a. introducing the nurse to the client
   b. planning the visit
   c. observing for nursing problems
   d. contracting with client on goals

4. Home health nurses consider key safety issues on their first visit to a client's home. Select the issue that applies to Mrs. Boyd, a woman with left-sided weakness because of a stroke and moderate obesity.

   a. infection control
   b. mobility and the home
   c. caregiver involvement
   d. condition of the neighborhood

5. Which of the following is an important consideration when the nurse IMPLEMENTS nursing interventions?

   a. establishing a plan of care that reflects the medical treatment plan
   b. identifying goals and outcomes that are measurable
   c. integrating the nursing care intervention into the client's lifestyle and culture
   d. documenting precisely the need for services rendered

Critical Thinking Exercises

1. Discuss how nursing education can better prepare students for the competencies that will be essential for nurses in the year 2005.

2. Ms. T. is an 82-year-old woman who had been living in the "old family farmhouse." She is recovering from a stroke with right hemiplegia. She is discharged with a quadripod cane for ambulation. Discuss the assessment the nurse must employ and possible referrals for Ms. T.

References

American Nurses Association. (1991). *Nursing's agenda for health care reform*. Washington, DC: American Nurses Association.

American Nurses Association. (1995). *Nursing's social policy statement*. Washington, DC: American Nurses Association.

Bechtel, G. A., Garrett, C., & Grover, S. (1995). Developing a collaborative community partnership program in medical asepsis with tattoo studios. *Public Health Nursing, 12,* 348–352.

Campbell, L. (1986). History of the hospice movement. *Cancer Nursing, 9* (6), 333–338.

Clark, M. J. (1992). *Nursing in the community*. Norwalk, CT: Appleton & Lange.

Humphrey, C. J. (1994). *Home care nursing handbook*. Gaithersburg, MD: Aspen Publishers.

Jackson, L. E. (1996). Understanding, eliciting and negotiating clients' multicultural health beliefs. In B. W. Spradley & J. A. Allender (Eds.), *Readings in community health nursing* (pp. 530–541) Philadelphia: Lippincott-Raven.

Jaffe, M. S., & Skidmore-Roth, L. (1993). *Home health nursing care plans*. St. Louis: Mosby-Year Book.

Jenkins, M. L., & Sullivan-Marx, E. M. (1994). Nurse practitioners and community health nurses: Clinical partnerships and future visions. *Nursing Clinics of North America, 29* (3) 459–470.

Kelly, K., & McClelland, E. (1989). Discharge planning: Home care considerations. In I. M. Martinson & A. Widmer (Eds.), *Home Health Care Nursing* (pp. 13–22) Philadelphia: W. B. Saunders.

Kersten, D., & Hackenitz, E. (1991). How to bridge the gap between hospital and home? *Journal of Advanced Nursing, 16* (1), 4–14.

Kiser, M., Boario, M., & Hilton, D. (1995). Transformation for health: A participatory empowerment education training model in the faith community. *Journal of Health Education, 26,* 361–365.

Knollmueller, R. N. (1994). Thinking about tomorrow for nursing: Changes and challenges. *The Journal of Continuing Education, 25,* 196–201.

Pew Health Professions Commission. (1993). *Health professions education for the future: Schools in service to the nation*. San Francisco: University of California, San Francisco Center for the Health Professions.

Pew Health Professions Commission. (1993). *Resource book for health professions education strategic planning and policy development*. San Francisco: University of California, San Francisco Center for the Health Professions.

Pew Health Professions Commission (1995). Critical challenges: *Revitalizing the health professions for the twenty-first century*. San Francisco: The Pew Health Professions Commission.

Primomo, J. (1995). Ensuring public health nursing in managed care: Partnerships for healthy communities. *Public Health Nursing, 12,* 69–71.

Rice, R. (1996). *Home health nursing practice: Concepts & application*. St. Louis: Mosby-Year Book.

Rice, R., & Rappl, L. (1996). The patient receiving rehabilitation services. In R. Rice (Ed.), *Home health nursing practice: Concepts & application* (pp. 271–281). St. Louis: Mosby-Year Book.

Rogers, M., Riordan, J., & Swindle, D. (1991). Community-based nursing case management pays off. *Nursing Management, 22* (3), 30–34.

Scott, C. B., & Moneyham, L. (1995). Perceptions of senior residents about a community-based nursing center. *Image: Journal of Nursing Scholarship, 27,* 181–186.

U. S. Department of Health and Human Services–Public Health Service. (1990). *Healthy people 2000: National health promotion and disease prevention objectives*. (DDHS Publication No. PHS 91-50212). Washington, DC: US Government Printing Office.

Williams, C. A. (1997). Community health nursing—What is it? In B. W. Spradley & J. A. Allender (Eds.), *Readings in community health nursing* (pp. 101–109). Philadelphia: Lippincott-Raven.

Zerwekh, J. V. (1989). Home care of the dying. In I. M. Martinson & A. Widmer (Eds.), *Home health care nursing* (pp. 217–230). Philadelphia: W. B. Saunders.

Zotti, M. E., Brown, P., & Stotts, R. C. (1996). Community-based versus community health nursing: What does it all mean? *Nursing Outlook, 44,* 211–217.

Appendix ✦ A

Guideline for Isolation Precautions in Hospitals

✦

Introduction

To assist hospitals in maintaining up-to-date isolation practices, the Centers for Disease Control and Prevention (CDC) and the Hospital Infection Control Practices Advisory Committee (HICPAC) have revised the "CDC Guideline for Isolation Precautions in Hospitals."

The revised guideline contains two parts. Part I, "Evolution of Isolation Practices," reviews the evolution of isolation practices in US hospitals, including their advantages, disadvantages, and controversial aspects, and provides the background for the HICPAC-consensus recommendations contained in Part II, "Recommendations for Isolation Precautions in Hospitals." The guideline supersedes previous CDC recommendations for isolation precautions in hospitals.

The guideline recommendations are based on the latest epidemiologic information on transmission of infection in hospitals. The recommendations are intended primarily for use in the care of clients in acute-care hospitals, although some of the recommendations may be applicable for some clients receiving care in subacute-care or extended-care facilities. The recommendations are not intended for use in daycare, well care, or domiciliary care programs. Because there have been few studies to test the efficacy of isolation precautions and gaps still exist in the knowledge of the epidemiology and modes of transmissions of some diseases, disagreement with some of the recommendations is expected. A working draft of the guideline was reviewed by experts in infection control and published in the *Federal Register* for public comment. However, all recommendations in the guideline may not reflect the opinions of all reviewers.

Types of Isolation Precautions

The "Guideline for Isolation Precautions in Hospitals" was revised to meet the following objectives: (1) to be epidemiologically sound; (2) to recognize the importance of all body fluids, secretions, and excretions in the transmission of nosocomial pathogens; (3) to contain adequate precautions for infections transmitted by the airborne, droplet, and contact routes of transmission; (4) to be as simple and user friendly as possible; and, (5) to use new terms to avoid confusion with existing infection control and isolation systems.

The revised guideline contains two tiers of precautions.

In the first, and most important, tier are those precautions designed for the care of all clients in hospitals regardless of their diagnosis or presumed infection status. Implementation of these "Standard Precautions" is the primary strategy for successful nosocomial infection control. In the second tier are precautions designed only for the care of specified clients. These additional "Transmission-Based Precautions" are used for clients known or suspected to be infected or colonized with epidemiologically important pathogens that can be transmitted by airborne or droplet transmission or by contact with dry skin or contaminated surfaces.

Standard Precautions synthesize the major features of Universal (Blood and Body Fluid) Precautions (designed to reduce the risk of transmission of bloodborne pathogens) and Body Substance Isolation (designed to reduce the risk of transmission of pathogens from moist body substances). Standard Precautions apply to (1) blood; (2) all body fluids, secretions, and excretions *except sweat*, regardless of whether or not they contain visible blood; (3) nonintact skin; and, (4) mucous membranes. Standard Precautions are designed to reduce the risk of transmission of microorganisms from both recognized and unrecognized sources of infection in hospitals.

Transmission-Based Precautions are designed for clients documented or suspected to be infected or colonized with highly transmissible or epidemiologically important pathogens for which additional precautions beyond Standard Precautions are needed to interrupt transmission in hospitals. There are three types of Transmission-Based Precautions: Airborne Precautions, Droplet Precautions, and Contact Precautions. They may be combined for diseases that have multiple routes of transmission. When used either singularly or in combination, they are to be used in addition to Standard Precautions.

The revised guideline also lists specific clinical syndromes or conditions in both adult and pediatric clients that are highly suspicious for infection and identifies appropriate Transmission-Based Precautions to use on an empiric, temporary basis until a diagnosis can be made; these empiric, temporary precautions are also to be used in addition to Standard Precautions.

Recommendations

The recommendations presented below are categorized as follows:

- *Category IA.* Strongly recommended for all hospitals and strongly supported by well-designed experimental or epidemiologic studies.

- *Category IB.* Strongly recommended for all hospitals and reviewed as effective by experts in the field and a consensus of HICPAC based on strong rationale and suggestive evidence, even though definitive scientific studies have not been done.

● *Category II.* Suggested for implementation in many hospitals. Recommendations may be supported by suggestive clinical or epidemiologic studies, a strong theoretical rationale, or definitive studies applicable to some, but not all, hospitals.

● *No recommendation; unresolved issue.* Practices for which insufficient evidence or consensus regarding efficacy exists.

The recommendations are limited to the topic of isolation precautions. Therefore, they must be supplemented by hospital policies and procedures for other aspects of infection and environmental control, occupational health, administrative and legal issues, and other issues beyond the scope of this guideline.

Administrative Controls

A. Education
   Develop a system to ensure that hospital patients, personnel, and visitors are educated about use of precautions and their responsibility for adherence to them. *Category IB*
B. Adherence to Precautions
   Periodically evaluate adherence to precautions, and use findings to direct improvements. *Category IB*

Standard Precautions

Use Standard Precautions, or the equivalent, for the care of all patients. *Category IB*

A. Hand washing
   (1) Wash hands after touching blood, body fluids, secretions, excretions, and contaminated items, whether or not gloves are worn. Wash hands immediately after gloves are removed, between patient contacts, and when otherwise indicated to avoid transfer of microorganisms to other patients or environments. It may be necessary to wash hands between tasks and procedures on the same patient to prevent cross-contamination of different body sites. *Category IB*
   (2) Use a plain (nonantimicrobial) soap for routine handwashing. *Category IB*
   (3) Use an antimicrobial agent or a waterless antiseptic agent for specific circumstances (*e.g.,* control of outbreaks or hyperendemic infections), as defined by the infection control program. *Category IB* (See Contact Precautions for additional recommendations on using antimicrobial and antiseptic agents.)
B. Gloves
   Wear gloves (clean, nonsterile gloves are adequate) when touching blood, body fluids, secretions, excretions, and contaminated items. Put on clean gloves just before touching mucous membranes and nonintact skin. Change gloves between tasks and procedures on the same patient after contact with material that may contain a high concentration of microorganisms. Remove gloves promptly after use, before touching noncontaminated items and environmental surfaces, and before going to another patient, and wash hands immediately to avoid transfer of microorganisms to other patients or environments. *Category IB*
C. Mask, eye protection, face shield
   Wear a mask and eye protection or a face shield to protect mucous membranes of the eyes, nose, and mouth during procedures and patient-care activities that are likely to generate splashes or sprays of blood, body fluids, secretions, and excretions. *Category IB*
D. Gown
   Wear a gown (a clean, nonsterile gown is adequate) to protect skin and to prevent soiling of clothing during procedures and patient-care activities that are likely to generate splashes or sprays of blood, body fluids, secretions, or excretions. Select a gown that is appropriate for the activity and amount of fluid likely to be encountered. Remove a soiled gown as promptly as possible, and wash hands to avoid transfer of microorganisms to other patients or environments. *Category IB*
E. Patient-care equipment
   Handle used patient-care equipment soiled with blood, body fluids, secretions, and excretions in a manner that prevents skin and mucous membrane exposures, contamination of clothing, and transfer of microorganisms to other patients and environments. Ensure that reusable equipment is not used for the care of another patient until it has been cleaned and reprocessed appropriately. Ensure that single-use items are discarded properly. *Category IB*
F. Environmental control
   Ensure that the hospital has adequate procedures for the routine care, cleaning, and disinfection of environmental surfaces, beds, bedrails, bedside equipment, and other frequently touched surfaces, and ensure that these procedures are being followed. *Category IB*
G. Linen
   Handle, transport, and process used linen soiled with blood, body fluids, secretions, and excretions in a manner that prevents skin and mucous membrane exposures and contamination of clothing, and that avoids transfer of microorganisms to other patients and environments. *Category IB*
H. Occupational health and bloodborne pathogens
   (1) Take care to prevent injuries when using needles, scalpels, and other sharp instruments or devices; when handling sharp instruments after procedures; when cleaning used instruments; and when disposing of used needles. Never recap used needles or otherwise manipulate them using both hands or use any other technqiue that involves directing the point of a needle toward any part of the body; rather, use either a one-handed "scoop" technique or a mechanical device designed for holding the needle sheath. Do not remove used needles from disposable syringes by hand, and do not bend, break, or otherwise manipulate used needles by hand. Place used disposable syringes and needles, scalpel blades, and other sharp items in appropriate puncture-resistant containers, which are located as close as practical to the area in which the items were used, and place reusable syringes and needles in a puncture-resistant container for transport to the reprocessing area. *Category IB*
   (2) Use mouthpieces, resuscitation bags, or other ventilation devices as an alternative to mouth-to-mouth resuscitation methods in areas where the need for resuscitation is predictable. *Category IB*
I. Patient placement
   Place a patient who contaminates the environment or who does not (or cannot be expected to) assist in maintaining appropriate hygiene or environmental control in a private room. If a private room is not available, consult with infection control professionals regarding patient placement or other alternatives. *Category IB*

Airborne Precautions

In addition to Standard Precautions, use Airborne Precautions, or the equivalent, for patients known or suspected to be infected with microorganisms transmitted by airborne droplet nuclei (small-particle residue [5 μm or smaller in size] of evaporated droplets containing microorganisms that remain suspected in air and that can be dispersed widely by air currents within a room or over a long distance). *Category IB*

A. Patient placement

Place the patient in a private room that has (1) monitored negative air pressure in relation to the surrounding areas, (2) 6 to 12 air changes per hour, and (3) appropriate discharge of air outdoors or monitored high-efficiency filtration of room air before the air is circulated to other areas in the hospital. Keep the room door closed and the patient in the room. When a private room is not available, place the patient in a room with a patient who has active infection with the same microorganism (cohorting), unless otherwise recommended, but with no other infection. When a private room is not available and cohorting is not desirable, consultation with infection control professionals is advised before patient placement. *Category IB*

B. Respiratory protection

Wear respiratory protection when entering the room of a patient with known or suspected infectious pulmonary tuberculosis. Susceptible persons should not enter the room of patients known or suspected to have measles (rubeola) or varicella (chickenpox) if other immune caregivers are available. If susceptible persons must enter the room of a patient known or suspected to have measles (rubeola) or varicella, they should wear respiratory protection. Persons immune to measles (rubeola) or varicella need not wear respiratory protection. *Category IB*

C. Patient-transport

Limit the movement and transport of the patient from the room to essential purposes only. If transport or movement is necessary, minimize patient dispersal of droplet nuclei by placing a surgical mask on the patient, if possible. *Category IB*

D. Additional precautions for preventing transmission of tuberculosis

Consult CDC "Guidelines for Preventing the Transmission of Tuberculosis in Health-Care Facilities" for additional prevention strategies.

Droplet Precautions

In addition to Standard Precautions, use Droplet Precautions, or the equivalent, for a patient known or suspected to be infected with microorganisms transmitted by droplets (large-particle droplets [larger than 5 μm in size] that can be generated by the patient during coughing, sneezing, talking, or the performance of procedures). *Category IB*

A. Patient placement

Place the patient in a private room. When a private room is not available, place the patient in a room with a patient(s) who has active infection with the same microorganisms but with no other infection (cohorting). When a private room is not available and cohorting is not achievable, maintain spatial separation of a least 3 ft between the infected patient and other patients and visitors. Special air handling and ventilation are not necessary, and the door may remain open. *Category IB*

B. Mask

In addition to standard precautions, wear a mask when working within 3 ft of the patient. (Logistically, some hospitals may want to implement the wearing of a mask to enter the room.) *Category IB*

C. Patient transport

Limit the movement and transport of the patient from the room to essential purposes only. If transport or movement is necessary, minimize patient dispersal of droplets by masking the patient, if possible. *Category IB*

Contact Precautions

In addition to Standard Precautions, use Contact Precautions, or the equivalent, for specified patients known or suspected to be infected or colonized with epidemiologically important microorganisms that can be transmitted by direct contact with the patient (hand or skin-to-skin contact that occurs when performing patient-care activities that require touching the patient's dry skin) or indirect contact (touching) with environmental surfaces or patient-care items in the patient's environment. *Category IB*

A. Patient placement

Place the patient in a private room. When a private room is not available, place the patient in a room with a patient(s) who has active infection with the same microorganism but with no other infection (cohorting). When a private room is not available and cohorting is not achievable, consider the epidemiology of the microorganism and the patient population when determining patient placement. Consultation with infection control professionals is advised before patient placement. *Category IB*

B. Gloves and handwashing

In addition to wearing gloves as outlined under Standard Precautions, wear gloves (clean, nonsterile gloves are adequate) when entering the room. During the course of providing care for a patient, change gloves after having contact with infective material that may contain high concentrations of microorganisms (fecal material and wound drainage). Remove gloves before leaving the patient's environment and wash hands immediately with an antimicrobial agent or a waterless antiseptic agent. After glove removal and handwashing, ensure that hands do not touch potentially contaminated environmental surfaces or items in the patient's room to avoid transfer of microorganisms to other patients or environments. *Category IB*

C. Gown

In addition to wearing a gown as outlined under Standard Precautions, wear a gown (a clean, nonsterile gown is adequate) when entering the room if you anticipate that your clothing will have substantial contact with the patient, environmental surfaces, or items in the patient's room, or if the patient is incontinent or has diarrhea, an ileostomy, a colostomy, or wound drainage not contained by a dressing. Remove the gown before leaving the patient's environment. After gown removal, ensure that clothing does not contact potentially contaminated environmental surfaces to avoid transfer of microorganisms to other patients or environments. *Category IB*

D. Patient transport

Limit the movement and transport of the patient from the room to essential purposes only. If the patient is transported out of the room, ensure that precautions are maintained to minimize the risk of transmission of microorganisms to other patients and contamination of environmental surfaces of equipment. *Category IB*

E. Patient-care equipment

   When possible, dedicate the use of noncritical patient-care equipment to a single patient (or cohort of patients infected or colonized with the pathogen requiring precautions) to avoid sharing between patients. If use of common equipment or items is unavoidable, then adequately clean and disinfect them before use for another patient. *Category IB*

F. Additional precautions for preventing the spread of vancomycin resistance

Consult the HICPAC report on preventing the spread of vancomycin resistance for additional prevention strategies.

Adapted from Garner, J.S., Hospital Infection Control Practices Advisory Committee. (1996). *Guideline for isolation precautions in hospitals*. Public Health Service, US Department of Health and Human Services, Centers for Disease Control and Prevention, Atlanta, GA.

Appendix ◆ B

Clinical Laboratory Values

SYMBOLS AND UNITS OF MEASUREMENT

α	alpha
AU	arbitrary units
cc	cubic centimeter
cm	centimeter
dl	deciliter
fl	femtoliter
γ	gamma
g	gram
gm	gram
IU	international unit
kg	kilogram
L	liter
μg	microgram
mEq	milliequivalent
mg	milligram
mIU	milliinternational unit
ml	milliliter
mm	millimeter
mmHg	millimeters of mercury
mmol	millimole
mOsm	milliosmole
mu	micro (μ)
ng	nanogram
%	percentage
pg	picogram
SI	Système International (international system)
U	unit
μ	micro

NORMAL VALUES: WHOLE BLOOD, SERUM, AND PLASMA TESTS

Name of Test	Conventional Values	SI Units
Activated partial thromboplastin time		
Average value	25–35 s	Same
Newborn	<90 s	Same
Adrenocorticotropic hormone		
In A.M.	25–100 pg/ml	25–100 ng/L
In P.M.	0–50 pg/ml	0–50 ng/L
Adrenocorticotropic hormone stimulation test: A rise of plasma cortisol level within 30–60 min	≥18 μg/dl	≥497 nmol/L
Alanine aminotransferase		
Average adult range	10–35 IU/L at 37°C	Same
Newborn–1 y	13–45 IU/L at 37°C	Same
Albumin		
Adult >60 y	3.4–4.8 g/dl	34–48 g/L
Adult <60 y	3.5–5.0 g/dl	35–50 g/L
Child	3.2–5.4 g/dl	32–54 g/L
Newborn	2.8–4.4 g/dl	28–44 g/L

Table continued on following page

NORMAL VALUES: WHOLE BLOOD, SERUM, AND PLASMA TESTS *(Continued)*

Name of Test	Conventional Values	SI Units
Albumin:globulin ratio	>1.0	Same
Aldosterone		
Adult—Average sodium diet		
Supine	3–10 ng/dl	0.08–0.27 nmol/L
Upright	5–30 ng/dl	0.14–0.83 nmol/L
After fluorocortisone suppression or intravenous infusion	<4 ng/dl	<0.11 nmol/L
Adrenal vein	200–800 ng/dl	5.54–22.16 nmol/L
Child		
11–15 y	<5–50 ng/dl	<0.14–1.39 nmol/L
3–5 y	<5–80 ng/dl	<0.14–2.22 nmol/L
1 w–1 y	1–160 ng/dl	0.03–4.43 nmol/L
Alkaline phosphatase		
Adult	4.5–13.0 King-Armstrong units/dl 1.4–4.4 Bodansky units	32–92 U/L
Infant	10–30 King-Armstrong units/dl	71–213 U/L
Alkaline phosphatase isoenzymes	**Percent inactivation 16 min at 55°C**	**Fractional inactivation 16 min at 55°C**
Liver	50–70	0.5–0.7
Bone	90–100	0.9–1.0
Intestine	50–60	0.5–0.6
Placenta	0	0
Regan	0	0
Alpha$_1$-fetoprotein		
Adult	2–16 ng/ml	2–16 µg/L
Normal pregnancy	550 ng/ml	550 µg/L
Ammonia		
Adult	15–45 µg/dl	11–22 µmol/L
Neonate	90–150 µg/dl	64–107 µmol/L
Amylase		
Adult	60–180 Somogyi units	25–125 U/L
Neonate	5–65 U/L	Same
Androstenedione		
Adult male	75–205 ng/dl	2.6–7.2 nmol/L
Adult female	85–275 ng/dl	3.0–9.6 nmol/L
Child 10–17 y	8–240 ng/dl	0.3–8.4 nmol/L
Newborn	20–290 ng/dl	0.7–10.1 nmol/L
Angiotensin-converting enzyme		
Male	12–36 IU/L	Same
Female	10–30 IU/L	Same
Anion gap	10–15 mEq/L	10–15 mmol/L
Anti-DNA antibody	Negative	Same
Radioimmunoassay method	<10% binding	<0.1 binding fraction
Enzyme immunoassay method	<250 U/L	Same
Indirect immunofluorescent method	<1:10	Same
Antiglobulin test, direct	Negative	Same
Antiglobulin test, indirect	Negative	Same
Antinuclear antibody	Negative at a 1:20 dilution	Same
Antithrombin III	21–30 mg/dl 86–113%	210–300 mg/L 86–113 AU
Aspartate aminotransferase		
Adult	8–20 U/L	Same
Newborn	16–72 U/L	Same
Bilirubin, direct		
Adult	0.0–0.4 mg/dl	<5 µmol/L
Bilirubin, indirect		
Adult	0.2–0.8 mg/dl	3.4–13.6 µmol/L
Bilirubin, total		
Adult	0.3–1.0 mg/dl	5–17 µmol/L
Child	0.2–0.8 mg/dl	3.4–13.6 µmol/L
Full-term neonate	6–10 mg/dl	103–171 µmol/L
Premature neonate*	<12 mg/dl	<205 µmol/L

NORMAL VALUES: WHOLE BLOOD, SERUM, AND PLASMA TESTS *(Continued)*

Name of Test	Conventional Values	SI Units
Blood gases, arterial		
pH	7.35–7.45	7.35–7.45
Pco$_2$	35–40 mmHg	4.7–5.3 kPa
HCO$_3$$^-$	21–28 mEq/L	21–28 mmol/L
Po$_2$		
Adult	80–100 mmHg	10.6–13.3 kPa
Newborn	60–70 mmHg	0.8–10.33 kPa
Oxygen saturation		
Adult	>95%	Fraction saturated: >0.95
Newborn	40–90%	Fraction saturated: 0.4–0.9
Base excess	±2 mEq/L	±2 mmol/L
Blood gases, mixed venous		
pH	7.33–7.43	7.35 ± 0.05
Pco$_2$	40–45 mmHg	5.3–6.0 kPa
HCO$_3$$^-$	24–28 mmHg	24–28 mmol/L
Blood volume, total	60–80 ml/kg	Same
Calcitonin, serum		
Adult	150 pg/ml	150 ng/L
Infant (cord blood)	25–150 pg/ml	25–150 ng/L
Infant (7 d old)	70–350 pg/ml	70–350 ng/ml
Calcitonin, plasma		
Male	≤19 pg/ml	≤19 ng/L
Female	≤14 pg/ml	≤14 pg/L
Calcium, total		
Adult	8.2–10.2 mg/dl	2.05–2.54 mmol/L
Child, 1 mo–1 y	8.6–11.2 mg/dl	2.15–2.79 mmol/L
Newborn–1 mo	7.0–11.5 mg/dl	1.75–2.87 mmol/L
Calcium, ionized	44–55% of total serum calcium	0.45–0.55 fraction of serum calcium
Adult, serum	4.65–5.28 mg/dl	1.16–1.32 mmol/L
Child, serum	4.8–5.52 mg/dl	1.2–1.38 mmol/L
Cancer antigen 125	<35 U/ml	<35 kU/L
Carbohydrate antigen 19-9		
Adult	<37 U/ml	<37 kU/L
Carbon dioxide, total		
Adult, venous	22–26 mEq/L	22–26 mmol/L
Adult, arterial	19–24 mEq/L	19–24 mmol/L
Infant, capillary	20–28 mEq/L	20–28 mmol/L
Carcinoembryonic antigen		
Adult, nonsmoker	<2.5 ng/ml	2.5 μg/L
Adult, smoker	Up to 5 ng/ml	Up to 5 μg/L
Carotene		
Adult	40–200 μg/dl	0.7–3.7 μmol/L
Infants	<60 μg/dl	<1.52 μmol/L
Catecholamines (standing)†		
Epinephrine	<900 pg/ml	<4914 pmol/L
Norepinephrine	125–700 pg/ml	739–4137 nmol/L
Dopamine	<87 pg/ml	<475 pmol/L
Ceruloplasmin		
Adult	20–40 mg/dl	200–350 mg/L
Neonate–3 mo	5–18 mg/dl	50–180 mg/L
Choride		
Adult	98–107 mEq/L	98–107 mmol/L
Newborn	98–113 mEq/L	98–113 mmol/L
Premature infant	95–110 mEq/L	95–110 mmol/L
Cholesterol, total	120–200 mg/dl	3.11–5.18 mmol/L
Clot retraction time	1–24 h	Same
Average time	4 h	Same
Clotting time	8–15 min	Same
Coagulation factor assay (general values)	50–150%	50–150 AU
Complement, total	75–160 U/ml	75–160 kU/L

Table continued on following page

NORMAL VALUES: WHOLE BLOOD, SERUM, AND PLASMA TESTS (Continued)

Name of Test	Conventional Values	SI Units
Complete blood count		
Hematocrit		
Male	40–54%	0.4–0.59 (volume fraction)
Female	38–47%	0.38–0.47 (volume fraction)
Hemoglobin		
Male	13.5–18.0 g/dl	135–180 g/L
Female	12–16 g/dl	120–160 g/L
Red cell count		
Male	$4.6–6.2 \times 10^6/\mu l$	$4.6–6.2 \times 10^{12}/L$
Female	$4.2–5.4 \times 10^6/\mu l$	$4.2–5.4 \times 10^{12}/L$
Red cell indices		
Mean corpuscular volume	$80–96 \ \mu m^3$	80–96 fl
Mean corpuscular hemoglobin	27–31 pg	27–31 pg
Mean corpuscular hemoglobin concentration	32–36%	0.32–0.36 (mean concentration fraction)
Red cell distribution width	13.1%	—
White cell count	$4.5–11 \times 10^3/\mu l$	$4.5–11.0 \times 10^9/L$
Platelets		
Adult	150,000–450,000 cells/L	$150–450 \times 10^9/L$
Newborn	84,000–478,000 cells/L	$84–478 \times 10^9/L$
Cortisol		
8 A.M.–10 A.M.	5–23 μg/dl	138–635 nmol/L
4 P.M.–6 P.M.	3–13 μg/dl	83–359 nmol/L
C-reactive protein	<1 mg/dl	<10 mg/L
Creatinine		
Adult male	0.7–1.3 mg/dl	62–115 μmol/L
Adult female	0.6–1.1 mg/dl	53–97 μmol/L
Newborn	0.3–1.0 mg/dl	27–88 μmol/L
Creatine phosphokinase (CPK)		
Adult male	38–175 U/L	Same
Adult female	25–135 U/L	Same
Child, male	35–185 U/L	Same
Child, female	50–100 U/L	Same
Newborn	10–200 U/L	Same
Isoenzymes		
Creatine phosphokinase–MM	5–70 U/L	Same
	90–97% (of total CPK)	0.9–0.97 (fraction of total CPK)
Creatine phosphokinase MB	0.7 U/L	Same
	0–6% of total creatine phosphokinase	0.0–0.06 (fraction of total CPK)
Creatine phosphokinase–BB	0.3 U/L	Same
	0–3%	0.0–0.03 (fraction of total CPK)
D-Dimer	<250 ng/ml	<250 μg/L
	No D-dimer fragments are present	Same
Dexamethasone overnight, single dose suppression test		
Plasma cortisol	Suppression to <5 μg/dl	Suppression to <138 nmol/L
D-Xylose absorption test		
Child–1 h	>30 mg/dl	>2 mmol/L
Adult (2 h, 5-g dose)	>20 mg/dl	>1.33 mmol/L
Adult (2 h, 25-g dose)	>25 mg/dl	>1.67 mmol/L
Epstein-Barr titer		
Viral capsid antigen—IgM	<1:10	Same
Viral capsid antigen—IgG	<1:10	Same
Epstein-Barr antinuclear antibody	<1:5	Same
Early antigen	<1:10	Same
Erythrocyte sedimentation rate		
Adult		
<50-y-old male	0–15 mm/h	Same
<50-y-old female	0–20 mm/h	Same
Adult		
>50-y-old male	0–20 mm/h	Same
>50-y-old female	0–30 mm/h	Same
Child	0–10 mm/h	Same

NORMAL VALUES: WHOLE BLOOD, SERUM, AND PLASMA TESTS *(Continued)*

Name of Test	Conventional Values	SI Units
Erythropoietin	5–36 µU/ml	5–35 IU/L
Estradiol		
Premenopausal female	30–400 pg/ml	110–1468 pmol/L
Postmenopausal female	0–30 pg/ml	0–110 pmol/L
Male	10–50 pg/ml	37–184 pmol/L
Estriol, pregnancy		
28–30 wk	38–140 ng/ml	132–486 nmol/L
32–34 wk	35–260 ng/ml	121–902 nmol/L
36–38 wk	48–570 ng/ml	167–1978 nmol/L
40 wk	95–460 ng/ml	330–1596 nmol/L
Euglobin clot lysis	1.5–4.0 h	Same
Factor II	0.5–1.5 U/ml	0.5–1.5 kU/L
	60–150%	60–150 AU
Factor V	0.5–2.0 U/ml	0.5–2.0 kU/L
	60–150%	60–150 AU
Factor VII	65–135%	65–135 AU
Factor VIII	60–145%	60–145 AU
Factor IX	60–140%	60–140 AU
Factor X	60–130%	60–130 AU
Factor XI	60–135%	60–135 AU
Factor XII	60–150%	60–150 AU
Factor XIII	Clot is stable in 5 mol of urea for 24 h	Same
Ferritin		
Adult male	20–250 ng/ml	20–250 µg/L
Adult female	10–120 ng/ml	10–120 µg/L
Newborn	25–200 ng/ml	25–200 µg/L
Fibrinogen		
Adult	200–400 mg/dl	2–4 g/L
Newborn	125–300 mg/dl	1.25–3.0 g/L
Fibrin split products	<10 µg/ml	<10 mg/L
F-Nucleotidase (adult)	2–17 IU/L	Same
Follicle-stimulating hormone		
Adult male	1–7 mU/ml	1–7 U/L
Adult female		
Follicular phase	1–9 mU/ml	1–9 U/L
Midcycle peak	6–26 mU/ml	6–26 U/L
Luteal phase	1–9 mU/ml	1–9 U/L
Gamma-glutamyl transferase		
Average adult range	5–40 IU/L	Same
Adult male	22.1 ± 11.7 IU/L	Same
Adult female	15.4 ± 6.58 IU/L	Same
Gastrin		
Adult male	<100 pg/ml	<100 ng/L
Adult female	<75 pg/ml	<75 ng/L
Newborn	120–183 pg/ml	120–183 ng/L
Globulin	2.8–4.4 g/dl	28–44 g/L
Glucagon, fasting	50–100 pg/ml	25 ng/L
Glucose, fasting		
Adult		
Whole blood	60–110 mg/dl	3.3–6.1 mmol/L
Serum, plasma	70–120 mg/dl	3.9–6.7 mmol/L
Elderly	80–150 mg/dl	4.4–8.3 mmol/L
Child, <2 y old	60–100 mg/dl	3.3–5.6 mmol/L
Infant	40–90 mg/dl	2.2–5.0 mmol/L
Newborn	30–60 mg/dl	1.7–3.3 mmol/L
Glucose monitoring (capillary blood)	60–110 mg/dl	3.3–6.1 mmol/L
Glucose-6-phosphate dehydrogenase screen	Enzyme activity is present	Same
Glucose tolerance test, oral (adult fasting)		
Baseline fasting blood glucose	70–105 mg/dl	3.9–5.8 mmol/L
30-min fasting blood glucose	110–170 mg/dl	6.1–9.4 mmol/L
60-min fasting blood glucose	120–170 mg/dl	6.7–9.4 mmol/L

Table continued on following page

NORMAL VALUES: WHOLE BLOOD, SERUM, AND PLASMA TESTS *(Continued)*

Name of Test	Conventional Values	SI Units
90-min fasting blood glucose	100–140 mg/dl	5.6–7.8 mmol/L
120-min fasting blood glucose	70–120 mg/dl	3.9–6.7 mmol/L
Glucose, 2-h postprandial	<140 mg/dl	<7.78 mmol/L
Glycosylated hemoglobin assay	5–8% of total hemoglobin	0.05–0.08 fraction of total hemoglobin
Growth hormone		
Adult		
Male	0–5 ng/ml	0–5 μg/L
Female	0–10 ng/ml	0–10 μg/L
Child	0–16 ng/ml	0–16 μg/L
Growth hormone stimulation test		
With arginine	>7 ng/ml	>7 μg/L
With insulin	>20 ng/ml	>20 μg/L
Growth hormone suppression test	<3 ng/ml	<3 μg/L
Hematocrit		
Male	40–54%	0.4–0.59 (volume fraction)
Female	38–47%	0.38–0.47 (volume fraction)
Hemoglobin		
Male	13.5–18.0 g/dl	135–180 g/L
Female	12–16 g/dl	120–160 g/L
Hemoglobin electrophoresis		
Hb A	95–98%	0.95–0.98 Hb fraction
Hb A$_2$	1.5–3.5%	0.015–0.035 Hb fraction
Hb F	0–2%	0.0–0.02 Hb fraction
Hb C	Absent	Same
Hb S	Absent	Same
Hemoglobin, fetal		
Adult	<2% Hb F	<0.02 mass fraction Hb F
Newborn	77% ± 7.3% Hb F	0.77 ± 0.073 mass fraction Hb F
Hepatitis A antibody	Negative	Same
Hepatitis B core antibody	Negative	Same
Hepatitis Be antibody	Negative	Same
Hepatitis Be antigen	Negative	Same
Hepatitis B surface antigen	Negative	Same
Hepatitis C antibody	Negative	Same
Hepatitis delta antibody	Negative	Same
High-density lipoprotein cholesterol		
Male	44–45 mg/dl	1.24–1.27 mmol/L
Female	55 mg/dl	1.425 mmol/L
Histoplasmosis serologic study		
Complement fixation titer	<1:4	Same
Immunodiffusion test	Negative	Same
Human chorionic gonadotrophin		
Male and nonpregnant female	<5 mU/ml	<5 U/L
Pregnant female		
1 wk gestation	5–50 mU/ml	5050 U/L
4 wk gestation	1000–30,000 mU/ml	1000–30,000 U/L
6–8 wk gestation	12,000–270,000 mU/ml	12,000–270,000 U/L
12 wk gestation	15,000–270,000 mU/ml	15,000–270,000 U/L
Human immunodeficiency virus serologic study	Negative	Same
Human leukocyte antigen	No destruction of lymphocytes	Same
Insulin (fasting)		
Adult	5–25 μU/ml	34–172 pmol/L
Newborn	3–20 μU/ml	21–138 pmol/L
1 h after eating	50–130 μU/ml	347.3–902.8 pmol/L
2 h after eating	<30 μU/ml	<208.4 pmol/L
Intrinsic factor antibodies	Negative	Same
Iron		
Adult male	65–175 μg/dl	11.6–31.3 μmol/L
Adult female	50–170 μg/dl	9.0–30.4 μmol/L
Newborn	100–250 μg/dl	17.9–44.8 μmol/L
Iron-binding capacity, total	218–385 μg/dl	36–69 μmol/L
Ketones	Negative	Same

NORMAL VALUES: WHOLE BLOOD, SERUM, AND PLASMA TESTS *(Continued)*

Name of Test	Conventional Values	SI Units
Lactate dehydrogenase (LDH)	70–200 IU/L	Same
Lactate dehydrogenase isoenzymes		
LDH_1	14–26%	0.14–0.26 (fraction of total LDH)
LDH_2	29–39%	0.29–0.39 (fraction of total LDH)
LDH_3	20–26%	0.2–0.26 (fraction of total LDH)
LDH_4	8–16%	0.08–0.16 (fraction of total LDH)
LDH_5	6–16%	0.06–0.16 (fraction of total LDH)
Lactic acid	1–2 mEq/L	1–2 mmol/L
Lactose tolerance test, blood glucose	>20–30 mg/dl	1.1–1.7 mmol/L
Low-density lipoprotein : High-density lipoprotein	<3	Same
LE cell test	Negative	Same
Leucine aminopeptidase		
Adult male	80–200 U/ml (Goldberg-Rutenberg units)	19.2–48.0 U/L
Adult female	75–185 U/ml (Goldberg-Rutenberg units)	18–44 U/L
Lipase (adult)	<200 U/L	Same
Lipids, total	400–800 mg/dl	4–8 g/L
Long-acting thyroid stimulation	None; no long-acting thyroid stimulator present	Same
Low-density lipoprotein cholesterol	<130 mg/dl	<3.37 mmol/L
Luteinizing hormone		
Adult male	1–8 mU/ml	1–8 U/L
Adult female		
Follicular phase	1–12 mU/ml	1–12 U/L
Midcycle peak	16–104 mU/ml	16–104 U/L
Luteal phase	1–12 mU/ml	1–12 U/L
Postmenopausal	16–66 mU/ml	16–66 U/L
Child, 6 mo–10 y	1–5 mU/ml	1–5 U/L
Magnesium		
Adult	1.3–2.1 mEq/L	0.65–1.05 mmol/L
Child		
12–20 y	1.56 ± 0.21 mEq/L	0.78 ± 0.11 mmol/L
6–12 y	1.56 ± 0.18 mEq/L	0.78 ± 0.09 mmol/L
5 mo–6 y	1.65 ± 0.23 mEq/L	0.83 ± 0.12 mmol/L
Newborn–4 d	1.2–1.8 mEq/L	0.6–0.9 mmol/L
Malaria smear	No organisms identified	Same
Metyrapone stimulation test (11-deoxy-cortisol)	>7 μg/dl	>200 nmol/L
Microfilariae smear	No parasites visualized	Same
Mononucleosis tests		
Monotest	Negative; nonreactive	Same
Heterophil titer	<1:56	Same
Neutrophil alkaline phosphatase	Score: 40–130	Same
Osmolarity		
Adult	285–319 mOsm/kg H_2O	285–319 mmol/kg H_2O
Child	270–290 mOsm/kg H_2O	270–290 mmol/kg H_2O
Osmotic fragility		
Initial hemolysis of erythrocytes	0.45% NaCl	4.5 g/L NaCl
Compete hemolysis of erythrocytes	0.3% NaCl	3 g/L NaCl
Parathyroid hormone		
Intact parathyroid hormone	210–310 pg/ml	210–310 ng/L
N-terminal	230–630 pg/ml	230–630 ng/L
C-terminal	410–1760 pg/ml	410–1760 ng/L
Parietal cell antibody	Negative	Same
pH (fetal scalp)	7.25–7.35	Same
Phenylalanine		
Guthrie test	<2 mg/dl	121 μmol/L
Fluorometry method		
Adult	0.8–1.8 mg/dl	48–109 μmol/L
Normal newborn	1.2–3.4 mg/dl	73–206 μmol/L
Premature newborn	2.0–7.5 mg/dl	121–454 μmol/L

Table continued on following page

NORMAL VALUES: WHOLE BLOOD, SERUM, AND PLASMA TESTS *(Continued)*

Name of Test	Conventional Values	SI Units
Phosphate, plasma (adult)	8.2–14.5 mg/dl	0.85–1.5 mmol/L
Phosphorus, serum		
Adult		
12–60 y	2.7–4.5 mg/dl	0.87–1.45 mmol/L
>60 y	2.3–3.7 mg/dl	0.74–1.2 mmol/L
Child		
2–12 y	4.5–5.5 mg/dl	1.45–1.78 mmol/L
10 d–2 y	4.5–6.7 mg/dl	1.45–2.16 mmol/L
Infant 0–10 d	4.5–9.0 mg/dl	1.45–2.91 mmol/L
Premature infant	5.4–10.9 mg/dl	1.74–3.52 mmol/L
Cord blood	3.7–8.1 mg/dl	0.85–1.5 mmol/L
Plasma cell volume	40–50 ml/kg	Same
Platelet aggregation	3–5 min	Same
Platelet count		
Adult	150,000–450,000 cells/μl	150–450 $\times$ 10^9/L
Newborn	84,000–478,000 cells/μl	84–478 $\times$ 10^9/L
Potassium		
Adult	3.5–5.1 mEq/L	3.5–5.1 mmol/L
Newborn	3.7–5.9 mEq/L	3.7–5.9 mmol/L
Progesterone		
Adult male	13–97 ng/dl	0.4–3.1 nmol/L
Menstruating female		
Follicular phase	15–70 ng/dl	0.5–2.2 nmol/L
Luteal phase	200–2500 ng/dl	6.4–79.5 nmol/L
Pregnant female		
7–13 wk gestation	1025–4400 ng/dl	32.6–139.9 nmol/L
30–42 wk gestation	6500–22,900 ng/dl	206.7–728.2 nmol/L
Prolactin		
Adult	0–20 ng/ml	0–20 μg/L
Pregnancy		
Third trimester	34–306 ng/ml	34–306 μg/L
Lactating mother	<40 ng/ml	<40 μg/L
Newborn	<300 ng/ml	<300 μg/L
Prostate-specific antigen (male > 15 y)	0.81 ± 0.89 ng/ml	0.81 ± 0.89 g/L
Prostatic acid phosphatase 4-Nitrophen-ylphosphate method (male)	0.13–0.63 U/L	2.2–10.5 U/L
Protein C	71–142%	0.71–1.42 fraction of whole
	2.82–5.65 μg/ml	2.82–5.65 mg/L
Protein electrophoresis		
Adult		
Albumin	3.5–5.0 g/dl	35–50 g/L
Alpha$_1$-globulin	0.1–0.3 g/dl	1–3 g/L
Alpha$_2$-globulin	0.6–1.0 g/dl	6–10 g/L
Beta globulin	0.7–1.1 g/dl	7–11 g/L
Gamma globulin	0.8–1.6 g/dl	8–16 g/L
Child		
Albumin	3.6–5.2 g/dl	36–52 g/L
Alpha$_1$-globulin	0.1–0.4 g/dl	1–4 g/L
Alpha$_2$-globulin	0.5–1.2 g/dl	5–12 g/L
Beta globulin	0.5–1.2 g/dl	5–11 g/L
Gamma globulin	0.5–1.7 g/dl	5–17 g/L
Protein S	61–130%	0.61–1.3 fraction of whole
Protein, total		
Adult, ambulatory	6.4–8.3 g/dl	64–83 g/L
Adult, recumbent	6.0–7.8 g/dl	60–78 g/L
Newborn	4–7 g/dl	40–70 g/L
Prothrombin time		
Average	10–13 sec	Same
Newborn–6 mo	13–18 sec	Same
Red cell volume		
Male	25–35 ml/kg	Same
Female	20–30 ml/kg	Same

NORMAL VALUES: WHOLE BLOOD, SERUM, AND PLASMA TESTS *(Continued)*

Name of Test	Conventional Values	SI Units
Renin, plasma		
Supine	12–79 mU/L	Same
Upright	13–114 mU/L	Same
Reticulocyte count		
Adult	0.5–1.5%	0.005–0.015 number fraction
	25,000–75,000/μl	25–75 × 10⁹/L
Newborn	1.1–4.5%	0.011–0.045 number fraction
Rheumatoid factor	Negative	Same
Serotonin	50–175 ng/ml	0.28–0.99 μmol/L
Sickle cell tests	Negative	Same
Sodium		
Adult	136–145 mEq/L	136–145 mmol/L
Newborn	133–146 mEq/L	133–146 mmol/L
Syphillis serologic studies		
Venereal Disease Research Laboratory	Negative; nonreactive	Same
Rapid plasma reagin	Negative; nonreactive	Same
Fluorescent treponemal antibody absorption test	Negative; nonreactive	Same
Microhemagglutination assay—*Treponema pallidum*	Negative; nonreactive	Same
Testosterone, free		
Adult male	52–280 pg/ml	180.4–971.6 pmol/L
Adult female	1.6–6.3 pg/ml	5.6–21.9 pmol/L
Child 1–10 y	0.15–0.66 pg/ml	0.5–2.1 pmol/L
Testosterone, total		
Adult male	300–1000 ng/dl	10.4–34.7 nmol/L
Adult female	20–75 ng/dl	0.69–2.6 nmol/L
Child 1–10 y	<3–10 ng/dl	<0.1–0.35 nmol/L
Thyroid microsomal autoantibodies	Titer < 1 : 1000; negative	Same
Thyroglobulin autoantibodies	Titer < 1 : 1000; negative	Same
Thyrotropin		
Adult	0.4–8.9 μU/ml	0.4–8.9 mU/L
Newborn, whole blood	<20 μU/ml	<20 mU/L
Thyrotropin-releasing hormone test		
Thyroid-stimulating hormone value		
Male	14–24 μIU/ml	14–24 mIU/L
Female	16–24 μIU/ml	16–26 mIU/L
Thyroxine		
Adult	5–12 μg/dl	64.4–154.4. nmol/L
Child 1–10 y	6.4–15.0 μg/dl	82.4–193.1 nmol/L
Newborn	6.4–23.2 μg/dl	82.4–298.6 nmol/L
Thyroxine-binding globulin	16–34 μg/ml	16–34 mg/L
Thyroxine, free	0.9–1.7 ng/dl	11.5–21.8 pmol/L
Tolbutamide stimulation, serum insulin level	<195 μU/ml	1354 pmol/L
Toxoplasmosis serologic study	IgM antibody titer: <1 : 8	Same
Transferrin		
Adult <60 y	200–400 mg/dl	2–4 g/L
Newborn	130–275 mg/dl	1.3–2.75 g/L
Transferrin saturate	20–50%	Same
Triglycerides		
Male <40 y	46–316 mg/dl	0.52–3.57 mmol/L
Female <40 y	37–174 mg/dl	0.42–1.97 mmol/L
Male >50 y	75–313 mg/dl	0.85–3.54 mmol/L
Female >50 y	52–200 mg/dl	0.59–2.26 mmol/L
Triiodothyronine		
Adult	95–190 ng/dl	1.5–2.0 nmol/L
Child 1–10 y	94–269 ng/dl	1.4–4.1 nmol/L
Newborn	32–250 ng/dl	0.49–3.8 nmol/L
Triiodothyronine, free	0.2–0.52 ng/dl	3–8 pmol/L
Triiodothyronine resin uptake		
Adult	25–35% of total	0.25–0.35 fraction of total

Table continued on following page

NORMAL VALUES: WHOLE BLOOD, SERUM, AND PLASMA TESTS (*Continued*)

Name of Test	Conventional Values	SI Units
Free thyroxine index	1.3–4.2	Same
Free triiodothyronine index	24–67	Same
Urea nitrogen		
Adult	5–20 mg/dl	1.8–7.1 mmol/L
Newborn–infant	4–16 mg/dl	1.4–5.7 mmol/L
Uric acid		
Adult <60 y		
Male	4.5–8.0 ng/dl	0.27–0.47 mmol/L
Female	2.5–6.2 ng/dl	0.15–0.37 mmol/L
Adult >60 y		
Male	4.2–8.0 ng/dl	0.25–0.47 mmol/L
Female	2.7–6.8 ng/dl	0.16–0.4 mmol/L
Child <12 y	2.0–5.5 ng/dl	0.12–0.32 mmol/L
Vasopressin		
With osmolarity of >290 mOsm/kg	2–12 pg/ml	1.85–11.1 pmol/L
With osmolarity of <290 mOsm/kg	<2 pg/ml	<1.85 pmol/L
Vitamin D, activated	25–45 pg/ml	60–180 nmol/L
White blood cell differential (adult),		
Segmented neutrophils	56%	0.56 (mean number fraction)
	1800–7800/μl	1.8–7.8 × 10^9/L
Bands	3%	0.03 (mean number fraction)
	0–700/μl	0.0–0.07 × 10^9/L
Eosinophils	2.7%	0.027 (mean number fraction)
	0–450/μl	0.0–0.45 × 10^9/L
Basophils	0.3%	0.003 (mean number fraction)
	0–200/μl	0.0–0.2 × 10^9/L
Lymphocytes	34%	0.34 (mean number fraction)
	1000–4800/μl	1.0–4.8 × 10^9/L
Monocytes	4%	0.04 (mean number fraction)
	0–800/μl	0.0–0.8 × 10^9/L

NORMAL VALUES: URINE TESTS

Name of Test	Conventional Values	SI Units
Aldosterone	2–26 μg/24 h	6–72 nmol/24 h
Calcium (adult)		
Normal calcium intake	100–300 mg/d	2.5–7.5 mmol/d
Infant and child	<6 mg/kg/d	<0.15 mmol/kg/d
Catecholamines		
Norepinephrine	15–56 μg/24 h	88.6–331 nmol/24 h
Epinephrine	<15 pg/ml	<82 nmol/24 h
Dopamine	100–400 pg/ml	625–2750 nmol/24 h
Vanillymandelic acid	2–7 mg/24 h	10–35 μmol/24 h
Metanephrine	24–96 μg/24 h	131–524 nmol/24 h
Normetanephrine	75–375 μg/24 h	409–2047 nmol/24 h
Chloride		
Adult	110–250 mEq/24 h	110–250 mmol/24 h
Adult >60 y	95–195 mEq/24 h	95–195 mmol/24 h
Child 10–14 y		
Male	64–176 mEq/24 h	64–176 mmol/24 h
Female	36–173 mEq/24 h	36–173 mmol/24 h
Child 6–10 y		
Male	36–110 mEq/24 h	36–110 mmol/24 h
Female	18–74 mEq/24 h	18–74 mmol/24 h
Child <6 y	15–40 mEq/24 h	15–40 mmol/24 h
Infant	2–10 mEq/24 h	2–10 mmol/24 h
Cortisol, free (adult)	0–110 μg/24 h	0–303.6 nmol/24 h
Creatinine clearance		
Adult male	1–2 g/d	8.8–17.7 mmol/L
Adult female	0.8–1.8 g/d	7.1–15.9 mmol/L
Child	70–140 ml/min/1.73 m^2	1.17–2.33 ml/s/m^2

NORMAL VALUES: URINE TESTS *(Continued)*

Name of Test	Conventional Values	SI Units
Dexamethasone suppression test, low dose (adult)		
17-hydroxycorticosteroid	<4 ng/24 h	<138 nmol/L
Free cortisol	<4 ng/ml	<11.04 nmol/24 h
D-Xylose absorption test		
Child	16–33% of ingested dose/5 h	0.16–0.33 fraction of ingested dose/5 h
Adult, 5-g dose	>1.2 g/5 h	>8 mmol/L/5 h
Adult, 25-g dose	>4 g/5 h	>26.64 mmol/L/5 h
Adult, >65 y	3.5 g/5 h	>23.31 mmol/L/5 h
Estriol, pregnancy		
28–30 wk	5–18 mg/24 h	17–62 μmol/L
32–34 wk	2–26 mg/24 h	24–90 μmol/L
36–38 wk	10–36 mg/24 h	35–125 μmol/L
40 wk	13–42 mg/24 h	45–146 μmol/L
Estrogens		
Postmenopausal female	<20 μg/24 h	69 μmol/24 h
Premenopausal female	15–80 μg/24 h	52–277 μmol/24 h
Male	15–40 μg/24 h	52–139 μmol/24 h
Child	<10 μg/24 h	<35 μmol/24 h
Fibrin split products	<0.25 μg/ml	<0.25 mg/L
Follicle-stimulating hormone		
Adult male	4–18 U/24 h	Same
Female		
Follicular phase	3–12 U/24 h	Same
Midcycle peak	8–60 U/24 h	Same
Glucose	Negative	Same
Hemosiderin	Negative	Same
Human chorionic gonadotropin		
Male, nonpregnant female	Negative	Same
Pregnant female	Positive	Same
17-Hydroxycorticosteroids		
Adult male	4.5–12.0 mg/24 h	12.4–33.1 μmol/24 h
Adult female	2.5–10.0 mg/24 h	6.9–27.6 μmol/24 h
Child		
8–12 y	<4.5 mg/24 h	<12.4 μmol/24 h
<8 y	<1.5 mg/24 h	<4.14 μmol/24 h
5-Hydroxyindoleacetic acid, quantitative, adult	1–7 mg/24 h	5–37 μmol/24 h
17-Ketogenic steroids		
Male	4–14 mg/24 h	13–49 μmol/24 h
Female	2–12 mg/24 h	7–42 μmol/24 h
Child		
11–14 y	2–9 mg/24 h	7–31 μmol/24 h
<11 y	0.1–4.0 mg/24 h	0.3–14.0 μmol/24 h
Ketones	Negative	Same
17-Ketosteroids		
Male	10–25 mg/24 h	37–87 μmol/24 h
Female	6–14 mg/24 h	21–49 μmol/24 h
Child		
10–14 y	1–6 mg/24 h	3–21 μmol/24 h
<10 y	<3 mg/24 h	<10 μmol/24 h
Lactose tolerance test		
Urine lactose		
Adult	12–40 mg/dl/24 h	0.7–2.2 mmol/L
Child	<1.5 mg/100 dl	—
Leukocyte esterase	Negative	Same
Casts	0–4 hyaline casts/low-power field	Same
Crystals	Few	Same
Luteinizing hormone		
Adult male	9–23 U/24 h	Same
Female	4–30 U/24 h	Same
Male 1–10 y	<1.0–5.6 U/24 h	Same
Female 1–10 y	1.4–4.9 U/24 h	Same

Table continued on following page

NORMAL VALUES: URINE TESTS *(Continued)*

Name of Test	Conventional Values	SI Units
Magnesium	7.3–12.2 mg/dl/d	3–5 mmol/d
Osmolarity		
Normal diet and fluid intake	500–800 mOsm/kg H_2O	500–800 mmol/kg H_2O
Range	50–1400 mOsm/kg H_2O	50–1400 mmol/kg H_2O
Ova and parasites	Negative	Same
Phenylalanine	Negative	Same
Potassium		
Adult	25–125 mEq/24 h	25–125 mmol/24 h
Child 10–14 y		
Male	22–57 mEq/24 h	22–57 mmol/24 h
Female	18–58 mEq/24 h	18–58 mmol/24 h
Child 6–10 y		
Male	17–54 mEq/24 h	17–54 mmol/24 h
Female	8–37 mEq/24 h	8–37 mmol/24 h
Infant	4.1–5.3 mEq/24 h	4.1–5.3 mmol/24 h
Pregnanetriol		
Adult	<2 mg/d	<5.9 μmol/d
Child		
0–6 y	<0.2 mg/d	<0.6 μmol/d
7–16 y	<0.3–1.1 mg/d	<0.9–3.3 μmol/d
Protein	40–150 mg/24 h	Same
Protein electrophoresis	40–150 mg/24 h	40–150 mg/24 h
Schilling test		
Stage 1	10–40% cobalt-58, vitamin B_{12} excretion/24 h	0.1–0.4 fraction of dose excreted
Stage 2	0–42% cobalt-57, vitamin B_{12}, and intrinsic factor excretion/24 h	0.0–0.42 fraction of dose excreted
Cobalt-57 : cobalt 58 ratio	0.7–1.3	Same
Sodium		
Adult	40–220 mEq/24 h	40–220 mmol/24 h
Child 10–14 y		
Male	63–117 mEq/24 h	63–117 mmol/24 h
Female	48–168 mEq/24 h	48–168 mmol/24 h
Child 6–10 y		
Male	41–115 mEq/24 h	41–115 mmol/24 h
Female	20–69 mEq/24 h	20–69 mmol/24 h
Uric acid (adult, average diet)	250–750 mg/24 h	1.48–4.43 mmol/24 h
Urinalysis		
Specific gravity	1.003–1.029	Same
pH	4.5–7.8	Same
Protein	Negative	Same
Bilirubin	Negative	Same
Urobilinogen	Normal	Same
Glucose	Negative	Same
Ketone	Negative	Same
Occult blood	Negative	Same
Red blood cells (male)	0–3/high-power field	Same
Red blood cells (female)	0–5/high-power field	Same
White blood cells	0–5/high-power field	Same
Bacteria	Negative	Same
Urobilinogen		
Male	0.3–2.1 mg/2 h	0.5–3.6 μmol/2 h
Female	0.1–1.1 mg/2 h	0.2–1.9 μmol/2 h
Water deprivation		
Specific gravity	1.025–1.032	Same
Urine osmolarity	>800 mOsm/kg	>800 mmol/kg

NORMAL VALUES: BODY FLUIDS

Body Fluid	Name of Test	Conventional Values	SI Units
Amniotic fluid	Amniotic fluid analysis		
	Chromosome analysis	Normal karyotype	Same
	Alpha₁-fetoprotein	0.5–3.0 Multiples of median (MoM)	Same

NORMAL VALUES: BODY FLUIDS (*Continued*)

Body Fluid	Name of Test	Conventional Values	SI Units
	Acetylcholinesterase	Negative	Same
	Rh incompatibility	Negative/1+	Same
	Bilirubin	0.01–0.03 mg/dl	0.02–0.06 μmol/L
	Creatinine		
	36 wk gestation	1.6–1.8 mg/dl	141–159 μmol/L
	37–38 wk gestation	>2 mg/dl	>177 μmol/L
	Lecithin to sphingomyelin ratio	>2	Same
	37–38 wk gestation		
	Phosphatidylglycerol	Present	Same
	Pulmonary surfactant	Positive; foam stability index, >0.48	Same
	Meconium	Absent	Same
Cerebrospinal fluid	Cerebrospinal fluid analysis		
	Pressure	90–180 mm H_2O	Same
	Appearance	Clear, colorless	Same
	Leukocyte count		
	Adult	0–5 cells/μl	0–5 × 10^6/L
	Child 5–18 y	0–10 cells/μl	0–10 × 10^6/L
	Neonate–1 y	0–30 cells/μl	0–30 × 10^6/L
	Lymphocytes (adult)	40–80%	0.4–0.8 fraction
	Monocytes	15–45%	0.15–0.45 fraction
	Neutrophils	0–6%	0.0–0.06 fraction
	Lymphocytes (neonate)	5–35%	0.05–0.35 fraction
	Monocytes	50–90%	0.5–0.9 fraction
	Neutrophils	0–8%	0.0–0.08 fraction
	Lactate	10–22 mg/dl	1.1–2.4 mmol/L
	Glucose	50–80 mg/dl	2.75–4.4 mmol/L
	Total protein	15–45 mg/dl	150–450 mg/L
	Albumin	10–30 mg/dl	100–300 mg/L
	IgG	1–4 mg/dl	10–40 mg/L
	Protein electrophoresis		
	Prealbumin	2–7%	0.02–0.07 fraction
	Albumin	56–76%	0.56–0.76 fraction
	Alpha$_1$-globulin	2–7%	0.02–0.07 fraction
	Alpha$_2$-globulin	4–12%	0.04–0.12 fraction
	Beta globulin	8–18%	0.08–0.18 fraction
	Gamma globulin	3–12%	0.03–0.12 fraction
	Myelin-basic protein	0–5% μg/L	Same
Effusion fluid	Carcinoembryonic antigen		
	Adult, nonsmoker	<2.5 ng/ml	2.5 μg/L
	Adult, smoker	Up to 5 ng/ml	Up to 5 μg/L
Gastric secretion	Gastric analysis		
	pH	<2	<2
	Basal acid output		
	Male	4.2 mEq/h	4.2 mmol/h
	Female	1.8 mEq/h	1.8 mmol/h
	Maximal acid output		
	Male	22.6 mEq/h	22.6 mmol/h
	Female	15.2 mEq/h	15.2 mmol/h
	Peak acid output		
	Male	35 mEq/h	35 mmol/h
	Female	25 mEq/h	25 mmol/h
	Basal acid output:maximal acid output	<0.4 (40%)	<0.4 (40%)
Peritoneal fluid	Peritoneal fluid analysis		
	Appearance	Clear, odorless, pale, yellow, scanty	Same
	Ammonia	<50 μg/dl	—
	Amylase	138–404 amylase units/L	Same
	Bacteria, fungi	None present	Same
	Cells	No malignant cells present	Same
	Glucose	70–90 mg/dl	3.89–4.99 mmol/L
	Protein	0.3–4.1 g/dl	3–41 g/L

Table continued on following page

NORMAL VALUES: BODY FLUIDS *(Continued)*

Body Fluid	Name of Test	Conventional Values	SI Units
	Red blood cells	None	None
	White blood cells	$<300/\mu l$	$<300 \times 10^6/L$
Perspiration	Sweat test	5–40 mEq/L	5–40 mmol/L
Semen	Semen analysis		
	Appearance	Opalescent gray-white color	Same
	Volume	2–5 ml	0.002–0.005 L
	Liquefaction	10–60 min	Same
	pH	7.2–7.8	Same
	Acid phosphatase	>200 U/ejaculate	Same
	Citric acid	>52 μmol/ejaculate	Same
	Fructose	>13 μmol/ejaculate	Same
	Zinc	>2.4 μmol/ejaculate	Same
	Motility	$>50\%$	>0.5 number fraction
	Concentration	$20–250 \times 10^6/ml$	$20–250 \times 10^9/L$
	Morphologic characteristics	$>50\%$ normal, mature spermatozoa	>0.5 number fraction
	Viability	$>50\%$ live spermatozoa	>0.5 number fraction
	Leukocytes	$<1 \times 10^6/ml$	$<1 \times 10^9/L$
Synovial fluid	Synovial fluid analysis		
	Appearance	Crystal clear, transparent, pale yellow	Same
	Viscosity	High	Same
	Volume	<3.5 ml	Same
	Red blood cells	Absent	Same
	White blood cells	$0–200/mm^3$	$0–200 \times 10^6/L$
	Nucleated cell count	<200 cells/μl	$<200 \times 10^6$ cells/L
	Granulocytes	$<25\%$ of nucleated cells	$<25\%$ of nucleated cells; number fraction of granulocytes
	Protein	3 g/dl	30 g/L
	Uric acid	<8 gm/dl	476 mol/L
	Glucose (fasting)	70–110 mg/dl	3.9–6.1 mmol/L
	Blood-synovial fluid glucose difference	<10 mg/dl	<0.56 mmol/L
	Fibrin clot	Negative or absent	Same
	Mucin clot	Positive or abundant	Same
	String test	Formation of a long string	Same
	Culture	No growth	Same
	Rheumatoid factor	Negative	Same
Vaginal secretions	Prostatic acid phosphatase	<2 U/L	Same

* The values for premature neonates vary according to the degree of prematurity.

† Values are lower when the patient is in a supine position.

Modified from Malarkey, L. M. & McMorrow, M. E. (1996). *Nurses's manual of laboratory tests and diagnostic procedures* (pp 942–969). Philadelphia: W. B. Saunders.

Answers to Study Questions

Chapter 1

1. The National League for Nursing formed for purpose of control of nursing

   b. education

   Rationale: The National League for Nursing was organized in 1893 by the superintendents of the nurse training schools. These women formed the American Society of Superintendents of Training Schools for Nurses (forerunner of the National League for Nurses) to gain a strong collective voice over the development of nursing education in the United States.

2. The National Organization of Colored Graduate Nurses started as a result of racial

   c. inequity

   Rationale: Statewide nursing organizations, especially in many southern states, barred African-American nurses from membership based on color. This denial at the state level meant that these nurses would not be eligible for membership in the American Nurses Association or the National League for Nurses. Moreover, black nurses confronted discrimination in the job market, in admission to nursing schools, and in opportunity to sit for licensure examinations. As a result of such widespread discrimination, the National Association of Colored Graduate Nurses formed in 1908 to address racial issues as well as professional issues facing all nurses in the United States during that period.

3. Outcome measures in accreditation ensure

   c. quality

   Rationale: The 1990s brought about a movement in higher education calling for greater accountability for quality to the public. The higher education community instituted the use of outcome measures as a means of ensuring quality education and monitoring public funds.

4. An important function of the nurse practice act is to

   a. protect the public

   Rationale: The nursing profession has faced a long history of barriers to practice that persists late into the 20th century. Until state registration laws were passed at the beginning of the 20th century, anyone could call himself or herself a nurse whether or not he or she had graduated from a nursing program. Paramount to all nurse practice acts was the protection of the public from unqualified practitioners.

Chapter 2

1. Which client would require Orem's wholly compensatory nursing system?

   b. anesthetized woman in surgery

   Rationale: A woman who is anesthetized would be unable to participate in her care and would be totally dependent on the nurse.

2. What are the four concepts most important to nursing?

   d. person, health, environment, and nursing care activities

   Rationale: Even though all of the concepts included in this question may be part of one or more nursing theories, the four concepts included in *every* nursing theory are person, health, environment, and nursing care activities.

3. During which phase of Peplau's nurse-client relationship does implementation occur?

   c. exploitation

   Rationale: When comparing Peplau's theory with the nursing process, implementation occurs during the exploitation phase.

4. In using Roy's Adaptation Model to care for a mother who has just delivered her baby, what is the focal stimulus?

   a. the birth

   Rationale: In Roy's Adaptation Model, the focal stimulus is the event immediately confronting the system, which would be the birth for a new mother.

5. Which theorist developed a nursing theory that emphasizes culture?

   a. Leininger

   Rationale: Culture is emphasized by Madeleine Leininger's Culture Care Theory.

Chapter 3

1. A central theme of utilitarianism is

   c. the greatest good for the largest number of people

   Rationale: As developed by British philosophers Jeremy Bentham and John Stuart Mill, utilitarianism values actions and decisions that produce the greatest quantity of happiness (or "the greatest good") for the greatest number of people.

2. Which of the following ethical concepts is *most* consistent with the beliefs of deontology?

   a. autonomy

   Rationale: According to deontological thinking, people have the freedom, thoughtfulness, and sensibility to act in a moral manner. Autonomy in health care has come to mean a self-directing freedom and moral independence in which an individual is free to choose and implement his or her own decisions. The ethical concept of autonomy is thus most consistent with the beliefs of deontology.

3. Under what condition can the client's autonomy be restricted?

   b. when the client's rights clash with the rights of a community

   Rationale: A health care worker may justify infringing on a client's autonomy in the name of promoting what is "good" for the community as a whole, as in the case of mandated childhood immunizations.

4. The *first* step in the ethical decision-making process is

   c. to gain an overall understanding of the situation

   Rationale: Before determining the client's decision-making capacity, or the nurse's own ethical beliefs, it is important to develop an understanding of the situation—its context, the parties involved, and the clinical, social, and ethical issues connected to it. Only after the situation has been understood and properly analyzed can one begin to identify which ethical principles are involved.

5. The *second* step in the ethical decision making process is

   a. to state the problem in ethical terms

   Rationale: An ethical problem must be identified and stated in ethical terms before it is appropriate to seek consultation either with a clinical ethicist or an ethics committee. Determining the client's decision-making capacity is appropriate after the ethical problem has been stated and the desired goals of all involved parties (including the client and the nurse) have been articulated.

Chapter 4

1. Failing to provide care considered a standard for a client would be classified as

   b. negligence

   Rationale: Negligence involves actions that fall below the standard of care for that professional group.

2. An example of assault is

   c. restraining a client who wants to leave the hospital against medical advice

   Rationale: A client who wants to leave the hospital against medical advice cannot be prevented from doing so. Staff who restrain the client would be at risk for a charge of assault.

3. Which of the following situations would be considered a violation of a client's confidentiality?

   b. allowing a client's family to read the client's chart when they request to do it

   Rationale: A client's family does not have the right to read a client's medical chart. Information that may be included on the chart can only be divulged with the client's permission.

4. The responsibility for obtaining an informed consent rests with the

   a. physician

   Rationale: The physician is responsible for obtaining a consent and for ensuring that the client is adequately informed.

Chapter 5

1. The most important concept for the nurse to remember when discussing health and illness concerns with the client is to

   b. validate the meaning of health-related concepts with the client

   Rationale: The meaning that the client has for health-related concepts frames his or her participation in health care. Understanding the meaning of concepts from the client's perspective allows the nurse to provide care that the client will value.

2. Frequently, the needs of the individual compete with the needs of society because

   a. not enough resources are available to meet every need

   Rationale: Contemporary American society does not provide resources to meet certain health care needs. A national health plan could be instituted to meet more health needs but not all health needs.

3. The primary reason that various settings exist to provide health care is that

   c. people have changing needs for health care services

   Rationale: The needs of the people drive the development and location of services.

4. The major conflict in the ongoing health care reform is between the concepts of

   d. cost and quality of care

   Rationale: The concepts of cost and quality of services are not necessarily opposite but are often viewed as opposite concerns. Attempts to lower cost must be tempered with the concerns of maintaining quality of care.

5. Continuity of care means that services will be administered

   d. as they are necessary

   Rationale: Continuity of care suggests that services will be available whenever necessary. Some people need only sporadic care, while others need ongoing care for chronic conditions.

Chapter 6

1. Which of the following is a biofeedback technique?

   a. being aware of involuntary cues

   Rationale: Biofeedback is being aware of involuntary cues and practicing relaxation techniques to diminish stress reactions. Answers b, c, and d, are all helpful in reducing stress, but they do not respond to involuntary cues.

2. Sam, age 4 years, will start school for the first time tomorrow. What would you assess Sam for that would require new coping skills?

   d. signs of maturational crisis

   Rationale: Answers a and b are possible but would subside quickly. The beginning of school is not a situational crisis; therefore, c would not be a correct answer. You would really need to assess for a maturational crisis for Sam to develop the skills necessary to cope with his new environment.

3. All but one of the following is important when assessing a client's potential for crisis. Which of the following would not be included in your assessment?

   b. mental status

   Rationale: You would not assess the mental status of a client when determining crisis potential. It is important to determine the client's perception of the event, his or her support systems, and his or her coping skills.

4. Which of the following combinations of foods may magnify stress?

   b. caffeine, alcohol, sugar, preservatives

   Rationale: Caffeine, alcohol, sugar, and preservatives all contain substances that may magnify stress. Answers a, c, and d may not be nutritious as combinations, but they do not exacerbate stress reactions.

5. When a person is experiencing positive feedback

   b. he or she is moving away from a normal state of homeostasis

   Rationale: He or she is becoming more ill—moving away from a normal state of homeostasis. Answers a, c, and d would be true for negative feedback.

Chapter 8

1. The nurse collects all of the following data from a client. Which piece would be considered subjective data?

   c. client has periods of nausea before meals

   Rationale: Nausea is a subjective complaint experienced by the client but not seen by the nurse. Pulse, skin temperature, and breathing pattern are assessments that the nurse can make without input directly from the client.

2. Which of the following *best* describes the purpose of a nursing history?

   b. it provides the nurse with an initial database to plan care for the client

Rationale: The primary purpose of the nursing history is to provide the nurse with information to formulate an initial database for the client.

3. Which of the following statements about an interview is true?

   a. it should be conducted in a quiet setting that affords the client privacy

   Rationale: Interviews should be conducted in a quiet area to allow for the client to concentrate on providing information and not be distracted from other noises in the environment.

4. When a nurse is determining the temperature or texture of a client's skin, which of the following assessment techniques is being used?

   d. palpation

   Rationale: Palpation is using the sense of touch to determine temperature or texture of the client's skin.

5. A diagnostic test that involves direct visualization of an internal organ is an

   b. endoscopy

   Rationale: An endoscopy involves the use of a fiberoptic endoscope that is passed into a cavity or organ of the body to visualize the inside of that cavity or organ.

Chapter 9

1. Rape trauma syndrome

   b. is a one-part nursing diagnosis

   Rationale: Syndromes are one-part nursing diagnoses. Because of the symptoms and behaviors involved in a syndrome, the diagnosis includes all of the information needed to plan nursing actions. Therefore, two-part and three-part nursing diagnoses are not appropriate for a syndrome.

2. Gaps in the data collection are evident in all but one of the following situations

   b. multiple nursing diagnoses can be made

   Rationale: Multiple nursing diagnoses may be made when complete information is available. Gaps in data collection occur when information is lacking, conflicting information needs to be clarified, or the client is reluctant to share information.

3. The purpose of theoretical models in nursing diagnosis is to

   d. guide nursing actions

   Rationale: The purpose of theoretical models is to guide nursing actions. The way a nurse determines the plan of nursing actions depends on the theoretical model that is used.

4. The group that has made the largest contribution to developing nursing diagnoses is

   c. NANDA

   Rationale: The North American Nursing Diagnosis Association (NANDA) has made the largest contribution to developing nursing diagnoses. The American Nurses' Association (ANA) represents nurses throughout the country. The National League for Nursing (NLN) is an accrediting body for nursing programs. The National Organization of Nurse Practitioner Faculties (NONPF) represents nurse practitioners.

5. Which of the following would not be part of a nursing diagnosis?

   c. value judgments

   Rationale: It is imperative to have accurate information when making a nursing diagnosis, and value judgments create a bias in the diagnosis that might have a negative effect on nursing actions.

Chapter 10

1. When setting priorities of care, first priority is given to problems that

   c. involve a life-threatening event

   Rationale: When determining which problems require highest priority, the nurse should always focus on those that involve a life-threatening event.

2. Which of the following outcomes would be described as being in the cognitive domain?

   d. client will identify the signs and symptoms of hypoglycemia

   Rationale: The cognitive domain involves knowledge; therefore, identifying signs and symptoms of hypoglycemia is a cognitive activity.

3. Which of the following would be considered a dependent nursing intervention?

   a. administer acetaminophen, 650 mg, every 4 hours for temperature above 101°F

   Rationale: Dependent nursing interventions are those that are based on a physician's prescription.

4. Which of the following is a plan of care that is developed through a multidisciplinary approach?

   b. critical pathway plan

   Rationale: Critical pathways reflect activities of the multidisciplinary care team.

Chapter 11

1. Implementation is carried out by

   d. the client and the nurse

   Rationale: The client and the nurse carry out implementation of the nursing process. The client and the physician or the nurse and the physician do not carry out implementation.

2. When administering a medication, it is the responsibility of the nurse to monitor the client for side effects: This would be an example of

   c. a dependent nursing action

Rationale: Monitoring side effects of a medication is a dependent nursing action. The actual ordering of the medication is done by a physician, and the nurse carries out the order and monitors for side effects.

3. All but one of the following is considered essential information to be entered in the client record.

   c. visits by friends

   Rationale: It is not essential for visits by friends to be entered into the client record. It is essential to enter physical signs and symptoms, changes in behavior, and visits by health team members.

4. Records where professionals from each discipline keep data on separate forms are known as

   b. source-oriented records

   Rationale: Source-oriented records contain separate forms for each discipline. Problem-oriented records are organized around a client problem. Focus charting categorizes data, and flow sheets are used in charting by exception.

5. A potential complication for a medical diagnosis would be considered

   b. a dependent nursing problem

   Rationale: Complications of a medical diagnosis are considered a dependent nursing problem, as it is the medical diagnosis that will generate the problem, and the intervention will depend on the physician's orders.

Chapter 12

1. Nursing care is evaluated through

   c. outcome data

   Rationale: Evaluating nursing care through outcome data is the only accurate way to perform the evaluation. Managing time, use of equipment, and team cooperation are not appropriate means to evaluate nursing care.

2. A consumer of health care may be all but one of the following

   d. the health provider

   Rationale: A health care provider is the deliverer of care. A family, a community, or an individual client may all be a consumer of health care.

3. Evaluation occurs

   b. whenever a nurse interacts with a client

   Rationale: Evaluation is an ongoing process that occurs with each client interaction. It is not the end of the nursing process. Interactions with other health care providers do not provide evaluation of nursing actions. Evaluation can be done at any time and not just at the end of a shift.

4. Which organizations have developed guidelines and standards for quality assurance in nursing practice?

   c. ANA and JCAHO

   Rationale: The American Nurses' Association (ANA) and the Joint Commission for the Accreditation of Health Care Organizations (JCAHO) have developed guidelines for quality assurance in nursing practice. The National League for Nursing (NLN) has guidelines for educational programs but not for nursing practice. The American Medical Association (AMA) is an organization for physicians.

5. When an outcome is completely met
   b. both the short-term and long-term outcomes were met

   Rationale: An outcome is not completely met until both the short-term and long-term goals are met. If either the short-term or the long-term goal is not met, then the outcome is not met.

Chapter 13

1. Which of the following is true of a therapeutic relationship?
   b. It is client focused.

   Rationale: Answers a, c, and d are all aspects of a social relationship. Social relationships have a wide variety of nonspecific helping behaviors that the person engaged in the relationship can choose from. A therapeutic relationship is client focused; it is not reciprocal. The nurse does not share his or her personal beliefs and values with the client. In a therapeutic relationship, help is the primary focus of the relationship.

2. Raising your voice to a person who is hearing impaired will
   c. cause additional residual hearing loss

   Rationale: Answers a, b, and d are not always true. The client will not hear you better. Remember that he or she has a hearing loss. It is more difficult to lip read, when you raise your voice as your facial muscles may become distorted. It is for that reason that your speech would not be clearer. The correct answer is c because you can cause pain to the ear canal.

3. In what phase of the therapeutic relationship is trust established?
   c. orientation phase

   Rationale: Remember that the orientation phase is the first phase of the relationship, and it is necessary to build trust at the beginning of the relationship so that answers a and b can take place effectively. Answer d is a phase of the therapeutic relationship.

4. An example of a secondary group is
   b. Boy Scouts

   Rationale: This group comes together for a specific purpose. Answers a, c, and d are all primary groups; membership is automatic and spontaneously chosen.

5. The termination phase of a group parallels what phase of the nursing process?
   a. evaluation

   Rationale: It occurs after the group has met group goals, just as evaluation occurs after implementation has been performed. Assessment would be similar to the beginning phase, and planning and implementation would take place in the working phases of a group.

Chapter 14

1. When providing information to Mr. J. about his hypertensive medication, the nurse first
   b. assesses what the client and family/significant other want to know

   Rationale: Concerns of the client and family are addressed first, because anxiety, fear, and uncertainty generated from concerns may interfere with the learner's ability to process essential information effectively.

2. The nurse applies the unitary learning principle when he or she refers to the client as
   c. Mrs. Jones, who was just discharged home

   Rationale: When the nurse refers to the client by her name, Mrs. Jones, he or she recognizes the learner as a whole person with unique psychological strengths, weaknesses, and health care experiences that play a role in her learning, illness, and recovery.

3. When teaching the client and family/significant other, the nurse should
   a. document what was taught and the outcomes achieved

   Rationale: The nurse's documentation of what was taught and the outcomes achieved serves as a guide for further reinforcement or advancement of the instruction as indicated. Documentation encourages referrals and recommendations for further teaching as needed for safe discharge.

4. Following a teaching session on heart medications, the nurse asks Miss J. to explain the purpose of the heart medication she is taking. The nurse is attempting to
   a. evaluate the degree to which a learning outcome has been achieved

   Rationale: Evaluation considers the degree to which expected outcomes are met. Results are made known to the learner by the teacher. Evaluation includes documentation of results. Success or failure of the learner to meet mutually set outcomes is recorded and communicated to other professionals and agencies caring for the client. Recommendations and referrals are communicated in writing and orally.

5. Which of the following learning activities requires the most active participation on the part of the learner?
   d. practicing insulin administration

   Rationale: Practicing insulin administration emphasizes motor and procedural skills. In addition to comprehending essential information about insulin and sites of injection, the learner must be ready for this experience. The activity requires movement with fine coordination, certainty, adaptation to new situations and manipulating materials out of understanding and ability. The learner gives a return demonstration to the teacher. Errors are identified. Correct activities are reinforced. Practice is recommended.

Chapter 15

1. According to Piaget, language development is the main characteristic during the

   b. preconceptual stage

   Rationale: It is during the preconceptual stage that the child focuses on language and expression through verbalization. During the sensorimotor stage, the child is learning through reflexive, repetitive, and imitative behaviors, whereas the concrete operation stage is concerned with school-age children and logical thinking. The initiative stage is one of Erikson's psychosocial stages of preschoolers.

2. According to growth and development theorists, growth and development progresses

   c. in a predictable, sequential manner

   Rationale: Growth and development occur in a cephalocaudal, proximodistal, and simple-to-complex manner. Measurements of head circumference occur during infancy; however, height, weight, and vital sign measurements are necessary throughout childhood. All children progress at an individual rate; however, growth and development occur in a predictable and sequential manner.

3. On admission to the hospital, a nursing assessment should include

   d. all of the above

   Rationale: A complete assessment should be performed on all children admitted to the hospital. A complete assessment should include a history and physical, along with a developmental assessment.

4. The best way to prepare a 15-year-old child for a painful procedure is to

   d. a and b

   Rationale: An adolescent wants to understand why the procedure is being performed and may have many more questions regarding his or her illness. To gain the child's trust and cooperation, the nurse must be honest in answering questions. Although a procedure may be painful or uncomfortable, the nurse needs to reassure the child of measures that will be used to lessen the discomfort and support the child.

5. A 4-year-old child has been admitted to the hospital for asthma. The doctor has ordered an x-ray of the child's chest. The best way for the nurse to prepare the child for this procedure is to explain

   b. that a large machine is going to take a picture of his or her lungs to see how they are working

   Rationale: This child understands the world through learning and exploring with all of his or her senses. The nurse should explain in terms of what the child will see, hear, or feel. The best explanation is b because it explains what the child will see. The other choices do not explain the procedure.

Chapter 16

1. To stimulate the rooting reflex in a neonate, a nurse should

   c. stroke the newborn's cheek with a fingertip

   Rationale: The rooting reflex, a survival mechanism, is elicited when the infant's cheek is stroked. The infant turns the head toward the stimulus in search of a nipple for feeding.

2. A nurse should expect to assess which of these motor activities in a normal 6-month-old infant?

   a. sits on the floor without support

   Rationale: Infants begin to sit upright unsupported at approximately 6 months of age. They are not able to grasp objects with the thumb and forefinger, put three objects into a container, or pull self to a standing position until at least 8 months.

3. When providing anticipatory guidance during a health promotion visit, which piece of information should a nurse give to a parent of a 3-year-old child?

   d. "Your child may experience fearful reactions to the dark, animals, and unfamiliar noises"

   Rationale: Preschoolers do not have the ability to distinguish pretend from reality, and they have a strong sense of fantasy. This contributes to the fear they experience of the dark, unfamiliar noises, and animals.

4. Which of these behaviors, if observed in a school-age boy, indicates achievement of Erikson's task of industry versus inferiority?

   b. cooperatively participates with other children when playing his favorite board game

   Rationale: During the stage of industry versus inferiority, a school-age child takes initiative and spends energy toward achieving mastery at the risk of feeling incompetent. Playing a competitive game with peers best illustrates this.

5. A nurse can expect which of these pubertal changes to occur first in the young girl?

   d. breast buds form

   Rationale: The earliest pubertal changes seen in female children occur as early as age 8 years and include the secondary characteristics of breast growth and the appearance of pubic hair.

Chapter 17

1. Which of the following best describes what Erikson meant by *generativity?*

   b. tutoring children in an after-school program

   Rationale: Although a, c, and d may all be activities enjoyed by adults in their middle years, *generativity,* as Erikson used the term, refers to imparting knowledge and wisdom along with giving time to a younger generation. Answer b involves learning interaction between generations and is the correct response.

2. As middle-aged adults develop spiritually, they

a. become more tolerant of other people's perspectives

Rationale: With increased life experience and exposure to a wider variety of people and situations, the middle adult tends to be less likely to see things as "either or" and to tolerate differences.

3. Which of the following is *not* an example of primary prevention by the nurse when working with a young adult?

d. providing support after a substance-abuse relapse

Rationale: Primary prevention seeks to promote healthy habits to avoid health problems or to identify them earlier to enhance treatment outcomes. Once someone has a substance abuse diagnosis, secondary (actual treatment) or tertiary prevention (preventing relapse) is appropriate.

4. During which phase of the nursing process is the nurse most likely to say to the middle adult, "Tell me about the chest pains you have been feeling?"

a. assessment

Rationale: Gathering information from the client to plan care, develop therapeutic interventions, and evaluate the effectiveness of care is an assessment function.

5. Middle-aged adults may find themselves having to provide care for an ailing spouse or a parent. Which of the following is *not* a good strategy by the nurse to help the caregiver and the client manage care at home?

d. take over all decisions about care and treatment

Rationale: The nurse helping a family member provide care in the home should encourage full participation by the client and the caregiver so that their priorities, values, and needs are included. The nurse who assumes this knowledge and takes over the decision-making process is not being supportive to those directly involved, even though the nurse may be well intentioned.

Chapter 18

1. Which developmental stage is Mrs. H. currently experiencing?

a. ego integrity versus despair

Rationale: The nurse must first determine which developmental stage the client is experiencing. This client is experiencing Erickson's stage of integrity versus despair. Mrs. H. is exhibiting despair when she begins to isolate herself and expresses to the nurse feelings of loneliness and uselessness.

2. The best nursing intervention you could design is to suggest that Mrs. H.

c. volunteer her services at the local Meals on Wheels program

Rationale: Your goal is to design an intervention that brings Mrs. H. into contact with others and makes her feel useful by giving of herself to others, thus increasing her self-esteem. Social interaction with others, contributing positively to society, and maintaining a sense of control

over the changes one is experiencing are essential to adapt to the psychological changes of aging.

3. As you begin your physical assessment, you notice that Mrs. H. has a beautiful tan. She tells you that she takes daily walks on the golf course to stay fit. After you compliment on her exercise routine, you must further assess which of the following?

d. what type of skin protection she uses

Rationale: The most important factor in aging of the skin is exposure to the sun.

4. While interviewing Mrs. H., you become impatient and feel a sense of urgency to move the interview along. The most likely reason for this is that

b. sensory changes in aging include a slowing down of all sensory processes, including the ability to answer questions quickly

Rationale: Important factors when interviewing older persons include sensitivity to perceptual losses and an attitude of respect and caring. Elderly clients require more time to answer questions.

5. When Mrs. H. returns for a follow-up visit, she tells you that she recently was turned down for a job at a local fast food restaurant that "only hires kids." This is an example of

e. ageism

Rationale: This is an example of an ageist bias. The following statements are also examples of ageism: "Older people belong on the shelf. They shouldn't take a younger person's job. Old people should retire; they lost their skills. They cannot do a decent job."

Chapter 19

1. By viewing a family group in terms of how well it works together and performs its roles, the nurse is utilizing the following family theory:

b. structural-functional

Rationale: Structural-functional theory views families in the context of how well they are able to fulfill their functions, both within and outside the family unit.

2. Family member roles

c. change as the family grows

Rationale: Each family member has multiple roles; some are easy to identify, and others are much more complex. They change as the family changes, grows, and moves in and out of stressful situations.

3. Through completing a family assessment, the nurse is able to

a. identify health issues of the family

Rationale: The family and the nurse work together to mutually establish goals and to evaluate progress. The purpose of the assessment is to help the family in identifying health issues of concern for the entire family.

4. Cultural influences in a family are important to determine in order to assess differences in

c. coping patterns to stress

Rationale: Cultural differences are seen most readily in value differences and coping patterns. How a person deals with stress is most often determined by his or her cultural background.

5. A genogram is a useful tool to determine

b. patterns of health problems through multiple generations

Rationale: All other answers reflect uses of the ecomap. The genogram is a family tree depicting structure through multiple generations. Symbols are used to identify illness and death.

Chapter 20

1. A nurse has just finished dressing the wound of a client with AIDS. The nurse should

c. dispose of the dressing in a biohazard bag that is placed in the infectious waste container

Rationale: Wound dressings usually have blood on them, as well as purulent material. OSHA requires bloody dressings to be discarded as potentially infectious material—thus, in a biohazard bag. Use a smaller bag in the client's room for convenience, and then transport the small bag to the larger infectious waste bag.

2. In the event of a fire in the client's room, the nurse should

d. rescue the client, sound the alarm, close all doors, and evacuate or extinguish the fire

Rationale: Remember "RACE": rescue, alarm, confine, extinguish. Always rescue the client in immediate danger first. Then sound the alarm to get help and alert others. Closing the doors helps to confine the fire to one room. Finally, extinguish the fire if possible or evacuate the area.

3. Standard precautions stress that

a. all body fluids from the client are potentially infectious

Rationale: The CDC recommends treating all body fluids from all clients as potentially infectious. This is because not every client that enters the health care system has been adequately tested for all bloodborne pathogens.

4. The three communicable diseases that require a special private room with negative air flow are

b. measles, chickenpox, and tuberculosis

Rationale: Measles, chicken pox, and tuberculosis all use air currents or droplet nuclei to stay airborne for long periods. Meningitis, mumps, and rubella require close contact (within 3 feet). AIDS is transmitted by the bloodborne route.

5. The easiest, most effective way to prevent transmission of infections is to

a. wash hands

Rationale: Antibiotics and the personal protective equipment that accompanies isolation effectively prevent transmission of disease but are costly. Soap, water, and friction remove transient bacteria on the hands. If an antimicrobial soap is used, many surface pathogens also are destroyed.

Chapter 21

1. The name of a drug that is considered the permanent drug name and reflects the chemical name is

d. generic name

Rationale: The generic name of a drug is its official name and reflects the chemical makeup of the drug.

2. The process by which a drug is transported by the circulating body fluids to various areas of the body is called

b. distribution

Rationale: Distribution refers to the transfer of the drug through the body.

3. Which of the following is a unit of weight measurement in the metric system?

b. kilogram

Rationale: Kilogram is a unit of weight in the metric system.

4. Which of the following individuals is legally permitted to dispense drugs?

c. pharmacist

Rationale: Only the pharmacist is legally permitted to dispense drugs.

5. For an average-sized adult, which of the following needle sizes would be appropriate to use when administering a subcutaneous injection?

b. 5/8 in

Rationale: A 5/8-in needle is used to administer a subcutaneous injection to an average-sized adult.

Chapter 22

1. During a bath, the nurse observes that a diabetic client's feet are very dry and cracking. The nurse should plan to

c. assess feet daily and apply lotion to feet

Rationale: Feet should be assessed daily for problems, and lotion should be applied to keep feet soft and less susceptible to injury.

2. Performing hygiene measures allows the nurse to do the following:

d. all of the above

Rationale: While the nurse performs hygiene measures, he or she can also do an assessment of all systems.

3. The layer of the skin that contains blood vessels, nerves, lymph, connective tissue, and fat cells is the

   b. dermis

   Rationale: The dermis of the skin contains these elements.

4. Tartar on the teeth can

   a. only be removed by a dental professional

   Rationale: Tartar is hard build-up that cannot be removed without special dental instruments.

5. When performing hygiene measures, the first thing the nurse should do is

   a. explain the procedure to the client

   Rationale: Explaining the procedure to the client reduces anxiety and allows him or her to be more comfortable.

Chapter 23

1. The most appropriate nursing intervention for a preulcer is

   b. determine cause and alleviate

   Rationale: Vigorous massage is contraindicated, as damage may occur at the capillary level. The key to prevention is to ascertain the cause and alleviate it. Applying an occlusive dressing may or may not be appropriate—it depends on the cause of the preulcer. If the ulcer is on the coccyx, for example, ROM will not be effective.

2. The nurse notes that a client's skin is reddened, with a small abrasion and serous fluid present. The nurse classifies this stage of ulcer formation as

   b. stage II

   Rationale: Reddening of the skin, with small abrasions and the presence of serous fluid, is characteristic of a stage II pressure ulcer.

3. The thick, black, leather-like crust of dead tissue that covers the ulcer is called

   a. eschar

   Rationale: This is the definition of eschar. Slough tissue is not described as thick and may be a variety of colors such as yellow or tan. Undermining is a description of the wound edges—not the wound tissue. Stage 3 is a pressure ulcer that is full thickness, not a description of the wound tissue.

4. In assessing wound drainage on a dressing from an abdominal incision, the nurse notes the drainage to be yellow and thick and a foul odor. The nurse would describe the drainage as

   a. purulent

   Rationale: Purulent is drainage described as containing phagocytized bacteria, dead white blood cells, and other wound debris. Serosanguineous drainage is thin and watery and pink-tinged, which denotes presence of blood. Sanguineous is bloody drainage. Serous is thin, watery, clear, or slightly cloudy drainage.

5. When turning a client after 60 minutes, the nurse notices a reddened area on the coccyx that remains for 15 seconds after the client was turned. Which of the following should the nurse do after measuring the reddened area?

   b. turn the client every 30 minutes

   Rationale: If a client has a reddened area after 1 hour, more frequent turning is necessary.

Chapter 24

1. Joshua Smee, a 16-year-old client, has been admitted to the emergency department for possible hypothermia. Mr. Smee was camping in the mountains when an unexpected blizzard occurred. In normal everyday experiences, the regulation of body temperature to changing environmental temperatures is controlled by

   b. the anterior and posterior hypothalamus

   Rationale: The balanced homeotherm state of body temperature is regulated by both the posterior and anterior hypothalamus. The anterior hypothalamus controls heat dissipation, and the posterior hypothalamus controls heat conservation.

2. Heat loss in the operating room where the air temperature is considerably lower than the body's temperature, would primarily result from

   c. radiation

   Rationale: Radiation is responsible for the majority of heat loss that occurs in a cold room. Radiation occurs as heat is transferred from the client's warm body through infared heat rays to cooler objects in the room.

3. Norma Johnson, an 80-year-old client, was discovered in her unheated home during freezing weather. She is admitted for suspected moderate hypothermia. Which of the following symptoms support this?

   a. decreased respiratory and cardiac rate

   Rationale: Decreased cardiopulmonary function occurs when a client is experiencing moderate hypothermia. Shivering is no longer present due to impaired hypothalamic function.

4. When taking a rectal temperature in an infant, the thermometer should be inserted into the rectum

   c. 0.5 in

   Rationale: The thermometer should be placed no more than 0.5 in into the rectum. An incorrectly placed thermometer that is inserted too far into the rectum could puncture the colon or rectum.

5. Nancy Thomas injured her foot while riding a bike. She was seen in the emergency department and had multiple sutures for a large laceration and was also told she had a severe sprain of her ankle. She was instructed to use cold therapy during the next 24 hours. What is the reason for the use of cold?

   b. blood viscosity is increased, but a decrease of cellular metabolism occurs

   Rationale: Cold therapy results in an increased blood viscosity, which facilitates clotting and prevents further bleeding. It also slows cellular metabolism, decreasing inflammation, which causes tissue damage.

Chapter 25

1. The hip joint is an example of a
   b. ball-and-socket joint

   Rationale: The hip consists of a ball-shaped head fitting into a concave shape. One articulates around the other.

2. The center of gravity is
   b. the point at which the body's center of mass is located

   Rationale: The center of gravity is where the center of the mass of an object is located.

3. Risk factors for the immobilized elderly client include
   a. decreased cognition
   b. incontinence of the bladder
   c. incontinence of the bowel
   d. visual impairment
   e. multiple chronic diseases
   3. all of the above

   Rationale: These are factors that cause physiological responses that lead to deterioration in the elderly because of decreased reserve.

4. Which of the following statements are true?
   2. b, d

   Rationale: Hinge joints permit flexion and extension. Gliding joints allow abduction and adduction, as well as flexion and extension.

5. Mr. Smith is going home after having a hip joint replaced. He is able to partially bear weight and needs to use crutches. Which gait pattern is most appropriate for him?
   b. three-point-and-one gait

   Rationale: This gait is appropriate for clients who can participate in a partial–weight-bearing program.

Chapter 26

1. The stage of sleep that is necessary for psychological restoration and for learning and memory to occur is
   d. REM

   Rationale: REM sleep is the time in the sleep cycle when psychological restoration occurs. This stage of sleep is necessary for memory and learning to occur. The exact functions of the NREM portions of the sleep cycle are not understood completely.

2. A client reports that he is having difficulty falling asleep, is experiencing frequent awakenings, and feels that his sleep is totally inadequate. The sleep disorder the client is describing is
   b. insomnia

   Rationale: Insomnia is a perception of inadequate sleep

and includes difficulty in initiating sleep, frequent awakenings from sleep, and a perception of a nonrestorative sleep. Narcolepsy is a disorder characterized by a set of clinical symptoms including abnormal sleep; overwhelming episodes of sleep that occur at inappropriate times; excessive daytime sleepiness; hallucinations; disturbances in nighttime sleep; and paroxysmal muscle weakness, catalepsy, and sleep paralysis. *Sleep apnea* is a term that describes one of two syndromes: obstructive sleep apnea or central sleep apnea.

3. Nursing interventions for a client with a sleep pattern disturbance include all of the following *except*
   c. increasing environmental stimuli

   Rationale: Increasing environmental stimuli does not facilitate sleep. This action would serve to worsen the sleep pattern disturbance.

4. If a client is on 10 mg of intravenous morphine every 4 hours, what would be the 24-hour dose of hydromorphone to provide the same analgesic effect?
   d. 9 mg

   Rationale: One needs to use an equianalgesic conversion chart to determine the correct dose of hydromorphone. Begin by calculating the 24-hour dose of morphine that the client is taking (*i.e.,* 10 mg every 4 hours would be a total of 60 mg in 24 hours). The equianalgesic doses of hydromorphone and morphine are as follows: 1.5 mg of intravenous hydromorphone is equivalent to 10 mg of intravenous morphine. Therefore, this client would need to receive a total of 9.0 mg of hydromorphone in a 24-hour period.

5. Nurses who are caring for clients with cancer who are taking opioids on a chronic basis need to assess them for all of the following *except*
   d. addiction

   Rationale: Clients with cancer who are taking opioid analgesics on a regular schedule develop tolerance, constipation, and sedation. Addiction, or psychological preoccupation with procuring a substance for effects other than their analgesic effects, is not a problem for clients who are taking pain medication to relieve pain associated with cancer or cancer treatment.

Chapter 27

1. A community health nurse is evaluating possible malnutrition in the elderly. What parameters would the nurse investigate?
   c. support systems

   Rationale: If the elderly have support systems, they are more likely to obtain and eat food. Without support systems, the elderly are more likely candidates for malnutrition because of decreased intake from lack of obtaining or eating food.

2. For a nurse to perform a nutritional assessment, which behavior is necessary?
   a. gather anthropometric data

   Rationale: Assessment is gathering data and anthropometric measures, including height, weight, and skinfold and circumference measurements.

3. On performing a nutritional assessment, what finding would warrant notifying the doctor?

   a. weight went from 100 lb to 93 lb in 1 month

   Rationale: This is a weight loss of greater than 5% within the last month.

4. A nurse writes a nutritional goal as follows: "Client will eat 95% of meals within 3 days." After 1 day, the nurse observes that the client ate 45% of meals. What should the nurse do?

   b. continue to observe the client's intake

   Rationale: Continuing to observe the client's intake is indicated because the goal is to be met in 3 days, not in 1 day.

5. Which intervention would the nurse perform for a client with a diagnosis of Altered Nutrition: Less Than Body Requirements?

   d. encourage exercising on a regular basis

   Rationale: Exercise can stimulate the appetite and prevent nervous tension, which can cause an excessive use of kilocalories.

Chapter 28

1. The cation found in greatest concentration in the ECF and responsible for fluid balance is

   a. sodium

   Rationale: Sodium is the primary cation of ECF, and as the major determinant of ECF osmolarity, sodium also helps control fluid volume.

2. Water moves across a semipermeable membrane by the process of

   b. osmosis

   Rationale: Osmosis is the net movement of water across a semipermeable membrane in response to a concentration difference until equilibrium is obtained.

3. M. B., a 66-year-old client, is at risk for fluid volume overload. In planning care for M. B., the nurse should

   c. weigh daily

   Rationale: M. B. should be weighed daily at the same time using the same scale, as weight is the most sensitive indicator of change in fluid volume status.

4. Respiratory acidosis is associated with

   d. hypoventilation

   Rationale: Hypoventilation results in a decreased secretion of carbon dioxide, and, as carbon dioxide levels increase, the blood pH decreases, resulting in respiratory acidosis.

5. Your client has an intravenous solution infusing into the right hand. On assessment, you note that the hand is swollen, cool to the touch, and pale. Your first action would be to

   b. discontinue the IV catheter and restart in the other arm

   Rationale: Signs of IV fluid infiltration include swelling at the site, cool temperature, and pale color. To decrease further complications, the nurse removes the IV cannula and restarts the IV in the opposite extremity.

Chapter 29

1. An arterial blood gas is ordered for a 25-year-old woman in the emergency room with status asthmaticus. After obtaining the blood, which of the following measures is essential for the nurse to implement?

   b. hold pressure on the site for at least 5 minutes

   Rationale: Firm pressure must be applied for 5 minutes to prevent bleeding or hematoma formation. The artery has been entered to obtain the sample. Longer and firmer pressure must be applied to an artery than to a vein.

2. A 59-year-old man is admitted to the floor with a chest tube in the right midaxillary line. Essential equipment to be kept at the bedside includes

   d. clamps and petroleum gauze pads

   Rationale: Clamps and petroleum gauze are kept at the bedside in the event that the tubing becomes disconnected or dislodges. If the tube becomes disconnected, the clamp is applied proximal to the disconnection (close to the client). If the tube dislodges and is accidentally removed, the petroleum gauze is placed over the open wound. Both of these interventions are temporary until the system is reestablished.

3. The nurse assesses a client's respiratory rate at 36. This rate is termed

   a. tachypnea

   Rationale: The condition in which respiratory rates are greater than 20 in the adult is termed tachypnea. Less than 12 is bradypnea. No respirations is apnea.

4. A 56-year-old man is admitted to the emergency room with a complaint of shortness of breath. To promote respiratory expansion and comfort, the client should be placed in which position?

   c. high-Fowler's

   Rationale: High-Fowler's position places the client sitting upright at approximately 90 degrees. This allows for unrestricted movement of the chest, diaphragm, and other muscles of respiration.

5. The amount of air inhaled and exhaled during normal quiet breathing is termed

   d. tidal volume

   Rationale: Tidal volume is the total amount of air in milliliters during one cycle of inspiration and expiration. It is approximately 10 mm/kg in the adult.

Chapter 30

1. The nurse assesses Mr. Wilson's apical rate to be 90 beats per minute, but the radial pulse is 74 beats per minute. You know that this is indicative of

   b. pulse deficit

   Rationale: Pulse deficit is defined as a significant difference between apical and radial pulse.

2. Susan Hart, 35 years old, is on β-blocker medication to lower her blood pressure. Since β-blockers lower both blood pressure and heart rate, she is in need of learning how to take her pulse. Methods of teaching her this procedure include

   c. palpating her radial pulse for 30 seconds

   Rationale: Radial pulses should be palpated for 15 seconds to 1 minute. If the heart rate is irregular, the pulse should be checked for 1 minute.

3. Your client is nervous about the "cardiac catheterization" that she will be undergoing tomorrow. She tells you that her friend told her that it is a very dangerous procedure and that she will be incapacitated for 1 week afterward. You would want to teach her that following a cardiac catherization

   a. she may need to lie flat in bed for several hours but then will be allowed out of bed

   Rationale: Usually the groin area is used for access for the procedure. To promote hemostasis at the site and avoid clot disruption, the client is usually instructed to lie flat for several hours.

4. When taking a blood pressure, the nurse should first

   d. palpate a radial pulse

   Rationale: This identifies approximate systolic blood pressure.

5. When auscultating heart sounds, the nurse should:

   b. Use both the bell and the diaphragm

   Rationale: The diaphragm allows the nurse to hear high-pitched sounds, and the bell, low-pitched sounds.

Chapter 31

1. When administering enteral feedings, the head of the bed should be

   d. elevated 30 degrees

   Rationale: Maintaining a 30-degree position helps to prevent aspiration and offers a more natural position for the client.

2. Which one of the following reasons is NOT a purpose for enemas?

   a. to maintain bowel regularity

   Rationale: An enema should not be used for maintaining bowel regularity, as it would promote dependence.

3. Mrs. A. has a transverse colostomy, and she is very upset about "the awful odor." The nurse should suggest that

Mrs. A. consume which of the following vegetables to help decrease odor?

   b. spinach

   Rationale: Green vegetables, such as spinach, have a high chlorophyll content, which helps to alleviate odor.

4. Which of these conditions contributes to bowel elimination changes in the elderly?

   b. decreased chewing ability

   Rationale: As the elderly person loses his or her teeth, his or her chewing ability is decreased.

5. The correct order in which to assess the abdomen would be

   a. inspection, auscultation, percussion, palpation

   Rationale: Inspection is always the first assessment to be done. If percussion and palpation are done before auscultation, they could alter auscultation findings.

Chapter 32

1. What is the functional unit of the kidney?

   d. nephron

   Rationale: Each kidney has more than a million functional units, called nephrons. The function of the kidney is to filter the blood. Nutritional substances are reabsorbed into the plasma, and waste products are excreted via urine. Bowman's capsule is part of the nephron structure. Ureters are the two muscular tubes that transport urine from the renal pelvis of the kidney to the urinary bladder. The bladder's function is to store urine.

2. What is the minimum amount of urine required in an adult to maintain kidney function?

   b. 30 ml/hour

   Rationale: One of the indicators of kidney function is hourly urine output. The minimum amount of urine required to maintain kidney function is 30 ml/hour.

3. How do the kidneys change as the adult ages?

   a. the kidneys respond slower to changes in fluid and electrolyte composition

   Rationale: As a person ages, kidney function decreases and responds more slowly to changes in fluid and electrolyte composition. Several structural changes affect kidney function, such as a decrease in kidney size and reserve nephrons. Renal perfusion and glomerular filtration also decrease with age.

4. Which of the following drug classifications has a side effect of urinary retention?

   c. anticholinergics

   Rationale: Anticholinergics inhibit the parasympathetic nervous system, which controls the micturition reflex center (S2–S4). Voluntary control and reflex urination cannot occur. Diuretics increase urine volume and excretion by interfering with sodium reabsorption at the nephron tubular sites. Fecal impaction may block the urethral structures, thus contributing to urinary retention. Laxatives can help alleviate fecal impaction and urinary retention. Sedatives such as flurazepam (Dalmane) and diazepam (Valium) may contribute to confusion in the elderly, which may cause functional incontinence.

5. A client has had his Foley catheter removed 4 hours ago and has not voided. Which of the following nursing actions would the nurse perform FIRST?

d. palpate at the symphysis pubis

Rationale: Prior to nursing interventions, the nurse needs to assess for bladder distention. A bladder that can be percussed and palpated more than two finger breadths above the pubic symphysis indicates bladder distention. If the bladder is distended, the nurse would promote voiding by noninvasive measures. If these measures were ineffective, the nurse would call the physician and perform intermittent catheterization to alleviate the urinary retention.

Chapter 33

1. A person experiencing a severe degree of anxiety related to a health problem can be expected to

c. deny the problem and rationalize the presence of signs and symptoms

Rationale: Mild to moderate levels of anxiety may cause a person to mobilize his or her resources to seek appropriate care. Severe anxiety is more likely to overwhelm the person's ordinary coping skills and provoke the person to deny that a problem exists; in this way, the person's self-concept is protected from the awareness of any threat.

2. The client least likely to experience a crisis as a result of illness or injury is someone who

d. has an internal locus of control and low levels of trait anxiety

Rationale: A person with an internal locus of control is most likely to believe that he or she can positively influence the outcome of an illness. An individual with low levels of trait anxiety is not likely to perceive a change in health status as an overwhelming stressor and is more likely to mobilize his or her ordinary coping strategies.

3. George Donohue, a 79-year-old retired police detective, resides in a nursing home. He has mild dementia and loves to talk with people. He tells the nurse that he doesn't feel important anymore. The intervention that is most likely to enhance Mr. Donohue's self-esteem is

c. encouraging him to talk about his days on the police force

Rationale: Elders with mild dementia still recall events from earlier in their life. Encouraging Mr. Donohue to share his memories of his work will support his identity and self-concept. Flattery, distraction, and requesting that his relatives visit will have limited impact on his self-esteem.

4. Mary Lee is a registered nurse working in an area where the population is culturally diverse. It is important that she

c. respect the values and health care practices of her clients and their families

Rationale: The nurse who respects the values and health care practices of his or her clients and their families will deliver culturally appropriate and sensitive care. It is not necessary to know the specific practices of every cultural group. It is necessary to convey consideration of cultural differences and a willingness to learn from clients and families.

5. Mr. Stern, a 55-year-old, married, overweight businessman who smokes cigarettes, is brought by ambulance to the emergency department with crushing chest pain. Education about "heart smart" living is likely to be most effective if provided

c. at home with his wife present

Rationale: Clients learn best when they are relaxed, over the initial crisis, and supported by their significant others.

Chapter 34

1. Stimuli are

c. events or changes that provoke or excite a nerve

Rationale: Stimuli include anything that can be seen, heard, smelled, tasted, felt, or detected by the nervous system.

2. The stimulus-response process consists of

a. reception, transmission, interpretation, perception, and response

Rationale: Stimuli are received by sensory receptors (reception), transmitted across synapses from neuron to neuron, and routed to structures in the central nervous system (transmission), where they are defined (interpretation), assigned meaning (perception), and acted on (response).

3. Manifestations of altered sensory perception include

d. all of the above

Rationale: All of the above are examples of behaviors that may present when the amount, intensity, and quality of stimuli exceed a person's range of tolerance or perceptive capabilities.

4. Barriers to accurate sensory perception do not include

d. being able to see a clock

Rationale: Being able to see a clock and know the time of day provides environmental cues that promote orientation and appropriate behavior. Too much or too little stimulation, separation from familiar people, and poor oxygenation represent conditions or events that interfere with accurate perception and response to stimuli.

5. Which answer best describes services or methods appropriate for people with sensory organ impairments?

a. sign language interpreters, telecommunication devices for the deaf, note writing

Rationale: Sensory organ function should be augmented with services and devices that enhance the ability to give and receive information; *e.g.,* sign language interpretation, telecommunication devices for the deaf, and other assistive services or devices.

Chapter 35

1. An example of a theistic nursing intervention is

   c. prayer

   Rationale: The use of prayer is based on a belief in a personal god who answers prayer; the other interventions may be based on a pantheistic world view that states that everything is god.

2. *Pantheism* refers to

   b. a belief that we are all god

   Rationale: Pantheism holds that everything is god; therefore, we are all god.

3. Assessment of spiritual needs includes all of the following except

   a. finding out everything about the client's religion

   Rationale: It is not necessary to find out everything about the client's religion; it is essential to discover what meaning the client ascribes to his or her religion and religious practices.

4. The universal aspects of a spiritual world view include all of the following except

   b. a sense of connectedness with something greater than ourselves

   Rationale: The belief that there is one god is not a universal aspect of spiritual world views. In fact, there are spiritual world views that espouse belief in multiple gods or deities. The universal qualities of a spiritual world view include a sense of connectedness to something greater than self, a search for meaning and purpose, and a sense of connectedness to others.

5. Which of the following statements about spiritual development are incorrect?

   a. spiritual development somewhat parallels cognitive development

   Rationale: Children construct their own simplistic world views that tend to provide concrete explanations for abstract concepts such as spirit. As they mature, they tend to identify with the spiritual world views of their parents.

Chapter 36

1. You are caring for an Asian woman at home who is currently taking digoxin, Lasix (furosemide), and Slow-K (potassium chloride) for a heart condition. You notice that she drinks an herbal tea each morning. Which of the following is your most appropriate intervention?

   a. assess the contents of the tea

   Rationale: The nurse must assess the tea first before providing care. Assessment is the first stage of the nursing process and should be the cornerstone for all community health nursing activities, especially when the nurse is faced with a culturally specific behavior or practice. Full assessments will avoid false judgments or rushed judgments and can enhance effective interventions.

2. A community health nurse states that all people living in the United States should learn to speak English. The nurse is displaying signs of

   d. cultural imposition

   Rationale: Cultural imposition is when a person not only believes that his or her cultural practices are better than other but also expects immigrants to his or her country to adopt those practices in replacement of their own.

3. You have just given a talk on safe sex to a group of African-American teenagers. One of the young women yells from the back of the room, "It is against my religion to use birth control. How can I practice safe sex?" What is the proper response?

   d. "I understand that these are complicated issues. It is your choice to practice safe sex knowing what you learned in today's class about the transmission of HIV."

   Rationale: When conducting health education in the community, the nurse needs to be an expert in health education. Part of this expertise is when the nurse can adjust his or her knowledge of developmental stages. This nurse in this example acknowledges the student's response and then refocuses the group on the primary goals of the education.

4. Which cultural group is likely to use the services of *curanderos* (folk healers) and *parteras* (lay midwives)?

   c. Mexican Americans

   Rationale: These are Hispanic terms for folk healers.

5. The "culture shock" that many immigrants experience after coming to the United States can be relieved by which of the following community health services?

   d. small group meetings at a cultural-specific community center with acclimated immigrants and new arrivals

   Rationale: When developing nursing interventions for the prevention or reduction of cultural shock, the nurse should use settings and persons who are nonthreatening and can foster learning. In this example, the nurse uses a community center that is known to the cultural group and persons who have successfully assimilated into the dominant culture. These techniques will be supportive and very informative.

Chapter 37

1. Sexuality is defined as

   c. the holistic state of being male or female

   Rationale: Sexuality encompasses a person's entire being—not just biological aspects of being.

2. Which of the following is true regarding the role of the nurse in sexual health care?

   b. the nurse must be aware of his or her own sexual feelings in all client interactions

Rationale: Self-awareness on the part of the nurse regarding sexuality allows him or her to make decisions with full knowledge.

3. Which of the following is true of sexuality in adulthood?

   b. sexuality continues until death

   Rationale: Because sexuality is intertwined with all other aspects of the self, sexuality is a part of all phases of the life cycle.

4. Which of the following is true of homosexuality?

   c. it has existed in most recorded cultures

   Rationale: Historical and anthropological literature indicates that homosexuality has existed in most cultures and has been treated differently by different cultures.

5. The role of the nurse in treating persons with a sexual dysfunction is to

   a. provide education and support

   Rationale: Along with other health care professionals, nurses participate in the treatment of persons with sexual dysfunctions, primarily by providing education and social support.

Chapter 38

1. When a client is in denial about his or her terminal illness and is refusing chemotherapy, it is important for the nurse to

   a. clarify what the client has been told

   Rationale: This is a good place to start. Next you will want to know what meaning the client gives to what he or she has been told.

2. When coming on a tearful client who is dying, the nurse should

   c. inquire what the tears are about

   Rationale: Although many people cannot articulate the reason for their concerns, this is a place to start. If the person does not want to talk, he or she can always indicate this.

3. Which of the following behaviors might be considered a normal response to just learning of the death of a loved one?

   e. all of the above

   Rationale: There is a wide range of what is normal with acute grief—almost anything is normal.

4. You are caring for a dying client who whispers to you, "Am I going to die?" How might you respond?

   d. "Tell me more about your thoughts and concerns."

   Rationale: You want to know more about the question, and the client's own answer will be important.

5. Nurses dealing with dying clients need to

   e. know how to allow a person to deal with his or her own emotional pain

Rationale: This is perhaps the most vital piece of wisdom. One cannot take away the pain of grief.

Chapter 39

1. Surgery performed to relieve symptoms of an illness but that does not cure the disease is known as

   c. palliative

   Rationale: Palliative surgery relieves the symptoms of an illness but does not cure the disease. It can improve the quality of life and possibly ease chronic pain.

2. The anesthesia classification that describes a client as one with severe systemic disease without functional limitations: (cardiovascular disease that limits activity, severe diabetes with systemic complications, or poorly controlled hypertension) would be considered a class

   c. III

   Rationale: Class II includes severe systemic disease without functional limitation; cardiovascular or pulmonary disease that limits activity; severe diabetes with systemic complications, history of myocardial infarction, angina pectoris, or poorly controlled hypertension.

3. The anesthesia involving blocking a specific set of nerve fibers or an individual nerve is known as

   b. regional anesthesia

   Rationale: Regional anesthesia involves blocking a specific set of nerve fibers or an individual nerve. The more familiar types of regional anesthesia include spinal, epidural, caudal, and peripheral nerve blocks.

4. A complication of spinal anesthesia is

   b. spinal headache

   Rationale: Complications of spinal anesthesia include hypotension, spinal headaches, and urinary retention.

5. The scope of nursing practice throughout the surgical experience is

   a. perioperative nursing

   Rationale: The perioperative experience begins when the client decides to have a surgical procedure and ends when the client returns to an acceptable level of function or to some form of resolution of the initial problem.

Chapter 40

1. As a home health care nurse, you have been asked by the physician to evaluate Mr. Black's home. Mr. Black suffered a stroke that left him paralyzed on the left side, and he is being discharged home from the hospital with a quadripod cane tomorrow. Which of the following would you consider FIRST in your evaluation?

   c. location of throw rugs and electrical cords

   Rationale: Environmental adaptations are often necessary to ensure safety and the client's highest level of functioning. Throw rugs and electrical cords could cause the client to trip and fall.

2. Mrs. B., an 80-year-old woman with a hip replacement, is being evaluated for discharge from the rehabilitation unit in 4 days. To assess Mrs. B.'s cognitive functioning, the nurse will administer a mini mental examination. The nurse explains to Mrs. B. that she will be giving her a simple test. Mrs. B. starts to cry and says "I always do horrible on tests, please don't make me take this one." The MOST APPROPRIATE action for the nurse at this time would be to

c. incorporate the questions of the mini mental examination in the general interview

Rationale: It is important to evaluate the client's cognitive status to develop teaching plans tailored to meet the client's individual needs, but the evaluation need not be stressful for the client.

3. A home health care nurse is scheduled for a first visit to a 68-year-old client who is a newly diagnosed diabetic. Which of the following activities would need to be completed before the admission visit?

b. planning the visit

Rationale: The nurse needs to plan his or her visit using the nursing process to ensure that he or she has all the necessary information and equipment to meet the client's needs.

4. Home health nurses consider key safety issues on their first visit to a client's home. Select the issue that applies to Mrs. Boyd, a woman with left side weakness because of a stroke who is moderately obese.

b. mobility and the home

Rationale: The nurse needs to assist the client to be independent in the home, as well as to consider the client's safety in mobility when a stroke affects ambulation.

5. Which of the following is an important consideration when the nurse IMPLEMENTS nursing interventions?

c. integrate the nursing care intervention into the client's lifestyle and culture

Rationale: The nurse needs to be sensitive to the many cultural differences seen in practice so that plans are tailored to the clients' and families' preferences and needs.

Glossary

abortion: termination of a pregnancy, whether spontaneous (*i.e.,* the body rejects the fetus) or elective (*i.e.,* the woman chooses a medical procedure to remove the fetus), prior to the fetus reaching the age of viability.

absorption: the process by which the drug molecule is transferred from the site where it enters the body to the circulating body fluids.

accountability: a professional characteristic of nursing whereby nurses take responsibility for the outcomes and standards of practice.

acculturation: change process resulting from contact between cultural groups.

acid: any substance that releases a hydrogen ion into a solution.

acidosis: an increase in hydrogen ion concentration with a decrease in pH below 7.40.

acne: inflammation of the sebaceous glands, often characterized by pustular eruptions of the skin.

acrocyanosis: bluish discoloration of the hands and feet; a normal finding in the newborn.

active listening: listening in which the nurse takes an active part by eliciting details from the client and by inviting the client to think more about what is being said.

active transport: movement of substances against a concentration gradient, requiring energy in the form of the adenosine triphosphate as well as a carrier substance.

acute confusional state: a temporary condition characterized by sudden onset, confusion, agitation, disorientation, and impaired higher-level thought processes.

acute pain: a painful condition of limited duration (*i.e.,* usually less than 3 months) that usually signals an underlying problem. Once the problem is corrected, the pain abates.

adaptation: the adjustment of an organism to changes in its environment.

addiction: a state whereby an individual becomes physically and psychologically dependent on a chemical substance.

adjuvant analgesics: drugs that have a primary indication other than pain but produce analgesia in certain painful conditions.

advance directives: documents that express the wishes of clients regarding what they want done or not done in certain circumstances surrounding death or possible death. May include the designation of a person (health care proxy or durable power of attorney) to make decisions for them should they be rendered incapable of making such decisions.

advanced practice nurse: a licensed registered nurse who has completed a master's degree in nursing from a program that offers the clinical specialist track, nurse clinician track, nurse practitioner track, certified nurse-midwife track, and/or nurse anesthetist track.

adventitious: abnormal.

adverse effect: unintended or side effect of a drug.

advocate: one who defends, pleads case of, promotes right of, attempts to change the system on behalf of another person (Bower, 1982).

aerosolization: dispersion of a fine mist.

affective domain: learning that emphasizes feeling and emotion, such as interests, attitudes, appreciation, and methods of adjustment.

ageism: discrimination toward another person based on age; like racism.

airway resistance: the factors that impede airflow into the lungs.

alkalosis: a decrease in hydrogen ion concentration with an increase in pH above 7.40.

alopecia: loss of hair; acute condition often caused by chemotherapy, radiation, and certain disease processes.

Alzheimer's disease: the major cause of dementia. Changes in the brain affect memory and are characterized by loss of judgment, carelessness, and loss of interest.

ambulation: ability to walk.

anabolism: growth-producing; nutrients are utilized to build or synthesize larger compounds.

anesthetic: a chemical agent, *e.g.,* inhalation, injection, topical, that blocks sensation.

aneurysm: dilation or weakness of a blood vessel. It is often described as a localized ballooning of the vessel.

angina: abnormal chest sensation or pain resulting from decreased coronary blood flow or increased cardiac tissue demand.

anions: negatively charged electrolytes, including bicarbonate, chloride, phosphate, and sulfate.

anorexia nervosa: eating disorder characterized by compulsive undereating that results in starvation and sometimes death.

anthropology: the study of human origins from physical, social, and environmental aspects.

anthropometric measurements: measurement of size and weight of the body that can be used in assessing a client's nutritional status.

anticipatory grief: the responses (thoughts, feelings, behaviors) experienced in advance of an actual loss or separation. These may be as intense as the reactions related to an actual loss and can help to prepare a person as in a rehearsal of responses.

anticipatory guidance: preparation of parents regarding normal growth and development prior to the occurrence of an expected event.

antimicrobial agent: a chemical or biological agent that stops or destroys bacteria, fungi, or viruses.

antipyretic: a substance that relieves fever. An antipyretic drug aids the body in reducing temperature elevations.

antiseptic: a chemical used on living tissue that either inhibits or destroys the growth of microorganisms.

anuria: output of less than 100 ml of urine in 24 hours.

anxiety: the individual's response to perceived threats to the self-concept. The response involves physiological and psychological manifestations, including diffuse apprehension that is vague in nature and is associated with feelings of uncertainty and helplessness (May, 1950).

Apgar score: a rapid evaluation of the newborn at birth that assesses color, heart rate, reflex irritability, and muscle tone.

apocrine glands: located in axillary and genital areas. The secretions of the apocrine glands are responsible for body odor.

arterial blood gas (ABG): diagnostic laboratory study that reveals important information about the status of arterial oxygenation and acid-base balance.

arteriogram: an invasive procedure examining arterial blood flow to an area.

arteriosclerosis: thickening of arterioles due to fatty deposits and lesions with loss of vessel elasticity and contractility.

asepsis: absence of infection or infectious material.

aseptic technique: the practice of maintaining a sterile environment throughout the intraoperative phase of the surgical experience.

assessment: the organized, purposeful collection and validation of data about the client's health status.

assimilation: that which brings uniformity or agreement; conversion of specific cultural traits through absorption by the dominating culture; adoption by the minority group of the majority group mores (Marks *et al.,* 1987).

asthma: a condition of recurrent attacks of paroxysmal dyspnea, accompanied by wheezing due to spasmodic contractions of the bronchi.

atelectasis: blockage of bronchioles by an accumulation of secretions that result from decreased ventilation; can lead to lung collapse or incomplete lung expansion.

attending behaviors: behaviors that show that the nurse is paying attention to what the client is saying. Examples include facing the client, leaning toward the client, using appropriate eye contact, keeping eyes open with eyebrows raised, and maintaining an open body posture.

auscultation: involves the sense of hearing when listening to sounds produced by various organs and systems.

autologous blood: blood collected from the intended recipient.

autonomic nervous system (ANS): the portion of the nervous system consisting of parasympathetic systems and primarily controlling involuntary body functions.

autonomy: a condition whereby a person is free to choose, to decide, and to act.

bacteria: free-living, single-celled microorganisms that occur in nature and in the human body.

bacteriuria: bacteria in the urine.

barrel chest: abnormal configuration of the chest from chronic respiratory conditions, such as emphysema, in which the lateral measurements of the chest approximate the anteroposterior measurement.

barriers: risk factors or conditions that interfere with the perception of and response to stimuli.

basal metabolic rate: the amount of energy necessary for the body to function at a resting state.

base: any substance that sequesters a hydrogen ion when in solution.

bedtime rituals: specific routines (*e.g.,* putting on bed clothes, brushing one's teeth, reading, or watching television) that a person does prior to going to sleep.

beliefs: statements held as true although lacking in empirical evidence; highly valued by individuals and can motivate health care practices.

beneficence: the duty to promote what is good for clients.

benign prostatic hypertrophy: enlargement of the prostate gland; associated with aging.

bereavement: the state or fact of being without a loved one due to death.

bioavailability: extent to which the active ingredients of a drug are absorbed and transported to their sites of action.

biofeedback training: a process that involves using feedback methods to teach individuals to be sensitive to and aware of body cues so that they can cognitively control certain involuntary physiologic functions.

biotransformation: process by which a drug molecule is chemically altered through the action of enzymes and is converted to a less active, harmless substance.

body language: nonverbal communication behaviors that are accomplished by how we move our bodies or body parts, present ourselves to the world, and use the personal space around us.

body substance isolation: isolation protocols that focus on barrier precautions rather than disease identification.

body temperature: balance of heat produced and heat lost by the body. The average body temperature is 98.6°F.

breast self-examination (BSE): a routine, systematic procedure whereby a woman examines her breasts for evidence of change that could indicate a malignant process.

bulimia: an eating disorder characterized by repeated episodes of overeating following by elimination through either vomiting or the use of laxatives.

burnout: a condition of physical and emotional exhaustion experienced as a result of job stressors related to caring for the ill and troubled.

calculi (stone): an abnormal concentration of mineral salts occurring in any part of the urinary tract.

capillary refill: time required for blood to return to an area after pressure to a site is removed. Normal result is 3 to 5 seconds.

caput succedaneum: a localized pitting edema in the scalp of a newborn usually formed during labor. At birth the baby's head may appear deformed, but the swelling begins to resolve immediately and is usually gone in a few days. Compare **cephalhematoma; molding.**

cardiac catheterization: invasive procedure in which a catheter is inserted into the heart to examine coronary arteries and pressures within the heart.

cardiac cycle: the time from the initiation of cardiac filling to the completion of contraction.

cardiac output: amount of blood ejected from the left ventricle during a 1-minute period. Cardiac output is computed as stroke volume times heart rate (CO = SV × HR).

caries (cavity): progressive erosion and destruction of the outer enamel of the tooth.

catabolism: the breaking down of complex substances into simpler substances.

cathartic: a medication that causes bowel evacuation.

catheterization: insertion of a tube (catheter) into the bladder to obtain urine. The catheter may be left in place for a long time (indwelling catheter) or inserted intermittently (intermittent catheterization).

cations: positively charged electrolytes, including sodium, calcium, potassium, and magnesium.

Centers for Disease Control and Prevention (CDC): the principal public health agency of the federal government concerned with infectious and noninfectious disease control.

central nervous system: the division of the nervous system that contains the brain and spinal cord.

cephalocaudal development: the sequence of body growth and maturation that proceeds from head to foot.

cephalhematoma: swelling of the scalp caused by subcutaneous bleeding and accumulation of blood resulting from birth trauma, often from forceps. Large cephalhematomas may become infected, require surgical drainage, and take several months to resolve. Compare **caput succedaneum; molding.**

certification: nurses who have met specific requirements in education and functional practice in a specialized area and receive endorsement from peers are eligible to take an examination that will result in certification. Certification examinations are based on national standards set by an organization such as the American Nurses Association Congress for Nursing Practice.

cerumen: secreted by the ceruminal glands located in the ears. Cerumen is a golden-brown waxy substance that protects the ear by trapping foreign material entering the ear.

ceruminal gland: gland located in the ear that secretes cerumen (wax).

change of shift report: a report in which one nurse sums up for one or more other nurses all the information necessary for the other nurses to safely assume responsibility for continuing the care of the clients.

chemoreceptor reflex: response of sensory nerve cell activated by chemical stimuli, such as a chemoreceptor in the carotid artery that is sensitive to the carbon dioxide in the blood, signaling the respiratory center in the brain to increase or decrease respiration.

child maltreatment syndrome: child abuse; all factors involving intentional harm to, or avoidable endangerment of, someone less than 18 years of age.

chronic pain: a painful condition of indefinite duration (*i.e.*, usually greater than 3 months) that is associated with sleep disturbances, changes in the client's mood, and a decrease in the client's quality of life.

circulating nurse: team coordinator for the client's care and safety throughout the intraoperative phase of the surgical experience.

circumcision: surgical removal of the foreskin of the penis, frequently performed shortly after birth.

clean wound: a wound in which pathogens are not present.

climacteric: a critical period in one's life.

clinical nurse specialist: an advanced practice degree from a master's degree program designed to prepare the registered nurse as an expert in a specialty area, such as direct care, consultation, education, research, managerial, and/or administrative components. This role is similar in educational preparation and work to the nurse clinician and the nurse practitioner. Differences may be in the area of work and focus of the rule.

clinical reasoning: the process by which collected data are analyzed and diagnostic statements are made.

closed-system catheterization: process by which a catheterization is performed with a sterile bag. Urine drainage is confined within the attached drainage bag.

closed questions: those that are appropriate for obtaining specific factual information and that usually begin with "what," "how," and "which."

cognitive conceit: a trait of late school-age children whereby they think they know more than adults.

cognitive development: the mental process of knowing or understanding.

cognitive domain: Learning that emphasizes intellectual outcomes; *e.g.*, knowledge, understanding, and thinking skills.

colic: acute abdominal pain in infants, most commonly during the first 3 months.

collaborative problem: a problem that occurs in relation to pathology and is identified by another health provider.

colloids: intravenous solutions that have the ability to expand a depleted blood volume by exerting a colloidal pressure similar to that of plasma proteins.

colonization: a condition in the body whereby microorganisms are present and no invasion of surrounding tissue occurs.

colonoscopy: visualization of the large intestine with a flexible fiberoptic endoscope.

colostrum: the fluid secreted by the breast during pregnancy and the first days post partum before lactation begins; consists of immunologically active substances.

communicable: the ability of a disease to be transmitted from person to person.

community-acquired infections: infections brought into the hospital with the client at the time of admission.

community-based nursing: provision of episodic nursing services that are individual or family-focused and delivered outside traditional hospital settings.

complete bed bath: bathing activities that must be performed totally by a caregiver.

compression of morbidity: a shift in the pattern of disease in the oldest old as the result of modern medical care and healthy lifestyle. This produces a higher incidence of disease and injury in this age cohort.

concept: a mental image or idea to which a label or meaning is attached.

concrete operational stage: the third stage of piagetian cognitive development, during which children develop logical but not abstract thinking.

concurrent audit: the process of studying client responses when the nursing action occurs.

conduction: heat lost from the body by contact of the body with an object. Body heat is lost when the body is in contact with a cooler object or substance.

confidentiality: the statutorily protected right that is afforded specifically designated health professionals such as nurses not to disclose information obtained during consultation with a client.

contaminated: having unwanted microorganisms.

context: the conditions under which a communication occurs.

continuity of care: the monitoring of people who are sick or at risk of being sick, so that services can be adapted appropriately. Continuity of care does not mean that care must be given always at the same level of intensity; rather, it suggests continuous monitoring of the changing need for care.

contraception: the prevention of pregnancy through means varying from abstinence to sterilization.

contractility: force of contraction.

convection: the loss of heat from the body through air currents. Body heat that has been conducted to the skin is lost by the movement of air across the skin's surface.

coping: adjusting to or solving internal and external challenges.

core temperature: the temperature of the deep tissues of the body. The temperature of blood in the pulmonary artery is at core temperature.

credé maneuver: a technique used for manual expression of urine from the bladder.

crepitus: cracking sounds produced when air is present in the subcutaneous tissue.

criminal law: state and federal statutes that define criminal offenses and corresponding fines and/or punishment (Black, 1991, p. 784). Examples of criminal offenses seen in health care include forgery (*e.g.,* forging someone's name on the medication administration record [MAR]) and practicing a licensed profession without a license.

crisis: a state of disequilibrium that results when a person is confronted with what for him or her constitutes an important problem that he or she can, for the time being, neither escape nor solve with his or her customary problem-solving resources (Caplan, 1964).

criteria: specific measurable qualities, attributes, or characteristics.

crystalloids: intravenous solutions that contain electrolytes.

cue: a signal that indicates a potential problem that may need nursing care.

cultural adaptation: adjustment of an individual's behavior to the concepts, ideas, traditions, and institutions of a culture.

cultural diversity: a concept recognizing that every culture has developed a unique way of understanding health and responding to illness. It stresses that the dominant culture's ways are not the right ways and advocates increased appreciation, awareness, and inclusion of differing perspectives in care of clients.

cultural norms: traditions and expectations that are determined by the heritage of a family unit. Ways of life and expectations can be established from religious beliefs and cultural groups as well as from traditions of a single family unit.

cultural sensitivity: to enhance care, sensitizing oneself and others to the cultural and social differences that exist between groups. (Jezewski, 1993)

culture: differences in health beliefs and practices by gender, race, ethnicity, economic class, sexual identity, and age (Eliason, 1993); provides a pattern of human behavior for life situations, a way of life (Crow, 1993); learned values, beliefs, customs.

culture brokering: the act of bridging, linking, or mediating between groups and persons with different ethnocultural backgrounds. The purpose of the brokering is to remove conflicts, produce change, and promote acceptance.

culture shock: a necessary rite of passage in which one feels alienation (Bell, 1994); psychological effect of the drastic change in cultural environment; feelings of helplessness, discomfort, disorientation while attempting to adjust to change.

cyanosis: a bluish discoloration of mucous membranes and/or skin resulting from decreased oxygenation of blood.

cystitis: inflammation of the urinary bladder.

daily reference values: desired intake levels for certain nutrients considered important for health.

dandruff: diffuse scaling of the epidermis of the scalp.

database: all the subjective and objective information collected about a client.

data cluster: organizing information gained during assessment into categories that can be used to determine a client's health problems and strengths.

data collection: the process of collecting all the subjective and objective information about a client.

data validation: confirming the accuracy of collected data and ascertaining that there are adequate data to support a diagnosis.

deciduous teeth: any one of the set of 20 primary teeth that appear normally during infancy, consisting of four incisors, two canines, and four molars in each jaw.

decoder (receiver): the person to whom a message is aimed. This person must be able to decode the message sent so it is a clearly understood thought.

deglutition: the act of swallowing.

dementia: a chronic, organic mental syndrome. Consists of impaired recent memory, personality change, and brain damage.

Denver II: revised version of the Denver Developmental Screening Test (DDST), which is used to chart developmental progress of children up to age of 6 years.

deontology: a system of ethical beliefs that focuses on people's capacity to assume moral obligations. A central concept is the respect for the person as a moral agent.

dependent intervention: nursing action that is based on the physician's orders.

dermis: the second layer of the skin, which houses nerves, hair follicles, glands, arteries, veins, capillaries, and fibrous elastic tissue.

designated blood: blood collected from a donor designated by the intended recipient.

despair: a loss of hope; to give up.

detrusor muscle: smooth muscle of the bladder; the muscle of micturition.

development: a qualitative increase in complexity of function; to bring out one's potential or capabilities through growth, maturation, and learning.

developmental tasks: a set of learned behaviors imposed on one that are required or necessary to live and grow in all ages and stages of life.

diagnosing: making a clinical judgment; identifying problems that are the responsibility of the nurse.

diagnosis: the analysis of the assessment data in order to determine the patient's responses that are amenable to nursing intervention, the clustering of data into distinct patterns, and the formulation of appropriate nursing diagnoses.

diagnostic studies: all tests involving the analysis of blood or any body fluid or other bodily functions.

diastole: the phase of the cardiac cycle associated with the relaxation of the ventricle, usually in reference to blood pressure.

dietitian: a person specially educated to assist individuals to enhance the quality of life through diet.

diffusion: the movement of particles across a semipermeable membrane from an area of greater concentration to an area of lesser concentration.

dirty wound: a wound with microorganisms (also identified as contaminated or colonized).

disengagement: the act of releasing oneself from obligation; freedom.

disinfectant: chemical used to kill or destroy most disease-producing organisms.

distribution: the process by which a drug molecule is transported by the circulating body fluids to various areas of the body.

diurnal rhythm: body rhythm that consists of a cycle of 24 hours. The circadian rhythm is a diurnal rhythm.

documentation: process of communicating information about the client in writing.

drug: a chemical that is introduced into the body to act on body cells for an intended therapeutic effect.

drug effect: the observed manifestations of the actions of chemical substances on the body.

ductus arteriosus: a tubular structure in the fetal heart connecting the left ventricle and the aorta.

durable power of attorney: the power granted by a client to a person to make health care decisions if the client is unable to do so.

dynamic posture: a position that can be moved into and out of freely.

dyschezia: straining or difficult defecation.

dysphagia: difficulty swallowing.

dyspnea: shortness of breath.

dysrhythmia: abnormal cardiac rate or rhythm.

dysuria: pain or difficulty in urination.

eccrine glands: found throughout the skin; most prevalent in the forehead, palms, and soles. These glands secrete sweat.

echocardiogram: noninvasive cardiac test that examines the structures of the heart.

ecomap: a tool used in family assessment to determine how the family members interact with one another as a system as well as with outside groups in their environment.

economics of health and illness: the overarching financial status and attitude of the public related to health care agencies, systems, and policies. The current U.S. system is moving from the established one of fee-for-service to a system of managed care.

edema: an accumulation of fluid in the interstitial spaces.

educational groups: groups developed to teach participants skills and provide information.

electrolytes: chemical substances that dissociate into electrically charged particles called ions when placed into a solution.

emigrant: one who leaves his or her country, state, or region.

encoder (sender): the person who initiates a transaction to exchange information, convey thoughts and feelings, or engage another.

endogenous infections: infections that originate from within the body.

endoscopic procedure: a procedure performed by using an instrument for visualizing the interior of a hollow organ.

enteral: pertaining to the small intestine.

enteral nutrition: providing liquefied nutrients via the gastrointestinal tract or orally; in nursing, usually refers to tube feedings.

enuresis: involuntary or inappropriate voiding of urine in a child at an age when bladder control is expected.

environment: all the conditions and circumstances impacting a person; the setting in which nursing care occurs.

Environmental Protection Agency (EPA): an agency in the executive branch that endeavors to abate and control pollution in air and water, solid waste, noise, radiation, and toxic substances.

epidemiology: the study of disease and injury in various populations.

epidermis: the most superficial layer of the skin; composed of layers of stratified epithelial cells.

error of commission: incorrectly interpreted or incorrectly clustered data.

error of omission: incomplete data collection.

erythema: redness of skin usually due to local inflammation.

erythema toxicum: pink papular rash with vesicles superimposed on thorax, back, buttocks, and abdomen of newborn.

ethical dilemma: a moral problem with no comfortable solutions because all alternatives are equally unsatisfactory.

ethics: a study of the nature and reason of morality.

ethnicity: a defining feature or features pertaining to, or characteristic of, a people, speech, or culture.

ethnocentrism: belief that one's own race, customs, beliefs, or values are the best or the only acceptable ones.

ethnographic study: a study of people using their culture as the framework for data collection and analysis.

evaluation: the process of determining the extent to which expected outcomes are achieved by the client.

evaporation: The process of converting liquids to vapors, which can result in a loss of body heat; insensible water loss through the skin or lungs, which can result in a loss of body heat.

excretion: the process by which the less active, biotransformed drug molecule is removed from the body.

exogenous infections: infections that originate from outside the body.

exotoxin: a toxic protein excreted into the surrounding medium/tissue by a microorganism.

expiration: the movement of air out of the lungs.

external environment: the social and cultural systems we live in and interact with, including living things and objects.

faith development: a belief of trust or confidence that gives life meaning.

family: the unit of support that an individual identifies with through responsibility and caring as he or she mediates the world.

family as client: the family unit viewed as an integral part of the care planning process. In this philosophical approach, the individual is a part of a greater whole that must be considered when determining needs and responses to care provided.

family assessment: a process used by the nurse, working with the family, to determine the strengths and needs of the family. Patterns, environment, stressors, and supports are determined.

family theory: a framework or context for organizing thoughts about how the family unit functions. There are multiple theoretical frameworks to draw on to assist the nurse in studying family function. Examples include general systems theory, structural-functional theory, developmental theory, institutional historical theory, and eclectic theory.

feces: solid waste products of digestion.

feedback: a process that feeds some of the output of a system back into the system as input. This input of information then influences the behavior of the system and its subsequent output. The process by which effectiveness of communication is determined.

fever: an elevation of the body temperature above its normal range. Fever is frequently caused by pyrogens.

filtration: the transfer of water and dissolved substances through a semipermeable membrane in response to a pressure gradient.

fine motor development: acquisition of the ability to perform small, detailed tasks, such as picking up small objects using thumb and finger in opposition.

fissure in ano: a painful lineal ulcer at the margin of the anus.

flatulence: excessive air or gas in the intestines.

flatus: air or gas in the gastrointestinal tract.

folk illness: health disorder attributed to nonscientific causes, e.g., caused by yin-yan forces or the evil eye.

folk medicine: treatment of disease following traditions and usually involving use of herbs or other natural substances.

folklore: traditions, customs.

fontanelle: soft spot in the skull of a newborn at the junction of bones that have not fused.

foramen ovale: natural opening in the fetal heart that allows blood to pass from the right to the left atrium to bypass the lungs.

formal operational thought: the ability to think in abstract terms and draw logical conclusions.

frequency: an increase in the number of times per day that an individual voids (see **urinary frequency**).

functional hematuria: presence of blood in the urine (often identified only by urinalysis).

fungus: free-living microscopic organism of the class to which molds and yeasts belong.

gatekeeping: the functions that determine who gets services within a health care system. Gatekeeping was originally controlled by physicians and administrators, but currently other participants, such as advanced practice nurses (nurse practitioners and clinical nurse specialists) and insurance companies, are involved.

gender: a complex, culturally influenced, subjective experience of being male or female.

generativity: the state of being productive and contributing to society; may refer to the production of offspring as well.

genogram: a tool used in family assessment to determine the structure of the family system. Symbols are used to denote family members; lines indicate generations and bonds. Notations are made regarding ages, illnesses, causes of death. A box or circle can be used to depict members of a household.

geriatrics: a specialty within the health care system that specializes in providing care to older persons.

gerontology: the branch of science that deals with aging and the special problems of older persons; from the Greek *geras,* meaning old age.

gestation: period of time from conception to birth.

gingiva (gums): oral mucosa that covers the bone supporting the teeth.

gingivitis: inflammation of the gingiva (gums) caused by bacteria or other particles trapped under the gum tissue.

goals: the focus of nursing care.

gram-negative bacteria: bacteria that when stained using the Gram method retain the red dye (safranin).

gram-positive bacteria: bacteria that when stained using the Gram method retain the blue dye (crystal violet).

granulation tissue: connective tissue containing multiple small blood vessels that assists in rapid healing of the wound bed.

grief: the total response (thoughts, feelings, behavior) to the emotional suffering caused by an anticipated or threatened loss or separation. Includes internal responses as well as observable reactions.

gross hematuria: blood in urine visible to the naked eye.

gross motor development: acquisition of the ability to perform large-muscle tasks, such as sitting and walking.

group: two or more individuals who share one or more common characteristics and meet on a regular basis in face-to-face interactions to achieve a common goal.

group cohesion: all of the positive values that people hold about the group experience and the reasons that prompt them to remain with the group.

group culture: a set of common characteristics that help facilitate goal achievement. Shared characteristics may involve a common ethnic heritage, a similar health problem, or the need to complete a group project.

group dynamics: the conscious and unconscious forces or emotional flow operating in a group and facilitating or impeding the group process and progression toward goal achievement.

group goals: the outcomes, or end results, a group seeks to achieve through its common effort. Group goals represent a collective aim that may or may not be the same as the goals of individual group members.

group membership: an identified relationship between a person and designated other persons who make up a group.

group norms: standards of conduct that provide guidelines for acceptable behaviors in groups. Group norms are powerful written or unwritten laws about how members should relate with one another.

group process: the naturally progressive phases of group development.

group roles: sets of behaviors that individuals display in relation to the expectations of the rest of the group members.

group therapy: a form of psychotherapy designed to help clients gain insight into dysfunctional behaviors and develop more appropriate coping strategies.

growth: a quantitative increase in size or physical maturity.

guided imagery: a process that uses pleasant mental images to help a client relax and increase his or her level of comfort.

habituation: an acquired tolerance from repeated exposure to a particular stimulus.

halitosis: bad breath.

health: a dynamic state of being in which the developmental and behavioral potential of an individual is realized.

health and illness: relative states that pertain to a client's physical, psychological, emotional, and spiritual functioning and to his or her cultural needs. Beliefs about health and illness vary from group to group and so should be validated by the individuals, families, or groups seeking nursing care.

health care delivery systems: systems in which clients seek and providers administer health care services. Present-day health care systems include hospital-based care, home care, hospice care, long-term care, quick care (surgi-centers, emergi-centers), and ambulatory care. Traditional public health departments (units), previously restricted to population-based wellness services, now provide some illness-related services.

health care reform: an ongoing local, regional, and national movement that will affect access to and participation in health care services.

health-illness continuum: a way of viewing a person's condition: on a line between health and illness; it takes into consideration the physical and the emotional/spiritual status of the person.

health problem: a deviation or variation in the well-being of a client.

heat cramps: a disorder that occurs from overheating the body, resulting in muscle cramps.

heat exhaustion: a disorder resulting from overexposure to heat, frequently resulting in excessive sweating; pale, cool skin; and the experience of confusion and weakness.

hemoptysis: coughing up blood from the lungs.

hemorrhoids: abnormally distended veins at the anal sphincter; can be internal or external.

hesitancy: difficulty in initiating urination.

heterosexuality: preference for a partner of the opposite sex.

higher-level thought processes: the use of cognitive skills such as orientation, attention, concentration, memory, judgment, and reasoning.

hirsutism: excessive growth of body and facial hair.

holistic care: assessing and interacting with the whole person.

holistic model of humans: model of human functioning that considers the nature of people to consist of body, mind, and spirit united, indivisible, and in constant interaction (Carson and Arnold, 1996).

Holter monitoring: cardiac monitoring system in which each electrical cycle of the heart is recorded for a 24-hour (or determined) period and later reviewed. The client, if able, completes a self-reported diary while wearing the monitor. This diary allows for the correlation of any dysrhythmia or changes with any documented symptoms or activities.

homeopathy: system of therapeutics based on theories that some diseases can be treated by small amounts of medicine.

homeostasis: the maintenance of a stable or constant internal environment that is dependent on the regulation of oxygen, carbon dioxide, organic nutrients and wastes, inorganic ions, and temperature within the human body.

homeostatic mechanisms: processes of self-regulation that preserve an organism's ability to adapt to stressors while maintaining inner balance.

homeotherm: an animal able to maintain a stable body temperature during changing environmental conditions.

homologous blood: blood collected from a volunteer donor for transfusion into another individual.

homosexuality: preference for a partner of one's own sex.

horizontal integration of services: resources are conserved by the joining of similar units of service, such as a chain of community hospitals.

host: a living organism on which a parasite (bacterium, virus, fungus, etc.) lives.

h.s. care: care given to clients before they retire for the night. Includes toileting, oral care, and comfort measures.

human reduction: viewing the client as other than a human being.

humanism: a world view that places ultimate value on humans and what humans are able to accomplish; in its purest form does not recognize the transcendent (Carson and Arnold, 1996).

hydronephrosis: collection of urine in the kidney pelvis due to obstructed outflow of urine.

hydroureter: dilation of the ureter related to increased resistance to urine flow below the level of the ureter.

hypersensitivity: an allergic reaction that may be slight, with manifestations such as skin rash, hives, and itching, or very severe, resulting in anaphylaxis or death.

hypertension: recorded blood pressure of greater than or equal to 140 mmHg systolic and/or 90 mmHg diastolic.

hyperthermia: a considerable increase in body temperature.

hypertonic: a solution with an osmolality greater than that of extracellular fluid.

hypothermia: a considerable decrease in body temperature.

hypotonic: a solution with an osmolality less than that of extracellular fluid.

hypoxia: condition in which an inadequate amount of oxygen is available to tissues.

iatrogenesis: occurrence of illness as a result of the medical treatment or medical plan of care.

iatrogenic infections: infections resulting from medical treatment and the result of the patient's own microbial flora.

idiosyncrasy: an unexplainable, unique reaction that occurs when a client takes a drug that typically does not produce this type of reaction.

illness: the state of being sick.

immigrant: a person who enters a new country or region to start a new life.

immunity: resistance to a disease through either natural or artificial stimulation.

immunization: a process by which resistance to an infectious disease is induced or augmented.

impaction: prolonged retention or accumulation of fecal material that forms a hardened mass in the intestine.

implementation: the act of putting into action the nursing strategies (often referred to as nursing orders or nursing actions) identified in the nursing plan of care.

incontinence: the inability of the anal sphincter to control the discharge of feces and gas (also see **urinary incontinence**).

incubation period: the interval from the time of infection with an organism to the time of development of disease.

independent intervention: nursing actions that are based on the nursing diagnosis and that nurses are qualified to use without a physician's order.

individual learning: activity that is influenced by the ability, experience, and attitude of the particular learner.

individuation: the process by which individuals grow from a general state of being to being their unique selves.

infarction: death of tissue resulting from prolonged ischemia.

infected wound: determined by the number of microorganisms present, usually greater than 10^5 (100,000) organisms per gram of tissue.

infection: a condition in the body where microorganisms are present and invade surrounding tissues.

infertility: the inability to conceive.

informed consent: a person's voluntary agreement to a procedure after being informed of risks, benefits, and consequences. This implies disclosure, understanding, voluntariness, competence, and giving permission.

inner canthus: the medial aspect of the eye where the upper and lower eyelids meet.

insomnia: a perception of inadequate sleep, including difficulty in initiating sleep, frequent awakenings from sleep, and a perception of a nonrestorative sleep.

inspection: the close, visual observation of the client, first of the individual as a whole and then of the separate body systems.

inspiration: the movement of air into the lungs.

integrity: the state of being whole; becoming complete with oneself.

integument: skin.

integumentary system: includes the skin, hair, glands in the skin, and the nails.

interdependent intervention: nursing actions that are performed in collaboration with other members of the health care team.

internal environment: the structure and function of the organ systems and tissues inside the body.

interpretation: the process of translating sensory signals within specific structures of the nervous system.

interventions: nursing actions that are aimed at the prevention, maintenance, or restoration of a client's health.

interview: an interactive communication process involving a mutual or reciprocal exchange of information between the nurse and the client.

intraoperative: occurring between the time that the client is admitted to the operating room and admission to the postanesthesia care unit.

intrapulmonary pressure: pressure in the lungs.

ischemia: absence or reduction in blood flow to an area, resulting in anoxia to the affected tissues.

isolation: procedures that describe separating patients with communicable diseases from other patients.

isotonic solution: a solution with an osmolality equal to that of extracellular fluid.

joint: junction between two bony surfaces, supported by ligaments, muscles, and a joint capsule.

Joint Commission on Accreditation of Healthcare Organizations (JCAHO): an accrediting agency that monitors quality in health care agencies (hospitals, long-term care facilities, etc.).

justice: a condition of fairness and equality, or a state of being deserving based on some criteria.

Kegel exercises: exercises developed to strengthen the pelvic-vaginal muscles as a means of controlling stress incontinence in women.

kilocalorie: heat that is required to raise 1 kilogram of water 1°C.

knowledge deficit: the state in which specific information is lacking; the inability to explain or use self-care practices recommended to restore health or maintain wellness.

Korotkoff sounds: audible sounds present during assessment of blood pressure.

kyphosis: abnormal cervical curvature of the spine, commonly referred to as "humpback."

language: a set of words that have meanings that are comprehensible within a group.

lanugo: soft, downy hair covering all parts of the fetus except palms, soles, and areas where other types of hair are normally found.

law: a system for resolving disputes, composed of general rules of conduct required of all members of society and the procedures to resolve disputes when conformity with the rules of conduct does not occur (Pozgar, 1996, p. 2).

leadership: influential behavior, voluntarily accepted by other group members, that moves a group toward its recognized goal and/or maintains the group.

learning: a process that involves perceiving and acquiring new knowledge, information, and skills that may result in changes in one's behavior.

legal liability: a broad legal term that can be defined as an obligation one is bound in law or justice to perform. When the obligation is not performed or performed in an unacceptable manner, a court or other tribunal can enforce liability as between the parties (Black, 1991, pp. 621, 631).

licensure: a legal document that assures the public that a qualified professional has attained the minimal degree of competency to reasonably protect the public's health, safety, and welfare.

locus of control: the person's perception of who or what is in control of his or her circumstances and environment. A person who has an internal locus of control believes that what happens in his or her life is determined by his or her own actions. A person with an external locus of control believes that fate, chance, authority figures, or something other than himself or herself is responsible for what becomes of him or her.

lung compliance: the ease with which the lung can be inflated against its elastic forces.

magnetic resonance imaging (MRI): a diagnostic procedure whereby structures throughout the body may be visualized by an examination that creates images with magnetic energy. No ionizing radiation is used.

maintenance roles: the role functions that help build and maintain group morale. Group members assuming maintenance role functions draw attention to the relational aspects of group life needed to nourish and support members as they labor to achieve the group task.

malnutrition: a deficiency, imbalance, or excess of nutrients.

managed care: a health care system designed to provide safe, quality care to groups of people. It is based on "average" needs and is less flexible than a fee-for-service model of care.

massage: a form of cutaneous stimulation that provides physical and mental comfort and relaxation.

maturational crises: predictable, stressful events that occur during a person's developmental process and for which the person has no coping skills.

meconium: thick and sticky greenish-to-black material that collects in the intestines of a fetus and forms the first stools of a newborn. It is composed of secretions of the intestinal glands, some amniotic fluid, and intrauterine debris, such as bile pigments, mucus, lanugo, and blood.

medical asepsis: a technique used for health care delivery that involves using barrier precautions, handwashing, and gloving to decrease infection transmission.

medical diagnosis: determines and labels client limitations and the need for treatment directed by a physician.

menarche: a female's first menstrual period, occurring toward the end of puberty.

menopause: the cessation of a woman's monthly menstrual cycle.

menstrual cycle: recurring hormone-induced changes in the female body, from ovulation to development and later degeneration of the corpus luteum to menstruation. The onset of menstruation is called menarche; the end of menstruation is called menopause.

message: the content a sender wishes another person (the receiver) to receive in the process of communication.

metabolism: ongoing processes that the body performs to convert nutrients into energy, body structures, and waste (elimination).

micturition: the discharge of urine from the bladder (other terms are *voiding* and *urinating*).

middle adulthood: a period of life transition between being a young adult and an elder adult.

milia: minute white papules commonly found on the nose and cheeks of a newborn, caused by obstruction of sebaceous follicles.

mobility: state of moving; the facility of movement.

model: a symbolic representation that uses a minimal number of words to express the abstract concepts and propositions.

modern nursing movement: represents the period following the opening of nurses' training schools in 1873. The modern nursing movement trained and educated women into "spheres of action . . . making women socially useful outside of the domestic sphere, emancipating them and giving them a chance to grow" (Stewart, 1948, p. 78).

mongolian spot: benign, bluish-black macule, from 2 to 8 cm, occurring over the sacrum and on the buttocks of some newborns.

monism: a belief that everything that exists is one (Pacwa, 1992).

moral development: conforming to generally accepted ideas of what is right and just in human conduct; one's view of right and wrong.

morning care: care given to clients after they awaken and have breakfast. Care includes toileting, bathing, oral, foot, nail, and hair care. Also includes comfort measures and linen changes.

mourning: the period of intense emotion following the experience of loss. The period includes the struggle to adapt to changes in one's life prompted by the loss.

multiple-tier system of care: includes basic medical care for all who need it, and further care on a fee-for-service or availability basis. Because the need for services is greater than the available resources, care must be rationed with the aim of getting resources to those who need them the most, not to those with the most money or the most influence on decision-making.

murmur: abnormal turbulent blood flow audible over the involved valve.

myocardium: middle layer of cardiac muscle that forms the walls of the heart.

narcolepsy: a disorder characterized by a set of clinical symptoms including abnormal sleep, overwhelming episodes of sleep that may occur at inappropriate times, excessive daytime sleepiness, hallucinations, disturbances in nighttime sleep, and paroxysmal muscle weakness, cataplexy, and sleep paralysis.

narrative notes: paragraphs of information that are written sequentially and usually organized in chronological order as a means of relating observations, interventions, and client responses to care.

necrosis: death of tissue; may be eschar (leathery, black tissue) or slough (usually moist, stringy, yellow, green, or gray tissue).

negative feedback: feedback that leads to the initiation of a series of changes that negate and attempt to correct any radical change from the norm, either toward excess or deficiency. Negative feedback thus inhibits further change from the norm.

neural function: the basic nervous system functions of reception, transmission, interpretation, perception, and response to stimuli.

neural structure: any of the anatomic components of the nervous system, *i.e.,* neurons, sensory receptors, nerve fibers, the spinal cord, and brain structures.

neurogenic bladder: a bladder that had some damage to or interruption of sensory or motor nerves, causing bladder function impairment.

neuron: the basic structure in the nervous system that conducts nerve impulses.

neuropathic pain: pain syndromes associated with damage to some part of the nervous system.

New Age spirituality: an eclectic world view borrowing from Hinduism, Zen, Sufism, and Native American religion and mixed with humanistic psychology, Western occultism, and modern physics. A belief in monism (everything is the same) that leads to pantheism (everything is God; self is God); no absolute right or wrong; values and behavior are relative (Sire, 1994).

NIOSH: National Institute of Occupational Safety and Health. An agency of the federal government that conducts research on health and safety concerns, tests and certifies respirators, and trains occupational safety and health professionals.

nocturnal emission (sometimes called "wet dream"): an involuntary, unconscious release of seminal fluid during sleep.

nocturia: excessive urination at night; need to void two or more times at night.

nonmaleficence: the duty to refrain from doing harm.

nonnutritive sucking: sucking need of the infant not satisfied by breast- or bottle-feeding. It is such a strong need that infants who are deprived of sucking, such as those with a cleft lip repair, will suck on their tongue.

nonopioid analgesics: a diverse group of drugs (*i.e.,* aspi-

rin, acetaminophen, and the nonsteroidal antiinflammatory drugs) that produce their analgesic effects by interfering with pain processing in the peripheral nervous system.

nontherapeutic communication techniques: techniques that impair the flow of communication in what would otherwise be a progressive movement toward client growth.

normal flora: microorganisms that are routinely found on skin and mucous membranes.

nosocomial infections: infections occurring during hospitalization but were not incubating at the time of admission.

NPO: nothing by mouth.

NREM (non-rapid eye movement) sleep: characterized by a sleeping posture with the eyes closed and the pupils myotic. However, a certain degree of tone remains in all muscle groups. Electrical activity of the cerebral cortex is characterized by spindles and slow waves.

nurse clinician: an advanced practice degree requiring a master's preparation in a particular area in nursing.

nurse practice act: state law (statute) passed by the state legislative body to ensure that safe and competent nursing practice is provided to the public in that state. Most nurse practice acts are administered by a board of nursing that is given the power by the state legislature to administer and enforce the specific requirements of the nurse practice act.

nurse practitioner: an advanced practice degree requiring a master's preparation in a particular area in nursing, such as primary health care, disease prevention, health promotion, and health maintenance.

nursing: the diagnosis and treatment of human responses to actual or potential health problems.

nursing actions: nursing interventions that focus on assisting people to cope successfully with problems and to achieve outcomes desired.

nursing audit: the process of studying quality assurance.

nursing care conference: meeting of a group of nurses and sometimes the client, family, or other health professionals to discuss client problem(s); each nurse has the opportunity to contribute to solving the problem.

nursing care rounds: the action of a group of nurses visiting a client's bedside to discuss their interventions, with the client participating.

nursing centers: centers that are organized and run by nurses to provide a wide variety of nursing services.

nursing diagnosis: a clinical judgment about an individual, family, or community; responses to actual or potential health problems or situations whereby wellness can be enhanced.

nursing examination: an examination of the client in which the nurse collects all the information about the client's objective or overt physical signs.

nursing history: a detailed description of the client's health status, which is obtained through a planned, systematic interview with the client.

nursing orders: another term for **interventions** or **nursing actions**.

nursing plan of care: method of describing nursing actions planned to meet the outcomes for the client. It consists of the nursing diagnoses identified for the client, the outcomes for each nursing diagnosis, and the actions planned for the client.

nursing process: a deliberate, organized, systematic activity that is used by nurses to carry out their professional roles when interacting with clients.

nutrients: substances supplied by food that are required by the body to function.

objective data: data that are observable by an individual or that can be measured by an appropriate method.

Occupational Safety and Health Administration (OSHA): a federal agency formed in 1970 whose primary concern is the health and safety of America's work force.

oliguria: urine output in relation to intake; an output of less than 400 ml per 24 hours.

open system catheterization: catheter and catheterization procedure that are exposed to the environment. Although sterile technique is employed, the urine drains into an open collection container.

open-ended questions: questions that require the client to express feelings, concerns, opinions, or perceptions; questions that require more than a simple yes or no.

operating room: the room where sterile surgical procedures take place.

opioid analgesics: drugs that work in the central nervous system at the level of the spinal cord and midbrain to produce analgesia.

opportunistic organisms: microorganisms that flourish when the body's immune system or normal flora is altered.

oral care: hygiene measures aimed at maintaining the healthy state of the mouth, oral mucosa, teeth, gums, and lips (brushing, flossing, and rinsing mouth).

orthopnea: shortness of breath when supine.

osmolality: the total number of osmotically active particles in a volume of solution.

osmolarity: the concentration of solute in a volume of solution.

osmosis: the movement of water across a cell membrane in response to a concentration difference.

ostomy: a surgical procedure in which an artificial opening is formed, as in colostomy, ileostomy, etc.

outcome evaluation: collection and analysis of data about client responses.

outcome: statement of the behavior or human response that is expected after provision of nursing care. Also referred to as *objective*.

outer canthus: lateral aspect of the eye where upper and lower eyelids meet.

overflow incontinence: urine retained in the bladder lost involuntarily as a result of an increase in abdominal pressure greater than the high urethral pressure that inhibits voiding initially.

overshoot: to overcompensate during attempts at system self-correction.

oxygenation: the process whereby oxygen is made available to cells and carbon dioxide is eliminated from cells.

PACU (postanesthesia care unit): the place where the client recovers from the effects of anesthesia.

pain: an unpleasant sensory and emotional experience associated with actual or potential tissue damage, or described in terms of such damage.

palpation: the use of touch to determine temperature, texture, size, shape, pulsation, consistency, and movement.

pantheism: a world view that holds that everything is God (Pacwa, 1992).

paralanguage: nonverbal components of spoken language. These components give speech its rhythm and humanness and include stress, accents, pitch, pause, intonation, rate, volume, and quality.

partial bed bath: hygiene measures for which the client needs assistance from a caregiver while in bed

paternalism: the deliberate restriction of people's autonomy by health care professionals based on the idea that the professionals know what is best for clients.

pathogen: a microorganism that produces disease.

patient-controlled analgesia: a regimen that allows the patient to self-administer predetermined doses of an analgesic drug in sufficient amounts to maintain relatively constant plasma concentrations of the pain medication and a relatively constant amount of analgesia.

perception: the process of interpreting and assigning meaning to stimuli.

percussion: striking a body surface to produce sound in order to determine the size, position, and density of the underlying part.

percutaneous injury: an injury that breaks the skin, such as a cut or needlestick.

perfusion: the flow of blood through an area.

perineal care: hygiene care of vaginal, urethral, and anal areas.

periodontal disease: disease of the supporting structures of the teeth. It is the advanced stage of gingivitis and can lead to tooth loss.

perioperative nursing: the scope of nursing practice throughout the surgical experience.

peripheral nervous system: the division of the nervous system that contains the cranial and spinal nerves, the autonomic nervous system, and the somatic nervous system.

peristalsis: wavelike contractions of the gastrointestinal tract.

person: the recipient of care; may be an individual, family, or community.

personal hygiene: the activity of self-care, including bathing and grooming.

personal space: a private zone or "bubble" around our bodies that we feel is an extension of ourselves and belongs to us.

pH: the hydrogen ion concentration in solution; its value is expressed as the inverse of the hydrogen ion concentration.

pharmacokinetics: the study of the movement of drugs through the body from absorption to excretion.

pharmacy: the site where drugs are prepared, dispensed, and sold.

physical dependence: a condition that occurs in clients who take opioids chronically when the drugs are discontinued abruptly or an opioid antagonist like naloxone is administered. The result is the production of an abstinence syndrome.

physiologic homeostasis: the maintenance of a relatively stable and constant internal dynamic equilibrium.

planning: the systematic, deliberate determination of a individualized nursing plan of care that considers the holistic nature of the client

plaque: buildup of bacteria and other particles that adhere to the enamel surface of the teeth; a lesion within an artery that causes the intimal surface to bulge into the lumen.

pleura: a double-walled sac that encases the lungs.

p.m. care: afternoon care. Includes simple hygiene measures: washing hands and face, oral care, toileting, comfort measures, and environmental hygiene.

poisons: chemical substances that exist in the environment and that can be very harmful to human life if they come in contact with the body through inhalation, digestion, or absorption.

polytheism: a belief in many gods.

polyuria: excessive urination, greater than 3000 ml in 24 hours.

positioning schedule: arranging the body in specified postures in a planned, prescribed manner over time.

positive feedback: a response to stimuli that results in intensifying the initiating stimuli, leading the organism away from the normal state.

positive listening: simply understanding the auditory messages sent by a sender.

positron-emission tomography (PET): a diagnostic procedure that measures changes in tissues through a radioisotope-generated color image.

postoperative: beginning when the client is admitted to the PACU and ending when the client returns to function or has some type of resolution.

posture: attitude or position of the body. Standing, sitting, and lying postures have certain planes and positions that are considered normal.

prejudice: strongly held opinions about a topic or group of people; may be positive or negative; originates from ethnocentrism, ignorance, misinformation, past experiences (Eliason, 1993).

premenstrual syndrome: a specific set of physical and emotional effects (*e.g.,* headache, extreme irritability) directly related to the menstrual cycle.

preoperational thought: thought that characterizes children from the ages of about 2 to 7 years, in Piaget's second stage of cognitive development. Children use mental images but with no concrete, systematic, orderly means for arranging their thoughts.

preoperative: beginning when the client decides to have surgery and ending when the client is admitted to the operating room.

pressure ulcer (decubitus ulcer): trauma to the skin and underlying tissue caused by pressure, friction, or shear that leads to direct, ischemic tissue damage. Most commonly occurs in people with limited mobility.

primary groups: naturally occurring group formations with informal structures. Membership is automatic or spontaneously chosen.

primary prevention: activities, such as health education and immunizations, that are directed at preventing disease and disability from occurring.

priorities: in nursing, client problems or nursing actions that should be given preference over others.

privacy: the client's right to have all personal information safeguarded from unauthorized disclosure.

PRN care: care required by a client as needed: not regularly scheduled.

problem, actual: a deviation from health that requires intervention.

problem-oriented record: records that are focused on a client problem, with all disciplines collaborating on a plan of care.

problem, potential: a situation in which a problem may occur and intervention may be necessary to prevent the problem from occurring.

professional organization: a group that forms for purposes related to a particular profession. Such an association can provide a forum in which members set standards of practice, offer certification, accredit, debate professional issues, provide professional development, determine criteria for education and practice, and work politically to lobby for change.

PROM (passive range of motion): when assistance is provided to move an extremity and joint through an identified range. The goal is joint and muscle-length maintenance, not muscle strengthening.

proposition: statement that clarifies the relationships among concepts.

protocol: documents that specify nursing management of broad clinical issues, phases of hospitalization, or interdependent clinical issues.

proximal-distal development: sequence of body growth and maturation from the spine out toward the extremities.

proximodistal: directional growth from the center of the body to the periphery or from near to far.

psychologic homeostasis: a state of equilibrium characterized by a satisfying self-concept, emotional balance, and harmonious interactions with the environment.

psychomotor domain: learning that emphasizes motor skills such as handwriting, typing, swimming, and operating machinery.

psychosexual development: development of the personality through sexual exploration from infancy to sexual maturity.

psychosocial development: development of the personality through environmental and societal interactions.

puberty: period of hormone-induced changes leading from childhood to adulthood.

public health nursing: provision of care services focused on prevention of disease injury, disability, and premature death through prevention measures focused on specific populations.

pulmonary function tests: tests to measure the functional ability of the lungs by identifying either a restriction or an obstruction to airflow or a combination of both.

purposeful learning: learning activity that is directed by the learner toward attainment of a meaningful outcome.

purulent drainage: cloudy, perhaps foul-smelling, drainage from a wound that also contains the byproducts of phagocytosis.

pyorrhea: the formation of pus in the pockets between the roots of the teeth and their surrounding tissue. Can result in subsequent loss of the teeth.

pyrexia: a body temperature above the normal average.

pyrogen: an agent that causes fever.

pyuria: the presence of white blood cells in urine.

quality assurance program: evaluation of nursing care given to groups of clients.

race: group of people who share common physical characteristics; *e.g.,* skin pigmentation, hair texture.

radiation: the loss of body heat by transfer of infrared heat rays from one object to another.

reactive hyperemia: occurs when pressure is released from an area and blood and therefore oxygen flood the tissues that were previously compressed, resulting in a reddening of the skin.

readiness for learning: the physiological, cognitive, and emotional preparedness for learning a task.

reception: the process of receiving stimuli through sensory receptors in the eyes, ears, tongue, nose, skin, and tissues and organs inside the body. When stimuli are sensed by a sensory receptor, a sensory signal is created.

recommended dietary allowances (RDAs): levels of intake for essential nutrients that are adequate to meet the needs of healthy people.

reference daily intakes: a population-adjusted average for all age/sex groups of the RDAs used on food labels.

reflux of urine: the "backing up" of urine into the ascending structure; *e.g.,* urine backing up from the bladder to the ureters.

reframing: the ability to view a problem or issue differently, like using a different color lens in a pair of glasses.

refugee: a person who leaves his or her homeland, usually due to economic, political, or social strife or persecution, to seek safety and shelter.

registration: required in the state in which a licensed professional practices. Registration must be renewed according to the laws of that state, unlike licensure, which is granted one time and is not renewable.

regulation: in pulmonary function, neural and chemical processes of breathing.

religion: humanity's attempt to structure spiritual issues by imposing rules, specifying rituals and practices, and codifying beliefs (Carson, 1989).

REM (rapid eye movement) sleep: a distinct stage of sleep that occurs at the end of each sleep cycle. During this stage of sleep, sleepers are extremely difficult to arouse. Sleepers exhibit numerous physiological changes, including rapid eye movements, facial muscle twitching, decreased muscle tone, irregular respiratory pattern, irregular and rapid heart rate, increased metabolic rate, increased temperature, increased blood pressure, and increased gastric secretions.

residual urine: the amount of urine remaining in the bladder after voiding has occurred.

response: behavior elicited by a stimulus. It is an attempt to continue or stop the stimulus.

rest: a state of mental relaxation and decreased physical activity.

restraint: a physical or mechanical device that limits a client's movement.

retention of urine: the accumulation of more than 50 ml in the bladder. It is due to an inability to empty the bladder or an obstruction distal to the bladder.

reticular activating system: a center within the cerebral cortex that is responsible for maintaining arousal and wakefulness.

retrospective audit: the process of studying client responses after services have been provided.

risk factors: for families, particular issues in a family unit that decrease the overall strength or hardiness. These issues could be particular to the lifestyle, psychosocial, environmental, or developmental needs of the unit. Risks should be mutually determined by the family and the nurse as issues that can be focused on to alter and increase the wellness of the family.

role: the part or task carried out by a family member. Someone may have more than one role. For example: parent, grandparent, and a sick role.

sanguineous drainage: fluid that is bloody and thus indicates active bleeding.

scoliosis: abnormal lateral curvature of the spine usually resulting in two curves, the abnormal curve and a complementary one.

scrub nurse: one who assists the surgeon during the procedure and helps maintain a sterile field throughout the surgical procedure.

sebaceous glands: glands located in the dermal layer of the skin that secrete sebum.

sebum: the oily, odorous fluid secreted from the sebaceous glands into the hair follicles. Sebum assists in lubricating the skin and the hair.

secondary groups: group formations specifically developed by people for the purpose of achieving identified goals.

secondary prevention: activities, such as Pap smears and TB testing, focused on early detection of disease in high-risk groups.

self: a conception of one's own person as distinguished from other objects in the external world as a separate being; the total of characteristic-response patterns and physical attributes of a person.

self-active learning: personal involvement of the learner in the learning process.

self-care: ability to independently perform activities of daily living (ADLs).

self-concept: an individual's perception of himself or herself. The self-concept includes body image, personal identity, role performance, and interpersonal competence.

self-esteem: an individual's overall evaluative judgment of himself or herself; how much he or she likes his or her particular person (Corkill-Briggs, 1975).

sensory perceptual alteration: a state in which the ability to interpret stimuli accurately is impaired, which may lead to inappropriate responses to stimuli.

sensory receptor: the structure that receives various types of stimuli.

seroconversion: blood test that converts from a baseline negative to positive.

serosanguineous drainage: fluid that is watery but pink-tinged, indicating some bleeding.

serous drainage: clear, watery plasma.

set point: a temperature point at which the hypothalmus attempts to maintain the body's heat balance.

sex: the physical state of being male or female.

sexual abuse: instigation of sexual activity without a person's full understanding or consent; use of a child for sexual activity.

sexual dysfunction: a barrier, whether physical or emotional, to normal sexual functioning.

sexuality: the quality or state of being sexual.

sexually transmitted disease: a disease spread primarily through sexual contact or copulation.

situational crises: usually sudden, unexpected stressful events that happen to an individual at any point in life and that cannot be controlled by the individual.

sleep: a state of reduced responsiveness to external stimuli; an altered state of consciousness from which a person can be aroused only if the stimulus is of sufficient magnitude.

sleep apnea: a condition characterized by the cessation of respiration during sleep.

sleep deprivation: a condition in which an individual experiences a disruption in the normal sleep-wake cycle because of overstimulation and disruption of normal bedtime routines.

social adaptation: the adjustment of an individual's actions and conduct to the norms, conventions, beliefs, and pressures of various groups.

somatic pain: pain that occurs as a result of the activation of nociceptors in cutaneous and deep tissues.

source-oriented record: charting system in which each group of health care professionals has its own portion of the chart set aside for storing information about observations and care unique to that group.

spasticity: hyperactivity of the normal stretch reflex as a result of an insult to the central nervous system.

spermarche: a male's first ejaculation of seminal fluid that contains sperm.

spinal analgesia: analgesia that is achieved by the delivery of analgesic drugs through a temporary or permanent catheter that has been placed in the epidural or intrathecal space.

spirit: the intangible, nonmaterial dimension of persons, frequently associated with life itself; not visible to the naked eye but its presence or absence is easily discernible to the human heart; frequently referred to as the soul (Carson, 1989).

spiritual distress: the state in which an individual experiences a disturbance in religious belief, practices, or value system (NANDA, 1995).

spiritual needs: any factors necessary to establish and/or maintain a dynamic personal relationship with God (as defined by that individual) and out of that relationship to experience forgiveness, love, hope, trust, and meaning and purpose in life (Carson, 1989).

spiritual well-being: an affirmation of life in a relationship with God, self, community and environment that nurtures and celebrates wholeness (Cook, 1980)

spirituality: the quality of recognizing and responding to the spirit and to issues of the spirit, such as awareness of a transcendent power; concerned with meaning and what is most important (Carson, 1989).

stagnation: to stop developing or progressing; to become stale.

standard: a written rule describing what a client may expect from nurses.

stenosis: the narrowing of an opening or blood vessel.

stereotyping: generalizing about a group or individual, usually concerning some form of behavior.

sterile: free from all living organisms.

sterilization: the physical or chemical methods used to completely destroy microorganisms on inanimate objects.

stimuli: events or changes that provoke or excite a nerve.

stranger fear: as infants demonstrate attachment to one person, they correspondingly exhibit less friendliness to others.

strangury: slow and painful urination, accompanied by spasms.

stratum corneum: the top epidermal layer, which is composed of dead keratinized cells. These are the cells that are abraded by the daily mechanical and chemical trauma of hand washing, scratching, and bathing.

stress: the process of adjusting to circumstances that disrupt, or threaten to disrupt, a person's equilibrium.

stress incontinence: involuntary loss of urine associated with physical pressure, *e.g.,* coughing.

stress responses: physiological and psychological reactions to stress.

stress test: noninvasive cardiac test performed on a treadmill or other equipment to assess blood flow to the heart muscle.

stressors: agents or factors that challenge the adaptive capacities of an organism or person.

stroke volume: volume of blood ejected from the left ventricle per contraction. Normal stroke volume is 70 cc.

structure: the manner in which the roles come together as a unit determines the structure of the family. The members' ability to work together or how they function is the consequence of the structure.

subcutaneous layer: the third and innermost layer of skin, which contains blood vessels, nerves, lymph, and connective tissue filled with fat cells.

subjective data: information that only the individual can report and that cannot be verified by another.

substance abuse: use of a specific chemical substance on a regular basis to produce behavioral alterations that impair the individual's functioning, produce a lack of control over taking the substance, and bring about the presence of withdrawal symptoms after stopping the intake of the substance.

suffrage: achieving political freedom by having the right to vote. Women in the United States became legally enfranchised in 1920.

sundowning: becoming confused at day's end (when the sun goes down).

support group: a group of individuals who offer advice and emotional support to a person under stress.

surface temperature: the temperature of the skin and subcutaneous tissue.

synapse: a coupling or connection between two neurons.

synergy: an abnormal pattern of motor recovery following central nervous system damage.

synthesis: in data analysis, clustering and determining the pattern of data to be used in the diagnostic statement.

syrup of ipecac: a nonprescription liquid that, when given orally, induces vomiting.

systole: the phase of the cardiac cycle associated with the contraction of the ventricle, usually in reference to blood pressure.

talking: the act of verbalizing symbols in order to convey thoughts, feelings, or ideas.

tartar: dental plaque that has not been removed and has hardened. Tartar cannot be removed with brushing: it must be scraped off by a dental professional.

task groups: groups designed to further the goals of an organization (*e.g.,* standing committees, ad hoc task forces, and "quality circles").

task roles: the roles of group members that facilitate group processing of ideas. Task role functions help the group stay focused on the task and directly assist the group to achieve its identified goal.

teratogenicity: an effect that occurs when a drug crosses the placenta and produces abnormalities in fetal development resulting in deformities.

tertiary prevention: care given after an illness has occurred. Its purpose is to limit the disability that results from a medical condition.

testicular self-examination (TSE): a routine, systematic procedure whereby a man examines his testes for evidence of change that could indicate a malignant process.

tetany: a severe muscle spasm that may occur with greatly diminished calcium levels.

theism: a world view that espouses belief in a loving and personal creator God who created humankind in His own image to love and serve Him and our neighbor (Carson & Arnold, 1996).

theory: a set of interrelated concepts and propositions that explains some aspect of our reality.

therapeutic effect: the intended effect of the drug or intervention when introduced into the body.

therapeutic rapport: a special bond that exists between nurse and client because they have established a sense of trust and a mutual understanding of what will occur in their relationship with each other.

therapeutic relationship: a helping relationship.

therapeutic relationship—orientation phase: a time when the nurse and client make an agreement that they will be working together to solve one or more of the client's problems. This phase represents an oral contract between nurse and client. It signals the initiation of a working relationship. This part of the relationship lays the groundwork for the work they will do together in the future.

therapeutic relationship—termination phase: the time near the end of the relationship when the work of the client and nurse is coming to a close.

therapeutic relationship—working phase: mainly a time for completing nursing interventions that address expected nursing outcomes.

thermoregulation: the control of heat production and heat loss; specifically, the maintenance of body temperature through physiologic mechanisms activated by the hypothalamus.

thoracentesis: the surgical perforation of the chest wall and pleural space.

thrombus: a blood clot attached to a blood vessel.

tidal volume: the amount of air that moves into and out of the lungs during normal, quiet respiration.

tolerance: a state in which an individual requires an increased amount of a drug to achieve a desired effect because of physical dependence on the drug.

tone: state of readiness or degree of muscle tension occurring on a scale of high, medium, and low and rigid, hypertonic, normal, hypotonic, and flaccid.

tort: a civil offense, not including a breach of contract, against an individual or against property (*e.g.,* a house, clothing) for which a person can obtain monetary damages by filing a suit in court (Pozgar, 1996, p. 36). Examples of torts in health care include professional negligence and false imprisonment.

total parenteral nutrition: providing all essential nutrients by means of a special formula via a large vein.

toxicity: excessive accumulation of a substance within the body, as in drug overdosing.

transcultural nursing: nursing practice within a cultural context; administration of health care using a world view; vital to the understanding of health, illness, and care.

transfer: movement of client from one surface to another.

transfer of learning: whatever is learned in one context or situation will apply or affect another context or situation.

transient flora: microorganisms that temporarily inhabit the skin and mucous membranes.

transient ischemic attack (TIA): temporary cerebral ischemia due to temporary disruption in blood supply to a part of the brain.

transmission: the process of conducting the sensory signal to specific structures in the nervous system that process the signal.

transport: movement of oxygen and carbon dioxide to and from the cells.

turning schedule: a planned program of turning and positioning clients that takes into account the needs and limitations of the client.

tympanites: drumlike distention of the abdomen due to air or gas in the intestine or peritoneal cavity.

unconditional positive regard: a term coined by the psychologist Carl Rogers to describe respect that is not dependent on the client's behavior.

unitary learning: the response of the whole individual to the total situation.

ureterocele: prolapse of the urethra through the urinary meatus.

urge incontinence: loss of urine associated with a sudden and strong urge to urinate; inability to hold back urination.

urinary frequency: abnormally frequent voiding.

urinary incontinence: involuntary loss of urine (usually a disorder in the urinary bladder or urethra, in the structures that support or surround them, or in the neural regulatory mechanism that controls voiding).

urinary urgency: intense and immediate need to void.

urticaria: a cutaneous reaction usually accompanied by itching and the appearance of flaking, whitish scales.

utilitarianism: a system of ethical beliefs that focuses on the good consequences of actions. A central concept is the production of the largest possible amount of happiness or benefit for the greatest number of people.

Valsalva maneuver: increase of intrathoracic pressure by forcible exhalation against the closed glottis; occurs when one strains to defecate.

values: deeply held beliefs that provide people with reference points as they make judgments and set priorities in daily life.

varicosities: bulging, prominent, twisted veins, usually in the lower extremities.

ventilation: the movement of gases in and out of the lungs.

veracity: the duty to tell the truth.

verbal communication: the use of words to convey messages. This type of communication is achieved by writing or speaking in a code mutually understood by sender and receiver.

vernix caseosa: a grayish-white, cheeselike substance that covers the skin of the fetus and newborn. It acts as a protective agent during intrauterine life and is thought to have an insulating effect against heat loss.

vertical integration of services: the linking of different levels of care provided by different facilities. For example, a hospital, a home care department, a durable medical equipment company, and a hospice may be linked vertically to conserve resources and to provide a self-referral system.

vesicoureteral reflux: the "backing up" of urine from the bladder into the ureters and sometimes the kidney pelvis.

virtues: personal attributes of moral strength, good practical judgment, and temperance.

virulence: the extent to which an organism can produce disease.

virus: obligate intracellular parasites that take over the genetic mechanism of an infected cell in order to reproduce (replicate). Viruses have either RNA or DNA, but not both.

visceral pain: pain originating from injury to internal organs.

vital capacity: maximum amount of air that can be moved in and out of the lungs.

voluntary accreditation: a process of peer review that uses a set of professionally developed criteria to evaluate an educational program in nursing to assure the public of quality nursing education.

well-being: an individual's sense of optimal wellness physically, emotionally, spiritually, developmentally, and socioculturally.

wellness: a composite of factors that affect both physical and mental health, such as participation in self-care nutritional status, and stress reduction.

withdrawal: a state in which an individual manifests unpleasant physiological changes when there is an abrupt cessation of an addictive substance.

work groups: see **task groups.**

world view: an understanding of the relevance and persuasiveness of culture; knowledge of the demographics, vital statistics, and morbidity and mortality rates on a national level.

young adulthood: a stage of life following adolescence and preceding the middle adult years.

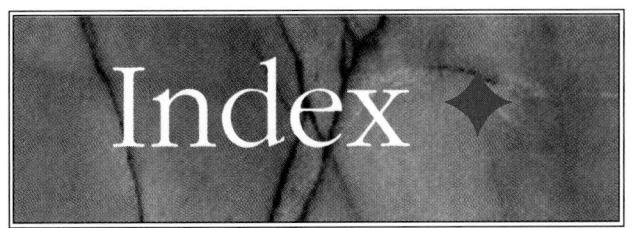

Index

Note: **Page numbers in** *italics* indicate illustrations; those followed by t indicate tables; those followed by b indicate boxed material; and those followed by p indicate procedures.

Biological safety *(Continued)*
implementation in, 425–435
planning in, 423, 425
Biopsy, lung, 853
Biotin, 740, 742t
Biotransformation, drug, 444
in children, 446, 446t
in elderly, 446, 447t
Birth control pills, 1130–1135, 1131t. See
also *Contraceptives.*
Bisexuality, 1136
Bismuth subsalicylate (Pepto-Bismol), for
diarrhea, 949
Bites, animal, 389
Blacks. See also under *Cultural; Culture.*
classification of, 1103
hair care for, 519
health status of, 1103t, 1103–1104
hypertension in, 895
in nursing, history of, 7–8
organizations for, 7
Bladder, examination of, 980
imaging of, 987–990, *988, 989*
irrigation of, 993–994, *998*
neurogenic, 972
radiography of, 987, *988*
structure and function of, 968–969
ultrasonography of, 990
Bladder catheterization. See *Urinary catheterization.*
Bladder control, bladder training for,
1009t
in toddlers. See *Toilet training.*
loss of. See *Urinary incontinence.*
Bladder decompression, 993–996
Bladder emptying, drugs for, 993, 997t
Bladder neck suspension, 1014t
Bladder storage, drugs for, 993, 997t
Bladder temperature, 622
Bladder training, 1009t
Bleach, for disinfection, 407
Blended family, 367, 367b, 369
Blindness. See *Vision impairment.*
Bloch Ethnic/Cultural Assessment Guide,
1099, 1100b–1102b
Blood, handling and disposal of, 406,
406b, *409,* 409–410
in sputum, 843, 844
in urine, 985t, 986–987
in vomitus, 844
occult, stool test for, 940, 941p–942p
pH of, 607t, 608t, 608–609
in acid-base disturbances, 849t
in respiratory disorders, 849, 849t
precautions for, 406–412. See also *Biological safety; Infection control.*
spills of, cleanup of, 410p
Blood cultures, 413–418
in respiratory assessment, 849
specimen collection for, 419p–420p
Blood glucose, regulation of, 112
Blood pressure. See also *Hypertension; Hypotension.*
factors affecting, 916
home monitoring of, 901
in adolescent, 311
in fluid and electrolyte imbalances, 803
in infant, 287
in preschooler, 299
in school-age child, 306
in toddler, 295
measurement of, 901, 902p–904p
in orthostatic hypotension, 916
postoperative, 1203

Blood specimen, 150
arterial, 849
collection of, 419p–420p
Blood studies, 150
chemistry, 150
hematological, 150
in cardiovascular assessment, 905–909,
911t
in respiratory assessment, 848–849
microbiology, 150
Blood transfusions. See *Transfusion(s).*
Blood urea nitrogen (BUN), 966
in fluid and electrolyte assessment, 806,
806t
in nutritional assessment, 757, 758t
Blood vessels, structure and function of,
894–895
Blood-borne infections, 405
prevention of, 407–411
Blood-borne pathogen standards, 407
Body alignment, 642, *642*
Body fluid. See also under *Fluid(s).*
Body fluid precautions, 407–412, 428,
433t. See also *Precautions.*
Body image, 1022–1023
in ostomy clients, 957–962
sexuality and, 1128–1129
Body language, 222
assessment of, 229
in interview, 143
Body mechanics, principles of, 644, 684b,
684–685
Body plethysmography, 853
Body proportions, age-related changes in,
302
Body sites, normally sterile, 418, 418b
Body substance isolation, 426–428, 433t
Body surface area (BSA), in dose calcula-
tion, 453, *454*
nomogram for, *454*
thermoregulation and, 612
Body temperature. See *Temperature.*
Body weight. See *Weight.*
Bolus injection, in intravenous drug administration, 486, 487, 493p–494p
Bonding, infant, 287, 291
Bone, 642
Bone density, decreased, in immobility,
645
Borborygmus, 935
Boston Training School for Nurses, 6
Bottle-feeding, 289t–290t, 759–761
microwave heating in, 388
of infants, 288, 289t–290t, 293
of neonates, 284–287, 289t–290t
stool in, 927
Bowel diversions, *957,* 957–962, 958p–
961p
Bowel elimination, 925–961
activity and, 929
age and, 927–928
assessment in, 934–940
assistive devices for, 943
bedpan for, 945–946, *946,* 947p–948p
bedside commode for, 540, 945–946,
946
bowel training for, 946–948, 949b
chronic illness and, 930
common problems in, 930–933
cultural factors in, 930
diagnosis in, 940
diagnostic procedures affecting, 928–929
diet and, 928, 943–945
enteral nutrition and, 930

Bowel elimination *(Continued)*
exercise and, 945
factors affecting, 927–930
fluid intake and, 928
health promotion for, 942–943, 943b
hygiene in, 540
immobility and, 645
implementation in, 940–962
in adults, 928
in children and adolescents, 927
in elderly, 928
in neonate, 282
in pregnancy, 930
lifestyle factors and, 929–930
medications and, 930
nursing process for, 934–962
assessment in, 934–940
abdominal auscultation in, 935
abdominal inspection in, 935
abdominal palpation in, 935
abdominal percussion in, 935
diagnostic studies in, 937–940, 940b
nursing history in, 934
physical assessment in, 934–940
diagnosis in, 940
evaluation in, 962
implementation in, 940–962
planning in, 940
pain and, 930
physiology of, 926–927
planning in, 940
positioning for, 945–946
postoperative, 929, 929b
privacy for, 943
psychological factors and, 929
timing of, 943
toilet training and, 297, 297b, 300t, 927
Bowel history, 934, 934b
Bowel incontinence, 932–933
bowel training for, 946–948, 949b
collector for, 580
in elderly, 928
nursing interventions for, 946–948
pouches for, 952–956, *956*
skin care in, 946
Bowel sounds, auscultation of, 935
Bowel training, 946–948, 949b
Braces, orthodontic, 310t
Brachial pulse. See also *Pulse.*
assessment of, 905, 907p
in blood pressure measurement, 903p
Brachioradialis reflex, assessment of, *1057,*
1058t
Braden scale, 570, 572t–573t
Bradycardia, postoperative, 1203, 1208
Bradypnea, 842t, 846
Brain, age-related changes in, 354b, 354–
355
structure and function of, 1041t
Brain stem, 1041t
Brand name, of drug, 441, 442t
Breast cancer, sexuality and, 1128–1129
surgery for, home care after, 1204b
terminal, nursing care plan for, 1157
Breast self-examination, 332b–333b, 332–
333
Breast-Feeding, Effective, 767, 768
Ineffective, 767, 768
Breast-feeding, 289t–290t, 759
as family planning method, 1134–1135
colostrum in, 282, 289t
maternal nutrition in, 764
nursing diagnoses for, 767, 768
of infants, 288, 289t–290t, 293

Ethical theories, 46
Ethicists, clinical, 56
Ethics, 45
  definition of, 45
  need for, 45–46
  normative, 46–54
  transcultural, 52b
  values-oriented, 54–55
  virtue, 55
  vs. morals, 45
Ethics committee, 56
Ethmoid sinuses, drug instillation in, 492, 498p–499p
Ethnic groups. See also under *Cultural; Culture.*
  elderly population in, 348, 349t
Ethnicity, 1095
Ethnocentrism, 1095
Etodolac (Lodine), 723, 725t
Etomidate (Amidate), 1172t
Eupnea, 842t, 846
Evaluation, 202–208. See also under *Outcome.*
  by Joint Commission on Accreditation of Healthcare Organizations (JCAHO), 208
  by Professional Review Organizations, 208
  communication in, 231
  criteria for, 203
  definition of, 135, 202
  nursing audit and, 206–208
  outcomes and, 202, 203–206
  purpose of, 202–203
  quality assurance and, 206–208
  standards for, 203, 208
Evaporation, 611
Evisceration, wound, 576
Exchange system diet, 776
Excitement phase, of sexual response cycle, 1124
Excretion, drug, 444
  in children, 446, 446t
  in elderly, 446, 447t
Excretory urography, 988
Exercise. See *Activity and exercise.*
Exercise stress testing, 911–912
Exercises, breathing, 867
  for bowel elimination, 945
  for muscle strength, 678–679, 679
  isometric, 678–679
  leg, postoperative, 1187–1188, 1188
  pelvic floor (Kegel), 1010t, 1015
  range of motion, 654–669, 656–671, 657p–667p. See also *Range of motion exercises.*
  resistance, 679, 679
Exertional heat injury, 626b
Existential Well-Being scale, 1085
Exogenous infection, 403
Exotoxin, 404
Expectorants, 872
Expiration, 838–839
Expiratory reserve volume, 839, 840
Explanatory theory, 22, 23
Expressive aphasia, 1068b
Extended family, 367b, 369
External meatus, examination of, 980
External urethral sphincter, 968
Extracellular fluid, 109, 792, 792. See also under *Fluid(s).*
  electrolyte concentration in, 792–793, 793t

Extracellular fluid *(Continued)*
  shifts of, 793, 972
Extraocular muscles, assessment of, 1052t
Extremities, inspection of, in cardiovascular assessment, 899
Extrusion reflex, 288
Exudate, assessment of, 566–567
  purulent, 567
Eye, age-related changes in, 515b
  artificial, 554
  assessment of, 513
  dry, 513
  in fluid and electrolyte imbalances, 804
  lazy, 1047
  structure of, 513, 514
Eye care, 513
  for artificial eye, 554
  for contact lens wearers, 551–554, 552p–554p
Eye drops, instillation of, 487–490, 495p–496p
Eye movements, assessment of, 1052t
Eye ointments, instillation of, 487–490, 495p–496p
Eye protection, in laser surgery, 1169

F
Face mask, oxygen, 874t, 876p
Facial nerve, assessment of, 1053t
Faith development. See also *Spiritual development.*
  Fowler's theory of, 271–272, 272t
Fallopian tubes, 1119t, 1120
Falls, in elderly, in hospital, 648
  prevention of, 395, 396
    critical pathway for, 397t
    in children, 285t–286t
    in elderly, 390, 391b
    nursing care plan for, 396
    restraints for, 395, 398, 398–400, 399t
      false imprisonment and, 68, 68
False imprisonment, 68, 68
Family, adaptation of to stress, 372–373
  adjustment of to new baby, 287
  American, 367–369
  as client, 372–373
  as data source, 139–140
  as primary group, 232
  as system, 370–372
  blended, 367, 367b, 369
  childless, 369
  cohabiting, 367b, 369–370
  common law, 367b, 369–370
  communal, 367b, 369–370
  cultural norms and, 367
  current trends in, 369–370
  definition of, 367
  developmental stages of, 371t, 371–372
  dual worker, 370
  extended, 367b, 369
  functions of, 370, 371
  nontraditional, 367b, 369–370
  nuclear, 367, 367b
  nursing care plan for, 379, 381
  nursing process for, 373–382, 381
    assessment in, 373–376. See also *Family assessment.*
    evaluation in, 380–382
    nursing diagnoses in, 376–379
    planning in, 379, 380b, 381
  of homosexuals, 1136
  same-sex, 369

Family *(Continued)*
  single adult, 367b, 369
  single parent, 367, 367b, 369
  social context for, 367
Family assessment, 373–376
  areas of concern in, 374
  case study of, 376, 377b–379b
  cultural factors in, 373
  data collection for, 374
  ecomap in, 374, 375
  environmental and lifestyle concerns in, 373, 376
  genogram in, 373–374, 374
  medication history in, 375
  purpose of, 373
  risk factor identification in, 376
  support system in, 373
Family Coping: Compromised, 376
Family history, 141
Family planning. See also *Contraceptives.*
  natural, 1133
Family Processes: Altered, 376
  birth of newborn and, 287
Family roles, 370
Family structure, 367b, 370
Family theory, 370–372
Farsightedness, 1044b
Fast food, nutritional content of, 337t
Fat, dietary, colon cancer and, 945
  subcutaneous, thermoregulation and, 612
Fatigue, hospitalization and, 707b, 711
Fats, dietary, 737–738
Fatty acids, 738–739
Fears, in preschooler, 303t
  in toddler, 300t
Fecal impaction, 933. See also *Bowel elimination.*
  digital removal of, 952, 956
  enemas for, 950–952, 953p–955p
  urinary retention and, 973
Fecal incontinence, 932–933. See also *Bowel elimination.*
  bowel training for, 946–948, 949b
  in elderly, 928
  nursing interventions for, 946–948
  skin care in, 578–580, 580b, 946
Fecal incontinence collector, 580
Fecal incontinence pouches, 952–956, 956
Feces, 926. See also *Stool.*
  expulsion of, 927, 927
  in breast-fed vs. bottle-fed infants, 927
  liquid, measurement of, 804b
Feedback, 24, 111–112, 215–216
  negative, 111–112
  positive, 112
Feeding, assistance with, 771, 772p–773p
  by blind clients, 771
  of infants, 288, 289t–300t, 293, 759–762
  of neonates, 282, 284–287, 289t, 759–761
  of toddlers, 290t, 296, 762
  tube, 776, 777p–780p, 777–780
Feeding tube. See also *Enteral nutrition.*
  drug administration via, 464, 468p
  insertion of, 777p–780p
Feet. See *Foot* entries.
Felony, 65
Female circumcision, 1106, 1106b
Femininity, cultural definitions of, 1118
Feminism, 1118
Femoral pulse, assessment of, 905, 908p
Fenoprofen (Nalfon), 723, 725t
Fentanyl, transdermal, 732

Heat lamp, 624, *624*
Heat loss, 610–611
in neonate, 284
Heat production, 610–611
in neonate, 631
Heat stroke, 626b
Heat syndromes, 626b
Heat therapy, 622–624
assessment for, 623
implementation of, *623,* 623–624, *624*
in pain management, 730, *731*
methods of, 623–624
Heat-conserving mechanisms, 630
Heating pad, 624
Heaves, 899
Heel protectors, 581, *581*
Height. See also *Length.*
measurement of, in nutritional assessment, 754
of adolescent, 311–312
of preschooler, *280–281,* 299
of school-age child, *280–281,* 306
of toddler, 295, 296
Height and weight charts, for children, *280, 281, 282*
Heimlich maneuver, 860p, 863
Hematemesis, 844
Hematocrit, 806, 806t
Hematologic studies, 413
Hematuria, 985t, 986–987
Hemiplegia, 648
Hemoccult test, 940, 941p–942p
Hemoglobin count, in nutritional assessment, 757, 758t
Hemoglobinuria, 985t, 987
Hemolytic reaction, transfusion-related, 824, 825t
Hemoptysis, 843, 844
Hemorrhoids, 933. See also *Bowel elimination.*
Hemovac, 575–576
Henderson, Virginia, 13, 28
Henry Street Settlement, 7–8
HEPA filters, 412
HEPA respirators, for tuberculosis prevention, 412, *412,* 433–434
Heparin, subcutaneous administration of, *470,* 470–477, 474p–477p
Hepatitis, occupational transmission of, 408–409, 409t
Hepatitis B, 1138–1139, 1139t
immunization for, 292t
Herbal remedies, 1099, 1103t
Hering-Breuer reflex, 841
Herpes genitalis, 1138–1139, 1139t
High colonic enema, 952, 953p–955p
High-density lipoproteins (HDLs), 739, 909, 911b
Higher-level thought processes, 1040
High-risk behavior, in adolescence, 314–316, 319t, 320t
Hinduism, 1083
Hinge joint, 641
Hip, range of motion exercises for, 664p–665p, 668, *669, 670*
Hirsutism, 519
Hispanics, 1096, *1097.* See also under *Cultural; Culture.*
health status of, 1103t, 1103–1104
History, diet, 753
family, 141
medical, 141
medication, 141, 461
nursing, 140–141

History *(Continued)*
social, 141
Holistic health care, 85–86, *86,* 260
Holistic model of humanity, 1077–1078, *1078*
Holmes and Rahe's stress model, 103–104, *105*
Holter monitor, 913–914, *914*
Home, childproofing of, 397–398
Home assessment, 520b
in discharge planning, 1225, 1227b
Home care, 87–88. See also *Community-based care.*
activities of daily living evaluation for, 1224, 1225t, 1226b
after breast cancer surgery, 1204b
assistive aids in, 1225–1226
blood pressure monitoring in, 901
case study of, 1230–1232
client's rights in, 45b
cultural competence in, 1110b
discharge planning for, 1209–1210, 1223–1228. See also *Discharge planning.*
documentation in, 1220b
drug administration in, 502b
enteral nutrition in, 780, 783b, 784b
environmental adaptations for, 1226–1228
environmental assessment for, 520b
equipment needed for, 1225–1226
for Alzheimer's disease, 1045b
for constipation, 932b
for urinary catheterization, 1015b
for wounds, 574b
functional assessment for, 1224, 1225t, 1226b
funding for, 1219
home assessment for, 1225, 1227b
hospice, 88–89, 1159–1160, 1160b, 1221–1222
in impaired mobility, 695–696
in terminal illness, 1159–1160
intravenous infusion in, 823b
medical waste disposal in, 406, 406b
nurse case manager in, 372b
nursing process for, 1228–1230
oxygen administration in, 874–889
sleep and rest in, 707b
spiritual needs in, 1085, 1085b
total parenteral nutrition in, 785, 785b
Home remedies, 1099, 1103t
Home safety. See *Safety.*
Homeodynamics, 29–30, 30t, 38t
Homeostasis, 109–112
adaptation and, 107. See also *Adaptation.*
compensatory mechanisms in, 111
definition of, 107
feedback in, 111
normal deviations from, 111–112
overshooting in, 112
physiological, 109, *110*
autonomic nervous system in, *110,* 110–111
endocrine system in, 103, *104,* 109, *110*
psychological, 109–110
self-regulation in, 111–112
Homeostatic mechanisms, 108–109
Homeotherm, 610
Homicide, in adolescence, 315
Homologous blood, 830
Homosexuality, 1136

Homosexuals, in families, 369–370
human immunodeficiency virus (HIV) in, 1136
Hopelessness, in cardiovascular disease, 917
Horizontal integration of services, 89–90, *90*
Hormonal changes, in middle age, 339
pubertal, 312, 313, 313t
Hormone replacement therapy, 341, 352
Hormones, adaptation and, 109, *110*
stress and, 103, *104,* 109, *110*
Hospice care, 88–89, 1159–1160, 1160b
Hospital, environmental hazards in, for employees, 390–391, 393–394, 394b
for patients, 651
environmental hygiene in, 519–521
medication distribution systems in, 453
safety in, 651
Hospital beds. See *Bed.*
Hospital practice settings, 16–17
Hospital-acquired infections. See *Nosocomial infections.*
Hospital-based diploma programs, 8
Hospitalization, 87
decline in, 1216
environmental structuring in, for sensory impaired clients, 1056–1068
immobility in, 644–648
sensory deprivation in, prevention of, 1059–1060
sensory overload in, prevention of, 1060–1068
sleep deprivation in, 707b, 711
stress of, 123–125, 124t
Host susceptibility, 406, 406b
Hot flashes, 355–356, 612
Hot pack, chemically activated, 624
Hot water bottle, 624
Household measurements, for drug dosage, 451, 452t
H.S. care, 507
Hubbard tank, 623
Human immunodeficiency virus (HIV) infection, 1138–1139, 1139t
in adolescents, 316
in homosexuals, 1136
nutrition in, 750
occupational transmission of, incidence of, 407, 408t
prevention of, 407–411
risk of, 409, 409t
tuberculosis in, 411, 412, 432–433
Human papillomavirus infection, 1138–1139, 1139t
Human response patterns framework, 147t
Humanism, 1076
Humanity, holistic model of, 1077–1078, *1078*
Humor, communication and, 224
Hyaline membrane disease, 858
Hydrating solutions, 811, 811t
Hydration, 791–831. See also under *Fluid.*
disturbances in, 795–796
Hydrocodone, 723–728, 726t, 727t
Hydrocolloid dressings, 590t, 592t, 594t, 596t, 597t, 598. See also *Dressings.*
application of, 603p
Hydrogel dressings, 591t, 594t. See also *Dressings.*
Hydrogen ion concentration, regulation of, 799–800
Hydrogen peroxide, for wound cleansing, 583, 583t

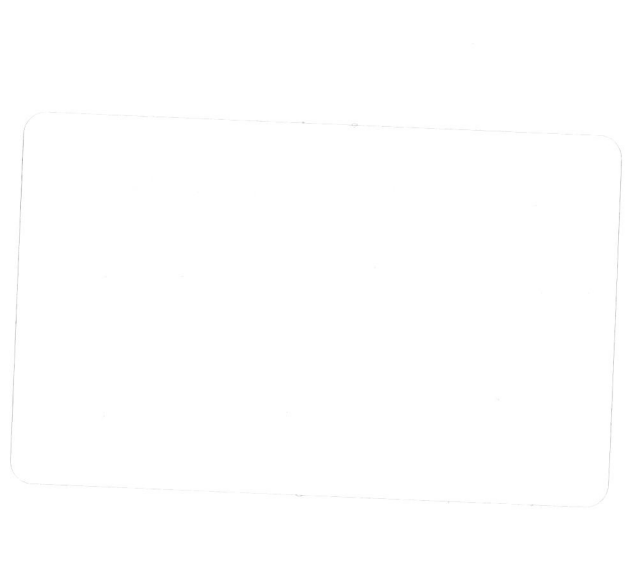

COMMON ABBREVIATIONS AND SYMBOLS

ABBREVIATION/ SYMBOL	TERM	ABBREVIATION/ SYMBOL	TERM
	Assessment Data		
abd	abdomen	neg	negative
ax	axillary	NG	nasogastric
BM	bowel movement	OTC	over-the-counter (medicine without a prescription)
BP	blood pressure	P	pulse
BSA	body surface area	PE	physical examination
bx	biopsy	PMH	past medical history
C&DB	coughing and deep breathing	R	respiration
c/o	complains of	R/O	rule out
cc	chief complaint	ROM	range of motion
DOA	dead on arrival	ROS	review of systems
dx	diagnosis	RX	treatment
F	Fahrenheit (temperature scale)	SOB	shortness of breath
h/o	history of	sx	signs; symptoms
HR	heart rate	T	temperature
in	inch	TPR	temperature, pulse, respiration
LMP	last menstrual period	VS	vital signs
LOC	level of consciousness	WNL	within normal limits
	Disease-Related Terms		
AIDS	acquired immune deficiency syndrome	fx	fracture
ASHD	arteriosclerotic heart disease	GI	gastrointestinal
BPH	benign prostatic hyperplasia	GU	genitourinary
CA	cancer	HTN	hypertension
CAD	coronary artery disease	MI	myocardial infarction
CHF	congestive heart failure	PVC	premature ventricular contraction
COPD	chronic obstructive pulmonary disease	PVD	peripheral vascular disease
CVA	cerebrovascular accident	STD	sexually transmitted disease
DM	diabetes mellitus	URI	upper respiratory infection
FUO	fever of unknown origin	UTI	urinary tract infection
	Orders		
$\bar{a}$	before	IU	international unit
ac	before meals	IV	intravenous
ad lib	at will; as desired	ko	keep open (IV)
AMA	against medical advice	noc	night
bid	two times a day	NPO	nothing by mouth
$\bar{c}$	with	NS	normal saline
CPR	cardiopulmonary resuscitation	OD	right eye
D/C	discontinue	OS	left eye
D/W	dextrose in water	O.T.	Occupational Therapy
DNR	do not resuscitate	$\bar{p}$	after
DSD	dry sterile dressing	po	by mouth (per os)
gtt	drop	post op	postoperative
h	hour	pre op	preoperative
hs	hour of sleep; bedtime	prep	preparation
I&O	intake and output	prn	as needed; whenever necessary
IM	intramuscular	pt	patient
IPPB	intermittent positive-pressure breathing	P.T.	Physical Therapy